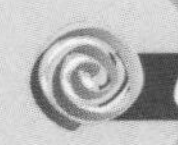

Cultural Cues

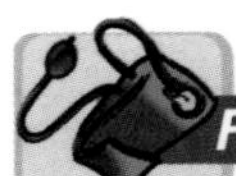

Focused Assessment

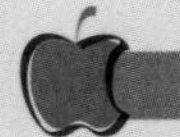

Health Promotion Points

Continued on the next page

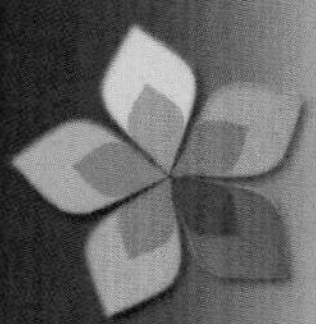

SPECIAL FEATURES—cont'd

Home Care Considerations

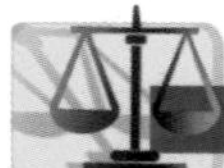

Legal & Ethical Considerations

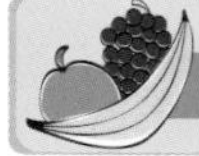

Nutritional Therapies

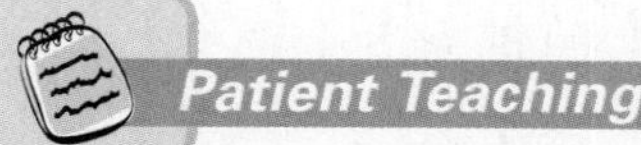

Patient Teaching

Safety Alert

Continued on the next page

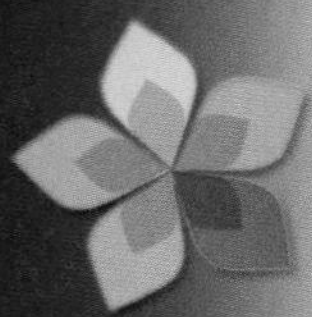

SPECIAL FEATURES—cont'd

NURSING CARE PLANS

Skills

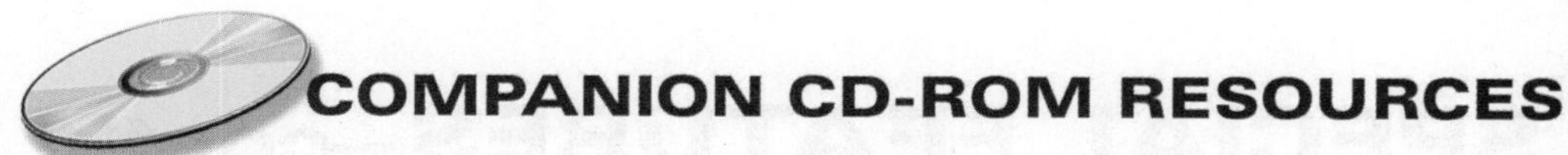

COMPANION CD-ROM RESOURCES

DORLAND'S AUDIO PRONUNCIATIONS

BONUS REVIEW QUESTIONS

FLUIDS AND ELECTROLYTES MODULE

HELPFUL PHRASES FOR COMMUNICATING IN SPANISH

MATHEMATICS REVIEW

Roman Numerals
Fractions
Decimals
Percentage
Proportion
Fahrenheit and Celsius
Systems of Measurement
Answers to Exercises and Review Questions

ANIMATIONS

Abdominal Examination
Acute Coronary Syndrome (ACS), Acute Myocardial Infarction (AMI), Coronary Ischemia, Coronary Artery Disease (includes use of aspirin and nitroglycerides)
Adrenal Function
Alzheimer's Disease
Anatomy of Eye
Ankle Fracture
Appendicitis, Symptoms
Asthma
Bleeding Ulcer, Pathophysiology, Symptoms; Hematemesis
Blood Clot Leading to Stroke
Blood Flow: Circulatory System
Brain Abscess
Brain Anatomy: Temporal Lobe, Brainstem, Cerebral Peduncle, Thalamus
Brain Lobes
Breast Cancer Spread; Metastasis
Cardiac Arrest, Ventricular Fibrillation, External Heart Monitor
Cerebellar Infarct; Stroke
Chemotherapy
Chest Pain Radiating to Arm
Cirrhosis
Congestive Heart Failure
Cranial Nerves
Diverticulitis
Eye: Aqueous Humor, Vitreous Humor
Function of Heart
Generalized Seizure
Hemothorax
Hip Fracture, Femur Fracture, Femoral Fracture
Lymphocyte Function
Meningitis
Normal Cardiopulmonary Physiology
Normal Cardiopulmonary System
Organ Systems 3D
Parkinson's Disease
Passage of Food Through Digestive Tract (various parts of digestive tract–esophagus to rectum)
Pelvic Inflammatory Disease
Pulmonary Embolus
Quadriplegia; Spinal Cord Injury
Radiation Therapy
Renal Anatomy and Function
Retinal Detachment
Sickle Cell Anemia
Simple Pneumothorax and Tension Pneumothorax
Spine Structure
Structure of the Heart
Subarachnoid Hemorrhage
TIA: Transient Ischemic Attack; CVA: Cerebrovascular Accident; Stroke; Brain Blood Clot
Tuberculosis
Vascular Tree: Heart, Aorta, Major Branches
Ventricular Fibrillation
Visual Pathway

AUDIO CLIPS

Aortic Ejection Sound Related to S1
Bronchial Breath Sounds
Bronchovesicular Breath Sounds
Diastolic Murmur
High-Pitched Crackles
High-Pitched Wheeze
Low-Pitched Crackles
Low-Pitched Wheeze
Midsystolic Click Sound Related to S1
Murmurs: Blowing, Harsh or Rough, and Rumble
Murmurs: High, Medium, and Low
Paradoxical Split Sound Related to S2
Pericardial Friction Rub
Pleural Friction Rub
Pulmonic Ejection Sound Related to S1
S1 at Various Locations
S2 at Various Locations
Single S1
Single S2
Stridor
Systolic Murmur
The Fourth Heart Sound (S4)
The Fourth Heart Sound (S4) with Bell Held Lightly then Applied Firmly
The Third Heart Sound (S3)
Vesicular Breath Sounds
Wide Split Sound Related to S2

VIDEO CLIPS

Inspection and Palpation: Breathing and Respiratory Excursion, Anterior Chest (adult male)
Inspection and Palpation: Respiration, Respiratory Excursion and Tactile Fremitus
Posterior Chest (adult male)
Palpation: Tactile Fremitus, Posterior Chest (adult female)
Inspection and Percussion: Diaphragmatic Excursion (adult male)
Percussion: Anterior Thorax (adult male)
Inspection and Palpation: Cardiac, Anterior Chest (adult female)
Inspection and Palpation: Cardiac Auscultory Landmarks (adult male)
Auscultation: Cardiac with Diaphragm (adult male)
Auscultation: Cardiac with Bell (adult male)
Auscultation: Cardiac with Diaphragm and Bell (adult female)

Continued on the next page

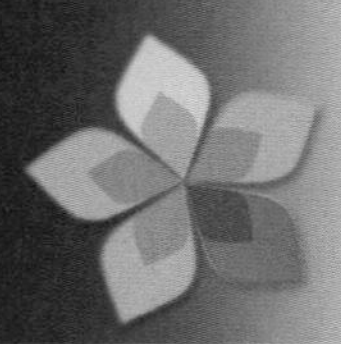

SPECIAL FEATURES—cont'd

COMPANION CD-ROM RESOURCES—cont'd

Auscultation: Carotid Artery (adult male)
Inspection and Palpation: Pulses, Lower Extremities (adult female)
Evaluation: Smell, Cranial Nerve I—Olfactory Nerve (adult male)
Evaluation: Central Vision and Visual Acuity (adult male)
Evaluation: Pupil Responses, Direct and Accomodation, Cranial Nerves III, IV, and VI—Oculomotor, Trochlear and Abducens Nerves (adult male)
Evaluation: Light Touch; Face, Upper and Lower Extremities, Cranial Nerve V –Trigeminal Nerve (older adult female)
Inspection: Fine Motor Coordination, Upper Extremities (older adult male)
Inspection: Fine Motor Coordination, Lower Extremities (older adult female)
Inspection and Palpation: External Ear (adult male)
Inspection: Ear Canal (adult male)
Inspection and Palpation: External Eye (adult male)
Evaluation: Central Vision and Visual Acuity (adult male)
Evaluation: Pupil Responses, Direct and Consensual (older adult female)
Inspection: Nose (adult female)
Auscultation: Abdomen, Bowel Sounds (adult male)
Percussion: Abdomen (adult male)
Percussion: Liver (adult male)
Percussion: Spleen (adult male)
Palpation: Abdomen Superficial and Deep (adult male)
Gait (older adult female)
Inspection: General Muscular Strength (adult male)
Inspection and Palpation: Muscular Development (adult male)
Inspection: Female Breasts (sitting position) (adult female)
Palpation: Female Breasts (supine position) (adult female)
Inspection: External Genitalia (younger adult female)
Inspection: Speculum Examination (younger adult female)
Inspection and Palpation: Standing Position (younger adult male)
Inspection and Palpation: Standing Position (younger adult male)
Palpation: Inguinal Hernia Evaluation (younger adult male)

FORMS

Chapter 2
- Adult Admission History
- Daily Physical Assessment
- Interdisciplinary Plan of Care
- Medication Reconciliation Form
- Daily Basic Care Worksheet

Chapter 4
- Special Consent to Operation, Postoperative Care, Medical Treatment, Anesthesia/Sedation, or Other Procedure
- Pre-op/Pre-procedure Checklist/Report form

Chapter 9
- Minimum Data Set, form 2.0
- Sections P 3 and H 3 a, b that apply specifically to the rehabilitation patient from Minimum Data Set, 2.0 forms, USDHHS, 1/30/98
- Katz Index of Independence in Activities of Daily Living
- Hospital Team Conference Report
- Transdisciplinary Initial Assessment Form
- Team Kardex Form

Chapter 21
- Adult/Pediatric Neuro Flow Record

Chapter 23
- Transient Ischemic Attack/Acute Ischemic Stroke Admission Form
- Plan of Care Form for Transient Ischemic Attack/Acute Ischemic Stroke Clinical Path

ADDITIONAL NURSING CARE PLANS

Nursing Care Plan 34–1: Care of the Patient with Renal Lithiasis
Nursing Care Plan 45–2: Care of the Patient with Bipolar Disorder (Manic Phase)
Nursing Care Plan 45–3: Care of the Patient with Depression
Nursing Care Plan 45–4: Care of the Patient with Anorexia Nervosa

SKILLS AND STEPS WITH PERFORMANCE CHECKLISTS

Skill 3–1: Starting the Primary Intravenous Infusion
Skill 3–2: Adding a New Solution to the Intravenous Infusion
Skill 3–3: Administering Intravenous Piggyback Medication
Skill 3–4: Administering Medication via Saline or PRN Lock
Skill 3–5: Administration of Medication with a Volume-Controlled Set
Skill 3–6: Administration of Blood Products
Steps 3–1: Adding Medication to an Intravenous Solution
Steps 3–2: Administering an IV Bolus Medication (IV Push)
Steps 3–3: Discontinuing an Intravenous Infusion or PRN Lock
Skill 13–1: Endotracheal and Tracheostomy Suctioning
Skill 13–2: Providing Tracheostomy Care
Skill 15–1: Phlebotomy and Obtaining Blood Samples with a Vacutainer System
Skill 28–1: Administering a Nasogastric/Duodenal Tube Feeding or Feeding via a PEG Tube
Skill 29–1: Steps for Changing an Ostomy Appliance
Steps 37–1: Combining Insulins
Skill 38–1: Assisting with a Pelvic Examination and Pap Test (Smear)

MEDICAL-SURGICAL NURSING

CONCEPTS & PRACTICE

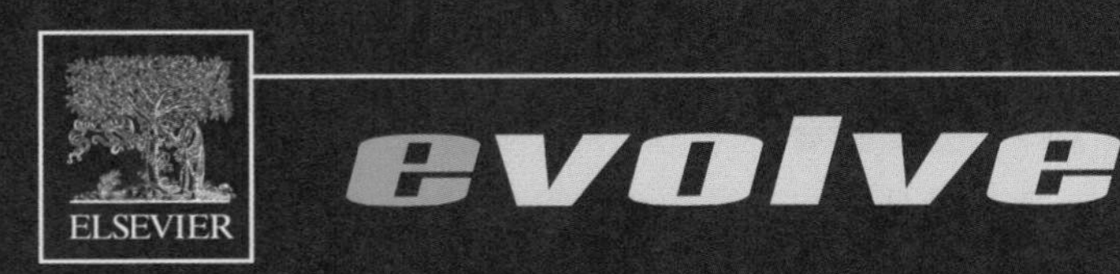

To access your Student Resources, visit the web address below:

http://evolve.elsevier.com/deWit

Evolve® Student Resources for deWit: Medical-Surgical Nursing: Concepts and Practice, offer the following features:

Student Resources

- **NCLEX-PN® Exam Style Interactive Review Questions**
  Test your knowledge with interactive activities
- **Bonus Review Questions**
  Test your knowledge with multiple-choice questions
- **Mathematics Review**
  Build a solid foundation for medication administration with this review of basic arithmetic skills
- **3D Animations**
  Learn through vivid visualizations of anatomy and physiology and physiologic processes
- **Video and Audio Clips**
  Content comes alive with enriching audio and visual assessments
- **Dorland's Audio Pronunciations**
  Learn to pronounce difficult medical terms with this helpful tool
- **Forms, additional Nursing Care Plans, Skills and Steps with Performance Checklists**
  Useful hospital forms and tools, and additional care plans and skills
- **WebLinks**
  An exciting resource that lets you link to hundreds of websites carefully chosen to supplement the content of the textbook; the WebLinks are regularly updated with new ones added as they develop
- **Additional Resources**
  Body Spectrum Electronic Anatomy and Physiology coloring book, Helpful Phrases for communicating in Spanish, and more!

http://evolve.elsevier.com/deWit

MEDICAL-SURGICAL NURSING

CONCEPTS & PRACTICE

Susan C. deWit, MSN, RN, CNS, PHN

Formerly, Instructor of Nursing
El Centro College
Dallas, Texas

Photographs by Jack Sanders, Portland, Oregon

SAUNDERS

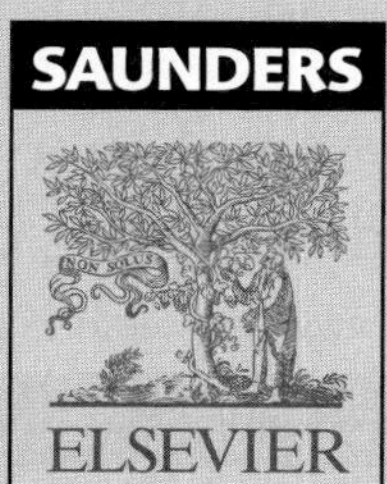

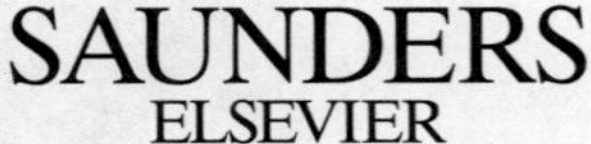

11830 Westline Industrial Drive
St. Louis, Missouri 63146

MEDICAL-SURGICAL NURSING: CONCEPTS AND PRACTICE ISBN: 978-1-4160-3223-6

Notice

Neither the Publisher nor the Author assume any responsibility for any loss or injury and/or damage to persons or property arising out of or related to any use of the material contained in this book. It is the responsibility of the treating practitioner, relying on independent expertise and knowledge of the patient, to determine the best treatment and method of application for the patient.

The Publisher

ISBN: 978-1-4160-3223-6

Vice President, Publishing Director: Sally Schrefer
Executive Publisher: Tom Wilhelm
Managing Editor: Robin Levin Richman
Developmental Editor: Mayoor Jaiswal
Publishing Services Manager: Jeffrey Patterson
Senior Production Editor: Mary G. Stueck
Book Designer: Teresa McBryan
Marketing Group Segment Manager: Kathy Mantz
Marketing Project Manager: Jamie Kitsis

Printed in the United States

Last digit is the print number: 9 8 7 6 5 4 3

To my daughter and son-in-law,
Kristen and Scott Webster, who are very special people

To all the students who will use this book
to learn the art and science of nursing,
who one day may be taking care of me

To my contributors, colleagues, and editors who lend
insight, support, and humor to the writing process

To my special cousins who include me in everything
and bring fun and companionship to my life

and

To the memory of my aunt, "Bogie,"
who will always be in my heart

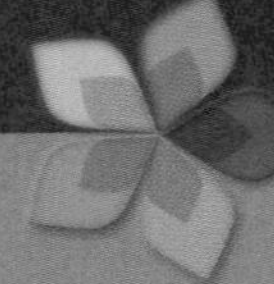

Contributors/Reviewers

CONTRIBUTORS

JIMMIE C. BORUM, MSN, RN
Clinical Instructor
Harris College of Nursing and Health Sciences
Texas Christian University
Fort Worth, Texas

CAROL DALLRED, MSN, RNC, WHCNP
Advanced Practice Nurse
University of Texas
M.D. Anderson Cancer Center
Houston, Texas

SIGNE S. HILL, BSN, RN, MA
Formerly, Instructor, Practical Nurse Program
Northeast Wisconsin Technical College
Green Bay, Wisconsin

HELEN STEPHENS HOWLETT, BSN, RN, MS
Formerly, Instructor, Practical Nurse Program
Northeast Wisconsin Technical College
Green Bay, Wisconsin

CANDICE K. KUMAGAI, MSN, RN
Clinical Instructor
Dallas County Community College District
Dallas, Texas

GLORIA LEIFER, RN, MA
Associate Professor
Riverside Community College
Riverside, California

PATRICIA A. O'NEILL, MSN, RN, CCRN
Nursing Instructor
DeAnza College
Cupertino, California

TRENA L. RICH, MSN, ARNP, BC, CIC
Director, Infection Prevention and Control Department
Riverside County Regional Medical Center
Moreno Valley, California

HOLLY STROMBERG, MSN, RN, CCRN
Director of Nursing Programs
Allan Hancock College
Santa Maria, California

FRANCES M. WARRICK, RN, MS
Program Coordinator, Vocational Nursing
El Centro College
Dallas, Texas

REVIEWERS

NANCY ELIZABETH ARMSTRONG, BSN, RN
Assistant Professor, Practical Nursing
West Kentucky Community & Technical College
Paducah, Kentucky

LA VON BARRETT, MSN, RN
Assistant Professor and Coordinator, Vocational Nursing
Amarillo College
Amarillo, Texas

DIANE M. BLIGH, RN, MS, CNS
Instructor, Nursing
Front Range Community College
Westminster, Colorado

SUSIE CARTER BROWN, BSN, RN, CRRN
Instructor, Health Career Institute
Our Lady of the Lake College
Baton Rouge, Louisiana

KATHY LYNN BURLINGAME, MSN, RN, CCRN
Associate Dean of Nursing
Minnesota State Community and Technical College
Detroit Lakes, Minnesota

PATRICIA COLLINS, PhD, MSN, RN, MS Ed
Director of Nursing and Allied Health
West Shore Community College
Scottville, Michigan

PATRICIA H. CREELMAN, MSN, RN
Director of Nursing Education
Quinsigamond Community College
Worcester, Massachusetts

KAREN D. DANIELSON, MSN, RN
Associate Professor, Practical Nursing
North Central State College
Mansfield, Ohio

JUDITH A. DONNELLY, BSN, MBA, RN
Instructor, Practical Nursing
Lancaster County Career & Technology Center
Willow Street, Pennsylvania

MELISSA LYNN EDWARDS, MSN, RN
Assistant Professor, Nursing
Dabney Lancaster Community College
Clifton Forge, Virginia

CATHY P. FREEMAN, BSN, RN
Instructor, Practical Nursing
South Georgia Technical College
Americus, Georgia

MARY D. GORDON, RN, MS, CNS
Burn Clinical Nurse Specialist
Shriners Hospitals for Children–Galveston
Galveston, Texas

TERESA GROOMS, MSN, RN
Instructor, Nursing
Southern State Community College
Hillsboro, Ohio

ANNA ALLEN MILLER HAMILTON, RN, MS, BS
Retired faculty, McLennan Community College
Waco, Texas

JEANNE HATELY, PhD, MSN, RN
Regional Nursing Director
Corinthian Colleges, Inc.
Santa Ana, California

REBECCA A. KELLY, MSN, RN, CS
Program Coordinator, Practical Nursing
Greater Altoona Career and Technology Center
Altoona, Pennsylvania

DIANE M. KEMPER, MS, RN, CCRN-CMC CNE
Instructor, Nursing
Harrisburg Area Community College
Gettysburg, Pennsylvania

LINDA B. JOHNSON, MSN, RN, CRNP
Instructor, Practical Nursing
Mercyhurst College–North East Campus
Erie, Pennsylvania

VALERIE I. LEEK, RNC, MS, CMSRN
Instructor, Licensed Practical Nursing
Cumberland County Technical Education Center
Bridgeton, New Jersey;
Adjunct Clinical Instructor of Registered Nursing
Cumberland County College
Vineland, New Jersey

SHARON J. McGRAW, MSN, RN, CRNP
Assistant Professor, Nursing
Northampton Community College
Bethlehem, Pennsylvania

LAURO MANALO, JR., MSN, RN
Instructor, Associate Degree in Nursing Program
Allan Hancock College
Santa Maria, California

BELINDA BRUMFIELD MUNSON, BSN, RNC
Instructor, Health Career Institute
Our Lady of the Lake College
Baton Rouge, Louisiana

SALLIE NOTO, MSN, RN, MS
Program Director, School of Practical Nursing
Career Technology Center of Lackawanna County
Scranton, Pennsylvania

JENNIFER PONTO, BSN, RN
Instructor, Vocational Nursing
South Plains College
Levelland, Texas

SANDRA G. REIDER, MSN, RN, BA
Instructor, Practical Nursing
Reading Area Community College
Reading, Pennsylvania

REBECCA K. ROMAGNA, MSN, RN
Instructor, Practical Nursing
Greater Altoona Career and Technology Center
Altoona, Pennsylvania

JOANN SCHEU, MEd, BSN, RN
Medical-Surgical Clinical Educator
Hanover Hospital
Hanover, Pennsylvania

SUSAN SEIBOLDT, MSN, RN
Instructor, Associate Degree Nursing Program
Carl Sandburg College
Galesburg, Illinois

CASSIE M. SHAW, BSN, RN
Instructor, Vocational Nursing
Vernon College
Wichita Falls, Texas

BRENDA K. SNYDER, MSN, RNC
Instructor, Nursing
Harrisburg Area Community College
York, Pennsylvania

KATHY SOMMERS, EdD, BSN, RN, MBA
Instructor, School of Nursing
Columbus State Community College
Columbus, Ohio

RUSSLYN A. ST. JOHN, MSN, RN
Coordinator, Practical Nursing
Saint Charles Community College
Cottleville, Missouri

ERIN YESENOSKY, MSN, RN
Instructor, Practical Nursing
Greater Altoona Career and Technology Center
Altoona, Pennsylvania

To the Instructor

Medical-Surgical Nursing: Concepts and Practice is written solely for the LPN/LVN student. Today's LPN/LVN must be educated to work within the variety of settings in which LPN/LVNs are employed: hospitals, long-term care facilities, rehabilitation institutes, ambulatory clinics, physicians' offices, and home care agencies. This new textbook incorporates aspects of nursing in each of these settings.

All of the most common adult medical-surgical disorders are covered, but the most attention is devoted to those disorders most prevalent in our society today. Before studying medical-surgical nursing, every LPN/LVN student has a course in fundamentals of nursing. This text builds on the concepts and skills presented in every fundamentals of nursing course. Nursing students today are overwhelmed by both textbook size and cost. We endeavor to avoid duplicating material that students have already covered in every fundamentals text. We integrate legal and ethical issues, nutrition, care of the older adult, communication, cultural aspects, complementary and alternative therapies, patient teaching, home care, health promotion, and basic management throughout the text rather than including separate chapters on these subjects. The term "patient" is used rather than "client" because that is what is still used in hospitals. "Resident" is used for those residing in long-term care facilities.

Many states are expanding LPN/LVN practice, via certification, to include administration of intravenous (IV) fluids and medications. Other states do not have IV therapy within the scope of LPN/LVN practice. Information on IV therapy is included within this text and on the Companion CD-ROM so that schools in states where such certification is possible will have the necessary educational materials within the student's medical-surgical nursing text.

With the expanding role of the LPN/LVN there is an even greater need for **critical thinking** and the development of **clinical judgment.** These crucial skills are stressed throughout the clinical chapters. **Evidence-based practice** is designated with a special EB icon EB so that the student will see the thrust of nursing toward a foundation based in research. Evidence-based practice research within nursing is in its infancy. There is medical evidence-based research on which nurses often base patient teaching. Both types of evidence-based practice are marked with the EB. Practice in priority setting is included in the various exercises and is a special section in each chapter of the Student Learning Guide.

The **NCLEX-PN® Exam** has an essential role in this textbook. End-of-chapter NCLEX-PN® Exam Style Review Questions include alternate-format questions, which are also incorporated into the ExamView Test Bank on the TEACH Instructor Resources available on the Evolve website. Interactive NCLEX-PN® questions are included for students on the Evolve website.

Nursing process and its application to nursing care are illustrated throughout the text as a tool, while concepts are stressed, and patients' needs are the focus of nursing care. There is a heavy emphasis on practical assessment: data collection to determine problems, assessment to monitor for the onset of complications, and assessment to determine the effectiveness of care (evaluation). LPN/LVNs assist RNs with data collection so that appropriate nursing diagnoses may be chosen for each patient. Guidelines for **focused assessments** pertinent to the body systems in which disorders occur are provided throughout the text to guide data collection. The LPN/LVN role of being able to work with nursing diagnoses, although not formulating them, is addressed. A focus on using expected outcomes and how to evaluate nursing care to see if they have been met is part of each clinical chapter.

Planning holistic care must include consideration of the patient's **cultural background** and its impact on perception of health, illness, and health practices. Cultural sensitivity must be integrated into patient care by a culturally competent nurse. Psychosocial care is included throughout the chapters. **End-of-life issues** and **palliative care** are presented at the end of the chapter on cancer. Boxes stressing specific areas of cultural considerations and patient education are interspersed throughout the discussions of nursing care, and encompass discharge planning.

Implementation of nursing actions is the heart of patient care and LPN/LVN practice. Nursing actions presented are specific and comprehensive. They are organized by common care problems to decrease repetition of information within a chapter and help the student learn by mastering concepts rather than memorizing facts. Further interventions are discussed with each disorder as appropriate. Safe practice is emphasized throughout the text.

LPN/LVN nurse practice acts do not encompass **delegation** as a function. With a few exceptions, only RNs can delegate, although in many situations

LPN/LVNs can assign tasks. Collaboration with other health care workers and the use of basic management skills to provide coordinated, cost-effective patient care is essential. In this text we particularly speak to the LPN/LVN management role in working with nursing assistants and assigning tasks appropriately.

Caring for the older adult is a major thread throughout the chapters. Data collection from the geriatric patient requires greater ability to elicit pertinent information from the patient or family as well as a knowledge of normal physiologic changes. Each chapter includes specific Elder Care Points. Suggestions for assessment (data collection) and particular interventions for the long-term care and the home care patient are included.

Patient teaching for health promotion and the maintenance of wellness and self-care is a basic function of the LPN/LVN. Each clinical chapter points out ways in which nurses can teach the public how to prevent many of the problems discussed. Self-care guidelines for the major disorders are presented. *Healthy People 2010* goals and objectives are highlighted.

Chronic illness and **rehabilitation care** are growing areas. A chapter addresses the differences in care approaches and nursing care for these individuals. The interaction of the interdisciplinary health care team in the rehabilitation of those with respiratory, cardiac, musculoskeletal, neurologic, and other problems is a major thread.

Clear, ongoing **communication** among health care professionals is essential for collaborative care to be effective. The ability to communicate effectively with and assign tasks to ancillary personnel is essential when caring for multiple patients in any setting. Practical information on communication is integrated throughout.

National Patient Safety Goals are highlighted to help students integrate **safety measures** into their practice. **Safety Alerts** remind students of specific safety concerns. **Clinical Cues** are presented to share pointers or considerations for clinical practice with students.

A friendly writing style and language at an understandable level for today's student has been used to gain and retain student attention to reading assignments. Since there are both male and female nurses, physicians, and patients, the use of "he" and "she" for patient, physician, and nurse varies from chapter to chapter. An English-as-a-Second Language (ESL) consultant reviewed each chapter and provided ideas to make the text more user-friendly and understandable for the student with limited proficiency in English. A section in each chapter of the *Student Learning Guide* has been designed to assist this student to more easily master the chapter content and to enhance English skills.

ORGANIZATION OF THE TEXT

Organized logically by body systems, *Medical-Surgical Nursing* includes all the purely medical-surgical content with little duplication of information typically found in fundamentals books. Unit One addresses medical-surgical nursing settings, nursing roles and issues, health care trends, assignment considerations, nursing process, and critical thinking. Unit Two covers all the key medical-surgical nursing topics including fluids and electrolytes, surgical patient care, infections, pain, cancer and palliative care, and a separate chapter on chronic illness and rehabilitation. The next 12 units cover all the body systems and their disorders. Unit Fifteen addresses emergency and disaster management—including bioterrorism—as well as trauma and shock. Unit Sixteen is entirely devoted to mental health nursing.

Standard LPN Threads Features

The following LPN Threads features are found in *Medical-Surgical Nursing:*

- **Full-color design, cover, photos,** and **illustrations** are visually appealing and pedagogically useful.
- **ESL (English as a Second Language)** considerations figure prominently in both the textbook and its Student Learning Guide. An ESL specialist reviewed all chapters during development to make sure they will be clearly understood by the ESL student and the student with limited proficiency in English.
- **Key Terms with phonetic pronunciations and text page references** improve and supplement terminology and language skills of the ESL student and the student with limited proficiency in English before they enter clinical practice. Key Terms are in color at first mention and simply defined in the text (all Key Terms are in the Glossary). An in-text CD icon directs the students to audio pronunciations for Key Terms on the companion CD.
- **Objectives** (numbered) are given on the first page of the chapter and are divided into Theory and Clinical categories. The objectives provide a framework for content and are especially impor-

tant to the TEACH Lesson Plans for the book, which are structured around chapter objectives.

- **Critical Thinking Questions** are given at the end of each **Nursing Care Plan** and the answers are provided in the TEACH Instructor Resources on the Evolve website.
- **Critical Thinking Activities** at the end of chapters include a realistic clinical case scenario and a clinical situation, both of which provide ample opportunity for the student to hone critical thinking skills. Answers are found in the TEACH Instructor Resources on the Evolve website.
- **Skills** (numbered and titled) follow the nursing process and are presented in a clear Action/Rationale format. Performance checklists for these skills are found in the Student Learning Guide, Companion CD-ROM, and Evolve website. More skills with performance checklists are provided on the Companion CD and Evolve website.
- **Key Points** are located at the end of chapters and summarize chapter highlights.

Special Features

Special pedagogical features throughout help the student understand and apply the chapter content, as follows:

- **Overview of Anatomy and Physiology** at the beginning of each system overview chapter provides basic information for understanding the body system and its disorders.
- **Five-Step Nursing Process** provides the consistent framework for disorders chapters.
- **Focused Assessment** box for each body system is primarily located in each Overview chapter and includes history taking and psychosocial assessment, physical assessment, and guidance on how to collect data/information for specific disorders.
- **NCLEX-PN® Exam Style Review Questions** at the end of each chapter include alternate-format questions and help the student become familiar with the format and prepare for the exam. Answers are provided at the end of the textbook.
- **Unit on Mental Health Nursing** includes information on disorders of anxiety and mood, eating disorders, cognitive disorders, thought and personality disorders, and substance abuse.
- **Disaster Management** content includes material focusing on preparation and mitigation to avoid losses and reduce the risk of injury associated with both natural and bioterrorist disasters.
- **Assignment Considerations** are discussed in Chapter 1, then found in subsequent chapters in boxes that address situations in which the RN delegates tasks to the LPN/LVN or when the LPN/LVN assigns tasks to nurse assistants per the individual state nurse practice act.
- **Evidence-Based Practice** is highlighted throughout the narrative with a EB to flag cutting-edge references to research studies in nursing and medical practice.
- **Legal & Ethical Considerations** boxes focus on specific disorder-related issues.
- **Safety Alert** boxes highlight specific danger or dangers to patients related to clinical care. Located as appropriate throughout.
- **Clinical Cues** provide guidance and advice related to the application of nursing care.
- **Think Critically About...**boxes encourage students to synthesize information and apply concepts beyond the scope of the chapter.
- **Concept Maps** found in disorders chapters are learning tools designed to help students visualize difficult material and to illustrate how a disorder's multiple symptoms, treatments, and side effects relate to each other.
- **Health Promotion Points** boxes address wellness and disease prevention.
- **Communication Cues** provide guidance in therapeutic communication skills in realistic patient care situations.
- **Cultural Cues** related to biocultural variations as well as health promotion for specific ethnic groups are interspersed throughout the narrative.
- **Nutritional Therapies** related to nursing care for specific disorders address the need for holistic care and reflect the increased focus on nutrition in the NCLEX-PN® Exam.
- **Patient Teaching** boxes are step-by-step instructions and guidelines for post-hospital care.
- **Elder Care Points** boxes address the unique medical-surgical care issues that affect older adults.
- **Home Care Considerations** boxes focus on post-discharge adaptations of medical-surgical nursing care to the home environment.
- **Complementary & Alternative Therapies** boxes are rich with information on how nontraditional treatments for medical-surgical conditions may be used to complement traditional treatment.
- **Bolded text** throughout the narrative emphasizes key concepts and practice.

TEACHING AND LEARNING PACKAGE

We provide a rich, abundant collection of supplemental resources for both instructors and students.

For the Instructor

TEACH Instructor Resources

The new, comprehensive TEACH Instructor Resources on the Evolve website provides a wealth of material to meet your teaching needs, in addition to everything in the Student Resources, including NCLEX-PN® Exam Style interactive review questions and WebLinks:

- **Open-Book Quizzes** for each chapter in the textbook.
- **PowerPoint Presentation** provides approximately 2400 text and image slides.

- **Electronic Image Collection** includes all the illustrations and photographs from the book plus supplemental images from other Elsevier titles that can be easily incorporated into the PowerPoint presentations.
- **ExamView Test Bank** contains approximately 1200 NCLEX-PN® Exam Style questions as well as alternate-format questions.
- **iClicker Questions** promote interactivity and feedback in the classroom.
- **Answer Keys** to the Critical Thinking Activities and Critical Thinking Questions in the textbook, Student Learning Guide activities and exercises (both print and additional activities on Evolve Student Resources), and bonus review questions.
- **TEACH Lesson Plans with Lecture Outlines,** based on textbook chapter learning objectives, provide a roadmap to link and integrate all parts of the educational package. These concise and straightforward lesson plans can be modified or combined to meet scheduling and teaching needs.

For the Student

- **Companion CD-ROM** (bound with text) includes Audio and Video Clips; 3D Animations of Anatomy and Physiology; Dorland's Audio Pronunciations; Helpful Phrases for Communicating in Spanish; Mathematics Review; Fluids and Electrolytes Module; forms used in health care settings; additional Nursing Care Plans; additional Skills and Steps with Performance Checklists; and a wealth of bonus review questions.
- **Clinical Quick Reference** is a pocket-sized, saddle-stitched booklet, 4 × 6 inches, 64 pages, shrink-wrapped with the textbook. It includes some of the most commonly seen disorders, their key assessment and interventions, nursing diagnoses, and related medications; information on chart review, selected clinical tools, laboratory values, and psychiatric interventions for working with patients who have behavior issues.
- **Student Learning Guide** is patterned after the highly successful Student Learning Guide for this author's *Fundamentals of Nursing* text, and includes a wide range of exercises, activities, and questions keyed to the textbook. It incorporates priority-setting exercises for most chapters. Each chapter ends with "Steps to Better Communication" to assist students with less proficient English enhance their learning and communication skills. Additional Student Learning Guide activities and exercises are available on the Evolve web-site. Answers to the all exercises appear in the TEACH Instructor Resources on Evolve.
- **Evolve Learning System Student Resources** include everything on the Companion CD as well as WebLinks; tables and tools useful in health care settings; Anatomy and Physiology Body Spectrum Coloring Book; online bibliography, and additional Student Learning Guide activities and exercises. NCLEX-PN® Exam Style interactive review questions test their knowledge and help them prepare for certification.
- **Virtual Clinical Excursion (VCE)** is an interactive workbook CD-ROM that guides the student through a multifloor virtual hospital in a hands-on clinical experience.

• • •

Teaching nursing has been one of the most exciting and gratifying phases of my life. I hope this textbook and its ancillaries make your job as an instructor easier and class preparation more time-efficient. May your students find excitement and joy in learning and applying the information you impart in the clinical setting.

SUSAN C. deWIT, MSN, RN, CNS, PHN

LPN Threads

The new *Medical-Surgical Nursing: Concepts and Practice* shares some features and design elements with other LPN titles on the Elsevier list. The purpose of these LPN Threads is to make it easier for students and instructors to use the variety of books required by the relatively brief and demanding LPN curriculum.

The shared features in *Medical-Surgical Nursing: Concepts and Practice* include the following:

- A **reading level evaluation** performed on every manuscript chapter during the book's development. The purpose is to increase the consistency among chapters and to make the text easy to understand.
- Cover and internal **design similarities.** The colorful, student-friendly design encourages the reading and learning of the core content.
- Numbered lists of **Objectives** begin each chapter.
- **Key Terms** with phonetic pronunciations and page number references are provided at the beginning of each chapter. The key terms are in color the first time they appear in the chapter.
- **Critical Thinking Questions** are given at the end of every Nursing Care Plan.
- Bulleted **Key Points** that summarize critical concepts are listed at the end of each chapter
- The **Bibliography** follows at the end of the text, and an on-line Bibliography is provided on the Evolve website.
- A comprehensive **Glossary** appears at the end of the text.
- A wide variety of Special Features related to critical thinking, clinical practice, care of the older adult, health promotion, safety, patient teaching, complementary and alternative therapies, communication, home health care, legal and ethical considerations, delegation and assignment, and more!

And for instructors…

- An **ExamView Test Bank** with the following categories of information: Topic, Step of the Nursing Process, Objective, Cognitive Level, NCLEX® Category of Client Need, Correct Answer, Rationale, and Text Page Reference
- A **PowerPoint slide presentation** in the TEACH Instructor Resources on Evolve
- **Open-Book Quizzes** in the TEACH Instructor Resources available on the Evolve website
- **Student Learning Guide answer keys** in the TEACH Instructor Resources on Evolve; the Study Guide itself contains text page number references where students can find the answers
- **Tips for teaching English-as-a-Second-Language (ESL) students** in the TEACH Instructor Resources on Evolve

In addition to content and design threads, these LPN textbooks benefit from the advice and input of the Elsevier LPN Advisory Board.

LPN Advisory Board

SHIRLEY ANDERSON, MSN
Kirkwood Community College
Cedar Rapids, Iowa

M. GIE ARCHER, MS, RN, C, WHCNP
Dean of Health Sciences
LVN Program Coordinator
North Central Texas College
Gainesville, Texas

MARY BROTHERS, MEd, RN
Coordinator, Garnet Career Center School of Practical Nursing
Charleston, West Virginia

PATRICIA A. CASTALDI, RN, BSN, MSN
Union County College
Plainfield, New Jersey

MARY ANN COSGAREA, RN, BSN
PN Coordinator/Health Coordinator
Portage Lakes Career Center
Green, Ohio

DOLORES ANN COTTON, RN, BSN, MS
Meridian Technology Center
Stillwater, Oklahoma

LORA LEE CRAWFORD, RN, BSN
Emanuel Turlock Vocational Nursing Program
Turlock, California

RUTH ANN ECKENSTEIN, RN, BS, MEd
Oklahoma Department of Career and Technology Education
Stillwater, Oklahoma

GAIL ANN HAMILTON FINNEY, RN, MSN
Nursing Education Specialist
Concorde Career Colleges, INC
Mission, Kansas

PAM HINCKLEY, RN, MSN
Redlands Adult School
Redlands, California

DEBORAH W. KELLER, RN, BSN, MSN
Erie Huron Ottawa Vocational Education School of Practical Nursing
Milan, Ohio

PATTY KNECHT, MSN, RN
Nursing Program Director
Center for Arts & Technology
Brandywine Campus
Coatesville, Pennsylvania

LIEUTENANT COLONEL (RET.) TERESA Y. McPHERSON, RN, BSN, MSN
Adjunct Instructor
St. Philip's College LVN/AND Nursing Program
San Antonio, Texas

FRANCES NEU, MS, BSN, RN
Supervisor, Adult Ed Health
Butler Technology and Career Development Schools
Fairfield Township, Ohio

DIANNA DANCED SCHERLIN, MS, RN
National Director of Nursing
Lincoln Educational Services
West Orange, New Jersey

BEVERLEY TURNER, MA, RN
Director, Vocational Nursing Department
Maric College, San Diego Campus
San Diego, California

C. SUE WEIDMAN, RN, BSN
Brown Mackie College, Nurse Specialist
Forest, Ohio

SISTER ANN WIESEN, RN, MRA
Erwin Technical Center
Tampa, Florida

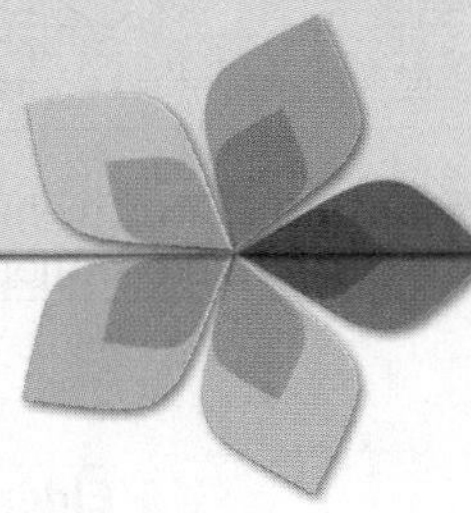

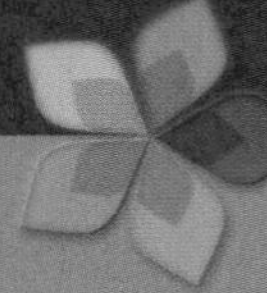

To the Student

Designed specifically for the LPN/LVN student, *Medical-Surgical Nursing: Concepts and Skills* has a visually appealing, easy-to-use format. Here are some of the numerous Special Features that will help guide you through medical-surgical nursing as you learn and apply the information:

Theory and Clinical Practice objectives highlight the chapter's main learning goals.

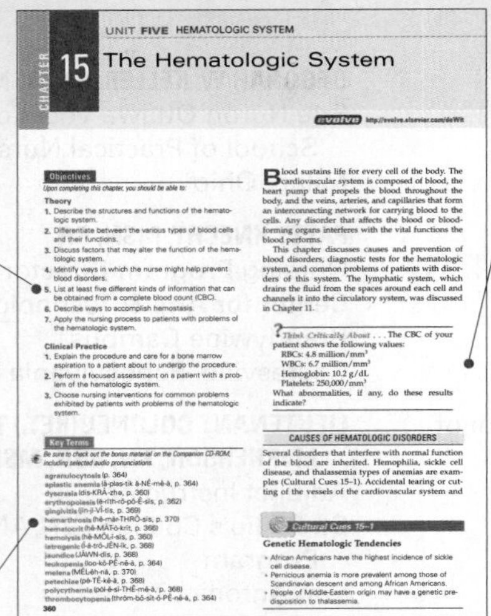

Think Critically about... boxes help you expand your knowledge and think "outside the box"

Overview of Anatomy and Physiology for body system chapters.

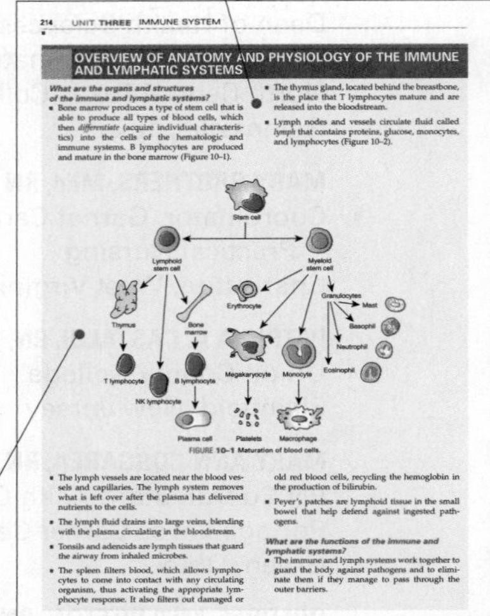

Key Terms with phonetic pronunciations and text page references are identified in color at first mention. Pronunciation Guide in Glossary.

Full-color photographs, design, and art enhance the text.

Focused Assessment boxes guide you in physical and psychosocial assessment and data collection

Complementary & Alternative Therapies boxes are rich with information on nontraditional treatments.

Safety Alert boxes highlight specific dangers related to clinical care.

Cultural Cues address the needs of culturally diverse patient populations.

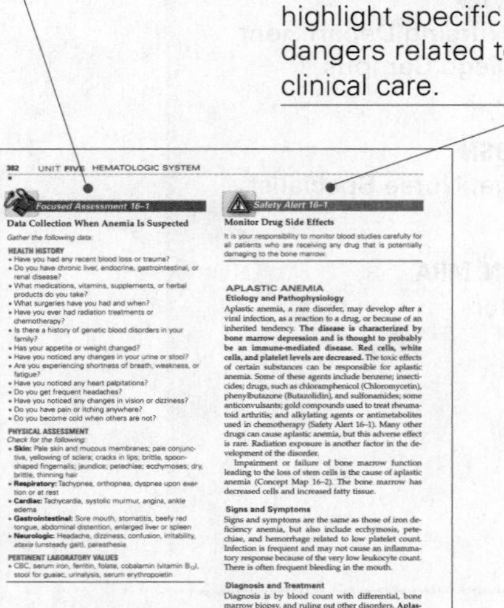

Health Promotion Points highlight wellness and disease prevention.

Elder Care Points address medical-surgical issues that affect older adults.

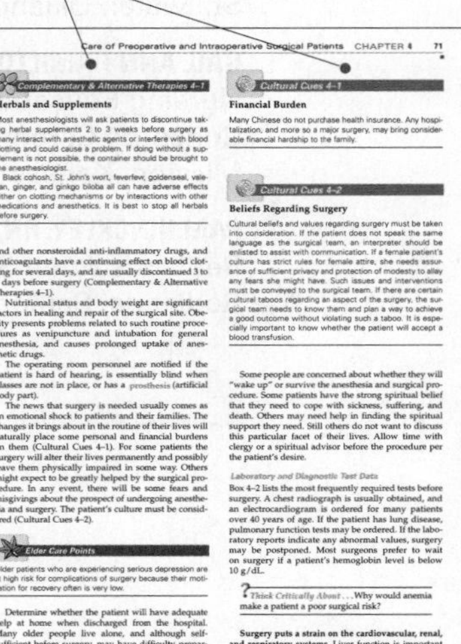

Evidence-Based Practice icon highlights cutting-edge research.

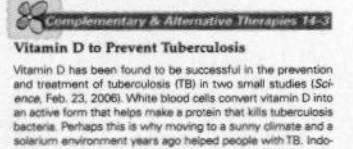

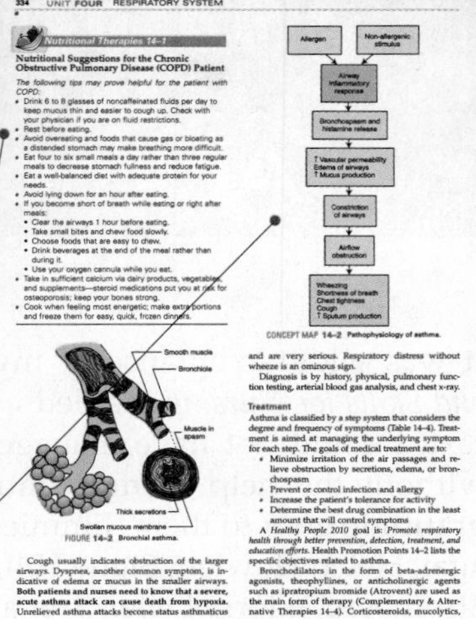

Legal & Ethical Considerations focus on specific disorder-related issues.

Nutritional Therapies address the need for holistic care.

Concept Maps help you visualize difficult content.

Assignment Considerations address delegation or assignment situations.

Patient Teaching boxes provide step-by-step instructions for post-hospital care.

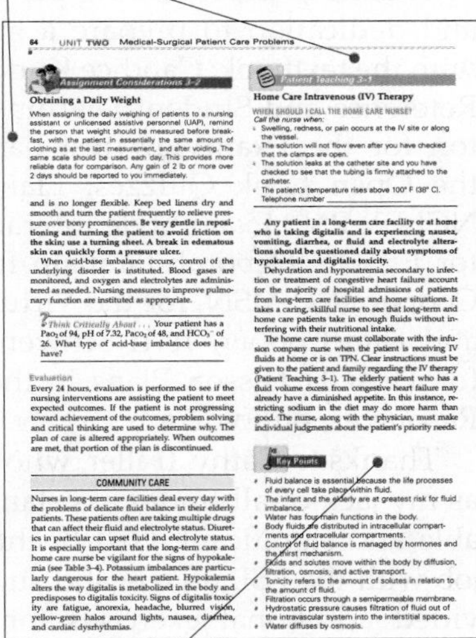

Communication Cues illustrate communication strategies through real-life nursing situations.

Nursing Care Plans with Critical Thinking Questions apply nursing process to clinical situations.

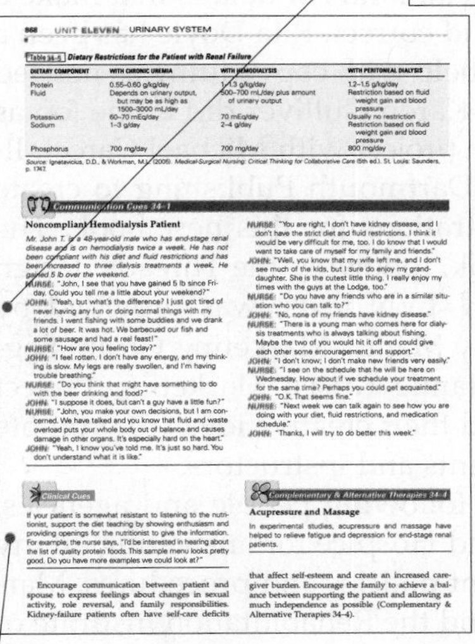

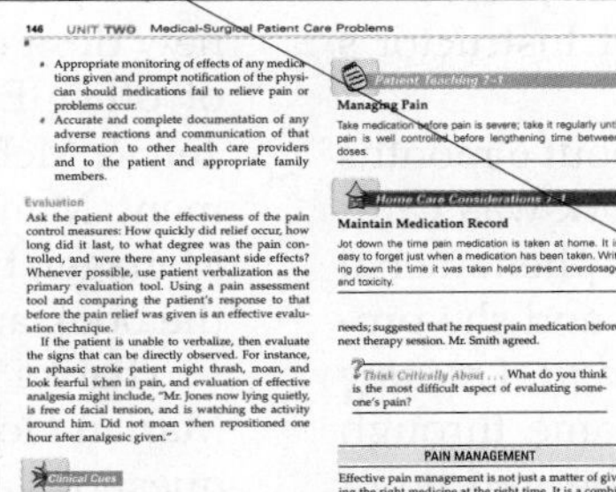

Home Care Considerations address patient and caregiver issues in the home care setting.

Key points summarize main concepts.

Clinical Cues serve as pointers in nursing situations.

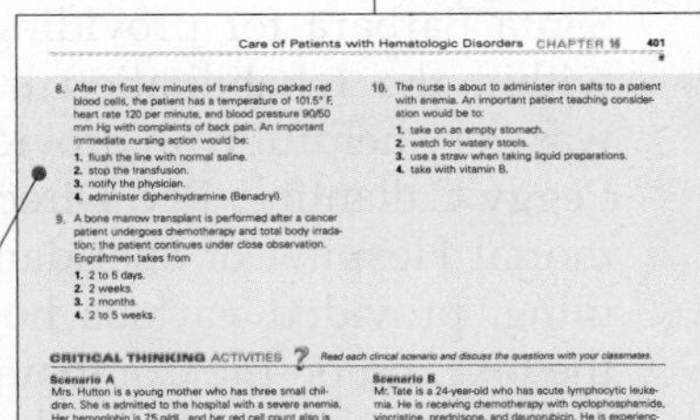

End-of-chapter NCLEX-PN® Exam Style Review Questions for student practice.

Critical Thinking Activities help you develop problem-solving skills.

FREE COMPANION CD!
Includes Audio and Video Clips, 3D Animations, Math Review, Fluid & Electrolytes Tutorial, bonus review questions, and more!

FREE CLINICAL QUICK REFERENCE!
Includes information regarding many common disorders, assessment, nursing diagnoses, interventions and treatment, chart review, clinical tools, laboratory values, and psychiatric interventions.

Acknowledgments

It was wide acceptance of my *Fundamental Concepts and Skills for Nursing* that led me to agree to write this text. I could not have managed to produce this text without the help of my contributors. My heart-felt gratitude goes to them: Jimmie Borum, Candice Kumagai, Helen Howlett, Signe Hill, Patricia O'Neill, Holly Stromberg, Gloria Leifer, Trena Rich, Frances Warrick, and Carol Dallred. Thanks go to the reviewers whose comments helped us to refine and clarify content as needed (see the list of Reviewers on pp. x and xi). The willingness of Larry Manalo to write the NCLEX-PN® Exam Style Review Questions at the end of the chapters and prepare the annotated PowerPoint presentation is greatly appreciated. He has done a commendable job.

Thanks to the following people for their hard work and dedication to prepare a great ancillary package with the textbook: Candice Kumagai for Clinical Quick Reference and Student Learning Guide; Allen Hamilton for the ExamView test bank; Dan Matusiak for the Open Book Quizzes; Elaine Princevalli for the NCLEX-PN® Exam Style interactive review questions for Evolve; Deborah Graham for the WebLinks; Kim Cooper, RN, MSN, for the Virtual Clinical Excursions; and Kim Cooper, Terri Schwenk, and Kelly Grosnell for TEACH Lesson Plans in the TEACH Instructor's Resources, on Evolve.

Thanks to Cathy Traller, who put in about 6 months as my jack-of-all-trades assistant. Her work was valuable and significant. Gail Boehme did a phenomenal job with the ESL review and suggestions and she provided additional exercises for the *Student Learning Guide* that accompanies the text. Gail came through like a champ even though she was in the middle of traveling between two locations to provide assistance and care for her elderly father. She reviewed every chapter in the text, making suggestions on how to make information more understandable for the ESL students. Kathy Stilling has assisted me with proofing pages and has been a tremendous help. Her expertise and friendship are highly valued.

Thanks to Southwestern Washington Medical Center for allowing us to photograph within their facility. Their patients, staff, and administration are so willing to help with whatever they can for the education of nursing students. Jack Sanders is a talented, creative, professional photographer whose beautiful photos are seen throughout this book. Ginger Navarro took on the job of photo coordination this time and has been a tremendous help.

Thanks to Robin Levin Richman, Managing Editor, and Mayoor Jaiswal, Developmental Editor at Elsevier who have brought this project to fruition. Their dedication and friendship have kept the project on track. Marie Thomas, Senior Editorial Assistant, has been, as usual, extremely efficient and helpful and has attended to every request very quickly. Mary Stueck, Senior Project Manager, always makes the production process pleasurable. Her sense of humor always gets us through the tough parts and lightens the days. Mary is extremely good at her job and has a talent for page layout that has really been challenged with this book. Megan Westerfeld is the most meticulous of copyeditors and is attentive to all kinds of details that make a book truly cohesive and correct. Rita Doyle has been a champ to step in and help with copyediting as needed while Megan moved. Karen Gulliver did a fine job as art coordinator for the project with Michael Carcel, Illustration Buyer and Dartmouth Publishing to create beautiful, useful illustrations for this new book. The new design of the book, following the Threads design of other Elsevier LPN/LVN texts, was provided by Teresa McBryan. Kathy Mantz, Marketing Group Segment Manager, and Jamie Kitsis, Marketing Project Manager, have applied their creative ideas to promote the book among students and instructors.

Thanks also to the following people and agencies: Marian Home Care and Hospice for answering all my questions about current policies and procedures. Marguerite Wordell, RN and the Rehabilitation Institute of Santa Barbara for providing the various forms used within the rehabilitation environment. Maggie also was very helpful with providing answers to questions. Peggy Callantine, RN, Director of Nursing at the Memorial Hospital of Sheridan County, Sheridan, Wyoming, provided various hospital forms used within the text and on the Companion CD-ROM.

Thanks to my gal friends here who make me take a break from the computer for a morning walk and then coffee a couple of times a week. They keep me sane.

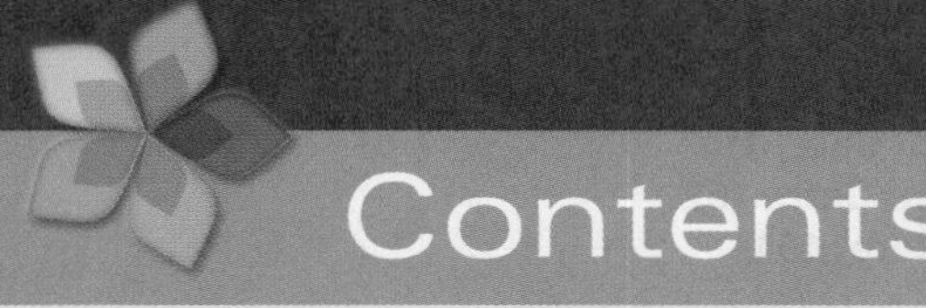

Contents

CHAPTER 1

Caring for Medical-Surgical Patients

evolve http://evolve.elsevier.com/deWit

Objectives

Upon completing this chapter, you should be able to:

1. Identify 10 sites of employment for licensed practical/vocational nurses (LPN/LVNs) in medical-surgical nursing.
2. Describe each of the roles of the LPN/LVN.
3. Explain the difference between a health maintenance organization (HMO) and a preferred provider organization (PPO).
4. Differentiate between Medicare and Medicaid in the areas of eligibility and services provided.
5. Describe how hospitals are reimbursed under the diagnosis-related group (DRG) system of Medicare.
6. Discuss four factors that contribute to rising health care costs.
7. Explain how *Healthy People 2010* could decrease health care costs as a health promotion and prevention of illness strategy.
8. Define and explain the importance of holistic care.
9. Explain how the nurse-patient relationship is established.
10. Discuss how psychological, social, cultural, and spiritual needs are incorporated in the LPN/LVN's plan of care.
11. Provide a general description of depressed and manipulative behavior.
12. Identify the relationship of unmet needs to withdrawn, dependent, hostile, and manipulative behavior.
13. Describe two nursing interventions to meet needs of patients exhibiting each of the following types of behavior: dependent, withdrawn, depressed, hostile, and manipulative.

Key Terms

Be sure to check out the bonus material on the Companion CD-ROM, including selected audio pronunciations.

acuity (ă-KŪ-ĭ-tē, p. 1)
biomedicine (BĪ-ō-MĔD-ĭ-sĭn, p. 12)
capitation (kă-pĭ-TĀ-shŭn, p. 5)
co-insurance (kō-ĭn-SHŪ-rĕnz, p. 5)
complementary and alternative medicine (CAM) (KŎM-plĕ-MĔN-tĕ-rē ănd ăl-TŬR-nă-tĭv MĔD-ĭ-sĭn, p. 13)
copayment (kō-PĀY-mĕnt, p. 5)
cost containment (kŏst kŏn-TĀN-mĕnt, p. 7)
deductible (dē-DŬK-tĭ-bŭl, p. 5)
delegation (DĔL-ĭ-GĀ-shŭn, p. 3)
dependent (dĕ-PĔN-dĕnt, p. 10)
diagnosis-related groups (DRGs) (dī-ăg-NŌ-sĭs rē-LĀ-tĕd grūpz, p. 6)
empathy (ĔM-pă-thē, p. 8)
fee-for-service (fē fŏr SĔR-vĭs, p. 5)
health maintenance organization (HMO) (hĕlth MĀN-tĕ-nĕnz ŏr-gă-nĭ-ZĀ-shŭn, p. 5)
Healthy People 2010 (HĔLTH -ē PĒ-pl, p. 7)
holistic care (hō-LĬS-tĭk kār, p. 8)
managed care (MĂN-ăjd kār, p. 5)
Medicaid (mĕd-ĭ-KĀD, p. 6)
Medicare (mĕd-ĭ-KĀR, p. 5)
nonjudgmental (NŎN-jŭj-MĔN-tăl, p. 12)
nurse practice act (nŭrz PRĂK-tĭs ăct, p. 2)
patient advocates (PĀ-shĕnt ĂD-vō-kătz, p. 3)
point-of-service (POS) option (point ŏv sĕr-vĭs ŏp-shŭn, p. 5)
preferred provider organization (PPO) (prĕ-FURD prō-vī-dĕr ŏr-gă-nĭ-ZĀ-shŭn, p. 5)
prospective payment system (PPS) (prŏs-PĔK-tĭv pā-ment sĭs-tĕm, p. 6)
provider (prō-vī-dĕr, p. 5)
retrospective payment system (rĕt-rŏs-PĔK-tĭv pā-mĕnt sĭs-tĕm, p. 5)
stereotypes (STĔR-ē-ō-tīps, p. 12)
unlicensed assistive personnel (un-LI-sĕnst ă-SĬS-tĭv pĕr-sō-NĔL, p. 3)

Medical-surgical nursing involves care for adult patients with medical and/or surgical conditions that affect either one or multiple body systems. Medical nursing involves caring for patients with diseases requiring a variety of treatments, including medication and diet therapy; surgical nursing involves caring for patients requiring operative procedures to treat diseases and/or trauma. Patients can have a single diagnosis of a medical or surgical condition or a combination of both.

EMPLOYMENT OPPORTUNITIES FOR LICENSED PRACTICAL/VOCATIONAL NURSES (LPN/LVNs) IN MEDICAL-SURGICAL NURSING

The traditional site of employment for medical-surgical nursing has been the hospital. Although many nursing jobs have moved to the community, a nursing shortage, an increase in the number of patients admitted, and an increase in **acuity** (severeness) of illness

Box 1–1 Various Sites of Employment for LPN/LVNs

AREAS WITHIN THE HOSPITAL
- Outpatient Surgery
- Intermediate Care Unit (Step-Down Unit)
- Intravenous (IV) Therapy Team*
- Emergency Department

ADDITIONAL SITES FOR EMPLOYMENT OPPORTUNITIES
- Ambulatory Care
- Long-Term Care Facility (Nursing Home)
- Rehabilitation Services (Extended Care, Postacute Care, Subacute Care)
- Home Health Care
- Ambulatory Clinics
- Medical Offices
- Hospice Care Agency
- Military Service
- Dialysis Center

*Requires postgraduate education and certification.

have increased demand for nurses in hospitals at this time. This site has a fast-paced environment and a rapid rate of patient turnover. Other sites of employment are listed in Box 1–1.

Think Critically About . . . What are the current medical-surgical opportunities for employment in your area of the country? Who will you contact for this information?

ROLES OF THE LPN/LVN

The state's **nurse practice act** (NPA) defines the role and scope of practice of LPN/LVNs. Administrative rules and regulations and interpretations of the state's board of nursing provide more *specific* details and clarification. Some NPAs list specifically what LPN/LVNs can do, but others are written to allow for changes in the evolving role of the LPN/LVN. This eliminates the need for state legislatures to reopen the act and revise it each time a change is required. It is your responsibility to be aware of the law of the state in which you are employed. The role of the LPN/LVN is to care for patients within the scope of the state's NPA while upholding clinical standards. The LPN/LVN provides safe patient care, serves as a patient advocate, teaches patients, and communicates effectively, all while functioning as a collaborative member of the health care team.

Think Critically About . . . Nurse practice acts vary considerably from state to state. Where can you obtain a copy of your state's NPA?

UPHOLD CLINICAL STANDARDS

Check your institution for guidelines and policies. The facility might restrict the LPN/LVN's role to less than the NPA allows, but no employer can give nurses permission to do what their license says they cannot do.

The National Association for Practical Nurse Education and Service, Inc. (NAPNES) and the National Federation of Licensed Practical Nurses, Inc. (NFLPN) are practical/vocational nursing organizations that provide standards that guide the role of the LPN/LVN. These standards of practice, which echo the values and priorities of the profession and provide guidelines for safe and competent nursing care, may be used as a basis of prosecution or defense in a court of law. Be sure to review the standards of your nursing organizations (see Appendices 1 and 2).

PROVIDE SAFE PATIENT CARE

In the hospital acute care setting, the LPN/LVN may be engaged in total care for assigned patients, under the supervision of a registered nurse (RN). This involves being responsible for giving care to meet patients' basic needs with the goal of making patients as independent as possible and preserving their ability to care for themselves. LPN/LVNs cannot assume the role of the professional (registered) nurse, but they participate in the nursing process by assisting the RN to assess (gather data on) patients and in planning and evaluating patient care. The LPN/LVN also assists with personal hygiene, performs ordered treatments, initiates nursing interventions, and administers drugs. In other situations, the LPN/LVN might be used as a medication and treatment nurse for all patients on a team, which includes performing more complex procedures. If asked to do a procedure or treatment that was not taught in their educational program but that is allowed by the NPA, LPN/LVNs can obtain further training and have their proficiency recorded in their file. An example of such a skill is monitoring blood transfusions (Spector, 2005).

TEACH PATIENTS

An important aspect of nursing care is to teach patients and families what they need to know to care for themselves or their loved ones, prevent complications, restore health, and prevent illness. LPN/LVNs also initiate teaching of basic hygiene and nutrition in the context of health promotion.

Examples of teaching include reinforcing what the registered nurse or physician teaches regarding scheduled diagnostic tests, upcoming surgery, how to treat a wound, or how to change a dressing. Other teaching activities concern how to take prescribed medication, what side effects to report, and the self-care activities necessary to promote rehabilitation and independence plus the lifestyle changes that may be required. LPN/LVNs contribute to the discharge plan and reinforce discharge instructions. They also provide information about community resources and self-help groups.

Think Critically About . . . Recall a time in clinical when you reinforced patient teaching. Rank your teaching on a scale of 1 to 10. How would you improve your performance in another patient teaching situation? Recall other patient situations in which you initiated health teaching and think about ways you might improve your teaching.

COMMUNICATE EFFECTIVELY

LPN/LVNs interact with patients and families in a therapeutic manner, give objective and thorough end-of-shift reports on assigned patients, and, using facility guidelines, maintain objective documentation of the care given and the status of patients. Nursing documentation is used to receive approval for hospitalization, length of stay, and reimbursement of facility charges.

WORK AS A COLLABORATIVE MEMBER OF THE HEALTH CARE TEAM

LPN/LVNs work with other members of the health care team (e.g., physician, RN, physical therapist, respiratory therapist, dietitian, pastoral care team, pharmacy personnel, and **unlicensed assistive personnel**) to provide the patient with an integrated, comprehensive plan of care.

Think Critically About . . . What is your role as a member of the team when on the clinical area? How can you improve?

ADVOCATE FOR THE PATIENT

Facility and unit routine can lead to an impersonal health care system impinging on patients' rights (see Appendix 3). LPN/LVNs as **patient advocates** stand up for patients' rights and intervene in their best interests to ensure the patients' needs are met. Advocating for a patient could be as simple as making arrangements for special food or meals at times other than within facility routine, or it may entail informing the personal physician of a patient concern. Conferring with more experienced team members can help a new nurse determine when routine can be altered in the patient's best interests.

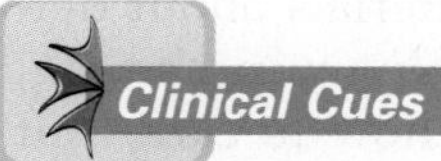

If a patient states that the morning bath really isn't wanted right now, you could postpone it for a while as your work schedule allows. However, you should fit in the bath before your shift is over. Leaving a bath to be done on the next shift upsets the oncoming staff and is not considered acceptable. Listen to the patient's reasons for not wanting the bath. If it appears that the bath really is being refused for that complete day, talk with the staff nurse or charge nurse about it. The patient has the right to refuse to bathe. Most often, if the benefits of the bath are explained, you can gain the patient's cooperation.

Think Critically About . . . If you have had the opportunity to advocate for an assigned patient, what happened and what did you do? How did you feel about the effectiveness of your action?

EXPANDED ROLE OF THE LPN/LVN

CHARGE NURSE/MANAGER OF CARE

The most common site of employment for the LPN/LVN is the nursing home or long-term care unit. In this setting, LPN/LVNs are frequently used in the role of charge nurse. Some NPAs specifically state that the LPN/LVN charge nurse functions in a nursing home under the general supervision (available by phone) of an RN.

Think Critically About . . . Does your state's nurse practice act place restrictions on the charge nurse position?

Delegating and Assigning

Delegation is transferring to competent unlicensed assistive personnel (UAPs) the authority to perform a selected nursing task/activity in a selected patient situation that is within the job description of the LPN/LVN. To delegate is to transfer authority. *Assignment* describes the distribution of work that each staff member is to accomplish on a given shift or work period. To assign is to direct a UAP to do nursing tasks/activities within his job description (National Council of State Boards of Nursing [NCSBN], *A Position Paper*, 2005b). See Box 1–2 for a comparison of assigning and delegating.

Not all states allow LPN/LVNs to delegate nursing tasks/activities, and state NPAs vary greatly concerning delegation. Check your state's NPA to determine whether you may delegate as an LPN/LVN charge nurse in your state. If your state gives you permission to delegate as a LPN/LVN, check if your place of employment gives permission for delegation in the written policies. Delegation is a *voluntary* function. You do not *have* to delegate because the NPA and the facility allow it.

Approximately half of the states allow LPN/LVNs to delegate when they are employed in the charge nurse

Box 1–2 *Comparison of Assigning and Delegating by the LPN/LVN Charge Nurse*

Ask the following questions:

1. Are tasks/activities in nursing assistant's job description?
   When assigning: Yes.
   When delegating: No. The tasks/activities delegated are in the job description of the LPN/LVN. Specific tasks/activities are not listed. Delegated tasks/activities depend on the nurse practice act and patient situation.
2. May nursing assistant refuse nursing task/activity?
   When assigning: No, unless staff person thinks he or she is unqualified for the task/activity assignment.
   When delegating: Yes. In addition, the nursing assistant must voluntarily accept the task/activity.
3. What accountability is held for nursing task/activity?
   When assigning: The nursing assistant is accountable for completing the task/activity and in a safe manner.
   When delegating: The LPN/LVN is accountable for delegating the right task/activity to the right person.

Adapted from Hill, S., & Howlett, H. (2005). *Success in Practical/Vocational Nursing: From Student to Leader* (5th ed.). Philadelphia: Saunders, p. 271.

position. Your nursing program might include class material on delegation. However, a position paper from the NCSBN (the group that develops your licensing examination) states that delegation is a complex skill that new graduates are not prepared to carry out. The skill must be developed in the clinical area after graduation by working with an experienced licensed nurse who serves as a role model and provides advice and support on delegation (NCSBN, 2005b).

In their 9-month to 1-year program, LPN/LVNs learn reasons for performing nursing tasks/activities and what could go wrong during their performance. LPN/LVNs learn their role in the nursing process. LPN/LVNs receive the authority to provide nursing care from their nursing license earned after graduating from a practical/vocational nursing program and successfully passing the NCLEX-PN examination. **Lists of tasks/activities to delegate do not exist. Such a list would eliminate considering the needs of each patient. A list of delegated tasks/activities would place some nursing care into the hands of unlicensed persons who do not have the knowledge and judgment for nursing care decisions.**

Each patient situation, regardless of complexity, determines which task/activity can be delegated. Patient condition can change rapidly, and an unlicensed person does not have the knowledge and judgment to detect such changes.

When allowed by the state's NPA and facility policies, delegation of tasks/activities within the LPN/LVN scope of practice involves *transferring the authority* to perform these functions. In certain states, some functions that are in the job description of the LPN/LVN charge nurse may be delegated to UAPs. See Box 1–3 for points to consider when for delegating nursing tasks/activities.

Box 1–3 *When the LPN/LVN Charge Nurse Delegates*

Ask unlicensed personnel to do part of the job to free you up to perform other responsibilities with the goal of improving resident care and meeting resident goals (outcomes):

- Because part of the charge nurse job is being given to unlicensed personnel, remember these personnel must *voluntarily* accept the delegation.
- You must provide unlicensed personnel with the necessary information, assistance, equipment, and monitoring to safely carry out the delegated task/activity.
- Although employers may suggest that certain tasks/activities be delegated, you are ultimately responsible for deciding *if* and *when* to delegate, *what* to delegate, to *whom*, and *under what circumstances.*

The National Council of State Boards of Nursing's position paper, *Delegation: Concepts and Decision-Making Process* (NCSBN, 1996), provides a decision-making process to be used by licensed persons in clinical settings as a guide for delegation of nursing duties. The National Council identifies Five Rights to include when delegating:

- Right Task—a task that can legally be delegated for a specific patient.
- Right Circumstances—the patient is stable, independent nursing judgment is not required for task, and resources to perform task are available.
- Right Person—the person asked to perform the task is competent and qualified to do so.
- Right Direction/Communication—objective and specific explanation of what should be done and when, and what to report to the charge nurse and when.
- Right Supervision—the charge nurse needs to monitor the performance of the task, intervene when needed, evaluate the results of the task, and provide feedback to the unlicensed person.

Additional National Council materials about delegation can be accessed at http://www.ncsbn.org. Additional information describing how to carry out delegation can be found in *Success in Practical/Vocational Nursing: From Student to Leader* (Hill and Howlett, 2005).

With heavy workloads, many tasks may need to be assigned to nursing assistants or other UAPs. Such tasks must be within the job description of the person to whom they are being assigned. You should always consider the advisability of assigning a task to another, as well as that person's ability to carry out the task, and provide information about how the task should be done and what should be recorded or reported to you.

HEALTH CARE FINANCING

TYPES OF HEALTH CARE FINANCING

The traditional method of financing health care services, **fee-for-service,** involves direct reimbursement by an insurance company to a **provider** (a licensed health care person such as a physician, dentist, or nurse practitioner) whose health care services are covered by a health insurance plan. To improve their profit, insurance companies charge a **deductible** (the yearly amount an insured person must spend out-of-pocket for health care services before a health insurance policy will begin to pay its share), a **copayment** (the amount an insured person must pay at the time of an office visit, prescription, or hospital service), and **co-insurance** (once a deductible is met, the percentage of the total bill paid by the insured person). The insurance company pays the remainder.

Capitation, as an alternative for fee-for-service payment, involves a set monthly fee charged by the provider of health care services for each member of the insurance group for a specific set of health care services. If services cost more than the monthly fee, the provider absorbs the cost of those services. At the end of the year, if any money is left over, the health care provider keeps it as a profit.

HOW PATIENTS PAY FOR HEALTH CARE SERVICES

The cost of health care services today discourages payment directly by the patient (private pay) as the primary method for payment of health care. Health insurance, as any insurance, spreads risk. The young and the healthy generally subsidize (support) the sick and older persons in the health insurance group.

GROUP HEALTH INSURANCE

Group health insurance is a method of pooling individual contributions with the goal of providing health care while protecting group members from financial disaster because of health care bills. When insured, an individual is said to have third-party coverage (a middleman). This financial middleman pays the individual's health care bills. Employers offer most group health insurance in the United States. Blue Cross/Blue Shield is an example of health insurance that may be obtained through an employer or by an individual. Many commercial insurance companies offer health insurance to individuals and groups.

MANAGED CARE

Managed care is a type of group health insurance developed to provide quality health care with cost and utilization (use) controls. This is accomplished by paying physicians to care for groups of patients for a set fee with limited services. Medical necessity and appropriateness of health care services are monitored by a utilization review system (Box 1–4).

Box 1–4 *Types of Managed Care Plans*

HEALTH MAINTENANCE ORGANIZATION (HMO)

- HMOs receive a prepaid fee to provide comprehensive care to members of the enrolled group.
- HMOs are generally located in buildings that are used solely for HMO business, and all physicians working in the HMO are hired specifically for the HMO.
- Encourage prevention of disease by the practice of preventive medicine.
- Discourage physicians from ordering excessive diagnostic tests and treatments.
- Patients may not have the option of choosing their physician each time treatment is needed.
- **Point-of-service (POS) option** allows a member to go outside the HMO to see a desired physician for an extra fee.

PREFERRED PROVIDER ORGANIZATION (PPO)

- Alternative to the strict utilization review system of some managed care plans.
- Fees are paid by fee-for-service arrangement.
- Health insurance companies contract with physicians and hospitals and negotiate discount fees.
- The members of the network are "preferred" providers. Patients may choose to see any physician in the network. If a patient chooses a preferred provider, a larger amount of the cost will be covered by the health care plan.
- Physicians remain in the same office in which their family practice is located. Part of their day is spent treating patients in their own family practice and part of the day is spent treating patients who are enrolled in the PPO.

GOVERNMENT-SPONSORED HEALTH INSURANCE

Medicare

Medicare is a federal program that helps to partially finance health care for all persons over age 65 years (and their spouses), who have at least a 10-year (40 quarters) record in Medicare-covered employment and are citizens or permanent residents of the United States. Coverage is also given to persons under age 65 who are victims of end-stage renal disease or who are permanently and totally disabled. Those eligible because of age or disability are entitled, by law, to the benefits of these programs. In November 2003, Congress passed the Medicare Prescription Drug, Improvement, and Modernization Act, which is the largest expansion of Medicare since Medicare started in 1965 (Box 1–5). Before 1983, hospitals submitted a bill to the government for the total charges they incurred for Medicare patients and were reimbursed for this amount. Payment was based on actual costs and was called a **retrospective payment system.** The federal

Box 1–5 *Basic Components of Medicare*

Medicare Part A *helps* pay for inpatient hospital care.

- Part A is available without cost to those eligible for the program.
- Helps pay for inpatient hospital care, including drugs, supplies, laboratory tests, radiology, and intensive care unit.
- Covers 20 days posthospitalization for skilled nursing facility care for rehabilitation services, home health care services under certain conditions, and hospice care.
- **Part A does not pay for** nursing home custodial services (e.g., patients only needing help with activities of daily living, feeding), private rooms, telephones, or televisions provided by hospitals or skilled nursing facilities.

Medicare Part B is similar to a major medical insurance plan and is funded by monthly premiums.

- At this time, all persons who elect to have this coverage pay the same monthly premium except for those with income over $80,000/year.
- Part B requires a deductible and pays 80% of most covered charges. The remaining 20% of charges are the responsibility of the patient.
- Part B helps pay for medically necessary physicians' services; outpatient hospital services (including emergency room visits); ambulance transportation; diagnostic tests, including laboratory services and mammography and Pap smear screenings; and physical therapy, occupational therapy, and speech therapy in a hospital outpatient department or Medicare-certified rehabilitation agency.
- **Part B does not pay for** most prescription drugs, routine physicals, services not related to treatment of illness or injury, dental care, dentures, cosmetic surgery, routine foot care, hearing aids, eye examinations, or glasses.

Medicare Part C refers to Medicare Advantage plans, such as HMOs or regional PPOs.

- Provides Part A, B, and D benefits to persons who elect this type of coverage instead of the original fee-for-service program.

Medicare Part D refers to the outpatient prescription drug benefit.

- Part D is available to all Medicare enrollees in the original fee-for-service program for an additional monthly fee.

government was the first group to try to stop the skyrocketing cost of health care. In 1983, the Health Care Financing Administration (now the Centers for Medicare and Medicaid Services [CMS]) adopted a system called **diagnosis-related groups (DRGs)** or illness groups. This system pays hospitals a flat rate for Medicare services by telling hospitals in advance how much they will be reimbursed and is called a **prospective payment system (PPS)**.

Under the DRG system, the fee the government will pay for hospitalization depends on the DRG category (illness) causing the patient's hospitalization. Hospitals receive a flat fee for each patient's DRG category regardless of length of stay in the hospital. Hospitals have an incentive to treat patients and discharge them as quickly as possible because if the hospital keeps the patient longer than the government's fee will cover, and the patient cannot be reclassified in the DRG system, the hospital has to make up the difference in costs. If the acute care facility can treat the Medicare patient for less than the guaranteed reimbursement, *the facility can keep the difference as profit*.

Because Medicare patients, as all patients, are discharged sooner from hospitals than they were in the past, extended care units or skilled care facilities and home care are frequently used to continue convalescence.

Box 1–6 *The Medicaid Program*

- Medicaid is the second largest item in state budgets and covers over 39 million low-income children and parents, many in working families.
- Medicaid is the largest source of health insurance for children in the United States. The State Children's Health Insurance Program (SCHIP) supplements Medicaid by providing coverage for low-income children who are not covered by health insurance and do not qualify for Medicaid.
- Medicaid is the primary source of health and long-term care coverage for low-income individuals with disabilities or chronic illnesses and those who need mental health services and substance abuse treatment.
- Medicaid covers services that Medicare does not cover for low-income Medicare beneficiaries, including long-term care and vision and dental care. Medicare beneficiaries who are also enrolled in Medicaid are known as "dual eligibles."

Think Critically About . . . Should Medicare pay for new, expensive, technological procedures that are developed to treat common medical problems of the elderly? Should cost-effectiveness enter the picture for treating Medicare patients? Explain the reason for your answer.

Medicaid

The **Medicaid** program, which is funded jointly by the federal and state governments, provides medical assistance for eligible families and individuals with low incomes and few resources. The federal government establishes broad national guidelines for the program. Each state establishes its own program services and requirements, including eligibility. Proportionally, Medicaid is the second largest item in state budgets (Box 1–6).

GOALS FOR HEALTH CARE

NEED FOR COST CONTAINMENT

The United States spends more on health care than any other country, yet 44 million persons remain uninsured. The increase in elderly, many with chronic illnesses requiring more frequent health care, taxes the Medicare system, and the impending retirement of "baby boomers" will tax that system even more. Medicare and Medicaid reimbursements to providers continue to decline. Many persons are unable to afford individual health insurance premiums. Some individuals covered by a health insurance plan find themselves unable to afford deductibles and copayments. Some retirees who received health insurance as part of retirement benefits have had these benefits taken away. Advances in technology make noninvasive diagnosis of some diseases and treatment of diseases possible with fewer complications and side effects, but are very expensive. The continually increasing costs of medications means that some patients cannot afford prescribed drugs.

The driving force today in all health care facilities is **cost containment** (the need to hold costs to within fixed limits while remaining competitive). Health care agencies are interested in improving their agency's "bottom line" with business principles that reduce waste and inefficiency. Consumers would like the cost of health care to be reduced while high-quality care and service are maintained.

Service, quality, and cost control are attributes of health care that need to be understood and considered in all clinical situations by the LPN/LVN, who has the opportunity to identify wasteful practices and inefficient routines in the work setting.

See Box 1–7 for the role you play as an LPN/LVN in containing health care costs in your work setting.

Box 1–7 *LPN/LVN Role in Containing Health Care Costs in the Work Setting*

1. Follow facility policy for charging patients for all supplies used in their care.
2. Follow facility policy for documenting patient care for reimbursement.
3. Organize patient care for effective and efficient use of time. If some aspect of care needs to be "redone," it would have been better and more time efficient to do it right the first time.
4. Decrease patient length of stay by implementing nursing care to help prevent complications.
5. Meet the patient's needs, not your needs.

From Hill, S., & Howlett, H. (2005). *Success in Practical/Vocational Nursing: From Student to Leader* (5th ed.). Philadelphia: Saunders, p. 304.

HEALTHY PEOPLE 2010 AND HEALTH PROMOTION

Healthy People 2010 is a nationwide health promotion and disease prevention agenda to improve the health of all Americans in the United States during the first decade of the 21st century. It includes a set of health objectives based on best scientific knowledge. *Healthy People* has the potential to affect the health of all Americans and reduce health care costs. The major goals for this decade are to:

- Increase the quality and years of healthy life
- Eliminate health disparities (inequality)

The goal is to eliminate by 2010 the differences in six areas of health status experienced by racial and ethnic minorities while trying to improve the overall health of all American individuals. The six target areas are infant mortality, cancer screening and management, cardiovascular disease, diabetes mellitus, human immunodeficiency virus (HIV) infection/acquired immunodeficiency syndrome (AIDS), and immunizations. There are 28 focus areas, including cancer, disability, and food safety.

Individuals, groups, and organizations must work as a team to incorporate *Healthy People 2010* into current programs, special events, publications, and meetings to improve the health of their communities. It is each LPN/LVN's responsibility to educate patients about healthy lifestyles by educating in their communities about health promotion. They should encourage patients to pursue healthier lifestyles and to participate in community-based health promotion programs. LPN/LVNs can also influence healthier lifestyles in their patients by modeling not smoking, healthy eating, weight management, and the like. Health Promotion Points 1–1 lists 10 health indicators that will be used to measure the health of the nation in 2010. These indicators reflect the major health concerns in the United States at the beginning of the 21st century.

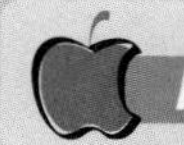

Health Promotion Points 1–1

Healthy People 2010 Ten Leading Health Indicators

Indicators that reflect the major health concerns in the United States at the beginning of the 21st century:

- Physical activity
- Overweight and obesity
- Tobacco use
- Substance abuse
- Responsible sexual behavior
- Mental health
- Injury and violence
- Environmental quality
- Immunization
- Access to health care

From National Center for Health Statistics. (2004). Healthy People 2010: *Leading Health Indicators at a Glance*. Rockville, Md: U.S. Department of Health and Human Services, Office of Disease Prevention and Health Promotion.

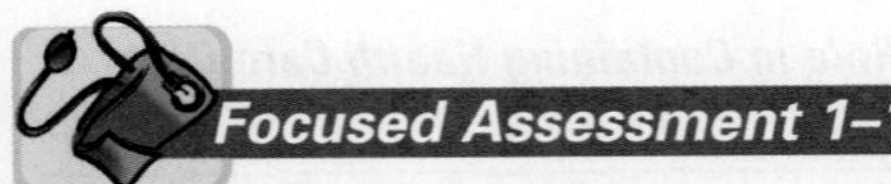

Focused Assessment 1–1

Data Collection for Holistic Assessment

PHYSICAL ASSESSMENT

- List and prioritize assessments/data to be collected for specific medical and/or surgical diagnoses and treatments for the patient.

PSYCHOLOGICAL ASSESSMENT

- What is your greatest concern about this hospitalization?
- Is there anyone you do not want to visit you while in the hospital?
- Who are the significant persons in your life?
- Who is your source of support, for help with problems?
- Do you have any fears that may get in the way of diagnosis and treatment? Closed spaces, darkness, needles, etc.?
- Do you experience problems with eating? Too much? Too little? If so, how much of a weight gain or loss have you had in the past 2 months?
- Do you smoke? How much every day?
- Do you drink alcohol? What and how often?
- What do you do to relieve stressful feelings?
- Do you experience feeling hopeless or very sad? How often and what triggers the feeling?
- Is there anyone in your life who abuses you? Verbally, physically? If so, describe how.
- Are you sexually active? If yes, are you satisfied with your sex life?

SOCIAL ASSESSMENT

- With whom do you live? How will your admission affect those with whom you live?
- Do you have a personal relationship with someone? If so, are you satisfied with this relationship?
- Do you have children? If so, who will care for your children while you are in the hospital?
- Are you employed? If so, how will your illness/accident/hospitalization affect your job? Do you have sick leave at work?
- Do you have health insurance?
- Who are the persons in your life who can be of help at this time?
- Will you be able to manage at home with bathing, meals, cleaning, laundry, errands, obtaining your medications and/or needed equipment for your treatments?
- Are there any physical impediments (stairs, tub but no shower, etc.) that will make it difficult at home?

CULTURAL ASSESSMENT

- What are your beliefs or practices for staying well?
- What foods do you have in your diet that help you stay well?
- What foods in your diet help you recover when you are sick?
- Do you use complementary and alternative (CAM) medicine?
- If you use CAM in addition to your physician, did you inform your physician of CAM use, including herbals?

SPIRITUAL ASSESSMENT

- How do you cope with problems or difficult situations?
- Do you believe in the power of prayer?
- Do you meditate or read spiritual materials?
- What are your beliefs about a higher power?
- If you have a relationship to a higher power, do you have a religious affiliation? If so, do you want a representative of your religious affiliation notified of your admission?
- Do you have any religious items that you wear on your person?

HOLISTIC CARE OF MEDICAL-SURGICAL PATIENTS

Holistic care involves dealing with the total person. Nurses need to be aware of the physiologic, psychological, social, cultural, and spiritual needs of patients. Data for many of these needs can be collected and interventions carried out while administering care and treatments (Focused Assessment 1–1). Assisting with bathing, feeding, ambulating, and other physical care provides an opportunity to find out about the dimensions of the patient's life besides his or her physical problems. The chapters in this text will teach you specific ways to gather data about problems that may occur in the various body systems. You will add this knowledge to what you learned about basic assessment and data collection in your prior course(s).

PSYCHOLOGICAL NEEDS

Nurse-Patient Relationship

An important part of the nurse-patient relationship is the nurse's ability to display empathy. No one can know or feel what another experiences. **Empathy** means the nurse accurately perceives the patient's current feelings and their meanings but does not experience the emotion with them. The nurse conveys the interpretation of the patient's feelings back to the patient for validation of their accuracy. This displays appreciation and awareness of the patient's feelings. In this way, the patient feels valued and accepted as a person. An example of an empathetic statement by the nurse is, "You seem upset about your surgery tomorrow." In contrast, sympathy involves entering into feelings with patients and is displayed by sorrow and concern (e.g., "You poor thing. I had that surgery.").

Some health care agencies judge their effectiveness by budgets and outcomes, but patients judge their experiences by the nature of the care they receive. Scores on patient satisfaction surveys drop when care is impersonal.

Therapeutic Relationship

The focus of the nurse-patient relationship is the patient and his problems and needs. The relationship is therapeutic because it provides the help needed for healing or return to wellness of the patient. In comparison, a social relationship is not goal directed, exists primarily for pleasure, and meets the needs of each person in the relationship. LPN/LVNs need to maintain boundaries when working with patients. They need to avoid using patient contact to meet personal needs (e.g., the need to be liked, the need for friendship or approval). LPN/LVNs need to develop awareness of their own needs and realize that those should be met within their personal lives.

The nurse-patient relationship ends when the patient is discharged. Avoid the temptation to continue the relationship on a social basis. This means no exchange of addresses, phone/cell numbers, or e-mail addresses. It is not beneficial to patients to stay in contact with their nurses after discharge. Sometimes patients want to present nurses with gifts at the time of discharge. Check school and facility policy regarding this practice.

Establish Trust. To develop a therapeutic relationship, trust needs to be established between patient and nurse. In today's health care system, time with patients is limited and each patient contact must be fully utilized. At each contact, knock before entering the room, give your name, identify yourself as a nursing student or LPN/LVN, and give the reason for your visit. Many older patients are not used to the informality of strangers addressing them by their given (first) name. Clarify how the patient would like to be addressed. Put the patient at ease with a pleasant, unhurried approach. Other behaviors to establish trust follow.

Use Therapeutic Communication Skills. Communicate at the level of the patient's understanding. Active listening helps the patient express needs and feelings. Ask patients what they think. Actively listen to their answers, as well as their concerns and fears. Avoid judging the message or the patient. Avoid forming a response while the patient is speaking. Rephrase the message when the patient is done to verify that you understand the message. Make sure the patient's and your verbal and nonverbal communication is congruent. Answer all patient questions when possible. Admit when you do not know the answer to a question and find out the answer as soon as possible. Avoid gossip, arguments, and complaints within patients' range of hearing. The focus needs to be the physical and mental well-being of patients and the development of trust. Patients may feel that if staff cannot get along with each other, how can staff focus on patients?

Maintain Patients' Self-Esteem. A major problem for patients of any age is the loss of self-esteem. Patients are sometimes dealt with as an illness (diagnosis) or behavior instead of a person who happens to have a particular illness or behavior. How often have you heard a patient referred to as "the gallbladder in 205" or "the depressed patient in 305"? Nurses and physicians are especially guilty of this demeaning practice. Some patients are treated differently: talked down to, in some cases coddled, and dealt with as though they have no strengths. You should identify the strengths of patients and find a way to support those strengths and thereby sustain patients' self-esteem.

? *Think Critically About . . .* If you have experienced an illness or injury or have a chronic illness, have you ever been treated in a demeaning way? How did it make you feel? How would you have liked to have been treated?

Display Nursing Competence. Nurses who are competent in their skills build patients' confidence, and this decreases patient anxiety. Focus on the patient and explain what procedures entail and what to expect before starting treatments. Patients expect nurses to be competent when performing treatments and to have the necessary equipment at hand before beginning a procedure. Leave the patient environment clean and orderly after procedures. Many nursing behaviors help to decrease patient stress, but pain control is especially important. Anticipate patients' pain control needs before they are expressed, for example, before painful procedures and before ambulating. Assess the need for further pain medication before the next dose is due; determine whether the medication is effective. If it is not doing the job, speak to the physician and get the order changed. Give a back rub along with pain medication when appropriate.

Display Compassion. Another name for compassion is "low-tech nursing," because no degree, advanced training, or increase in unit budget is required to display kindness and patience to patients. Treat them

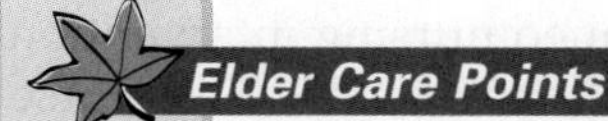

Elder Care Points

A Memo From Your Older/Elderly Patient

Avoid treating me as if I have a mental impairment until you clarify by looking on my chart that I do have one. Avoid shouting at me until you clarify that I have a hearing deficit. Regardless, speak in a normal volume and a medium to low pitch and enunciate clearly.

Be patient with me. It might take me longer to get out of bed, walk to the bathroom, or answer your repeated questions about my pain level. If you need to give me information, for example, for a diagnostic test, give me the information slowly and ask for feedback to see if I understand the information. It would help if you gave me information to read.

If my family or friends are with me and you want information about me, ask me and let me speak for myself. Also, I want to be included in decision making and planning for my care. Ask me if I would mind being hugged or touched before you do so. If I don't mind, avoid patting me on the head like a child. That is demeaning. Be patient when I talk too much. I may be lonely. Treat me in a way you would want your mother or father treated, or how you would want to be treated if you were in my situation.

with common courtesy, and see them as unique individuals worthy of respect. All health care workers need to be aware of the rights of the patient (see Appendix 3). A good starting point is to see the patient in the bed as someone's spouse, relative, friend, or parent. Touch can be reassuring, calming, and encouraging to patients. In this era of threats of sexual harassment, some nurses may be afraid to touch patients. Touch an arm or hand and be aware of the patient's reaction to see if this is acceptable. Be aware of cultural taboos about being touched.

Intervening with Patients Who Display Difficult Behaviors

A patient who is physically ill is also affected emotionally by illness or injury. It is not unusual for patients to display behavior that is not their usual behavior. Patients' emotional needs and resulting behaviors are usually temporary and related to the stresses of the illness. Occasionally the behavior is related to underlying disorders that will benefit from a psychiatric consultation or treatment. Psychiatric disorders and nursing care to promote mental health are discussed in Chapters 45 through 48. Even patients whose primary illness is a physical rather than psychological disorder can sometimes express emotional discomfort through dependent, withdrawn, hostile, or manipulative behavior. They may behave in ways that are confusing to the patient and uncomfortable for the nurse who is not prepared to intervene effectively.

Identifying and meeting a patient's emotional needs are part of the responsibility of the LPN/LVN in all care settings, from acute care to home care. A holistic and personalized approach to nursing care needs to respect a patient's need for both emotional and physical support and provide planned nursing intervention to meet each patient's emotional needs. The nurse needs to look for the emotion that underlies the behavior. If the patient is extremely dependent, he or she is often extremely frightened. Patients who are withdrawn and depressed frequently need help in increasing their coping techniques. Hostility is sometimes an expression of anger toward the illness or oneself. If anger is turned inward, it may be expressed as depression. If anger is turned outward, it may be expressed by striking out at others or physically attacking. Manipulation might be grasping for control over a part of life when everything else seems out of control.

It is easier to deal with patients' behavior if you understand that patients' responses to a particular situation are the best they are capable of at that particular time. The task of the nurse is to recognize that patients' behavior results from the demands being placed on them at the moment. This requires kindness, understanding, and sometimes firmness on the part of the nurse. People tend to become childlike and fearful when they are ill or act as if they are unaffected by their illness. Patients appreciate having someone with them who can guide them through their ordeal in a therapeutic manner. Make use of the interventions included in Box 1–8 when dealing with patients who display difficult behaviors.

The Patient with Dependent Behavior. Patients with **dependent** behavior attempt to satisfy an unmet need by depending on others rather than themselves. Patients with dependent behavior are unreasonably demanding of the nurse's time and attention, show little or no initiative in performing the simplest of self-care activities, or exhibit flirtatious behavior to attract attention to themselves.

The Patient with Withdrawn Behavior. Withdrawal from contact with others reflects a need to feel safe, secure, and trustful and can indicate feelings of anxiety, fear, anger, or depression. Patients with withdrawn behavior may exhibit silence, failure to make eye contact, recoiling from touch, superficial conversation without any self-disclosure or sharing of feelings, denial of feelings, and denial of reality, such as their own illness and its effects on their lives.

The Patient with Depressed Behavior. Depression can be situational or clinical. Hospitalization and being in a different environment are examples of circumstances that can result in situational depression. More than just feeling blue and sad manifests depressed behavior. Situational and clinical depression can be manifested by symptoms of unrelenting despair and wanting to die. Causes of clinical depression can include the inability to deal with angry feelings and negative feelings. Although some degree of depression might be expected in hospitalized patients, symptoms of depression should not be ignored. Patients who are depressed may exhibit loss of appetite, fatigue, vague aches and pains, insomnia, poor posture, gazing into space, and difficulty making decisions. Sometimes the patient with depression will make statements such as, "I didn't sleep all night," even though staff reported that it appeared the patient was asleep all during the 11 P.M. to 7 A.M. shift. Although the patient may have been asleep all night, the sleep does not feel satisfying to him.

The Patient with Hostile Behavior. Hostile behavior is an expression of patients' need to have control over what is happening to them. Illness inevitably represents some degree of loss. Patients may fear loss of independence, loss of control over body functions, or loss of the ability to care for and financially support themselves or their family. Family members who are upset over a serious, rapidly progressing, or perhaps fatal illness of a loved one may also display hostile behavior toward staff. The patient with hostile behavior may shout, criticize, threaten to "report" the nurse, and constantly complain about the care provided. Some may strike out physically. Some may turn anger toward themselves and may attempt to hurt themselves.

The Patient with Manipulative Behavior. Patients with manipulative behavior fear losing total control of themselves or their environment. Patients with ma-

Box 1–8 ***Nursing Interventions for Patients with Difficult Behaviors***

THE PATIENT WITH DEPENDENT BEHAVIOR

- Increase the amount of time spent with these patients, establish trust, anticipate needs and wants, and assure them that needs will be met if not medically contraindicated.
- Focus on these patients' abilities and encourage them to do for themselves. Encourage them to do one small task of daily care on their own, such as wash their own face or put on their gown. Praise them matter-of-factly when they comply.
- If constant ringing for the nurse is a problem, setting limits may discourage this behavior. Meet all patients' current requests and then tell them that you will check in 30 minutes if the call bell is not used. By returning as promised, you help dependent patients feel secure that personal care requested will be considered.
- Lengthen the time period between checks to 45 minutes and then to 1 hour. Inform patient of next time interval.

THE PATIENT WITH WITHDRAWN BEHAVIOR

- Provide a consistent routine of care so these patients know what to expect.
- Reduce environmental stress, confusion, and disorder and limit the number of health care providers these patients must interact with.
- Be alert to personal space needs and avoid violating these needs. Watch for cues as to changes in patients' need for personal space.
- Avoid whispering, secretive behavior, teasing, and joking.

THE PATIENT WITH DEPRESSED BEHAVIOR

- Sitting quietly next to the patient may be comforting to this patient.
- Encourage and assist the patient to engage in activities of daily living. Be aware that the pace of work will be slower.
- Information will be processed more slowly. Give directions for diagnostic tests, one at a time.
- Offer patients sincere feedback. Point out their accomplishments and strengths in a low-key manner.
- Sincerely emphasize patients' good qualities.
- Avoid stories that illustrate the patient's situation could be worse.
- Avoid being bright and cheerful in their presence or admonish them to "cheer up and look at the bright side of things."
- Show that you care by being with these patients and interacting with them.
- If the patient makes a threat of suicide, take this threat seriously.
- Clinical guidelines call for using both psychotherapy and medications.
- If the patient is on an antidepressant, the drug needs to be given as ordered. Many antidepressants are given at bedtime so the patient will benefit from the sedating side effect of the drug. These drugs are not stimulants. They elevate the mood of the patient. Annoying side effects (such as nervousness, insomnia, nausea, etc.) generally may appear before the drug is effective. Most of the time, the side effects subside as the drug begins to work. Encourage the patient to give the drug the time to take effect.

THE PATIENT WITH HOSTILE BEHAVIOR

- Take time to talk to these patients and ask what is bothering them. Listen and you may be able to intervene. It might be a situation that can be changed.
- Allow patients who are hostile to make reasonable suggestions and choices about their care and meet suggestions when they do not threaten recovery or interfere with their medical-surgical condition. Avoid empty promises.

THE PATIENT WITH MANIPULATIVE BEHAVIOR

- Avoid being flattered by compliments. Tell patients they may ask directly for something they need. Assure them that all direct, reasonable requests that are not harmful to their recovery will be considered.
- If patients have the call light on frequently, make a plan with them that you will check on them at an agreed upon interval (for example, on the half hour) throughout the shift. Requests can be made at that time. Tell patients that the call light may be put on in between times only if there is a real emergency. Be persistent in maintaining the schedule and remind patients of this agreement with you if necessary.
- Occasionally patients with manipulative behavior will take extreme measures to get your attention such as attempting suicide. Take any threats of suicide seriously.
- A patient may tell you something like, "I thought you were my friend, but you are just like the others." Avoid becoming defensive. Avoid trying to impress upon the patient how busy you are with other responsibilities.

nipulative behavior are focused on themselves and concerned with getting their own needs met.

Think Critically About . . . When you were assigned to a patient who had a manipulative pattern of behavior, think about whether the patient reminded you of someone you know personally. Then ask yourself, if you "hung that person's face" on this patient and responded to the patient accordingly?

SOCIAL NEEDS

Think Critically About . . . What impact would your admission today for an emergency appendectomy have on your life?

Inability to assume personal responsibilities can be a source of worry for patients and interfere with a positive outcome of illness or surgery. Some aging parents live with their adult children and depend on them for care. Some patients monitor their aging or infirm parents' ability to care for themselves in their own homes. Patients who are grandparents may play an active, daily role in caring for grandchildren. A patient may be needed to help a spouse or significant other meet daily needs. A single parent may have been admitted on an emergency basis while children are at school. If a patient lives alone, pets may be a concern. When employed, patients might have used all their sick leave, not have health insurance, or carry a high deductible. Some employed persons cannot afford the employee share of health insurance premiums. Some unemployed patients cannot afford the cost of an individual health insurance plan. Patients enrolled in an educational program might be concerned about having to drop a course or program because of loss of time due to hospitalization, diagnostic tests, or restrictions such as not being able to drive. In their excitement to be discharged, patients might not consider the restrictions/requirements of their condition in relation to treatments at home, obtaining supplies and medications, driving, cooking, cleaning, food shopping, doing laundry, and so forth.

> *Think Critically About . . .* Review your answer to the question at the beginning of social needs. How could you resolve your concerns? Who could help you in this situation?

CULTURAL NEEDS

Health care today and into the future needs to accommodate patients of many cultural backgrounds. Patients may think and behave differently because of social class, religion, ethnic background, minority group status, marital status, or sexual preference. Avoid making judgments about people who are culturally different. This does not mean nurses must adopt others' cultural practices. It means being open-minded and **nonjudgmental,** taking the difference at face value, accepting people as they are, and giving high-quality care. Quality of the care must not be decreased because of differences observed or imagined.

> *Think Critically About . . .* Can you give examples of judgmental behaviors you observed during your clinical rotation?

The philosophy of individual worth is the belief in the uniqueness and value of each human being who comes for care regardless of differences in that individual. Nurses need to realize that individuals have the right to live according to their personal beliefs and values *as long as those beliefs and values do not interfere with the rights of others and are within the law.*

Nursing students sometimes think that somewhere there is a recipe book that will tell them how to care for people who are different from them. Applying information to all individuals in a group can lead to assumptions, which are called **stereotypes.** A stereotype is a simplification used to describe all members of a specific group without exception. It is an expectation that all individuals in a group will act exactly the same in a situation just because they are a member of that group. Stereotypes ignore the individual differences that occur within every cultural group. Members of any culture may have modified the degree to which they observe the values and practices of their culture. Information about cultural groups can explain but not predict behavior (Cultural Cues 1–1).

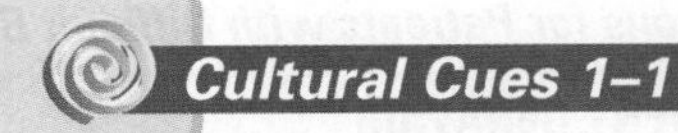

Cultural Preferences

People from the Philippines may be shy and feel awkward in unfamiliar surroundings. They may give little direct eye contact. A family member should be allowed at the bedside at all times. The patient may be reluctant to venture out of the room to ambulate.

Many Cambodians believe that the soul resides in the head and it is inappropriate to touch their heads without permission. Ask before touching the head when changing head dressings or applying eyedrops.

Hmong from Southeast Asia prefer their own relatives as interpreters. They may not trust a hospital-employed interpreter. The interpreter should be of the same sex as the patient as neither Hmong men or women may discuss or admit to intimate problems to an interpreter of the opposite sex.

When disease strikes, some people blame pathogens (germs), others blame spirits, and others blame an imbalance in the body. Some cultural groups have folk medicine practices such as rituals, special procedures (such as rubbing the skin with the edge of a coin to release toxins causing illness), and special persons in the group to cure disease (physician, herbalist, shaman, curandero). Some groups believe that special foods or food combinations ("cold" foods for "hot" illness) and herbs (echinacea, feverfew) can prevent or cure illnesses. Others see no relationship between the diet and health. Some patients look at prevention as an attempt to control the future. They may wonder about the necessity of making a trip to a health care provider for preventive care (e.g., immunizations). Different beliefs of patients need to be respected.

Biomedicine

Biomedicine, the dominant health system of the United States, focuses on symptoms. The goal of biomedicine is to find the cause of disease and then eliminate or correct the problem. Many Americans use methods that focus on the whole body and not just symptoms when treating disease.

Complementary and Alternative Medicine

Complementary (used in conjunction with biomedical treatments) **and alternative** (substitute for conventional medicine) ***medicine* (CAM)** focuses on assisting the body's own healing powers and restoring body balance. The National Center for Complementary and Alternative Medicine (NCCAM) of the National Institutes of Health researches and evaluates the effectiveness and safety of CAM therapies. Natural medicines often have not undergone scientific studies to determine correct dose, side effects, or risk of interactions with other medicines or certain foods. Patients need to be reminded that all herbals and supplements need to be included when they are asked for a list of drugs taken.

SPIRITUAL NEEDS

Spirituality is an essential part of being human. The spirit is the innermost part of a person, the very essence that provides animation. The spirit incorporates the beliefs and values that provide strength and hope, awareness of self (including inner strengths), and understanding of life's meaning and purpose. Patients have a spiritual self with spiritual needs and use personal spiritual practices to meet those needs. Examples of personal spiritual practices may include gardening, reading inspirational books, listening to music, meditating, praying, communing with nature, practicing breathing techniques, volunteering, expressing gratitude, and counting blessings.

Spirituality and *religion* are related terms but do not have the same meaning. Religion attempts to formalize and ritualize spiritual beliefs. Some patients help meet their spiritual needs by belonging to a specific religious denomination. The different rituals and practices of a religion can bring the security of the past into a crisis situation. Concrete symbols, such as books, pictures, icons, herb packets, beads, statues, jewelry, and other objects, can affirm the patient's connection with a higher power. The value of patients' rituals and religious practices is determined by their faith and not scientific evidence. Spirituality, one's life force, does not necessarily include religion.

Crisis situations frequently surface in acute health care situations. Patients' beliefs and values can profoundly affect their response to these crises, their attitude toward treatment, and their rate of recovery. The need for spiritual care for patients and families may be intensified by the following situations: hospitalization, pain experiences, having a chronic or incurable disease, a terminal illness, and the death of a loved one. See Box 1–9 for spiritual care interventions.

The pastoral care team allies with nurses in providing spiritual care for patients, but this team does not relieve nurses of their responsibility to provide spiritual care. Follow agency policy for arranging visits of patients' clergy or spiritual advisors, when visits are desired. Agency policies vary and are being tested nationwide.

Box 1–9 ***Spiritual Care Interventions***

- Ask open-ended questions—ones that cannot be answered by yes or no.
- Actively listen to the patient. Sit beside the patient. Make eye contact, if culturally appropriate.
- Be nonjudgmental of patients and their responses.
- Avoid giving advice or a lecture to the patient.
- Avoid being a proselytizer (a person who tries to convert another person to his or her own religion).
- Be aware of nonverbal messages from the patient.
- Understand the feelings of the patient but avoid adopting those feelings.
- Expect to learn from patients.
- Stay with the patient after the person has received an unfavorable diagnosis.
- When patients request help with prayer, offer to pray with them if you are comfortable doing so.
- When the patient requests help with specific readings, offer to read to the patient.
- Assist the patient to participate in desired spiritual/religious rituals.
- Protect the patient's spiritual/religious articles. Do not remove them if they are being worn unless required for an emergency.

Adapted from Hill, S., & Howlett, H. (2005). *Success in Practical/Vocational Nursing: From Student to Leader* (5th ed.). Philadelphia: Saunders, p. 197.

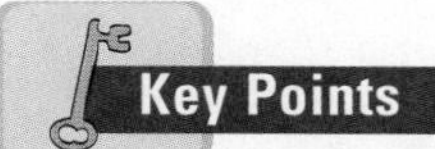

- Medical-surgical nursing is a vast nursing specialty that involves care for adult patients with medical and/or surgical conditions that affect either one or more body systems. Sites of employment include hospitals and varied facilities in the community.
- The most common site of employment of the LPN/LVN as charge nurse is the nursing home/long-term care facility.
- Qualities and skills needed by LPN/LVNs for use in medical-surgical nursing include the following: uphold clinical practice standards, provide safe patient care, teach patients, communicate effectively, work as a collaborative member of the health care team, and advocate for the patient.
- Each state's nurse practice act defines what the LPN/LVN can and cannot do in the practice of practical/vocational nursing, including delegating as a charge nurse.
- Assignment involves assigning tasks to unlicensed personnel that are in their job descriptions, once the patient situation has been declared stable.
- Delegation involves designating duties to unlicensed personnel that are in the job description of the LPN/LVN, are within the boundaries of the nurse practice act, and are dependent on the patient situation.
- The fee-for-service method of financing health care services has been challenged by the capitation method of financing those services.
- Medicare and Medicaid are examples of government-sponsored health insurance in the United States.

- To help curb rising health care costs, the federal government adopted a payment system called diagnosis-related groups (DRGs) as part of Medicare.
- The driving force in health care facilities is cost containment. LPN/LVNs play a role in containing health care costs in the work setting.
- Holistic care includes being aware of the physical, psychological, social, cultural, and spiritual needs of patients.
- The nurse-patient relationship is therapeutic and goal directed, and ends when the patient is discharged.
- Trust is established with patients by using therapeutic communication skills, maintaining the patient's self-esteem, displaying competence while providing care, and displaying compassion for patients.
- The patient with a physical illness is also affected emotionally by his or her illness or injury and may display dependent, withdrawn, depressed, hostile, or manipulative behaviors.

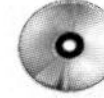
Go to your **Companion CD-ROM** for an Audio Glossary, animations, video clips, and bonus review questions.

evolve Be sure to visit the companion Evolve site at http://evolve.elsevier.com/deWit for interactive NCLEX-PN Exam Style Review Questions, WebLinks, and additional online resources.

NCLEX-PN® EXAM STYLE REVIEW QUESTIONS

Choose the best answer(s) for the following questions.

1. On initial assessment, the patient is found to be more interested in asking questions regarding the nurse and evading personal questions, and is often silent with no eye contact. These characteristics are more likely to be found in which of the following behaviors?
   1. Withdrawn
   2. Manipulative
   3. Dependent
   4. Hostile
2. Which of the following statements made by a patient strongly indicates dependent behavior?
   1. "I can do this by myself."
   2. "I will try to do this."
   3. "Would you help me if I am not able to do it myself?"
   4. "Would you do these things for me?"
3. A terminally ill patient states, "I find solace in communing with nature." An appropriate nursing action would be to:
   1. provide periods of rest and relaxation.
   2. place patient in a room with a view.
   3. turn the television to the Nature channel.
   4. take the patient outdoors whenever possible.
4. A patient with manipulative behaviors would most likely make which of the following statements?
   1. "I would need the pain medications in 2 hours."
   2. "Would you help me choose my meals?"
   3. "You are not helping me!"
   4. "I will report you to the charge nurse."
5. The nurse is caring for a patient with an indwelling urinary catheter. Which task can be delegated to the nursing assistant?
   1. Providing perineal care
   2. Collecting urine specimen for laboratory testing
   3. Irrigating the catheter to ensure patency
   4. Instilling antibiotics
6. In caring for patients with pressure ulcers, which task would be most appropriate to delegate to the nursing assistant?
   1. Provide assistance in making dietary choices
   2. Participate in determining the appropriate type of wound care
   3. Reposition the patient every 2 hours
   4. Describe wound condition
7. The nurse finds a confused elderly patient attempting to get out of bed. The patient has a history of falls. To maintain the patient's self-esteem and safety, the nurse should:
   1. apply physical restraints.
   2. administer sedatives.
   3. install a bed alarm.
   4. provide constant reassurance.
8. When providing discharge instructions to a patient after knee replacement, which of the following statements indicate a need for further teaching?
   1. "I will wash my hands prior to changing my dressing."
   2. "I will be on strict bed rest to allow my knee to heal."
   3. "I will take analgesics before the pain gets worse."
   4. "I will be able to eat a regular diet."
9. Which of the following should the nurse consider before delegating a specific task? *(Select all that apply.)*
   1. Know the scope of practice
   2. Be aware of the staff competency and experience
   3. Seek approval from the administration
   4. Determine stability of patient condition
   5. Provide adequate explanation and oversight of the task
10. Which of the following statements indicate therapeutic nurse-patient relationship? *(Select all that apply.)*
    1. "You poor thing. I had a similar surgery."
    2. "You seem upset regarding your procedure."
    3. "What do you mean when you say that?"
    4. "You will be fine."
    5. "May I hold your hand?"

CRITICAL THINKING ACTIVITIES

Read each clinical scenario and discuss the questions with your classmates.

Scenario A

Midway during your medical-surgical rotation, your instructor schedules a clinical evaluation. Using the daily clinical evaluations you both have worked on since the beginning of this clinical experience, she asks you to bring written documentation of the following to the meeting.

1. List your strong areas within the roles of the LPN/LVN with corresponding behaviors.
2. List the roles of the LPN/LVN and corresponding behaviors where you feel you need improvement.
3. Develop a plan with specific behaviors to improve the above roles during the rest of the medical-surgical rotation.

Scenario B

The federal government of the United States is faced with budget problems resulting in large deficits and the need to reduce spending. Congress suggests reducing spending by cuts in the Medicare and Medicaid programs. The congressperson of your district asks for your opinion and rationale for the answers for each of the following questions:

1. Should Medicare pay the cost of coronary bypass surgery for an active 85-year-old person?
2. Should Medicaid pay for care in an extended care facility for an 88-year-old person who has suffered a stroke and is long-term comatose?
3. Should Medicare or Medicaid pay for lifestyle prescription drugs (e.g., Viagra) for men eligible for these programs?

Scenario C

Bill Boyd, age 72, was surprised at the aloofness of the admission clerk as she "entered" him into the system by way of computer for admission for a total knee replacement, his first hospital experience. Two personnel who assisted him to his assigned room called him "Bill." Neither introduced themselves or indicated the role they played in his admission. While wearing a patient gown with the opening down the front and waiting for a nurse to interview him, people kept coming into his room without knocking. One asked his wife if he drank coffee or tea with his meals. That night, the sound of TVs, the click and beep of machines, and staff talking in the halls prevented him from getting a good night's sleep before surgery.

1. List the things that went wrong with Mr. Boyd's admission day experience.
2. Describe how you would have made admission day a better experience.
3. Explain the reasons for the things you chose to do differently.

CHAPTER 2

Critical Thinking and Nursing Process

evolve http://evolve.elsevier.com/deWit

Objectives

Upon completing this chapter, you should be able to:

Theory

1. Explain what critical thinking is in your own words.
2. Describe how critical thinking affects clinical judgment.
3. Discuss why nurses in all programs must learn to think critically.
4. Clarify your role in nursing process according to your state's nurse practice act.
5. Explain three fundamental beliefs about human life as the basis for nursing process.
6. Identify the source for LPN/LVN standards for nursing process.

Clinical Practice

1. Explain how factors that influence critical thinking are experienced by you during patient care.
2. Provide a clinical example of how nursing process is used in the care of medical-surgical patients.
3. Provide an example of each of the following techniques of physical examination: inspection and observation, olfaction, auscultation, and percussion.
4. Prepare a list for beginning-of-shift assessment for a specific patient.
5. Write an example of a patient goal that is realistic, measurable, and time referenced.
6. Differentiate between nursing orders and medical orders.
7. Explain the value of identifying the patient's actual problems that lead to nursing diagnoses.

Key Terms

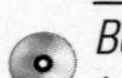

Be sure to check out the bonus material on the Companion CD-ROM, including selected audio pronunciations.

auscultation (ăw-skŭl-TĀ-shŭn, p. 23)
congruent (kŏn-GRŪ-ĕnt, p. 20)
critical thinking (p. 16)
data collection (assessment) (DĀ-tă, p. 17)
evaluation (ĭ-văl-ū-Ā-shŭn, p. 17)
expected outcomes (p. 28)
goals (p. 28)
implementation (ĭm-plĭ-mĕn-TĀ-shŭn, p. 17)
inspection (p. 19)
interdisciplinary (collaborative) care plans (kŏ-LĂB-ĕr-ă-tĭv plănz, p. 30)
measurable (p. 29)
North American Nursing Diagnosis Association International (NANDA-I) (p. 26)
nursing diagnosis (p. 27)
nursing interventions (p. 29)
nursing process (p. 18)
objective data (ŏb-JĔK-tĭv DĀ-tă, p. 19)
observation (p. 19)
olfaction (ol-FĂK-shŭn, p. 20)
palpation (păl-PĀ-shŭn, p. 23)
percussion (pĕr-KŬ-shŭn, p. 23)
planning (p. 17)
priority setting (p. 28)
realistic (p. 28)
subjective data (sŭb-JĔK-tĭv DĀ-tă, p. 19)
time-referenced (p. 29)

CRITICAL THINKING

Critical thinking is a problem-solving method that incorporates the scientific method and always asks, "Is there a better way?" Critical thinking is a lifelong process and, as you practice the knowledge you are gaining, you become more skilled at thinking critically and applying the knowledge to patient care.

CRITICAL THINKING AND CLINICAL JUDGMENT

Alfaro-Lefevre (2004) provided a definition of critical thinking applied to clinical judgment in nursing, which Hill and Howlett (2005) have adapted to practical/vocational nursing as follows:

- Purposeful, informed, outcome focused (results oriented). It requires careful identification of patient problems, issues, and risks, and makes accurate decisions about what is happening, what needs to be done, and prioritization of patient care.
- Driven by patient, family, and community health care needs.
- Based on principles of nursing process and the scientific method.
- Uses both logic and intuition, based on knowledge, skills, and experience of the LPN/LVN.
- Is guided by standards and ethical codes of the following organizations:

- National Association of Practical Nurse Education and Service, Inc. (NAPNES)
  - Standards of Practice for Licensed Practical/Vocational Nurses (see Appendix 1)
  - Code of Ethics (see Appendix 1)
- National Federation of Licensed Practical Nurses, Inc. (NFLPN)
  - Nursing Practice Standards for the Licensed Practical/Vocational Nurse, including the Code (see Appendix 2)
- National Council of State Boards of Nursing (NCSBN)
  - Definitions of the Four Phases of Nursing Process for Practical/Vocational Nurses (Box 2–1).
- Calls for strategies that make the most of human potential (e.g., using individual strengths), and compensate for problems created by human nature (e.g., overcoming the powerful influence of personal beliefs, values, and prejudices).
- Means constantly reevaluating, self-correcting, and striving to improve (e.g., practicing skills, learning new skills, attending classes, workshops, and reading nursing journals).

Critical thinking involves expanding thinking beyond the obvious. New ideas and alternatives are offered in a constructive way. The critical thinker is willing to consider other ideas and recognizes that there may be more than one way to do the right thing. The thinker realizes that there may not be a perfect solution. Judgments are based on facts (knowledge), not assumptions, which are synthesized and applied to a patient situation. A critical thinker recognizes the patient's primary problems and makes decisions on how to prioritize and deal with the problems or deviations from normal health status.

? *Think Critically About . . .* Can you list three examples in which you might use critical thinking in the classroom?

Box 2–1 ***NCSBN Definitions of Four Phases of Nursing Process for LPN/LVNs***

Phase 1—Data Collection: A systematic gathering and review of information about the patient, which is communicated to appropriate members of the health team.

Phase 2—Planning: Assisting the RN in the development of nursing goals, and interventions for a patient's plan of care and maintaining patient safety.

Phase 3—Implementation: The provision of required nursing care to accomplish established patient goals.

Phase 4—Evaluation: Compares the actual outcomes of nursing care to the expected outcomes, which are then communicated to members of the health care team.

From NCLEX-PN test plan for the National Council Licensure Examination for Practical/Vocational Nurses. (2001, effective date April 2002). Chicago: National Council of State Boards of Nursing.

Critical thinking is at its best when the brain is purposefully engaged. For example, while listening to report at the beginning of the shift, you pay attention to what the nurse is saying. Think about how you will apply the information you have gained. Observe the critical thinking activities that take place between the nurses during report, as they collaborate in solving a patient-related problem. Also observe the same thing later in the shift as the nurse(s) make decisions about patient care issues, when to notify the physician, and the like. Consider the following when receiving report:

- Do I understand what is being said?
- What will I be expected to do?
- What are the priorities of nursing care?
- What areas need further clarification?
- What procedures will require instructor supervision?

Examine your thinking and the thinking of others and apply the knowledge to patient care. Critical thinking is based on science and scientific principles and includes the following:

- Collecting data in an organized way
- Verifying data in an organized way
- Looking for gaps in information
- Analyzing the data

Apply critical thinking when developing a care plan with the patient's need(s) in mind.

As a student and a nurse, you will have to be able to access information, understand information, recall it, and use it as the basis for critical thinking in the clinical area. Much of what you learn as a student involves exposure to sources of information and how to locate the sources quickly. Of course, some information must be committed to memory, and the more you use this information, the easier it is to remember. As you practice putting information into your own words when planning patient care, you are reinforcing comprehension of information. Memorizing alone without comprehension is not critical thinking. Critical thinking allows the nurse to apply knowledge and principles to different patient care situations.

FACTORS THAT INFLUENCE YOUR THINKING AND NURSING CARE

Attitude

A major factor in learning and applying critical thinking is attitude. The critical thinker is humble and recognizes that he does not have all the answers and that his perceptions may be clouded by personal values and beliefs. The critical thinker will consider evidence that is presented.

Communication Skills

The critical thinker communicates effectively both verbally and in writing. Before speaking, the critical thinker thinks through what is going to be said. Information is presented in a clear, concise manner.

Box 2–2 Actual Examples of Student Charting (How Not to Chart)

- Vaginal packing out. Dr. Heffle in.
- Dr. Jones in. Had large formed brown stool.
- On the second day the knee was better, and on the third day it disappeared.
- She is numb from the toes down.
- Patient was alert and nonresponsive.

Written documentation through charting tells the other health team members what was planned, the patient's reaction to the care, and if expected outcomes were met. Sometimes students are so focused on getting information into the nurse's notes that attention is not paid to how the total message reads (Box 2–2).

Think Critically About . . . Recall the first time you gave report on a patient. What was the general feedback you received? Had feedback changed with the most recent report you gave, and if so, in what way?

It is helpful to identify a nurse who is skilled at thinking critically and communicates clearly both verbally and through charting. This might be an instructor or a nurse who works on the medical-surgical unit. This person can serve as a mentor to you as you are learning to apply critical thinking knowledge. The most effective mentor will be one who coaches by asking questions rather than just giving answers.

INTEGRATING CRITICAL THINKING AND NURSING PROCESS

The NCSBN integrated critical thinking and nursing process into all aspects of the practical/vocational licensing examination (NCLEX-PN) in 2002. The NCSBN also clearly defined the LPN/LVN role in nursing process.

Think Critically About . . . What does your state's nurse practice act (NPA) indicate about the role of the LPN/LVN? What questions do you have regarding clarification of the law?

If in doubt about the role of the LPN/LVN in the nursing process, direct your questions to your state's board of nursing. It is important to have studied the NPA of the state in which you work. According to NCSBN research with LPN/LVNs, all U.S. states and territories identify a scope of practice for either LPNs or LVNs. However, the practices allowed by those scopes vary widely. While most LPN/LVN scopes of practice stipulate a directed role under the supervision of a registered nurse (RN), many differ in the areas of care planning, assessment, intravenous therapy, teaching, and delegation (Spector, 2005).

NURSING PROCESS AND MEDICAL-SURGICAL NURSING

Nursing process is the language of nursing. It is an orderly way to assess a patient's response to current health status and to plan, implement, and evaluate the patient's response to nursing care. It is a way to communicate to all nursing personnel what is to be done and by whom during all shifts. It provides a way to make changes in patient care if progress is not being made. The nursing process utilizes and builds on a patient's strengths and partners the nurse with the patient whenever possible. The goal of nursing process is to alleviate, minimize, or prevent real or potential health problems.

FUNDAMENTAL BELIEFS AS THE BASIS FOR NURSING PROCESS

The nursing process is based on some fundamental beliefs about human life, the role of nursing, and the delivery of health care:

- Every person is endowed with worth and dignity.
- Every person has basic needs common to all humans, and these needs must be met to some degree if a person is to survive and enjoy an acceptable level of wellness.
- Meeting one's basic human needs may require assistance from someone else until one is able to resume responsibility for oneself.
- Every person has the right to high-quality service regardless of his or her socioeconomic status, cultural background, race, religious belief, or sexual orientation.
- Patients and their families prefer a patient-centered approach that actively seeks input and respects their thoughts, feelings, and needs.
- The focus of nursing should be on maintaining health, preventing disease, and helping the sick and injured.
- The nurse engaged in the nursing process will continue to work toward self-fulfillment by studying, learning, and improving competence.

APPLYING LPN/LVN STANDARDS IN MEDICAL-SURGICAL NURSING

The five basic steps of the nursing process are (1) assessment (data collection), (2) nursing diagnosis, (3) planning, (4) implementation, and (5) evaluation.

The NCSBN states that four of these steps (phases) apply to the LPN/LVNs in medical-surgical nursing (see Box 2–1). The four phases describe the LPN/LVN in an assisting role.

ASSESSMENT (DATA COLLECTION)

The LPN/LVN acts in a more independent role when participating in data collection (assessment) and the implementation phases of the nursing process. LPN/LVNs systematically gather and review data about the patient and communicate it to appropriate members of the health care team. A complete database includes a thorough health history, physical assessment, psychosocial assessment, and cultural and spiritual assessment. Most health facilities use a standardized form to follow when developing the admission database so it is as complete as possible. Both **subjective data** (data that the patient gives that cannot be seen or felt by another, such as pain) and **objective data** (that which can be verified by sight, smell, touch, or sound) are included.

The purpose of data collection is to have a relevant database from which patient problems and potential problems are identified. It is the basis for developing a problem list from which nursing diagnoses will be developed. If there is an immediate life-threatening problem, determine immediately what action must be taken and if additional expertise is needed to deal with the problem. Once the patient's physical condition is stabilized, a formal care plan can be developed.

Sources of Information

Review of Admission Forms. The admission form generally accompanies a patient to the unit (Figure 2–1; refer to the CD-ROM for the complete form). It has the basic information such as the patient's name, reason for admission, and other important information. If the patient has been hospitalized in the past, previous records may be included. The physician's history and medical examination, if available, will focus on the patient's physical and mental status. The medical diagnosis will guide the nurse in collecting assessment data and identifying patient problems. Check to see if results of preliminary laboratory work, x-rays, or other test results are included. If available, read the current information before entering the patient's room. It will enhance your critical thinking and observation skills during your initial contact. It will also help you not to repeat obvious questions unless you are trying to verify data that are unclear.

> ? *Think Critically About . . .* How many sources can you identify that would provide information for a nursing database on a patient who has been admitted to a long-term care facility?

Interview. The patient is the primary source of information because she knows more about herself than anyone else (Focused Assessment 2–1).

If for some reason the patient is incapacitated, then secondary sources are useful (e.g., a spouse, significant other, relative, friend, or patient advocate). The secondary source can also help verify information that was provided by the patient. Box 2–3 provides suggestions for interviewing. The remainder of the admission form is filled out by the nurse and includes such items as status of advance directives, assessments for fall risk, pain level, pressure ulcer risk, nutrition requirements, and ability to perform activities of daily living. Psychosocial, cultural, and spiritual assessment data are gathered.

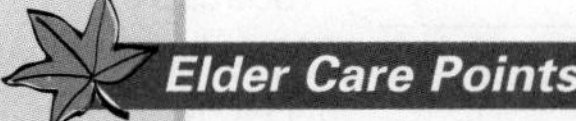

Plan extra time for an interview with a patient who is elderly. The elderly person who is ill may think and speak more slowly and often has a longer health history to relate than a younger person.

Numerous hospitals are including a Medication Reconciliation form (see the CD-ROM for this form) to identify and prevent polypharmacy (multiple drugs prescribed for the same condition by different physicians). It also reduces the risk of medication ordering errors and adverse interactions between drugs. Patient allergies and medications—prescription, over-the-counter, and herbal preparations and supplements—are included. Both the physician and the pharmacist review the form.

Patients need to know that the information gathered will be recorded and used in planning their care. Ask patients what they think is their major problem or "chief complaint." Other questions concern the present level of pain; when the last bowel movement occurred; problems with urination, appetite, difficulty sleeping; and whether they have any additional concerns or complaints.

Physical Assessment. Measuring the patient's blood pressure, pulse, respiration, temperature, weight, and height usually begins physical data collection. Accuracy is essential. These are truly "vital signs" that are indicators of what is happening at any given moment. In addition to measuring vital signs, correlate current readings with the baseline data, trends of past readings, the patient's current clinical status, and the medical care that has been provided. Such data yield significant information about the patient's condition and response to medication and other treatments. Complete assessments are performed daily (Figure 2–2; see the CD-ROM for the complete form).

Inspection and Observation. **Inspection** (looking) and **observation** (looking and noting) are important aspects of nursing assessment. Use your eyes to pick up

PATIENT INFORMATION

Date/time: ____________

Information given by: ☐ Patient ☐ Spouse ☐ Other: ____________

Accompanied by: ☐ Self ☐ Spouse ☐ Relative ☐ Other: ____________

Person/organization having legal responsibilities: ☐ Self ☐ Spouse ☐ Parent ☐ Other: ____________

Emergency contact name: ____________ Phone: ____________

Language spoken: ☐ English ☐ Other: ____________ Interpreter arranged: date/time/initials: ____________

Chief complaint/reason for hospitalization/procedure: ____________

Height: ______ Weight: ______ ☐ Actual Type of scale: ______ ☐ Stated

PAST MEDICAL HISTORY

☐ Heart/circulatory problems ______
☐ High blood pressure ______
☐ Kidney/bladder problems ______
☐ Breathing problems ______
☐ Liver problems ______
☐ Vision/hearing problems ______
☐ Stomach problems ______
☐ Infectious disease (TB, hepatitis) ______
☐ Recent exposure to infectious disease ______
☐ Blood transfusion reaction ______
☐ Diabetes
☐ Cancer
☐ Seizures

☐ Stroke ______
☐ Arthritis ______
☐ Mammogram date ______
☐ Pneumovax date ______
☐ Flu shot date ______

☐ Pregnant:
If yes, LMP: ___/___/___
☐ Depression
☐ Anxiety
☐ Other psychiatric or mental illness

Tobacco

What types do you use: (check all that apply)

☐ None ☐ Cigarettes ☐ Cigars ☐ Chewing tobacco

How long have you used? ______

How much do you use? ______

If yes, enter referral for Tobacco Awareness Program (TAP)

Alcohol/drugs

Do you use alcohol or drugs? ☐ Yes ☐ No

If yes, how much do you use? ______

How long have you used alcohol/drugs? ______

Do you want to quit using drugs or alcohol? ☐ Yes ☐ No

*IF yes, consult Psychiatric Services and/or Case Management via computer for referral

Are there any other significant family medical problems we should be aware of: ☐ Yes ☐ No ______

Past hospitalizations: ______

Allergies: ☐ None known ☐ Please refer to Medication Reconcilation Form (#1001987)

LATEX SENSITIVITY

Have you ever been told you have a latex allergy?

☐ Yes ☐ No

If no, have you ever had (check if yes):

☐ A reaction after handling balloons, band aids, poinsettias, rubber or elastic products?

☐ Itching, tearing, sneezing or runny nose after a dental procedure?

☐ A reaction to avocados, bananas, kiwi, or chestnuts?

If yes to any of the above, initiate Latex Sensitivity protocol

Addressograph

FIGURE **2–1** Adult admission history. This is the first page of a four-page form; the entire form is included on your Companion CD-ROM. (Courtesy of Sheridan Memorial Hospital, Sheridan, WY.)

clues about the patient's physical and mental condition. Note the patient's facial expression, posture, grimaces, movements, and whether answers are **congruent** (answers match the feeling tone of what is said). Inspect the hair, skin, nails, and oral mucous membranes for data about hydration and dental hygiene. Observe the patient's state of personal care. Is the hair combed, and are the nails clean and reasonably trimmed? Is there anything in the room that gives evidence of support systems, family, or friends?

Olfaction. **Olfaction** (smelling) can provide data about a patient's personal hygiene as well as clues to possible illness. The sweet, fruity odor of acetone can be indicative of diabetic acidosis. The smell of newly mown clover can be present with hepatic coma. The smell of alcohol indicates the patient has been drinking.

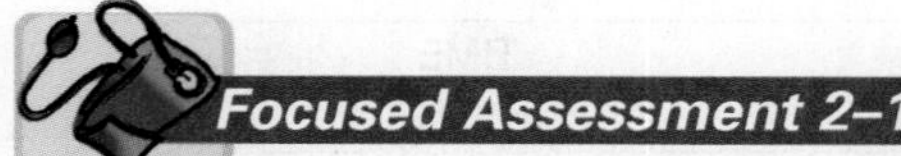

Focused Assessment 2–1

Abbreviated General Patient Interview Guide

SOCIAL ASSESSMENT

- What is your marital status? Who lives with you?
- What is your occupation?
- Are you an active church member, or do you belong to any organization?
- Do you have health insurance?
- How are things at home with you here in the hospital?
- Are there any medical problems that run in the family?
- Have you had previous surgeries or serious injuries?
- Whom do you have in your life who is supportive to you?
- What prescription drugs do you take? What over-the-counter medicines?
- Do you smoke? How much?
- Do you drink wine or alcohol? When and about how much do you drink?
- Are you allergic to any drug? Foods? Other substances?
- What do you like to eat? Describe yesterday's meals and snacks.

PHYSICAL ASSESSMENT

- What brought about your admission here?
- What health problems do you have?
- Do you routinely see other physicians? For what?

REVIEW OF SYSTEMS

Ask questions about the presence of the following:

- **Head and neck**

  Frequent headaches; dizziness, ringing of the ears, problems hearing; visual problems, glaucoma, cataracts, glasses or contact lenses; surgery of the brain, eyes, or ears; frequent colds; nasal allergies; sinus infections; frequent sore throats; hoarseness; trouble swallowing; swollen glands; mouth sores; date of last dental examination; history of thyroid problems; use of a hearing aid; difficulty sleeping; napping

- **Chest**

  Cough, sputum production; asthma, wheezing, frequent bronchitis; history of pneumonia; tuberculosis, exposure to tuberculosis; exposure to occupational respiratory hazards; palpitations, chest pain; shortness of breath; history of heart problems, murmurs, hypertension; anemia; surgery

  Female: frequency of breast examinations; date of last mammogram; nipple discharge; breast lumps

- **Abdomen (gastrointestinal tract)**

  Indigestion; pain; nausea; vomiting; excessive thirst or hunger; frequency of bowel movements; change in bowel movements; rectal bleeding; black or tarry stools; constipation; diarrhea; excessive gas; hemorrhoids; history of gallbladder or liver problems

- **Genitourinary**

  Problems with urination; up at night to urinate; dribbling of urine; history of urinary tract infection; stones

  Female: sexually active; sexual problems; menstrual cycle and any problems; last menstrual period; bleeding between periods or after menopause; vaginal discharge; date of last Pap smear; history of herpes or other vaginal disorders

  Male: sexually active; genital problems or penile discharge; history of herpes or other sexually transmitted diseases, any sexual problems.

- **Extremities and musculoskeletal system**

  Joint pain or stiffness; back problems; muscle pain; limited range of motion; vascular problems in legs or arms; easy bruising; skin lesions; history of phlebitis; thrombophlebitis; gout, arthritis, fractures, injury

PSYCHOLOGICAL ASSESSMENT

- Are you experiencing anxiety? Depression?
- Do you have unusual memory problems?
- Do you have difficulty thinking?
- Are you ever confused?

NCLEX-PN test plan for the National Council Licensure Examination for Practical/Vocational Nurses. (2001; effective date April 2002). Chicago: National Council of State Boards of Nursing.

Sometimes patients with acute alcoholism may smell like aftershave, mouthwash, vanilla, Sterno, or other substances containing a high percentage of alcohol.

Foul or metallic mouth odors usually indicate poor oral hygiene or periodontal disease. Odor from the nose may be indicative of chronic sinusitis with postnasal drip or an obstruction in the passages.

Patients with anemia, an endocrine problem, or a central nervous system abnormality may be trying to cover up unpleasant body odor with bath powder or heavy perfume. An unpleasant genital odor may indicate an infection, poor hygiene, or insufficient fluid intake. This is more commonly found in female patients in long-term care facilities. Without additional attention, body areas will become reddened, irritated, and sometimes infected.

Palpation. **Palpate** (touch) the patient's skin to learn if it feels healthy, or it is coarse, dry, swollen, cold, or clammy. Dryness may be related to dehydration. Swelling may indicate edema (fluid in the tissues). If you

Box 2–3 ***Interview Suggestions***

- Introduce yourself to the patient by name and as an LPN/LVN student.
- Be respectful.
- A patient is entitled to be addressed by his surname. Do so, unless the patient asks you to address him differently.
- Pull up a chair so that the patient can see and hear you.
- Speak slowly and clearly.
- Ask your questions without dropping your voice at the end of the sentence. Be alert to any hearing difficulty the patient may have.
- Give time for the patient to respond.
- Attempt to resolve incongruence in body language and responses.
- Ask for clarification if you are unsure what is meant by a particular statement or response.
- Summarize for the patient what you think you heard during the interview.
- Ask the patient for any corrections or additions.

DATE:	TIME:
	Initials:
NEUROLOGIC When awake is alert and oriented to person, place, time and situation. Speech clear, follows commands. Appropriate neurologic response to auditory, visual and tactile stimuli.	**WNL**
	WNL Except
	Reassess: No Change - time
	Disoriented: Person
	Place
	Time
	Situation
	LOC: Lethargic
	Agitated
	Unresponsive
	Communication Pattern: WNL
	WNL Except
PUPILS Equal, round, with prompt reaction to light.	**WNL**
	R ___ L ___ B ___ Fixed
	R ___ L ___ B ___ Dilated
	R ___ L ___ B ___ Sluggish
	R ___ L ___ B ___ Pinpoint
PSYCHOSOCIAL Affect and emotional state appropriate to situation, age and developmental level.	**WNL**
	Describe
	Education: Refer to Education Record
RESPIRATORY Respirations with regular pattern and depth. Unlabored and symmetrical chest wall expansion. Clear bilateral breath sounds heard. Pink mucous membranes. No cough. No sputum production.	**WNL**
	WNL except
	Reassess: No Change - time
	Breath Sounds:
	Location:
	Crackles
	Rhonchi
	Wheezes
	Diminished
	Respiratory Pattern:
	Irregular
	Labored
Location Key:	Dyspneic
RUL = Rt upper lobe	Tachypneic
RML = Rt middle lobe	Diminished
RLL = Rt lower lobe	**Cough:** Productive
LUL = Lt upper lobe	
LLL = Lt lower lobe	Nonproductive
BLL = Bilat lower lobes	**Secretions:** Clear
	Yellow
Bil = Bilateral lobes	Green
All = All lobes	Blood-tinged
	Thick
	Thin
Chest tube Location Key:	**Chest Tube:**
RM = Rt mediastinal	**Location**
LM = Lt mediastinal	**Suction** ________ **mmHg**
RP = Rt pleural	**Drainage:** See Key Page 2
LP = Lt pleural	**Air Leak:**
P = Pericardial	**Dressing:**

Key for Assessment: ✔ Assessment completed; ☐ Assessment not Applicable; * Refer to Annotation/Frequent Monitoring Sheet

	TIME:
	Initials:
AIRWAY CARE Type: ☐ Oral ☐ Nasal ☐ Trach ☐ Stoma	O_2 Mode:
	Liters:
	Humidified:
	Pulse Oximetry% if ordered
O_2 MODE KEY NC = Nasal Cannula M = Mask NRB = Non-Rebreather PRB = Partial Rebreather	**Incentive Spirometry:** q ___ hrs Volume Goal: _____
	TCDB: q _____ hrs
	Trach Care
	Trach Size _________
	Trach Type _________
	Suction
	BIPAP:
CARDIOVASCULAR MED/SURG: Rate reg. Radial pulse palpable. Absence of cyanosis, edema. Capillary refill less than 2 seconds. S_1S_2 heard. Normal sinus rhythm with tele. No JVD.	**WNL**
	WNL except
	Reassess: No Change - time
	Capillary Refill >2 sec
PULSE SCALE: 0 = Not palpable 1+ = Faintly Palpable 2+ = Palpable (normal) 3+ = Bounding (hyperdynamic)	**Pulses:**
	Location _____ Scale _____
	Edema:
	Location _____ Scale _____
	Telemetry w/ alarms on
PITTING EDEMA: 0 = None. 0 depth of indentation 1 = Trace. 0 - ¼" depth of indent 2+ = Mild. ¼ - ½" depth of indent 3+ = Moderate. ½-1" depth of indent 4+ = Severe. >1" depth of indent	Heart Sounds:
	Homans' Sign
	TED stockings
GASTROINTESTINAL No difficulty chewing or swallowing. Abdomen soft, non-tender and non-distended. Bowel sounds present. Absence of nausea, vomiting, diarrhea. Bowel movements within own norm.	**WNL**
	WNL except
	Reassess: No Change - time
	Bowel Sounds:
	Location:
	Hyperactive
	Hypoactive
	Absent
Key Location:	
RUQ - Right Upper Quadrant	**Abdomen:** Distended
	Tender
LUQ - Left Upper Quadrant	Feeding Tube Type: _______
	Placement Verified: _______
RLQ - Right Lower Quadrant	Site Care: _______
	Date of last BM _______
LLQ - Left Lower Quadrant	**Incontinent:**
AQ - All Quadrants	Diapers/Briefs
	Bowel Program:
	Nausea
	Vomiting
	Diarrhea
	Constipation
	Difficulty Swallowing:
	Appetite: NPO
	Poor
	Absent

FIGURE **2–2** Daily physical assessment. This is the first page of a six-page form; the entire form is included on your Companion CD-ROM. (Courtesy of Sheridan Memorial Hospital; Sheridan, WY.)

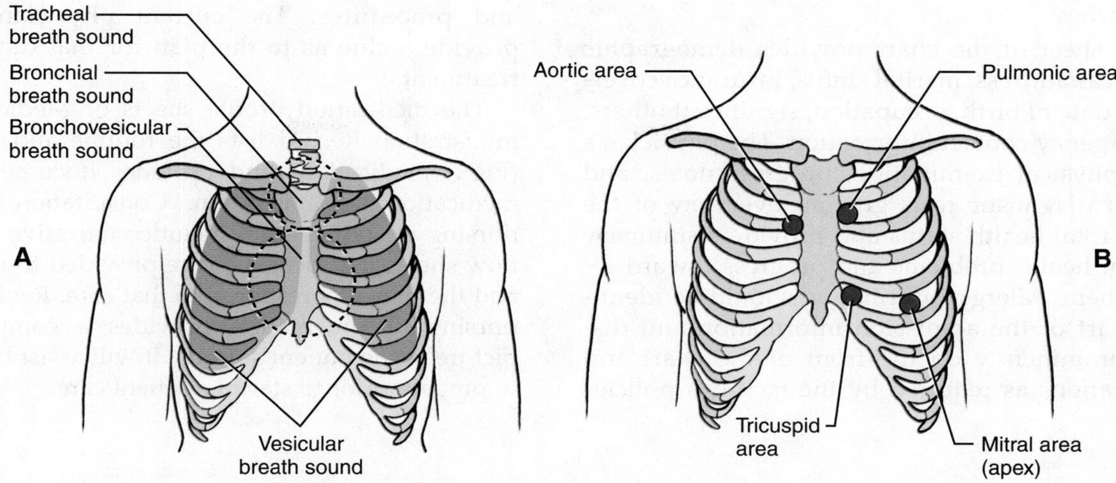

FIGURE **2–3** **A,** Place the stethoscope on the bare skin at these locations to hear the lung sounds. **B,** Place the stethoscope at the apex of the heart to listen to the apical pulse.

depress the skin with your fingers and your touch leaves pitting (indentation) on the skin, edema is present. Measure and record the depth of pitting and the length of time the tissue remains indented. **Palpation** of the skin can provide additional information. Cold extremities may indicate poor circulation. Hot tissue may be the result of localized inflammation, and you will want to examine the area more carefully. Use your fingertips, not your thumb, to palpate the pulses. Use the flat of the hand to palpate the abdomen to determine whether it is soft or hard or if there are any tender areas. Palpate the breasts for abnormal growths. Premenopausal women may have masses in their breasts, making it difficult to determine which lumps are significant. This is a good time to ask assistance from your instructor, the staff RN, or the clinical nurse specialist.

Auscultation. **Auscultation** (listening) is an important skill in gathering data. Listen to the sounds of the patient's breathing with and without a stethoscope. You may hear wheezing from constricted bronchi or stridor caused by a partial airway obstruction. Listening to the quality of a patient's cough will determine whether it is dry or moist. With the stethoscope, the sounds are amplified and you can auscultate normal, abnormal, or adventitious breath sounds (Figure 2–3). Listen to the apical pulse at the apex of the heart. Auscultate the abdomen for bowel sounds, listening carefully in each quadrant (Figure 2–4).

Percussion. Physicians, nurse practitioners, and physician assistants use **percussion** much more. By using a light, quick tapping on different surfaces of the body, they are able to tell the size, location, and density of different organs, especially in the chest, abdomen, and kidney areas. Percussion of the abdomen will reveal areas of excessive gas in the bowel.

Practical Daily Assessment (Data Collection)

A general abbreviated assessment (data collection) is completed on each assigned patient at intervals, and

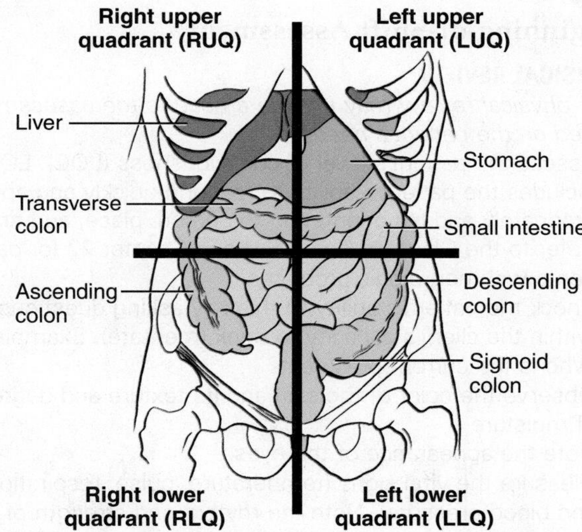

FIGURE **2–4** Listen for bowel sounds in all four quadrants of the abdomen.

then a focused assessment is directed to areas in which the patient is experiencing health problems. This is done to augment the complete admission assessment of the patient. It is based on the identified problems, data from report, and the medical diagnoses and treatment. Many hospitals have standardized forms for collecting head-to-toe data on the patient. Information from reviewing the patient's chart and care plan is used to identify areas in which focused assessment data should be collected. Ask for a demonstration of an appropriate head-to-toe assessment. Focused Assessment 2–2 presents a guide for the beginning-of-shift assessment.

Think Critically About . . . Can you develop your own basic daily assessment (data collection) list? What specific points should be added to the identified problems and medical diagnoses of the patient to whom you are assigned?

Chart Review

The face sheet of the chart provides demographic data such as address, marital status, insurance coverage, age, date of birth, occupation, significant others, and emergency contact information. The physician's history, physical examination, progress notes, and results of diagnostic tests give an overview of the patient's total health status and provide a summary of current health problems and progress toward resolving them. Allergy information should be identified as part of the admission information and displayed prominently on the front of the chart and other locations as required by the facility's policies and procedures. The current physician's orders provide a clue as to the plan for that day (tests or treatments).

The medication profile sheets or Medication Administration Record lists the routine and as-needed (PRN) medications and provides documentation of medication administration. Consultation sheets or nursing documentation includes narrative notes and flow sheets that describe care provided to the patient and the patient's response to that care. Reviewing the nursing documentation provides a comprehensive picture of the patient's needs. It will assist the student to prepare prior to starting patient care.

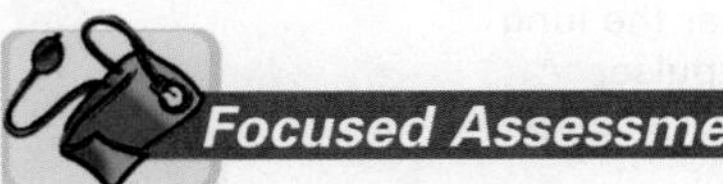

Focused Assessment 2–2

Beginning-of-Shift Assessment

PHYSICAL REVIEW

The physical review may include a head-to-toe assessment based on the patient's needs.

- Assess the patient's level of consciousness (LOC). LOC includes the patient's ability to respond quickly and appropriately and his orientation to person, place, and time. Refer to the Glasgow Coma Scale in Chapter 22 for patients with neurologic problems.
- Check the patient's ability to think by asking questions within the client's capacity to think (mentate). Example: Who is the current president?
- Observe the color of the skin and its texture and degree of moisture.
- Note the appearance of the eyes.
- Measure the vital signs (temperature, pulse, respiration, and blood pressure). Note the rhythm and strength of the pulse and the rhythm and depth of respiration. Also observe the patient's respiratory effort.
- Ask the patient to describe any pain. If necessary, ask questions to determine the location, severity, quality, and precipitating and alleviating factors.
- Auscultate the chest using the stethoscope. Listen for breath sounds, noting normal, abnormal, and adventitious breath sounds. Listen at the apex of the heart, checking for regularity of rhythm. Auscultate the apical pulse for 60 seconds to count the rate and observe the rhythm of the heartbeat. It is difficult for the new nurse to pick up extra heart sounds, but you can determine if there is an increase or decrease in the heart rate.
- Assess the skin turgor (elasticity of the skin) by gently lifting the skin on the upper chest with your thumb and forefinger and observing the speed with which it snaps back when you let go.
- Observe the contour of the abdomen, noting whether it is flat, round, or distended.
- When the patient is in a supine position or low Fowler's position, auscultate bowel sounds in all four quadrants.
- Gently palpate the abdomen with the palm side of the fingers, noting whether the abdomen is soft or firm. Also ask the patient whether he experiences any pain or discomfort, indicating areas of tenderness. Inquire about appetite and weight changes.
- Assess the patient's bowel and bladder status. Note when the patient had his last bowel movement (from the chart or by asking the patient) and whether or not flatus is being passed. Review the intake and output (I&O) for the past 24 hours. Observe and palpate the pubic area to assess bladder distention, especially if there is a discrepancy between the current and previous I&O. If the patient has an indwelling catheter, observe the characteristics of the urine in the drainage tube and the rate of drainage.
- Ask the patient to move each extremity. Observe the ability to actively move the joints through the range of motion and the coordination of the movements. If the patient is unable to actively move any joints, assist the patient with passive motion and note the degree of flexibility. Ask the patient to move extremities against resistance to determine extremity strength. The nurse can also determine the patient's level of cooperation and ability to follow directions during the exercises.
- Compare the peripheral pulses bilaterally.
- Note the presence of any edema.

TUBES AND EQUIPMENT STATUS

- *Intravenous catheter:* Condition of site; fluid in progress, rate, additives; time next fluid is to be hung.
- *Nasogastric tube:* Suction setting; amount and character of drainage; patency of tube; security of tube.
- *Urinary catheter:* Character and quantity of drainage; tubing not under patient.
- *Dressings:* Location; drains in place; wound suction devices; amount and character of wound drainage.
- *Pulse oximeter:* Intact probe; readings.
- *Patient-controlled analgesia pump:* Properly functioning; correct medication infusing; amount of solution remaining.
- *Traction:* Correct weight; body alignment; weights hanging free.
- *Equipment:* Applied properly; functioning as ordered.

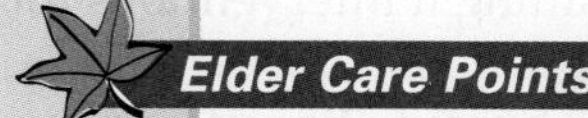

Elder Care Points

You walk into your patient's room and find Mrs. Nethers, age 72, has been restrained because she pulled out her oxygen tube, intravenous line, and urinary catheter earlier in the morning. She has also attempted to get out of bed several times. Yesterday she was alert and had a lucid conversation with you. Mrs. Nethers had surgery yesterday after you left the unit to go to class and has been receiving codeine for pain. You recall when you looked up medications that codeine could have a severe behavioral side effect, especially for an older patient. You inform the medication nurse and request that he discuss the information with the physician before giving additional doses.

Other clinicians such as the dietitian, respiratory therapist, and social worker also contribute documentation to the patient's chart. Information provided by these clinicians completes the comprehensive picture of the patient. You must keep all information you gather private (Legal & Ethical Considerations 2–1).

After obtaining patient information, preparation entails:

- Formulating a care plan or a list of patient care activities **in order of priority.**
- Developing a time management plan for care that is flexible and can be adjusted to accommodate changes in the patient's condition.
- Listing focused assessments you will make during the initial assessment and data that will be collected at intervals during care and before you go off duty.
- Reviewing procedures that will be performed and listing the equipment needed for each.
- Looking up required drug information for each routine and PRN drug listed on the profile, including intravenous solutions and additives.
- When reporting for clinical practice, reviewing the patient's chart for current information.
- Obtaining a current care profile if the agency uses this type of document. The document can be used during report, while providing care, and when charting and reporting information.

Your notes and lists are an excellent organization tool for reporting vital signs, medications given, and treatments performed. Your care plan is necessary for evaluating patient progress toward attaining goals and outcomes. Your care plan can identify issues not yet addressed on the chart problem list that might be added to it.

? *Think Critically About . . .* How will you use the patients' care plans to effectively receive and give report? What are the items to which you will pay greatest attention or will emphasize?

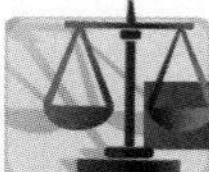

Legal & Ethical Considerations 2–1

Protected Health Information

Any protected health information that the student collects from a patient's chart must be carefully guarded to avoid violating the confidentiality component of the Health Insurance Portability and Accountability Act (HIPAA). Information that is retained by the student for educational purposes must be devoid of identifying information. Student preparation paperwork that contains protected health information must be destroyed following the policies and procedures of the facility.

Diagnostic Tests

Review laboratory and test data to identify general concerns and confirm assessment findings. Most often the diagnostic data help chart the patient's progress. Tests commonly ordered include the following.

White Blood Cell Count. When the patient has an infection, an increased number of white blood cells (WBCs) are sent from the bone marrow to attack bacteria or viruses causing the infection. An increased number of WBCs may occur with mild infections, appendicitis, pregnancy, leukemia, hemorrhage, and other conditions. Strenuous exercise, emotional distress, and anxiety can also cause an increase in WBCs. A low WBC count makes it harder for a patient to fight off colds and other infections. Low counts are also seen with illnesses such as mumps, lupus, cirrhosis of the liver, and cancer. In addition, radiation therapy and certain types of drug therapy tend to lower the WBC count. When looking up medications before giving them to the patient, notice if a potential side effect is a reduction in WBCs. If you have a cold or other infection, be aware that the patient with an already compromised immune system will respond more severely to any infection that might be contracted from you. It is not prudent for a staff member with a cold or other infection to work with a patient who has a low WBC count. If you must care for such a patient, then isolation barrier precautions should be maintained (gown, mask, gloves, etc.). Check with your instructor before beginning to provide care.

Red Blood Cell Count. Red blood cells (RBCs) contain hemoglobin and carry oxygen and carbon dioxide in the blood. The RBC count determines if the number of RBCs in your body is low (anemia) or high (polycythemia). Common causes of an abnormal RBC count are iron deficiency anemia due to chronic blood loss (i.e., menstruation, small amounts of bleeding due to colon cancer), acute blood loss (i.e., acute bleeding, ulcer, trauma), hereditary disorders (i.e., sickle cell anemia), or improper diet. Polycythemia is relatively uncommon. Relate the laboratory value of the RBC count to what you have read in your text about the underlying disorder. Note any difference in vital signs that correlate with a high or a low RBC count.

Hemoglobin. Low hemoglobin (Hb) levels often indicate anemia, and usually the patient will also have a low RBC count and a low hematocrit (Hct). Signs and symptoms of anemia (paleness, shortness of breath, fatigue) will start to show when the Hb is too low. Are these symptoms you have noted when collecting data? If so, has there been any change? Women tend to normally have a lower RBC count and Hb than men. Be sure to check all three values (RBC count, Hb, and Hct) when scanning a lab report and see if you can correlate the results with your observations of the patient.

Hematocrit. Hematocrit measures how much of the patient's blood is made up of RBCs. This measurement is useful in identifying anemia, the presence of liver disease, and RBC production in the bone marrow. Hematocrit increases during dehydration and, along with Hb, increases in polycythemia. Observing all three measurements (RBC count, Hb, and Hct) will make a difference in planned observations and data gathering. For example, if the patient has polycythemia, there is a risk of a stroke or myocardial infarction from a clot. Watch for signs of these problems.

Platelet Count. Platelets help stop bleeding after injury or surgery. The platelet count may change with bleeding disorders, heart disease, diabetes, inflammatory disease, and anemia. If your patient has bruising or is prone to bruising, a platelet count may be ordered. Patients may have brought in their own supply of over-the-counter medications such as aspirin and herbal products such as ginkgo biloba that may affect the platelet count. Be alert to what is in the bedside table drawers. Sometimes you will find the answer to what is causing the problem.

Glucose. High blood glucose after fasting for 12 hours is suggestive of diabetes. Additional tests will be done to confirm the diagnosis. If the patient does have diabetes, you will be involved in coaching the patient to test her own glucose level with a blood glucose meter. For some patients, the glucose level readings determine the amount of insulin they receive after each reading. The glucose level must be checked as ordered and the correct amount of insulin must be given on time. Once again, you will be able to track patient progress toward stabilizing the illness. A slightly elevated glucose is sometimes related to stress.

A low glucose level occurs with hypoglycemia. The patient will experience symptoms such as weakness, nausea, sweating, and confusion. A high-protein snack such as cheese may sustain the patient longer than a sweet treat. A sweet treat raises the blood sugar quickly, but the increase is not sustained. A protein food raises the level more slowly and sustains the increase for a longer period of time.

Hemoglobin A_{1C}. An Hb A_{1C} test provides an average blood sugar for the past 2 to 3 months. It is considered the "gold standard" in determining if interventions for diabetes are working.

Thyroid-Stimulating Hormone. Thyroid-stimulating hormone testing is the most sensitive way to identify both hypothyroidism and hyperthyroidism. TSH increases in primary hypothyroidism and decreases in hyperthyroidism. Check to see if the TSH is within normal limits.

Other Resources

When collecting patient data, the student has more time than the staff nurses. Take advantage of the time. Course textbooks are the primary resource. Other texts, journal articles, and the Internet can provide a wealth of information. Since there is no control over information placed on the World Wide Web, Internet resources should be evaluated carefully in light of information provided in print resources. Human resources such as your instructor, pharmacists, dietitians, social workers, occupational therapists, physical therapists, physicians, and other specialists can provide valuable information about specific aspects of the patient. Work to gain a comprehensive picture of the patient's situation.

ANALYSIS AND NURSING DIAGNOSIS (LPN/LVN ROLE)

The LPN/LVN reports data collection findings to the RN and assists in verifying and categorizing the collected data and grouping it in logical order. The LPN/LVN also assists in determining significant relationships between data, patient needs, and problems. A *prioritized* list of patient problems is developed. The focus is on actual and potential patient problems that can be addressed with independent nursing interventions. From the analysis, the RN chooses nursing diagnoses from the current **North American Diagnosis Association International (NANDA-I)** list (see inside back cover). The nursing diagnoses are general statements or stems labeling patient problems. The stem is then linked with the etiology (cause) and evidence (signs and symptoms) of the problem, making the nursing diagnosis statement specific to the patient. Nursing care is based on the *priority* of patient problems. High-priority problems are dealt with first. Lesser problems will be dealt with as there is time. The nursing diagnosis statements are based on all of the available patient data, including, but not limited to, the nursing assessment (subjective and objective) data, diagnostic test data, and the medical diagnosis. Placing a nursing diagnosis in the care plan means that the nurse is accepting accountability for accuracy of the statement. If a problem is permitted to continue without a correct nursing diagnosis designated, the patient could be harmed (Alfaro-Lefevre, 2004) (Nursing Care Plan 2–1).

Think Critically About . . . What is important in choosing the correct nursing diagnosis for a care plan? How would you determine that a nursing diagnosis on a facility care plan is appropriate for the patient?

It is important for a nurse to differentiate between a **nursing diagnosis** and a medical diagnosis. The physician is concerned with medical diagnosis: health problems that can be treated with surgery, medications, and other forms of therapy provided or prescribed by the physician. Nursing diagnoses identify the patient's response to her illness or health condition. Nursing practice addresses physical, psychological, social, cultural, and spiritual comfort and well-being; the prevention of complications; and patient education. Nursing care focuses on preventing, minimizing, and alleviating specific health problems. Although the physician is responsible for managing medical problems, the nurse

NURSING CARE PLAN 2–1

Care of the Patient with Imbalanced Nutrition

SCENARIO Martha Nielson, age 82, was admitted because of continued loss of weight and weakness. She is a frail-looking woman who walks slowly and with hesitation. The patient has experienced loss of appetite, loss of weight, and loss of energy since her right mastectomy 3 years ago.

PROBLEM/NURSING DIAGNOSIS *Eats only 5% of each meal*/Imbalanced nutrition, less than body requirements, related to loss of appetite and weakness.

Supporting assessment data *Objective:* Ht. 5′7″, Wt. 100 lb, loss of 35 lb.

Goals/Expected Outcomes	Nursing Interventions	Selected Rationale	Evaluation
Patient will eat 1500 calories of soft diet and drink 2000 mL of liquids each 24-hr period	Six small meals at 8 A.M., 10 A.M., noon, 2 P.M., 4 P.M., and 6 P.M. Patient seated in chair with minimal assistance. Encourage self-feeding. Assist only if needed. Likes chicken, mashed potatoes, gravy, sweet potato, creamed peas, and lemon pie.	Small, attractively arranged soft diet of favorite foods will entice patient to eat without feeling too full.	By day 2, patient will be able to consume 1000 calories in a 24-hr period.
	Set up tray for easy reach. Open packages and milk carton. Remove lids. Cut meat.	Preserves strength and helps her overcome weakness.	By day 4, patient will be able to remove lids and cut most of her meat.
	Offer 240 ml liquids at 6 A.M., 9 A.M., 11 A.M., 3 P.M., 5 P.M., 7 P.M., and 9 P.M. Vary choices. Likes apple juice, orange juice, ice cream, water, Jell-O. Likes 7-UP at lunch and dinner. Enjoys tea at breakfast and 3 P.M. Record time, amount, and liquids taken.	A variety of favorite liquids in small amounts alternating between meals will be easier to consume.	By day 2 will drink 1000 mL during 24-hr period.
Patient will verbalize that she has more energy and spend more awake time during the day	Collect data on amount of hours patient is awake and the length and number of naps.	Provide objective data as a baseline.	Patient states that she feels more energetic and will decrease the length of morning and afternoon nap times to ½ hr each.

CRITICAL THINKING QUESTIONS

1. What practical methods can the nurse use to entice the patient to eat without actually feeding her?
2. What are measures that the nurse can use to encourage activity without tiring patient excessively?

often uses clues from the medical diagnosis to identify patient problems and to develop accurate nursing diagnoses.

The NANDA-I approved stems, chosen by the RN based on an analysis of available data, label patient problems that can be independently treated using nursing interventions. The other two components of each nursing diagnosis make the statements specific to the patient's situation and direct the planning and implementation phases of the nursing process. A complete nursing diagnosis includes the problem (NANDA-I stem), the etiology (related causes of the problem), and the signs and symptoms (evidence of the problem).

The etiology component describes the known or suspected cause or causes of a problem. For example, a patient's ineffective breathing patterns could be related to reduced lung capacity, anxiety, or pain. The signs and symptoms of the problem describe the subjective and objective evidence of the problem. The diagnosis is supported (evidenced) by the assessment data. A patient's ineffective breathing pattern might be evidenced by her statement of shortness of breath or the nurse's observation of dyspnea (difficulty breathing), changes in respiratory rate or rhythm, or decreased oxygen saturation levels. The RN, after considering all of the available data relevant to the patient's respiratory function, might develop the following diagnosis statement: Ineffective breathing related to abdominal incision pain as evidenced by shallow respirations and low pulse oximeter readings (89% to 92%).

Actual problems are problems that the patient currently exhibits and should include all three components of the diagnosis statement. The patient does not currently exhibit evidence of potential problems, but the data demonstrate that a problem could occur. Potential problems begin with the phrase, "risk for" and include the NANDA-I stem and the etiology. An example of a potential problem is: Risk for fluid volume deficit related to vomiting and diarrhea. In this example, the patient is not currently showing signs of dehydration, but is at risk because of the fluid loss associated with vomiting and diarrhea. Identifying potential problems allows the nurse the opportunity to be alert for and take measures to prevent problems and complications rather than waiting for a problem to materialize before taking action. The LPN/LVN is expected to be familiar with the NANDA-I list of nursing diagnoses.

PLANNING

The LPN/LVN standard indicates that the LPN/LVN will utilize the nursing process in planning nursing care and will assist the RN in the identification of health goals and interventions for a patient's plan of care. In order to develop an effective care plan, the patient should be involved in determining priorities. The nurse should collect data to determine the patient's opinion of her situation, as well as her knowledge and deficits. Data regarding desired information and what the patient is willing and able to do to improve the situation are gathered also. Sometimes, something that the nurse might consider minor is very important to the patient.

Setting Priorities of Care

Priority setting is a method of handling problems and tasks according to the importance (priority) of the patient's problems. Maslow's hierarchy of needs is one way to prioritize nursing care (Figure 2–5). The lowest level of needs—those needed to sustain life, such as an airway and breathing—must be attended to immediately, even before a formal care plan is developed. All problems might not be included in the initial plan. As problems are dealt with successfully, they are modified or discontinued. Other problems are added to the plan as they arise. Priority setting is a skill that must be developed in order to work efficiently and safely. Along with prioritization is the need to recognize when assignment of some tasks to others should occur. Nursing diagnoses are listed on the care plan in order of priority.

Goals and Expected Outcomes

All stated goals must be patient centered, realistic, measurable, and include a time frame. The goals are set by the patient and nurse, and are achievable by the patient. Goals and expected outcomes relate to the following: (1) restoring health when there is a health problem, and (2) promoting health when the patient's resources can and should be directed at regaining or maintaining health. For example, the patient is eager to learn how to live with the diagnosis of diabetes. You instruct the patient about the illness, how to monitor the glucose level, action needed to stabilize the glucose level, how to administer insulin, how to maintain a supportive diet, the kinds and frequency of appropriate exercise, how to prevent infections, and when to seek additional medical help.

Goals state a general intent about what the patient will achieve. **Expected outcomes** describe a specific result at a certain point. The terms are used interchangeably in some agencies, although the American Nurses Association prefers the term *outcomes*. The focus of outcomes is what the patient, not the nurse, will do. An outcome is written as: The patient will . . . Patient input is important in order for motivation to occur to do what needs to be done to accomplish the outcome. Outcome statements are derived from the signs and symptoms included in the nursing diagnosis statement. The nurse, in conjunction with the patient, reverses the "evidenced by" component of the problem into an achievable, positive outcome statement. All outcome statements must have the following characteristics:

- **Realistic** (attainable, based on the patient's condition and desire)

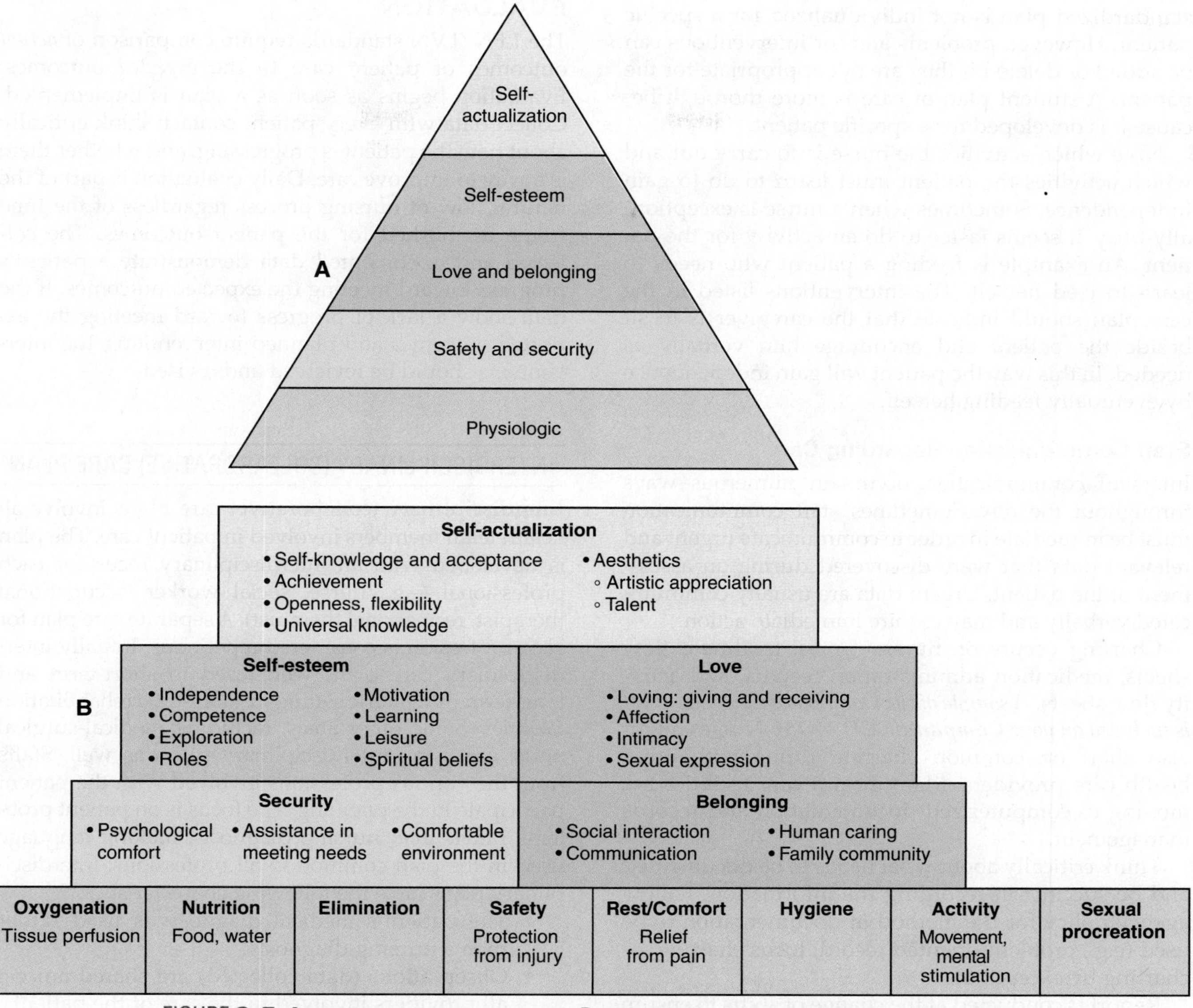

FIGURE 2–5 **A,** Maslow's hierarchy of needs. **B,** Evolving hierarchy of needs adapted by nursing to help determine priorities of care.

- **Measurable** (tells how you will know that the outcome is reached)
- **Time-referenced** (an educated guess as to how long it will take to attain the outcome)

The word "patient" is used as the subject of the statement. The time stated is realistic for the patient or the problem. It includes a time frame for reevaluation. The outcome statements are written with a subject, an action verb, conditions or modifiers, and the criterion (standard) for desired performance. Expected outcomes should include:

- Patient activity that can be observed by the nurse or patient knowledge that can be assessed. Consider how "the patient will select *[action verb—can be measured or observed]* low-sodium foods from a list" provides a better indicator of knowledge than "the patient will understand *[passive verb]* a low sodium diet."
- Description of how the patient's behavior will be measured, including the accuracy and quality of performance and the time frame within which the objective is to be met.

Nursing Interventions

Nursing interventions are nursing actions and patient activities chosen to achieve the goals and expected outcomes. Independent nursing interventions can be initiated and implemented without a physician's order. They are written on the nursing care plan.

IMPLEMENTATION

The LPN/LVN standards require providing care within the scope of practice to accomplish established goals. Standardized care plans are frequently found on medical-surgical units and include generic nursing care for frequently encountered patient problems. The standardized plan is not individualized for a specific patient. However, problems and/or interventions can be added or deleted if they are not appropriate for the patient. A student plan of care is more thorough because it is developed for a specific patient.

Note which activities the nurse is to carry out and which activities the patient must learn to do to gain independence. Sometimes when a nurse is exceptionally busy, it seems faster to do an activity for the patient. An example is feeding a patient who needs to learn to feed herself. The interventions listed in the care plan should indicate that the caregiver is to sit beside the patient and encourage him verbally as needed. In this way the patient will gain independence by eventually feeding herself.

Staff Communication Regarding Care

Interstaff communication occurs in numerous ways throughout the day. Sometimes staff communication must be immediate in order to communicate urgent and relevant data that were discovered during an assessment of the patient. Urgent data are usually communicated verbally and may require immediate action.

Charting occurs on nurses' notes, treatment flow sheets, medication administration records, and activity flow sheets. *A sample of the Daily Basic Care worksheet is included on your **Companion CD-ROM**.* Nurses might also chart on common charting forms with other health care providers. Many health care facilities are moving to computerized documentation and records management.

Think critically about what needs to be documented and be succinct in recording the information. Follow agency policy for the method of documentation to be used (e.g., problem-oriented record, focus charting, or charting by exception).

Report is conducted at the change of shifts to ensure continuity of care for the patients and is conducted according to facility protocol. On some medical-surgical units, all the staff listens to report on all of the patients. The advantage of this method is that all of the nurses and nursing assistants are aware of the needs of every patient. Other units use an individualized report system in which only the assigned nurse receives report on his assigned patients. Walking rounds are another method for change-of-shift report. The nurses go to the various patient rooms and the departing nurse and patient describe what happened during the previous shift. They discuss what the departing nurse and patient see as priorities for the next shift. An advantage of walking rounds is that the patient has direct input into his care. It is more time consuming than other methods, but provides a sense of partnering for the patient, and the arriving nurses have an opportunity to see and hear the patient before beginning care. It is especially helpful and saves time if the arriving nurse has the Kardex sheet or computer care plan printout in hand.

EVALUATION

The LPN/LVN standards require comparison of *actual* outcomes of patient care to the *expected* outcomes. Evaluation begins as soon as a plan is implemented. Collect data with every patient contact; think critically about how the patient is progressing, and whether there is a way to improve care. Daily evaluation is part of the natural flow of nursing process regardless of the time frame established for the patient outcomes. The collected and documented data demonstrate a patient's progress toward meeting the expected outcomes. If the data show a lack of progress toward meeting the expected outcomes and planned interventions, the interventions should be reviewed and revised.

INTERDISCIPLINARY (COLLABORATIVE) CARE PLAN

Interdisciplinary (collaborative) care plans involve all health team members involved in patient care. The plan is developed with an interdisciplinary focus for each professional (e.g., nurse, social worker, occupational therapist, recreational therapist). A separate care plan for each profession is considered repetitious. Initially interdisciplinary care plans were used in short-term and long-term psychiatric settings and in some rehabilitation facilities. Some other areas, including medical-surgical units, are using interdisciplinary plans as well. Staffs from the various professions involved with the patient participate in the planning. The focus is on patient problems rather than nursing diagnosis, making language used in the plan common to all professions. Interdisciplinary plans have the following characteristics:

- The patient's medical diagnosis is used rather than a nursing diagnosis.
- Observations (data collected) are shared among all providers involved in the care of the patient.
- A problem list is developed and prioritized. The patient's statement of problem(s) that led to admission is considered. **Priorities are those that are most important for life-saving/physiologic needs.**
- A shared care plan is created, identifying specific and shared responsibilities for all professions represented.
- The plan is discussed with the patient (when possible) or patient advocate. After all, these are patient goals based on patient needs. The team plays a supportive role during implementation of the plan.

Documentation of progress is usually on a common form or computer record to allow easy access for all team members involved with the patient (Figure 2–6). *The complete two-page form is located on your **Companion CD-ROM**.*

Evaluation is ongoing, with periodic in-depth evaluation by the team on agreed-upon dates. Interventions are deleted, added, and changed as needed (Bauer and Hill, 2000).

Plan of Care Select appropriate focus. Add interventions as needed. Check the appropriate box(es) in the Evaluation column to indicate daily progress.							
				Evaluation M: Goal met C: Continue plan NM: Goal not met R: Goal/plan revised/reviewed w/pt			
Date Started/ Initials	Focus	Expected Patient Outcome	Interventions	Date	Date	Date	Date
	Safety	Risk of injury will be minimized	• Bed in low position • Side rails up PRN • Call bell within reach • Clean, organized, well-lit environment • Use non-slip footwear • ADL needs evaluated/offered q 2 hr	☐ M ☐ C ☐ NM ☐ R Initial	☐ M ☐ C ☐ NM ☐ R Initial	☐ M ☐ C ☐ NM ☐ R Initial	☐ M ☐ C ☐ NM ☐ R Initial
	Fall risk	Risk of falls will be minimized	• Follow Safety Interventions above • Pt on Fall Prevention Protocol • Instruct patient to call for ADL assist • Bed alarm on • Posey alarm PRN • Sitter utilized • Frequent reorientation	☐ M ☐ C ☐ NM ☐ R Initial	☐ M ☐ C ☐ NM ☐ R Initial	☐ M ☐ C ☐ NM ☐ R Initial	☐ M ☐ C ☐ NM ☐ R Initial
	Psycho-social	Patient will have feelings validated and addressed	• Allow patient to express feelings • Provide emotional support • Address questions and concerns • Make appropriate referrals	☐ M ☐ C ☐ NM ☐ R Initial	☐ M ☐ C ☐ NM ☐ R Initial	☐ M ☐ C ☐ NM ☐ R Initial	☐ M ☐ C ☐ NM ☐ R Initial
	Prevention of infection and/or cross-infection	Patient will not develop an infection and/or will not transmit infection to others	• All patients placed in standard precautions	☐ M ☐ C ☐ NM ☐ R Initial	☐ M ☐ C ☐ NM ☐ R Initial	☐ M ☐ C ☐ NM ☐ R Initial	☐ M ☐ C ☐ NM ☐ R Initial
	Skin integrity	Patient will be assessed for skin risk per Braden Scale and remain free of skin breakdown	• Assess skin integrity • Assist with turning/positioning q 2 hr and prn • Encourage mobility • Attention to bony prominences • Elevate heel prn • Reduce friction • Skin care • Prompt attention to incontinence	☐ M ☐ C ☐ NM ☐ R Initial	☐ M ☐ C ☐ NM ☐ R Initial	☐ M ☐ C ☐ NM ☐ R Initial	☐ M ☐ C ☐ NM ☐ R Initial
	Skin integrity impaired	Patient's wounds will be assessed; an optimal environment for healing will be provided	• Skin integrity interventions as above • Waffle mattress prn • Chart wound assessment • Dressing changes prn • Wound care referral	☐ M ☐ C ☐ NM ☐ R Initial	☐ M ☐ C ☐ NM ☐ R Initial	☐ M ☐ C ☐ NM ☐ R Initial	☐ M ☐ C ☐ NM ☐ R Initial
	Nutritional status	Nutritional status will be maintained and/or improved	• Nutritional screen • Monitor I/O and nutritional intake • Assist with meals and fluids • Provide snacks and/or supplement	☐ M ☐ C ☐ NM ☐ R Initial	☐ M ☐ C ☐ NM ☐ R Initial	☐ M ☐ C ☐ NM ☐ R Initial	☐ M ☐ C ☐ NM ☐ R Initial

FIGURE 2–6 Interdisciplinary plan of care. This is the first page of a two-page form; the entire form is included on your Companion CD-ROM. (Courtesy of Sheridan Memorial Hospital, Sheridan, WY.)

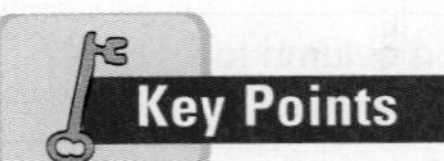

Key Points

- Critical thinking generates new ideas and judges the worth of those ideas. It prompts the LPN/LVN to ask what could be improved and what measures would prevent further harm to the patient.
- Clinical judgment is a proactive reasoning skill that uses critical thinking in the clinical area to determine the appropriate actions to take in a specific situation.
- Factors that influence critical thinking and decisions about nursing care include our culture, personal motivation, attitude, and verbal and written communication ability.
- The National Council of State Boards of Nursing (NCSBN) has defined the role of the LPN/LVN in regard to nursing process.
- Know the nurse practice act (NPA) of the state in which you are employed: The LPN/LVN scope of practice is specific for that state.
- Nursing process is an advanced problem-solving method used to collect and analyze data in order to plan, implement, and evaluate patient care in an orderly way. It is the language of nursing and provides a method for nurses to communicate with regard to patient care.
- Goals and expected outcomes are patient centered and describe what the patient will do to achieve the desired results. They are realistic, time referenced, and measurable.
- The American Nurses Association has developed medical-surgical nursing standards for RNs. Standards for LPN/LVNs are based on the NCSBN definitions for nursing process.
- Receiving a patient assignment and preparing a preliminary care plan prior to beginning patient care is considered safe practice for student nurses as the NPAs in all states mandate student nurses to function equivalent to an LPN/LVN.
- Techniques of physical examination used by the LPN/LVN include inspection and observation, olfaction, palpation, and auscultation. Percussion is a more advanced method generally used by nurse practitioners and physicians.
- Nurses need to be aware of common laboratory and other diagnostic tests and their relationship to common illness. Laboratory and diagnostic tests also provide a way to track the effectiveness of treatments and the emergence of side effects of select medications.
- Interdisciplinary (collaborative) care plans are used in health facilities where it is more convenient for all professions involved to have their plan of care interwoven with others. Medical diagnosis, rather than nursing diagnosis, is used because of the number of disciplines involved.
- Staff communication takes place both verbally and by charting. Urgent communication is done verbally as soon as possible.

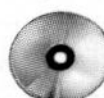

Go to your **Companion CD-ROM** for an Audio Glossary, animations, video clips, and bonus review questions.

evolve Be sure to visit the companion Evolve site at http://evolve.elsevier.com/deWit for interactive NCLEX-PN Exam Style Review Questions, WebLinks, and additional online resources.

NCLEX-PN EXAM STYLE REVIEW QUESTIONS

Choose the best answer(s) for the following questions.

1. Which of the following is considered critical in assessing sleep disturbance of the patient? *(Select all that apply.)*

1. Family history of sleep disorders
2. Rituals associated with sleep
3. Feelings of restfulness
4. Diet choices
5. Urinary habits

2. When caring for an older woman who developed a 5-cm pressure ulcer on her sacrum because of being immobilized and incontinent, an appropriate patient goal would be:

1. the patient will be able to ambulate to the bathroom with minimal assist.
2. the nurse will be able to provide turning and repositioning schedules for the nursing staff.
3. the patient will verbalize importance of using pressure-reducing devices and frequent repositioning schedules during her stay.
4. the family will be able to provide protein-rich foods during the hospital stay.

3. While dangling at bedside, the patient suddenly complains of "faintness and dizziness." An immediate nursing action would be to:

1. check vital signs.
2. assist the patient back to lying position.
3. open airway.
4. provide reassurance.

4. A nursing diagnosis addressing risk for falls would be most appropriate for which types of patients?

1. An immobilized patient
2. A patient with rashes
3. A patient on antihypertensive medications
4. A patient having elective surgery

5. Which of the following patient statements indicates the need for further teaching regarding the use of an incentive spirometer?

1. "I will inhale as deeply as possible each time I use the spirometer."
2. "I need to slightly tilt the incentive spirometer to reduce effort."

3. "To monitor progress, I will record the top volume achieved."
4. "I may have trouble sealing the mouthpiece due to mouth dryness."

6. Which of the following nursing actions should be implemented when addressing the needs of an elderly patient with the nursing diagnosis: Imbalanced nutrition: less than body requirements related to poor dental condition? *(Select all that apply.)*
   1. Encourage fluid intake if not contraindicated by the medical condition.
   2. Inspect oral cavity and condition of mucous membranes and teeth.
   3. Assist with swallowing.
   4. Initiate speech therapy and dietitian consult.
   5. Monitor daily caloric intake and weekly weights.

7. The nurse is collecting data from an older adult with a history of fractures. Appropriate nursing assessment would include which of the following?
   1. Determining orientation to person, place, and time
   2. Auscultating for heart sounds
   3. Checking pulse oximetry
   4. Testing passive and active range of motion

8. While obtaining the health history, the nurse finds that the patient is on long-term anticoagulant therapy. Which of the following patient statements would strongly correlate with excessive anticoagulant therapy? *(Select all that apply.)*
   1. "I have noticed some blood streaking in my bowel movements."
   2. "I have been embarrassed by frequent, uncontrollable gassiness."
   3. "My urine has been cloudy with occasional clots."
   4. "I readily bruise whenever I bump into anything."
   5. "Flossing my teeth has been painful and bloody."

9. Which of the following would be considered an appropriate goal for a patient with risk for sleep pattern disturbance related to aging-related sleep stage shifts?
   1. The patient will be able to perform personal hygiene with minimal assistance.
   2. The patient will be able to identify measures to promote sleep at the end of the shift.
   3. The patient will be able to schedule periods of activity and rest after adequate instruction.
   4. The patient will be able to consider taking multiple naps during the day.

10. As a treatment for hypertension, the nurse reinforces instruction regarding the prescribed medication, hydrochlorothiazide. Which of the following patient statements indicates a need for further education regarding the prescribed medication?
    1. "I will need to decrease my intake of coffee and tea."
    2. "Relaxation techniques render the medication more effective."
    3. "I look forward to sunbathing."
    4. "Quitting smoking is one of my priorities."

CRITICAL THINKING ACTIVITIES 

Read each clinical scenario and discuss the questions with your classmates.

Scenario A

Critical thinking points are listed on pages 16 and 17. Consider each point.

1. Write one real example from personal experience: patients or family or friends.
2. Is there more you could have done, or could it have been done in a better way?
3. Did your action prevent harm to the person?

Scenario B

Mr. Nash, age 68 years, describes himself as a tough guy. He is currently on bed rest with his right leg in traction. He had fallen from his house roof while adjusting the TV antenna. His main theme is, "What do I have to do to get outta here?" Although grumpy, Mr. Nash's positive attribute is that he will do whatever will get him released from the hospital. "I've gotta smell my own air and I want my nightly martini!"

1. Write an example of a patient-centered expected outcome for Mr. Nash that is realistic, time referenced, and measurable.

Scenario C

Since no jobs are currently available in the medical-surgical unit at the local hospital, you have applied at the mental health facility. You know that your medical-surgical observation skills will be useful in data collection (assessment). The mental health facility uses interdisciplinary care plans.

1. Explain the major differences in a nursing process–focused plan and an interdisciplinary plan.
2. What is the responsibility of each medical specialist involved in developing and carrying out the interdisciplinary plan?

CHAPTER 3

Fluids, Electrolytes, Acid-Base Balance, and Intravenous Therapy

evolve http://evolve.elsevier.com/deWit

Objectives

Upon completing this chapter you should be able to:

Theory

1. Recall the various functions fluid performs in the body.
2. Identify the body's mechanisms for fluid regulation.
3. Review three ways in which body fluids are continually being distributed among the fluid compartments.
4. Distinguish the signs and symptoms of various electrolyte imbalances.
5. Discuss why the elderly have more problems with fluid and electrolyte imbalances.
6. Recognize the disorders that cause specific fluid and electrolyte imbalances.
7. Compare the major causes of acid-base imbalances.
8. State correct interventions to correct an acid-base imbalance.
9. Discuss the steps in managing an intravenous infusion.
10. Describe the measures used to prevent the complications of intravenous therapy.
11. Identify intravenous fluids that are isotonic.
12. Discuss the principles of intravenous therapy.

Clinical Practice

1. Assess patients for signs of dehydration.
2. Correctly assess for and identify edema and signs of overhydration.
3. Apply knowledge of normal laboratory values in order to recognize electrolyte imbalances.
4. Carry out interventions to correct an electrolyte imbalance.
5. Determine if a patient has an acid-base imbalance.
6. Carry out measures to prevent the complications of intravenous therapy.
7. Compare interventions for the care of a patient receiving total parenteral nutrition with one undergoing intravenous therapy.

Key Terms

Be sure to check out the bonus material on the Companion CD-ROM, including selected audio pronunciations.

acidosis (ă-sĭ-DŌ-sĭs, p. 53)
active transport (ĂK-tĭv, p. 38)
aldosterone (p. 35)
alkalosis (ăl-kă-LŌ-sĭs, p. 49)
anions (ĂN-ī-ŏnz, p. 45)
antidiuretic hormone (ăn-tĭ-dī-ū-RĔT-ĭk HŎR-mōn, p. 35)
ascites (ă-SĪ-tēz, p. 45)
atrial natriuretic peptide (p. 35)
carpopedal spasm (spăzm, p. 49)
cations (KĂT-ī-ŏnz, p. 45)
dehydration (dē-hī-DRĀ-shŭn, p. 38)
diffusion (dĭ-FŪ-zhŭn, p. 36)
edema (ĕ-DĒ-mă, p. 43)
electrolytes (ĕ-LĔK-trō-līts, p. 45)
extracellular (ĕks-tră-SĔL-ū-lăr, p. 35)
filtration (fĭl-TRĀ-shŭn, p. 37)
hydrostatic pressure (hī-drō-STĂ-tĭk PRĔ-shŭr, p. 37)
hypercalcemia (hī-pĕr-kăl-SĒ-mē-a, p. 49)
hyperchloremia (hī-pĕr-klŏr-Ē-mē-ă, p. 50)
hyperkalemia (hī-pĕr-kă-LĒ-mē-ă, p. 48)
hypermagnesemia (hī-pĕr-măg-nĕ-SĒ-mē-ă, p. 50)
hypernatremia (hī-pĕr-nă-TRĒ-mē-ă, p. 46)
hyperphosphatemia (hī-pĕr-fŏs-fă-TĒ-mē-a, p. 50)
hypertonic (hī-pĕr-TŎN-ĭk, p. 37)
hyperventilation (hī-pĕr-vĕn-tĭ-LĀ-shŭn, p. 54)
hypervolemia (hī-pĕr-vō-LĒ-mē-a, p. 43)
hypocalcemia (hī-pō-kăl-SĒ-mē-ă, p. 49)
hypochloremia (hī-pō-klŏr-Ē-mē-a, p. 50)
hypodermoclysis (hī-pō-dĕrm-ŏk-LĪ-sĭs, p. 61)
hypokalemia (hī-pō-kă-LĒ-mē-ă, p. 48)
hypomagnesemia (hi-pō-măg-nĕ-SĒ-mē-ă, p. 50)
hyponatremia (hī-pō-nă-TRĒ-mē-a, p. 45)
hypophosphatemia (hī-pō-fŏs-faw-TĒ-mē-a, p. 50)
hypotonic (hī-pō-TŎN-ĭk, p. 37)
hypovolemia (hī-pō-vō-LĒ-mē-ă, p. 43)
hypoxemia (hī-pŏk-SĒ-mē-ă, p. 54)
insensible (p. 38)
interstitial (ĭn-tĕr-STĬSH-ăl, p. 36)
intracellular (ĭn-tră-SĔL-ū-lăr, p. 35)
intravascular (ĭn-tră-VĂS-cū-lăr, p. 36)
ions (ī-ŏnz, p. 36)
isotonic (ī-sō-TŎN-ĭk, p. 37)
ketoacidosis (kē-tō-ă-sĭ-DŌ-sĭs, p. 53)
osmolality (ŏs-mō-LĂ-lĭ-tē, p. 45)
osmosis (ŏz-MŌ-sĭs, p. 36)
stridor (STRĪ-dŏr, p. 54)
tetany (TĔT-ă-nē, p. 49)
transcellular (trăns-SĔ-lū-lăr, p. 36)
turgor (TŬR-gŏr, p. 38)

Over half of the body's weight is water. The actual percentage depends on a number of factors, including age, sex, nutritional status, and state of wellness. Throughout life there is a gradual decline in the amount of body water. An infant's body is approximately 77% water, and an elderly person's body is about 45% water. **The elderly and the very young are more likely to experience severe consequences with even minor changes in their fluid balance.** The greater the amount of fat in the body, the less the percentage of body water as fatty tissue does not contain as much water as other tissues. People of all ages and states of wellness need a normal fluid balance to survive.

Keeping body fluids within a normal range is necessary because the life processes of each cell of every organ take place within fluid. The nutrients needed for life, reproduction, and the normal functioning of a cell must be dissolved or suspended in water. Moreover, the largest part of each cell is fluid. For all of the cell's life processes to take place, there must be a continuous exchange of water, glucose, oxygen, nutrients, electrolytes, and waste products.

The four main functions of water in the body are to:

- Be a vehicle for the transportation of substances to and from the cells.
- Aid heat regulation by providing perspiration, which evaporates.
- Assist in maintenance of hydrogen (H^+) balance in the body.
- Serve as a medium for the enzymatic action of digestion.

Table 3–1 shows sources of water and avenues of water loss.

DISTRIBUTION AND REGULATION OF BODY FLUIDS

Body fluids are continually in motion, moving in and out of the blood and lymph vessels, the spaces surrounding the cells, and the bodies of the cells themselves. Fluid within the cell is considered to be in one compartment **(intracellular)** and fluid outside the cell in another **(extracellular)** (Figure 3–1). The extracellular fluid (ECF) is further divided into three types (Box 3–1). Fluid excretion is mainly achieved via the kidney.

Control of fluid balance is managed by:

- The **thirst mechanism**. The osmoreceptors in the hypothalamus sense the internal environment and promote the intake of fluid when needed.
- **Antidiuretic hormone** (ADH), which controls how much fluid leaves the body in the urine. ADH causes reabsorption of water from the kidney tubules.
- **Aldosterone** and **atrial natriuretic peptide** (ANP), which regulate the reabsorption of water and sodium ions from the kidney tubules.
- Baroreceptors in the carotid sinus and aortic arch, which detect pressure changes indicating an increase or decrease in blood volume. They stimulate the sympathetic or parasympathetic nervous system to return the pressure to normal.

When body fluid is more concentrated, receptors in the hypothalamus stimulate nerve impulses that travel to the brain and are interpreted as thirst, motivating the person to drink. When the blood volume decreases, ADH is secreted by the posterior pituitary. This signals the renal tubules to reabsorb more water, thereby increasing blood volume, and urine output decreases. Pain, nausea, and stress can cause the release of ADH by the pituitary also. When the ECF volume is low, or when sodium concentration is elevated, aldosterone is released by the adrenal cortex. This hormone causes reabsorption of sodium from the renal tubules. The release of aldosterone is regulated by the renin-angiotensin-aldosterone system. Renin is released when there is decreased blood flow to the kidney. Baroreceptors in the atrium of the heart detect fluid overload and atrial natriuretic peptide is released from the myocardium. Atrial naturetic peptide helps protect the body from fluid overload.

To be normally distributed within the body, water and the substances suspended or dissolved in it must move from compartment to compartment. As blood flows through the capillaries, fluid and solutes can move into the interstitial spaces, where substances such as nutrients and wastes can be exchanged by the cells of the body. The movement of fluids, electrolytes, nutrients, and waste products back and forth across the cell membranes is accomplished by several processes (Figure 3–2).

Table 3–1 ***Sources of Water and Avenues of Water Loss***

SOURCES	24 HOURS (AVERAGE INTAKE)	AVENUE OF LOSS	AMOUNT OF LOSS (AVERAGE OUTPUT)
Oral fluids	1500 mL	Urine	1500 mL
Food	800 mL	Perspiration	400 mL
Metabolism	200 mL	Feces	200 mL
		Expired air	400 mL
Total	2500 mL		2500 mL

Adapted from deWit, S.C. (2005) *Fundamental Concepts and Skills for Nursing* (2nd ed.). Philadelphia: Elsevier Saunders, p. 420.

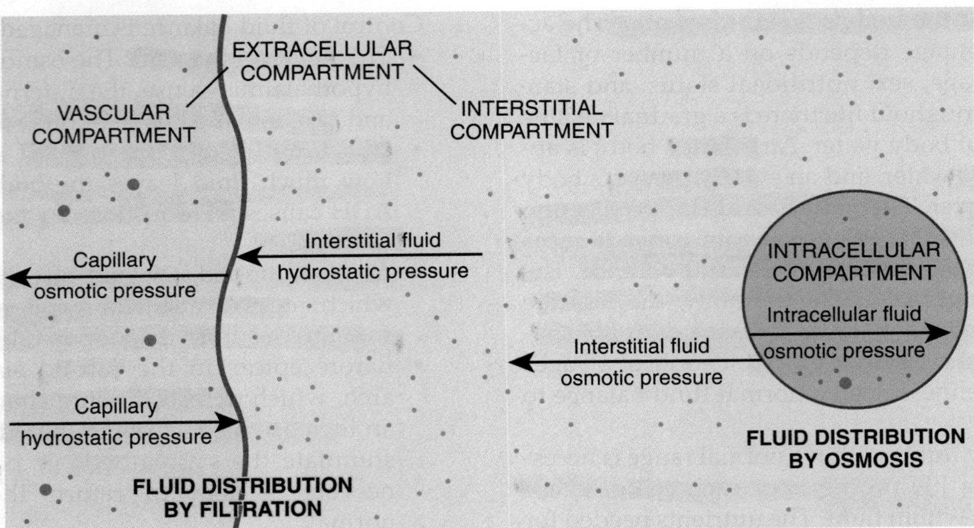

FIGURE **3–1** Factors that influence body fluid distribution.

Box 3–1 ***Body Fluid Distribution***

Extracellular Fluid: Approximately ⅓ of total body water. Transports water, nutrients, oxygen, waste, etc., to and from the cells. Regulated by renal, metabolic, and neurologic factors. **High in sodium (Na^+) content.**

- **Intravascular Fluid:** Fluid within the blood vessels. Consists of plasma and fluid within blood cells. Contains large amounts of protein and electrolytes.
- **Interstitial Fluid:** Fluid in the spaces surrounding the cells. High in sodium (Na^+) content.
- **Transcellular Fluid:** Includes aqueous humor, saliva, cerebrospinal, pleural, peritoneal, synovial, and pericardial fluids, gastrointestinal secretions, and fluid in urinary system and lymphatics.

Intracellular Fluid: About ⅔ of total body fluid. Fluid contained within the cell walls. Most cell walls are permeable to water. **High in potassium (K^+) content.**

From deWit, S.C. (2005). *Fundamental Concepts and Skills for Nursing* (2nd ed.). Philadelphia: Elsevier Saunders, p. 421.

MOVEMENT OF FLUID AND ELECTROLYTES

Passive Transport

Diffusion. **Diffusion** is the process by which substances move back and forth across the membrane until they are evenly distributed throughout the available space. As the plasma moves along a capillary, large amounts of fluid filter through pores in the capillary walls. The fluid moves into and out of the capillaries. It does this by filtering through the permeable capillary wall or cell membrane walls. There is a capillary hydrostatic pressure inside the capillary that pushes against the wall of the capillary. When the solution on one side of the membrane is more concentrated than the solution on the other side of the membrane, the particles in the more concentrated solution travel through the membrane to the less concentrated side in an attempt to equalize the concentration of the two solutions. Diffusion is possible because of *kinetic* motion, which diffuses the molecules in the intracellular fluid (ICF) and the plasma. These molecules literally bounce off one another, mixing and stirring the body fluids.

Diffusion, then, is a spontaneous mixing and moving that allows the exchange of molecules, **ions** (electrically charged particles), cellular nutrients, wastes, and other substances dissolved or suspended in body water. The direction of water flow depends on which side of the membrane has the greatest concentration of solutes. Substances will move from a high to a low concentration until the concentration on both sides of the membrane is equal. This is called movement down a concentration gradient. **Glucose, oxygen, carbon dioxide, water, and other small ions and molecules move by diffusion.** It is a process of equalization.

Diffusion may occur by movement along an electrical gradient as well. The attraction between particles of opposite charge and the repellent action between particles of like charge comprise an electrical gradient. Many intracellular proteins have a negative charge that tends to attract the positively charged sodium and potassium ions from the ECF.

Osmosis. **Osmosis** refers to the movement of pure solvent (liquid) across a membrane. **Water diffuses by osmosis.** When there are differences in concentration of fluids in the various compartments, osmotic pressure will move water from the area of lesser concentration of solutes to the area of greater concentration until the solutions in the compartments are of equal concentration. The process takes place via a semipermeable membrane—a membrane that allows some substances to pass through but prevents the passage of other substances. **Fluid moves between**

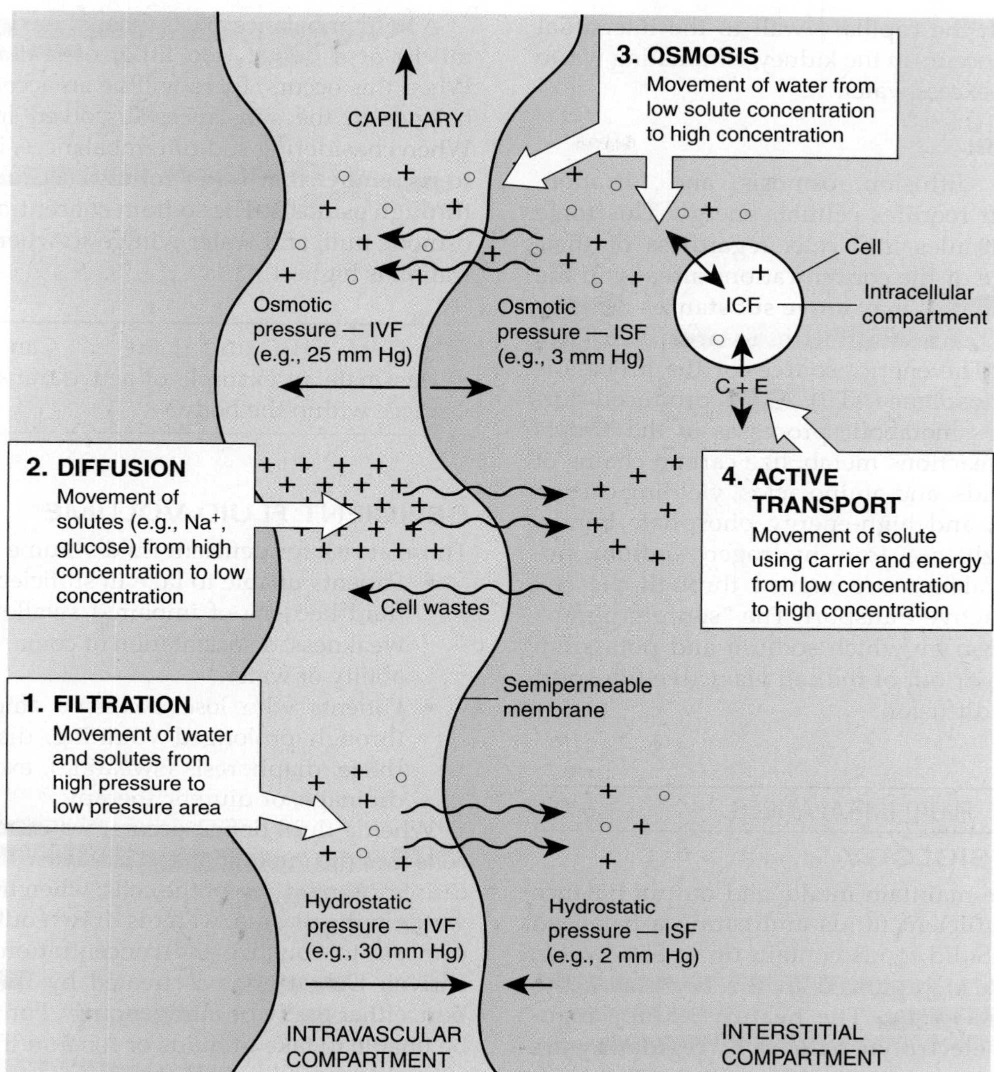

FIGURE 3–2 Movement of water and electrolytes between compartments.

the interstitial and intracellular and the interstitial and intravascular compartments by osmosis. When living cells are surrounded by a solution that has the same concentration of particles, the water concentration of the ICF and the ECF will be equal. Such a solution is termed **isotonic** (of equal solute concentration). If cells are surrounded by a solution that has a greater concentration of solute than the cells, the water in the cells will move to the more concentrated solution and the cells will dehydrate and shrink. The solution is **hypertonic** (of greater concentration) in relation to the cells. If the cells are surrounded by a solution that has less solute than the cells, the solution is **hypotonic** (of less concentration) in relation to the cells. The particles within the cells exert an osmotic pressure drawing water inward through the semipermeable membrane. The cells swell from the extra fluid (overhydrate). These concepts are important to the administration of intravenous fluids. Solutions are classified as isotonic, hypertonic, or hypotonic according to their concentration of electrolytes and other solutes. **Osmotic pressure is what holds fluid in the vascular space.** (See the discussion of intravenous fluid therapy later in the chapter for further discussion.)

> *Think Critically About . . .* Can you describe to a classmate the difference between osmosis and diffusion?

Filtration. **Filtration** is the movement of water and suspended substances outward through a semipermeable membrane. The pumping action of the heart creates **hydrostatic pressure** (pressure exerted by fluid) within the capillaries. Hydrostatic pressure causes fluid to press outward on the vessel. That force promotes filtration, forcing movement of water and electrolytes through the capillary wall to the interstitial fluid. Filtration occurs in the kidney, eliminating waste substances and excess water.

Active Transport

In contrast to diffusion, osmosis, and filtration, active transport requires cellular energy. This force can move molecules into cells regardless of their electrical charge or the concentrations already in the cell. Active transport **may move substances from an area of lower concentration to an area of higher concentration.** The energy source for the process is adenosine triphosphate (ATP). ATP is produced during the complex metabolic processes in the body's cells. Enzyme reactions metabolize carbon chains of sugars, fatty acids, and amino acids, yielding carbon dioxide, water, and high-energy phosphate bonds. Amino acids, glucose, iron, hydrogen, sodium, potassium, and calcium are moved through the cell membrane by active transport. The "sodium pump" is the mechanism by which sodium and potassium are moved into or out of the cell via active transport rather than by diffusion.

FLUID IMBALANCES

PATHOPHYSIOLOGY

Healthy people maintain intake and output balance by drinking sufficient fluids and eating a balanced diet each day. Solid foods contain up to 85% water, and water is also produced in the body as a by-product of metabolism. **The healthy kidney regulates fluid and electrolyte balance by regulating the volume and composition of extracellular fluid.** Illness affects fluid balance in many ways. The patient may be unable to ingest food or liquids, there may be a problem with absorption from the intestinal tract, or there may be a kidney impairment that affects excretion or reabsorption of water and electrolytes. Any disease that affects circulation (e.g., congestive heart failure) will ultimately affect the distribution and composition of body fluids. Extra fluid is lost when the metabolic rate is accelerated, such as occurs in fever, thyroid crisis, burns, severe trauma, and states of extreme stress. Perspiration can account for a fluid loss of a maximum of 2 L/hr in an adult. For every degree of fever on the Celsius scale, an **insensible** (not aware of) water loss of 10% may occur. Perspiration and water lost in respiration are insensible losses. When the weather is hot and dry, water loss from the body is greater. Patients on mechanical ventilators, those with rapid respirations, and those with severe diarrhea or excessive amounts of fistula drainage also lose greater quantities of water. **In fact, any seriously ill patient is at risk for a fluid and electrolyte imbalance.**

A fluid imbalance exists when there is an excess (too much) or a deficit (too little) of water in the body. When this occurs, there will be an accompanying imbalance in the substances dissolved in body water. When considering sodium imbalances, **it is important to remember that water follows sodium in the body through osmosis.** The sodium concentration causes an osmotic pull, and water will go to where that concentration is highest.

? *Think Critically About . . .* Can you give a classmate an example of active transport taking place within the body?

DEFICIENT FLUID VOLUME

Those at risk for deficient fluid volume are:

- Patients unable to take in sufficient quantities of fluid because of impaired swallowing, extreme weakness, disorientation or coma, or the unavailability of water.
- Patients who lose excessive amounts of fluid through prolonged vomiting, diarrhea, hemorrhage, diaphoresis (sweating), excessive wound drainage, or diuretic therapy.

When a fluid deficit occurs, water moves from the cells into the interstitial and intravascular spaces. This causes **dehydration** of the cells; when there is too little water in the plasma, water is drawn out of the cells by osmosis to equalize the concentration and the cells shrivel. Dehydration is treated by fluid administration, either orally or intravenously. For those who will be unable to take in fluids or food on their own for an extended period, a feeding tube must be placed or total parenteral nutrition (TPN) started. Care of the patient with a feeding tube and patients undergoing TPN is discussed in Chapter 29.

Signs and symptoms of dehydration are presented in Box 3–2. **Turgor** (degree of elasticity) is checked by gently pinching up the skin over the abdomen, forearm, sternum, forehead, or thigh (Figure 3–3). In a person with normal fluid balance, the skin when pinched will immediately fall back to normal when released. If a fluid deficit is present, the skin may remain elevated or tented for several seconds after the pinch. This test measures skin elasticity as well and is not a valid indicator of fluid status in the elderly. In the infant, dehydration is evident by sunken fontanels.

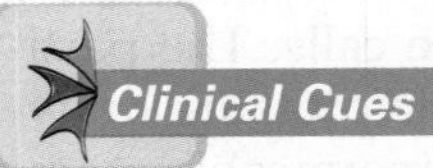

The most accurate measure of fluid gain or loss for any age group is weight change. A weight gain or loss of 2.2 lb (1 kg) in 24 hours indicates a gain or loss of 1 L of fluid.

Box 3–2 Signs and Symptoms of Fluid Deficit and Fluid Excess

SIGNS AND SYMPTOMS OF DEHYDRATION (FLUID VOLUME DEFICIT)

- Thirst
- Poor skin turgor
- Weight loss
- Weakness
- Complaints of dizziness
- Postural hypotension
- Decreased urine production
- Dark, concentrated urine
- Dry, cracked lips and tongue
- Dry mucous membranes
- Sunken, soft eyeballs
- Thick saliva
- Dry, scaly skin
- Flat neck veins when lying down
- Rapid, weak, thready pulse
- Elevated temperature ≥100.6° F (38.1° C)
- Increased hematocrit
- High urine specific gravity with low volume

SIGNS AND SYMPTOMS OF OVERHYDRATION (FLUID EXCESS)

- Weight gain
- Slow, bounding pulse
- Elevated blood pressure
- Firm subcutaneous tissues
- Possibly edema
- Possibly crackles in lungs upon auscultation
- Lethargy, possible seizures
- Possibly visible neck veins when lying down
- Decreased serum sodium
- Decreased hematocrit from hemodilution
- Low urine specific gravity with high volume

From deWit, S.C. (2005). *Fundamental Concepts and Skills for Nursing,* (2nd ed.). Philadelphia: Elsevier Saunders, p. 424.

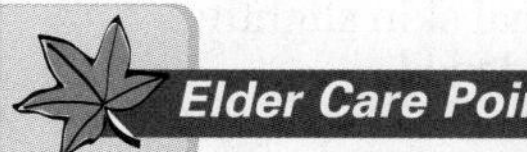

Elder Care Points

Fluid volume deficit is a very common problem in the elderly. There is an age-related decline in total body water and a decrease in thirst sensation and taste that causes elderly people to become dehydrated more easily. If urinary incontinence problems are present, the person becomes reluctant to drink extra fluids. Thirst is a late sign of dehydration in the elderly.

Many elderly people rely on laxatives and enemas to clear the bowel. This practice can cause fluid volume deficit along with sodium and potassium loss. **Fluid volume deficit contributes to constipation and orthostatic hypotension with related dizziness and falls and makes the person more susceptible to infection.**

A furrowed, dry tongue that is not the result of drug therapy indicates a fluid deficit. If the person has fever, this adds to the fluid loss. Because of the fluid and accompanying electrolyte losses, the person may become confused. Offering the patient small amounts of liquid frequently, if it can be kept down, or an electrolyte solution such as Gatorade, helps prevent additional problems.

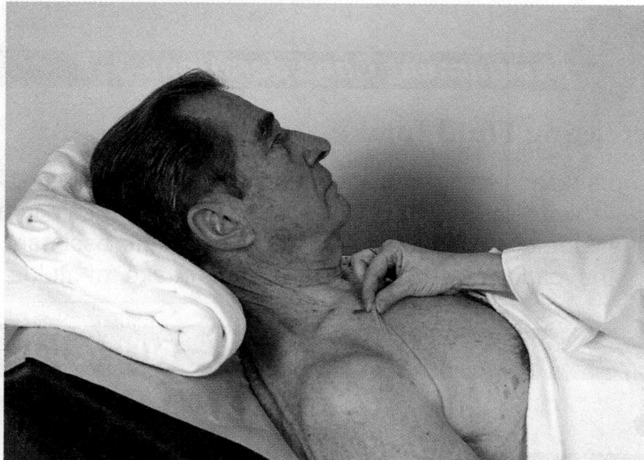

FIGURE **3–3** Testing tissue turgor.

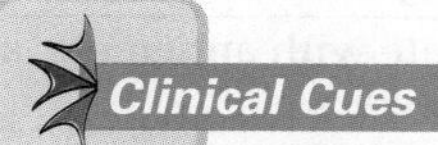

Clinical Cues

Measure the blood pressure and pulse in the lying, sitting, and standing positions. If there is a systolic blood pressure drop of 20 mm Hg accompanied by a pulse rate increase of 10 bpm at 1 minute after the position change, fluid volume deficit is suggested. This is termed *orthostatic* or *postural hypotension.*

Nursing Management

Provide an adequate intake for those who are unable to do this for themselves. Include the patient's preferences for liquids on the plan of care (Assignment Considerations 3–1). Water alone will not restore a fluid deficit. The patient also needs electrolytes and therefore should receive fruit juices, bouillon, and any other nutritious liquid he is able to tolerate (Nursing Care Plan 3–1).

A frequent cause of excessive loss of fluids is abnormally rapid excretion of intestinal fluids, such as that which occurs in vomiting and diarrhea.

Think Critically About . . . Why does increasing fluid intake for the patient with fever lower the body temperature?

NAUSEA AND VOMITING

Nausea is a feeling of discomfort or an unpleasant sensation vaguely felt in the epigastrium and abdomen. It is a symptom of illness. Nausea is often accompanied by a tendency to vomit. Nausea is experienced when nerve endings in the stomach and other

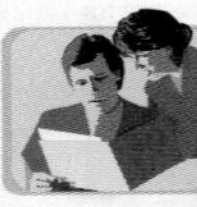

Assignment Considerations 3–1

Increasing Fluid Intake

If a nursing assistant or unlicensed assistive personnel (UAP) is available to assist, *assign* the task of increasing fluid intake to that person. Work out a timed plan for the assistant to help the patient with regular, periodic intake of fluids by mouth. Ask that the patient drink 4 oz of fluid every hour. Advise of any safety precautions regarding difficulty swallowing, need for assistance to the bathroom, etc. Review the need for accurate intake and output recording.

NURSING CARE PLAN 3–1

Care of the Patient with Deficient Fluid Volume

SCENARIO A 78-year-old female is admitted to the hospital after 3 days of vomiting and diarrhea. She is confused, disoriented, dehydrated, and very weak.

PROBLEM/NURSING DIAGNOSIS *Vomiting and diarrhea*/Deficient fluid volume related to fluid loss and inability to take in sufficient fluids.

Supporting assessment data *Subjective:* Hx of vomiting and diarrhea for 3 days; unable to keep anything in stomach. Had eaten food at a church picnic on a hot day. *Objective:* Furrowed tongue, tenting of skin on sternum, thick saliva, and dry mucous membranes. 3-lb weight loss from normal. Urine sp. gr. 1.030; scant urine; temp. 101.4° F (40° C).

Goals/Expected Outcomes	Nursing Interventions	Selected Rationale	Evaluation
Diarrhea and vomiting will stop within 24 hours	Medicate with antiemetic as ordered.	Antiemetic should stop vomiting.	IM injection of Vistaril given Z-track as ordered. Has not vomited in last hour.
Patient will be able to eat normally before discharge	Initiate IV therapy as ordered.	IV therapy will replenish fluids and electrolytes in the body.	IV fluids infusing. Site clean, dry without redness.
Fluid balance will be reestablished within 72 hours	Monitor IV site and fluid every hour.		
	Initiate I&O recording. Keep patient clean and dry.	I&O record provides data to determine degree of fluid imbalance.	Two liquid stools. Continue plan.
	Reduce odors in room to decrease nausea.	Odors contribute to nausea.	No odor in room.
	Provide assistance to bathroom as needed.	Assistance helps prevent falls in weak patients.	Assistance provided.
	Protect perianal skin with ointment as ordered.	A barrier cream or ointment will protect the perianal skin from excoriation from diarrhea.	Perianal skin slightly reddened.
	When vomiting stops, administer medication for diarrhea as ordered.	Medication will slow or stop the diarrhea.	Took Lomotil tab with a sip of Gatorade.
	When able to take PO fluids, offer sips of electrolyte solution, and progress to a clear liquid diet.	Small sips of fluid are easier to keep in the stomach. Electrolyte solution replenishes low electrolytes.	Taking sips of Gatorade.
	Offer mouth care after vomiting and at least q 2 hr.	Mouth care promotes comfort and reduces nausea.	Mouth care provided.
	Monitor mucous membrane status and skin turgor. Weigh daily.	Provides data about rehydration status.	Mucous membranes more moist.
	Monitor electrolyte values.	Provides data about electrolyte imbalances.	Laboratory results not back yet. Continue plan.

? CRITICAL THINKING QUESTIONS

1. What would be other concerns that should be addressed in her care plan?
2. What do you think is the cause of her confusion and disorientation?

Key: *Hx*, history; *I&O*, intake and output; *IM*, intramuscular; *IV*, intravenous; *PO*, oral; *sp. gr.*, specific gravity.

Complementary & Alternative Therapies 3–1

Preventing Nausea

Sea bands (acupressure wrist bands) are very helpful to many people who suffer from nausea and vomiting. They are available at most drugstores. Ginger tea is another alternative therapy that has proven helpful.

parts of the body are irritated. The irritated nerve endings in the stomach send messages to the part of the brain that controls the vomiting reflex, but nerve cells in other parts of the body can trigger the same response. An example is intense pain in any part of the body. Pain can trigger the nausea-vomiting mechanism. Nausea and vomiting are an automatic response of the involuntary autonomic nervous system to unpleasant stimuli (Complementary & Alternative Therapies 3–1).

Nausea and vomiting may occur from gastrointestinal irritation from foods, viruses, radiation irritation of the mucosa, and some drugs and other chemicals. Certain types of anesthetics, and pregnancy may trigger nausea. **Prolonged vomiting can lead to sodium and potassium deficits and metabolic alkalosis due to the loss of electrolytes and stomach acids.**

The patient may complain of nausea or feeling "sick to my stomach," queasiness, abdominal pain, epigastric discomfort or burning, and vomiting. The patient also exhibits pallor; mild diaphoresis; cold, clammy skin; excessive salivation; and attempts to remain quiet and motionless. **If vomiting occurs, the vomitus should be observed for odor, color, contents (e.g., undigested food), and amount.** Noting and recording vomiting patterns, conditions that trigger vomiting, and quality of nausea as described by the patient can be helpful in planning treatment.

Medical treatment consists of administering one of the antiemetic drugs (Table 3–2). Antihistamines, sedatives and hypnotics, anticholinergics, phenothiazines, and other drugs are used to control nausea and vomiting. The patient is given nothing by mouth (kept NPO) until vomiting has stopped and then is started back on clear liquids, progressing slowly to a regular diet. Sips of carbonated drinks are usually tolerated well at first.

Have the patient lie down and turn his head to one side or sit and lower the head between the legs so that vomitus is not aspirated into the respiratory tract. An emesis basin is held close to the side of the face. A cool, damp washcloth can be used to wipe the patient's face and the back of the neck. Breathing through the mouth may also help. Provide mouth care after the episode. Sucking on ice chips helps reduce nausea in some patients.

A quiet, cool, odor-free environment helps. If nausea and vomiting persist, observe for dehydration.

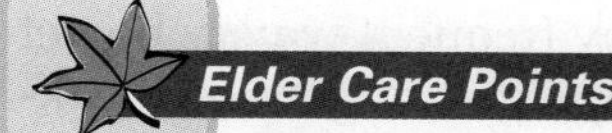

Elder Care Points

Older patients must be rehydrated cautiously. Patients who have cardiac problems are at risk for fluid overload from intravenous (IV) infusions. If a liter of fluid infuses too fast, it can cause the patient to go into congestive heart failure. **If an IV infusion falls behind, it should not be regulated to make up for lost time by infusing fluid at a rate faster than ordered.**

DIARRHEA

Diarrhea is defined as the rapid movement of fecal matter through the intestine. It results in the loss of water and electrolytes and poor absorption of nutrients. These substances, especially the potassium needed by the body to prevent alkalosis, are lost in large amounts.

Major diarrhea is related to local irritation of the intestinal mucosa, especially that caused by infectious agents, such as *Salmonella, Clostridium difficile,* and *Escherichia coli;* gastrointestinal flu; and chemicals. Chronic and prolonged diarrhea is typical of such disorders as ulcerative colitis, irritable bowel syndrome, allergies, lactose intolerance, and nontropical sprue. Obstruction to the flow of intestinal contents, such as from a tumor or a fecal impaction, also can produce diarrhea.

In acute diarrhea, the stomach and intestines are rested by limiting the intake of foods. Once oral feedings are allowed, clear liquids are begun and progressed to bland liquids and then solid foods with increased calories and high-protein, high-carbohydrate content. Rehydrating solutions containing glucose and electrolytes are given first. Iced fluids, carbonated drinks, whole milk, roughage, raw fruits, and highly seasoned foods are to be avoided.

Medications prescribed for diarrhea depend on the cause of the disorder and the length of time the condition has been present (see Table 3–2). Mild cases usually respond well to kaolin and bismuth preparations, (e.g., Kaopectate), which coat the intestinal tract and make the stools more firm. Antispasmodic drugs such as belladonna or paregoric reduce the number of stools by decreasing the peristaltic rate and relaxing the intestinal musculature. Bismuth subsalicylate (Pepto-Bismol) is helpful in that it soothes the mucosa and binds water. It is the recommended treatment for "traveler's diarrhea" and can also be used for prevention of this type of diarrhea. Codeine, diphenoxylate (Lomotil), or loperamide (Imodium) are useful to decrease the peristaltic action that causes the frequency of stools. Diarrhea caused by infections may be treated with drugs that are specific for the causative organism. If metabolic acidosis occurs, it is treated by giving buffer solutions. Depending on the organism responsible, drugs may not be given initially to allow the toxins to be eliminated from the body.

Diarrhea is characterized by frequent watery bowel movements, abdominal cramping, and general weakness. The watery stools often contain mucus and are blood-streaked. It is the consistency rather than the number of stools per day that is the hallmark of diarrhea. In some cases the number can be as high as 15 to 20 liquid stools. If the condition is chronic, the patient can suffer from dehydration, malnutrition, and anemia. Bowel sounds are likely to be loud gurgling and tinkling sounds that come in waves and are hyperac-

Table 3–2 ***Drugs Commonly Prescribed for Vomiting and Diarrhea***

CLASSIFICATION	ACTION	NURSING IMPLICATIONS	PATIENT TEACHING
ANTIEMETICS			
Hydroxyzine (Vistaril, Atarax) Promethazine (Phenergan)	Antihistamine-antiemetic used to stop nausea and vomiting. Depresses the central nervous system (CNS).	Give by Z-track injection. Never give IV or Subcut. Monitor vital signs. Check compatibility before mixing with other drugs. Monitor for dizziness and hypotension. Observe for urinary retention.	Avoid concurrent alcohol ingestion or other CNS depressants. Avoid activities that require alertness. Rise slowly to prevent dizziness. Avoid prolonged sunlight.
Prochlorperazine maleate (Compazine)	Blocks chemoreceptor trigger zone, which in turn acts on vomiting center. Stops nausea and vomiting.	Monitor vital signs and for respiratory depression, especially in elderly. Check compatibilities before mixing with other drugs. Watch for seizures, muscle stiffness, and untoward reactions.	Avoid hazardous activities; avoid alcohol and other CNS depressants. Advise urine may be pink to reddish brown. Avoid the sun or wear sunscreen and protective clothing. Report bleeding, rash, bruising, blurred vision, or clay-colored stools.
Ondansetron (Zofran)	Blocks serotonin peripherally, centrally, and in the small intestine.	Monitor for extrapyramidal signs (shuffling gait, tremors, grimacing, rigidity). Observe for rash or bronchospasm.	Report diarrhea, constipation, rash, change in respiration or discomfort at IV insertion site.
ANTIDIARRHEALS			
Diphenoxylate atropine (Lomotil)	Slows intestinal motility. Slows or stops diarrhea.	Assess bowel pattern and monitor for constipation. Discontinue if not effective after 2 days of treatment.	Do not use alcohol or CNS depressants. Do not exceed the prescribed dosage. May be habit forming. Avoid hazardous activities.
Loperamide HCl (Imodium)	Works on intestinal muscles to decrease peristalsis; reduces volume and increases stool bulk. Slows or stops diarrhea.	Monitor stools and for electrolyte imbalances. Monitor for dehydration. Discontinue if not effective after 2 days of treatment.	Drowsiness may occur; do not operate machinery. Do not take other over-the-counter preparations.
Kaolin-pectin (Kaopectate)	Decreases gastric motility and water content of stool; acts as adsorbent and demulcent.	Monitor bowel pattern. Monitor for dehydration and electrolyte imbalances.	Do not exceed recommended dosage. Shake suspension well. Take other medications 2 hr before or after administration.
Bismuth salts (Pepto-Bismol)	Inhibits prostaglandin synthesis responsible for gastrointestinal hypermotility; stimulates absorption of fluid and electrolytes. Prevents or stops diarrhea.	Monitor bowel pattern. Do not give to children under age 3.	Shake liquid before using. The tongue may darken and stools may turn black. Do not take other salicylates along with this medication. Stop taking if diarrhea has not stopped in 2 days.
Camphorated opium tincture (paregoric)	Opiate that acts to decrease intestinal motility.	Controlled substance. Addictive with long-term use. Monitor bowel function. May cause nausea and vomiting.	Do not exceed prescribed dosage. Causes CNS depression; do not operate machinery.

tive. Note and record the number of stools during the shift and the characteristics of each stool and any associated pain.

> ***Think Critically About . . .*** What type of fluid and electrolyte imbalances is the patient who has food poisoning and is suffering from both vomiting and diarrhea likely to have?

Nursing Management

Nursing measures are aimed at providing physical and mental rest, preventing unnecessary loss of water and nutrients, protecting the rectal mucosa, and eventually replacing fluids. Diarrhea can be associated with nervous tension and anxiety. The patient often is embarrassed by his condition and inconvenienced by frequent trips to the bathroom or the need to request a bedpan. This emotional stress only serves to aggravate the condition and make it worse. Help break the vicious cycle by maintaining a calm and dignified manner, accepting and understanding the patient's behavior, and providing privacy and a restful environment for him.

> ***Think Critically About . . .*** How would you assess the patient with diarrhea for signs of dehydration?

EXCESS FLUID VOLUME

An excessive amount of *body water* usually occurs first in the extracellular compartment because the water enters and leaves the body from this compartment. Normally, an excess of water alone is not a problem. Healthy people do not ordinarily drink too much water. When people become ill, they may receive more water than they excrete. This can happen if they receive intravenous fluid too quickly, are given tap water enemas, or are persuaded to drink more fluids than they can eliminate. If these events happen, the patient will suffer a fluid volume excess. When any of these conditions is present, the patient is likely to suffer from *water intoxication*.

Impaired elimination, such as occurs in renal failure, is an important cause of fluid volume excess. Signs and symptoms of overhydration are presented in Box 3–2. An objective measure of water excess and circulatory overload is the hematocrit. This is a measurement of the volume percentage of red blood cells in whole blood. When fluid volume excess occurs, **hypervolemia** (excessive blood volume) may also occur. Hypervolemia causes an elevation of blood pressure. **Normal hematocrit values range from 35 to 54 mL of red blood cells per 100 mL of whole blood, depending on age and sex. If there is an excess of water, the proportion of red blood cells to milliliters of blood will be lower, and the hematocrit will be below the normal values because of dilution by the water.**

Urine concentration provides another clue to the fluid status. Urine concentration is commonly measured by the specific gravity. The concentration of urine is compared with the specific gravity of distilled water, which is 1.000. Urine contains urea, electrolytes, and other substances, so its specific gravity will exceed 1.000. Urine specific gravity ranges between 1.003 and 1.030. The average range is 1.010 to 1.025.

EDEMA

A more common fluid imbalance is associated with the retention of water, sodium, and chloride, which produces edema. **Edema** is defined as an accumulation of freely moving interstitial fluid, that is, fluid in the spaces surrounding the cells. Look for puffy eyelids and swollen hands. Edema also can occur in body cavities, as in the peritoneal cavity (ascites) and the cranial cavity. The accumulation of body fluids can affect almost all of the tissue spaces, in which case it is known as *generalized edema*, or it can affect a limited area, in which case it is called *localized edema. Generalized edema* occurs when the body's mechanisms for eliminating excess sodium fail. It becomes life threatening when it overloads the circulatory system, as in congestive heart failure, and when it involves the lungs, as in pulmonary edema.

There are four general causes of edema:

- An increase in capillary hydrostatic pressure
- A loss of plasma proteins
- Obstruction of lymphatic circulation
- An increase in capillary permeability

An increase in hydrostatic pressure is what causes pulmonary edema. A loss of plasma proteins decreases osmotic pressure in the vascular system. A tumor or infection can damage a lymph node, or lymph nodes may be removed during cancer surgery. Lymphedema of the arm may be a consequence of mastectomy surgery in which lymph nodes are removed.

When an inflammatory response or infection occurs, histamine and other chemical mediators are released from the cells involved in the tissue injury. These chemicals cause increased capillary permeability, and more fluid moves into the interstitial spaces. Proteins leak into the interstitial spaces also, decreasing the osmotic pressure in the capillaries. This causes the extra fluid to be held in the interstitial spaces rather than moving back into the capillaries. When fluid shifts from the vascular space (from the plasma) to the interstitial space, dehydration and **hypovolemia** (too little blood volume) can occur. This occurrence often is termed *third spacing*. It may occur with extensive trauma, burns, peritonitis, intestinal obstruction, nephrosis, sepsis, and cirrhosis of the liver where there is an increase in capillary hydrostatic pressure or increased capillary membrane permeability.

? *Think Critically About* . . . What characteristics would you expect to find in a urine specimen from a patient who is dehydrated? How would it differ from a urine specimen from a patient who has a fluid volume excess?

Localized edema often occurs with inflammation. Localized edema usually is nonpitting, does not come and go, and is characterized by tight, shiny skin that is stretched over a hard and red area. Causes of localized edema include trauma, allergies, burns, obstruction of lymph flow, and liver failure.

Dependent edema is noted in the feet, ankles, and lower legs or in the sacral region of patients confined to bed or chair. It is an effect of gravity and therefore can be somewhat relieved by elevating the affected part 18 inches or above heart level when possible and repositioning the patient frequently. Pitting edema is common in patients with dependent edema. The name is derived from the fact that a pit or depression can be created by pressing a fingertip against the swollen tissue. **To check for pitting edema, the thumb is pressed into the patient's skin at a bony prominence, such as the tibia or malleolus, and held for 5 seconds.** If the depression, or "pit," remains for a while after the pressure is released, the patient has pitting edema. Assessing the severity and progress of pitting edema in the feet and ankles (pedal edema) can be done more accurately by rating the findings and comparing assessments from one shift to another (Figure 3–4).

The scale rating system that is often used for pedal edema is as follows:

- 1+, Mild pitting—slight indentation with no swelling of the leg
- 2+, Moderate pitting—indentation subsides quickly
- 3+, Deep pitting—indentation remains for a short time, leg looks swollen
- 4+, Very deep pitting—indentation lasts a long time and leg is very swollen

Treatment

Treatment of a fluid imbalance involves correcting the underlying cause and assisting the body to rebalance fluid content. For conditions of edema, fluid may be restricted or diuretic drugs may be administered to facilitate excretion of the excess fluid. A diuretic is a drug that prompts the kidneys to increase the excretion of fluid. Bed rest may be ordered to facilitate fluid excretion.

The patient is placed on a low-sodium diet. Elastic stockings or sequential compression devices are ordered for foot and leg edema. Intake and output recording is requested.

? *Think Critically About* . . . Can you describe the assessments you would make to determine whether your 68-year-old patient is experiencing edema?

Home Care

For the patient with a fluid deficit, it is important to teach the patient and family to measure intake and output and to keep a log of the amounts. The patient should be encouraged to take small amounts of liquid every hour while awake. If the patient has been vomiting, it is better to let carbonated beverages go flat before drinking them to decrease stomach distention.

If an elderly patient has been vomiting considerably for several hours or has had constant diarrhea and no intake of fluid, a visit to the emergency department is in order so that intravenous fluids can be given to prevent serious dehydration.

When the patient has a fluid excess, he should be weighed daily and a chart kept. The patient and family should be taught how to assess edema and to record findings. If edema is worsening or weight is rising, the physician should be notified.

ELECTROLYTES

Solutes are electrolytes and other substances that are dissolved in the body fluids. Some molecules, when placed in solution, undergo a separation of their atoms

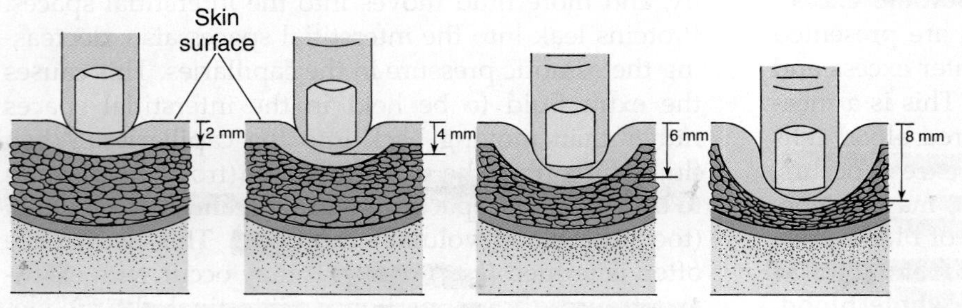

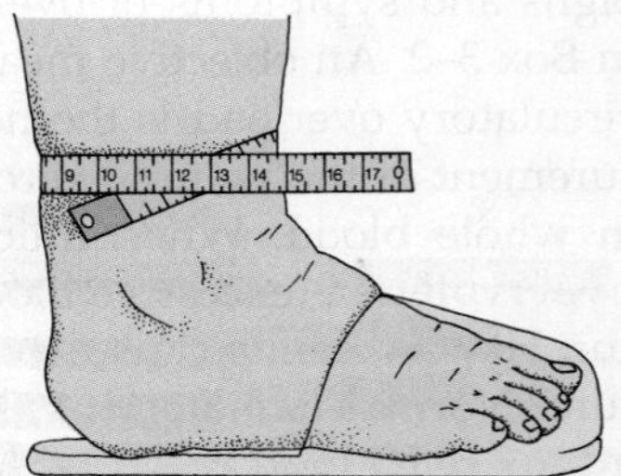

FIGURE **3–4** Measuring pedal edema.

into electrically charged ions. These molecules are called **electrolytes** because their atomic particles are capable of conducting an electric current. The molecules of electrolytes break up into atomic particles that are either negatively charged **(anions)** or positively charged **(cations)**. For example, when sodium chloride (table salt) is dissolved in body water, its molecules separate into sodium ions, which are positively charged (Na^+), and chloride ions, which are negatively charged (Cl^-).

Because some electrolytes are positively charged and some are negatively charged, they are chemically active. **This chemical activity allows for the creation of an electrical impulse across the cell membrane, making possible the transmission of nerve impulses, contraction of muscles, and excretion of hormones and other substances from glandular cells.** It is thus apparent that electrolytes are essential to the normal functioning of the body.

OSMOLALITY

Nonelectrolyte solutes include protein, urea, glucose, creatinine, and bilirubin. Along with the electrolytes, these solutes contribute to the **osmolality** (concentration of the solution determined by the number of solutes in it) of the body fluid. Osmolality controls water movement and the body fluid distribution in the intracellular and extracellular compartments. The osmolality of the ICF is maintained primarily by potassium. The osmolality of the extracellular fluid is controlled by sodium. Normal osmolality of body fluids is 280 to 294 milliosmoles per kilogram (mOsm/kg).

? *Think Critically About* . . . Why should you watch for signs of fluid imbalance in any patient who has a serious infection or who has suffered considerable physical trauma?

ELECTROLYTE IMBALANCES

Electrolytes have many functions in the body. In order to determine if there is an electrolyte imbalance, you must know the normal range for each electrolyte (Table 3–3). Many disorders can cause a shift in electrolytes and an imbalance with too much or too little of an electrolyte circulating in the bloodstream or inside the cells of the body.

SODIUM IMBALANCES

Hyponatremia

Hyponatremia, a deficit of sodium in the blood **(Na^+ less than 135 mEq/L)**, is the most common electrolyte imbalance patients experience. This can occur from either a sodium loss or an excess of water. Decreased secretion of aldosterone results in sodium loss. Congestive heart failure, liver disease with **ascites** (abnor-

Table 3–3 *The Major Electrolytes: Normal Ranges and Functions*

ELECTROLYTE	NORMAL RANGE	SI UNITS	FUNCTION
Sodium (Na^+)	135–145 mEq/L	135–145 mmol/L	**Major cation of the extracellular fluid.** Major role in regulation of water balance. Regulates extracellular fluid volume through somatic pressure. **Water follows sodium concentration in the body.** Essential to the transmission of nerve impulses and helps maintain neuromuscular irritability. Important in controlling contractility of the heart. Helps maintain acid-base balance. Aids in maintenance of electroneutrality.
Potassium (K^+)	3.5–5.0 mEq/L	3.5–5.0 mmol/L	**Major intracellular cation.** Important to nerve transmission and muscle contraction. Helps maintain normal heart rhythm. Helps maintain plasma acid-base balance.
Calcium (Ca^{2+})	8.4–10.6 mg/dL	2.10–2.65 mmol/L	Involved in formation of bone and teeth. Necessary for blood coagulation. Essential for normal nerve and muscle activity.
Magnesium (Mg^{2+})	1.3–2.5 mg/dL	0.65–1.05 mmol/L	Necessary for building bones and teeth. Necessary for nerve transmission and is involved in muscle contraction. Plays an important role in many metabolic reactions, where it acts as a cofactor to cellular enzymes.
Phosphate (PO_4^-)	2.5–4.5 mg/dL	1.0–1.5 mmol/L	Necessary for formation of adenosine triphosphate (ATP). Cofactor in carbohydrate, protein, and lipid metabolism. Activates B-complex vitamins.
Chloride (Cl^-)	96–106 mEq/L	96–106 mmol/L	Helps maintain acid-base balance. Important to formation of hydrochloric acid for secretion to the stomach. Aids in maintaining plasma electroneutrality.
Bicarbonate (HCO_3^-)	22–26 mEq/L	23–29 mmol/L	A buffer that neutralizes excess acids in the body. Helps regulate acid-base balance.

From deWit, S.C. (2005). *Fundamental Concepts and Skills for Nursing* (2nd ed.). Philadelphia: Elsevier Saunders, p. 420.

mal accumulation of fluid within the peritoneal cavity), and chronic renal failure result in excessive water retention without concurrent sodium retention. This results in a hypervolemia combined with hyponatremia. The decrease in osmotic pressure in the extracellular compartment may cause a fluid shift into the cells. A decrease in blood pressure may occur. The average intake of sodium is 4 to 5 g/day. If there is a problem with water balance, sodium may be restricted in the diet. The consequence of hyponatremia is impaired nerve conduction. Signs and symptoms of hyponatremia are:

- Fatigue, lethargy, muscle weakness
- Muscle cramps
- Abdominal cramps and nausea and vomiting
- Headache, confusion, seizures
- Decreased blood pressure

Table 3–4 presents the risk factors for hyponatremia along with the nursing interventions to correct the condition.

Hypernatremia

Hypernatremia occurs when the sodium level rises above 145 mEq/L. Water loss from fever, respiratory

Table 3–4 ***Electrolyte Imbalances and Nursing Interventions***

SERUM VALUE	SIGNS AND SYMPTOMS	CAUSES/RISK FACTORS	NURSING INTERVENTIONS
SODIUM—NORMAL RANGE: 135–145 mEq/L			
Hyponatremia <135 mEq/L	Central nervous system and neuromuscular changes resulting from failure of swollen cells to transmit electrical impulses. Mental confusion, altered level of consciousness, anxiety, coma, anorexia, nausea, vomiting, muscle cramps, seizures, decreased sensation.	Inadequate sodium intake, as in patients on low-sodium diets. Excessive intake or retention of water (kidney failure and heart failure). Loss of bile, which is rich in sodium as a result of fistulas, drainage, gastrointestinal surgery, nausea and vomiting, and suction. Loss of sodium through burn wounds. Administration of intravenous (IV) fluids that do not contain electrolytes.	Restrict water intake as ordered for patients with congestive heart failure, kidney failure, and inadequate antidiuretic hormone production. Liberalize diet of patient on low-sodium diet. Closely monitor patient receiving IV solutions to correct hyponatremia. Replace water loss with fluids containing sodium.
Hypernatremia >145 mEq/L	Dry mucous membranes, loss of skin turgor, intense thirst, flushed skin, oliguria, and possibly elevated temperature; weakness, lethargy, irritability, twitching, seizures, coma, intracranial bleeding.	High-sodium diet, inadequate water intake as in comatose, mentally confused, or debilitated patient. Excessive sweating, diarrhea, failure of kidney to reabsorb water from urine. Administration of high-protein, hyperosmotic tube feedings and osmotic diuretics.	Encourage increased fluid intake; measure intake and output (I&O); give water between tube feedings; restrict sodium intake; monitor temperature.
POTASSIUM—NORMAL RANGE: 3.5–5.0 mEq/L			
Hypokalemia <3.5 mEq/L	Abdominal pain, gaseous distention of intestines; cardiac dysrhythmias, muscle weakness, decreased reflexes, paralysis, paralytic ileus, urinary retention, lethargy, confusion, electrocardiogram (ECG) changes, increased urinary pH.	Inadequate intake of potassium-rich foods. Loss of potassium in urine when kidneys do not reabsorb the mineral. Loss of potassium from intestinal tract as a result of diarrhea or vomiting, drainage from fistulas, overuse of gastric suction. Improper use of diuretics.	Instruct patients (especially those taking diuretics) about foods high in potassium content; encourage intake. Observe closely for signs of digitalis toxicity in patients taking this drug. Teach patients to watch for signs of hypokalemia. Administer potassium chloride supplement as ordered. Monitor I&O and cardiac rhythm.
Hyperkalemia >5.0 mEq/L	Muscle weakness, hypotension, paresthesias, paralysis, cardiac dysrhythmias, ECG changes.	Conditions that alter kidney function or decrease kidney's ability to excrete potassium. Intestinal obstruction that prevents elimination or potassium in the feces. Addison's disease, digitalis toxicity, uncontrolled diabetes mellitus, insulin deficit, crushing injuries and burns.	Decrease intake of foods high in potassium. Increase fluid intake to enhance urinary excretion of potassium; provide adequate carbohydrate intake to prevent use of body proteins for energy. Carefully administer proper dose of insulin to diabetic patients. Instruct patient in proper use of salt substitutes containing potassium.

From deWit, S.C. (2005). *Fundamental Concepts and Skills for Nursing* (2nd ed.). Philadelphia: Elsevier Saunders, pp. 425–427.

Table 3–4 *Electrolyte Imbalances and Nursing Interventions—cont'd*

SERUM VALUE	SIGNS AND SYMPTOMS	CAUSES/RISK FACTORS	NURSING INTERVENTIONS
CALCIUM—NORMAL RANGE: 8.4–10.6 mg/dL			
Hypocalcemia <8.4 mg/dL	Paresthesias, seizures, muscle spasms, tetany, hand spasm, positive Chvostek's sign, positive Trousseau's sign, cardiac dysrhythmia, wheezing, dyspnea, difficulty swallowing, colic, cardiac failure.	Inadequate dietary intake of calcium and vitamin D. Impaired absorption of calcium from intestinal tract, as in diarrhea, sprue, overuse of laxatives and enemas containing phosphates (phosphorus tends to be more readily absorbed from the intestinal tract than calcium and suppresses calcium retention in the body). The parathyroid regulates calcium and phosphorus levels. Hyposecretion of parathyroid hormone can result in hypocalcemia.	Encourage adults to consume sufficient calcium from cheese, broccoli, shrimp, and other dietary sources. Have 10% calcium gluconate solution at bedside of patient having thyroidectomy in case of surgical damage to the parathyroid glands. Give all oral medicines containing calcium 30 min before meals to facilitate absorption.
Hypercalcemia >10.6 mg/dL	Anorexia, abdominal pain, constipation, polyuria, confusion; renal calculi, pathologic fractures, cardiac arrest.	Excess intake of calcium, as in patient taking antacids indiscriminately. Excess intake of vitamin D. Conditions that cause movement of calcium out of bones and into extracellular fluid (e.g., bone tumor, multiple fractures). Tumors of the lung, stomach, and kidney, and multiple myeloma. Immobility and osteoporosis.	Administer diuretics as prescribed to increase urinary output and calcium excretion. Monitor I&O; encourage high fluid intake (3000–4000 mL/day).
MAGNESIUM—NORMAL RANGE: 1.3–2.1 mEq/L			
Hypomagnesemia <1.3 mEq/L	Insomnia, hyperactive reflexes, leg and foot cramps, twitching, tremors; seizures, cardiac dysrhythmias, positive Chvostek's sign, positive Trousseau's sign, vertigo, hypocalcemia and hypokalemia.	Chronic malnutrition, chronic diarrhea. Bowel resection with ileostomy or colostomy; chronic alcoholism; prolonged gastric suction; acute pancreatitis; biliary or intestinal fistula; osmotic diuretic therapy; diabetic ketoacidosis.	Diet counseling to help patients at risk increase their level of magnesium (e.g., milk and cereals). Monitor intravenous infusions of magnesium closely. Monitor I&O.
Hypermagnesemia >2.1 mEq/L	Hypotension, sweating and flushing, nausea and vomiting; muscle weakness, paralysis, respiratory depression; cardiac dysrhythmias.	Overuse of antacids and cathartics containing magnesium; aspiration of sea water, as in near-drowning. Chronic kidney failure.	Teach patients to avoid abuse of laxatives and antacids; instruct patients with renal problems to avoid over-the-counter drugs that contain magnesium. Encourage fluid intake to increase urinary excretion of magnesium if not contraindicated. Monitor I&O. Administer diuretics as ordered.
PHOSPHATE—NORMAL RANGE: 3.0–4.5 mg/dL			
Hypophosphatemia	Confusion, seizures, numbness, weakness, possible coma. Chronic state may cause rickets and osteomalacia.	Vitamin D deficiency or hyperparathyroidism; use of aluminum-containing antacids.	Assess for vitamin D deficiency, hyperparathyroidism, or overuse of aluminum-containing antacids.
Hyperphosphatemia	Anorexia, nausea, vomiting.	Renal insufficiency.	Assess for restlessness, confusion, chest pain, and cyanosis. Monitor respirations. Check all electrolyte levels.

Nutritional Therapies 3–1

Foods High in Sodium

The patient experiencing a fluid volume excess or needing to decrease sodium intake should avoid the following foods:

- Buttermilk
- Canned meats or fish
- Canned soups
- Canned vegetables
- Casserole and pasta mixes
- Catsup
- Cheese (all kinds)
- Delicatessen meats
- Dried fruits
- Dried soup mixes
- Foods containing monosodium glutamate (MSG)
- Frozen vegetables with sauces
- Gravy mixes
- Ham
- Hot dogs
- Olives
- Pickles
- Prepared mustard
- Preserved meats
- Processed foods
- Salted nuts
- Salted popcorn
- Salted snack foods
- Softened water
- Soy sauce
- Tomato or vegetable juice

Note: Check all packaged food labels for sodium content.

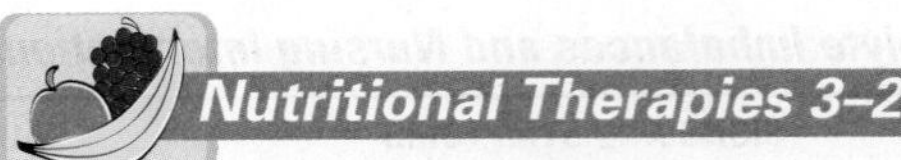

Nutritional Therapies 3–2

Common Foods High in Potassium

Counsel the patient taking a potassium-wasting diuretic to add some of these foods to the daily diet:

- Avocado
- Baked potato
- Banana
- Cantaloupe
- Codfish
- Meats
- Milk
- Oranges
- Raisins
- Salmon
- Tuna

Safety Alert 3–1

Potassium Precaution

Urine output must be at least 30 mL/hr before intravenous potassium is administered. **Intravenous potassium must always be diluted before administration and is never given as a "push" (rapid undiluted) injection.**

infection, or watery diarrhea is the usual cause. Excessive administration of sodium bicarbonate for the treatment of **acidosis** (excess of acid or depletion of alkaline substances in the blood and body tissues) is another cause. Decreased water intake may occur in immobile, confused, or dependent patients as well as in those who have sustained damage to the thirst center in the hypothalamus. The body tries to correct the situation by conserving water through reabsorption in the renal tubules. **Hypernatremia causes an osmotic shift of fluid from the cells to the interstitial spaces, causing a cellular dehydration and interruption of normal cell processes.** Signs and symptoms of hypernatremia are:

- Decreased urine output if compensatory ADH is being secreted
- Increased thirst with dry mucous membranes
- Weakness and agitation
- Good tissue turgor and firm subcutaneous tissues

Sodium intake is restricted for the patient with hypernatremia (Nutritional Therapies 3–1).

POTASSIUM IMBALANCES

Hypokalemia

Hypokalemia occurs when the potassium level falls below 3.5 mEq/L. Hypokalemia may occur due to poor diet, illness causing a shift of potassium from ECF to ICF, or increased potassium loss. Vomiting, diarrhea, gastrointestinal suction, excessive sweating, and diuretic therapy may deplete potassium levels. Hypokalemia can cause serious problems. Signs and symptoms of hypokalemia are:

- Cardiac dysrhythmias and electrocardiographic (ECG) changes
- Muscle weakness and decreased reflexes
- Urinary retention and increased urine pH
- Abdominal pain, gaseous distention, and paralytic ileus
- Lethargy and confusion

It is important to teach patients taking diuretics that are not potassium-sparing to increase the potassium in the diet, take potassium supplements as prescribed, and watch for signs of hypokalemia (Nutritional Therapies 3–2). **Severe hypokalemia (K^+ less than 2.5 mEq/L) may cause cardiac arrest.** Extra potassium must be given to help correct the imbalance (Safety Alert 3–1).

Hyperkalemia

Hyperkalemia occurs when the serum potassium level rises above 5.0 mEq/L. The mechanical disruption of cell membranes causes a shift of potassium from the ICF to the ECF. This happens when extensive tissue damage occurs in burns or crush injuries. Hyperkalemia occurs in renal failure, overuse of potassium-sparing diuretics, digitalis toxicity, overuse of potassium-containing salt substitutes, uncontrolled diabetes mellitus, and a variety of other illnesses. **Hyperkalemia can cause life-threatening cardiac dysrhythmia.** Signs and symptoms of hyperkalemia include:

- ECG changes and cardiac dysrhythmias that may progress to cardiac arrest
- Paresthesias and muscle weakness progressing to paralysis
- Fatigue and nausea

Oral intake of potassium is curtailed and fluids are administered to increase the excretion of potassium (see Table 3–4). A potassium exchange resin (Kayexalate) may be given when hyperkalemia is caused by renal failure.

CALCIUM IMBALANCES

Hypocalcemia

Hypocalcemia occurs when the calcium level drops below 8.4 mg/dL. This can occur from nutritional deficiency of either calcium or vitamin D. Hypocalcemia occurs in disorders in which there is a shift of calcium into the bone. Metastatic cancer invading bone is one such cause. Removal or injury of the parathyroid glands during thyroidectomy causes parathyroid hormone deficiency and consequent hypocalcemia. Excessive infusion of bicarbonate solution, **alkalosis** (excess of alkaline or decrease of acid substances in the blood and body fluids), blood transfusions, and hypoparathyroidism may cause hypocalcemia. Malabsorption and deficient serum albumin may cause hypocalcemia. Hypocalcemia in renal failure results from retention of phosphate ions, which causes a loss of calcium ions. In addition, vitamin D is not activated, causing the loss of absorption of calcium from the intestinal tract.

Calcium ions are needed for a variety of metabolic processes and enzyme reactions. It is essential for blood clotting. Calcium deficit upsets the stability of nerve membranes, causing abnormalities in nerve conduction and muscle contractions.

Signs and symptoms of hypocalcemia are:

- Paresthesias and abdominal cramps
- Spontaneous stimulation of skeletal muscle with muscle twitching, **carpopedal spasm** (a characteristic contraction of the fingers, also called Trousseau's sign) and hyperactive reflexes
- Chvostek's sign, a spasm of the lip or face when the spot on the face in front of the ear is tapped
- **Tetany** (skeletal muscle spasm where the muscles are in sustained contraction and causing spasm)
- Weak heart contractions with weak pulse, decreased blood pressure, and dysrhythmias
- Laryngospasm if deficit is severe

Check for Trousseau's sign and Chvostek's sign when calcium or magnesium deficit is a possibility. A blood pressure cuff is placed on the arm and inflated above systolic pressure for 3 minutes to test for Trousseau's sign. If a spasm of the hand occurs, the reaction is positive (Figure 3–5). Chvostek's sign is assessed by tapping the facial nerve about an inch in front of the earlobe. A unilateral twitching of the face is a positive response (Figure 3–6). Deep tendon reflexes are tested by tapping a partially stretched muscle tendon with a percussion hammer. The extent of the reflex is scored from 0 to 4+, with 0 representing no response, 2+ a normal response, and 4+ a hyperactive response.

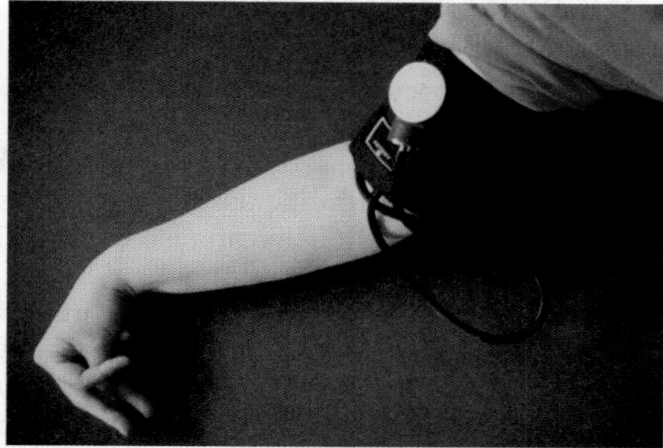

FIGURE 3–5 Palmar flexion (carpopedal spasm) indicating positive Trousseau's sign in hypocalcemia.

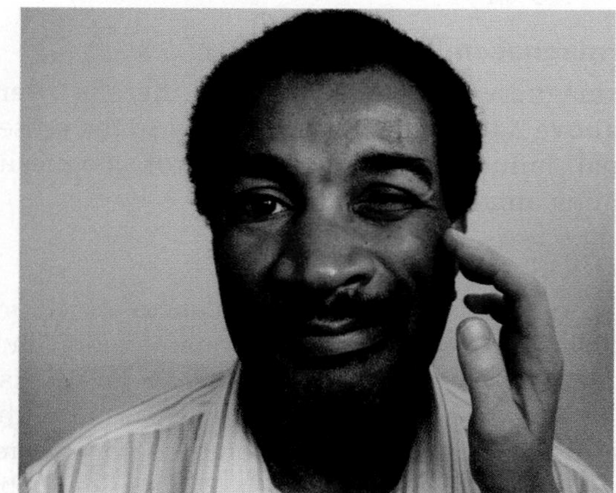

FIGURE 3–6 Facial muscle response indicating positive Chvostek's sign in hypocalcemia.

Hypercalcemia

Hypercalcemia occurs when the serum calcium level is above 10.6 mg/dL. This can occur during periods of lengthy immobilization when calcium is mobilized from the bone or when an excess of calcium or vitamin D is taken into the body. Most cases are related to hyperparathyroidism or malignancy in which there is metastasis with bone resorption. Such malignancies include multiple myeloma and lung or renal cancers.

Signs and symptoms of hypercalcemia are:

- Muscle weakness, lethargy, stupor, and personality change
- Anorexia and nausea
- Polyuria because ADH action is interfered with in the kidney and more fluid is excreted
- Dysrhythmias; cardiac arrest can occur if the calcium level is severely high
- Decreased bone density and spontaneous fractures if increased parathyroid hormone is the cause of the hypercalcemia

Diuretics are administered to increase calcium excretion. A high fluid intake is encouraged (see Table 3–4).

MAGNESIUM IMBALANCES

Hypomagnesemia

Hypomagnesemia occurs when the serum level drops below 1.3 mEq/L. This may result from malabsorption, malnutrition, or increased loss from renal tubular dysfunction or thiazide diuretic use. Extensive gastric suction, diarrhea, or alcoholism can also cause it. **Hypomagnesemia usually is present when hypokalemia and hypocalcemia occur.** Magnesium is important in DNA and protein synthesis and in many enzyme reactions. Magnesium imbalances are rare, but hypomagnesemia is associated with malabsorption or malnutrition such as occurs with alcoholism. Diuretic use, diabetic ketoacidosis, hyperparathyroidism, and hyperaldosteronism may cause a deficit of magnesium. Signs and symptoms are listed in Table 3–4.

Hypermagnesemia

Hypermagnesemia is present when there is a serum level above 2.1 mEq/L. It occurs rarely, in the presence of renal failure or from overuse of magnesium-containing antacids and cathartics.

ANION IMBALANCES

Because of electroneutrality, imbalances of chloride, phosphate, and bicarbonate accompany cation imbalances. **Hypochloremia, a level below 95 mEq/L, is associated with hyponatremia.** It can also occur with severe vomiting and is seen as a compensatory decrease in acid-base disorders. **Hyperchloremia, a level above 103 mEq/L,** occurs along with hypernatremia and a form of metabolic acidosis. **Hypophosphatemia occurs when the level falls below 3.0 mg/dL.** It may result from use of aluminum-containing antacids that bind phosphate, from vitamin D deficiency, or from hyperparathyroidism. **Hyperphosphatemia, a level above 4.5 mg/dL, commonly occurs in renal failure.** See Table 3–4 for signs and symptoms of phosphate imbalance.

ACID-BASE SYSTEM

Acid-base balance is crucial to maintain in the body as cell enzymes only function within a very narrow pH range. To understand the concept of acid-base balance and how it is maintained in the body fluids, one should be familiar with some basic facts about biochemistry and the terms commonly used in discussions of hydrogen ion concentration (Box 3–3).

Nutrients in the blood diffuse into the cells, where various metabolic processes take place. Metabolic wastes, including acids, from those cellular processes diffuse back from the cells to the blood. There are three mechanisms that control or try to rebalance pH:

- Buffer pairs circulating in the blood respond to pH changes right away. The bicarbonate–carbonic acid buffer system is responsible for more than half of the buffering. There are three other buffer systems in the body as well, the phosphate system, the hemoglobin system, and the protein system.
- The respiratory system alters the respiratory rate and depth. Because carbon dioxide dissolves in the blood and combines with water to form carbonic acid, retaining or blowing off carbon dioxide helps retain or eliminate acids from the body.
- The kidneys change the excretion rate of acids and the production and absorption of bicarbonate ion. The kidneys are slow to compensate, but are the most effective compensating mechanism (Figure 3–7).

The bicarbonate–carbonic acid buffer system links an acid, carbon dioxide, with water and a bicarbonate ion, a base. A buffer is a substance that increases the amount of acid or alkali in the solution to produce a unit change in pH. The balance of the bicarbonate ions and carbonic acid ions is controlled by the respiratory system and the kidneys. The carbon dioxide produced by cell metabolism diffuses into the blood. There it reacts with water and forms carbonic acid. The carbonic acid dissociates (separates) to form hydrogen ions and bicarbonate ions as needed.

The process can be reversed in the lungs, freeing up carbon dioxide so it can be expired along with water, thereby reducing the total acid in the body.

Box 3–3 *Chemistry Facts Related to Acid-Base Balance*

Some of the more important facts about acid-base balance are:

- An *acid* is defined as a substance capable of giving up a hydrogen ion during chemical exchange.
- A *base* is a substance capable of accepting a hydrogen ion.
- Acids react with bases to form water and a salt.
- **A reaction of an acid and a base to form water and a salt is a *neutralization reaction because both the acid and the base are neutralized.***
- Acids react with carbonates and bicarbonates to form carbon dioxide gas.
- The term *pH* refers to the concentration of hydrogen (H) in a solution. The "p" represents a *negative* logarithm, which is an inverse proportion. This means that **the higher the concentration of hydrogen ions in a solution, the lower the pH.** A higher pH indicates the opposite, that is, a lower concentration of hydrogen ions.
- A chemically neutral solution has a pH of 7.00.
- **The pH of the body's fluids is normally somewhat alkaline (between 7.35 and 7.45).**
- A pH below 7.25 or above 7.55 is considered life threatening.
- A pH above 7.8 ***(alkalosis)*** or a pH below 6.8 ***(acidosis)*** usually is fatal.
- A blood pH of 7.4 indicates a ratio of 1 part carbonic acid to 20 parts bicarbonate (base).
- Acidosis is the result of either a loss of base or an accumulation of acid.

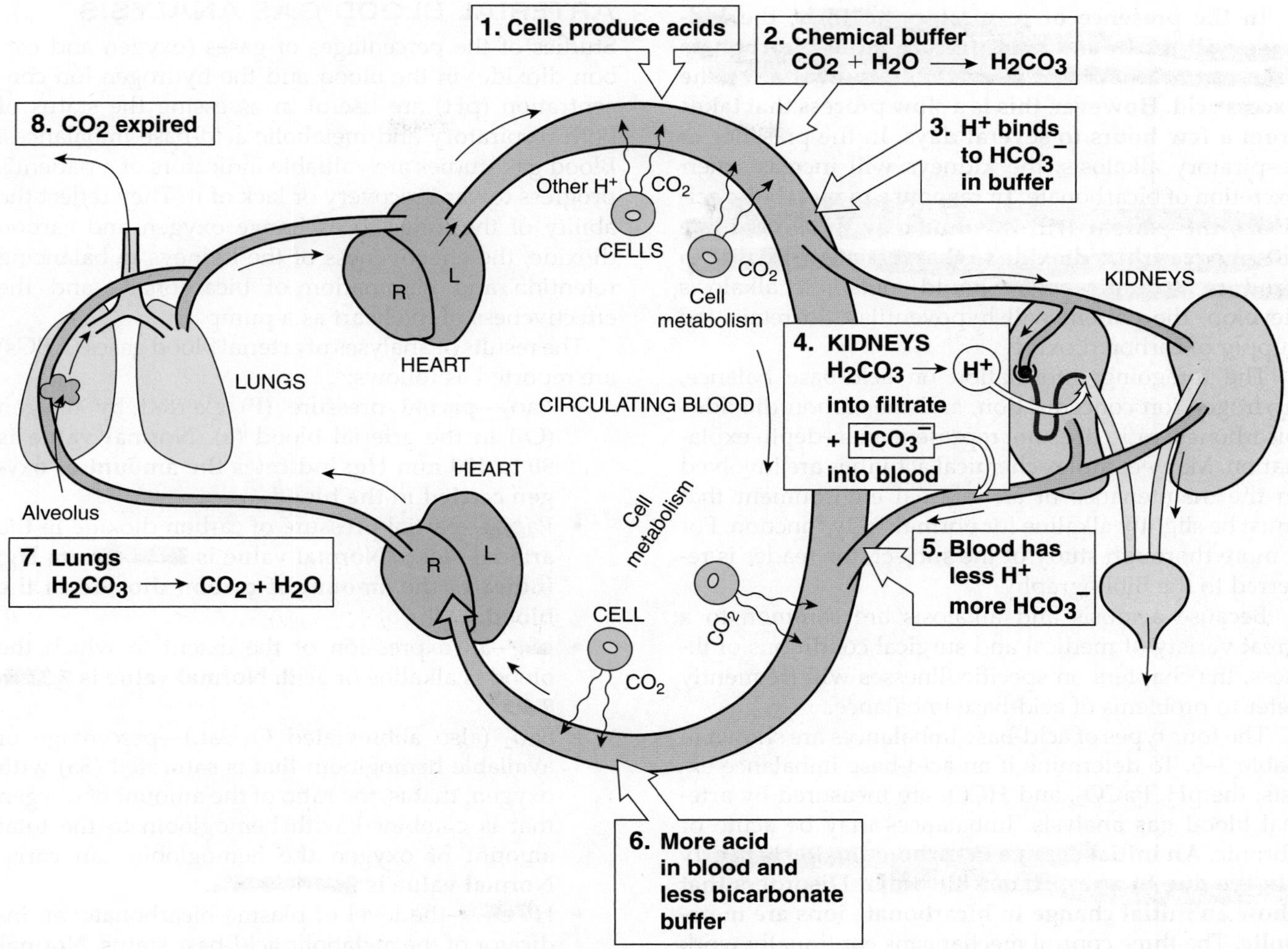

FIGURE 3–7 Regulation of acid-base balance by chemical buffers, respiratory system, and renal system.

Enzymes in the kidney promote the formation of hydrogen ions, which are excreted in the urine while the bicarbonate ions are returned to the blood. The kidneys, through the influence of aldosterone, can exchange hydrogen ions for sodium ions. Acids can be removed in the kidney by combining them with ammonia and other basic chemicals. Urine pH can vary from 4.5 to 8.0 as kidney compensation occurs.

ACID-BASE IMBALANCES

PATHOPHYSIOLOGY

Most of the body's metabolic activities produce carbon dioxide gas, which moves from the tissues into the blood, where it combines with water to form carbonic acid ($CO_2 + H_2O = H_2CO_3$). The body deals with this constant manufacture of acid in a number of ways so that the correct ratio of carbonic acid to bicarbonate can be maintained and an alkaline environment provided for normal cellular activities. If the ratio is not maintained, the acid-base balance is upset. The pH will either fall below the normal range and acidosis will occur, or it will rise above normal range and alkalosis will be present. As long as the ratio of carbonic acid to bicarbonate is maintained at 1:20, the pH remains within normal limits.

There are four acid-base imbalances:

- Respiratory acidosis
- Metabolic acidosis
- Respiratory alkalosis
- Metabolic alkalosis

The role played by the lungs in a respiratory imbalance is concerned with the retention or "blowing off" (excretion) of carbon dioxide (CO_2). In *hypoventilation,* the lungs do not eliminate enough CO_2, and it remains in the body, unites with water, and forms carbonic acid. The opposite is *hyperventilation,* in which too much CO_2 may be blown off.

The kidneys are the principal organs of control in maintaining a normal pH during metabolic activities because they either reabsorb or excrete bicarbonate. If they eliminate too much bicarbonate, acidosis will develop. Conversely, if they fail to eliminate enough bicarbonate and allow it to be reabsorbed into the bloodstream, alkalosis will develop.

In the presence of respiratory acidosis, the kidneys will retain and manufacture more bicarbonate than normal so that it is available to neutralize the excess acid. However, this is a slow process that takes from a few hours to several days. In the presence of respiratory alkalosis, the kidneys will increase their excretion of bicarbonate. **In response to metabolic acidosis, the patient will involuntarily hyperventilate to remove carbon dioxide so that it is not available to produce carbonic acid.** Should metabolic alkalosis develop, the patient will hypoventilate to retain the supply of carbon dioxide.

The foregoing information on acid-base balance, hydrogen ion concentration, and the carbon dioxide–bicarbonate ratio does not represent an in-depth explanation. Many complex chemical activities are involved in the maintenance of an internal environment that must be slightly alkaline for normal body function. For a more thorough study of the subject, the reader is referred to the Bibliography.

Because acidosis and alkalosis are common to a great variety of medical and surgical conditions of illness, the chapters on specific illnesses will frequently refer to problems of acid-base imbalance.

The four types of acid-base imbalances are shown in Table 3–5. To determine if an acid-base imbalance exists, the pH, $PaCO_2$, and HCO_3 are measured by arterial blood gas analysis. Imbalances may be acute or chronic. **An initial change in carbon dioxide is nearly always due to a respiratory disorder. Disorders that show an initial change in bicarbonate ions are metabolic.** The three control mechanisms continually work together to maintain acid-base balance: the respiratory system, the kidneys, and the bicarbonate buffer system. When an imbalance occurs, the lungs and kidneys try to *compensate* by working to bring the pH back toward normal limits.

Table 3–5 ***The Four Acid-Base Imbalances***

IMBALANCE	CAUSES	BLOOD GAS VALUES
Respiratory acidosis	Slow, shallow respirations Respiratory congestion/obstruction	pH <7.35 $Paco_2$ >45 mm Hg
Metabolic acidosis	Shock (poor circulation) Diabetic ketoacidosis Renal failure Diarrhea	pH <7.35 HCO_3^- <22 mEq/L
Respiratory alkalosis	Hyperventilation	pH >7.45 $Paco_2$ <35 mm Hg
Metabolic alkalosis	Vomiting Excessive antacid intake Hypokalemia	pH >7.45 HCO_3^- >26 mEq/L

From deWit, S.C. (2005). *Fundamental Concepts and Skills for Nursing* (2nd ed.). Philadelphia: Elsevier Saunders, pp. 425–427.

ARTERIAL BLOOD GAS ANALYSIS

Studies of the percentages of gases (oxygen and carbon dioxide) in the blood and the hydrogen ion concentration (pH) are useful in assessing the status of both respiratory and metabolic acid-base imbalances. Blood gas studies are valuable indicators of a patient's progress toward recovery or lack of it. They reflect the ability of the lungs to exchange oxygen and carbon dioxide, the effectiveness of the kidneys in balancing retention and elimination of bicarbonate, and the effectiveness of the heart as a pump.

The results of analyses of arterial blood gases (ABGs) are reported as follows:

- Pao_2—partial pressure (P) exerted by oxygen (O_2) in the arterial blood (a). **Normal value is 80 to 100 mm Hg; indicates the amount of oxygen carried in the blood.**
- $Paco_2$—partial pressure of carbon dioxide in the arterial blood. **Normal value is 35 to 45 mm Hg; indicates the amount of carbon dioxide in the blood.**
- pH—an expression of the extent to which the blood is alkaline or acid. **Normal value is 7.35 to 7.45.**
- Sao_2 (also abbreviated O_2 Sat.)—percentage of available hemoglobin that is saturated (Sa) with oxygen, that is, the ratio of the amount of oxygen that is combined with hemoglobin to the total amount of oxygen the hemoglobin can carry. **Normal value is 94% to 100%.**
- HCO_3^-—the level of plasma bicarbonate; an indicator of the metabolic acid-base status. **Normal value is 22 to 26 mEq/L.**
- Base excess or deficit—indicates the amount of blood buffer present. Alkalosis is present when this value is abnormally high. Abnormally low values indicate acidosis. Measured in "+" or "−" values.

RESPIRATORY ACIDOSIS

An increase in carbon dioxide levels occurs in a variety of disorders. It is seen in several conditions:

- Acute problems such as airway obstruction, pneumonia, asthma, chest injuries, or pulmonary edema
- Chronic obstructive pulmonary disease (COPD), such as emphysema
- With opiate use that depresses the respiratory rate

Think Critically About . . . What could you do to help your home care patient who has pneumonia prevent respiratory acidosis?

A patient with COPD is most likely to develop acute acidosis when an infection of the respiratory tract further impairs his breathing capacity and the removal of carbon dioxide.

Signs and symptoms of respiratory acidosis include complaints of increasing difficulty in breathing, a history of respiratory obstruction (acute or chronic), dyspnea, weakness, dizziness, restlessness, sleepiness, and change in mental alertness.

The treatment for respiratory acidosis is establishment or maintenance of an airway. A tracheostomy or the insertion of an endotracheal tube may be necessary. Oxygen administration may be needed, and ventilation may need the assistance of a mechanical ventilator. Conservative treatment is by postural drainage, deep-breathing exercises, bronchodilators, and antibiotics if indicated. Care must be taken when administering certain drugs that depress the respiratory center. These include narcotics, hypnotics, and tranquilizers.

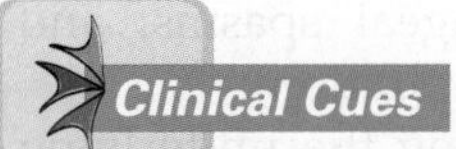

In patients with COPD, the respiratory drive mechanism is altered, and oxygen can act as a respiratory depressant. Oxygen should be administered with great care to these patients (no more than 2 to 3 L/min) because it can cause respiratory arrest.

If a patient's history is unknown, oxygen is begun at a rate of 2 to 3 L/min until it is determined that a higher flow rate can be tolerated.

The patient must be watched closely for respiratory and cardiac arrest. Should either occur, it will be necessary to maintain respiration and circulation artificially through cardiopulmonary resuscitation.

METABOLIC ACIDOSIS

An excessive loss of bicarbonate ions or an increased production or retention of hydrogen ions leads to metabolic acidosis. The main causes of metabolic acidosis are:

- Excessive loss of bicarbonate ions from diarrhea
- Renal failure
- Diabetic ketoacidosis
- Hyperkalemia

In diabetes mellitus, excessive burning of fats occurs because of insulin insufficiency, and the end product is fatty acids. When more energy than usual is expended, as in athletic competition, lactic acid builds up in the body as oxygenation of tissue falls. In kidney disease there is decreased excretion of acids and decreased production of bicarbonate.

The symptoms of metabolic acidosis include weakness, lethargy, headache, and confusion (Concept Map 3–1). If the acidosis is not relieved, these symptoms progress to stupor, unconsciousness, coma, and death. The breath of the patient may have a fruity odor owing to the presence of ketone bodies (ketoacidosis). Vomit-

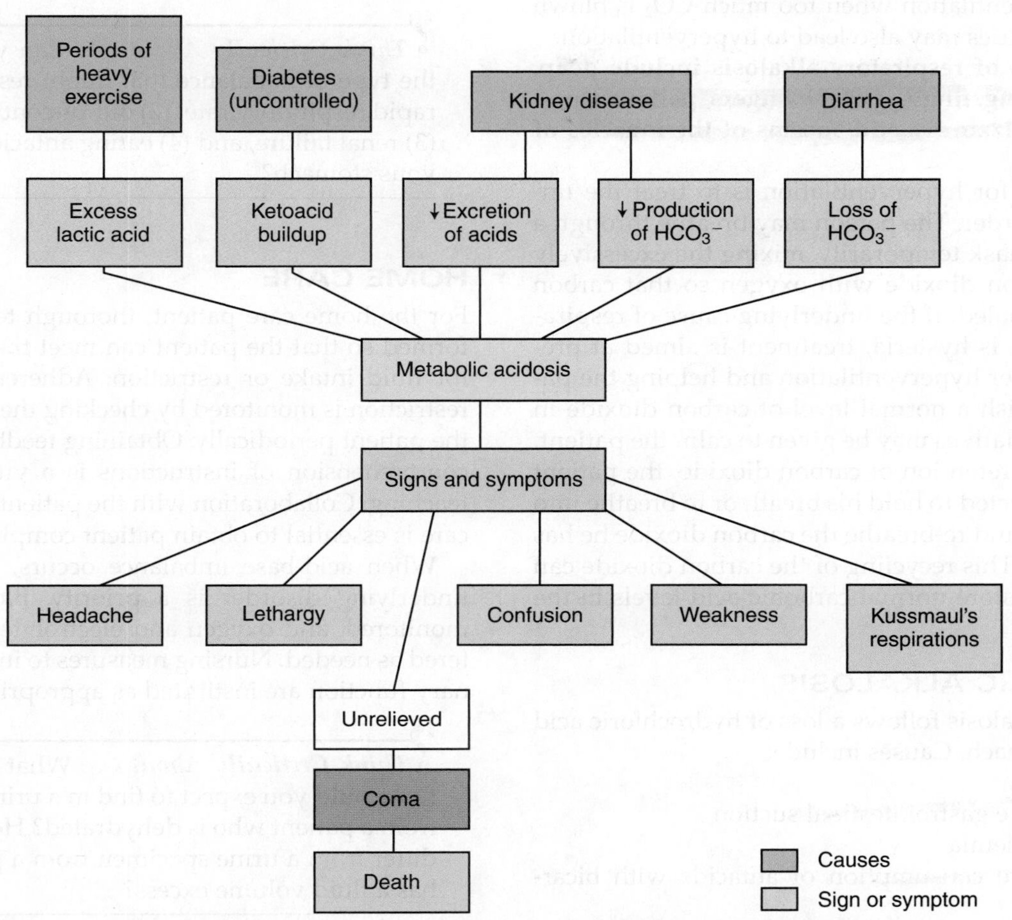

CONCEPT MAP **3–1** Causes, signs, and symptoms of metabolic acidosis.

ing and diarrhea may occur and aggravate the problem because of the loss of fluids and electrolytes, which are essential to restoring the acid-base balance.

Evidence that the compensatory mechanisms are at work in metabolic acidosis are deep rapid breathing (Kussmaul's respirations) and secretion of urine with a low pH.

Treatment of metabolic acidosis is aimed at the underlying cause. Insulin is administered if the patient is in diabetic ketoacidosis. Dialysis may be necessary to correct the problem in the patient with kidney failure. **Immediate treatment of severe metabolic acidosis requires administration of intravenous (IV) bicarbonate or lactate.**

RESPIRATORY ALKALOSIS

Alkalosis occurs less frequently than acidosis. **Hyperventilation** (a rapid respiratory rate) results in respiratory alkalosis. It is usually caused by:

- Anxiety
- High fever
- An overdose of aspirin

Patients hyperventilate for a variety of reasons; these include **hypoxemia** (insufficiency of oxygen, which triggers an automatic increase in respiration), reactions to certain drugs, pain, and hysteria. The overzealous use of mechanical ventilation also can cause hyperventilation when too much CO_2 is blown off. Head injuries may also lead to hyperventilation.

Symptoms of respiratory alkalosis include deep, rapid breathing, tingling of the fingers, pallor around the mouth, dizziness, and spasms of the muscles of the hands.

Treatment for hyperventilation is to treat the underlying disorder. The person may breathe through a re-breather mask temporarily, mixing the excessively exhaled carbon dioxide with oxygen so that carbon dioxide is inhaled. If the underlying cause of respiratory alkalosis is hysteria, treatment is aimed at preventing further hyperventilation and helping the patient reestablish a normal level of carbon dioxide in his blood. Sedatives may be given to calm the patient. To aid in the retention of carbon dioxide, the patient may be instructed to hold his breath or to breathe into a paper sack and re-breathe the carbon dioxide he has just exhaled. This recycling of the carbon dioxide can eventually restore normal carbonic acid levels in the blood.

METABOLIC ALKALOSIS

Metabolic alkalosis follows a loss of hydrochloric acid from the stomach. Causes include:

- Vomiting
- Extensive gastrointestinal suction
- Hypokalemia
- Excessive consumption of antacids with bicarbonate

Hypokalemia causes this disorder because the kidney then retains K^+ while excreting H^+.

Other causes include drainage from intestinal fistula, diuresis resulting from potent diuretics that increase potassium loss in the urine, and steroid therapy, which causes retention of sodium and chloride and loss of potassium and hydrogen.

Signs and symptoms of metabolic alkalosis include such neurologic signs as **irritability, disorientation, lethargy, muscle twitching, tingling and numbness of the fingers, and convulsions;** and respiratory manifestations such as **slow, shallow respirations, decreased chest movements, and cyanosis.** In addition, there may be symptoms of potassium and calcium depletion. If the alkalosis progresses, tetany will occur and seizures and coma result. Tetany is characterized by severe muscle cramps, carpopedal spasms, laryngeal spasms, and **stridor** (shrill, harsh sound upon inspiration).

Treatment is directed at correcting the underlying cause and attempting to restore the body fluids to a less alkaline state. Fluids and electrolytes are replaced orally and parenterally as needed. Emergency measures include the administration of an acidifying solution such as ammonium chloride.

Figure 3–8 compares the causes, physiologic effects, and compensatory mechanisms for acidosis and alkalosis.

> ? *Think Critically About . . .* Can you identify the type of imbalance that might result from (1) rapid respiratory rate, (2) out-of-control diabetes, (3) renal failure, and (4) eating antacids for a nervous stomach?

HOME CARE

For the home care patient, thorough teaching is performed so that the patient can meet the requirements for fluid intake or restriction. Adherence to sodium restriction is monitored by checking the food intake of the patient periodically. Obtaining feedback regarding comprehension of instructions is a vital part of the teaching. Collaboration with the patient on the plan of care is essential to obtain patient compliance.

When acid-base imbalance occurs, control of the underlying disorder is a priority. Blood gases are monitored, and oxygen and electrolytes are administered as needed. Nursing measures to improve pulmonary function are instituted as appropriate.

> ? *Think Critically About . . .* What characteristics would you expect to find in a urine specimen from a patient who is dehydrated? How would it differ from a urine specimen from a patient who has a fluid volume excess?

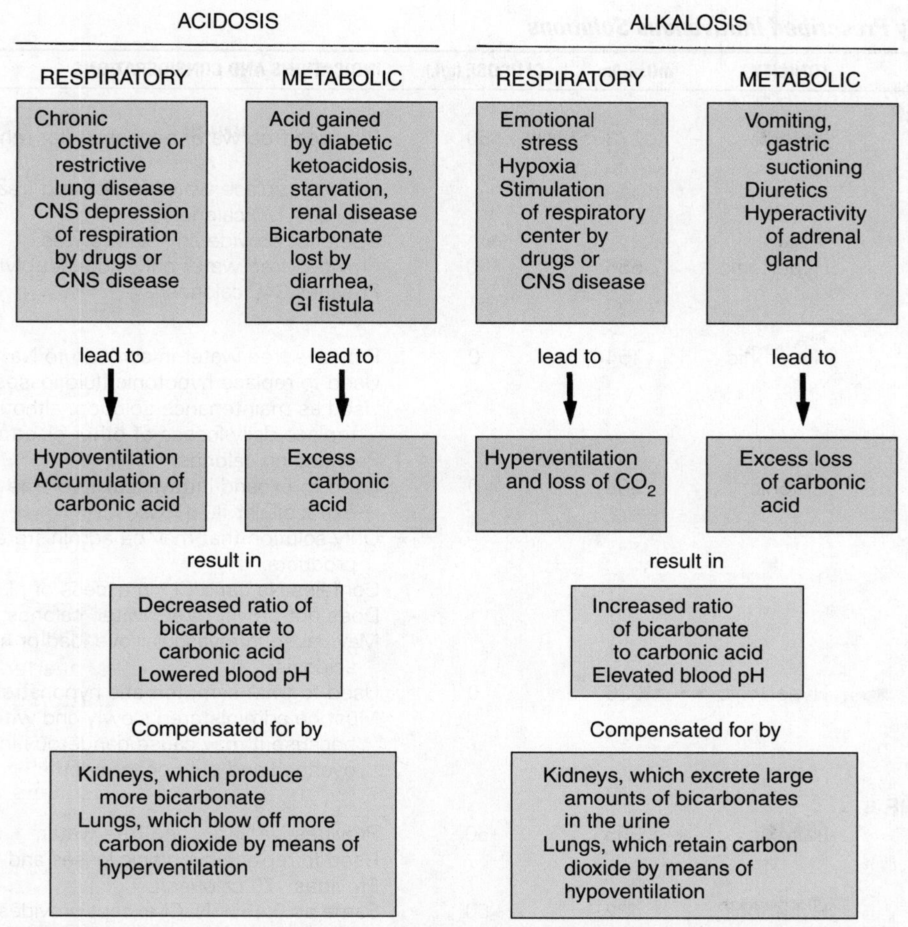

FIGURE 3–8 Comparison of causes, physiologic effects, and compensatory mechanisms for acidosis and alkalosis.

INTRAVENOUS FLUID THERAPY

The administration of fluids through the veins is the most common means by which water, electrolytes, nutrients, and some drugs may be given when oral intake is not possible or must be supplemented. Intravenous therapy is often used when a fluid deficit is present or when there are electrolyte imbalances. Intravenous fluids may also be used to help reestablish acid-base balance. Medications may be administered in an IV solution when rapid action is required. Total parenteral nutrition (TPN) is used for the parenteral administration of nutrients for patients with gastrointestinal problems who cannot take in nutrients in any other way.

Some terms related to the concentration of an IV fluid and the effect this has on cells are:

- **Isotonic**—a solution that has the same osmotic pressure as ICF. Body cells can be bathed in an isotonic solution without net flow of water across the cell membrane.
- **Hypotonic**—a solution that has a lower osmotic pressure (is less concentrated) than that of body fluids. Cells bathed in a hypotonic solution will swell as water passes from the less concentrated solution across the cell membrane and into the cell. *Note:* Sterile distilled water is hypotonic and is never added to an IV solution.
- **Hypertonic**—a solution that has a higher osmotic pressure than that of body fluids. Cells bathed in a hypertonic solution will shrink as water passes out of the cell into the fluid surrounding it.

An example of an isotonic solution is 0.9% normal saline. Hypotonic solutions are those with less than 5% glucose or with anions less than 150 mEq/L. Fluids commonly used in IV therapy are presented in Table 3–6.

Blood-related fluids that are given IV include whole blood, packed cells from which the plasma has been removed leaving only the red blood cells, and plasma. Whole blood is sometimes given to replace that which has been lost through hemorrhage. Packed cells may be administered to patients with anemia or some other blood disorder or to patients who cannot tolerate a large volume of fluid very well, such as those with renal disease or congestive heart failure. Plasma is given to increase blood volume (as in shock), to provide protein, and to treat disorders of coagulation.

Table 3–6 ***Commonly Prescribed Intravenous Solutions***

SOLUTION	TONICITY	mOsm/kg	GLUCOSE (g/L)	INDICATIONS AND CONSIDERATIONS
DEXTROSE IN WATER				
5%	Isotonic	278	50	Provides free water necessary for renal excretion of solutes. Used to replace water losses and treat hypernatremia. Provides 170 calories/L. Does not provide any electrolytes.
10%	Hypertonic	556	100	Provides free water only, no electrolytes. Provides 340 calories/L.
SALINE				
0.45%	Hypotonic	154	0	Provides free water in addition to Na^+ and Cl^-. Used to replace hypotonic fluid losses. Used as maintenance solution, although it does not replace daily losses of other electrolytes. Provides no calories.
0.9%	Isotonic	308	0	Used to expand intravascular volume and replace extracellular fluid losses. Only solution that may be administered with blood products. Contains Na^+ and Cl^- in excess of plasma levels. Does not provide free water, calories, other electrolytes. May cause intravascular overload or hyperchloremic acidosis.
3.0%	Hypertonic	1026	0	Used to treat symptomatic hyponatremia. Must be administered slowly and with extreme caution because it may cause dangerous intravascular volume overload and pulmonary edema.
DEXTROSE IN SALINE				
5% in 0.225%	Isotonic	355	50	Provides Na^+, Cl^-, and free water. Used to replace hypotonic losses and treat hypernatremia. Provides 170 calories/L.
5% in 0.45%	Hypertonic	432	50	Same as 0.45% NaCl except provides 170 calories/L.
5% in 0.9%	Hypertonic	586	50	Same as 0.45% NaCl except provides 170 calories/L.
MULTIPLE ELECTROLYTE SOLUTIONS				
Ringer's solution	Isotonic	309	0	Similar in composition to plasma except that it has excess Cl^-, no Mg^{2+}, and no HCO_3^-. Does not provide free water or calories. Used to expand the intravascular volume and replace extracellular fluid losses.
Lactated Ringer's (Hartmann's) solution	Isotonic	274	0	Similar in composition to normal plasma except does not contain Mg^{2+}. Used to treat losses from burns and lower gastrointestinal tract. May be used to treat mild metabolic acidosis but should not be used to treat lactic acidosis. Does not provide free water or calories.

Modified from Lewis, S.M., Heitkemper, M.M., Dirksen, S.R., et al. (2007). *Medical-Surgical Nursing: Assessment and Management of Clinical Problems* (7th ed.). St. Louis: Mosby.

Blood product administration is presented in Chapter 16 along with the blood disorders.

In the treatment of shock, fluids called *plasma expanders* are administered to increase the volume of plasma. Examples of plasma expanders are low-molecular-weight dextran, albumin, Hespan, and Plasmanate.

NURSING RESPONSIBILITIES IN ADMINISTERING IV FLUIDS

Responsibility for the safe and effective administration of IV fluids rests with every member of the nursing staff (Legal & Ethical Considerations 3–1). As with any therapeutic measure, IV therapy is not without its hazards to the patient. Many complications can be avoided through careful handling of equipment and meticulous monitoring of the patient's reaction to the fluids he is receiving (Safety Alert 3–2).

The four goals of nursing care for a patient receiving an IV infusion are:

- Preventing infection
- Minimizing physical injury to the veins and surrounding tissues
- Administering the correct fluid at the prescribed time and at a safe rate of flow (Box 3–4)
- Observing the patient's reaction to the fluid and medications being administered

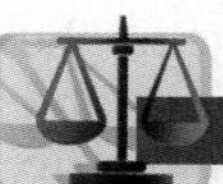

Legal & Ethical Considerations 3–1

Intravenous Therapy Guidelines

Check your state's nurse practice act to determine what aspects of intravenous therapy, if any, your state will allow the LPN/LVN to perform. With the continuation of the nursing shortage, a few states have expanded their LPN practice act to allow licensed LPNs to perform a variety of intravenous therapy functions. Other states are considering expanding their practice acts accordingly.

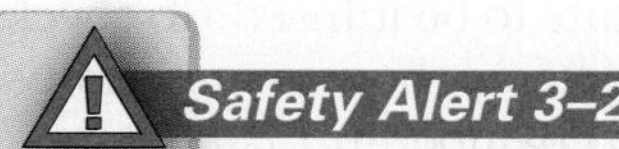

Safety Alert 3–2

Intravenous (IV) Line Connection Safety

When connecting an IV solution or disconnecting a line, always trace the line to where it connects to the patient to make certain that it is an IV line and connects to an IV device. Many mistakes have been made by connecting an IV fluid to the wrong device.

All equipment and fluids used for IV therapy must be sterile and safe for administration. Before any plastic bag or bottle of solution is added to an IV set, it must be checked for leaks and possible contamination (Safety Alert 3–3).

When a new bottle of fluid or additional medication is added to an IV infusion already in progress, strict surgical asepsis must be observed. Each time a new unit of solution or medication is added to an IV setup, there is a danger of introducing bacteria into the patient's blood system. Because of the danger of incompatibility, it is essential that the nurse check each drug and each solution to be certain they can be mixed. *Always wash your hands just before handling IV fluids and equipment.* **The port on the IV tubing into which the administration set of a piggyback medication is to be attached must be carefully and thoroughly wiped with a fresh alcohol swab before the tubing is attached to the container.**

There should be a clear occlusive (airtight) dressing over the IV insertion site. The edges of the dressing should adhere to the skin on all sides. Tubing should be secured so that accidental pulling on the tubing will not affect the IV cannula. Dressings are changed according to agency protocol, but usually are changed at least every 72 hours. If a dressing becomes loose, it should be removed and a new dressing applied (Box 3–5).

The site of venipuncture should be watched closely for signs of inflammation. Redness, swelling, and heat in the area should be reported as they are possible signs of phlebitis. Chills and an elevation of body temperature may indicate a bacterial infection. Table 3–7 presents the complications of IV therapy.

When an IV is discontinued, the tubing is clamped, all tape is removed, and the needle or catheter is gently, but quickly, withdrawn using Standard Precautions. A dry, sterile gauze is held on the site with enough pressure to control the leakage of blood and to avoid the formation of a hematoma. If possible, raising the patient's limb for a minute or two to drain blood from the site of insertion will help prevent leakage of blood from the punctured vein.

In 2007, National Patient Safety Goals were revised by The Joint Commission. Goal 1 is to Improve the accuracy of patient identification. This means that at least two patient identifiers (neither being the patient's room number) must be used whenever intravenous fluid is administered (Safety Alert 3–4). The nurse should check the patient's armband with the medication administration record for the correct name and the correct agency identification number as well as asking patients to state their name.

Box 3–4 *The Five Rights Applied to Intravenous (IV) Therapy*

Be sure you have:

- The right solution with or without additives as ordered; the correct solution to follow what has been infusing
- The right dose (amount) of solution and additive as ordered
- The right route (peripheral IV, peripherally inserted central catheter [PICC], central line, port)
- The right time (to infuse)
- The right patient as identified with two identifiers

Additionally,

- Teach the patient the reason for administration of the fluid and/or drug and signs and symptoms of problems to report to you.
- Check for drug and latex allergies.
- Be aware of potential interactions with IV medications or irrigating solutions.
- Maintain sterility of all solutions, tubing, and connections.

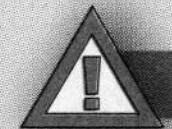

Safety Alert 3–3

Intravenous (IV) Solution Safety

A plastic bag of solution may be squeezed to check for leaks. Any solution that is discolored or has small particles, a white cloud, or film in it should not be used. If there is no vacuum in a bottle when it is opened, the solution may be contaminated. Gently invert the bag or bottle and hold it up to the light so you can see if there are any particles floating in it.

RATE OF FLOW

Rate of flow is an important factor in safe and effective IV therapy. Intravenous setups should be checked once an hour to be certain that the fluid is running correctly and there are no problems. When possible, an IV pump that

Box 3–5 *Intravenous Therapy Guidelines*

- **Keep IV fluid sterile.** Make sure that everything coming in contact with the solution is sterile, including the inside surface of the cannula hub, and all connecting points between the bag and drip chamber and between the tubing and the needle.
- **Protect the cannula site from contamination to avoid possible infection.** An airtight, transparent dressing is used over the cannula site; some agencies apply an antibiotic ointment to the site.
- **Keep tubing free of air.** Clear tubing of air before connecting to the cannula. Do not allow the current bag to run dry before changing to the next one.
- **Hang fluids at the correct height.** Fluids flow through the tubing by the force of gravity. If there is negative pressure in the IV line, blood will flow back into the tubing. Keep the bag of fluid sufficiently above the level of the cannula site to maintain flow, but avoid having it too high because this significantly increases the effect of gravity.
- **Carefully regulate the rate of flow.** If the IV is behind schedule, do not open up the clamp and run in a large amount of fluid at one time to catch up. Rather, recalculate either (1) the span of time for the infusion or (2) the rate of drops per minute for the fluid to run at the ordered rate.
- **Track intake and output when a patient is receiving IV fluids or blood.** Keep accurate intake and output records and compare intake with output over 24 hours.
- **The solution to run in first should be hung the highest.** When a second bag is attached piggyback to a primary IV line, lower the primary bag without clamping the tubing so it will begin to flow when the piggyback has run in. Attach the piggyback beneath the roller clamp on the primary tubing.
- **Assess the site frequently for signs of complications.** Infiltration, swelling at the IV site, irritation of the vein, formation of a clot stopping the flow, or systemic reaction should be identified quickly. Signs of infiltration are pain or discomfort at the site caused by dislodgement of the needle or puncture of the vein. Vital signs should be taken several times a day to detect early signs of infection or adverse reaction.

is set for the specific rate of flow is used to administer IV fluids. IV pumps, although not infallible, keep IV fluids flowing at the desired rate and act as safeguards should a problem arise. Even when a pump is used, you must check to see that it is delivering the solution accurately as prescribed. Principles that affect the rate of flow for IVs not administered by a pump are as follows:

- The higher the container is placed above the level of the patient's heart, the faster the rate of flow.
- The fuller the container, the faster the rate of flow.
- The more viscous (thicker) the fluid, the slower the flow; for example, packed red cells will flow more slowly than 5% dextrose in water.
- The larger the diameter of the needle and tubing, the faster the flow.
- The higher the pressure within the vein, the slower the flow. As an infusion progresses and the veins become fuller, the IV solution may drip more slowly.
- Fluid will pass through a straight tube faster than through one that is coiled or hanging below the level of the cannula.

There usually is a chart available to the nurse who needs to determine the number of drops that should be given per minute to administer a given amount of fluid in a specified time. The IV tubing package will contain information about the number of drops the set will deliver per milliliter. If a chart is not available, calculate the number of drops per minute to be infused. To check the rate of flow, you must know how many drops should pass through the drip chamber in *1 minute.*

Once the number of drops per minute has been set and the IV infusion is flowing, the IV setup must be checked at 30- to 60-minute intervals to be sure that it continues to flow at the prescribed rate. As explained in the list of principles that affect the rate of flow, any number of factors can speed up or slow down the infusion.

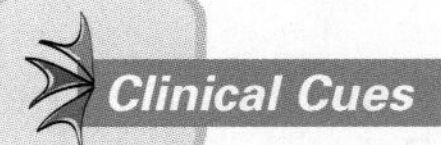

Whenever the patient who has an IV infusing is up out of bed, recheck the drop rate once he is settled back in bed. The fluid drop rate often changes when the patient is up and moving around.

If the IV slows down and has not been checked and readjusted for some time, **no attempt should be made to "catch up"** a large volume of fluid by speeding up the rate of flow beyond that ordered. This can lead to circulatory overload and a volume excess that may produce pulmonary edema in susceptible people. Table 3–8 presents points to check when an IV solution will not run at the prescribed rate.

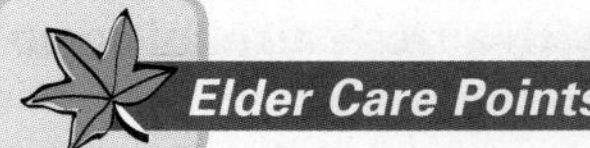

Elderly people and those with either renal or cardiac conditions cannot tolerate rapid administration of fluids. Check an infusing IV for these patients every 30 minutes.

Think Critically About . . . How would you calculate the rate of flow for an order for "1000 mL of D_5W [dextrose 5% in water] over 8 hours" using a drip set that delivers 15 gtt/mL? How would the rate differ if the drip set delivers 20 drops (gtt)/mL? How would you calculate the flow rate for an order for "250 mL NS [normal saline] at 50 mL/hour" using a microdrip set (60 gtt/mL)?

Table 3–7 Complications of Intravenous (IV) Therapy and Nursing Interventions

COMPLICATION	SIGNS AND SYMPTOMS	NURSING INTERVENTIONS
LOCAL		
Infiltration	Arm swollen, tender, cool to touch; may or may not have blood return.	Remove IV catheter and restart IV in the other extremity.
Extravasation	Pain at insertion site, tender and cool to touch, IV flow slows, edema, burning, pale, fluid leaking around catheter. Tissue sloughing may occur in 1–4 wk.	Stop infusion immediately. Remove the IV catheter and restart in the other extremity. If drug is involved, aspirate from short cannula. Administer antidote if available. Apply cold compresses if not contraindicated. Photograph site. Monitor site in 24 hr. Provide written instructions for patient and family.
Phlebitis	Vein hard with skin red, swollen, tender, warm; blood return present; IV infusion may or may not be sluggish.	Remove IV catheter, document; apply warm moist pack to the IV site. Restart IV in other extremity. Monitor frequently.
Thrombophlebitis	Site red, tender, warm; IV infusion sluggish.	Never irrigate the IV catheter; remove the IV catheter, notify the physician, restart IV in opposite extremity. Apply cool compresses initially, followed by warm.
IV site skin infection	Site hot, red, painful but not hard or swollen; IV infusion sluggish.	Remove IV catheter, restart in opposite extremity, change entire administration system. Clean site with alcohol. Apply warm compresses. May send tip of catheter for culture.
Venous spasm	Slowing of infusion rate; cramping or pain at or above the insertion site. Numbness in the area. Inability to withdraw peripherally inserted central catheter (PICC) or midline catheter.	Slow infusion rate and apply warm compresses. Do not apply tension to catheter or forcibly remove it. Encourage consumption of warm liquids. Keep extremity covered and dry.
Nerve damage	Tingling, "pins and needles" feeling, or numbness at or below the catheter insertion site.	Immediately stop the cannula insertion if patient complains of severe pain. If sensations do not go away once the catheter is secured, remove the catheter.
Catheter embolus	Decrease in blood pressure (BP); pain along vein; weak, rapid pulse; cyanosis of nail beds; loss of consciousness.	Remove IV catheter and inspect, place a tourniquet high on limb of IV site, notify physician, obtain x-ray, prepare for surgery to remove pieces.
SYSTEMIC		
Infection	Fever, chills, general malaise.	Change the infusion system, notify the physician, obtain cultures as ordered.
Speed shock	Light-headedness or dizziness; flushed face, irregular pulse, decreased BP, loss of consciousness, cardiac arrest.	Stop the infusion, notify the physician, monitor vital signs frequently. Run dextrose 5% in water at a keep-vein-open rate.
Circulatory overload	Shortness of breath, tachypnea, increased BP, moist cough, crackles, puffiness around eyes and dependent edema.	Elevate head of the bed, keep patient warm, assess for edema, slow the infusion rate, notify the physician. Administer oxygen and diuretic as ordered.

INTRAVENOUS INTAKE

The total amount of IV fluid infused during the shift is calculated at the end of the shift. For example, if the beginning count was 350 mL (amount in the container at the beginning of the shift) and a new solution of 1000 mL was added after the 350 mL was infused, then the 350 mL infused is added to whatever amount of the 1000 mL that was added has infused by the end of the shift:

	COUNT	INFUSED
Count at beginning of shift	350 mL	
New solution added at 11:30	1000 mL	350 mL
Count left at end of shift	525 mL	475 mL
Total amount of IV intake for shift		825 mL

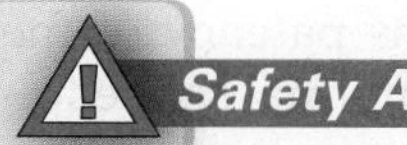

Five Rights for Intravenous (IV) Therapy

The IV administration of fluids requires the same safety precautions as any other medication does. Follow the Five Rights and the additional rules for drug administration (see Box 3–4). The label must be read and compared to the order or the medication administration record (MAR) three times to ensure that the correct solution is being given to the correct patient. The patient's ID band must be checked each time a solution is administered.

Table 3–8 Troubleshooting: IV Flow

CHECK	RATIONALE
Height of infusion container	Patient may have changed position. The container should be at least 36 inches above the heart.
System vent	Air vent may be absent or occluded, which will prevent the flow.
Position of tubing	Tubing may be kinked, obstructing flow. Tubing may be hanging below the bed, interfering with the gravity flow.
Position of the extremity where the site is located	Flexion of the extremity may have compressed the vein, slowing the flow.
Any possible obstruction to flow	A protective device on the limb may be too tight. Tape may be compressing the circumference of the extremity.
When filter was changed	Filter may be occluded.
Position of the cannula within the vessel	Cannula may be lying against the vessel wall, obstructing flow. Slightly turning the cannula to reposition the tip may cure the problem.
If other measures have not opened the line, attempt to aspirate blood from the cannula	A small clot may be obstructing the cannula. Aspiration may withdraw the clot.

Intravenous therapy may become such a commonplace procedure to nurses that they are tempted to be complacent about it. However, it should never be thought of as a routine procedure that requires little attention. **Any fluid or medication that enters a vein has an immediate effect. There is no margin for error in its administration.**

FLUSHING PRN LOCKS OR CENTRAL INTRAVENOUS LINES

Flushing the catheter or line prevents contact and reactions between the fluid that was last infused and incompatible drugs. Flushing maintains patency of the lumen. Either normal saline alone or normal saline followed by a heparin solution is used.

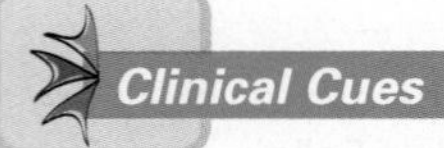

When a heparinized saline is required to keep the lumen of a catheter patent, use a volume of the solution that is equal to twice the volume of the catheter lumen with the extension set or connectors added on. This will usually be between 5 and 10 mL; check your facility policy.

Before using a PRN (as-needed) lock, you should flush the catheter according to agency policy to determine patency (openness) of the lumen and to flush out any heparinized solution. The procedure will depend on the type of valved catheter or positive fluid-displacement needleless device in place. When flushing, apply slow, gentle pressure to the syringe plunger. **If you feel any resistance, stop the procedure immediately.** Proceeding may force a clot into the venous circulation that will become an embolus that could cause severe damage to the patient. Aspirate for a brisk blood return from the catheter lumen, and then flush the blood from the catheter with the flush solution. Three to 10 mL of normal saline is used depending on the length of the catheter that is in place (Safety Alert 3–5).

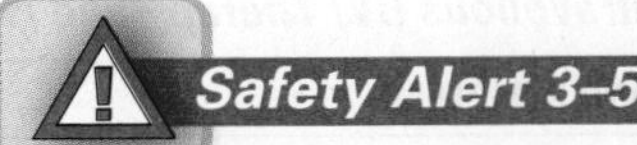

Flushing Intravenous Catheters

Do not use more than 30 mL of bacteriostatic normal saline within a 24-hour period to flush the catheter. Always use single-dose vials or syringes of solution for flushing. Do not use a multiple-dose vial for this purpose as it may be contaminated and could cause infection.

PRN locks and catheters should be flushed immediately following use or when an IV piggyback medication infusion is completed. Delay in disconnecting the intermittent infusion administration set and flushing the lock could allow blood backflow into the catheter lumen because the infusion pressure drops lower than the venous pressure when the infusion is complete. A clot can form, occluding the lumen. **Be aware of when an intermittent infusion should be completed and be at the bedside prepared to remove the piggyback infusion set and flush the PRN lock.**

CENTRAL LINE CARE

Provide site care every 24 to 48 hours per agency protocol if a gauze dressing is in place. Transparent dressings require site care every 3 to 7 days. Every central line dressing should be examined once each shift, and the dressing should be changed if it is soiled. A central line dressing change and site care is a sterile procedure. The old dressing is removed using nonsterile gloves. Box 3–6 presents the guidelines for the dressing change.

Blood Drawing

Blood drawing from a central line is not recommended unless venipuncture is not advisable. If a blood draw is performed, strict aseptic technique must be used. It is preferable to use needleless connectors and vacuum tubes for the procedure rather than a needle and syringe or vacuum tube with needle. Box 3–7 presents the guidelines for a blood draw.

Subcutaneous Infusion

Subcutaneous infusion is often used in home care or during hospice palliative care. Subcutaneous therapy is useful when the patient cannot tolerate oral medica-

Box 3–6 Guidelines for a Central Line Dressing Change

- Use Standard Precautions. Wear a mask.
- Old dressing is removed using clean, nonsterile gloves.
- With sterile gloves, inspect the site and cleanse it according to agency protocol. (Usually the site is cleansed with antiseptic swabs, circling outward from the catheter. This is repeated twice more. Allow to dry completely. Next the site is cleansed using an alcohol swab circling outward. Repeat twice. Allow to dry completely. Alternatively one set of combination antiseptic swabs may be used.)
- Apply a new occlusive dressing, or a sterile gauze dressing.
- Tape down the dressing.
- Coil the extension tubing for a peripherally inserted central catheter (PICC) or mid-line catheter and tape it to the patient's arm.
- Note the date, time, and your initials on the label for the dressing.
- Clamp lumens to catheter one at a time and remove the injection caps; cleanse the port with povidone-iodine and allow to dry completely.
- Place new caps over the ports; open the clamp for the infusion.

Box 3–7 Guidelines for a Blood Draw from a Central Line*

- Use Standard Precautions.
- Cleanse the injection cap with povidone-iodine and allow to dry completely.
- Stop IV infusion, if running, temporarily.
- Aspirate for blood flash.
- Flush the catheter port with 5 to 10 mL of normal saline depending on the length of the catheter.
- Using a Vacutainer tube, withdraw 5 mL of blood and discard in a biohazard container.
- Withdraw the amount of blood required in the correct color-top Vacutainer tubes.
- Flush catheter with 5 to 10 mL of sterile normal saline solution depending on length of catheter.
- If an infusion will not be continued, flush the catheter port with the correct amount of heparin solution (usually at least 3 mL, but follow agency protocol).
- Clamp the lumen, remove the cap, and cleanse the port with povidone-iodine; allow to dry completely.
- Place a new cap on the port; open the clamp, and resume the IV infusion.†

*LPNs in some states are being trained to perform blood draws from central lines.
†New guideline of Intravenous Infusion Nurses' Society.

tions, when injections are too painful, or when vascular access is too difficult to obtain. Pain management is the primary use, although several other types of drugs are infused in this manner.

Hypodermoclysis, the slow infusion of isotonic fluid into subcutaneous tissue, may be used for small volumes of fluid. Generally, the front and sides of the thighs, the hips, the area under the clavicle, and the upper abdomen are the sites used. A butterfly needle or a special subcutaneous infusion device is used to provide access for the fluid.

Intraosseous Infusion

Intraosseous infusion utilizes the rich vascular network located in the long bones. Even large volumes of fluid can be absorbed from this site. However, this type of infusion site is only used during the immediate period of burn or severe trauma resuscitation and should not be used for more than 24 hours. In adults, a 15- or 16-gauge needle is used to gain access to the medullary area in the bone. Sites used are the distal or proximal tibia and the distal femur. This method of infusion is sometimes used in pediatrics. Only a physician or advanced practice practitioner performs this procedure.

Epidural Infusion

Epidural infusion is used for administration of medication for pain control or for anesthesia (see Chapter 7).

Partial or Total Parenteral Nutrition

Many patients with fluid and electrolyte imbalances are nutritionally depleted. Partial parenteral nutrition (PPN) is given when a patient cannot maintain an adequate nutritional status with oral intake. PPN is given through a large peripheral vein in the arm. If sufficient nutrition cannot be delivered by oral intake and PPN, or by enteral feedings, TPN is begun. Figure 3–9 shows placement of a peripherally inserted central catheter and of a central venous catheter.

TPN solution is made up of a nitrogen (protein) source, hypertonic dextrose, and supplementary vitamins and minerals. The solution is hypertonic and contains 1 calorie/mL or 1000 calories/L. Some solutions also contain lipids. Because of its degree of concentration, it must be infused through a central vein, usually the subclavian, where the high rate of blood flow quickly dilutes it. The Hickman, Broviac, and Groshong catheters are the most frequently used central line catheters, and they can be used for long-term therapy. TPN solution is administered with a pump or an infusion controller device so that the rate is constant (Safety Alert 3–6).

TPN solutions and catheters must be handled with strict asepsis, as the solution is an ideal medium for bacterial growth. Infection is a major complication of TPN. The TPN solution is mixed in the pharmacy under sterile conditions. There are many complications of TPN in addition to infection, including glucose intolerance, electrolyte imbalance, phlebitis, allergic reaction, and fluid overload. The port through which TPN is administered is not used for any other solution. The patient must be carefully monitored. When TPN is begun, the flow rate is slowly started at about 60 to 80 mL/hr, and gradually increased in increments of 25 mL/hr until the maintenance rate is reached. This allows the body to adjust to the glucose load. Blood

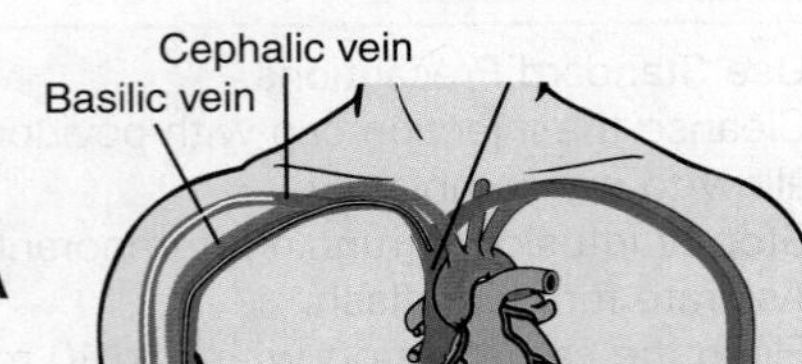

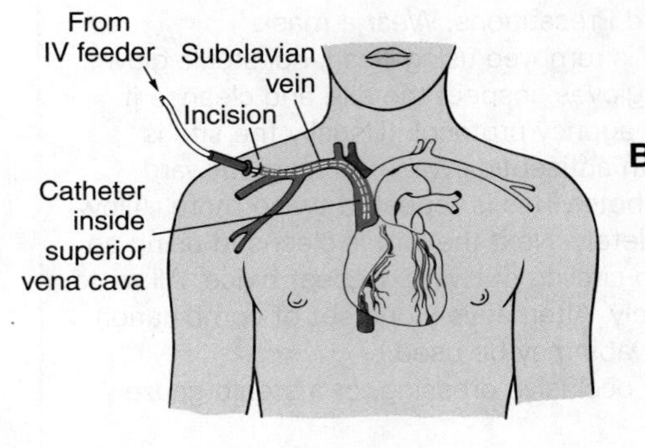

FIGURE **3–9** **A,** Placement of a peripherally inserted central catheter (PICC) through the antecubital fossa. **B,** Placement of a central venous catheter inserted into the subclavian vein.

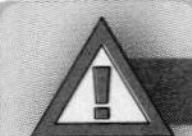

Safety Alert 3–6

Total Parenteral Nutrition (TPN) Safety Precaution

The flow rate for TPN solution is never changed to "catch up" on the amount of fluid that should have been infused if the flow has slowed for some reason. The hypertonic solution can draw fluid into the vascular system, causing fluid overload.

sugar determinations are performed frequently during the stabilization period, which is usually the first week. If the patient's body has difficulty with glucose tolerance, insulin may be ordered and is added to the TPN solution. At the end of therapy, the flow rate is tapered down for 1 to 2 hours before stopping the fluid to allow the body to adjust.

PPN is used for patients in whom central venous access is not possible or who will need IV nutritional support for only 7 to 10 days. The concentration of the solution given is less because it does not flow into a vessel with a large blood flow, which would dilute it. Box 3–8 summarizes the principles for administering TPN.

Free-flow protection must be used on all general-use and patient-controlled analgesia infusion pumps. Alarms should be tested regularly and are to be activated with appropriate settings, and be sufficiently audible at all times an infusion pump in use. Although important for any intravenous infusion, an alarm system is vitally important when TPN is being administered.

NURSING MANAGEMENT

Assessment (Data Collection)

First, assess the patient for risk of fluid, electrolyte, or acid-base imbalance. Then assess for physical signs and symptoms of alterations in normal balance. Question the patient about subjective signs and symptoms (Focused Assessment 3–1).

Box 3–8 ***Principles for Administration of Total Parenteral Nutrition (TPN)***

- Placement of a central venous catheter must be verified by x-ray before beginning the infusion of the TPN solution.
- Use an infusion pump to administer TPN solution; start infusion slowly at first and increase to desired rate over a 24-hour period.
- If solution is administered cyclically (e.g., at night only), taper to the desired flow over 1 to 2 hours and taper flow down to 1 to 2 hours before completion.
- Check the amount actually infusing every 30 to 60 minutes; do not rely solely on the pump functioning accurately.
- Before administering other solutions or drugs through another lumen of the central line, check compatibility with the TPN solution.
- Monitor continuously for signs of complications such as glucose intolerance, infection, fluid volume excess, phlebitis, and sepsis.
- Record the intake and output accurately.
- Never speed up the solution flow rate beyond that ordered even though it falls behind for some reason.

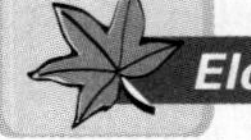

Elder Care Points

Checking for tenting is not an accurate way to assess dehydration in the elderly because their skin loses elasticity with aging and will tent with normal hydration. It is better to check for dry mucous membranes, concentrated urine, and other signs and symptoms in these patients.

Nursing Diagnosis

Using critical thinking, the assessment database is analyzed, problem areas are identified, and nursing diagnoses are chosen. Nursing diagnoses commonly used

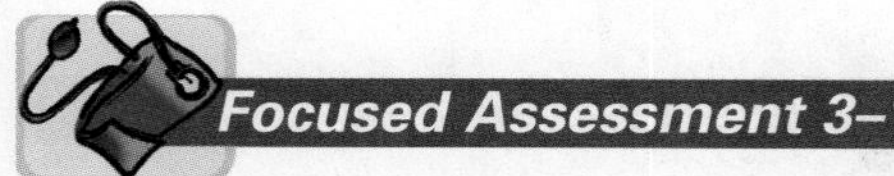

Data Collection for Problems of Fluid, Electrolyte, and Acid-Base Imbalance

Assess the following areas:

CURRENT ILLNESS

Head

- Alertness, orientation, dizziness, signs of confusion, irritability, restlessness
- Appearance of eyes and eyelids
- Condition of oral mucous membranes, tongue, fluidity of saliva

Skin and Extremities

- Color, moisture, temperature, areas of discoloration
- Turgor
- Tightness of rings
- Evidence of and degree of edema
- Strength of handgrip
- Cramping of muscles
- Reflexes
- Chvostek's sign
- Trousseau's sign

Laboratory and Diagnostic Tests

- Hematocrit changes
- Urine amount, color, odor, and specific gravity
- Electrolyte values
- Blood gas values
- Electrocardiogram T-wave changes

Vital Signs

- Blood pressure changes
- Pulse rate, rhythm, and character
- Temperature
- Respirations
- Change in weight

Lungs

- Breath sounds (any crackles?)

INTAKE AND OUTPUT

KNOWN DISEASE CONDITIONS

MEDICATIONS

---

for patients with fluid, electrolyte, or acid-base imbalances are:

- Deficient fluid volume
- Excess fluid volume
- Risk for imbalanced fluid volume
- Ineffective tissue perfusion
- Decreased cardiac output
- Impaired gas exchange
- Ineffective breathing pattern
- Risk for injury related to IV fluid administration

Other nursing diagnoses may be appropriate as a result of the fluid, electrolyte, or acid-base imbalance or may be related to the cause of the imbalance, for example, diarrhea.

Planning

Collaboration with the patient and family or caregiver allows the best plan to be devised. Priorities of care are set. The goal is to restore the patient's fluid, electrolyte, or acid-base balance. Individual expected outcomes are written as appropriate. Expected outcomes might be:

- Patient will exhibit normal skin turgor.
- Patient's weight will stabilize at normal baseline.
- Intake and output will be balanced.
- Blood gases will return to normal.
- Breath sounds will be clear to auscultation.
- There will be no evidence of edema.
- Electrolyte values will be within normal limits.
- Patient will not experience complications of IV therapy.

A specific time frame would be incorporated into the expected outcome. Nursing interventions are chosen to help the patient achieve the outcomes. Nursing Care Plan 3–1 presents examples of expected outcomes and nursing interventions.

Implementation

When patients are unable to take in sufficient fluids on their own, work with the physician to provide adequate fluid and electrolytes. If patients can swallow and retain fluid, assist them frequently with taking small amounts of fluid. Establish a plan for assisting with both hot and cold liquid consumption. With conscientious care, the need for IV feeding can be avoided. Assessment of what the patient prefers is helpful. In addition to water, fruit juices, bouillon, Popsicles, soft drinks, or Jell-O can be offered.

Think Critically About . . . What type of fluid and electrolyte imbalances is the patient who has intestinal flu and is suffering from both vomiting and diarrhea likely to have?

The patient with a fluid volume excess may have an order for fluid restriction. This means that the patient may have only a certain amount of fluid over a 24-hour period. Work out a schedule of fluid intake so that liquids are spaced evenly and the patient does not receive all the allotted liquids in a short time. A typical schedule would be day, 600 mL; evening, 400 mL; night, 200 mL. If not prohibited, sugarless hard candies and chewing gum can help relieve thirst. Frequent oral care is essential.

Diuretics are often prescribed, particularly when there is a potential for congestive heart failure or pulmonary edema. Daily weight and electrolyte status must be monitored along with intake and output for these patients (Assignment Considerations 3–2).

Skin care is particularly important in preventing a breakdown over an edematous area. The stretched skin is extremely fragile, has a decreased blood supply,

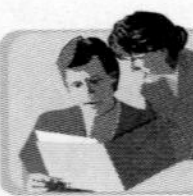

Assignment Considerations 3–2

Obtaining a Daily Weight

When assigning the daily weighing of patients to a nursing assistant or unlicensed assistive personnel (UAP), remind the person that weight should be measured before breakfast, with the patient in essentially the same amount of clothing as at the last measurement, and after voiding. The same scale should be used each day. This provides more reliable data for comparison. Any gain of 2 lb or more over 2 days should be reported to you immediately.

and is no longer flexible. Keep bed linens dry and smooth and turn the patient frequently to relieve pressure over bony prominences. **Be very gentle in repositioning and turning the patient to avoid friction on the skin; use a turning sheet. A break in edematous skin can quickly form a pressure ulcer.**

When acid-base imbalance occurs, control of the underlying disorder is instituted. Blood gases are monitored, and oxygen and electrolytes are administered as needed. Nursing measures to improve pulmonary function are instituted as appropriate.

Think Critically About . . . Your patient has a PaO_2 of 94, pH of 7.32, $PaCO_2$ of 48, and HCO_3^- of 26. What type of acid-base imbalance does he have?

Evaluation

Every 24 hours, evaluation is performed to see if the nursing interventions are assisting the patient to meet expected outcomes. If the patient is not progressing toward achievement of the outcomes, problem solving and critical thinking are used to determine why. The plan of care is altered appropriately. When outcomes are met, that portion of the plan is discontinued.

COMMUNITY CARE

Nurses in long-term care facilities deal every day with the problems of delicate fluid balance in their elderly patients. These patients often are taking multiple drugs that can affect their fluid and electrolyte status. Diuretics in particular can upset fluid and electrolyte status. It is especially important that the long-term care and home care nurse be vigilant for the signs of hypokalemia (see Table 3–4). Potassium imbalances are particularly dangerous for the heart patient. Hypokalemia alters the way digitalis is metabolized in the body and predisposes to digitalis toxicity. Signs of digitalis toxicity are fatigue, anorexia, headache, blurred vision, yellow-green halos around lights, nausea, diarrhea, and cardiac dysrhythmias.

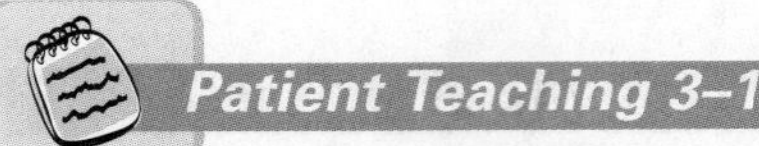

Patient Teaching 3–1

Home Care Intravenous (IV) Therapy

WHEN SHOULD I CALL THE HOME CARE NURSE?

Call the nurse when:

- Swelling, redness, or pain occurs at the IV site or along the vessel.
- The solution will not flow even after you have checked that the clamps are open.
- The solution leaks at the catheter site and you have checked to see that the tubing is firmly attached to the catheter.
- The patient's temperature rises above 100° F (38° C).

Telephone number ____________

Any patient in a long-term care facility or at home who is taking digitalis and is experiencing nausea, vomiting, diarrhea, or fluid and electrolyte alterations should be questioned daily about symptoms of hypokalemia and digitalis toxicity.

Dehydration and hyponatremia secondary to infection or treatment of congestive heart failure account for the majority of hospital admissions of patients from long-term care facilities and home situations. It takes a caring, skillful nurse to see that long-term and home care patients take in enough fluids without interfering with their nutritional intake.

The home care nurse must collaborate with the infusion company nurse when the patient is receiving IV fluids at home or is on TPN. Clear instructions must be given to the patient and family regarding the IV therapy (Patient Teaching 3–1). The elderly patient who has a fluid volume excess from congestive heart failure may already have a diminished appetite. In this instance, restricting sodium in the diet may do more harm than good. The nurse, along with the physician, must make individual judgments about the patient's priority needs.

Key Points

- Fluid balance is essential because the life processes of every cell take place within fluid.
- The infant and the elderly are at greatest risk for fluid imbalance.
- Water has four main functions in the body.
- Body fluids are distributed in intracellular compartments and extracellular compartments.
- Control of fluid balance is managed by hormones and the thirst mechanism.
- Fluids and solutes move within the body by diffusion, filtration, osmosis, and active transport.
- Tonicity refers to the amount of solutes in relation to the amount of fluid.
- Filtration occurs through a semipermeable membrane.
- Hydrostatic pressure causes filtration of fluid out of the intravascular system into the interstitial spaces.
- Water diffuses by osmosis.

- Diffusion moves water from the interstitial spaces into the cells.
- The kidney is a major factor in the regulation of fluid and electrolyte balance in the body.
- Fluid may be lost from the body in many ways (see Table 3–1).
- Fluid volume deficit may occur due to fluid losses or because of lack of fluid intake.
- A fluid deficit causes dehydration.
- Checking skin turgor is one way to assess for dehydration.
- Check the tongue and mucous membranes of the elderly to assess for dehydration.
- Weight change is the most accurate measure of fluid gain or loss.
- Fluid deficit is a common problem in the elderly.
- Electrolytes need to be replaced along with fluid when there has been a fluid deficit.
- Nausea, vomiting, and diarrhea are causes of fluid deficit.
- Prolonged vomiting leads to sodium and potassium deficits and metabolic alkalosis.
- Position the vomiting patient so that aspiration of vomitus does not occur.
- Rehydrate the elderly dehydrated patient cautiously so that overhydration does not occur.
- There are a variety of causes of vomiting and diarrhea.
- Medications help stop vomiting and diarrhea (see Table 3–2).
- Fluid volume excess leads to hypervolemia, edema, and possible pulmonary edema.
- Assessment will reveal elevated blood pressure and a full, bounding pulse.
- Edema may be localized or general; pitting edema may occur.
- Loss of plasma proteins may cause edema.
- When fluid shifts from the intravascular space to the interstitial spaces, hypovolemia may occur.
- With fluid excess, sensorium may be clouded.
- Edema may be treated with diuretic medications, a low-sodium diet, and elastic stockings or sequential compression devices.
- A nurse must know normal ranges for the major electrolytes in the body (see Table 3–3).
- Electrolytes are responsible for the transmission of nerve impulses, contraction of muscles, and excretion of hormones.
- The nurse must be familiar with the signs and symptoms of electrolyte imbalances (see Table 3–4).
- Urine output must be at least 30 mL/hr before IV potassium is given.
- Intravenous potassium is always diluted and never given as a bolus injection.
- Most functions of the body require a slightly alkaline environment.
- Acid-base imbalances upset the normal function of the body's systems.
- The kidneys are the principal organ in controlling a normal pH; the lungs also assist.
- Too much carbonic acid in the body causes acidosis; too much bicarbonate in the body causes alkalosis.
- Maintenance of acid-base balance is a very complex process.
- Changes in carbon dioxide are usually respiratory; changes in bicarbonate are usually metabolic.
- Diabetic ketoacidosis causes metabolic acidosis and can be life threatening.
- Arterial blood gases are analyzed to determine if there is an acid-base imbalance and to see what type of imbalance is present.
- Each acid-base imbalance has its own signs and symptoms and probable treatments.
- Every ill patient should be assessed for a fluid, electrolyte, and acid-base imbalance.
- Intravenous therapy can provide the patient with fluid, electrolytes, and nutrients.
- Intravenous fluids are isotonic, hypotonic, or hypertonic.
- There are many nursing responsibilities in administering intravenous therapy (see Box 3–5).
- Intravenous therapy must be administered in a strict aseptic manner.
- The five rights should be used when administering any IV fluid or drug.
- Monitoring for complications of IV therapy is a top priority (see Table 3–7).
- Rate of IV flow must be monitored closely; never rely solely on an IV pump.
- The elderly can become fluid overloaded very quickly.
- Follow agency procedure for flushing PRN locks and central lines.
- Subcutaneous infusion is mostly used for pain control.
- Total parenteral nutrition is utilized when a patient cannot obtain adequate nutrition by other means.

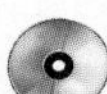

Go to your **Companion CD-ROM** for an Audio Glossary, animations, video clips, and bonus review questions.

evolve Be sure to visit the companion Evolve site at http://evolve.elsevier.com/deWit for interactive NCLEX-PN Exam Style Review Questions, WebLinks, and additional online resources.

NCLEX-PN EXAM STYLE REVIEW QUESTIONS

Choose the best answer(s) for the following questions.

1. Spironolactone (Aldactone) 50 mg orally daily has been prescribed for a patient. Based on the nurse's understanding of the mechanism of action of this medication, appropriate nursing action would include which of the following:

1. monitoring for hypokalemia.
2. reducing dietary intake of salt substitutes.
3. supplementing meals with vitamin D.
4. encouraging fluid intake.

2. The nurse is gathering data regarding the patient's risk for fluid volume deficit. Which of the following factors put the patient at additional risk?
   1. Liver failure
   2. Viral gastroenteritis
   3. Lymph node dissection
   4. Protein-calorie malnutrition

3. The nurse appropriately elicits a sign of hypercalcemia by:
   1. tapping the face about 1 inch from the earlobe.
   2. palpating a partially stretched tendon.
   3. inspecting facial symmetry.
   4. applying pressure on the radial pulse.

4. An elderly female is in the emergency department for severe anxiety. Her respirations are 30 per minute with deep excursions. She is pale with spasms of the hands. The patient most likely manifests signs and symptoms of:
   1. hypercalcemia.
   2. respiratory alkalosis.
   3. dehydration.
   4. hyperparathyroidism.

5. Which of the following patients are considered at high risk for fluid and electrolyte imbalance? *(Select all that apply.)*
   1. A 45-year-old woman with thyroid crisis
   2. A 35-year-old trauma victim on ventilator
   3. A 60-year-old woman with temperature of 98.6° F (37° C)
   4. A 70-year-old man on anticoagulant therapy
   5. A 30-year-old woman complaining of persistent diarrhea

6. While taking the clinical history, the female patient who was admitted for severe gastroenteritis starts vomiting. An appropriate nursing action would include the following, except to:
   1. have the patient lie down on her back.
   2. encourage mouth breathing.
   3. turn head toward one side.
   4. wipe patient's face and back with a cool damp washcloth.

7. In planning care for a patient with congestive heart failure, the nurse formulates the nursing diagnosis: Excess fluid volume related to inadequate cardiac output. The nursing diagnosis would mostly likely be evidenced by which of the following signs or symptoms?
   1. Temperature of 101.5° F (38.6° C)
   2. Hematocrit 35%
   3. Fine crackles in the lung sounds
   4. Clear yellow urine

8. Which of the following would be most accurate in monitoring effective fluid resuscitation in a patient with severe dehydration?
   1. Weight
   2. Urine output
   3. Respirations
   4. Serum sodium

9. An elderly man is admitted for severe disorientation, confusion, and general weakness. His spouse reports that the patient is not able to tolerate any food or fluids and has had several episodes of vomiting and diarrhea. The patient is most likely to have:
   1. hypokalemia.
   2. metabolic acidosis.
   3. hyponatremia.
   4. respiratory alkalosis.

10. The nurse responds to a patient complaining of pain, burning, and wetness over the peripheral intravenous site. On assessment, the nurse finds that the intravenous insertion site is tender and cool to touch. These are signs and symptoms of:
    1. phlebitis.
    2. infiltration.
    3. infection.
    4. venous spasm.

CRITICAL THINKING ACTIVITIES  *Read each clinical scenario and discuss the questions with your classmates.*

Scenario A

Mrs. Thompson, age 64, is admitted to the hospital for congestive heart failure. She is very edematous. She is slightly confused upon admission, and although she is not on absolute bed rest, she tells you she is too weak to get out of bed.

1. What type of diet would you expect the physician would order for Mrs. Thompson? Why?
2. Why are daily weights ordered for Mrs. Thompson, and why are those data important?
3. Mrs. Thompson is on fluid restrictions. How would you schedule her fluid intake?

Scenario B

Mr. Mendez, age 76, is admitted with dehydration and diarrhea. He is confused and listless.

1. What parameters would you assess to see if his fluid balance is improving?
2. What electrolyte imbalances would you expect to find?
3. Why would you need to keep a close eye on Mr. Mendez's IV that is ordered?
4. What acid-base imbalance is he likely to be experiencing?
5. What assessment data would tell you that Mr. Mendez's plan of care is working to rebalance his fluid and electrolytes?

CHAPTER

4 Care of Preoperative and Intraoperative Surgical Patients

evolve http://evolve.elsevier.com/deWit

Objectives

Upon completing this chapter, you should be able to:

Theory

1. Discuss the advantages of current technological advances in surgery.
2. Identify the types of patients most at risk for surgical complications, and state why each patient is at risk.
3. Explain the preparation of patients physically, emotionally, and psychosocially for surgical procedures.
4. Plan and implement patient and family teaching to prevent postoperative complications.
5. Analyze the differences in the various types of anesthesia and list the advantages and disadvantages to the surgeon and the patient.
6. Compare the roles of the scrub nurse and the circulating nurse.

Clinical Practice

1. Perform a thorough nursing assessment for a preoperative patient.
2. Teach the patient postoperative exercises during the preoperative period.
3. Prepare a patient for surgery using a preoperative check list.
4. Administer preoperative medications.
5. Document preoperative care and assessment data.
6. Observe during a patient's surgery.

Key Terms

Be sure to check out the bonus material on the Companion CD-ROM, including selected audio pronunciations.

anesthesia (ăn-ĕs-THĒ-zē-ă, p. 85)
atelectasis (ă-tē-LĔK-tă-sĭs, p. 73)
autologous (aw-TŎL-ō-gŭs, p. 69)
capnography (kăp-NŎG-ră-fē, p. 86)
dehiscence (dē-HĬS-ĕntz, p. 73)
palliative (p. 68)
perioperative (pĕr-ē-OP-ĕr-ă-tĭv, p. 69)
pneumonia (nū-MŌ-nē-ă, p. 73)
prosthesis (prŏs-THĒ-sĭs, p. 71)
robotics (rō-bŏ-tĭks, p. 67)
stasis (STĀ-sis, p. 77)
thrombophlebitis (thrŏm-bō-flĕ-BĪ-tĭs, p. 77)

REASONS FOR SURGERY

Surgery is performed for a variety of reasons (Table 4–1). No matter what type of surgery the patient is undergoing, it is a serious event. Knowing terminology specific to surgical procedures will help you to envision what the patient will undergo (Box 4–1).

Laparoscopic and endoscopic procedures have taken the place of many "open" surgeries in which a large incision is necessary. Minimally invasive laparoscopic surgery (done through small openings in the abdomen) can be performed more quickly, with less trauma to tissue, resulting in less inflammatory response and therefore less pain. There is a quicker recovery time for the patient as well. Laparoscopic cholecystectomy has reduced time off work for gallbladder removal from 6 weeks down to approximately 1 week.

Surgery may be performed as a same-day or outpatient procedure or an inpatient procedure in a hospital or surgery center. Minor surgery is often performed in a physician's office. Preparation for surgery is usually begun before admission. The patient has diagnostic tests done in the days just before the scheduled surgery. The ability to deliver and reinforce teaching for postoperative and home care is crucial to the well-being and quick recovery of patients.

TECHNOLOGICAL ADVANCES IN SURGERY

Surgeries are being transmitted via videoconferencing to locations around the world to enhance capabilities and skill levels of surgeons everywhere. Now that endoscopic surgery, which uses an instrument to visualize interior structures of the body, as well as the use of operating microscopes and lasers, is commonplace in the surgical suite, robots have entered the operating room. **Robotics** (design of computerized, mechanical instruments) is seen as a key to less invasive, less trau-

Table 4–1 Selected Categories of Surgical Procedures

CATEGORY	DESCRIPTION	CONDITION OR SURGICAL PROCEDURE
REASONS FOR SURGERY		
Diagnostic	Performed to determine the origin and cause of a disorder or the cell type for cancer	Breast biopsy Exploratory laparotomy Arthroscopy
Curative	Performed to resolve a health problem by repairing or removing the cause	Laparoscopic cholecystectomy Mastectomy Hysterectomy
Restorative	Performed to improve a patient's functional ability	Total knee replacement Finger reimplantation
Palliative	Performed to relieve symptoms of a disease process, but does not cure	Colostomy Nerve root resection Tumor debulking Ileostomy
Cosmetic	Performed primarily to alter or enhance personal appearance	Liposuction Revision of scars Rhinoplasty Blepharoplasty
URGENCY OF SURGERY		
Elective	Planned for correction of a nonacute problem	Cataract removal Hernia repair Hemorrhoidectomy Total joint replacement
Urgent	Requires prompt intervention; may be life threatening if treatment is delayed more than 24–48 hours	Intestinal obstruction Bladder obstruction Kidney or ureteral stones Bone fracture Eye injury Acute cholecystitis
Emergent	Requires immediate intervention because of life-threatening consequences	Gunshot or stab wound Severe bleeding Abdominal aortic aneurysm Compound fracture Appendectomy
DEGREE OF RISK OF SURGERY		
Minor	Procedure without significant risk; often done with local anesthesia	Incision and drainage (I&D) Implantation of a venous access device (VAD) Muscle biopsy
Major	Procedure of greater risk, usually longer and more extensive than a minor procedure	Mitral valve replacement Pancreas transplant Lymph node dissection
EXTENT OF SURGERY		
Simple	Only the most overtly affected areas are involved in the surgery	Simple/partial mastectomy
Radical	Extensive surgery beyond the area obviously involved; is directed at finding a root cause	Radical prostatectomy Radical hysterectomy

From Ignatavicius, D.D., & Workman, M.L. (2005). *Medical-Surgical Nursing: Critical Thinking for Collaborative Care* (5th ed.). Philadelphia: Elsevier Saunders, p. 295.

matic surgeries in the future. The robot is operated from a nearby computer while the surgeon views magnified three-dimensional images of the surgical field on the computer's screen. The robot's tiny camera has multiple lenses that allow magnification up to 12 times that of normal vision. There are assistants and a second surgeon next to the patient, but the primary surgeon performs the surgery at the computer. For heart surgery, the robot's needle-like "fingers" are introduced through pencil-sized holes in the chest to perform certain heart surgery techniques. Remote-controlled instruments are inserted through small incisions. A big advantage of using the robot is that it has "rock-steady" hands, providing precision that is beyond human dexterity. Because only small incisions are needed, the patient has less pain postoperatively and requires less time to heal. There is less scarring, and fewer infections develop with this new surgical technique.

One of the most recent innovations in robotics is Penelope, the Surgical Instrument Server (SIS). This robot functioned in June 2005 at New York Presbyte-

Box 4–1 Terminology Used for Surgical Procedure

Suffixes are often attached to a stem word to describe a surgical procedure. For example, appendectomy *means cutting out the appendix.*

- -ectomy: Cutting out or off (col*ectomy:* cutting out a part of the colon)
- -lysis: Removal or destruction of (neuro*lysis:* freeing a nerve from adhesions)
- -oma: Tumor (excision of a fibr*oma:* removal of a connective tissue tumor)
- -ostomy: To furnish with an outlet (col*ostomy:* creating an outlet for the colon from the body)
- -otomy: Cutting into (thorac*otomy:* cutting into the chest cavity)
- -plasty: Revision, molding, or repair of tissue (mammo*plasty:* revision of the breast)
- -pexy: Fixation, anchoring in place (orchio*pexy:* fixation of an undescended testicle in the scrotum)

rian Hospital as an independent surgical assistant by handing and retrieving surgical instruments. It uses voice recognition software and machine vision technology to identify surgical instruments and to hand them to surgeons as they ask for them, and to retrieve the instruments and place them back on the instrument table. Penelope is expected to be a common part of the surgical team within 5 years.

AUTOLOGOUS BLOOD FOR TRANSFUSION

Since the mid-1980s, patients undergoing elective surgery have had the option of donating their own blood prior to surgery in case a transfusion is needed during or after surgery. The blood is withdrawn at the blood bank several weeks before the surgery, prepared, and stored for future transfusion to the patient. This is called an **autologous** (related to self) transfusion. The ability to do this has greatly decreased the anxiety of many patients who feared transfusion with blood that might possibly be contaminated with a blood-borne virus, such as human immunodeficiency virus or hepatitis B or C. Cell savers are used to collect and salvage blood during and after surgery, and that blood can be reinfused if the patient needs it.

BLOODLESS SURGERY

Many patients are opting for bloodless surgery these days. This means that they may not want the risk that is inherent in a blood transfusion. A combination of techniques to minimize blood loss and maximize blood volume and function are used. Epoetin alfa (Epogen, Procrit) may be given to stimulate red blood cell production 3 weeks before surgery. Anemic patients may be treated with hyperbaric oxygen preoperatively to improve cell oxygenation. Hemostatic agents may be given before or during surgery to promote clotting. During surgery, the surgeon may request induced hypotension or hypothermia to decrease oxygen demand. Hemodilution, in which several units of the patient's blood are removed and replaced with crystalloids or colloids to expand vascular volume, is another technique. This method decreases blood viscosity, improving oxygen transport, and, if bleeding occurs during surgery, fewer red cells are lost. Autotransfusion from blood collected via a cell saver may be employed. The blood is prevented from clotting, and can be prepared and infused at a later time.

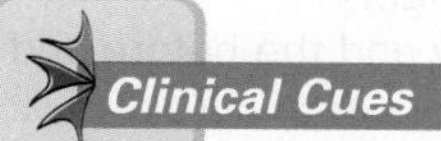

Clinical Cues

Followers of Jehovah's Witness will not accept a blood transfusion from another person because of their religious beliefs. They believe that there are eternal consequences from receiving blood not their own. In the past, this precluded them from having certain major surgeries. Now bloodless surgery is one option for them.

NURSING MANAGEMENT

Perioperative nursing refers to the care of the patient before, during, and after surgery. The nurse plays a key role during this period.

Assessment (Data Collection)

The patient should be in the best possible physical condition before surgery. In emergencies, of course, this cannot be controlled, but planned surgery might be postponed until the patient is physically able to withstand the stress of anesthesia and major surgery. To determine the patient's readiness for surgery, a thorough health assessment is conducted and risk factors are considered. In addition to the admission assessment data that are gathered when the patient is first admitted (refer to Chapter 2), the perioperative nurse gathers data specific to the surgical procedure and postoperative course. Thorough assessment facilitates planning of care during and after surgery (Focused Assessment 4–1).

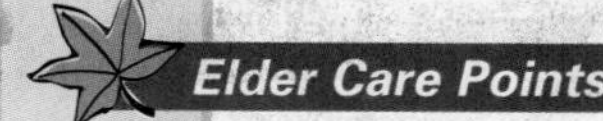

Elder Care Points

Patients over the age of 75 have surgical complication rates three times higher than younger adults. The elderly patient is less able to adjust and compensate for the stress of surgery as physiologic reserves (cardiac, respiratory, renal) have declined. The elderly patient is more likely to have impaired renal, hepatic, respiratory, and cardiac function and chronic diseases that cause patient vulnerability to fluid and electrolyte imbalances during and after surgery.

Any significant deviations from normal range should be brought to the attention of the surgeon. For example, an elevated temperature might indicate an

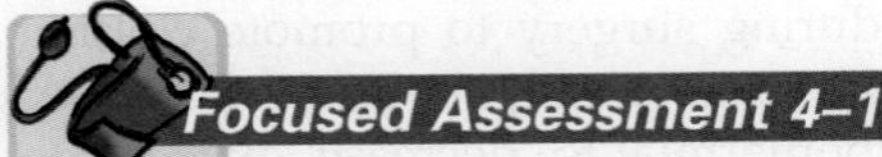

Preoperative Data Collection

In addition to the admission assessment data that are gathered when the patient is first admitted (see Chapter 2), the perioperative nurse gathers data specific to the surgical procedure and postoperative course.

HEALTH HISTORY AND PSYCHOSOCIAL ASSESSMENT

- Have you previously had surgery? What was your experience?
- What is the reason for this surgery?
- How do you feel about having this surgery?
- What do you know about this surgery and the before and after care?
- What are your expectations of this surgery?
- Have you or any family members ever experienced any problems with surgery or anesthesia?
- Will this surgery create any problems in your usual roles or relationships?
- Do you have any chronic illnesses?
- Have you gained or lost considerable weight recently?
- Do you have any allergies to medications, iodine, shellfish, adhesive tape, or latex?
- What medications, over-the-counter preparations, vitamins, herbs, and supplements do you take?
- Do you smoke? How much and for how many years?
- What is your usual use of alcohol?
- When was your last bowel movement?
- Do you have any problems with urination?
- Do you currently have an upper respiratory infection?
- Do you have any musculoskeletal problems that need to be addressed during positioning for surgery?
- Do you have health insurance?
- What people will be able to help you during your recovery?
- Will you be able to cope with inconveniences during your recovery without additional help?
- How do you usually cope with pain?
- Are there any particular concerns or fears that you have regarding the surgery now?

CULTURAL ASSESSMENT

- What is your primary language?
- Do you have any cultural or spiritual practices that you would like to observe during this period of surgery and recovery?
- What are your cultural customs regarding privacy, blood transfusions, and disposal of body parts?

SPIRITUAL ASSESSMENT

- Do you have spiritual or religious beliefs?
- Do you wish to talk with or see your spiritual or religious advisor?
- Is there any conflict between your value or belief system and this planned surgery?

PHYSICAL ASSESSMENT

- Measure height and weight
- Measure vital signs
- Auscultate the lungs and heart
- Listen for bowel sounds
- Check pulses and compare bilaterally
- Gather basic neurologic data: level of consciousness, orientation to time, place, and person; ability to think, answer questions, and follow instructions
- Assess skin status, integrity, moisture, and temperature
- Assess for recent tattoos, piercings, and body jewelry
- Assess for limitations in joint range of motion
- Assess for muscle weakness
- Assess for loose teeth, dentures, bridges, contact lenses, hearing aid, and other prostheses

LABORATORY AND DIAGNOSTIC TEST DATA

- Verify that test results are in the chart
- Note any abnormal findings

infection that would need to be brought under control before surgery. Knowing the patient's usual blood pressure reading is necessary for comparison after surgery when postoperative shock is a concern. Height and weight are measured and charted before surgery so the anesthesiologist can accurately calculate anesthetic dosages. Allergies must be identified and noted on the front of the patient's chart. An allergy bracelet should be located on the patient's arm (Safety Alert 4–1).

Think Critically About . . . Why would a localized infection be a contraindication for surgery in some instances?

Of particular importance is whether or not the patient is taking a corticosteroid. Patients should be questioned about medicines and eyedrops that may contain a corticosteroid. Corticosteroids may delay wound healing, can alter fluid and electrolyte balance, and affect several metabolic functions in the body. Corticosteroids should be tapered slowly before surgery and never stopped abruptly. Vitamin E, aspirin

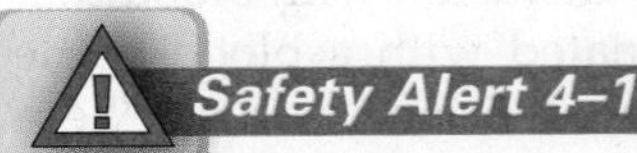

Latex Allergy

The patient who is allergic to latex is at high risk of exposure during surgery when unconscious and unable to monitor the environment. The perioperative nurse must be constantly vigilant to keep anything with latex on it out of the patient's environment. Even rubber stoppers on medication bottles or IV containers can be a problem. The operating room must be prepared to be "latex free." A "latex-free" crash cart is kept at hand in case of emergency.

Complementary & Alternative Therapies 4–1

Herbals and Supplements

Most anesthesiologists will ask patients to discontinue taking herbal supplements 2 to 3 weeks before surgery as many interact with anesthetic agents or interfere with blood clotting and could cause a problem. If doing without a supplement is not possible, the container should be brought to the anesthesiologist.

Black cohosh, St. John's wort, feverfew, goldenseal, valerian, ginger, and ginkgo biloba all can have adverse effects either on clotting mechanisms or by interactions with other medications and anesthetics. It is best to stop all herbals before surgery.

---

and other nonsteroidal anti-inflammatory drugs, and anticoagulants have a continuing effect on blood clotting for several days, and are usually discontinued 3 to 7 days before surgery (Complementary & Alternative Therapies 4–1).

Nutritional status and body weight are significant factors in healing and repair of the surgical site. Obesity presents problems related to such routine procedures as venipuncture and intubation for general anesthesia, and causes prolonged uptake of anesthetic drugs.

The operating room personnel are notified if the patient is hard of hearing, is essentially blind when glasses are not in place, or has a **prosthesis** (artificial body part).

The news that surgery is needed usually comes as an emotional shock to patients and their families. The changes it brings about in the routine of their lives will naturally place some personal and financial burdens on them (Cultural Cues 4–1). For some patients the surgery will alter their lives permanently and possibly leave them physically impaired in some way. Others might expect to be greatly helped by the surgical procedure. In any event, there will be some fears and misgivings about the prospect of undergoing anesthesia and surgery. The patient's culture must be considered (Cultural Cues 4–2).

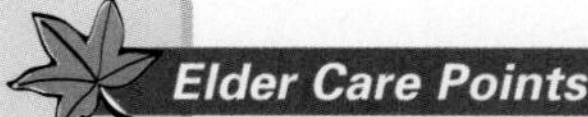

Elder Care Points

Older patients who are experiencing serious depression are at high risk for complications of surgery because their motivation for recovery often is very low.

Determine whether the patient will have adequate help at home when discharged from the hospital. Many older people live alone, and although self-sufficient before surgery, may have difficulty preparing meals, bathing, or performing wound care while recovering from surgery.

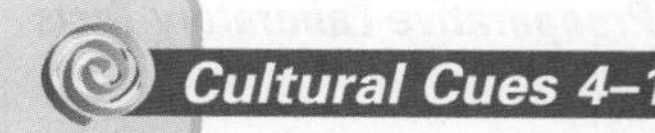

Cultural Cues 4–1

Financial Burden

Many Chinese do not purchase health insurance. Any hospitalization, and more so a major surgery, may bring considerable financial hardship to the family.

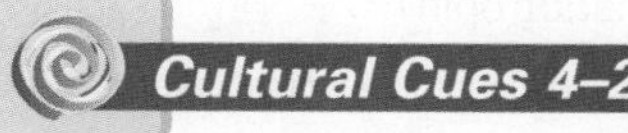

Cultural Cues 4–2

Beliefs Regarding Surgery

Cultural beliefs and values regarding surgery must be taken into consideration. If the patient does not speak the same language as the surgical team, an interpreter should be enlisted to assist with communication. If a female patient's culture has strict rules for female attire, she needs assurance of sufficient privacy and protection of modesty to allay any fears she might have. Such issues and interventions must be conveyed to the surgical team. If there are certain cultural taboos regarding an aspect of the surgery, the surgical team needs to know them and plan a way to achieve a good outcome without violating such a taboo. It is especially important to know whether the patient will accept a blood transfusion.

Some people are concerned about whether they will "wake up" or survive the anesthesia and surgical procedure. Some patients have the strong spiritual belief that they need to cope with sickness, suffering, and death. Others may need help in finding the spiritual support they need. Still others do not want to discuss this particular facet of their lives. Allow time with clergy or a spiritual advisor before the procedure per the patient's desire.

Laboratory and Diagnostic Test Data

Box 4–2 lists the most frequently required tests before surgery. A chest radiograph is usually obtained, and an electrocardiogram is ordered for many patients over 40 years of age. If the patient has lung disease, pulmonary function tests may be ordered. If the laboratory reports indicate any abnormal values, surgery may be postponed. Most surgeons prefer to wait on surgery if a patient's hemoglobin level is below 10 g/dL.

? *Think Critically About . . .* Why would anemia make a patient a poor surgical risk?

Surgery puts a strain on the cardiovascular, renal, and respiratory systems. Liver function is important because the liver is involved in synthesizing clotting factors, producing albumin, and metabolizing and

Box 4–2 Commonly Ordered Preoperative Laboratory Tests

- Complete blood count (CBC)
- Urinalysis (UA)
- Blood glucose*
- Electrolytes
- Prothrombin time (PT)
- Partial thromboplastin time (PTT)
- Blood type and crossmatch
- Liver function tests (AST, ALT, bilirubin)*
- Renal function tests (BUN, creatinine)*
- Beta-human chorionic gonadotropin†

Key: *ALT,* alanine aminotransferase; *AST,* aspartate aminotransferase; *BUN,* blood urea nitrogen.
*May be ordered as part of a metabolic panel or sequential multiple assay (SMA)-6 or SMA-12.
†To check for pregnancy in women of childbearing age.

detoxifying drugs. Although requesting preoperative diagnostic tests is the responsibility of the physician, you will need to explain to the patient why these tests have been ordered.

Assessment of Surgical Risk Factors

Carefully assess the patient before surgery for risks of complications. The infant and the elderly person are at higher risk for complications of surgery due to either immature body systems or a decline in function of various body systems. Maintaining core body temperature is one concern when caring for these patients. Table 4–2 summarizes a variety of factors that impose an added risk during surgery or for postoperative complications.

> *Think Critically About . . .* What points would you make when explaining to a patient how smoking is harmful to the surgery patient?

Assessment of Learning Needs

There is some general information the surgical patient should have about what will be happening immediately before, during, and after surgery (Patient Teaching 4–1). There also are specific preventive measures to be learned. Instruction in these and other pre- and postoperative procedures is discussed later in the Implementation section. If it is expected that members of the family or supportive friends will assist the patient during the postoperative period, they need to be included in teaching sessions as well.

Nursing Diagnosis

Nursing diagnoses in the preoperative stage include actual and potential problems based on your assessment. Examples of common nursing diagnoses are as follows:

- Anxiety related to the surgical experience and outcome
- Fear related to risk for death, effects of impending surgery, or loss of control due to anesthesia
- Grieving related to impending loss of a body function or body part
- Deficient knowledge related to preoperative and postoperative routines
- Insomnia related to stress or unfamiliar environment
- Ineffective coping related to lack of problem-solving skills or adequate support
- Ineffective role performance related to inability to care for children during hospitalization or perform job duties

Each diagnosis is supported by data obtained during the nursing assessment.

Planning

Specific expected outcomes will be written for each nursing diagnosis (Nursing Care Plan 4–1). However, there are general *nursing goals* for all preoperative patients. The expectation is that the patient will be:

- Prepared for surgery physically and emotionally
- Able to demonstrate deep breathing, coughing, and leg exercises
- Able to verbalize understanding of the procedure and the expectations of her in the postoperative period
- Able to maintain fluid and electrolyte balance throughout the perioperative period

When preoperative patients are assigned, you must plan your work for the shift carefully to have the patients ready for surgery without neglecting the needs of other assigned patients.

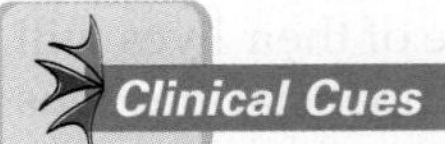

At the beginning of the shift, check to see that all preoperative medications are on hand. Check the surgery schedule and estimate the time needed to prepare the patient for surgery. If preoperative medications are ordered, calculate the dosages of preoperative medications ahead of time so that you will be prepared to quickly draw them up when the call comes from the operating room (OR) nurse to "pre-op" the patient.

Implementation

Preoperatively your time is divided between preparing the patient for surgery and teaching about what will happen and how to hasten recovery. The same-day surgery patient receives teaching from the physician's office nurse or a surgical intake nurse. Teaching sessions may be scheduled when the patient comes for diagnostic testing. Sending written instructions home with the patient reinforces what has been taught. The patient should be given a phone number to call for answers to questions that arise before entering the hospital for surgery. Protocol may differ from one facility to another.

Table 4–2 ***Surgical Risk Factors***

FACTOR	KEY POINTS
Diabetes mellitus and other chronic diseases	Stress of surgery may cause swings in blood glucose levels that are difficult to control. Patient may receive intravenous insulin during and after surgery. Wound healing tends to be delayed in the diabetic patient, making the risk of **dehiscence** greater. There is a higher incidence of infection in surgical wounds in diabetic patients. Liver and kidney disease make it more difficult to metabolize and eliminate anesthesia and waste products.
Advanced age with inactivity	Healing is slower in elderly patients. The risk of disuse syndrome, hypostatic **pneumonia**, and thrombus formation is higher in an inactive elderly person.
Very young person	Infants have difficulty with temperature control and in maintaining normal circulatory blood volume; they are at risk of dehydration.
Malnutrition	Inadequate nutritional stores lead to poor wound healing and skin breakdown.
Dehydration	Reduced circulating volume reduces kidney perfusion and predisposes to a reduced urine output and thrombus formation. Dehydration also alters electrolyte values. The dehydrated patient is more at risk for problems with pressure areas during surgery.
Obesity	The extremely heavy patient does not breathe as deeply and is at risk of hypostatic pneumonia. Excessive fatty tissue also is a factor in poor wound healing.
Cardiovascular problems	Patients with hypertension, left ventricular hypertrophy, cardiac dysrhythmias, or history of congestive heart failure are at a higher risk for myocardial infarction from the stresses of surgery and anesthesia.
Peripheral vascular disease	Poor circulation in the extremities predisposes the patient to possible thrombus formation and pressure sores on the lower legs and feet. Antiembolism stockings or devices are generally prescribed for use during and after surgery.
Liver disease	Interferes with normal blood clotting; liver cannot properly detoxify anesthetics and other drugs.
Respiratory disease	Inhaled anesthetics may irritate the respiratory mucosa, creating more secretions. With immobility there is greater probability of accumulated secretions and inflammation of the lungs and bronchial tree. Impaired oxygen–carbon dioxide exchange may cause acid-base imbalance.
Substance abuse or alcohol dependence	May alter reaction to anesthetic agents. Alcohol dependence may cause withdrawal symptoms if the use of alcohol is discontinued abruptly.
Smoking	Causes increased lung secretions from anesthesia and predisposes the patient to **atelectasis** and pneumonia postoperatively. Smokers are more prone to thrombus formation.
Regular use of certain drugs	Aspirin, nonsteroidal anti-inflammatory drugs, and anticoagulants make the patient more prone to excessive bleeding. Corticosteroids reduce the body's response to infection and delay the healing process.
Excessive fear	Stimulates the sympathetic nervous system and causes the release of hormones, causing swings in the body's chemistry and vital signs. Increased muscle tension makes surgery more difficult. Physical manifestations of fear can interfere with achieving the desired state of anesthesia.

Adapted from deWit, S.C. (2005). *Fundamental Concepts and Skills for Nursing* (2nd ed.). Philadelphia: Elsevier Saunders, p. 731.

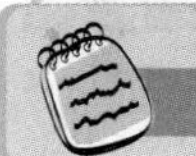

Patient Teaching 4–1

General Preoperative Teaching

General information that almost all surgical patients should receive includes information related to:

- **Preoperative procedures:** Enemas, skin preparation, care of belongings, restriction of food and liquid intake, and administration of bedtime sedatives and preoperative medication; time to come to the hospital
- **Technical information:** Anticipated surgical procedure; location of incisions; dressings, tubes, drains, catheters, or equipment that are expected
- **Day of surgery:** Time surgery is scheduled, time to arrive at hospital or time patient is to leave her room, probable length of procedure, effects of preoperative medications, where family will wait, when and where they can see the patient after surgery, pain control, and postoperative routine
- **Postanesthesia care unit** (PACU): General environment (noise, lights, equipment), frequent taking of vital signs, pulse oximetry, and administration of oxygen
- **Surgical intensive care unit** (SICU) (if patient is to go there from PACU): Location of the unit, expected length of stay, and visiting privileges

NURSING CARE PLAN 4–1

Care of the Patient Scheduled for a Simple Mastectomy

SCENARIO A married 38-year-old woman, the mother of two children ages 16 and 14, is scheduled for a simple mastectomy as treatment for a localized malignant tumor that was detected by self-examination of her breasts.

PROBLEM/NURSING DIAGNOSIS *Cancer diagnosis*/Fear related to cancer, disfigurement, and possible death.
Supporting assessment data *Subjective:* Grandmother died of breast cancer. *Objective:* Malignant tumor by biopsy, crying at intervals; states is worried about husband's reaction to the loss of the breast.

Goals/Expected Outcomes	Nursing Interventions	Selected Rationale	Evaluation
Patient will discuss fears openly by day 2	Establish rapport and trust.	Establishing trust helps patient express fears and concerns.	Spent time with patient answering questions.
Patient will look at incisional area before discharge	Encourage her to discuss fears with nurse and family.	Expressing fears decreases anxiety.	
Patient will identify spiritual support before discharge	Encourage her to think of cancer as a challenge.	A positive perspective empowers the patient.	
Patient will talk about having cancer by postop day 2	Help her to identify specific fears and deal with each one separately.	Decreases the fear of the unknown. Dispelling fear and anxiety makes learning easier.	Stated is afraid of chemotherapy. Is now using the word "cancer" when discussing her surgery. Discussed ways to meet the challenges of chemotherapy.
	Teach relaxation exercises to decrease anxiety.	Relaxation exercises help decrease anxiety.	Expressed willingness to learn a relaxation exercise. Tried relaxation exercises twice.
Patient will join support group for cancer patients after discharge Patient will utilize community resources after discharge	Advise of community resources available to her.		Expressed appreciation for information about a support group.

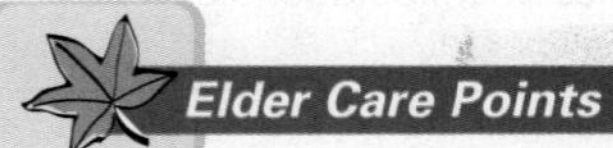

It is particularly important to reinforce instruction and information given to the elderly patient. The anxiety of surgery, unfamiliar surroundings, diminished hearing and vision, and forgetfulness make learning more difficult and may decrease retention of information. Seek specific feedback periodically of points that are important for the patient to remember. Treat all patients with respect and dignity.

Obtaining Consent for Surgery

Before the surgeon can perform an operation, written permission signed by either the patient, her guardian, on whoever holds power of attorney must be obtained. This written consent protects the surgeon against claims of unauthorized surgery and provides the patient an opportunity to exercise her right of *informed consent*. In most hospitals, the "contract" is a printed form that the patient signs before surgery. The correct procedure is written into the contract. The surgeon explains the procedure, risks, and benefits; the nurse only witnesses the patient's signature. The patient must be mentally competent and give consent freely and without coercion. The consent form is attached to the patient's chart and is sent to the operating room (OR) with the patient. **The nurse must always check that a consent form has been signed before giving the preoperative medication** (Legal & Ethical Considerations 4–1). Figure 4–1 shows an example of a standard consent form.

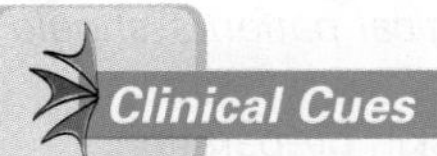

Patients have the right to change their minds and revoke consent up until the time of surgery. If a patient tells you the surgery isn't wanted, delay preoperative preparations and explore the issue with the patient. If it appears the consent for surgery really is being revoked, notify the charge nurse and the surgeon.

NURSING CARE PLAN 4–1

Care of the Patient Scheduled for a Simple Mastectomy—cont'd

PROBLEM/NURSING DIAGNOSIS *Simple mastectomy scheduled*/Knowledge deficit about preoperative routine and postoperative care.

Supporting assessment data *Subjective:* States "I've never had surgery before. What will I need to do?" *Objective:* Puzzled expression on face.

Goals/Expected Outcomes	Nursing Interventions	Selected Rationale	Evaluation
Patient will verbalize understanding of preoperative procedures and requirements before surgery Family will express understanding of what will happen preoperatively, where they will stay during surgery, and what to expect after surgery by end of teaching session	Do preoperative teaching for patient and family: routine procedures, NPO status, expected tubes and drains, equipment to expect in room, probable length of surgery, where family will wait, pain relief measures, handling of arm on operative side, coughing, deep breathing and leg exercises, ambulation, diet, daily postoperative routine.	Knowledge reduces fear of the unknown and anxiety.	Performed return demonstrations and verbalized understanding of routine and procedures. Family verbalized understanding of what to expect.
	Call pastor or chaplain if patient desires a visit.	Clergy can be a positive support in time of stress.	A pastoral visit is scheduled for this afternoon.
	Provide private time for patient and husband and patient and family.	Private time is necessary for serious discussions.	Will have private talk with husband and one with daughters later today. Continue plan.

? CRITICAL THINKING QUESTIONS

1. How would you specifically assess this patient's learning needs?
2. How could you assess for any cultural factors that would affect her learning or your teaching?

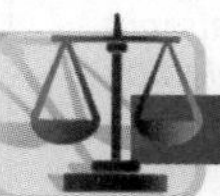

Legal & Ethical Considerations 4–1

Giving Surgical Consent

Mrs. Jones, age 66, was slightly confused due to dehydration when she was brought to the hospital. She has signed a surgical consent for a hip replacement. Her daughter feels she was confused when she signed the form and questions its validity. What would you do? How would the surgeon verify that Mrs. Jones was not confused when she signed the form?

? *Think Critically About . . .* Why should the consent be signed before giving preoperative medication? What happens if a patient has been given the preoperative medication and then it is discovered that the surgical consent form has not been signed?

Restriction of Food and Fluid

Food and fluids will often be restricted for 6 to 8 hours before surgery, and the patient is placed on NPO (nothing by mouth, or *nil per os*) status. A light meal such as toast and clear fluids may be allowed up to 6 hours before surgery and a regular meal may be allowed 8 hours prior to surgery. Clear liquids such as black coffee, tea, apple juice, or carbonated beverages may be consumed up to 2 hours before surgery in some elective cases. Sometimes the surgeon or anesthesiologist will allow an oral blood pressure medication, heart medication, or anticonvulsant to be taken with a sip of water the morning of surgery. Always check the physician's order before giving anything by mouth in the immediate preoperative period. The purpose of the restriction is to prevent nausea, vomiting, and aspiration, which can occur, but is rare with modern anesthesia. Confirm with the patient that the NPO order has been heeded. Insulin may or may not be given; check the orders.

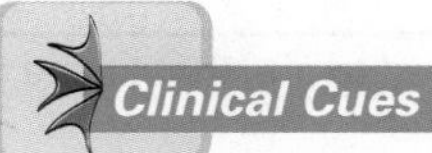

Clinical Cues

If a patient has not remained NPO for the prescribed period, surgery may be cancelled.

Elimination

If the patient is having abdominal or colon surgery, enemas may be ordered to be given until clear. Sometimes GoLYTELY solution is utilized orally instead. The pa-

SPECIAL CONSENT TO OPERATION, POSTOPERATIVE CARE, MEDICAL TREATMENT, ANESTHESIA/SEDATION, OR OTHER PROCEDURE

PATIENT LABEL

1CPROC

Patient ______________________

Patient No. ______________________

State law guarantees that you have both the *right* and *obligation* to make decisions concerning your health care. Your physician can provide you with the necessary information and advice, but as a member of the health care team, you must enter into the decision-making process. This form has been designed to acknowledge your acceptance of treatment recommended by your physician.

1. I hereby authorize Dr. ______________________ and/or such associates or assistants as may be selected by said physician to treat the following condition(s) that has (have) been explained to me. (Explain the nature of the condition[s] in professional and lay language.)

____

____

____

2. The procedures planned for treatment of my condition(s) have been explained to me by my physician. I understand them to be as follows. (Describe procedures to be performed in professional and lay language.)

____

____

____

____

At: ______________________
(NAME OF HOSPITAL OR MEDICAL FACILITY)

3. I recognize that during the course of the operation, post-operative care, medical treatment, anesthesia/sedation, or other procedure unforeseen conditions may necessitate additional or different procedures than those above set forth. I therefore authorize my above named physician, and his or her assistants or designees, to perform such surgical or other procedures as are in the exercise of his, her, or their professional judgment necessary and desirable. The authority granted under this paragraph shall extend to the treatment of all conditions that require treatment and are not known to my physician at the time the medical or surgical procedure is commenced.

4. I have been informed that there are significant risks such as severe loss of blood, infection, and cardiac arrest that can lead to death or permanent or partial disability, that may be attendant to the performance of any procedure. I acknowledge that no warranty or guarantee has been made to me as to result or cure.

IMPORTANT: HAVE PATIENT SIGN FULL OR LIMITED DISCLOSURE BOX AND SIGNATURE LINE AT BOTTOM.

Full Disclosure

I certify that my physician has informed me of the nature and character of the proposed treatment, of the anticipated results of the proposed treatment, of the possible alternative forms of treatment, and the recognized serious possible risks, complications, and the anticipated benefits involved in the proposed treatment and in the alternative forms of treatment, including nontreatment.

____
(PATIENT/OTHER LEGALLY RESPONSIBLE PERSON SIGN IF APPLICABLE)

Limited Disclosure

I certify that my physician has explained to me that I have the right to have clearly described to me the nature and character of the proposed treatment, the anticipated results of the proposed treatment, the alternative forms of treatment, and the recognized serious possible risks, complications, and anticipated benefits involved in the proposed treatment, and in the alternative forms of treatment, including nontreatment.
I do not wish to have these risks and facts explained to me.

____
(PATIENT/OTHER LEGALLY RESPONSIBLE PERSON SIGN IF APPLICABLE)

Any sections below which do not apply to the proposed treatment may be crossed out. All sections crossed out must be initialed by both physician and patient.

5. I consent to the administration of anesthesia/sedation by my attending physician, by an anesthesiologist, or other qualified party under the direction of a physician as may be deemed necessary. I understand that all anesthetics involve risks of complications and serious possible damage to vital organs such as the brain, heart, lung, liver, and kidney and that in some cases may result in paralysis, cardiac arrest, and/or brain death from both known and unknown causes. I understand there is a risk of dental injury during airway management.

6. I consent to the use of transfusion of blood and blood products as deemed necessary, and potential complications associated with this procedure have been explained to me by my physician.

7. Any tissues or parts surgically removed may be disposed of by the hospital or physician in accordance with accustomed practice.

I certify this form has been fully explained to me, that I have read it or have had it read to me, that the blank spaces have been filled in, and that I understand its contents.

DATE ______________ TIME ______________ A.M. P.M.

____
PATIENT/OTHER LEGALLY RESPONSIBLE PERSON SIGN

WITNESS ______________________

____
RELATIONSHIP OF LEGALLY RESPONSIBLE PERSON TO PATIENT

450 4/06

FIGURE 4–1 Surgical consent form. (Courtesy of Southwest Washington Medical Center, Vancouver, WA.)

tient may be on a special soft or liquid diet for the 3 days prior to surgery to decrease the content of the bowel.

Ask the patient to empty the bladder, unless a catheter is in place, just before administering any ordered preoperative sedative medications. The bladder should not be distended when abdominal surgery is performed because of the danger of perforating it. Relaxation induced by medications and anesthesia causes the urge to urinate if the bladder is not empty. The patient is not allowed out of bed to use the bathroom after receiving sedation.

Expected Tubes and Equipment

If a nasogastric tube will be inserted during surgery for postoperative use, explain its purpose, its care, and what it will feel like to the patient. Give an estimate of how long the tube will remain in the stomach. The tube is usually removed when bowel sounds return, and nausea has passed. If surgery has occurred in the stomach or intestinal tract, the tube may remain longer. Explain the function of other tubes such as drains, an intravenous (IV) line, oxygen delivery and monitoring devices, a chest tube, and a urinary catheter, as well as their care and probable duration of use.

Rest and Sedation

It is desirable for the patient to be as well rested as possible prior to surgery so the body is not compromised in meeting the stresses of anesthesia and the surgical procedure. A sedative may be ordered for the patient the night before surgery, but the inpatient often must ask for it. If the patient was admitted the day before surgery, check on her frequently during the night. If the patient awakens and is restless, sit and listen and try to dispel fears, offer a soothing back rub, or give backup sedation as ordered. The patient scheduled for same-day surgery should take the sedative at home and retire early the night before because it may be necessary to arise early to enter the hospital.

Pain Control

Many surgeons will order a patient-controlled analgesia (PCA) pump for their patients postoperatively. If a PCA pump is ordered, patients should receive instruction about the pump and how to operate it prior to surgery. If patients will be receiving injections for pain control, explain that this type of medication is ordered on an as-needed basis every 3 to 4 hours and that they must ask for it. Oral pain medication is usually ordered for every 4 to 6 hours as needed. Explain that asking for the pain medication before the pain becomes severe makes it easier to control the pain level. Teach the patient about the pain scale that is used at the facility and how it is used.

Skin Preparation

The patient may be asked to shower with a special antibacterial cleanser the night or morning before surgery to remove as many microorganisms from the skin as possible. Removing hair from the operative site may be done the morning of surgery either in the patient room or the OR. Explain the process, the area to be prepared, and timing of the preparation to the patient (Figure 4–2). Nail polish is removed so that the pulse oximeter can function correctly when attached to the finger. Makeup is removed; note the presence of permanent makeup on the preoperative checklist. Ask about contact lenses and have them removed as well.

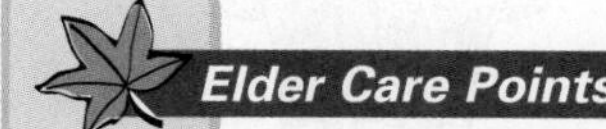

Elder Care Points

The elderly patient should be taught needed information in short segments to prevent confusion and increase the patient's comprehension. Written reminders of the instructions should be given to the patient.

Preoperative Teaching

Teaching the patient correct breathing, coughing, turning, and leg exercises is a high priority during the preoperative period. Venous return is often hampered during the surgical procedure due to the position assumed on the operating table and pooling of blood in the lower extremities. The **stasis** (slowing of flow) of blood places the patient at risk for **thrombophlebitis** (blood clot and inflammation of a vessel). Specific leg exercises help to prevent this complication (Figure 4–3). Explain the importance of doing the exercises and show the patient how to do each one and ask for a return demonstration (Patient Teaching 4–2). One way for patients to remember to do the exercises is to remind them to exercise whenever a commercial comes on if they watch TV. The exercises should be done after surgery at least 5 to 10 times every hour while awake until the patient is up and about normally.

For deep breathing and coughing, it is preferable for the patient to sit up with the back away from the mattress or chair. This allows for full lung expansion. The surgical chest or abdominal incision should be splinted with a pillow (Figure 4–4).

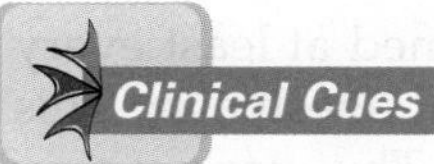

Clinical Cues

A small, firm "coughing pillow" can be made by folding a bath towel or a light blanket and securing it inside a pillow case with the ends tucked inside over the towel or blanket.

It is helpful to have a significant other present for these teaching sessions so that coaching and encouragement can later be given to the patient. Deep breath-

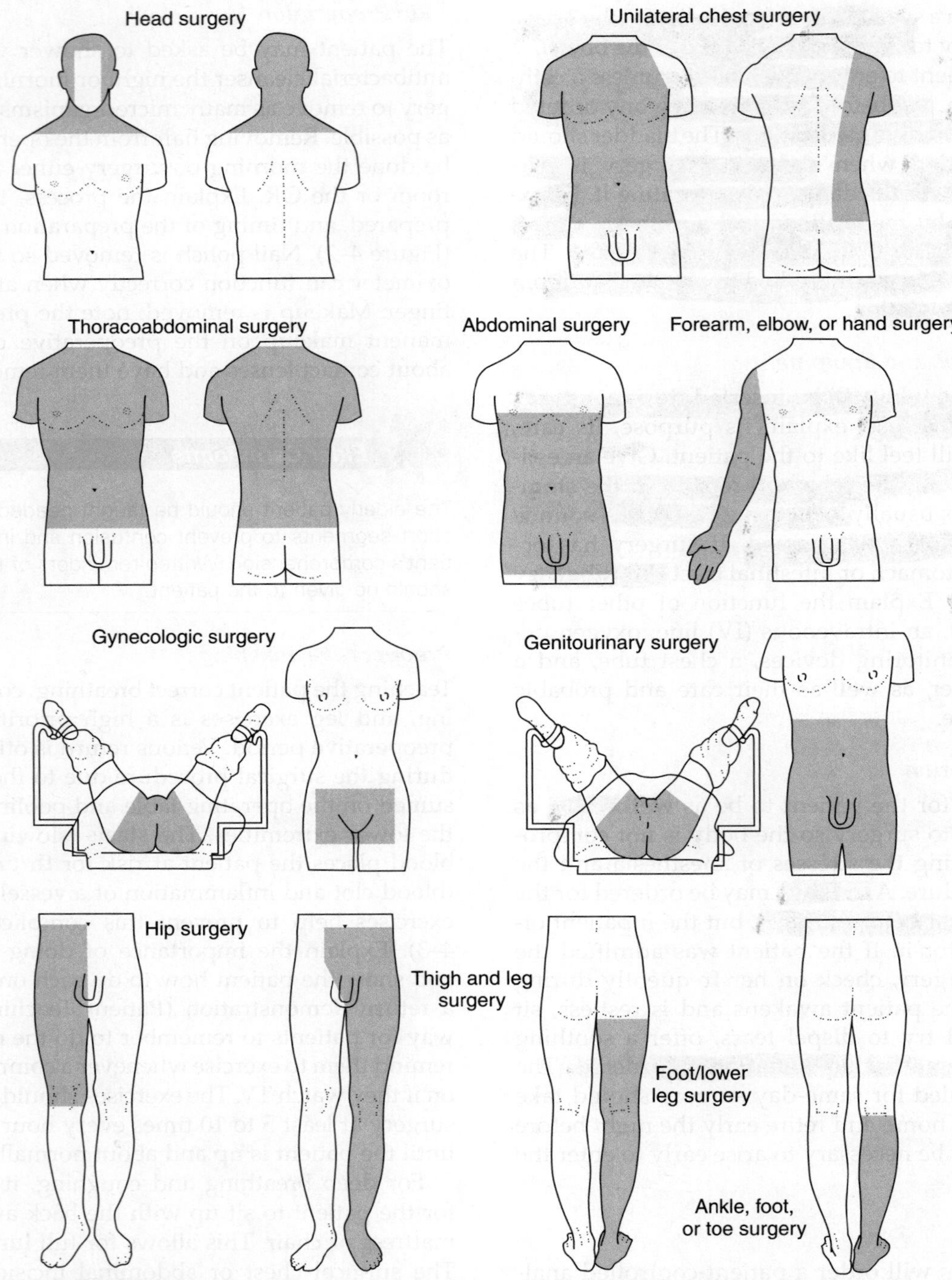

FIGURE 4–2 Skin preparation of common surgical sites. Shaded areas indicate areas of hair removal.

ing and coughing should be performed at least every 2 hours for 3 to 7 days after general anesthesia. This does not require a physician's order. The surgeon may order use of an incentive spirometer. Instruct the patient in its use and supervise until the patient has mastered the technique (Patient Teaching 4–3). Help the same-day surgery patient devise a schedule for doing the exercises.

Show the patient how to turn in bed by flexing the legs to relax the abdominal muscles, placing a pillow between the legs, grabbing on to the side of the bed, and slowly turning to the side. This maneuver is also used for getting up out of bed. The patient is also instructed in what to expect before, during, and after surgery. A trapeze bar for orthopedic patients is very helpful for turning and repositioning.

Family Instructions. The family of the patient scheduled for surgery should be advised to come to the hospital 1 to 1½ hours before surgery. They should be told about the usual routines, where to wait, the approximate time the patient may be expected to return, and what to anticipate in the way of tubes, equipment, and patient appearance after surgery. This knowledge keeps them from thinking the patient has

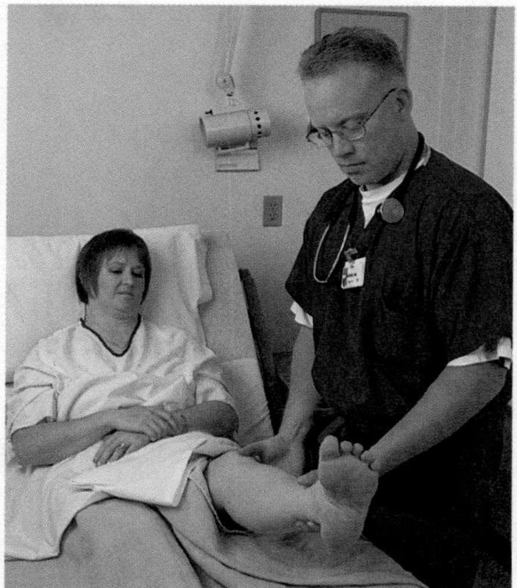

FIGURE 4–3 Teaching foot and leg exercises.

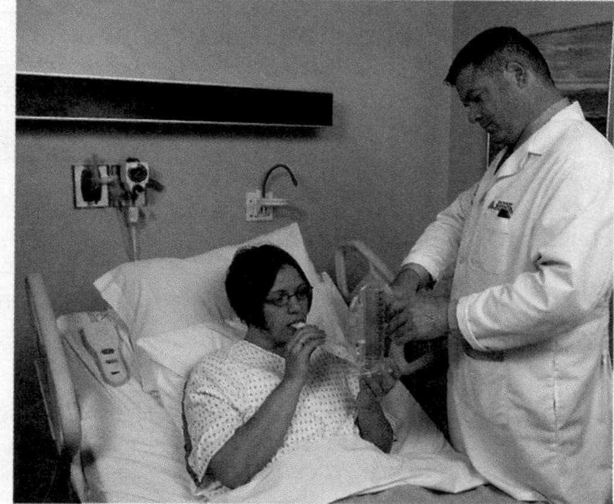

FIGURE 4–4 Teaching deep breathing and coughing while splinting the incision.

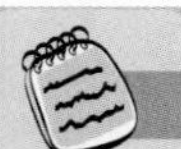

Patient Teaching 4–2

Postoperative Foot and Leg Exercises

- Flex and extend the right foot, moving the toes upward and downward, four or five times.
- Repeat with the left foot.
- Trace circles to the right with the right foot five times; repeat with circles to the left.
- Trace circles to the right with the left foot five times; repeat with circles to the left.
- Bend the right leg at the knee, sliding the foot back toward the buttocks as far as possible; raise the bent leg off the bed, extend the leg and dorsiflex the foot; extend the foot and lower the leg to the bed.
- Bend the left leg at the knee, sliding the foot back toward the buttocks as far as possible; raise the bent leg off the bed, extend the leg and dorsiflex the foot; extend the foot and lower the leg to the bed.
- Tighten the buttocks muscles for a count of 10 and release to exercise the quadriceps muscles.
- Repeat each exercise four more times.

"taken a turn for the worse" when they see the extra equipment for suction, oxygen, or IV therapy in use after surgery. A warning about the occasional delays in starting surgery can keep the family from becoming excessively anxious if the patient is not back at the expected time.

Immediate Preoperative Care

The patient is usually dressed in a clean hospital gown, without underwear, for the operating room. Hair is covered with a surgical paper cap. Long hair should be fixed so that it will tangle minimally; all hairpins and barrettes must be removed. Ask about body piercings and the presence of piercing jewelry, including the tongue and genital areas. Explain why *all* jewelry must be removed for safety due to electro-

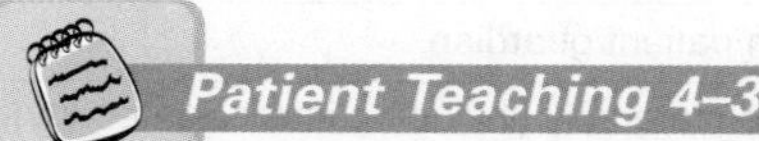

Patient Teaching 4–3

Lung Exercises

Postoperatively you will be asked to deep breathe and cough to open the lungs and clear secretions. Sit up away from the mattress when you do these exercises. The exercises should be performed every 2 hours during waking hours and at night when awakened to measure vital signs.

DEEP BREATHING

- Take a deep breath in through the nose, hold for a few seconds, and slowly exhale.
- Repeat four more times.

FORCED EXHALATION COUGHING

Splint the abdominal or chest incision and:

- Take a deep breath through the nose and cough as you exhale with the mouth open but covered with a tissue.
- If you cannot move secretions with your cough, use a forced exhalation cough.
- Take a deep breath through the nose and forcibly quickly exhale, producing a "huff" cough.
- Repeat the process.
- Repeat again four more times, using three short "huffs" as you exhale to bring the secretions to the mouth, where they can be expectorated.

USING AN INCENTIVE SPIROMETER

- Insert the mouthpiece, covering it completely with the lips.
- Take a slow deep breath and hold it for at least 3 seconds.
- Exhale slowly, keeping the lips puckered.
- Breathe normally for a few breaths.
- Try to increase the inspired volume by at least 100 mL with each breath on the spirometer.
- Once maximal volume is achieved, attempt to inspire this volume 10 times, resting a few breaths in between each attempt.
- Clean the mouthpiece of the spirometer when finished. During the first 3 postoperative days, try to do this every hour.

PREOP/PREPROCEDURE CHECKLIST/REPORT FORM

PATIENT LABEL

1SURG

Date	Time	
Surgery/procedure		YES
Correct patient ID band on		☐
	On chart	☐
	Dictated	☐

History and Physical
H&P 24 hours to 30 days: update with "No Pertinent Change in History & Physical" stamp
H&P 31-180 days: H&P update form #2396
OB H&P Update for Surgery/Procedures form #2543

	YES	N/A
Initiate Anesthesia Preop order 101.S09. As appropriate initiate OB Anesthesia Order 144.P11	☐	
Include at least one page of patient ID stickers	☐	
Procedural consent: Signed/On Chart	☐	
Procedural site verified with patient/guardian	☐	
Procedural site marked when laterality (including internal laterality), multiple structures (fingers, toes, lesions) or multiple levels (spine). Specify site: ______	☐	☐
Preop antibiotic given	☐	☐
Interpreter if needed	☐	☐
HBOC transfer report on chart (when applicable)	☐	☐
Acuscan MAR-LOS custom report on chart (when applicable)	☐	☐

OB ☐ The Department of Social and Health Services consent for sterilization completed and on chart dated ≥ than 30 days prior to procedure (*unless meets exception criteria, listed in Standards of Care Notebook)
☐ Notify anesthesia provider

Diagnostic ☐ Labs on chart ☐ X-rays with patient (when appropriate) ☐ When applicable Glucose: ______/time ______
☐ Type and screen ☐ ECG (when applicable) Blood units available: # ______

Medications/IV ☐ MAR on chart ☐ IV/Saline lock in place ☐ If TPN running, start second peripheral IV site

Belongings	Labeled	With Patient/Family	To OR
Contacts			
Glasses			
Hearing aids R L Both			
Dentures ☐ Upper ☐ Lower ☐ Partial			

Prep ☐ Personal clothing removed ☐ Prep completed
☐ Snap gown ☐ Voided, time: ______ ☐ Foley
☐ Jewelry/body piercings: ☐ None ☐ Taped ☐ Family ☐ Patient registration safe
☐ Preop teaching done Last oral/fluid intake: Time:

Unit based or bedside procedures: FINAL VERIFICATION
☐ Correct patient ☐ Correct side/site ☐ Correct position
☐ Correct procedure ☐ Correct equipment/trays

REPORT USING SBAR: Provide an opportunity to ask and answer questions. Include significant history/special needs.

INITIALS/SIGNATURE IF SIGNATURE PAGE NOT USED

2067 4/06

FIGURE 4–5 Preoperative checklist. (Courtesy of Southwest Washington Medical Center, Vancouver, WA.)

cautery used during surgery and the danger of an electrical burn from conduction of electricity through metal. Jewelry, along with money and credit cards, is given to a significant other to keep or is secured in a valuables envelope and placed under lock and key according to facility policy. If a wedding band is to be worn to surgery, tape the ring to the finger without restricting circulation. Dentures are removed, placed in a labeled cup, and kept in a designated place according to hospital policy. Sometimes the anesthesiologist will order the dentures left in place to facilitate the administration of anesthesia by mask. If a hearing aid is left in place, a very visible note should be placed on the front of the chart cover and it should be noted on the preoperative checklist sheet.

The patient's identification bracelet is checked with the chart for accuracy to avoid any error or mix-up of patients in the operating room. Verify that the procedure site indicated on the surgical consent form is the same as what the patient states. The site will be verified and marked in the preoperative holding area.

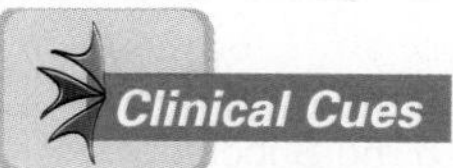

Attend to all items on the preoperative checklist that can be handled ahead of time (Figure 4–5). This prevents hurrying, which can increase mistakes, and prevents delaying administration of the preoperative medications while the list is completed.

Drugs sometimes ordered by injection may include a sedative, an antihistamine-antiemetic, an anticholinergic to decrease secretions, a tranquilizer, and a narcotic analgesic (Table 4–3). A medication to inhibit gastric acid secretion may be administered intravenously. Check that the surgical consent is signed and give any ordered medications on time (Safety Alert 4–2). Ask the patient to empty the blad-

Table 4–3 Commonly Prescribed Preoperative Medications

DRUGS	AVERAGE DOSE	PURPOSES	NURSING IMPLICATIONS
SEDATIVES			
Nembutal sodium Seconal sodium	100 mg IM 90 min before surgery	Decrease anxiety; lower blood pressure and pulse; enhance action of anesthetic	Be alert for opposite effect in certain patients, particularly the elderly, who may become restless and confused. Must be given at precise time ordered.
TRANQUILIZERS			
Thorazine	12.5–25 mg IM up to 2 hr before surgery	Reduce anxiety; promote relaxation	Patient should be confined to bed after injection because of danger of fainting. Sensitive children and adults may exhibit motor restlessness and opisthotonos. Check blood pressure for signs of extreme hypotension.
Hydroxyzine pamoate (Vistaril)	25–50 mg IM	Reduce anxiety and tension; promote relaxation	Raise side rails. Give IM by Z-track method.
Diazepam (Valium)	5–10 mg IM	Reduce tension and anxiety, promote relaxation, decrease muscle spasm	Reduce dosage of narcotics. Monitor respirations.
Lorazepam (Ativan)	Adults: 2–4 mg PO at bedtime	Prevent anxiety and insomnia before surgery	Watch for orthostatic hypotension and dizziness; prevent falls.
Droperidol (Inapsine)	0.22–0.275 mg/kg IM	Promote tranquilization and sleep; prevent nausea and vomiting	Take vital signs 30 min after administration. Assist with ambulation. May need to decrease postoperative analgesia doses until fully metabolized.
Midazolam (Versed)	0.07–0.08 mg/kg IM	Induce drowsiness and relieve apprehension	Moderate sedation; sedation before short-term diagnostic or endoscopic procedures; amnesic effect.

Key: *ac,* (Lat. *ante cibum*) before meals; *IM,* intramuscular; *IV,* intravenous; *PO,* oral.

Continued

Table 4–3 Commonly Prescribed Preoperative Medications—cont'd

DRUGS	AVERAGE DOSE	PURPOSES	NURSING IMPLICATIONS
Drying Agents			
Atropine sulfate Scopolamine (Hyoscine)	0.03–0.6 mg IM 0.03–0.6 mg Subcut	Diminish secretions from mucous membranes of mouth and respiratory tract	Do not give to patients with glaucoma. Observe for rash, flushing of skin, and elevated temperature, which are common side effects, particularly in children. Raise bed rails and maintain close supervision of patient who has received scopolamine; may become very drowsy or restless and injure self.
Glycopyrrolate (Robinul)	0.004 mg/kg IM	Diminish secretions; block cardiac vagal reflexes	Contraindicated in glaucoma. Check dosage carefully. Use smaller doses in elderly. Watch for adverse reaction in elderly patients. Monitor for urinary hesitancy.
Analgesics			
Morphine sulfate Meperidine (Demerol)	8–15 mg Subcut 50–100 mg IM	Reduce anxiety; promote relaxation; not necessarily to relieve pain when given preoperatively	Check respiratory rate before giving. Nausea, vomiting, and constipation may result. Observe patient for increased restlessness, tremors, and delirium, which may occur as side effects.
Fentanyl (Sublimaze)	0.7–2 mcg/kg IV q 2–3 min	Moderate sedation, analgesia/anesthesia	Monitor vital signs; observe for rash, urticaria; monitor respiratory function. Keep resuscitative equipment on hand.
Hydromorphone hydrochloride (Dilaudid)	1–6 mg IM/Subcut/IV	Reduce anxiety; promote relaxation	Check vital signs before giving. Raise side rails.
Antiemetics			
Promethazine hydrochloride (Phenergan)	12.5–25 mg IM up to 2 hr before surgery	Prevent nausea and vomiting, sedation, prevent allergic reactions	Watch for hypotension; monitor vital signs.
Ondansetron (Zofran)	4 mg bid	Prevent nausea and vomiting postoperatively	Observe for hypersensitivity reaction. Watch for extrapyramidal symptoms.
Metoclopramide (Reglan)	1–2 mg/kg IV or 10–15 mg PO qid 30 min ac	Antiemetic; promote gastric emptying	Give gum or hard candy for dry mouth if allowed. Monitor mental status. Watch for tardive dyskinesia, especially in the elderly.
Prochlorperazine (Compazine)	5–10 mg IM 1–2 hr prior to anesthesia	Antiemetic; antipsychotic	Monitor respirations closely. Watch for untoward reactions and extrapyramidal symptoms.
Granisetron hydrochloride (Kytril)	1 mg IV	Antiemetic	May affect taste. Watch for headache. Check frequency and consistency of stools.

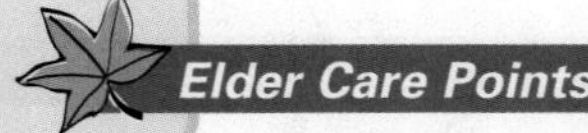

Because of decreasing liver and kidney function that occurs with age, elderly patients, especially those over 75, will need reduced dosages of preoperative narcotics and sedatives. Observe for signs of toxicity.

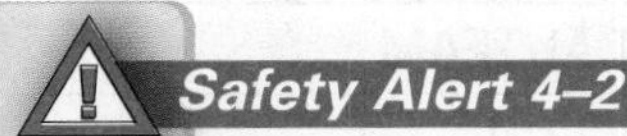

Preventing Falls

If the patient has received a sedative preoperatively, remember to put up the side rails of the bed per facility protocol, and to lower the bed. Remind the patient not to get up without assistance. This is an important patient safety measure after administering sedation.

der before giving medications. Often no medication is given before the patient is in the surgical area.

Preoperative medications may be given for the following reasons:

- To reduce anxiety and promote a restful state (Cultural Cues 4–3)
- To decrease secretion of mucus and other body fluids
- To counteract nausea and reduce emesis
- To enhance the effects of the anesthetic

Assist in transferring the patient to the stretcher when the transport person comes to take the patient to surgery. Compare the patient's identification bracelet name and numbers with the transport request sheet. Check the chart to make certain that everything ordered has been done and complete final documentation.

? *Think Critically About . . .* How would you handle a situation in which a patient scheduled for an abdominal procedure has put back on underwear or jewelry after you finished doing the preoperative checklist?

Preparation of the Patient Unit

While patients are in surgery, prepare the room for their return. Make the bed with fresh linen, including a draw sheet placed between the shoulder and the knee area that can be used as a lift sheet to reposition the patient. For abdominal or perineal surgery, an underpad is placed at the hip area to catch excess drainage. Fan-fold the top covers to the far side of the bed or to the bottom of the bed. Have the bed in a raised

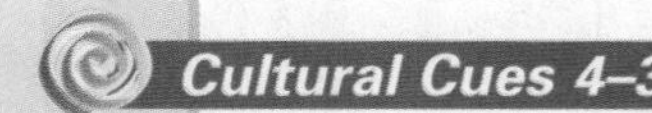

Differences in Drug Metabolism

Asians, and particularly the Chinese, metabolize psychotropic drugs differently than other ethnic groups. Valium causes greater sedation with normal doses. Atropine is also metabolized differently and can greatly accelerate the heart rate. These patients should be monitored closely when receiving these drugs.

position at the height of the stretcher that will return the patient, and arrange furniture so that the stretcher can be pulled up alongside the bed. Place the IV pole at the head of the bed.

Gather an emesis basin, tissues, a frequent vital signs sheet or postoperative record, an intake and output sheet, a small towel and washcloth, and a pen and place them on the bedside table or console (Figure 4–6). Connect oxygen and suction equipment if their need is anticipated. A thermometer, sphygmomanometer, pulse oximeter, and stethoscope should be close at hand upon the patient's return to the unit. If a PCA pump, sequential pneumatic compression devices, or a passive range-of-motion machine will be needed, see that they are obtained and ready.

Evaluation

Evaluation is accomplished by determining if the nursing goals have been met. If the patient is properly prepared for surgery, is kept NPO, is reasonably calm, and is knowledgeable about the procedure and what is expected of her, then the general goals have been met. If the preoperative medications were not given on time or the patient was not ready for transport at the appointed time, then you need to review your steps to see where improvement can occur. Data are gathered to determine if expected outcomes written for individual nursing diagnoses are being met (see Nursing Care Plan 4–1 on p. 74).

INTRAOPERATIVE CARE

In the surgical holding room, the circulating nurse will verify the patient's identification, verify that all preoperative orders have been accomplished, and verify that all relevant documents and diagnostic studies are available. The anesthesia care provider will start an IV line if one is not already in place. The surgical site will be verified and marked if it involves a left/right distinction, multiple structures, or multiple levels as in spinal procedures. When the OR is ready, the patient is transferred to the operating table. Patient identification is verified again by the circulat-

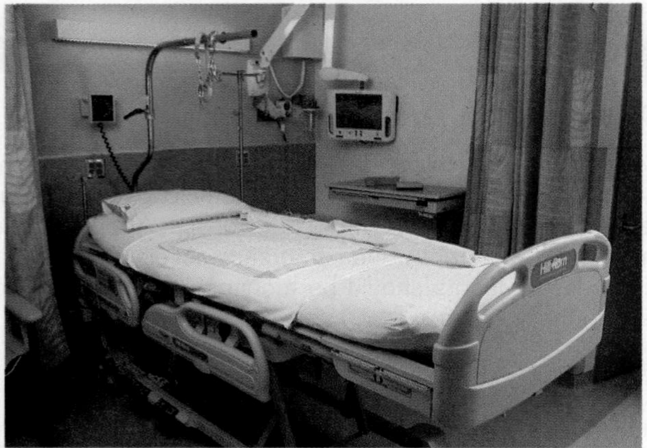

FIGURE 4–6 Room prepared for surgical patient's return.

ing nurse (Safety Alert 4–3). The patient is positioned with padding to prevent injury to nerves and to minimize pressure over bony prominences (Figure 4–7). Serious injury and pressure ulcers can develop from improper positioning or lack of padding for a surgical procedure. Safety straps are secured to safeguard the patient.

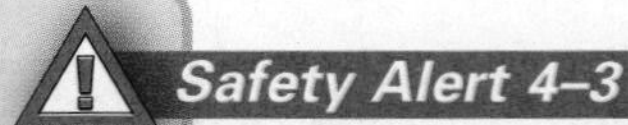

Time Out

Before surgery begins, a "time out" occurs and a final verification of the correct patient, procedure, site, and (as applicable) implants is performed. Any questions or concerns must be resolved before the procedure begins.

THE SURGICAL TEAM

The surgical team consists of the surgeon, surgical assistants, the anesthesia care provider, the circulating nurse, and the scrub person. The surgeon is the head of the surgical team. The surgeon may be a physician, oral surgeon, or podiatrist. The *first* surgical assistant is another physician, a surgical resident, or a specially trained and authorized registered nurse. Other assistants may be RNs or LPN/LVNs. The surgeon, the surgical assistants, and the scrub nurse are sterile members, perform a surgical scrub or rub, and wear sterile gowns and gloves. They work within the sterile field.

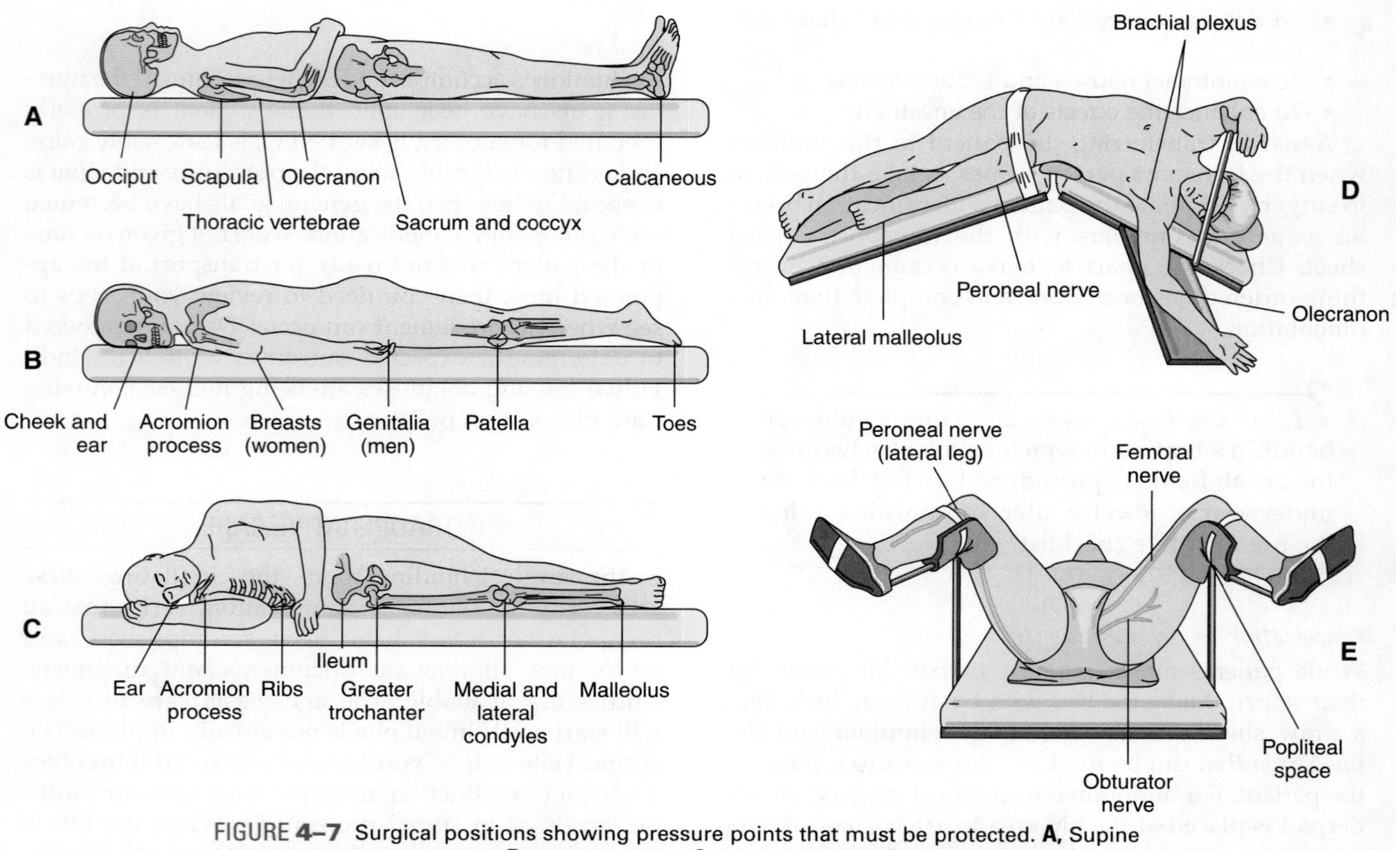

FIGURE 4–7 Surgical positions showing pressure points that must be protected. **A,** Supine (dorsal recumbent) position. **B,** Prone position. **C,** Lateral position. **D,** Lateral (kidney) position. **E,** Lithotomy position.

Box 4–3 Major Functions of the Scrub Person

- Gathers all equipment for the procedure.
- Prepares all sterile supplies and instruments using sterile technique.
- Gowns and gloves surgeons upon entry into operating room.
- Assists with sterile draping of the patient.
- Maintains sterility within the sterile field during surgery.
- Hands instruments and supplies to the operating team during surgery.
- Maintains a neat instrument table.
- Labels and handles surgical specimens correctly.
- Maintains an accurate count of sponges, sharps, and instruments on the sterile field; verifies counts with the circulating nurse before and after surgery.
- Monitors for breaks in sterile technique and points them out.
- Cleans up after the surgery is over.

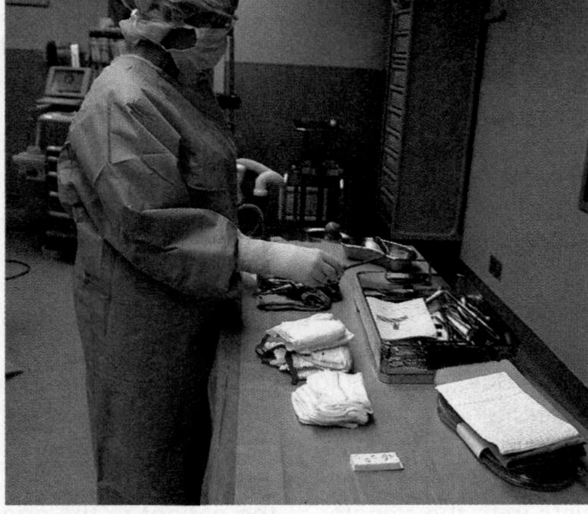

FIGURE 4–8 Scrub nurse setting up the instrument table in the operating room.

THE SURGICAL SUITE

The operating rooms are removed from other areas of the hospital. Access to the surgical suite area is restricted so that only OR personnel and surgical patients are allowed there. The OR is maintained as a positive pressure environment to reduce the entrance of microbes that might cause infection. The surgical suite is divided into three distinct areas to help keep the ORs as microbe free as possible. The unrestricted zone is essentially the control desk area. Street clothes may be permitted here. Semirestricted zones include the hallways and outer regions of the operating rooms. The circulating nurse and anesthesia care providers work in these areas. Clean scrub clothes and caps are required. The restricted zone is the area surrounding the operating table and instrument trays and table. Personnel wear scrub cloths, sterile gowns, caps, shoe covers, masks, and sterile gloves within this area. Asepsis is the responsibility of all surgical personnel.

The temperature in the operating room is kept at 66° to 70° F (18.9° to 21.1° C) to discourage microbial growth and to keep the surgical team comfortable under the bright lights and in the layers of surgical clothing. Cabinets, instrument tables, instrument trays, and disposal buckets are usually made of stainless steel that can be easily cleaned and disinfected. The restricted area is scrubbed down with disinfectant after each procedure. The entire room is kept scrupulously clean.

ROLES OF THE CIRCULATING NURSE AND THE SCRUB PERSON

A surgical technician or a specially trained nurse (LPN/LVN or RN) may be the scrub person. This person functions within the sterile area of the operating room (Box 4–3, Figure 4–8). **Sterile technique is maintained at all times. Any break in sterile technique should be immediately pointed out and remedied.**

The circulating nurse is responsible, along with the anesthesia care provider, for maintaining the safety and dignity of the patient (Box 4–4). The circulating nurse is the communication link between the OR and those outside the surgical suite.

ANESTHESIA

Anesthesia (the loss of sensory perception) has been in use for surgical procedures since the 1840s. Newer anesthetics and techniques make anesthesia safer than ever, but **there is still a risk any time a patient is anesthetized.** The goals of anesthesia administration are (1) to prevent pain; (2) to achieve adequate muscle relaxation; and (3) to calm fear, ease anxiety, and induce forgetfulness of an unpleasant experience. Anesthetics are administered in a number of ways to achieve these goals. Patients are classified according to their age, physical condition, and risk status and assigned a risk potential. The choice of anesthesia depends on the type of surgical procedure to be performed and the risk potential. What is used is the choice of the anesthesia care provider, although it is discussed with the patient (Table 4–4). The anesthesia care provider may be an anesthesiologist, another physician, or a certified registered nurse anesthetist (CRNA) who is supervised by an anesthesiologist.

GENERAL ANESTHESIA

General anesthesia is induced by the administration of an inhalant gas or by medication introduced intravenously. During general anesthesia, the patient is in

Box 4–4 Major Functions of the Circulating Nurse

- Coordinates care, oversees the environment, and cares for the patient in the operating room.
- Verifies that consent is signed and accurate and that surgical site is correctly marked.
- Greets patient and performs patient assessment.
- Checks medical record and preoperative forms for completeness.
- Sets up the operating room; adjusts lights, stools, and discard buckets; and ensures supplies and diagnostic support are available.
- Gathers and checks all equipment that is anticipated to be used, ensuring its safe function.
- Opens sterile supplies for scrub nurse.
- Provides needed padding and warming or cooling devices for the operating table.
- Assists with ties of surgical team's gowns.
- Assists with the transfer of the patient to the operating table and positions the patient.
- Places electrocautery ground pad under patient if electrocautery is to be used.
- Assists the anesthesia induction provider with anesthesia.
- May prep the patient's skin before sterile draping occurs.
- Handles labeling and disposition of specimens.
- Coordinates activities with radiology and pathology departments.
- Monitors urine and blood loss during surgery and reports findings to the surgeon.
- Observes for breaks in sterile technique and announces them to the team.
- Monitors traffic and noise within the operating room.
- Communicates information on the surgery's progress to family during long procedures.
- Documents care, events, interventions, and findings.
- Helps transfer patient to gurney and accompanies patient to recovery area, providing report of the surgery and patient condition to the recovery nurse.

Table 4–4 Types of Anesthesia: Uses, Advantages, and Disadvantages

ROUTE OF ADMINISTRATION	AGENTS COMMONLY USED	ACTION AND SIDE EFFECTS	NURSING IMPLICATIONS
GENERAL ANESTHESIA			
Inhalation	Methoxyflurane	Renal toxicity: related to total dose	Contraindicated in patients with actual or potential kidney disease. Rarely used now. Can reduce need for narcotics during immediate postoperative period.
	Halothane	Possible liver damage	Monitor respiratory rate and pulse for signs of respiratory depression.
	Nitrous oxide (laughing gas)	Relatively nontoxic; can cause hallucinations and dreams	None
	Ethrane	Rapid induction, possible respiratory depression and cardiac dysrhythmia; similar to halothane, but does not cause kidney or liver damage	Monitor for possible seizure activity.
	Isoflurane (Forane)	Rapid induction and recovery; enhances muscle relaxants; does not depress myocardium; causes respiratory depression	Monitor respiration and blood pressure.
Intravenous	Combination of fentanyl and droperidol (Innover), or fentanyl and thiopental (Sublimaze)	Not as easily controlled as inhalation anesthesia	Do not give in combination with other sedatives, hypnotics, or other strong analgesics because of possible additive effects, chiefly hypotension and respiratory depression.
		Major dangers are laryngospasm and bronchospasm	Monitor closely for signs of laryngospasm.
	Morphine sulfate	Increases cardiac output; agent of choice for open-heart surgery and vascular surgery	Observe for respiratory depression.
	Ketamine (Ketalar) used alone or with nitrous oxide	Onset brief; suitable for short procedure.	Given with caution to elderly patients with atherosclerosis and contraindicated in patients with hypertension because of increased cardiac output and elevation of blood pressure.
		Postoperative hallucinations in adults	Protective safety measures to prevent injury during irrational behavior, excitement, and confusion.
		Airway obstruction and vomiting may occur	Provide quiet environment; avoid visual, auditory, and tactile stimulation.

Table 4–4 ***Types of Anesthesia: Uses, Advantages, and Disadvantages—cont'd***

ROUTE OF ADMINISTRATION	AGENTS COMMONLY USED	ACTION AND SIDE EFFECTS	NURSING IMPLICATIONS
GENERAL ANESTHESIA—cont'd			
Intravenous—cont'd	Methohexital sodium (Brevital)	Very short acting; five times stronger than sodium pentothal; less likely to cause bronchospasm	Monitor respiration closely.
	Etomidate (Amidate)	Little effect on cardiovascular system; may cause nausea and vomiting, hiccoughs, myoclonia, and inhibition of adrenal activity	Observe for adverse effects such as transient skeletal muscle movements, hypoglycemia, hypotension, nausea, and hiccoughs.
	Remifentanil (Ultiva)	Short acting; lasts 5 min Metabolized by enzymes outside the liver; provides fog-free recovery Causes less nausea and vomiting	Pain reduction properties also last only a short time (5 min).
	Bupivacaine (Marcaine)	Available with epinephrine to decrease bleeding May cause tremors, twitching, shivering; respiratory arrest can occur if absorbed systemically	Mixed with epinephrine, and may cause ischemia of anesthetized area, so monitor for adequate blood flow postoperatively; protect area until full sensation has returned.
NEUROMUSCULAR BLOCKING AGENTS			
Intravenous	Succinylcholine (Anectine) Pancuronium (Pavulon) Vecuronium (Norcuron) Atracurium (Tracrium) Pipecuronium (Arduan) Tubocurarine (Tubarine) Mivacurium (Miracron) Rocuronium (Zemuron) Doxacurium (Nuromax) Cisatracurium (Nimbex) Rapacuronium (Raplon)	Facilitate endotracheal intubation; promote skeletal muscle paralysis to make access to surgical sites easier; cause apnea requiring mechanical ventilation; cause prolonged muscle relaxation; some cardiac alterations may occur	Maintain patent airway until patient is able to breathe and cough on own; ensure availability of reversal drugs and respiratory support equipment. Some drugs are long acting.
PROCEDURAL (MODERATE) SEDATION			
Benzodiazepines	Midazolam (Versed)	Sedative, hypnotic, and antianxiety effect Causes retrograde amnesia May cause tremors, weakness, chills, or hiccoughs Potential for cardiac arrest	Monitor for hypotension and hypoventilation or apnea.
	Diazepam (Valium)	Relaxes skeletal muscle, decreases anxiety, prevents seizure May cause respiratory depression, tachycardia, and hallucinations	Observe for electrocardiogram changes. Monitor respiratory status closely. Observe intravenous line site for phlebitis.
Opioids	Fentanyl (Sublimaze)	Provides long-acting analgesia; may cause respiratory depression several hours after administration Cardiovascular depression can occur	Monitor respiratory rate and depth; monitor for hypotension. Keep atropine, naloxone (Narcan), vasopressors, and resuscitation equipment close at hand.
	Morphine	Depresses pain impulse transmission May cause bradycardia, cardiac arrest, respiratory depression or apnea	Monitor vital signs closely; keep resuscitation equipment at hand. Watch for nausea and vomiting.
Nonbarbiturate	Propofol (Diprivan)	Short acting with minimal postoperative nausea, vomiting, or sedation May cause allergic skin reaction. Patient becomes aware of postoperative pain quicker than with other anesthetics	Administer analgesia when patient emerges in pain.

a deep sleep state with muscle relaxation and is not aware of the surroundings. An endotracheal tube or nasal endotracheal catheter may be placed to maintain the airway. Placement of a laryngeal mask is another option. There are three stages of general anesthesia:

- Induction—unconsciousness is induced
- Maintenance—period during which the surgical procedure is performed
- Emergence—surgery is completed and the patient is prepared to return to consciousness; neuromuscular blocking agents are reversed

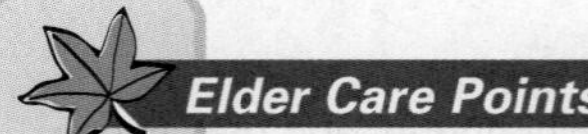

Elder Care Points

- An accurate height and weight of the elderly patient are very important for calculation of anesthetic agents and medication dosages.
- Kidney function is declining in the elderly person, and drugs are not eliminated from the body as quickly. Reduced dosages are often needed.

REGIONAL ANESTHESIA

Regional anesthesia is accomplished by administering a nerve block. It is often more economical than general anesthesia. This may be accomplished by injecting the spinal, epidural, caudal, or peripheral nerve area. The block anesthetizes the local area or the area distal to the block. Spinal or epidural blocks are frequently used for high-risk patients undergoing pelvic or lower extremity surgery; epidural blocks are widely used in obstetric procedures.

PROCEDURAL SEDATION ANESTHESIA (MODERATE SEDATION)

A local anesthetic agent or regional anesthesia to numb the area plus IV sedation is used to provide systemic analgesia and sedation during a surgical procedure. The combination can be used for any procedure that can be done with local or regional anesthesia and is being used more and more frequently (Complementary & Alternative Therapies 4–2). The patient is monitored closely for blood pressure changes, oxygen saturation levels, and heart activity. Recently carbon dioxide levels have begun to be monitored by **capnography** (measurement of inhaled and exhaled carbon dioxide). Capnography provides a tracing that is a graphic representation of exhaled CO_2. The Microstream machine allows monitoring without intubation with a nasal cannula–like device.

LOCAL ANESTHESIA

Local anesthesia is used for minor procedures such as superficial tissue biopsies, surface cyst excision, insertion of pacemaker, and insertion of vascular access devices. The patient who has had local anesthesia is transferred directly to the nursing unit and does not need care in the postanesthesia care unit (PACU, also called the postanesthesia recovery room [PAR or PARR] or postanesthesia recovery unit [PARU]). Postanesthesia care is covered in Chapter 5.

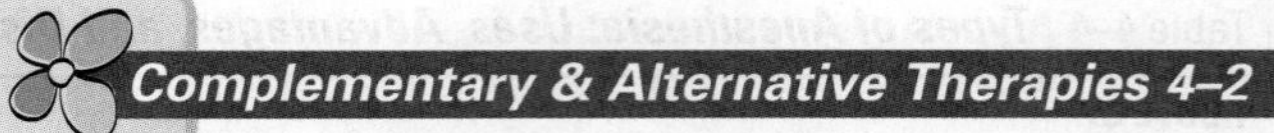

Complementary & Alternative Therapies 4–2

Music's Effects

Music that the patient likes is known to have a calming influence on the preoperative patient. Research studying the use of music delivered by earphones to the patient during surgery is showing that music may reduce the amount of anesthesia and analgesia needed. The patient appears to become more relaxed and less anxious. Before and after surgery, listening to a blank CD through earphones appears to lower anxiety and pain, probably because the earphones decrease outside sensory stimulation.

POTENTIAL INTRAOPERATIVE COMPLICATIONS

Potential intraoperative complications of surgery include:

- Infection
- Fluid volume excess or deficit
- Hypothermia
- Malignant hyperthermia
- Injury related to positioning

No person with an active infection should be in the operating room. Surgical asepsis is practiced with great care to prevent contamination of the surgical site. Counts of sponges, needles, and instruments are performed to verify that no equipment has been left in a wound where it might cause a postoperative infection or complication.

Fluids are carefully regulated by the anesthesia care provider and the surgeon. The circulating nurse keeps a running tally of fluid input, urine output, and blood drainage and keeps the team aware of fluid status.

Temperature of the patient is monitored during surgery to ensure that it does not drop dangerously. The cool atmosphere, cool IV fluids, inhalation of cool anesthetic gases, and exposure of body surfaces will lower a patient's normal temperature. Sometimes the hypothermia is desirable for certain lengthy procedures to decrease metabolic needs of the body. If the patient's temperature drops too low, warmed IV fluids may be administered, or a body warming device may be used. Hypothermia can adversely affect cardiac function.

Malignant hyperthermia is an inherited disorder. Muscle metabolism and heat production increase rapidly and uncontrollably in response to the stress of surgery and some anesthetic agents. Fever, tachycardia, cyanosis, tachypnea, muscle rigidity, diaphoresis, hypotension, and irregular heart rate develop. If not treated quickly, cardiac arrest can occur. The circulating nurse monitors the patient's temperature along with the anesthesia care provider. If the temperature begins to rise rapidly, anesthesia is discontinued and the surgical team takes measures to correct the physiologic problems.

The patient is placed in one position for an extended period of time during a surgical procedure. Such positioning places the person at risk for injury such as problems of immobility and pressure damage to the skin and underlying tissue. A variety of materials are used for padding pressure areas and stabilizing the patient's body. The circulating nurse must understand the risk factors for each surgical position and position and pad joints and pressure areas accordingly. Joint problems and pressure ulcers can develop days after surgery from damage that occurred during the surgical procedure.

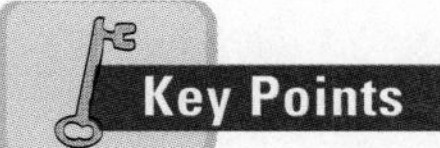

Key Points

- Surgical procedures may be elective, emergency, palliative, diagnostic, curative, exploratory, or reconstructive (see Table 4–1).
- The use of lasers, fiberoptic endoscopes with high-resolution video cameras and operating microscopes, and robotic technology has revolutionized surgery.
- Autologous transfusion or bloodless surgery techniques are reducing problems that can be caused by blood transfusions from outside donors.
- A thorough assessment is performed by the nurse, and any risk factors for surgery are identified (see Focused Assessment 4–1).
- The elderly patient is at much greater risk from surgery and anesthesia than a younger adult.
- Cultural factors and preferences should always be assessed and considered.
- An appropriate individual nursing care plan is formulated for the preoperative period.
- The surgeon must obtain informed consent from the patient before surgery is performed.
- A variety of preoperative procedures are used to prepare the patient for surgery.
- The method to be used for postoperative pain control is explained and discussed with the patient.
- Preoperative teaching of exercises to be performed postoperatively is very important; the patient is taught leg exercises and deep breathing and coughing exercises.
- Immediate preoperative care includes checking to see that all jewelry and metal objects have been removed from the patient.
- A signed surgical consent form is checked before preoperative medication is administered.
- Once preoperative sedation, if ordered, is administered, the patient is cautioned to stay in bed.
- The patient's identity and the correct surgical site are carefully checked before the patient is transported to surgery.
- After the patient leaves for surgery, the room is prepared for postoperative care.
- The operating room is kept as microbe-free as possible.
- Surgical asepsis is the responsibility of the entire operating room staff.
- A "time out" occurs just prior to the start of the surgical procedure to recheck the patient's identity, the surgical procedure to be performed, and the site of the surgery.
- The scrub person and the circulating nurse, along with the surgeon and anesthesiologist or CRNA, provide care for the patient while in the operating room.
- The circulating nurse and the scrub person have distinctly different roles.
- Anesthesia is used to prevent pain; achieve adequate muscle relaxation; and calm fear, allay anxiety, and induce amnesia of an unpleasant experience.
- Inhalant gases and intravenous medications are used to induce general anesthesia, and the patient progresses through stages of induction to total anesthesia.
- Regional anesthesia, procedural (moderate) sedation, or local anesthesia is used for many surgical procedures.
- There is a risk of several complications during the intraoperative period.
- Patients are positioned carefully and pressure points and joints are padded to prevent injury.
- The circulating nurse, the anesthesia care provider, and the surgeon observe for symptoms of complications, and measure are taken immediately to avert a problem the minute a symptom is discovered.

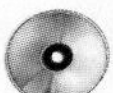

Go to your **Companion CD-ROM** for an Audio Glossary, animations, video clips, and bonus review questions.

evolve Be sure to visit the companion Evolve site at http://evolve.elsevier.com/deWit/for interactive NCLEX-PN Exam Style Review Questions, WebLinks, and additional online resources.

NCLEX-PN EXAM STYLE REVIEW QUESTIONS

Choose the best answer(s) for the following questions.

1. Regarding informed consent for surgical procedure, the nurse is responsible for which of the following?
   1. Explanation of the procedure
   2. Determination of risks and benefits of the procedure
   3. Assessment of mental competency of the patient
   4. Administration of medications after the patient completes the consent

2. Which of the following nursing interventions are critical in preoperative preparation of the patient? *(Select all that apply.)*
   1. No oral intake for at least 6 hours.
   2. Allow clear liquids up to 2 hours prior to major procedures.
   3. Ensure timely administration of insulin injections at all times.
   4. Withhold all cardiac medications, antihypertensives, and anticonvulsants.
   5. Confirm patient compliance with the nothing by mouth *(nil per os;* NPO) status.

3. The nurse reinforces the importance of turning, coughing, and deep breathing to a preoperative patient. Which of the following patient statements indicates a need for further instruction?
   1. "I could place a pillow to brace my abdominal incision to reduce pain with coughing."
   2. "I would lie still in bed to reduce the risk of injuring my surgical wound."
   3. "Coughing would help reduce pneumonia."
   4. "Immediately getting out of bed speeds up recuperation."

4. While administering promethazine hydrochloride (Phenergan), the preoperative patient requests clarification for the indication for the medication. An appropriate nursing response would be:
   1. "This reduces mucous secretion."
   2. "The medication helps prevent allergic reactions."
   3. "The medication serves to reduce pain."
   4. "This prevents anticipated infection associated with invasive procedures."

5. While reviewing the clinical history of a preoperative patient, which of the following patient information warrants immediate notification of the physician?
   1. Temperature 101.5° F (38.6° C)
   2. Serum sodium 135
   3. Diminished breath sounds
   4. Blood pressure 135/80

6. While transferring the patient from the preoperative area to the surgical suite, the patient says, "Am I going to make it?" An appropriate response by a nurse would be:
   1. "Everything will be all right."
   2. "Didn't your physician discuss the possible adverse outcomes of the procedure?"
   3. "You seem anxious. Tell me more about how you are feeling."
   4. "Your physician has performed the procedure several times."

7. During a preoperative teaching session, the patient asks the nurse, "What is general anesthesia?" An accurate explanation would be:
   1. provision of a nerve block.
   2. administration of inhalant gas to produce deep sleep.
   3. resultant local anesthesia.
   4. mild sedation and systemic analgesia.

8. During a major surgery, the patient is considered at risk for which of the following?
   1. Injury related to placement in one position for extended period of time
   2. Altered nutrition: less than body requirements related to prolonged fasting
   3. Infection related to hypothermia in the surgical suite
   4. Deficient fluid volume related to continuous infusion of fluids

9. In discussing options for fluid resuscitation during major surgery, the physician indicated availability of bloodless surgery. The nurse would include which of the following interventions? *(Select all that apply.)*
   1. Administration of erythropoietin
   2. Provision of postoperative hyperbaric oxygen therapy
   3. Induction of hypothermia
   4. Banking blood prior to surgery
   5. Autologous transfusion

10. The preoperative patient asks for clarification regarding instructions for preoperative skin preparation. Which of the following statements by the nurse is correct?
    1. "Contact lenses can be worn during the procedure."
    2. "Shaving over potential operative areas is recommended."
    3. "Shower with the prescribed antibacterial soap."
    4. "Preserve skin tone with mild makeup."

CRITICAL THINKING ACTIVITIES  *Read each clinical scenario and discuss the questions with your classmates.*

Scenario A

Your patient is scheduled for abdominal surgery this morning. You are assigned two other patients to care for as well. One of these patients is stable and will be going home. The other patient is going for a computed tomography (CT) scan at 9:30 A.M.

1. Describe in detail how you would plan your morning care for these three patients.
2. Your surgical patient shares with you that she is having second thoughts about having this surgery. How would you handle the situation?
3. Your surgical patient has the following preoperative medications ordered:
   - Meperidine (Demerol) 50 mg
   - Hydroxyzine (Vistaril) 25 mg
   - Midazolam (Versed) 0.07 mg/kg

   Describe the equipment you would use to administer the medications and where and how you would administer the medications.

Scenario B

On your first day on the surgical unit, you are assigned a patient who is scheduled for surgery at 10:00 A.M. The following preoperative medication is ordered intramuscularly (IM):

- Meperidine 75 mg IM (on hand, meperidine 50 mg/mL)
- Promethazine HCl 25 mg IM (on hand, promethazine 50 mg/mL)
- Atropine 0.4 mg IM on call (on hand, atropine 0.4 mg/mL)

1. What would you check in the patient's chart as part of her preoperative preparation?
2. What steps would you take to complete the preoperative checklist and charting for this patient before administering the preoperative medications?
3. Describe how you would draw up and administer the preoperative medications.

CHAPTER 5

Care of Postoperative Surgical Patients

evolve http://evolve.elsevier.com/deWit

Objectives

Upon completing this chapter, you should be able to:

Theory

1. Describe the care of the patient in the postanesthesia care unit (PACU).
2. Identify the necessary points for the PACU nurse to cover when giving report to the floor nurse for the postoperative patient.
3. Formulate a plan of care for a postoperative patient returning from the PACU.
4. Determine assessment factors for each of the potential postoperative complications.
5. Prepare the surgical patient for discharge.

Clinical Practice

1. Identify how to promote adequate ventilation of the lungs during recovery from anesthesia in the PACU.
2. Prepare to perform an immediate postoperative assessment when a patient returns to the nursing unit.
3. Apply interventions to prevent potential postoperative complications.
4. Assess for postoperative pain and provide comfort measures and pain relief.
5. Promote early ambulation and return to independence in activities of daily living.
6. Perform discharge teaching necessary for postoperative home self-care.

Key Terms

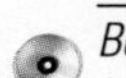

Be sure to check out the bonus material on the Companion CD-ROM, including selected audio pronunciations.

anaphylaxis (ă-nă-fă-LĂK-sĭs, p. 104)
atelectasis (ă-tĕ-LĔK-tă-sĭs, p. 95)
dehiscence (dĕ-HĬS-ĕntz, p. 102)
embolus (ĔM-bō-lus, p. 99)
evisceration (ē-vĭs-ĕr-Ā-shŭn, p. 102)
hematoma (hē-mă-TŌ-mă, p. 100)
Homans' sign (HŌ-mănz sīn, p. 96)
malignant hyperthermia (hī-pĕr-THĔR-mē-ă, p. 104)
paralytic ileus (păr-ă-LĬT-ĭk ĬL-ē-ŭs, p. 98)
pneumonia (nū-MŌ-nē-ă, p. 97)
purulence (PŪ-roo-lĕns, p. 101)
seroma (sĕ-RŌ-mă, p. 100)
thrombophlebitis (thrŏm-bō-flĕ-BĪ-tĭs, p. 96)
thrombosis (thrŏm-BŌ-sĭs, p. 96)

IMMEDIATE POSTOPERATIVE CARE

POSTANESTHESIA CARE UNIT

When surgery with general anesthesia is completed, the patient is transferred to the postanesthesia care unit (PACU) adjacent to the surgical suites (Figure 5–1). Patients who have had spinal anesthesia for a major procedure go to the PACU also. Very critically ill patients, such as those recovering from open heart surgery, are often taken directly to the intensive care or critical care unit for anesthesia recovery. Recovery from a major surgical procedure is a critical time, and specially trained nurses closely monitor each patient. Surgical patients who had procedural sedation or a local or regional anesthetic are usually recovered in the ambulatory surgery area. The PACU nurse receives a verbal report from the anesthesia care provider about the procedure, blood loss, anesthesia administered, fluids infused, medications administered, and any problems encountered.

The patient is immediately attached to the cardiac and pulse oximeter monitors, and oxygen is usually administered if the patient had general anesthesia or if it is ordered. Oxygen helps eliminate the anesthetic gases and helps meet the increased metabolic demand for oxygen caused by surgery. Any respiratory problems are immediately addressed as maintenance of airway and adequate ventilation takes priority. The sedation and relaxation often cause the tongue to occlude the airway. For that reason an oral airway may be in place. Alternatively, the airway can be opened by moving the jaw forward (Figure 5–2). Suction is on and readily available to clear secretions. If needed, mechanical ventilation is provided. Warm blankets are placed over the patient. Vital signs are assessed and compared with baseline readings, and a full assessment is performed. Neurologic assessment includes level of consciousness, orientation, sensory and motor status, and size, equality, and reactivity of the pupils. The patient may be asleep, drowsy but arousable, or awake.

Intake and output is determined to assess function of the urinary system. Urinary output is monitored closely. All intravenous (IV) lines are checked for patency, the correct solutions are verified along with the

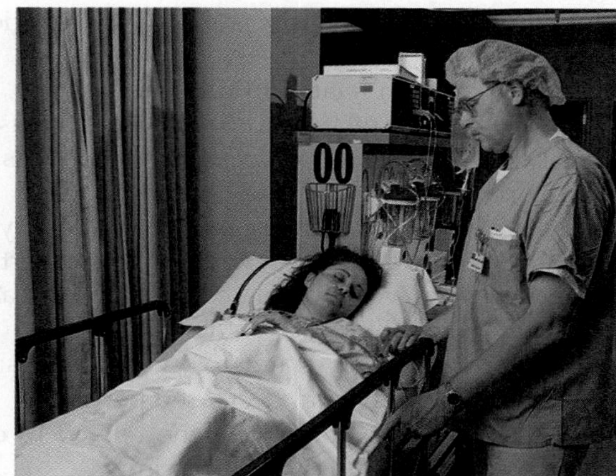

FIGURE 5–1 Nurse attends to patient in postanesthesia recovery unit.

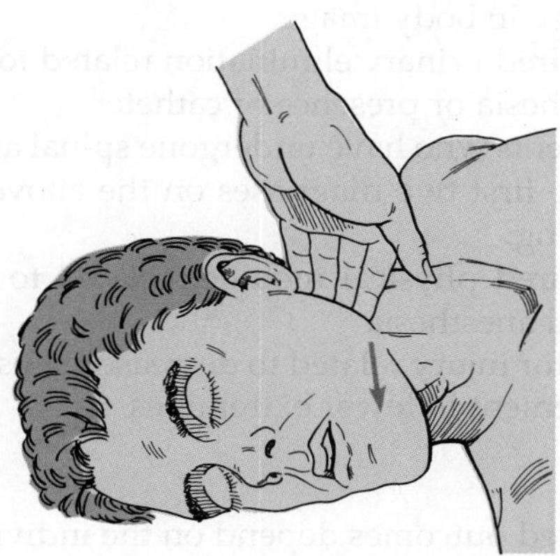

FIGURE 5–2 Jaw-thrust maneuver to open the airway. The fingers are placed behind the angle of the jaw, lifting the jaw forward. As the jaw moves, the tongue comes forward, opening the airway.

correct drip rate, and wound drains and evacuation devices are inspected for proper function. Dressings are inspected for unexpected drainage.

Recovery can take from 2 to 6 hours. Because patients are coming out of anesthesia through the various anesthesia stages and are unstable, the environment is kept as quiet as possible. Communication among the staff is done in hushed tones and kept to a minimum. The patient may wake up confused and need reorientation and reassurance that the surgery is over, that he is in the recovery room, and that his family or significant other has been notified. Once the patient is awake, family members are sometimes allowed to visit for a few minutes so that they are assured that their loved one is all right and recovering.

The PACU nurse performs assessments every 15 minutes or according to the status of the patient. Assessment for complications of the particular surgery and anesthesia are ongoing. The patient remains in the PACU until the vital signs are stable and the patient is awake and able to respond to stimuli. A form

Box 5–1 Postanesthesia Care Unit (PACU) Discharge Criteria

The Aldrete scoring system is commonly used to determine if the patient is stable enough for discharge from the PACU. Activity, respiration, circulation, consciousness, and oxygen saturation level are each scored from 0 to 2. A total score of 9 to 10 indicates criteria for discharge. That score level indicates that:

- There is only moderate or light drainage from the operative site.
- Urine output is at least 30 mL/hr (0.5 mL/kg/hr) for an adult.
- All essential immediate postoperative care has been completed.

Box 5–2 Postanesthesia Care Unit Report to Nursing Unit Nurse

GENERAL INFORMATION

- Patient name, age
- Diagnosis
- Allergies
- Stability level

SURGICAL DATA

- Surgeon's name
- Surgical procedure performed
- Length of surgery time
- Unexpected surgical events
- Vital sign trends during surgery
- Anesthetic administered
- Medications administered during surgery and recovery
- Amount of blood loss and replacement

POSTANESTHESIA CARE COURSE

- Vital signs and oxygen saturation
- Urine output
- Intravenous solutions and blood products administered, with amounts
- Tubes, drains, and equipment in use
- Results of any intraoperative lab or diagnostic tests (Note whether patient/family has been told pathology results)
- Pain status and time of last dose of analgesia
- Any problems encountered

of the Aldrete scoring system may be used to determine readiness for transfer (Box 5–1). Activity, respiration, circulation, consciousness, skin color, and oxygen saturation are each given a score of 0 to 2. A total score of 9 or 10 usually indicates the patient is ready for transfer. When the discharge criteria for the PACU are met, the patient is transferred back to the nursing unit and report is given to the staff nurse (Box 5–2).

? *Think Critically About . . .* What is the number one priority of care for the patient in the PACU?

For many procedures the patient may be transferred from the operating room (OR) directly back to the same-day surgery unit. The nurse monitors the patient's respiration, circulation, vital signs, neurologic status, fluid balance, wound drainage and dressings, and comfort level. When the vital signs are stable, the patient is allowed to sit up and then is ambulated. When able to ambulate unassisted, and to empty the bladder, the patient may be discharged if discharge criteria are met. Recovery time in the same-day surgery unit usually takes 1 to 3 hours. Discharge teaching is begun before the surgery and continues once the patient is again alert. Written instructions are always sent home with the patient. If the patient has undergone sedation, another adult driver must provide transportation home after same-day surgery. Surgery patients who have received anesthesia or procedural sedation are advised not to resume normal activities or make important decisions for at least 24 hours after surgery. The phone number of the surgeon, along with signs and symptoms to report, is written on the postoperative instruction sheet in case complications arise.

? *Think Critically About . . .* How would you assess a patient to determine whether or not the gag reflex has returned sufficiently after being sedated to allow him to have a few ice chips?

NURSING MANAGEMENT

Assessment (Data Collection)

After the patient returns from the PACU, the nurse checks identity, settles the patient in bed, and performs an initial postoperative assessment. **Airway, breathing, and circulation are always the top priorities.** This provides a baseline against which frequent postoperative assessment data can be compared to prevent or quickly detect signs of complications (Focused Assessment 5–1). Vital signs are taken more frequently if they are unstable; this is a nursing judgment (Assignment Considerations 5–1).

Monitoring for signs of the various complications that may occur as a result of surgery is a major nursing responsibility. **The first 72 hours after surgery require frequent observations to detect signs of postoperative complications.** Reassessment is performed frequently while providing nursing care.

Nursing Diagnosis

Nursing diagnoses commonly used for postoperative patients who have undergone general anesthesia are as follows:

- Impaired gas exchange related to the effect of anesthesia on the lungs
- Ineffective breathing pattern related to analgesia and pain
- Impaired skin integrity related to surgical incision
- Risk for infection related to surgical wound
- Risk for injury related to sedation, decreased level of consciousness, or excessive blood loss
- Acute pain related to disruption of tissue
- Ineffective airway clearance related to inability to breathe deeply and cough without discomfort
- Deficient fluid volume related to fluid loss and nothing by mouth (NPO) status
- Risk for constipation related to opioid analgesics, decreased mobility, and decreased peristalsis
- Self-care deficit, bathing/hygiene related to decreased mobility, tubes, and dressings
- Ineffective tissue perfusion related to surgery, anesthesia, and positioning in the OR
- Ineffective coping related to loss of body part or change in body image
- Impaired urinary elimination related to effects of anesthesia or presence of catheter

For patients who have undergone spinal anesthesia, include the first two diagnoses on the above list plus the following:

- Impaired physical mobility related to effects of spinal anesthesia
- Risk for injury related to decreased sensation and movement in lower extremities

Planning

The expected outcomes depend on the individual specific nursing diagnoses. General *nursing* goals are as follows:

- Maintain patent airway and adequate respiratory exchange.
- Maintain adequate tissue perfusion.
- Promote normal physiologic body function.
- Prevent injury.
- Promote comfort and rest.
- Promote wound healing.
- Promote psychological adjustment to lifestyle or body image changes.
- Prevent complications.

When planning your work for the shift, allow time for frequent postoperative assessments. Careful planning is essential to care for the early postoperative patient properly and not neglect the needs of other assigned patients.

Implementation

Maintain Ventilation

Oxygen saturation is monitored closely and oxygen is administered as ordered. The postoperative patient is at risk for respiratory problems from the effects of anesthesia on the lungs, from being in one position on the OR table for the duration of surgery, and from limited mobility in the immediate postoperative period. **Maintaining a patent airway is a priority measure.** The patient must be positioned on the side or with the

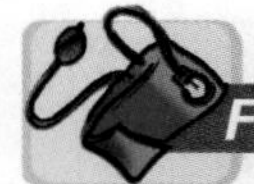

Focused Assessment 5–1

Postoperative Assessment

AREA	ASSESSMENT	SCHEDULE
Airway	• Lung sounds, depth and quality of air movement; respiratory rate	• Auscultate lungs initially; respiratory rate q 15 min until fully aroused from anesthesia; then assess quality of respirations with vital signs assessment
	• Oxygen saturation	• Note per vital signs schedule and whenever in room
	• Oxygen delivery at rate ordered and patent system	• Check oxygen delivery system with initial assessment and each shift
Circulation	• Auscultate heart; check peripheral pulses and sensation, especially distal to surgical site. Assess skin color.	• Initially, q 4 hr × 2, then with vital signs. If surgery was on an extremity, assess each time vital signs are measured.
Mental status	• Level of consciousness and orientation	• Initially and then with full vital signs
Vital signs	• Temperature	• Check initially; then q 8 hr once stable
	• Blood pressure, pulse, and respirations	• Check q 15 min × 1 hr; q 30 min × 4; q 1 hr × 4; q 4 hr × 24–48 hr; or per agency protocol
Fluid status and hydration	• Intravenous infusion site and flow rate	• Check initially and when in room
	• Intake and output	• Check each shift
	• Skin turgor; oral membranes	• Check initially and each shift
Surgical site	• Check for bleeding; mark drainage on dressing; assess wound drainage in containers	• Initially and q 1 hr × 4; then with vital signs
Gastrointestinal	• Auscultate bowel sounds; assess abdomen	• Initially, then q 8 hr
	• Check nasogastric drainage color, character, amount	• Check drainage whenever in room
Tubes	• Check for patency and function of each	• Initially; then with vital signs after 1 hr
Kidney function	• Assess urine output from Foley catheter; must void within 8 hr if no Foley in place	• Initially and q 1 hr × 4; then if >30 mL/hr, q 4 hr
Pain	• Use a pain scale and observation of nonverbal behaviors	• Initially and with vital signs; assess at least q 3 hr
Skin	• Pressure areas over bony prominences	• Initially and q 2 hr

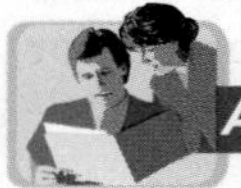

Assignment Considerations 5–1

Postoperative Vital Signs

Because postoperative patients need close vigilance in the early postoperative period, it is best not to assign the taking of frequent vital signs to unlicensed assistive personnel (UAPs) for the first couple of hours. Other parameters besides the measurement of vital signs need to be checked on a frequent schedule. After the first couple of hours, the vital sign measurement task can be assigned to a UAP if you know the person is proficient in obtaining accurate measurements. Remind the UAP of exactly what you want reported to you: temperature elevation above 99.8° F (37.1° C), blood pressure alteration of a specific amount down or up from the baseline; tachycardia, and respiratory rate increase above or below normal range.

head turned to the side to prevent aspiration, if not contraindicated, until fully recovered, alert, and with the swallowing (gag) reflex intact.

Some degree of **atelectasis** (collapse of alveoli in the lungs) exists after anesthesia. A mild hypoxia is usually present for about 48 hours after surgery. A large percentage of all patients who have had either abdominal or thoracic surgery suffer from increasing atelectasis and pneumonitis. **If any area of the lung remains atelectic for more than 72 hours, hypostatic pneumonia from retained secretions is likely to occur.** Auscultate the lungs carefully for abnormal sounds indicating retained secretions, assess the rate and depth of breathing, and encourage the patient to deep breathe and cough every 2 hours. *Hypostatic pneumonia* occurs when lack of movement or of position change causes stasis of secretions, which become a breeding ground for bacteria. Coughing to remove secretions may be contraindicated for patients who have had a hernia repair or eye, ear, brain, jaw, or plastic surgery. Check the physician's orders. If the patient cannot cough effectively, instruct to "huff" cough (see Patient Teaching 4-3). Be certain the patient turns every 2 hours as well because this changes the distribution of gas and blood flow in the lungs and helps move secretions. Early ambulation is ordered to promote ventilation. **Signs of complications for procedures other than thoracic surgery are complaints of shortness of breath, pain on inspiration, and extreme fatigue, which is related to hypoxemia.** The use of an incentive spirometer is especially helpful to prevent atelectasis and hypoventilation and should be used every hour while the patient is awake for the first 24 hours following surgery and then every 2 hours. The elderly patient may need extra coaching to master the technique.

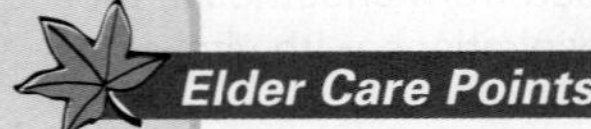

Elder Care Points

The risk of hypoventilation is greater in the elderly because lung expansion may be hampered by calcification of costal cartilage and weakened respiratory muscles.

A pulse oximeter may be utilized to determine blood oxygenation. Monitor the readings periodically and report oxygen saturation (Sao_2) readings below 95% to the physician. Pulse oximetry is covered in Chapter 12.

Maintain Circulation and Tissue Perfusion

When considerable blood is lost during surgery, a blood transfusion may be ordered. Autologous blood may be transfused if the patient donated blood several weeks prior to surgery or if the patient's blood was collected as it was lost during surgery. This blood is can be filtered and returned to the patient.

If a procedure involves an extremity or the pelvic area, the distal or peripheral pulse is checked during each full assessment. Swelling at the surgical site can compress vessels and decrease blood flow distal to the area. The skin distal to the surgical site should be warm to the touch, and there should be brisk capillary refill in the fingers or toes. Color, movement, and sensation of the fingers and toes should be checked to detect nerve compression from swelling and edema.

Blood pressure and pulse should be compared with preoperative values to determine if there are significant changes. An increase in pulse may indicate that internal bleeding is occurring, but it can also signify incomplete pain control. Blood pressure falling below the patient's normal baseline level may indicate major bleeding.

The use of antiembolic (elastic) stockings increases venous return from the legs and helps prevent stasis of blood in the lower extremities. The stockings should be checked frequently to ensure that they fit smoothly. They may be removed for 15 to 30 minutes per shift for bathing and to allow air circulation to the skin. If the patient is at considerable risk of venous **thrombosis** (blood clot), the surgeon may order sequential pneumatic compression devices (SCDs) to be applied to the legs. SCDs alternately compress and release, squeezing the legs and propelling blood along the vessels (Figure 5–3). Orders for ambulation are written as soon as the patient is able to be up and walking.

Low-dose subcutaneous heparin injections may be ordered for any patient who has a history of

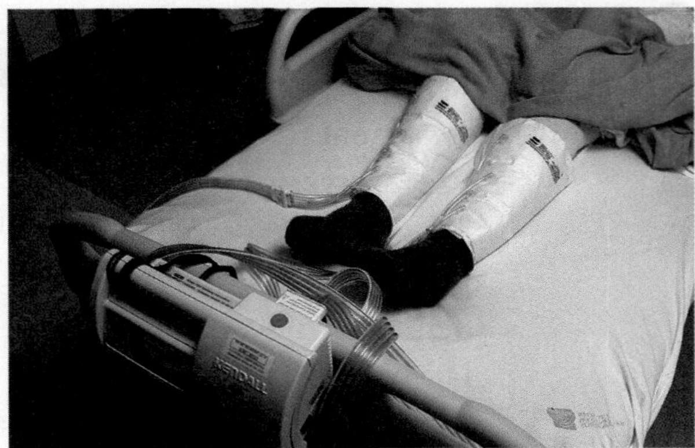

FIGURE **5–3** Sequential compression devices in place to prevent thrombus formation.

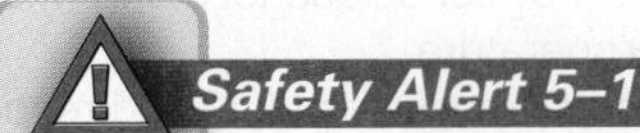

Safety Alert 5–1

Preventing Embolus

The patient's legs should never be massaged, as this might dislodge a blood clot and cause an embolus that could lodge in the lungs, heart, or brain, causing a pulmonary embolus, myocardial infarction, or stroke.

thrombophlebitis (clot and inflammation in a blood vessel). Thrombophlebitis does not usually occur until after the fifth day of bed rest, when stasis has allowed a clot to form and irritate the vein. Question the patient about pain or tenderness in the legs. Assess for **Homans' sign** (pain in the calf when the leg is raised with the knee bent and then straightened while dorsiflexing the foot). If the patient complains of leg pain, the area should be gently palpated for increased warmth, and the physician must be notified (Safety Alert 5–1).

Think Critically About . . . The initial vital sign readings for your patient at return from surgery were blood pressure (BP) 138/86, pulse 76, respirations 14, temperature 97.7° F (36.5° C). An hour later they were BP 126/74, pulse 80, respirations 14, temperature 98.0° F (36.7° C). What action, if any, should you take?

Prevent Injury

Safety is a primary concern until the patient is fully recovered from anesthesia. Always leave the bed in the low position after administering care. Remind the patient to call for assistance as needed and be certain the call bell is within reach. Remember that you are the patient's advocate while he is still recovering from surgery and anesthesia or under the influence of narcotic analgesia. Be certain that all appropriate safety measures are listed on the patient's care plan.

Reassure the patient who has had spinal anesthesia that it is normal for the legs to feel numb and heavy and that feeling will soon return to normal. A flat position with only a pillow is maintained until feeling returns. Sense of position in space will return to the legs first, then sensation to deep pressure, then voluntary movement, and finally feeling of superficial pain and temperature. A feeling of "pins and needles" in the legs is common. The patient is prone to hypotension until all effects of the spinal anesthesia are gone. Lying flat for 6 to 8 hours may decrease the chance of post–spinal anesthesia headache. Observe for a spinal headache. If a headache develops, staying flat in bed reduces the pain. Keep IV fluid running as ordered. **Encourage the patient to drink a lot of fluids, including those containing caffeine.** The patient can turn the head to the side and sip from a straw while someone else holds the container. The fluids and caffeine raise the vascular pressure at the spinal puncture site and help to seal the hole.

? *Think Critically About . . .* How would your care for the patient who has had spinal anesthesia differ from that of the patient who has had general anesthesia?

Many surgical procedures extend over several hours, which means that the patient has been lying motionless, in a fixed position, on a hard table for a considerable time. The nurse should check pressure points related to the position that the patient was in during surgery and provide padding and appropriate positioning for areas that are painful.

? *Think Critically About . . .* Your postoperative patient was placed in a right side-lying position during surgery. Which specific places should you check for signs of pressure problems? How would you position the patient who is complaining of pain in the right hip as well as pain in the left flank where the surgery occurred?

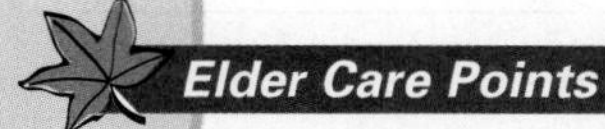

Elder Care Points

Because skin is fragile and there is less subcutaneous tissue in an elderly person, check bony prominences carefully for signs of breakdown. Joint strains can occur from positioning necessary for certain types of surgery; perform position changes slowly and gently.

Prevent Infection

Use aseptic technique when caring for the postoperative patient. Good handwashing is the primary means of preventing infection. Dressing changes are performed with strict sterile technique while the patient is in the hospital; the patient may use clean technique at home. Encouraging fluid intake in order to flush the bladder will help prevent a bladder infection for the patient who was catheterized or has an indwelling catheter. Turning, coughing, and deep breathing, plus ambulation, will assist in preventing **pneumonia** (inflammation and accumulation of exudate in the lung) from retained secretions and lack of movement. Handling drains and emptying closed wound drainage devices aseptically prevents the entry of microorganisms.

Assess the surgical wound area each shift and assess for signs of infection: local pain, increased tenderness, warmth, redness, or drainage of purulent material. Monitor the blood count for increasing leukocytes (white blood cells), and the body temperature for unexpected increase.

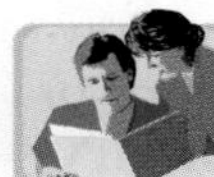

Assignment Considerations 5–2

Urinary Output

When a UAP is assigned to turn the patient every 2 hours, remind the person to check that the tubing of any indwelling catheter is not under the patient or crimped. If the UAP is assigned the task of emptying the Foley catheter bag at the end of the shift, ask that you be notified if there is less than 30 mL of urine per hour for the shift in the output. Verify that the UAP knows to maintain sterility of the urinary catheter system and to wipe the spout with an alcohol sponge after emptying the urine bag.

Maintain Fluid Balance

The urine output is closely monitored after surgery. If the patient has an indwelling catheter, the urine in the bag is observed every hour in the early postoperative period. If the urine flow is less than 30 mL/hr, it is reported to the charge nurse. **If flow is less than 60 mL over a 2-hour period, the surgeon is notified.** The catheter is checked to ensure that it is not kinked and that the connecting tubing is not lying beneath the patient (Assignment Considerations 5–2). If no catheter is present, the patient must void within 4 to 8 hours depending on the type of surgery undergone. If the patient is unable to empty the bladder spontaneously, obtain an order for catheterization.

Patients usually return from surgery with an IV infusion running. Depending on the type of surgery, IV fluids may be continued for a few days or may be discontinued after the fluid has infused. Check orders to see that the correct solution is running. **No potassium additive should be given until the urine flow is at least 30 mL/hr.** Potassium may cause hyperkalemia if kidney function is not adequate. Assess the IV site for patency and lack of complications once an hour. Recheck the IV flow rate as well. All IV fluid administered is recorded as intake on the intake and output record.

As soon as the patient is conscious and the swallowing (gag) reflex has returned, offer a few ice chips or sips of water unless there is an order to maintain NPO status. All intake is recorded on the intake and output record. At the end of each shift, the difference between the intake and output is noted. The body will initially retain fluid due to fluids lost during the procedure and the stress reaction from surgery. Postoperatively, the output will slowly increase until it is more than the intake; after 2 to 3 days, a balance should again occur.

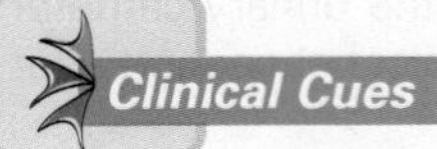

A cup of ice equals ½ cup of water.

Anesthesia may cause the patient to be nauseated, and vomiting is not uncommon. The emesis basin is kept close by, and the patient is positioned on his side to prevent aspiration. Check the orders to determine on which side the patient can be positioned. The surgeon usually writes an order for medication in the event of excessive nausea or vomiting. **It is best to medicate the patient before actual vomiting occurs to prevent stress on the incision and sutures.**

Applying a cool cloth to the forehead and back of the neck, rinsing the mouth, ridding the room of odors, and providing a quiet environment also help to reduce nausea. After emesis, mouth care should be provided. If vomiting is uncontrolled with medication, a nasogastric (NG) tube may need to be inserted to suction stomach contents and prevent further fluid and electrolyte loss.

Surgeons often leave in an NG tube after most abdominal procedures because handling of the gastrointestinal tract, and general anesthesia, causes peristalsis to halt and secretions will not flow through the system properly. When an NG tube is in place, check that is positioned properly and that the suction is set according to orders, and is functioning. Assess the amount of drainage produced every 1 to 2 hours. If the drainage turns dark brown and grainy, it should be checked for blood with a special reagent. The presence of blood should be reported to the surgeon.

Elder Care Points

Fluid and electrolyte shifts may cause confusion in the elderly patient after surgery. The skin and vessels are more fragile, and the IV site must be assessed frequently for signs of infiltration. Adjustment of the body to fluid shifts is more difficult, and the elderly patient is very prone to postural hypotension when changing to a standing position. Be sure to adequately support the patient.

Promote Gastrointestinal Function

A healthy surgical patient may be kept on nothing but IV fluids for several days without developing a serious nutritional problem. If extensive tissue repair is required for healing, supplemental nutrition by enteral or parenteral feeding may be started (see Chapters 3 and 28 for details of enteral and total parenteral nutrition). A patient who is kept on IV fluids only will lose some weight as there are insufficient calories in the IV fluids to meet total daily requirements. A liter of 5% dextrose in water contains only 200 calories.

Eating after surgery with general anesthesia is not allowed until bowel sounds have returned due to the risk of development of **paralytic ileus** (failure of forward movement of bowel contents). Listen for bowel sounds in all four quadrants at least once per shift. When diet progression is indicated, the surgeon usually orders clear liquids, followed by full liquids, then a regular diet if the preceding diets have been tolerated. After spinal anesthesia, the patient may be allowed to eat right away.

Discomfort from abdominal distention and considerable flatus may occur after general anesthesia because peristalsis ceases. Ambulating is helpful in moving and evacuating gas. Taking only small amounts of liquid or food at a time, drinking only tepid liquids, and refraining from drinking with a straw helps keep flatus to a minimum. If permitted, the patient can try resting in a slight Trendelenburg's position, with the legs and rectum higher than the stomach; this may assist in the evacuation of flatus.

Once the patient is eating again, a bowel movement should occur within 2 to 3 days. If this does not occur, an order for a suppository or laxative may be needed to stimulate a bowel movement. Patients receiving narcotic analgesics may become constipated and require stool softeners or laxatives to produce normal bowel movements.

Think Critically About . . . Name four specific interventions you might try to prevent constipation in your postoperative patient who is receiving narcotic analgesics for pain.

Promote Comfort

Pain and discomfort interfere with rest and inhibit the processes of healing and repair. Although analgesic drugs are almost always prescribed for the postoperative patient, comfort measures also should be used. Nonsteroidal anti-inflammatory drugs and non-narcotic analgesics may be used to augment opioids, as they work on both the peripheral and the central nervous system to control pain. Opioids tend to depress respirations and the cough reflex and therefore may contribute to the development of pulmonary problems as described previously. They also can increase the possibility of nausea and vomiting. Using other drugs in combination with opioids helps to control pain with the least amount of side effects. Pain must be reduced so that the patient will rest, turn, cough, and deep breathe frequently. Pain medication should be given consistently for the first 24 to 48 hours postoperatively. The nurse should assess the pain level and the effectiveness of analgesia using a pain scale at least every 3 hours. Remind the patient to request medication before the pain becomes severe.

If the patient is complaining of pain upon return to the unit, refer to the notes from the PACU nurse and see if any pain medication was given. Note what preoperative medications were administered. **When droperidol plus fentanyl (Innovar) is given as a preoperative medication, narcotic pain medication is reduced by half for the 8 hours after the preoperative medication, or the narcotic analgesic may gravely depress respirations.** If respirations are within normal limits and there is no contraindication to doing so, medicate the patient promptly with the ordered analgesic. If it is too soon to give more analgesia, reposition the patient, be sure the bladder is not distended and causing discomfort, check that the patient is warm enough, and use other comfort measures to relieve the pain, such as distraction and imagery. Note when analgesia is due and have it ready to administer at the appointed time.

Relaxation techniques also can help to decrease the patient's discomfort. Teach about relaxation exercises (see Chapter 7). Pain medication may be administered by subcutaneous or intramuscular injection, intravenously, epidurally, or by intermittent administration of local anesthetic into the pleural space via an intrapleural catheter. Two methods very commonly used for pain control are the epidural catheter and the patient-controlled analgesia pump. The problem of pain, methods of pain control, pain medications, and their administration are discussed in greater detail in Chapter 7.

Operating rooms are kept very cool so that the staff members working under the bright lights do not become overheated. The patient's temperature in this environment often decreases, especially during prolonged abdominal surgery in which the peritoneal cavity has been open for a long period. The patient may feel cold and should be kept warm with extra blankets or warmed bath blankets applied under the top covers. Placing socks on the feet may help. Some anesthetic agents may cause tremors as they are metabolized. If uncontrollable shivering occurs, contact the physician for medication orders.

Dressings on extremities should be checked to be certain that they are not so tight that circulation is impaired. Check the pulse, skin temperature, sensation, and movement distal to the surgical site to evaluate circulation (neurovascular assessment). A little finger should be able to slip between a dressing and the extremity.

Occasionally continuous hiccups will occur after surgery, making the patient quite uncomfortable. Having the patient breathe into a paper bag will often relieve the hiccups (Complementary & Alternative Therapies 5–1). Sedatives and tranquilizers are sometimes prescribed to promote relaxation and reduce irritation of the phrenic nerve. Severe, persistent cases may require surgical interruption of impulses along the nerve pathways so as to remove the cause of the spasms of the diaphragm.

Promote Rest and Activity

The patient needs to sleep after surgery. The room should be kept quiet and nursing activities grouped to prevent waking the patient more than necessary. At least every 2 hours the patient must do leg exercises and change position. Orders for ambulation may begin within several hours after surgery. Raise the head of the bed first and let the body adjust to the position change. Then sit the patient on the side of the bed, allowing the legs to dangle over the side with the feet on the floor. After a few minutes, slowly assist the patient to stand. Assist the patient to walk around the room, or for at least a few steps. Use a gait belt and have someone assist you if the patient is very weak. Pain medication can be timed to decrease pain during ambulation if it does not make the patient too groggy. Emphasize to the patient that exercise is vital to prevent circulatory problems. Keeping blood from pooling in the extremities helps prevent thrombus formation and **embolus** (a thrombus or clot that travels and lodges elsewhere in the body). Offer praise for all efforts. Continue to ambulate on a set schedule until the patient is up and about independently. In many hospitals, physical therapy orders will be written and the physical therapist will be responsible for ambulating the patient and overseeing range-of-motion exercises.

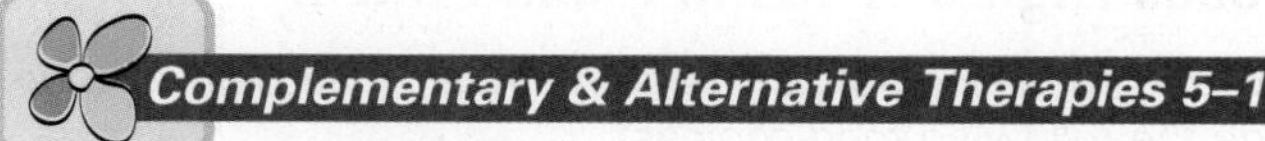

Stopping Hiccups

An alternate treatment for hiccups is to massage the earlobes. Massage activates the acupressure points, interrupting the hiccup reflex.

Other commonly used remedies include:

- Fill a glass with at least 4 oz of water. Lean over a sink and drink the water from the back side of the glass. Drink continuously until the glass is empty.
- Stick a finger in each ear, and hold your breath.
- Drink from a glass that someone else is holding for you.
- Breathe into a paper bag deeply 20 times.
- Place a teaspoon of sugar or peanut butter on the tongue and let it slowly dissolve; the hiccups will be gone when the sugar or peanut butter has dissolved.

If the patient is on strict bed rest, range-of-motion exercises must be performed at least four times a day. The patient may do active range of motion on most joints, but passive range of motion on joints the patient is unable to exercise must be done unless physical therapy visits have been ordered. Family members may help with these exercises.

Promote Wound Healing

Adequate rest, sufficient blood supply, and proper nutrition all promote wound healing. Rest decreases the metabolic rate and allows nutrients to be available for healing rather than being used for the energy of activity. Blood contains the amino acids and other elements needed for rebuilding tissue and is essential to healing. Good circulation ensures that the blood reaches the wound. *Vitamin C* is necessary for collagen production, the formation of capillaries that bring blood to the healing tissues, and resistance to infection. The minerals zinc, copper, and iron assist in the formation of collagen. *Proteins* provide the amino acids that are the building blocks of tissue and are vital to the healing process (Nutritional Therapies 5–1).

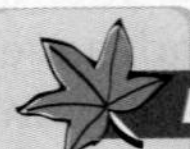

Elder Care Points

- The elderly person often has chronic diseases that interfere with oxygenation and transport of nutrients to the cells and removal of wastes from the cells.
- Vitamin and mineral deficiencies are common in the elderly, contributing to poor wound healing.
- Regeneration of tissue takes more time, partially because of the slower metabolic rate that occurs with age.

Nutritional Therapies 5–1

Foods High in Vitamin C and Protein

When counseling surgical patients about their diet, encourage the following food choices:

FOODS HIGH IN VITAMIN C

Citrus fruits and juices	Turnip or collard greens
Strawberries	Broccoli
Cantaloupe	Mangos
Tomatoes	Peaches
Bell peppers	Pineapple
Cabbage	Potatoes

FOODS HIGH IN PROTEIN

Meats: chicken, beef, pork, lamb*	Beans
Cottage cheese	Eggs
Milk*	Ice cream
Cheese	Grain products: breads, pasta
Peanut butter	Tofu; soy products

*Meats and milk products contain the highest amounts of protein.

Surgical incisions most often heal by primary, or first, intention (Table 5–1).

Factors Interfering with Wound Healing. **Smoking produces a decrease in the amount of hemoglobin available to carry oxygen to the healing tissues. Healing time in cigarette smokers is prolonged.** Mechanical injury from friction, pressure, or abrasion, such as can occur when tape is removed, disrupts the healing tissue and prolongs wound healing. Physical injury destroys granulation tissue, which is the framework on which new cells grow and mature to form a covering for the wound. All healing wounds should be handled gently and shielded from injury. When dressings are removed from a wound, care must be taken not to dislodge granulation tissue. The presence of pathogenic organisms in a wound prolongs the inflammatory process and delays healing. Anti-infective drugs are sometimes given postoperatively to prevent wound infection, and they should be administered at the times ordered to maintain appropriate blood levels of the drugs.

Excessive stress, apprehension, and emotional disturbances seem to make the body more vulnerable to invasion by foreign organisms by depressing the immune system. When it is under excessive stress, the body also is less able to mobilize the elements and cells that promote healing.

Corticosteroids taken for a chronic condition will slow the healing process because they suppress the immune and inflammatory response.

Interventions for Wound Care. The surgical wound should be inspected during dressing changes or at least once a day. Assessment includes observing the incision line for signs of excessive swelling, formation of a **hematoma** (blood-filled swelling), **seroma** (serum-filled swelling), redness, and tearing of the skin or other signs of separation of the edges of the skin that have been sutured together. Normally, a surgical wound is sealed

Table 5–1 *Phases of Primary Intention Wound Healing**

PHASE	ACTIVITY
Phase I Acute inflammatory reaction (3–4 days)	Process of hemostasis. Constriction of blood vessels, platelet aggregation and the formation of fibrin, and epithelial cell migration. Phagocytosis occurs. Scab forms.
Phase II Proliferation and granulation (3rd or 4th day to 2–3 wk)	Macrophages clear debris, fibroblasts synthesize collagen, capillary networks are built, granulation tissue is formed. Closure by contracture begins.
Phase III Scar maturation and contracture (3–6 wk)	Remodeling with collagen lysis and synthesis; scar tissue thins and becomes paler, but stronger.

*A surgical incision most often heals by primary intention. Many accidental wounds and some infected wounds heal by secondary or tertiary intention.

within hours and little drainage is expected. If there is evidence of bleeding, **purulence** (pus), or any other sign that the wound is not healing as it should, this should be reported and documented. Include the appearance of any drainage in your charting. Drainage may be serous (clear or very light yellow), serosanguineous (reddish yellow), or sanguineous (blood red). Documentation should include whether sutures or staples are intact and the wound edges are well approximated.

The best way to prevent hospital-acquired infection of a surgical wound is always to wash your hands before doing wound care or touching the patient, use aseptic technique and Standard Precautions for dressing changes, and change the dressings as ordered.

Additional factors that may slow wound healing in a postoperative patient include vomiting, abdominal distention, and strenuous respiratory efforts, such as coughing and forcefully exhaling breaths of air without proper splinting of the incision. The wound should be properly splinted for coughing to prevent dehiscence of the incision (see Figure 4–4).

Dressings. **Surgical dressings should be checked each time vital signs are taken for the first 24 hours after surgery, every 4 hours during the next 24 hours, and then at least every 8 hours as long as the surgical wound is covered with a dressing.** If a wound is not expected to drain, but drainage is evident, the surgeon should be notified. If drainage is outlined and the time and date noted, the nurse can tell if the wound is draining more than it should be over a period of hours. The surgeon usually does the first dressing change. If the dressing becomes saturated before this, it should be reinforced by placing more dressing material over the area. If within the orders, the outer dressings may be removed, leaving those in direct contact with the wound, and new outer dressings secured in place. When there is excessive drainage, the dressing probably will require reinforcing every 4 hours. Changing the dressing more often than once a shift is not recommended because of the danger of introducing infectious agents, traumatizing the wound, and interfering with the regeneration of tissue.

Each time the dressing is changed, the amount and characteristics of drainage on it should be noted and documented. If the wound is infected, the odor of the drainage can give a clue as to the kind of organism causing the infection. A musty odor is characteristic of aerobic organisms. An acrid (sharp, stinging) or putrid (foul) odor is characteristic of anaerobes. Anaerobic infections are frequently seen in colorectal and vaginal surgery. An infected wound should be cultured to see what organism is causing the infection.

Drains. Drains are used to remove fluid and air from around the operative site. Drains are used to (1) prevent accumulation of fluids or air at the operative site; (2) protect suture lines; and (3) remove specific fluids, such as bile, cerebrospinal fluid, or drainage from an abscess. Drains that do not attach to a suction device either are attached to a drainage bag or have dressings placed to catch the fluid. An example of a drain is the *Penrose,* which is inserted into the abdominal cavity or any other area where an abscess, fistula, or other condition requires drainage (Figure 5–4). A T-tube drain may be placed in the common bile duct after surgery on the gallbladder or liver.

Some drains require continuous suction and are therefore connected to some type of apparatus that creates suction to facilitate removal of drainage. If a drain is kinked, the accumulated fluid and gas can cause pain, create dead air space (which delays healing), damage the healing tissue at the suture lines, and delay healing by compressing surrounding capillaries and cutting off oxygen supply to the cells.

One kind of drain system is the closed-wound suction device (e.g., Hemovac). The drainage catheter is connected to a spring-loaded drum, collapsed at least once a shift to create the desired suction, which pulls fluid into a collection area of the device. Jackson-Pratt suction devices are about the size of the bulb on a blood pressure cuff. They have a valve on top that is opened to allow removal of fluid and collapse of the bulb and then is closed to create negative pressure, which provides the suction. As drainage accumulates in the bulb, it is emptied and recompressed (Figure 5–5). This should be done at least once per shift.

Removing Sutures and Staples. When an order is written to remove sutures or staples, check the order, gather the proper equipment, inform the patient about the procedure, correctly identify the patient, wash hands, glove, and inspect the incision carefully. For a long incision or an incision over a joint, remove every other suture or staple first (Figure 5–6). If the edges of the incision do not pull apart, remove the rest of the sutures or staples. Often Steri-Strips (small, reinforced strips of adhesive) are applied to hold the incision together until healing is complete.

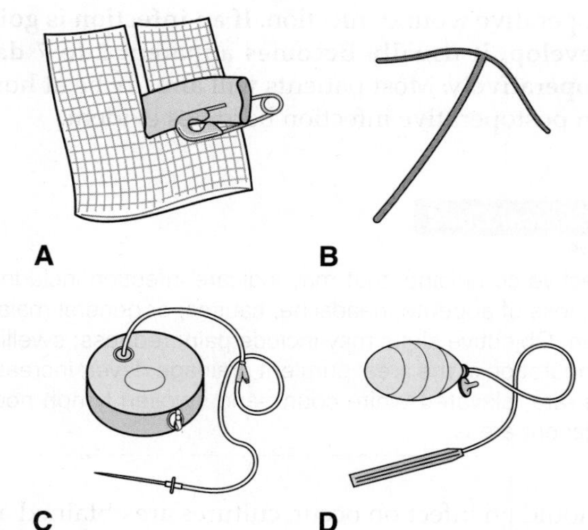

FIGURE 5–4 Wound drain and suction devices. **A,** Penrose drain. **B,** T-tube drain. **C,** Hemovac drainage system. **D,** Jackson-Pratt drain and reservoir.

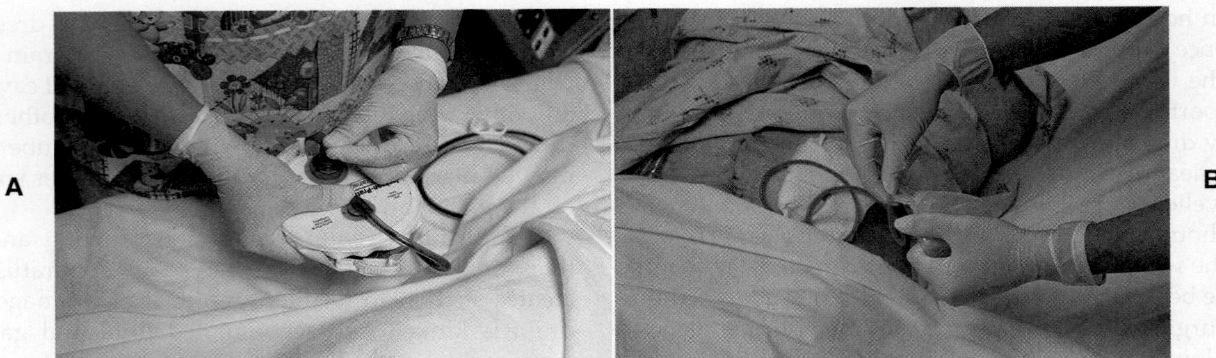

FIGURE 5–5 Reactivating surgical wound suction devices by compressing the suction device after emptying the reservoir. **A,** Hemovac. **B,** Jackson-Pratt.

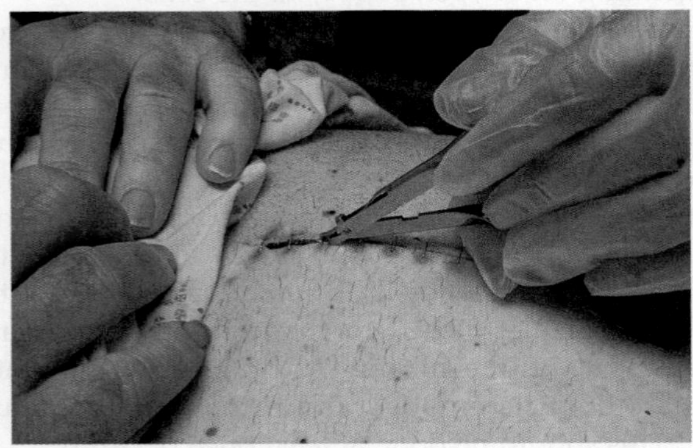

FIGURE 5–6 Surgical staples are removed with a special implement.

Prevent Postoperative Complications

Table 5–2 summarizes the major postoperative complications and nursing interventions to prevent them. Some complications are immediately life threatening.

Wound Infection. Infection of a wound can occur in any surgical procedure, but it is more common in wounds caused by accidental injury and in those that were infected at the time of surgery. A prophylactic antibiotic may be ordered to prevent the occurrence of postoperative wound infection. **If an infection is going to develop, it usually becomes apparent 2 to 7 days postoperatively.** Most patients will already be at home when postoperative infection becomes evident.

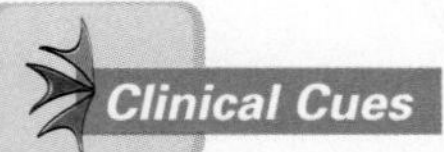

Subjective complaints that may indicate infection include fatigue, loss of appetite, headache, nausea, or general malaise or pain. Objective signs may include pain; redness; swelling, and induration in the area; purulent drainage; fever; increased pulse rate; elevated white count; and swollen lymph nodes in adjacent areas.

Should an infection occur, cultures are obtained and appropriate antibiotics are given for a specific time. Wound irrigations may be ordered for an open, infected wound. Sterile normal saline is the most common solution for this purpose. The wound may be packed with dressings moistened with the sterile saline solution.

A noninfected wound should not be cleaned or irrigated with anything but sterile normal saline as other substances irritate the tissue and slow healing.

Transmission-based isolation precautions or Contact Precautions are instituted when a wound is infected. Gowns, as well as gloves, are worn when performing dressing changes or wound irrigations on infected wounds. If splattering is likely, protective eyewear and masks are also worn. Soiled dressings and supplies are bagged in plastic barrier bags and deposited in a biohazard trash receptacle. **Dressings from an infected wound should never be placed in the patient's room trash container.**

Dehiscence and Evisceration. Throughout the period following abdominal surgery, the nurse must be alert for possible disruption or separation of some or all the layers of the surgical wound. This is called **dehiscence.** If the wound completely separates and the contents of the abdominal cavity (viscera) protrude through the incision, the condition is called **evisceration** (Figure 5–7).

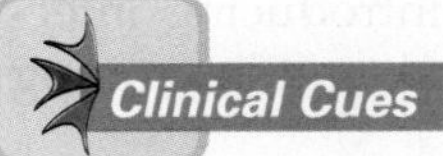

Dehiscence can occur at any time during the postoperative period, but it most commonly occurs between the 5th and 12th postoperative day. This is when the patient is feeling stronger and more active, but healing is not complete, or when infection has occurred. When checking an abdominal surgical wound, be particularly aware of any drainage on the dressing. There is often a noticeable increase in the amount of serosanguineous drainage on the wound dressing before the separation of the wound layers becomes apparent. Subjectively, the patient may not notice any symptoms until he feels something "give way" in the wound.

The separation or disruption usually is brought on by a sudden strain or stress on the suture lines, as, for example, when the patient sneezes, coughs, or has an episode of retching and vomiting. **Patients who are**

Table 5–2 **Postoperative Complications**

PROBLEM	SIGNS AND SYMPTOMS	PREVENTIVE INTERVENTIONS
Atelectasis	Decreased breath sounds over areas not aerating; dyspnea	Deep breathing and coughing; use of incentive spirometer; early ambulation; teach to cough properly.
Pneumonia: hypostatic, aspiration, or bacterial	Fever, malaise, increased sputum, purulent sputum, cough, flushed skin, dyspnea, pain on inspiration; abnormal breath sounds, crackles, rhonchi	Deep breathing, coughing, and frequent turning; early ambulation; incentive spirometer use; range-of-motion exercises if unable to ambulate; medication if bacterial.
Paralytic (adynamic) ileus	No bowel sounds 24–36 hr after surgery or fewer than 5 sounds/min	Monitor bowel sounds; encourage early ambulation; nothing by mouth as ordered. Do not feed until bowel sounds return.
Thrombophlebitis	Pain or warmth in calf of leg, swollen leg, warm area to touch on leg; possible temperature elevation	Encourage leg exercises; keep the patient well hydrated; encourage ambulation; use antiembolic stockings or devices.
Urinary retention	Distended bladder; inability to void spontaneously	Palpate bladder; encourage voiding, catheterize if unable to void within 8 hr per order; medicate to increase urinary sphincter tone as ordered.
Urinary tract infection	Dysuria, frequency, foul-smelling urine	Force fluids when allowed; encourage frequent voiding; keep catheter clean and patent; use aseptic technique to empty drainage bag.
Wound infection	Redness, swelling, pain, warmth, drainage, fever, increased leukocytes, rapid pulse and respirations (fever 72 hr after surgery indicates infection in some system or in the wound)	Assess wound characteristics and drainage. Monitor white blood cell count and temperature. Use aseptic technique for wound care; encourage adequate nutrition and fluids; encourage activity.
Pulmonary embolus	Shortness of breath, anxiety, chest pain, rapid pulse and respirations, cyanosis, cough, bloody sputum	Antiembolism stockings, adequate fluid intake, frequent turning or ambulation, preventive anticoagulant if ordered; leg exercises.
Hemorrhage and shock	Evidence of copious bleeding; decreased blood pressure, elevated pulse, cold clammy skin, decreased urinary output	Give blood or volume expander; stop bleeding. Place in shock position with feet and legs elevated and head flat; administer ordered medications to raise blood pressure; administer oxygen; frequent vital signs measurement.
Wound dehiscence or evisceration	Discharge of serosanguineous drainage from wound and sensation that "something gave"; separation of wound edges with intestines visible through abdominal incision	Teach to splint properly for coughing. Place patient supine; cover wound with sterile saline-soaked gauze or towels; return to operating room for repair; monitor for shock.
Fluid imbalance	Signs of overhydration: crackles in lungs, edema, weight gain. Signs of dehydration: weight loss, diminished pulse, dry mucous membranes, decreased tissue turgor.	Control intravenous flow rate. Monitor intake and output; correct imbalances. Output will be less than intake for first 72 hr after surgery with general anesthesia. Auscultate lungs each shift. Monitor weight; check for edema.
Malignant hyperthermia	High temperature, cardiac dysrhythmias, muscle rigidity, hypotension, tachypnea, and dark cola-colored urine.	Genetic predisposition; can only monitor and treat symptoms; apply cooling blanket and ice packs. Give dantrolene as ordered.

Adapted from deWit, S.C. (2005). *Fundamental Concepts and Skills for Nursing* (2nd ed.). Philadelphia: Elsevier Saunders, p. 750.

most at risk for dehiscence and evisceration are those who are diabetic, obese, malnourished, or dehydrated; have a malignancy; have experienced multiple traumas to the abdomen; or have an infected wound. Abdominal distention, strenuous coughing, and broken sutures also are factors in wound disruption, but dehiscence can occur with any surgical wound. Wound dehiscence and evisceration create an emergency that requires immediate surgery and are very serious complications. Between the time the dehiscence and exposure of the intestines occur and surgery is done, the patient should lie supine with the knees flexed. The wound should be covered with either a sterile towel or sterile dressings moistened with sterile normal saline. With early discharge after surgery, the wound may disrupt at home (Home Care Considerations 5–1).

? *Think Critically About . . .* Can you identify seven assessment findings that together would indicate that the patient most likely has a wound infection?

Hemorrhage and Shock. The two most common complications of anesthesia and surgery are shock and infection. Of these, shock presents the most immediate danger to the patient, as it can quickly develop into a life-threatening emergency condition. The person in shock is suffering from a disruption of normal physio-

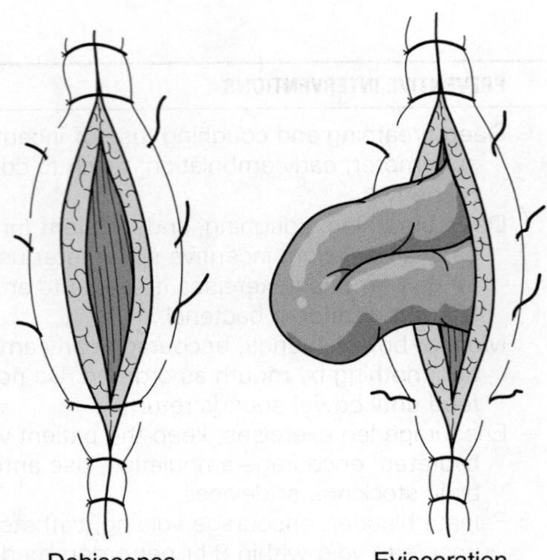

FIGURE 5–7 Complications of wound healing: dehiscence and evisceration.

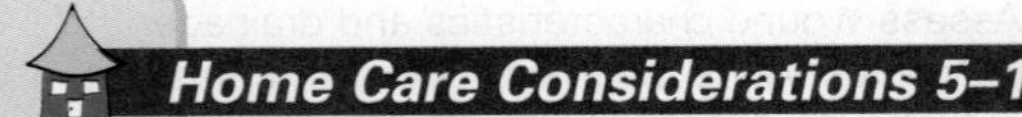

Home Care Considerations 5–1

In Case of Dehiscence or Evisceration

If dehiscence or evisceration occurs at home, a sterile gauze moistened with sterile water or, if that is unavailable, fresh water should be placed over the exposed bowel. The object is to keep the bowel membrane moist. Immediately notify the home care agency or the physician, call someone to help, and have the patient lie supine with the moistened dressings in place.

logic function. This disruption can result from (1) failure of the heart to function as a pump *(cardiogenic shock)*, as in cardiac arrest (see Chapter 20); (2) a low volume of blood *(hypovolemic shock)*, as in hemorrhage; (3) collapse of the blood vessels as a result of faulty nervous system regulation *(neurogenic shock)* (see Chapter 22); (4) **anaphylaxis** (severe, allergic reaction), as in hypersensitivity to a drug or other allergen (see Chapter 11); and (5) sepsis, occurring when the toxins from bacteria bring about a relaxation and dilation of blood vessels with a resultant drop in blood pressure (see Chapters 6 and 44).

In the immediate postoperative period, the patient is most likely to suffer from cardiogenic, hypovolemic, or neurogenic shock. However, any of the five kinds of shock are a possibility after anesthesia and surgery. The symptoms of shock depend to some degree on the cause of circulatory failure.

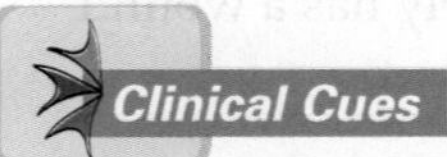

Clinical Cues

Early signs of impending hypovolemic shock from hemorrhage are:

- Thirst
- Restlessness
- Tachycardia
- Tachypnea

Patients with neurogenic and cardiogenic shock may not present any warning signs of impending shock other than changes in the vital signs.

As the shock progresses, the blood pressure begins to drop. The pulse rate increases and may be bounding at first, but becomes thready and indistinct as circulatory collapse occurs. The skin becomes cold and clammy, and pallor becomes evident. There may be air hunger, with cyanosis of the lips and nail beds as a result of tissue hypoxia. As shock deepens, the blood pressure continues to fall, and the patient loses consciousness, eventually becoming comatose. Untreated shock ultimately is fatal.

Both general and local anesthesia can bring about circulatory collapse. If there is evidence that the patient is in the early stage of shock, he should be placed in the supine position with the lower extremities elevated to add blood volume to the vital organs. **Patients in cardiogenic shock are placed in Fowler's position to lower the diaphragm and increase oxygenation as long as they do not become too hypotensive.** Pain contributes to the progression of shock, but large doses of narcotics can decrease blood pressure further.

Sometimes patients who develop shock also develop disseminated intravascular coagulation. This is a life-threatening disorder evidenced by bleeding from many sites, and it is discussed in Chapter 44.

Intravenous fluids and medications are important to prevent and treat shock. Supplemental oxygen also is usually given to combat tissue hypoxia and cardiac response. Chapter 44 discusses the specific treatment for shock.

Malignant Hyperthermia. **Malignant hyperthermia** (MH) is a complication of general anesthesia that is life threatening. Anesthetic agents that may trigger MH include halothane, isoflurane, enflurane, and succinylcholine. MH occurs from a biochemical reaction in genetically predisposed persons. Signs of MH include high temperature, cardiac dysrhythmia, muscle rigidity of the jaw or other muscles, hypotension, tachypnea, and dark cola-colored urine. The temperature may rise up to 111.2 F° (44° C). The extremely high temperature is a late sign of MH. The anesthesiologist and surgeon should be notified immediately if any of these signs occurs. If it is not treated swiftly and effectively, MH will kill the patient. Dantrolene sodium (Dantrium) is the medication used to treat MH and is infused rapidly. The patient is immediately placed on a hypothermia blanket, ice bags are applied to the armpits and groin to cool the core of the body, and iced saline IV solutions may be administered. Cold-solution enemas may be given as well.

Promote Psychological Adjustment

The patient may be concerned about the ability to perform self-care postoperatively or acceptance of an altered body or health status by family and friends. Depending on the type of surgery performed, the patient may experience considerable change in body image. If there is extensive scarring, a body image change is likely. If part of an extremity, an organ, or part of a breast has been surgically removed, the necessary psychological adjustment is considerable. Such adjustment takes a lot of time. The patient should be assessed for signs of ineffective coping, such as withdrawn, depressed behavior; less attention to grooming than before; and poor communication efforts. If these signs occur, work with the patient to identify areas of concern and then collaborate with the other health team members to develop a plan of assistance.

Help the patient by encouraging discussion of feelings regarding what has been removed and the effect it might have on the patient's life. Being an active listener, and gradually having the patient focus on the positives in life rather than on the loss incurred, is helpful. Referral to an appropriate community support group of people who have undergone a similar experience and are learning to cope can be very helpful (Communication Cues 5–1).

Evaluation

Evaluation is based on whether goals and expected outcomes have been met. Evaluative statements regarding previously stated general goals might be as follows:

- Lungs clear to auscultation; respirations 18
- Pulse 82, BP 136/86, peripheral pulses present
- Pain controlled for 4 hours with analgesia; states pain medication controls pain for about 4 hours
- Incision clean, dry, and without redness
- States is glad that periods of pain and malaise will be gone
- No signs of thrombophlebitis or infection

Each nursing care plan is evaluated on whether the individual specific outcomes have been met. Further examples of evaluation are in the nursing care plan for this chapter (Nursing Care Plan 5–1).

Discharge Planning

With same-day surgery and early release from the hospital after inpatient surgery, it is vital that discharge planning be started at admission or several days before the surgery. Needs for home care must be assessed. Will the patient need assistance with bathing? Meals? Dressing changes (Cultural Cues 5–1)? It may be necessary to arrange home health care with an aide to assist with bathing and a nurse to assess the patient's condition and provide wound care. Equipment, such as oxygen, suction, or an IV pump, may need to be ordered before discharge so that the transition to home goes smoothly.

The family or significant others must be included in discharge planning and teaching. Often it is a family member who will do the dressing changes, monitor for side effects of medication, alert the physician to signs of complications, and be generally supportive to the patient during recovery.

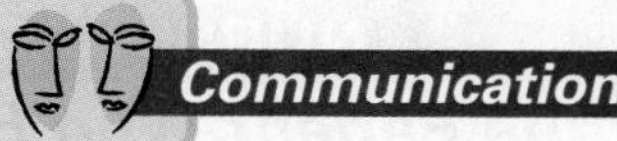

Communication Cues 5–1

Recovering from Abdominal Surgery

Mrs. Wilson is a 74-year-old who is recovering from abdominal surgery. Although her body language tells her nurse she is experiencing pain, she has denied any need for pain medication since she administered her patient-controlled analgesia dose 3 hours before.

NURSE: "Mrs. Wilson, I would like to see you able to cough more vigorously, move about in bed more, and ambulate more frequently. I think that if you would use your pain pump more often you would be more comfortable doing your exercises and coughing."

MRS. WILSON: "I'm not that uncomfortable and those medications always cause problems for me."

NURSE: "Problems?"

MRS. WILSON: "Yes, I get really constipated."

NURSE: "The doctor has a stool softener ordered for you to help to prevent constipation, and by increasing fluids, we should be able to control that. Do you have other problems with the pain medication?"

MRS. WILSON: "Yes, it makes me light-headed and unsteady on my feet."

NURSE: "If the medication makes you light-headed, we can switch you to a different medication. One of us will stay with you when you are out of bed to see that you do not fall."

MRS. WILSON: "I'm very afraid of falling, breaking a hip, and adding to my troubles."

NURSE: "By taking the medication and being more comfortable, you'll feel more like doing your exercises. That's how you can help prevent postoperative complications such as pneumonia or blood clots."

MRS. WILSON: "I certainly don't want pneumonia or a blood clot!"

NURSE: "Moving about more will also increase circulation and help your wound to heal faster."

MRS. WILSON: "O.K., I'll take the pain medication if it will help me prevent complications."

When the patient is discharged, review specific instructions regarding care at home, including care of the incision or wound, diet, activity level, medications, and signs and symptoms of complications to report to the health care provider (Patient Teaching 5–1). Make certain that it is understood when to see the physician for follow-up. Send home sufficient supplies of items needed for dressing changes, and tell the patient and family where such items can be obtained. Make every attempt to see to it that the patient does not go home with unanswered questions.

? *Think Critically About . . .* Which health care professionals would it be necessary to collaborate with to plan appropriate continuing care for the elderly patient who has had a hip replacement (and also has chronic lung disease) and is being discharged home to the care of a 76-year-old spouse?

NURSING CARE PLAN 5–1

Care of the Patient Who Has Had a Simple Mastectomy

SCENARIO A married 38-year-old woman and the mother of two children ages 16 and 14 underwent a simple mastectomy as treatment for a 4.5-mm malignant tumor.

PROBLEM/NURSING DIAGNOSIS *Surgical incision*/Impaired skin integrity related to surgical wound.

Supporting assessment data *Objective:* Right mastectomy; dressing on right chest.

Goals/Expected Outcomes	Nursing Interventions	Selected Rationale	Evaluation
Wound will be free of signs of infection at discharge.	Keep Jackson-Pratt suction functioning properly.	Suction is needed to pull drainage from operative site.	No signs of infection. Incision clean, dry, and without reddening.
Wound will heal completely within 6 weeks.	Note character and amount of drainage; document.	Helps detect excessive bleeding.	Draining small amounts of serosanguineous fluid.
	Reinforce dressing as needed.		No need for dressing reinforcement.
	Assess for excessive bleeding q hr for 4 hr, then q 2 hr for first 24 hr.		Small amount of serosanguineous drainage in Jackson-Pratt.
	Assess pulses in arm q 2 hr to detect excessive swelling in arm.	Swelling in arm can cause nerve damage.	Minimal swelling in arm; pulses are 2+.
	Monitor temperature, and white blood cell (WBC) count.	Temperature and WBC count trends will show if infection is developing.	No increase in temperature or WBC count.
	Assess wound for signs of infection with each dressing change.	Sterile dressing helps prevent infection.	Wound clean and dry without signs of infection.
	Change dressing q 8–24 hr as needed.		Surgeon changed dressing this afternoon. Continue plan.

PROBLEM/NURSING DIAGNOSIS *Surgery*/Pain related to surgical incision.

Supporting assessment data *Subjective:* Complains of incisional pain and discomfort. *Objective:* Right mastectomy; rates pain at 4 on pain scale.

Goals/Expected Outcomes	Nursing Interventions	Selected Rationale	Evaluation
Pain will be controlled by analgesia as noted by patient.	Instruct on use of patient-controlled analgesia (PCA).	Knowledge is needed to use PCA effectively.	Using PCA appropriately.
	Assess pain level q 3–4 hr.	Assessing pain level will demonstrate whether pain is adequately controlled.	Pain level consistently below 4.
	Provide comfort measures.	Comfort measures increase effect of analgesia.	Straightened bed; brought warmed blanket. Continue plan.
Pain is controlled by oral analgesia by discharge.	Administer analgesics as ordered.		

COMMUNITY CARE

The patient may be given follow-up care at an outpatient clinic, physician's office, subacute care unit, rehabilitation unit, extended-care unit, or the home. The nurse assesses the patient's condition and progress and performs treatments and procedures such as wound care. The nurse case manager will coordinate the care of the whole team, collaborating with the social worker, physical therapist, respiratory therapist, nurse's aide, dietitian, pharmacist, physician, and other health care professionals. The quality of nursing care delivered often is the factor that prevents complications and rehospitalization of the patient.

The home care, office, or outpatient clinic nurse must reinforce teaching about the signs and symptoms of complications, such as infection, dehiscence, pulmonary embolus, or thrombophlebitis, and verify that the patient can adequately perform his own self-

NURSING CARE PLAN 5–1

Care of the Patient Who Has Had a Simple Mastectomy—cont'd

PROBLEM/NURSING DIAGNOSIS *Anesthesia*/Potential for impaired gas exchange related to inhalation anesthesia.

Supporting assessment data *Objective:* Had general anesthesia. Restricted mobility. *Subjective:* "I don't like using the incentive spirometer. Do I have to cough? It hurts."

Goals/Expected Outcomes	Nursing Interventions	Selected Rationale	Evaluation
Patient will not have atelectasis by end of postop day 2.	Have patient use incentive spirometer q hr while awake.	Incentive spirometer use opens alveoli, decreasing atelectasis.	Using incentive spirometer; barely diminished breath sounds in lung bases.
	Have patient cough q 2 hr.	Coughing clears secretions from lung irritation due to anesthesia.	Coughed secretions are clear.
Lung sounds will be clear at discharge.	Auscultate lungs q 8 hr.	Auscultation determines status of breath sounds.	Lungs clear.
	Encourage ambulation.		Ambulated ×2.
	Monitor temperature, respirations, and oxygen saturation.		Continue plan.

PROBLEM/NURSING DIAGNOSIS *Loss of breast*/Risk for grieving related to loss of body part and perception of femininity.

Supporting assessment data *Objective:* Right mastectomy. *Subjective:* Expresses concern about husband's reaction to surgery.

Goals/Expected Outcomes	Nursing Interventions	Selected Rationale	Evaluation
Patient will verbalize feelings of self-worth and confidence.	Have patient list her strengths and positive attributes.	Focusing on strengths can help counter feelings of loss.	Is patient verbalizing feelings of confidence and self-worth? Not yet.
Patient will discuss sadness over loss of breast.	Encourage sharing of sad feelings and fears with husband.	Talking openly with husband may provide reassurance.	Expressed sadness over breast loss to husband.
	Talk with husband privately about his feelings.	Involvement will show her he still cares for her.	Husband reluctant to speak about the surgery or his feelings so far.
	Involve husband in patient's care.		
	Encourage daughters to discuss their feelings and fears with patient.		Daughters have not been in yet today.
	Encourage independence in patient.	Independence increases self-confidence.	Brushed her teeth. Continue plan.

? CRITICAL THINKING QUESTIONS

1. You auscultate the patient's lungs the evening after surgery, and sounds are diminished in the bases. What do you think it means?
2. What would you do if the radial pulse in the arm on the same side as the breast surgery becomes weaker and harder to detect?

care (Home Care Considerations 5–2). Some physicians discharge patients who are ambulatory and normally self-sufficient, thinking that they can do complicated wound care. This is often not the case; most patients need assistance with anything more than a simple dressing change. This is particularly true if the patient lives alone. The nurse collaborates with the patient, physician, social worker, and community agencies to secure the assistance the patient needs.

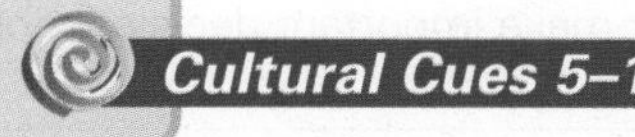

Cultural Cues 5–1

Performing Wound Care

Traditional Chinese, although not overly modest, may have a cultural hesitance about touching their own bodies. For this reason, it is important to assess who will perform wound care and change dressings at home. A home health nurse may need to be accessed, or teaching of another family member may be important.

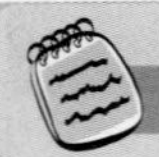

Patient Teaching 5–1

Discharge Instructions for the Same-Day Surgery Patient

The following points should be covered for the same-day surgery patient before discharge.

Diet

- Type of diet and importance of proper nutrition for healing
- Dietary restrictions, if any
- Avoiding alcohol for first 24 hours after anesthesia
- Special dietary recommendations
- Recommended fluid intake

Activity

- Recommended exercise and frequency
- Instructions for special equipment: crutches, walker, cane, splint, etc.
- Schedule for deep breathing, coughing, and leg exercises; how long to continue these activities; remember to splint the incision when coughing and getting out of bed
- Recommended rest periods
- Activity restrictions (i.e., driving, intercourse, and lifting)
- Application, use, and care of antiembolism stockings

Wound care

- Hand hygiene
- Dressing changes and frequency
- Cleansing of wound; irrigations
- Drainage observations
- Signs to report
- Use of heat or cold packs
- Supplies and where to obtain them

Temperature monitoring

- Record time and temperature
- Report temperature >100° F (38° C)

Type of bath and frequency

Medications

- Analgesics
- Antibiotics
- Sedatives
- Vitamin supplements
- Other medications

Precautions related to anesthesia or side effects of medication

- Caution regarding using machinery
- Caution regarding making decisions for 24 hours
- Drug interactions
- Potential for constipation
- Potential for urinary retention

Next scheduled appointment with the physician

Signs and symptoms to report

- Elevated temperature
- Increasing malaise
- Severe pain or swelling
- Bleeding through bandage
- Decreased sensation below surgical site
- Severe nausea and vomiting

Expectation for return to usual activities

Expectation for return to feeling normal

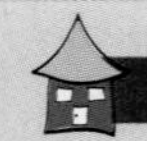

Home Care Considerations 5–2

Home Care for Postsurgical Patients

Discharge planning begins at the time of admission. Whether the patient is a same-day surgery patient or an inpatient, the same general points will need to be covered before discharge.

- The patient must know about each medication to be taken and when to take it.
- The diet, any restrictions, and guidelines for fluid intake are discussed. Alcohol must be avoided for 24 hours after surgery.
- Any restrictions on activity are listed and instructions for use of any special equipment such as crutches, splint, walker, and so forth are presented.
- Patients should not drive or make important decisions for 24 hours after anesthesia.
- The type of bath permitted is explained.
- Cleansing and dressing of the wound are discussed along with where to obtain supplies.
- Signs and symptoms to report to the surgeon, such as temperature above 100° F (38° C), increasing malaise, severe pain or swelling, bleeding through the bandage, decreased sensation below the surgical site, or severe nausea and vomiting, are listed.
- Instructions as to when to schedule a follow-up appointment with the physician are essential.
- Written instructions should be sent home with the patient for all essential points of care.

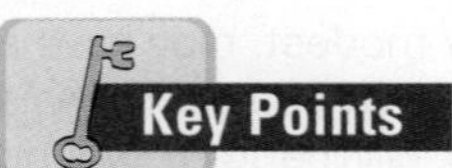

- The PACU monitors patients very closely until they are fully aroused from anesthesia.
- Maintaining a patent airway is the highest priority.
- The nurse is vigilant for signs of complications and performs frequent assessments during the postoperative period.
- Nursing interventions are aimed at providing pain control, comfort, and fluid balance; protecting the pa-

tient from injury; maintaining vital functions; and preventing infection.
- The nurse tries to prevent or intervene in the many potential complications of surgery.
- Discharge planning begins at admission and covers all areas of basic needs, wound care, and activity restrictions.
- Written instructions regarding all aspects of postoperative care should be sent home with the patient.

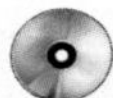

Go to your **Companion CD-ROM** for an Audio Glossary, animations, video clips, and bonus review questions.

evolve Be sure to visit the companion Evolve site at http://evolve.elsevier.com/deWit for interactive NCLEX-PN Exam Style Review Questions, WebLinks, and additional online resources.

NCLEX-PN EXAM STYLE REVIEW QUESTIONS

Choose the best answer(s) for the following questions.

1. While taking care of a postoperative patient, the nurse must reinforce which of the following to reduce complications associated with any major surgery?
   1. Use incentive spirometer sparingly
   2. Ambulate as soon as possible
   3. Cough every 4 hours
   4. Turn and deep breathe

2. A 32-year-old woman who has undergone bilateral radical mastectomy is withdrawn and quiet. She is afebrile with no apparent complaints of pain. Her dressings are dry and intact. Pulses are full on both upper extremities. A priority nursing diagnosis for this patient would be:
   1. Acute pain related to surgical incision.
   2. Risk for infection related to surgery.
   3. Disturbed body image related to loss of body parts.
   4. Impaired communication related to unknown.

3. In planning care for an elderly patient who had open reduction and internal fixation of the right femur, the nurse formulates the nursing diagnoses of risk for infection related to surgical incision and compromised immunity associated with advanced age. An appropriate expected outcome would be:
   1. the nurse will monitor changes in temperature and laboratory values during the shift.
   2. the patient will be able to state the signs and symptoms of wound infections before discharge.
   3. the caregiver will be able to teach aseptic techniques to the patient before discharge.
   4. the nursing assistant will be able to demonstrate proper hand washing technique when taking the patient's vital signs.

4. Which of the following statements indicates patient understanding regarding the use of patient-controlled analgesia (PCA) pump?
   1. "I can readily become addicted to pain medication."
   2. "To a certain extent, I control the amount of pain medication I can have."
   3. "I will be completely pain-free."
   4. "I need to call the nurse when I need pain medication."

5. To promote wound healing, the postoperative patient is instructed to consider eating foods high in protein. Which of the following patient food choices warrant further patient teaching?
   1. Chips and bean dip
   2. Chicken quesadilla
   3. Green salad
   4. Tofu stir fry

6. After a series of instructions and demonstrations in preparation for home discharge, the postoperative patient is allowed to administer his own Subcut enoxaparin (Lovenox). Which of the following patient behaviors warrant further patient teaching?
   1. Wiping the injection site with alcohol
   2. Aspirating blood before Subcut injection
   3. Retaining the air bubble in the prefilled syringe
   4. Applying bandage on the site after administration

7. Upon arrival from the postanesthesia care unit, the patient complains of severe thirst. The nurse finds that the patient is increasingly restless, tachypneic, and tachycardic. The nurse would likely suspect which of the following?
   1. Hypovolemia
   2. Cardiogenic shock
   3. Normal response to anesthesia
   4. Pain medication overdose

8. The patient is prescribed antiembolism stockings. The patient asks, "Why do I need these leg stockings?" An appropriate nursing response would be:
   1. "Your physician ordered these stockings."
   2. "These prevent formation of clots."
   3. "These massage your legs to make you feel better."
   4. "You sound upset. Do these stockings bother you?"

9. Regarding the care of a postoperative patient with a Jackson-Pratt wound drain, which of the following are appropriate nursing actions? *(Select all that apply.)*
   1. Assess the wound drain for seal and patency.
   2. Measure amount of drainage.
   3. Compress the bulb to reestablish pressure.
   4. Remove the drain from the insertion site.
   5. Notify the physician immediately when there is no drainage.

10. The nurse is taking care of a postoperative patient. On initial assessment, the nurse notes the following: temperature 106° F (41.1° C); blood pressure 90/60; pulse 58; respirations 30. There is muscle rigidity of the jaw muscles. Urine is dark. An priority nursing action would be to:
    1. instruct patient to relax and take deep breaths.
    2. notify the physician immediately.
    3. administer pain medications.
    4. give a tepid sponge bath.

CRITICAL THINKING ACTIVITIES 

Read each clinical scenario and discuss the questions with your classmates.

Scenario A

Ms. Simpson just had a colon resection for a tumor. You are assisting with her care in the PACU. She is waking up, but is still groggy. Her breathing is somewhat shallow. She has a large dressing on the left side of the abdomen.

1. What would you do to improve her respiratory status?
2. Describe the method used to ensure an open airway.

Scenario B

You are assigned to care for a 37-year-old man who just had a surgical repair of a ventral hernia. The patient had spinal anesthesia. He is a same-day surgery patient.

1. How does the care of this patient differ from that of a patient who had inhalation or general anesthesia?
2. If this patient has difficulty voiding after surgery, how could you assist him?
3. If he develops a spinal headache, what measures could be taken to decrease his discomfort?

Scenario C

Mrs. Stinson, 78 years old, returned to the nursing unit from surgery 1 hour ago. She underwent an abdominal hysterectomy and exploration for cancer of the uterus. She has an IV infusion running into the right forearm. Her blood pressure has gradually fallen from 138/88 to 102/62. She is restless, complains of thirst, and is anxious.

1. What assessments would you make?
2. What actions would you take? In what order would you perform these actions?

CHAPTER

6 Infection Prevention and Control

evolve http://evolve.elsevier.com/deWit

Objectives

Upon completing this chapter, you should be able to:

Theory

1. Describe what factors increase the risk of infection.
2. Discuss how the body uses its natural defensive mechanisms to protect against infection.
3. Explain how fever plays a role in the prevention of infection.
4. Describe the classic signs of infection.
5. Identify when expanded precautions are to be used.
6. List the types of personal protective equipment and when they should be used.
7. Describe factors that make the elderly more susceptible to infections.
8. Identify factors that may impair the process of healing and repair of damaged tissue.

Clinical Practice

1. Care for a patient whose condition requires extended precautions.
2. From a day's patient assignment, determine the factors present for each patient that are risk factors for infection.

Key Terms

Be sure to check out the bonus material on the Companion CD-ROM, including selected audio pronunciations.

acquired (p. 115)
agent (Ā-gĕnt, p. 111)
communicable (kō-MŪ-nĭ-kă-b'l, p. 111)
disease (dĭ-ZĒZ, p. 111)
Expanded Precautions (prē-KAW-shŭns, p. 120)
exudate (ĔKS-ū-dāt, p. 116)
hand hygiene (HĪ-gēn, p. 119)
health care–associated infection (ĭn-FĔK-shŭn, p. 122)
host (hōst, p. 112)
immunity (ĭ-MŪ-nĭ-tē, p. 115)
infection (ĭn-FĔK-shŭn, p. 111)
inflammation (ĭn-flă-MĀ-shŭn, p. 117)
innate (ĭ-NĀT, p. 115)
macrophages (MĂK-rō-faj-ĕz, p. 116)
multidrug-resistant organism (MDRO) (MŬL-tĭ-drŭg rē-zĭs-tĕnt ŌR-găn-ĭz-ĕm, p. 128)
normal flora (p. 111)
pathogen (PĂTH-ō-gĕn, p. 112)
personal protective equipment (PPE) (p. 121)
phagocytosis (făg-ō-sī-TŌ-sĭs, p. 116)
sepsis (SĔP-sĭs, p. 126)
shedding (p. 111)
Standard Precautions (STĂN-dĕrd prē-KĂW-shŭnz, p. 120)
susceptible (p. 111)
vaccines (p. 111)
vectors (VĔK-tĕrz, p. 119)

Entering the world from an essentially sterile environment, an infant is quickly colonized with a variety of microorganisms called normal flora. This **normal flora** (microorganisms that normally exist in the body and provide natural immunity against certain infections) is most often found on or in body systems that have some form of contact with the outside environment (Table 6–1). This flora prevents the most harmful microorganisms from colonizing the body. **Vaccines** and antimicrobial agents have made the prevention and/or treatment of infectious diseases more efficient, yet they are not always effective. Understanding how the body defends itself against infection, and how to prevent further exposure to *pathogenic* (disease-producing) microorganisms, is crucial in order to provide safe and effective nursing care.

THE INFECTIOUS PROCESS AND DISEASE

An **infection** is the presence and growth of pathogenic microorganisms, in a **susceptible** (lacking resistance) host, to the extent that tissue damage occurs, such as pulmonary tuberculosis. Infection can be **communicable** (can be passed from one person to another directly, through touch, or indirectly, by using a contaminated glass) and noncommunicable. **Disease** is one possible outcome of an infection. Once an infection has occurred, the person is considered communicable until the organism is no longer **shedding** (to lose by natural process) infectious organisms from the body. This period of communicability varies by the type of pathogen involved and the host's ability to fight off the infecting **agent** (any power, principle, or substance capable of producing an effect, whether physical, chemical, or biologic). Bacteria, for example, upon entering the body, must find a way to attach to a

Table 6–1 ***Normal Flora of the Body****

SITE	NORMAL FLORA	
Eye	*Corynebacterium* species *Neisseria* species *Staphylococcus aureus*	*Staphylococcus epidermidis* *Streptococcus* species
Upper respiratory tract (nose, mouth, throat)	*Corynebacterium* species *Enterobacter* species *Haemophilus* species *Klebsiella* species *Lactobacillus* species	*Neisseria* species *Staphylococcus* species *Streptococcus viridans* Various types of anaerobes
Skin	*Corynebacterium* species *Staphylococcus aureus* *Staphylococcus epidermidis*	*Streptococcus* species Yeasts such as *Candida* and *Pityrosporum*
Small bowel and colon	*Bacteroides* species *Clostridium perfringens* *Enterobacter* species (i.e., coliform)	*Escherichia coli* *Streptococcus faecalis*
Vagina	*Corynebacterium* species *Klebsiella* species *Lactobacillus* species *Proteus* species	*Pseudomonas* species *Staphylococcus* species *Streptococcus* species

Adapted from deWit, S.C. (2005). *Fundamental Concepts and Skills for Nursing* (2nd ed.). Philadelphia: Elsevier Saunders.
*The central nervous system, lower respiratory tract, and upper and lower urinary tracts are normally sterile. This table lists only those organisms most commonly found in the various body systems. They can also cause illness or infection if they are able to invade another system within the body.

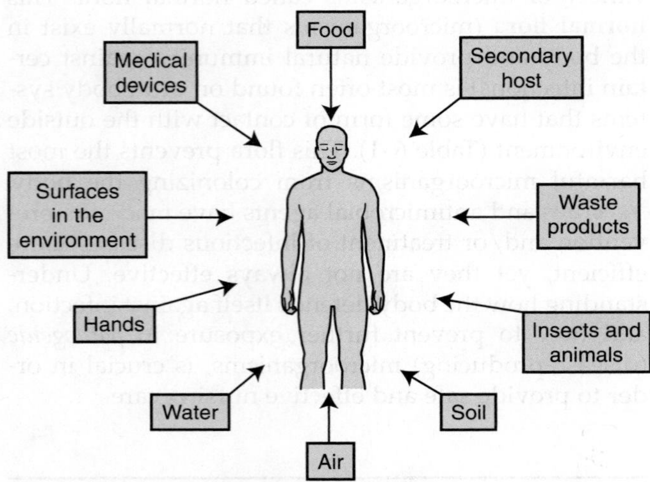

FIGURE 6–1 The environment and the spread of infection.

host (an organism in which another, usually parasitic organism, is nourished and harbored) cell in order to multiply. Once the organisms have found a place to multiply, they can then spread through the body via the circulatory or lymphatic system.

The development of an infection is dependent upon the interrelationship between the *host*, the *agent*, and the *environment*.

FACTORS THAT INFLUENCE INFECTIOUS DISEASE

Many factors concerning the host determine the type of response the body will have to an invading pathogen. *Risk* of exposure is influenced by the lifestyle, occupation, and socioeconomic status of the host. The underlying disease state, as well as the immunologic and nutritional status of the host, influences the *degree* of resistance or susceptibility the body will have to the pathogen. Environmental factors can also increase the likelihood of developing an infection (Figure 6–1). Other factors that influence infection or disease are listed in Table 6–2.

DISEASE-PRODUCING PATHOGENS

Any microorganism capable of producing disease is known as a **pathogen.** Once pathogens have entered the body, many are able to adapt to their new environment, enhancing survival and increasing their likelihood of causing illness or disease. Pathogens can be transmitted from one person to another through one of three routes: *airborne*, *contact*, or *droplet*. Hand hygiene is the number one way to prevent the spread or transmission of pathogenic microorganisms. Following respiratory etiquette by covering your cough/sneeze and performing hand hygiene afterward is another method to use in preventing the spread of infection.

Categories of Microorganisms

Today there are nine categories of microorganisms that are known to cause infection in humans. They are bacteria, viruses, protozoa, rickettsia, chlamydia, fungi, mycoplasmas, helminths, and prions.

Bacteria. Bacteria are classified into three major categories, according to their shape, gram-staining properties, and requirements for oxygen. Round or spherical bacteria are referred to as *cocci*, rod-shaped bacteria are referred to as *bacilli*, and spiral or corkscrew-shaped bacteria are called *spirochetes*. Some bacteria grow in chains (streptococci), some grow in pairs (diplococci), and some grow in clusters (staphylococci). In order to identify the type of bacteria, the microbiologist will place a body fluid sample on a slide and stain it with

Table 6–2 ***Factors That Influence Infection and Disease***

THE HOST	THE AGENT	THE ENVIRONMENT*
Intrinsic (genetic predisposition or born with it) Age, sex, race Chronic diseases (i.e., diabetes mellitus)	Dosage and duration of exposure to the infecting agent(s)	Coexisting chronic disease (i.e., hypertension, diabetes mellitus)
Extrinsic (environmental): Personal behaviors (i.e., drugs, alcohol, hygiene, sexual practices)	Biologic—bacterial, fungal, viral, protozoal microbes can be involved	Living environment—overcrowded, lives in a dormitory or prison setting
Occupation	Chemical—organic and inorganic, pesticides, pharmaceuticals	Travel to country with endemic diseases such as tuberculosis or HIV/AIDS
Socioeconomic status	Physical—ionizing radiation, cold, heat, electricity, noise	Vectors (i.e., mosquitoes, flies, ticks, fleas)

Adapted from Mandell, G.L., Bennett, J.E., & Dolin, R. (Eds.). (2005). *Mandell, Douglas, and Bennett's Principles and Practice of Infectious Disease* (6th ed.). Philadelphia: Elsevier Saunders; Arias, K.M. (2000). *Quick Reference to Outbreak Investigation and Control in Health Care Facilities.* Gaithersburg, Md: Aspen; and Evans, A.S., & Brachman, P.S. (1998). *Bacterial Infections of Humans: Epidemiology and Control* (3rd ed.). New York: Plenum.
Key: *HIV/AIDS,* human immunodeficiency virus/acquired immunodeficiency syndrome.
*Environment includes not only the body, but also where one lives and works.

crystal violet and iodine. The dyes are then "washed" away with alcohol or acetone. If the body fluid sample stays violet or purple, it is gram positive. If it becomes pink or red, it is gram negative. This information is important for the medical team to know, in that it helps them to identify what type of broad-spectrum antimicrobial drug to prescribe for the patient until final microbiology culture results are available.

Bacteria that require oxygen to live and reproduce are *aerobic;* those that cannot tolerate the presence of oxygen are *anaerobic.* When bacteria enter the body, they trigger the immune system to produce *antibodies* (proteins that fight and destroy antigens). Some bacteria produce poisonous substances called *endotoxins* (toxins that are found within the bacteria and are released when the cell breaks apart); others produce *exotoxins* (excreted by both gram-negative and gram-positive bacteria).

Different bacteria thrive under different environmental conditions. Some form *spores* (a protective covering over the original cell) to protect themselves against destruction from heat, cold, lack of water, toxic chemicals, and radiation. Examples of spore-forming infectious diseases are anthrax and botulism. Other bacteria thrive best in water, such as *Pseudomonas* species or *Legionella.* The bacterium that causes tuberculosis can survive for years in many environments. Some bacteria, such as *Staphylococcus aureus,* can survive in very high temperatures.

Different methods can be used to prevent infection and its spread. The physiologic response of the body can be to stimulate the immune system to produce a fever or, through the exposure of the body to an antimicrobial drug, the body's immune response is triggered to destroy the invading pathogenic microorganism through phagocytosis. Another method is to clean, sterilize, or boil inanimate objects, such as a glass or surgical instrument, to prevent the spread of infection if the items are used by or on a patient. If these items are not properly treated, cleaned, or sterilized, infection may result. If the wrong antimicrobial agent is given or not completed as prescribed, the patient is at increased risk for developing infection with a multidrug-resistant organism.

Viruses. Viruses are not cells. They do not have cell walls and do not reproduce like other microbes. They can only be seen through electron microscopy, and cannot be treated with antibiotics or antifungals. They are composed of either DNA or RNA; have an outside coating made of protein; and are dependent upon the cell they have invaded in order to survive and reproduce. Some viruses will use the cytoplasm from the cell they have attacked to develop an "envelope" that makes it harder for the body's immune system to destroy them. Viruses have the ability to keep changing their protein markers, called antigens, making it difficult for the virus to be neutralized or killed by white blood cells (WBCs). Once viruses have established themselves in the body, they can trigger an immune response that is harmful to the cells. They can also damage cells by preventing protein synthesis from occurring. New viral elements can be released into the circulation either by the virus breaking down the wall of the cell it has invaded and releasing itself or from small offshoots that have burst, thereby infecting other cells.

Viruses are classified as one of three types: (1) latent—because they can reside in the body for years without producing symptoms and then suddenly cause an acute flare-up of symptoms (e.g., herpes simplex); (2) *oncogenic* (cancer causing)—because they have the ability to alter the cell walls to the point where the cells become malignant; and (3) active—where the virus enters the body, invades a number of cells, and infects the body (e.g., influenza and severe acute respiratory syndrome, which are discussed in Chapter 14).

Viruses, as well as bacteria, vary in their resistance to destruction by chemical disinfectants, but most are easily inactivated or destroyed by heat. However, some of the hepatitis viruses must be boiled as long as 30 minutes before they can be considered nonpathogenic. It is important to note that antibiotics do not help in a viral infection but antiviral agents, such as acyclovir, can help prevent a more virulent viral infection from occurring if taken at the first signs of illness.

Protozoa. Protozoa are one-celled parasitic organisms that have the ability to move. There are four main types, named by their method of travel within their environment. They are called either amebas, ciliates, flagellates, or sporozoa. These microorganisms are typically found in water and soil. Many protozoa species have the ability to lie dormant, especially when the environment is hostile. Although thousands of species exist, only a few are pathogenic to humans. In order to cause disease, some protozoans have to be ingested while others are introduced into the body through the bite of a vector, such as a mosquito.

Rickettsia and Chlamydia. Rickettsia are small, round or rod-shaped bacteria that are often transmitted by the bites of body lice, ticks, and fleas. *Chlamydia* is also a bacterium, but it is even smaller than the Rickettsia species and is typically transmitted via close contact, especially sexual. Both are dependent on a living host; therefore, they are more like a parasite than actual bacteria.

Think Critically About . . . A patient you are providing care to has chlamydia. She asks you how she may have contracted it, how it can be treated, and what can she do to prevent spreading the infection. What do you tell her?

Fungi. Fungi are very small, primitive organisms that grow on living plants, animals, and other decaying organic material. They also thrive in warm, moist environments. Fungal infections in humans are called *mycoses* and are classified into three main types: (1) cutaneous mycoses, which grow in the outer layer of the skin; (2) subcutaneous mycoses, which involve the deeper layers of the skin, subcutaneous tissues, and sometimes bone; and (3) systemic or deep mycoses involving internal organs.

Fungal infections are difficult to eradicate once they have invaded a host. This is because fungi tend to form spores that are resistant to ordinary antimicrobial agents. Antifungal agents can be given topically or systemically, but can be toxic to the liver and the nervous system; therefore, the course of treatment must be carried out cautiously and over a long period.

Fungal infections commonly found in immune-competent hosts includes coccidioidomycosis (caused by *Coccidioides immitis*), histoplasmosis (caused by *Histoplasma capsulatum*), and blastomycosis (caused by *Blastomyces dermatitidis*). They are all systemic mycoses caused by inhalation of airborne spores. Once in the lung, the spores take root and then can spread to any part of the body. However, it is important to note that the majority of fungal infections are self-limited and do not cause clinical disease.

Opportunistic fungal infections (infections that occur in a person with a depressed immune system) are more typically found in patients who have some form of immune compromise and typically includes species from *Candida, Cryptococcus* (can infect any organ in the body, including the brain and the meninges), and *Aspergillus* (found in soil, dust, and decomposing organic material).

Mycoplasmas. Mycoplasmas, once thought to be a virus, are very small organisms that do not have a cell wall. They are more like an extracellular parasite because they attach themselves to epithelial cells that line the body cavities and outer surfaces, such as the skin. They tend to be slow growing. For example, *Mycoplasma pneumoniae* can take up to 3 weeks to incubate before signs or symptoms begin to appear.

Other Infectious Agents

Helminths. Helminths are worms (either round, flat, or hook-like) and flukes. All are parasitic and are typically spread via the fecal-oral route. Pinworms are most commonly found in children and cause significant itching in the perianal area due to the eggs being laid outside the rectum. Flatworms, such as a tapeworm, can grow up to 50 feet long and live in the intestines. Hookworm and fluke infestations can easily penetrate the skin, and are found in the blood and invade organs such as the liver and lungs. Flatworms and flukes can cause significant weight loss and debilitation.

Prions. Prions, although quite rare (one case per 1 million persons), are usually spread through eating meat, especially brain tissue that has been infected, or in even rarer cases, through corneal transplantation from a donor who had a prion infection (Brown et al., 2000). Prions are extremely resistant to the typical methods used for killing most viruses, bacteria, and fungi. These organisms require a type of special cleaning and sterilization that can be especially hard on surgical instruments.

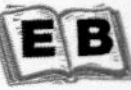

THE BODY'S DEFENSE AGAINST INFECTION

The four primary lines of defense the body has against infection are (1) the skin, (2) normal flora, (3) the inflammatory response, and (4) the immune response.

SKIN

Think Critically About . . . Your work environment and the usual activities performed throughout your shift: where do you think you are most likely to come in contact with pathogens that might cause infection? What precautions can you take to prevent or lessen your risk of exposure? Be specific.

Mechanical and Chemical Barriers to Infection

Mechanical Barriers. Mechanical barriers are intact skin and mucous membranes. They are the primary defense the body has against invading microorganisms and infection. Skin, being the largest organ of the body, serves as a first line of defense against harmful agents in the environment. It functions as a protective covering for the more delicate and vulnerable underlying tissues and organs.

The portals of exit and entry provide the means by which pathogens move in and out of the body. For example, pathogens most frequently exit or enter the body where the skin and mucous membranes meet, such as through the mouth, nose, and gastrointestinal or genitourinary tracts, as well as through a cut in the skin.

Chemical Barriers. Chemical barriers assist the skin and mucous membranes in fighting off invasive organisms by the secretion of tears, saliva, and mucus. Lactic and fatty acids, which inhibit the growth of bacteria, are excreted via sweat and the sebaceous glands. Secretions from the mucous membranes lining the respiratory, gastrointestinal, and reproductive tracts contain an abundance of a bactericidal enzyme called *lysozyme*. This same enzyme is found in tears and saliva. Stomach acid and digestive enzymes kill off most swallowed microorganisms. Mucus produced by the respiratory tract helps capture a variety of inhaled particles. *Cilia* (tiny hairs), which line the respiratory tract, trap organisms and debris and then propel them up and out of the body with a wavelike action.

Think Critically About . . . What effect might medications such as Nexium and Prilosec (proton pump inhibitors), which reduce stomach acid, have on a person's general health? How will this impact a patient's ability to fight off pathogenic microorganisms that may be swallowed?

Protective and Defensive Mechanisms Against Infection

Our bodies have two forms of **immunity** (the body's ability of being unaffected by a particular disease or condition) against infections. They are **innate** (born with/natural) and **acquired** (develops throughout life) (Box 6–1 or see Chapter 10 for more detail). When the body's defense mechanisms are stressed or exhausted, it is more susceptible to infection. Heredity, the degree of natural resistance, and one's own immune status are the greatest determinates of infection, but personal habits and behaviors are also factors to consider. General health, state of nutrition, hormone balance, immune status, and the presence of a chronic disease, such as diabetes mellitus, may influence the degree of susceptibility a person may have to infection.

Box 6–1 ***Innate and Acquired Immunity***

INNATE IMMUNITY
- The body senses the presence of pathogenic microorganisms.
- Genetic predisposition to respond to invasion in a specific way
- Responds rapidly to invasion of pathogenic microorganisms
- Elements consist of antibodies, phagocytes, natural killer cells, and mast cells

ACQUIRED IMMUNITY
- Cellular and humoral immunity are activated through T-cell and B-cell receptors.
- Genetic rearrangement occurs throughout life.
- Develops slowly once the body has been initially invaded
- Provides the body with protection with each subsequent exposure to the same pathogens
- Is the basic component for immunity induced via vaccination
- Elements consist of antibodies and cytotoxic and helper T cells

Adapted from Munford, R.S. (2005). Sepsis. In G.L. Mandell, J.E. Bennett, & R. Dolin (Eds.). *Mandell, Douglas, and Bennett's principles and Practice of Infectious Disease* (6th ed.). Philadelphia: Elsevier Saunders, pp. 906–926.

Fever. Fever is one of the primary mechanisms the body has to prevent infection from an invading microorganism. Once the immune system has determined that an invasion is trying to occur, it signals the hypothalamus in the brain to raise the body temperature. In an effort to fight off the infection, the body increases the heart rate and respiratory rate due to the increased metabolic and oxygen demand at the cellular level. Shivering occurs to increase the core body temperature, but the surrounding environment feels cooler than the new core body temperature, and the patient may complain that she is "freezing to death." It is at this point in the inflammatory response that fever is noticeably increased. In an attempt to decrease the body's temperature via evaporation, *diaphoresis* (sweating) occurs, and it is not unusual for the patient to not want to be covered by a blanket or sheet. This increased heat in the body creates a hostile environment to the microorganisms, and a person whose immune system is intact is able to destroy them more efficiently. Once the threat of infection is no longer present, the immune system again signals the hypothalamus and the body is able to start cooling down on its own.

Think Critically About . . . A patient who comes to the clinic and asks you to explain what causes a person to have a temperature. When is it wise to take medication to decrease the temperature? At what point would it be considered dangerous *not* to try to reduce the fever? Would the age of the patient be a factor you should consider in your teaching?

Nutrition. Poor nutrition predisposes a person to developing an infection because the body may not have sufficient protein stores to generate enough antibodies to help fight off an infection. The very young and the elderly have a less efficient immune system, and that is why it is important to ensure that these age groups have received the appropriate vaccinations and immunizations. Excessive stress, whether emotional, physical, or both, is another factor that influences a person's immune status. Stress can increase blood cortisol levels, which will decrease the antiinflammatory response of the body. Therefore, it is important to keep the body's protective mechanisms intact and in good working order so that susceptibility to infection is decreased.

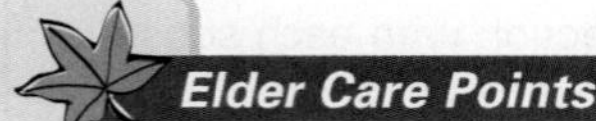

Elder Care Points

It is important that the elderly population's diet contains sufficient protein to maintain a healthy immune system. Many elderly do not eat sufficient protein because of monetary concerns or because of physical limitations that interfere with their ability to prepare a proper meal. Referral to a home delivery meal program may assist in providing appropriate dietary intake of protein and other essential nutrients to help fight off infection.

Antigen. An antigen is a form of protein found on the outside of cells that has the ability to identify it as "self" (native) or "non-self" (foreign). Antigens can stimulate the immune response to wipe out microorganisms.

Antibodies. Antibodies, also known as immunoglobulins (Ig), are one part of acquired immunity. They have many functions, such as neutralizing toxins and killing invading pathogens. There are five types of antibodies. IgM appears first if the body is exposed to an antigen. It will bind to the antigen and work to clear the pathogen from the body. IgG is the most abundant immunoglobulin found in the body and is the only one that crosses the placental barrier, reaching the developing fetus. It can also be given to provide passive immunity until the body's own immune system can defend itself. IgA is found in tears, mucus, saliva, gastric fluid, colostrum, and sweat. This immunoglobulin prevents pathogens from attaching to or penetrating epithelial cells, such as the skin. IgE has the ability to bind to mast cells and basophils and when triggered, releasing histamine and heparin. This in turn stimulates a hypersensitive reaction, as seen in bronchial asthma or systemic anaphylaxis. IgD works together with IgM, and one of its functions is to stimulate certain cells in the immune system; however, its overall role in the immune response is still unclear.

Bone Marrow. The bone marrow is a major component in the body's defense system. Bone marrow plays an important role in the manufacturing of blood products that help the body defend itself against infection. These products are called *leukocytes, neutrophils, macrophages,* and *lymphocytes.*

Leukocytosis. Leukocytosis is an increased number of *leukocytes* (white blood cells), usually seen at the beginning of an infection when the person's immune system has not been overly stressed. Leukocytosis is seen more often with bacterial than viral infections. When infection does occur, the bone marrow is stimulated to produce and release more leukocytes to help the body fight off, inactivate, and destroy the invading pathogens.

Phagocytosis. The process of **phagocytosis** (the ingestion and digestion of bacteria), also a form of innate immunity, assists the body in destroying invading pathogens. This is the body's first line of defense at the cellular level. Within the first few hours of the onset of the inflammatory process, the monocytes swell up (becoming macrophages) and migrate to the site of inflammation. Neutrophils, which are a type of leukocyte, are also released and have the ability to kill both aerobic and anaerobic organisms. After the macrophages and neutrophils engulf and destroy bacteria and other foreign matter, they die, producing an **exudate** (discharge) that is composed of tissue, fluid, dead cells, and their by-products. This exudate, usually yellow or green in color, is commonly known as *pus* and is a sign of infection.

Macrophages. **Macrophages** are *monocytes* (large leukocytes) that have left the bloodstream and have migrated into the tissues. They ingest and destroy pathogens and clear away the cellular debris and dead neutrophils in the latter stages of an infection. Macrophages cleanse the lymphatic fluid as it passes through the lymph nodes and perform a similar action on the blood as it passes through the liver and spleen.

Liver Cells. As part of the innate immune system, about 50% of all macrophage cells can be found in the liver's Kupffer cells. These macrophages act either to prevent invasion by pathogens mechanically or to neutralize the pathogen chemically (through the pH of body secretions). Macrophages also have the ability to destroy bacteria that have found their way into the blood circulation through the liver's portal system. The body's defense mechanisms against pathogens are summarized in Table 6–3.

NORMAL FLORA

The flora that is normally present on the skin and in the mucous membranes, gastrointestinal tract, and vagina coexist with the body and control the growth of harmful pathogens. When the amount of the normal flora is diminished, other pathogens may cause infection. When the body's immune system is suppressed for whatever reason, normal flora may grow out of control and cause infection. For example, *Candida albicans* causes a yeast infection (thrush) that frequently occurs after treatment with antibiotics, because the normal flora has been destroyed, allowing the *Candida* to flourish. Table 6–4 shows changes in the natural

Table 6–3 ***The Body's Mechanism of Defense Against Infection***

MECHANISM	FACTORS INVOLVED IN PROTECTION
Innate (natural) immunity	Determined by age, ethnicity, and genetics. Greater resistance to disease.
Antibody-mediated (humoral) immune response, (antigen-antibody; B lymphocytes)	Antibodies are produced against invading pathogens and inactivate or destroy them.
Cell-mediated immune response (T lymphocytes)	Sensitized T cells kill or inactivate antigens by chemical release or secretion of substances that destroy the antigen.
Inflammation	Cells damaged by pathogens release enzymes, and leukocytes are attracted to the area; the damaged area is "walled off" and phagocytosis disposes of the microorganisms and dead tissue.
Phagocytosis by white blood cells	Leukocytes, neutrophils, and macrophages (large monocytes) engulf, ingest, kill, and dispose of invading microorganisms.
Fever	May not always have fever with an infection, such as seen with immunocompromised or debilitated patients or in patients who have been on long-term corticosteroid therapy. Causes surface blood vessels to constrict, which leads to shivering in order to hold heat in the body (to kill the invading organisms). Increases metabolic rate, so can be problematic for patients with cardiorespiratory problems due to increased workload on the heart/circulatory system. Fever stops once the antiinflammatory agents have helped to restore homeostasis.
Normal flora	Present on skin and in mucous membranes of oral cavity, gastrointestinal tract, and vagina. Helps prevent excessive growth of pathogens.
Intact skin	Skin is the first defense; slightly acid pH and normal flora present unfavorable environment for colonization of pathogens.
Mucous membranes	Mucous membranes, with their mucociliary action, provide mechanical protection against invasion of pathogens. Mucous secretions contain enzymes that inhibit many microorganisms. Respiratory system clears about 90% of introduced pathogens.
Gastrointestinal tract	Peristaltic action empties the gastrointestinal tract of pathogenic organisms. Acid pH of stomach secretions, bile, pancreatic enzymes, and mucus protects against invasion by harmful pathogens.
Genitourinary tract	Flushing of urine through the system washes out microorganisms. The acid pH of urine helps maintain a sterile environment in the system.

Table 6–4 ***Changes in Natural Defense Mechanisms that Occur with Age***

CHANGE	CONSEQUENCE
Decreased skin turgor and greater skin friability	Skin is more susceptible to friction damage and tearing.
Decreased elasticity and atherosclerosis of peripheral vessels	Decreased blood flow to extremities produces slower wound healing.
Calcification of heart valves	Provides a location for bacteria to attach and cause endocarditis.
Stiffness of thorax from arthritis or aging changes, weakened respiratory muscles, decreased ciliary action from smoking or exposure to air pollution	Decreased ability to maintain good oxygenation leads to less respiratory reserve; greater tendency to retain secretions as cilia cannot move foreign substances and secretions as easily; cough reflex and effort are diminished.
Gastrointestinal tract motility is decreased as muscles weaken; acid production is decreased	Insufficient acid to inhibit growth of pathogens; decreased motility allows organisms to remain in gastrointestinal tract and multiply.
Prostate changes, bladder prolapse, and urethral strictures	Bladder is not completely emptied at each voiding, which allows for stagnation; provides medium for growth of pathogens.
Immune response decreases as bone marrow does not produce new blood cells as rapidly	Mobilization of body defenses to fight infection and heal wounds is slower.

defense mechanisms that occur with age and cause the elderly to become more susceptible to infection.

THE INFLAMMATORY RESPONSE

Inflammation is an immediate, localized, protective response of the body to any kind of injury or damage to its cells or tissues. It is considered to be the second line of defense to infection at the cellular level. Almost all tissues of the body respond to injury by initiating this inflammatory process (Figure 6–2). Three basic purposes of the inflammatory response are to (1) neutralize and destroy harmful agents, (2) limit their spread to other tissues in the body by walling off the organisms, and (3) prepare the damaged tissues for repair.

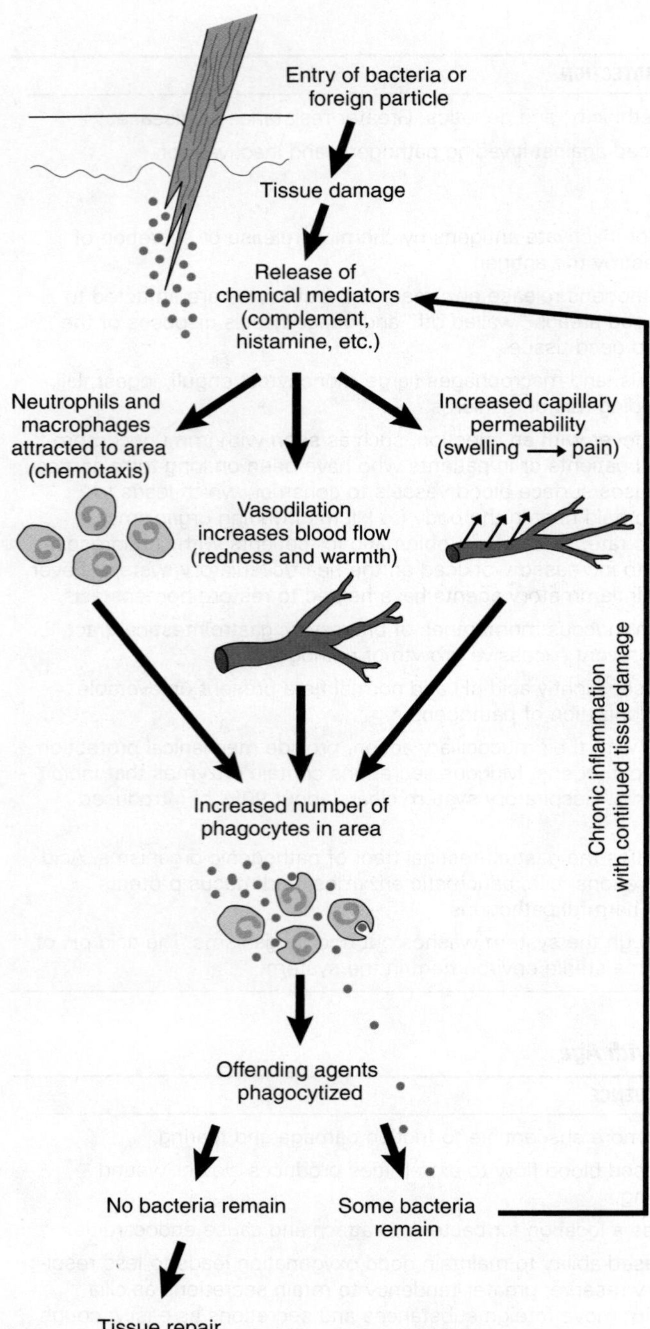

FIGURE 6–2 Steps in the inflammation process.

Inflammatory Changes

Changes that are part of the inflammatory response can occur locally, at the site of injury, and systemically. These changes involve (1) the cells of the damaged tissues and adjacent connective tissues; (2) the blood vessels in and near the site of injury; (3) the blood cells, particularly the leukocytes; (4) the macrophages and phagocyte activity; (5) the immune system; and (6) the hormonal system. If there is an inadequate inflammatory response, for whatever reason, the pathogens may cause active, systemic infection in the patient.

Signs and Symptoms of Inflammation

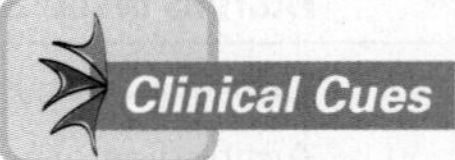

The five local signs and symptoms of inflammation are heat, redness, swelling, pain, and limitation or loss of function.

Local Reactions. *Redness* and *heat* are caused by the increased blood flow to the affected area. *Swelling* is the result of the increased permeability of the capillaries and the leakage of fluid from the blood into the tissue spaces around the cells. Blockage of lymphatic drainage from the site also contributes to the local swelling. *Pain,* caused by the chemicals released by the defensive cells and the accumulation of fluid in the area, irritates the nerve endings. To lessen pain, a person avoids pressure to the affected area or holds it immobile.

Systemic Reactions. Systemic reactions to inflammation are familiar to any of us who have had the flu or some other kind of generalized infection. Headache, *myalgia* (muscle aches), fever, diaphoresis, chills, *anorexia* (loss of appetite), and *malaise* (weakness) are some of the more common signs/symptoms a person may experience if she has a systemic infection. (Note: An inflammatory response can occur in the absence of an infection, such as rheumatoid arthritis or a histamine response due to an insect bite.)

Nursing care for patients who have a systemic infection includes providing for a balanced fluid intake and output, pain relief, and temperature control. Measures ensuring adequate nutrition and rest are employed. If there is an inadequate inflammatory response to a systemic infection, the patient may have an increased susceptibility to bacterial infections spreading elsewhere in the body, which can further delay tissue repair and wound healing.

Chemical Release and Vascular Changes

The complement system is a group of proteins that lie dormant in the body until they have been activated through an encounter with a foreign substance. The activation of these proteins enhances phagocytosis and the inflammatory process. If viral invasion has occurred, the chemical *interferon* is released in order to protect the cells against further viral invasion. As soon as damage occurs, the blood vessels in the injured area briefly constrict and, as histamine and serotonin are released, they dilate so that more blood is brought to the damaged cells. The walls of the capillaries become more *permeable* (i.e., their pores enlarge) so that water, proteins, and defensive cells can seep into the fluid surrounding the damaged cells. One of the classic outward signs of inflammation is leakage of fluid into the spaces around the cells, producing a localized swelling or *edema.* This results in a "walling off" of the area and delays the spread of pathogens, toxins, and other harmful agents to the rest of the body.

THE IMMUNE RESPONSE

The third line of defense is the immune response, which attempts to defend and protect the body. The immune response is a remarkable series of complex chemical and mechanical activities that take place within the body. These activities involve (1) the detection of entry by foreign agents as soon as they gain access to the body's cells; (2) immediate recognition of the agents as foreign or alien; and (3) the ability to distinguish one kind of foreign agent from another and to "remember" that particular agent if it appears again years later.

While the phagocytes are engulfing and destroying bacteria and other harmful agents, the specific antibodies and antitoxins produced by the immune response are transported by the circulatory system to the tissue spaces that are surrounding the site of inflammation. It is here where they attack the foreign cells and neutralize the toxins those cells produce. The immune response is discussed more fully in Chapter 10.

Hormonal Response

Some hormones, such as cortisone, have an *antiinflammatory* action that limits inflammation to the locally damaged tissues. Other hormones, such as aldosterone, are *proinflammatory,* which means that they stimulate the body's protective inflammatory response. Thus the hormones have a regulatory effect on the inflammatory process so that the response is well balanced and provides maximum benefit. Other hormones, such as those excreted by the adrenal glands, can interfere with healing, and in some cases of severe inflammation, the physician may prescribe an antiinflammatory drug to relieve these symptoms.

The Chain of Infection

For an infectious disease to be spread from one person to another, certain conditions must be met. As seen in the links of a chain, infection occurs through a cyclical process and each part of this cycle is interrelated (Figure 6–3). Prevention or control of infection is aimed at interrupting this cycle at any point within the chain of infection. This can include the performance of hand hygiene or the wearing of gloves to protect the hands or a cover gown to protect one's clothing.

The mechanism of transmission of a pathogenic agent within the environment or to another person is by either direct or indirect contact. **Vectors** such as mosquitoes, fleas, ticks, and flies, can transmit pathogens through their bites or stings. (Refer to Chapter 14 for information on West Nile virus and avian flu, which are spread via a vector [mosquitoes or birds].)

The three most important aspects in the infection chain are the interaction of the *agent*, the *host*, and the *mode of transmission*.

A reservoir is any place a pathogen is normally found. The reservoir can be *animate* (living) such as people, animals, and insects, or it can be *inanimate* (nonliving), as found in soil, in water, and on surfaces

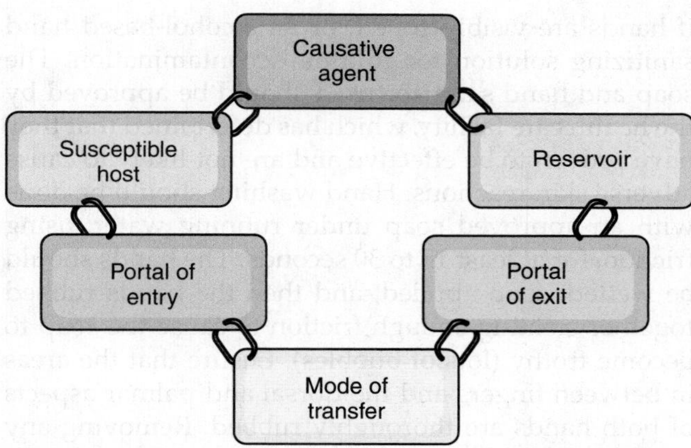

FIGURE 6–3 The cyclical process of infection. Each link of the infection cycle must be present and in the proper sequence to produce disease.

Box 6–2 *Human Reservoirs*

Carrier: Person has the actual infection but does not show any obvious signs or symptoms; typically does not take precautions to prevent the spread of infection and can transmit it to others

Colonized: Can transmit the pathogenic organisms by either direct or indirect contact with inanimate objects or within her own environment

Infectious (symptomatic): Has obvious signs and symptoms of infection; less likely to spread infection as precautions are usually taken

of objects such as a cup or bed rails. The body can be a reservoir because pathogenic organisms can grow and multiply *(colonize)* on the skin or inside the body without causing a specific immune response or an infection. Infectious agents can also be found in body excretions or secretions such as saliva, sputum, urine, feces, and wound drainage. Someone who has become colonized with a specific pathogen, such as methicillin-resistant *Staphylococcus aureus* (MRSA) or vancomycin-resistant *enterococci* (VRE), can be an asymptomatic carrier (a *reservoir*) and unknowingly spread the infection to others because they are not aware that they have been exposed and are now colonized with an organism that is known to be multidrug resistant (see Box 6–2 for more information on human reservoirs). In the home or community, contaminated or improperly cooked food, stagnant water, or sewage can also be a source of infection.

INFECTION PREVENTION AND CONTROL

PREVENTING AND CONTROLLING THE SPREAD OF INFECTION

Hand Hygiene

Hand hygiene is the primary intervention any health care provider can use to control the spread of infection. Hand hygiene can be performed with soap and water, if hands are visibly soiled, or an alcohol-based hand sanitizing solution for routine decontamination. The soap and hand sanitizer used should be approved by the health care facility, which has determined that they have proven to be effective and are not likely to cause adverse skin reactions. Hand washing should be done with an approved soap under running water, using friction, for at least 15 to 30 seconds. The hands should be wetted, soap applied, and then the hands rubbed together creating enough friction to cause the soap to become frothy (lots of bubbles). Ensure that the areas in between fingers and the dorsal and palmar aspects of both hands are thoroughly rubbed. Removing any rings or other forms of jewelry prior to washing hands with soap and water is an important step in performing this vital process. It is important to note that hand hygiene must be performed *regardless* of whether gloves were worn while providing care to a patient. The wearing of artificial fingernails or extenders is not recommended for those health care providers who have direct patient contact because pathogens can be found beneath the nails.

Box 6–3 *Standard Precautions*

1. Use barrier precautions, such as gloves, gown, face mask, and protective eyewear, to prevent exposure of skin or mucous membranes to a patient's blood, body fluid, or other potentially infectious materials while providing care or assisting with a procedure with your patient.
   a. Change gloves between contact with one body part and another (i.e., respiratory and urinary).
   b. Perform hand hygiene immediately after removing gloves.
   c. Discard used gloves in the appropriate waste container; do not wash or reuse them.
2. Prevent injury by needle stick or cut from sharp instruments.
   a. Be cautious and attentive any time you are handling a needle or sharp instrument.
   b. Do not recap a used needle by hand; scoop the cap onto the needle on a flat surface or deploy the safety device attached to the needle.
   c. Immediately dispose of a used needle or other sharp instrument in the puncture-resistant container provided for that purpose in the room.
   d. Replace puncture-resistant containers when they are three quarters full and as needed; do not attempt to push needles into a container that is too full.
3. Prevent possible self-contamination or exposure through broken skin.
   a. If you have open lesions or weeping dermatitis, do not give direct patient care or handle patient care equipment until the condition has resolved.
4. Prevent possible self-contamination during cardiopulmonary resuscitation.
   a. Use disposable mouthpiece or resuscitation bag for emergency mouth-to-mouth breathing.
   b. Wear the appropriate personal protective equipment (PPE) whenever possible.

PRECAUTION CATEGORIES FOR INFECTION PREVENTION AND CONTROL

Standard Precautions

Standard Precautions have been in place in all health care delivery systems since they were mandated by the Centers for Disease Control and Prevention (CDC) in the 1980s (see Appendix 5). These precautions are designed to prevent the transmission of microorganisms from one patient to another as well as to protect the health care worker from unnecessary exposure to infection. Standard Precautions are to be used on all patients because their potential for being colonized, or actually infectious, is not always known. Barrier precautions, such as gloves or isolation techniques that include the proper handling and disposal of secretions, excretions, and exudates, can prevent the transmission of pathogens from one person, or object, to another (Box 6–3).

Expanded Precautions

Expanded Precautions incorporate Standard Precaution techniques with additional protective actions specific to the organism and location involved. These safety measures are to be implemented for patients with a suspected or confirmed infection or who are known to be colonized with a highly transmissible organism. These additional precautions are known as category-specific precautions and include the following: Airborne Infection Isolation, Contact Isolation, and Droplet Isolation. Health care facilities have information cards that are usually placed on the door to the patient's room to ensure that all who enter the room are made aware of the safety precautions and the personal protective equipment (PPE) that must be used prior to entry. Depending on the microorganism involved, the nurse verifies which types of Expanded Precautions are to be used. If the nurse is unsure as to what type are needed, she should contact the hospital infection control professional for guidance. The effectiveness of Standard Precautions and Expanded Precautions depends on the nurse's knowledge of the microorganism involved, the ways in which it can be transmitted, and the compliance with the infection prevention and control precautions. See Table 6–5 for more information regarding category-specific isolation methods.

Think Critically About . . . What type of expanded precautions would be necessary for a patient who is admitted with complications of varicella? What PPE would you need in order to assist this patient with activities of daily living?

Table 6–5 ***Category-Specific Isolation Precautions (Expanded Precautions)***

ISOLATION CATEGORY	PRIVATE ROOM*	MASKS	GOWNS	GLOVES	COMMON DISEASES PLACED INTO ISOLATION CATEGORY
Airborne Infection Isolation	Always; door to room must be kept closed at all times	Must wear a fit-tested NIOSH-approved N95 respirator	No, unless draining wounds	No, unless draining wounds	Pulmonary or laryngeal tuberculosis, or draining tuberculous skin lesions; smallpox, viral hemorrhagic fever, SARS; measles; varicella, disseminated zoster
Contact Precautions	Preferred; cohorting of patients with same type of infection is acceptable	Situation dependent	Always; if patients are cohorted, staff must perform hand hygiene and change PPE *between* patients	Always; if patients are cohorted, staff must perform hand hygiene and change PPE *between* patients	Open or draining wounds, history of MRSA, VRE, ESBL positive; diarrhea; MDRO infections
Droplet Precautions	Preferred; cohorting of patients with same type of infection is acceptable	Wear a surgical mask when entering room; patient should wear mask during transport and observe cough etiquette	Not usually	When helping with cough-inducing procedures or discarding of used tissues	Pneumonia, influenza, rubella, pertussis, streptococcal pharyngitis, meningitis caused by *Neisseria meningitidis* or *Haemophilus influenzae* type B

Key: *ESBL,* extended spectrum beta lactamase; *MDRO,* multidrug-resistant organism; *MRSA,* methicillin-resistant *Staphylococcus aureus; NIOSH,* National Institute of Occupational Safety and Health; *PPE,* personal protective equipment; *VRE,* vancomycin-resistant enterococci.

*In most cases when a private room is required, patients infected with the same organism may share a room. For any patient in Expanded Precaution isolation, limit the time the patient is out of the room; notify receiving unit or department that the patient is in isolation so that appropriate measures can be taken prior to the arrival of the patient.

Personal Protective Equipment

Personal protective equipment (PPE) is the use of some type of barrier to protect a person from exposure to blood-borne pathogens, body fluids, or other potentially infectious materials. These barriers include, but are not limited to, gloves, cover gowns, face masks, eye protections, and respirator masks. By law, health care facilities are required to provide PPE at no expense to the staff (Occupational Safety and Health Administration Bloodborne Pathogens Standards, 1910.132). If a latex allergy is suspected, the nurse should contact her Occupational/Employee Health Services department so that a more detailed assessment can be made. If it is determined that a latex allergy does exist, that facility is required to provide the staff member with the appropriate PPE. Figure 6–4 shows methods for donning and removing PPE.

Protective Environment

Not all health care facilities care for patients who have had hematopoietic stem cell transplantation; this is why only a brief introduction to protective environments is presented in this text. For those facilities that do provide this service, this type of patient requires highly specialized forms of expanded isolation techniques. Nurses and other health care staff who provide care to the transplant recipient receive detailed education and training on the appropriate care and interventions that are required. Special airflow and filtration rooms with positive air pressure, smooth surfaces to aid in disinfection, minimizing the length of time the patient is outside of the protective environment, and ensuring staff are free from signs/symptoms of illness are only some of the interventions required. For additional information, refer to the facility's policy and procedure manuals or the CDC's website, www.cdc.gov, for further guidance.

Respiratory Hygiene and Cough Etiquette

Two methods of preventing droplets from spreading to others include teaching people to cover the mouth when sneezing or coughing and turning one's head away to prevent coughing into the face of another (Figure 6–5). In addition, educating patients and families to dispose of soiled tissues in waste containers and to perform hand hygiene after contact with actual or potentially contaminated items is important. To prevent the transmission of pathogenic microorganisms to a patient, instruct her to avoid contact with others who may have an infection.

Transmission of an infectious organism can be interrupted at the portal of entry by using only clean or sterile items when caring for patients. Use of effective hand hygiene techniques by health care workers, visitors, and patients is key in the prevention of infection. Immunization and measures to boost immunity through proper nutrition and a healthy lifestyle also increase a

DONNING AND REMOVING PPE
Donning Personal Protective Equipment (PPE)
The type of PPE will vary based on the level of precautions required, such as Standard and Contact, Droplet, or Airborne Isolation Precautions.

Gown
- Fully cover torso from neck to knees, arms to end of wrist, and wrap around the back
- Fasten in back at neck and waist

Mask or respirator
- Secure ties or elastic band at middle of head and neck
- Fit flexible band to nose bridge
- Fit snug to face and below chin
- Fit-check respirator

Goggles or face shield
- Put over face and eyes and adjust to fit

Gloves
- Extend to cover wrist of isolation gown

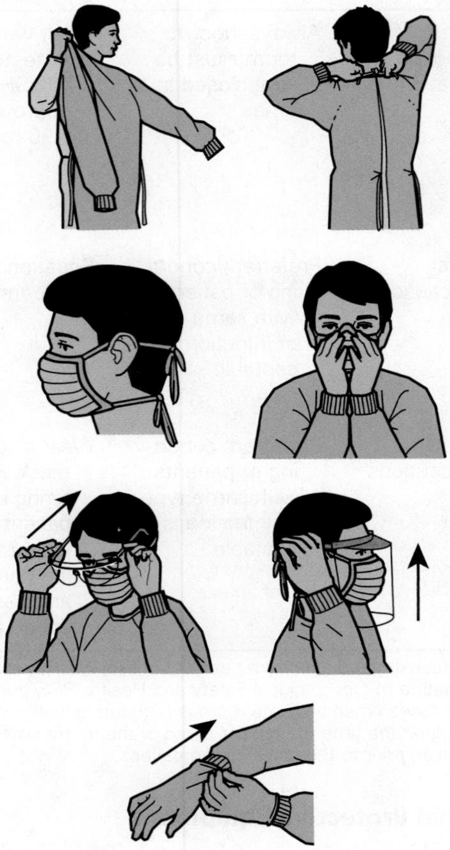

SAFE WORK PRACTICES
- Keep hands away from face
- Limit surfaces touched
- Change gown and gloves when torn or heavily contaminated
- Perform hand hygiene

FIGURE **6–4** Donning and removing personal protective equipment (PPE).

person's resistance to infection. Table 6–6 lists factors that can make a host more susceptible to pathogens.

> *Think Critically About . . .* What you would do if, while taking a blood pressure reading, you have a patient who sneezes or coughs and does not cover her nose or mouth? How would you respond? What type of education would benefit the patient? What additional precautions would you need to institute once the patient has left the examination room?

HEALTH CARE–ASSOCIATED INFECTIONS

A **health care–associated infection** (HAI), formerly known as a *nosocomial* infection, occurs when a patient is cared for in any kind of health care setting and acquires an infection. There are specific criteria that must be met in order for the infection to be classified as an HAI, such as length of time in the facility before the onset or appearance of the infection. Because health services are provided in a wide variety of locations, such as acute care facilities, outpatient surgery or dialysis centers, homes, and mobile clinics, it is sometimes difficult to determine just where the patient may have become infected.

Although inanimate objects such as needles, contaminated surgical instruments, and linens are major sources of infection in these settings, every patient is directly and indirectly in contact with large numbers of health care workers, each of whom could be the source of infection. That is why it is important to ensure that appropriate precautions, such as hand hygiene and Expanded Precaution techniques, are followed at all times. Table 6–7 presents HAI risk factors.

Removing Personal Protective Equipment (PPE)

Remove PPE at doorway before leaving patient room, or in anteroom; remove respirator outside of room.

Gloves
- Outside of gloves are contaminated!
- Grasp outside of glove with opposite gloved hand; peel off
- Hold removed glove in gloved hand
- Slide fingers of ungloved hand under remaining glove at wrist

Goggles or face shield
- Outside of goggles or face shield is contaminated!
- To remove, handle by "clean" head band or ear pieces
- Place in designated receptacle for reprocessing or in waste container

Gown
- Gown front and sleeves are contaminated!
- Unfasten neck, the waist ties
- Remove gown using a peeling motion; pull gown from each shoulder toward the same hand
- Gown will turn inside out
- Hold removed gown away from body, roll into a bundle, and discard into waste or linen receptacle

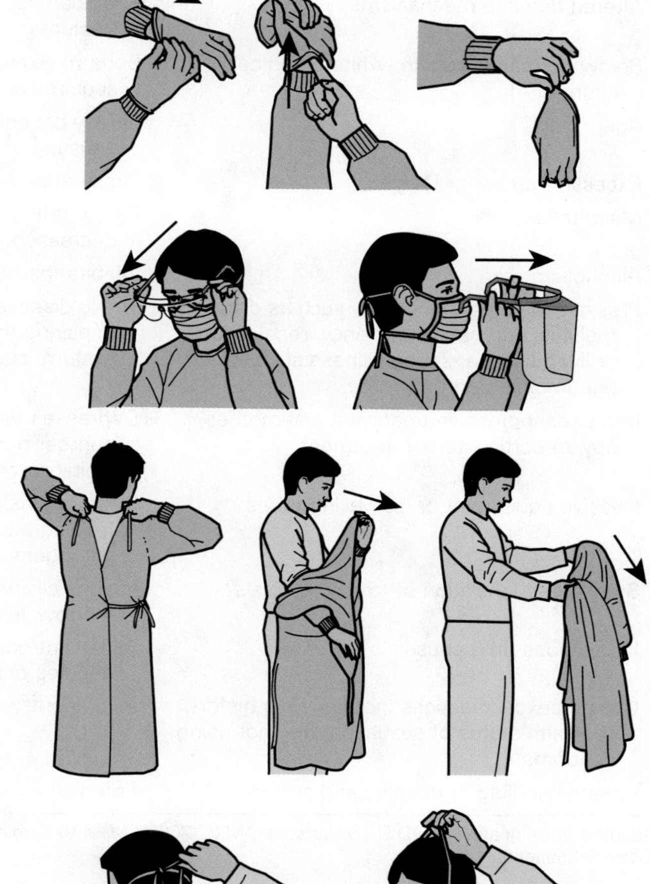

Mask or respirator
- Front of mask/respirator is contaminated—DO NOT TOUCH!
- Grasp bottom then top ties/elastics and remove
- Discard in waste container

Hand hygiene
- Perform immediately after removing all PPE!

FIGURE **6–4, cont'd** Donning and removing personal protective equipment (PPE).

THE COST OF HEALTH CARE–ASSOCIATED INFECTIONS

Human suffering, prolonged hospital stays, and time lost from work are some of the concerns with an HAI. Another cost is the increased expense of health care delivery. For example, the cost of treating a catheter-related bloodstream infection in a patient in the surgical intensive care unit averages $56,167 and can extend the hospital stay by as much as 21 days (Dimick et al., 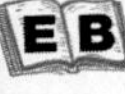 2001). Because of the escalating cost of HAIs, Congress is working with multiple agencies to help design a more appropriate method of tracking and reporting HAIs so that there will be uniformity across the country and, hopefully, less confusion on behalf of the health care consumer. Many states have already enacted mandatory reporting of HAIs to their state health departments, and others are soon to follow.

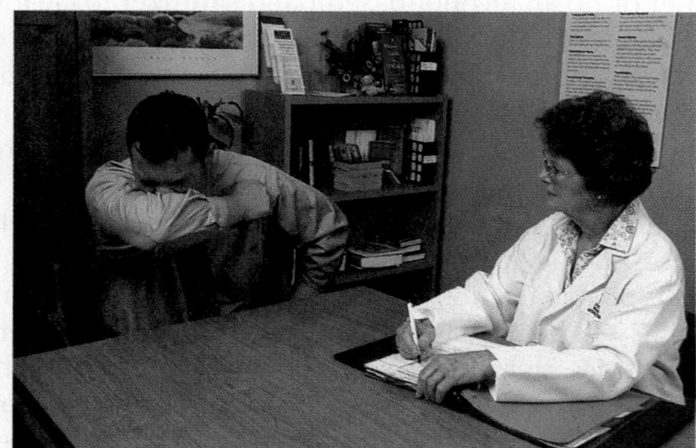

FIGURE **6–5** Covering your cough to help prevent the spread of infection.

Table 6–6 Risk Factors for Increased Susceptibility to Infection

RISK FACTOR	CONSEQUENCE
Altered defense mechanisms	Body damage from trauma, breaks in the skin or mucous membranes; fractures.
Below normal leukocyte (white blood cell) count	Bone marrow suppression from chemotherapy or toxic agents; genetic or acquired agranulocytosis, such as what is seen with chemotherapy drugs.
Age	Elderly patients and the very young are more susceptible to infection, probably because of declining or immature immune function.
Excessive stress or fatigue	These states seem to interfere with the body's normal defense mechanisms.
Malnutrition	Poor nutrition interferes with cell growth and replacement, which contributes to decreased immune function.
Alcoholism	Inhibits the immune system.
Preexisting chronic illnesses, such as diabetes mellitus, adrenal insufficiency, renal failure, or liver disease; serious illness such as pneumonia, peritonitis, etc.	These disease states upset the normal homeostatic balance within the body, impairing the normal defense mechanisms. Serious illness taxes the immune system, causing greater susceptibility to other pathogens.
Immunosuppressive treatment, chemotherapy, or corticosteroid treatment	Depresses the immune system or harms the bone marrow, decreasing the number of leukocytes. Corticosteroids depress the inflammatory response, inhibiting one of the body's defense mechanisms.
Invasive equipment or indwelling tubes	Fracture pins, endotracheal or tracheostomy tubes, intravenous cannulas, feeding tubes, and urinary catheters provide a potential route of entry for pathogens.
Smoking or inhalation of toxic chemicals	Inhibits ciliary action of the respiratory tract. Toxic chemicals may damage bone marrow, inhibiting the production of leukocytes.
Intravenous drug abuse	Allows introduction of microorganisms into the bloodstream from contaminated needles or from lack of aseptic technique.
Unsafe sexual practices (not knowing history or health status of sexual partner, not using condoms)	Allows entry of pathogenic organisms through the genital mucosal tissue.
Unsafe handling of needles and sharps	Potential for breaks in the skin through which pathogens may enter.

Adapted from Ignatavicius, D.D., & Workman, M.L. (2006). *Medical-Surgical Nursing: Critical Thinking for Collaborative Care* (5th ed.). Philadelphia: Elsevier Saunders.

NURSING INTERVENTIONS TO PREVENT HEALTH CARE–ASSOCIATED INFECTIONS

Hand hygiene is the key to breaking the chain of infection; however, for it to be effective, you need to know what to use. For example, if the patient has an *S. aureus* infection, the health care worker can use (1) soap and water or (2) an alcohol-based hand sanitizer to cleanse the hands. However, if the patient has a *C. difficile* or *Candida albicans* infection, the health care worker must use only soap and water to cleanse the hands. The alcohol in alcohol-based sanitizers only makes the spores for these organisms "sticky"; it does not kill them. In addition, if a patient with *C. difficile* is discharged, the housekeeping staff needs to know that the patient had this type of infection so that the appropriate cleaning agents will be used. Careful attention to hand hygiene before and after any direct patient contact, before and after any invasive or sterile procedure, after contact with infectious materials (e.g., wound drainage, feces, urine, or sputum), and before contact with immunocompromised patients is the primary method by which infection can be prevented.

Soiled or contaminated items should not be placed on the floor or remain in an uncovered trash container in the patient's room. Disposing of infectious materials, such as tissues, used dressings, soiled linens, and contaminated equipment, in covered, moisture-resistant biohazard containers helps contain the organism, as well as odors. Protecting patients from others with respiratory infections and from visitors with other communicable diseases is also appropriate. Table 6–8 reviews the major sites of HAIs, the infectious agents most often responsible, and some of the interventions nurses may take to prevent or control the spread of infection at each site.

Along with preventive interventions and appropriate treatments, the nurse must continuously assess the patient to identify early signs of infection or its spread. It is also helpful to review each patient's immunization status against such infections as tetanus, pertussis, influenza, hepatitis B, pneumococcal pneumonia, and varicella. The findings must then be documented in the medical record.

INFECTION SURVEILLANCE AND REPORTING

Surveillance demands that the nurse be alert for signs or symptoms of infection in patients under their care. For example, the nurse should routinely assess the

Table 6–7 Risk Factors for Health Care–Associated Infections

RISK	SOURCE OR CAUSE
Impaired host defenses	Invasive tubes (i.e., endotracheal, nasogastric, enteral feeding) Position of the patient (i.e., supine vs. head of bed >30 degrees) Impaired or altered mental status; sedation Malnutrition, malignancy; immunosuppression
Large dose or introduction of microorganisms	Bacterial colonization Gastric pH neutralized due to H_2-receptor-blocking agents Lack of oral hygiene Acute vs. chronic sinusitis Invasive procedures; open wounds Contaminated respiratory equipment
Overgrowth of virulent organisms	Prolonged or inappropriate antibiotic use Iatrogenic (inadequate hand hygiene); multidrug-resistant organism infection Central venous lines (i.e., subclavian, femoral, peripherally inserted central catheter) Comorbid illness (i.e., diabetes mellitus, peripheral vascular disease) Frequent hospitalizations or exposure to invasive therapies Prolonged hospital stays

Adapted from Flanders, A.S., Collard, H.R., & Saint, S. (2006). Nosocomial pneumonia: State of the science. *American Journal of Infection Control, 34*: 84-93.

patient for unexpected elevation of temperature; malaise; cough; loss of appetite; foul-smelling urine; new-onset diarrhea; and wounds that are red, swollen, painful, or have a foul-smelling discharge. It is important to note the color of the purulent drainage as it is helpful in identifying the kind of organism that may be causing an infection (i.e., *S. aureus* produces a golden discharge and *Pseudomonas aeruginosa* has bluish green discharge).

The nurse should pay particular attention to those patients who are more susceptible to infection. These patients include those who (1) are weakened by severe illness or injury; (2) have drainage tubes or catheters, intravenous cannulas, or other invasive devices for monitoring or treatment; (3) are very young or very old; (4) have had recent surgery; or (5) are immunocompromised. When an infection is suspected, the nurse reports this to the patient's health care provider. In certain situations, Expanded Precautions may need to be instituted even before culture results are available. If there is a question as to what type of Expanded Precautions to initiate, the nurse should contact the facility's infection control department.

Table 6–8 Nursing Interventions to Prevent Health Care–Associated Infections

MOST COMMON SITES	NURSING INTERVENTIONS
Urinary tract	Catheterize only when absolutely necessary. Observe sterile technique when catheterizing. Keep drainage system for indwelling catheter closed, off the floor, and below bladder level at all times to avoid urine reflux. Empty urine drainage bag into clean container, without contaminating spout. Wipe spout with alcohol pad before securing it. Remove indwelling catheter as soon as possible to decrease risk of infection.
Surgical wounds	Administer prophylactic antimicrobials as ordered. Change soiled dressing and linens promptly. Dispose of them in the correct container. Ensure that patient has adequate nutrition and sufficient fluid intake.
Respiratory tract	Encourage the patient to cough, deep breathe, and move. Perform suctioning, tracheostomy care, and other procedures under aseptic technique. Protect patient from others with colds or other signs of infection.
Bloodstream (bacteremia)	Maintain meticulous aseptic technique in the administration of intravenous (IV) fluids. Follow recommended procedure for daily care of insertion site (including the dressing) and IV tubing and catheters. Assess site for increased redness, pain, or infiltration. Remove and insert new IV set per facility policy, and when indicated.

DESTROYING AND CONTAINING INFECTIOUS AGENTS

The goals of destroying and containing infectious microorganisms are achieved by techniques and methods that (1) either kill the organisms or render them harmless or (2) isolate the sources of infection, so that they cannot be spread to others. This is accomplished through medical or surgical aseptic technique.

MEDICAL ASEPSIS AND SURGICAL ASEPSIS

Medical Asepsis

Medical asepsis (the goal is to reduce microorganisms) includes hand hygiene, separation or isolation of the patient, use of appropriate precautions for the handling and disposing of contaminated articles, and other techniques devised to contain and destroy infectious agents, such as cleansing and disinfection.

Surgical Asepsis

Surgical asepsis (the goal is to completely eliminate microorganisms) involves the sterilizing of instruments, skin, linens, and other articles that will be used to perform surgery or other types of sterile procedures. This is because a surgical procedure typically requires that the first line of defense (i.e., the skin) be compromised in some way. Surgical asepsis must also be used when placing an intravenous catheter into a vein, when inserting a Foley catheter into the urinary bladder, during the placement of internal monitoring devices, or during other invasive procedures such as a cardiac angiogram. Hand hygiene for surgical asepsis is more vigorous and must be done according to the facility's policy and procedure. In a surgically aseptic environment, surgical gowns, face masks, and sterile gloves are necessary and must be put on and removed in a specific way. Procedures being performed at the bedside that require surgical asepsis, such as a central line placement, require that all persons in the room wear a face mask and head cover. The person performing the procedure must also wear sterile gloves and a sterile cover gown. The patient must be covered with sterile drapes, and only sterile equipment and supplies are to be used. The door to the room must be closed throughout the procedure (CDC, 2002).

SEPSIS AND SEPTIC SHOCK

If a patient's HAI or community-acquired infection is not adequately treated, the pathogen may enter the bloodstream, causing a bacteremia and a systemic inflammatory response syndrome (SIRS), commonly referred to as **sepsis.** When microorganisms enter the bloodstream, they are carried throughout the body and may invade any tissue or body system. Symptoms of SIRS or sepsis include, but are not limited to, tachycardia (heart rate >90 beats/min), increased cardiac output, *tachypnea* (rapid breathing), fever (core temperature 100.4° F [38° C]), and an elevated WBC count. An altered level of consciousness may also occur. Sepsis is most commonly associated with bacterial invasion from gram-negative bacteria, such as *Pseudomonas aeruginosa, Escherichia coli,* and *Klebsiella pneumoniae,* or gram-positive bacteria such as *Staphylococcus aureus* and *Streptococcus pneumoniae.* The toxins secreted into the blood from these pathogens react with the blood vessels and cell membranes, stimulating a massive inflammatory and immune response. Increased capillary permeability that results in loss of fluid from the vascular space, cellular injury, and greatly increased cellular metabolic rates can occur if the sepsis is not aggressively treated.

Septic shock is a critical manifestation of an infection that has not responded to treatment. This state can then lead to multiorgan system failure, and death can result if the symptoms are not quickly recognized in the earlier stages of sepsis and treatment is not instituted immediately. Patients who have sepsis and have progressed to septic shock present with decreased cardiac output, increased systemic vascular resistance, increased tissue damage, and profound hypotension. This leads to hypoxemia and acidosis. The sympathetic nervous system then tries to compensate by causing pronounced vasoconstriction in an effort to get sufficient blood flowing back to the heart and brain. Septic shock often is accompanied by massive clot formation (due to the vasoconstriction and hypovolemia) throughout the body, called disseminated intravascular coagulation (DIC), which is considered life threatening. Treatment of DIC involves controlling and eliminating the infection; supporting the patient with intravenous fluids, blood pressure control, and supplemental oxygen; and providing supportive care that prevents further complications.

There are four primary types of shock; however, this section focused only on septic shock. Refer to Chapter 44 for further information on the other types of shock.

NURSING INTERVENTIONS FOR PATIENTS WITH SEPSIS OR IN SEPTIC SHOCK

Each nurse, through the assessment process, must consider which patients are at greatest risk for developing sepsis. When a patient has been identified as being at risk for sepsis, it is important to monitor for changes from the baseline assessment, such as a change in mental status; the development of warm, dry, flushed skin; peripheral edema; a full, bounding pulse; normal to high blood pressure; and decreased urine output. The temperature may be normal or elevated, depending on the organism(s) that are causing the sepsis. Pneumonia and postsurgical wound infections are two conditions that can lead to sepsis if not correctly treated, and some patients, often the elderly, experience *hypothermia* (below normal temperature) when septic.

Sepsis is diagnosed from the clinical presentation of the patient as well as the results of laboratory tests, such as elevated leukocyte count, decreased platelets, and serial blood cultures that may be positive for invading organisms. Antimicrobial sensitivities are done on these pathogens to determine which drugs would be most appropriate to treat the infection. Ensuring that the correct antimicrobial agents are prescribed in a timely manner decreases the risk of the patient developing a multidrug-resistant infection and eliminates the pathogens as quickly as possible.

When the patient is known to have sepsis, the nurse must be vigilant for signs of septic shock (Table 6–9). If any of these signs and symptoms is noted, the charge nurse and the physician are notified immediately. It is also important to know whether there are standing

Table 6–9 ***Signs and Symptoms of Septic Shock and Nursing Interventions***

SIGN OR SYMPTOM	NURSING INTERVENTION
NEUROLOGIC	
Altered mental status Early: anxious or restless Late: lethargic to coma	Ensure patient's safety is not at risk due to the mental state; have a sitter at the bedside.
CARDIAC	
Diminished peripheral pulses Decreasing blood pressure	Ensure patient has patent intravenous (IV) access and an IV fluid pump is at the bedside.
Decreased cardiac output Increasing heart rate with "thready" pulse	This is a sign that the sepsis is worsening and immediate action must be taken.
Postural hypotension Low central venous pressure Delayed capillary filling time	
RESPIRATORY	
Complaints of increasing fatigue	Assist the patient with repositioning; provide supplemental oxygenation.
Increased respiratory rate, shallow breaths, cyanosis around lips and in nail beds	Start supplemental oxygen.
Adventitious breath sounds (i.e., crackles)	
Arterial blood gases show decreased PaO_2, decreased $PaCO_2$ due to hyperventilation; however, in the final stages of shock, arterial blood gases will show an increased $PaCO_2$, low pH and bicarbonate levels	
INTEGUMENTARY/MUCOUS MEMBRANES	
Cool or clammy skin Pale to cyanotic in color Dry mouth, sometimes with a "geographic tongue"	
URINARY	
Decreasing urinary output	A Foley catheter may need to be inserted in order to obtain a more accurate measurement.
Increasing urine specific gravity, glucose and acetone in urine	

Key: $PaCO_2$, arterial partial pressure of carbon dioxide; PaO_2, arterial partial pressure of oxygen.
Adapted from Ignatavicius, D.D., & Workman, M.L. (2006). *Medical-Surgical Nursing: Critical Thinking for Collaborative Care* (5th ed.). Philadelphia: Elsevier Saunders.

protocols that the nurse can implement while awaiting further instructions from the attending physician. There are some interventions, such as providing supplemental oxygen or implementing cooling measures, that may help alleviate some of the symptoms that the patient is experiencing; however, these may help for only a short period of time.

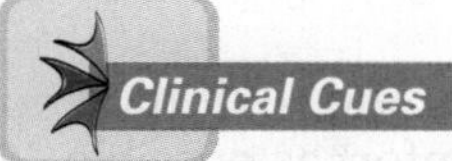

Clinical Cues

If sepsis is discovered early, the chance of a full recovery is good. If septic shock progresses to the stage of tissue damage from microthrombus formation and DIC, the prognosis is poor and death may soon occur. Closely monitoring the patient who has an infection for signs of sepsis, and reporting any such signs to the physician, are extremely important.

NURSING MANAGEMENT

Assessment (Data Collection)

Detecting infection in a patient requires a thorough nursing assessment. Subjective data can be obtained by asking the patient questions such as what symptoms is she having and when did they begin? Assessment questions should be directed toward the signs and symptoms the patient is experiencing. Questions should also include whether the patient is or has had any of the following: pain, headache, stiff neck, fever, or chills. A way to ensure that the correct questions are being asked is to think of what body system appears to be the problem and focus the interview accordingly. For example, if the patient states that it hurts to go to the bathroom, ask if she is having any urgency or burning when trying to empty the bladder. With some signs and symptoms, it may be appropriate to ask if patients have traveled outside the country recently (i.e., amebic dysentery), or if they have been bitten by any insects prior to onset of symptoms (i.e., West Nile virus), or if they have a compromised immune system, either from disease or from drug exposure (i.e., chemotherapy agents). (Refer to Chapter 14 for more information on West Nile virus.)

Subjective complaints that may indicate infection include fatigue, loss of appetite, headache, nausea, general malaise, and pain.

Objective data often point to the specific body system affected by the infection, but may also include systemic signs such as fever, increased pulse, or increased respiratory rate. Data collection includes assessing vital signs; auscultating the lungs to check for abnormal breath sounds; inspecting the skin for lesions or rashes; and checking the urine for cloudiness, discoloration, abnormal odor, and increased specific gravity. Bowel sounds are auscultated in all four quadrants, and then the abdomen is gently palpated for signs of tenderness. In addition, look for signs of local infection such as redness, swelling, pain or tenderness on palpation or movement, heat in the affected area, and possibly loss of function of the affected body part.

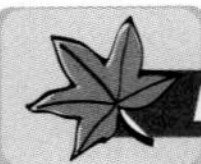

Elder Care Points

Many elderly people, especially those over the age of 80, have a normally low body temperature. Because of decreased inflammatory and immune response, there may be very little rise in temperature in the presence of infection. Small increases in temperature in these patients may be quite significant. Signs of inflammation may not be present or may be less than what is typically seen in a younger person. A decrease in mental alertness, increased fatigue, or sudden onset of confusion, irritability, or apathy may be clues that an infection is present.

Diagnostic Tests

Laboratory data that may indicate infection include an elevated WBC count, changes in the distribution and number of the various types of leukocytes, an elevated erythrocyte sedimentation rate (ESR), and microbiology cultures that test positive for microorganisms.

Bacteriologic tests are done by culturing blood, body fluids, or waste products such as feces. Cultures are grown from specimens collected. When obtaining a culture, the nurse must be careful to (1) use aseptic technique, where indicated and with sterile equipment; (2) only collect fresh material from the suspected site, avoiding contamination by microbes from nearby tissues and fluids; (3) and use the appropriate container for the sample, making sure the container is correctly labeled and tightly covered to avoid spilling and contamination during transport to the laboratory.

Sensitivity tests are done in conjunction with microbiology cultures to determine which antimicrobials can most effectively destroy or inhibit the multiplication and growth of the specific infecting microbe. Once this has been determined, the drug that is most likely to kill the invading microorganism needs to be started as soon as possible. Inadequate dosages or delays in administration can lead to a genetic mutation of the pathogen involved or the development of a **multidrug-resistant organism** (MDRO).

With some infectious diseases, intradermal skin tests are done to determine the presence of certain active or inactive diseases, such as tuberculosis, coccidioidomycosis, and candidiasis. Radiography (x-rays), computed tomography (CT), or magnetic resonance imaging (MRI) may be used to detect changes in the tissues or organs, and to locate abscesses anywhere within the body.

Nursing Diagnosis

The specific type of infection and the problem it presents determine the correct nursing diagnosis. For example, if the patient has a urinary tract infection, the more specific nursing diagnosis would be Alteration in urinary elimination; if there were a wound infection, the specific nursing diagnosis would be Impaired skin integrity. In some cases, collaboration with other health team members helps establish the correct nursing diagnosis. Appropriate nursing diagnoses for patients with infection always include Risk for infection and Risk for injury. Any patient entering the hospital for surgery or an invasive procedure is at risk for an HAI. Therefore, Risk for infection should be listed as a nursing diagnosis on the patient's care plan. The nursing diagnosis of Deficient knowledge related to lack of knowledge about the disease, prevention of infection, or self-care should always be considered.

Planning

The planning phase of the nursing process should take into account the physical strength of the patient and the need for rest. Every effort should be made to maintain the integrity of the skin and mucous membranes so that they continue to serve as effective barriers to infectious agents. This means planning and implementing good skin care, oral hygiene, and personal cleanliness. The psychological impact of Expanded Precautions must be addressed as some patients may feel "dirty" or that people are avoiding them because they have an infectious disease.

The nursing goals for recovery from infection include measures to help the patient:

- Use the body's own defensive and healing processes
- Obtain adequate rest, nutrition, and hydration
- Be as free from physical discomfort as possible
- Be free of as much mental anxiety or depression as possible
- Ensure that sufficient oxygen and blood are supplied to the infected tissues

These measures aid in the healing process. Write specific expected outcomes once the individual nursing diagnoses are chosen.

Implementation

Providing a quiet environment with nursing care planned to provide extended uninterrupted rest periods is important in the recovery process. Relieving the discomforts of fever and muscle aches is accomplished by tepid sponge baths, ice bags, antipyretics, and massage. Warm compresses and the application of heat, as appropriate, can also promote healing. Mild physical exercise promotes circulation and helps some patients to relax. It can also increase blood circulation to an infected area. This ultimately will help to remove the metabolic wastes that were produced from the body.

Provide patient and family teaching regarding the infection, including the following:

- The purposes of diagnostic tests, treatments, and special precautions
- Why the family must help maintain medical asepsis to prevent the spread of infection to themselves and others

Administering Antimicrobial Agents

The administration of antiinfective drugs is an important nursing responsibility. The nurse must also give the drugs on time to maintain effective blood levels. In addition, the nurse must monitor the patient for drug side effects and evaluate the progress of the patient to determine whether the drug is effective in eradicating the infection. General nursing actions for the administration of an antimicrobial medication are shown in Table 6–10.

The nurse must be familiar with the different antimicrobial classifications prior to administering the

Table 6–10 ***General Nursing Implications for the Administration of Antimicrobial Drugs***

NURSING IMPLICATIONS	RATIONALE
PRIOR TO GIVING THE ANTIMICROBIAL	
• Check all drugs patient is receiving for drug interactions with the antimicrobial prescribed.	To prevent toxicity or lack of absorption
• Know the reason why the patient is to receive an antimicrobial drug (question the health care provider if the drug does not seem appropriate for the patient).	To help prevent drug administration errors
• Check that dosage of an antimicrobial drug is appropriate for the patient who may have decreased kidney or liver function.	To ensure drug levels do not build up to a toxic level
• Verify allergies with the patient before administering an antimicrobial drug.	To prevent allergic reaction or adverse outcomes
• Ensure cultures have been obtained prior to administering the antimicrobial agent. If culture and sensitivity results are available, verify that the drug that was ordered is one to which the organism is sensitive. If it is not, clarify the order with the health care provider.	To ensure medication being given is appropriate for the microorganism involved
• Check precautions for administration of the antimicrobial drug, especially when the patient is pregnant or lactating.	To prevent harm to the developing fetus or infant
WHEN GIVING AN ANTIMICROBIAL DRUG	
• Follow the five rights of medication administration.	To prevent errors and injury to the patient
• Give each dose of an antimicrobial drug as close to the scheduled time as possible.	To maintain a consistent blood level of the drug
• Check to see if serum drug levels have been ordered. Ensure that they are drawn as specified by the physician.	To ensure drug dosage is effective and to ensure toxicity will not occur
MONITOR FOR POSSIBLE SIDE/ADVERSE EFFECTS OF THE ANTIMICROBIAL AGENT	
• The most common general side effects are gastrointestinal upset, anorexia, nausea, diarrhea, rash, and photosensitivity.	Knowing what the side effects are aids the nurse in effectively teaching the patient about what to observe for and report to the physician.
• Monitor patient for signs of allergic reaction, such as rash, hives, itching, drug fever, swelling of the mucous membranes, difficulty breathing, or anaphylaxis.	To ensure appropriate interventions are instituted quickly and to prevent more severe outcomes up to, and including, death
• Check for signs of superinfection in patients taking high doses of an antimicrobial drug for an extended period of time (i.e., oral thrush, vaginal itching or discharge, diarrhea).	To ensure appropriate countermeasures can be instituted in a timely manner
TEACH THE PATIENT TAKING AN ANTIMICROBIAL DRUG TO	
• Take the medication with a full glass of water.	To aid with absorption
• Take all of an antimicrobial drug prescription, regardless of whether the patient feels better and has no obvious signs or symptoms of infection.	To prevent the development of multidrug-resistant microorganisms
• Take the medication in relationship to meals. (Different drugs vary in this respect; some need to be taken with food and some should be taken on an empty stomach.)	For best absorption of the drug with minimal gastrointestinal side effects
• Discontinue the drug and notify the health care provider if an allergic reaction occurs.	To ensure treatment is instituted quickly and to prevent more severe outcomes up to, and including, death. May require an alternate type of antibiotic to be prescribed.
• Use a sunblock and protective clothing when sun exposure is unavoidable when taking an antimicrobial agent that is known to cause photosensitivity.	To decrease the risk of sunburn
• Unless contraindicated, increase fluid intake to 2500–3000 mL/day, especially when taking a sulfa-type drug.	To prevent crystallization in the kidneys and promote drug excretion

Table 6–11 *Antimicrobial Agent Classifications*

CATEGORY	ANTIMICROBIAL AGENT
Antibacterial Agents: work by inhibiting the replication and growth of bacterial organisms. *Most common side effects:* nausea, vomiting, and diarrhea.	
Narrow Spectrum	**Gram-positive cocci and gram-positive bacilli**
	Penicillins G and V
	Vancomycin
	Erythromycin
	Clindamycin
	Gram-negative aerobes
	Aminoglycosides—gentamicin, tobramycin, neomycin, and azithromycin
	Cephalosporins:
	1st generation (e.g., cefazolin [Ancef], cephalexin [Keflex])
	2nd generation (e.g., cefaclor [Ceclor], cefotetan [Cefotan], cefuroxime [Zinacef])
	Mycobacterium tuberculosis
	Ethambutol
	Isoniazid
	Pyrazinamide
	Rifampin
Broad Spectrum	**Gram-positive cocci and gram-negative bacilli**
	Broad-spectrum penicillins (i.e., ampicillin)
	Cephalosporins:
	3rd generation (e.g., cefipime [Maxipime], cefixime [Suprax], cefotaxime [Claforan], ceftriaxone [Rocephin])
	Tetracyclines (e.g., doxycycline, minocycline)
	Carbapenems (e.g., imipenem and meropenem)
	Sulfonamides (e.g., sulfasalazine, sulfisoxazole)
Antiviral Agents: work by interfering with DNA or RNA synthesis required for the virus to duplicate itself. *Most common side effects:* headache, nausea, vomiting, anorexia, diarrhea. More severe side effects include acute renal failure, encephalopathy, and bleeding disorders.	
	Acyclovir
	Amantadine
	Azidothymidine
	Saquinavir
Antifungal Agents: work by increasing the permeability of the cell membrane by binding with certain components, leading to decreased nutrients to the cell. *Most common side effects:* headache, fever, chills, nausea, vomiting, and anorexia. More severe side effects include acute kidney and/or liver failure, hemorrhagic gastroenteritis.	
	Amphotericin B
	Ketoconazole
	Itraconazole
Antihelmintic Agents: work by causing paralysis of the invading parasite. *Most common side effects:* dizziness, headache, fever, nausea, vomiting, anorexia, diarrhea and rash.	
	Pyrantel

Adapted from Lehne, R.A. (2006). *Pharmacology for Nursing Care* (6th ed.). Philadelphia: Saunders; and Skidmore-Roth, L. (2006). *Mosby's Nursing Drug Reference*. Philadelphia: Elsevier Mosby.

*As with any other drug, it is important for the nurse to know what the drug is and what it is being given for, and to provide close nursing observation, especially if the patient has never received the drug in the past. Teaching the patient signs and symptoms to report is also an important part of providing safe and effective nursing care.

prescribed drug. For antibiotic agents, there are two primary categories, narrow spectrum and broad spectrum. There are also antiviral, antifungal, and anthelmintic agents (Table 6–11). The narrow-spectrum agents primarily work on a select type of microorganism such as a gram-positive organism that is susceptible to penicillin. A broad-spectrum antibiotic can attack a larger group of organisms. However, these agents can also cause superinfections because they wind up killing off many of the "good bacteria" in the body. A narrow-spectrum antibiotic is the preferred choice for treatment over a broad-spectrum agent because it primarily goes after the pathogenic organism and also reduces the risk of developing an MDRO infection.

Meeting Psychosocial Needs

For any patient, it is advisable to assess what her cultural beliefs are and then work with the family to provide the foods that they believe will assist in the patient's recovery (Cultural Cues 6–1). This information needs to be documented in the nursing care plan so that other health care providers will know how to ensure that nutritional needs are being met.

Supporting Coping Mechanisms

Stress seems to make the body more vulnerable to invasion by foreign organisms by depressing the immune system. When under excessive stress, the body also is less able to mobilize the elements and cells that promote healing. The nurse should realize that the at-

Cultural Cues 6–1

Hot and Cold Foods

Some Asian cultures believe that a balance of hot and cold foods should be eaten when a fever or infection is present. They believe that cold foods, such as watermelon or white radish soup, will help the body fight off the infection and retain its balance.

Many Hispanic cultures believe that "hot" and "cold" forces are thrown out of balance when illness strikes. They may prefer cold foods such as dairy products, honey, or fresh vegetables when they are suffering from infection.

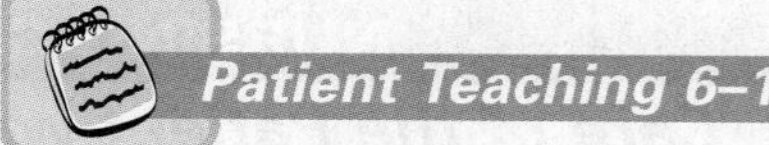

Patient Teaching 6–1

How to Prevent and Control Infection

Teach the patient and family about the measures that should be used when the patient has an infection.

- The ways in which the infection is transmitted.
- How to perform proper hand hygiene.
- Correct techniques for wound care.
- The approved method for disinfecting or sanitizing equipment, supplies, and linens.
- The correct method for proper handling and disposal of contaminated articles.
- Any specific precautions for the type of infection the patient has.

titude shown toward a patient and the ways in which the nurse strives to meet the patient's needs could reduce stress and promote healing in ways that are not yet completely understood.

If the illness is lengthy, concerns about work and home responsibilities may cause anxiety or increase the patient's stress levels. Therefore, collaboration with the social worker or case manager for solutions to such problems may be needed.

Patient Teaching for Preventing and Controlling Infection

Appropriate teaching is essential so that the patient and her family will understand why specific precautions are necessary. Before beginning teaching, the nurse needs to find out how much the patient or family knows about the patient's condition and the problems that may arise. Nurses have an obligation to teach the patient how to care for herself and how to avoid infection through good personal hygiene (Patient Teaching 6-1).

If a patient is to take antimicrobial medications at home, she must be taught how to take them. She must also be cautioned to take all the medication as prescribed and to not discontinue taking any antimicrobial medication, even if she begins to feel better. Explain to the patient and the family that if she stops before the full amount has been taken, it can lead to a second outbreak of the infection and possibly a return to the hospital. Other aspects of teaching will depend on each patient's learning needs and home situation.

Evaluation

Evaluation is determined by how well the goals of care and expected outcomes have been met (Nursing Care Plan 6–1). Laboratory values showing the absence of infection and the patient showing a greater sense of well-being are other criteria that determine the effectiveness of nursing care (see Chapter 10 for more information on diagnostic tests and normal laboratory values). Evaluation of the success of interventions includes data indicating:

- Temperature, pulse, and respirations are within normal range
- WBC count and ESR are within normal limits and cultures are negative
- Ability to rest comfortably
- Absence of or decrease in severity of pain and discomfort
- Fluid and nutritional needs are being met

COMMUNITY CARE

As more nurses work in community settings, opportunities to educate the public about preventing the spread of infection become even more important. Controlling the spread of infectious diseases within the community is accomplished in conjunction with public health officials. Their major goals, and those of nurses who work with them, are to (1) promote sanitary standards in communities, (2) identify persons who are highly susceptible to infection and reduce their chances of developing an infectious disease, and (3) provide immunization programs to protect people against certain infectious diseases.

HOME CARE

The home care nurse must work with the patient and family members to prevent the transmission of pathogens from the environment outside and inside of the house. All people living in the home should be instructed to wash their hands as soon as they return home from being out in a public place. Microorganisms are picked up on the hands from a variety of items, such as shopping cart handles, elevator buttons, door handles, and telephone receivers. The incidence of colds and flu might be decreased if, during the heavy respiratory illness season, people who are at increased risk for infection would stay away from crowded stores and theaters where pathogens are likely to be airborne.

The home care nurse must teach the techniques of medical asepsis to patients and family members to prevent cross-infection from one person to another or

NURSING CARE PLAN 6–1

Care of the Patient with an Abdominal Wound

SCENARIO Patient is a 28-year-old male who has been diagnosed with a lower abdominal wound infection that is culture positive for methicillin-resistant *Staphylococcus aureus* (MRSA). He is going to be discharged in 2 days.

PROBLEM/NURSING DIAGNOSIS *Wound infection*/Impaired skin integrity related to infected abdominal wound.

Supporting assessment data *Objective:* Drainage from abdominal wound is culture positive for MRSA, a multidrug-resistant organism (MDRO).

Goals/Expected Outcomes	Nursing Interventions	Selected Rationale	Evaluation
Infection will be controlled and not spread	Place in Contact Precautions and explain purpose and requirement to patient and visitors.	To prevent the spread of infection to other patients and staff.	No evidence of spread of infection.
	Assist patient with bath to ensure skin has been cleaned. Change wound dressing as ordered and as needed.	Enables the nurse to do a thorough skin assessment. Ensures that the wound is assessed at least daily and nurse can track progression of wound treatment.	Bathed. Dressing changed, less drainage and redness.
	Monitor vital signs, complete blood count, microbiology cultures.	Indicates progress in resolving the infection.	Vital signs stable. WBC decreasing. Outcomes met.

PROBLEM/NURSING DIAGNOSIS *Has never cared for a wound*/Deficit knowledge related to proper wound care at home.

Supporting assessment data *Subjective:* States, "I don't know how to change the dressing."

Goals/Expected Outcomes	Nursing Interventions	Selected Rationale	Evaluation
Prior to discharge, the patient and family member will be able to: Demonstrate proper hand hygiene techniques.	Demonstrate proper hand hygiene technique and observe patient and family member perform this task.	Providing opportunities for education and training throughout the hospital stay increases the knowledge base the patient or the caregiver can build upon.	Patient verbalizes reasons for contact precautions; patient and family member demonstrate proper hand hygiene, wound cleansing, and dressing change techniques using medical asepsis; patient and family member verbalize signs and symptoms to report to physician and states that he understands how to take medication and why he must finish the prescription.
State reasons for using contact precautions for dressing change. Demonstrate dressing change, maintaining medical asepsis before discharge.	Demonstrate dressing change and wound cleansing procedure; obtain return demonstration from patient and family member before discharge.	Providing hands-on training increases the understanding of wound healing and need for appropriate wound care.	
List signs and symptoms that should be reported to physician.	Instruct patient and family to watch for elevated temperature, increased redness, swelling, pain, or purulent discharge from wound, and to report any such findings to the physician.	Knowing what to look for and report decreases the risk of adverse outcomes.	
State why it is important to complete the course of antibiotic therapy exactly as directed.	Explain importance of taking medication exactly as prescribed and of finishing entire prescription.	Taking antimicrobials as prescribed decreases the risk of the patient developing an MDRO infection.	Outcomes being met.

? CRITICAL THINKING QUESTIONS

1. What other nursing methods could you implement that would promote healing?
2. How would you recommend the patient's linens be laundered at home?

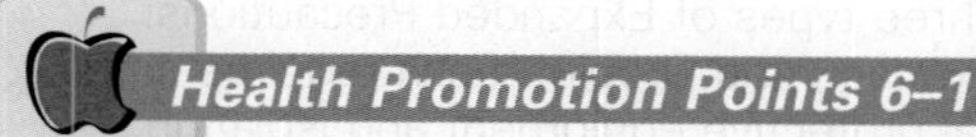

What You Can Do to Prevent Infections at Home

1. Wash your hands often.
   - **When:** Before eating; before, during, and after handling/preparing food; before dressing a wound, giving medicine, or inserting contact lenses; after contact with bodily fluids or blood; after changing a diaper; after using the bathroom; after handling animals, their toys, leashes, or waste; after handling anything contaminated, such as trash, drainage, soil, etc.
   - **How:** Wet hands and apply soap, briskly rub hands together for 20 seconds, rinse thoroughly with warm water, and dry with a clean towel.
2. Routinely clean surfaces.
   - **In Kitchen:** Clean counters, cutting boards, and all other surfaces before, during, and after preparing food, especially meat and poultry. Use hot, soapy water and scrub cutting boards well.
   - **In Bathroom:** Clean and disinfect all surfaces routinely.
3. Handle and prepare food safely.
   - **Clean:** Clean hands and work surfaces often.
   - **Separate:** Don't cross-contaminate one food with another; use separate cutting boards for meat and fresh produce and keep food separate in the refrigerator.
   - **Cook:** Cook foods to proper temperatures; use a food thermometer. Find recommended food cooking temperatures at *www.fightbac.org/heatitup.cfm* or *www.isitdoneyet.gov*
   - **Chill:** Refrigerate foods promptly.
4. Get immunized.
   - Make sure you and your loved ones get the necessary shots suggested by your health care provider at the proper time, and maintain immunization records for the family. Ask your physician about special programs that provide free shots for your child.
5. Use antibiotics appropriately.
   - Take antibiotics exactly as prescribed by your health care provider. Antibiotics do not work against viruses such as colds or flu.
6. Be careful with pets.
   - Follow the immunization schedule for your pets as recommended by the vet.
   - Clean litter boxes daily.
   - Make sure your child does not put any object or hands in the mouth after touching animals.
   - Wash hands thoroughly after contact with animals, especially after visiting farms, petting zoos, and fairs.
   - Use flea and tick prevention treatment on cats and dogs.
7. Avoid contact with wild animals.
   - Do not leave food around and keep garbage cans sealed around your home.
   - Clear brush, grass, and debris around your home.
   - Seal any entrance holes to animal dens, if any are found inside or outside of your home.
   - Use insect repellent to prevent ticks.

Compiled from information on www.cdc.gov.

the spread of infection in the patient. Hand hygiene is stressed, and family members are taught not to share personal items, especially toothbrushes or razors that might be contaminated by blood. Dishes and eating utensils are washed with soap and water or in the dishwasher. The patient's soiled linens, clothing, and towels should be washed as soon as possible or stored in sealed plastic bags until washed. Surfaces contaminated with traces of blood, urine, feces, or vomitus should be sanitized using a clean cloth, soap, and hot water, and then recleaned with a 1:10 solution of chlorine bleach and hot water. Within the home, the patient and family are taught to contain infectious wastes such as dressings and soiled tissues in a sealed, impermeable plastic bag. The bags can then be disposed of in the garbage cans outside of the home.

Meats, poultry, and dairy products are to be handled properly during cooking preparation and stored in the refrigerator. Thawing frozen food products on the countertop increases the likelihood of bacterial contamination. Kitchen surfaces such as countertops and cutting boards must be disinfected after poultry, meat, and fresh vegetables are prepared for cooking. Wooden cutting boards tend to hold more bacteria than plastic or glass boards. Regardless of the type of board used, it needs to be scrubbed thoroughly with hot soapy water, rinsed, and dried with a clean towel (Health Promotion Points 6–1).

Maintaining a healthy lifestyle that promotes an intact immune system increases a person's resistance to infection. Obtaining adequate sleep, eating properly, and exercising regularly all contribute to increased resistance to illness or infection. Adopting effective stress reduction techniques and using them regularly can also be beneficial.

LONG-TERM CARE

The elderly are more susceptible to infection. Those in long-term care facilities often have chronic illnesses that add to their susceptibility. Many elderly have low-grade infections of the urinary, respiratory, or gastrointestinal tract that can be easily passed on to others if hand hygiene is not consistently practiced. Providing assistance to residents to wash their hands before meals and after toileting, after being in community rooms such as the dining room or social activities lounge, and any time their hands become soiled will greatly reduce the incidence of HAIs. Cleaning incontinent patients promptly and maintaining skin integrity is an essential nursing function. Also, to help decrease the odors caused by incontinence, it is important to secure soiled linens in plastic linens bags prior to removal from the patient's room.

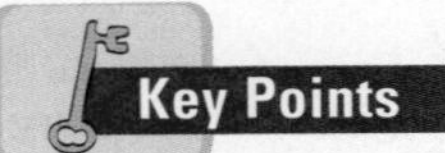

Key Points

- Normal flora is needed to help prevent harmful microorganisms from colonizing or infecting the body.
- An infection is the presence and growth of pathogenic microorganisms, in a susceptible host, to the extent that tissue damage occurs.
- The relationship between the host, the agent, and the environment is what determines whether an infection will or will not occur.
- A pathogen is any organism that, if allowed to grow, can cause infection or disease.
- There are multiple types of antimicrobial drugs that can be used to fight infection: antibiotics for bacterial infections, antivirals for viral infections, and antifungals for fungal infections.
- The body has mechanical barriers, such as the skin and mucous membranes, and chemical barriers, such as tears or saliva, that help fight against infection.
- The overall health of a person helps determine the body's ability to initiate an inflammatory response to fight off invading pathogens.
- Fever is one of the primary immune responses to fighting off invading microorganisms.
- Septic shock occurs when the body is unable to mount an effective defense against invasion. If septic shock is not recognized early, death can occur.
- Hand hygiene is the number one way to prevent the spread of infection.
- There are three types of Expanded Precautions: Airborne, Contact, and Droplet. Each requires different personal protective equipment and isolation protocols.
- Protective environment isolation is used for patients who have received hematopoietic stem cell transplantation.
- Using respiratory hygiene and cough etiquette helps to prevent the spread of infection.
- To ensure appropriate antimicrobial agents are being given to a patient with an infection, it is important to ensure that blood or other body fluid specimens for culture have been collected prior to the start of any antimicrobial agent.
- In teaching a patient about methods to prevent the spread of infection, it is important to determine how much the patient already knows so that the nurse can assist the patient in learning what is needed to prevent the spread of infection, such as hand hygiene, the correct use of antimicrobial agents, cleaning of wounds, and keeping the home environment clean.
- Patients and their families learn by example. If they see the nurse and other health care workers following hand hygiene protocols, they are more likely to do the same.

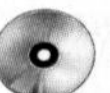
Go to your **Companion CD-ROM** for an Audio Glossary, animations, video clips, and bonus review questions.

evolve Be sure to visit the companion Evolve site at http://evolve.elsevier.com/deWit for interactive NCLEX-PN Exam Style Review Questions, WebLinks, and additional online resources.

NCLEX-PN EXAM STYLE REVIEW QUESTIONS

Choose the best answer(s) for the following questions.

1. The nurse is admitting a patient with an infected abdominal wound. Wound cultures are positive for methicillin-resistant *Staphylococcus aureus*. Appropriate nursing care for this patient includes:
   1. monitoring temperature and white blood count.
   2. placing the patient on strict intake and output.
   3. instituting respiratory precautions.
   4. encouraging ambulation along the hallways.

2. During an assessment, the nurse notes the following signs and symptoms: fever, fatigue, general weakness, cold and clammy skin, nausea, vomiting, and diarrhea. What is an appropriate nursing diagnosis?
   1. Pain
   2. Deficient fluid volume
   3. Deficient knowledge
   4. Ineffective coping

3. Which of the following patient instructions is most critical to a patient being discharged on antibiotic therapy?
   1. Wash your hands.
   2. Monitor urine color.
   3. Reduce stress.
   4. Take all the antibiotics as prescribed.

4. Cross-infection among members of the household who take care of a relative with a severe infection can be prevented by which of the following behaviors? *(Select all that apply.)*
   1. Share personal items.
   2. Practice hand hygiene.
   3. Use bleach to clean surfaces.
   4. Seal used dressings in impermeable bags.
   5. Wash soiled linens weekly.

5. While taking care of a Latin American patient with pneumonia, the nurse reinforces the need to meet nutritional requirements. Which of the following should be most encouraged to promote healing?
   1. Fresh vegetables and corn bread
   2. Chicken broth
   3. Fish and rice with vegetables
   4. Bread and pastries

6. When determining the most appropriate antibiotic for an infection, the physician is likely to rely on which of the following?
   1. Elevated white blood cells
   2. Culture and sensitivity
   3. Erythrocyte sedimentation rate
   4. Fever

7. The nurse assumes the care of a patient with active pulmonary tuberculosis. Before entering the patient's room, what is an appropriate nursing action?
   1. Keep the door open to maintain continuous airflow.
   2. Wear a properly fit-tested N95 mask.
   3. Don sterile gloves.
   4. Observe strict Standard Precautions.

8. While explaining the need for reverse isolation, the 52-year-old postchemotherapy patient wails, "How can I hug my children when I am locked up in this room?" A likely nursing diagnosis would be:
   1. Pain.
   2. Altered nutrition.
   3. Deficient knowledge.
   4. Social isolation.

9. Which of the following interventions would the nurse implement for a patient with active pulmonary tuberculosis who has social isolation related to imposed airborne precautions?
   1. Limit the number of visitors to immediate family.
   2. Provide alternative means of maintaining social contact like electronic mail and phone calls.
   3. Plan adequate periods of rest and relaxation.
   4. Reinforce rationale for airborne precautions.

10. A plan of care for an older adult with a urinary tract infection should include strategies for:
    1. enabling the body to use natural defenses.
    2. obtaining adequate, rest, nutrition, and hydration.
    3. reducing urinary signs and symptoms.
    4. developing coping strategies.

CRITICAL THINKING ACTIVITIES

Read each clinical scenario and discuss the questions with your classmates.

Scenario A

Mrs. Compton, age 44, is admitted to the hospital for a hysterectomy. During the admission assessment procedure, you notice a large, draining abscess in her axillary region. She also has a temperature of 100° F, and she tells you that she has not felt well for the past few days.

1. What would be your course of action following this assessment?

Scenario B

Mr. Lopez, age 18, has been admitted to the orthopedic unit following an automobile accident. He has sustained an open fracture of the femur and has been placed in traction.

1. What would be some expected signs and symptoms of inflammation that he might experience?
2. What specific problems might his care present for the nurse?

CHAPTER

7 Care of Patients with Pain

evolve http://evolve.elsevier.com/deWit

Objectives

Upon completion of this chapter, you should be able to:

Theory

1. Demonstrate an understanding of the current view of pain as a specific entity requiring appropriate intervention.
2. Review the "gate theory" of pain and its relationship to nursing care.
3. Compare nociceptive pain and neuropathic pain and the nursing care for each type.
4. Explain how pain perception is affected by personal situations and cultural backgrounds.
5. Describe the false perceptions that underlie many current ideas about pain and pain management and assist patients to achieve a clearer, more factual understanding.
6. List the different pharmacologic approaches to pain management, with examples of each.
7. Analyze the major differences between acute and chronic pain and their management.

Clinical Practice

1. Effectively utilize the nursing process for pain management.
2. Use appropriate pain evaluation tools for a variety of patients.
3. Recognize common side effects of analgesics and describe techniques for addressing them.
4. Employ nonpharmacologic approaches to pain management with a variety of patients.

Key Terms

Be sure to check out the bonus material on the Companion CD-ROM, including selected audio pronunciations.

acute pain (ă-KŪT pān, p. 139)
adjuvant (ĂJ-ŭ-vănt, p. 139)
buccal mucosa (BŬK-ăl MŪ-cō-să, p. 147)
chronic pain (KRŎN-ĭk pān, p. 139)
endorphins (ĕn-DŎR-fĭnz, p. 137)
epidural (Ĕ-pĭ-DŪ-rŭl, p. 147)
intractable pain (ĭn-TRĂC-tă-bŭl pān, p. 147)
modulation (p. 137)
neuropathic pain (nū-rō-PĂTH-ĭk pān, p. 139)
nociceptive pain (nō-sē-SĔP-tĭv pān, p. 137)
pain threshold (pān, p. 139)
pain tolerance (pān TŎL-ŭr-ŭns, p. 139)
perception (pĕr-CĔP-shŭn, p. 137)
phantom pain (FĂN-tŏm pān, p. 139)
placebos (plă-SĒ-bōz, p. 145)
referred pain (rĭ-FŬRD pān, p. 141)
transduction (trănz-DŬK-shŭn, p. 137)
transmission (trăns-MĬ-shŭn, p. 137)

A common link among people who require health care is pain, or the fear of pain. The causes of pain are varied. An illness or injury may cause pain. Surgical intervention and other treatments may cause pain. Anticipation of treatment may foster a fear of pain. People frequently fear that they will not be able to get relief from pain that is occurring or may occur during treatment. Traditionally, pain was seen as a *symptom* of the illness or injury, something that was temporary and would go away as healing occurred. The physician decided what pain control drug *(analgesic)* was needed and the nurse administered it according to the physician's order. It was the role of the physician and nurse to determine the presence of pain and to administer appropriate treatment.

Current thinking views pain not as just a symptom, but as a specific problem that needs to be treated. Today we also recognize that the patient must be part of the management team. Although we have equipment that accurately measures such things as blood pressure, heart rhythm, or brain waves, there is no such equipment for measuring pain. Pain is a subjective experience. Only the patient knows the location of the pain and its degree of intensity. Only the patient knows what treatment regimen works and how long it is effective.

THE THEORY OF PAIN

Pain can be defined as a neurologic response to unpleasant stimuli. Pain receptors are abundantly distributed throughout the skin and in many deeper structures of the body. Receptors for pain do not become dulled with repeated stimulation. Indeed, studies indicate that under some conditions, repeated stimulation results in an increase in the acuteness of the pain sensation.

The actual mechanism of pain is still poorly understood. It is known that pain results from the release of various chemicals from damaged cells. It may be helpful to think of pain as being controlled by a "gate" in the central nervous system (Figure 7–1). When the gate is open, the pain sensation is allowed through, and when it is closed the pain sensation is blocked. The gate control theory also recognizes that stimuli other than pain pass through the same gate. When a large volume of nonpainful stimuli are competing for the gate, pain impulses may be blocked. A high volume of pain, however, may override other stimuli and pass through the gate, causing the individual to perceive the pain.

Aspects of this theory relate to nursing practice in several ways:

- Two types of nerve fibers carry pain stimuli: small diameter and large diameter.
- Activity in the small-diameter nerve fibers seems to open the gate, and activity in the large-diameter nerve fibers seems to close it. Massage and vibration produce activity in the large-diameter nerve fibers.
- High levels of sensory input create brainstem impulses that seem to close the gate. Distraction in the form of activity or social interaction produces these kinds of impulses.
- An increase in anxiety seems to open the gate, and a decrease seems to close it. The fear that pain will not be controlled may actually increase pain intensity, and knowing that pain can or is being controlled may reduce it.

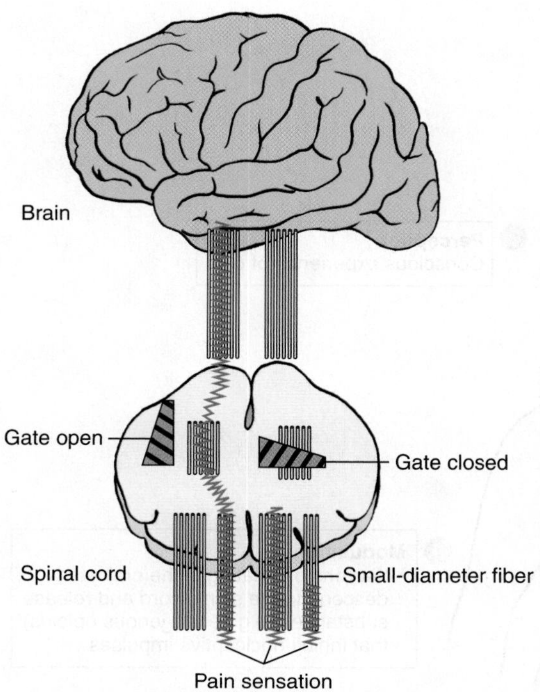

FIGURE 7–1 The gate control theory of pain.

Another way of looking at pain and its management is the idea of "pieces of pain." The more intense the pain, the greater the number of pieces, and therefore a greater number of "pieces" of analgesia will be required to control it. This idea states that inadequate analgesia results in leftover, untreated pain, and relief or control is not achieved.

It is also known that the body produces substances called **endorphins** (endogenous morphine) that can attach to pain receptors and block pain sensation. There are still many questions about endorphins and how they work. Their properties appear to include modification and inhibition of unpleasant stimuli, reduction of anxiety, and relief of pain. They also may produce feelings of euphoria and well-being. For example, the "runner's high" is believed to occur because endorphins are released after physical exercise.

? *Think Critically About . . .* Describe the differences between the old view of pain and the new view of pain.

THE CLASSIFICATION OF PAIN

There are two pathophysiologic classifications of pain: nociceptive and neuropathic. **Nociceptive pain** is associated with pain stimuli from either *somatic* (body tissue) or *visceral* (organs) structures. Somatic nociceptive pain arises from injury to tissue where pain receptors called nociceptors are located. These nociceptors may be found in skin, connective tissue, bones, joints, or muscles. Trauma, burns, or surgery may cause injuries triggering somatic nociceptive pain. Visceral nociceptive pain arises from pathophysiology in visceral organs such as the organs of the gastrointestinal tract. Pathologic conditions triggering visceral nociceptive pain include tumors and obstructions of the organs (Table 7–1).

There are four phases of pain associated with nociceptive pain (McCaffery and Pasero, 1999). **Transduction** is the first phase and begins when tissue damage causes the release of substances that stimulate the nociceptors and initiate the sensation of pain. **Transmission** is the second phase and involves movement of the pain sensation to the spinal cord. **Perception,** the third phase, occurs when impulses reach the brain and the pain is recognized. The fourth phase, **modulation,** occurs when neurons in the brain send signals back down the spinal cord by release of neurotransmitters (Figure 7–2).

Aspects of nociceptive pain relate to nursing practice in several ways:

- Treatment of nociceptive pain may be directed toward one or all of the four phases.

- Nonsteroidal anti-inflammatory drugs (NSAIDs) work by blocking the production of the substances that trigger the nociceptors in the transduction phase.
- Opioids interfere with the transmission phase.
- Nonpharmacologic treatments, such as distraction and guided imagery, may be effective during the perception phase.
- Drugs that block neurotransmitter uptake work in the modulation stage.

Table 7–1 ***Physiologic Sources of Pain***

PHYSIOLOGIC STRUCTURE	CHARACTERISTICS OF PAIN	SOURCES OF ACUTE POSTOPERATIVE PAIN	SOURCES OF CHRONIC PAIN SYNDROMES
NOCICEPTIVE PAIN			
Somatic Pain			
Cutaneous or superficial: skin and subcutaneous tissues	Sharp, burning Dull, aching, cramping	Incisional pain, pain at insertion sites of tubes and drains, wound complications, orthopedic procedures, skeletal muscle tissue	Bony metastases, osteoarthritis and rheumatoid arthritis, low back pain, peripheral vascular diseases
Deep somatic: bone, muscle, blood vessels, connective tissues			
Visceral Pain			
Organs and the linings of the body cavities	Poorly localized Diffuse, deep cramping or splitting, sharp, stabbing	Chest tubes, abdominal tubes and drains, bladder distention or spasms, intestinal distention	Pancreatitis, liver metastases, colitis, appendicitis
NEUROPATHIC PAIN			
Nerve fibers, spinal cord, and central nervous system	Poorly localized Shooting, burning, fiery, shocklike, sharp, painful numbness	Phantom limb pain, postmastectomy pain, nerve compression	HIV-related pain, diabetic neuropathy, postherpetic neuralgia, chemotherapy-induced neuropathies, cancer-related nerve injury, radiculopathies

Adapted from Ignatavicius, D.D., & Workman, M.L. (2006). *Medical-Surgical Nursing: Critical Thinking for Collaborative Care* (5th ed.), Philadelphia: Elsevier Saunders, p. 132.

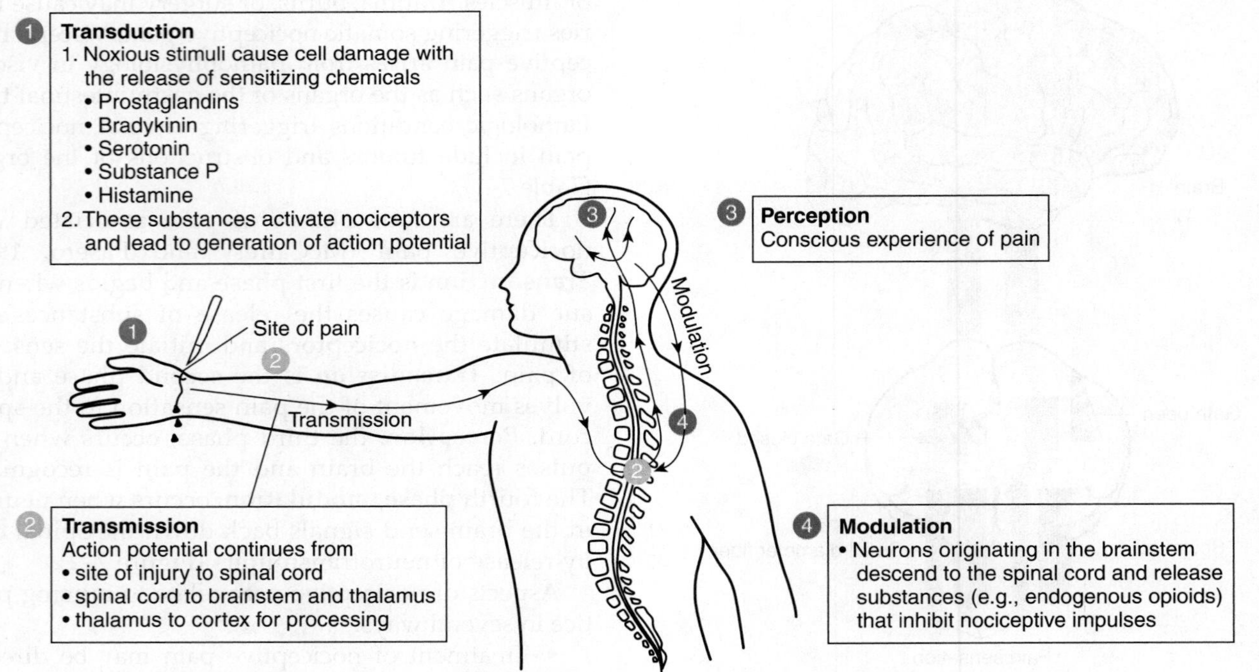

FIGURE **7–2** Nociceptive pain originates when tissue is injured. *1,* Transduction. *2,* Transmission. *3,* Perception. *4,* Modulation.

Neuropathic pain is associated with a dysfunction of the nervous system that involves an abnormality in the processing of sensations. These dysfunctions in the nervous system are often associated with medical conditions rather than tissue damage. The dysfunction may occur in the peripheral or central nervous system. In peripheral nervous system neuropathic pain, it is believed that pain receptors become sensitive to stimuli and send pain signals more easily. Nerve endings grow additional branches that send stronger pain signals to the brain. As the branches grow, they influence touch and warmth receptors. Other peripheral nervous system conditions may cause neuropathic pain. Neuropathic pain may be the result of damage to nerve roots such as compression or entrapment. Examples of such conditions include diabetes mellitus and Guillain-Barré syndrome. Another dysfunction of the central nervous system occurs when the pain signal that would normally move from the periphery toward the brain reverses and the signal is sent in the opposite direction. **Phantom pain,** the pain felt in a limb after amputation, is an example.

Aspects of neuropathic pain relate to nursing practice in several ways:

- Analgesics and opioids usually do not relieve neuropathic pain.
- **Adjuvant** medications such as NSAIDs, tricyclic antidepressants, anticonvulsants, and corticosteroids relieve neuropathic pain.

PERCEPTION OF PAIN

The ways in which humans react to pain can vary widely from person to person and in the same individual under different circumstances. Pain threshold and pain tolerance are concepts that are used when discussing the perception of pain. **Pain threshold** is the point at which pain is perceived. Research indicates that the threshold of pain does not vary significantly among people. **Pain tolerance** is the length of time or the intensity of pain a person will endure before outwardly responding to it. Research indicates that tolerance varies among people. Factors that affect pain tolerance include culture, pain experience, expectations, and role behaviors. People with **acute pain** (of recent onset, lasting less than 6 months) may have physiologic symptoms such as increased pulse and respiratory rates, increased blood pressure, diaphoresis, and increased muscle tension. They may also experience nausea and vomiting. People with **chronic pain** (lasting months or years) may have learned adaptive methods that allow them to have some control over it. Symptoms associated with chronic pain include irritability, depression, withdrawal, and insomnia. Coping with pain takes a lot of energy, and patients who are debilitated are less able to withstand pain than are strong, robust people. Fatigue caused by pain can lead to an increase in pain perception.

Pain can cause a variety of physiologic responses, including increased respiratory rate, pulse, or blood pressure; muscle tension; sweating; flushing or pallor; and frowning or grimacing. Although the presence of any of these factors may indicate pain, their absence does not prove the absence of pain.

A person's cultural background influences feelings about pain (Cultural Cues 7–1). In much of Western culture it is considered valuable to have a high pain tolerance, particularly among men. Some cultures allow for free expression of pain, and moaning, crying, and other actions are considered appropriate. A nurse whose cultural background approves the "stiff upper lip" approach to handling pain may see the patient who outwardly expresses pain as weak or manipulative. Those patients whose cultural upbringing causes them to hide and deny pain may suffer needlessly unless the nurse can intervene by helping them to understand that analgesia will aid the healing process by encouraging movement and decreasing fatigue. Learning to accept without judgment the various ways of coping with and expressing pain is a very necessary process for nurses.

NURSING MANAGEMENT

Assessment (Data Collection)

Evaluation of another person's pain is a major nursing challenge. Because there is no technology for accurate measurement, a combination of evaluation methods is used. The complete assessment of a person's pain should include information about the pain's location, characteristics, quantity, and pattern. In addition, the assessment should include data concerning other symptoms that occur when the person is in pain, what factors alleviate the pain, and what factors aggravate the pain (Focused Assessment 7–1).

Observation

Appearance. The face may look tense, drawn, or pale. There may be a grimace or even a look of fear.

Behavior. A normally verbal patient may become quiet or withdrawn. One who is normally pleasant may become irritable, demanding, or argumentative. The individual may protect or "cradle" the painful area with the hands or arms. Tears, refusal of food or drink, or any behavior that is out of the ordinary for the individual may be an indication of pain.

Activity Level. A person in pain often reduces activity to a minimum. Staying in bed, creeping slowly from place to place, stooping over during ambulation, and stopping frequently to rest or lean against a support can all indicate pain.

Verbalization. Many individuals in pain may verbalize their discomfort. However, it is not always easy to interpret the degree of pain from what is said. Limited

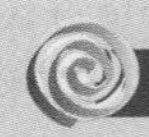

Cultural Cues 7–1

Cultural Beliefs Affecting Pain Perception and Treatment

Various groups from different cultures may have beliefs about pain that differ from yours. Do recall, however, that just because a person is linked to a particular cultural group, it doesn't mean that he participates in the cultural practices of that group. Proper assessment of beliefs is very important.

CULTURE	PAIN EXPRESSION AND MEANING	PREFERENCES AND ACTION
Caucasian (Whites)	Men display strong stoicism. Narcotic use brings fear of addiction for many. May minimize pain and continue to work and carry out usual activities. May decrease use of pain medication quickly.	Prefer to use non-narcotic medications. Many prefer to use relaxation and distraction techniques rather than medication, or just to "tough it out."
Hispanics	Mexican-Americans often feel that pain is "God's will" and are stoical. Pain may be seen as a consequence of immoral behavior. For the "macho" male, expressing pain shows weakness and may cause lack of respect. Other Hispanic groups tend to be expressive of pain and discomfort and may moan, groan, or cry, and this is seen as acceptable.	Many feel that injectable medication is better treatment for pain than a pill. Prayer, heat, and herbs may be used to treat pain.
Africans (Blacks)	Pain is often seen as a sign of sickness. May express pain openly, but this varies. Pain may be seen as something to just be endured.	Laying-on of hands and prayer are thought to help relieve pain. May rely on spiritual or religious belief to help endure pain.
Asians	Varies among subgroups, but generally tend to be stoical. Bearing pain may be seen as a matter of family honor. May describe pain obliquely in terms of body symptoms. Some Filipinos view pain as a part of life and to endure it is honorable. Elders may fear addiction to pain medication.	May prefer oral or intravenous pain medication; injections may be seen as too invasive of privacy. May use applications of moist heat. Family may request pain medication for the patient.
American Indians	Many believe that pain is something to be endured and will not ask for pain medication. Pain is often described in general body terms such as "I don't feel good." May not be aware that they can ask for medication for pain.	Many use traditional medicine men and rely on herbal preparations. May tell family or visitors about the pain rather than the health care provider.
Arabs	View pain as something to be controlled and expect prompt treatment. May describe pain in terms of hot and cold. May express pain more openly to family than to health care providers.	Usually prefer injectable medication over pills.

vocabulary, lack of experience in verbalizing abstract concepts, fear of disbelief or disapproval from the caregiver, and fear of becoming addicted to the analgesic can all impair the person's ability to communicate his pain.

Physiologic Clues. Physiologic clues to pain include rapid, shallow, or guarded respirations, pallor, diaphoresis, increased pulse, elevated blood pressure, dilated pupils, and tenseness of the skeletal muscles. However, remember that problems other than pain can also cause these to occur. All physiologic changes must be fully assessed to determine the cause.

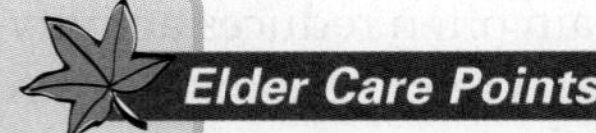

Elder Care Points

Older patients may not report pain for a variety of reasons. They may think pain is an expected part of aging. They may deny pain because it means they are getting older. They may not report pain because they feel they cannot afford the cost of tests or treatments.

Assessment Tools

A variety of scales and evaluation methods have been developed for use in pain management. Some of the more commonly used tools are briefly described.

Number Scales. These use a scale, such as 0 to 5 or 0 to 10, with 0 indicating no pain and the highest number indicating the greatest amount of pain imaginable. The numbers in between show graduated levels of pain. The scale may be simply verbal, or it may actually be drawn on a piece of paper so the person can mark or point to the degree of pain. These can be used very effectively with people who have a good understanding of the numerical concept and who like a strictly logical approach. They are not effective with young children, anyone who has difficulty with numbers, or anyone who is confused or disoriented. Also, some patients have reported that they cannot relate a numerical scale to something as intensely personal as pain.

Visual Scales. A variety of these scales are available. Some use photographs or simple drawings of faces with expressions showing a pain-free state (happy and smil-

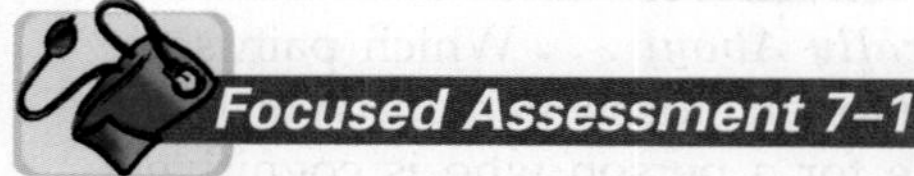

Focused Assessment 7–1

Data Collection for the Patient with Pain

The nurse asks the following questions while assessing a patient with pain:

LOCATION
- Where is your pain?
- Can you point to the pain?

CHARACTERISTICS
- Can you describe your pain?
- What words would you use to describe the pain? (aching, burning, gnawing, sharp, stabbing, shooting, etc.)
- Is the pain constant or does it come and go?

QUANTITY
- How strong or intense is your pain?
- Use pain scale.

PATTERN
- How long have you had this pain?
- Did the pain begin during activity, before eating, after eating?
- Did the pain start suddenly?
- Has the pain increased over time?

ASSOCIATED FACTORS
- Have you had other symptoms such as nausea and vomiting, shortness of breath, rapid heart rate, sweating?

ALLEVIATING FACTORS
- What have you tried to relieve the pain? (medication, certain position, application of heat or cold, distraction)
- Did it work?

AGGRAVATING FACTORS
- What, if anything, makes the pain increase?

ing) and then progress through a series of faces showing increased discomfort. The final picture shows a face either crying or with an intense grimace (Figure 7–3).

Color Scale. A color scale allows the patient to select the colors that represent varying degrees of pain. Colored pieces of paper, crayons or markers, or colored pieces of plastic such as poker chips can be used. The patient selects a color that represents no pain, a color that represents severe pain, and then one, two, or three other colors for pain levels in between. This scale is often used with children, but very young children cannot understand more than three or four possible choices.

Pieces of Pain Scale. This scale uses five poker chips or other identical, plain objects, each one representing a "piece" of pain. The patient can indicate the degree of pain by selecting the number of chips that equals the intensity of pain being experienced.

Behavioral Pain Scale. This scale is used with patients who are cognitively impaired or cannot speak. The nurse assesses the patient's behavior in categories such as facial expression, limb movement, and activity level (Figure 7–4). A score from 0 to 2 is obtained for each category, and the category scores are added together to arrive at a pain score total of 0 to 10. It is useful when assessing the pain of infants, young children, or older adults.

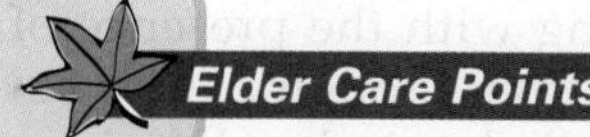

Elder Care Points

A more accurate assessment of pain in the elderly is obtained when several types of pain scales are used, such as a number scale, a visual scale, and a behavioral scale.

When using a pain assessment scale, it is important that the nursing staff use it consistently and that the patient fully understands how to use it. The type of scale being used and any pertinent information about how the patient uses the scale must be included in the patient care plan.

? *Think Critically About . . .* Can you explain the difference between acute and chronic pain to someone.

Difficulties in Data Gathering

Much of the data gathered when assessing pain comes from conversation with the patient, and this presents a variety of problems. The first is language itself. Concepts of the true meaning of words in the language may vary greatly from person to person. It is important to discuss the words used to describe pain and to agree upon their meaning (Table 7–2). It also is important that documentation include the patient's exact words.

The need to work through an interpreter or deal with language difficulties when the patient speaks a foreign language compounds the problem of communication. Whenever possible, the nurse should use a medical professional with a good knowledge of both languages as an interpreter. Most hospitals have a list of approved interpreters to assist in these situations. People who do not have a medical background may not give accurate meanings in the translation, and patients may hide personal, embarrassing, or painful information if the interpreter is a family member or personal friend.

Describing the location of pain can be made difficult by the problem of **referred pain** (pain felt in a different part of the body from where it actually originates). Heart pain may be felt in the jaw or radiating down the arm. Gastric pain may center in the area of the heart rather than the stomach. Pain in one area of the body is frequently referred to another area (Figure 7–5). **There also is a tendency not to believe an individual's statement of pain if there is**

no outward appearance of pain. For example, a patient watching an exciting football game with a friend may enjoy the game even if his surgical incision is quite painful. The lack of a grimace or physiologic changes indicative of pain may be viewed as an absence of pain, when in fact the patient is using distraction as a way of coping with the presence of pain. People may fall asleep even though pain is severe, particularly if uncontrolled pain has left them in a state of exhaustion.

? ***Think Critically About . . .*** Which pain scale would you use for an elderly person? Which one would you use for a person who is cognitively impaired?

Nursing Diagnosis

The nursing diagnosis for pain is frequently "Pain related to" the cause of the pain. An example would be "Pain related to fractured pelvis and fractured left femur."

WONG-BAKER FACES PAIN RATING SCALE

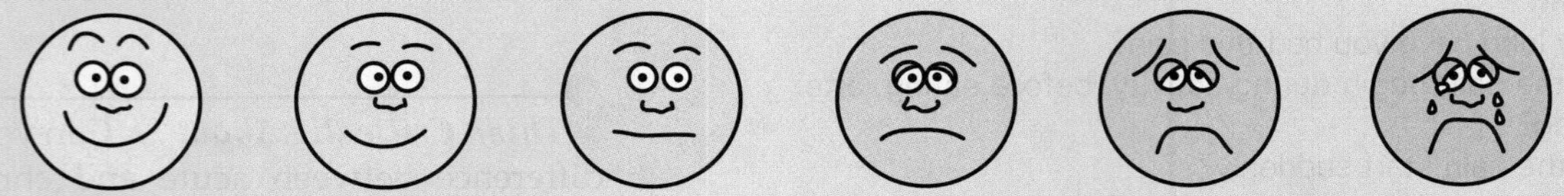

0–5 coding	0	1	2	3	4	5
0-10 coding	0	2	4	6	8	10

Explain to the client that each face is a person who feels happy because he or she has no pain (hurt) or sad because he or she has some or a lot of pain. Face 0 is very happy because there is no hurt. Face 1 hurts just a little bit. Face 2 hurts a little more. Face 3 hurts even more. Face 4 hurts a whole lot. Face 5 hurts as much as you can imagine, although you don't have to be crying to feel this bad. Ask the client to choose the face that best describes how he or she is feeling. Recommended for persons 3 years of age and older.

Translations:

ENGLISH	No hurt	Hurts little bit	Hurts little more	Hurts even more	Hurts whole lot	Hurts worst
SPANISH	No duele	Duele un poco	Duele un poco más	Duele mucho	Duele mucho más	Duele el máximo
FRENCH	Pas mal	Un petit peu mal	Un peu plus mal	Encore plus mal	Très mal	Très très mal
ITALIAN	Non fa male	Fa male un poco	Fa male un po di piu	Fa male ancora di piu	Fa molto male	Fa maggior-mente male
PORTUGUESE	Não doi	Doi um pouco	Doi um pouco mais	Doi muito	Doi muito mais	Doi o máximo
BOSNIAN	Ne boli	Boli samo malo	Boli malo više	Boli još više	Boli puno	Boli najviše
VIETNAMESE	Không dau	Hỏi dau	Dau hỏn chút	Dau nhiêu hỏn	Dau thât nhiêu	Dau qúa dô
CHINESE	無痛	微痛	較痛	更痛	很痛	劇痛
GREEK	Δεν Πονάϊ	Πονάϊ Λιγο	Πονάϊ Λιγο Πιο Πολν	Πονάϊ Πολν	Πονάϊ Πιο Πολν	Πονάϊ Παρα Πολν
ROMANIAN	No doare	Doare puţin	Doare un pic mai mult	Doare şi mai mult	Doare foarte tare	Doare cel mai mult

FIGURE 7–3 Wong Baker FACES Pain Rating Scale.

Planning

The overall goal is relief of pain. If that will be impossible to achieve, then control of pain is the goal. Plan the goals of nursing care by indicating actions that will promote the comfort of the patient during treatment and recovery. Planning should be a team effort, and both pharmacologic and nonpharmacologic interventions should be considered. Physician input comes as written orders and progress notes and may also be available through direct discussion. In pain management, input

Table 7–2 *Common Terms to Help Patient to Describe Pain*

Degree of pain (from least to most severe)	Absent, minimal, mild, moderate, fairly severe, severe, very or extremely severe, exquisite
Quality of pain	Crushing, tingling, itching, throbbing, pulsating, twisting, pulling, burning, searing, stabbing, tearing, biting, blinding, nauseating, debilitating
Frequency of pain	Constant, intermittent, occasional, related to something specific (e.g., only when coughs)

	0	1	2
Face	No particular expression or smile	Occasional grimace or frown, withdrawn, disinterested	Frequent to constant frown, clenched jaw, quivering chin
Legs	Normal position or relaxed	Uneasy, restless, tense	Kicking, or legs drawn up
Activity	Lying quietly, normal position, moves easily	Squirming, shifting back and forth, tense	Arched, rigid, or jerking
Cry	No cry (awake or asleep)	Moans or whimpers, occasional complaint	Cries steadily, screams or sobs, frequent complaints
Consolability	Content, relaxed	Reassured by occasional touching, hugging, or talking to; distractible	Difficult to console or comfort

FIGURE 7–4 FLACC Scale for pain assessment used for cognitively impaired persons.

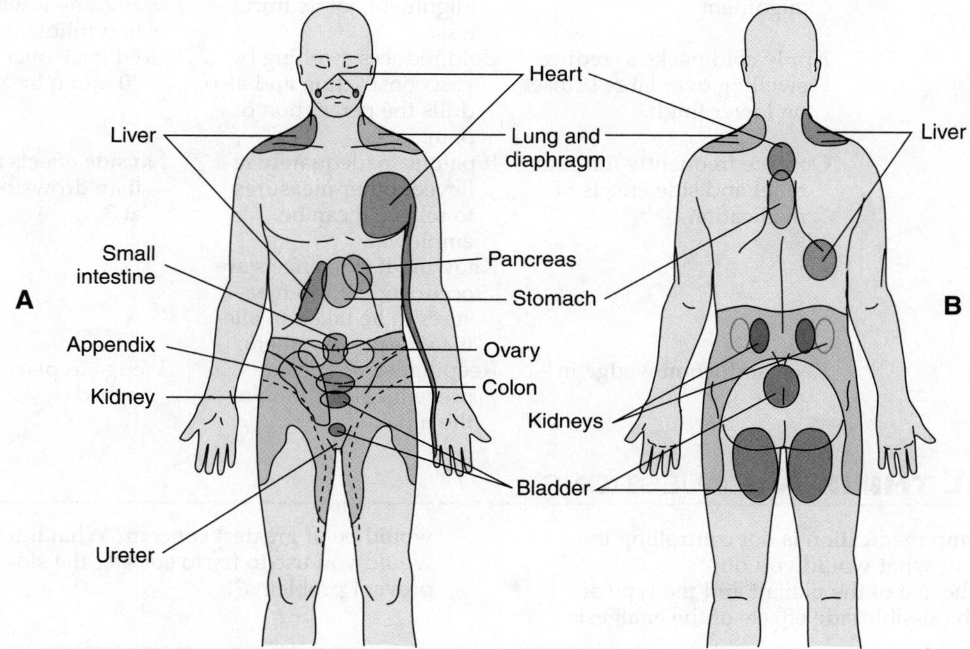

FIGURE 7–5 Usual sites of referred pain. **A**, Front. **B**, Back.

from pharmacists, therapists, and other health care professionals should be included. As recovery progresses, the nursing care plan is updated. The type of medication, method of delivery, and comfort measures will change as the patient's needs change.

Planning must address all areas that affect the patient's pain management needs, including family situation, cultural influences, financial constraints, and whether pain is acute or chronic in nature (Nursing Care Plan 7–1).

Implementation

Actions are always implemented based on the current patient assessment. Therefore, all patients must be reassessed at the beginning of each hospital shift, clinic, or home visit. Appropriate actions would include providing an analgesic as ordered, using nonpharmacologic measures such as repositioning or massage (adjunctive measures), and reporting to the physician when measures are not effective or have unwanted side effects. Implementation also includes monitoring effects of treat-

NURSING CARE PLAN 7–1

Care of the Patient with Pain

SCENARIO Mr. Osbourne, an 82-year-old patient with a history of cerebrovascular accident, has been admitted via the emergency room after a fall and left hip fracture. A total hip replacement was performed this morning. Orders include morphine sulfate via patient-controlled analgesia (PCA), which has just been started. Mr. Osbourne has complained of pain at 8 on a 0–10 scale. His blood pressure and pulse are slightly elevated, but his temperature and respirations are normal. He has been restless and moaning. You implement the following portion of his plan of care.

PROBLEM/NURSING DIAGNOSIS *Pain and muscle aching in left hip and leg*/Pain related to surgical incision and replacement of hip.

Supporting assessment data *Subjective:* Grimaces and moans when moves in bed; moves very cautiously; states muscles feel sore. *Objective:* Incision at left hip; hip replacement on 5/17.

Goals/Expected Outcomes	Nursing Interventions	Selected Rationale	Evaluation
Patient will report pain at 0–3 on a 0–10 scale within 2 hr	Teach to use the PCA pump.	Knowledge of how to use the pump allows the patient to use it correctly.	Using pump correctly, but without good relief.
	Encourage relaxation techniques, provide diversionary activities such as television and electronic games.	Relaxation and diversion are known to lessen pain by focusing the mind elsewhere.	Taught relaxation exercise. Does not wish to watch TV at present. Will have someone bring his GameBoy.
	Encourage use of the PCA before ambulation, exercise, or repositioning.	Medicating before activity reduces pain from the activity.	Medicated before physical therapy visit.
	Position in good body alignment.	When the body is in correct alignment, joints hurt less.	Repositioned in correct alignment with abduction pillow q 2 hr.
	Apply cold packs to reduce swelling over large bruise on lower thigh.	Cold reduces swelling by vasoconstriction and also dulls the perception of pain.	Cold pack over thigh for 20 min q hr × 8 hr.
	Observe frequently for pain relief and side effects of medication.	If pain is inadequately relieved, other measures to relieve it can be employed. Knowing if side effects are occurring allows measures to be taken to alleviate or prevent them.	No side effects noted other than drowsiness. Pain at 3.
	Keep abduction wedge in place.	Keeping leg abducted prevents dislocation of the hip.	Wedge in place when in bed.

? CRITICAL THINKING QUESTIONS

1. If the PCA pump medication is not controlling the pain adequately, what would you do?
2. Considering the age of the patient and the type of surgery, which possible side effects of the analgesia would be of greatest concern? What interventions would you use to try to counter the side effects and prevent problems?

ment and patient and family teaching. You may need to deal with false perceptions about pain (Box 7–1).

Preventing complications from medications is an important aspect of implementation. Specific actions would include:

- Prominent documentation on the chart and medication record of any known drug allergies, and updating of this information should the patient show an adverse reaction to a current medication.
- Accurate recording of pertinent information obtained during the initial assessment phase, such as current medications, previous experience with pain, analgesics, and adjuncts to pain relief.
- Patient and family teaching regarding dose, frequency, and the need to first consult with the physician or nurse before taking any other medications to avoid dangerous interactions.

Box 7–1 ***False Perceptions About Pain***

There are many misconceptions regarding pain, and these can affect the ability of the physician and nurse to effectively assess the patient's pain and provide adequate pain relief.

- **False perception:** If pain is really present, there must be a demonstrable cause.
  - **Fact: Pain can be present even though no cause can be found.** Although damage to the cells does lead to the release of chemicals that stimulate the pain receptors, in many cases pain may be present although no cellular abnormality can be found. The patient with a migraine headache may or may not suffer less than one with a brain tumor. We cannot say that just because the brain tumor can be shown on a brain scan and the headache cannot, the person with the brain tumor has greater pain than the person with the migraine headache.
- **False perception:** The person who has a low tolerance for pain has no self-control and probably is emotionally immature or childish.
  - **Fact: Pain tolerance is a physiologic response to pain that is made more complex by psychosocial factors, many of which can be beyond the control of the patient.** Tolerance for pain is defined as that duration or intensity of pain the person is *willing* to endure without seeking relief. **Pain tolerance varies greatly from one individual to another and in the same individual from time to time.** Nurses often place a high value on a patient's ability to feel pain without complaining or asking for relief. Those who value a high pain tolerance usually impose their own values on their patients by ignoring or belittling their reports of pain. The person who should decide how willing he ought to be to tolerate pain is the one who is suffering.
- **False perception:** The neonate is too neurologically immature to perceive or remember pain, so analgesia is unnecessary in this age group.
  - **Fact: *Neonates do perceive and maintain memory of pain.* They cry and pull away from procedures such as heelstick blood tests. Male infants cry and struggle when they are circumcised. Neonates with medical conditions that require repeated blood tests begin to cry and pull away as soon as someone grasps the foot as if to perform a blood test, indicating a memory of pain from previous heelsticks. Analgesia is appropriate during procedures or situations that would be known to cause pain in more mature clients.**
- **False perception:** Elderly patients have a decreased ability to perceive pain, and pain medicines are dangerous for them because of their age.
  - **Fact: *Ability to express pain may be impaired by decreased cognitive function, but acute pain is still perceived.* Age combined with physical impairments such as decreased kidney or liver function may reduce tolerance for various medications, but with appropriate dosage and monitoring, geriatric patients can have good pain management without severe side effects. Untreated pain will interfere with sleep, nutrition, healing, and general well-being.**
- **False perception:** Reactions to acute pain and chronic pain are the same.
  - **Fact: In general, acute pain is more often associated with anxiety and chronic pain with depression.** The emotional reaction does not cause the pain, but it can intensify it. The management of acute and chronic pain is not the same, as discussed in the chapter text.
- **False perception:** Addiction to pain-relieving drugs is always a hazard, and for the sake of the patient, nurses often must withhold a drug even though the patient asks for it.
  - **Fact: A very small percentage of patients (probably less than 1% and no more than 3%) become addicted to drugs administered for the purpose of relieving acute pain.** In spite of an abundance of evidence to the contrary, this mistaken belief about the dangers of addiction persists, causing needless suffering among patients who are denied adequate pain relief.
- **False perception: Placebos** (substances prescribed that contain no medication, such as sterile saline or sugar pills) are very useful in assessing whether a patient actually has pain.
  - **Fact: There is no basis for believing that a patient who finds relief from pain after receiving a placebo is pretending to have pain or that it is "all in his mind."** The question of how placebos affect people and why they have a positive response in some and not in others still is poorly understood. However, there has been sufficient study of the subject to show that actual pain is sometimes well relieved by placebos.

- Appropriate monitoring of effects of any medications given and prompt notification of the physician should medications fail to relieve pain or problems occur.
- Accurate and complete documentation of any adverse reactions and communication of that information to other health care providers and to the patient and appropriate family members.

Evaluation

Ask the patient about the effectiveness of the pain control measures: How quickly did relief occur, how long did it last, to what degree was the pain controlled, and were there any unpleasant side effects? Whenever possible, use patient verbalization as the primary evaluation tool. Using a pain assessment tool and comparing the patient's response to that before the pain relief was given is an effective evaluation technique.

If the patient is unable to verbalize, then evaluate the signs that can be directly observed. For instance, an aphasic stroke patient might thrash, moan, and look fearful when in pain, and evaluation of effective analgesia might include, "Mr. Jones now lying quietly, is free of facial tension, and is watching the activity around him. Did not moan when repositioned one hour after analgesic given."

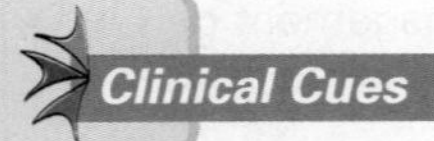

Evaluation of the effectiveness of the pain control medication used should be based on the route of administration. Medications given by mouth may take 60 minutes to be effective. Injections are effective in 30 to 45 minutes. Intravenous medications are effective in 15 minutes.

Documentation

All measures to control pain must be accurately documented:

- Initial pain assessment: Document the location, intensity, duration, and method used to assess (e.g., pain scale, patient verbalization); aggravating factors; alleviating factors
- Measures taken (e.g., analgesic medication, adjunctive measures)
- Evaluation of effectiveness of measures
- Physician notification of problems or concerns and physician response, if applicable
- Related patient or family education (Patient Teaching 7–1)

Example. Mr. Smith states that his pain level following physical therapy is 7 on a 0-to-10 scale. Morphine sulfate 10 mg intramuscularly (IM) in the right deltoid is given. Forty-five minutes after injection, Mr. Smith states that his pain level is now 2 to 3. Pulse 72, respirations 16, moving freely in bed. Discussed pain relief needs; suggested that he request pain medication before next therapy session. Mr. Smith agreed.

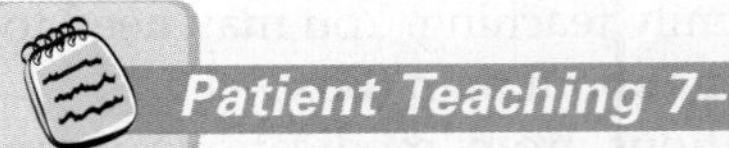

Managing Pain

Take medication before pain is severe; take it regularly until pain is well controlled before lengthening time between doses.

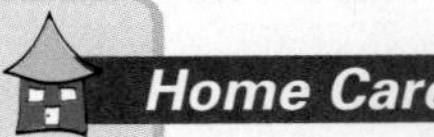

Home Care Considerations 7–1

Maintain Medication Record

Jot down the time pain medication is taken at home. It is easy to forget just when a medication has been taken. Writing down the time it was taken helps prevent overdosage and toxicity.

? ***Think Critically About . . .*** What do you think is the most difficult aspect of evaluating someone's pain?

PAIN MANAGEMENT

Effective pain management is not just a matter of giving the right medicine at the right time. It is a combination of pharmacologic and nonpharmacologic approaches that together give the individual the greatest possible degree of comfort for the longest possible time (Home Care Considerations 7–1). The World Health Organization has made recommendations for a step approach to pharmacologic pain control (Figure 7–6).

PHARMACOLOGIC APPROACHES

Analgesics and Routes of Administration

Oral Analgesics. An oral analgesic is any substance taken by mouth for the control of pain. These include over-the-counter (OTC) medications such as acetaminophen (Tylenol), aspirin (Bayer), and ibuprofen (Motrin), and prescription medications such as codeine and morphine (Safety Alert 7–1). Oral analgesics are available in extended-release forms that can provide 12 to 24 hours of pain relief.

Intramuscular Analgesics. Intramuscular (IM) analgesics are substances that are injected into the muscular tissue to control pain.

Intravenous Analgesics. Intravenous (IV) analgesics are substances injected or infused over a prescribed time directly into the vascular system.

Subcutaneous Analgesics. Subcutaneous analgesics are medications that are injected or infused into the

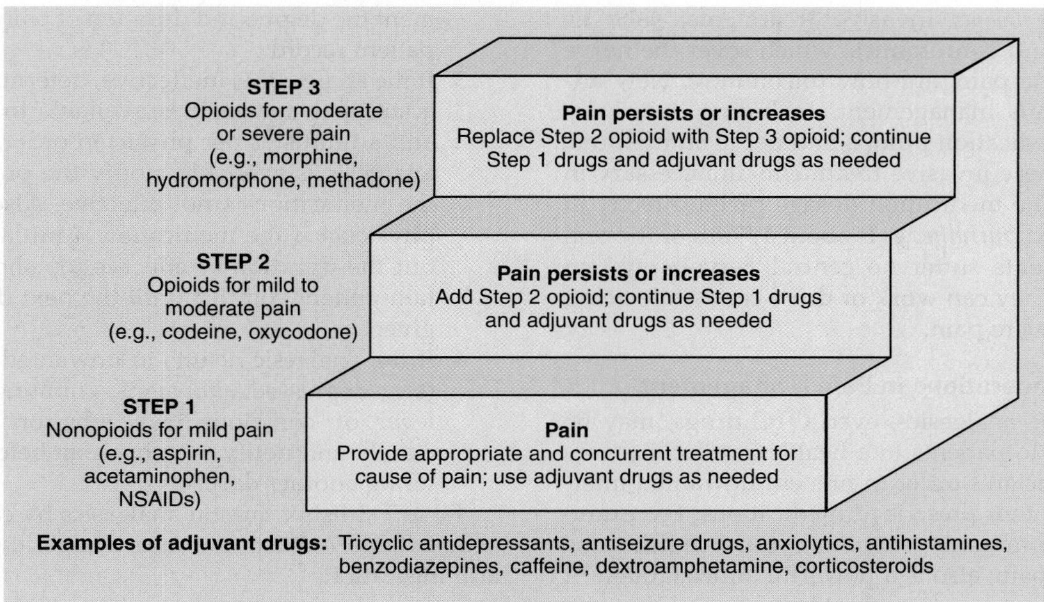

FIGURE 7–6 The analgesic ladder proposed by the World Health Organization.

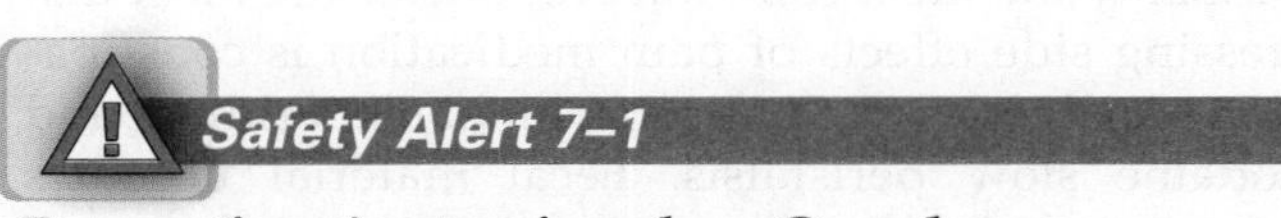

Preventing Acetaminophen Overdose

Check all other medications and over-the-counter (OTC) drugs the patient is receiving when administering doses of acetaminophen. Many OTC drugs consist of a combination containing this drug. Toxicity may occur if more than the total recommended safe dosage is ingested.

subcutaneous (fatty tissue just beneath the skin) tissue to control pain.

Topical Analgesics. Topical analgesics are medications placed in a specific area on the skin that are absorbed via the vascular system. Topical anesthetics are used to treat pain from minor procedures such as venipunctures.

Transdermal Patches. Transdermal patches placed on the skin rely on vascular uptake of pain medication. These patches can provide relief from systemic pain and are commonly used with patients who have chronic pain. Transdermal patches containing lidocaine may be used for local pain.

Buccal Swabs. Buccal swabs contain medication that is absorbed through the **buccal mucosa** (mucous membrane lining the inside of the mouth) and provides rapid relief from pain. Buccal swabs are commonly used with hospice patients.

Patient-Controlled Analgesia. Patient-controlled analgesia (PCA) is an infusion device controlled by the patient that injects the prescribed dose of analgesia. The PCA machine is programmed so that the patient can decide when a dose is given, but cannot exceed the maximum dose or minimum time interval ordered by the physician. PCA analgesia is usually given IV, but may also be administered Subcut. Make certain that free-flow protection is in use on the PCA pump so that overdosage is not possible.

Epidural Analgesic. An epidural analgesic is medication infused directly into the **epidural** space near the base of the spine using a programmable pump. An anesthesiologist inserts the infusion catheter. Patients receiving epidural analgesia need to be monitored for possible delayed respiratory suppression or apnea, bradycardia, hypotension, urinary retention, nausea and vomiting, and allergic reactions such as itching or hives. Report adverse symptoms to the anesthesiologist immediately. The insertion site should be monitored for signs of infection, localized allergic reaction, and leaking.

Peripheral Nerve Catheter. A peripheral nerve catheter is used to deliver local anesthetic to the sheath of a nerve. These catheters are typically used for patients who have had total joint replacement.

Nonanalgesic Medications Used for Pain Control

Antidepressants. A number of antidepressant medications have been found effective in controlling some specific types of pain, such as nerve root pain. They may be given alone or in combination with other analgesic medications.

Chemotherapeutic Agents and Other Immunosuppressants. Occasionally drugs such as methotrexate (Rheumatrex) are used for **intractable pain** in rheumatoid conditions.

Anticonvulsants. Newer anticonvulsants, such as gabapentin (Neurontin), have been approved for treatment of neuropathic pain.

Invasive Treatments. Invasive treatments, such as rhizotomies and cordotomies, which sever the nerve conducting the pain, are now uncommon. New advances in pain management, including surgically implanted medication pumps and nerve stimulators, have made these invasive treatments unnecessary in most cases. The medication dosage given directly to the spinal cord *(intrathecal)* is about 1/70th of the oral dose, so patients suffer no central nervous system side effects. They can work or drive cars while being relieved of severe pain.

Special Considerations in Pain Management

Pharmacologic analgesics, even OTC drugs, may be administered to patients in a health care facility only under a physician's order to prevent unwanted interactions with other prescribed medications. For example, aspirin, commonly taken for occasional headache and arthritis pain, also is a powerful anticoagulant. It can lead to dangerous complications for someone who has a bleeding disorder or who is also on an anticoagulant medication. Acetaminophen in high doses is toxic to the liver, and may therefore be contraindicated in patients with a liver disorder. Alerting patients that OTC drugs can have serious interactions with their prescribed drugs is an important part of patient education in home care and ambulatory care.

Elderly patients also suffer pain. The idea that pain perception diminishes with age is false. In fact, perception of pain may actually increase with age, as the individual becomes frail and has fewer resources for tolerating pain.

The very elderly frequently have reduced tolerance for medications. Smaller doses of analgesics may give effective relief without causing overwhelming sedation or disorientation. Elderly patients on analgesics must be monitored carefully.

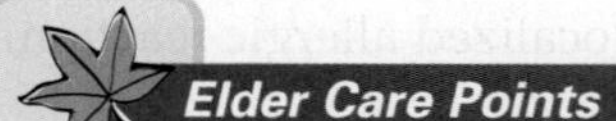

Elder Care Points

The route of administration matters in the elderly. Intramuscular injections are not recommended for the elderly because diminished muscle and fatty tissue may affect the bioavailability of drugs.

Nurses' Responsibilities

In addition to following the "five rights" (right patient, right drug, right dose, right route, right time), the nurse has a variety of responsibilities when giving analgesic medications:

1. Document drug, dose, route (including location of injection site for IM or Subcut injections), and reason for giving.
2. Monitor the effectiveness of pain relief after 15 to 30 minutes and at 1- to 2-hour intervals. Document the degree and duration of pain relief in the patient record.
3. If the analgesic is ineffective, determine whether a stronger analgesic is available to the patient and administer per physician order. If no other analgesic is available, notify the physician that the medication is not effective. Also notify the physician if the medication is initially effective but the duration of effect is too short to maintain patient comfort until the next dose may be given.
4. If the analgesic results in unwanted side effects (e.g., depressed vital signs, vomiting, or altered level of consciousness), monitor the patient closely and notify the physician before administering another dose.

Table 7–3 lists common analgesics by category and action. Table 7–4 lists common analgesics by route of administration.

SIDE EFFECTS AND COMPLICATIONS OF PAIN MEDICATION

Probably the most common and one of the most distressing side effects of pain medication is constipation. Analgesics such as morphine, meperidine, and codeine slow peristalsis. Fecal material becomes compacted and dry because of the extended time of passage through the intestines. Patients receiving these medications for any length of time should be monitored carefully for regular, normal bowel movements. **Oral fluids must be increased if possible.** Stool softeners and fiber-based laxatives, such as psyllium (Metamucil), can be helpful if approved by the physician.

Some side effects, such as drowsiness and euphoria, generally only last for the first few days and then spontaneously disappear. However, the nurse must always be alert to the possibility of a more serious adverse reaction. Allergic reactions, such as itching and hives, need to be reported immediately. The medication needs to be discontinued and an alternative order obtained. The patient may also need an antihistamine such as diphenhydramine (Benadryl) for relief of symptoms. Narcotic analgesics can depress the respiratory system to the point of apnea (no respiration). Should this occur, resuscitation must begin immediately. In the hospital setting this means providing respiratory support and calling the code team. In settings such as the home, physician's office, or clinic, it means respiratory support and calling 911. The standard treatment for respiratory suppression from narcotics is naloxone (Narcan), an effective narcotic antagonist that can be given IM or IV.

The most feared side effect, that of addiction to narcotics, in reality almost never occurs. **Patients in pain have a right to expect that effective analgesia will be available to them.**

Table 7–3 Analgesic Medications by Type, Primary Action, and Nursing Implications

TYPE OF DRUG AND PRIMARY ACTION	EXAMPLES	NURSING IMPLICATIONS
Non-narcotic analgesics, including nonsteroidal anti-inflammatory drugs (NSAIDs) *Action:* Block pain at the peripheral nervous system level.	Over-the-counter aspirin, acetaminophen, ibuprofen,* ketoprofen,* naproxen.* Prescription naproxen, indomethacin, ibuprofen, ketoprofen.	May be present in combination drugs. Various possible side effects of which to be aware.† Educate patients not to use in combination with over-the-counter dosage of same medication.
Narcotics (opioids) *Action:* Block pain at the central nervous system level.	Morphine, meperidine, hydromorphone, codeine, fentanyl.	Constipation common, can be severe. Can cause respiratory depression; antidote is naloxone (Narcan).
Medications with nonanalgesic primary actions used as adjuncts to pain control. *Action:* Various mechanisms of action.	Antidepressants: Amitriptyline, imipramine, trazodone hydrochloride. Anticonvulsants: Phenytoin, carbamazepine, gabapentin, pregabalin. Stimulants: Caffeine, dextroamphetamine. Muscle relaxants: Carisoprodol, baclofen. Chemotherapeutic agents: Methotrexate.	Varied due to varied mechanisms of action. Always be aware of side effects and possible adverse reactions.

*Nonprescription dose.

†*Note:* Combination drugs are often used. These may combine two forms of analgesic (e.g., acetaminophen and codeine) or an analgesic with another type of medication, such as an antihistamine. It is important to be aware of what is in combination drugs to prevent administration of excessive amounts of one of the components.

Table 7–4 Common Analgesic Medications by Route*

ORAL	INJECTABLE
Acetaminophen	Baclofen
Acetaminophen with codeine	Buprenorphine
Aspirin	Butorphanol
Baclofen	Fentanyl
Carisoprodol	Hydromorphone
Gabapentin	Meperidine
Hydrocodone	Morphine sulfate
Hydromorphone	Nalbuphine
Propoxyphene	
Ibuprofen	
Ketoprofen	
Morphine sulfate, time-released	
Naproxen	
Oxycodone	

*The number of medications available for the control of pain is large and varied. This table gives only some of the more common generic analgesics, including adjunctive medications, currently used.

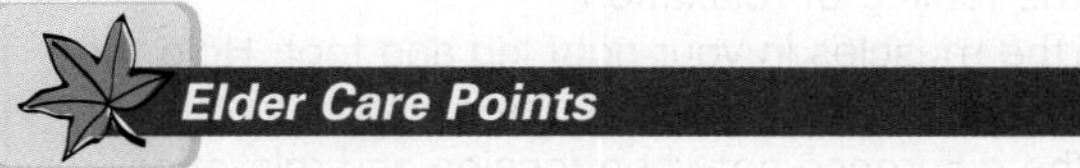

Some drugs are considered especially risky for elderly patients. Propoxyphene (contained in Darvon and Darvocet) can be toxic to elderly patients. Tramadol (Ultram) and meperidine (Demerol) lower the seizure threshold and should be used cautiously in the elderly.

NONPHARMACOLOGIC APPROACHES

A variety of methods exist for relieving pain without medication or as an adjunct to medication. It is probable that the first treatment for pain was the automatic vigorous rubbing of the painful area, as when we rub our head or elbow if we bump it. Using adjuncts can increase the effectiveness of pain medication and may decrease the frequency at which it is needed.

Sleep

Adequate sleep and rest are major factors in healing. Rest increases pain tolerance and improves response to analgesia. Allow adequate time between treatments and other care for naps, and plan night care so interruptions in sleep are kept to a minimum. For instance, take vital signs when the patient is awake to use the bathroom or requests pain medication. It is important to remember that exhaustion will cause a patient to sleep despite severe pain, but such sleep is not as therapeutic. Appropriate analgesia combined with adequate rest promotes healing.

Warmth

Gentle heat is very soothing for many types of pain. Gentle heat promotes vasodilation of the area, which promotes increased blood supply and movement of nutrients to the affected area. Sources include warm compresses, warm blankets, water-filled heating devices, Hydrocollator pads, whirlpools, tub baths, heat lamps, and chemical self-heating packs. Compresses and packs are usually left in place for 15 to 20 minutes, although gentle heat sources such as water-filled heating devices may be used over longer periods. Always check the temperature before applying, and monitor the patient closely for tolerance. To prevent injury to the skin, never apply a warm compress directly to the surface of the skin. The very young and the very old are particularly sensitive to heat. Anyone with an altered level of consciousness or loss of normal sensation may not realize something is too hot, and those with loss of movement may not be able to move away from the heat source when necessary.

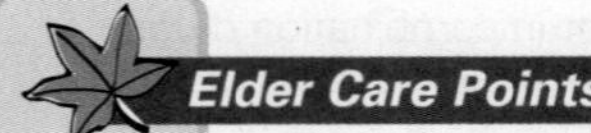

Elder Care Points

The skin of the elderly is thin and burns more easily. Stroke patients frequently have areas of lost or diminished sensation. Patients with senile dementia may not recognize that something is too hot. Even the alert and oriented elderly person frequently falls asleep and may be burned without being aware of it. Monitor any heat application very carefully. Do not apply heat to any areas where nerve damage or decreased sensation has occurred.

Distraction

Any activity that takes a person's attention away from pain is termed a *distraction*. This includes watching TV, talking with friends, or playing a board game. People have an innate ability to distract themselves from their surroundings or situation. Health care workers may mistakenly interpret the patient's ability to do this as proof that there is no pain. Distracting activities can take the patient's mind off the pain momentarily, but they do not stop it. Distraction can be helpful in bridging the time gap between giving an analgesic and the onset of pain relief.

Relaxation

Relaxation also is called "tension release" and involves the conscious relaxation of muscle groups. It is frequently done as a progression, beginning at the feet and moving up the body, ending with the neck and facial muscles. Initially, the nurse can guide the patient verbally, slowly directing the attention to the next muscle group to be relaxed. After one or two sessions, many patients can effectively provide their own relaxation sequence (Box 7–2).

Imagery and Meditation

These methods use mental techniques to induce relaxation. Guided imagery involves assisting the patient to form mental images of a pleasant environment where they are comfortable and happy. For some, the experience is visual; in their minds they "see" a beautiful place. For others, it is a process of achieving a feeling of comfort and peace. Either is highly effective in giving the patient a brief mental "vacation" from pain. These methods often are used during painful procedures, such as bone marrow extraction.

Meditation involves the use of a focus point, which may be a sound or a repeated phrase (sometimes called a *mantra*), or the sound of the breath as it moves in and out of the body, or a visual image. The visual

Box 7–2 Relaxation Exercise

This exercise is performed by recording the script onto audiotape or CD and following the instructions as the tape is played. Using the exercise regularly over a period of weeks makes it easier to call on these techniques to induce relaxation during an examination or at other times you feel particularly tense.

Slowly read the script in a soft, firm voice. Allow sufficient pauses between segments for the instructions to be followed. Sit in a chair or lie down to do the exercise. Decrease outside noise and distractions as much as possible.

SCRIPT

- Close your eyes and find something to focus on mentally. It might be a spot of light, your pulse, a visual image, or whatever you choose. Try to hold it constant.
- Breathe in slowly and deeply; hold it a moment, and slowly breathe out. Now breathe normally, slowly, in and out.
- Tighten your face and neck muscles as firmly as you can, while clenching your teeth. Feel the tension. Hold it; slowly relax the muscles. Feel the relaxation in your face, jaw, and neck.
- With less tension, tighten the muscles in the face, jaw, and neck again. Feel this level of tension. Let go and relax. Notice the feeling of relaxation.
- Tighten your chest muscles firmly. Hold it; feel the tension. Let the chest muscles relax. Notice the difference between the tension and relaxation.
- Tighten the chest muscles again with less tension. Now let the muscles relax. Feel the relaxation.
- Tighten the fists and arm muscles as hard as possible. Hold the tension a moment. Slowly relax the muscles. Notice the difference in feeling between tension and relaxation
- Tighten the fists and arm muscles again with less tension. Hold it. Let the muscles relax. Feel the relaxation.
- Tighten the abdominal muscles firmly. Hold the tension, noting the feeling. Relax the muscles, noting the difference between tension and relaxation.
- Tighten the abdominal muscles again with less tension. Hold it. Allow the muscles to relax completely. Notice the feeling of relaxation.
- Tighten the muscles in your right leg and foot. Hold the tension. Note the feeling. Allow the muscles to relax. Notice the difference between tension and relaxation.
- Tighten the muscles in your right leg and foot again with less tension. Hold it. Completely let go of the tension in the muscles and relax. Feel the relaxation.
- Tighten the muscles in your left leg and foot firmly. Hold it. Note the tension. Allow the muscles to relax. Focus on the difference between tension and relaxation.
- Tighten the muscles in your left leg and foot again with less tension. Hold it. Completely let go of the tension in the muscles and relax. Notice the feeling of relaxation.
- Breathe in and out deeply and slowly five times, focusing on your breathing.
- When you are ready, open your eyes.

image may be a picture or object that the patient gazes at, or it may be an imagined image.

Hypnosis

Hypnosis, or therapeutic suggestion, should be done by someone trained in the technique. It involves the use of focusing and relaxation to induce a trance-like state during which a patient receives suggestions that may be helpful after returning to a normal level of consciousness. Although people under hypnosis cannot be induced to do things they would ordinarily feel were wrong, this remains a common fear. Reassurance may help the patient to be more accepting, but hypnosis should be used only if the subject is comfortable with the idea and open to its use.

Biofeedback

This specialized technique requires the use of a machine that measures the degree of muscular tension with skin electrodes. The machine has colored lights that change (usually red to yellow to green) and a tone that changes in pitch from higher to lower as the patient relaxes. The patient receives visual and auditory confirmation of self-induced relaxation. This technique is particularly effective with people who are highly competitive because it rewards success and allows them to "win" the game.

Music

Music used alone can be highly effective in bringing about relaxation. It also can be used as a focal point for meditation or to enhance other distracting activities. Nature sounds also can be used to induce relaxation, including audiotapes of the ocean, running streams, breezes, rain, and birds singing. Headphones allow the patient to be immersed in sound without disturbing others. Headphones with music can be used during loud or long diagnostic procedures such as magnetic resonance imaging.

Cold

Cold is particularly helpful in reducing swelling. Cold applied to an area reduces swelling by vasoconstriction. It also can be effective in relieving muscle spasms and some types of joint pain. Ice massage of sore muscles can be done by freezing water in a paper cup, then tearing away the edge of the cup to expose the ice, leaving the base of the cup as a handle. Some individuals, however, are very sensitive to cold. If cold applications cause shivering, tensing of the muscles, or an increase in pain or spasm, discontinue their use.

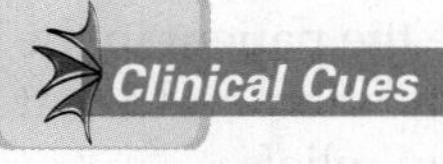

Clinical Cues

The effectiveness of cold is maximized in 15 to 20 minutes; therefore, remove the source after that time.

Binders

Binders are helpful for strains, sprains, and wounds or surgical incisions that are packed. They support the tissues during movement, such as ambulation or coughing, which reduces the pain.

Massage (Cutaneous Stimulation)

Once a mainstay of nursing comfort measures, massage is enjoying a return to popularity. It uses long firm strokes, short soft circular strokes, and occasionally gentle pounding with the sides of the hands. It stimulates the circulation, relaxes the muscles, and increases the general sense of well-being. When the painful area has inflammation, or consists of a wound or an incision, massaging another area of the body with gentle but firm pressure helps the patient direct attention away from the pain. Always be guided by the patient's sense of comfort. Use only the degree of pressure that is pleasant and relaxing.

Simple massage can be done by a family member with just a little instruction, giving them an opportunity to assist in the care in a positive and loving way. Massage should not be used on any area that has been reddened by pressure. This tissue is already compromised and massage can cause further damage through "shearing," the traumatic pulling of tissue layers away from one another.

Acupuncture/Acupressure

Acupuncture originated centuries ago in China and involves the use of tiny needles inserted into the skin at specific points along lines called *meridians,* a concept similar to that of nerve pathways. In recent years it has gained favor in the United States as a pain control measure. Acupressure involves the use of external finger pressure at the meridian points to achieve similar effects. Both acupuncture and acupressure require extensive training for proper use and should only be done by someone fully trained in these procedures (Complementary & Alternative Therapies 7–1).

Transcutaneous Electrical Nerve Stimulation

Transcutaneous electrical nerve stimulation (TENS) utilizes a small electrical stimulator attached to the skin with electrodes placed around the area of pain. A

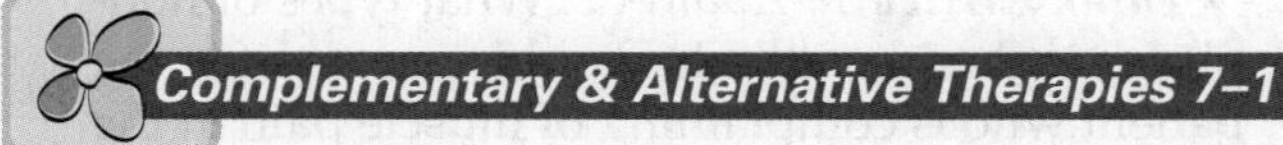

Complementary & Alternative Therapies 7–1

Pain Relief

Complementary and alternative therapies are used more for pain relief than for anything else. Therapies used include relaxation, meditation, biofeedback, yoga, hypnosis, imagery, chiropractic, acupuncture, acupressure, massage, aromatherapy, and herbal preparations and supplements. Research from the National Institutes of Health has proven that acupuncture is effective for many patients for various pain problems.

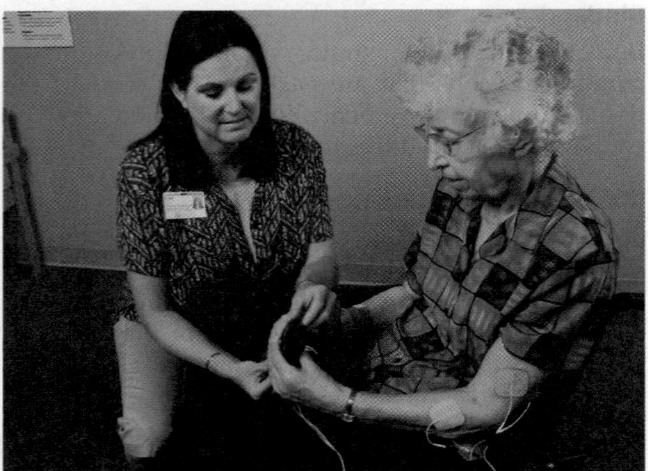

FIGURE 7–7 Instructing the patient on how to use a TENS unit.

low current running between them acts to block pain sensation. The degree of stimulation can be controlled by the patient using dials on the stimulator. The application of TENS requires specific training and must be ordered by a physician (Figure 7–7). Occasionally a patient will find TENS unpleasant rather than helpful. In such cases, the physician should be notified and an alternative method of pain control selected.

Spinal Cord Stimulator

The spinal cord stimulator is implanted in the epidural space adjacent to nerves that innervate the affected body area. This device is used for patients with chronic pain who have not responded to medications.

Menthol

When applied to the skin, menthol causes warming and this may have an analgesic effect. Mentholated products are usually massaged into the skin, giving the individual the benefit of both massage and warmth. They are available over the counter, but require a physician's order in a hospital or clinic setting. Do not use with external heating devices, to avoid overheating the skin surface. Caution the patient to wash his hands well after applying and to avoid contact of the menthol with the eyes or mucous membranes.

? • *Think Critically About . . .* What types of nonpharmacologic methods would you use for the patient who is complaining of muscle pain in the shoulder after an auto accident?

ACUTE VERSUS CHRONIC PAIN

Patients with acute pain are frequently anxious and fearful. This fear and anxiety can take many forms. They may fear something is seriously wrong, that they will not get relief from the pain, or that, if they do, they will become addicted to the pain medication. The anxiety and fear of these patients frequently are alleviated by first providing adequate analgesia to relieve the pain and then educating them about their pain and the methods that can be used to control pain safely. Being made part of the pain management team reassures patients that health care professionals believe them and want to make them comfortable so they can focus on getting well and back to normal activity. Nurses should rely upon the patient's report of pain and intervene to promote comfort. Some nurses hesitate to administer pain medication to patients with a history of drug abuse. Such patients may experience acute pain, for example, following surgery. The postoperative period is not the time to withhold pain medication from any patient. Concept Map 7–1 shows the various types and causes of pain.

Chronic pain, on the other hand, is most commonly associated with depression. People who hurt most or all of the time frequently resign themselves to the idea that they can never again live a normal life. New research and the work of several outstanding pain centers and nurse and physician specialists now offer much to sufferers of chronic pain. Many people whose lives were previously dictated by their pain now experience good control and have returned to normal, productive lives. Table 7–5 compares the two types of pain.

COMMUNITY CARE

Community care can take place in a variety of settings, with varying levels of training among direct caregivers. Nurses working in a hospital setting may be called upon to teach pain management techniques to those who provide care in the community setting. Nurses working in areas that serve the community directly need a clear understanding of pain care management to assist their patients best.

EXTENDED CARE

Extended-care facilities may provide rehabilitative services, long-term care services, or both. Each type of care may include specific pain management needs.

Patients undergoing rehabilitation often have acute pain related to therapy, particularly in the early phases. It is important that therapy be scheduled to allow for adequate rest and recovery time. It also is important that analgesic medication be given on a schedule that provides the patient with the greatest freedom from pain during therapy sessions. This assists the patient to cooperate with therapy, which in turn encourages a more rapid recovery. Always include the patient in the planning. He knows best what medication and what time schedule are giving the best pain relief.

Long-term care facilities, also called nursing homes, skilled nursing facilities, transitional care

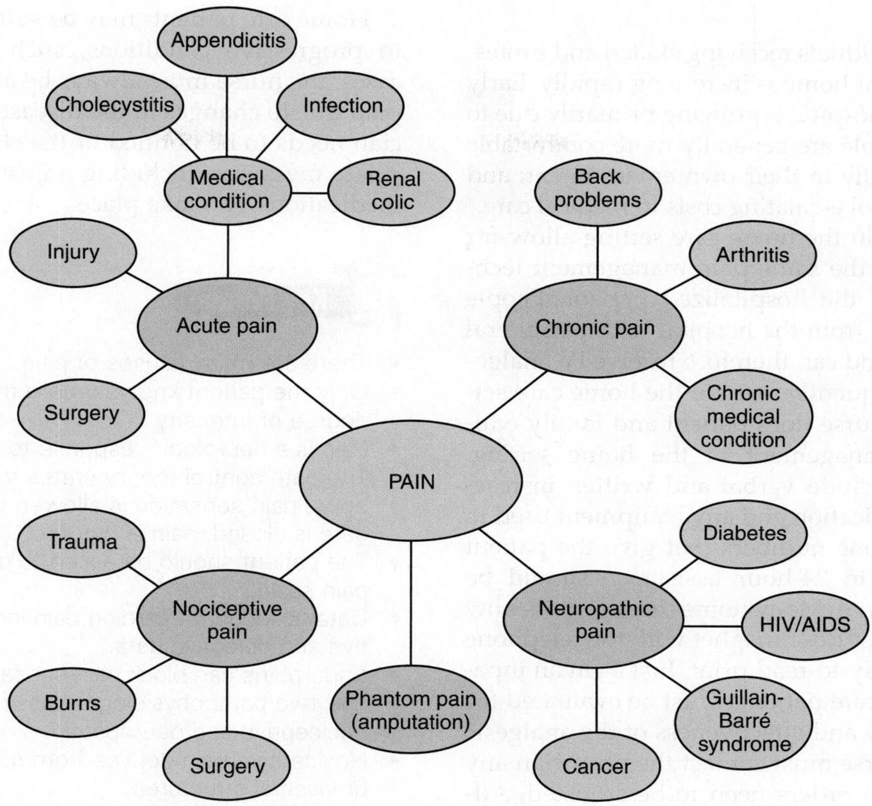

CONCEPT MAP 7–1 The various types and causes of pain.

Table 7–5 *Acute Versus Chronic Pain*

	ACUTE	CHRONIC
Duration	Hours to days.	Months to years.
Prognosis for relief	Good; may resolve spontaneously or in response to analgesic therapy.	Poor unless complicating factors removed; spontaneous relief unusual.
Cause	Relatively easy to identify.	Sometimes cause is known, but diagnosis may be complex or undetermined.
Psychosocial effects	Usually transient or none. May temporarily disrupt normal activities or routine.	Can affect ability to earn a living, enjoy social activities, maintain self-esteem.
Effect of therapy	Medication usually beneficial, surgery often helpful.	Medications may be helpful, but patient may become dependent. Multiple medication regimen may be used. Surgery may help, but also may worsen the problem.

units, and board and care homes, often have patients who live there for the last weeks, months, or even years of their lives. In this setting, the term *resident* is used, rather than patient. They may have pain following a fall, after dental work, or during a period of illness; and they may have chronic pain from such conditions as arthritis, degenerative disorders, or cancer. Residents in these settings may be mentally alert and oriented, or be alert and confused, or have a decreased level of consciousness. However, each of these individuals can perceive pain and should be given appropriate analgesics when pain exists. The nurse can be of great assistance to the physician in ordering analgesia by providing accurate information about the type of pain, the frequency, the intensity, and precipitating factors. For instance, a resident with degenerative arthritis may have chronic joint pain and benefit from a routine oral analgesic such as acetaminophen (Tylenol) or ibuprofen (Motrin). Those with more severe chronic problems, such as cancer, may benefit from routine time-released medications such as MS Contin (oral morphine sulfate in a time-released tablet). As pain increases, more narcotic may be needed to gain relief, but also remember that the very elderly or debilitated may be more drug sensitive. Monitor all medications carefully and work with the physician to ensure that the resident's pain is being appropriately addressed. Ideally, the resident is comfortable as well as alert and able to participate in activities of choice.

HOME CARE

The number of individuals receiving skilled and professional nursing care at home is increasing rapidly. Early discharge from the hospital is growing primarily due to (1) the fact that people are generally more comfortable and heal more rapidly in their own environment; and (2) the need to control escalating costs in medical care.

Licensed nurses in the home care setting allow for the use of many of the same pain management techniques available to the hospitalized patient. People frequently go home from the hospital with peripheral or central IV lines and can therefore receive IV analgesia. PCA is now frequently used in the home care setting. The licensed nurse does patient and family education on pain management in the home setting. Teaching should include verbal and written instructions about the medication and any equipment used to dispense it. Telephone numbers that give the patient and family access to 24-hour assistance should be prominently displayed. Many home care agencies now provide a refrigerator door magnet with the telephone number in large, easy-to-read print. Just as in an inpatient setting, home care patients must be evaluated for the continued safety and effectiveness of the analgesic medication. The nurse must contact the physician any time the medication orders need to be adjusted. Adjuncts to pain management, such as simple massage, relaxation techniques, and the use of pillows, warmth, repositioning, or soft music, are readily taught to patients and families for use in the home care setting.

PCA medications are on occasion given by Subcut rather than IV infusion, particularly for those patients with poor peripheral venous access who are not candidates for a central line. A tiny needle is placed in the subcutaneous tissue on the abdomen and taped in place. Sites are changed at regular intervals to maintain good absorption of the medication and avoid damage to the tissues. However, the increased use of central IV catheters and ports and the availability of oral timed-release analgesics are making Subcut PCA devices much less common.

Current guidelines for home care by agencies such as Medicare require that case management be done by a licensed professional. This is usually an RN, although the registered physical therapist may fill this role for patients whose only acute need is continued restorative therapy. The role of the LPN/LVN is that of direct patient care under the guidance of the case manager. In many states, LPNs/LVNs may insert peripheral IV lines and infuse standard IV solutions without any additives, but cannot begin an infusion of medications, blood products, or solutions with additives. The LPN/LVN may monitor an ongoing infusion and discontinue the infusion as needed, but must report any difficulties immediately to the RN case manager for intervention. Some states offer IV therapy certification for LPNs/LVNs that allows them to infuse medications.

Home care patients may be suffering from pain due to progressive conditions, such as cancer. In such cases, the nurse must always be alert to an increase in pain due to changes in the disease process. The physician needs to be notified of the change so that appropriate measures, including adjusting or changing the medications, can take place.

- There are many causes of pain.
- Only the patient knows where the pain is and its degree of intensity.
- Pain is a neurologic response to unpleasant stimuli.
- The gate control theory states that when the gate is open, pain sensation is allowed through; when the gate is closed, pain is blocked.
- The patient should be asked to use an appropriate pain scale.
- Data collection regarding pain includes both subjective and objective data.
- Endorphins can block pain sensation.
- The two pathophysiologic classifications of pain are nociceptive and neuropathic.
- Nociceptive pain derives from stimulation of somatic or visceral structures.
- There are four phases of nociceptive pain: transduction, transmission, perception, and modulation.
- Neuropathic pain is from dysfunction of the nervous system.
- Neuropathic pain is relieved with NSAIDs, tricyclic antidepressants, anticonvulsants, and corticosteroids.
- Pain tolerance varies from one individual to another.
- Pain threshold is the point at which pain is perceived.
- Cultural factors and beliefs affect the perception of pain by each person.
- Pain assessment/data collection includes the areas of appearance, behavior, activity level, verbalization, and physiologic clues.
- An interpreter may be required to gather correct data about a non–English-speaking patient's pain.
- Goals of care are (1) relief of pain, and (2) control of pain.
- Pharmacologic and nonpharmacologic methods are used to treat pain.
- False perceptions about pain may affect care (see Box 7–1).
- Accurate documentation of pain assessments and interventions is essential.
- If pain is not being relieved by the current plan of care, the plan must be changed.
- Evaluation of the effectiveness of measures used to relieve pain is a primary nursing responsibility.
- Pain management is complex and utilizes many methods.
- Always follow the "five rights" when administering pain medication.
- It is important to know all about the commonly used analgesics (see Table 7–4).
- Constipation is a common side effect of narcotic analgesia, and preventive measures should be used.

- Adequate sleep assists in controlling pain.
- Hypnosis and biofeedback have been proven to be effective for many people for a variety of types of pain.
- Become familiar with the various nonpharmacologic methods of treating pain.
- Chronic pain is common among the elderly in long-term care facilities.
- Home care patients need good patient teaching and follow-up.

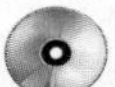
Go to your **Companion CD-ROM** for an Audio Glossary, animations, video clips, and bonus review questions.

evolve Be sure to visit the companion Evolve site at http://evolve.elsevier.com/deWit for interactive NCLEX-PN Exam Style Review Questions, WebLinks, and additional online resources.

NCLEX-PN EXAM STYLE REVIEW QUESTIONS

Choose the best answer(s) for the following questions.

1. An appropriate expected outcome for a patient with acute pain related to recent surgical procedure would be:
   1. the patient will demonstrate use of patient-controlled analgesia pump.
   2. the nurse will administer adequate amounts of pain medications.
   3. the family will be able to identify the patient's need for pain medications.
   4. the physical therapist will be able to encourage early ambulation.

2. In determining the patient's perception of pain, which of the following questions would be useful in assessing pain? *(Select all that apply.)*
   1. "Where are you hurting?"
   2. "What pain control measures have worked in the past?"
   3. "How would you describe your pain?"
   4. "What were you doing before the onset of the pain?"
   5. "Did another person witness your pain?"

3. The nurse caring for an elderly female patient who appears to be withdrawn and quiet. She grimaces whenever she is touched. An appropriate nursing action would be to:
   1. administer pain medications.
   2. assess for underlying causes of the patient's behavior.
   3. encourage coughing and deep breathing.
   4. notify the physician.

4. A 25-year-old patient complains of moderate pain at his incision site. The nurse administers morphine sulfate intramuscularly. The next appropriate nursing action would be to:
   1. evaluate the effectiveness of the pain medication.
   2. provide opportunities for adequate nutrition.
   3. teach importance of increasing tolerance to pain.
   4. reinforce the addictive nature of the pain medication.

5. A patient with continuous epidural analgesia asks, "Why do I feel cold and wet at the small of my back?" An appropriate response would be:
   1. "Let me take a look at your epidural site dressing."
   2. "You have a small catheter at the small of your back that provides pain medication."
   3. "Your physician administered a numbing solution on your back."
   4. "No need to worry. You will be all right."

6. A patient with chronic pain asks, "What is a TENS unit?" What is the best nursing response?
   1. "It is an implant in the epidural space adjacent to nerves that innervate the affected body area."
   2. "It provides a small electrical stimulus to the skin around the area of pain."
   3. "It involves the use of external finger pressure at the meridian points."
   4. "It supports the tissues during movement."

7. Which of the following statements by a nurse promote(s) the use of massage in reducing pain? *(Select all that apply.)*
   1. Family members can perform it safely and effectively.
   2. It stimulates the circulation in reddened areas.
   3. It relaxes the muscles.
   4. It increases the patient's general sense of well-being.
   5. It uses short, mild strokes.

8. The nurse reinforces the need for safe administration of gentle heat to the nursing assistant. Which of the following actions by a nursing assistant indicates understanding of the safe application of gentle heat?
   1. Covering the heating pad before applying to the pain site
   2. Encouraging fluid intake
   3. Repositioning the patient for comfort
   4. Assisting with coughing and deep breathing

9. After administering ketorolac (Toradol) 30 mg intramuscularly, an immediate nursing action would be:
   1. recap the needle.
   2. massage the area.
   3. apply sterile dressing.
   4. encourage coughing.

10. The nurse is assigned to care for a patient with an epidural for analgesia. Which of the following signs and symptoms would require immediate physician notification?
   1. Blood pressure 80/60 mm Hg
   2. Temperature 98.6° F (37° C)
   3. Respirations 12/min
   4. Urinary output less than 30 mL/hour

CRITICAL THINKING ACTIVITIES 

Read each clinical scenario and discuss the questions with your classmates.

Scenario A

Ann Jefferson, a 43-year-old, has suffered from shoulder pain from an old healed fracture for several years. Her physician has prescribed an oral narcotic analgesic for her when the pain becomes too severe to be controlled with acetaminophen, but Ann does not want to continue taking drugs that she "might become addicted to."

1. How would you respond to Ann's statement regarding her fear of addiction to the pain medication?
2. What other measures could you suggest for management of Ann's pain?

Scenario B

Fred Hickson had a bowel resection 3 days ago. He is determined to get back to work quickly and is very cooperative about ambulation. He refuses pain medication, stating, "I don't need it." You note that he stops frequently to lean against the wall, walks stooped over, and grimaces when no one is looking.

1. Why might Fred be refusing pain medication?
2. What information might you share regarding pain control and getting well after major surgery?
3. What suggestions might you make to Fred regarding his comfort?

CHAPTER

8 Care of Patients with Cancer

evolve http://evolve.elsevier.com/deWit

Objectives

Upon completing this chapter you should be able to:

Theory

1. Identify characteristics of neoplastic (abnormal tissue) growth.
2. Identify at least five factors that may contribute to the development of a malignancy.
3. State at least four practices that can contribute to prevention and early detection of cancers.
4. Describe ways to include the recommendations of the American Cancer Society for routine checkups and detection of cancers into patient education.
5. Discuss the pros and cons of the various treatments available for cancer.
6. State the major problems and appropriate nursing interventions for a patient coping with expected side effects of radiation or chemotherapy.
7. State the stages of the grieving process experienced by the dying cancer patient.

Clinical Practice

1. Devise a general plan of nursing care for the patient receiving chemotherapy.
2. Discuss the teaching necessary for the patient who has bone marrow suppression from cancer treatment.
3. Institute nursing interventions to help the patient cope with the common problems of cancer and its treatment.
4. Utilize appropriate nursing interventions to help patients and families deal with the psychosocial effects of cancer and its treatment.
5. Identify nursing interventions to help the patient cope with death and dying.

Key Terms

Be sure to check out the bonus material on the Companion CD-ROM, including selected audio pronunciations.

benign (bē-NĪN, p. 158)
biopsy (BĪ-ŏp-sē, p. 167)
carcinogen (kăr-SĬN-ō-jĕn, p. 160)
carcinoma (kăr-sĭ-NŌ-mă, p. 159)
cytology (sī-TŎL-ō-jē, p. 165)
cytotoxic (sī-tō-TŎK-sĭk, p. 176)
deoxyribonucleic acid (DNA) (dē-ŏx-ē-rī-bō-noo-KLĀ-ĭc ĂS-ĭd, p. 158)
encapsulated (ĕn-KĂP-sū-lāt-ĕd, p. 158)
hematoma (hē-mă-TŌ-mă, p. 159)
incidence (p. 157)
leukemia (loo-KĒ-mē-ă, p. 159)
lymphoma (lĭm-FŌ-mă, p. 159)
malignant (mă-LĬG-nănt, p. 158)
melanoma (mĕl-ă-NŌ-mă, p. 159)
metastasis (mĕ-TĂS-tă-sĭs, p. 159)
mutation (mū-TĀ-shŭn, p. 160)
neoplasm (NĒ-ō-plăzm, p. 158)
occult blood (ŏ-KŬLT blŭd, p. 166)
oncogene (ŎNGK-ō-jĕn, p. 160)
palliative care (PĂL-ē-ă-tĭv, p. 185)
promoters (p. 162)
prognosis (prŏg-NŌ-sĭs, p. 159)
sarcoma (săr-KŌ-mă, p. 159)
TNM staging (p. 160)
transformation (p. 162)
tumor markers (TOO-mŏr, p. 168)
vesicant (p. 177)

THE IMPACT OF CANCER

Cancer is a group of diseases that characteristically grow in an uncontrolled manner with the spread of abnormal cells. That does not mean that the growth cannot be controlled in many instances by specific treatment. In the early 1900s, there was little hope for survival once cancer was detected. This year, 4 of 10 people who are diagnosed with cancer will be alive in 5 years.

About 1,444,920 new cases of cancer will be diagnosed in 2007. In addition, it is estimated that more than 1 million people will be told that they have squamous cell skin cancer. That's about the same as in 1977. The **incidence** of lung cancer in men has declined during this time and the incidence in women has stabilized. However, the incidence of breast cancer has increased overall. This is mostly attributed to improved detection. Death rates for many other major cancers have held steady or declined since the 1930s. Although cancer treatment has made progress, cancer still accounts for one in four deaths in the United States. About 559,650 people will die from it in 2007. On the other hand, there are 10.1 million living Americans who have a history of cancer, and 6.5 million of them were diagnosed over 5 years ago. **That means that 64% of cancer patients are surviving.** Because of im-

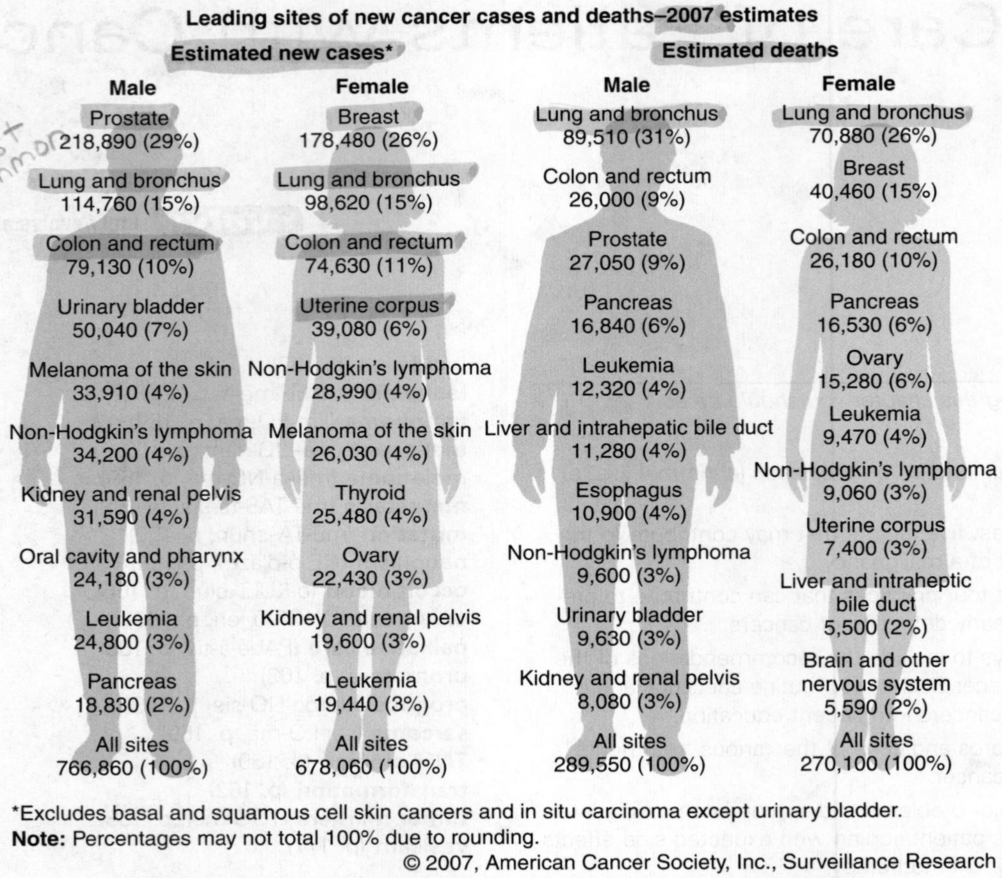

Leading sites of new cancer cases and deaths–2007 estimates

Estimated new cases*		Estimated deaths	
Male	**Female**	**Male**	**Female**
Prostate 218,890 (29%)	Breast 178,480 (26%)	Lung and bronchus 89,510 (31%)	Lung and bronchus 70,880 (26%)
Lung and bronchus 114,760 (15%)	Lung and bronchus 98,620 (15%)	Colon and rectum 26,000 (9%)	Breast 40,460 (15%)
Colon and rectum 79,130 (10%)	Colon and rectum 74,630 (11%)	Prostate 27,050 (9%)	Colon and rectum 26,180 (10%)
Urinary bladder 50,040 (7%)	Uterine corpus 39,080 (6%)	Pancreas 16,840 (6%)	Pancreas 16,530 (6%)
Melanoma of the skin 33,910 (4%)	Non-Hodgkin's lymphoma 28,990 (4%)	Leukemia 12,320 (4%)	Ovary 15,280 (6%)
Non-Hodgkin's lymphoma 34,200 (4%)	Melanoma of the skin 26,030 (4%)	Liver and intrahepatic bile duct 11,280 (4%)	Leukemia 9,470 (4%)
Kidney and renal pelvis 31,590 (4%)	Thyroid 25,480 (4%)	Esophagus 10,900 (4%)	Non-Hodgkin's lymphoma 9,060 (3%)
Oral cavity and pharynx 24,180 (3%)	Ovary 22,430 (3%)	Non-Hodgkin's lymphoma 9,600 (3%)	Uterine corpus 7,400 (3%)
Leukemia 24,800 (3%)	Kidney and renal pelvis 19,600 (3%)	Urinary bladder 9,630 (3%)	Liver and intraheptic bile duct 5,500 (2%)
Pancreas 18,830 (2%)	Leukemia 19,440 (3%)	Kidney and renal pelvis 8,080 (3%)	Brain and other nervous system 5,590 (2%)
All sites 766,860 (100%)	All sites 678,060 (100%)	All sites 289,550 (100%)	All sites 270,100 (100%)

*Excludes basal and squamous cell skin cancers and in situ carcinoma except urinary bladder.

Note: Percentages may not total 100% due to rounding.

FIGURE **8–1** Leading sites of new cancer cases and deaths (2007 estimates).

provements in treatment methods, patients who are diagnosed today may have much higher survival rates. More people can survive cancer if it is treated in its earliest stages. In fact, the American Cancer Society (ACS) estimates that if all the cancers that can be detected early were diagnosed in localized stages, the 5-year survival rate would be 95%. Figure 8–1 shows the leading sites of new cancer cases and deaths.

This chapter discusses the prevention and control of cancer; current diagnostic and screening techniques that help detect cancer in its earliest stages; therapeutic procedures that greatly improve a cancer victim's chances for survival; ethical issues in treatment of cancer patients; palliative care; cancer rehabilitation; and the role of the nurse in the control and treatment of malignant diseases.

PHYSIOLOGY OF CANCER

The human body is continuously producing new cells to replace those that are worn out and to repair damage done by illness and injury. An abnormal replication of cells results in a **neoplasm** (new growth of tissue), which is not beneficial and often is harmful to the body.

The word **benign** indicates a neoplasm that is usually harmless. Benign growths are almost always **encapsulated** (surrounded by a fibrous capsule). The capsule prevents the release of cells and their spread to other parts of the body. These growths can, however, create problems if they obstruct the passage of fluid and air. If they grow to such a size that they press against and interfere with the normal structure and function of nearby organs, that presents problems too.

The cells of **malignant** (uncontrolled growth that can lead to death) growths are quite different from normal cells. Cancer cells are the result of a change in normal body cells, probably due to some alteration in the normal cells' **deoxyribonucleic acid (DNA)**. DNA is the material that contains the genetic makeup of all future generations of the cell. The change in the DNA alters the structure and function of the cancer cell and of those it creates. Hence cancer cells do not look like or behave like normal cells (Figure 8–2).

The nucleus of a malignant cell is large and irregular. As the cell divides and duplicates, it fails to follow the rules that regulate the reproduction of normal cells. Malignant cells do not seem to "know" when to stop multiplying. Their offspring *proliferate* (multiply) in great numbers and grow more and more disorganized and uncontrollable. Some take on new charac-

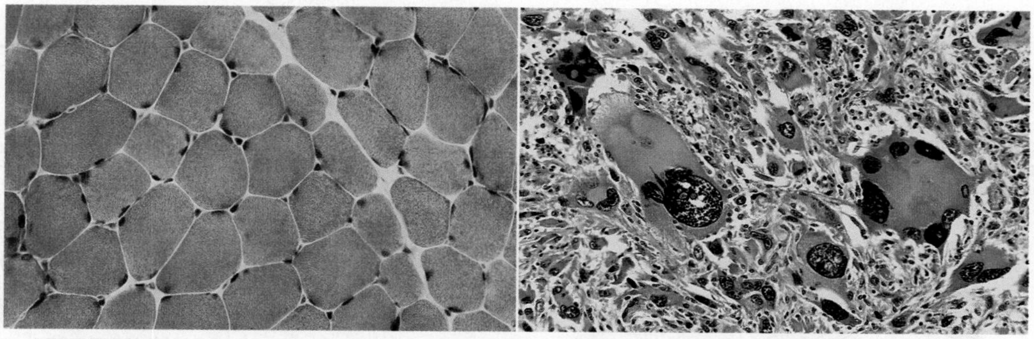

A B

FIGURE 8–2 Normal and malignant skeletal muscle cells. **A,** Normal skeletal muscles cells. Note that cells are well differentiated and similar in appearance. **B,** Malignant tumor cells in skeletal muscle (rhabdomyosarcoma).

teristics so that they do not in any way resemble the cells of the original tissue. Because malignant cell growth is not regulated as it is in normal cells, the malignant cells multiply and form tumorous masses. They invade neighboring tissues and travel to other parts of the body. There they establish another colony of malignant cells. Their demand for nutrients depletes the supply of nourishment available for normal cells. This spread of tumor cells is called **metastasis** (movement of cancer cells from the original cancer site to other areas of the body). **Not all malignant cells metastasize, but the great majority of them do.** This is true because malignant cells are easily broken off from their original mass of tissue and are able to survive on their own until they reach their new home.

? *Think Critically About* . . . Can you compare and contrast the aspects of a benign and malignant tumor for a classmate?

CLASSIFICATION OF TUMORS

Tumors are often classified according to the organs or tissues from which they first began to grow or the substances of which they are formed. The suffix *-oma* means tumor and is used in the names of various kinds of growths or swellings. However, remember that *-oma* simply means tumor, not malignant tumor. The suffix can designate any swelling, including one in which there is a collection of fluids, as well as one containing malignant cells. For example, **hematoma** (another word for bruise) is a combination of *hema-*, meaning blood, and *-oma,* meaning a swelling or collection of fluid or cells.

The prefixes used in classifying *neoplasms* (another name for tumors) indicate the kind of tissue in which they originate. For example, a tumor arising from fatty (lipid) tissue is called a *lipoma.* A *fibroma* is a tumor composed of fibrous tissue. A *leiomyofibroma* contains both smooth-muscle tissue and fibrous connective tissue. Lipomas, fibromas, and leiomyomas are the most frequently occurring types of benign growths.

Malignant growths are divided into four main types. **Sarcomas** arise from mesenchymal tissues, that is, bone, muscles, and other connective tissues. **Carcinomas** originate in epithelial tissues (skin and mucous membranes). These kinds of cancers make up the majority of glandular cancers of the stomach, uterus, lungs, skin, and tongue. **Leukemias** and **lymphomas** comprise the cancers of the blood-forming system. Malignancies of the pigment cells of the skin are called **melanomas.**

These are the main groups of cancers. More accurate naming can be done by adding modifying prefixes. For example, *osteosarcomas* arise from bone *(osteo-),* and *adenocarcinomas* arise from glandular *(adeno-)* structures.

METASTASIS

The word *metastasis* means the movement of cells from one part of the body to another. Bacterial cells metastasize, and so do malignant cells. Malignant growths can invade normal body tissue by attacking nearby tissues. They destroy normal cells and take their place. Malignant cells also may separate from the original tissue mass and travel to distant parts of the body. **Metastasis refers to the moving of these cells to another site.** Malignant cells can metastasize by traveling in the blood and body fluids, in much the same way as bacterial cells. It also is possible for free malignant cells to be directly transplanted from one organ to another during surgery, when gloves and instruments that have these cells on them serve as vehicles for their transportation. Another way in which malignant cells can "contaminate" normal tissues and organs is by entering a body cavity and coming in contact with a healthy organ. For example, malignant cells may break off from a diseased organ, enter the abdominal cavity, and attach themselves to an ovary or the *mesentery* (tissues that connect the internal organs to the abdominal cavity wall) (Figure 8–3).

The prognosis (prediction of survival) for a patient with a malignancy depends on how much the

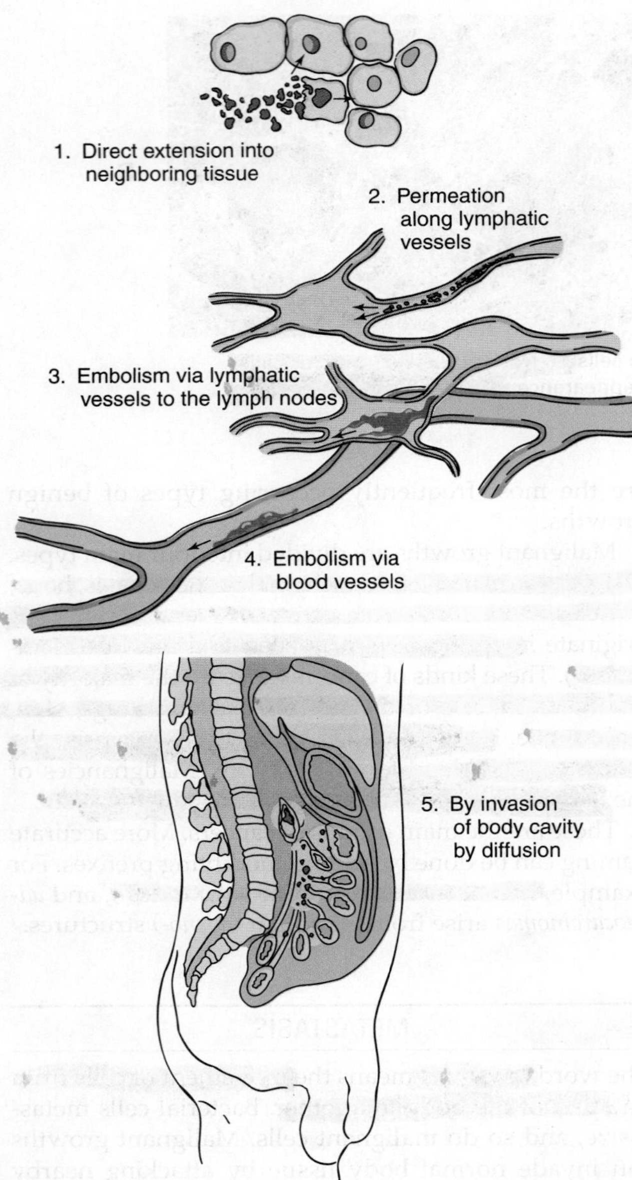

FIGURE 8–3 Modes of dissemination of cancer.

malignant cells have attacked body tissues. A localized growth is one that remains at the original site *(in situ)* and has not yet released its cells, even though the growth may have invaded underlying tissues. As long as all of the cells are in the area in which the new growth started, the cancer is said to be *localized*. At this stage the disease is much more easily destroyed.

A *regional* malignancy is one in which cells from the original malignancy have spread to the body area right around the tumor. This might include nearby lymph nodes. The spread has been limited, however, by the body's protective mechanisms. These cells may continue to grow and multiply, and if the regional cancer is not successfully treated, they will eventually break away and spread throughout the body. This creates an *advanced* cancer that is usually fatal.

Table 8–1 TNM Staging System for Cancer

TUMOR	
T0	No evidence of primary tumor.
TIS	Carcinoma in situ.
T1, T2, T3, T4	Progressive increase in tumor size and involvement.
TX	Tumor cannot be assessed.
NODES	
N0	Regional lymph nodes not demonstrably abnormal.
N1, N2, N3	Increasing degrees of demonstrable abnormality of regional lymph nodes.
NX	Regional lymph nodes cannot be assessed clinically.
METASTASIS	
M0	No evidence of distant metastasis.
M1, M2, M3	Ascending degrees of distant metastasis, including metastasis to distant lymph nodes.
M4	Multiple organ involvement.

One system that identifies cancers by how much the malignancy has spread is the TNM staging system. The three basic parts of the system are *T* for primary tumor, *N* for regional nodes, and *M* for metastasis. The number written beside each letter indicates how much the malignancy has spread and attacked other tissues (Table 8–1). For example, T1, N0, M0 means that the tumor is small and localized (no involvement of regional lymph nodes and no metastasis). A label of T1, N2, M0 indicates a small (T1) tumor with moderate regional involvement (N2) but no metastasis to distant sites (M0).

CAUSATIVE FACTORS

All cancer results from defects in the DNA of genes. These defects either are inherited or are caused by **mutation** (a permanent change in the DNA sequence of a gene) during a person's lifetime from exposure to chemicals or radiation. Several cancer-causing genes **(oncogenes)** are discovered each year. Oncogenes are mistakes in the instructions inside a cell. New cells are no longer normal. The defective gene tells the new cells to multiply at a higher rate. Also, it prevents the new cells from dying and being reabsorbed. This results in a tumor, or mass.

Likewise, *tumor suppressor genes* are being discovered. These are healthy, normal genes that control the growth of cells in the body. Each person's body has a different ability to withstand the effects of cancer-causing substances **(carcinogens)**, to mount a healthy immune response, and to repair damaged DNA. It is hoped that someday discoveries in molecular biology will allow individual risk profiles to be drawn that could be used to counsel people to avoid certain occupational and environmental exposures.

Many harmful agents exist in the external environment that are known to be carcinogenic, and others are strongly suspected. **Among these harmful agents are certain chemicals, sources of radiation, and viruses.**

In addition to these external causative factors, there are some internal factors that affect an individual's ability to cope with malignant cells. Hormones play an undetermined role in the development and progress of cancer, and several inherited genes have been discovered that increase a person's chance of getting some types of cancer. In some families there is a tendency to develop cancer in certain organs. This is shown in certain high-risk groups, which are described later in this chapter.

Another factor that enters into the development of a malignancy is age. Although cancer can strike at any age, older people are more susceptible. This is because they have a weakened immune system, their powers of adaptability are weakened, and they have been exposed to carcinogens over a longer period than have younger people. *Immunocompetence,* or the capability of one's immune system to deal with foreign cells—bacterial, viral, or malignant—is an important factor in the development of cancers.

CHEMICAL CARCINOGENS

More than 200 years ago (1775), Sir Percival Pott linked the occurrence of cancer to a substance in the environment when he observed that cancer of the scrotum was common among the chimney sweeps of London. He attributed this high incidence of cancer to repeated accumulations of soot on the skin of these young men, whose occupation required continuous contact with the coal soot in the chimneys they cleaned. Since that time, almost 500 different chemical carcinogens have been identified.

? *Think Critically About . . .* Can you identify three chemicals used in your home or your garden that are carcinogenic? How can you reduce your exposure to them and decrease the risk of cancer?

Many of the cancer-producing substances in the environment are related to occupations that involve repeated exposure to certain substances that are handled or inhaled. **Petrofluorocarbons (polychlorinated biphenyls or PCBs) and some pesticides (e.g., DDT) are known carcinogens.** These and other such chemicals decrease immunocompetence. For example, cancer of the skin often is related to the handling of pitch, asphalt, crude paraffin, and petroleum products. Lung cancer is linked to irritating substances in the air, such as tobacco smoke, asbestos, and chemical wastes from industry and automobiles. Cancer of the bladder is associated with certain substances in aniline dyes, which are present in the environment of workers in that industry. Vinyl chloride, nickel, arsenic, and chromate are linked to cancers in workers in industries that utilize those chemicals. Benzene, an ingredient in older unleaded gasoline, is linked to leukemia. These are but a few of the chemical agents that can contribute to the development of cancer in humans.

Chewing tobacco has been directly related to cancer of the tongue and structures of the mouth and throat. **Cigarette smoking is a known direct cause of cancer of the lung and is thought to be linked to esophageal, pancreatic, bladder, and kidney cancers** (Health Promotion Points 8–1).

Immunosuppressive drugs used to suppress organ transplant rejection are a cause of non-Hodgkin's lymphoma. Synthetic estrogens are linked to a higher incidence of endometrial cancer. Many of the drugs used to treat cancer affect the immune system and can predispose to other types of cancer. Table 8–2 shows carcinogens that are commonly encountered in the environment.

Table 8–2 ***Common Carcinogenic Substances***

SUBSTANCE	TYPE OF CANCER
Asbestos	Lung, peritoneal, pericardial
Benzene	Acute myelocytic leukemia
Tobacco	Lung, mouth, pharynx, larynx, esophagus, pancreas, bladder, kidney
Alcoholic beverages	Mouth, pharynx, larynx, esophagus, liver
Ionizing radiation	Leukemia, tumors of most organs
Sunlight (ultraviolet rays)	Skin
Diethylstilbestrol (prenatally)	Vagina
Estrogens, synthetic	Endometrial
Androgens, synthetic	Liver
Vinyl chloride	Liver
Aromatic amines	Bladder
Arsenic (inorganic)	Lung, skin
Chromium	Lung
Nickel dust	Lung, nasal sinuses
Chronic hepatitis B or C infection	Liver
Human T-cell lymphotropic virus type I (HTLV-1)	Adult T-cell leukemia and lymphoma
Human papillomavirus	Cervix
Phenacetin	Renal pelvis, bladder
Alkylating agents (used for chemotherapy)	Acute myelocytic leukemia
Cyclosporine (used to prevent transplant rejection)	Non-Hodgkin's lymphoma

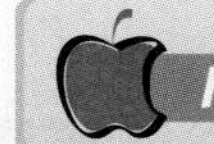

Health Promotion Points 8–1

Effects of Smoking

Encourage those who smoke to quit. Ninety percent of lung cancers in men and 79% in women are related to smoking. Use of tobacco in conjunction with the intake of alcohol is related to several other types of cancer.

PROMOTERS

Some substances are not carcinogenic when found alone, but when they are in a person's body with a known carcinogen, cancer occurs faster. These substances are called **promoters**. Alcohol is such a substance. When nicotine is present, cancers occur at a faster rate in those who are heavy consumers of alcohol than in someone who uses nicotine but does not drink alcohol. It is thought that about 90% of all head and neck cancers are tobacco plus alcohol related.

CHRONIC IRRITATION

In one of the earliest theories about the causes of cancer, a skin cancer was attributed to long-term chronic irritation of the skin and mucous membranes. Although this condition may be a *contributing cause* of cancer, chronic irritation alone usually does not lead to malignancy. There must be other factors present, particularly a mole on the skin and/or exposure to a chemical carcinogen or ultraviolet rays, in order for the cancer process to begin.

Research on a variety of chemicals that may have this same type of influence is ongoing. The link is most likely that the second substance involved, although not directly carcinogenic, has a depressant or harmful effect on the immune system, making the person more susceptible to growth of malignant cells.

PHYSICAL CARCINOGENS

Radiation

Radiation may originate from x-ray machines and radioactive elements or from the ultraviolet rays of the sun. These rays are capable of penetrating certain body tissues and causing the development of malignant cells in the affected area. The relationship of intense and prolonged exposure to these rays and the production of cancer cells was first discovered when it was noted that there was a high incidence of cancer, particularly leukemia, among people who pioneered studies of x-rays, radium, and uranium. Later it was found that survivors of atomic blasts at Hiroshima and Nagasaki at the end of World War II suffered an unusually high incidence of leukemia.

There is continued concern about the dangers that excessive radiation in the environment presents, especially the long-term effects that are not immediately apparent but may eventually prove to be related to malignancy. In addition to leukemia, cancers of the skin, bone marrow, breast, lung, and thyroid are believed to be closely linked to exposure to radiation.

The ultraviolet rays of the sun can produce skin cancer. The deterioration of the Earth's ozone layer is causing more ultraviolet rays to reach the earth than in the past, which compounds the problem. The susceptibility of the individual also is a factor. People with fair complexions have less protective pigment and therefore are more likely to develop skin cancer from ultraviolet radiation than are people with darker skin.

Radon Gas

People who live in areas that have more radon emission from the earth have a higher incidence of malignancy in the population than people in areas that are low in radon.

Viruses

In recent years, intensive research has been directed toward establishing a link between viruses and malignancy. Experiments involving animals have demonstrated that a number of cancers can be produced in animals by injecting them with a filtrate from virus-infected malignant growths. **The hepatitis B virus is carcinogenic for liver cancer.** The Epstein-Barr virus causes Burkitt's lymphoma. Cases of adult T-cell leukemia and lymphoma are caused by human T-cell lymphotropic virus. A form of the human papillomavirus causes cervical carcinoma and is related to throat cancer in nonsmokers. These viruses are known as *oncoviruses* because of their ability to cause cancer.

After the **transformation** (change into something else) of a normal cell into a precancerous state, the malignant cell probably requires many conditions favorable to its multiplication and growth into a cancerous tumor. **Viruses are capable of introducing new genetic material into a normal cell and transforming it into a malignant one.** Furthermore, cell reproduction can be altered when viruses interact with carcinogens. Viruses such as the human immunodeficiency virus (HIV) can damage the immune system and decrease immunocompetence, causing the body to become more susceptible to the growth of abnormal cells. Some cancers, such as Kaposi sarcoma are only seen in HIV-infected or severely immunocompromised patients (see Chapter 11 for more information).

GENETIC PREDISPOSITION

All cancers are caused by genes that malfunction and cause overgrowth of cells. Research is revealing that there is a genetic predisposition to various types of cancer. It has been known for many years that breast cancer is more likely to occur in women who have a close female relative who developed breast cancer before the age of 50. Gene markers have been found for colon cancer, breast cancer, and leukemia. However, only 5% to 10% of cancers are directly inherited. The remaining cancers are caused by genes that are damaged (mutated) throughout the lifetime and are not inherited. Some people are more susceptible to these mutations (Cultural Cues 8–1). With the completion of the Human Genome Project, the genes that are related to specific cancers are being identified. In the next decade, genetic markers, or oncogenes, will be found for many other forms of cancer. Such markers, or the proteins they produce, could identify high-risk individuals who then might undergo more vigorous, regular diagnostic testing to

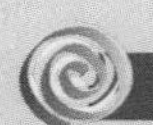

Cultural Cues 8–1

Race Factors

Some populations are at a higher risk for certain types of cancer. For example, of the four types of melanoma, African Americans are most susceptible to the acral lentiginous type while whites are least susceptible to it. Lentigo maligna melanoma is found most often in Hawaii.

detect any malignancy in the very earliest stages. Since several cancers have precursor lesions, such as adenomatous polyps in the colon, such early discovery would greatly increase survival rates.

CONTRIBUTING FACTORS

INTRINSIC FACTORS

Age, sex, and race are considered "predisposing factors" for certain types of cancers. This simply means that, statistically, certain types of cancer strike particular age, sex, or racial groups more frequently than others. For example, prostate cancer is far more common in black males than in white males. The incidence of cervical cancer is higher in black women than in white women. Breast cancer is more prevalent in white women than in Asian women. As for age factors, approximately 76% of cancers occur in people age 55 and older.

STRESS

Another factor that seems to play a role in the development of cancer is stress. Considerable stress over long periods has an adverse effect on the immune system, making it less effective in ridding the body of invading organisms and decreasing the body's ability to destroy abnormal cells. Stress is one more factor that can perhaps tip the scales in favor of growth of malignant cells. When one partner of a long-term relationship dies, the stress of the loss and adjustment to life without the person seems to increase the likelihood of cancer in the surviving partner.

DIET

Most experts agree that approximately 30% of cancers could be reduced through proper nutrition and exercise. There is strong evidence that healthy diet and normal body weight are crucial in the control of cancer. Cancers of the breast, colon, rectum, endometrium, esophagus, uppermost abdomen, gallbladder, pancreas, liver, and kidney are all related to excess weight and obesity. Although there is no universal agreement about the role of fiber in the prevention of malignancy, high-fiber foods such as fruits, vegetables, and cereals are recommended as a wholesome substitute for fatty foods.

Nutritional Therapies 8–1

Dietary Recommendations to Minimize Risk for Cancer

- Eat a varied diet and avoid obesity.
- Reduce total saturated and unsaturated fat intake to 30% of total caloric intake.
- Eat more high-fiber foods: whole-grain cereals, breads, pastas, fresh fruits, and vegetables.
- Include foods rich in vitamins A and C in the daily diet.
- Eat cruciferous vegetables and those containing beta-carotene daily: cabbage, broccoli, Brussels sprouts, kohlrabi, cauliflower, carrots, yellow squash.
- Avoid smoked, salt-cured, nitrite-cured, and charred (blackened) foods.
- Keep alcohol consumption moderate: no more than two drinks or two glasses of wine or beer per day (one drink for women).

MEASURES TO PREVENT CANCER

The nurse can be very instrumental in educating the public about ways to prevent cancer. Each nurse should teach patients the following measures at every opportunity.

DIET AND NUTRITION

Encourage maintenance of normal weight. Obesity is considered a risk factor in many cancers. It also makes early detection of many cancers difficult. One study noted that men and women who were overweight by 40% or more have a 33% and 35% greater risk, respectively, for developing cancer than do persons with normal weight.

Nitrite and nitrate food additives are also known to be cancer *stimulators* (encourage cancer). However, research has indicated that if foods containing nitrites are eaten in combination with foods containing vitamin C (ascorbic acid), the formation of nitrosamines is blocked. This means, for example, that if orange juice is consumed along with a meal containing bacon, there is less chance of carcinogenic nitrosamines damaging the body. In this instance, the vitamin C is a cancer *inhibitor.*

? *Think Critically About . . .* If you saw that a package of meat contained nitrates, what other chemical would you expect to find in the package?

The ACS has issued nutritional recommendations that are believed to reduce the risk for certain cancers. These recommendations, summarized in Nutritional Therapies 8–1, are from a report by a special committee on nutrition and cancer and are based on studies conducted for more than 20 years by the ACS's Re-

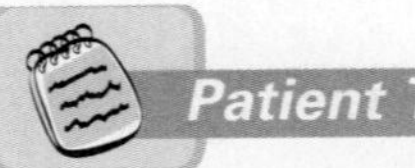

Patient Teaching 8–1

Avoiding and Limiting Exposure to Carcinogens

- Knowing which substances used in the household, yard, and areas of recreation and at the place of work are carcinogenic and using protective measures against them can decrease exposure.
- The use of protective clothing, gloves, and mask as appropriate when spraying pesticides or chemicals or using chemical cleaners or strippers greatly decreases exposure.
- Being certain the area is well ventilated when using chemical cleaners indoors is protective.
- Thoroughly washing the hands and any exposed skin after using compounds containing carcinogenic chemicals provides protection.
- Utilizing an appropriate sunscreen and protective clothing when outdoors, avoiding sunburns, and avoiding tanning salons and sun lamps greatly decreases the incidence of skin cancer.
  - Australians have the highest rate of skin cancer in the world and have developed a message that is a good way to instruct your patients: **slip, slap, slop, strap—slip** on protective clothing, **slap** on a hat, **slop** on some sunscreen, and **strap** on sunglasses.
- Avoiding swimming and water sports in contaminated waters and avoiding eating fish from waters that have chemical contamination limit exposure.
- Washing or rinsing fruits and vegetables before preparing them for eating or cooking decreases exposure to agricultural pesticides.

search Program. Although no direct cause-and-effect relationship between diet and cancer has been demonstrated, there is ample evidence that avoidance of obesity and modification of the diet can help prevent some types of cancers.

? *Think Critically About* . . . Can you identify three specific changes you could make in your personal diet that might decrease your cancer risk? What would you add to the diet or what would you stop eating?

ALCOHOL

Moderation in the drinking of alcohol is recommended, because drinking often is accompanied by cigarette smoking or the use of smokeless tobacco. It also can lead to liver damage and possibly to liver cancer.

ENVIRONMENT

Because ground water is so often contaminated with chemicals that have leached into it from fertilizers, pesticides, and industrial wastes, it is wise to know the chemical makeup of the local water supply. If the geographic area is highly contaminated, bottled water might help prevent further damage to immunocompetence and thereby decrease the incidence of cancer (Patient Teaching 8–1).

IDENTIFYING HIGH-RISK PEOPLE

Studies of individuals who have developed cancer—their medical history, lifestyle, and family history—have shown that some people are more likely to develop certain kinds of cancer than others. Table 8–3 shows information on high-risk groups published by the ACS in order to develop an awareness of the need for frequent and thorough examinations to detect cancer early in those who are susceptible to developing a malignancy.

DETECTION OF CANCER

The purpose of screening large segments of a population is to identify as many susceptible people as possible. Screening clinics often identify individuals who already have developed malignancies but have no symptoms and are not aware that they are suffering from cancer.

Cancer sometimes is called the "great masquerader" because it is capable of causing symptoms similar to those of a variety of diseases. Cancer is, after all, a group of diseases. It can strike any organ of the body, affecting different organs with different functions, and therefore can present an untold number of symptoms as it progresses. To be able to identify the symptoms of cancer in its earliest stages, it is important to be aware of its warning signals (Box 8–1).

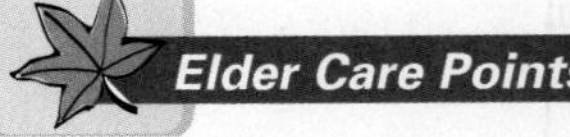

Elder Care Points

- Elderly patients are at increasingly higher risk for developing cancer.
- Many of the cancer screening programs are suggested to begin at age 50 or older.

Because the incidence of cancer is so much higher in the person over age 50, and because those who have reached old age have been exposed to more carcinogens for a longer period of time, annual screening for cancer is even more important as people age.

In addition to the medical history and thorough physical examination that are essential components of

Table 8–3 *Major Risk Factors for Cancer*

TYPE OF CANCER	RISK FACTORS	SIGNS
Lung	• Heavy smoker over age 50 • Smoked a pack a day for 20 years • Started smoking at age 15 or before • Exposure to environmental smoke • Exposure to asbestos, arsenic, certain chemicals in the workplace • Radiation or radon exposure • History of tuberculosis	Persistent cough, blood in the sputum, chest pain, recurring pneumonia or bronchitis
Breast	• History of breast cancer • History of some forms of breast biopsy • Close relatives with history of breast cancer • Early menarche; late menopause • Never had children; first child after age 30 • Lengthy exposure to cyclic estrogen • Higher educational and socioeconomic status	Lump in breast, nipple discharge, thickening, dimpling, nipple retraction, pain or tenderness of the nipple
Colon-rectum	• History of rectal polyps • Rectal polyps run in family • History of inflammatory bowel disease	Blood in stool; alteration in bowel pattern (e.g., constipation alternating with diarrhea)
Uterine-cervical	• Frequent sex in early teens or with many partners • History of HPV • Low socioeconomic status • Poor care during or following pregnancy	Unusual bleeding or discharge
Uterine-endometrial	• Estrogen therapy • Tamoxifen therapy • Late menopause (after age 55) • History of infertility or failure to ovulate • Diabetes, high blood pressure, gallbladder disease, and obesity • Pelvic irradiation	Unusual bleeding or discharge
Skin	• Excessive exposure to sun or tanning booth • Fair complexion • Work with coal tar, pitch, or creosote	Change in the size, color, or appearance of a mole or spot on the skin; scaliness, oozing, bleeding or change in appearance of a bump or nodule; spread of pigmentation beyond the border; change in sensation of any skin lesion
Oral	• Heavy smoker and drinker • Use of smokeless tobacco • Poor oral hygiene	White patch in the mouth or on the tongue; nodules
Ovary	• History of ovarian cancer among close relatives • History of breast cancer • History of never having children	None until well advanced
Prostate	• Over age 65 • Black ancestry	Difficulty urinating; hesitancy, blood in the urine; need to urinate frequently; pain in lower back, pelvis, or upper thighs
Stomach	• History of stomach cancer among close relatives • Diet heavy in smoked, pickled, or salted foods • Some link with blood group A	Nonspecific; indigestion, feeling of fullness or pressure; pain and weight loss are late signs
Pancreas	• Smoking	No signs
Bladder	• Smoking	Painless blood in the urine; need for frequent urination
Leukemia	• Down syndrome • Exposure to excessive radiation • Exposure to benzene (unleaded gas) • HTLV-1 infection • Philadelphia chromosome	Frequent infections, easy bruising, fatigue, weight loss, nosebleeds, paleness

Key: *HPV,* human papillomavirus; *HTLV-1,* human T-cell lymphotropic virus type 1.

any health status evaluation, the health care professional also conducts certain tests to determine whether a malignancy is present. Recommendations of the ACS for routine checkups and early detection of cancer are shown in Box 8–2.

One widely used technique to detect cancer is to examine cells under a microscope to determine whether they are malignant or premalignant. This technique is called cytology, and the most widely used cytologic test is the Papanicolaou smear. A *cytologic examination* can be done by obtaining a sample of secretions in which there are cells that have been released from adjacent tissue. The technique involves either scraping or brushing a sample of cells from the area or collecting body secretions that contain cells. These secretions may be cervical discharges, sputum, gastric washings, pleural fluid, or urinary washings. The specimen is placed on a slide and sent to a laboratory, where a specially trained technologist or pathologist examines the cells microscopically. If "suspicious" cells are found, the patient is referred to a health care professional for more extensive diagnostic tests. The "Pap smear," named after Dr. George Papanicolaou, who first developed the procedure, is used in screening for cancer of the uterine cervix.

Another screening technique, used for colorectal cancer, is the simple test for **occult blood** (hidden blood) in the stool. This can be obtained through a fecal occult blood test (FOBT) or a newer test called the fecal immunochemical test (FIT). The person simply collects one or more stool specimens, depending on the particular test being used, applies a thin smear on the container provided, and returns the slides to the health center, clinic, or clinical laboratory. In one of the

Box 8–1 ***The Seven Warning Signs of Cancer***

CAUTION

- **C**hange in bowel or bladder habits
- **A** sore that does not heal
- **U**nusual bleeding or discharge
- **T**hickening or lump in breast or elsewhere
- **I**ndigestion or difficulty in swallowing
- **O**bvious change in wart or mole
- **N**agging cough or hoarseness

Box 8–2 ***Routine Measures Recommended by the American Cancer Society for the Early Detection of Cancer***

BREAST

- Regular monthly self-examination of breasts for lumps, nodules, or changes in contour; check by physician every 3 years until age 40, then every year.
- Beginning at age 40, a mammogram is recommended yearly.

COLON-RECTUM

At age 50, begin screening with one of the following:

- Yearly fecal occult blood test (FOBT) or fecal immunochemical test (FIT).*
- Flexible sigmoidoscopy every 5 years.*
- Both FOBT/FIT and flexible sigmoidoscopy (better than either alone)
- Double-contrast barium enema every 5 years.
- Colonoscopy every 10 years.

CERVIX AND UTERUS

- Pelvic examination every year.
- Yearly Pap test (or every 2 years if liquid based) beginning by age 21 or 3 years after initiation of sexual intercourse.
- Beginning at age 30, after three consecutive normal Pap tests, the test may be performed every 2 to 3 years at the discretion of the physician. Women at high risk for cervical cancer should continue with annual Pap tests.
- Beginning at age 70, low-risk women with three normal Pap tests in a row and no abnormal Pap test in the last 10 years may discontinue screening.
- Endometrial screening is not recommended. However, those at high risk for endometrial cancer should have an endometrial tissue biopsy taken yearly beginning at age 35 at the discretion of their primary care clinician.

TESTICLES AND PROSTATE

- At age 14, begin performing testicular self-examination (TSE) once a month.
- Beginning at age 50, digital rectal examination (DRE) and prostate-specific antigen (PSA) test should be performed annually to men who have at least a 10-year life expectancy.
- Men at high risk (African American men and men with a strong family history of one or more first-degree relatives [father, brothers] diagnosed before age 65) should begin testing at age 45.
- Those with even higher risk may begin screening at age 40.

SKIN

- Self-examination of skin by all adults once a month to detect new lesions and monitor appearance of moles.
- Consultation with a dermatologist if pale, wax-like, pearly nodules, or red, scaly, sharply outlined patches are found.
- Melanoma may present as a mole that is asymmetrical one half to the other, or may have an irregular border, pigmentation that is not uniform throughout the mole, or a diameter greater than 6 mm. A dermatologist should be consulted if any of these changes are found.

ORAL

- Regular dental examinations.
- Consult physician or dentist if a white patch remains in mouth for more than a week, or a nodule is felt on the gums, tongue, or mucous membranes.
- Inspect the sides and bottom of the tongue every few months.

HIGH-RISK EXCEPTIONS

More frequent and thorough examinations recommended for:

- Women with personal family histories of breast cancer.
- Women who began having sexual intercourse at an early age or those with many partners.
- Women who have a history of obesity, infertility, failure of ovulation, abnormal uterine bleeding, or estrogen therapy.
- Men and women who have a personal family history of cancer of the rectum, familial polyposis, Gardner's syndrome, ulcerative colitis, or a history of polyps, and those with a family incidence of melanoma.

Each person is encouraged to confer with a physician and determine whether these recommendations are adequate in light of his or her personal history and risk factors.

*These tests should be combined.

tests (FOBT) directions for withholding meat and other foods, vitamins, and drugs from the diet for several days before the test must be clear to the patient. Otherwise, a false-positive or false-negative reading might be obtained. **Occult blood in the stool is not always an indication of cancer of the bowel or rectum.** Other conditions also can produce this symptom.

Research continues on identifying proteins produced by mutated DNA that might be used to diagnose various types of cancer. These tests may soon be available for those at high risk for bladder, cervical, lung, breast, colon, and prostate cancer. If these tests prove reliable, they may well be incorporated into a normal part of routine medical care.

Other procedures used to identify lesions that are possibly malignant include radiologic studies, endoscopy, sonography, magnetic resonance imaging, computed tomography, clinical laboratory testing of enzymes and other substances in the blood, and studies specific to the system in which the cancer is suspected.

DIAGNOSTIC TESTS

Biopsy

Biopsy of a tumor and examination of the cells so obtained are the most certain techniques for establishing a diagnosis of malignancy in most neoplasms. Malignancies involving blood cells, as in leukemia, are diagnosed by examining these cells.

A **biopsy** is the removal of living cells for the purpose of examining them under a microscope. The cells may be removed by surgical *excision* (cutting out) of a small part of a tumor, by the *aspiration* (suction) of cells through a needle introduced into the growth, or by brush biopsy. If the tumor is small, the entire growth may be removed. The specimen obtained is examined under the microscope.

Ordinarily, the specimen is prepared in the laboratory by placing it in paraffin and waiting 24 hours before examining it. However, if the sample is taken in the operating room and the surgeon is waiting for the results to determine the extent of surgery needed to remove all the malignant cells, the tissues may be frozen for quick examination. This technique is called *preparing a frozen section.*

New procedures, such as fine-needle aspiration (FNA) and *percutaneous* (through the skin) large-core breast biopsy, are used for diagnosing breast cancer without the disfigurement of traditional surgical breast biopsy. Breast biopsy is combined with imaging techniques such as ultrasound to verify correct placement of the biopsy needle. Then FNA is combined with computer analysis of the samples obtained.

Radiologic Studies

Mammography is a radiologic examination of the breast that is useful in diagnosing malignant growths, and x-ray films are particularly helpful in diagnosing bone and hollow organ tumors. Mortality can be cut by 31% when routine mammography screening is performed (Tabar et al., 2003). The respiratory, digestive, and urinary tracts can be visualized by x-ray if a *radiopaque* (not penetrated by the x-rays) substance is used. The substance passes through the hollow organ and, since it is radiopaque, the inner structure of the organ is clearly demonstrated on the x-ray film. A radiopaque substance commonly used is barium, which may be swallowed by the patient or given in an enema.

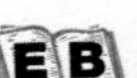

Another radiologic technique involves the use of a radioactive substance (*radionuclide* or *isotope*) that is given to the patient prior to the x-ray filming. The isotope is a "tumor-seeking" chemical that searches for the tumor and may or may not concentrate around it. A special scanning apparatus moves back and forth over the subject's body; as it moves, it records information about the concentration of the isotope in the area being examined. If the substance is concentrated in the tumor, the growth shows up as a "hot spot" on the screen of the scanning apparatus. If the tumor does not accept the isotope, the normal tissue around the tumor concentrates the isotope, and the tumor shows up as a "cold spot." This technique is commonly used in the investigation of thyroid tumors.

A commonly used radiologic scanning technique is *computed tomography (CT) scanning*. This method is noninvasive and involves relatively small amounts of radiation exposure for the subject. The term *noninvasive* means that no surgical procedures are needed to reveal the size, shape, contour, and density of an organ. The procedure is not uncomfortable for the patient and requires minimal preparation.

In CT scanning, the x-ray source moves past the subject in one direction while the film moves in another. In this way, three-dimensional cross sections, or "slices," of tissue can be obtained. The scanner rotates an entire 180 degree (half circle) around the area being examined, filming as it rotates 1 degree at a time. Information received by the scanner is relayed to a computer, which presents an image of the tissues one slice at a time. The "picture" presented by the computer is an interpretation of the varying densities of tissues, fluids, and bones. Tumors, as well as other abnormal structures within the body tissues, can be seen in this way.

Another imaging technique is called *magnetic resonance imaging* (MRI). As in CT scanning, MRI produces views of "slices" of tissue. MRI can sometimes "see" tumors and abnormalities that other techniques miss. It can also be used in real time to monitor cancer treatments. However, not everyone can use MRI. Patients with pacemakers, certain metal fragments or clips, or shrapnel in the body cannot use MRI because the powerful magnets used in this technique can bend and twist metal and can damage the body.

Endoscopy

An endoscope is an instrument used for direct visualization of internal body parts. It is designed so that it can be inserted and passed along the interior of hollow organs and cavities. The endoscope has a flexible fiberoptic tube fitted with a lens system so the examiner can view tissues in more than one direction. It has a light to illuminate the area being examined.

Types of endoscopes include the colonoscope for the colon, the bronchoscope for the trachea and bronchi, the laparoscope for the ovaries or the contents of the abdominal or pelvic cavity, and the cystoscope for the interior of the bladder. During an endoscopy, the physician may take a sample of cells from a suspicious area so they can be examined more precisely under a microscope (biopsy).

LABORATORY TESTS

Although no one blood test can establish a definite diagnosis of cancer, certain tests are used to ascertain specific information. A complete blood count is helpful in diagnosing leukemia. The presence of a high level of prostate-specific antigen (PSA) may indicate prostate cancer. The PSA test is a recommended part of the routine physical for the male over age 50, or earlier if the patient is at high risk. Instructions for this test are found in Box 8–3.

Specialized tests for tumor markers have been developed in the past few years. These tests detect biochemical substances synthesized and released into the bloodstream by tumor cells. However, these are not 100% accurate for diagnosing tumors because many of these substances also are produced by normal or embryonic cells and are also found in benign conditions. **Therefore, tumor markers are mainly used to confirm a diagnosis or the response to therapy, or to detect a relapse.** CA-125 is used to detect the presence of ovarian cancer or its recurrence after therapy. Carcinoembryonic antigen (CEA) and CA 19-9 are tumor marker tests used to detect the recurrence of gastrointestinal, pancreatic, and liver cancer after initial treatment, and CA 27-29 is used most frequently to follow the progress in breast cancer treatment and later to check for recurrence.

Box 8–3 *Prostate-Specific Antigen (PSA) Test*

- No sexual activity for 24 to 48 hours prior to the test
- Avoid test until after urinary tract infection is cleared
- Do not perform test after recent urinary tract surgery
- Collect blood sample prior to digital examination
- Prostatic acid phosphatase (PAP) is collected to confirm an elevated PSA
  - *Phosphatase* gives information about extent of disease
  - Alkaline phosphatase often elevated with bone cancer and liver metastasis

NURSING MANAGEMENT

Assessment (Data Collection)

The first step is to find out whether the patient has been informed of her diagnosis and what is known about the illness and treatment. Some patients may suspect they have cancer but do not want to discuss it. Even those who have been informed may choose not to talk about it or ask any questions about their treatment. The fact that a patient cannot discuss her illness and seek help in dealing with the problems it presents should indicate how very frightened she is and how much she needs help and understanding. The nurse must assess how the disease is affecting the patient's body and life to plan comprehensive care.

A thorough assessment of the system in which the cancer is located and a good general physical assessment provide a baseline upon which changes in physical function caused by the cancer can be evaluated. A psychosocial assessment of the patient and family or significant others provides data that point out psychosocial needs, coping abilities and techniques, and resources for support and care.

Finally, the nurse should determine how he can assist the patient to make the most of the personal resources and abilities that the patient currently possesses. This could mean helping with adjustment to the emotional impact of only recently learning the diagnosis of cancer, or it could require helping the patient to deal with the pain and discomfort of advanced malignancy and to prepare for a peaceful death.

Nursing Diagnosis

Patients with cancer, depending on the stage of the disease, can have a great number of problems, and a large number of nursing diagnoses may be appropriate. Specific diagnoses are chosen for the body systems and functions in which the disease or tumor is causing disruption of homeostasis. Common general nursing diagnoses associated with a diagnosis of cancer can be found in Box 8–4.

Planning

Specific expected outcomes are written for each nursing diagnosis chosen as appropriate for the patient. Examples are included in Nursing Care Plan 8–1. Planning is a collaborative process that includes the patient, the family, the physician, the oncologist, the nurse manager, the social worker, and other specialists on the health care team. The home care nurse, the infusion therapy company nurse, and the pharmacist often are involved in care and should be included in the planning process. The nurse manager usually is the one who consults with the others of the team and coordinates the plan of care.

Implementation

Specific interventions are included in Nursing Care Plan 8–1 and in the following sections.

Box 8–4 Common Nursing Diagnoses Used for Patients with Cancer

- Imbalanced nutrition (less than body requirements) related to increased metabolic demand and nausea, vomiting, diarrhea, or mucositis.
- Risk for infection related to bone marrow depression from therapy.
- Pain, acute or chronic, related to effects of tumor on body structures or cancer therapy.
- Impaired skin integrity related to surgical or radiation therapy.
- Disturbed body image related to weight loss or hair loss.
- Risk for injury to patient, staff, and visitors related to exposure to a radioactive implant.
- Impaired physical mobility related to restricted activity secondary to a radioactive implant.
- Diarrhea related to effects of cancer treatment.
- Constipation related to effects of chemotherapy.
- Impaired urinary elimination related to radiation therapy or secondary to effects of chemotherapy.
- Activity intolerance related to fatigue.
- Deficient knowledge related to drugs and side effects.
- Self-care deficit related to weakness and fatigue.
- Fear related to the possibility of dying.
- Ineffective individual coping related to denial of significance of cancer.
- Ineffective family coping related to inability to function as a result of anxiety over patient's prognosis.

Evaluation

Evaluation is based on determining whether the expected outcomes specified for the patient are being or have been met. Constant assessment for signs of complications, side effects of therapy, nutritional status, and pain status is necessary. The nursing care plan must be changed when the interventions initially chosen are not effective in meeting the desired outcomes. Collaboration with the patient and the other members of the health care team is important to the success of care plan changes.

COMMON THERAPIES, PROBLEMS, AND NURSING CARE

There are three traditional modes of therapy for malignancies: *surgery, radiation,* and *chemotherapy. Hormone manipulation, immunotherapy with biologic response modifiers,* and *bone marrow transplantation* are treatments combined with traditional therapies.

Each of the modes of treatment may be used singly or in combination with one or more of the other methods available. For example, chemotherapy may be used as an *adjuvant* (assisting treatment) after surgical removal of a tumor. No one method is necessarily better or more effective than another except in regard to the location of the malignancy, its type and extent of spread, and the reaction of the tumor itself and the individual patient. The methods of treatment are chosen after due consideration of many factors and are prescribed with the best interest of the patient in mind.

SURGERY

Surgery may be performed to obtain a biopsy specimen; as *prophylaxis* (preventive treatment), such as in the removal of the ovaries of a woman whose mother had ovarian cancer; to determine the effectiveness of therapy by looking to see whether the initial tumor is reduced in size; for *palliation* (offering relief), as in *debulking* (removing as much as possible) a tumor to prevent pressure on adjacent structures or obstruction of vessels or the gastrointestinal tract; or as an attempt at cure. Reconstructive surgery also is associated with cancer treatment. The woman who has lost a breast to mastectomy may have the breast reconstructed. Other extremely mutilating forms of cancer surgery require reconstructive procedures after the initial procedure. Flap grafts in a patient who underwent radical neck surgery for cancer of the throat are an example.

Surgical removal of a malignant growth is the oldest method of treatment. It works very well for tumors that are easily accessible. Adjacent tissues that may contain malignant cells also are excised. Regional lymph nodes often harbor malignant cells, and these can then travel to distant parts of the body and establish a new cancer site if not removed. Newer surgical procedures and techniques have significantly reduced the need for extensive surgical removal of adjacent tissues and structures. Radical mastectomy, for example, involves removal of the entire breast along with underlying pectoral muscle tissues and lymph nodes under the arm on the affected side. This procedure has been replaced almost completely by a modified radical mastectomy, or lumpectomy, combined with radiation and/or chemotherapy, which is far less traumatic and mutilating. If there is no evidence of metastasis, some patients are good candidates for simple removal of the tumor *(lumpectomy).* The use of radiation and/or chemotherapy during, after, and sometimes before surgery has decreased the need for extensive removal of adjacent tissues and is associated with decreased recurrence.

RADIATION THERAPY

The source for radiation therapy is either a linear accelerator or a radioactive element or substance. The purpose of radiation is to destroy malignant cells (which are more sensitive to radiation than are normal cells) without permanent damage to adjacent body tissues.

Ionizing radiation can have both an immediate and a delayed effect on malignant cells. It can damage the cell membrane immediately, causing *lysis* (bursting) or decomposition of the cell, or it can cause a break in both strands of the DNA in the cell's nucleus. **When a cell is damaged in this way, it will not die until it attempts to divide and replicate itself. The rate at which a particular kind of cell undergoes mitosis**

determines whether the effects of radiation will occur in a matter of days, months, or years. This explains the delayed effects and side effects of radiation that might not be evident at the time of treatment but appear later. Normal cells have a greater ability to repair the DNA damage than malignant cells. Some tissues are more sensitive to radiation than others, and this is taken into account when the physicist-physician calculates the dose of radiation needed to eradicate the tumor. The other factors considered are the sensitivity of the tumor to radiation, its location, and its size. Once calculated, the dose is *fractionalized,* meaning it is

NURSING CARE PLAN 8–1

Care of the Patient with Cancer

SCENARIO Mr. Pole is receiving chemotherapy for leukemia. This is his third round of weekly intravenous treatments. His platelet count is down to 185,000; he has had difficulty eating as a result of mucositis and anorexia. He states that he is mildly nauseated most of the time. He is 15 lb underweight.

PROBLEM/NURSING DIAGNOSIS *Undergoing chemotherapy*/Risk for infection related to bone marrow suppression.

Supporting assessment data *Objective:* Receiving chemotherapy drugs that suppress bone marrow.

Goals/Expected Outcomes	Nursing Interventions	Selected Rationale	Evaluation
Patient will remain free of infection	Monitor WBCs (more susceptible to infection when <3000 and granulocyte count is <2000).	Neutropenia is a sign of immunosuppression.	WBCs 3200.
	Assess for signs of infection every shift.	Elevated temperature may indicate infection.	Temp. 98.8° F (37.1° C); no signs of infection.
	Teach good hygiene, mouth care, hand washing before meals and after using bathroom.	Hand hygiene prevents spread of infection.	Patient washing hands appropriately and using good hygiene.
	Restrict visitors; allow no one to visit who has an infection.	Visitors may introduce infection.	Visitors monitored.
	Use protective isolation techniques if needed.	If neutrophil count <500, initiate protective isolation.	Isolation not yet initiated.
	Encourage good nutrition and hydration.	Good nutrition and hydration minimizes irritation.	Taking sufficient food and fluid; continue plan.
	Give Neupogen as ordered.	Neupogen raises the WBC and neutrophil count.	Neupogen 300 mcg Subcut given 1 time/day.

PROBLEM/NURSING DIAGNOSIS *Receiving chemotherapy*/Risk for injury related to impaired blood clotting ability.

Supporting assessment data *Objective:* Receiving chemotherapy. (Chemotherapy treatment lowers platelets and extends bleeding time.)

Goals/Expected Outcomes	Nursing Interventions	Selected Rationale	Evaluation
Patient will remain free from hemorrhage	Monitor blood count; assess for bleeding of gums or bruising and bleeding into joints q shift.	Blood count plays an important role in blood clotting and bleeding.	WBCs 3200; platelet count 180,000.
	Observe for signs of bleeding: hematuria, melena, etc.		No signs of bleeding.
	Refrain from needle sticks as much as possible.		
	Give stool softener as ordered to prevent straining at stool and bleeding.	Hard stools can initiate bleeding in the rectum.	BM soft; continue plan.
	Avoid rectal bleeding.		Stool softener administered.
	Do not take temperature rectally.		Oral temp: 98.8° F (37.1° C).
	Brush teeth with very soft brush or tooth sponge. Do not floss.	Avoid bleeding gums.	Appropriate dental hygiene.

NURSING CARE PLAN 8–1

Care of the Patient with Cancer—cont'd

PROBLEM/NURSING DIAGNOSIS *Nauseated with no appetite*/Alteration of nutrition (less than body requirements), related to nausea, vomiting, and mucositis.

Supporting assessment data *Subjective:* "I feel nauseated." *Objective:* Chemotherapy administration.

Goals/Expected Outcomes	Nursing Interventions	Selected Rationale	Evaluation
Patient will verbalize relief from nausea	Keep room odor free; give mouth care before meals.	Odors may aggravate nausea.	
Patient will be able to eat with minimal discomfort	Give ordered antiemetic before and during chemotherapy.	Antiemetics help prevent chemotherapy-induced nausea and vomiting (N&V).	Antiemetic 45 min before meals.
Patient will maintain present weight	Assess mouth and mucous membranes q shift.	Sore mouth may reduce food intake.	Mucous membranes reddened, but intact.
	Give meticulous mouth care q 2 hr.		Mouth care: 7, 9, 11, 1, and 3 o'clock.
	Use distraction, meditation, relaxation techniques.	N&V may be reduced with behavioral interventions.	Has not vomited this shift.
	Give small, frequent feedings.	Experts recommend these dietary interventions.	Enriched shake taken between meals.
	Encourage added calories in meals and food supplements between meals.		

PROBLEM/NURSING DIAGNOSIS *Balding from chemotherapy*/Body image disturbance related to alopecia and weight loss.

Supporting assessment data *Subjective:* "I look awful; I don't want any visitors to see me." *Objective:* Loss of considerable amount of hair from head.

Goals/Expected Outcomes	Nursing Interventions	Selected Rationale	Evaluation
Patient will adjust to new body image within 3 wk as evidenced by verbalization	Encourage him to maintain sense of humor.	Humor is a positive coping strategy.	
	Use caps, head bandana, and eyebrow pencil as needed.	Hair covering may reduce negative body image.	Has not yet lost hair; checking on purchase of wig; family is bringing head scarves.
	Assure him that hair will eventually grow back.		
	Encourage verbalization of feelings; focus on strengths.	Verbalization is a positive coping technique.	Talking more about feelings regarding weight loss and appearance.
	Establish and maintain trusting relationship.		
	Assess spiritual needs; help patient achieve spiritual consolation.		Continue plan.
	Encourage him to obtain clothing that fits.		

Continued

divided over many days, to deliver the optimum dosage with the least amount of effects to normal tissues. The course of radiation is spread over a period of days to weeks. The *rad,* or *radiation absorbed dose,* is the unit used for measuring dosages of radiation.

Teletherapy and brachytherapy are the two types of radiation delivery for use to treat cancer. Teletherapy is *external,* in which the source of radiation is outside the patient. Brachytherapy is *internal,* in which the source of radiation is a radioactive element or substance that has been implanted or injected into the body.

Because of improvements in tumor localization, beam direction, megavoltage machines, planning and prescribing the field to be irradiated, and determining the precise dosage needed, radiation therapy is far more beneficial and less harmful than it was when it was first pioneered. With the *linear accelerator,* and its

NURSING CARE PLAN 8–1

Care of the Patient with Cancer—cont'd

PROBLEM/NURSING DIAGNOSIS *Expressing fear of dying*/Fear related to diagnosis of cancer.

Supporting assessment data *Subjective:* "Do you really think the treatment will cure my cancer? I'm afraid that I'll go through all this and it will just come back in a few months."

Goals/Expected Outcomes	Nursing Interventions	Selected Rationale	Evaluation
Patient will verbalize fears and develop coping mechanisms to decrease fear	Encourage verbalization and identification of specific fears.	Verbalizing fears makes them easier to face.	Is verbalizing fears; encouraged to do same with family.
	Help him to explore ways to cope with fears.	Knowing what to expect helps people plan.	Used to meditate; encouraged to do so.
	Assess spiritual needs; contact minister or other as patient desires.	Patients have their own beliefs about death.	Began teaching imagery techniques.
	Offer support by active listening, offering hope in some form, and be there for patient.	Active listening provides comfort and strength.	
	Encourage expression of fears to significant others.	When significant others are aware of the patient's fears they have a better understanding of behavior.	Continue plan.

? CRITICAL THINKING QUESTIONS

1. What is another nursing diagnosis that may apply to a patient who is receiving chemotherapy?
2. Why should the nurse be concerned about infection in a patient who is receiving chemotherapy?

partner, the *cyclotron*, the damage to normal tissue can be minimized by keeping the dosage or degree of penetration accurate and by aiming the rays from several different angles. The latter technique increases the concentration of the rays in the area of the tumor with a minimum of damage to overlying tissues. Cobalt-60 machines deliver gamma rays and are much more efficient and precise than in the early years of radiation therapy. Also, today's techniques result in painless radiation administration.

External Radiation Therapy

The linear accelerator used for external radiation therapy produces a voltage many times higher than machines used for diagnostic purposes. It produces extremely high-energy x-ray and electron beam irradiation that bombards the malignant cells and destroys them. Because malignant cells are dividing at an abnormally high rate, they are more susceptible to destruction than are normal cells.

Modern radiation therapy has improved immensely since the mid-1980s. The use of computers in planning accurate radiation dosage and projectory distributions has decreased the side effects considerably. Since DNA is the critical target for radiation damage, the increased knowledge about DNA gained from the Human Genome Project has also helped streamline radiation therapy. The use of *stereotactic* (exact positioning in space) surgery is effective for small brain tumors (Figure 8–4). Many cancer research institutions have lead-lined surgical suites where intraoperative radiation therapy may be delivered directly to the affected area after tumor removal and before the incision is closed. Depending on the dosage (rads) given, the patient may not need to receive further radiation. This method has proven beneficial for cancers of the head and neck, abdomen, pelvis, and extremities and for patients with operable pancreatic cancer.

Nursing Care of Patients Undergoing External Radiation Therapy. Nursing care goals related to radiation therapy for cancer include (1) helping the patient and family or significant others cope with the diagnosis of cancer and its treatment with radiation therapy; and (2) teaching the patient and significant others how to recognize and manage the expected side effects of radiation.

Helping Patients Cope with Radiation Therapy for Cancer. A lack of knowledge about the side effects of radiation and how to cope with them can greatly add to the anxiety and stress that the patient feels. It is not unusual for a layperson to have some misconceptions about how radiation works, whether a patient can present a hazard to others while undergoing treat-

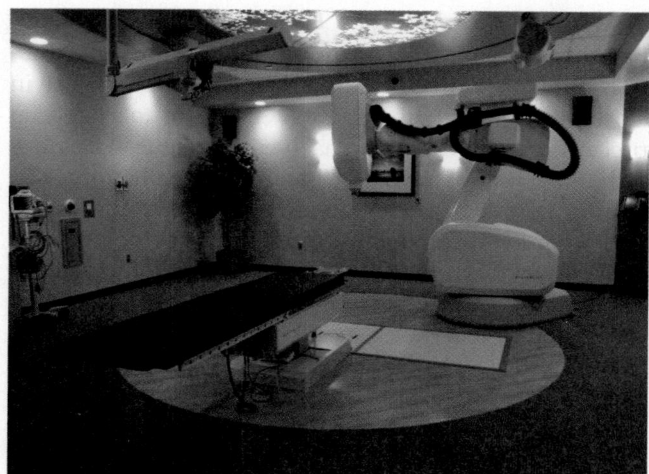

FIGURE 8–4 Cyberknife used to deliver radiation to a small brain tumor. It is particularly useful for recurrence of tumor.

ment, when she will begin to experience its effects, and how long it will be before she begins to recover from them.

Before the first treatment, the patient is told what therapeutic effects are anticipated, what it is like to have a treatment, and what is expected of her during the course of therapy. Because the patient will probably be treated on an outpatient basis, she should be encouraged to keep her scheduled appointments and notify the clinic if cancellation is necessary. Assurance that the source of radiation is in the machine only and that it is not possible to "contaminate" others with radioactivity should be provided. Someone should accompany the patient for initial treatments, preferably a family member or a close and trusted friend, who can provide emotional support. It is essential that time be set aside for the nurse to establish a trusting relationship with the patient, to prompt and answer any questions about therapy, and to provide an avenue for communication throughout the course of treatment.

Skin Care During Radiation Treatment. With the advanced methods and computerized delivery of radiation, there is much less trauma to the skin from radiation therapy than in previous years. The patient should understand that should skin damage occur, it is usually only temporary.

In preparation for radiation therapy, the physician will outline the area to be exposed to radiation by marking it with indelible ink. The exposed area will need special care. Most clinics and hospitals have written procedures and precautions to be used to avoid unnecessary trauma to the exposed areas of skin.

In general, the area is washed with warm water and mild soap throughout the course of treatments (McQuestion, 2006). 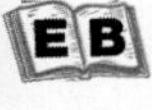 Only the hand is used, rather than a wash cloth. The area is gently patted dry with a clean, soft, towel; it is never rubbed. Alcohol, lotions, salves, powder, and makeup must not be used, unless prescribed by the physician, as they either dry out the skin or magnify any radiation damage. The patient should be advised to not remove any of the markings for radiation treatments.

The patient should be instructed to avoid lying on the area as much as possible and to avoid wearing tight clothing over it. Only 100% cotton clothing should be worn over the area. She also should avoid exposing it to sunlight and extremes of cold as well as heat, including hot shower water. Patients should not shave the treated area, or if they must, an electric razor should be used. Although skin damage is rare now, the degree of reaction of the skin to radiation is individual and should be assessed daily, either by the patient or some knowledgeable person.

? *Think Critically About* . . . Can you list the points to be covered for care of the skin when teaching the patient who is to undergo external radiation therapy?

Teaching the patient and significant others how to recognize expected side effects and take an active part in their management is particularly important when the patient is not hospitalized. She will feel less helpless and more in control if she is able to participate in assessing her condition and planning and implementing her care at home. It is unfair to expect either the patient or her significant others to remember everything they are told about her care. Therefore, it is essential that they have some written information to refer to once they leave the clinic. They also should be encouraged to write down any questions they might have before the next visit or note any points on which they feel they need more information.

Internal Radiation Therapy

Radiation from *radioactive elements* has the same ionizing effect as that from linear accelerators; the only difference is the source of radiation. The nuclei of radioactive elements are unstable for differing reasons. These nuclei spontaneously decay in an effort to become stable, and in the process they emit various particles as well as radiant energy. Some elements, such as radium and uranium, are naturally unstable and therefore radioactive. These elements are used as sealed implants. Other elements such as cobalt and iodine can be made unstable by being bombarded with high-energy particles in a nuclear reactor.

Internal radiation therapy involves introducing a radioactive element into the body. The material may be administered in different ways: (1) it can be placed in a *sealed* container and inserted into a body cavity at the site of the tumor or placed directly into the tumor; or (2) it may be administered in an *unsealed* form and taken orally or injected by syringe.

To be effective, the radiation source must come into direct contact with the tumor tissue for a specified time. Most implants emit a lower level of radiation than is effective because they are in constant contact with the tumor cells. **Because the radiation source is within the patient, radiation is emitted for a period and can be a hazard to others.**

As soon as an element becomes radioactive, it begins to lose its characteristic of radioactivity. The rate at which it becomes less radioactive is called its *half-life*, which is the amount of time it takes for half of its radioactivity to dissipate. The half-life of radium is about 1600 years, whereas the half-life of iodine is only about 8 days. It is important that the nurse caring for a patient receiving sealed or unsealed sources of radiation know the element used, its half-life, and the ways in which it might be eliminated from the body. Cesium is a radioactive element frequently used to treat malignancies of the mouth, tongue, vagina, and uterine cervix.

Some isotopes are given orally and others are administered into a body cavity. The isotopes are unsealed sources of radiation. If radioactivity is a hazard, it is a problem only for the duration of the half-life of the isotope. The substance is eliminated through body secretions such as sweat, sputum, vomit, urine, or feces. Examples of unsealed sources include iodine-131, which is in a solution and is swallowed by the patient, phosphorus-32, and gold-198, which is administered by injection. Radioactive iodine is useful in the treatment of thyroid malignancies because that gland readily takes up iodine. Thus the radioactive element is delivered to the site of the tumor, where it can be more effective. The major hazard from radioactive iodine is in the patient's urine, but iodine is also excreted in the feces and sweat; therefore, special precautions must be taken according to hospital policy. **The nurse must know the half-life of the isotope given to plan appropriate safety precautions. Hospital policies and procedures must be followed when caring for a patient receiving an unsealed source of radiation.**

Nursing Care of Patients Receiving Internal Radiation. Patients who are treated by internal sources of radiation can be a source of radioactivity. Those who are in close contact with them must therefore take special precautions to protect themselves against unnecessary radiation. Radioactivity is a frightening phenomenon to most people because they do not fully understand it and are misinformed about how it affects the body.

It is important that the nurse know whether the radioactive element is sealed and inserted into the body to remain for a certain time, or it is an unsealed source that may be eliminated through body secretions and excreta. Unsealed sources usually have a very short half-life, which means they are not radioactive for as long as sealed sources are.

Principles of Radiation Protection

In general, the amount of radiation a nurse might receive while caring for a patient being treated with internal radioactive elements depends on three factors: (1) the distance between the nurse and the patient; (2) the amount of time spent in actual proximity to the patient; and (3) the degree of shielding provided.

Distance is an important factor in reducing exposure to radiation. Doubling one's distance from a radioactive element, reduces the exposure to one fourth, and tripling the distance reduces it to one ninth (Figure 8–5).

Time spent near the source of radiation can be controlled by the nurse who plans his nursing care carefully so that he can spend less time with the patient without sacrificing the quality of care given. The total time should be less than 30 minutes per 8-hour shift.

Shielding from radiation exposure must take into account the type of rays being emitted. The denser the shielding material, the less the possibility of penetration by the rays and the better the protection. A lead

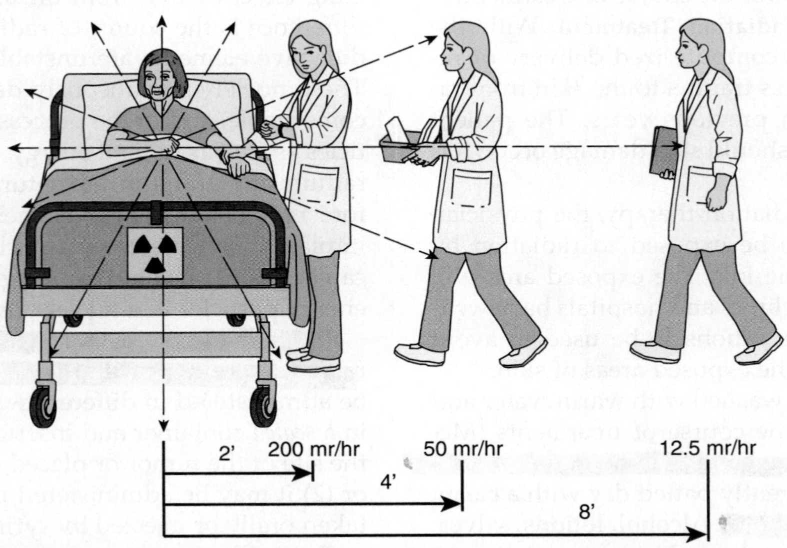

FIGURE 8–5 Time, distance, and shielding in radiation exposure. The nurse nearest the source of radioactivity (the patient) is more exposed; at 2 feet, exposure is more than 15 times than at 8 feet.

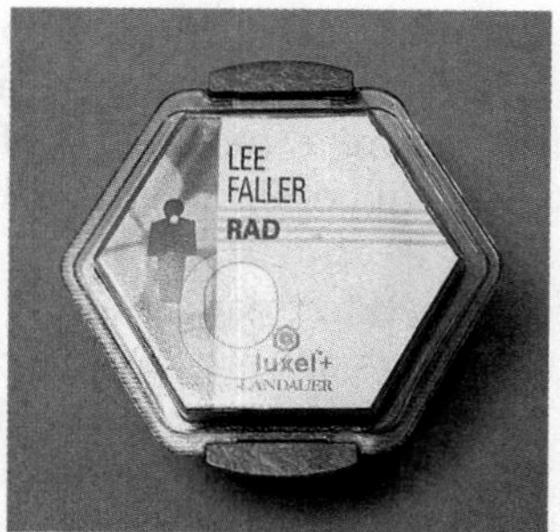

FIGURE 8–6 Radiation counter badge worn by personnel who might be exposed to radiation.

shield that is 1 cm thick offers the same amount of protection as 5 cm of concrete or 30 cm of wood. Lead aprons give protection from diagnostic x-rays, but do not provide adequate shielding from the *gamma rays* emitted by radium, cesium-137, and cobalt-60. Anyone coming into contact with or in proximity to a source of radiation should wear a radiation dosimeter badge (Figure 8–6). This badge measures the radiation dose that the individual has received through exposure to the source.

Hospitals where sealed sources of radiation are implanted into the body tissues to treat malignancies usually have written policies and procedures to guide personnel who are responsible for patient care. General precautions for the patient with a sealed source of radiation are in Box 8–5. After the physician removes the source, the patient is no longer in need of special precautionary care. Special observations are necessary, however, in the event a systemic reaction develops.

Box 8–5 *Precautionary Measures When a Patient Is Receiving Internal Radiation Therapy from a Sealed Source*

- Place the patient in a private room.
- Place a sign on the patient's door indicating that the patient is receiving internal radiation therapy.
- Observe principles of time and distance. Limit time spent in the room. Work as quickly and as efficiently as possible. Avoid standing near the part of the patient's body where the radioactive element is located; stand at the shoulders or the feet depending where the implant is located.
- Check all linens, bedpans, and emesis basins routinely to see if the sealed source has been accidentally lost from the tissue.
- If a sealed source is dislodged, but has not fallen out of the patient's body, notify the x-ray department at once. If the source has fallen out, *do not pick it up with your bare hands.* Use forceps and place it in a lead container.
- Most patients are placed on bed rest and instructed to remain in certain positions so that emanations from the element will reach the correct area.
- Visitors will spend limited time in the room.
- No children or pregnant women should visit.

Box 8–6 *Precautions When Caring for the Patient Receiving Internal Radiation from an Unsealed Source*

- Observe the principles of time, distance, and shielding for radiation protection.
- Wear gloves when handling bedpans, bed linens, and patient's clothes.
- Dispose of urine, feces, and vomitus according to policy.
- Handle dressings with forceps and dispose of them according to policy.
- Follow hospital procedure for disposal of patient's bed linens and clothing.

Some special precautions that should be observed when caring for a patient receiving internal radiation therapy from an unsealed source are found in Box 8–6. Table 8–4 shows the side effects most commonly experienced by patients undergoing radiation therapy.

Appropriate nursing care for problems related to radiation therapy is presented in the section on common problems related to cancer or cancer therapy.

CHEMOTHERAPY

The oncologist has a wide variety of drugs from which to choose when planning a course of treatment for a patient with cancer. He may choose to give a particular drug alone or in combination with other drugs. Chemotherapy may be used with other forms of therapy,

Table 8–4 *Common Side Effects of Radiation Therapy*

TYPE AND AREA	EFFECT
EXTERNAL RADIATION	
Head and neck	• Irritation of oral mucous membranes with oral pain and risk of infection • Loss of taste • Irritation of the pharynx and esophagus with nausea and indigestion • Increased intracranial pressure
Chest	• Inflammation of lung tissue with increased susceptibility to infection
Abdomen	• Nausea, vomiting, diarrhea, anorexia
Pelvis	• Diarrhea • Cystitis • Sexual dysfunction • Urethral and rectal stenosis
General side effects	• *Skin:* Change in texture and/or color; moist desquamation (rare); alopecia • *Blood:* Bone marrow depression with leukopenia, anemia, and thrombocytopenia • Depressed immune function • Fatigue
INTERNAL RADIATION	
General effects	• Elevated temperature • *Cervical implant:* Urinary frequency, diarrhea, nausea, vomiting, anorexia • *Head and neck implant:* Mucositis, oral pain and risk of infection, anorexia

for example, following surgery and before, during, or after radiation treatments, or with immunotherapy.

Among the drugs used to treat malignancies are the *antineoplastic* agents (Table 8–5). **The overall effect of antineoplastic drugs is to decrease the number of malignant cells in a generalized malignancy, such as leukemia, or to reduce the size of a localized tumor and thereby lessen the severity of symptoms.** Antineoplastic drugs are cytotoxic (poisonous to cells), and their damaging effects are not limited to malignant cells. However, normal cells do not reproduce in exactly the same way as malignant cells and are able to repair themselves more rapidly and effectively. Steroids often are used in combination with antineoplastic drugs for cancer treatment.

Drugs are combined to treat certain types of cancers because different drugs are effective at different times in the growth and replication cycle of the tumor cell. This method offers the best chance of killing the most malignant cells. Chemotherapy is the preferred treat-

Table 8–5 *Common Antineoplastic Drug Classes, Their Action, and Major Side Effects*

CLASSIFICATION AND EXAMPLES	ACTION	MAJOR SIDE EFFECTS*
ALKYLATING AGENTS		
Cyclophosphamide Cisplatin Mechlorethamine Busulfan Chlorambucil Dacarbazine Melphalan Streptozocin Lomustine Thiotepa	Attach "alkyl groups" or organic side chains to the proteins in the cell, poisoning it; inhibit cell division.	Bone marrow depression, nephrotoxicity, with some. Nausea, vomiting, diarrhea, dermatitis; hyperpigmentation. Cisplatin: Hearing loss.
ANTIMETABOLITES		
Methotrexate 6-Mercaptopurine 6-Thioguanine 5-Fluorouracil Floxuridine Gemcitabine Cytarabine	Interfere with a specific cell phase, thereby preventing replication. Some inhibit enzymes that make essential cellular constituents; others attach to DNA, interfering with replication.	Bone marrow depression, stomatitis, intestinal ulceration, nausea, vomiting, diarrhea.
ANTITUMOR ANTIBIOTICS		
Bleomycin Carboplatin Dactinomycin Doxorubicin Daunorubicin Plicamycin Mitomycin-C Mitoxantrone	Injure cells by direct interaction with DNA, causing distortion. Interfere with DNA or RNA synthesis.	Bone marrow depression, some cause cardiotoxicity; stomatitis, alopecia. Bleomycin causes pneumonitis and pulmonary fibrosis.
MITOTIC INHIBITORS		
Vincristine Vinblastine Vinorelbine Etoposide	Interfere with mitosis. Act during M phase of cell cycle to prevent cell division.	Vincristine: Peripheral neuropathy, constipation. Vinblastine: Bone marrow depression.
MISCELLANEOUS AGENTS		
Altretamine Asparaginase Etoposide Hydroxyurea Procarbazine Mitotane Teniposide Paclitaxel Imatinib mesylate Epirubicin Docetaxel Cladribine	These drugs work in a variety of ways; consult information for each drug.	Bone marrow depression is the major side effect of all except asparaginase and mitotane. Asparaginase: Pancreatic dysfunction. Mitotane: Central nervous system depression. Paclitaxel: Peripheral neuropathy.
HORMONE-RELATED AGENTS		
Tamoxifen	Lowers circulating hormone levels to prevent hormone-related tumors	Hot flushes; deep venous thrombosis; cancer

*Each drug has specific side effects. Consult information regarding each individual drug before administration.

ment for various kinds of leukemias, some lymphomas, multiple myeloma, and many types of tumors resulting from metastasis.

Techniques of administration of antineoplastic agents include intra-arterial, intraperitoneal, intraventricular, and *intrathecal* (within a space of the spine) as well as intravenous infusion. Cancers of the liver, ovary, and brain have sometimes shown better remission with intraventricular or intraperitoneal infusion treatment. An advance in chemotherapy has been the use of lower doses of multiple drugs to treat various types of malignancies. Because side effects are lessened when lower doses of a drug are used, several drugs can be used in combination to hit all phases of the cell cycle, destroying more malignant cells.

Often a central line or implanted injection port is used to administer chemotherapy drugs that are to be given over several weeks or months (Figure 8–7). The nurse cares for the central line and its insertion site according to hospital policy using strict aseptic technique.

Many antineoplastic drugs are **vesicants** (chemicals causing tissue damage upon direct contact) that can cause severe local injury if they escape from the vein into which they are administered. Administration should be only into veins that have good blood flow. If *extravasation* (escape from the vein into the tissue) occurs, the infusion is stopped immediately. The type of treatment required depends on the drug that extravasated and the amount that escaped into the tissue. **Consult the pharmacist, the policy and procedures manual, and the physician should extravasation occur.**

Some antineoplastic drugs have toxic effects that must be monitored. Table 8–6 presents the assessments necessary to detect various types of organ toxicity. One drug, dexrazoxane (Zinecard), appears to be heart protective for patients receiving the cardiotoxic drug doxorubicin (Adriamycin). If a drug is toxic to the reproductive system, the patient should make a decision about banking sperm or eggs before beginning chemotherapy.

Nursing Care of Patients Receiving Chemotherapy

Nursing management of the patient receiving chemotherapy requires special knowledge and skills beyond those of basic nursing. The nurse oncologist is a specialist who is able to give comprehensive nursing care because of years of study and experience. A full discussion of care of the patient receiving chemotherapy is therefore beyond the scope of this text. There are, however, some general principles that can be helpful to the nurse who encounters a patient receiving a course of chemotherapy for cancer or experiencing some of the toxic side effects of antineoplastic drugs.

Not all antineoplastic drugs produce every toxic side effect, and the oncologist plans therapy so that destruction of malignant cells is maximized and toxicity is kept at a minimum. **The toxicity associated with chemotherapy is most evident in the cells of the body that have a short life span and must continuously reproduce to provide the body with the normal cells it needs. These include the blood cells, hair follicles, and epithelial cells of the mucous membranes lining the digestive tract. Most chemotherapeutics are excreted in the body fluids, so precautions should be taken. Remember, most of these drugs are *teratogenic* (can cause birth defects), so they should be avoided during pregnancy.**

The more common side effects of chemotherapy and their implications for nursing are summarized in Table 8–5. Some of the side effects of chemotherapy are similar to the expected effects of radiation. Although the causes of the problems are different, assessment of

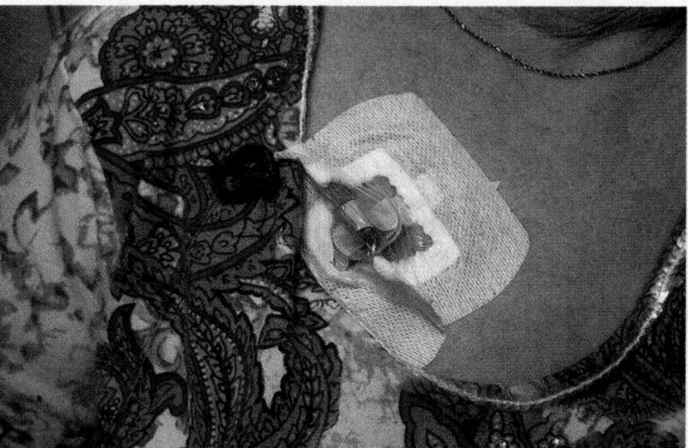

FIGURE 8–7 Implanted infusion port for administration of chemotherapy drugs or continuous morphine drip.

Table 8–6 Assessment for Toxic Effects of Chemotherapy*

SIDE EFFECT	INTERVENTION
Bone marrow suppression	Monitor red and white blood cell count and differential count for numbers of neutrophils and granulocytes; check platelet count.
Cardiotoxicity	Monitor for signs of congestive heart failure, such as pulmonary crackles, shortness of breath, tachycardia, weight gain, and peripheral edema. Monitor ECG.
Neurotoxicity	Monitor for weakness, paresthesias, sensory loss (particularly in feet), and decreased reflexes. Constipation and urinary hesitancy are other signs.
Pulmonary toxicity	Evidenced by pulmonary infiltrates and pulmonary fibrosis on x-ray. Monitor respiratory status closely; auscultate for decreased breath sounds and for crackles.
Hepatotoxicity	Monitor liver function tests: AST, ALT, bilirubin.
Nephrotoxicity	Monitor kidney function tests: creatinine and blood urea nitrogen; monitor urine output.
Ototoxicity	Monitor for tinnitus or hearing loss.

Key: *ALT,* alanine aminotransferase; *AST,* aspartate aminotransferase; *ECG,* electrocardiogram.

*Many antineoplastic drugs are toxic to various organs of the body. Whenever a specific drug has one of these toxicities, include the specific assessment parameters for that toxicity in your regular assessment.

the patient and symptomatic relief measures are the same. Nursing interventions for selected problems in a patient receiving chemotherapy for cancer are summarized in Nursing Care Plan 8–1 (see p. 170).

HORMONE THERAPY

Hormone therapy is used as an adjunct to other types of cancer therapy. It can slow tumor growth or prevent recurrence. When a hormone is added to the body, it alters the balance of naturally produced hormones. **Giving large amounts of one hormone prevents the uptake of other hormones. So if the tumor growth is aided by one type of hormone, giving another type prevents the uptake of the growth-promoting hormone and slows the progress of the tumor.** Tamoxifen used against certain types of breast cancer is an example. Tamoxifen has been shown to be chemopreventive for women with high risk factors and for recurrence for certain types of breast cancer (Smith et al., 2005).

EB

Side effects of hormone therapy depend on the type of hormone used. Androgens and anti–estrogen receptor drugs produce masculinizing effects, such as facial and chest hair. Menses may stop and breast tissue will shrink. These drugs cause fluid retention in women. Acne is another side effect of the androgens. Hypercalcemia and liver dysfunction can occur with prolonged therapy. Women taking estrogens and progestins have irregular heavy menses, fluid retention, and tenderness of the breasts. These drugs increase the risk for thrombus formation in both men and women. In men taking estrogens or progestins to combat prostate cancer, there is a feminizing effect with decreased facial hair, a redistribution of body fat, breast development (*gynecomastia*), and smoothing of the facial skin. Over time, some testicular and penile atrophy may occur, and it may become more difficult to attain and maintain an erection.

IMMUNOTHERAPY USING BIOLOGIC RESPONSE MODIFIERS

Biologic response modifiers (BRMs) are agents that manipulate the immune system in the hope of controlling or curing a malignancy with little or no toxic effect on normal cells. These agents either stimulate or suppress immune activity. The BRMs include interferons, interleukins, colony-stimulating factors, monoclonal antibodies, vaccines, gene therapy, and nonspecific immunomodulating agents. They essentially make the immune system function better. BRMs stimulate the immune system to recognize cancer cells and to institute action to destroy them. Some BRMs, such as colony-stimulating factor (CSF), work by enhancing a quicker recovery of the bone marrow after radiation or chemotherapy. CSF stimulates bone marrow to function more quickly. Neumega (interleukin-11) is a drug that stimulates thrombocyte (platelet) production. This drug is used to decrease the bleeding tendencies induced by chemotherapy and could help create new chemotherapy protocols that are more effective against cancer cells.

There are two types of BRMs used to fight cancer: interleukins and interferons. **Interleukins help the immune system cells recognize and destroy abnormal cells. Interferons slow down cell division in cancer cells, stimulate natural killer cells, hold back the appearance of oncogenes, and assist cancerous cells to revert back to more normal cells.** Both interleukins and interferons are manufactured using *recombinant* (artificial DNA sequence) DNA technology. Interleukins are undergoing clinical trials on patients with melanoma, renal cell carcinoma, and colorectal cancer. Alfa-2b, an interferon, is used mainly against hairy cell leukemia, but it has been somewhat effective to treat ovarian cancer, renal cell cancer, and cutaneous T-cell lymphoma. Both interleukins and interferons are very expensive to manufacture.

A second group of BRMs includes monoclonal antibodies (MoAbs) and tumor necrosis factor, both of which have direct antitumor effects. Genetic engineering techniques can produce the monoclonal antibodies, and thus this form of therapy holds much promise for the future. Rituximab (Rituxan) and trastuzumab (Herceptin) are examples of MoAbs that have been approved by the U.S. Food and Drug Administration. Rituxan is used in the treatment of non-Hodgkin's lymphoma, and Herceptin is used for the treatment of metastatic breast cancer in patients who produce an excess amount of a protein called HER-2.

The third group contains miscellaneous agents that have different functions. This group includes cancer vaccines, which may stimulate the immune system to attack the cancer cells (therapeutic) or stimulate the production of antibodies against a cancer-causing virus (prophylactic). Also included are nonspecific immunomodulating agents that may stimulate the immune system and either restore depressed immune function or increase immune inflammatory responses. Epoetin (Epogen) and filgrastim (Neupogen) are given when the red or white blood cell count, respectively, is low. These drugs have no antitumor activity, but they assist the cancer patient by stimulating erythrocyte production, thus helping to avoid blood transfusions.

BONE MARROW TRANSPLANTATION

Bone marrow transplantation (BMT) is mainly used to correct the severe bone marrow damage caused by chemotherapy or radiation. Sometimes whole-body irradiation is used to treat a hematopoietic cancer such as leukemia or Hodgkin's disease. Irradiation of this sort totally incapacitates the body's bone marrow, and the patient would die if blood cells could not again be manufactured. BMT is discussed in Chapter 16.

GENE THERAPY

As research reveals the genes thought to be responsible for various types of cancers, the possibility of gene splicing or replacement becomes a reality. Genetic engineering is still in its infancy, but many scientists are hard at work hoping to make it a reality for cancer patients. The genes *BRCA1* and *BRCA2* are implicated in approximately half of the cases of inherited breast and ovarian cancer. Research has shown that when healthy *BRCA1* genes are injected into mice that have faulty *BRCA1* genes, tumor growth is slowed. This has proven true for other genes implicated in other types of cancer. Some day gene therapy may be the major treatment for cancer.

EVALUATING THE EFFECTIVENESS OF MEDICAL TREATMENT

The oncologist conducts an ongoing evaluation of each patient's status to determine how effective the prescribed treatment has been and to plan for a future course of therapy should it be needed. It is particularly important to know whether there has been a reduction in the size of the tumor and an abatement of the patient's symptoms. This is the purpose of "second-look surgery."

A test for monitoring the effectiveness of treatment is a measurement of CEA levels. This particular antigen is a glycoprotein that is produced during fetal life but is not normally present after birth. Its production may resume again, however, and CEA levels can be increased by some kinds of liver disease, heavy cigarette smoking, and especially gastrointestinal and colorectal cancers. Because of the many and diverse conditions that can elevate CEA levels, the test cannot be used to diagnose cancer. However, it can be used as a tumor marker to evaluate the effectiveness of treatment, because CEA levels usually fall to within the normal range about 1 month after successful treatment of cancer. Other tumor markers, such as PSA for prostate cancer and CA-125 for ovarian cancer, are used to track the success of treatment and recurrence in those cancers.

COMMON PROBLEMS RELATED TO CANCER OR CANCER THERAPY

The problems that occur in the cancer patient are complex and depend on both the location and type of cancer and the therapy used to treat it. A discussion of the most common problems and the related nursing care is presented here.

ANOREXIA, MUCOSITIS, AND WEIGHT LOSS

Many cancer patients experience an alteration in taste. Often the first thing noticed is that red meat does not taste good. The taste of sweets also is altered. *Anorexia* (loss of appetite) often is associated with changes in taste and with inflammation of the mouth and tongue, which can cause the patient great difficulty in eating and drinking. The loss of appetite can quickly lead to deficiencies of protein and calories. **The patient with anorexia can experience a significant weight loss (2 or more pounds per week) and suffer from severe malnutrition.** A synthetic substance derived from the female hormone progesterone, megestrol (Megace), has proven to work well to stimulate the appetite. A thorough routine for mouth care to minimize damage and anorexia should be started several days before the beginning of chemotherapy or radiation therapy to the head and neck. Radiation to the head or neck will produce some inflammatory changes in the mouth and often also in the pharynx and esophagus. Measures to combat this expected reaction include frequent oral intake of liquids that are not irritating chemically, the use of artificial saliva, and frequent and consistent mouth care.

Patients are encouraged to drink water as often as they can to help alleviate the discomfort of dryness of the mouth and tongue. However, drinking water will not completely resolve the problem. Artificial saliva combats mouth dryness in a different way and helps keep the mucous membranes soft and moist. It also helps buffer the acidity in the mouth and thus reduce irritation of the oral mucosa. It is available in the form of a spray (Salivart) and a gel (Biotene Oral Balance) and can be used by the patient as often as desired. If artificial saliva cannot be found at a local pharmacy, it can be obtained online from most of the online drugstores.

The patient undergoing chemotherapy may experience *mucositis* (irritation and inflammation of the mucosa) in the mouth. A major goal of mouth care, other than protection of the mucosa, is preservation of the teeth and prevention of infections of the gums. To accomplish this, the patient should be encouraged to accept as much responsibility as she can for frequent and consistent oral hygiene. She probably will need to be taught how to brush her teeth using a soft brush or tooth sponges (toothettes) and gentle strokes. She also should be taught how to irrigate her mouth to remove debris and counteract acidity. The solutions most often used for this are normal saline, mild solutions of peroxide (1:5 ratio), or a bicarbonate of soda and salt solution (¼ to ½ tsp of baking soda and ⅛ to ¼ tsp salt in an 8-oz glass of water). Fluid intake must be increased to 3000 mL/day. Because of the risk of infection, toothbrushes should be rinsed with a bleach solution or hydrogen peroxide and then rinsed with water before reuse. Running them through the dishwasher is another option.

Relief of the mouth pain of mucositis or *stomatitis* (inflammation of the mouth) is provided by special topical compounds, such as Xylocaine Viscous, that are "swished and spit." Such compounds contain a topical anesthetic and an anti-inflammatory agent. **The patient is instructed not to swallow this solution.** The patient should avoid spicy foods, alcohol, and tobacco.

The metabolic demand of malignant growth, anorexia, and mucositis that makes eating difficult all contribute to weight loss. Weight loss also can occur in cancer patients because of disturbances in their metabolism in which the body metabolizes its own proteins for energy instead of using the carbohydrates available in the diet or in body fat. The body has to work hard to repair normal cells after cancer treatment. Initially, the patient's current weight should be noted and recorded and compared with her ideal weight. Her protein intake should be increased to compensate for the fact that cancer patients often metabolize their own tissues for energy, even though glucose may be readily available in the blood. Small, frequent feedings, attention to preferences for foods, and a pleasant and restful environment during meals are often helpful. Supplemental feedings to provide additional protein and calories can help avoid excessive weight loss and protein deficiency (Nutritional Therapies 8–2). These taste better if they are served in glass or plastic rather than out of a metal container. The ACS has patient pamphlets available on ways to increase nutritional intake.

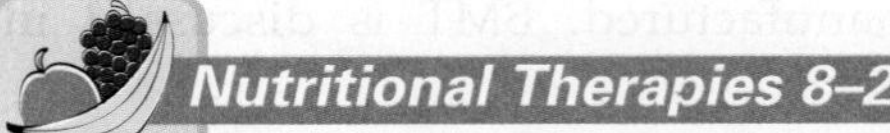

Nutritional Therapies 8–2

Nutritional Formulas and Preparations for Supplemental Feedings

PRODUCT	COMPANY
Carnation Instant Breakfast	Clintec/Carnation
Delmark Instant Breakfast	Sandoz
Forta Shake	Ross
Meritene Powder	Novartis
Sustacal Powder, Sustacal Liquid	Mead, Johnson
Ensure	Abbott
Promote	Ross
Isocal	Novartis
Prosobee	Mead, Johnson
Resource	Sandoz

NOTE: Other protein products and "energy" booster products are available at health food stores and sporting goods stores. Patients should sample various supplements in liquid and bar form to find the ones that are most pleasing.

NAUSEA, VOMITING, AND DIARRHEA

Radiation therapy of the abdomen or lower back often produces nausea, vomiting, and diarrhea starting 7 to 10 days after the beginning of treatment. Various antineoplastic drugs also can produce these side effects. Antiemetic regimens should be chosen based on the potential of the chemotherapy regimen to cause nausea. Dose and timing vary for the antiemetic agents, but the regimen (consisting of several different drugs) is usually started 30 minutes to an hour prior to doses of chemotherapy and continued 1 to 2 days afterward. Antiemetics are used for nausea and vomiting resulting from radiation therapy as well. A class of antiemetics commonly used, serotonin antagonists, acts on the chemoreceptor trigger zone for vomiting and has proven very beneficial to the chemotherapy patient. These drugs are working for previously resistant chemotherapy-induced nausea and vomiting.

Eating before treatment seems to decrease nausea. Eating toast or crackers before arising or engaging in activity during periods of nausea may decrease vomiting. Liquids, liquid supplements, or easily digested foods are given at 3- to 4-hour intervals in small amounts. Foods and liquids should be high in protein and calories, bland, lukewarm, and to the patient's taste. Meals should be eaten slowly and food chewed thoroughly. Carbonated drinks or tea is tolerated better than other liquids, but should be taken 1 hour before or after meals, not with meals. It is best not to lie down for at least 2 hours after a meal. Caffeine and rich or fatty foods should be avoided. The patient's environment should be free of bothersome smells, sights, or sounds. If food odor is nauseating, consider serving cold meals. Chewing gum or sucking on hard or sour candy, or ice, helps reduce nausea in some patients. Nursing care involves providing comfort measures and mouth care. If nausea strikes, breathing slowly and deeply through the mouth may prevent vomiting. The patient is monitored for dehydration and electrolyte imbalances when excessive vomiting occurs.

Diarrhea may occur from radiation to the abdomen, lower back, or pelvis. Many of the chemotherapy drugs cause diarrhea because they affect the cells of the intestinal mucosa, causing inflammation. Treatment involves avoiding high-fiber foods that encourage rapid evacuation from the bowel and adding low-fiber foods such as bananas and cheese to the diet. Cleansing the rectal area and applying petroleum jelly, A&D ointment, or Desitin cream helps decrease discomfort and protects the skin from breakdown. The physician may prescribe a medication to decrease the number and frequency of bowel movements. The nurse must monitor the patient for signs of dehydration and electrolyte imbalance.

CONSTIPATION

Certain antineoplastic drugs, such as vincristine, vinblastine, and taxol, cause constipation. Increasing fluids (as allowed), adding fiber to the diet, administering stool softeners and fiber laxatives, exercise, and monitoring vigilantly for the beginning signs of constipation are the usual measures taken. Suppositories or enemas may be necessary.

CYSTITIS

Cytoxan and ifosfamide may cause cystitis. The nurse monitors for hesitancy, urgency, and pain on urination. The urine is checked for cloudiness and signs of *hematuria* (blood in the urine). Fluids are increased to 2 to 3 L/day. The patient is encouraged to empty the bladder frequently. The antineoplastic drug is administered in the morning and/or early afternoon so that most of it can be flushed from the bladder before bedtime, so that the patient sleeps through the night.

IMMUNOSUPPRESSION, BONE MARROW SUPPRESSION, AND INFECTION

Suppression of the bone marrow is the major reason that doses of chemotherapy must be limited. When the marrow is suppressed, meaning its cell production is slowed, few new erythrocytes, leukocytes, or platelets are produced. The reduction of erythrocytes decreases oxygen-carrying power and the patient experiences hypoxia and fatigue. Decreased platelets bring an increased risk of bleeding. A low leukocyte count means lower immune function and lower ability to fight infection.

All antineoplastic drugs cause some degree of bone marrow suppression, but some can cause severe suppression. The amount of suppression is dose related. This is a life-threatening side effect for the patient. The suppression usually is temporary, and improvement in bone marrow function occurs within weeks to months of therapy completion. The white blood cell (WBC) count is monitored for a count of less than 3000/mm^3, indicating neutropenia. Neupogen or Leukine is given to raise the neutrophil count and the WBC count. Often it is started before the count drops so low.

The resultant anemia places an increased workload on the heart and lungs as they attempt adequately to oxygenate the body. When the platelet count reaches a low of 50,000/mm^3, any small injury can lead to an episode of prolonged bleeding. At 20,000/mm^3, spontaneous bleeding that is difficult to control may occur. Therefore, at a count of 100,000/mm^3, the next dose of chemotherapy is withheld. If the count is less than 50,000/mm^3, bleeding precautions are observed (no invasive procedures), and if the count is less than 10,000 to 15,000/mm^3, the patient is transfused. As described earlier, the drug Epogen may be helpful to stimulate red blood cell production and avoid transfusion.

The increased danger of infection is an indication to the nurse to become very attentive to good, frequent, and thorough hand washing and to maintain strict asepsis in all aspects of patient care. If the neutrophil count is below 500 mm^3, follow the policy and procedures for protective isolation to prevent infection. Patient Teaching 8–2 shows the guidelines for teaching the patient ways to decrease the risk of infection after discharge.

Patients with thrombocytopenia can take measures to help lower the risk of bleeding (Patient Teaching 8–3). An infusion of platelets may be administered if

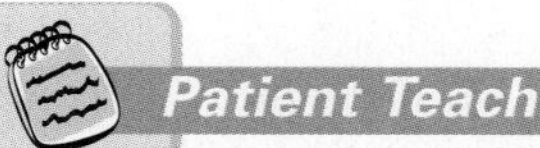

Patient Teaching 8–2

Guidelines for the Patient Prone to Infection Because of Cancer Treatment

- Wash your hands well with an antimicrobial soap or alcohol-based hand rub:
  - Before eating.
  - After using the toilet.
  - After blowing your nose.
  - After handling items many people have handled, such as railings, money, shopping carts, library books, newspapers, and pieces of mail.
  - After touching a pet.
  - After spending time out in public.
- Do not share personal care items (razor, toothbrush, toothpaste, washcloth, towels, deodorant, hand lotion, lipstick, etc.).
- Clean toothbrush by running it through the dishwasher or soaking it in a bleach or hydrogen peroxide solution.
- Stay away from people with respiratory or other infections.
- Bathe daily if possible; use an antimicrobial soap.
- Examine the mouth daily for sores or white patches; perform mouth care frequently.
- Examine the skin, especially the feet, for signs of broken areas daily.
- Wash dishes, utensils, and items used in cooking in hot sudsy water or run them through a dishwasher.
- Drink only fresh, bottled water.
- Do not reuse drinking cups or glasses without washing them.
- Keep lips moist with lip ice or petroleum jelly to avoid cracking.
- Stay out of crowded places.
- Eat only canned or cooked foods.
- If leukocyte count is extremely low, maintain a low-bacteria diet by avoiding salads, raw fruits and vegetables, undercooked meat, pepper, or paprika.
- Do not handle garden flowers, plants, or earth.
- Do not clean out cat litter boxes or bird cages.
- Have someone change water in flower arrangements if such are allowed.
- Monitor temperature daily.
- Be careful not to nick or scratch the skin.
- Report the following signs of infection to the physician immediately:
  - Temperature over 100° F (38° C).
  - Persistent cough.
  - Colored or foul-smelling drainage from wound or nose.
  - Presence of a boil or abscess.
  - Cloudy, foul-smelling urine or burning on urination.

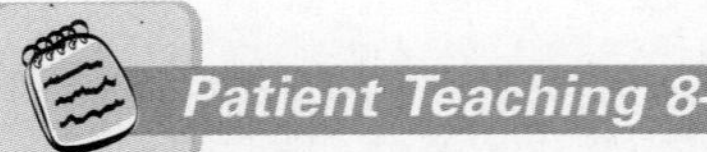

Patient Teaching 8–3

Guidelines to Prevent Bleeding and Bruising in the Patient with a Low Platelet Count

- Use a soft toothbrush and brush lightly; do not floss.
- Use only an electric razor or depilatory for shaving.
- Avoid constipation by increasing fluid and roughage in the diet; take a stool softener if needed.
- Caution health care workers not to use a tourniquet to obtain blood specimens.
- Tell health care workers what normal blood pressure is so that cuff is not pumped up excessively.
- Avoid nonprescription drugs that inhibit platelet function: aspirin, ibuprofen (Motrin, Advil), Alka-Seltzer. Check for salicylates that inhibit platelet function in all analgesic and cold medicines.
- Move around carefully to avoid bumping into things; avoid contact sports or any sport where falling is a risk.
- If a bump or injury occurs, apply ice to area for 1 hour.
- Avoid tight, constricting clothing or shoes.
- Do not wear jewelry with sharp edges.
- Use ample lubrication for intercourse; avoid anal intercourse.
- Avoid blowing the nose or picking at it; if you must blow, blow gently without occluding either nostril.

the count falls to 20,000/mm^3. The patient must be handled gently. Using a lift sheet helps in turning and repositioning the patient. Needle sticks for injections, laboratory specimens, and intravenous line starts are kept to a minimum. The smallest gauge needle possible for the task should be used. Pressure is applied to the site for 5 to 10 minutes or until bleeding stops. All urine and stool should be tested for the presence of blood. Abdominal girth is measured daily to check for internal bleeding. Ice is applied to any area that is bumped or injured.

The diet is modified to avoid irritating foods. Stool softeners are given to keep the stool soft and to prevent the Valsalva maneuver that occurs with constipation. No rectal suppositories or enemas are given, and rectal temperatures are contraindicated.

Immunosuppression may be treated with colony-stimulating factors (CSFs), such as granulocyte-macrophage colony-stimulating factor (GM-CSF), granulocyte colony-stimulating factor (G-CSF), or epoetin (EPO), to increase leukocytes, granulocytes, and erythrocytes. Granulocyte-stimulating factors are questionable for patients with a cancer of the blood-forming organs, such as leukemia, unless whole-body irradiation has occurred, as there is a possibility that more abnormal cells will be produced. These agents are used after total body irradiation for Hodgkin's disease, acute lymphocytic lymphoma, and non-Hodgkin's lymphoma. They are given after the BMT has been completed.

Think Critically About . . . What would you do in this situation? You came to work with a slightly scratchy throat and a drippy nose this morning. The charge nurse has assigned you to a cancer patient who has bone marrow suppression.

HYPERURICEMIA

The antimetabolite drugs cause an increase in uric acid in the blood as cancer cells are destroyed. A high fluid intake helps prevent problems of *hyperuricemia* (high uric acid in the blood) that occurs. Allopurinol may be prescribed to decrease the incidence of gout caused by the hyperuricemia; it is started at the beginning of therapy in an effort to prevent the problem.

FATIGUE

The fatigue occurring from immunosuppression treatment itself requires an adjustment of lifestyle. Physically, the patient may feel tired and without energy. She may find she is impatient and irritable and withdraws from her social environment. This decrease in activity may lead to a decline in function that is irreversible.

The nurse must instruct the patient in good fatigue management. This would include minimal unnecessary bed rest, a good balance of energy and expenditure, minimizing emotional distress, maintaining activities of daily living, using energy-saving devices, and prioritizing activities. Maintaining a good nutritional status with high protein intake will help keep up energy levels. Supplemental feedings between meals often are necessary to ensure adequate calorie intake. Fluids should be increased to 3 L/day on day 3 of chemotherapy, unless contraindicated, to help flush the waste materials from killed cancer cells from the body and to decrease the toxicities of the antineoplastic drugs. Explain that fatigue is a normal result of cancer treatment and that it may continue for 2 to 3 months after completion of therapy. Light exercise such as walking tends to increase energy level (Kornmehl, 2007). 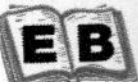

ALOPECIA

Hair loss *(alopecia)* resulting from chemotherapy is temporary. Occasionally radiation therapy to the head causes permanent hair loss. Although some techniques, such as using ice caps or a tourniquet around the scalp during the administration of chemotherapy, have been somewhat effective, they are not recommended by oncologists. The reduction of circulation of the drug to the area may prevent the killing of cancer cells that are harbored in the blood or lymph vessels in the scalp and head.

Hair begins regrowth about a month after the chemotherapy ends. The patient must be told that the new hair may be different in texture and color from the original. Meanwhile the patient should choose a wig

Table 8–7 ***Common Drugs Known to Be Effective for Cancer Pain***

DRUG	BRAND NAME	DURATION (hr)	DOSAGE (mg)	SIDE EFFECTS
COMMON ORAL PAIN RELIEVERS—MILD TO MODERATE INTENSITY				
Acetaminophen	Tylenol	3–4	650	Hepatic
Aspirin	Many brands	3–5	550	GI
Codeine	Many brands	3–5	32	CNS, GI
Hydrocodone	Vicodin	3–4	5	CNS, GI
Ibuprofen	Motrin, Advil	3–5	400	GI
Ketoprofen	Orudis	5–7	50	GI
Naproxen	Naprosyn	2–8	250	GI
Oxycodone	Roxicodone	3–6	5	CNS, GI
Piroxicam	Feldene	24	20	GI
Propoxyphene	Darvon	4–6	65	CNS
DRUG	**BRAND NAME**	**DURATION (hr)**	**PARENTERAL DOSE (mg)**	**ORAL DOSE (mg)**
COMMON OPIOID PAIN RELIEVERS—MODERATE TO SEVERE INTENSITY				
Morphine	Generic	4–5	10	30
Controlled-release morphine	MS Contin	6–12	—	30
Hydromorphone	Dilaudid	3–4	1.5	4
Methadone	Dolophine	5–6	10	20
Fentanyl	Duragesic	1–2	0.1	0.025
Oxycodone	Roxicodone	3–6	—	5
Controlled-release oxycodone	OxyContin	12	—	10
Codeine	Generic	2–4	120	200

Key: *CNS*, central nervous system; *GI*, gastrointestinal.

or head cover, before hair loss occurs, to wear until the hair is regrown. Some offices of the ACS have wigs available for loan that have been donated by former patients. In today's times, it is popular to "sport" the baldness that results from treatment. Singer Melissa Etheridge made her first stage appearance after cancer treatment without any wig or cap. Whatever your patient decides, help her understand that society supports her as a unique individual.

PAIN

For many cancer patients, pain is a daily reality. Pain reduces appetite, limits activity, and interferes with sleep. Most cancer pain (90%) can be relieved or at least controlled by a combination of measures. Often, however, the pain of cancer is undertreated. The Agency for Healthcare Research and Quality (AHRQ) has published guidelines for the control of cancer pain. To obtain a copy of *Quick Reference Guide for Clinicians* and a consumer's guide called *Managing Cancer Pain,* call 1-800 4-CANCER or visit the AHRQ website (www.ahrq.gov/clinic/epcsums/canpainsum.htm), where the guideline may be viewed in its entirety. The guidelines direct health professionals to use the assessment techniques and modalities discussed in Chapter 7 to control the patient's pain. Acupuncture has been validated as being useful to

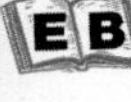

help control cancer pain (Evans & Rossner, 2005).

Nonpharmacologic Interventions

Nonpharmacologic interventions are combined with oral, topical, and parenteral analgesia to achieve relief or good control of pain. Pain must be (1) assessed and documented regularly; (2) discussed openly with family and family reports believed and understood; (3) addressed with options that are appropriate for the setting and for family; and (4) treated with interventions in a timely fashion. **The main factor in pain treatment is to continue to seek a combination of interventions or different treatments until the pain is under control.** Pain should be reassessed 15 to 30 minutes after parenteral drug administration and 1 hour after oral drugs are given. Medication doses should be scheduled regularly and around the clock to maintain a therapeutic drug level to prevent pain recurrence. The pain medication employed should be known to be effective for cancer pain. Table 8–7 gives a list of current oral and intravenous medications known to be effective against cancer pain. By putting aside worries about addiction to opiates, believing the patient's reports of pain and what relieves it, and concentrating on humane treatment of cancer patients, the nurse can be the instrument for helping the patient achieve a pain-free or pain-controlled existence. Pain control or relief greatly increases the quality of life for the cancer patient.

? *Think Critically About . . .* The pain control regimen for an assigned cancer patient is not working well. Can you write a role-play situation that would show your classmates how you would interact with the physician to obtain better pain control for your patient?

PATIENTS WITH METASTATIC DISEASE

A percentage of cancer patients experience metastasis. Table 8–8 shows the most common locations for metastasis for major cancers. Treatment options are usually

Table 8–8 Common Sites of Metastasis for Different Cancer Types

CANCER TYPE	SITES OF METASTASIS
Breast cancer	Bone* Lung* Liver Brain
Lung cancer	Brain* Bone Liver Lymph nodes Pancreas
Colorectal cancer	Liver* Lymph nodes Adjacent structures
Prostate cancer	Bone (especially spine and legs)* Pelvic nodes
Melanoma	Gastrointestinal tract Lymph nodes Lung Brain
Primary brain cancer	Central nervous system

From Ignatavicius, D.D., & Workman, M.L. (2006). *Medical-Surgical Nursing: Critical Thinking for Collaborative Care* (5th ed.). Philadelphia: Elsevier Saunders, p. 475.
*Most common site of metastasis for the specific malignant neoplasm.

the same as for primary cancer. Nursing care becomes more complex as more body systems are affected. All nurses caring for cancer patients should be aware of the possibility of metastasis and be alert for signs that might indicate it has occurred. Periodic assessment of the patient is done by the physician to rule out metastasis. Bone scans are periodically performed to detect metastasis to locations in the skeleton.

FEAR AND INEFFECTIVE COPING

The patient newly diagnosed with cancer faces enormous stress. **Knowledge about the disease, treatment options, and what will be experienced during each type of treatment greatly decreases fear in patients and families.** Knowing what to expect allows people to plan and feel confident that they will have some control over what is happening to them. An assessment of the patient's and family's usual coping techniques is important in formulating the overall plan of care.

When a patient has been diagnosed with cancer, pay attention to the patient's partner. Give the partner enough knowledge to decrease anxiety and the patient will be calmer. Be honest about the adverse effects of chemotherapy, immunotherapy, radiation therapy, and other treatments, but take a positive approach. Indicating that many patients feel a little nauseated with chemotherapy, but that there is medication that controls nausea very well, is better than telling the patient that there won't be any problems with the chemotherapy.

The nurse must consider psychosocial and spiritual care when working with the cancer patient as the disease will affect every aspect of life in some way. The nurse's job is to be supportive, to assist the patient to use strengths in planning and fighting the disease, and to coordinate family strengths in order to support the patient to continue with daily life.

Box 8–7 Internet Resources for the Cancer Patient

The following resources provide information about various types of cancer, treatments, financial support, caregiver concerns, and clinical trials of new drugs and treatments.

- American Cancer Society: www.cancer.org/docroot/home/index.asp
- American Leukemia and Lymphoma Society: www.leukemia-lymphoma.org/hm_lls
- Cancer Care: www.cancercare.org
- Cancer Clinical Trials: www.cancer.gov/clinicaltrials
- Cancer Index: www.cancerindex.org/clinks6.htm
- Cancer Information Network: www.cancerlinksusa.com/support/index.asp
- Financial Resources for Cancer Patients: http://cancer.about.com/b/a/225745.htm
- National Cancer Institute: www.cancer.gov
- National Coalition for Cancer Survivorship: www.canceradvocacy.org
- National Hospice and Palliative Care Organization: www.nhpco.org/templates/1/homepage.cfm
- National Institutes of Health—Cancer: http://health.nih.gov/result.asp/103
- Oncolink: www.oncolink.com
- United Ostomy Association: www.uoa.org

Speak with the patient and partner about sexual concerns. Intimacy is to be encouraged. Unless the patient is recovering from surgery, has pathologic fractures, or is severely immunosuppressed, sexual intercourse should not be a serious problem. If sexual function has been altered by surgery or treatment, help the patient find other means of sexual expression and gratification.

Referral to a social worker may be needed to coordinate resources for treatment and care assistance. Care of the cancer patient is a collaborative process that involves many members of the health care team. Family, friends, individuals, and community groups are among the sources of support and encouragement that the cancer patient might need to care for herself and attain some level of independence and peace of mind.

Local chapters of the ACS and American Lung Association have a wide variety of services available to professionals and laypersons interested in caring for the cancer patient. These include an annotated bibliography of public, patient, and professional information and education materials, pamphlets and booklets, and audiovisual programs. To obtain materials from the ACS, one can write or call the nearest ACS division. There are more than 3000 local ACS unit offices in the United States and Puerto Rico. Box 8–7 lists websites for some of the organizations that can provide assistance.

Learning as much as possible about the particular kind of cancer advises the patient of available options.

Knowledge of the latest and most effective treatments should be gained before making a decision about treatment. Contacting the National Cancer Institute for the latest information is wise.

Throughout treatment, the patient should be actively seeking information. The patient must trust the physician and the hospital or treatment facility. Trust is not developed on the basis of someone else's recommendation alone. Encourage the patient to maintain a sense of humor and to look for a little pleasure and enjoyment in life on a daily basis to counteract the hours consumed by treatment.

Nurses working in the radiation oncology center, the oncology floor of the hospital, the oncology outpatient clinic, the home, or the physician's office can be instrumental in providing support, direction, and hope for the cancer patient.

Box 8–8 Kübler-Ross' Stages of Dying

- **D**enial (This can't happen to me!)
- **A**nger (Why *me*?)
- **B**argaining (Yes me, *but* . . .)
- **D**epression (It *is* me, I give up . . .)
- **A**cceptance (*I'm ready* . . .)

Box 8–9 Common Fears of the Dying Patient

Almost all dying patients face varying levels of fear. Specifically, these fears may include:

- Fear of the unknown
- Fear of abandonment and loneliness
- Fear of loss of relationships
- Fear of loss of experiences in the future
- Fear of dependency and loss of independence
- Fear of pain

CARE FOR THE DYING CANCER PATIENT

PSYCHOLOGICAL PROCESS OF DEATH

Although many more cancer patients are being cured, cancer is still the second leading cause of death in the United States. Sometimes cancer cannot be eliminated. In 2006, it is anticipated that 564,830 Americans will die from cancer. That amounts to 1500 patients who die from cancer every day. Oncology nurses need to understand the grief process and the process of death and dying and apply knowledge about these processes compassionately when caring for cancer patients.

Grieving

Elisabeth Kübler-Ross introduced the world to the stages of grief and dying when her landmark book, *On Death and Dying*, was published in 1969. Kübler-Ross suggested that people go through several predictable junctures as they learn to adapt to the processes of loss or impending death. Not everyone goes through all the stages, nor do people go through stages in any set order. These five stages may apply to the grieving process when a body function or part is lost (such as a lost breast from cancer), a loved one dies, or one's own death is approaching (Box 8–8).

Fear

The patient feels and expresses many powerful emotions as she grieves the loss of her life. Almost all dying patients face varying levels of fear. Specifically, these fears may include those found in Box 8–9.

Caregivers are almost never successful in directly making patients less afraid of death through talk. The nurse is most helpful to the patient in just "being there" for the patient and telling her he cares. A nurse who is compassionate and soothing provides comfort and strength for the patient.

In the same way, when a patient displays behavior that is upsetting to the family, the nurse can explain to the family that patients go through these stages and the behavior is not because the family has done something wrong. These are times that both the patient and family are in great need, and nursing support can be profoundly comforting.

When nurses care for dying patients regularly, they can't help but reflect upon their own mortality. It is important for the nurse to review his beliefs about death and dying and reaffirm those beliefs. In this way, the nurse is then able to support patients who may have their own beliefs about the mysteries of death. Table 8–9 provides some common spiritual beliefs and practices.

The nurse should take a periodic inventory of his continued ability to provide care without "burnout." If a nurse has come to the point where he can only provide care as a detached and distant individual, he can no longer be supportive, compassionate, and understanding. It is time to take a break or move on and let others provide care for the dying patient.

PALLIATIVE CARE

Patients are living longer with cancer than they have in the past. This means steps must be taken to maintain as high a quality of life as possible in the dying cancer patient.

Palliative care, also called *comfort care*, is directed at meeting the needs of the dying patient by providing comfort while maintaining a high quality of life. Nurses who care for the dying patient have a unique opportunity to become an intimate part of the patient's life. Nurses can support the dying patient physically and emotionally while maintaining a professional role.

Whether assisting the patient in the hospital or at home, certain comfort measures are required. Palliative care requires a specialized body of knowledge and skill that can be difficult to obtain, and also to maintain if the nurse is not routinely applying the skills. Clinical issues across the settings involve the following.

Table 8–9 ***Spiritual Beliefs and Practices Regarding Death***

BELIEF SYSTEM	EXISTENCE OF DEITY	END-OF-LIFE (EOL) RITUALS	AFTERLIFE?	SPECIAL BELIEFS SURROUNDING EOL
Christianity Catholic	One unified deity—trinity of Father, Son and Holy Spirit	Last Rites ("Anointing of the Sick").	Soul goes to purgatory followed by eternity—heaven or hell.	Catholics may be cremated, but the cremains must be interred, not scattered or kept.
Protestant	One unified deity—trinity of Father, Son and Holy Spirit	No special rituals. Minister may perform extreme unction.	Consequences of actions on Earth dictate whether soul goes to heaven or hell and it happens immediately after death.	Beliefs vary among sects. In general, cremation and autopsies are allowed.
Judaism	One God	*Halakhot* (contains accepted Jewish laws and customs of death and mourning).	Immortality of the soul; belief in afterlife among the Orthodox.	Euthanasia, suicide, and assisted suicide are strictly forbidden. The body is never left alone until burial. Autopsy is discouraged. The body must not be cremated.
Buddhism	No	Rituals to ensure that the conciousness leaves the body.	Progression of the soul.	Sick patients must not know they are dying.
Hinduism	Multitudes of gods and goddesses—being of ultimate oneness	*Antyesti samskara* (death rites). The Hindu dies at home, if possible. Family member chants a mantra at moment of death.	Progression of the soul—cycles of rebirth.	*Mahaprasthana* (a vision of a tunnel of light). Death is a blissful time. Avoidance of excessive drugs. Body is cremated. Only men go to cremation site.
Islam	One God (Allah) powerful but unknowable	Family members or an Imam (clergy) read Koran and offer prayers.	Another world after death.	Dying person should face Mecca before and after death.
American Indian/ Alaska Native	Common concept is dual divinity—creator and mythical individual	May have Christian or Aboriginal traditions. May smoke ceremonial pipe.	In general, no precise belief. May believe in reincarnation, or progression to another world.	Traditional natives object to incorporation of their religious beliefs into other spiritual paths or into commercial affairs.
African American	Most believe in one deity	Important to incorporate prayer in coping with illness.	Depends upon actual religion, but most believe in an afterlife.	More likely to request life-sustaining therapies. Spiritual beliefs incorporated into treatment. Physician is God's instrument.

NURSING MANAGEMENT OF THE DYING PATIENT

Anticipatory Guidance

Anticipating the death assists the nurse in preparing the family and patient by giving them guidance about physical changes, symptoms, and complications that may arise. This may also aid the patient and family in deciding about possible hospice care.

Terminal Hydration

A dying patient gradually reduces fluid intake. Dehydration can also be increased by the disease process. Also, a dry mouth and feeling of thirst may be induced by the drugs being administered. The nurse must help educate the patient and family as to both the benefits and burdens of hydration. Many times the course is for patients to choose what to take and be allowed to refuse further nourishment. This is termed *"patient-endorsed intake."*

End-Stage Symptom Management

There are many expected symptoms that are related to metabolic changes at the end of life. The last few days of patient life has been studied extensively. The nurse must recognize these symptoms and be able to either alleviate them or help explain them to the patient and family. Since comfort is the goal of palliative care, administering only oral medications is the preferred choice. However, this may not be possible as death draws near, and it is also the goal to allow a pain-free death. In some cases it may be possible to administer transdermal and/or rectal pain medications.

Pain. Transdermal fentanyl has helped eliminate the burden of pain at the end of life. Sometimes this regimen is supplemented with rescue doses of morphine. Whatever the regimen, studies have shown that pain relief, either total or at least enough to make the pain tolerable, is possible 75% to 97% of the time.

Dyspnea. When patients are near death, they often subjectively feel as if they cannot get enough air. It is difficult to determine what causes this feeling, but several measures can be taken. The patient can be placed in Fowler's position, activities reduced, and air temperature adjusted, and medications such as bronchodilators can be given. It is important for the nurse to remember that this feeling can be very frightening for both the patient and family members, and aggressive treatment to lessen discomfort is important.

Death Rattle. Noisy ventilation is heard when patients can no longer clear their throats of normal secretions. Family members are often alarmed and are afraid the patient will choke to death. In these cases, scopolamine or atropine, drugs that are known to reduce secretions, may be used to quiet the patient and bring breathing back to normal.

Delirium. Dying patients may experience hallucinations and/or altered mental status. Nurses must first search for causes such as pain, positional discomfort, or bladder distention and address those physical problems. Next, the nurse should discuss the delirium with the patient's family and encourage the family to talk to the patient in quiet tones while remaining calm.

NURSING RESOURCES

Palliative care is a fairly new field, and many nurses have chosen to undertake this specialty. The palliative care nurse is an important element for the patient's and family's comfort during this transition. In September 2004, a certification examination for LPN/LVNs was launched by the National Board for Certification of Hospice and Palliative Nurses (NBCHPN). Detailed information is available by calling 1-888-519-9901 or visiting the NBCHPN website (www.nbchpn.org).

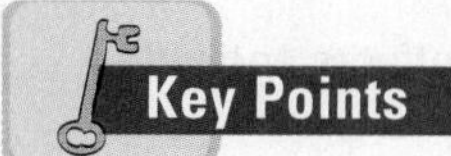

Key Points

- Cancer is a large group of over 100 diseases.
- More lives could be saved by early detection and prompt treatment.
- Cancer cells begin growing as a result of a change in normal body cells, probably a mutation in their DNA.
- Malignant cells can spread to other areas of the body.
- Tumors are classified according to the organs or tissues from which they first begin.
- All cancer results from defects in the DNA of genes.
- Harmful agents that are carcinogenic exist in the environment.
- Some people may have a genetic predisposition to some types of cancer.
- Age, sex, and race are considered predisposing factors for certain types of cancers.
- Changing certain lifestyle characteristics, such as quitting smoking, maintaining normal weight, reducing alcohol usage, avoiding and limiting exposure to carcinogens, and eating a varied diet, can lower the risk of cancer.
- It is important to be aware of the seven warning signs of cancer.
- Cytology, biopsy, radiologic studies, and laboratory tests are common methods used to diagnose cancer.
- Tumor markers detect biochemical substances synthesized and released into the bloodstream by tumor cells and are used mainly to confirm a diagnosis or response to a cancer therapy.
- There are three traditional modes of therapy for malignancies: surgery, radiation, and chemotherapy.
- The nurse must protect himself from overexposure to radiation.
- One of the most important areas of the patient's body to protect from radiation is the skin.
- Antineoplastic chemotherapy drugs are effective at different times in the growth and replication phases of the tumor cell cycle.
- Many antineoplastic drugs can cause tissue damage upon direct contact, so the nurse must take care to protect the patients from extravasation and administer the drugs into veins that have good blood flow.
- Nursing management of the patient receiving chemotherapy requires special knowledge and skills beyond those of basic nursing.
- Biologic response modifiers manipulate the immune system to stimulate or suppress activity. These drugs assist the body in destroying cancer cells with minimal effect on normal tissue.
- Bone marrow transplantation is used to correct damage caused by chemotherapy or radiation.
- The most recent approach to cancer therapy is gene therapy and genetic engineering.
- Problems related to cancer or cancer therapy are complex and often require knowledgeable nursing care.
- Nausea, vomiting, diarrhea, and constipation are frequent complaints of cancer patients and require vigilant care.
- Cancer treatment may suppress the patient's bone marrow and the patient may develop thrombocytopenia, requiring her to cease therapy for a period of time. This is a common occurrence, and nurses need to be able to explain the problem to the patient so that she does not become unnecessarily anxious.
- While pain is not unique to cancer, it is a common occurrence in cancer patients. The main factor in pain treatment is to continue to seek a combination of interventions or different treatments until the pain is under control.
- Cancer is still the second leading cause of death in the United States. Many cancer patients and their

families will go through the five steps of grief that are recognized in patients experiencing loss.
- Steps must be taken to maintain as high a quality of life as possible in the dying cancer patient.
- Palliative care is providing comfort for the dying patient and maintaining a high quality of life throughout the death process.
- Palliative care is a specialty for which LPN/LVNs may seek certification.

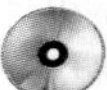

Go to your **Companion CD-ROM** for an Audio Glossary, animations, video clips, and bonus review questions.

evolve Be sure to visit the companion Evolve site at http://evolve.elsevier.com/deWit/ for interactive NCLEX-PN Exam Style Review Questions, WebLinks, and additional online resources.

NCLEX-PN EXAM STYLE REVIEW QUESTIONS

Choose the best answer(s) for the following questions.

1. The patient who is recently diagnosed with a metastatic cancer cries, "Am I going to die?" An appropriate nursing response would be:

1. "You will be all right."
2. "Do you want me to call for a priest or minister?"
3. "I will stay with you for a while."
4. "Do you have family members who could help you as you go through this?"

2. The nurse reinforces patient instructions regarding neutropenic precautions. Important topics should include the following except:

1. pregnancy.
2. diet restrictions.
3. hand washing.
4. social isolation.

3. A patient who recently had chemotherapy for lung cancer complains of uncontrollable nausea and vomiting with accompanying loss of appetite. An appropriate nursing diagnosis would be:

1. Ineffective coping.
2. Deficient knowledge.
3. Anticipatory grieving.
4. Imbalanced nutrition: less than body requirements.

4. The family members attending to the needs of a dying patient express distress regarding the noisy breathing. An important nursing action would be to:

1. increase pain medications.
2. administer atropine.
3. reassure family members.
4. consult a priest or a minister.

5. A terminally ill female patient reminiscing about the "good old days" becomes increasingly confused. She talks of seeing relatives who have died. Which of the following are appropriate nursing interventions? *(Select all that apply.)*

1. Discuss the patient's behaviors with the family.
2. Force oral fluids.
3. Encourage the family to talk to the patient in quiet tones.
4. Promote a calm environment.
5. Apply physical restraints.

6. The patient is scheduled for bone marrow biopsy to confirm the diagnosis of leukemia. As the nurse reinforces physician instructions regarding the procedure, an appropriate nursing statement regarding bone marrow biopsy would be:

1. "It is performed in the operating room."
2. "It is a painless procedure."
3. "It introduces a needle to aspirate tissue samples."
4. "It requires a surgical incision."

7. The patient is notified by the physician as having a "hot spot" on a thyroid scan. Which of the following patient statements indicates understanding of the physician's findings?

1. "Everything will be all right."
2. "I need to put my affairs in order."
3. "I have a mass that takes up the radioisotope."
4. "I have a normal thyroid gland."

8. Before chemotherapy, a female patient expresses concerns regarding hair loss. She says that her partner would no longer love her because she will not be as attractive. An appropriate nursing diagnosis would be:

1. Disturbed body image related to anticipated loss of hair.
2. Ineffective coping due to perceived loss of relationship.
3. Powerlessness related to chemotherapy.
4. Risk for impaired skin integrity related to hair loss.

9. A 40-year-old female patient is scheduled for external radiation therapy for breast cancer. In helping the patient cope with her illness and the effects of radiation therapy, the nurse should help her focus on which of the following? *(Select all that apply.)*

1. Complying with scheduled radiation therapies
2. Taking precautions on exposing other family members
3. Protecting the skin by applying lotion
4. Wearing snug-fitting clothing
5. Understanding the therapeutic effects and side effects

10. A patient had chemotherapy for non-Hodgkin's lymphoma 2 weeks ago. Based on the understanding of the effects of chemotherapy, the nurse would anticipate which of the following clinical findings?

1. Temperature 101.5° F (38.6° C)
2. Elevated white blood cell count
3. Easy bruising
4. Change in hair color

CRITICAL THINKING ACTIVITIES 

Read each clinical scenario and discuss the questions with your classmates.

Scenario A

An acquaintance tells you that she has had a mole on her back for several years and it appears to be getting larger and darker. She states she is worried about the fact that it is getting bigger, but says that she is scared to go to the physician. She doesn't have health insurance and is worried about paying for the visit.

1. What is your obligation as a nurse in encouraging this person to see a physician at once?
2. What suggestions could you make about obtaining a medical opinion without incurring a lot of expense?

Scenario B

Ms. Allen went to her physician for a regular physical checkup and was told that she had malignant cells in the cervical secretions obtained from her Pap test. She had a biopsy of the cervix, and this, too, proved to contain malignant cells. She was admitted to the hospital, cesium was implanted in the cervix, and Ms. Allen was kept in bed in a private room during the treatment.

1. If you were assigned to give A.M. care to this patient, what special precautions would you take to protect yourself from excessive radiation?
2. What would be some signs and symptoms that you would watch for to determine whether Ms. Allen is having either a local or a systemic reaction to radiation?

Scenario C

Mary is a 19-year-old college student receiving chemotherapy for Hodgkin's disease.

1. Identify psychosocial problems you would expect Mary to have, and state the measures you would suggest to help her deal with them.

CHAPTER 9

Chronic Illness and Rehabilitation

evolve http://evolve.elsevier.com/deWit

Objectives

Upon completing this chapter, you should be able to:

Theory

1. Discuss relevant nursing issues for patients with chronic illness.
2. Identify patients at risk for problems associated with immobility.
3. Describe the effect of immobility on each of the major systems of the body.
4. Discuss the general goals for the resident in a long-term care facility and how to meet those goals.
5. Identify differences in the role of the LPN/LVN in a long-term care facility versus the hospital setting.
6. Describe the types of rehabilitation programs that might be found in a large city.
7. State the goals of rehabilitation.
8. Identify the members of the rehabilitation team and the collaborative care–giving process and state the role of each.
9. Explain the differences in philosophy and required attitude between the home care setting and the hospital.

Clinical Practice

1. Choose specific interventions to assist the patient with a chronic illness who is home-bound and has issues of loneliness.
2. When in a long-term care facility, discuss with the charge nurse the measures that are used for safety and fall prevention in that facility.
3. Observe a rehabilitation team conference to see how a collaborative care plan is created or updated.
4. From assessment data, identify areas of psychosocial need for a home care patient and family.

Key Terms

Be sure to check out the bonus material on the Companion CD-ROM, including selected audio pronunciations.

disability (p. 190)
handicap (p. 190)
hemiparesis (hĕm-ē-pă-RĒ-sĭs, p. 199)
impairment (ĭm-PĂR-mĕnt, p. 190)
orthostatic hypotension (ŏr-thō-STĂT-ĭk hī-pō-TĔN-shŭn, p. 196)
rehabilitation (rē-hă-bĭl-ĭ-TĀ-shŭn, p. 200)
sundowning (SŬN-doun-ĭng, p. 198)

Patients with chronic illnesses and disabilities are cared for in long-term care facilities, rehabilitation institutes, at home, at outpatient clinics, at rehabilitation agencies, and in physicians' offices. Nurses who work with patients who have a chronic illness, or are disabled, need to be skilled in providing care and comfort, promoting coping skills and adaptive living capabilities, promoting self-care for independent living, and fostering quality of life. This chapter discusses the patient with chronic illness, nursing in the long-term care facility, how rehabilitation nursing differs in philosophy from acute care nursing, and the role of the LPN/LVN in home care.

CHRONIC ILLNESS

Chronic illness affects millions of people. Diabetes, hypertension, heart disease, cancer, neurologic disorders (such as multiple sclerosis and stroke), asthma, arthritis, back disorders, and musculoskeletal deformities and disorders all require continuous care. Although many people with a chronic illness can lead an active and productive life, about 46 million people in the United States have chronic illnesses or disabilities that interfere with normal function. People, and particularly the elderly, may have more than one chronic illness. This makes treatment and care very complicated. Many health insurance companies have a case management department that oversees services for those with chronic illnesses. When working with patients who have a chronic illness, the terms *impairment*, *disability*, and *handicap* are encountered. **Impairment** refers to dysfunction of a specific organ or body system. **Disability** indicates a difficulty in performing certain tasks because of impairment, and having a **handicap** means that there is a physical or mental defect or characteristic that prevents or restricts a person from participating in a normal life or limits the capacity to work; a handicap is usually related to a disability.

Because of the loss of function, usual roles may be changed. The person may no longer be able to be the primary breadwinner, music teacher, church elder, or hold whatever positions in the work force or community formerly held. Changes in the person's role affect the family as well. Daily patterns are altered to accommodate treatments and therapy and to cope with the problems of disability. Sorrow is felt for all that has been lost. The patient may wonder, why did this happen to me? Spiritual distress may be experienced as the person is faced with the limitations of the illness or disability that has occurred. Holistic care that addresses spiritual and psychosocial needs as well as physical needs is essential.

Patients with a chronic illness often feel powerless, especially in the phases of diagnosis and early treatment. Patients realize that the chronic illness will dictate much of their course in life now, and that they have less control over what is happening to their body. Support of usual coping techniques and teaching new ways to cope help the patient effectively deal with the illness and the changes in life patterns it has brought. Nurses can be instrumental in instilling hope for a good quality of life despite the illness.

PREVENTING THE HAZARDS OF IMMOBILITY

Patients are immobilized to varying degrees and for different amounts of time. The multiple trauma patient may be on bed rest for several weeks. The patient with advanced multiple sclerosis may be able to move around only with a wheelchair. The patient who experiences great difficulty breathing from advanced lung disease or heart disease may have very little energy and does not move around much for that reason. The patient with spinal cord injury or brain damage from a stroke may be immobile for the rest of the lifetime. Patients who have pain or who have arthritic joints that cause pain with movement also tend to be less mobile. Patients who have any disorder requiring bed rest are at risk. All of these patients are subject to the problems of immobility.

You must evaluate each patient situation and determine whether the patient is at risk for problems related to immobility. **Even if the patient is going to be immobile for only a few days, measures should be taken to prevent secondary problems.** Box 9–1 presents a list of common disorders that often cause some degree of immobility. Patients with these disorders should be assessed for the degree of risk for the various problems of immobility, and interventions to prevent them should be initiated.

The prevention of problems related to immobility begins the moment a patient first becomes ill or injured. Preventive actions must continue as long as the patient needs health care. The systems of the body work together as a whole. Lack of activity affects more than one system. The effects vary depending on the general health of the individual, his age, the degree of immobility, and the length of time of inactivity or bed rest. Lack of mobility may begin a vicious cycle that can lead only to an ever-increasing loss of independence for the patient. As he becomes less able to move, the patient becomes more dependent, and as he becomes more dependent, he is less able to care for himself—which in turn leads to even more adverse effects from immobility. It is the responsibility of the nurse to avoid the beginning of such a cycle by helping the patient maintain normal functioning of each body system to the highest degree possible (Nursing Care Plan 9–1).

Box 9–1 ***Disorders that May Cause Immobility***

- Multiple sclerosis
- Stroke
- Spinal cord injury
- Lower extremity amputation
- Head injury
- Multiple trauma
- Fractures of the knee, leg, ankle, hip, pelvis, or spine
- Neuromuscular disorders: muscular dystrophy, amyotrophic lateral sclerosis, poliomyelitis, cerebral palsy, myasthenia gravis, etc.
- Congenital deformities
- Burns
- Advanced metastatic cancer
- Advanced stages of chronic disorders such as Parkinson's disease, Alzheimer's disease, or Huntington's chorea
- Severe rheumatoid arthritis, osteoarthritis, and other forms of arthritis

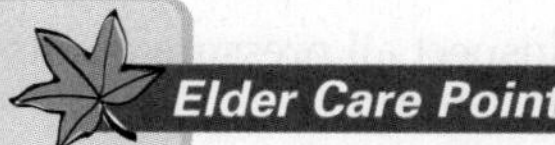

Elder Care Points

Although a lot of elderly people are active in their daily lives, many do not engage in much exercise activity. When immobilized, these patients quickly lose what strength and flexibility they had as muscle fibers atrophy quickly. It is much more difficult for these patients to regain mobility.

Early effects of immobility include a decrease in muscle strength, generalized weakness, easy fatigue, joint stiffness, decreased coordination, abdominal distention, and various metabolic changes detectable by laboratory test. Table 9–1 presents the more severe problems with measures for prevention when lack of activity occurs for more than a few days.

Assess the patient daily, looking closely at each body system in which a problem related to immobility might occur. Know the signs and symptoms of each type of problem and understand how to intervene to decrease or prevent it. Discussion of the pathophysiology of the problems of immobility, including the signs and symptoms, medical treatment, and nursing care for each problem, is provided in the relevant chapters of this text.

NURSING CARE PLAN 9–1

Care of an Immobilized Resident

SCENARIO Carl Sanders is an 83-year-old male with weakness and debilitation and who has several chronic diseases. He has been transferred to the long-term care facility following a hospitalization for pneumonia.

PROBLEM/NURSING DIAGNOSIS *Cannot walk, turn, or reposition self*/Impaired physical mobility related to weakness, debility, illness, and age.

Supporting assessment data *Objective:* Needs assistance to turn, reposition in the bed, or walk.

Goals/Expected Outcomes	Nursing Interventions	Selected Rationale	Evaluation
Resident will maintain present joint mobility	Perform ROM on joints tid.	Regular ROM prevents frozen joints.	Active ROM done twice this shift.
Resident will perform active ROM of arms by discharge	Assist to turn and reposition q 2 hr.	Repositioning helps prevent pressure ulcers and hypostatic pneumonia.	Repositioned q 2 hr.
	Place in high Fowler's position for meals; assist to chair for lunch.		Up in chair for meals. Breath sounds clear right; slightly diminished in left base.

PROBLEM/NURSING DIAGNOSIS *Break in skin with redness on left hip*/Impaired skin integrity related to immobility and pressure over left trochanter.

Supporting assessment data *Subjective:* "I can't move very much." *Objective:* Too weak to reposition self; stage I pressure ulcer over left trochanter.

Goals/Expected Outcomes	Nursing Interventions	Selected Rationale	Evaluation
Resident will have no evidence of more pressure damage to skin	Turn at least 2 q hr and more frequently if possible.	Relieves pressure on dependent areas.	Position adjusted q 1 hr.
	Use supports for positioning and cushioning for relief of pressure.	Prevents pressure ulcers and keeps body in good anatomical alignment.	On pressure relief mattress; pressure relief cushion in chair.
Stage I pressure ulcer will heal within 3 wk	Keep reddened area clean, with clear film dressing in place; inspect q shift.	Cleanliness prevents infection. Clear film dressing seals in moisture while allowing inspection.	Clear dressing in place; reddening decreasing.
	Inspect all pressure points q 4 hr.	Identifies skin problems.	Pressure points inspected q 4 hr. No new reddened areas.
	Use turning sheet to turn patient.	Helps prevent shearing injuries from sliding resident on sheet.	Turning sheet used for turning.

PROBLEM/NURSING DIAGNOSIS *Little stool passed*/Constipation related to immobility.

Supporting assessment data *Subjective:* "I feel constipated." *Objective:* Only small amount of hard, dry stool passed once in last 4 days.

Goals/Expected Outcomes	Nursing Interventions	Selected Rationale	Evaluation
Resident will have normal bowel pattern by discharge	Administer oil retention enema as ordered followed by suppository; monitor results.	Oil will soften stool. Suppository stimulates bowel movement.	Oil retention given; held for 20 min. Had large BM; suppository not needed.
	Assist to bedside commode after breakfast every day. Provide privacy.	Sitting on commode and privacy promote ease of bowel movement.	Assisted to commode after enema. Privacy provided.
	Give stool softener daily as ordered.	Keeps stool soft.	Received stool softener.
	Increase fluids to 8 oz every hour while awake.		Took in at least 6 oz of fluid each hour; continue plan.
	Increase fiber in diet.	Adds bulk, helping to prevent constipation.	Ate a bran muffin at breakfast.
	Offer warm prune juice each morning.	Stimulates bowel and softens stool.	Warm prune juice taken before enema.

NURSING CARE PLAN 9–1

Care of an Immobilized Resident—cont'd

PROBLEM/NURSING DIAGNOSIS *Unable to walk*/Risk for injury related to possible falls.

Supporting assessment data *Objective:* Unable to walk without falling, gets confused after dark and tries to get out of bed.

Goals/Expected Outcomes	Nursing Interventions	Selected Rationale	Evaluation
Resident will not sustain fall in hospital	Place call light and personal items within reach. Answer call light promptly.	Helps prevent him from trying to get out of bed without assistance.	Call bell and personal items on bed and bedside table within reach.
	Place an alarm device on the bed.	Alerts staff to attempt to get out of bed without assistance.	Bed alarm in place and functioning.
	Frequently reinforce instructions not to get up without assistance.		Reinforced not to get up without assistance every 2 hr.
	Assist to bedside commode and back to bed.	Prevents falling.	Assisted to bedside commode after enema.
	Keep low light on in room at night to decrease confusion.	Light helps maintain orientation to room.	Placed instruction on Computer Care Plan.
	Check on resident frequently; anticipate needs.	Anticipating needs helps keep resident from arising without assistance.	Checked on resident every hour during this shift.

PROBLEM/NURSING DIAGNOSIS *Recovering from pneumonia*/Impaired mobility related to weakness and debility.

Supporting assessment data *Subjective:* "I've really been sick; I'm so weak." *Objective:* Lungs just cleared of secretions; breathes shallowly.

Goals/Expected Outcomes	Nursing Interventions	Selected Rationale	Evaluation
Resident will perform breathing exercises q 2 hr while awake	Assist to sitting position for deep-breathing exercises, use of spirometer, and coughing q 2 hr.	Lungs can expand better when thoracic cage is not against the mattress.	Assisted to sit up and perform deep breathing and coughing. Used spirometer q 2 hr.
Lung fields will remain clear	Encourage adequate fluid intake.	Keeps secretions more liquid and easier to expectorate.	Taking more fluid per hour (6 oz).
	Encourage to take deeper breaths during each commercial break when watching TV.	Aerates lower alveoli.	Encouraged to remember to take deep breaths during commercials on TV.
	Auscultate lungs each shift.	Detects changes in lungs.	Lungs clear right; slightly diminished sounds at left base.
	Turn q 2 hr.	Helps prevent hypostatic pneumonia.	Turned q 2 hr while in bed.

PROBLEM/NURSING DIAGNOSIS *Immobile for many days*/Risk for ineffective tissue perfusion related to venous stasis.

Supporting assessment data *Subjective:* "I've been mostly in bed for over a week." *Objective:* Has been inactive and in bed most of the time for the past 10 days. History of previous thrombophlebitis in right leg.

Goals/Expected Outcomes	Nursing Interventions	Selected Rationale	Evaluation
Resident will not have evidence of thrombophlebitis or deep venous thrombosis	Encourage active ROM of legs, feet, and ankles q 2 hr while awake.	Muscle movement compresses blood vessels, propelling blood to the heart.	Performing active ROM of legs, feet, and ankles after breathing exercises q 2 hr.
	Keep TED hose smoothly in place except for 30 min while bathing.	Elastic hose place pressure on vessels, encouraging venous return to the heart.	TEDs reapplied after bath.
	Encourage extra fluid intake.	Fluid prevents dehydration and hemoconcentration.	Offered fluid each time care provided.
	Assess for Homans' sign once per shift.	Homans' sign may indicate a thrombus (clot).	No positive Homans' sign.

Continued

NURSING CARE PLAN 9–1

Care of an Immobilized Resident—cont'd

Goals/Expected Outcomes	Nursing Interventions	Selected Rationale	Evaluation
	Visually inspect legs for reddening or swelling.	Reddening, swelling, or pain may indicate a thrombus or thrombophlebitis.	No reddening or swelling of legs and ankles.

PROBLEM/NURSING DIAGNOSIS *Immobile for 10 days*/Risk for infection of the urinary tract related to immobility.
Supporting assessment data *Subjective:* "I've had several bladder infections in the past." *Objective:* Urine is concentrated and slightly cloudy.

Goals/Expected Outcomes	Nursing Interventions	Selected Rationale	Evaluation
Resident will not develop a urinary tract infection	Increase fluid intake to at least 3000 mL/day.	Promotes more urine flow.	Is increasing fluid intake this shift.
	Encourage fluid intake every hour until 2 hr before bedtime.		Offering fluids each time care is provided (q 1–2 hr).
	Assess for bladder distention q 4 hr.	Helps determine if bladder is being emptied sufficiently.	No bladder distention; voiding sufficient quantities.
	Observe characteristics of urine for signs of infection.	Cloudy, foul-smelling urine may indicate infection.	Urine is yellow, clear, and without foul odor.
	Measure intake and output.	Helps evaluate fluid intake.	Intake 1800 mL this shift. Output 1465 mL this shift.

PROBLEM/NURSING DIAGNOSIS *In bed in room most of time; roommate not able to communicate*/Risk for loneliness related to lack of social interaction.
Supporting assessment data *Subjective:* "I'm really sick of being in bed." *Objective:* Roommate is aphasic and cannot communicate verbally.

Goals/Expected Outcomes	Nursing Interventions	Selected Rationale	Evaluation
Resident will maintain social contact	Bring phone to resident and assist to call family members and friends.	Phone calls maintain contact with family and friends.	Phoned wife this morning. Says will call friend later this evening.
	Ask volunteers to play cards with him.	Playing cards with another provides social interaction.	Requested volunteer to play cards for late afternoon.
	Visit his room frequently.	Stopping in room provides social contact.	In room q 1 hr.
	Set up a schedule with family members for visits.	Spread out visits help dispel loneliness.	Wife is trying to set up visiting schedule.

? CRITICAL THINKING QUESTIONS

1. What other psychosocial problems might this resident have?
2. Once he is stronger and able to walk with assistance, what measures could you take to help prevent him from falling?
3. What type of activities will help him to restore muscle strength?

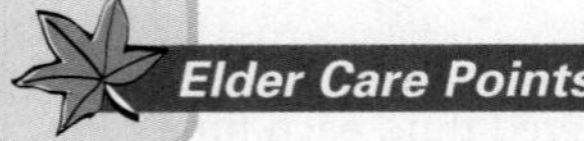

Elder Care Points

Because of the changes in the various body systems that normally occur with aging, the elderly patient is at much greater risk for problems of immobility. Monitor closely for hypostatic pneumonia, constipation, urinary problems, and inadequate nutritional intake due to anorexia. Attention to range-of-motion exercises is very important and often neglected.

CHRONIC ILLNESS AND REHABILITATION CARE

A chronic illness may follow an acute illness or an accident. Some patients are transferred to a transitional unit or long-term care facility for a period of weeks for recovery after the most acute phase of illness or injury has passed. Many elderly who have several chronic problems and deficits in self-care enter long-term care

Table 9–1 ***Prevention of the Common Hazards of Immobility***

COMPLICATION	PREVENTION
MUSCULOSKELETAL	
Contractures	Range-of-motion exercises
Foot drop	Foot support while in bed, range-of-motion exercises, high-top tennis shoes
Osteoporosis	Range-of-motion exercises, ambulation if possible (walking)
Susceptibility to fractures	Weight-bearing exercises
Muscular atrophy	Passive or active range-of-motion exercises
GASTROINTESTINAL	
Constipation	Increased activity level Increased fluid intake, fiber
CARDIOVASCULAR	
Decreased cardiac output	Range-of-motion exercises
Increased venous stasis	Exercise, support hose, or antiembolism stockings
Thrombus formation	Exercise, support hose, or antiembolism stockings
Embolism	Avoidance of leg massage, low-molecular-weight heparin
NEUROLOGIC	
Disorientation	Sleep-wake schedule in accord with light-dark pattern Reorientation (to person, place, and time) Control of sensory stimulation Avoidance of sudden position changes, tilt table
RENAL/URINARY	
Calculi	Decreased dietary calcium level Increased fluid intake Maintenance of acidic urine
Infection	Increase fluids Use intermittent catheterization instead of indwelling if possible
RESPIRATORY	
Pneumonia	Frequent repositioning in wheelchair or bed Respiratory exercises

facilities for the remainder of their lives. Other patients may enter a rehabilitation facility for an extended time. Some patients are discharged home to continue with rehabilitation services as an outpatient.

Long-Term Care

In the long-term care facility, an RN usually is the director of nurses. An LPN/LVN often is the charge nurse, and certified nursing assistants (CNAs), patient care assistants, or restorative aides provide much of the basic direct care to the residents. An occupational therapist, physical therapist, speech pathologist, respiratory therapist, activity therapist, or other professional provides services as needed. A physician or advanced-practice nurse supervises each resident's care program. Although the RN ultimately is responsible for the nursing care plan of each resident, the LPN/LVN charge nurse often is the person who admits the resident and initiates the plan of care. If the LPN/LVN initiates a plan of care, collaboration with the RN is necessary to ensure that the plan is appropriate and complete. The LPN/LVN performs treatments and wound care, assists with gathering assessment data from the residents regularly, organizes the shift's workload, administers medications, documents assessment findings and care given, assists with updating the nursing care plans, and assigns care tasks to patient care assistants. The LPN/LVN oversees care for a group of residents for a shift. The RN supervisor manages the care for the entire facility on a 24-hour basis and delegates tasks to the LPN/LVN. The LPN/LVN assigns tasks to the patient care assistants. Those tasks may include assistance with toileting, bathing, feeding, ambulation, or range-of-motion (ROM) exercises; care of the resident unit; and transfer of residents from bed to chair (Assignment Considerations 9–1). Patient care assistants are the core caregivers of the long-term care facility. The skillful LPN/LVN will establish rapport, harmony, and respect among the work team by valuing these workers, appreciating their contributions, and listening to their concerns.

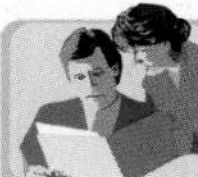

Assignment Considerations 9–1

Appropriate Assignments

When assigning tasks to unlicensed assistants (certified nursing assistants, patient care assistants, restorative aides), you must know that the person has shown competence at performing the task. Competencies of assistive personnel should be documented in their personnel files. Evaluation of task competence must be done at least annually. Give specific directions about what you want the person to do, how it is to be done, and what needs to be reported to you. You are responsible for the care of any resident or patient assigned to you.

Do not assign unlicensed personnel to perform tasks for unstable patients.

When planning care for residents in a long-term care facility, the LVN/LPN must keep in mind that the overall goals of care for the facility are to provide a safe environment, assist the resident to maintain or attain as much function as possible, promote individual

Box 9–2 National Patient Safety Goals

The 2007 National Patient Safety Goals that specifically pertain to long-term care and rehabilitation facilities include:

- Reduce the risk of patient harm resulting from falls.
- Implement a fall reduction program including an evaluation of the effectiveness of the program.
- Encourage the patients' active involvement in their own care as a patient safety strategy.
- Define and communicate the means for patients and their families to report concerns about safety and encourage them to do so.

Box 9–3 Problems and Disorders That Increase the Risk of Falls

- Musculoskeletal disorders that impair normal ambulation or balance
- Neurologic problems such as peripheral neuropathy affecting the feet
- Balance or gait problems resulting from stroke or inner ear problems
- Postural hypotension or dizziness caused by medications
- Impaired vision
- Impaired hearing
- Extreme weakness
- Oxygen deficit that may cause dizziness and loss of balance
- A history of previous falls

independence, and **allow the resident to maintain or achieve as much autonomy as possible.**

Safety. Providing a safe environment for a group of residents, many of whom may not be totally mentally competent, while allowing autonomy and independence is a great challenge. Two of the greatest safety problems often are to keep confused residents within the boundaries of the facility and to prevent falls. Those with physical disabilities need other measures to ensure safety. National Patient Safety Goals have been developed specifically for long-term care and rehabilitation facilities (Box 9–2). Meeting resident safety and independence needs without resorting to chemical or physical restraints requires caring, commitment, and ingenuity on the part of the nurse.

Fall Prevention. The first step in the prevention of falls is to recognize which residents are at greatest risk (Box 9–3). All residents are assessed for the risk of a fall upon admission and whenever their condition changes (Box 9–4). The next step to prevent a fall is to recognize hazards in the environment that could precipitate a fall (Box 9–5).

Restorative programs focus on muscle strengthening and balance. Residents who are at risk for orthostatic hypotension (blood pressure that falls with position change from supine to sitting or standing) are taught ways to decrease the risk of falling. Be alert to the fact that a resident who was previously ambulating safely may be weakened if he has been recently sick with fever, urinary tract infection, flu, a cold, vomiting, or diarrhea. The resident who is receiving diuretic therapy must be assessed frequently for fluid and electrolyte imbalance that could cause weakness, dizziness, or confusion (Safety Alert 9–1). Residents on diuretic therapy must receive prompt assistance for toileting when assistance is requested. The resident who needs narcotic therapy for pain or sedatives to sleep must be safeguarded. Instruct the resident to ring for assistance should the need to arise from the bed or chair occur. The bed should be kept in the low position.

Box 9–4 Fall Risk Assessment

Place a check mark in front of the items that apply to the patient

GENERAL INFORMATION

___ Age over 70
___ History of falls*
___ Confusion at times
___ Confused most of the time*
___ Impaired memory or judgment
___ Unable to follow directions*
___ Needs assistance with elimination
___ Visual impairment
___ Feels physically weak*

MEDICATIONS

___ Central nervous system suppressants (narcotic, sedative, tranquilizer, hypnotic, antidepressant, psychotropic, anticonvulsant)
___ Medication that causes orthostatic hypotension (antihypertensive, diuretic)*
___ Medication that may cause diarrhea (cathartic)
___ Medication that may alter blood glucose levels (insulin, hypoglycemics)

GAIT AND BALANCE

___ Poor balance when standing*
___ Balance problems when walking*
___ Swaying, lurching, or slapping gait*
___ Unstable when making turns*
___ Needs assistive device (walker, cane, holds on to furniture)*

Note: A check mark on any starred item indicates a risk for falls. A combination of four or more of the unstarred items indicates a risk for falls.
From deWit, S.C. (2005). *Fundamental Concepts and Skills for Nursing* (2nd ed.). Philadelphia: Elsevier Saunders, p. 311.

? ***Think Critically About . . .*** Can you describe how you would determine just how at risk a new resident is for falls? Can you identify points that should be included in the assessment of a high risk for a fall?

Box 9–5 *Interventions to Help Prevent Falls*

- Keep pathways free of objects.
- Remove loose rugs or secure with a nonslip pad.
- Place shoes and slippers underneath the bed or chair rather than in the pathway.
- Provide lighting without glare or deep shadows.
- Provide adequate night lighting for the pathway from the bed to the bathroom.
- Wipe up spilled liquids immediately.
- Keep wheels locked on all equipment when stationary.
- Place belongings within easy reach to prevent leaning from the bed or chair.
- Check to see that the call bell is within reach before leaving the room.
- Promptly answer call light to prevent the resident's arising without assistance.
- Encourage the use of supportive, sturdy footwear with nonslip soles for ambulation.
- Floor covering should not be slippery or highly patterned, and should be easily navigated when ambulating in common footwear or with assistive devices.
- Encourage residents to crouch down rather than bending over to pick up something, and to sit to dry the feet and pull on underwear and pants.
- Place grab bars by the toilet, in the bath or shower, along each set of stairs, and in the hallways.
- Provide chairs that are the proper height and depth to prevent "falling" into the chair or leaning far forward to arise from the chair.

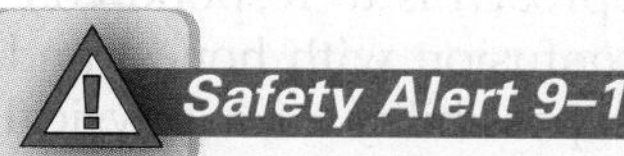

Safety Alert 9–1

Medication Assessment

Assessing all medications a resident is taking to determine the risk of medication-induced postural hypotension or dizziness is a must. Medications that cause dizziness are a frequent contributor to falls. Over-the-counter medications should be considered along with prescriptions.

Use of Security Devices and Alternative Measures. When a resident frequently forgets instructions to call for assistance, repeatedly attempts to get up and falls, or interferes with medical treatment by pulling out ordered tubes or scratching at wounds, the use of security devices may be necessary. Chemical restraints are tranquilizers or sedatives that calm a resident and alter behavior. Physical and chemical restraint use is restricted by law and is applied only as a last resort for safety when a resident is a proven threat to self or others (Legal & Ethical Considerations 9–1). **The purpose of such statutes is to ensure that restraints are used to protect residents, not to hinder their movements for the staff's convenience.** Alternative measures are always tried first (Box 9–6). When a security device is used, the least restrictive device is chosen. A variety of techniques help provide a restraint-free, yet safe, environment. The techniques depend on the type of population present in a

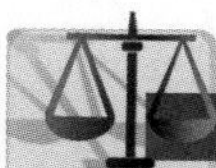

Legal & Ethical Considerations 9–1

Considering Restraints

Patient deaths have occurred due to improperly applied restraints. Laws require that they be used only as a last resort for safety after all other measures, such as sitters, family at the bedside, alarms, or distractions, have been attempted and failed. Documentation must be thorough, indicating alternative measures that have been tried and that the measures have failed. The time the restraint is applied, the condition of the patient at that time, interim assessments, and the time the restraint is removed and the condition of the patient at that time must be documented.

Box 9–6 *Measures Helpful to Prevent the Need for Security Devices*

- Explore what may be upsetting the resident and causing agitation.
- Place the restless or high-risk resident in a room or location close to the nurses' station where he can be checked frequently and attempts to get up will be most likely observed.
- Reorient the acutely confused resident as frequently as possible.
- Use validation to reaffirm feelings and concerns of the resident with dementia.
- Provide distraction activities that keep the resident busy; give the person a "job" to do.
- If the resident is agitated, turn off the television and provide soft, soothing music.
- Provide familiar and cherished items that the resident can handle.
- Ask a family member to stay with the resident.
- Use a bed or chair alarm to alert nursing staff that the resident is attempting to get out of bed or chair unassisted.
- Remain with the unsteady, agitated, or confused resident when he is up and about.
- Leave another person in charge of your residents when leaving the unit for a meal break or other reason; specifically mention which residents need to be visually checked frequently.
- If a resident needs to get up at night frequently to urinate and does not call for assistance, restrict fluid intake after 6 P.M. if appropriate.
- Provide social and diversional activities to a resident confined to a wheelchair or bed so that boredom does not cause the person to try to get up and seek activity.
- Move the mattress onto a low platform or the floor so that it is easier for the resident to get in and out of bed without the risk of a fall.

facility. **All security devices must only be used as a last resort and must be ordered by a physician.** If a qualified, licensed nurse determines the need for a chemical or physical security device in an emergency, the need is specifically documented when the security device is ap-

Box 9–7 Principles Related to the Use of Security and Safety Devices

- The use of safety or security devices must help the resident or be needed for the continuation of medical therapy.
- All devices that limit movement or immobilize must be ordered by a physician.
- Use the least amount of immobilization needed for the situation. For example, use mitts rather than wrist restraints if the resident cannot otherwise be prevented from pulling out tubes or lines.
- Apply the device snugly but not so tightly as to interfere with blood circulation or nerve function.
- If a security device is applied, check on the resident at least every hour. Assess for breathing, circulation, and possible nerve or skin impairment.
- An immobilization device must be removed and the resident's position changed at least every 2 hours. Active or passive exercises are performed for immobilized joints and muscles.
- Reassess need for the security measure every 4 to 8 hours.
- Meet needs for food, fluids, and toileting and assess these needs every 2 hours.
- Assess pain/comfort level and provide interventions as necessary.
- Document alternative measures taken and their success or failure. Document all pertinent data related to assessments when security devices are in place, when they were applied, and when removed.
- The physician should be notified as soon as the security device is deemed no longer necessary.

plied. All measures taken to try to correct the situation without the use of a security device prior to its application also are documented. A physician's order for the security device must be written within 24 to 48 hours. Box 9–7 presents the principles related to the use of security and safety devices.

The resident who is immobilized with a security device must be checked visually at least every 30 minutes to ensure that his body is in good alignment and that there are no problems. These checks must be documented. A check of skin color for circulation in the affected body parts is important whenever you are in the room. Residents must be turned or repositioned every 2 hours. Thorough assessment of skin and circulation is done at that time.

Managing Confusion and Disorientation. For the resident with mild confusion and disorientation, various techniques and measures are used to help maintain orientation. Reality orientation involves both the environment and the people who interact with the resident and should be followed 24 hours a day. The environment is structured so that the resident has concrete and continual reminders of the year, day, and time of day. Environmental aids include a readable, up-to-date calendar, a clock, and the daily newspaper or local television or radio news (Figure 9–1).

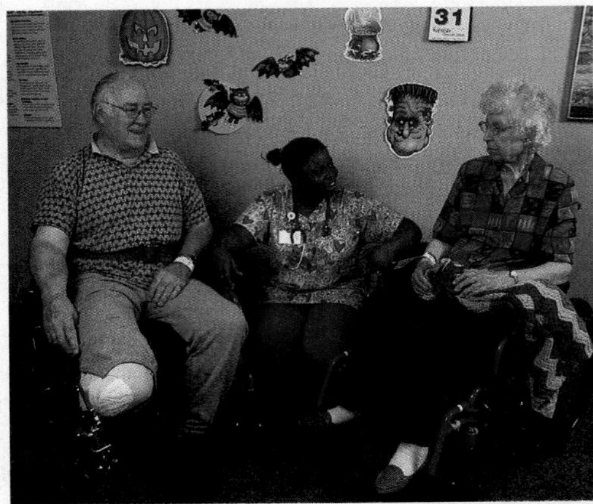

FIGURE 9–1 Long-term care environment promotes reality orientation.

Consistency in mealtimes, scheduled activities, treatments, and daily personal care routine also can be helpful. Limit the number of choices to be made during these activities. A time schedule for activities and events within the facility is posted in large type where the resident can refer to it frequently. Decorations for the next upcoming holiday give clues as to the current season of the year. Try to assign caregivers who are familiar to the resident, avoid unfamiliar situations, and limit visitors to one or two people at a time.

A positive and helpful approach is to respond continuously to the resident's confusion with honest and real information. Assess the possibility of a physical cause for the confusion, such as urinary tract infection, constipation, dehydration, or suboptimal pain control.

Nocturnal confusion (**sundowning**) occurs often among some elderly long-term care residents. Sensory deficits, such as impaired sight and hearing, add to the resident's confusion and anxiety at night when the environment becomes different because of darkness. A night light that gives illumination without shining in the resident's eyes or causing frightening shadows can be used. Keep the call bell within reach and visit the resident frequently to calm and reassure. Moving the resident closer to the nurses' station, touching, and other signs of caring are all ways in which you can intervene to minimize nocturnal confusion. A bed alarm that alerts staff when the resident attempts to get out of bed is helpful. Door alarms that announce when the resident has left his room, or designated area, may be used in place of security devices and prevent wandering in unsafe areas. Keeping the resident active during the day and encouraging physical exercise helps promote sleep at night. **Listening to the resident to try to determine any possible cause of unrest or fear can help solve the problem.**

Promoting Independence. The move to a long-term care facility is a major upheaval for the resident, par-

Table 9–2 Uses of Common Assistive-Adaptive Devices

DEVICE	USE
Buttonhook	Threaded through the buttonhole to enable patients with weak finger mobility to button shirts. Alternative uses include serving as a pencil holder.
Sock puller	Assists in putting on socks and compression stockings. Is placed in sock; then pulling on the strings pulls up the sock.
Extended shoe horn	Assists in putting on shoes for patients with decreased mobility. Alternative uses include turning light switches off or on while the patient is in a wheelchair.
Plate guard	Applied to a plate to assist patients with weak hand and arm mobility to feed themselves.
Gel pad	Placed under a plate or a glass to prevent dishes from slipping and moving. Alternative uses include placement under bathing and grooming items to prevent their movement.
Foam buildups	Applied to eating utensils to assist patients with weak handgrasps to feed themselves. Alternative uses include the application to pens and pencils to assist with writing, or over a buttonhook to assist with grasping the device.
Hook and loop fastener (Velcro) straps	Applied to utensils, a buttonhook, or a pencil to slip over the hand and provide a method of stabilizing the device when the patient's handgrasp is weak.
Long-handled reacher	Assists in obtaining items located on high shelves or at ground level for patients who are not able to change positions easily.
Elastic shoelaces or Velcro shoe closure	Prevents the need for tying shoes.

Adapted from Ignatavicius, D.D., & Workman, M.L. (2006). *Medical-Surgical Nursing: Critical Thinking for Collaborative Care* (5th ed.). Philadelphia: Elsevier Saunders, p. 127.

ticularly when it is for the rest of the person's lifetime. Specific goals should be set with the resident to encourage independence in activities of daily living (ADLs) and in recreational activity. Perhaps a resident can pursue a former hobby, such as knitting or playing the piano, if one is available. Adaptive devices and a consult with the dietitian may provide all the assistance that is necessary for self-feeding once again. Other adaptive devices can make daily living considerably easier (Table 9–2). **To promote a resident's independence, the staff should refrain from doing tasks that the resident is capable of doing himself.** For the resident who has had a stroke or suffers from debilitating arthritis or other musculoskeletal problem, use of adaptive devices can assist in the promotion of independence, provide some autonomy, and help to maintain function (Figure 9–2).

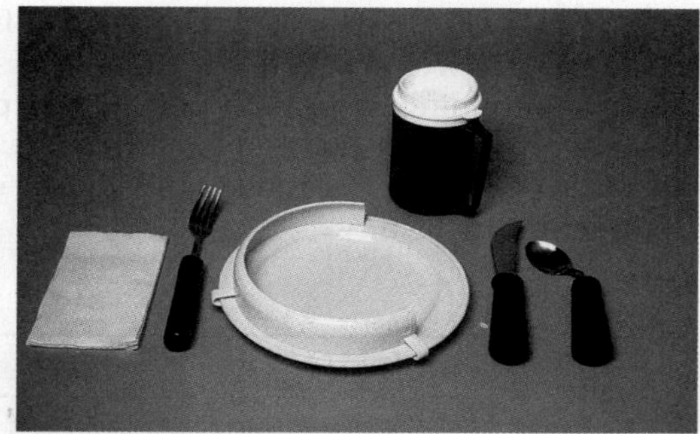

FIGURE 9–2 Adaptive devices to promote independence in eating.

? *Think Critically About . . .* Can you think of three ways to foster independence in the new resident who is still quite weak, has suffered a stroke, and has right-sided **hemiparesis** (weakness)? He is right-handed.

Maintaining Function. Once a functional assessment has been completed, specific goals should be written to maintain the highest level of function possible for the resident. If the resident is ambulatory, exercise should be encouraged daily on a planned basis. If the resident is not ambulatory, ROM exercises should be performed several times a day. Measures to promote continued bowel and bladder continence are essential. Assessing patterns of elimination and providing assistance for toileting as needed is a basic part of promoting continued function and protecting the resident's dignity. If the resident has been temporarily incontinent because of illness or surgery, then a bowel or bladder retraining program is appropriate. Chapters 29 and 34 discuss such programs.

Mental stimulation is essential to maintaining a high level of cognitive functioning. Although resident preference should be considered in group television viewing areas, the staff should consider planning segments of time to turn on informational programs that are interesting. Scientific shows, travel shows, public television specials, and similar programs can stimulate thinking and encourage the sharing of thoughts on a variety of subjects. Assisting residents to work crossword puzzles is another way to help them keep an active mind. When a resident cannot write or read because of poor vision, group work on a puzzle is an option. Card games promote mental stimulation as well as social interaction. Group activities such as bingo, group singing, holiday celebrations, and entertainment acts provide socializa-

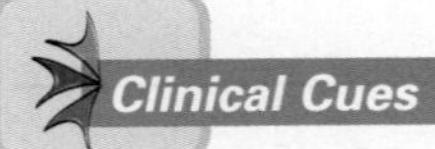

Activity theory states that people will be happiest in direct proportion to how much activity they are able to maintain as they grow older. Continuity theory proposes that participating in activities and relationships that have been maintained over a long period of time contributes to a sense of well-being and allows a sense of integrity and continuity with the past.

Finding out what activities have a lot of meaning for the resident and seeing how those might be continued or adaptations made so that there still is enjoyment in the activities can greatly enhance the quality of the resident's life.

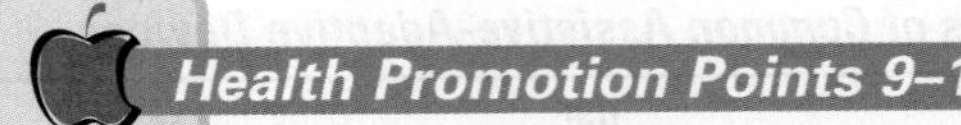

Healthy People 2010 Rehabilitation

Relevant goals for rehabilitation set by Healthy People 2010 *are:*

- Reduce the proportion of adults with disabilities who report feelings such as sadness, unhappiness, or depression that prevent them from being active.
- Increase the proportion of adults with disabilities who participate in social activities.
- Increase the proportion of adults with disabilities reporting sufficient emotional support.
- Increase the proportion of adults with disabilities reporting satisfaction with life.
- Increase the proportion of health and wellness and treatment programs and facilities that provide full access for people with disabilities.
- Reduce the proportion of people with disabilities who report not having the assistive devices and technology needed.
- Reduce the proportion of people with disabilities reporting environmental barriers to participation in home, school, work, or community activities.

tion and stimulation. Continuing interest in lifelong activities is a factor in successful aging for many.

Documentation. Documentation in a long-term care facility is somewhat different from that in the hospital or in home care. An admission assessment and an extensive eight-page Minimum Data Set (MDS) form that is required by the federal government are filled out (Figure 9–3). Bowel and bladder training assessment forms and training program forms, weekly pressure ulcer reports, and 24-hour intake and output records are some of the other documentation forms used in the long-term care facility.

REHABILITATION

Rehabilitation is the process whereby a disabled person is helped to achieve optimal function. A primary goal of rehabilitation is to minimize the deficit from the condition and maximize the abilities that are intact. It involves measures to achieve the highest level of physical, emotional, psychological, and social function and well-being possible. Vocational rehabilitation is job retraining for the disabled under the Americans with Disabilities Act (ADA) to provide a means of contributing to self-support. Rehabilitation is concerned with achieving a better quality of life. The majority of patients who require rehabilitation services are disabled as a result of a chronic illness. Others have become disabled from trauma incurred during an accident. Several of the objectives for *Healthy People 2010* are rehabilitation oriented (Health Promotion Points 9–1). One objective seeks to increase formal education for people with chronic and disabling conditions by including information about community and self-help resources as a part of managing their condition.

Each year about 8000 spinal cord injuries occur in the United States, and one out of four of the more than 2 million people who suffer head injuries annually have residual deficits. Another objective of *Healthy People 2010* is to reduce the incidence of secondary disabilities associated with injuries of the head and spinal cord. As the population ages, more people suffer heart attacks and strokes, which often leave the person with residual deficits. The need for rehabilitation services will continue to grow rapidly.

REHABILITATION PROGRAMS

There are rehabilitation services offered in freestanding rehabilitation hospitals, rehabilitation units in general hospitals, and skilled nursing home units where the patient stays for a few weeks.

Patients who have had a hip replacement often are placed in a skilled nursing facility for rehabilitation before returning home. Many communities have a hospital with an outpatient rehabilitation program for patients with cardiac and respiratory problems. Rehabilitation services are scarce in rural areas, and patients who have suffered neurologic injury or loss of musculoskeletal function due to amputation, trauma, or disease often have to go to a rehabilitation center miles away from home. Programs within large cities are often available for vision or hearing rehabilitation. YMCAs often have rehabilitation programs with water exercise for patients with severe arthritis. Most burn centers have comprehensive rehabilitation programs available for the burn patient. Rehabilitation programs have a philosophy that is based on three beliefs:

- Each person is unique, whole within himself, and interdependent with his own environment.
- Independence can be achieved within the limits of disability when the person is a full participant in managing his own life.

Numeric Identifier________________

MINIMUM DATA SET (MDS) — *VERSION 2.0*
FOR NURSING HOME RESIDENT ASSESSMENT AND CARE SCREENING

BASIC ASSESSMENT TRACKING FORM

SECTION AA. IDENTIFICATION INFORMATION

1.	**RESIDENT NAME***	**a.** (First) **b.** (Middle Initial) **c.** (Last) **d.** (Jr/Sr)
2.	**GENDER***	1. Male 2. Female
3.	**BIRTHDATE***	Month — Day — Year
4.	**RACE/* ETHNICITY**	1. American Indian/Alaskan Native 2. Asian/Pacific Islander 3. Black, not of Hispanic origin 4. Hispanic 5. White, not of Hispanic origin
5.	**SOCIAL SECURITY* AND MEDICARE NUMBERS* [C in 1st box if non med. no.]**	**a.** Social Security Number **b.** Medicare number (or comparable railroad insurance number)
6.	**FACILITY PROVIDER NO.***	**a.** State No. **b.** Federal No.
7.	**MEDICAID NO. ["+" *if pending,* "N" *if not a Medicaid recipient*]***	
8.	**REASONS FOR ASSESS-MENT**	[Note—Other codes do not apply to this form] **a. Primary reason for assessment** 1. Admission assessment (required by day 14) 2. Annual assessment 3. Significant change in status assessment 4. Significant correction of prior full assessment 5. Quarterly review assessment 10. Significant correction of prior quarterly assessment 0. *NONE OF ABOVE* ***b. Codes for assessments required for Medicare PPS or the State*** *1. Medicare 5-day assessment* *2. Medicare 30-day assessment* *3. Medicare 60-day assessment* *4. Medicare 90-day assessment* *5. Medicare readmission/return assessment* *6. Other state required assessment* *7. Medicare 14-day assessment* *8. Other Medicare required assessment*

9.	**Signatures of Persons Who Completed a Portion of the Accompanying Assessment or Tracking Form**		
	I certify that the accompanying information accurately reflects resident assessment or tracking information for this resident and that I collected or coordinated collection of this information on the dates specified. To the best of my knowledge, this information was collected in accordance with applicable Medicare and Medicaid requirements. I understand that this information is used as a basis for ensuring that residents receive appropriate and quality care, and as a basis for payment from federal funds. I further understand that payment of such federal funds and continued participation in the government-funded health care programs is conditioned on the accuracy and truthfulness of this information, and that I may be personally subject to or may subject my organization to substantial criminal, civil, and/or administrative penalties for submitting false information. I also certify that I am authorized to submit this information by this facility on its behalf.		
	Signature and Title	Sections	Date
a.			
b.			
c.			
d.			
e.			
f.			
g.			
h.			
i.			
j.			
k.			
l.			

GENERAL INSTRUCTIONS

Complete this information for submission with all full and quarterly assessments (Admission, Annual, Significant Change, State or Medicare required assessments, or Quarterly Reviews, etc.)

* = Key items for computerized resident tracking
[ ] = When box blank, must enter number or letter [a.] = When letter in box, check if condition applies

FIGURE 9–3 Sample page of Minimum Data Set form 2.0, U.S. Department of Health and Human Services.

Continued

Resident______________________ Numeric Identifier______________________

MINIMUM DATA SET (MDS) — *VERSION 2.0*
FOR NURSING HOME RESIDENT ASSESSMENT AND CARE SCREENING

BACKGROUND (FACE SHEET) INFORMATION AT ADMISSION

SECTION AB. DEMOGRAPHIC INFORMATION

1.	DATE OF ENTRY	*Date the stay began. Note — Does not include readmission if record was closed at time of temporary discharge to hospital, etc. In such cases, use prior admission date* Month — Day — Year	
2.	ADMITTED FROM (AT ENTRY)	1. Private home/apt. with no home health services 2. Private home/apt. with home health services 3. Board and care/assisted living/group home 4. Nursing home 5. Acute care hospital 6. Psychiatric hospital, MR/DD facility 7. Rehabilitation hospital 8. Other	
3.	LIVED ALONE (PRIOR TO ENTRY)	0. No 1. Yes 2. In other facility	
4.	ZIP CODE OF PRIOR PRIMARY RESIDENCE		
5.	RESIDENTIAL HISTORY 5 YEARS PRIOR TO ENTRY	***(Check all settings** resident **lived in** during 5 years prior to date of entry given in item AB1 above)*	
		Prior stay at this nursing home	a.
		Stay in other nursing home	b.
		Other residential facility—board and care home, assisted living, group home	c.
		MH/psychiatric setting	d.
		MR/DD setting	e.
		NONE OF ABOVE	f.
6.	LIFETIME OCCUPATION(S) [Put "/" between two occupations]		
7.	EDUCATION *(Highest level completed)*	1. No schooling 2. 8th grade/less 3. 9-11 grades 4. High school 5. Technical or trade school 6. Some college 7. Bachelor's degree 8. Graduate degree	
8.	LANGUAGE	*(Code for correct response)* **a.** Primary Language 0. English 1. Spanish 2. French 3. Other	
		b. If other, specify	
9.	MENTAL HEALTH HISTORY	Does resident's RECORD indicate any history of mental retardation, mental illness, or developmental disability problem? 0. No 1. Yes	
10.	CONDITIONS RELATED TO MR/DD STATUS	***(Check all conditions** that are related to MR/DD status that were manifested before age 22, and are likely to continue indefinitely)*	
		Not applicable—no MR/DD (Skip to AB11)	a.
		MR/DD with organic condition	
		Down's syndrome	b.
		Autism	c.
		Epilepsy	d.
		Other organic condition related to MR/DD	e.
		MR/DD with no organic condition	f.
11.	DATE BACKGROUND INFORMATION COMPLETED	Month — Day — Year	

SECTION AC. CUSTOMARY ROUTINE

1.	CUSTOMARY ROUTINE *(In year prior to DATE OF ENTRY to this nursing home, or year last in community if now being admitted from another nursing home)*	***(Check all that apply.** If all information UNKNOWN, check last box only.)*	
		CYCLE OF DAILY EVENTS	
		Stays up late at night (e.g., after 9 PM)	a.
		Naps regularly during the day (at least 1 hour)	b.
		Goes out 1+ days a week	c.
		Stays busy with hobbies, reading, or fixed daily routine	d.
		Spends most of time alone or watching TV	e.
		Moves independently indoors (with appliances, if used)	f.
		Use of tobacco products at least daily	g.
		NONE OF ABOVE	h.
		EATING PATTERNS	
		Distinct food preferences	i.
		Eats between meals all or most days	j.
		Use of alcoholic beverage(s) at least weekly	k.
		NONE OF ABOVE	l.
		ADL PATTERNS	
		In bedclothes much of day	m.
		Wakens to toilet all or most nights	n.
		Has irregular bowel movement pattern	o.
		Showers for bathing	p.
		Bathing in PM	q.
		NONE OF ABOVE	r.
		INVOLVEMENT PATTERNS	
		Daily contact with relatives/close friends	s.
		Usually attends church, temple, synagogue (etc.)	t.
		Finds strength in faith	u.
		Daily animal companion/presence	v.
		Involved in group activities	w.
		NONE OF ABOVE	x.
		UNKNOWN—Resident/family unable to provide information	y.

SECTION AD. FACE SHEET SIGNATURES

SIGNATURES OF PERSONS COMPLETING FACE SHEET:

a. Signature of RN Assessment Coordinator		Date

I certify that the accompanying information accurately reflects resident assessment or tracking information for this resident and that I collected or coordinated collection of this information on the dates specified. To the best of my knowledge, this information was collected in accordance with applicable Medicare and Medicaid requirements. I understand that this information is used as a basis for ensuring that residents receive appropriate and quality care, and as a basis for payment from federal funds. I further understand that payment of such federal funds and continued participation in the government-funded health care programs is conditioned on the accuracy and truthfulness of this information, and that I may be personally subject to or may subject my organization to substantial criminal, civil, and/or administrative penalties for submitting false information. I also certify that I am authorized to submit this information by this facility on its behalf.

Signature and Title	Sections	Date
b.		
c.		
d.		
e.		
f.		
g.		

[ ] = When box blank, must enter number or letter [a.] = When letter in box, check if condition applies

FIGURE **9–3, cont'd** Sample page of Minimum Data Set form 2.0, U.S. Department of Health and Human Services.

- The goal is to enable patients to mobilize their own resources, choose goals, and attain them through their own efforts. Rehabilitation involves the whole person and is a team effort involving a variety of disciplines.

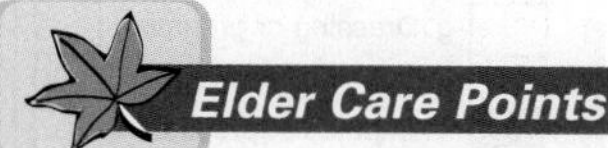

Elder Care Points

An elderly patient who has suffered a major loss of body function may not be initially receptive to rehabilitation efforts. It takes a skillful nurse to help motivate the patient to want to improve his functional ability. Sometimes introducing the patient to someone close to his own age who has been through a similar illness and has managed to regain some functions is the best "medicine." Gentle encouragement with praise for small efforts and accomplishments is better than trying to force the patient to perform exercises or practice tasks.

A respiratory rehabilitation program teaches self-care techniques to the patient that will help him attain a better quality of life. There are generally three components to a respiratory rehabilitation program:

- Breathing exercises
- Paced walking exercise
- Correct use of inhaled medications

Patients are enrolled in the program for a number of weeks and interact with other patients who have the same problems. A nurse or respiratory therapist teaches the various breathing techniques, paced walking, and use of inhalers. The nurse conducts motivational group activities to increase the desire to participate in an exercise program and to display the benefits of following the program. Teaching on how to avoid respiratory infections is reinforced. The nurse or respiratory therapist is available to encourage the patient and to evaluate progress on using the techniques taught while exercising. Vital signs are monitored periodically to determine the effect of exercise on cardiac and respiratory function. Some rehabilitation centers provide respiratory services by weaning the patient from the ventilator and then working with him to improve respiratory function and functional capacity for ADLs.

Cardiac rehabilitation programs are usually outpatient based and consist of:

- Monitored exercise to increase strength and endurance and build collateral circulation to the heart
- Diet counseling and education to lower cholesterol, triglycerides, and body fat
- Medication counseling regarding the purpose, administration, and side effects of the prescribed medications
- Vital sign monitoring to determine the effect of exercise on the cardiovascular system
- Group sessions on stress reduction techniques

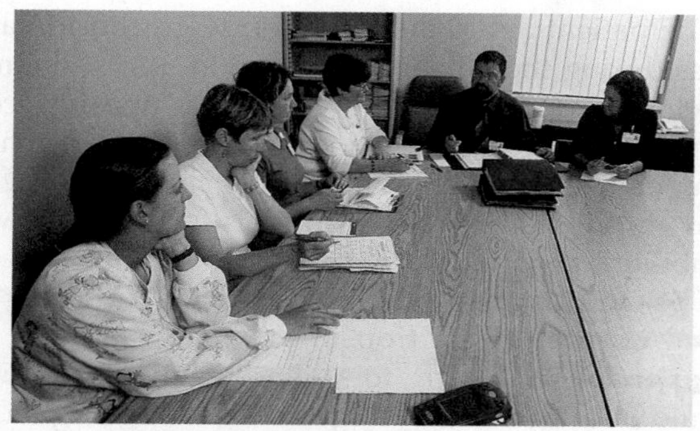

FIGURE 9–4 The rehabilitation team conferring about the client's care.

- Support group sessions for those experiencing depression or anxiety after surgery or a myocardial infarction

Such cardiac rehabilitation programs usually have a physician, nurses, physical therapist, dietitian, and psychologist or social worker on staff.

Rehabilitation after knee surgery and other musculoskeletal injuries is often performed on an outpatient basis. Either the physical therapist goes to the home or the patient travels to the physical therapy facility. Supervised exercise is performed to increase ROM, decrease pain, strengthen muscles, promote ambulation, and improve balance.

Patients with neurologic damage from a spinal cord or head injury may need to spend several months in a rehabilitation facility. Because of insurance limitations, inpatient treatment is not always possible. Rehabilitation efforts then need to be continued at home.

THE REHABILITATION TEAM

The nurse who works with rehabilitation patients must be flexible and creative and recognize that the patient is the "captain" of the rehabilitation team. The nurse's function is to assist the patient to achieve an optimal state of wellness as *defined by the patient.* It is very important that the nurse be nonjudgmental and not impose her own values and attitudes on the patient.

The rehabilitation nurse must be able to work collaboratively with other health team members. Besides the physician, occupational, physical, speech, cognitive, and recreational therapists, vocational counselors, and social workers are part of the team. The nurse assists in seeing to it that the patient correctly performs exercises and activities as instructed by such therapists and reinforces their teaching. A collaborative or interdisciplinary care plan is followed so that each member of the team is aware of what treatment and education the patient is receiving. Both short- and long-term goals are set. This provides for continuity of interdisciplinary care, recognizing the critical importance of each discipline in promoting positive outcomes for the patient. Team conferences are scheduled regularly for members to collaborate on the patient's care and evaluate rehabilitation progress (Figure 9–4).

The patient and family both undergo considerable stress during the rehabilitation period. Assist them in developing positive coping techniques and in recognizing their strengths. A good sense of humor, gentle, firm people skills, patience, and the ability to provide solid encouragement are good tools for working with rehabilitation patients.

The philosophy of rehabilitation nursing is based on the recognition of the patient's need for independence. Learn to judge when the patient should be allowed to struggle to do something on his own and learn to recognize when the patient's frustration is reaching a level at which you should step in and assist.

The LPN/LVN Role in Rehabilitation

There are often two levels of LPNs/LVNs employed in rehabilitation facilities. One is the licensed LPN/LVN I and the other is the licensed LPN/LVN II with intravenous therapy and Functional Independence Measure (FIM) certification. The LPN/LVN I does not infuse intravenous therapy, but does all other nursing activities except for assessments. The LPN/LVN II performs the same functions as the LPN/LVN I plus the tasks involved with intravenous infusions. At least a year of medical-surgical experience is the usual requirement for employment at a rehabilitation facility. The LPN/LVN initiates and participates in updating the team plan of care in collaboration with the RN to meet the patient's needs. The LPN/LVN assists with patient and family education by supporting the outlined teaching plan and reinforcing teaching. Any barriers to patient/caregiver readiness to learn are reported to the supervisor. Recommendations are made to team members on how to facilitate patient/caregiver learning. Learning outcomes are evaluated and documented. The LPN/LVN is an active participant and facilitator of both structured and nonstructured learning experiences. Leadership functions are to supervise the patient care assistants, the certified nursing assistants, and the nursing rehabilitation technicians. The LPN/LVN acts as a preceptor for unlicensed personnel as needed and appropriate. As a member of the team, all normal patient care nursing duties are carried out, and input and feedback are provided to the team. When assigned to do so, the LPN/LVN carries out quality improvement activities.

NURSING MANAGEMENT

Assessment (Data Collection)

After obtaining a thorough history, a physical and psychosocial assessment are performed for each patient to establish a baseline; to determine physical limitations, ability to perform ADLs, and amount of assistance needed; and to identify present psychosocial difficulties (Focused Assessment 9–1). A skin risk assessment and fall risk assessment are performed (see Chapter 42 for the pressure ulcer risk assessment tool). Patients covered by Medicare will have data filled in on the section of the MDS pertinent to rehabilitation (Figure 9–5). The patient's home environment is examined before discharge to determine whether physical features of the home, such as stairs, narrow doorways, or access to bathroom facilities, will present a problem. Questions about the neighborhood, such as the location of shopping centers and types of transportation available, are asked. Inquire about who does the grocery shopping, cooking, errands, and housework for the patient.

The patient's usual daily schedule and habits of everyday living are explored, including sleeping and waking patterns, eating, elimination patterns, hygiene, grooming, sexual activity, working, and leisure activities. A *functional assessment* of how the patient's disability has affected his former usual patterns (Box 9–8) focuses on the patient's present ability to perform ADLs, such as toileting, bathing, dressing, grooming, and ambulating, as well as his ability to use the telephone, shop, prepare food, and perform housekeeping chores. Various assessment tools are used to determine the patient's ability to function. A common one, the Katz Index of Independence in Activities of Daily Liv-

SECTION P. SPECIAL TREATMENTS AND PROCEDURES

3.	NURSING REHABILITATION/ RESTORATIVE CARE	*Record the NUMBER OF DAYS each of the following rehabilitation or restorative techniques or practices was **provided to the resident for more than or equal to 15 minutes per day in the past 7 days*** *(Enter 0 if none or less than 15 min. daily.)*			
		a. Range of motion (passive)		f. Walking	
		b. Range of motion (active)		g. Dressing or grooming	
		c. Splint or brace assistance		h. Eating or swallowing	
		TRAINING AND SKILL PRACTICE IN:	■	i. Amputation/prosthesis care	
		d. Bed mobility		j. Communication	
		e. Transfer		k. Other	

SECTION H. CONTINENCE IN LAST 14 DAYS

3.	APPLIANCES AND PROGRAMS				
		Any scheduled toileting plan	a.	Did not use toilet room/ commode/urinal	f.
		Bladder retraining program	b.	Pads/briefs used	g.
		External (condom) catheter	c.	Enemas/irrigation	h.
		Indwelling catheter	d.	Ostomy present	i.
		Intermittent catheter	e.	*NONE OF ABOVE*	j.

FIGURE 9–5 Sections P 3 and H 3 a, b that apply specifically to the rehabilitation patient from Minimum Data Set 2.0 forms, U.S. Department of Health and Human Services, January 30, 1998.

Box 9–8 *Functional Independence Measure Scoring Categories*

- Self-care
- Sphincter control
- Transfers
- Locomotion
- Communication
- Social cognition

A score of 0 or 1 is given in each category. Totaled scores indicate Independent (6–7), Modified Dependence (3–5), or Complete Dependence (1–2).

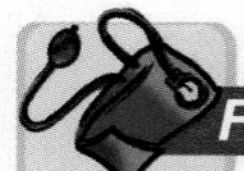

Focused Assessment 9–1

Data Collection for the Rehabilitation Patient

After reviewing the patient's history, the following data are collected by asking pertinent questions for each body system or function:

CARDIOVASCULAR
- Fatigue
- Chest pain
- Arrhythmia
- Fear of cardiac event

RESPIRATORY
- Activity tolerance
- Shortness of breath
- Fear of not being able to breathe

GASTROINTESTINAL/NUTRITION
- Dysphagia
- Anorexia, nausea, vomiting
- Eating pattern; amount of oral intake
- Weight loss or gain
- Bowel status; change in stool
- Serum albumin levels

URINARY
- Urinary pattern
- Fluid intake
- Retention
- Self-catheterization status
- Urinalysis and/or culture

NEUROLOGIC
- Motor function
- Sensation
- Cognitive abilities
- Assistive devices

MUSCULOSKELETAL
- Muscle strength
- Range of motion
- Endurance
- Fall risk assessment
- Assistive devices
- Safety measures

INTEGUMENTARY
- Skin condition
- Skin risk of breakdown
- Presence of lesions
- Measures to decrease risk of breakdown

DEGREE OF INDEPENDENCE
- Functional Independence Measure scores per certified personnel assessment
- Ability for activities of daily living (Katz assessment)

PSYCHOSOCIAL
- Alteration in roles
- Financial concerns
- Support people
- Self-concept status
- Coping mechanisms
- Sexual concerns
- Employment/educational concerns
- Family strain
- Home environment alterations needed

MEDICATIONS
- Scheduled medications
- PRN (as-needed) medications
- Over-the-counter preparations

ing (Figure 9–6), helps evaluate how much assistance the patient needs for various activities.

Psychosocial assessment includes evaluating self-esteem and body image. The Baird Body Image Assessment Tool is often used. Use of defense mechanisms, level of anxiety, and usual coping techniques are explored. To ascertain the patient's response to loss, the nurse asks the patient to describe feelings related to the loss of a body part or body function. The patient's support systems and the family's coping abilities also are determined. As rehabilitation progresses, the nurse performs a vocational assessment so that the vocational counselor can assist the patient in finding appropriate training, education, or employment after discharge from the rehabilitation program.

Patients with life-changing illness or injury, those who have suffered major loss of body function or former roles, and those who have lost most of their independence and social contacts may suffer from anger and depression. Assessing mental outlook is an ongoing nursing function. Should several signs of severe depression become evident, consult with the physician. The patient must be kept safe. Determining suicide potential in the depressed patient is important. Chapter 48 discusses assessment and intervention for depression and suicidal thought.

Sexual concerns should be addressed during the rehabilitation period. Help the patient identify problems and concerns and work to assist in finding means for sexual expression and gratification. If you are not comfortable or knowledgeable in this role, an appropriate referral to a psychologist or sex therapist should be made.

? ***Think Critically About . . .*** Can you explain the difference between a physical assessment and a functional assessment?

Nursing Diagnosis

Nursing diagnoses appropriate for the patient undergoing rehabilitation are located in Box 9–9. Individual nursing diagnoses are chosen based on the data collected.

KATZ INDEX OF INDEPENDENCE IN ACTIVITIES OF DAILY LIVING

Activities Points (1 or 0)	**Independence** (1 Point) NO supervision, direction, or personal assistance	**Dependence** (0 Points) WITH supervision, direction, personal assistance or total care
Bathing Points: _______	Bathes self completely or needs help in bathing only a single part of the body such as the back, genital area, or disabled extremity	Needs help with bathing more than one part of the body, getting in or out of the tub or shower; requires total bathing
Dressing Points: _______	Get clothes from closets and drawers and puts on clothes and outer garments complete with fasteners; may have help tying shoes	Needs help with dressing self or needs to be completely dressed
Toileting Points: _______	Goes to toilet, gets on and off, arranges clothes, cleans genital area without help	Needs help transferring to the toilet, cleaning self, or uses bedpan or commode
Transferring Points: _______	Moves in and out of bed or chair unassisted; mechanical transfer aids are acceptable	Needs help in moving from bed to chair or requires a complete transfer
Continence Points: _______	Exercises complete self-control over urination and defecation	Is partially or totally incontinent of bowel or bladder
Feeding Points: _______	Gets food from plate into mouth without help; preparation of food may be done by another person	Needs partial or total help with feeding or requires parenteral feeding

Total Points: _______

Score of 6 = High; patient is independent.
Score of 0 = Low; patient is very dependent.

FIGURE **9–6** Katz Index of Independence in Activities of Daily Living. (From Katz S, Down TD, Cash HR, et al. [1970]. Progress in the development of the Index of ADL. *Gerontologist,* 10:20–30. Copyright © The Gerontologist Society of America. Reproduced with permission of the publisher.)

Box 9–9 ***Nursing Diagnoses Commonly Used for Rehabilitation Patients***

- Impaired physical mobility related to neuromuscular impairment, sensory-perceptual impairment, and/or pain
- Self-care deficit *(specify deficits)* related to perceptual or cognitive impairment and/or neuromuscular impairment
- Risk for impaired skin integrity related to alteration in sensation or nutritional status
- Risk for injury related to musculoskeletal weakness, perceptual or cognitive impairment
- Impaired urinary elimination related to neurologic dysfunction or trauma or disease affecting spinal nerves
- Constipation related to neurologic impairment
- Ineffective coping related to added stressors or situational crisis
- Compromised family coping related to situational crisis and/or added stressors
- Impaired home maintenance related to neuromuscular impairment, perceptual or cognitive impairment
- Deficient knowledge related to self-care and techniques for rehabilitation
- Disturbed body image related to loss of normal function or traumatic injury and/or scarring
- Sexual dysfunction related to neuromuscular impairment, pain, or impaired mobility

Planning

An interdisciplinary plan of care is devised for each rehabilitation patient. Often there will be five or more health professionals involved. Periodic care conferences are essential for the members of the health care team to evaluate the progress of the patient, share perceptions and ideas, and revise the plan of care if it is not helping the patient to meet established expected outcomes (Figure 9–7). Other forms used for interdisciplinary care and tracking progress are located on the student CD-ROM that is included with this text. Depending on the situation, care conferences may occur once every 1 or 2 weeks or once a month. Both long-term and short-term goals will be

Patient name: Payer: Date: / / ☐ Intro ☐ Interim ☐ Discharge

Medical status — Precautions ___ Infections ___ Seizure ___ Aspiration ___ Cardiac ___ Fall ___ Ortho ___ Dysreflexia ___ Bleeding ___ Code Green

Discharge plan — **Education plan (Peds)**

Key discharge goals — Goal — Date Met

Psychologic adjustment

Team goals/Treatment planning
- Home evaluation needed Y N In next 2 weeks
- Daily living trial date ___/___/___
- Therapeutic community evaluation date ___/___/___
- Work/school evaluation date ___/___/___

1. Patient/caregiver activities/issues

2. Return to school/Work issues N/A___

3. Obstacles to discharge

4. Area of potential handicap
- Vocation/Avocation: Y N
- Family role: Y N
- School: Y N
- Community involvement: Y N

5. Key weekly goals (3-4) to achieve discharge plan
1.
2.
3.
4.

6. Strategies to achieve key weekly goals

7. Continuity of care ELOS:

TEAM MEMBER SIGNATURES/DATE				OTHER/DATE	
Phys	/ /	OT	/ /		/ /
Case Mgr.	/ /	PT	/ /		/ /
Coun/Psyc	/ /	TR	/ /		/ /
Nurse	/ /	SLP	/ /		/ /

HOSPITAL TEAM CONFERENCE REPORT

FIGURE 9–7 Hospital team conference report form used in a rehabilitation facility.

set. Expected outcomes are written for each nursing diagnosis.

Implementation and Evaluation

Interventions are carried out in a manner that encourages the patient to do as much for himself as possible. Praise is given for even small accomplishments or attempts at self-care. When working with the patient, observe for undue fatigue. Pace activities according to the patient's fatigue level. Physical and occupational therapists work closely with rehabilitation patients to help them adapt so that they can perform ADLs (Figure 9–8). Speech therapists, activity therapists, and others will be involved in the implementation of the

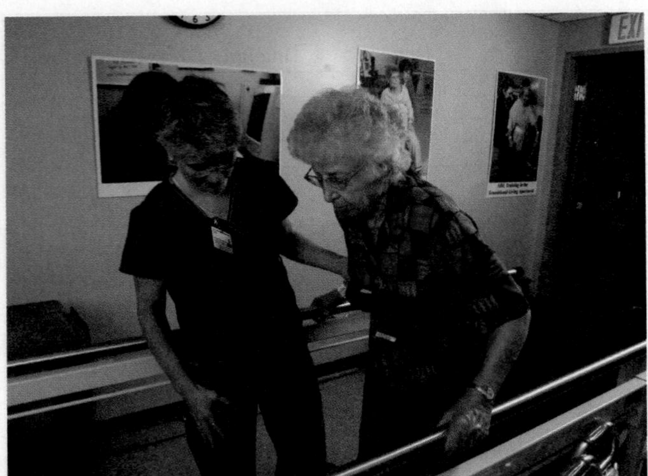

FIGURE **9–8** Physical therapist working with a patient on ambulation and muscle strengthening.

care plan. The patient will be kept very busy during rehabilitation.

Discharge planning is implemented from the time the patient enters rehabilitation. The family and patient will need resources within the community and the nation (Box 9–10).

Evaluation is performed by gathering data that show whether the goals and expected outcomes have been met.

(Refer to the companion CD for the "Transdisciplinary Initial Assessment" and "Team Kardex" forms.)

HOME CARE

The majority of care in the community setting is given by home health and hospice agencies. Home health care is the preferred and most cost-effective method of health care delivery. Recent innovations in medical equipment have allowed more complex, high-technology care to be given at home. For the patient there are many benefits, both physically and psychologically. **The goal of home care is to keep the patient as well and independent as possible and enable him to stay at home.** The LPN/LVN must have 1 year's experience working in an acute care facility before being hired for home care in most states.

The RN acts as case manager and coordinates the care of all of the health care providers involved in the patient's care. The RN is responsible for the plan of care and for seeing that care is delivered in an uninterrupted manner. She must act as a liaison with the other care providers to see to it that all efforts effectively complement one another. The LPN/LVN may perform treatments, perform appropriate delegated duties of the RN, or be employed to provide care in the home on a daily shift basis.

Home care nursing can prevent an expensive readmission to a hospital or entry into a long-term care facility. Home health care is family centered, and the family members or significant other are responsible for the ongoing care of the patient. The nurse visits to intervene and see that the patient is provided comfort, complications are prevented and health is improved, and to assist with rehabilitation (Figure 9–9). Because home health care is family centered, **the philosophy of the nurse must have a different focus. In the home care setting, the patient and family are in charge. The nurse is a guest in the home, and acts as a consultant, coordinator of care, provider of skilled care, teacher, and advocate.** This is an instance in which the patient and family are truly "patients." They are seeking the nurse's services and must be treated as valued customers. Learn to be nonjudgmental of the patient, the family, and the living arrangements. Together set goals for care, and then establish boundaries of your role. Should the living situation not be ideal, furnishings and equipment lacking, or the home dirty, establish trust with the patient and family before trying to accomplish major changes. Be sensitive to the patient and family's cultural values, financial resources, and specific ways of doing things and try not to impose your own views. Work together with the patient and family to improve home safety. Share knowledge of available resources (see Box 9–10). **A home care nurse must be very flexible and creative in teaching patients and families ways to accomplish care of the patient while abiding by the principles of asepsis and safety.**

A large percentage of the home care nurse's time with the patient is spent evaluating physical and psychosocial status, signs of complications, side effects of medications, and effects of therapy. Both the safety of the home and the quality of nutritional and basic care are evaluated. The nurse is with the patient and is able to gather considerable useful data for the physician. Considerable time is spent consulting with physicians by phone, updating them on the patient's condition, seeking new orders, and collaborating about care needs. Each visit to the patient includes a physical assessment of the identified problems and of nutritional, home safety, elimination, skin, and psychosocial status. All findings are documented. The nurse also documents data indicating that home health nursing care is still needed. Between visits, the nurse may contact the patient or family to check on various aspects of care or to see whether there are any concerns. The patient and family may contact the agency or the nurse at any time, and phone calls are encouraged.

Other functions of the home health nurse include performing wound care and dressing changes, organizing medications for scheduled administration, monitoring blood sugar levels, drawing blood samples for laboratory testing, giving injections or teaching injection technique, monitoring pain control, and moni-

Box 9-10 ***Resources for Rehabilitation Patients and Families***

Administration on Developmental Disabilities,
U.S. Department of Health and Human Services,
370 L'enfant Promenade, S.W.,
Washington, DC 20447
(202) 690-6590
www.acf.hhs.gov/programs/add

American Diabetes Association,
1701 North Beauregard St.,
Alexandria, VA 22311
(800) 342-2383
www.diabetes.org/home.jsp

American Heart Association National Center,
7272 Greenville Avenue, Dallas, TX 75231;
American Stroke Association National Center,
7272 Greenville Avenue,
Dallas TX 75231
www.americanheart.org

American Lung Association, 61 Broadway, 6th Floor,
New York, NY 10006
www.lungusa.org

Clearinghouse on Disability Information,
Office of Special Education and Rehabilitation Services,
550 12th Street, S.W., Room 5133,
Washington, DC 20202-2550
(202) 245-7307
www.ed.gov/about/offices/list/osers/index.html

Information Center for Individuals with Disabilities,
P. O. Box 750119,
Arlington Heights, MA 02475
e-mail: contact@disability.net

Mainstream Living, Inc.,
333 SW 9th Street,
Des Moines, IA 50309
(515) 243-8115
www.mainstreamliving.org

National Amputation Foundation,
40 Church St.,
Malverne, NY 11565
(516) 887-3600
http://home.comcast.net/~n2fc/natamp/naf.html

National Clearinghouse on Postsecondary Education for Individuals with Disabilities, HEATH Resource Center,
2121 K Street, N.W.,
Washington, DC 20037
(800) 544-3284
www.heath.gwu.edu

National Council on Disability,
1331 F Street, S.W.,
Suite 850,
Washington, DC 20004
(202) 272-2004
www.ncd.gov

National Rehabilitation Information Center,
4200 Forbes Blvd., Suite 202,
Lanham, MD 20706
(800) 346-2742

Office of Vocational and Adult Education,
U.S. Department of Education,
400 Maryland Ave., S.W.,
Washington, DC 20202-7100
(202) 245-7700
www.ed.gov/about/offices/list/ovae/index.html

MORE INTERNET RESOURCES FOR PATIENTS AND FAMILIES

Esmerel's Rehabilitation Resources
www.esmerel.org/misc/rehab.htm

Moss Rehab Resource Net
Links to accessible travel, daily living aids, assistive technology, state assistive technology centers, etc.
www.mossresourcenet.org

Rehabilitation Research Center
Lists of resources for traumatic brain injury and spinal cord injury
www.tbi-sci.org/main.html

Disability Resource Management Web Watcher—Vocational Rehabilitation
www.disabilityresources.org/VOC-REHAB.html

NATIONAL ASSOCIATION WEBSITES—DISABILITY AND REHABILITATION

Brain Injury Association
www.biausa.org

National Arts and Disability Center
www.nadc.ucla.edu

National Council on Disability
www.ncd.gov

National Dissemination Center for Children with Disabilities
www.nichcy.org

National Organization on Disability
www.nod.org

National Spinal Cord Injury Association
www.spinalcord.org

National Rehabilitation Organization
www.Nationalrehab.org/website/index.html

CAREGIVER RESOURCES

Family Village—Disability-Related Resources
Information resources on specific diagnoses, communication connections, adaptive products and technology, adaptive recreational activities, education, worship, health issues, disability-related media and literature, and much, much more! Has specific resources for Latinos, African Americans, and Asian Americans with disabilities.
www.familyvillage.wisc.edu/living/index.html

Family Caregiver Alliance
A variety of resources, including a long-distance caregiver handbook.
www.caregiver.org/caregiver/jsp/home.jsp

National Family Caregivers Association
www.nfcacares.org

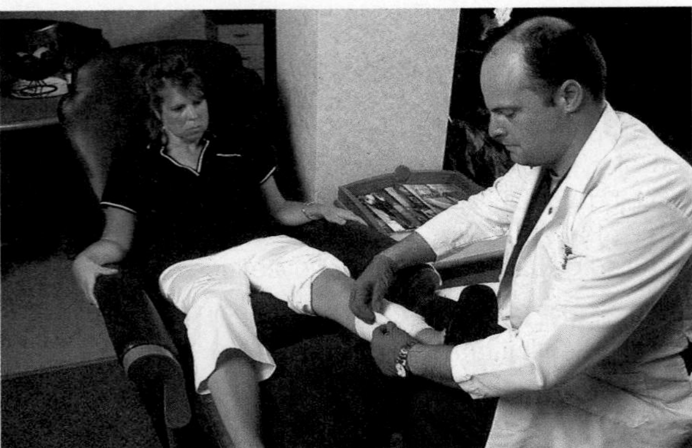

FIGURE 9–9 Home health nurse changing a dressing.

toring enteral feedings. Teaching self-care and rehabilitation techniques and monitoring progress and compliance with treatment are primary nursing functions that help control health care costs and keep the patient from needing hospitalization. The home care nurse needs to be a strong advocate for the patient regarding needs and treatment.

The home care nurse provides considerable psychosocial care for the patient and family. Sometimes, the nurse is the only visitor the patient has. In this instance, the nurse becomes a sort of friend, providing social interaction as well as needed health care. The nurse must become knowledgeable about negotiating the complex medical care system and obtaining supplies, medications, or services when the patient does not have money for them. A full knowledge of the community's resources available to the patient is essential. Most home health agencies have lists of resources available. The medical social worker who has a liaison with the agency also can be of help. Where the hospital nurse stays out of financial concerns, other than referrals to the social worker, the home care nurse must try to help the patient find remedies to financial problems so that stress will be reduced and energies can be directed at healing and techniques of self-care.

Think Critically About . . . Can you explain how you would go about trying to obtain a shower chair for a patient who cannot afford to buy or rent one?

THE LPN/LVN IN HOME CARE

Generally the LPN/LVN working in home care is under the supervision of the RN case manager. The LPN/LVN may be providing "private-duty" services for an unconscious patient who needs skilled care such as tracheal suctioning or tube feedings, performing home visits to change dressings or monitor blood sugar levels, or acting as an in-agency supervisor by coordinating home health aide visits and supervising their

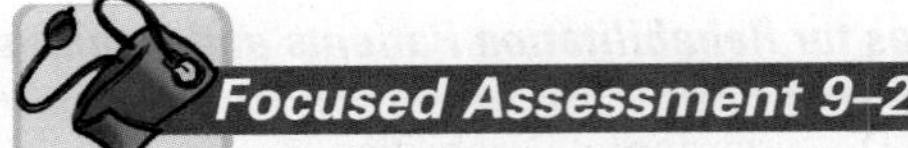

Focused Assessment 9–2

Assessing Caregiver Stress

The following questions provide data to determine when a caregiver's stress is reaching unhealthy levels.

- What help do you have in caring for your spouse/relative?
- Are there more family members who might help out?
- Is your sleep often disturbed to meet your spouse/relative's needs?
- Do you feel strained with all your family and caregiving responsibilities?
- Have you been feeling edgy or irritable lately?
- Are you feeling overwhelmed?
- Do you feel you cannot leave your relative alone?
- Have you been having crying spells?
- Are you having difficulty making decisions?
- Do you find you have trouble keeping your mind on what you are doing?
- Are you having frequent headaches, backaches, or muscle or stomach pain?
- Do you have any social contact?

work. The role of the LPN/LVN in home care is growing. The family provides assistance with personal care, and a home health aide may visit a few times a week to bathe the patient and shampoo hair. Homemaking is provided by family members, significant others, or a homemaker aide. "Sitters" may be hired to attend to the patient's needs at night if the family is not able to provide this service.

Nursing care plans are formulated in collaboration with the patient, the family or significant other, and all other health care providers. Teaching and 24-hour needs are considered and often form a large part of the plan. Case conferences are conducted regularly, even if they are done by the case manager on the telephone with the others involved in the patient's care. Medicare requires a case conference every 60 days when more than one discipline is involved in the patient's care.

THE FAMILY CAREGIVER

When a patient has considerable disability and cannot function independently, a family member often becomes the main caregiver. Depending on the degree of dependence of the patient, the caregiver may have an overwhelming task in caring for the patient, maintaining the house, obtaining food and supplies, cooking, and coordinating therapy or physician appointments. The caregiver's usual life is disrupted and social contacts are limited by time constraints and fatigue. The nurse must assess the caregiver's stress levels regularly (Focused Assessment 9–2). Some home care agencies have an assessment tool for this purpose. When caregiver stress is high, calling the agency social worker for a consult can provide either more help for the caregiver, or a respite program that might provide a few days of needed rest and relaxation. A respite program provides room, meals, and care for an individual while the caregiver is relieved of all responsibility.

Key Points

- Chronic illness interferes with normal function for about 43 million people in the United States.
- Hazards of immobility are many and can occur within just a few days for the immobile patient.
- It is a nursing responsibility to prevent hazards of immobility.
- The elderly are especially prone to develop problems of immobility.
- Long-term care facilities attend to the care of many people who have chronic illness.
- The LPN/LVN often works as a charge nurse in a long-term care facility.
- The LPN/LVN supervises the nursing assistants in the long-term care facility.
- Safety of residents is a primary goal in the long-term care facility.
- Much attention is directed to preventing resident falls.
- Security devices are only used to protect the resident, or others, and only as a last resort.
- Frequent assessment is essential when a security device is applied to a resident.
- Techniques to minimize confusion and disorientation are used consistently.
- Keeping the resident active during the day helps decrease nocturnal confusion.
- A goal of long-term care is to promote as much independence as possible for the resident.
- Long-term care facilities must help residents to maintain or regain function.
- Rehabilitation helps a disabled person to achieve optimal function.
- There are rehabilitation programs for patients with respiratory, heart, and musculoskeletal problems.
- Rehabilitation is a team effort of the patient and many health professionals.
- The nurse assists with determination of rehabilitation needs.
- Rehabilitation is carried out with a collaborative plan of care.
- Home care agencies provide continuing care in the community.
- LPNs/LVNs are supervised by the physician or RN in the home care environment.
- In the home care setting, the patient and family are in charge; you are a guest in the home.
- Home care nurses must be flexible and creative in order to accomplish needed care of the patient in the home.

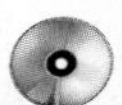

Go to your **Companion CD-ROM** for an Audio Glossary, animations, video clips, and bonus review questions.

evolve Be sure to visit the companion Evolve site at http://evolve.elsevier.com/deWit/ for interactive NCLEX-PN Exam Style Review Questions, WebLinks, and additional online resources.

NCLEX-PN EXAM STYLE REVIEW QUESTIONS

Choose the best answer(s) for the following questions.

1. A 78-year-old female patient is admitted with sudden onset of confusion and disorientation during the early evenings. Her family indicates that she is generally alert and oriented during the day. The nurse would likely recommend which of the following?
   1. Keep all the lights brightly lit the whole day.
   2. Promote activity and physical exercise during the day.
   3. Encourage napping during the day.
   4. Medicate with sleeping pills.
2. The nurse is assessing a patient's spouse for caregiver distress. Which of the following questions would be appropriate?
   1. "How long have you been married?"
   2. "What television shows do you watch?"
   3. "Are there any available resources to help you take care of your spouse?"
   4. "Do you love your spouse?"
3. After careful consideration of less restrictive measures, the nurse decides to apply physical restraints to a confused elderly man. Which of the following measures must the nurse include to ensure safe use of physical restraints? *(Select all that apply.)*
   1. Promptly attend to the toileting needs of the patient.
   2. Reevaluate use of the restraints every shift.
   3. Ensure adequate nutrition and hydration.
   4. Administer scheduled doses of sedative-hypnotics.
   5. Provide frequent range-of-motion exercises.
4. A 56-year-old male patient is admitted with a torn rotator cuff. Upon transfer to the medical surgical unit, the patient complains of pain when he raises his arm. The dressing is dry and intact. Vital signs are: 120/60, HR 55, RR 12, and temperature 99° F (37° C). An appropriate nursing diagnosis would be:
   1. Self-care deficit
   2. Ineffective coping
   3. Risk for infection
   4. Impaired physical mobility

5. The nurse gives discharge instructions to a 65-year-old Asian woman who had open-heart surgery. After detailing the importance of increasing activity, the patient smiles and nods her head. The nurse understands that the patient:
   1. understood the instructions.
   2. acknowledged the efforts of the nurse.
   3. demonstrated enthusiasm with increasing activity.
   4. approved of the current treatment regimen.

6. During a home visit, the nurse finds scatter rugs all over the house, the kitchen sink full of dirty dishes, the toilet has a strong odor, and the pantry and refrigerator have several outdated food items. The 76-year-old patient is coherent with occasional forgetfulness, disheveled with stained clothing, and generally emaciated. An appropriate nursing diagnosis would be:
   1. Decisional conflict
   2. Powerlessness
   3. Self-care deficit
   4. Imbalanced nutrition: less than body requirements

7. The nurse reinforces the use of incentive spirometer to a patient with blunt chest injury. Which of the following patient actions indicates understanding of nursing instructions?
   1. The patient exhales normally.
   2. The patient takes rapid, shallow breaths.
   3. The patient seals the mouthpiece during exhalation.
   4. The patient tilts the incentive spirometer.

8. The nurse suspects early complications of immobility in a 45-year-old patient admitted for multiple stab wounds to the chest. The nurse would most likely find: *(Select all that apply.)*
   1. increased muscle strength.
   2. generalized weakness.
   3. shortness of breath.
   4. limited range-of-motion.
   5. imbalance.

9. The nurse provides discharge instructions regarding home safety to a 60-year-old woman. Which of the following patient statements indicate a need for further teaching?
   1. "Scatter rugs would be useful in decreasing glare from shiny floors."
   2. "My favorite slippers can be stored underneath my bed."
   3. "I need to have a handyman install grab bars in the bathroom."
   4. "I need to be really careful when picking up something."

10. The nurse admits a 70-year-old female patient who has a history of falls. She is hard-of-hearing with bilateral cataracts. She is taking antihypertensive medications. A priority nursing diagnosis would be:
    1. Risk for falls
    2. Impaired verbal communication
    3. Deficient knowledge
    4. Activity intolerance

CRITICAL THINKING ACTIVITIES  *Read each clinical scenario and discuss the questions with your classmates.*

Scenario A

Mr. Porter has been discharged home and transferred to a home health nursing agency for continued care after suffering a stroke that has left him with left-sided hemiplegia and dysphagia. His wife will be taking care of him, but she has severe arthritis and cannot perform many needed tasks. You are assigned to provide "private-duty" care to him as he must have tube feedings.

1. What assessments would you make each day?
2. How would you collaborate with the case manager and the physical therapist?
3. How would you plan care for rehabilitation?
4. What would you teach Mr. Porter's wife about taking care of the equipment for his tube feeding?

Scenario B

Mrs. Robbins is a new resident in the long-term care facility in which you work. She is mentally alert, but needs assistance with bathing, dressing, and toileting because of arthritis and weakness and fatigue from heart failure. She can use a walker to ambulate short distances, but does not like to do so.

1. How would you promote independence and autonomy for this resident?
2. How can maintenance of function be promoted for her?
3. How would you promote socialization for Mrs. Robbins?

The Immune and Lymphatic Systems

evolve http://evolve.elsevier.com/deWit

Objectives

Upon completing this chapter, you should be able to:

Theory

1. Describe the body's innate (natural) immune response.
2. Contrast the characteristics of innate and acquired immunity.
3. Describe the role of the lymphatic system in the immune response.
4. Identify the various ways in which immunity to disease occurs.
5. List the factors that interfere with normal immune response.
6. Explain the role of immunizations in relation to immunity.

Clinical Practice

1. Identify assessments that indicate immune system function.
2. Describe precautions to be taken for patients with an impaired immune system.

Key Terms

Be sure to check out the bonus material on the Companion CD-ROM, including selected audio pronunciations.

acquired immunity (ă-KWĪRD ĭ-MŪ-nĭ-tē, p. 220)
antibodies (ĂN-tĭ-bŏ-dēz, p. 217)
antigen (ĂN-tĭ-jĕn, p. 216)
antigen-antibody response (ĂN-tĭ-jĕn ĂN-tĭ-bŏ-dē rē-SPŎNS, p. 218)
antitoxin (ĂN-tĭ-tŏk-sĭn, p. 218)
autoimmune (ăw-tō-ĭ-MŪN, p. 220)
autoimmune disease (ăw-tō-ĭ-MŪN dĭ-ZĒZ, p. 216)
cell-mediated immunity (sĕl MĒ-dē-ā-tĕd ĭ-MŪ-nĭ-tē, p. 219)
complement system of proteins (PRŌ-tēnz, p. 220)
cytokines (SĪ-tō-kīnz, p. 217)
homeostasis (hō-mē-ō-STĀ-sĭs, p. 213)
humoral immunity (HŪ-mŏr-ăl ĭ-MŪ-nĭ-tē, p. 217)
hyperpyrexia (hī-pĕr-pī-RĔX-ē-ă, p. 231)
iatrogenic (ī-ăt-rō-JĔN-ĭk, p. 221)
immune deficiency (ĭ-MŪN dĕ-FĬSH-ĕn-sē, p. 216)
immunization (ĭm-ū-nĭ-ZĀ-shŭn, p. 221)
immunoglobulin (ĭm-ū-nō-GLŎB-ū-lĭn, p. 218)
immunoscintigraphy (ĭm-ū-nō-sĭn-TĬG-ră-fē, p. 226)
innate immunity (ĭ-NĀT ĭ-MŪ-nĭ-tē, p. 220)
lysis (LĪ-sĭs, p. 218)
neutropenia (nū-trō-PĒ-nē-ă, p. 231)
passive immunity (PĂ-sĭv ĭ-MŪ-nĭ-tē, p. 220)
stromal cells (STRŌ-măl sĕlz, p. 217)
toxin (TŎK-sĭn, p. 218)

The immune and lymphatic systems work together to defend the body against threats from multiple sources. The sensory nervous system interacts by helping to alert the body to outside physical threats. Internally, the immune and lymphatic systems are constantly protecting against microscopic threats to **homeostasis (tendency to maintain internal stability and balance)**. The hematologic system interacts in the production of specialized white blood cells that help fight infection and rid the body of foreign invaders. A review of the structure and functions of the immune and lymphatic systems is necessary to understand immune responses.

PROTECTIVE MECHANISMS OF THE IMMUNE AND LYMPHATIC SYSTEMS

The human body has multiple protective mechanisms. The skin, nasal membranes, and urinary tract all provide external barriers to foreign substances and organisms. If one of the barriers is penetrated, the *natural immune system* is activated. Natural nonspecific immunity is present in the body even before exposure to any antigens, which means the body recognizes certain organisms as harmful without ever having encountered that organism before. This recognition allows the body to defend against the intruder immediately. The system responds the same way each time to repeated encounters with the same organism. The defensive cells, proteins, and chemicals of the innate (natural) immune system are located in the blood and are readily available for activation. When foreign microorganisms penetrate the external barriers, damaged cells release chemicals that initiate the inflammatory response.

INFLAMMATORY RESPONSE

Inflammation or the inflammatory response occurs with any tissue injury and with any encounter of foreign organisms. It is the first step in the body's defense

OVERVIEW OF ANATOMY AND PHYSIOLOGY OF THE IMMUNE AND LYMPHATIC SYSTEMS

What are the organs and structures of the immune and lymphatic systems?

- Bone marrow produces a type of stem cell that is able to produce all types of blood cells, which then *differentiate* (acquire individual characteristics) into the cells of the hematologic and immune systems. B lymphocytes are produced and mature in the bone marrow (Figure 10–1).
- The thymus gland, located behind the breastbone, is the place that T lymphocytes mature and are released into the bloodstream.
- Lymph nodes and vessels circulate fluid called *lymph* that contains proteins, glucose, monocytes, and lymphocytes (Figure 10–2).
- The lymph vessels are located near the blood vessels and capillaries. The lymph system removes what is left over after the plasma has delivered nutrients to the cells.
- The lymph fluid drains into large veins, blending with the plasma circulating in the bloodstream.
- Tonsils and adenoids are lymph tissues that guard the airway from inhaled microbes.
- The spleen filters blood, which allows lymphocytes to come into contact with any circulating organism, thus activating the appropriate lymphocyte response. It also filters out damaged or old red blood cells, recycling the hemoglobin in the production of bilirubin.
- Peyer's patches are lymphoid tissue in the small bowel that help defend against ingested pathogens.

What are the functions of the immune and lymphatic systems?

- The immune and lymph systems work together to guard the body against pathogens and to eliminate them if they manage to pass through the outer barriers.

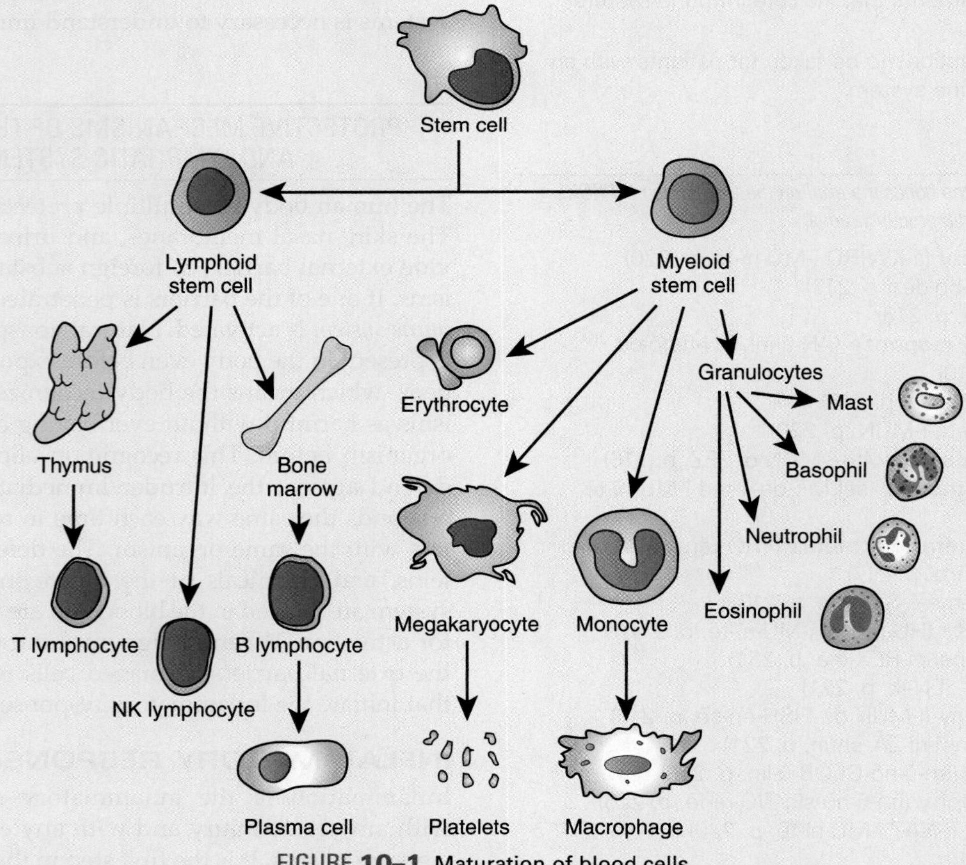

FIGURE **10–1** Maturation of blood cells.

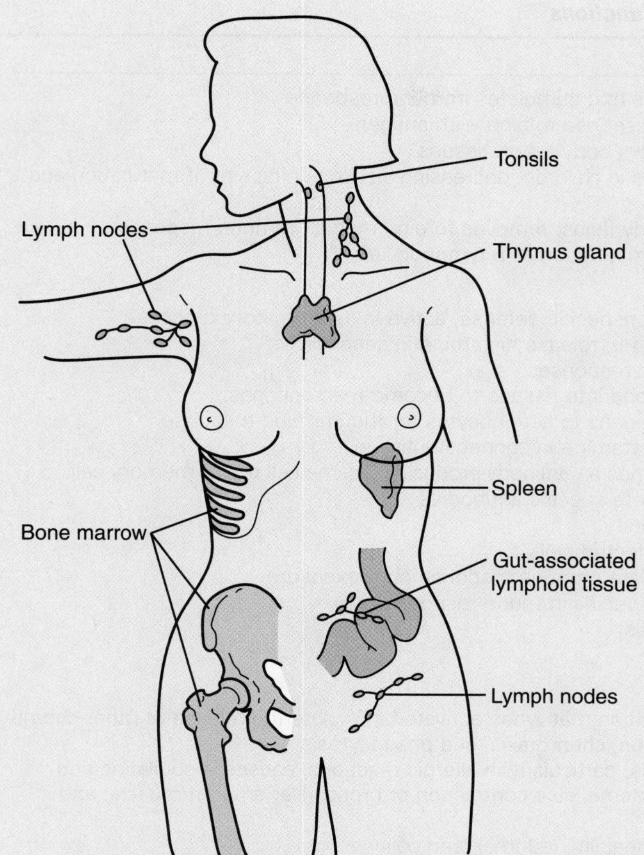

FIGURE 10–2 Organs of the immune system.

- The neutrophils and macrophages of the hematologic system assist the immune system by phagocytosis when an antigen is encountered.
- Chemical mediators, plasma cells, and B and T lymphocytes play active roles in the immune response (Table 10–1).
- Both humoral and cellular immunity is carried out by the lymphocytic cells, a specialized type of white blood cell that originates in the bone marrow.
- T lymphocytes, which provide cellular immunity, pass through the thymus and migrate to the lymph tissues throughout the body.
- B lymphocytes migrate to lymphoid tissue, where they wait in readiness to form either sensitized lymphocytes or antibodies.
- The lymph system in addition to facilitating the work of lymphocytes, also drains tissue fluid and puts it back into the circulation.
- Innate (natural) immunity is nonspecific immunity that is in humans when they are born, making them not susceptible to diseases of other species.
- Immunity can be acquired actively or passively.

What effects does aging have on the immune and lymphatic systems?

- Neonates are susceptible to infection due to an immature immune system.
- The thymus gland is largest during childhood and adolescence. After adolescence it begins to shrink in size and its production of T lymphocytes lessens.
- Aging causes skin to become thin, less elastic, and more prone to injury. The skin is the first barrier encountered by pathogens.
- Decreased ciliary action in the respiratory system and gastrointestinal tract results in decreased removal of potentially harmful organisms.
- Presence of chronic diseases can decrease the immune response.

mechanisms (see coverage of the inflammatory response in Chapter 6). Trauma, infectious organisms, chemicals, or heat may injure tissue. If the injury is to external tissues, there will be redness and swelling, and the area will be warm and tender. This is due to cells, proteins, and chemicals being sent to the affected tissue. These substances increase blood flow to the area by dilating upstream vessels, resulting in warmth and redness. The substances also affect downstream vessels, causing vasoconstriction that results in swelling. The swelling compresses nerves, causing pain.

The inflammatory response alone may be adequate in killing the invading organism by creating a hostile environment (refer to Figure 6–2). Protective proteins that are activated in the inflammatory response include the *complement system of proteins.* Several of these protein enzymes, when sequentially activated, form a "membrane attack complex" (MAC) that embeds itself into the cell membrane of the attacker microbe. This activation occurs when there is exposure of complement-binding sites on antibodies after they attach to antigens. This break in the cell wall allows salt to enter the cell, followed by water, which causes swelling and bursting of the microbe.

The same cells, proteins, and chemicals respond to internal tissue injury. The results are not as readily visible, but are detectable if appropriate assessments are conducted. The mechanisms of the inflammatory response combine with the immune response to eliminate foreign invaders (Figure 10–3).

Table 10–1 Major Components of the Immune System and Their Functions

COMPONENT	FUNCTION
Antigen	Foreign substance or component of cell that stimulates immune response
Antibody	Specific protein produced in humoral response to bind with antigen
Autoantibody	Antibodies against "self" antigen; attacks body's own tissues
Thymus	Gland located in the mediastinum, large in children, decreasing size in adults; site of maturation and proliferation of lymphocytes
Lymphatic tissue	Contains many lymphocytes; filters body fluids, removes foreign matter, immune response
Bone marrow	Source of stem cells, leukocytes, and maturation of B lymphocytes
CELLS	
Neutrophils	White blood cells: For phagocytosis; nonspecific defense; active in inflammatory process
Basophils	White blood cells: Bind immunoglobulin E; release histamine in anaphylaxis
Eosinophils	White blood cells: Participate in allergic responses
Monocytes	White blood cells: Migrate from the blood into tissues to become macrophages
Macrophages	Phagocytosis; process and present antigens to lymphocytes for the immune response
Mast cells	Release chemical mediators such as histamine in connective tissue
B lymphocytes	Humoral immunity–activating cell becomes an antibody-producing plasma cell or a B memory cell
Plasma cells	Develop from B lymphocytes and secrete specific antibodies
T lymphocytes	White blood cells: Cell-mediated immunity
Cytotoxic or killer T cells	Destroy antigens, cancer cells, virus-infected cells
Memory T cells	Remember antigens and quickly stimulate immune response on reexposure
Helper T cells	Activate B and T cells; control or limit specific immune response
Natural killer (NK) lymphocytes	Destroy foreign cells, virus-infected cells
CHEMICAL MEDIATORS	
Complement	Group of inactive proteins in the circulation that when activated stimulate the release of other chemical mediators, promoting inflammation, chemotaxis, and phagocytosis
Histamine	Released from mast cells and basophils, particularly in allergic reactions; causes vasodilation and increased vascular permeability or edema, also contraction of bronchiolar smooth muscle, and pruritus
Kinins (e.g., bradykinin)	Cause vasodilation and increased permeability (edema), and pain
Prostaglandins	Group of lipids with varying effects; some cause inflammation-vasodilation and increased permeability, and pain
Leukotrienes	Group of lipids, derived from mast cells and basophils, that cause contraction of bronchiolar smooth muscle and have a role in development of inflammation
Cytokines (messengers)	Includes lymphokines, monokines, interferons, and interleukins; produced by macrophages and activated lymphocytes; stimulate activation and proliferation of B and T cells (communication between cells); involved in inflammation, fever, and leukocytosis
Chemotactic factors	Attract phagocytes to area of inflammation

From Gould, B.E. (2002). *Pathophysiology for the Health Professions* (2nd ed.). Philadelphia: Saunders, p. 37.

IMMUNE RESPONSE

The immune response is a remarkable series of complex chemical and mechanical activities that take place in the body. These activities involve (1) constant surveillance to detect the entry of foreign agents **(antigens)** as soon as they gain access to the body's cells; (2) immediate recognition of the agents as "non self" (i.e., foreign or alien); and (3) the ability to distinguish one kind of foreign agent from another and to remember that particular agent if it appears in the body again at a later time. The lymphatic system, thymus, spleen, lymph nodes, bone marrow, and Peyer's patches in the small intestine play a major role in the immune response (see Figure 10–2). Many different cells, proteins, and chemicals assist in defending the body against invaders.

The immune response is usually triggered by the body's identification of something as foreign or non self. This recognition is key to the body responding to the threat in an appropriate manner and in not reacting to tissues or cells that are "self." When an inappropriate response happens, one of two types of disorders occurs. If there is a lack of appropriate response, an **immune deficiency** is present. The second type of disorder occurs when the body produces an immune response to a "self" cell or tissue, causing an **autoimmune disease.**

While injury activates the immune system, massive trauma and chronic illness can inhibit the ability of the system to respond.

TYPES OF IMMUNITY

Once a particular kind of foreign substance has been detected and identified, the body responds in two general ways. **It immediately produces a protein (called**

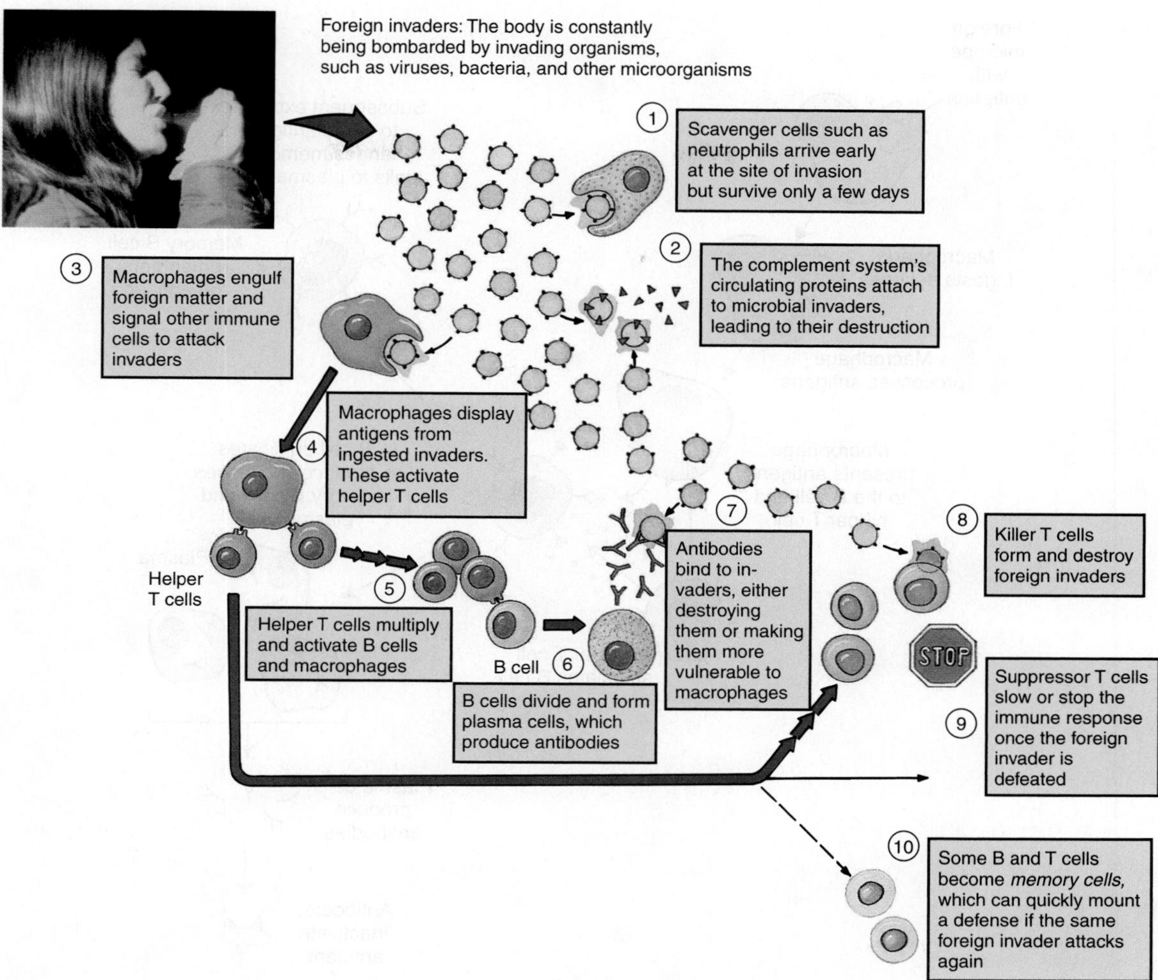

FIGURE **10–3** Action of the immune response against foreign invaders.

an *antibody*) that is specifically designed to do battle with the *antigen*. The immediate response is called a *humoral response*. *Humoral* refers to any fluid or semifluid. There is also a delayed response that involves the use of sensitized lymphocytes to attack whole cells, such as those of bacteria and viruses, and malignant cells. This second kind of response is called a *cellular* or *cell-mediated*, response.

The cells that mediate the response are the T lymphocytes. Examples of antigens include the cells of bacteria, viruses, fungi, and other infectious organisms, as well as the toxins they produce. Nonliving matter such as pollen, dust, and the chemicals in detergent also can be antigens. For some people, certain foods are perceived by the body as antigens and result in a reaction when the particular food is eaten.

T cells and B cells interact with each other in complex ways. Helper T cells must interact with B cells before the B cells can become plasma or memory cells. The suppressor T cells regulate the amount of antibody that B cells produce. Both T cells and B cells are necessary for a normal immune response to occur. Acquired and inherited disorders can inhibit T and B cell activity.

PRIMARY HUMORAL RESPONSE

Lymphocytic B cells are involved in humoral immunity and the production of antibodies. They arise from stem cells in the bone marrow and undergo a maturation process that involves bone marrow **stromal cells** (cells that contribute to the development of multiple tissues and blood cells) and their **cytokines** (messenger hormones). When mature, the B cells migrate to the lymph nodes. When stimulated by an antigen, a B cell becomes a plasma cell that secretes antibody molecules into the bloodstream. B cells secrete immunoglobulins called **antibodies** in response to the specific antigen they encounter (Figure 10–4). This is antibody-mediated or **humoral immunity.** Some of the antigen-stimulated B cells become memory cells. This mechanism is the basis for acquired immunity. The memory cells reactivate the plasma cells to produce large quantities of the specific type of antibody needed to fight

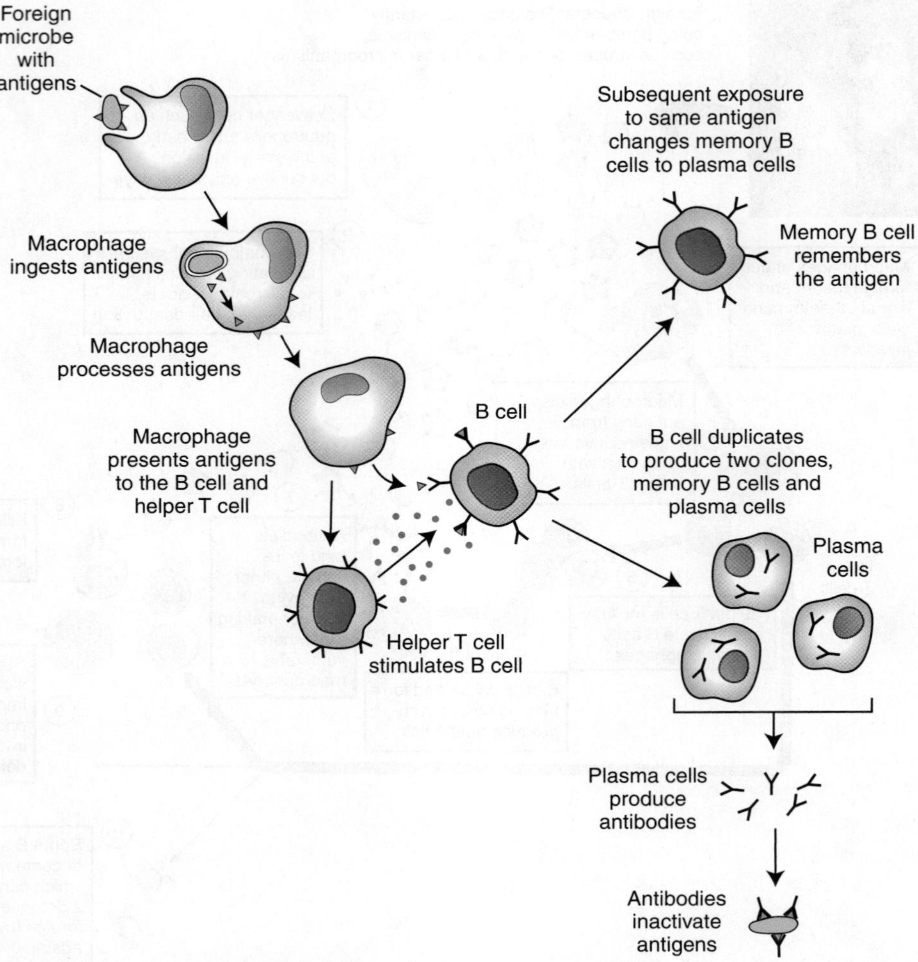

FIGURE **10–4** Humoral (antibody)-mediated immunity.

the particular type of antigen, when the same antigen enters the body a second time. It is an immediate and potent response, and antibodies continue to be produced for many months.

Antibodies are a kind of protein synthesized by plasma cells. They are called **immunoglobulins.** There are five classes of immunoglobulins (Igs): IgA, IgD, IgE, IgG, and IgM. Each antibody is able to attach to the kind of antigen for which it is made (Table 10–2). This ability of an antibody to form a bond with its antigen is important to the destruction of the antigen, but it can sometimes result in damage to the body's own cells. Antibodies are found in the serum of blood and in other body fluids and tissues, including the urine, saliva, tears, breast milk, interstitial fluid, spinal fluid, lymph nodes, and spleen. An antibody can either destroy or inactivate its particular antigen by (1) mechanically harming it, (2) activating a complement system, or (3) causing the release of chemicals that affect the environment of the antigen.

In some instances, the antibody prepares the antigen for ingestion by phagocytes. It does this by a process called **lysis,** in which the antibody damages the membrane of the antigen's cell, causing it to rupture and making its contents accessible for digestion.

If the antigen is a **toxin** (poison) produced by a bacterial or viral cell, the antibody produced is called the **antitoxin** that is capable of neutralizing the poisonous chemical of the antigen by covering the toxic sites of the antigenic agent. An antitoxin is, therefore, a specific type of antibody that acts through the process of *neutralization.*

When a bacterium or other antigen enters the body, it may encounter a B lymphocyte that is specific for that bacterium or antigen. The B lymphocyte becomes a plasma cell that secretes IgM (antibody), which attacks the bacterium or antigen. After the particular bacterium or antigen is encountered for the first time, it takes 4 to 8 days for the B lymphocyte to produce immunoglobulins that can attack. If the same bacterium or antigen enters the body a second time at a later date, the immunoglobulin response by the memory cells is quicker, occurring in 1 to 2 days. The major function of the humoral **antigen-antibody response** is to provide protection against acute, rapidly developing bacterial and viral diseases. The antigen-antibody response also is involved in allergies and transfusion reactions.

Table 10–2 Immunoglobulins and Their Functions

CLASS	PERCENT OF TOTAL*	LOCATION	FUNCTION
IgG	75–85	Blood plasma	Major antibody in primary and secondary immune responses; inactivates antigen; neutralizes toxins; crosses placenta to provide immunity for newborn; responsible for Rh reactions
IgA	5–15	Saliva, mucus, tears, breast milk	Protects mucous membranes on body surfaces; provides immunity for newborn
IgM	5–10	Attached to B cells; released into plasma during immune response	Causes antigens to clump together; responsible for transfusion reactions in the ABO blood typing system
IgD	0.2	Attached to B cells	Receptor sites for antigens on B cells; binding with antigen results in B-cell activation
IgE	0.5	Produced by plasma cells in mucous membranes and tonsils	Binds to mast cells and basophils, causing release of histamine; responsible for allergic reactions

From Applegate, E. (2006). *The Anatomy and Physiology Learning System* (3rd ed.). Philadelphia: Saunders, p. 299.
*Immunoglobulins.

SECONDARY CELLULAR RESPONSE

The second type of immunologic response of the body involves various interactions with antigens by T lymphocytes. Unlike the humoral response, which takes place in the plasma, the cellular response involves whole cells called *sensitized lymphocytes* and occurs out in the tissues. They are said to be *sensitized* because they have been made sensitive to a specific antigen after their first contact with it. Subsequent exposure to the antigen to which they are sensitive triggers a host of chemical and mechanical activities, all designed to either destroy or inactivate the offending antigen.

Those lymphocytes destined to provide cellular immunity pass through the thymus and migrate to the lymph tissues throughout the body. These are called the *T lymphocytes* (the "T" is for thymus) and they are further divided into helper T cells, memory T cells, suppressor T cells, and sensitized T cells (killer cells) (Figure 10–5). T cells provide defense against viral infections. Viruses are difficult to get rid of because they inject themselves into host cells and reproduce themselves. *T cells respond to foreign or abnormal molecules on the surface of cells.* Host cells containing virus have small fragments of the virus slightly protruding from the cell membrane. T cells identify the virus fragment as foreign and kill the host cell. T cells and macrophages produce a variety of substances called *lymphokines* that help destroy antigens. Killer T cells attach themselves to cells bearing antigen and secrete toxic substances that kill the antigen-bearing cells. This cell-to-cell contact response is called **cell-mediated immunity** or cellular immunity.

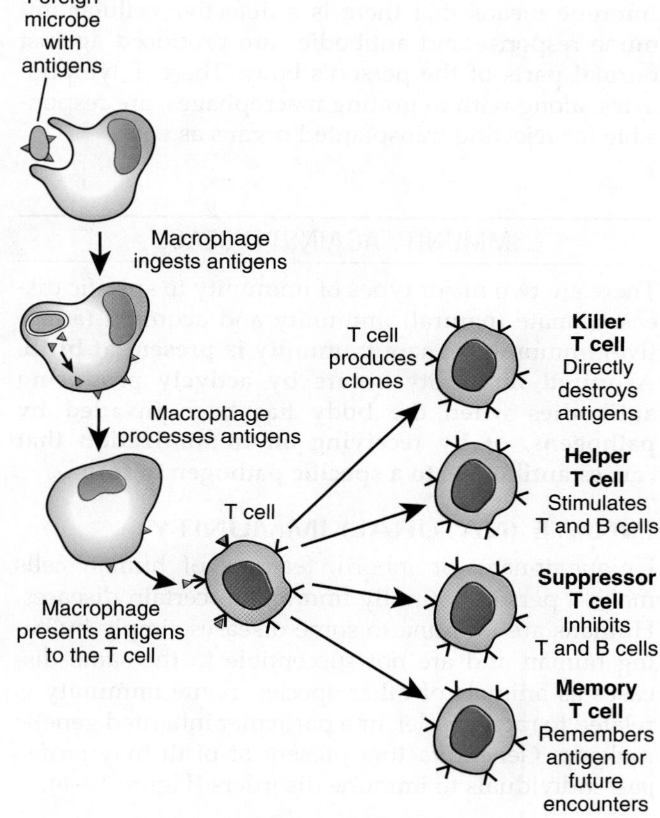

FIGURE 10–5 Cell-mediated immunity.

The T lymphocytes mediate (indirectly accomplish) the cellular response. When an antigen is complex (e.g., a bacterium or another type of living cell), T lymphocytes that are specifically reactive with the particular antigen mediate the cellular response in several ways. These specific T lymphocytes enter the circulating fluids of the body from the lymphoid tissues, migrate widely, and react anywhere in the body where they encounter the particular antigen. Destruction of the antigen may occur by release of chemicals into the membrane of the target cell, by secretion of lymphokines such as interleukin-2 or T-cell growth factor, or by other processes. This direct contact by the T lymphocytes with an antigen is called *killer activity,* and such lymphocytes are named *killer T cells.* Cellular immune response is often termed *delayed hypersensitivity.* The larger the amount of antigen present, the greater the response of sensitized T lymphocytes.

The **complement system of proteins** is a series of proteins produced in the liver that work with antibodies to destroy antigens. The complement system directly kills microbes by attaching to the cell wall and allowing salt and water into the cell, causing it to burst. It also assists in the inflammatory and immune response. The proteins of the system "complement" or assist the immune system.

The T lymphocytes perform immune surveillance for the body by detecting cells that enter the host and have foreign antigens on their surface. T lymphocytes are defensive cells that patrol the blood and tissues. This is why transplanted tissue must have surface antigens that are very similar to those of the host tissue to be accepted by the host body. Sensitized T lymphocytes are the cause of allergic reactions. T cells are responsible for the inflammatory response present in people with a variety of autoimmune diseases. **Autoimmune** means that there is a defective cellular immune response and antibodies are produced against normal parts of the person's body. These T lymphocytes, along with migrating macrophages, are responsible for rejecting transplanted organs as well.

IMMUNITY AGAINST DISEASE

There are two major types of immunity to specific disease: innate (natural) immunity and acquired (adaptive) immunity. **Innate immunity is present at birth. Acquired immunity occurs by actively producing antibodies when the body has been invaded by pathogens, or by receiving an immunization that causes antibodies to a specific pathogen to form.**

INNATE (NATURAL) IMMUNITY

Unique innate, or inborn, features of human cells make a person naturally immune to certain diseases. Humans are immune to some diseases simply by being human and are not susceptible to the same diseases as animals of other species. Some immunity is related to race, gender, or a particular inherited genetic makeup. Genetic factors present at birth may *predispose* individuals to immune disorders (Figure 10–6).

ACQUIRED IMMUNITY

In acquired immunity, a person can either actively produce his or her own antibodies or passively receive antibodies produced by another person or animal (**passive immunity**). *Passive natural immunity* is the type that is transmitted from mother to baby. The mother passes antibodies to the fetus in utero or after birth through breast milk. When the fetus is in utero, it passively receives some natural immunity when antibodies from the mother's bloodstream pass through the placenta and mix with the blood of the fetus. Those maternal antibodies are then present in the infant's blood at birth. More immunity can be passed to the infant through breast milk. Breast-feeding is the best way to protect the newborn from infectious disease. Depressed immune function in the mother will limit the benefit to the baby.

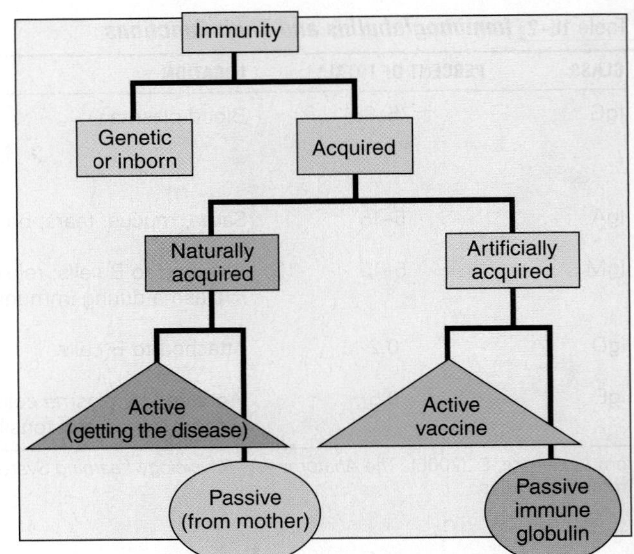

FIGURE **10–6** Types of immunity.

Administration of human immune globulin to boost the immune system is an example of *passive artificial immunity.* Human immune globulin, formerly called gamma globulin, contains antibodies against not just one, but many infectious diseases. It is used when an unimmunized person contracts one of the common childhood diseases because it is assumed that adults, from whom it has been taken, have been exposed to and developed antibodies against these diseases during their lifetime.

The serum from the blood of a horse contains ready-made antibodies and antitoxins against tetanus when the horse has been prepared with increasingly strong injections of that antigen. Antivenins that contain antibodies against snake venoms and the poisons produced by the black widow spider are available. Injections that provide passive immunity should be given as early as possible in the disease as they only protect against further tissue damage. They cannot reverse damage already done.

Passive immunity is usually time limited as the antibodies provided only last for a specific period.

? *Think Critically About . . .* What type of immunity is provided by a "flu shot"? How does an injection of human immune globulin protect a world traveler from hepatitis A?

Active naturally acquired immunity occurs when a person contracts and survives a disease. Once survival from a particular disease has occurred, the person is immune and need not fear that particular disease.

Active artificially acquired immunity occurs by vaccination or immunization. To provide active immunity to diseases by artificial means, the actual pathogenic microorganisms are grown and cultured in the laboratory. They are divided into single doses under rigid controls and made into vaccines. These specially treated microorganisms are weakened (attenuated), or killed, so that they will stimulate the production of antibodies but will not cause the disease itself. Vaccines from cowpox, viruses, tetanus and tubercle bacilli, polio, influenza, pneumonia bacteria, measles, mumps, chickenpox, and hepatitis viruses are examples of agents used to produce an active immunity in humans.

This method of stimulating the production of immunizing substances in the body is successful in situations in which there is time to wait for the person to build up her own defenses. This immunity does not last indefinitely. The body must be reminded of the need to produce more antibodies. To achieve this, a booster dose of an immunizing agent is given to jog the memory of the specific B cells and cause them to actively produce more antibodies.

CAUSES OF IMMUNE AND LYMPHATIC SYSTEM DISORDERS

With all of the complexity of the human immune response, there are multiple natural areas of dysfunction that occur, as has been discussed. One of the more commonly encountered reasons for alteration in immune function not caused by pathogenic factors, is **iatrogenic**—a condition caused by treatment. Current therapies for asthma, inflammatory disorders, autoimmune disorders and organ transplantation are all aimed at suppressing or attenuating the body's natural response. While this effect is helpful in addressing the primary disorder, it also makes the patient more vulnerable to infection. Many over-the-counter medications have anti-inflammatory effects and are used to decrease pain caused by inflammation. The inflammation is the initiation of the immune process. Suppression of this response can hinder the body's ability to fight infection.

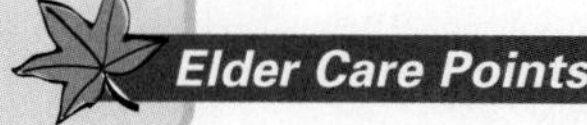

Elder Care Points

The older patient is at risk for problems with immunity due to decreased immune function. The older patient is more likely to have chronic illness and have decreased nutritional intake. For those in long-term care facilities, living in close proximity to others makes transmission of diseases more likely.

Consumption of alcohol can alter the body's ability to launch an immune response. There are both long- and short-term effects of alcohol on the immune system. Two drinks can impair the ability of the B lymphocytes to produce antibodies and can affect T-cell activity. Long-term alcohol use leads to alteration in liver function and impaired nutrition, also altering immune function. Many other drugs, including cocaine, marijuana, and amphetamines, also compromise the immune system.

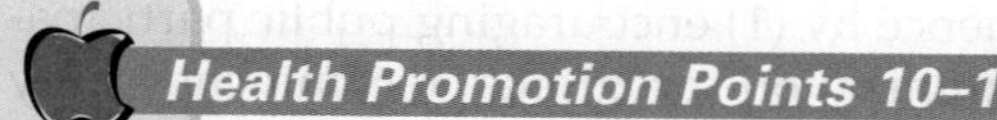

Health Promotion Points 10–1

Maintaining a Healthy Immune System

A healthy immune system is a function of a healthy body. Eating right and getting enough rest and exercise are all key in maintaining resistance to infection and disease. Frequently skipping meals, eating unhealthy meals, sleeping too little, or not exercising weakens the immune system and makes people more susceptible to pathogens.

Autoimmune disorders are caused by a malfunction of the body's immune system. When the body does not recognize tissues as "self," an autoimmune disorder occurs and the defense mechanisms are launched against the body's own tissues. The trigger for this dysfunction is unknown. Some conditions are thought to be initiated by a systemic infectious process, and others by inherited factors (Health Promotion Points 10–1).

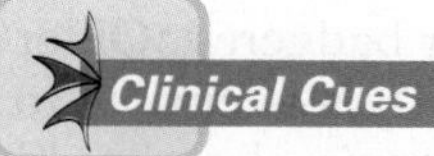

Clinical Cues

Treat any patient with chronic substance abuse as immunocompromised until proven otherwise.

PREVENTION OF IMMUNE AND LYMPHATIC SYSTEM PROBLEMS

IMMUNIZATION

Before **immunization** and inoculation became commonplace, the only way an individual could acquire immunity was to suffer an attack of the disease and, owing to a strong constitution and good fortune, manage to survive. Immunity from immunizations is usually achieved by administering the vaccine in divided doses over weeks or months. This sets in motion the more powerful, longer lasting secondary response. For example, infants are given immunizations at intervals during infancy and then periodically after that. To stimulate continued immunity, adults should have immunizations against tetanus and diphtheria every 10 years.

Nursing Implications

The nurse plays a major role in providing education regarding the importance of immunizations to public health. Diseases preventable by immunization cause deaths and disability every year. Nurses can have significant influence by (1) encouraging public participation in immunization programs recommended by health officials, (2) helping to identify people in need of immunization, and (3) preventing and minimizing sensitivity reactions to immunizing agents.

Healthy People 2010 goals include Goal 14: Prevent disease, disability, and death from infectious diseases, including vaccine-preventable diseases.

An important aspect of health teaching is to improve the general public's awareness of the importance of immunization as a means of avoiding certain diseases and their consequences. In spite of the availability of vaccines against poliomyelitis, measles, rubella, mumps, and other potentially dangerous diseases, there still are many children who have not been adequately immunized. This is particularly true in areas that have a large recent immigrant population and in areas populated by the poor, who do not have easy access to the health care system. Nurses have a responsibility to inform the public of the purpose of immunization in terms the layperson can understand (Legal & Ethical Considerations 10–1). Figure 10–7 shows the secondary response and longer lasting immunity provided by a second injection of an antigen.

Parents should be told why immunization is best for their children and be warned of the dangers faced by children who are not adequately immunized. The nurse must present this information in such a way that the parents do not feel threatened or badgered. Older adults and others who are particularly susceptible to influenza and pneumococcal pneumonia also should be immunized according to the recommendations of public health officials. Health care workers should be immunized annually for influenza so they do not transmit the disease to susceptible populations. The Centers for Disease Control and Prevention (CDC) has recommended immunization schedules for all ages, including those who have never been vaccinated. The CDC website at www.cdc.gov/nip has the most up-to-date information (Table 10–3).

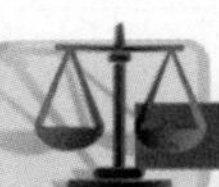

Legal & Ethical Considerations 10–1

Immunizations

Immunizations are a proven way to decrease illness for individuals and the spread of diseases in communities. Some religious and cultural practices forbid immunizations. How can the needs of society be balanced with the rights of individuals?

Circumstances that require postponing immunization include fevers, pregnancy, immune deficiency disease, immunosuppressive therapy, and administration of serum immune globulin, plasma, or whole blood transfusion 6 to 8 weeks before the immunization. Immunization also is contraindicated when a person is taking certain drugs. Brochures accompanying these drugs will state whether they prohibit the administration of an immunizing agent. The vaccine for tuberculosis (TB), bacille Calmette-Guérin (BCG), is not routinely used in the United States due to the low incidence of TB. In countries where TB is more prevalent, BCG is given. Individuals who have received BCG will have a positive TB skin test.

Whenever an immunizing agent is to be administered, precautions must be taken to ensure as far as possible that the patient is not hypersensitive to the components of the agent. Many times chick embryo, horse serum, and other substances are used to make the vaccine or immune serum. These substances can produce a serious allergic reaction in people who are hypersensitive to them. Immunizing agents that are most often associated with anaphylaxis, a potentially fatal reaction, include tetanus antitoxin, diphtheria antitoxin, rabies antitoxin, and antilymphocyte globulin.

It is imperative that a history of allergies in the patient and her family be obtained before administering an immunizing agent. It also should be determined whether the patient has an immune deficiency disease of any kind that would prevent a normal immune response to the immunizing agent. If a patient does have a history of allergies or an immune deficiency, the physician should be made aware of this fact before the immunizing agent is given. If the patient has had an allergic reaction to the specific agent she is supposed to receive, the drug must not be given.

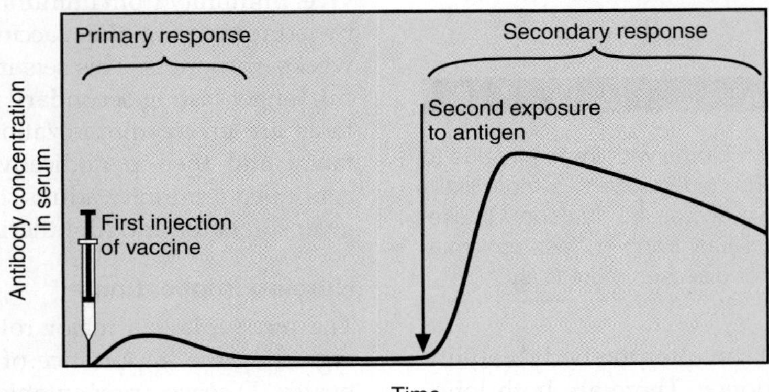

FIGURE 10–7 Comparison of primary and secondary immune response.

Complementary & Alternative Therapies 10–1

Garlic Assists Immune Action

Garlic has been used for centuries to increase resistance to the common cold and other infections. It has a variety of actions, including antilipidemic, antitriglyceride, antiplatelet, antioxidant, cancer preventive, and antimicrobial. It inhibits both gram-positive and gram-negative organisms and is effective against fungi, virus, and helminths. Because it interacts with many drugs, the physician should be consulted before administration. It should not be used by pregnant women as it may induce early labor. Those patients on anticoagulants need to know that it may extend the action of their drugs.

There are times when a skin sensitivity test is indicated before any serum is administered to a patient. Skin testing for sensitivity should not be confused with skin testing for diagnostic purposes. Testing for sensitivity is done to determine whether a minute amount of the immunizing agent will produce a local reaction. If it does, chances are the patient will have a severe reaction if the agent is given systemically.

In spite of these precautions, it is possible that a patient will suffer from hypersensitivity to an immunizing agent. To avoid serious problems, the nurse should always be prepared to act quickly and effectively in such an emergency. In all patient care areas where immunizing agents are administered, emergency equipment should be readily available. As an extra precaution to ensure prompt treatment of a hypersensitivity reaction if one occurs, it is advisable for people receiving immunizing agents to remain in the clinic or office for 15 to 20 minutes after an injection.

In addition to augmenting the immune system by administering immunizations, the nurse should instruct the patient in other measures for maintaining a healthy immune system (Complementary & Alternative Therapies 10–1). Keeping the body healthy is the best way to preserve immune function. Not smoking, staying active, getting adequate rest, and eating a balanced diet are all measures that should be encouraged.

NURSING MANAGEMENT

Assessment (Data Collection)

If the immune system is functioning normally, there will be an absence of physical signs and symptoms. It is when the system is active, doing its job, or unable to mount an active defense that detectable physical signs will be apparent.

Since the function of the immune system is to guard the body against microbial invasion and to fight infection that cannot be prevented, it is important to assess for signs and symptoms of infection. These include fever, redness, swelling, and exudate from open skin areas. Patients who have a known infection and do not exhibit signs and symptoms of infection should be evaluated for an immune deficiency. Another indicator

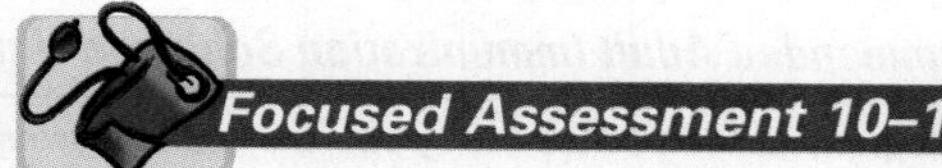

Focused Assessment 10–1

Data Collection for the Lymphatic and Immune Systems

When gathering data, ask the following questions:

- What immunizations have you had? When were you last immunized for tetanus, diphtheria, and influenza?
- Have you had a recent infection? Or recurring infections?
- Do you have any allergies?
- Do you have any chronic illnesses such as diabetes, rheumatoid arthritis, inflammatory bowel disease, Crohn's disease, lung disease, renal disease, or acquired immunodeficiency syndrome?
- Have you ever had cancer? Undergone radiation therapy or chemotherapy?
- Have you recently had surgery or a blood transfusion?
- Do you get sick frequently?
- Have you traveled out of the country?
- What do you usually eat in a day?
- Has your weight changed lately?
- Do you smoke, drink, or use recreational drugs?
- Have you been exposed to industrial or agricultural chemicals?
- Have you been exposed to industrial radiation?
- Are you on any medications?
- Do you take any supplements or herbal preparations?
- Do you see a physician regularly?
- Are you under excessive stress at home or in your job?
- Are you sexually active? Are you monogamous? (Try to determine sexual orientation.)

of a depressed or inadequate immune response is recurrent infections or infections of common organisms to which individuals with normal immune systems are not susceptible.

History Taking

A thorough history should be gathered (Focused Assessment 10–1). Previously diagnosed diseases affecting the immune system, immunizations, medications (including herbal supplements), allergies, and nutritional status are important areas to explore. The patient should also be questioned about any recent surgeries, blood transfusions, and diagnoses of chronic illnesses. Habits and lifestyle questions are also important but may not be as comfortable for the nurse to discuss with the patient. Since important diseases affecting the immune system are transmitted by transference of blood and body fluids, sexual history is very important. Information regarding smoking history and exposure to environmental and industrial radiation or pollutants should also be obtained.

Physical Assessment

The skin is a major defense against access to the body by microorganisms. It is important to do a thorough assessment of the skin to identify any potential entry-

Table 10–3 Recommended Adult Immunization Schedule United States, October 2006–September 2007

Recommended adult immunization schedule, by vaccine and age group

<table>
<tr><th>Age group (yrs) ▶
Vaccine▼</th><th>19–49 years</th><th>50–64 years</th><th>≥65 years</th></tr>
<tr><td rowspan="2">Tetanus, diphtheria, pertussis (Td/Tdap)[1]*</td><td colspan="3">1-dose Td booster every 10 yrs</td></tr>
<tr><td colspan="2">Substitute 1 dose of Tdap for Td</td><td></td></tr>
<tr><td>Human papillomavirus (HPV)[2]*</td><td>3 doses (females)</td><td></td><td></td></tr>
<tr><td>Measles, mumps, rubella (MMR)[3]*</td><td>1 or 2 doses</td><td colspan="2">1 dose</td></tr>
<tr><td>Varicella[4]*</td><td>2 doses (0, 4–8 wks)</td><td>2 doses (0, 4–8 wks)</td><td></td></tr>
<tr><td>Influenza[5]*</td><td>1 dose annually</td><td colspan="2">1 dose annually</td></tr>
<tr><td>Pneumococcal (polysaccharide)[6,7]</td><td colspan="2">1–2 doses</td><td>1 dose</td></tr>
<tr><td>Hepatitis A[8]*</td><td colspan="3">2 doses (0, 6–12 mos, or 0, 6–18 mos)</td></tr>
<tr><td>Hepatitis B[9]*</td><td colspan="3">3 doses (0, 1–2, 4–6 mos)</td></tr>
<tr><td>Meningococcal[10]</td><td colspan="3">1 or more doses</td></tr>
</table>

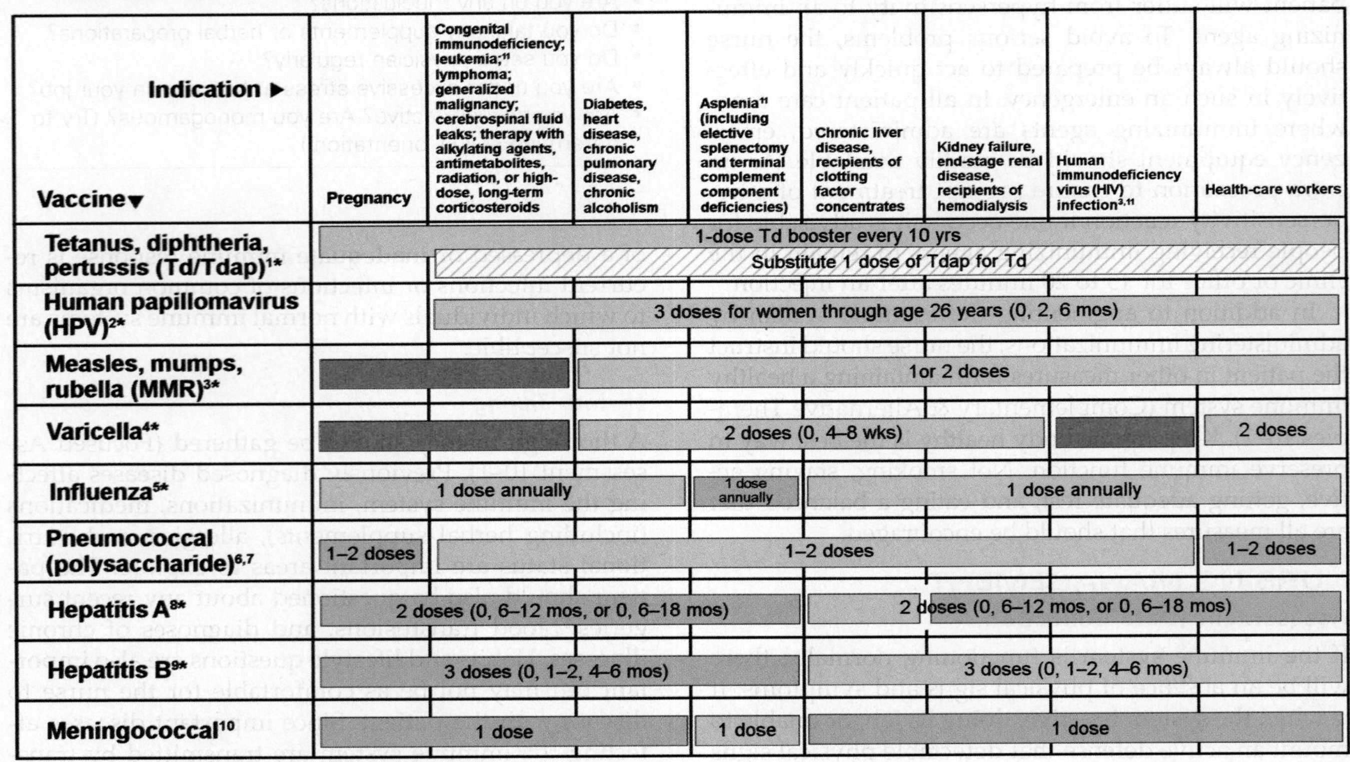

Recommended adult immunization schedule, by vaccine and medical and other indications

<table>
<tr><th>Indication ▶
Vaccine▼</th><th>Pregnancy</th><th>Congenital immunodeficiency; leukemia;[11] lymphoma; generalized malignancy; cerebrospinal fluid leaks; therapy with alkylating agents, antimetabolites, radiation, or high-dose, long-term corticosteroids</th><th>Diabetes, heart disease, chronic pulmonary disease, chronic alcoholism</th><th>Asplenia[11] (including elective splenectomy and terminal complement component deficiencies)</th><th>Chronic liver disease, recipients of clotting factor concentrates</th><th>Kidney failure, end-stage renal disease, recipients of hemodialysis</th><th>Human immunodeficiency virus (HIV) infection[3,11]</th><th>Health-care workers</th></tr>
<tr><td rowspan="2">Tetanus, diphtheria, pertussis (Td/Tdap)[1]*</td><td colspan="8">1-dose Td booster every 10 yrs</td></tr>
<tr><td></td><td colspan="7">Substitute 1 dose of Tdap for Td</td></tr>
<tr><td>Human papillomavirus (HPV)[2]*</td><td></td><td colspan="7">3 doses for women through age 26 years (0, 2, 6 mos)</td></tr>
<tr><td>Measles, mumps, rubella (MMR)[3]*</td><td colspan="2"></td><td colspan="6">1or 2 doses</td></tr>
<tr><td>Varicella[4]*</td><td colspan="2"></td><td colspan="4">2 doses (0, 4–8 wks)</td><td></td><td>2 doses</td></tr>
<tr><td>Influenza[5]*</td><td colspan="3">1 dose annually</td><td>1 dose annually</td><td colspan="4">1 dose annually</td></tr>
<tr><td>Pneumococcal (polysaccharide)[6,7]</td><td>1–2 doses</td><td colspan="6">1–2 doses</td><td>1–2 doses</td></tr>
<tr><td>Hepatitis A[8]*</td><td colspan="4">2 doses (0, 6–12 mos, or 0, 6–18 mos)</td><td colspan="4">2 doses (0, 6–12 mos, or 0, 6–18 mos)</td></tr>
<tr><td>Hepatitis B[9]*</td><td colspan="4">3 doses (0, 1–2, 4–6 mos)</td><td colspan="4">3 doses (0, 1–2, 4–6 mos)</td></tr>
<tr><td>Meningococcal[10]</td><td colspan="3">1 dose</td><td>1 dose</td><td colspan="4">1 dose</td></tr>
</table>

* Covered by the Vaccine Injury Compensation Program

These recommendations must be read along with the footnotes.

- For all persons in this category who meet the age requirements and who lack evidence of immunity (e.g., lack documentation of vaccination or have no evidence of prior infection)
- Recommended if some other risk factor is present (e.g., on the basis of medical, occupational, lifestyle, or other indications)
- Contraindicated

From www.cdc.gov.

Table 10–3 ***Recommended Adult Immunization Schedule United States, October 2006–September 2007—cont'd***

Footnotes

Recommended Adult Immunization Schedule, UNITED STATES, OCTOBER 2005–SEPTEMBER 2006

1. **Tetanus and Diphtheria (Td) vaccination.** Adults with uncertain histories of a complete primary vaccination series with diphtheria and tetanus toxoid-containing vaccines should receive a primary series using combined Td toxoid. A primary series for adults is 3 doses; administer the first 2 doses at least 4 weeks apart and the third dose 6–12 months after the second. Administer 1 dose if the person received the primary series and if the last vaccination was received ≥10 years previously. Consult ACIP statement for recommendations for administering Td as prophylaxis in wound management (www.cdc.gov/mmwr/preview/mmwrhtml/00041645.htm). The American College of Physicians Task Force on Adult Immunization supports a second option for Td use in adults: a single Td booster at age 50 years for persons who have completed the full pediatric series, including the teenage/young adult booster. A newly licensed tetanus-diphtheria-acellular pertussis vaccine is available for adults. ACIP recommendations for its use will be published.
2. **Measles, Mumps, Rubella (MMR) vaccination.** *Measles component:* adults born before 1957 can be considered immune to measles. Adults born during or after 1957 should receive ≥1 dose of MMR unless they have a medical contraindication, documentation of ≥1 dose, history of measles based on healthcare provider diagnosis, or laboratory evidence of immunity. A second dose of MMR is recommended for adults who 1) were recently exposed to measles or in an outbreak setting, 2) were previously vaccinated with killed measles vaccine, 3) were vaccinated with an unknown type of measles vaccine during 1963–1967, 4) are students in postsecondary educational institutions, 5) work in a healthcare facility, or 6) plan to travel internationally. Withhold MMR or other measles-containing vaccines from HIV-infected persons with severe immunosuppression. *Mumps component:* 1 dose of MMR vaccine should be adequate for protection for those born during or after 1957 who lack a history of mumps based on healthcare provider diagnosis or who lack laboratory evidence of immunity. *Rubella component:* administer 1 dose of MMR vaccine to women whose rubella vaccination history is unreliable or who lack laboratory evidence of immunity. For women of child-bearing age, regardless of birth year, routinely determine rubella immunity and counsel women regarding congenital rubella syndrome. Do not vaccinate women who are pregnant or might become pregnant within 4 weeks of receiving the vaccine. Women who do not have evidence of immunity should receive MMR vaccine upon completion or termination of pregnancy and before discharge from the healthcare facility.
3. **Varicella vaccination.** Varicella vaccination is recommended for all adults without evidence of immunity to varicella. Special consideration should be given to those who 1) have close contact with persons at high risk for severe disease (healthcare workers and family contacts of immunocompromised persons) or 2) are at high risk for exposure or transmission (e.g., teachers of young children; child care employees; residents and staff members of institutional settings, including correctional institutions; college students; military personnel; adolescents and adults living in households with children; nonpregnant women of childbearing age; and international travelers). Evidence of immunity to varicella in adults includes any of the following: 1) documented age-appropriate varicella vaccination (i.e., receipt of 1 dose before age 13 years or receipt of 2 doses [administered at least 4 weeks apart] after age 13 years); 2) born in the United States before 1966; 3) history of varicella disease based on healthcare provider diagnosis or self- or parental report of typical varicella disease for non–U.S.-born persons born before 1966 and all persons born during 1966–1997 (for a patient reporting a history of an atypical, mild case, healthcare providers should seek either an epidemiologic link with a typical varicella case or evidence of laboratory confirmation, if it was performed at the time of acute disease); 4) history of herpes zoster based on healthcare provider diagnosis; or 5) laboratory evidence of immunity. Do not vaccinate women who are pregnant or might become pregnant within 4 weeks of receiving the vaccine. Assess pregnant women for evidence of varicella immunity. Women who do not have evidence of immunity should receive dose 1 of varicella vaccine upon completion or termination of pregnancy and before discharge from the healthcare facility. Dose 2 should be given 4–8 weeks after dose 1.
4. **Influenza vaccination.** *Medical indications:* chronic disorders of the cardiovascular or pulmonary systems, including asthma; chronic metabolic diseases, including diabetes mellitus, renal dysfunction, hemoglobinopathies, or immunosuppression (including immunosuppression caused by medications or by HIV); any condition (e.g., cognitive dysfunction, spinal cord injury, seizure disorder or other neuromuscular disorder) that compromises respiratory function or the handling of respiratory secretions or that can increase the risk of aspiration; and pregnancy during the influenza season. No data exist on the risk for severe or complicated influenza disease among persons with asplenia; however, influenza is a risk factor for secondary bacterial infections that can cause severe disease among persons with asplenia. *Occupational indications:* healthcare workers and employees of long-term care and assisted living facilities. *Other indications:* residents of nursing homes and other long-term care and assisted living facilities; persons likely to transmit influenza to persons at high risk (i.e., in-home household contacts and caregivers of children birth through 23 months of age, or persons of all ages with high-risk conditions); and anyone who wishes to be vaccinated. For healthy nonpregnant persons aged 5–49 years without high-risk conditions who are not contacts of severely immunocompromised persons in special care units, intranasally administered influenza vaccine (FluMist®) may be administered in lieu of inactivated vaccine.
5. **Pneumococcal polysaccharide vaccination.** *Medical indications:* chronic disorders of the pulmonary system (excluding asthma); cardiovascular diseases; diabetes mellitus; chronic liver diseases, including liver disease as a result of alcohol abuse (e.g.,cirrhosis); chronic renal failure or nephrotic syndrome; functional or anatomic asplenia (e.g., sickle cell disease or splenectomy [if elective splenectomy is planned, vaccinate at least 2 weeks before surgery]); immunosuppressive conditions (e.g., congenital immunodeficiency, HIV infection [vaccinate as close to diagnosis as possible when CD4 cell counts are highest], leukemia, lymphoma, multiple myeloma, Hodgkin disease, generalized malignancy, organ or bone marrow transplantation); chemotherapy with alkylating agents, antimetabolites, or high-dose, long-term corticosteroids; and cochlear implants. *Other indications:* Alaska Natives and certain American Indian populations; residents of nursing homes and other long-term care facilities.
6. **Revaccination with pneumococcal polysaccharide vaccine.** One-time revaccination after 5 years for persons with chronic renal failure or nephrotic syndrome; functional or anatomic asplenia (e.g., sickle cell disease or splenectomy); immunosuppressive conditions (e.g., congenital immunodeficiency, HIV infection, leukemia, lymphoma, multiple myeloma, Hodgkin disease, generalized malignancy, organ or bone marrow transplantation); or chemotherapy with alkylating agents, antimetabolites, or high-dose, long-term corticosteroids. For persons aged ≥65 years, one-time revaccination if they were vaccinated ≥5 years previously and were aged <65 years at the time of primary vaccination.
7. **Hepatitis A vaccination.** *Medical indications:* persons with clotting factor disorders or chronic liver disease. *Behavioral indications:* men who have sex with men or users of illegal drugs. *Occupational indications:* persons working with hepatitis A virus (HAV)-infected primates or with HAV in a research laboratory setting. *Other indications:* persons traveling to or working in countries that have high or intermediate endemicity of hepatitis A (for list of countries, visit www.cdc.gov/travel/diseases.htm#hepa) as well as any person wishing to obtain immunity. Current vaccines should be given in a 2-dose series at either 0 and 6–12 months, or 0 and 6–18 months. If the combined hepatitis A and hepatitis B vaccine is used, administer 3 doses at 0, 1, and 6 months.
8. **Hepatitis B vaccination.** *Medical indications:* hemodialysis patients (use special formulation [40 μg/mL] or two 20-μg/mL doses) or patients who receive clotting factor concentrates. *Occupational indications:* healthcare workers and public-safety workers who have exposure to blood in the workplace; and persons in training in schools of medicine, dentistry, nursing, laboratory technology, and other allied health professions. *Behavioral indications:* injection-drug users; persons with more than one sex partner in the previous 6 months; persons with a recently acquired sexually transmitted disease (STD); and men who have sex with men. *Other indications:* household contacts and sex partners of persons with chronic hepatitis B virus (HBV) infection; clients and staff of institutions for the developmentally disabled; all clients of STD clinics; inmates of correctional facilities; or international travelers who will be in countries with high or intermediate prevalence of chronic HBV infection for >6 months (for list of countries, visit www.cdc.gov/travel/diseases.htm#hepa).
9. **Meningococcal vaccination.** *Medical indications:* adults with anatomic or functional asplenia, or terminal complement component deficiencies. *Other indications:* first-year college students living in dormitories; microbiologists who are routinely exposed to isolates of *Neisseria meningitidis;* military recruits; and persons who travel to or reside in countries in which meningococcal disease is hyperendemic or epidemic (e.g., the "meningitis belt" of sub-Saharan Africa during the dry season [Dec–June]), particularly if contact with the local populations will be prolonged. Vaccination is required by the government of Saudi Arabia for all travelers to Mecca during the annual Hajj. Meningococcal conjugate vaccine is preferred for adults meeting any of the above indications who are aged ≤55 years, although meningococcal polysaccharide vaccine (MPSV4) is an acceptable alternative. Revaccination after 5 years may be indicated for adults previously vaccinated with MPSV4 who remain at high risk for infection (e.g., persons residing in areas in which disease is epidemic).
10. **Selected conditions for which *Haemophilus influenzae* type b (Hib) vaccine may be used.** *Haemophilus influenzae* type b conjugate vaccines are licensed for children aged 6 weeks–71 months. No efficacy data are available on which to base a recommendation concerning use of Hib vaccine for older children and adults with the chronic conditions associated with an increased risk for Hib disease. However, studies suggest good immunogenicity in patients who have sickle cell disease, leukemia, or HIV infection, or have had splenectomies; administering vaccine to these patients is not contraindicated.

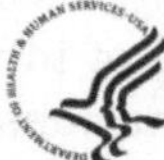

DEPARTMENT OF HEALTH AND HUMAN SERVICES
CENTERS FOR DISEASE CONTROL AND PREVENTION

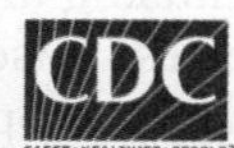

Approved by the Advisory Committee on Immunization Practices (ACIP), the American College of Obstetricians and Gynecologists (ACOG), and the American Academy of Family Physicians (AAFP)

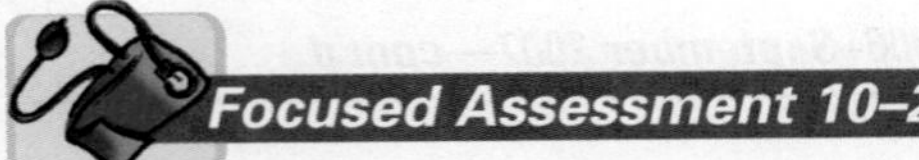

Physical Assessment of the Lymphatic and Immune Systems

Assess the following:

- Take vitals signs, noting if there is an increase in temperature or pulse rate.
- Measure height and weight.
- Inspect the skin for color, turgor, texture, and presence of lesions.
- Assess extremities for edema.
- Inspect ears, eyes, nose, and throat for drainage, redness, or exudate.
- Palpate lymph nodes in the neck to identify enlargement or tenderness.
- Auscultate lung fields and assess work of breathing.
- Analyze laboratory results such as CBC, C-reactive protein, and antibody screening tests.

ways for organisms. Remember to assess those areas where catheters, tubes, and other medical devices may bypass the skin barrier. The skin may show excessive immune reaction, as in an allergic response resulting in hives or other skin eruptions.

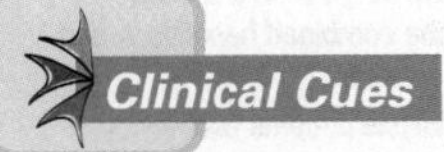

Latex allergy can be another cause of redness at tube sites if the tube contains latex.

When the immune response is activated, lymph nodes may become swollen and tender and can be assessed by palpation. Nodes in the neck, axillae, and groin areas are those most commonly examined.

Data obtained from a head-to-toe physical assessment provide important information regarding immune and lymphatic system function (Focused Assessment 10–2).

Diagnostic Tests, Procedures, and Nursing Implications

Skin Testing. *Skin testing* is one of the most commonly used techniques to measure immunity and to identify people who may have a dormant infectious disease. These tests include the *Schick test* to determine susceptibility to diphtheria and the *tuberculin skin test* (Mantoux test) to identify those who might need treatment for TB. The Mantoux test and other tests for TB are covered in Chapter 14.

Several types of skin testing may also be done to identify allergens that are causing allergic symptoms in an individual. A scratch test (also called prick or puncture test) may be done by dropping extracts of allergens into scratches made on the skin. Intradermal injection of allergens is used to detect allergies to insect venom or penicillin. Patches containing allergens that might cause contact dermatitis are placed in direct contact with the skin. Inflammation and itching identify those allergens that provoke the immune system.

Laboratory Tests. Laboratory tests on blood and serum also give important information regarding the status of the immune system. A complete blood count (CBC) gives information regarding the number of circulating white blood cells. The differential indicates what percentage of the total white cell count is accounted for by the different cells. An increased white count indicates that the immune system has been activated (Table 10–4). If a specific disease or condition is suspected, blood testing can determine if antibodies to that disease or condition are present.

Imaging Studies. **Immunoscintigraphy** is a nuclear medicine imaging procedure in which antibodies labeled with radioactive isotope are injected into the bloodstream. The isotope emits gamma rays that can be detected by the imaging equipment. Computers construct a picture of sites in the body where the antibody accumulates. Primary use of this technique is for identification of neoplasms, but studies are showing promise in locating areas of infection. Current research is investigating techniques for "tagging" other cellular components of the immune system with radioactive substances that can then be visualized with nuclear medicine equipment.

Computed tomography (CT), magnetic resonance imaging (MRI), and positron emission tomography (PET) can all be utilized to evaluate the thymus gland and other tissue structures of the immune system.

Nursing Diagnosis

Nursing diagnoses commonly encountered for patients with immune and lymphatic disorders are numerous. They are chosen based on the problems identified during data collection (Table 10–5).

Planning

Planning is based on the particular problems identified for the individual patient. General nursing goals include:

- Protect from infection
- Improve health status
- Maintain high degree of wellness to promote optimal immune function

Expected outcomes are written for each nursing diagnosis (see Table 10–5).

Implementation

Nursing interventions include all methods for prevention of spread of infection. Meticulous adherence to Standard Precautions, including appropriate hand hygiene, is essential (Assignment Considerations

Table 10–4 ***Diagnostic Tests for Disorders of the Immune and Lymphatic Systems***

TEST AND NORMAL RANGE	PURPOSE	DESCRIPTION	NURSING IMPLICATIONS
Complete blood count (CBC)	Determine whether abnormalities are present in the numbers of blood cells or types of blood cells; assess the amount of hemoglobin present Useful to diagnose anemia	Fill a lavender-top tube containing EDTA with a venous sample of blood. Use a site where there is little chance of dilution from intravenous solution. Mix the blood and the EDTA by gently rotating the tube.	Warn the patient that a "stick" is about to occur, but that the pain will be short-lived. Apply pressure directly to the puncture site after withdrawing the needle; at the antecubital space, do **not** have the patient flex the arm as this tends to cause a hematoma.
Erythrocytes Hemoglobin: Females: 12.0–16.0 g/dL; males: 13.0–18.0 g/dL Red blood cell count: Females: 4.2–5.4 million/mm^3; males: 4.6–6.2 million/mm^3 Hematocrit: Female: 37%–47%; male: 40%–54% **Leukocytes** White blood cell (WBC) count: 4500–11,000/mm^3 **Differential Count** Granulocytes Neutrophils: 54%–62% of WBCs Eosinophils: 1%–3% of WBCs Basophils: 0%–1% of WBCs Agranulocytes Lymphocytes: 25%–33% of WBCs Monocytes: 3%–7% of WBCs Thrombocytes (platelets): 150,000–400,000/mm^3 of blood Mean corpuscular hemoglobin (Hb) (MCH): 26–34 pg/cell Mean corpuscular Hb concentration (MCHC): 32–36 gm/dL Mean corpuscular volume (MCV): 80–96 μm^3			
Lymphangiogram Normal-size vessels and nodes without filling defects	Detect abnormalities in the lymphatic system, especially cancer	Dye is injected intradermally between the first three toes of each foot while the patient is supine. Local anesthesia is injected, and an incision is made in the dorsum of the foot to inject iodine contrast material directly into a lymphatic vessel over a 1½-hr period. X-rays are taken of the abdomen, pelvis, and upper body.	Repeat films are taken in 24 hr. Obtain written consent. Assess for allergy to iodine or shellfish. Explain procedure. Postprocedure, elevate legs for 24 hours to decrease swelling. Assess for signs of infection and oil embolism q 4 hr × 24 hr.
Spleen sonogram Proper size, shape, and position	Detect structural abnormalities of the spleen	An ultrasound wand is moved over the abdomen in the area of the spleen with the patient supine on the examining table.	Explain that the test takes about 30 min.
Spleen scan Even distribution of labeled erythrocytes throughout the spleen	Detect anatomical changes in the spleen; determine invasion of Hodgkin's or metastatic disease Usually done in conjunction with a liver scan	A radioactive nuclide colloid is injected intravenously. After about 20 min, a minimum of three views are obtained. Radiation exposure is about 0.5 rad (equal to about 1 yr of natural radiation exposure to the body). Schedule scan before tests using barium.	Explain that a substance will be injected and, after about 20 min, scanning begins. Radiation exposure is minimal. The test takes about 60 min.

*Diagnostic tests for human immunodeficiency virus are presented in Chapter 11. Bone marrow aspiration is covered in Chapter 15.

Continued

Table 10–4 ***Diagnostic Tests for Disorders of the Immune and Lymphatic Systems—cont'd***

TEST AND NORMAL RANGE	PURPOSE	DESCRIPTION	NURSING IMPLICATIONS
Immunoglobulins, serum IgG: 640–1350 mg/dL IgA: 70–310 mg/dL IgM: 90–350 mg/dL IgD: 0.0–6.0 mg/dL IgE: 0.0–430 ng/dL	Used to detect and monitor quantities of antibodies circulating in the blood Useful for monitoring hypersensitivity diseases, immune deficiencies, autoimmune diseases, and chronic infections	Serum is placed on a slide containing agar gel and an electric current is passed through the gel. The immunoglobulins are separated out and electrophoresed according to the quantity and difference in electrical charge.	No fasting or special preparation is required. Requires drawing 7–10 mL of blood.
Complement assays Total serum complement (CH_{50}): 150–250 units/mL C3 (mature T cells): 85–175 mg/dL C4 (T helper cells): 15–45 mg/dL	Used to monitor immune disorders	In the presence of antibody/antigen complexes, the complement system is overly activated, and the complement components are "consumed" or used up.	No fasting or special preparation is required. Requires drawing 7–10 mL of blood.
C-Reactive protein (CRP) <1.0 mg/dL	Detect the presence of an inflammatory process	CRP is initiated by antigen-immune complexes, bacteria, fungi, and trauma. It interacts with the complement system.	Explain that fasting may be required for 4–12 hr. Water is permitted. Requires drawing a blood sample. Cigarette smoking can cause increased levels. Alcohol consumption can decrease levels. Estrogens and progesterones may cause increased levels. Statins, fibrins, and niacin may cause decreased levels.
Lymph node biopsy Negative for abnormal cells or infectious agents	Detect changes in tissue; identify autoimmune disease or detect the spread of malignancy	Tissue is obtained by needle aspiration, excision, or needle punch using aseptic technique.	Fasting may be required. Sedation and/or local anesthesia will be administered. Biopsied material is placed in formaldehyde. Label and transport to the laboratory immediately. A dry sterile dressing is applied to the biopsy site. Instruct the patient to watch for signs of infection: increasing pain, redness, swelling, purulent drainage, or fever >101° F. (38.3° C).
Culture	Determine organism responsible for infection	A sample of exudate, fluid, or tissue is taken from the suspected infected area.	The procedures for collecting bacterial, viral, and fungal samples are different. Consult the agency protocol. Gather the correct culture tubes and culture media. Label all containers before collection of the specimen(s). Transport the specimen(s) to the laboratory immediately.

10–1, p. 231). Additional protection from infection may include implementation of protective isolation. Promotion of balanced, adequate nutrition is essential in maintaining or regaining optimal immune function. Reducing the risk of health care–associated infections (ones that are acquired while a patient is in the hospital) is one of the objectives of the 2007 Hospital National Patient Safety Goals.

The National Patient Safety Goals for 2007, set by The Joint Commission (TJC), includes Goal 7, which emphasizes the need to "reduce the risk of health care–associated infections."

Table 10–5 ***Common Nursing Diagnoses and Interventions for Patients with Alteration in Immune and Lymphatic Function***

NURSING DIAGNOSIS	GOALS/EXPECTED OUTCOMES	NURSING INTERVENTIONS
EXCESSIVE IMMUNE RESPONSE		
Risk for ineffective breathing pattern related to excessive immune response	Patient will maintain a patent airway and adequate oxygenation	Maintain patent airway Assess respiratory function q 2–4 hr. Provide supplemental oxygen as needed and ordered.
Risk for hyperthermia secondary to inflammatory response	Patient will maintain core temperature within normal range	Monitor temperature. Administer antipyretics as indicated. Initiate cooling measures if indicated. Monitor intake and output. Encourage fluid intake.
Risk for impaired skin integrity secondary to allergens	Patient's skin will be intact and without redness or rash or hives	Assess for rash or hives. Administer topical and systemic medications as ordered. Keep skin clean and dry, use lotions for lubrication. Refrain from bathing in hot water. Suggest use of ice to decrease itching. Keep nails short to reduce risk of injury from scratching. Provide distraction activities to shift focus from itching.
Anxiety related to threatened health status	Patient will assist with lessening symptoms through various techniques Patient's anxiety will decrease by discharge	Assess level of anxiety. If patient is having respiratory difficulty, stay with the patient. Explain to the patient what is being done to help her and what she can do to lessen the symptoms. Teach relaxation exercises.
DEFICIENT IMMUNE RESPONSE		
Infection, either actual or risk for, secondary to decreased resistance	Patient will remain free of infection or, if infection occurs, it will be promptly identified and treated	Maintain infection control standards to prevent hospital-acquired infections. Assess for signs and symptoms of infection. Aggressively treat infection if it occurs. Instruct patient in techniques to prevent acquisition of infection.
Risk for impaired social interaction resulting in social isolation	Patient will participate in social activities within ability	Encourage interaction utilizing technology to maintain relationships and prevent infections. Provide positive reinforcement when the patient participates socially. Provide education regarding modes of transmission so that social interactions can be safely undertaken.
Risk for imbalanced body temperature secondary to illness	Maintain body temperature within normal range	Monitor core body temperature. Maintain a comfortable ambient temperature. Restore/maintain temperature within patient's normal range.
Risk for imbalanced nutrition: less than body requirements secondary to loss of appetite	Maintain stable weight	Assess presence and degree of nausea or loss of appetite. Assist patient to make a dietary plan including favorite foods. Consult with dietitian and health care team. Offer frequent small meals. Promote an odor-free, relaxing atmosphere for meals.

Continued

Table 10–5 Common Nursing Diagnoses and Interventions for Patients with Alteration in Immune and Lymphatic Function—cont'd

NURSING DIAGNOSIS	GOALS/EXPECTED OUTCOMES	NURSING INTERVENTIONS
DEFICIENT IMMUNE RESPONSE—cont'd		
Deficient knowledge regarding disease process and prevention of infection transmission	Patient and family will verbalize understanding of disease process, treatment, and necessary precautions	Assess readiness to learn. Provide information in multiple formats: verbal, visual media, written. Teach necessary precautions to prevent infection. Provide positive reinforcement. Use team and group teaching as appropriate. Provide access to other information sources. Refer to community agencies and support groups.
LYMPH SYSTEM DISORDERS		
Acute pain related to disease process	Patient's pain will be reduced and kept within range acceptable to patient	Teach patient use of pain scale for reporting of pain. Accept patient's report of pain. Monitor vital signs. Provide comfort measures. Instruct and encourage relaxation, imagery, and diversional activities. Administer analgesics as needed to maintain acceptable comfort level. Encourage adequate rest periods. Work with patient and family to identify effective strategies for pain management.
Imbalanced nutrition: less than body requirements secondary to disease process	Patient will maintain present or ideal body weight	Determine ability to chew and swallow. Identify patient food preferences. Offer frequent small meals. Weigh daily. Promote relaxing meal environment. Provide oral care before and after meals.
Powerlessness related to disease process	Patient will become actively involved in care and will make choices related to care	Assess patient's knowledge and perception of condition. Identify patient support systems. Listen to patient's expressions of feelings. Show concern for patient as an individual. Treat patient's decisions with respect. Encourage realistic goal setting. Provide opportunities for the patient to control as many events as restrictions allow.
Body image disturbance related to lymphedema	Patient will verbalize understanding of body changes	Teach patient and family about pathophysiology of lymphedema. Institute measures to reduce lymphedema: elevation of extremity and use of pressure sleeve as ordered. Teach measures to prevent lymphedema recurrence. Support patient decision making. Refer to appropriate support groups.

Psychosocial care to decrease fear, help deal with lifestyle changes or role changes, and reduce stress is important in caring for the whole person. Patient teaching regarding the disorder, treatment, signs of complications, and self-care is an effective way to reduce stress and fear. Nursing care for specific disorders of the immune and lymphatic system is presented in the next chapter.

Evaluation

Determination of whether expected outcomes are being met includes assessing for signs and symptoms of immune function. This includes gathering physical data as well as monitoring laboratory test values for improvement. Temperature and other vital signs are good indicators of immune function. General well-being and side effects of medications are also param-

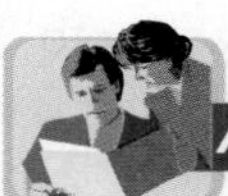

Assignment Considerations 10–1

Brief Certified Nursing Assistants (CNAs) and Unlicensed Assistive Personnel (UAPs)

When assigning patients or tasks to CNAs or UAPs remember to share that a patient is *immunocompromised* (very susceptible to infection) and that it is important to be extra diligent about hand hygiene. Ask them to help restrict the presence in the room of people who have an infection. Remind them that it is important that the patient obtain sufficient rest and not be continually disturbed. Ask the assistant to report any new skin lesion, irritation, or redness that is noticed during bathing. State that you want to know if the urine has a foul odor. Remember at the end of the shift to thank the person for the help provided.

eters to be monitored in evaluation of effectiveness of nursing and medical interventions.

COMMON PROBLEMS RELATED TO THE IMMUNE AND LYMPHATIC SYSTEMS

FEVER

A rise in body temperature signals a normal immune system response to infection. The rise in temperature is one of the facets of fighting off the invaders and promoting a hostile environment. There is clinical evidence that fever is helpful and there is controversy about treating an elevation in body temperature. *Hyperthermia* or fever related to infections can cause discomfort, and excessive fever can lead to complications such as seizures. Decreasing body temperature by physical or pharmaceutical means promotes comfort for the individual but may decrease the effectiveness of the body's efforts to eliminate microorganisms.

Excessive fever **(hyperpyrexia)** is usually treated with antipyretics and cooling measures.

Nursing Management

Cooling measures can be as simple as removing excess coverings or as complex as utilization of mechanical cooling blankets. Usual nursing measures for decreasing body temperature include sponging with tepid water. Cold water is contraindicated because rapid cooling can induce shivering, which will drive the temperature back up.

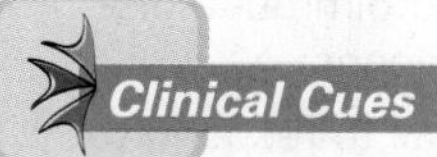

Clinical Cues

Sometimes temperature can be lowered by placing ice bags in the armpits and groin. Be sure to insulate the packs with cloth before placing them. These areas have good blood circulation that the cold can reach. Cooling the blood cools the core temperature.

The ideal treatment for fever is to address the cause. Appropriate antibiotic therapy can reduce fever by fighting the infection. Allergic inflammatory responses can be treated with corticosteroids. Anti-inflammatory medications such as aspirin, ibuprofen or acetaminophen may be administered to lower the temperature.

NUTRITION

Anorexia (alteration in desire for food) often accompanies fever, infection, and use of antibiotics. Adequate nutrition is essential in maintaining the immune system and rebuilding tissues affected by infection. Calories, vitamins, and protein are all needed as building blocks. Adequate fluid intake is also important. Increased body temperature is caused by increased metabolic rate. This increase in cellular metabolism utilizes more water than under normal circumstances. That water must be replenished in order for the body to function at an optimum level.

Nursing Management

Frequently offering favorite fluids and foods in small portions can tempt the appetite. When febrile, individuals often enjoy cold or frozen items. Easily digested food items are usually more tempting. Increased fluid intake is important. Fluids with nutrients and calories may be more attractive than solid food. Soups and juices are most often well tolerated.

IMMUNOSUPPRESSION

Many patients are immunosuppressed either from the disease process or from the treatment for it. This makes the person very susceptible to common organisms. Patients taking corticosteroids for any reason, such as for asthma or following organ transplantation, are immunosuppressed. Patients on chemotherapy and individuals with diabetes also have a depressed immune system. Hospital settings are known for having a high concentration of pathogens just due to the illnesses of the inpatients.

Nursing Management

In the hospital environment, **it is critical that all standard infection control procedures be implemented without fail.** Patients with **neutropenia** (less than normal amount of white blood cells) may need additional precautions. Reverse isolation, protective isolation, and neutropenia precautions are terms referring to procedures that may be implemented to protect immunosuppressed patients from infection. This may include restrictions on fresh fruits, vegetables, and flowers. Also restricted are visitors who may have an infectious disorder. Regardless of the term utilized, the principle is the same—prevention of transmission of a potentially infective agent to a patient with an impaired immune system. These measures may include specially constructed rooms with positive airflow, monitoring of water purity, and monitoring of air conduits for presence of microorganisms. The degree to which these measures are implemented is determined by the degree of immunosuppression. Any patient who is ill and hospitalized has an immune system under stress. Health care workers meticulously adhering to Standard Precautions will help protect patients. Chapter 16 presents neutropenia precautions.

Think Critically About . . . What devices, tools, equipment, or other objects are routinely carried from patient room to patient room without disinfection? Where do they fit in the chain of infection? What can you, as a health care provider, do about reducing transmission of microorganisms?

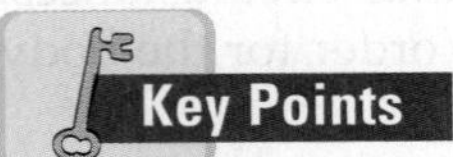

Key Points

- The immune and lymphatic systems protect the body against microscopic threats to homeostasis.
- The inflammatory response is the first step in the immune response.
- Antibodies are proteins that fight antigens.
- T and B lymphocytes are major forces in fighting infection.
- The body produces a humoral (immediate) and cellular (delayed) response to antigens.
- Consumption of alcohol can alter the body's ability to launch an immune response.
- Active artificially acquired immunity occurs by vaccination or immunization.
- Immunizations introduce pathogens to the body in a controlled way, allowing the body to produce antibodies to prevent future illness.
- The nurse plays a major role in providing education regarding the importance of immunizations to public health.
- Decreased immune response puts the patient at risk for infection.
- Measures should be instituted to prevent hospital-acquired infections.
- ALWAYS use Standard Precautions and meticulous hand hygiene to help prevent the spread of organisms among hospitalized patients.
- Good nutrition and healthy lifestyle choices are important for a healthy immune system.
- Immunosuppression can be caused by treatment for conditions such as cancer and asthma.

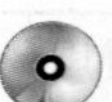

Go to your **Companion CD-ROM** for an Audio Glossary, animations, video clips, and bonus review questions.

evolve Be sure to visit the companion Evolve site at http://evolve.elsevier.com/deWit/ for interactive NCLEX-PN Exam Style Review Questions, WebLinks, and additional online resources.

NCLEX-PN EXAM STYLE REVIEW QUESTIONS

Choose the best answer(s) for the following questions.

1. The administration of weak or attenuated microorganisms to stimulate the production of antibodies without causing a full-blown disease is referred to as:
   1. active naturally acquired immunity.
   2. active artificially acquired immunity.
   3. passive natural immunity.
   4. passive artificial immunity.
2. The nurse demonstrates understanding of natural immunity when he makes which of the following statements?
   1. "Breastfeeding is the best way to enhance the infant's immunity."
   2. "Timely vaccination could easily provide protection from hepatitis."
   3. "The skin provides the first line of defense in warding off diseases."
   4. "Administration of human immune globulins boosts the immunity."
3. Before administering antibodies against tetanus, which of the following patient statements would indicate a need for further nursing assessment?
   1. "I have reactions to horse serum."
   2. "I cannot have any seafood."
   3. "I have lactose intolerance."
   4. "I do not like eggs."
4. During a health promotion outreach for older adults, the nurse discusses the physiological changes in aging that increase susceptibility to infection. Which of the following statements is true?
   1. "With advanced age, the shin becomes tough and leathery."
   2. "Decreased cilia in the lung provides a more hospitable to harmful organisms."
   3. "Decreased normal flora in the intestines potentially causes the harboring of pathogens."
   4. "Repeated infections build up immune responses."
5. The patient is newly diagnosed with an autoimmune thyroid disease. When the nurse discusses the patient's questions and concerns, the patient asks, "What did the physician mean by autoimmune disease?" The nurse appropriately responds:
   1. "The body's immune defenses fail to respond to the pathogenic agents."
   2. "Immune defenses are attacking the normal body cells."
   3. "There is a break in the body's defenses."
   4. "The physician was able to identify the underlying cause of the disorder."

6. The nurse assesses the condition of a sacral pressure ulcer on an immobilized patient. Which of the following signs and symptoms indicate the presence of infection?

1. Warm to touch
2. Pink wound surface
3. Wound culture <10,000 colonies
4. Purulent drainage

7. While taking care of an immune-compromised patient, which action by a nursing assistant indicates a need for instruction and supervision by a nurse?

1. Reporting changes in the physical characteristics of the urine
2. Allowing all family members in the patient's room at all times
3. Meticulous hand hygiene before entering the patient's room
4. Turning the patient while bathing the patient

8. The patient indicates, "I take garlic pills to reduce my risk for cancer." Which of the following is an appropriate nursing response?

1. "How much and how often do you take your garlic pills?"
2. "Have you been screened for cancer?"
3. "What other herbal medications are you taking?"
4. "You sound worried. Could you talk more about it?"

9. The nurse prepares the patient for a blood draw for C-reactive protein. An important patient instruction before the procedure includes:

1. Hormone replacement therapy can increase the level of C-reactive protein.
2. An increased level of C-reactive protein is associated with cigarette smoking and alcohol.
3. Niacin enhances production of C-reactive protein.
4. The procedure requires a 4- to 12-hour fast with no water intake.

10. Before receiving antivenin, the patient asks, "How does the antivenin work?" You demonstrate knowledge of the medication when you make which of the following statements?

1. "The antivenin provides a life-long protection from any snake bite."
2. "The antivenin must be given as early as possible to afford immediate reversal of the subsequent effects of the venom."
3. "The antivenin reverses the effects of the poisonous snake bite."
4. "The antivenin cannot be given to patients who are allergic to eggs."

CRITICAL THINKING ACTIVITIES 

Read each clinical scenario and discuss the questions with your classmates.

Scenario A

Mr. Green, an 80-year-old farmer, is admitted with pneumonia. VS: T 103° F (oral), BP 136/78, HR 100, RR 28, and no complaint of pain.

1. What assessment data indicate that the immune system is active?
2. Describe how the body is reacting to the lung infection. Which type of immunity will help fight the infection?
3. List appropriate nursing interventions for Mr. Green.

Scenario B

Mrs. Hope brings her newborn into the pediatrician's office. She is seeking information.

1. Mrs. Hope asks when she should bring her baby in for immunizations. What will you tell her?
2. Explain how immunizations help protect the body.
3. Discuss what information should be given so that Mrs. Hope could identify if her baby has had a reaction to an immunization.

CHAPTER 11

Care of Patients with Immune and Lymphatic Disorders

evolve http://evolve.elsevier.com/deWit

Objectives

Upon completing this chapter, you should be able to:

Theory

1. Describe the modes of transmission for HIV.
2. Identify the signs and symptoms exhibited by a person with AIDS.
3. Discuss the risks to individuals with an immune deficiency disorder.
4. Explain how an allergic reaction occurs when a patient experiences an excessive immune response.
5. Explain why tissue matching is so important for organ and tissue transplants.
6. Describe the methods used to prevent transplant rejection.
7. Explain how autoimmune disorders are thought to occur.
8. Compare systemic lupus erythematosus with other autoimmune diseases.
9. Discuss the two types of lymphoma and how they are diagnosed.
10. Describe nursing interventions for lymphedema.

Clinical Practice

1. List nursing measures taken to prevent the spread of infection to an immunocompromised patient.
2. State the signs and symptoms of an anaphylactic reaction and the usual measures that would be taken to treat it.
3. Formulate a nursing care plan for a patient who has systemic lupus erythematosus.

Key Terms

Be sure to check out the bonus material on the Companion CD-ROM, including selected audio pronunciations.

acquired immunodeficiency syndrome (AIDS) (ă-KWĪRD ĭm-ū-nō-dĕ-FĬSH-ĕn-sē SĬN-drōm, p. 235)
anaphylaxis (ă-nă-fă-LĂK-sĭs, p. 258)
anasarca (ăn-ă-SĂR-kă, p. 249)
angioedema (ăn-jē-ō-ĕ-DĒ-mă, p. 263)
atopy (ĂT-ō-pē, p. 258)
autoimmune disease (aw-tō-ĭ-MŪN dĭ-ZĒZ, p. 234)
depression (of immune function) (de-PRĔSH-ŭn, p. 234)
dermatome (DĔR-mă-tōm, p. 245)
disseminated (dĭ-SĔM-ĭ-nāt-ĕd, p. 246)
human immunodeficiency virus (HIV) (ĭm-ū-nō-dĕ-FĬSH-ĕn-sē VĪ-rŭs, p. 235)
immune deficiency (ĭ-MŪN dĕ-FĬSH-ĕn-sē, p. 234)
lymphedema (lĭm-fĕ-DĒ-mă, p. 249)
opportunistic infections (OIs) (ŏp-pŏr-tū-NĬS-tĭk ĭn-FĔK-shŭnz, p. 237)
prodrome (PRŌ-drōm, p. 244)
protease inhibitor (PRŌ-tē-ās ĭn-HĬB-ĭ-tŏr, p. 239)
replicate (RĔP-lĭ-kāt, p. 237)
retrovirus (rĕ-trō-VĪ-rŭs, p. 237)
reverse transcriptase (rē-VĔRS trănz-SCRĬP-tās, p. 237)
sentinel infections (SĔN-tĭ-nĕl ĭn-FĔK-shŭnz, p. 237)
suppression (of the immune response) (sŭ-PRĔ-shŭn, p. 237)
urticaria (ŭr-tĭ-KĀ-rē-ă, p. 263)
wheals (wēlz, p. 263)

Abnormal responses of the immune system are divided into two basic categories: (1) **immune deficiency**, that is, insufficient production of either antibodies or immune cells or both; and (2) inappropriate response, which involves overreaction or hypersensitivity to antigens from the external environment and results in **autoimmune diseases**. An autoimmune disease occurs when the immune system is unable to tell the difference between foreign cells and the body's own cells.

Inadequate function of the immune system can affect either the *humoral* (fluid) or cellular components of the system. Insufficient production of these components can be present at birth *(congenital)* or acquired during life as discussed in Chapter 10. In some cases the acquired deficiency is a primary condition; in others it is secondary to some other disorder or treatment. In all cases, a deficiency of immune system response leaves its victims unable to resist invasion of foreign microbes and therefore susceptible to overwhelming infection.

Acquired immune deficiency can result from any of a number of factors. Administration of chemotherapy for treatment of some cancers can temporarily reduce the ability of the bone marrow to produce white cells. Common viral infections, including influenza, infectious mononucleosis, and measles, can cause **depression** of short-term immune function. Other conditions that can decrease immune response include smoking, malnutrition, surgery, and stress. The immune system may be therapeutically suppressed to prevent a tissue transplant rejection.

DISORDERS OF THE IMMUNE SYSTEM

DISORDERS OF IMMUNE DEFICIENCY

ACQUIRED IMMUNE DEFICIENCY SYNDROME

Etiology

Contraction of the **human immunodeficiency virus (HIV)** and the subsequent development of **acquired immunodeficiency syndrome (AIDS)** is the most serious of the immune deficiency disorders. There is no cure for AIDS, but medications can slow the progression of the disease and research is progressing on a vaccine. The International AIDS Vaccine Initiative, a network of professionals in 23 countries, is helping with research efforts. While the advance of the disease may be slowed with treatment, at this time AIDS is still a fatal disease. People who become HIV positive develop AIDS after varying periods of time. Drug therapy may keep the person relatively healthy and AIDS free for many years. Research is ongoing for effective treatments for AIDS, but primary emphasis is on prevention of the disease.

Transmission and Prevention

Gaining knowledge about HIV and educating others—patients, colleagues, and community—are important parts of the nurse's role (Cultural Cues 11–1). There must be an understanding of the virus to dispel fears associated with becoming infected with HIV/AIDS. The nurse must be able to assess the risk behaviors practiced by patients in order to provide appropriate education. The goal is to slow and eventually stop the transmission of this virus. The first step in the prevention of HIV infection is knowledge, and nurses can provide that knowledge. Current medical research has shown that HIV cannot be transmitted by casual contact. Additional information can be found in the Centers for Disease Control and Prevention (CDC) fact sheet, "HIV and Its Transmission" (CDC, 2007). The ONLY mode of transmission is by exposure to HIV-infected blood, body fluids, or tissue (Box 11–1).

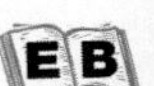

There have been no documented cases of HIV transmission from tattoos and piercings. There have been documented cases of hepatitis B transmission with these activities, and HIV is transmitted in a similar manner as hepatitis B. There may be a possibility of transmission in these settings if needles and instruments are not properly sanitized. Since March of 1985, all blood and blood products are screened for blood-borne pathogens. Prospective organ donors are also screened. According to the CDC, the current risk of contracting HIV from receiving a blood transfusion, blood products, or a donated organ is extremely small, even in populations with a high incidence of HIV infection.

Health education agencies, as well as the gay community, have made a major effort to educate people about the possibility of exposure through unprotected sex, which is the primary mode of transmission. There is a push to encourage monogamous sexual relationships and discourage casual sex, as well as to avoid anal or vaginal intercourse with a partner who is seropositive with HIV. Nonoxynol-9, an ingredient in spermicidal jelly, has been shown in studies to inactivate or kill HIV in a test tube. It also causes tissue irritation and may promote HIV exposure by disrupting the tissue barrier. It is currently not recommended as a deterrent to HIV exposure. Avoidance of anal intercourse prevents microscopic tears in the lining of the anus, which is thinner than the walls of the vagina. Any break in the skin is an entry portal for HIV (Health Promotion Points 11–1 and 11–2).

There is no reason for HIV-infected individuals to completely discontinue sexual activity. Touch and intimacy are important parts of any relationship. However, there is a need to reduce the risk of transmitting the virus to others and at the same time prevent exposure to any other sexually transmitted infections (also

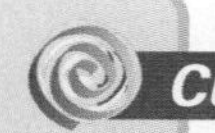

Cultural Cues 11–1

HIV and Minorities

HIV reporting in the United States indicates that more than 73% of new HIV infections occur in minorities. The highest incidence among this group occurs in African Americans and Hispanics (CDC, 2003). It is thought that the following factors increase the incidence of HIV infection and progression to AIDS among minority groups:

- Lack of culturally sensitive and high-quality information about HIV risk and prevention
- Socioeconomic status and limited access to health care
- Health beliefs concerning sexual practices, roles of women, the value of children, and HIV treatment
- The high cost of antiretroviral combined therapy

Box 11–1 *Modes of Human Immunodeficiency Virus (HIV) Exposure*

Modes of HIV exposure may include:

- Unprotected sexual contact with an HIV-infected partner (sexual transmission)
- Sharing needles with an HIV-infected drug user
- Occupational exposure through a needle stick with an HIV-contaminated needle
- Maternal transmission to an infant through vaginal delivery or breast milk
- Receiving a transfusion of HIV-infected blood or blood products
- Receiving an organ transplant from an HIV-infected person

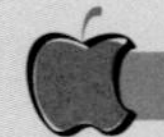

Health Promotion Points 11–1

Safer Sexual Practices

Safer sex practices prevent transmission by putting a barrier, a condom, or another impermeable barrier between the body fluids of one partner and the other. However, the only guaranteed way to prevent transmission sexually is through abstinence. When safer sex is discussed, reference is made to methods that reduce the possibility of exposure. The use of latex condoms is recommended because they are more impermeable than other types of condoms that may allow penetration of the virus through the membrane of the material used (polyurethane and deproteinized latex condoms are available for those allergic to latex).

known as sexually transmitted diseases). Sexually transmitted infections are more difficult to treat when the immune system is suppressed.

An unsafe practice that is a known method of HIV transmission is being the receptive partner in anal or vaginal intercourse without a latex condom, or being the insertive partner. Another unsafe practice is orogenital (fellatio or cunnilingus) or oroanal (rimming) stimulation without a barrier (dental dam). Contact with all body fluids, such as semen or vaginal secretions and blood, must be avoided. The key to being less prone to becoming infected with HIV, or other sexually transmitted infections (e.g., syphilis, gonorrhea, cytomegalovirus, chlamydia, hepatitis B, herpes, and condyloma), is to know methods of protection and to use them consistently. Barrier sex must be practiced with every sexual encounter to prevent transmission of HIV.

HIV infection is transmitted primarily by contact with blood containing HIV through broken skin or mucous membranes. Sexual contact provides the avenue for the majority of cases. Data provided by the CDC indicate that in the United States there are more males than females with HIV or AIDS. The primary mode of transmission in males is male-to-male sexual contact. In females it is heterosexual contact. The other significant mode of transmission is sharing needles and syringes for drug injection. HIV can be transmitted to babies from their mothers before or during birth. In some cases, HIV has been shown to be transmitted to newborns through breast milk. Today all blood products for transfusion are tested and are an extremely rare source of the virus. Health care workers are at risk for exposure through needle sticks or contaminated blood and body fluids getting into an open cut or a mucous membrane such as the eyes or inside of the nose. Proper use of personal protective equipment such as gloves, gowns, and masks can greatly reduce exposure to pathogens. Activation of safety features on needles and other sharps, with proper disposal, will also protect health care workers (Safety Alert 11–1).

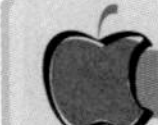

Health Promotion Points 11–2

Healthy People 2010 HIV

GOAL 13: HIV—PREVENT HIV INFECTION AND ITS RELATED ILLNESS AND DEATH

Objective 21.10: Confine annual incidence of diagnosed AIDS cases among adolescents and adults to no more than 12 per 100,000 population.

- Include questions regarding sexual activity and use of safer sex practices whenever obtaining a health history from all patients.
- Assess all patients for exposures to blood-borne or sexually transmitted diseases.
- Encourage knowledge of the patient's own, and his partner's, HIV status.
- Encourage people who are HIV positive to:
  - Avoid sharing toothbrushes, razors, or other items that could become contaminated with blood.
  - Not donate sperm, blood, plasma, or body organs or other body tissues.
  - Inform all contacted health care practitioners of their HIV status.
  - Clean blood or other body fluid spills on household or other surfaces with freshly diluted household bleach: 1 part bleach to 10 parts water.

Objective 21.11: Increase years of healthy life of an individual infected with HIV by extending the interval of time between an initial diagnosis of HIV infection and AIDS diagnosis and between AIDS diagnosis and death.

- Teach HIV-positive people who have no signs or symptoms of immunodeficiency to seek regular medical evaluation and follow-up.
- Encourage HIV-positive people to adhere to drug regimen, especially highly active antiretroviral therapy (HAART).
- Teach HIV-infected people to begin or maintain behaviors known to assist in maintaining or improving immune function.
- Encourage HIV-positive people to use safer sex practices.
- Encourage HIV-positive women to avoid pregnancy.

Pathophysiology

The disease is caused by infection with HIV, a retrovirus that integrates itself into the genetic material of the cell it infects, changing the DNA of the host cell. This causes the host cell to be unable to fulfill its normal functions in the immune system. The primary host cell for HIV is the CD4 lymphocyte, the "quarterback" of the immune system. HIV seriously impairs the ability of the cell-mediated immune response to work as effectively as it would normally. The disease presents many clinical problems and involves multiple systems (Figure 11–1).

The most recent revision of the CDC definitions of AIDS and HIV infection was done in 1993, and those definitions are still currently in use. The change in definitions added the use of CD4 T lymphocyte counts in the classification of HIV infection and modified the

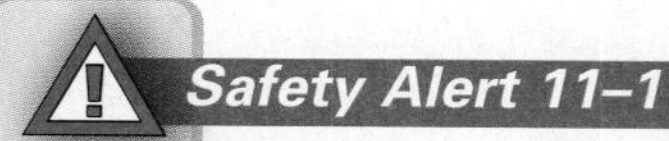

Disposal of Sharps

- Place all disposable sharp instruments, or "sharps," directly into a special biohazard container immediately after use.
- Never place your fingers down into a sharps container.
- Shake the container to settle the contents and make room for more if necessary.
- Replace sharps containers when they are three quarters full.
- Seal and send the full sharps container to be sterilized before its disposal or incineration.
- If a needle stick occurs, wash the area of puncture thoroughly with soap and water, report to charge nurse immediately afterward, complete an incident/occurrence report, and follow the agency-instituted protocol for treatment and follow-up.
- Develop a conscious awareness of where contaminated needles might be left or carried in the immediate environment by other health care workers to prevent needle stick injuries.

definition of AIDS to include HIV-infected persons with CD4 T lymphocyte count less than 200 cells/mm^3 (Table 11–1). **Suppression** of the immune response as a result of HIV infection is the cause of AIDS. Two types of HIV have been identified, HIV type 1 (HIV-1) and HIV type 2 (HIV-2). Within each type of HIV are groups and subtypes. HIV-1 is the most common cause of HIV infection in the United States, Europe, and Asia. HIV-2 is widespread in western Africa.

HIV-1 and HIV-2 are both **retroviruses.** Retroviruses differ from other viruses because of an enzyme called **reverse transcriptase,** which helps the virus reproduce in the host cell. HIV types 1 and 2 have only ribonucleic acid (RNA) as their genetic material. When they **replicate** (reproduce), their genetic material is placed in the deoxyribonucleic acid (DNA) of the host cell. The resulting new DNA continues the process of replication, and its RNA produces larger numbers of viral particles, as many as 50 million to 2 billion a day. These viral particles are released from the host cell into the circulatory system, where they infect other cells, such as macrophages and lymphoid tissue.

The T cells that have the protein CD4 on their surface are known as CD4 positive or CD4+ and as T helper cells. Normally CD4+ T cells activate B cells, natural killer cells, and phagocytes. These cells participate in both cellular and humoral immunity. The CD4 receptor site is where HIV attaches and begins the process of infecting the CD4 lymphocytes. When these cells are infected, they are either unable to function normally or are destroyed. This immune dysfunction makes the infected person more prone to **opportunistic infections (OIs),** organisms commonly found in the environment (discussed later in this chapter).

Signs and Symptoms

The time span from infection with HIV to the actual onset of AIDS is extremely variable among individuals. Some people infected with HIV have no symptoms for many years. As the immune system is less and less functional, symptoms appear of **sentinel infections** (infections that may indicate underlying immunosuppression), such as oral thrush, recurrent vaginal yeast infection, or a skin disorder. The initial signs and symptoms of AIDS are similar to flulike symptoms: fever, fatigue, diarrhea, and loss of appetite. In addition, some people also have skin rashes, night sweats, swollen lymph glands, and significant weight loss. Memory or movement problems may also be present. Some individuals do not have any symptoms to indicate onset of infection.

Diagnosis

Testing is available from a physician or local public health clinic, or by home test kit. Most home test kits do not provide results immediately at home, but allow the individual to buy the kit anonymously, collect a specimen in the privacy of his home, and receive results at home that are coded with a number and are anonymous. Self-test kits that offer results at home are on the market, but at this time, none is approved by the Food and Drug Administration (FDA). Testing is usually done on a blood specimen, but can also be done with oral fluids and in some cases with urine. Whether blood or another body fluid is tested, a second test is done on the same specimen to confirm that the results are correct. The follow-up test is done using a different test method than that used for the initial testing to confirm the findings. HIV tests search for antibodies to the virus; there is no test to detect the actual virus. After exposure to HIV, there may be a delay before antibodies appear in the blood. Therefore, a negative HIV test after initial exposure is not considered the final word until a second negative test is conducted 1 to 3 months later. The most common test used is the enzyme-linked immunosorbent assay (ELISA), which is a form of enzyme immunoassay. If the first test is positive, it is followed by the Western blot (Box 11–2).

The CDC is recommending that physicians offer HIV testing to individuals ages 13 to 64 as part of routine medical examinations. It is estimated that 25% of people who are HIV positive are unaware of their status. By not knowing their condition, they could be unintentionally infecting others.

Management of Early HIV Infection

When an individual tests positive for HIV and the diagnosis is confirmed by repeat testing, a comprehensive examination of health status is conducted. Particular attention is paid to eye and mouth condition, neurologic status, skin and lymph nodes, and any signs of OIs. A psychological assessment is added to help determine the patient's present and long-term needs. The

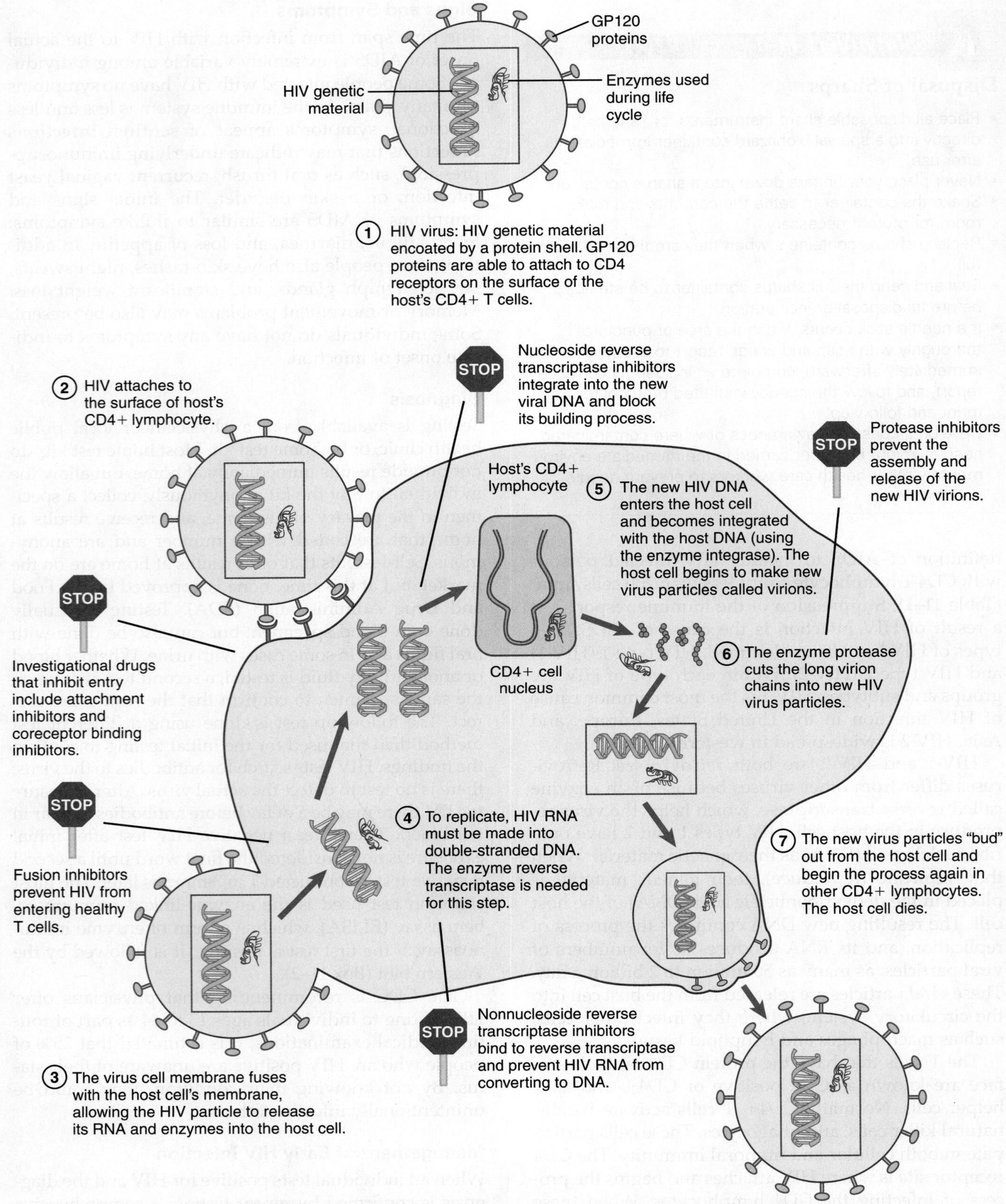

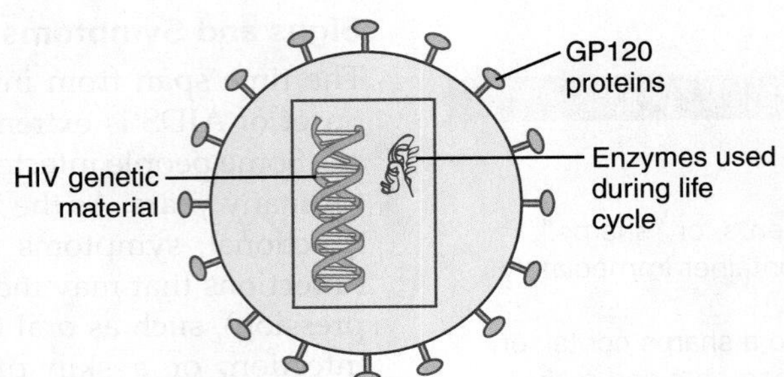

FIGURE 11–1 The steps in the life cycle of the HIV virus with correlation to medications.

Table 11–1 ***Classification System for HIV Infection***

CD4 T-CELL CATEGORIES	CLINICAL CATEGORIES (A) ASYMPTOMATIC, ACUTE (PRIMARY) HIV OR PERSISTENT GENERALIZED LYMPHADENOPATHY	(B) SYMPTOMATIC, NOT (A) OR (C) CONDITIONS	(C) AIDS-INDICATOR CONDITIONS
Category 1 >500/mm³	A1	B1	C1
Category 2 200–499/mm³	A2	B2	C2
Category 3 <200/mm³	A3	B3	C3

1993 CDC SURVEILLANCE CASE DEFINITION

CATEGORY A: ASYMPTOMATIC HIV

- Asymptomatic HIV infection
- Persistent generalized lymphadenopathy
- Acute HIV infection with accompanying illness or history or HIV infection

CATEGORY B: SYMPTOMATIC HIV

- Bacillary angiomatosis
- Candidiasis: oropharyngeal (thrush), vulvovaginal (>1 mo)
- Cervical dysplasia
- Fever >38° C or diarrhea >1 mo
- Hairy leukoplakia
- Herpes zoster involving at least two distinct episodes or more that one dermatome
- Idiopathic thrombocytopenic purpura
- Listeriosis
- Pelvic inflammatory disease
- Peripheral neuropathy

CATEGORY C: AIDS-DEFINING INFECTIONS

- Candidiasis of bronchi, trachea, or lungs
- Candidiasis, esophageal
- Cervical cancer, invasive
- Coccidioidomycosis, disseminated or extrapulmonary
- Cryptococcosis, extrapulmonary
- Cryptosporidiosis, chronic
- Cytomegalovirus disease or retinitis
- Encephalopathy, HIV related
- Herpes simplex virus
- Histoplasmosis, disseminated or extrapulmonary
- HIV-associated dementia
- Isosporiasis, chronic intestinal
- Kaposi sarcoma
- Lymphoid interstitial pneumonia
- Lymphoma, Burkitt's, immunoblastic, primary of brain
- *Mycobacterium avium-intracellulare* complex
- *Mycobacterium tuberculosis,* pulmonary or extrapulmonary
- Nocardiosis
- *Pneumocystis jiroveci* (formerly *carinii*) pneumonia
- Pneumonia, recurrent
- Progressive multifocal leukoencephalopathy
- *Salmonella* septicemia, recurrent
- Toxoplasmosis of internal organs
- Wasting syndrome due to HIV

From Centers for Disease Control and Prevention. (1992; revised 1993). Revised classification system for HIV infection and expanded surveillance case definition for AIDS among adolescents and adults. *MMRW Morbidity and Mortality Weekly Report,* 41(RR-17).

assessment includes a sexual history and a substance use history. A CD4 lymphocyte count is performed to establish the stage of HIV infection and to decide the timing of initiation of antiretroviral therapy and prophylaxis for OIs. Selecting optimal therapy is based not only on clinical data but also on individual factors, such as past health status, medication history, quality-of-life issues, and patient expectations of therapy. The World Health Organization (WHO) recommends the following criteria for starting treatment with antiretroviral therapy: WHO stage IV of HIV disease (clinical AIDS), regardless of the CD4 count; WHO stages I, II, or III of HIV disease, with a CD4 count below 200/mm³; or WHO stages II or III of HIV disease with total lymphocyte count below 1200/mm³ (Box 11–3).

Treatment

Various classes of antiretroviral drugs are specifically used to fight HIV infection and act directly on the virus itself. Great advances have been made in drug treatment of HIV-positive individuals. Because of the quantity of research being conducted, recommendations for drug therapies are adjusted as new combinations are proven more effective. To check the latest recommendations, see the National Institutes for Health website (www.aidsinfo.nih.gov/guidelines). Table 11–2 presents the most current list of antiretroviral medications.

Nonnucleoside reverse transcriptase inhibitors (NNRTIs) act by binding to and disabling reverse transcriptase, a protein that is needed for replication of HIV. Nucleoside reverse transcriptase inhibitors (NRTIs) are defective versions of building blocks needed by HIV to replicate. When NRTIs are used in place of the normal building block, reproduction of the virus is hindered. **Protease inhibitors** (PIs) work at the last stage of the viral reproduction cycle. They prevent HIV from being successfully assembled and released from the infected CD4 cell by disabling a protein needed for replication. Currently the most effective

Box 11–2 HIV Tests

ENZYME-LINKED IMMUNOSORBENT ASSAY (ELISA), A TYPE OF ENZYME IMMUNOASSAY (EIA)

Normal value: Negative

- HIV-antibody screening test (positives must be confirmed with a Western blot).
- Antibody assays do not detect HIV antibody in the earliest stages of the infection. (HIV antibody may be detected normally from 2 weeks to 6 months after the acute infection.)
- False-positive ELISA may be seen in the presence of maternal antibodies.

Sensitivity: 98%

WESTERN BLOT (WB)

Normal value: Negative

- HIV-antibody test used to confirm a positive ELISA.
- False-positive WB may be seen in the presence of maternal antibodies.

POLYMERASE CHAIN REACTION (PCR)

Normal value: Negative

- A qualitative measurement of cell-associated proviral DNA.

Sensitivity: 100%

IMMUNOFLUORESCENT ANTIBODY ASSAY (IFA)

Normal value: Negative

Sensitivity: 99.8%

CD4 CELL COUNT

Normal value: 500 to 1500 cells/mm^3

- Values below 200 cells/mm^3 prompt treatment.

treatment seems to be a combination of drugs. Highly active antiretroviral therapy (HAART) is a combination of available drugs and is recommended as HIV treatment. It has been shown that this therapy is also effective against some of the other conditions common to HIV/AIDS. New antiretroviral and protease inhibitor drugs are quickly becoming available, and different combinations are being evaluated for effectiveness. It is estimated that therapy may cost $16,000 or more per year, per patient. Many patients with chronic conditions are unable to afford the prescribed drug therapies. OIs are treated with drugs specific to their cause, and sometimes antimicrobials are given to prevent infection, all of which adds up to an ongoing expense to maintain the best possible health.

? *Think Critically About . . .* How would you go about helping an AIDS patient find a way to afford the medications needed to control the disease?

Complications

Opportunistic Infections. OIs are defined as diseases caused by microorganisms commonly present in the environment or the body that only cause disease when there is a weakening or suppression of the immune system. The major OIs are the herpes family viruses, hepatitis, cytomegalovirus (CMV), *Mycobacterium tuberculosis* (MTb), *Mycobacterium avium* complex (MAC), *Cryptococcus neoformans,* histoplasmosis (Histo), candidiasis, *Pneumocystis jiroveci* (formerly *Pneumocystis carinii*) pneumonia (PCP), toxoplasmosis (Toxo), and cryptosporidiasis (Crypto) (Table 11–3).

Box 11–3 World Health Organization Classification System for HIV Infection and Staging

CLINICAL STAGE I

- Asymptomatic infection
- Persistent generalized lymphadenopathy
- Acute retroviral infection

Performance scale 1: Asymptomatic, normal activity

CLINICAL STAGE II

- Unintentional weight loss <10% of body weight
- Minor mucocutaneous manifestations (e.g., dermatitis, prurigo, fungal nail infections, angular cheilitis)
- Herpes zoster within previous 5 years
- Recurrent upper respiratory tract infections

Performance scale 2: Symptoms, but nearly fully ambulatory

CLINICAL STAGE III

- Unintentional weight loss >10% body weight
- Chronic diarrhea >1 month
- Prolonged fever >1 month (constant or intermittent)
- Oral candidiasis
- Oral hairy leukoplakia
- Pulmonary tuberculosis within the previous year
- Severe bacterial infections
- Vulvovaginal candidiasis

Performance scale 3: In bed more than normal but <50% of normal daytime during the previous month

CLINICAL STAGE IV

- HIV wasting syndrome
- *Pneumocystis jiroveci* (formerly *carinii*) pneumonia
- Toxoplasmosis of the brain
- Cryptosporidiosis with diarrhea >1 month
- Isosporiasis with diarrhea >1 month
- Cryptococcosis, extrapulmonary
- Cytomegalovirus disease of an organ other than liver, spleen, or lymph node
- Herpes simplex virus infection, mucocutaneous
- Progressive multifocal leukoencephalopathy
- Any disseminated endemic mycosis (e.g., histoplasmosis)
- Candidiasis of the esophagus, trachea, bronchi, or lung
- Atypical mycobacteriosis, disseminated
- Non-typhoid *Salmonella* septicemia
- Extrapulmonary tuberculosis
- Lymphoma
- Kaposi sarcoma
- HIV encephalopathy

Performance scale 4: In bed >50% of normal daytime during previous month

Table 11–2 Medications Used for HIV/AIDS Therapy

TRADE NAME	GENERIC NAME	NURSING IMPLICATIONS AND SIDE EFFECTS
NUCLEOSIDE REVERSE TRANSCRIPTASE INHIBITORS (NRTIs)		
Combivir	Lamivudine/zidovudine	Assess for dizziness; monitor CBC, hepatic and renal function. May cause nausea and nasal congestion.
Emtriva	FTC, emtricitabine	Oral solution dosing is different from capsules and should be refrigerated. Tell patient to avoid fatty foods. Monitor for abdominal pain. Monitor vision, hearing, touch, and balance.
Epivir	Lamivudine, 3TC	Teach patient to avoid fatty foods. Assess vision, hearing, touch, balance, and for abdominal pain. May cause acute pancreatitis and peripheral neuropathy.
Epzicom	Abacavir/lamivudine	As above plus assess for fever, rash, headache, nausea, sore throat, fatigue, shortness of breath. If such flulike symptoms develop, drug must be stopped permanently.
Hivid	Zalcitabine, DDC (dideoxycytidine)	Monitor for signs of peripheral neuropathy; numbness, tingling. See individual drug information.
Retrovir	Zidovudine, AZT	Monitor CBC for neutropenia and anemia. Assess for dizziness.
Trizivir	Abacavir, lamivudine/zidovudine	See implications for drugs of the combination.
Truvada	Tenofovir disoproxil/emtricitabine	Monitor renal and liver function. Dosing is adjusted according to creatinine clearance. Give on an empty stomach. See implications for individual drugs.
Videx	Didanosine, DDI (dideoxyinosine)	Give on an empty stomach. Monitor vision, hearing, touch, and balance; monitor CBC.
Viread	Tenofovir disoproxil fumarate	May need 2 hr between taking other drugs. Monitor liver and renal function.
Zerit	Stavudine, d4T	Monitor vision, hearing, touch, and balance. Monitor for generalized pain.
Ziagen	Abacavir	Watch for allergic reactions. Monitor for flulike symptoms; stop drug if they appear.
NONNUCLEOSIDE REVERSE TRANSCRIPTASE INHIBITORS (NNRTIs)		
Rescriptor	Delavirdine, DLV	Monitor for rash or headache. Give 1 hr before or after antacids. May be taken without regard to food. Store at room temperature.
Sustiva	Efavirenz	Nervous system symptoms may occur. Monitor for headaches, dysphoria, dizziness, insomnia, and nightmares. Contraindicated in pregnancy.
Viramune	Nevirapine, BI-RG-587	Monitor for rash, headache, and abdominal pain. May potentiate anticoagulants. May cause liver toxicity.
PROTEASE INHIBITORS (PIs)		
Agenerase	Amprenavir	May cause hyperglycemia. High-fat food will decrease absorption. Tell patient not to take supplemental vitamin E.
Aptivus	Tipranavir	Take with food.
Crixivan	Indinavir, IDV, MK-639	Ensure adequate hydration. May cause kidney stones. Give on an empty stomach. Monitor for jaundice, flank or back pain and hematuria. May cause kidney stones.
Invirase	Saquinavir mesylate, SQV	Invirase must be given with ritonavir. Should be given with, or right after a high-calorie, fatty meal. Instruct patient to wear sunscreen as may cause photosensitivity.
Kaletra	Lopinavir/ritonavir	Administer with food. Do not give to patients with known sulfonamide allergy.
Lexiva	Fosamprenavir calcium	Monitor serum lipid levels.
Norvir	Ritonavir, ABT-538	Check medications that SHOULD NOT be given with Norvir. Give with a light meal. Monitor serum lipid levels.
Reyataz	Atazanavir sulfate	Give with food. Monitor bilirubin levels; monitor for jaundice as may cause hyperbilirubinemia.
Viracept	Nelfinavir mesylate, NFV	Give with a meal for full effect.
FUSION INHIBITORS		
Fuzeon	Enfuvirtide, T-20	Rotate Subcut injection sites from upper arm to inner thigh to abdomen. Local reaction at injection site is common. Dose must be reconstituted before injection. Monitor for skin reactions at injection site.

Table 11–3 Opportunistic Infections

CLASSIFICATION	SIGNS AND SYMPTOMS	DIAGNOSTIC TESTS	TREATMENT/MEDICATIONS	NURSING CONSIDERATIONS
VIRAL DISEASES				
Herpes viruses Herpes simplex 1 (HSV-1) Herpes simplex 2 (HSV-2)	Painful skin blisters preceded by itching and/or tingling for 24 hours HSV-1 and HSV-2 occur in oral, genital and perirectal areas; HSV-2 more common in genital and rectal areas	Viral culture if needed for diagnosis	Acyclovir (Zovirax), famciclovir (Famvir) 500 mg PO tid for 7-10 days *or* valacyclovir (Valtrex) 1 g PO q 8 hr for 7 days	Lesions near the eyes or complaints of change in vision, require immediate treatment Hospitalization for treatment with IV acyclovir is recommended Fluid from herpes vesicles is highly infectious
Herpes zoster (HZV, VZV, shingles)	Herpes zoster occurs along dermatomes of the body and is very painful		Sometimes cortisone is added for herpes zoster No known cure	Patients with herpes zoster may develop a post-herpetic neuralgia
Cytomegalovirus (CMV)	*Retinitis:* Blurry vision or loss of central vision that can lead to blindness	*Retinitis:* Ophthalmology examination	*Retinitis:* Ganciclovir implants + oral ganciclovir (1000 mg tid); IV ganciclovir (5 mg/kg q 12 hr for 14–21 days); IV foscarnet (Foscavir) (90 mg/kg q 12 hr for 14–21 days); *or* oral valganciclovir (900 mg bid for 21 days then 900 mg daily for 7 days) IV Cidofovir (Vistide) with oral probenecid for ganciclovir strains	CMV retinitis is the most common form of CMV in HIV+ individuals The incidence of CMV has decreased due to better therapies for HIV+ individuals CD4 counts are less likely to be low enough for the infection to take hold Cidofovir requires IV hydration before administration
	Esophagitis: Ulcerations; pain; difficulty in swallowing *Colitis:* Fever; diarrhea; stomach pain	*Esophagitis and colitis:* endoscopy and/or biopsy	*Esophagitis and colitis:* IV ganciclovir or IV foscarnet for 3–6 wk	
	Pneumonitis: Pneumonia-like symptoms	*Pneumonitis:* diagnose for other organisms first, such as bacteria, *Pneumocystis jiroveci;* if negative, then bronchoscopy with bronchoalveolar lavage and/or biopsy	*Pneumonitis:* IV ganciclovir or IV foscarnet for 3–6 wk	
	Encephalitis: Confusion; fever; tiredness	*Encephalitis:* brain MRI, spinal tap	*Encephalitis:* IV ganciclovir, IV foscarnet, or combination of both until clinical improvement	
Hepatitis Hepatitis B virus (HBV) Hepatitis C virus (HCV)	Fatigue; nausea; vomiting; arthralgias; fever; right upper quadrant pain; jaundice; dark urine; clay-colored stools	Alanine aminotransferase (ALT); albumin; bilirubin; prothrombin time; platelet count; complete blood count; HBeAg	The optimal treatment strategies for patients with HIV/HBV co-infection have not been defined It is recommended to treat HIV infection before tackling HCV infection	Boosting the immune system with HIV medications helps the body fight HCV more effectively. Most HIV medications can cause liver damage

Table 11–3 Opportunistic Infections—cont'd

CLASSIFICATION	SIGNS AND SYMPTOMS	DIAGNOSTIC TESTS	TREATMENT/MEDICATIONS	NURSING CONSIDERATIONS
BACTERIAL/MYCOBACTERIAL				
Mycobacterium tuberculosis (MTb)	High fever; night sweats; loss of appetite and weight loss; chronic productive cough sometimes with hemoptysis; shortness of breath occurs late in the disease	Chest x-ray; AFB sputum analysis	Isoniazid, rifampin, pyrazinamide, ethambutol Four antiTB drugs are given for the first 2 mo; then two drugs are administered for an additional 4 mo (if the organism is susceptible to standard medications)	Respiratory precautions for hospitalized patients include use of HEPA filtration and fit-tested masks for health care providers The health department is notified of each TB case and provides the required follow-up care
Mycobacterium avium complex (MAC)	Persistent fever; night sweats; fatigue; weight loss; anemia; abdominal pain; dizziness; diarrhea; weakness	Culture from blood, bone marrow, or cerebrospinal fluid	Azithromycin (500–600 mg daily); *or* clarithromycin (500 mg bid) + ethambutol (15 mg/kg/day) + rifabutin (300 mg daily).	In HIV+ individuals treatment should be continued for life
FUNGAL DISEASES				
Cryptococcal meningitis	Fever, headaches, malaise worsening over several weeks; confusion, personality or behavior changes; blindness; deafness	Cryptococcal antigen (CrAg) of peripheral blood (which usually is positive); blood cultures, including acid-fast bacilli (AFB); fungal cultures; CT head scan; spinal tap	IV amphotericin B (0.7 mg/kg/day) + PO flucytosine (25 mg/kg) q 6 hr	Hydrocephalus can be a complication Maintenance therapy should be continued until CD4 cells can be maintained at ≥100 cells/μL
Histoplasmosis	Fever; fatigue; weight loss; difficulty in breathing; swollen lymph nodes; pneumonia-like symptoms	Test for *Histoplasma* antigen in urine and blood, bone marrow, or blood culture; biopsy of lesion (skin, mouth, lymph node)	Amphotericin B (0.7–1.0 mg/kg/day for 3–14 days) *or* the lipid formulations of amphotericin B (3 mg/kg/day for 3–14 days)	Ongoing maintenance therapy is needed Prophylactic treatment is recommended in regions with high instances of histoplasmosis infections
Candidiasis (thrush, vaginal yeast infection)	White patches on gums, tongue, lining of mouth; pain; difficulty in swallowing; loss of appetite Cheesy consistency white vaginal discharge; itching	Visual examination; smear; culture	Mild forms can be treated with topical nystatin Moderate cases are treated with fluconazole, itraconazole, or ketoconazole	Thrush can make eating and swallowing difficult Have patient avoid acidic, spicy, or hot foods as well as cigarettes, alcohol, and carbonated drinks as they may irritate mouth tissues Soft, cool, and bland foods (e.g., oatmeal, mashed beans, apple sauce) are recommended Medicated cream or ointment can be used on the vulva to decrease itching during vaginal treatment

Continued

Table 11–3 ***Opportunistic Infections—cont'd***

CLASSIFICATION	SIGNS AND SYMPTOMS	DIAGNOSTIC TESTS	TREATMENT/MEDICATIONS	NURSING CONSIDERATIONS
FUNGAL DISEASES—cont'd				
Pneumocystis jiroveci (formerly *carinii*) pneumonia (PCP)	Shortness of breath; dyspnea on exertion; fever; dry, nonproductive cough	Chest x-ray; bronchoscopy; sputum culture; pulmonary function tests	Trimethoprim-sulfamethoxazole (Bactrim, Septra, Co-trimoxazole) (TMP/SMX) (two double-strength tablets q 8 hr; *or* IV TMP 5 mg/kg and SMX 25 mg/kg q 8 hr	Sulfamethoxazole is a sulfa drug and almost half of the people who take it have an allergic reaction. PCP can be prevented; it is recommended that anyone whose CD4 cell count is >200 should be on PCP prophylaxis
PARASITIC DISEASES				
Toxoplasmosis	Altered mental state (confusion, delusional behavior), severe headaches, fever, seizures and coma Can also affect the eye causing eye pain and reduced vision.	MRI brain lesions, antibody titer, tissue culture, CSF culture	Pyrimethamine (200 mg loading dose, then 50–75 mg daily) + leucovorin (10–20 mg daily) + sulfadiazine (1 g q 6 hr); *or* clindamycin (600 mg q 6 hr)	Medications given to treat Toxo can interfere with vitamin B and cause anemia Folic acid is usually given with treatment Individuals with CD4 counts >100 should be on prophylactic medications
Cryptosporidiosis	Chronic diarrhea with frequent watery stools; stomach cramps; nausea; fatigue; weight loss; appetite loss; vomiting; dehydration and electrolyte imbalance (especially sodium and potassium)	Detection of eggs (called oocysts) in the stool or biopsy of small intestines	There is no proven treatment	For persons with AIDS, antiretroviral therapy that improves immune status will also decrease or eliminate symptoms of Crypto infection Crypto is usually not cured and may come back if the immune status worsens

MTb may present as a pulmonary infection, but in approximately 50% of people infected with HIV, MTb is found in sites other than the lungs. Locations outside the respiratory tract, such as bone, skin, liver, central nervous system (CNS), spleen, and the gastrointestinal tract (GI) can all be infected by MTb.

Viral Infections. The herpes family of viruses consists of many well-known members. Herpes simplex types 1 and 2, herpes zoster (shingles), CMV, Epstein-Barr virus (EBV), and varicella (chickenpox) all can be a problem to patients with AIDS.

In HIV-infected individuals, herpes usually presents as outbreaks in the oral, genital, and perirectal areas. Patients experience a **prodrome** (early symptoms) of itching and tingling 24 to 48 hours prior to the actual outbreak of vesicles at the site of infection. As with any of the herpesviruses, the clear liquid from the vesicles is highly infectious and the lesions are very painful. The pain decreases as the lesions get to the crusting stage. Chronic ulcerative lesions may form after the vesicles rupture. Symptoms of fever, pain, bleeding, lymph node enlargement, headache, myalgia, and malaise may occur if the infection becomes systemic.

The clear liquid from herpes lesions is highly infectious, and great care must be taken not to infect other areas of the body. Because herpes zoster appears at times of immune suppression, further outbreaks may occur in times of increased stress. If the eruptions occur on the face, they may involve the eye. A herpes eye infection should be promptly treated as it can cause scarring on the cornea and affect vision.

Herpes Simplex Virus Type 1 and Type 2. Herpes simplex virus type 1 and type 2 (HSV-1 and HSV-2, respectively) may be transmitted sexually. HSV-1 usually occurs in the nose, mouth, pharynx, and esophagus. HSV-2 generally appears in the genital, perineal, and perirectal areas. Because of cross-infection, HSV-2 may be cultured from the usual HSV-1 sites and vice versa.

Herpes Zoster. Varicella-zoster virus, a member of the herpes family, causes shingles and chickenpox.

Once thought to be separate disorders, the organism was given two names. Currently, the primary infection that causes chickenpox is called varicella and the reactivation of the virus that causes shingles is called herpes zoster. After infection with chickenpox, the virus becomes dormant in the base of nerve pathways, and when immune suppression become severe enough, it reactivates. Sometimes called zoster and sometimes shingles, the virus manifests itself with a prodrome of itching or tingling, usually 24 to 48 hours prior to the appearance of vesicles. The vesicles usually appear along a **dermatome** (nerve tract). Varicella pneumonia and varicella encephalitis also have been reported. The vesicles fill with a clear liquid that is highly infectious. As they rupture, they shed virus that can infect the individual in other areas of the body. It is especially important to caution the patient regarding transmission of the varicella virus to the eyes, nose, or oral cavity. Cross-infection can be prevented by using good hand hygiene practices (Safety Alert 11–2).

Recurrent herpes zoster virus (HZV) infections may occur because of immune suppression. **It is usually at times of increased stress that the outbreaks occur.** Reactivation of the infection in HIV-infected individuals may signal the onset of other OIs and may lead to widespread disease in skin and abdominal organs.

Complications of HZV infection include scarring and postherpetic neuralgia that presents as prolonged pain at the site of the outbreak. Shingles eruptions that occur on the face usually involve the seventh cranial nerve and may involve the eye. The symptoms of shingles are itching and tingling along the affected nerve accompanied by burning and shooting pain, headache, and low-grade fever. If vesicles are present, the virus shed in the draining fluid can cause chickenpox in susceptible individuals. HZV infections of the eye need to be promptly diagnosed and treated. The infection can cause scarring on the cornea and affect vision.

The drug of choice is acyclovir (Zovirax). The initial treatment is with oral dosing. Severe infections may be treated with intravenous acyclovir. Acyclovir-resistant strains of the virus have been isolated, and the treatment for them is usually with foscarnet (Foscavir). It should be noted that foscarnet is only given intravenously and is nephrotoxic; therefore, monitoring of the patient's creatinine and blood urea nitrogen is necessary. Foscarnet is very irritating to the peripheral veins and therefore is given via a central venous access catheter or diluted as recommended by the manufacturer. Because of its nephrotoxicity, it requires preinfusion hydration with normal saline. Some patients require postinfusion hydration as well.

Cytomegalovirus. Cytomegalovirus, another member of the herpesvirus family, is commonly found in all geographic areas. The virus is carried by people and transmitted by close contact between people. It is not associated with food, water, or animals. CMV is spread by contact with body fluids and is most commonly spread in situations in which person-to-person contact is common. In households and child care centers, CMV is spread through hand-to-mouth contact with infected body fluids. CMV is also transmitted sexually and by intimate contact. Blood transfusions, organ transplants, and breast-feeding are also mechanisms of transmission. CMV can also be passed from an infected pregnant woman to her baby in utero or during the birth process. CMV is commonly found in the urinary and respiratory tracts.

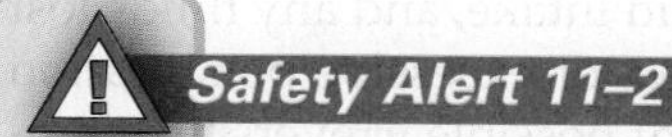

Chickenpox Transmission

The herpes zoster virus that causes shingles is highly infectious. Any nurse who has not had chickenpox, or been successfully immunized against chickenpox, should not be assigned to care for a patient with herpes zoster. Pregnant nurses should not care for any patient with herpes lesions as the virus may damage the fetus.

Cytomegalovirus may infect the retina, lung, GI tract, liver, CNS, or circulatory system. Pulmonary infections produce shortness of breath, dyspnea on exertion, and nonproductive cough. The two most common sites of infection are the retina (may cause blindness) and the GI tract (causing abdominal cramps, diarrhea, weight loss, and anorexia). These symptoms are severe and long lasting. CMV infection in the GI tract is more easily treated than infection in the eye, and may afford long periods of remission. Treatment for CMV in the eye is more complicated. If treatment for CMV retinitis is not continuous, there is a possibility that vision will be lost. The first sign in the eye is loss of peripheral vision. CNS symptoms may cause memory loss, muscle weakness, paralysis, lethargy, headache, numbness in the extremities, and personality changes. Ganciclovir is indicated in the treatment of CMV retinitis. Valganciclovir (Valcyte), an oral treatment for AIDS-related CMV retinitis, has been shown to provide more ganciclovir available for use in the bloodstream than any other preparation. It is also used in post–organ transplantation patients as a treatment for CMV. Ganciclovir can also be delivered via an intravitreal implant, which is placed by a surgeon in the posterior segment of the eye and delivers the drug directly to the site of infection. There are ganciclovir-resistant strains of the virus, and the treatment for them is usually with foscarnet.

Another drug used for treatment of CMV retinitis is cidofovir (Vistide). Its renal side effects are similar to those of foscarnet. It also is given only intravenously. To minimize the potential for nephrotoxicity, probenecid and intravenous hydration with normal saline should be administered with each infused dose of cidofovir. Patient instructions must include recommendations to increase oral fluid intake, and any fluids lost through vomiting, diarrhea, or excessive perspiration must be replaced to prevent possible irreversible damage to the kidneys.

Think Critically About . . . If you saw a lesion on the thigh of a female patient and were not certain if it was a herpes lesion, what would you do?

Hepatitis. Infection with hepatitis C is common in HIV-positive individuals. The co-infection makes each disease more difficult to treat. Many of the medications used for treatment of HIV have the potential to damage the liver. Careful monitoring and drug dosing must be used in managing the care of these patients. See Chapter 30 for information on hepatitis.

Bacterial Infections

Mycobacterium *Tuberculosis.* MTb may present as a pulmonary infection, but in approximately 50% of people infected with HIV, MTb is found in sites other than the lungs. Locations outside the respiratory tract, such as bone, skin, liver, CNS, spleen, and GI tract, can all be infected by MTb.

Symptoms of pulmonary tuberculosis (TB) include dyspnea, cough, fever, chest pains, weight loss, night sweats, and anorexia. Symptoms of systemic infection are fever, chills, weight loss, night sweats, and anorexia. *Extrapulmonary* (outside of the lung) infection symptoms are site related.

Treatment of MTb includes the use of rifampin (RIF), isoniazid (INH), pyrazinamide (PZA), and ethambutol (EMB) or streptomycin (SM). The recommended dosing regimens require continual medication administration for 6 to 12 months.

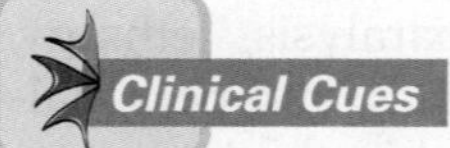

The National Guideline Clearinghouse, a branch of the Department of Health and Human Services, recommends directly observed therapy for MTb. This means that health care staff should observe the consumption of medications. This is to ensure compliance since therapy must continue for many months.

MTb is transmitted via airborne particles. If a patient with active TB is hospitalized, TB respiratory isolation should be implemented, which includes use of HEPA (high-efficiency particulate arresting) filtration for room air and use of fitted respirator masks for health care personnel.

Mycobacterium avium *Complex.* MAC infections are caused by *M. avium* and *M. intracellulare.* The sites generally infected by these bacteria are the respiratory system and GI tract. However, they may infect the bone marrow and thus the circulatory system as well. Symptoms may include fevers, night sweats, weight loss, lymphadenopathy, malaise, and organ disease. MAC becomes a threat when the immune system is seriously depleted, for example, when the CD4 count is extremely low. At this point, many primary care providers will initiate prophylaxis for MAC and/or serial blood cultures to identify acid-fast bacilli in the blood. A bone marrow examination also may be performed if MAC is suspected and anemias of unknown etiology are present.

Fungal Infections

Cryptococcosis. Cryptococcosis often presents as meningitis and is the fourth most common OI in HIV-infected individuals. The causative agent is *Cryptococcus neoformans.* In HIV-infected individuals with a low CD4 count, generally about 100 cells/mm^3, cryptococcosis may manifest as a fungal meningitis or **disseminated** (widespread) disease. Usual sites of infection are the CNS and circulatory system. It also may appear in the lung, heart, GI tract, bone, prostate, lymphatic system, and skin. Symptoms are any or all of the following: fever, headache, visual changes, nausea, vomiting, nuchal rigidity, confusion, and altered mental status. Neurologic changes and seizures may also occur. This fungus is found in pigeon droppings and in the soil. The usual entry point is the lungs, where it causes an asymptomatic infection. Because of severe immune suppression, the cell-mediated immune response does not destroy the fungi. The infection reactivates in immunosuppressed individuals because the T lymphocytes and macrophages cannot destroy the organism.

Treatment is generally with intravenous (IV) amphotericin B, an antifungal drug. This drug can cause renal toxicity, which is generally reversible if the drug is stopped. Common side effects with amphotericin B include fever and shakes *(rigors).* To prevent these, the primary care provider may premedicate the patient prior to the infusion with antipyretics, antiemetics, or antihistamines. Meperidine (Demerol) may be given to prevent rigors. Initially the patient receives treatment daily. Treatments may be reduced to 3 to 5 days a week to decrease the incidence of renal toxicity. The medication is best given via a central venous access device, as phlebitis may occur if the medication is given via a peripheral vein.

Fluconazole (Diflucan) is used for long-term management. Fluconazole is an antifungal that may be given orally or IV. In the oral form it does not cause the renal toxicity and depletion of potassium magnesium, and phosphate that occur commonly with amphotericin B.

Histoplasmosis. The causative agent for histoplasmosis (Histo) is *Histoplasma capsulatum.* This infection is generally related to the environment or region of the country where the patient has lived. The northeastern region of the United States and along the Canadian border is called the "Histo belt" because of the higher incidence of histoplasmosis found there. Generally histoplasmosis presents as a pulmonary infection, but may become disseminated. Symptoms may include dyspnea, weight loss, fever, and cough. The affected sites of disseminated disease are commonly the liver, spleen, and other lymphoid tissue. This infection can also involve the skin.

Candidiasis. *Candida albicans* can affect the skin, mucous membranes in the mouth, vagina, GI, or urinary tract. In HIV-infected individuals, oral infections usually present as white patches on the surface of the tongue and buccal mucosa. When involving the pharynx, esophagus, and hard palate, symptoms of sore throat and altered taste sensation are present. This condition is commonly referred to as *thrush.* Esophageal candidiasis can be characterized by difficulty or pain when swallowing. Nystatin (Mycostatin) swish and swallow is the treatment for oral and esophageal thrush. Repeated outbreaks of vaginal candidiasis (yeast infection) may be the initial presenting symptom of HIV infection in women. Fluconazole (Diflucan) orally or vaginally is the most common treatment.

Pneumocystis jiroveci *(Formerly* carinii*).* *Pneumocystis carinii* pneumonia (PCP) is also called pneumocystosis. The causative agent was originally thought to be a protozoan *(Pneumocystis carinii),* but more current research has resulted in its reclassification as a fungus *(Pneumocystis jiroveci).* The organism is present in the environment and is introduced into most individuals during childhood by inhalation. When the CD4 count is 200 cells/mm^3 or less, *P. jiroveci* is deactivated. The presenting symptoms may be a dry, nonproductive cough, fever and night sweats, malaise, shortness of breath, dyspnea on exertion, and weight loss. This infection may become disseminated, and the symptoms will be site related. It may infect the kidneys, eyes, liver, spleen, and lymph nodes.

There are now multiple effective treatment regimens for pneumocystosis as well as mechanisms to prevent the inactive infection from becoming active. Trimethoprim-sulfamethoxazole (Bactrim, Septra) is recommended for first-line therapy. For prevention, dapsone is used alone, but for treatment of active PCP, dapsone is used together with trimethoprim.

PCP also is seen in patients who have received chemotherapy for cancer as well those who have had organ transplants and have been therapeutically immune suppressed to prevent organ rejection.

Parasitic Infections

Toxoplasmosis. Toxoplasmosis (Toxo) is caused by a *protozoan* (a unicellular organism) called *Toxoplasma gondii.* The organism is found everywhere around the world. It is present in raw meats. Cats become infected by eating raw meats, and they excrete the organism in their feces. In the feces, the oocysts (Toxo eggs) become spores within 24 hours. The spores remain in the environment for about a year. In the individual with a normal immune system, an infection can cause flulike symptoms or may cause a severe inflammatory response, and if the Toxo survives, cysts are formed (Health Promotion Points 11–3). If that person then becomes immunosuppressed, the cysts break down and infect the patient's body. Most commonly toxoplasmosis infects the CNS, although it may also infect the lungs, heart, peritoneum, GI tract (especially the colon), and skin.

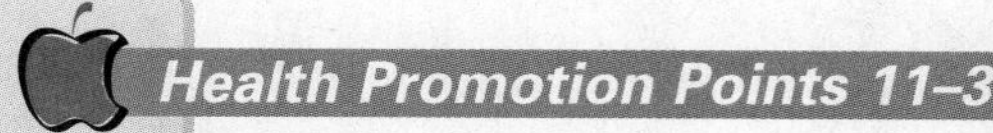

Health Promotion Points 11–3

Preventing Toxoplamosis

Toxoplasma gondii, the organism that causes toxoplasmosis, is found in poorly cooked meats, particularly pork, venison, and mutton. It is also found in cat feces. Immunosuppressed or pregnant individuals should not empty cat litter boxes or eat undercooked meat. Children's sand boxes and dirt play areas are frequently used by outdoor cats as litter boxes. Gardeners routinely come in contact with soil that could be contaminated. *Toxoplasma* is transmitted by the individual swallowing the organism. Good hand hygiene after contact with contaminated items can help prevent the spread of the organism.

The clinical manifestations may be nonspecific and include fever, headache, nausea and vomiting, and malaise. Usually CNS symptoms predominate, such as focal neurologic symptoms or seizures, fever, and headache. Altered mental status, confusion, lethargy, cognitive impairment, and coma may also be CNS symptoms of toxoplasmosis. Treatment includes pyrimethamine, folinic acid, and sulfadiazine for as long as 6 weeks. Lifelong suppressive therapy consists of the same medications in doses different from treatment of the acute disease.

Cryptosporidiosis. Cryptosporidiosis is caused by a microscopic parasite, *Cryptosporidium parvum,* and is commonly known as "Crypto." *Cryptosporidium,* an intestinal protozoan, presents in HIV-infected individuals with severe, large-volume, foul-smelling, watery diarrhea. The diarrhea is self-limiting in some cases to anywhere from 4 to 20 days. It can cause severe abdominal cramping, malaise, and electrolyte imbalance, especially of sodium, potassium, and chloride from the loss of large volumes of intestinal fluids. It may cause weight loss, dehydration, malnutrition, skin breakdown, and debilitation. It may cause the individual to withdraw socially because of the fear of foul-smelling, involuntary bowel movements, the inconvenience of frequent trips to the restroom, an emotional reaction to the change in body image, and worry about what friends may think.

The best treatment is prevention. Crypto is easily spread by contaminated food or water, or direct contact with an infected person or animal. People with healthy immune systems can be infected, but the symptoms are usually self-limiting. Individuals with AIDS can be severely ill with Crypto. There are no

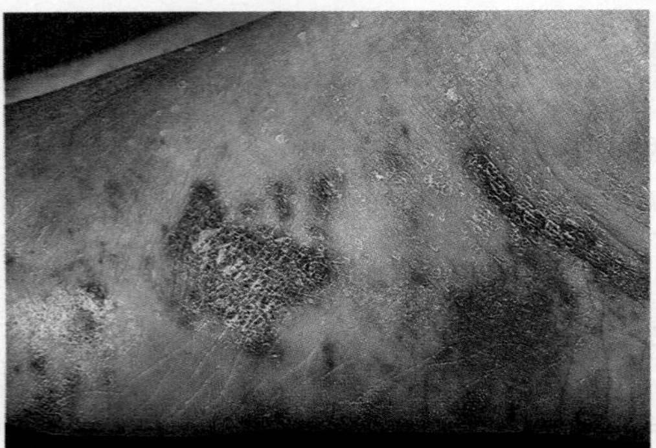

FIGURE 11–2 Kaposi sarcoma.

pharmacologic therapies that will eliminate the parasite. Most therapies are aimed at symptom control and replacement of lost fluid and electrolytes.

Neoplasms

Kaposi Sarcoma. Kaposi sarcoma (KS) is still the most commonly seen neoplasm in HIV-infected men, even though statistically the numbers have decreased. Cervical cancer is the most common cancer among women who have sexually transmitted HIV. In a study reported in 2004, the most common malignancies in men were KS, non-Hodgkin's lymphoma (NHL), and lung cancer. In women, cervical cancer, NHL, and lung cancer were most common (Nutankalva, McNeil, Reddy, 2004).

KS appears as discolored areas on the skin, but can also form on internal organs (Figure 11–2). The skin discoloration may range from pink to red or purple. The lesions tend to darken over time. In people with olive or black skin, the lesions may appear dark brown or black. The discoloration is caused by the formation of many tiny blood vessels under the skin. Current research is indicating that KS may be initiated by a herpesvirus called human herpesvirus 8. Although KS does not usually cause death, it is a contributor to illness in the HIV-infected individual.

Highly active antiretroviral therapy (HAART) has been shown to be the best treatment for active KS. In some individuals, HAART can halt the progression of skin lesions and even eliminate them. In addition to drug therapy, skin lesions can be treated with liquid nitrogen, surgically removed, or injected with anticancer drugs. Radiation therapy is probably the most commonly used local therapy. Low-dose radiation is used for small skin lesions. Larger doses are required for internal organs and lymph node involvement. Radiation treatment has been effective in reducing the size of tumors near lymph nodes, thus allowing release of lymph that was trapped by the pressure on the node, resulting in a decrease in distal lymphedema.

If KS has spread into internal organs and HAART treatment is not enough, doxorubicin (Doxil), daunorubicin (DaunoXome), or paclitaxel (Taxol) may be added to the treatment regimen.

Lymphomas. Lymphomas are tumors of the immune system, specifically the tissues and cells of the lymphatic system. There are many types of lymphomas. NHL is the most commonly seen in people with HIV or AIDS. NHL may occur after the occurrence of other OIs, or it may be the primary symptom in unsuspecting individuals who believe that they are at low risk for HIV infection. The exact cause is unknown, but there is a high correlation of people with HIV/AIDS and development of NHL. This condition is discussed in more detail later in the chapter.

Neurologic Complications. AIDS dementia and HIV encephalopathy result from HIV infection and may occur at any point in the HIV disease process. In some individuals it may be the presenting symptom. The etiology of the neurologic signs and symptoms displayed is uncertain. They are thought to arise from HIV itself or could be a result of infections, tumors, or drug-related complications. The presenting symptoms have a very subtle beginning and are difficult to differentiate from depression, Parkinson's disease, and Alzheimer's disease.

Treatment with HAART appears to be the most effective intervention by targeting the primary cause of the problem. Nursing interventions focus on preventing the individual from doing harm to himself or others. Safety issues become paramount, and referral to a home care agency for skilled nursing assessment of the patient, of the home environment for safety, and of home maintenance status is needed. The nurse should assess the individual's ability to perform personal care, activities of daily living (ADLs), food preparation, and ability to remember to eat and to take medications. Referral to community-based AIDS organizations is appropriate with the patient's or responsible party's consent.

NURSING MANAGEMENT

Assessment (Data Collection)

Assessment in the adult with HIV infection, including symptomatic AIDS, is very important. It is during the assessment that a determination of the patient's physical, mental, and psychosocial status is made. This basic data collection step becomes the basis for the plan of care for the each patient, appropriate to his condition. A complete head-to-toe physical assessment should be performed, and any deviations from normal findings should be documented and considered significant (Focused Assessment 11–1). The assessment should include an evaluation of signs and symptoms, physical status, functional level (ability to perform ADLs), self-care abilities, support systems, financial status, and living environment. The assessment of the functional level of the patient must be an ongoing assessment.

History and Physical Assessment

The history should include a general assessment of the patient's past and present status to help determine specific teaching needs as well as any risk behaviors the patient may practice. Obtain a sexual history to

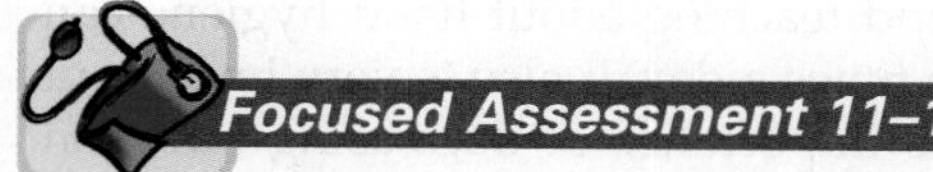

Data Collection for the HIV-Positive Patient

First gather a general health history, then:

- Determine level of consciousness, orientation to time and place, cognition, and concentration ability.
- Assess for visual changes.
- Obtain height, weight; note any weight loss from usual weight.
- Determine if there has been a change in eating pattern.
- Evaluate ability to swallow.
- Determine presence of nausea, vomiting, or diarrhea. If diarrhea is present, note the volume and quality.
- Assess for dehydration and electrolyte imbalances (see Chapter 3).
- Obtain vital signs. Assess for orthostatic hypotension and fever.
- Auscultate the heart.
- Assess for peripheral and periorbital edema and lymphedema.
- Assess condition of skin and mucous membranes.
- Assess neurologic function, cognition, and neurovascular status.
- Assess quality of respirations; auscultate breath sounds.
- Determine character of the cough and sputum if cough is present.
- Identify any psychosocial issues that may complicate or enhance care.

ascertain the risk of transmission and possible exposure to other sexually transmitted diseases. Current medications and treatments should also be included, as well as whether the patient is on any experimental or complementary therapies. If the patient was previously diagnosed as HIV positive, ascertain if any OIs have been acquired. Also ask if any of the community-based AIDS service organizations have been accessed. If not, referral should be made prior to discharge. The nutritional history is very important. Obtain current weight, not stated weight. Compare the patient's past and present weight for any recent weight loss or gain. Present nutritional status should be compared to the patient's past pattern to note any changes in eating habits that exist. Ask if the patient is experiencing nausea, vomiting, or diarrhea. These states not only can affect the patient's ability to take in sufficient calories, nutrients, and fluids, but also may lead to problems with electrolyte balance. If the patient is experiencing diarrhea, the volume and quality should be noted. Assess for signs of dehydration such as leg cramps and potassium depletion, which can cause cardiac arrhythmias. If the patient is vomiting, hyponatremia may occur and make the hypokalemia worse. Assess for pale mucous membranes and dry flaky skin. Wasting syndrome in HIV disease causes a loss of lean muscle mass and subcutaneous adipose tissue, so skin turgor is not a good sign of dehydration in this population.

Obtain vital signs. Especially significant are pulse and blood pressure. Observe for signs of hypotension and orthostatic hypotension. Also assess for signs of peripheral and periorbital edema and lower extremity **lymphedema** (abnormal collection of lymph fluid). In advanced HIV disease, observe the patient for **anasarca** (generalized massive edema) resulting from severe depletion of albumin caused by inadequate nutritional intake.

Assess cognition, concentration abilities, level of consciousness and orientation to place and time. Assess for mood changes, irritability, and depression. Situational depression related to the HIV/AIDS diagnosis may be noted. However, it may be an appropriate response, considering the HIV seropositive status. Clinical depression and other behavioral changes also may be noted. The patient may experience changes in motor and sensory function, such as gait changes, imbalance, and changes in vision, particularly in peripheral visual fields. The neurologic history is the initial time to question the patient about any pain or numbness in the extremities, any changes in ability to walk, or any balance problems. It is important to obtain baseline information since HIV/AIDS can cause neurologic changes during the disease process.

Ask about the patient's history of respiratory illnesses that may put him at risk for current problems, such as pneumonia, chronic obstructive pulmonary disease, or asthma. Observe for any abnormal breath sounds. Cough is a very important symptom to assess in HIV disease. Question whether the patient smokes, how much, and for how long. If the patient is experiencing a cough, is it dry and nonproductive or moist and productive? Is the patient experiencing any drenching night sweats? Any shortness of breath or dyspnea on exertion? These questions may indicate the possibility of pulmonary tuberculosis or pneumonia.

Psychosocial History. HIV infection causes stress in HIV-infected healthy persons and in those with clinical disease. It generates a unique series of stresses for the infected person, sexual partners, family members, and health care professionals. By collecting data during psychosocial assessment, the nurse is better able to anticipate the needs and vulnerabilities of the patient and is in a better position to plan and implement interventions.

This assessment should include a substance use history and a history of interpersonal relationships, educational level, and career information. Look at the past coping skills to see what coping techniques may be useful in the present situation. Learn about the social support system. Has the patient experienced multiple losses of friends? What is the living situation? Does someone live with the patient? Is there any community organization membership? Church, mosque, or synagogue attendance? Identify the patient's social set. Is there support available within that community? The answers to these questions will provide information to enable development of a functional plan of interventions and referrals.

> ***Think Critically About . . .*** A diagnosis of HIV affects a person's self-concept. How could you help a patient to voice his feelings about the diagnosis and to cope with it?

Nursing Diagnosis

Table 11–4 identifies common nursing diagnoses, expected outcomes, and interventions used for patients with AIDS. As with any other disease process, the patient with HIV/AIDS can have nursing diagnoses formulated specifically for any of his problems. However, some of the North American Nursing Diagnosis Association (NANDA) nursing diagnoses occur in this population frequently. These diagnoses may be associated with systemic, psychosocial, or specific body system responses to HIV. Specific nursing diagnoses are chosen for the particular problems the patient is having. That often depends on the stage of the patient's disease.

Planning

Planning is a very important part of the nursing process. To develop a plan that will work, collaboration with other members of the health care team is essential. The health care team includes the patient, other nurses, physicians, the dietitian, the pharmacist, the discharge planner and the primary caregiver at home. Additional health care providers may be involved for specific needs. If the patient is to adhere to the plan, he must have ownership of it, and the way to get the patient to own the plan is to give him every chance to make the decisions that will affect the outcome of his nursing care. The patient also must believe that the plan will be evaluated and reassessed along the way, so changes can be made when necessary. The nurse should supply information, education, and support, as well as assist the patient to decide on goals and expected outcomes for the plan of care. The major nursing goals are listed in Box 11–4 and are considered along with the individual patient problems. When these steps are included in the planning stage, the implementation of the plan will be much easier. Expected outcomes are written individually for each nursing diagnosis chosen for the care plan.

Implementation

Standard Precautions must be consistently used when caring for all patients (Chapter 6). For prevention of secondary infections, hand hygiene is very important not only in the inpatient setting for health care providers, but at home for the patient and family (Assignment Considerations 11–1). An important strategy in implementing the plan of care is making the most of the teaching opportunities that present themselves. Role modeling and teaching about hand hygiene can happen multiple times a day. It also is very important to emphasize the importance of decreasing infection risk in the home setting during meal preparation. Not only should hands be routinely washed, but also cutting surfaces, knives, and food preparation areas where raw poultry, meat, and seafood were touching. Raw fruits and vegetables should be rinsed thoroughly before consuming (Patient Teaching 11–1). For the patient at home, there are suggestions for infection control in Patient Teaching 11–2.

Wasting syndrome is a physiologic problem associated with HIV infection. The more knowledgeable the patient and caregiver are about methods to maintain adequate nutritional status, the less of a problem will be the effects of wasting (Nutritional Therapies 11–1). Referral to a nutritionist or dietitian is helpful. Do not delay in providing information while waiting for the "experts." Instruct the patient in the basis of a nutritious balanced diet using the USDA MyPyramid as a guide. Provide written materials for future reference at home. *Anorexia* (loss of appetite) is a common problem that leads to wasting. Suggest to the primary meal server that the patient be served six small meals a day and be offered food supplements between meals.

Instruct the patient in the appropriate method of medication administration. By taking antibiotic and antiretroviral medications consistently as ordered, less resistance to the drugs occurs, and the effectiveness of the drugs is prolonged. Make sure the patient understands when to take medications in relation to meals.

Encourage social interaction and independence in activities as tolerated and refer to support groups to boost the patient's self-esteem and feelings of self-worth. This may reduce the effects of situational depression and empower the patient. Consistency in promoting a positive attitude also will reduce the powerlessness the patient might experience.

Evaluation

The evaluation of nursing actions is performed to determine whether the expected outcomes have been met. Data indicating that the outcomes have been met must be collected and analyzed. The patient's ability to participate in the care must be factored into the plan. A regular time frame should be set to evaluate the outcomes as a team with input from the patient. The patient's expectations may not be the same as those of the health care team or the primary caregivers, so when outcomes are evaluated, variations in expectations should be addressed.

Monitoring laboratory testing to determine immune status, blood cell status, and effects of medications is a large part of the evaluation process.

HIV Risk and the Older Person

Elder care is an area that often is forgotten when discussing HIV infection. This may be a result of the focus

Table 11–4 *Nursing Diagnoses and Interventions for the Patient with HIV/AIDS*

NURSING DIAGNOSIS	EXPECTED OUTCOMES	NURSING INTERVENTIONS
Risk for infection Elevated body temperature Depressed immune function	Patient will exhibit no signs of infection; normal temperature	Monitor for outward signs of infections and for symptoms of opportunistic infection Monitor body temperature daily Assess for signs of dehydration and altered mental status
Impaired gas exchange Excessive lung secretions Use of respiratory accessory muscles for breathing	Patient's oxygenation will improve to within normal levels within 3 wk	Monitor breath patterns and sounds q 4 hr Position to allow for maximum chest expansion Provide supplemental oxygen as ordered Encourage deep breathing and coughing as need indicates Conserve strength and oxygen by assisting with activities of daily living Monitor blood gases as ordered Suction airway PRN as ordered
Impaired skin integrity Multiple areas of skin abrasion State of dehydration	No further areas of skin breakdown will occur Areas of abrasion will heal within 2 wk	Assess skin status q 4 hr; assess for areas of excoriation, lesions, rashes, and discoloration Report changes from baseline findings. Keep skin clean and dry Change linens as needed if diaphoresis or incontinence is present Use elbow and heel protectors and special mattress while patient is immobilized Apply lotion to dry skin Assess for dehydration q 4 hr Encourage adequate fluid intake per physical status Assess for signs of fluid overload/edema Monitor input and output
Impaired oral mucous membrane Fungal infection Irritation from drug therapy	No evidence of fungal infection at the end of 3 wk	Assess and monitor the status of the mouth, tongue, and teeth; refer for dental care Teach proper dental hygiene Refer for nutritional counseling as need indicates
Imbalanced nutrition: less than body requirements	Patient will not experience further weight loss	Assess patient's ability to take in food, chew, and swallow Assess for pain in throat, loss of taste sensation
Weight loss	Patient will gain at least 0.5 lb/wk	Monitor weight twice a week Record input and output Administer antiemetics as ordered Assess the availability of food within living situation Assess ability of caregiver to meet patient's nutritional needs Assist with planning for small frequent meals Administer dietary supplements if required
Loss of appetite Impaired swallowing		
Pain		
Pressure on nerves from Kaposi sarcoma Discomfort from peripheral neuropathy	Pain will be controlled within tolerable levels within 4 days	Assess levels of pain; assess patient's methods to relieve it Relieve causes of pain by correcting underlying condition if possible. Administer pain medications as ordered; assess amount of relief provided by medication; if relief is not adequate, consult with physician for more effective protocol for pain relief; explore use of NSAIDs and antidepressant medications for pain relief in conjunction with other analgesics Implement adjunctive therapies to assist with pain relief: massage, cold or hot applications, repositioning, distraction, meditation, imagery Teach relaxation techniques

Key: *CNS,* central nervous system; *NSAIDs,* nonsteroidal antiinflammatory drugs; *PRN,* as needed.

Continued

Table 11–4 *Nursing Diagnoses and Interventions for the Patient with HIV/AIDS—cont'd*

NURSING DIAGNOSIS	EXPECTED OUTCOMES	NURSING INTERVENTIONS
Activity intolerance	Level of activity intolerance will improve within 1 mo	Encourage periods of rest alternated with periods of activity; plan activities according to usual stamina levels; change schedule of activities as degree of fatigue indicates need; assist with activities of daily living as needed to conserve energy
Weakness Central nervous system and peripheral nerve involvement		Encourage self-care in small increments as condition improves
Disturbed thought processes	Oxygenation will be improved, if possible, within 2 days	Assess mental and thought processes to establish a baseline
Drug side effects	Electrolyte imbalances contributing to problem will be corrected within 3 days	Monitor for causes of interference in thought processes: anemia, electrolyte imbalances, drug side effects, impaired oxygenation or dementia
Impaired oxygenation		Orient patient to person, time, and place frequently
Effects of disease process		Utilize techniques to assist with memory lapses: calendar, clock, labels for things Structure the environment per patient's wishes; do not move placement of belongings and frequently used items such as eyeglasses, tissues, book, etc Decrease outside stimuli when patient is trying to concentrate
Chronic low self-esteem	Patient will verbalize personal strengths within 3 wk	Encourage socialization to prevent withdrawal and social isolation.
Considerable weight loss Altered physical appearance Inability to maintain employment	Patient will take action to find ways to increase feelings of worth within 2 mo	Refer to support group for strengthening of self-concept. Refer to nutritionist to improve nutrition and physical appearance Encourage volunteer work to increase self-worth and feelings of accomplishment
Sexual dysfunction HIV status Decreased physical well-being Fatigue Presence of anogenital lesions	Patient will develop methods of sexual expression and intimacy that will not endanger self or others	Instruct patient to plan periods of rest around periods of sexual activity Offer referral to support groups or therapy to deal with issues of altered body image Instruct patient and significant other in the effective practice of abstinence, use of condoms, and barrier sex Discuss alternative methods of intimacy until anogenital lesions are healed
Ineffective coping Diagnosis of life-threatening illness Fatigue Anxiety	Patient will marshal usual effective coping techniques to meet challenges of the illness	Establish rapport with the patient, significant other, and family Assess past methods of effective coping. Assess patient's strengths Schedule activities that may cause stress when the patient is most rested or has support person available Review effective methods for problem solving
Powerlessness Diagnosis of life-threatening illness Increasing fatigue	Patient will maintain control over treatment and lifestyle choices	Show patient respect Allow patient control of daily schedule, activity, and treatment choices Foster independence in patient by allowing to do as much self-care as possible Reinforce behaviors that indicate the patient is planning for the future
Grieving HIV status Diagnosis of life-threatening illness	Patient will express feelings within 3 wk	Encourage verbalization of feelings; provide nonthreatening, supportive environment; be an active listener Refer to support group to facilitate grief process Refer to social services and pastoral care to assist with directives to physicians, living will, and designation of power of attorney Encourage positive thinking for increased energy level and constructive handling of grief

Table 11–4 Nursing Diagnoses and Interventions for the Patient with HIV/AIDS—cont'd

NURSING DIAGNOSIS	EXPECTED OUTCOMES	NURSING INTERVENTIONS
Disturbed sensory perception (visual) Loss of visual fields HIV damage to CNS	Patient will develop methods of dealing with visual changes within 1 mo	Assess amount of visual deficit Orient patient to the environment Speak to and touch patient frequently while in the room Keep patient informed of what you are doing and what will be happening to decrease fear and anxiety Instruct to report any further change in vision Assist with methods to enhance remaining vision and to prevent injury
Self-care deficit Fatigue Deterioration of physical condition Mental changes Neurological impairment	Patient will accomplish as many activities of daily living as possible without undue fatigue Patient will accept assistance with activities of daily living within 2 wk	Assess ability to perform own activities of daily living Provide assistance for activities the patient is unable to perform Refer to occupational and physical therapy for assistive devices and home equipment needed Instruct significant other and family members how to assist with activities of daily living
Impaired home maintenance Fatigue Activity intolerance Inadequate finances	Patient will achieve adequate home maintenance within 1 wk	Assess availability of caregiver in the home to assist with shopping, cleaning, meal preparation, and transportation Assess income for adequacy to support living and needed medical care Refer to social services and community agencies for help and other resources

Box 11–4 Major Nursing Goals for Adults with HIV/AIDS

- Prevent secondary bacterial, viral, and fungal infections.
- Prevent wasting due to malnutrition.
- Maintain or improve the present level of immune function.
- Maintain adequate social functioning.
- Maintain or improve current mental status.

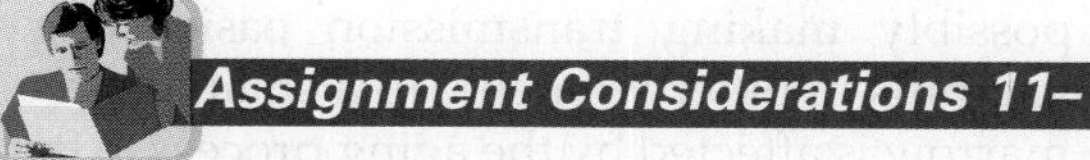

Assignment Considerations 11–1

Protecting the Patient

When working with immunocompromised patients, be aware of the physical health of co-workers. If a nursing assistant or other health care team member states that she feels like she is coming down with a cold or the flu, make sure she is not assigned to care for patients with alterations in immune function. For everyone's health, this person should not be at work at all, but if symptoms appear during the work shift, it may not be practical to replace her immediately.

Patient Teaching 11–1

The Patient with Compromised Immunity

Teach the patient who has a compromised immune system to:

- Assess for signs of infection on a daily basis and report such signs immediately.
- Take the temperature at least once a day.
- Seek an antimicrobial therapy prescription at the first signs of infection.
- Take all prescribed medications per instructions.
- Wash hands frequently and particularly before eating, after toileting, after petting an animal, after shaking hands or dancing with someone, and when returning home from shopping or errands.
- Refrain from mingling in crowds.
- Avoid others who have an infection.
- Avoid sharing of personal items such as toothbrushes, deodorant sticks, and razors.
- Wash the armpits, groin, genitals, and anal area at least twice a day with an antimicrobial soap.
- Cook foods well and avoid eating raw foods.
- Wash dishes in the dishwasher or with hot, soapy water.
- Do not dig in the soil or work with houseplants.
- Obtain adequate rest daily to allow the body to function as well as possible.
- Explore the use of stress reduction techniques and encourage regular implementation of the ones that are most attractive.
- Avoid travel to areas with poor sanitation or inadequate health care facilities.

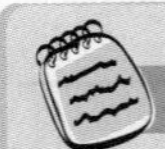

Patient Teaching 11–2

Infection Control in the Home of the Person Who Is HIV Positive

Consistent hand hygiene should be practiced by everyone in the home. Personal care items such as razors and toothbrushes should not be shared.

HOUSEKEEPING

- Clean up urine, blood, feces, vomitus, or other body fluids and the area with soap and warm water. Disinfect the area by wiping with a fresh 1:10 solution of household bleach (1 part bleach to 10 parts water). Dispose of solid wastes and solutions used for cleaning by flushing down the toilet.
- Soak rags, mops, and sponges used for cleaning in a fresh 1:10 bleach solution for at least 5 minutes to disinfect them.
- Clean bathroom surfaces with regular household cleaners and then disinfect with a 1:10 bleach solution.

LAUNDRY

- Rinse clothes, towels, or bedclothes if they become soiled with urine, blood, feces, vomitus, sputum, or other body secretions. Flush the water used for rinsing down the toilet. Launder the items with hot water and detergent with 1 cup of bleach added per load.
- Keep soiled clothes in a closed plastic bag before laundering.

BIOHAZARD DISPOSAL

- Dispose of "sharps" in a labeled puncture-proof container with a lid, using Standard Precautions to avoid needle sticks. When the container is full, decontaminate contents by adding a 1:10 bleach solution. Seal the container with tape and place it in a plastic biohazard bag. Return it to the home care nurse for proper disposal.
- Flush solid waste from incontinence pads, paper towels, toilet tissue, etc. down the toilet. Place the items and all disposable gloves in tied plastic bags and dispose of them in the regular trash.

Adapted from Ignatavicius, D.D., & Workman, M.L. (2005). *Medical-Surgical Nursing: Critical Thinking for Collaborative Care* (5th ed.). Philadelphia: Elsevier Saunders, p. 447.

on youth in the United States. Age is no barrier to becoming infected with HIV, and in some cases may actually predispose people to infection. A myth that must be discarded is that older adults, generally considered to be people over the age of 65, are no longer interested in a sexual relationship. This is simply not true. Many older adults are single as a result of death of a spouse/partner or divorce. Life expectancy has increased to greater than 75 years, with increased years of health. Times and values are changing, and older people may not have the comfort level to negotiate safer sex. Because pregnancy is not a consideration in this age group, condoms are not used as often as they should be. It is imperative to give older patients the appropriate information while respecting their

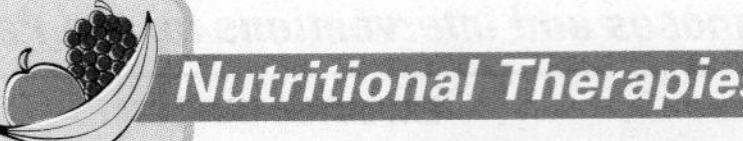

Nutritional Therapies 11–1

Improving Food Intake for the AIDS Patient

Attempt to minimize factors related to difficulty in chewing, swallowing, or inflamed oral mucosa.

Encourage the following measures:

- Eat small amounts frequently
- Eat high-calorie snacks or commercially available liquid supplements or "power" bars
- Eat foods at room temperature
- Soften dry grain foods such as breads, crackers, and cookies in milk, tea, or other nonacidic beverage before eating them
- Incorporate nonabrasive foods that are easy to swallow such as pasta, well-cooked eggs, baked fish, soft cheese, pudding, and ice cream
- Suck on Popsicles to numb mouth pain

The patient should avoid:

- Raw fruits and vegetables
- Spicy, acidic, or salty foods
- Alcohol
- Excessively hot food

feelings. Women, in general, are more vulnerable to HIV infection from sexual transmission because semen has far higher concentrations of the virus than infected vaginal secretions. A woman's male sex partner is statistically more likely to have had multiple other sexual contacts, increasing the likelihood of HIV infection. HIV testing for *both* partners before entering into a new sexual relationship should be encouraged, along with recommendations to use barrier techniques.

There are normal aging processes that put older women and men at higher risk as well. Skin and mucous membranes are more fragile in the elderly person, possibly making transmission easier (e.g., atrophic vaginitis in older women). To a small degree, the bone marrow is affected by the aging process. After the age of 70, there is a definite decline in the functioning of the immune system as evidenced by the increase in neoplasms and the decreased ability to fight infections. People in this age group often have had transfusions for surgery done some years ago; this puts them at greater risk of having contracted HIV from this source.

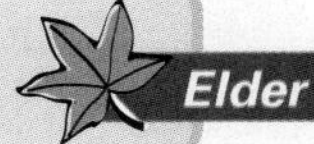

Elder Care Points

New diagnoses of HIV infection are growing faster in the over-50 age group than in the under-50 age group. All health care providers must remember to ask the same questions regarding behaviors that put people at risk of patients in all age groups. Age-specific referrals to a geriatric nurse practitioner or counselor with experience working with older adults may also be appropriate.

Community Education and Care

Nurses are on the front lines of the AIDS epidemic. The skill and ability to educate and care for the patients and community are part of nursing responsibility. Each nurse should be alert to the possibility of transmission of HIV and the methods of prevention and take every opportunity to share this information with at-risk populations, not only the patients, but also their significant others, families, and friends, as well as professional colleagues. Most people living with HIV or AIDS are not inpatients; they are in community settings.

Nurses provide care in many different places: the neighborhood school, churches, nursing homes, homeless shelters, or the patient's home. In each of these situations, the nursing process is used to assess and refer for care. Assessment should include evaluating the patient and family for risk of infection due to high-risk behaviors or reduced immune function. The identified need may be education about infection control, preventing transmission of HIV, or providing a referral to community agencies for further information. Nurses have the opportunity to meet the challenge of care for the person with HIV/AIDS. Information on the care of the pediatric patient with HIV/AIDS can be found in pediatric textbooks.

HIV Confidentiality and Disclosure Issues

Confidentiality is essential for all patients. In the case of a patient with HIV, it becomes very important to prevent discrimination and to comply with the Health Insurance Portability and Accountability Act (HIPAA). Knowledge of a patient's HIV status should not have any influence on the care delivered other than to provide condition-appropriate, supportive, safe care. Standard Precautions are to be utilized for all patients. No additional precautions are needed for HIV-positive patients.

Confidentiality is an ethical requirement for health care professionals. When interviewing patients, some very personal and sensitive information about themselves and their families or significant others is obtained. If this information is released inappropriately, there may be severe penalties such as legal or financial sanctions because of existing laws in most states. A lawsuit may be the consequence for the nurse who is indiscreet. For the patient, the consequences may be loss of job, loss of housing, and loss of insurance benefits, as well as job and social discrimination and rejection by families and friends (Legal & Ethical Considerations 11–1).

Since 1983, all states have been required to report AIDS cases, including patient demographic information, to the federal government for tracking like all other contagious diseases. HIV-positive status has not been tracked in the same way. Most states have reported HIV status using a coded system allowing for anonymity of the patient. In July of 2005, the CDC formally recommended that all states adopt a confidential name–based reporting system (Legal & Ethical Considerations 11–2).

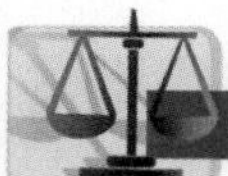

Legal & Ethical Considerations 11–1

Confidentiality and HIV

The right to disclose HIV status is regulated by the state in which you are working. It is important for every licensed nurse to be aware of the state regulations and of the policies in the employing agency or institution.

When a patient's family member asks what is wrong with the patient, if the patient has given permission for explanations to the family, explain the symptoms and what progress or lack thereof is occurring. Leave it to the patient to disclose diagnostic information and HIV status to the family.

The diagnosis of AIDS is a medical diagnosis and can be discussed among health care personnel like any other medical diagnosis, for the purpose of rendering care to the patient.

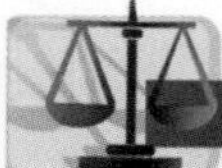

Legal & Ethical Considerations 11–2

When a Nurse Is HIV Positive

If a health care provider is HIV positive, there is a risk of transmitting the virus to others. What is the ethical, moral, and legal responsibility to the patients in such a situation?

Occupational Exposure to HIV

The first question that comes to mind when caring for an individual with HIV infection has to be, "How can I protect myself from becoming infected and still provide care?" In response to this continually asked question, the CDC, the American Nurses Association, the Occupational Safety and Health Administration (OSHA), and many health care agencies, private and governmental, have developed research-based guidelines to prevent exposure and infection with HIV and other blood-borne pathogens (CDC, 1998). 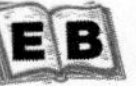

Follow the CDC's Standard Precautions and the policies and procedures of the employer for the prevention of transmission of blood-borne pathogens (see Chapter 6). There are standard policies in all institutions. Second, review the personal protective equipment provided by the institution, where it is located, and how to use it properly. Consistently use personal protective equipment as required during every patient contact. Know what your rights and responsibilities are according to the state and institutional policy, should there be an accidental occupational exposure (Safety Alert 11–3). Report any exposure to your manager or supervisor immediately and to the employee health department, and follow through with the protocols that are in place. Infection control is the key to

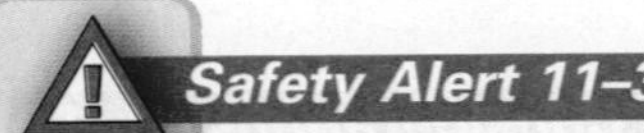

Safety Alert 11–3

Possible Exposure to HIV

Upon an accidental exposure to blood or body fluids of a person who either is HIV positive or whose HIV status is unknown, use of postexposure prophylaxis is essential. Exposure can be from a needle stick, mucosal contact with body fluids, or contact with body fluids via a break in the skin unprotected by a latex glove. The goal is to prevent conversion to an HIV-positive status. The facility nurse or infection control officer should be immediately notified. Two-drug or three-drug therapy, depending on the degree of determined risk, will be initiated as soon as possible after the exposure event. The medications will need to be taken for 4 weeks. The drugs used are each from a different class (NRTI, NNRTI, and PI classes).

safety in any health care setting. Health care workers need to review the CDC standards and take the precautions listed in Table 6–5.

THERAPEUTIC IMMUNOSUPPRESSION

Patients may become immunosuppressed as a result of deliberate treatment. The patient who has received an organ transplant may suffer from total rejection of the organ by his own body cells if they react to the organ as if it were a harmful agent. To avoid rejection of the transplanted organ, the patient may receive certain drugs that inhibit the action of his immune system. Certain cytotoxic drugs, as well as x-rays used to produce radiographs, can be immunosuppressive. Hence these agents can be used to benefit the patient when immunosuppression is desirable. The use of immunosuppressive agents requires the maintenance of a delicate balance between control of the immune response and control of infections that occur when the immune response is suppressed.

Multiple medications are used to prevent rejection after organ transplantation. The most commonly given include methylprednisolone (a corticosteroid), lymphocyte immune globulin (reduces the number of circulating thymus-dependent lymphocytes), antithymocyte globulin (immunosuppressive agent that selectively destroys T lymphocytes), muromonab-CD3 (blocks the function of CD3 molecules in the membrane of human T cells), basiliximab (binds and blocks the interleukin-2 receptor chain on the surface of activate T lymphocytes), daclizumab (inhibits the function of white cells), and rapamycin (an antibiotic that demonstrates antifungal, anti-inflammatory, antitumor, and immunosuppressive properties).

Azathioprine (Imuran) and cyclosporine (Sandimmune) continue to be the most commonly used antirejection medications in combination with the ones already discussed. The doses of these drugs are adjusted according to the immune response of each patient. This type of therapy increases the risk for bacterial and fungal infections in the patient. Cyclosporine acts as a selective immunosuppressant, leaving intact some of the body's defenses against infection. There is evidence that use of the drug increases the survival rate of patients with certain organ transplants, but it does not completely eliminate the danger of organ rejection. It has been shown that the immunosuppression tends to allow the growth of some cancers.

In addition to preventing the rejection of transplanted organs, immunosuppressive therapy also may be employed to manage multiple myeloma, rheumatoid arthritis, other kinds of neoplastic growths, and other autoimmune diseases.

Whatever the reason for the immune deficiency, the patient will require special nursing care so that the possibility of an overwhelming infection is kept at a minimum.

TREATMENT OF IMMUNE DEFICIENCIES

The management of immune deficiency depends on its degree of severity and its primary cause. Some patients have virtually no ability to synthesize antibodies or sensitized lymphocytes, whereas others experience only a temporary minor defect in humoral immune response and cell-mediated immunity.

Injections of immune globulin may be given on a regular basis to provide passive immunity for those who are unable to produce their own antibodies. Antibiotics are used in large doses as soon as an infection is evident. These drugs should rarely be used as a preventive measure because antibiotics themselves can be immunosuppressive. Inappropriate use of antibiotics in some cases can lead to the development of drug-resistant strains of the organism.

In some types of immune deficiency, passive immunization can be accomplished by transfusing specifically sensitized lymphocytes to help the patient resist an infection. When function of the bone marrow is involved, as in leukemia, the patient may receive a bone marrow transplant to provide the stem cells that will eventually become immune bodies.

To help prevent or combat infection in immunosuppressed patients, granulocyte colony-stimulating factor—filgrastim (Neupogen)—is used to promote the growth of neutrophils. This drug is used for both AIDS patients and some types of cancer patients who have immunodeficiency. It is a challenge to prevent infection while therapeutically suppressing the immune response.

Whenever possible, treatment is aimed at controlling the disease or eliminating the condition that is the primary cause of an inadequately functioning immune system. Sometimes, as in cases of nephrosis, liver disease, drug toxicity, and viral infections, this may be possible. In other instances, however, treatment consists of minimizing the effects of the immune deficiency.

Experimental drugs continue to be developed for use in the treatment of AIDS. These same medications offer hope for other types of immune deficiency disorders.

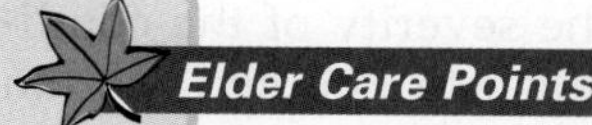

Elder Care Points

Aging does not affect the bone marrow to a significant degree. It does cause the thymus gland to become smaller, and T cells apparently diminish in the circulation; B-cell numbers remain the same. All the mechanisms involved in decreased immune function are not yet clear, but it is apparent that after age 70 there is a definite decline in the function of the immune system.

NURSING MANAGEMENT

Assessment (Data Collection)

When an immune deficiency is suspected, the patient is questioned about frequent infections, exposure to HIV, immunosuppressive drug therapy, and family history of genetic immune disorders. Nutritional status is assessed by measuring weight and height, inspecting the skin, hair, and general appearance of the patient, and inquiring about weight loss. Information is gathered about the current physical status of the patient, such as his general state of health, any infections he may have at the time, and how these infections are affecting him. Inquiring about occupational or environmental exposure to agents that might harm the bone marrow also is important. Excessive alcohol intake depresses the immune system, so gathering a drinking history is indicated. Determining whether or not the patient is on corticosteroid therapy is essential.

Physical assessment includes palpating the superficial lymph nodes to detect abnormalities and assessing the body systems involved in complaints. The abdomen is palpated to detect organ enlargement, such as an enlarged liver or spleen.

Diagnostic Tests

A complete blood count with differential is obtained to determine the numbers of circulating lymphocytes. Other tests used to ascertain immune status include bone marrow studies, serum protein, protein electrophoresis, immunoelectrophoresis, T-cell and B-cell assays, and enzyme-linked immunosorbent assays (ELISAs). Other tests specific to the type of disorder suspected may be performed.

Nursing Diagnosis and Planning

Nursing diagnoses for patients with immune deficiency always include risk for infection. Other nursing diagnoses are written according to the particular problems and complaints of the patient.

The primary nursing goals when caring for a patient who has an immune deficiency are to (1) protect the patient from infection, (2) improve health status, and (3) promote as high a degree of wellness as possible so that the immune system can function at an optimal level. Planning care for the patient with an immune deficiency focuses on preventing exposure to pathogens. If a patient's immune deficiency is severe, he will need to be placed in protective (reverse) isolation sometimes called Neutropenic Precautions. Working with patients in this type of isolation requires more time because of the precautions involved. Integrating care of this patient with the rest of the assignments for the shift needs to be carefully planned. Nurses caring for immunodeficient patients should not be caring for patients with active infections at the same time. Expected outcomes are written based on the nursing diagnoses chosen for the patient and might include:

- Patient will remain free from infection.
- B-cell and T-cell counts are within normal limits.

Implementation

Adequate nutrition with sufficient protein is important, as proteins are needed to synthesize antibodies. If the patient is on corticosteroid therapy, appetite control may be a problem and the patient must be watched for continuous weight gain. If the patient has a condition or is on medications that suppress appetite or cause nausea, implementing strategies to improve nutritional intake is necessary. Nutritional supplements may be added, and multiple small meals of high-protein foods chosen by the patient may be scheduled during the day.

? *Think Critically About . . .* How would you explain to a patient why good-quality protein is important in the diet when an immunodeficiency is present?

Psychosocial care to assist the patient to deal with the fear associated with the knowledge that he may contract a serious infection at any time is a nursing responsibility. The lives of patients with immune disorders often are disrupted by infections and by the therapy to control the disorder (Safety Alert 11–4). They may have trouble remaining in school or at work because of frequent illness or malaise. Collaboration with the social worker is often indicated to assist with role changes and financial constraints. In many instances, financial, family, transportation or job issues may be stressors. Stress can be a negative factor in fighting the disease process. Appropriate nursing interventions and referrals to resources can greatly assist the patient.

The nurse can be instrumental in teaching the patient techniques to reduce stress. Excessive stress further depresses immune function. Light exercise, meditation, relaxation techniques, and imagery are all appropriate interventions for stress management

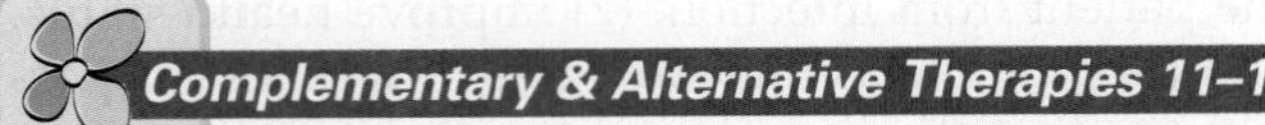

Complementary & Alternative Therapies 11–1

Use of Alternative Therapies by Patients with HIV

Complementary and alternative therapies are routinely used by HIV patients. Relaxation, meditation, Reiki, and imagery are helpful in decreasing stress. Acupressure and acupuncture may help control pain. Some herbal therapies and supplements can be dangerous because they can interfere with the drug therapy, and the primary health care provider should be consulted before using them. There are many therapies that have been studied and are safe to use. Others do not treat a specific disease, but are used for relaxation and health promotion.

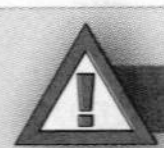

Safety Alert 11–4

Preventing Infection Among Immune-Deficient Patients

Hospitalized patients with deficient immune function must be protected from exposure to infectious organisms. Protective isolation may be indicated (see Chapters 6 and 16). For any patient with immune deficiency, meticulous hand hygiene is essential before and after each contact with the patient, and disinfection of any object that may serve as a source of infection is necessary. Strict observance of surgical aseptic technique is essential during the performance of invasive nursing care procedures such as catheterization, dressing changes, intravenous infusions, and all other activities that might lead to the introduction of pathogenic microorganisms into the body.

(Complementary & Alternative Therapies 11–1). See the relaxation script in Box 7-2 in Chapter 7.

Patient education regarding the immune disorder and any therapy that the patient is to receive should be provided (see Patient Teaching 11–1). The patient is taught continuously to assess for signs of infection and to report them immediately.

Evaluation

Evaluation of nursing actions is performed to determine whether expected outcomes are being met. Laboratory test results are checked to assess whether immune function is improving. B-cell and T-cell assays are particularly important. The patient is evaluated for recovery from any infection that might have been present. Temperature is monitored for elevations, **although immune deficient patients may not have a temperature elevation even in the presence of infection.** The patient also is evaluated for general well-being, appetite, and weight maintenance, and for side effects of the medications he is taking.

DISORDERS OF INAPPROPRIATE IMMUNE RESPONSE

HYPERSENSITIVITY AND ALLERGY

Hypersensitivity reactions, better known as allergic reactions, are the body's excessive response to a normally harmless substance. The severity of the condition can range from a mild rash to **anaphylaxis** (an extreme allergic reaction that is life threatening). Allergens can enter the body in several ways and can have either a local or a systemic effect. The tendency to develop allergies, known as **atopy,** affects about 10% of the population.

Etiology and Pathophysiology

An allergy is an abnormal, individual response to certain substances that normally do not trigger such an exaggerated reaction. Allergies are divided into two major categories: (1) immediate hypersensitivity reactions that are mast cell mediated (type I hypersensitivity) and (2) delayed-reaction allergies involving T cells (type II hypersensitivity). As with all types of immune response, abnormal as well as normal, a full-blown reaction will not occur until an individual's immune cells have been sensitized to the specific substance that triggers the response. This means that, on first contact with the allergen, there will be very little specific antibody in the circulating blood or in the lymphoid tissues. The body then produces antibodies to the allergen. On the second and subsequent contacts, the antibody specific to the allergen is present in large quantities, circulating in the body fluids, where it can be transported to the location of the allergen, causing an allergic reaction.

Type I or rapid reactions result from the increased production of immunoglobulin E antibodies. During this reaction, histamine and other chemicals toxic to the body's cells are released. The chemicals cause dilation of blood vessels, which increases the transport of antibody and chemicals to the site of battle. Type I reactions include anaphylaxis, allergic asthma, and atopic allergies such as hay fever. Allergies to latex, bee venom, peanuts, iodine, drugs, shellfish, and many other environmental antigens are type I reactions (Figure 11–3). Type II or delayed reactions result from increased production of immunoglobulin G.

Types of Allergens. Identifying allergens by categories can help the patient recognize less obvious allergic substances. Four broad types of allergens may be distinguished according to the way in which they gain access to the body. *Inhalants* enter the body through the nose and mouth; they include dust, molds, pollen, fragrances, animal dander, and some chemicals. *Contactants* come in direct contact with the skin. These include detergents and soaps, cosmetics, plants such as poison ivy, and dyes such as those used in shoe leather.

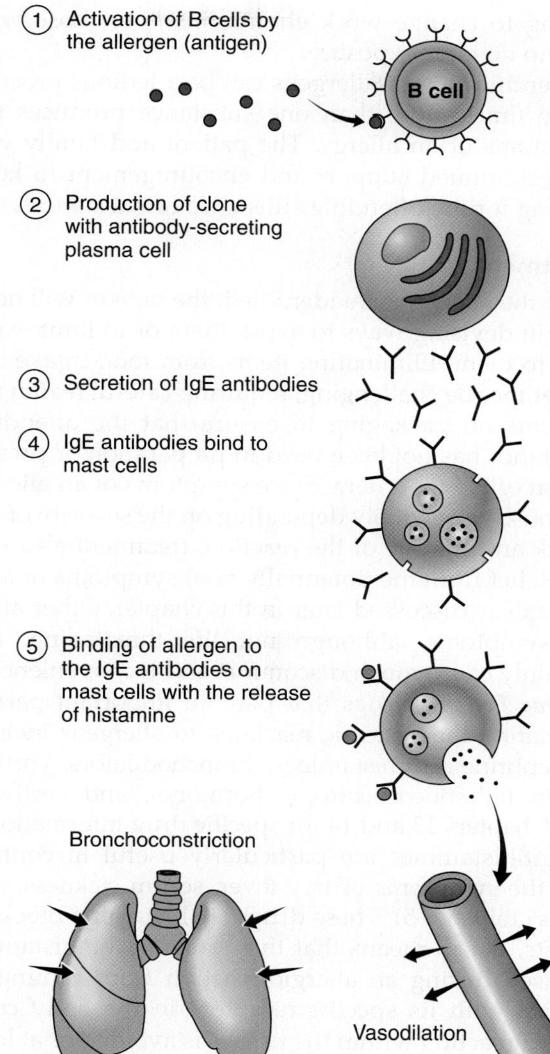

FIGURE **11–3** Immediate-reaction allergy.

Metals in jewelry and latex in gloves and other products that come in contact with skin can also produce a reaction. *Ingestants* are swallowed and are usually food or medications. Citrus fruits, tomatoes, strawberries, cow's milk, wheat, eggs, dairy products, seafood, chocolate, nuts, and colas are common food offenders. Monosodium glutamate, other preservatives, and artificial food coloring can be potent allergens for some people.

Among the drugs, the most likely to cause an allergic reaction are aspirin, barbiturates, anticonvulsants, and antibiotics, but any drug may cause an allergic reaction. *Injectables* enter the body through hypodermic, intramuscular, and intravenous injections or by snake and other animal bites or insect stings. Immunizing agents such as vaccines, animal saliva, and venoms are the allergens that most commonly enter the body by this route.

Box 11–5 *Substances Known to Cause Hypersensitivity and Possible Anaphylaxis*

DRUGS
- Aspirin
- Cephalosporins
- Chemotherapy agents
- Insulins
- Local anesthetics
- Nonsteroidal anti-inflammatory drugs (NSAIDs)
- Penicillins
- Sulfonamides
- Tetracyclines

DIAGNOSTIC AND TREATMENT AGENTS
- Allergenic extracts for desensitization
- Blood products
- Iodine-containing contrast media used for x-rays

ANTITOXIN SERA
- Diphtheria antitoxin
- Poisonous spider antitoxin
- Snake venom antitoxin
- Tetanus antitoxin

FOODS
- Chocolate
- Eggs
- Fish
- Milk
- Nuts (especially peanuts)
- Shellfish
- Strawberries
- Wheat

INSECT STINGS
- Ants (particularly fire ants)
- Bees
- Hornets
- Wasps
- Yellow jackets

Signs and Symptoms

The chemical release may affect all blood vessels, causing widespread blood vessel dilation and swelling of tissues and congestion in mucous membranes. The release of histamine may cause the contraction of smooth-muscle tissues in the bronchioles. These internal changes produce the symptoms of allergy, notably redness, swelling, increased exudate, and breathing difficulties such as wheezing and dyspnea. Rhinorrhea, sneezing, and itchy, red, watery eyes are common when the nose and eyes are exposed to a contact allergen.

Diagnosis

Identification of Allergens. Identification of the specific allergen or allergens causing the allergic reaction may be fairly easy or extremely difficult. A list of substances commonly known to cause allergic responses is listed in Box 11–5. The patient is questioned about exposure to known substances that may cause an allergic response. Reaction to stings, drug allergies, and other conditions that are not routine occurrences in the life of the patient are readily noticed because the cause-and-effect relationship is apparent, but vague symptoms, such as a stuffy nose from allergy to inhalants, may be less obvious.

Prior to administration of some medications that are known to be allergenic, a test dose of the drug may be given. For medications given IV, a very small dose can be given and then, at 10-minute increments, increasing amounts of the drug are infused until the full dose is administered. The patient is monitored closely for signs and symptoms of a reaction during this process, with resuscitation drugs and equipment immediately available.

Skin testing to identify specific allergens can be done in a number of ways. In the scratch test, the skin is slightly scratched so that only its upper layer is broken and no blood appears. A sampling of the suspected allergen is applied to the scratched area. In the intracutaneous or intradermal method, the sample of allergen is injected just below the epidermis. In the patch test, a small amount of the allergen is simply placed on the surface of the skin and covered with an airtight dressing (patch). A positive reaction to these tests is indicated by the appearance of a small (dime-size) wheal at the site of contact with the allergen. Once the allergen has been identified, measures can be taken to eliminate it or lessen exposure.

A helpful tool for identifying suspected allergens in foods is the elimination diet. It usually starts with foods that are known to be frequent offenders. The patient is asked to eliminate one food at a time and to record in a food diary all the foods eaten each day. This includes additives and preservatives in processed foods that were eaten. If the patient's symptoms persist for a week to 10 days after eliminating one food (e.g., milk and dairy products), he is allowed to resume his intake of that particular food, and another one is chosen for elimination.

Latex Allergy. Many health care providers as well as patients have developed latex allergies. Most items that have been routinely manufactured with latex now are produced with non-latex alternatives including gloves, Foley catheters, surgical drains, Band-Aids, condoms, and many other supplies. Nurses need to be aware of all patient allergies, including latex, so that appropriate interventions can be initiated. OSHA requires that employers furnish personal protective equipment for employees. For those employees with latex allergy, non-latex items are made available.

The ideal solution to any allergy is to avoid or eliminate the allergen. In some cases it is not possible to completely eliminate the source, and the individual must remove herself from the environment. Severe latex allergies have resulted in some health care workers having to change work environments to those with little to no latex exposure.

Identification of allergens can be a tedious process. Many times more than one substance produces the symptoms of an allergy. The patient and family will need continued support and encouragement to keep looking for the offending substance or substances.

Treatment

Once the allergens are identified, the patient will need help in devising ways to avoid them or to limit exposure to them. Eliminating items from food intake can sometimes be challenging, requiring careful reading of contents on packaging to ensure that the offending substance has not been used in preparation or preservation of the food item. Since symptoms of an allergic response vary widely depending on the severity of the attack and the site of the reaction, treatment also varies. Relief from the potentially fatal symptoms of anaphylaxis is discussed later in this chapter. Other allergic symptoms, although not life threatening, can certainly cause much discomfort and inconvenience.

Drug Therapy. Drugs that play an important part in alleviating the systemic reactions to allergens include epinephrine, antihistamines, bronchodilators, corticotropin (adrenocorticotropic hormone), and cortisone (see Chapters 13 and 14 for specific drug information).

Antihistamines are particularly useful in controlling the symptoms of hay fever, serum sickness, and hives (Table 11–5). These drugs are histamine-blocking agents, which means that they prevent the histamine released during an allergic reaction from coming in contact with its specific receptors in the body cells. Thus a reaction within the tissues is avoided or at least greatly reduced. The result of this blocking action includes relief from itching, decrease in swelling of mucous membranes, decrease in production of secretions, and reduction in other symptoms of an allergic reaction. Diphenhydramine (Benadryl) is commonly used orally and topically to counteract allergic symptoms.

Patients requiring antihistamines are warned of the side effects of drowsiness and impaired coordination, both of which require restrictions on driving an automobile and operating machinery during the beginning of therapy. Other side effects, such as dryness of the mouth, urinary retention, weakness, and blurred vision, are not uncommon. Antihistamines and decongestants can aggravate hypertension and should be used cautiously in patients with high blood pressure.

Many elderly men experience hesitancy, urinary retention, and difficulty with ejaculation when they take antihistamines. Bladder distention must be monitored in these patients, and the drug discontinued if the problem cannot be resolved.

Anti-inflammatory agents such as corticotropin and cortisone are administered to reduce the inflammatory response that occurs in an allergic reaction. Bronchodilators help relieve the respiratory distress that may be

Table 11–5 ***Drugs Commonly Used in the Treatment of Allergy***

CLASSIFICATION	ACTION	SIDE EFFECTS	NURSING IMPLICATIONS
ANTIHISTAMINES			
First-Generation Agents			
Ethanolamines Carbinoxamine (Clistin) Clemastine (Tavist Allergy) Diphenhydramine (Benadryl) **Ethylenediamines** Tripelennamine (PBZ) **Alkylamines** Brompheniramine (Dimetane) Chlorpheniramine (Chlor-Trimeton) Dexchlorpheniramine (Polaramine) Triprolidine (Actidil) **Piperidine** Azatadine (Optimine) **Phenothiazines** Promethazine (Phenergan)	Bind with H_1 receptors on target cells, blocking histamine binding. Relieve acute symptoms of allergic response (itching, sneezing, excessive secretions, mild congestion).	First-generation agents cross blood-brain barrier, bind to H_1 receptors in brain, cause *sedation* (diminished alertness, slow reaction time, somnolence) and *stimulation* (restless, nervous, insomnia). Some drugs (e.g., ethanolamines) are more likely to cause sedation. Patients vary in their sensitivity to these side effects. The next most common side effects involve the GI system and include loss of appetite, epigastric distress, constipation, and diarrhea. May cause palpitations, tachycardia, urinary retention or frequency.	First-generation agents: • Warn patient that operating machinery and driving may be dangerous because of sedative effect. Drowsiness usually passes after 2 wk of treatment. • Teach patient to report palpitations, change in heart rate, change in bowel/bladder habits. • Instruct patient not to use alcohol with antihistamines because of additive depressant effect. • Rapid onset of action, no drug tolerance with prolonged use.
Second-Generation Agents Loratadine (Claritin) Cetirizine (Zyrtec) Fexofenadine (Allegra) Desloratadine (Clarinex)		Second-generation agents have limited affinity for brain H_1 receptors. Cause minimal sedation, few effects on psychomotor activities or bladder function.	Second-generation agents: • Teach patient to expect few, if any, side effects. • More expensive than classic antihistamines. • Rapid onset of action, no drug tolerance with prolonged use. General interactions: • Do not take with alcohol or any form of tranquilizer or sedative. • Do not take with any monoamine oxidase inhibitor.
DECONGESTANTS			
Oral Pseudoephedrine (Sudafed) Phenylpropanolamine	Stimulate adrenergic receptors on blood vessels, promote vasoconstriction, and reduce nasal edema and rhinorrhea.	CNS stimulation, causing insomnia, excitation, headache, irritability, increased blood and ocular pressure, dysuria, palpitations, tachycardia.	• Advise patient of adverse reactions. • Advise that some preparations are contraindicated for patients with cardiovascular disease, hypertension, diabetes, glaucoma, prostate hyperplasia, hepatic and renal disease.
Topical (nasal spray) Oxymetazoline (Dristan) Phenylephrine (Neo-Synephrine)	Same as above.	Same as above, plus rhinitis medicamentosa (rebound nasal congestion).	• Teach patient that these drugs should not be used for >3 days or more than 3–4 times a day. Longer use increases risk of rhinitis medicamentosa.
Azelastine (Astelin)	Blocks action of histamine.	Headache, bitter taste, somnolence, nasal irritation.	

Key: *CNS*, central nervous system; *GI*, gastrointestinal.

a symptom of involvement of the respiratory tract. Tranquilizers and sedatives promote the rest needed for repair of body tissues from a severe reaction and relieve the stress that aggravates an allergic reaction. Local reactions involving widespread and deep skin lesions are treated with salves, wet compresses, and soothing baths. The patient also must be protected from a secondary bacterial infection.

Desensitization. When it is not possible for a patient to avoid exposure to allergens, or if the symptoms cannot be managed successfully, the physician may suggest desensitization. The purpose of this form of therapy is to render the patient less sensitive to the allergens. The program involves regular injections of extremely small quantities of selected antigens on a daily, weekly, or monthly schedule. The amount given is gradually increased until there is noticeable clinical improvement, and then a maintenance dose is given. The program may last for years, but improvement should be noted in about 6 to 24 weeks after it is begun.

Successful management of hypersensitivity depends in large measure on the ability of the patient to understand the allergy and to follow the prescribed regimen of treatment. Support from health caregivers and family can encourage the patient to stay with the lengthy process.

Nursing Management

To track down the allergens causing the patient's symptoms requires time and diligence. To gather data for the initial assessment, see Focused Assessment 11–2. The patient may need to keep a diary of foods eaten and chemicals that are used (i.e., soaps, cleaners, garden products, cosmetics, etc.) for a few weeks. Recalling family history of allergy and types of allergy symptoms may prove helpful. Repeated assessments may need to be planned over a period of weeks or months if the patient is reactive to a variety of allergens. The major goals for the patient with hypersensitivity and allergic reactions are presented in Health Promotion Points 11–4.

Many substances that are commonly found in households are allergens that are not easily eliminated from the environment. Pet dander, dust, and molds are all common sources of allergies. Overstuffed furniture, heavy draperies, and thick carpets serve as excellent reservoirs for these substances. Removal of carpeting, routine cleaning as well as daily dusting and vacuuming, and elimination of dust-harboring furnishings can help remove some allergens. A great deal of teaching about keeping the home and work environment as allergen free as possible is required. Compliance with daily dusting and vacuuming is very difficult unless the person's allergy is severe, prompting every effort to control it. Electrostatic filters and top-quality vacuum cleaners with filters are essential for those with severe inhalant allergies. In some cases, it may be necessary to part with a cherished family pet, or to overcome the habit of smoking and to ask others not to smoke in one's presence. Purchase of an air-conditioning unit that effectively filters out airborne allergens may be very beneficial. Other common allergens found in the home include cleaning compounds, cosmetics, and dyes in fabrics and materials used in home furnishings. Wearing rubber gloves when washing dishes, laundering clothes, or performing other chores requiring contact with cleansing agents helps prevent contact with the offending agent.

Controlling household mold is another area for allergy prevention. If there is an allergy to mold, houseplants should be removed to eliminate this possible source. Molds grow in moist environments. Showers and bathing areas are moist more often than other ar-

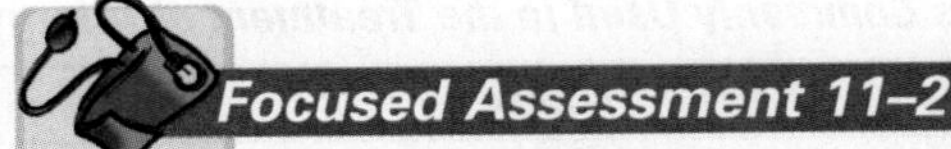

Focused Assessment 11–2

Data Collection for Patients with Allergy

Look for the following indicators of allergic responses:

GENERAL

- History of food intolerances, colic, abdominal cramping, bloating or pain, vomiting, and diarrhea in the absence of general illness
- History of unusual reaction to any drug, insect sting, odor, or fumes
- History of recurrent respiratory problems or seasonal flare-ups of any symptoms
- History of fatigue, wheezing, or shortness of breath upon exertion

SKIN

- Itching, burning, dryness, scaling, irritations, inflammations, hives, rash (note symmetry and location), scratches, or urticaria

EYES

- Burning, itching, tearing, history of styes
- Redness, discoloration below eyes (allergic shiners), conjunctivitis, rubbing, or excessive blinking

NOSE

- History of nose twitching, stuffiness, recurring nosebleeds, sudden episodes of sneezing or snorting
- Allergic salute (pushing nose upward and backward with heel of hand), nasal polyps, nasal voice

MOUTH AND THROAT

- Open-mouth breathing, continual throat clearing, shiny bald patches on tongue with slightly elevated borders, mouth wrinkling with facial grimaces, redness of throat, swollen lips or tongue

EARS

- History of hearing loss, drainage from ears

NECK

- Palpable, enlarged lymph nodes

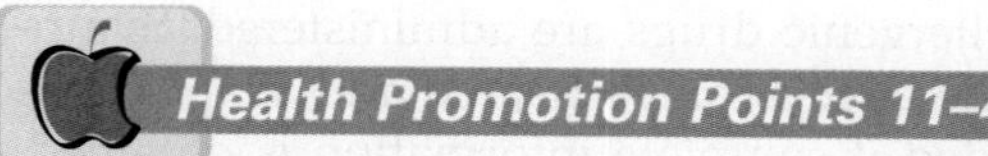

Nursing Goals for Patients with Hypersensitivity Reactions

The major goals in managing hypersensitivity and allergic reactions are to:

- Assist in the diagnosis of hypersensitivity.
- Help the patient identify the particular substance or substances that trigger an allergic response.
- Assist the patient in devising ways to avoid or at least limit exposure to these allergens.
- Relieve the symptoms of an allergy.
- Decrease the exaggerated response to the allergen(s).
- Provide health teaching.

eas of the house and typically are prone to mold growth. Basements and foundation structures also are at risk for mold growth. Routine cleaning and adequate ventilation can help reduce or eliminate mold growth in homes. Good drainage and restricting moisture around foundations can help decrease structural mold. Dehumidifiers can reduce moisture in basements. Successful compliance with recommendations should reduce the frequency, severity, and symptoms of the allergic reaction.

Nurses and others who handle certain drugs may develop allergies to these drugs. For example, penicillin and streptomycin can cause contact dermatitis in some people who are regularly exposed to them. Hands should be washed thoroughly after handling antibiotics.

As with the control of the spread of infectious agents, avoiding exposure to allergens requires knowledge of the nature of the allergen, how it is transmitted, its source or reservoir, and its portal of entry. Once these have been established, the nurse and the patient work together to eliminate the allergen from the patient's environment insofar as this is feasible. Alteration in habits and location may also help eliminate exposure.

Patients with skin allergic conditions should be taught that a warm environment and sweating increase the sensation of itching. Advise the patient to keep cool without chilling and not to take hot showers or hot baths. Another important aspect of care for these patients is prevention of scratching and excoriation of the skin. Over-the-counter topical lotions as well as prescription medications and salves can help relieve itching.

? *Think Critically About . . .* What actions would you suggest for removing allergens from the home environment for someone allergic to man-made fibers?

ANAPHYLACTIC REACTION AND ANAPHYLACTIC SHOCK

Etiology and Pathophysiology

Anaphylaxis is a serious, life-threatening, whole-body allergic reaction. Any agent that causes a severe hypersensitivity reaction can cause anaphylaxis. When it occurs, there is swelling and rupture of the affected cells, with the release of histamine. This chemical substance causes dilation of small blood vessels, a pooling of blood, and release of fluid into tissues. These changes in turn may produce circulatory collapse and profound shock (Figure 11–4).

Avoidance of anaphylaxis requires an awareness of previous allergic reactions and identification of those people who are likely to experience a serious reaction. It is extremely important to question each patient who is about to receive drugs that are likely to produce an allergic reaction about allergies before the medication is given. Charts should be checked and patients questioned about allergies before (1) giving medications or immunizations, (2) dispatching them for x-ray studies using contrast media, and (3) minor or major surgery. **It is wise to check for allergies in several places, including the front of the chart, the physician's history, and the nurse's admission history, as well as verbally with the patient and the family.** When people are ill or experiencing the stress of being hospitalized, they often forget about allergies or fail to mention an allergy that they do not think is significant.

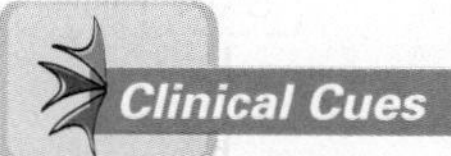

Allergies to seafood indicate an intolerance to iodine. This means there is potential for an allergic reaction to iodine-based contrast agents used in radiologic imaging studies. Be certain that the shellfish/iodine allergy is noted on the front of the chart, on the medication administration record, and in other locations where allergies are to be noted in the medical record.

Signs and Symptoms

The patient also suffers from difficult breathing as a result of the narrowing of the air passages and accumulation of mucus. The appearance of hives **(urticaria)** or swelling beneath the skin **(angioedema)** may signal the onset of an anaphylactic episode. Hives, or sudden outbreaks of **wheals** (small areas of swelling) on the skin that itch and burn, may appear without subsequent anaphylaxis.

The patient with an anaphylactic reaction is in a very serious condition requiring immediate attention. Circulatory collapse can occur very rapidly, leading to fatal anaphylactic shock. The heart muscle does not function as it should, causing decreased output of blood and a drop in blood pressure. The patient also experiences dyspnea of increasing severity, and convulsions may occur. If these conditions are not relieved immediately, the patient can die within 5 to 10 minutes.

Emergency supplies should be readily available whenever vaccines, serum for passive immunization, and highly allergenic drugs are administered. Symptoms from side effects can be treated and anaphylaxis may be avoided if complete information is obtained. Premedication with steroids and/or antihistamines can be administered if a substance needs to be given that the patient has shown sensitivity to in the past.

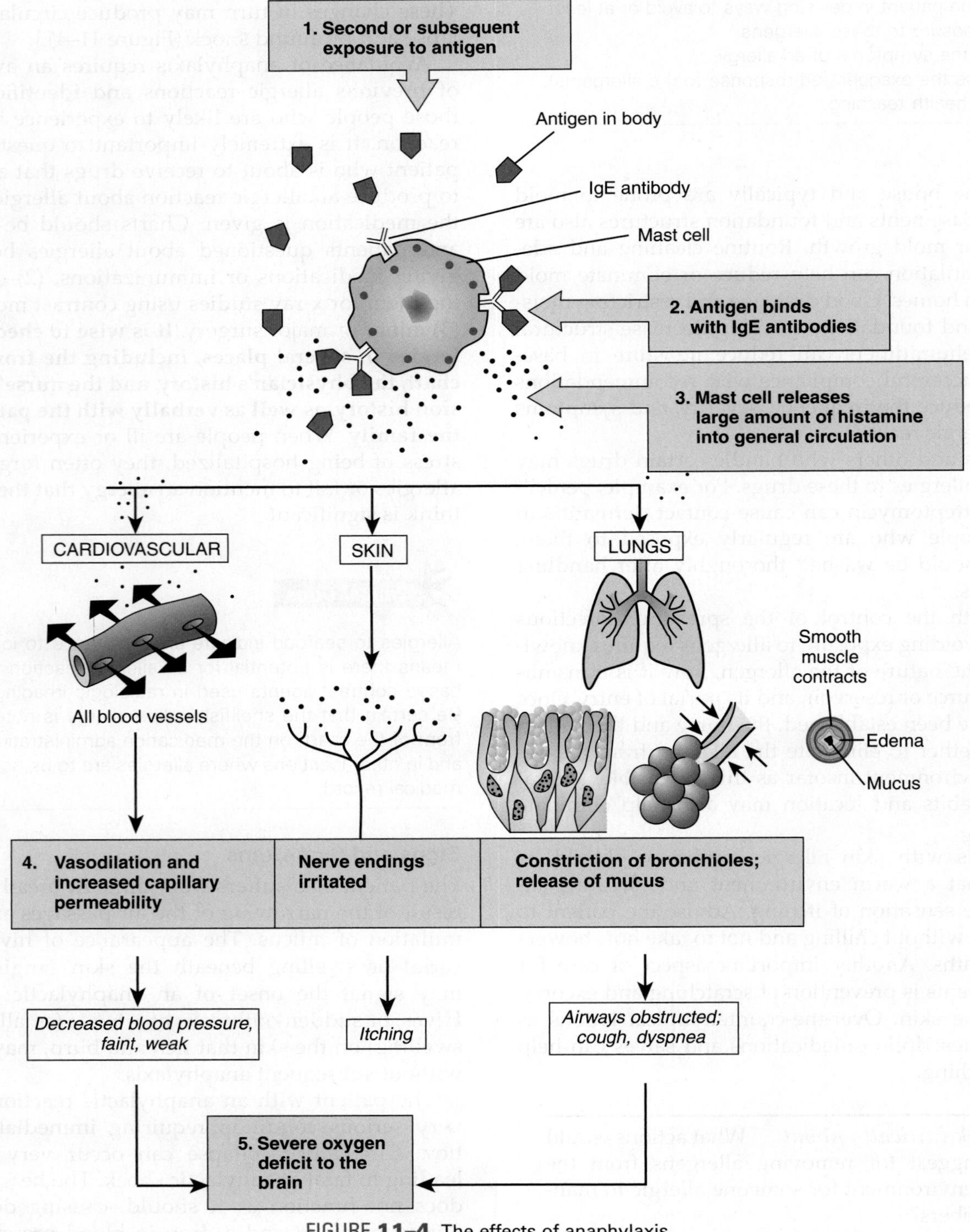

FIGURE 11–4 The effects of anaphylaxis.

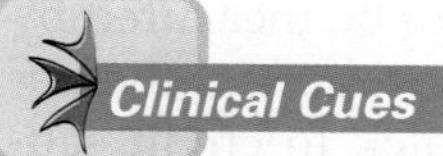

Many patients report allergies to medications that are actually manifestations of side effects, intolerance, or nonallergic adverse reactions. Nausea, constipation, diarrhea, coughing, or drowsiness may be side effects of medications not intended to cause any of these symptoms. Reactions to drugs that do not involve the immune system are considered nonallergic adverse reactions. Careful questioning of the patient can help distinguish what kind of reaction the patient has experienced in the past.

? *Think Critically About . . .* What is the first thing you would do if a patient starts complaining of shortness of breath and wheezing just after you have administered an antibiotic by injection?

Diagnosis

Anaphylaxis is a syndrome—a collection of signs and symptoms—and not a distinct disease process. There is no universally accepted definition, but features have been identified that allow for recognition of the syndrome. The diagnosis is made from the presenting clinical symptoms that include a sudden onset involving one or more body systems, producing one or more symptoms such as hives, itching, stridor, wheezing, or shock. These signs and symptoms lead to the clinical diagnosis of anaphylaxis. Laboratory and other diagnostic tests may be done to rule out other possible causes for the symptoms, but there is no test to confirm the diagnosis of anaphylaxis.

Treatment and Nursing Management

Treatment of anaphylaxis includes:

- Establishing a patent airway and administering oxygen to relieve the symptoms of dyspnea and hypoxia.
- Administering aqueous epinephrine to counteract the effect of histamine: relax the bronchioles, increase the cardiac output, and elevate the blood pressure.
- Administering antihistamine (diphenhydramine hydrochloride [Benadryl]) to stop the effects of the histamine released by the body cells.
- Instituting measures to control shock.
- Providing psychological support during the course of the problem and its treatment.

People who are aware of their extreme sensitivity to certain substances should wear an identification giving that information. In this way, any health care provider will be forewarned if the person requires emergency treatment and is unable to communicate with medical personnel. Multiple companies offer "medical jewelry" that can relay pertinent information. It also is advisable for individuals who are highly allergic to stings from bees, wasps, or other insects, or severely allergic to nuts or some other food, to carry with them a small kit containing epinephrine, syringe, needle, tourniquet, and diphenhydramine hydrochloride. These kits are available, by prescription, from a pharmacy and are recommended by allergists due to how quickly a bee sting or similar event can be fatal to someone who is highly sensitive.

When there is difficulty with breathing due to swelling in the airway, high-flow oxygen is provided if the patient is breathing on his own. Assisted breathing is provided for those not able to breathe effectively. While the patient is still able to move air in and out, administration of inhaled medications to relax the airways is used to maintain breathing. If these measures are not effective, then an emergency tracheotomy or cricothyrotomy may need to be performed.

Epinephrine is given to counter the allergic reaction. It can be given intravenously, intramuscularly, or subcutaneously, depending on what route is most readily available. **If the patient is taking beta blockers, they will hinder the effectiveness of the epinephrine.** Diphenhydramine is also used to alleviate the symptoms of the allergic reaction. Corticosteroids may also be used to control the inflammatory response and reduce symptoms.

Diligent patient monitoring is essential. Any change in breathing or vital signs needs immediate intervention. The process of anaphylaxis can lead to shock. These events all may occur very rapidly. Adequate pharmacologic support and IV fluids are important in order to maintain perfusion and an adequate blood pressure. See Chapter 44 for information on treating shock.

The patient will experience extreme anxiety in the presence of a compromised airway. The nurse should make sure that a health care provider is with the patient at all times, for reassurance and to make certain that prompt actions are taken when indicated.

SERUM SICKNESS

Serum sickness is another type of generalized, widespread reaction to an antigenic substance. Usually the antigen is a drug or a foreign serum such as the immunizing sera that confer passive immunity.

Serum sickness develops more slowly, occurring over a period of 2 to 3 weeks after injection of the drug. It presents with less serious symptoms and usually is self-limiting. Symptoms commonly associated with serum sickness include skin rash, edema, joint pain and swelling, renal vasculitis, swelling of lymph nodes, and sometimes high fever and prostration. Treatment most often involves administration of antihistamine and aspirin, the latter being helpful in reducing the inflammatory reaction that often affects the joints. More serious symptoms require treatment similar to that for anaphylaxis.

AUTOIMMUNE DISORDERS

Autoimmune disorders not mentioned in this chapter are discussed in chapters dealing with the system in which the symptoms are most prevalent. For example, rheumatoid arthritis and similar disorders are discussed in Chapter 32, psoriasis is discussed in Chapter 42, and multiple sclerosis is covered in Chapter 24 with the degenerative neurologic disorders.

Etiology and Pathophysiology

Autoimmune disorders are thought to be caused by the immune system reacting against the body's own cells. Intense research is being conducted to increase understanding of the immune system and how the process starts that results in damage to and alteration in function of the body's own tissues. Autoimmune disorders have been categorized according to how extensively the disorder affects tissues (Table 11–6). The categories are referred to as systemic autoimmune diseases and localized autoimmune diseases. As implied by their names, disorders that affect many organs or tissues are considered systemic and disorders affecting only a single organ or tissue are considered local. The different diseases are covered within the system chapter of the body system most affected by the disease.

Signs and Symptoms

Since multiple tissues and organ systems may be involved, presenting signs and symptoms are variable. A specific disease may be identified that has as an autoimmune disorder as a root cause. Table 11–6 gives a partial list of diseases thought to be caused by autoimmunity. Not all experts agree on which diseases belong on the list, but at this time more than 80 diseases are thought to be triggered by an alteration in immune function. Some of the diseases have other etiologies in addition to autoimmunity, and some are thought to be primarily a disorder of the immune system.

Diagnosis

The diagnosis of autoimmune disorders can be very difficult. Symptoms tend to be vague and intermittent in early stages of some conditions. A complete physical examination should be conducted. Symptoms such as pain, fatigue, and dizziness cannot be measured by a test and must be evaluated by the report of the patient. Some clinicians are not as quick to credit self-reporting that cannot be validated by an objective test. This can be frustrating for patients looking for a diagnosis. Many tests are done to rule out conditions that have similar symptoms.

Blood tests that evaluate immune function, including a complete blood count with differential, will be performed. Some immune disorders are associated with a specific antibody that can be detected in the blood. Other laboratory tests evaluating inflammation, such as sedimentation rate and C-reactive protein levels, are not specific to immune disorders, but may help confirm the diagnosis when used with other information. For disorders that are organ specific, a biopsy of the affected tissue may be done.

Treatment and Nursing Management

Treatment falls into two categories: (1) replacement or support of lost or ineffective function, and (2) therapies targeted to halt the destructive process. In medication therapy for autoimmune disorders, the chemical treatment is aimed at altering cell function to prevent further harmful effects, not kill the cells. Identification and treatment of autoimmune disorders is a rapidly growing field. Current research should be consulted regularly to stay abreast of new developments.

SYSTEMIC LUPUS ERYTHEMATOSUS

Etiology and Pathophysiology

Systemic lupus erythematosus (SLE) is also known as lupus. There are several forms of the disease, but the most commonly known type is the systemic form. As with most autoimmune disorders, the cause is not known. Research indicates that genetics as well as environmental influences play a role in the development of the disease. A variety of drugs can cause a lupus-like syndrome, including oral contraceptives, hydralazine, and procainamide.

SLE occurs from an abnormal reaction of the body against serum proteins and its own cells; it is an autoimmune disease. Inflammation, blood vessel abnormalities, and immune complex deposition in tissues occur throughout the body. SLE usually waxes and

Table 11–6 ***Autoimmune Disorders and Body Systems Affected***

SYSTEMIC AUTOIMMUNE DISEASES	LOCALIZED AUTOIMMUNE DISEASES
Rheumatoid arthritis (joints; less commonly lungs, skin)	Type 1 diabetes mellitus (pancreatic islet cells)
Systemic lupus erythematosus (skin, joints, kidneys, heart, brain, red blood cells)	Hashimoto's thyroiditis, Graves' disease (thyroid)
Scleroderma (skin, intestine; less commonly lungs)	Celiac disease, Crohn's disease, ulcerative colitis (gastrointestinal tract)
Sjögren syndrome (salivary glands, tear glands, joints)	Multiple sclerosis, Guillain-Barré syndrome (central nervous system)
Goodpasture syndrome (lungs, kidneys)	Addison's disease (adrenal glands)
Wegener's granulomatosis (nasal sinuses, lungs, kidneys)	Primary biliary sclerosis, primary sclerosing cholangitis, autoimmune hepatitis (liver)
Polymyalgia rheumatica (large muscle groups)	Raynaud's phenomenon (fingers, toes, nose, ears)
Temporal arteritis/giant cell arteritis (arteries of the head and neck)	

wanes throughout the course of the disease. Some individuals have a very mild form of the disorder and have infrequent flare-ups with minimal symptoms. Others have severe, debilitating symptoms sometimes leading to death. Individuals of all ages have been diagnosed with SLE. However, African American women of childbearing age in the United States are affected the most frequently. Most patients are diagnosed between the ages of 20 and 45. Prior to 1955, the 5-year survival rate was less than 50%. In 2006, the 10-year survival rate is reported at 90%.

Signs and Symptoms

Signs and symptoms include painful or swollen joints and muscle pain, unexplained fever, red rash usually on the face, unusual loss of hair, sensitivity to the sun, extreme fatigue and weakness, mouth ulcers, and swollen glands (Figure 11–5). Because the symptoms are similar to those for other conditions and they come and go, it can be difficult to diagnose the disorder. All body systems can be affected (Figure 11–6). If the kidneys are affected, it may result in nephrotic syndrome or acute or chronic renal failure that leads to dialysis. (see Chapter 34). Neurologic symptoms may range from headaches to seizures and cognitive disorders. Pleurisy may develop, or shortness of breath and pulmonary hypertension. Heart failure, pericarditis, and coronary disease may also be symptomatic of SLE (see Chapters 19 and 20).

Diagnosis

There is no one test that confirms a diagnosis of SLE. A complete medical history is very important for diagnosing SLE. Typically the patient shows evidence of a multiorgan disorder. Blood tests that will be done to help confirm the diagnosis include antinuclear antibody levels, complete blood count, urinalysis, and tests for renal and liver function. A syphilis test measures antiphospholipid antibodies in the blood, which are known to be present in lupus, so a false-positive syphilis test is another indicator of SLE. Tests for signs of inflammation include obtaining an erythrocyte sedimentation rate and C-reactive protein level. Current research is focusing on identifying biomarkers that indicate SLE is present. This will allow for development of laboratory tests for diagnostic purposes and may provide a better understanding of the nature of the disease for treatment development.

Treatment

Current treatments are targeted at symptom control. There is no intervention that is curative. Medications including nonsteroidal anti-inflammatory drugs are used for pain control. The antimalarial drugs chloroquine and hydroxychloroquine are used for treatment of joint and skin problems. Hydroxychloroquine is currently the only antimalarial drug approved by the FDA for use in lupus. Glucocorticoids such as prednisone are used for major flare-ups. Long-term use of steroids causes multiple complications. Immunosuppressives, including azathioprine and cyclophosphamide, are used to control systemic symptoms of lupus. Mycophenolate mofetil, an antirejection drug devel-

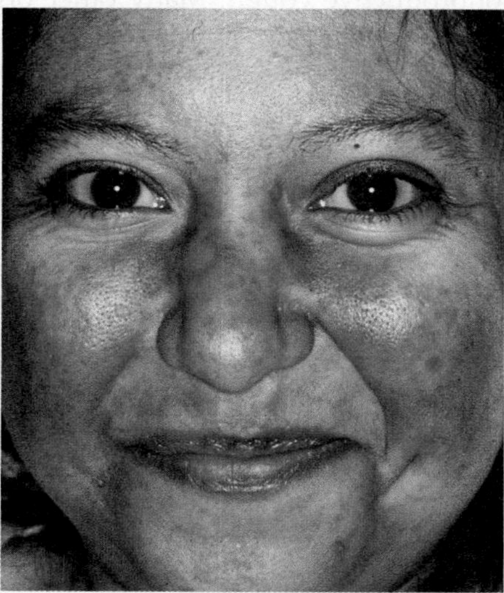

FIGURE 11–5 The characteristic "butterfly" rash of systemic lupus erythematosus.

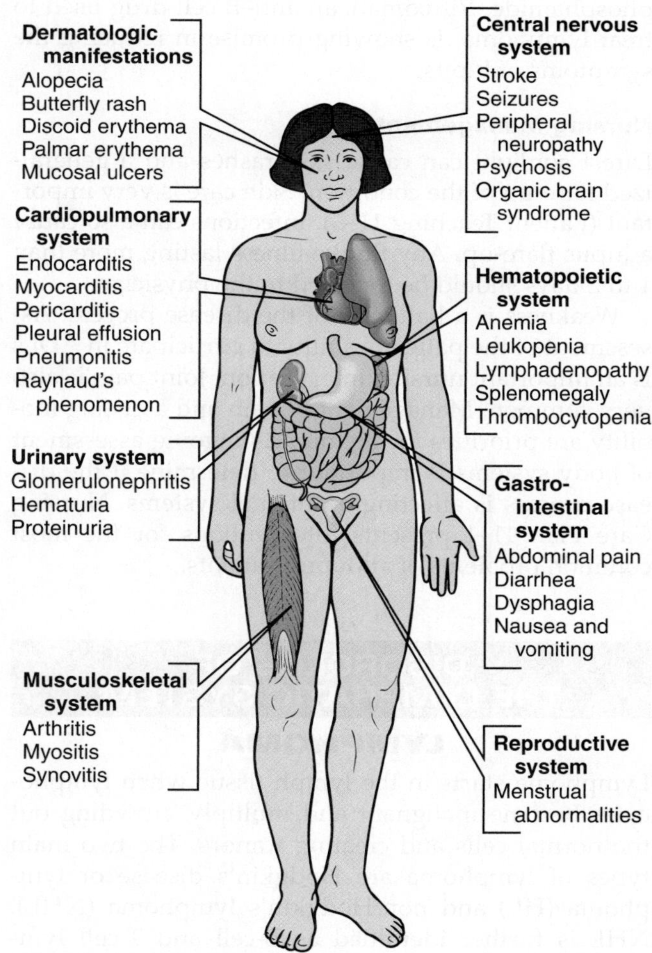

FIGURE 11–6 Multisystem involvement in systemic lupus erythematosus.

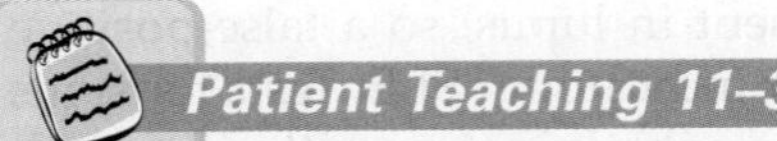

Patient Teaching 11–3

Skin Protection for Patients with Systemic Lupus Erythematosus

The patient with systemic lupus erythematosus should be taught the following:

- Avoid direct sunlight and any other type of ultraviolet lighting, including tanning beds.
- Use an SPF 30 or higher sunblock when outdoors.
- Wear long pants, a long-sleeved shirt, and a wide-brimmed hat when in the sun.
- Cleanse the skin only with a mild soap such as Ivory.
- Dry the skin thoroughly by patting rather than rubbing it.
- Apply lotion liberally to dry skin areas at least twice a day.
- Avoid using alcohol-based skin care products, face powder, or other astringent agents.
- Use cosmetics that contain moisturizers.
- Inspect the skin daily for rashes and open areas.

Adapted from Ignatavicius, D.D., & Workman, M.L. (2006). *Medical-Surgical Nursing: Critical Thinking for Collaborative Care* (5th ed.). Philadelphia: Elsevier Saunders, p. 412.

oped to prevent heart transplant rejection, is showing promise in treatment of lupus in the place of cyclophosphamide. Rituximab, an anti–B cell drug used to treat lymphoma, is showing promise in reducing the symptoms of lupus.

Nursing Management

Direct sunlight can cause skin rashes and a generalized flare-up of the condition. Skin care is very important (Patient Teaching 11–3). Infections can also cause a lupus flare-up. Any flulike illness lasting more than 1 to 2 days should be reported to the physician.

Weakness is a hallmark of the disease process. Assessment of the patient's ability to participate in ADLs is an important nursing intervention. Joint pain is also very common. Management of pain and assisting mobility are priorities for the nurse. Ongoing assessment of body systems is important to determine if the disease process is affecting additional systems. Nursing Care Plan 11–1 presents interventions for the most common problems of all lupus patients.

DISORDERS OF THE LYMPHATIC SYSTEM

LYMPHOMA

Lymphoma starts in the lymph tissue when lymphocytes become malignant and multiply, crowding out the normal cells and creating tumors. The two main types of lymphoma are Hodgkin's disease or lymphoma (HL) and non-Hodgkin's lymphoma (NHL). NHL is further identified as B-cell and T-cell lymphoma. There are five subtypes of HL and 30 subtypes of NHL. Because there are so many variations of these diseases, classification is complicated and relies on microscopic examination of tissues and the known extent of the disease. Many of the NHL subtypes look similar, but they are quite different and respond to different therapies with different success rates.

HODGKIN'S DISEASE

Etiology and Pathophysiology

Hodgkin's disease primarily affects young adults, but also occurs in those over 55 years of age. The cause is not known, but research shows that there is possibly a genetic component as well as environmental factors that in combination trigger the onset of the disease. Implicated as possible triggers are viral infections, particularly with the Epstein-Barr virus, and previous exposure to various chemical agents. The American Cancer Society estimates 8190 new cases will be diagnosed in 2007. The current survival rates are 85% at 5 years and 77% at 10 years. It is one of the most curable of cancers when diagnosed early.

The malignant lymph cells multiply and replace normal cells in the nodes and lymph tissue. It is not know how the disease spreads from one area to another. The disease is staged depending on the area of the body, with affected nodes or tissues, and whether involvement is above or below the diaphragm or both (Figure 11–7).

Signs and Symptoms

The disorder often is discovered when swollen lymph nodes are found on a routine examination or an employment physical examination. Some patients experience remittent fever, night sweats, or unexplained weight loss. Severe pruritus is an early sign. A small percentage of patients affected by Hodgkin's disease will experience pain in the lymph nodes after consumption of alcohol. While not a common finding, when present it is considered diagnostic for Hodgkin's disease. If there is a mediastinal mass of involved lymph tissue, the patient may have a nonproductive cough. Many other organs can become affected, as displayed in Figure 11–8.

Diagnosis, Treatment, and Nursing Management

A definitive diagnosis is made by the presence of Reed-Sternberg cells in the tissues obtained by biopsy of the lymph nodes. X-rays, computed tomography scans, and positron emission tomography scans are used to help diagnose the disease.

Treatment depends on how far the disease has progressed. Box 11–6 presents the classification of stages for Hodgkin's disease. Remission and cure often are achieved with the use of radiation, chemotherapy, or both. For stages I and II, administration of doxorubicin (Adriamycin), bleomycin, vinblastine, and dacarbazine, or ABVD therapy, has proven the most successful. With proper treatment, the 20-year disease-free survival rate is 70% to 80%. Stage III and IV disease shows better improvement with mechlorethamine, vincristine (Oncovin), procarbazine, and prednisone, or MOPP therapy, in combination with ABVD therapy. The number of cycles of chemotherapy depends on the stage of the disease and the response of the patient. Patients may experience many complications from the disease itself or from the chemotherapy and radiation.

A thorough health history should be obtained from the patient, including family history. Documentation of symptoms, their severity, and how long they have been present is important. Nursing care focuses on symptoms and the side effects of the therapy. The nursing diagnoses, expected outcomes, and interventions for

NURSING CARE PLAN 11–1

Care of the Patient with Systemic Lupus Erythematosus (SLE)

SCENARIO Julie Hansen, age 37, has just been diagnosed with SLE. She has flat erythema in a butterfly pattern over the face, is complaining of joint pain in her knees and elbows, and has experienced constant fatigue and weakness for the past 6 months. Her ESR is elevated and she has a positive ANA. Other tests helped confirm the physician's diagnosis. She lives with her husband and 12- and 14-year-old son and daughter.

PROBLEM/NURSING DIAGNOSIS *Weakness and fatigue*/Activity intolerance related to inflammatory nature of the disease as evidenced by need for increased rest and sleep and inability to keep up with household chores along with work.

Supporting assessment data *Subjective:* States she cannot keep the laundry done or the house clean as she is so tired when she comes home from work. Has been using more and more "fast food" for family dinners.

Goals/Expected Outcomes	*Nursing Interventions*	*Selected Rationale*	*Evaluation*
Patient will be able to manage household along with work with help within 6 wk.	Explore chores that other family members may be able to take over.	Husband and children could help with cleaning, laundry, errands, and meal preparation.	Daughter will wash the clothes and son will fold and put them away. Husband will do errands. All members will assist with meal preparation and cleanup.
	Assist to work out a schedule for rest periods at lunchtime, after work, and on the weekends.	Resting for 30 min at lunchtime eases fatigue.	Will try to find a place at or near her workplace where she can rest at lunchtime. Continue plan.
	Assist to plan meals for the week and to cook large quantities of items on the weekend that can be divided into individual meals and frozen for family dinners.	It is less fatiguing to cook large quantities of entrees once a week and to freeze portions than to prepare a dinner every day.	Will consider what meals might be cooked ahead on the weekends and frozen. Continue plan.

PROBLEM/NURSING DIAGNOSIS *Painful knees and elbows*/Chronic pain related to inflammation from disease process.

Supporting assessment data *Subjective:* "My knees and elbows ache whenever I have walked for more than a block or used my arms to lift things frequently during a day." *Objective:* Tenderness around elbow and knee joints.

Goals/Expected Outcomes	*Nursing Interventions*	*Selected Rationale*	*Evaluation*
Patient will experience fewer days of pain with regular use of anti-inflammatory.	Instruct to take 400 mg of ibuprofen tid on a regular basis.	Keeping a steady blood level of the drug will help decrease and prevent inflammation.	States will begin taking the prescribed regimen of ibuprofen. Continue plan.
	Advise to let family lift heavy items and do chores requiring repetitive elbow motion or squatting.	Refraining from lifting, repetitive joint motion, and squatting helps prevent joint strain and added inflammation.	States will let family bring in groceries and put them away. Will remind family to pick up around the house every other day. Will refrain from gardening down on her knees. Continue plan.

Key: *ANA*, antinuclear antibody; *ESR*, erythrocyte sedimentation rate; *SPF*, sun protection factor.

Continued

NURSING CARE PLAN 11-1

Care of the Patient with Systemic Lupus Erythematosus (SLE)—cont'd

PROBLEM/NURSING DIAGNOSIS *Reddened area over much of face*/Risk for impaired skin integrity related to "butterfly" rash and sun sensitivity from disease process.

Supporting assessment data *Subjective:* States sunburns very easily. *Objective:* Inflamed rash in butterfly pattern over large part of face.

Goals/Expected Outcomes	Nursing Interventions	Selected Rationale	Evaluation
Patient's skin will remain intact.	Instruct in proper skin care with mild soap and alcohol/astringent-free products.	Avoiding harsh skin care products will help prevent excoriation and breaks in the skin.	States will check her skin-care products for alcohol and astringents.
	Instruct to moisturize the skin twice daily.	Moisturizing products will help keep skin supple and prevent breaks.	Will begin moisturizing a second time a day before bedtime. Continue plan.
	Instruct to inspect the skin closely for any breaks or new lesions.	Finding breaks in the skin promptly and caring for them properly will help prevent infection.	Will begin to inspect skin after shower daily. Continue plan.
	Instruct to cover skin when out in the sun and to avoid ultraviolet rays as much as possible.	Protecting the skin from sunlight will help prevent flare-ups of the disease and will protect the skin from further damage.	Will wear suggested clothing of long sleeves, long pants, and a wide-brimmed hat when out in the sun.
	Instruct to use an SPF sunblock product of 30 or more when outdoors.	Sunblock helps prevent the damage that can occur from ultraviolet rays.	States will use sunblock on a daily basis on exposed parts of skin.
	Instruct to stop going to the tanning salon.	Ultraviolet light damages the skin and can cause a flare-up or progression of SLE symptoms.	States hates to give it up, but will refrain from going to tanning salon.

? CRITICAL THINKING QUESTIONS

1. What types of entrees could you suggest that could be fixed ahead in large quantities and then frozen in family-sized portions?
2. What might you suggest as ways to rest at lunchtime when the patient is at work on weekdays?

the patient with Hodgkin's disease are the same as those for the patient with leukemia (see Chapter 16).

NON-HODGKIN'S LYMPHOMA

Etiology, Pathophysiology, and Signs and Symptoms

The American Cancer Society predicts 63,190 new cases of NHL will be diagnosed in 2007. Part of the increase over previous years is related to its occurrence in AIDS patients. There is an abnormal proliferation of neoplastic lymphocytes in patients with NHL. The cause of lymphoma is unknown, but viruses, immunosuppression, and age are all thought to be possible contributors. Since the 1970s, the incidence has increased in those over age 65. NHL is the sixth most common cancer in males and the fifth most common cancer in females in the United States.

This type of lymphoma tends to have more widespread involvement of lymphoid tissue than found in Hodgkin's disease. NHL tumors can occur in the bone, GI tract, spleen, respiratory system, brain, or other parts of the body. NHL usually presents as a unilateral, painless enlargement of a lymph node that may progress to generalized, painless lymphadenopathy. The cervical lymph nodes are the most commonly affected initially. Other symptoms are nonspecific but may include fever, night sweats, and weight loss greater than 10% of baseline body weight. As the tumor enlarges, it spreads to adjacent lymph nodes or organs. Symptoms related to other organs are site specific and include nausea, vomiting, elevated liver enzymes, cough, shortness of breath, high fevers, chills, night sweats, and elevated intracranial pressure. Hepatomegaly or splenomegaly occurs in about one third of patients.

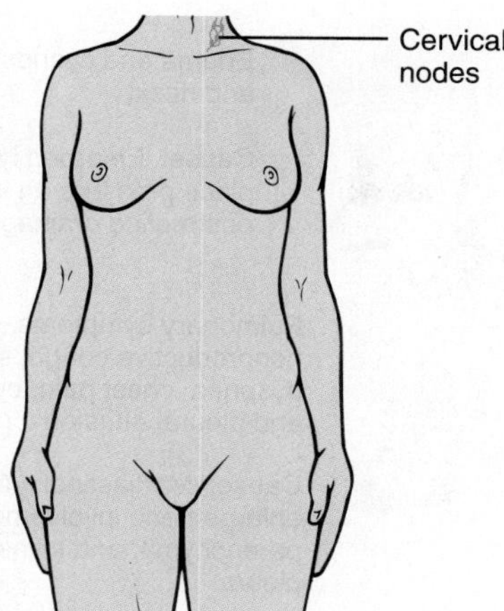

Stage I
Involvement of a single lymph node or a single extranodal site

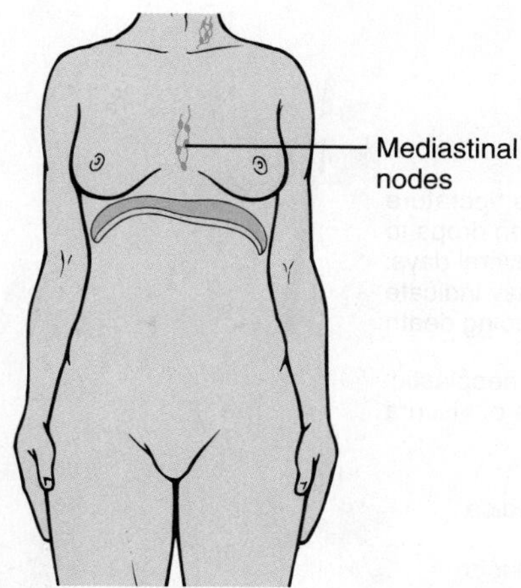

Stage II
Involvement of two or more lymph node regions on the same side of the diaphragm or localized involvement of an extranodal site and one or more lymph node regions of the same side of diaphragm

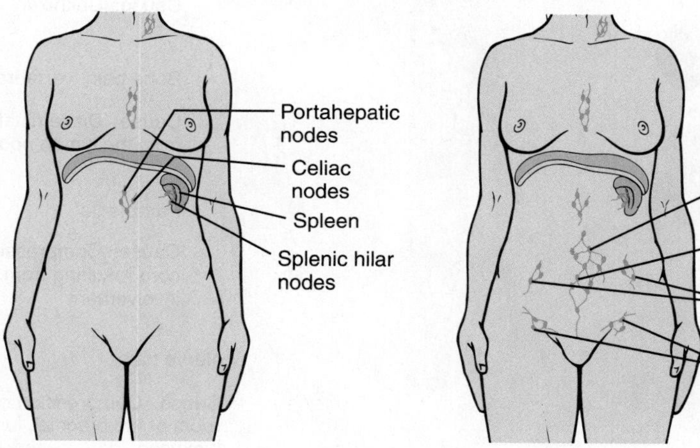

Stage III
Involvement of lymph node regions on both sides of the diaphragm. May include a single extranodal site, the spleen, or both; now subdivided into lymphatic involvement of the upper abdomen in the spleen (splenic, celiac, and portal nodes) (*Stage* III_1) and the lower abdominal nodes in the para-aortic, mesenteric, and iliac regions (*Stage* III_2)

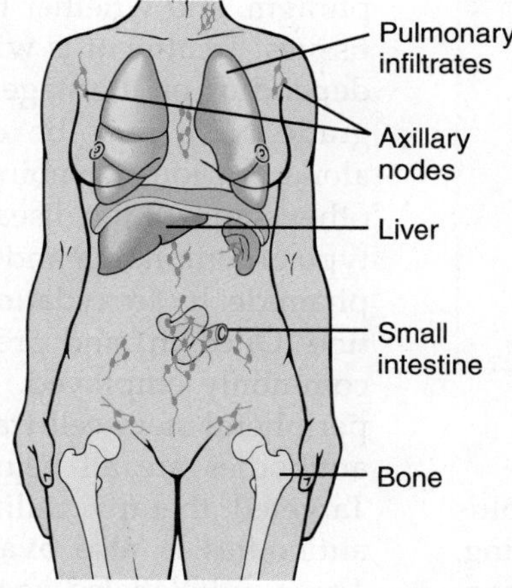

Stage IV
Diffuse or disseminated disease of one or more extralymphatic organs or tissues with or without associated lymph node involvement; the extranodal site is identified as *H*, hepatic; *L*, lung; *P*, pleura; *M*, marrow; *D*, dermal; *O*, osseous

FIGURE 11–7 Staging of Hodgkin's lymphoma.

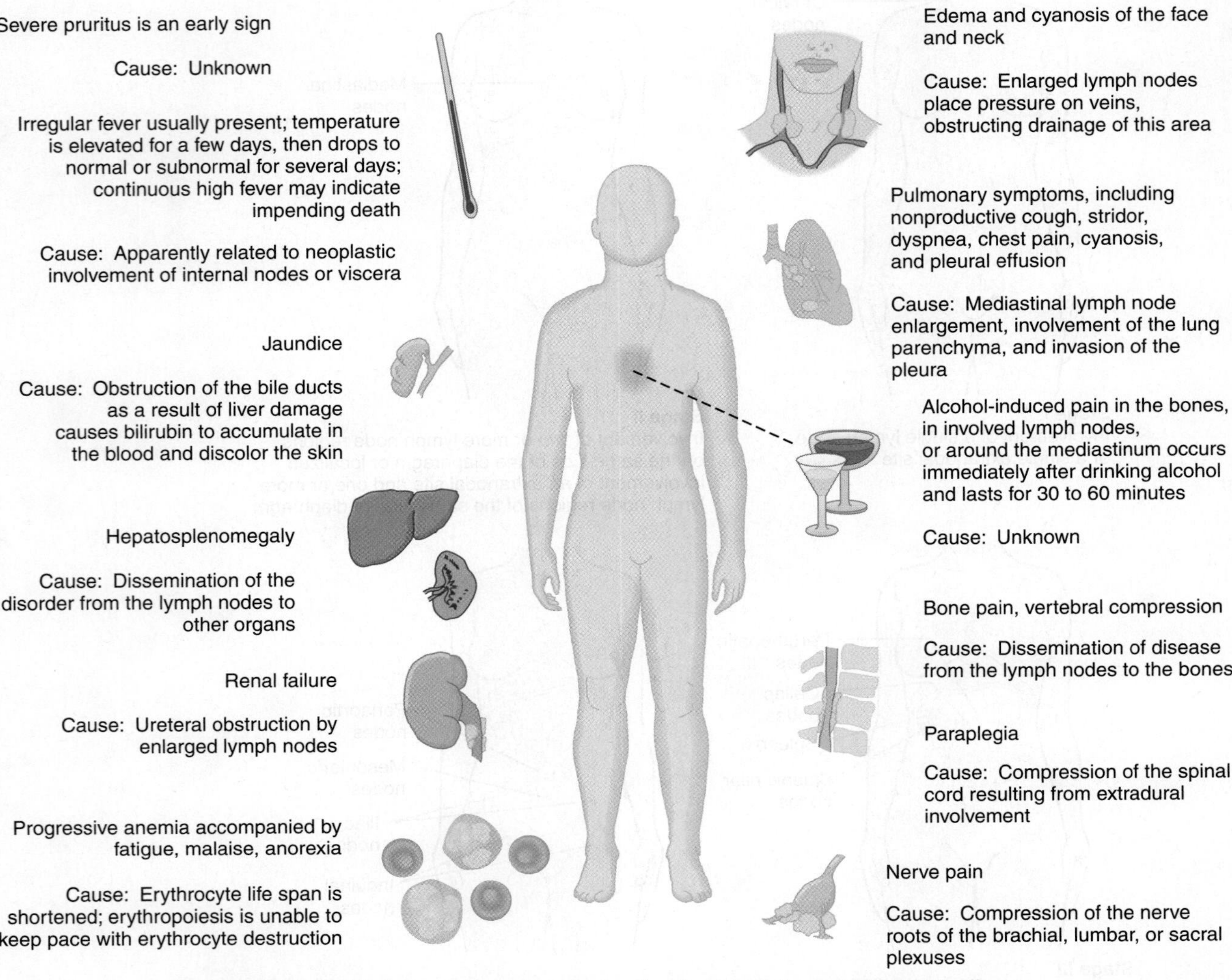

FIGURE **11–8** Clinical manifestations and pathophysiologic basis of Hodgkin's disease.

Box 11–6 ***Stages of Hodgkin's Disease***

- **Stage I** indicates one lymph node region is involved (e.g., the right neck).
- **Stage II** indicates involvement of two lymph nodes on the same side of the diaphragm (e.g., both sides of the neck).
- **Stage III** indicates lymph node involvement on both sides of the diaphragm (e.g., groin and armpit).
- **Stage IV** involves the spread of cancer outside the lymph nodes (e.g., to bone marrow, lungs, or liver).

Diagnosis and Treatment

Diagnosis is by history and physical examination, plus blood studies and lymph node biopsy. During staging, computed tomography and magnetic resonance imaging are used to determine the extent of tissue involvement. Bone marrow biopsy is an important tool.

The effectiveness of treatment depends on the stage of the tumor when diagnosed and the aggressiveness of the type of lymphoma present. Staging considers the number and location of affected lymph nodes, whether the nodes are on one or both sides of the diaphragm, and whether the disease has spread to other tissues. Treatment is with chemotherapy or radiation, depending on the stage of disease. Stage I or II or low-grade NHL may be cured with radiation therapy alone. Various combinations of drugs are used for other stages of the disease depending on the identified type of lymphoma and its aggressiveness. Cyclophosphamide, hydroxydaunomycin (doxorubicin), vincristine (Oncovin) and prednisone, or CHOP therapy, is commonly employed. Bone marrow transplantation, peripheral stem cell transplantation, and monoclonal antibodies are all being used as treatment options. Targeted therapy utilizing radiolabeled monoclonal antibodies is also available for treatment of NHL. These radiolabeled agents recognize and react to kill specific tumor cells. The drug used is ibritumomab tiuxetan labeled with yttrium-90 (Zevalin). Other experimental therapies are under study.

Surgery may be employed if the tumor is localized. Radiation is used together with chemotherapy or surgery. HAART in conjunction with anticancer drugs seems to hold promise even for AIDS patients with advanced NHL. Vaccines are currently in clinical trials. They are being used to prevent a recurrence of the disease after it has been treated with chemotherapy. Overall, the 1-year relative survival rate for NHL is 70% and the 5-year survival rate is 51%.

Nursing Management

Nursing care is directed toward supporting the patient through the diagnostic process and observing and treating the side effects of radiation and chemotherapy. If bone marrow or stem cell transplants are performed, nursing care and patient education must focus on prevention of infection and other complications. Chapter 8 contains information on specific nursing diagnoses and interventions for the patient with cancer. Common nursing diagnoses for the NHL patient include:

- Risk for infection related to neutropenia from chemotherapy or radiation
- Ineffective protection/risk for hemorrhage related to thrombocytopenia secondary to treatment
- Fatigue
- Imbalanced nutrition: less than body requirements
- Disturbed body image
- Risk for ineffective therapeutic regimen management

Expected outcomes might include:

- Patient will not experience infection.
- Patient will not experience hemorrhage.
- Fatigue will lessen after 6 weeks of treatment.
- Patient will gain 2 lb per week until desired weight is reached.
- Patient will join a support group and work to incorporate his body image.
- Patient will maintain his therapeutic regimen during treatment cycles.

Nursing interventions are similar to those for the problems of leukemia (see Chapter 16).

LYMPHEDEMA

Swelling of the tissues drained by the lymphatic system occurs as a result of obstruction to the flow of lymph along the vessels. The primary form is especially common in the lower extremities and other dependent organs. The obstruction is the result of a congenital condition in which there is deficient growth of the lymphatic system in a lower extremity. This condition chiefly affects females and most often becomes apparent during the middle teens to early 20s.

Lymphedema may also be secondary to an obstruction caused by trauma to the lymph vessels and nodes, such as occurs during mastectomy when lymph nodes are removed. Other causes of obstruction include extensive soft-tissue injury and scar formation and, in tropical countries, parasites that enter lymph channels and block them. Regardless of the etiology, treatment goals are to minimize the impact of the disease process on the individual. There is no cure for the condition.

The lymphatic system drains water, proteins, and lipids from the interstitial spaces and returns it to the blood vessels. Proteins are large molecules and attract water. When the lymph system is unable to transport the proteins, large amounts of fluid accumulate, causing swelling. This fluid causes further damage to surrounding tissues. The area of the body affected by lymphedema is prone to infection and possible malignancy. The skin overlying the swollen area thickens and often develops cracks and furrows.

Lymphedema that involves an extremity often can be treated conservatively using simple nursing measures. Prevention and treatment of lymphedema of the arm and hand following mastectomy are covered in Chapter 38. Surgical intervention is palliative at best and is controversial as a treatment option. A compression sleeve or legging is often useful (Patient Teaching 11–4).

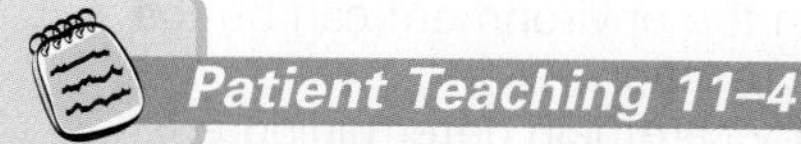

Measures to Prevent or Decrease Lymphedema

Teach the patient to:

- Elevate the extremity to the level of the heart. This reduces hydrostatic pressure within the veins.
- Cleanse and dry the skin thoroughly and regularly, applying gentle skin moisturizers to prevent cracking.
- Perform active exercise of the skeletal muscles. This promotes massage of the lymph vessels and the movement of lymph.
- Apply elasticized stockings or gloves when up and active. This increases pressure on vessels and encourages venous return. (Garments may be removed when the extremity can be elevated.)
- Avoid as much as possible even minor trauma to the area.
- Avoid constrictive clothing.
- Not allow blood pressure to be taken on the affected extremity or blood to be drawn from it.

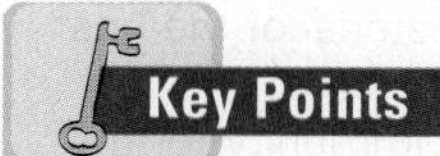

- Disorders of the immune system involve a deficiency or an inappropriate response.
- AIDS is caused by infection with the human immunodeficiency virus.
- Opportunistic infections secondary to AIDS cause increased morbidity and mortality.
- Management of AIDS includes controlling symptoms and preventing the spread of infection.
- Health care workers must implement standard precautions when working with any patient.
- Immunosuppression may be used therapeutically for patients undergoing tissue transplants.
- Special precautions must be taken for patients who are immunosuppressed.

- Many substances in the environment can be the cause of an allergic reaction.
- Nurses must be very careful in determining a patient's existing allergies prior to medication administration.
- Anaphylaxis is a life-threatening condition.
- Emergency equipment and medications must be available when potentially allergenic substances are administered.
- Autoimmune disorders are thought to be caused by the immune system reacting to the body's own cells.
- Autoimmune disorders are treated by suppressing the immune system.
- Lymphoma starts in the lymph tissue when malignant lymphocytes multiply and crowd out normal cells.
- Hodgkin's disease and non-Hodgkin's lymphoma are thought to be possibly triggered by environmental factors.
- The Epstein-Barr virus is linked to many cases of Hodgkin's disease. A genetic factor may be present as well.
- Non-Hodgkin's lymphoma is growing in incidence as the population achieves greater age.
- Treatment for lymphoma depends on staging and aggressiveness of the particular type of the disease.
- Nursing care for lymphomas focuses on preventing infection and managing the symptoms of the disease and the side effects of the therapies.
- Lymphedema may be congenital or secondary to injury or surgical removal of lymph nodes.

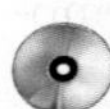
Go to your **Companion CD-ROM** for an Audio Glossary, animations, video clips, and bonus review questions.

evolve Be sure to visit the companion Evolve site at http://evolve.elsevier.com/deWit/ for interactive NCLEX-PN Exam Style Review Questions, WebLinks, and additional online resources.

NCLEX-PN EXAM STYLE REVIEW QUESTIONS

Choose the best answer(s) for the following questions.

1. Which of the following statements are true regarding human immunodeficiency virus transmission? *(Select all that apply.)*

1. Breast milk can harbor the virus.
2. Proper use of personal protective equipment reduces the risk of disease transmission.
3. Needle exchange programs facilitate the spread of the virus.
4. Needle-stick injuries place health professionals at risk.
5. Monogamous relationships provide the best defense from the virus.

2. The nurse reinforces the physician's order to draw blood for a human immunodeficiency virus test. The patient asks, "What is the human immunodeficiency virus?" She explains that:

1. the test confirms the presence of the autoimmune disease.
2. the virus changes the genetic material of the host cell.
3. the test would ensure a lifelong immunity to the virus.
4. presence of the virus indicates full-blown acquired immunodeficiency syndrome.

3. A patient who is known to be positive for human immunodeficiency virus is admitted with oral thrush, recurrent vaginal yeast infections, and skin infections. The nurse suspects that these signs indicate:

1. opportunistic infection.
2. antibiotic resistance.
3. immunosuppression.
4. sentinel infection.

4. The nurse anticipates that the physician would order which of the following laboratory tests to determine the stage of human immunodeficiency virus status, the timing of the initiation of therapy, and the prophylactic management of opportunistic infections?

1. Blood culture and sensitivity
2. Western blot test
3. T-cell count
4. Enzyme-linked immunospecific assay

5. In determining the optimal therapy for a patient infected with the human immunodeficiency virus, the physician considers which of the following? *(Select all that apply.)*

1. Clinical data
2. Compliance with therapy
3. Medication tolerance
4. Insurance coverage
5. Physician expectations

6. The nurse explains the mechanism of action of the zidovudine, a nucleoside reverse transcriptase inhibitor (NRTI) to a patient who is newly diagnosed with acquired immunodeficiency syndrome. An accurate statement by the nurse would be:

1. "It cures the viral infection."
2. "It inhibits viral reproduction by disabling conversion of RNA to DNA."
3. "It prevents formation of viral protein precursors."
4. "It facilitates the production of immature, noninfectious viral particles."

7. A patient with cytomegalovirus retinitis was prescribed foscarnet (Foscavir). Which of the following requires immediate nursing attention before this medication is administered?

1. Elevated serum creatinine
2. Decreased CD4 lymphocytes
3. Fever
4. Acyclovir-resistant viral infection

8. A patient presents with difficulty breathing associated with cough, fever, weight loss, and night sweats. An appropriate nursing action would be to:
   1. initiate extended precautions.
   2. prohibit visitors.
   3. administer antiparasitic medications.
   4. monitor intake and output.

9. The physician gives instructions to a patient with a transplant regarding the use of immunosuppressive drugs. Which of the following patient statements indicates a need for further instructions?
   1. "These medications put me at risk for various types of infections."
   2. "Organ rejection is no longer my concern."
   3. "Some of my body's defense would remain intact."
   4. "My physician would adjust the dosage of these medications, depending on my response."

10. The nurse admits an elderly man with acute alcoholism. On initial assessment, the nurse notes that the patient is slightly confused, irritable, emaciated, has poor dentition, and is homeless. A likely nursing diagnosis would be:
    1. Risk for infection.
    2. Ineffective coping.
    3. Disturbed body image.
    4. Deficient knowledge.

CRITICAL THINKING ACTIVITIES

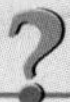

Read each clinical scenario and discuss the questions with your classmates.

Scenario A

Mark Johnson is an 80-year-old patient being admitted to the hospital for pneumonia. Five years ago he had a blood transfusion for treatment of injuries suffered in an automobile accident during a trip to Africa. He is now HIV positive, which was recently discovered. He has no other health problems. He is married and has three grown children and eight grandchildren.

1. What symptoms are displayed by someone who is HIV positive?
2. What should be discussed with his family regarding his HIV status?
3. How should his HIV infection be treated?

Scenario B

Mr. Watson is a 45-year-old patient who is admitted to the hospital for an abdominal hernia operation. You notice that he has cold symptoms, and you ask him about them. Mr. Watson replies that he is allergic to something and often has these symptoms.

1. How might you help Mr. Watson determine the airborne substance(s) to which he is allergic?
2. What techniques are used to determine foods that may be allergens?
3. What role does histamine play in the symptoms of an allergic reaction?
4. Why are antihistamines helpful in managing allergy symptoms?
5. What measures should be taken to avoid a fatal allergic reaction to drugs that are administered in a hospital or clinic?

Scenario C

Marilyn Jost, age 15, is a young friend of yours who is highly allergic to penicillin and bee stings. The last time she experienced a reaction to a bee sting on her leg, the entire limb became swollen. Marilyn is active in the teen church group and frequently goes on camping trips. Her physician has suggested that she wear an identification bracelet stating her allergies and that she carry an emergency kit when she is on a camping trip. Her mother sees no need for these precautions because Marilyn is a perfectly healthy girl. Marilyn says she wouldn't know what to do with the kit if she did get stung by a bee or wasp.

1. How would you explain to Marilyn and her mother the need for the identification bracelet and the kit?
2. How would you go about teaching Marilyn to use the emergency kit?

Scenario D

Cindy Lee, a 45-year-old single mother of two, is 4 months post left radical mastectomy. She works in an office full time and is having problems with lymphedema in her left arm.

1. What is the cause of lymphedema?
2. What will you recommend to Cindy to help reduce the problems she is having?
3. What resources are available for her?

CHAPTER 12 The Respiratory System

evolve http://evolve.elsevier.com/deWit

Objectives

Upon completion of this chapter, you should be able to:

Theory

1. Recall the structure and function of the respiratory system.
2. Identify three causative factors related to disorders of the respiratory system.
3. Provide instructions to patients on measures to prevent long-term problems of the respiratory system.
4. Employ proper techniques for assessing the respiratory system.
5. List nursing responsibilities for patients undergoing diagnostic tests and procedures for disorders of the respiratory system.

Clinical Practice

1. Verify that nursing diagnoses chosen for patients with problems of the respiratory system are appropriate.
2. Propose interventions for a patient who has a problem with oxygenation.
3. Teach a patient to cough effectively.

Key Terms

Be sure to check out the bonus material on the Companion CD-ROM, including selected audio pronunciations.

adventitious (ăd-vĕnt-TĪ-shŭs, p. 285)
antitussive (ăn-tĭ-TŬS-ĭv, p. 292)
aphonia (ă-FŌ-nē-a, p. 282)
apnea (ĂP-nē-a, p. 279)
bradypnea (brăd-ĕp-NĒ-ă, p. 283)
compliance (kŏm-PLĪ-ăns, p. 279)
crackles (KRĂK-ŭlz, p. 284)
dyspnea (DĬSP-nē-ă, p. 279)
hypercapnia (hī-pĕr-KĂP-nē-ă, p. 293)
hypocapnia (hī-pō-KĂP-nē-ă, p. 293)
hypoxia (hī-PŎK-sē-ă, p. 295)
kyphosis (kĭ-FŌ-sĭs, p. 279)
orthopnea (ŏr-thŏp-NĒ-ă, p. 293)
perfusion (pĕr-FŪ-zhŭn, p. 276)
rhonchi (RŎNG-kī, p. 284)
sequelae (sē-KWĒL-ă, p. 287)
sputum (SPŪ-tŭm, p. 283)
stridor (STRĪ-dŏr, p. 284)
tachypnea (tăk-ĭp-NĒ-ă, p. 283)
wheeze (wēz, p. 284)

When a problem interferes with the ability to breathe or with the diffusion of oxygen or carbon dioxide across the alveolar membranes into the capillaries, homeostasis of the whole body is affected. **Perfusion** (blood flow into cellular tissue) is also an essential part of respiration because the bloodstream carries the oxygen to the cells of the body. Blood must be pumped past the alveolar membrane for oxygen and carbon dioxide diffusion to take place. Then the blood must circulate to all parts of the body for the oxygen taken in through the lungs to reach the cells. Many problems can interfere with a healthy respiratory system. Trauma or disease can affect the structures of the respiratory system or the nerves controlling respiration. To understand these problems, a basic knowledge of the anatomy and physiology of the respiratory system is essential. A brief overview is provided to refresh the student's memory.

CAUSES OF RESPIRATORY DISORDERS

The respiratory system is particularly susceptible to harmful substances in the environment. Inhalation of bacteria and other organisms can quickly produce an infection in either the upper or lower respiratory tract. Tobacco smoke, allergens, poisonous gases, and other toxic substances cause irritation and inflammation of the air passages and can eventually lead to chronic inflammation, obstructive diseases, and tumors. There may be a familial tendency toward allergies, asthma, or other lung problems.

Because adequate exchange of oxygen and carbon dioxide depends on sufficient blood supply to lung tissues, cardiac disease, emboli, and other disorders of the heart and pulmonary blood vessels eventually cause problems in the respiratory system. Aside from infection of the respiratory tract, there are two major types of ventilatory diseases: *restrictive* and *obstructive*. Each group has different causative factors and pathophysiologic effects.

Restrictive diseases are a group of disorders characterized by decreased lung capacity. They are not necessarily primarily lung disorders, but their eventual effect is to limit expansion of the lung and chest wall, and they

Text continued on p. 280

OVERVIEW OF ANATOMY AND PHYSIOLOGY OF THE RESPIRATORY SYSTEM

What are the functions of each of the structures of the upper respiratory system?

- On its way to the lungs, air passes through the nose, mouth, pharynx, larynx, and trachea (Figure 12–1).
- The nasal cavity is lined with mucous membrane that warms and moistens the air as it passes through; moisture protects the cilia.
- The mucous membrane secretes mucus, which traps dust particles and bacteria.
- The *cilia* (small, hairlike projections) propel the mucus toward the larynx, where it can be swallowed or expectorated.
- The paranasal sinuses (maxillary, frontal, sphenoid, and ethmoid) are air-filled cavities lined with mucous membrane and situated among the facial bones around the nasal cavity (Figure 12–2).
- The sinuses reduce the weight of the skull, produce mucus, and influence voice quality.
- The pharynx is about 5 inches long and extends from the back of the mouth to the esophagus.
- The pharynx serves as a passageway for the respiratory tract and the gastrointestinal system, moving air to the lungs and food to the esophagus.
- The tonsils, which are part of the lymphatic system, are located in the pharynx; if they become inflamed and enlarged, they may interfere with breathing.
- The larynx is important to the formation of the sounds of speech.
- The epiglottis forms a hinged "door" at the entrance to the larynx.
- The larynx sits between the pharynx and the trachea. The vocal cords are located in the larynx.
- The trachea extends from the larynx to the bronchi; it is the "windpipe" and carries air to the lungs.
- The trachea is made up of cartilage, smooth muscle, and connective tissue and is lined with mucous membrane.

How does the epiglottis protect the airway?

- When swallowing is initiated, the epiglottis closes over the larynx, preventing food from entering it. The food is then directed into the esophagus.
- The epiglottis prevents aspiration of food and secretions into the lungs.
- When the swallowing reflex is weak or missing, aspiration is a risk.

How is speech produced in the larynx?

- The vocal cords are made up of mucous membrane attached to the front and back of the larynx.
- The glottis is the space between the folds of the vocal cords.

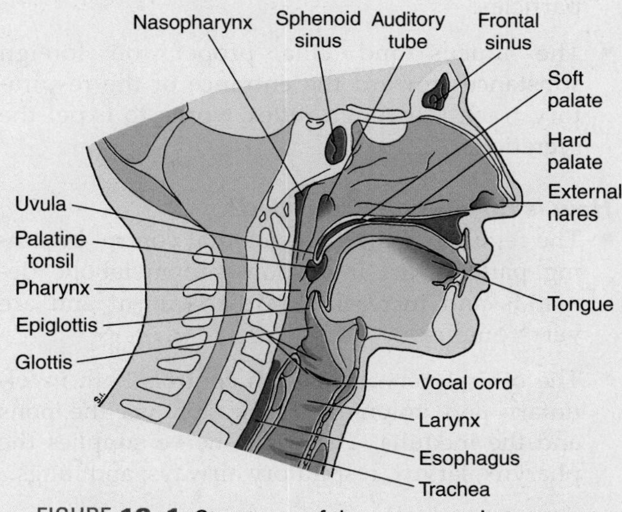

FIGURE **12–1** Structures of the upper respiratory tract.

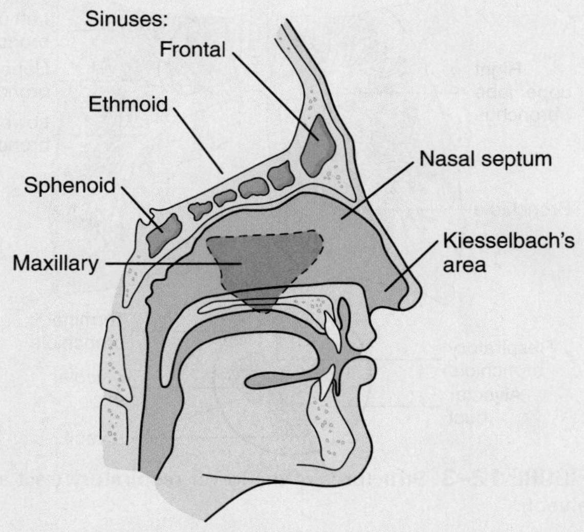

FIGURE **12–2** The paranasal sinuses.

Continued

OVERVIEW OF ANATOMY AND PHYSIOLOGY OF THE RESPIRATORY SYSTEM—cont'd

- When air from the lungs exits through the larynx, it causes rapid opening and closing of the glottis.
- Movements of the mouth, lips, jaws, and tongue convert the sounds made by the rush of air into speech sounds.

What are the functions of the structures of the lower respiratory system?

- After passing through the nose, pharynx, larynx, and trachea of the upper respiratory system, air enters the left and right bronchi, which branch off of the trachea.
- The bronchi carry air into the lungs; the right lung has three lobes, and the left lung has two lobes.

How is oxygen delivered to the alveolar membrane, where it can diffuse into the blood?

- The main bronchi divide into smaller, and smaller bronchi and then divide into bronchioles that deliver the air to the alveoli (Figure 12–3).
- The right bronchus angles off to the right; inhaled foreign objects tend to lodge here.
- Alveoli are tiny air sacs that come into contact with the pulmonary arterioles and venules.

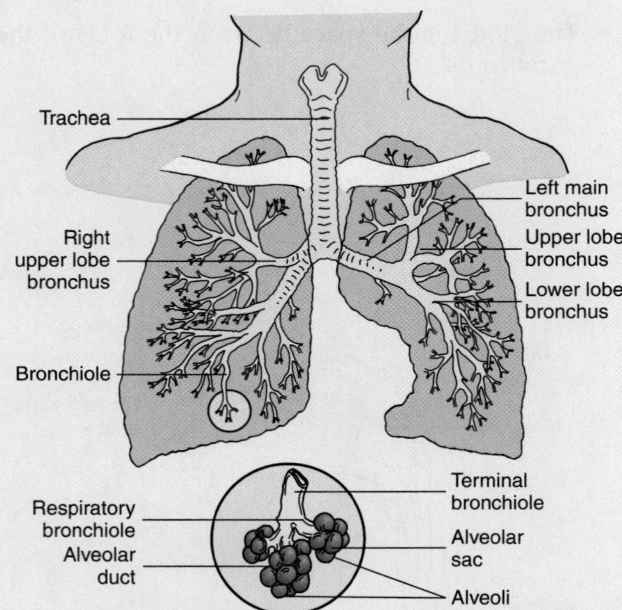

FIGURE **12–3** Structures of the lower respiratory tract and alveoli.

- The alveoli are lined with membrane that allows the passage of oxygen into the blood and the passage of carbon dioxide from the blood into the alveoli.

How is the lung protected?

- The pleural sac, which encloses each lung and protects it, is an airtight compartment. Pressure within the pleural cavity is negative, being less than that of the outside atmosphere. **If the pleural sac is punctured, air will rush into the pleural cavity and collapse the lung.**
- The *pleura* is a serous membrane of two layers. One layer, the parietal pleura, covers each lung, and the visceral pleura lines the inner wall of the chest cavity.
- A small amount of fluid between the two layers of pleura lubricates the pleural cavity and prevents friction between the pleural layers from occurring when the lungs expand and deflate.
- The pleural cavity is a potential space between the pleural layers where there is normally only a small amount of fluid.
- The mucous membrane lining the many small branches of the bronchial tree contains tiny hairlike projections (cilia) that trap and help remove small foreign particles that are inhaled.
- The mucous membrane secretes mucus, which assists the cilia in cleansing foreign substances from the respiratory tract by trapping them.
- The alveoli contain macrophages that quickly destroy inhaled bacteria and other foreign particles.
- The mucus and cilia propel the foreign substances toward the entrance of the respiratory tract; the cough reflex works to expel the secretions.

How is respiration controlled?

- The regulatory mechanisms that control breathing patterns act in response to metabolic demands and increasing cardiac output and are very complex.
- The central nervous system controls both involuntary and voluntary respiration via the pons and the medulla. The vagus nerve supplies the pharynx, larynx, respiratory airways, and lungs.

- The brainstem chemoreceptors are sensitive to changes in carbon dioxide (CO_2) and hydrogen ions in the cerebrospinal fluid; the chemoreceptors in the aorta and the carotid arteries are sensitive to low oxygen (O_2) levels in the blood.
- The signals of changing levels of hydrogen ions (measured by pH), CO_2, and O_2 trigger the respiratory center to send signals through the spinal cord. The signals travel along the peripheral nervous system to the phrenic and intercostal nerves that control the diaphragm and respiratory muscle contractions.
- When CO_2 and hydrogen ion levels in the cerebrospinal fluid become higher than normal, the central receptors in the brainstem signal the nerves to initiate faster respiration to "blow off" the excess CO_2. Carbon dioxide levels give the primary signals for respiration.
- When arterial blood O_2 levels fall below normal, the respiratory centers in the aorta and carotid arteries signal the nerves to cause the lungs to inflate more fully, making the person breathe more deeply and at a faster rate. **Chemoreceptors respond to changes in arterial blood gases.**
- **When CO_2 levels are constantly high, as occurs with chronic lung disease such as emphysema, the respiratory drive comes from the receptors for low arterial O_2 instead of high levels of CO_2. If these patients are given too much oxygen, their respiratory drive is suppressed and they will stop breathing** (Normal blood gas levels are in Table 12–3 later in the chapter.)

How do the bones of the thorax and the respiratory muscles affect the respiratory process?

- Inspiration (inhalation) and expiration (exhalation) occur by movement of the diaphragm and the intercostal muscles in the chest wall.
- When the diaphragm contracts, it moves downward. The other chest muscles contract, pulling the rib cage up and out expanding the lungs and creating a greater area of negative pressure. Air from the atmosphere, which has a positive higher pressure, flows into the lungs.
- When the muscles relax, the lungs are allowed to return to a resting position that has a smaller internal volume and air is pushed out in exhalation.
- During normal breathing, about 500 mL of air moves in and out of the lungs with each breath.
- The respiratory muscles depend on nerve impulses from the spinal cord. **If damage to the spinal cord occurs above the level where the respiratory nerves are located (T1), voluntary respiration ceases.**
- If the muscles of the diaphragm and chest are paralyzed, **apnea** (absence of breathing) occurs.
- The thoracic cage, composed of the thoracic vertebrae, the sternum, and the ribs, forms a stable unit that allows the respiratory muscles to function correctly.
- If the ribs, the sternum, or any bones of the thorax or chest wall are injured or fractured, breathing becomes harder and **dyspnea** (difficult breathing) occurs.
- **Arthritis of the rib cage may cause decreased ability of the thorax to expand and contract.**
- **Compliance** describes the elasticity of the lungs. It refers to how easily the lungs inflate; when compliance is decreased, the lungs are more difficult to inflate. Chronic obstructive pulmonary disease (COPD) and aging alter compliance due to damage in the alveoli.
- **Weakness of the respiratory muscles, such as occurs with neuromuscular diseases, also causes decreased lung capacity.**
- **Kyphosis** (inward curvature and collapse) of the spine constricts the thoracic cavity and restricts the capacity of the lungs to expand fully.

What factors can affect the exchange of oxygen and carbon dioxide?

- Oxygen mixed in air enters the alveoli through the alveolar ducts that extend from the bronchioles.
- The alveoli are lined with a permeable membrane.
- Surfactant is secreted by cells in the alveoli; surfactant decreases surface tension on the alveolar wall, allowing it to expand more easily with inspiration and preventing alveolar collapse upon expiration. This provides an adequate surface across which diffusion of O_2 and CO_2 can take place.
- When surfactant levels are low, alveoli cannot properly expand and O_2 and CO_2 cannot cross the membrane adequately.
- When interstitial edema occurs in the lung tissue, the alveolar membrane is thickened and gases cannot diffuse across the membrane as easily. If fluid fills the alveoli, such as occurs with an inflammatory process in the lung, the gases cannot diffuse across the membrane. Tumor may block access for gas exchange.

Continued

OVERVIEW OF ANATOMY AND PHYSIOLOGY OF THE RESPIRATORY SYSTEM—cont'd

- Edema in the lungs occurs with infectious processes such as pneumonia and in disorders such as congestive heart failure.

How does oxygen get to the tissues, and how does carbon dioxide travel from the cells to be exhaled by the lungs?

- The blood transports both O_2 and CO_2. *Erythrocytes* (red blood cells) play the major role in transporting these gases. The plasma also transports a portion of each gas; about 3% of O_2 is dissolved in the plasma. About 7% of CO_2 is transported dissolved in the plasma.
- The major portion of the O_2, about 97%, attaches to the heme portion of the hemoglobin molecule carried by the erythrocytes and forms *oxyhemoglobin.*
- Oxyhemoglobin carries the majority of the oxygen to the cells of the body.
- CO_2, a cellular waste product, combines with water in the red blood cell, forming carbonic acid; *dissociation* (uncombining) occurs, forming hydrogen ions and bicarbonate ions.
- About 77% of CO_2 is transported in the blood plasma in the form of bicarbonate ions.
- The remaining 23% of CO_2 combines with hemoglobin and is carried to the lungs in that manner.
- In the lung, the process reverses and the bicarbonate ions reenter the red blood cells and combine with hydrogen ions to form carbonic acid, which then dissociates into water and CO_2. The CO_2 diffuses across the alveolar membrane and is exhaled.

What age-related changes affect the respiratory system?

- The decrease in the immune system's efficiency makes the elderly more susceptible to upper respiratory infections.
- The cough reflex is weaker because of weakened respiratory muscles, thoracic wall rigidity, and decreased ciliary movement, making the potential for aspiration greater.
- Osteoporosis may cause kyphosis, which impinges on lung expansion.
- Adults age 70 and older have some degree of changes in connective tissue that cause decreased elasticity and affect lung function and ventilation.
- Total body water decreases to 50% after age 70, which means that the mucous and respiratory membranes are not as moist as in younger individuals. Mucus becomes much thicker.
- There is some degree of impairment of the ciliary action in the airways, which makes it more difficult to remove mucus, and retained mucus provides a breeding ground for bacterial infection.
- There is a loss of normal elastic recoil of the lung during expiration, and the patient must use muscle action to complete expiration. This increases the work of breathing.
- Muscle atrophy may affect the respiratory muscles, diminishing their strength.
- Connective tissue changes and loss of elastic tissue in the alveoli cause the alveolar membranes to become thickened, decreasing the ease with which gases can diffuse across the membranes. Oxygen saturation decreases, with partial pressure of oxygen (Po_2) dropping to 75 to 80 mm Hg from the usual 80 to 100 mm Hg.
- Essentially these changes mean that the elderly patient has less respiratory reserve. The body cannot meet demands made for increased oxygenation.

can include a large variety of illnesses. Examples include scoliosis and kyphosis, both of which **decrease the size of the chest cavity;** arthritis, which increases stiffness of the chest wall; *pneumothorax* (collapsed lung), which diminishes lung surface; neuromuscular disorders that weaken the strength of the muscles of respiration (e.g., myasthenia gravis); and disorders of the lung that increase stiffness and decrease lung volume (e.g., pneumonia, atelectasis, and fibrosis).

Obstructive pulmonary diseases **are characterized by problems moving air into and out of the lungs.** Narrowing of the openings in the tracheobronchial tree increases resistance to the flow of air, making it difficult for oxygen to enter and contributing to air trapping, as exhalation also is difficult. Asthma, emphysema, and chronic bronchitis are examples of obstructive lung diseases. Tumor in the lung can also obstruct air flow to the alveoli.

PREVENTION OF RESPIRATORY DISORDERS

The best ways to prevent infection and inflammation of the respiratory system are to:

- Practice hand hygiene frequently.
- Stay out of crowds, especially during cold and flu season.
- Refrain from smoking.
- Avoid known allergens as much as possible.

Maintaining adequate nutrition and obtaining sufficient rest help keep the immune system healthy and thereby decrease the frequency of infections. Tobacco smoke is not only irritating to the mucous membranes, but also is a cofactor in the occurrence of throat cancer (Health Promotion Points 12–1). **About 90% of throat cancer occurs in people who both smoke and immoderately drink alcohol. Refraining from excessive alcohol intake is very important in preventing throat**

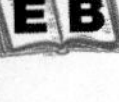

cancer (American Cancer Society, 2007).

Allergy to substances that are airborne causes the mucous membranes of the nose and sinuses to become irritated and inflamed. When these membranes are inflamed, bacteria and viruses can more easily invade the cells and cause infection. Control of inhalant allergies decreases the incidence of upper respiratory infection (URI).

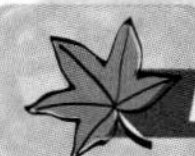

Elder Care Points

The elderly should not be exposed to children with colds and coughs. The elderly person who is mostly confined to the house or a long-term care facility and does not mingle with the public much does not have the immunity to common viruses and bacteria that younger, more socially active people do.

Elimination of such widespread respiratory diseases as the common cold and influenza is hardly possible, considering the many daily contacts a person has with viruses and other infectious organisms. Practicing good hand hygiene and utilizing *Standard Precautions* and airborne or droplet precautions when working with patients with respiratory infections will decrease contagion. For certain groups such as the elderly and the chronically ill, immunization against influenza is an effective means of reducing the incidence of respiratory disease (CDC, 2005c).

The U.S. Public Health Service Advisory Committee on Immunization recommends annual immunization for high-risk persons. Immunization against pneumococcal infection that occurs secondary to viral infection also is recommended for high-risk persons (Box 12–1). Physicians, nurses, and others involved in providing health care, and therefore often exposed to influenza viruses, also should be immunized.

Although there is some danger in taking the vaccine, the benefits far outweigh the risks. Among the more serious reactions to influenza vaccine are allergic reactions, fever, malaise, muscle soreness, and possibly the development of Guillain-Barré syndrome. This latter reaction occurs in only about 1 in 100,000 individuals. **People who are allergic to eggs, chicken protein, or feathers should not be given the vaccine because it is prepared from chicken embryos.**

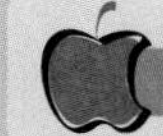

Health Promotion Points 12–1

Sore Throat

Teach people to seek medical assessment when hoarseness or a sore throat lasts longer than 2 weeks, as this will assist in the early detection of throat malignancy.

Box 12–1 *Individuals at High Risk for Respiratory Infection*

People considered at "high risk" are:

- more than 65 years of age
- living in extended-care facilities
- with chronic respiratory disorders
- with congenital or chronic cardiovascular disorders
- with chronic renal disease
- with diabetes mellitus or a chronic metabolic disorder
- with a compromised immune response

Other actions that can be taken to avoid serious respiratory disease include prompt treatment of upper respiratory infections, especially in children.

Perhaps one of the most important preventive measures is to avoid prolonged and repeated inhalation of irritating substances. Such substances include tobacco smoke, industrial gases, coal dust, soot and other carbons, and air polluted by automobile exhaust. **Stopping smoking does decrease the incidence of respiratory ailments.**

Think Critically About . . . Can you think of three changes in lifestyle that might prevent you or a family member from developing a chronic or serious respiratory disorder?

Box 12–2 presents terms specific to the respiratory system.

NURSING MANAGEMENT

Assessment (Data Collection)

History Taking

The patient is questioned about frequency of URI, known inhalant allergies, and sinus problems (Focused Assessment 12–1). Patients with sinus problems may complain of headache, malaise, a bad taste in the

Box 12–2 ***Terms Commonly Used in Respiratory Care***

As with other specialties in health care, some terms are used almost exclusively in respiratory care. A selection of these terms and their definitions follow.

- **Diffusion:** The movement of oxygen and carbon dioxide across the alveolar-capillary membrane. It takes place between the gas in the alveolar spaces and the blood in the pulmonary capillaries.
- **Elastance:** The extent to which the lungs are able to return to their original position after being stretched or distended.
- **Lung compliance:** The ability of the lungs to distend in response to changes in volume and pressure of inhaled air. Lung compliance first increases and then decreases with age as the lungs become stiffer and the chest wall more rigid.
- **Hypoxia:** A broad term meaning diminished availability of oxygen to the body tissues.
- **Hypoxemia:** Deficient oxygenation of the blood.
- **Resistance:** The force working against the passage of air. The major determinant is the radius of the airway.
- **Respiratory failure:** An abnormality of gas exchange with either an excess of carbon dioxide or a deficit of oxygen, or both.
- **Perfusion:** The passage of a fluid through the vessels of a specific organ.
- **Shunting:** Turning aside or diverting. **Intrapulmonary shunting is the diverting of blood so that it does not take part in the gas exchange at the alveolar sites.** When intrapulmonary shunting occurs, blood enters the left side of the heart without being oxygenated. It is, therefore, a possible cause of hypoxemia.
- **Surfactant:** A complex lipoprotein produced by cells lining the alveoli and essential to ventilatory function. Its primary purpose is to lower surface tension within the alveoli. It prevents collapse of the lung by stabilizing the alveoli and decreasing capillary pressures.
- **Ventilation:** The movement of air from the external environment to the gas exchange units of the lung. It can be spontaneous or done by a mechanical ventilator.

mouth, nasal congestion or obstruction, purulent drainage from the nose, and painful upper teeth. Those with pharyngitis often report a sore or "scratchy" throat, malaise, headache, and sometimes a cough. Dysphagia also might be a problem for patients with pharyngitis, because swallowing involves pushing the food back against the inflamed oropharynx. **Hoarseness and loss of the voice (aphonia) are common symptoms of laryngitis.**

When assessing the elderly male, it is important to obtain a thorough smoking history and a history of alcohol intake throughout adulthood. The male older than age 60 who has consumed alcohol very regularly or immoderately and who also has a history of smoking is at high risk for cancer of the larynx. If the patient is in obvious respiratory distress, only a few questions about his present illness and chief complaint are asked. Later, during a formal admission interview and informal discussions with the patient and his family, more information can be obtained to plan individualized nursing care.

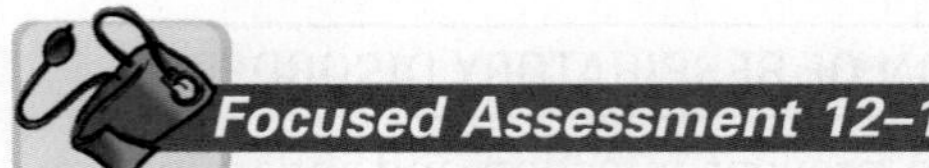

Data Collection for the Respiratory System

DURING HISTORY TAKING

Ask About

- Smoking history
- History of alcohol consumption
- Asthma
- Pneumonia
- Hay fever
- Allergies
- Sinusitis
- Bronchitis
- Tuberculosis
- Other lung diseases
- Influenza and pneumonia immunization
- Occupational respiratory hazards
- Night sweats
- Medications, over-the-counter medicines, supplement use

Ask About Present Status

- Chief complaint and precipitating factors
- Cough frequency
- Sputum production
- Dyspnea, orthopnea
- Measures used for symptom relief

WHEN GATHERING PHYSICAL DATA

Observe for

- Nose: deviation, flaring of nostrils, discharge, patent nares
- Trachea position
- Sinus pain upon palpation
- Skin color
- Posture: need to be upright or to lean forward
- Shape of chest
- Use of accessory muscles for respirations: intercostal retractions
- Shape of fingers
- Rate of respiration, depth, rhythm
- Character of respiration: how deep are the breaths?
- Restlessness or agitation
- Symmetric chest expansion
- Cough: frequency, characteristics
- Sputum: amount, character, color, presence of blood

Auscultate the Lungs

- Systematic pattern of auscultation
- Listen for abnormal breath sounds or absence of breath sounds
- Any wheezes, crackles, rhonchi, or "rubs"?
- Do abnormal sounds clear up when patient coughs?

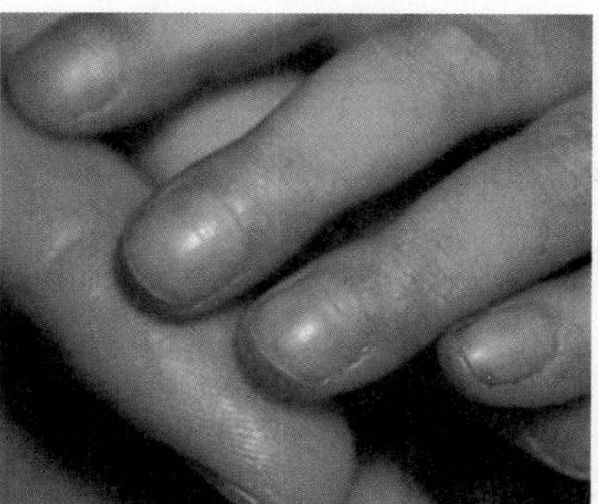

FIGURE **12–4** Clubbing of fingers.

Physical Assessment

Start the assessment at the head and end with lung auscultation. There may be facial puffiness over the affected sinus. Palpation of the neck may reveal enlarged lymph nodes.

Note skin color, as it can be significant in a respiratory assessment; however, cyanosis of the skin is not a reliable indicator of hypoxemia. Cyanosis occurs late in the process of oxygen depletion and could indicate problems of circulation or hemoglobin deficiency. Look at the hands to see whether there is clubbing of the fingers (Figure 12–4), which is frequently seen in patients with chronic respiratory or heart disease. The fingers are wider than normal at the distal end, similar in shape to a club. There also is marked rounded curvature of the fingernails. These physical changes result from inflammatory changes in the bones of the fingers from prolonged oxygen deficiency.

A *productive* cough is moist and deep, often accompanied by bronchial crackles or wheezing, and ends in producing quantities of sputum. A *nonproductive* cough is dry and harsh and no sputum is produced. **Sputum** refers to material brought up from the bronchial tree. It is not mucus from the sinuses, nasal secretions, or saliva. Table 12–1 shows various characteristics of sputum and the implications of each.

Note the posture of the patient, the amount of effort exerted to breathe, the way abdominal muscles and other accessory muscles of respiration are used, the number of words that can be said between breaths, and, of course, the rate and depth of breaths.

A patient with chronic obstructive pulmonary disease (COPD) may lean forward in a sitting position and use the abdominal muscles to force air out of the lungs. Other movements during ventilation indicating difficulty are elevating the shoulders and ribs, tensing the neck and shoulder muscles, and flaring of the nostrils. Exhaling through pursed lips is another clue to obstructive disorders. A retraction of the spaces below and around the sternum also might be observed in a patient in respiratory distress. Note the number of pillows the patient uses to prop up in bed or if the head of the bed needs to be raised to facilitate breathing. This position indicates orthopnea. **Other indications of respiratory difficulty are extreme restlessness and agitation.**

Table 12–1 ***Characteristics of Sputum and Possible Causes****

CHARACTERISTIC	POSSIBLE CAUSE
Thick, tenacious, and "ropey"; difficult to cough up	Chronic bronchitis, emphysema
Scant, sticky, rust colored	Pneumococcal pneumonia
Frothy, pinkish or blood tinged	Pulmonary edema
Yellow, yellow-green, or grayish yellow, with foul odor or taste	Pulmonary infection
Blood tinged, bloody, or blood streaked	Tuberculosis, or ulcerated pulmonary vessel, or bronchogenic carcinoma
Large amounts	Pneumonia or bronchitis
Scanty	Asthma
Very thick and viscous	Inadequate hydration

*Normal sputum is white and slightly viscous and has no odor or taste.

Next, auscultate the lungs. Have the patient sit up, if possible, so that the bed or back of the chair is not interfering with chest expansion. Ask the patient to remain quiet and to breathe slowly and deeply through the mouth. Turn off the radio or television. Listen to one full breath in each location (Figure 12–5). Place the stethoscope diaphragm against the skin with moderate pressure. Move from one side of the midline of the chest to the equivalent location on the other side of the midline, comparing one side's sounds with the other. Begin above the clavicles and progress downward in the intercostal spaces to above the sixth rib. On the back, start above the scapula and progress along the sides of the spine, inside the scapular area, on down and then toward the lateral areas above the 10th thoracic vertebra. Laterally, listen in the midaxillary line in three descending locations to just above the diaphragm. If the patient is short of breath, begin posteriorly at the bases of the lungs and work upward as the patient may not be able to cooperate for the full sequence. Table 12–2 presents sounds normally heard in various locations.

Note the rate and character of respirations. Is respiration rapid (**tachypnea**) or slow (**bradypnea**)? Are there any signs of respiratory distress? Note whether both sides of the chest expand equally when a breath is taken. Is the patient using any accessory respiratory muscles to breathe? Are there intercostal retractions? Does the patient seem restless or confused? **If so, this may indicate an oxygen deficit.**

Is the shape of the chest normal, or is it "barrel" shaped (Figure 12–6)? Obstructive disorders can cause enlargement of the front-to-back (anterior-posterior) measurement of the chest wall, giving a barrel-like appearance to the chest because of the presence of trapped

Table 12–2 ***Normal Lung Sounds***

TYPE OF SOUND	LOCATION WHERE NORMALLY HEARD*	DESCRIPTION OF SOUND
Vesicular breath sounds	Over lung tissue to level of sixth intercostal space.	Low to medium pitch with a soft whooshing quality; inspiration is two to three times the length of expiration.
Bronchovesicular breath sounds	Over the mainstem bronchi, below the level of the clavicles, beside the sternum; posteriorly: between the scapulae.	Moderate to high pitch with a hollow, muffled quality; equal time of inspiration and expiration.
Bronchial breath sounds	Over the trachea above the sternal notch (these sounds are abnormal elsewhere and often indicate atelectasis).	High pitch with a loud, harsh, tubular quality; inspiration half as long as expiration.

*See Figure 2–3.

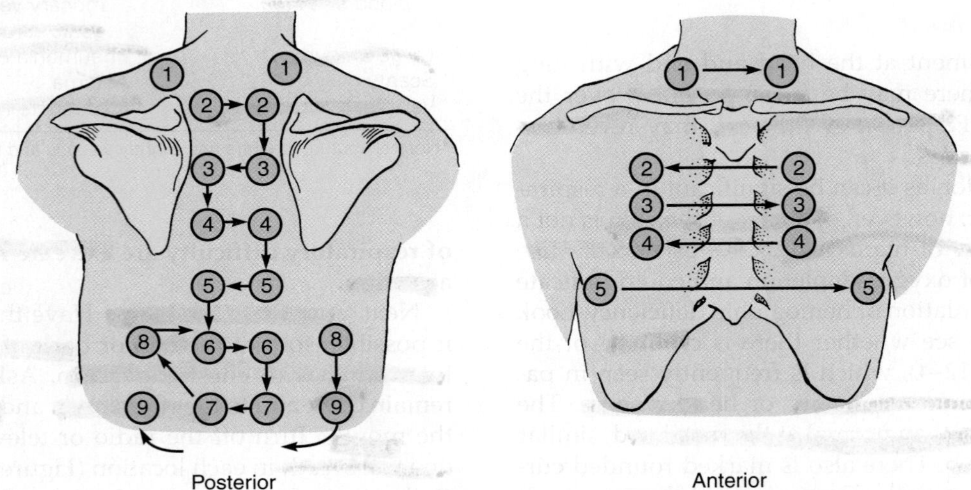

FIGURE **12–5** Sites for auscultation of the lungs.

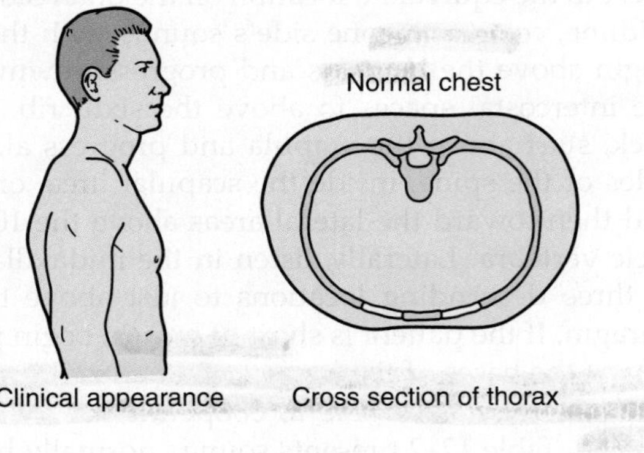

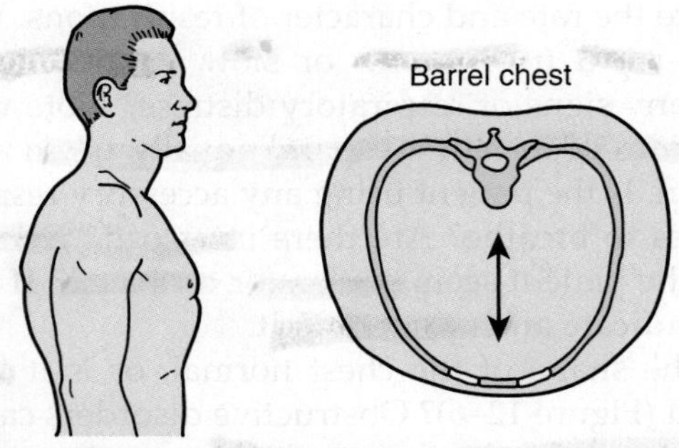

FIGURE **12–6** Barrel chest typical of a patient with chronic obstructive pulmonary disease.

air in the lungs and inadequate recoil. These forces prevent the chest from returning to its original position at the end of each expiration. Over time there is a gradual elevation of the resting level of the diaphragm, which produces an increase in the size of the chest wall. Is there kyphosis or scoliosis, which may cause restriction of the thoracic cavity?

Listen for abnormal sounds. Are there any **wheezes**? Wheezes are a whistling, musical, high-pitched sound produced by air being forced through a narrowed airway. It is common in patients with asthma. **Rhonchi** are coarse, low-pitched, sonorous, rattling sounds caused by secretions in the larger air passages. **Crackles** are produced by air passing through moisture in the smaller airways. Crackles are either fine or coarse. Fine crackles are high in pitch and can be heard in patients who have atelectasis, fibrosis, pneumonia, or early congestive heart failure. **Crackles sound similar to the sound produced by rubbing hairs between the fingers close to the ear.** Coarse crackles are louder and low in pitch and are heard in patients with bronchitis, pulmonary edema, and resolving pneumonia.

Stridor ("croaking" sounds) can be heard when there is partial obstruction of the upper air passages. These sounds are typically heard in children with croup, but can also occur in adults with some kind of

Table 12–3 Diagnostic Tests for Respiratory Problems

TEST	PURPOSE	DESCRIPTION	NURSING IMPLICATIONS
Laryngoscopy	*Direct:* To detect or remove lesions, polyps, or foreign bodies in the larynx or to obtain biopsy specimens or tissue for culture. *Indirect:* To assess function of the vocal cords or obtain tissue by biopsy.	*Direct:* A fiberoptic laryngoscope is used; sedation and local or general anesthetic is administered. *Indirect:* A laryngeal mirror, head mirror and light source are used. Inspection is performed at rest and during phonation.	*Direct:* Patient should be NPO for several hours prior to procedure. Administer preprocedure medications; ensure that respiratory status will be monitored closely. Advise that the room will be darkened. An ice collar may be applied postprocedure. A mild sore throat and hoarseness may occur. *Indirect:* Patient will be upright for procedure. *Postprocedure:* Keep patient NPO until gag reflex has returned. Encourage fluid intake.
Mediastinoscopy	To inspect the mediastinum and biopsy mediastinal lymph nodes Biopsies give information about lung metastasis, sarcoidosis, and granulomatous infections	Mediastinoscope is inserted via a small incision made at the suprasternal notch.	Informed consent is required. Preoperative and postoperative care are the same as for other surgeries. Keep patient NPO after midnight the night before the procedure. Administer preoperative sedation 1 hr prior to the procedure. *Postprocedure:* Observe for crepitus around insertion site indicating air from pneumothorax. Observe for distended veins and pulsus paradoxus as a hematoma may be preventing cardiac filling.
Chest x-ray	To determine pathologic conditions in the lungs, such as pneumonia, lung abscess, tuberculosis, atelectasis, pneumothorax, and tumor. Also gives indication of heart size	Front, back, and lateral views are taken; fluoroscopy may be used to visualize lung and diaphragm movement. Tomograms, which give enhanced pictures of "slices" of lung tissue, may be done; tomograms better define location and size of known lesions in the lung. More sophisticated tomograms can be obtained by CT.	Tell patient to remove clothes down to the waist and put on an x-ray gown so that it ties in back. Will be asked to take a deep breath and hold it while the radiograph is taken. Radiographs take 15–45 min.

Key: HCO_3^-, bicarbonate ion; *IV,* intravenous(ly); *NPO,* nothing by mouth; *$Paco_2$,* partial pressure of arterial carbon dioxide; *Pao_2,* partial pressure of arterial oxygen.
Note: For tuberculosis test, refer to Chapter 14.

Continued

obstruction. The inflammation that is producing the obstruction often also affects the larynx, producing hoarseness.

Another abnormal, or **adventitious,** sound is that of a *pleural friction rub,* which is a grating or scratchy sound similar to creaking shoe leather or an opening, squeaky door that occurs when irritated visceral and parietal pleura rub against each other.

Learning to detect abnormal breath sounds takes practice, and the only way to get that is by listening to lungs. Practice on friends and relatives and listen to each patient available. Chest pain can occur with frequent coughing, pleurisy, or trauma to the lungs. However, you must always rule out a cardiac cause. Remember to observe respiratory function while you are talking with the patient.

Diagnostic Tests and Procedures

Table 12–3 presents the most common diagnostic tests performed for problems of the respiratory system. A complete blood cell count with hemoglobin and hematocrit determinations is done to detect any deficiency in

Table 12–3 ***Diagnostic Tests for Respiratory Problems—cont'd***

TEST	PURPOSE	DESCRIPTION	NURSING IMPLICATIONS
Computed tomography (CT)	To visualize soft tissue densities, tumors, and blood clots	Chest CT with 5- to 10-mm cross-sectional views of the entire thorax with 1-mm scans of suspicious areas. Contrast agent may be utilized.	Check for sensitivity to iodine, shellfish, or the specific contrast media. Provide information about the test.
Lung ventilation and perfusion scan (V-Q scan)	To assess lung ventilation and lung perfusion; to locate pulmonary embolism and diagnose tumor, emphysema, bronchiectasis, or fibrosis	*Perfusion scan:* An IV injection of radioactive dye is given. Decreased blood flow to any part of the lung is shown by decreased radioactivity in that area. *Ventilation scan:* Radioactive gas is inhaled and, when scanned, presents a pattern of ventilation in the lungs.	Assess for allergy to iodine. Ask patient to remove all metal jewelry from around the neck. Assure patient that amount of radioactivity used is very small and is not harmful. Either iodine- or technetium-based dye is used. An IV access will be inserted. Patient will be asked to hold breath for a short period for the ventilation scan. Images are viewed by use of a scintillation scanner.
Pulmonary angiography	To visualize pulmonary vasculature; to locate pulmonary embolus or other abnormality	Radiopaque dye is injected via a catheter into the right side of the heart or the pulmonary artery. Radiographs are taken; fluoroscopy is used.	Check consent form. Assess for allergy to dye. Explain that patient may feel warm flush as dye is injected. *Posttest:* Monitor vital signs and check pressure dressing for signs of hemorrhage.
Bronchoscopy	To inspect bronchi; to remove foreign objects or mucous plugs; to biopsy lesions	Preoperative sedation (benzodiazepine) is usually given. Throat is sprayed with local anesthetic. With neck hyperextended, a flexible fiberoptic bronchoscope is guided into bronchi; biopsies are taken if needed. Oxygen is administered; a patent IV line is necessary in case emergency drugs are needed.	Keep patient NPO for 6 hr prior to test. Check consent form; administer preoperative sedative. Give mouth care just before test. *Posttest:* Monitor vital signs and for bleeding, dyspnea, and swelling of face and neck; sputum will be slightly blood-tinged at first. Position patient on side until gag reflex has returned. Check for return of gag reflex by having patient take small sips of water. When gag reflex has returned, throat lozenges may be used for sore throat.
Pulmonary function tests (PFTs)	To determine integrity of mechanical function and gas exchange function of the lungs: volume of air lung can hold, rate of flow of air in and out of the lung, and elasticity, or compliance, of lung	Patient breathes in as much air as possible and then breathes out as much air as possible into a spirometer, indicating the forced vital capacity (FVC); forced expiratory volume in 1 second (FEV_1) is measured. Other measurements include total lung capacity (TLC), vital capacity (VC), tidal volume (TV), functional residual capacity (FRC), and residual volume (RV).	Should not be done within 1–2 hr of eating. No smoking for 4–6 hr prior to test. Patient is not to take any drugs causing sedation. Explain procedure to patient. *Posttest:* Monitor vital signs and allow patient to rest, as test can be fatiguing.

Table 12–3 ***Diagnostic Tests for Respiratory Problems—cont'd***

TEST	PURPOSE	DESCRIPTION	NURSING IMPLICATIONS
Arterial blood gas (ABG) analysis	To determine if there is adequate exchange of carbon dioxide and oxygen across alveolar membrane; to determine acid-base balance within the body; to determine hypoxemia	Useful for patients with respiratory disorders, problems of circulation and of blood distribution, body fluid imbalances, and acid-base imbalances. Arterial blood sample is drawn and tested for pH, PaO_2, $PaCO_2$, and HCO_3^-.	Explain procedure to patient; arterial puncture is briefly painful. Apply firm pressure for 5–10 min after specimen is drawn. Compare lab results to normal values: pH: 7.35–7.45 PaO_2: 80–100 mm Hg $PaCO_2$: 35–45 mm Hg HCO_3^-: 22–26 mm Hg
D-dimer	To assess thrombin and plasmin activity. Useful for diagnosing pulmonary embolism and disseminated intravascular coagulation (DIC)	Blood test that provides assay of fibrin degradation.	No fasting is required. Collect blood sample in a blue-top tube.
Sublingual CO_2 level	Detect early perfusion problems	Probe of handheld device is placed under the tongue.	Reading takes 60–90 sec. Explain the procedure to the patient.
Capnography	Detect hypoventilation	Monitors CO_2 in every breath by aspirating breaths from the airway using infrared technology. Plots a waveform on the monitor.	Uses a nasal cannula and a finger probe. Explain the procedure and purpose.
Sputum analysis	To examine sputum from lower respiratory tract for bacteria, bacilli, or malignant cells; to determine color, consistency, and sensitivity of bacteria to specific antibiotics	Sputum specimen is examined and cultured for bacteria; acid-fast stain and Gram stain are done for tuberculosis bacillus; cytologic studies may be done to search for malignant cells. If bacteria are present, sensitivity studies to antibiotics are performed.	Explain that specimen is desired from lower areas of lungs; may require respiratory therapy to obtain proper specimen or coaching in proper coughing technique. Best specimen is obtained in A.M. before eating or mouth care. Provide mouth care after obtaining specimen. Specimen is expectorated into sterile container.
Oximetry (O_2 sat)	To noninvasively monitor arterial oxygen saturation (SaO_2) To allow comparison of oxygenated hemoglobin to total hemoglobin	Device attaches to earlobe, pinna of ear, or fingertip. Sensor warms skin, increasing capillary blood flow. Light beam is used to obtain reading, which is displayed by number on oximeter monitor.	Explain equipment to the patient. Keep sensor intact on patient. Monitor SaO_2 readings and record. Report readings persistently below 95% to physician.

Continued

oxygen-carrying capacity of the blood. An elevated white blood cell count may indicate the presence of infection.

Diagnostic Visual Examination of the Nose, Mouth, and Throat. The interior of the nose, mouth, and pharynx and the tonsils can be inspected by an examiner using a tongue blade and a good source of light. The nose is inspected for redness, swelling, discharge, and lumps. With the head tilted upward, the inside of the nares is inspected for pallor, redness, swelling, and polyps and for mucus color, consistency, odor, and amount. The examiner obtains a better view if a nasal speculum is used. The hard and soft palates are inspected, and the mobility of the soft palate is evaluated by asking the patient to say "ah." The pharynx can be brought into view by asking the patient to say "ee." The examiner is looking for signs of inflammation, lesions, plaques, or exudates. The paranasal sinuses are assessed by observing for purulent discharge in the nares and by palpating over the sinus areas for tenderness. Sometimes sinus x-rays are ordered. Magnetic resonance imaging may be ordered to locate tumors and pathologic abnormalities of the esophagus and larynx.

Throat Culture. The most common reason for culturing pharyngeal secretions is to establish a definitive diagnosis of infection with *Streptococcus pyogenes* (strep throat). A culture permits prompt and appropriate treatment of a potentially dangerous infection that can have such **sequelae** (following result) as rheumatic heart disease and glomerulonephritis. A throat culture also is sometimes done to identify carriers of various organisms or to establish a diagnosis of diphtheria, meningitis, or whooping cough. These

Table 12–3 *Diagnostic Tests for Respiratory Problems—cont'd*

TEST	PURPOSE	DESCRIPTION	NURSING IMPLICATIONS
Thoracentesis	To remove pleural fluid, instill medication, or obtain fluid for diagnostic studies	With local anesthetic, a large-bore needle is inserted through the chest wall into the pleural space, and fluid is withdrawn with a large-bore syringe. Aseptic technique must be used. Specimens are obtained for culture, microscopic examination, and stains. Medication may be instilled. Usually done at the bedside.	Requires signed consent. Explain procedure to patient. Take baseline vital signs. Position patient sitting, facing side of bed, and leaning over the overbed table with arms crossed on it; pillows or the back of a chair can also be used. Monitor respirations and skin color during procedure. Assist patient to remain still. Chest radiograph may be ordered after procedure. Monitor vital signs q 15 min for 1 hr or until stable, then routinely. Auscultate breath sounds frequently. Rapid breathing, cyanosis, hemoptysis, changes in breath sounds, and tachycardia should be reported immediately. Chart amount and appearance of fluid and condition of patient.

Thoracentesis position.

diseases can be particularly harmful to elderly, debilitated, or very young patients and therefore require prompt diagnosis and treatment. A quick "strep screen" is frequently done in the physician's office or ambulatory clinic.

Lung Function Tests. A chest x-ray is usually ordered when the patient is experiencing a lower respiratory problem that does not quickly resolve. Usually two views are taken: an anterior-posterior and a lateral view. Sputum testing for acid-fast bacilli is ordered for patients when tuberculosis is suspected. Sputum specimens should be collected just after the patient awakens in the morning. Suctioning may be required to obtain the specimen. A quicker, more accurate test for tuberculosis drug susceptibility is called MODS. It is less expensive to perform than current culture-based tests (Moore, 2006). A new simple blood test may replace the tuberculin skin test used for tuberculosis screening. The QuantiFERON-TB Gold test is more reliable and has been indicated in the new guideline from the CDC on tuberculosis testing (CDC, 2005a).

Pulmonary function tests (PFTs) are useful in screening gross abnormalities in the respiratory system (Figure 12–7). The *forced vital capacity* (FVC) is affected by diseases that restrict lung motion. *Forced expiratory volume in 1 second* (FEV_1) gives some estimate of the amount of *obstruction* to the patient's airflow. The FEV_1 is lower in obstructive pulmonary diseases such as emphysema and chronic bronchitis.

The results of pulmonary function tests often are recorded in the following terms:

- *Total lung capacity (TLC):* The volume (amount) of gas the lung can hold at the end of a maximal inspiration
- *Vital capacity (VC):* The volume of gas that a person can exhale after inhaling as much air as possible (maximal inspiration)
- *Tidal volume (TV):* The volume of gas either inspired or exhaled during each breath
- *Functional residual capacity (FRC):* The volume of gas remaining in the lungs when the lungs and chest wall are at resting end-expiratory position (i.e., at rest at the end of a normal expiration)
- *Residual volume (RV):* The volume of gas remaining in the lungs after a person has exhaled as much air as possible (maximal expiration)

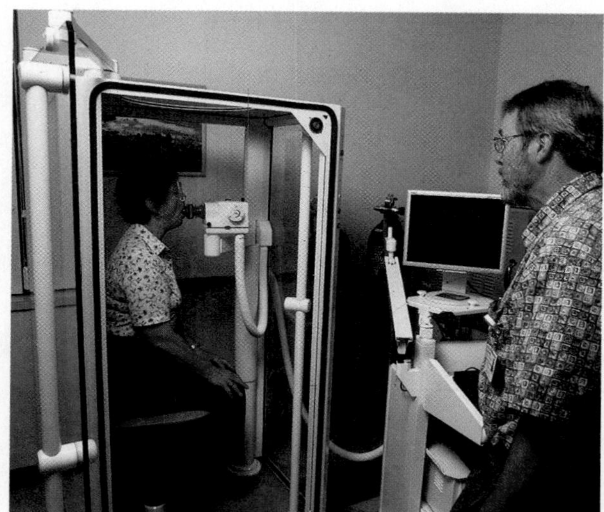

FIGURE **12–7** Patient undergoing pulmonary function testing by respiratory therapist in the pulmonary laboratory.

Figure 12–8 shows the various subdivisions of total lung capacity.

Peak Flowmeter. Asthma and COPD patients are often asked to check their peak expiratory flow with the use of a peak flowmeter (Figure 12–9). Normal peak flow values for adults are based on age, gender, height, and underlying lung disorder. Normal values range from 300 to 700 L/min but are assessed by comparison against a patient's baseline values. While standing, the patient exhales into the mouthpiece and a small arrow points to the maximum expiratory flow volume. The device is useful for knowing when additional medications are needed to prevent acute exacerbation of disease.

Lung Biopsy. When tumor is suspected, a lung biopsy may be obtained during bronchoscopy or by open thoracotomy (Figure 12–10). Postprocedure care includes observing sputum for blood and monitoring vital signs closely. Nothing is given by mouth until the gag reflex returns. An open surgical biopsy will require usual postoperative care, including monitoring for bleeding, shortness of breath, and infection.

Think Critically About . . . Your patient is to have a direct laryngoscopy. She wants to know what she will feel. What would you tell her about the procedure?

Nursing Diagnosis

Appropriate *nursing diagnoses* for patients with respiratory disorders, or respiratory surgery, depend on the type of problem and the stage of the disorder. The most commonly used nursing diagnoses include:

- Ineffective breathing pattern related to constricted airways
- Impaired gas exchange related to alveolar damage from chronic inflammation
- Ineffective airway clearance related to physical alteration in airway (presence of tenacious secretions or tracheostomy)
- Fatigue related to hypoxemia
- Activity intolerance related to hypoxemia
- Anxiety related to dyspnea
- Ineffective health maintenance related to inability to stop smoking
- Risk for infection related to chronic inflammation or surgical procedure
- Pain related to inflammation and constant cough
- Risk for imbalanced body temperature related to infection
- Impaired verbal communication related to surgical procedure (laryngectomy)
- Ineffective coping related to changes in body image and roles
- Disturbed body image related to loss of voice or disfiguring surgical procedure

Other diagnoses may be included in the care plan as they relate to secondary problems.

Planning

Planning for the patient with a respiratory disorder should consider comfort measures, time needed for eating or feeding, use of strict asepsis for wound and tracheostomy care, provision of measures to provide a means of communication, time for patient education, and consideration of psychosocial needs. Working with patients who have dyspnea requires that the nurse plan extra time to accomplish treatments and care. A patient who is *hypoxic* (oxygen deficient) moves more slowly, takes more time to answer questions, and has less energy.

The nursing goals for the patient with a respiratory disorder are to:

- Promote oxygenation
- Prevent infection
- Prevent further lung damage
- Promote rehabilitation

Specific *expected outcomes* are individualized for each patient (see the nursing care plans in Chapters 13 and 14).

Implementation

Examples of interventions and teaching necessary for the patient with respiratory disorders are presented in Table 12–4. Interventions are discussed in the section Common Respiratory Patient Care Problems that appears later in this chapter, and in the sections Treatment and Nursing Management and Common Therapeutic Measures for the specific disorders discussed in Chapters 13 and 14. Rest periods between treatments or activities of daily living are often necessary. Teaching is a major part of nursing care for the respiratory patient.

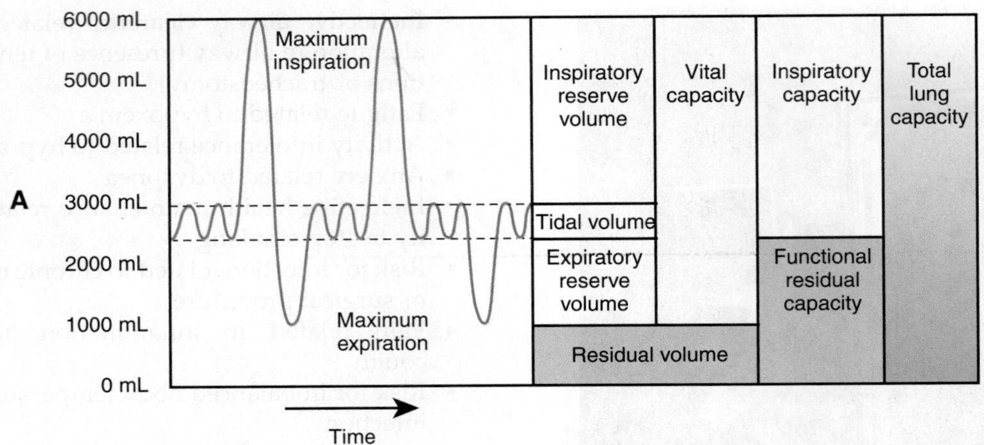

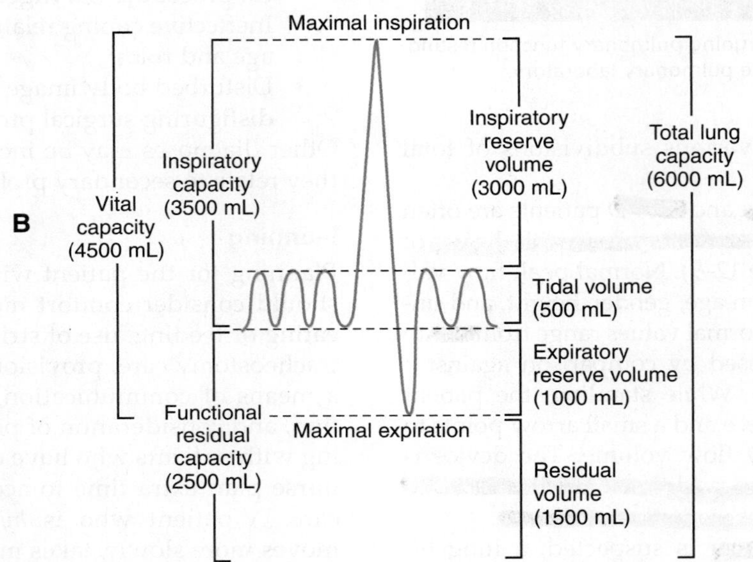

FIGURE **12–8** **A**, Comparison of respiratory volumes and capacities as measured by spirometry. **B**, Amounts of lung volumes and capacities.

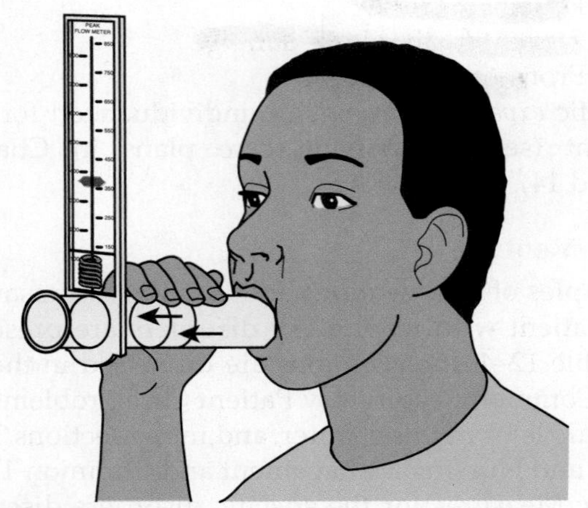

FIGURE **12–9** Use of a peak flowmeter to measure peak expiratory flow volume.

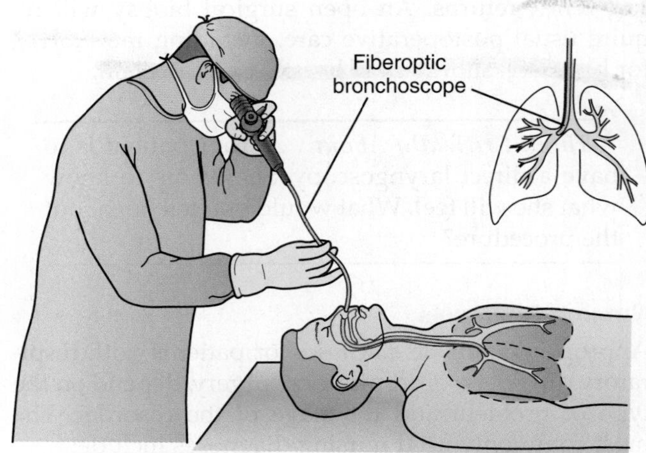

FIGURE **12–10** Fiberoptic bronchoscopy.

Table 12–4 *Common Nursing Diagnoses, Expected Outcomes, and Nursing Interventions for Patients with Respiratory Disorders*

NURSING DIAGNOSIS	GOALS/EXPECTED OUTCOMES	NURSING INTERVENTIONS
Impaired gas exchange related to decreased airflow and respiratory muscle fatigue.	Patient will use modified breathing techniques to facilitate ventilation.	Instruct in techniques of pursed-lip, diaphragmatic breathing, deep breathing, and effective coughing; teach relaxation techniques. Review medication dosages and schedule with patient and proper technique for use of measured-dose inhaler; assess effectiveness and compliance. Encourage use of incentive spirometer.
	Patient will display increased ability to tolerate nonstrenuous activity by walking short distances without breathlessness.	Begin stepped exercise program to improve muscle function and promote efficient oxygen use by muscles. Help formulate plan for pacing activities of daily living. Assess sputum and obtain culture for infective organism if need indicated.
Ineffective airway clearance related to viscous sputum.	Thinner mucus that is easier to cough up. Fluid intake will increase to 3000 mL/day Patient will demonstrate proper use of nebulizer.	Explain effect of inadequate fluid intake on liquidity of mucus; assess what fluids patient likes, advise to drink 8 oz of fluid every hour while awake, suggest use of room humidifier at home; review technique for using nebulizer and mucolytic agents. Obtain peak flow readings before and after nebulizer treatment.
Risk for respiratory infection related to compromised respiratory system and decreased resistance.	Patient will have no more than one respiratory infection per year.	Review ways to decrease contact with respiratory infectious organisms: avoiding people with colds, flu, and other infections; frequent hand hygiene. Teach to avoid respiratory irritants; stay in house when air pollution index is high; avoid smoke, dust, and cold air. Observe sputum for changes in color, consistency, odor, and amount; call clinic promptly if signs of infection occur. Give influenza and Pneumovax vaccines. Encourage to maintain adequate nutrition.
Situational low self-esteem related to inability to do much of anything	Patient will express improvement in self-concept within 3 mo. Patient will be able to resume favorite hobby within 3 mo.	Allow to verbalize concerns; assist to focus on activities possible; explore ways of continuing favorite activities using modifications. Give encouragement and praise for efforts in stepped exercise program.
Activity intolerance related to dyspnea.	Patient will be able to perform bathing and dressing without dyspnea within 3 mo.	Encourage use of pursed-lip and diaphragmatic breathing.
	Patient will participate in and comply with stepped exercise program.	Begin stepped exercise program as soon as acute respiratory infection has resolved. Alternate activity with rest periods, beginning with small increments of activity. Utilize oxygen as prescribed at 2–3 L/min during acute episodes of dyspnea.
Anxiety related to hypoxia and dyspnea.	Patient will verbalize that anxiety has lessened within a week.	Allow to verbalize concerns within ability to speak without becoming dyspneic. Encourage use of pursed-lip and diaphragmatic breathing to decrease dyspnea. Teach best positions to decrease dyspnea. Teach relaxation techniques; encourage practice. Interact with calm, reassuring manner.
Ineffective health maintenance related to continued smoking.	Patient will look at alternative ways to quit smoking within 1 wk. Patient will begin a stop smoking program within 3 wk.	Explain the harmful effects of continued smoking. Motivate patient to quit smoking by emphasizing benefits of increased stamina and decreased dyspnea if smoking is halted. Introduce to various methods and programs for quitting smoking. Introduce to people with equivalent lung disease who have quit smoking. Praise any effort at decreasing or quitting smoking.

Evaluation

Evaluation is performed by gathering data and determining if the specific expected outcomes have been met. Effectiveness of interventions for and treatment of the patient with a respiratory disorder is based on improved breathing pattern, arterial blood gas values, and lung sounds. Decreases in coughing, sputum production, wheezing, and signs of infection are other parameters that indicate improvements. Lessened dyspnea, as well as more energy and ability to perform more self-care and other activities, indicates that interventions are effective. Reassessment is an ongoing nursing activity for the patient with a respiratory problem. The plan must be changed if the selected interventions are not assisting the patient to meet the expected outcomes.

COMMON RESPIRATORY PATIENT CARE PROBLEMS

INEFFECTIVE AIRWAY CLEARANCE

A cough is usually a reflex triggered by a foreign substance or some other irritant in the respiratory tract. Coughing can be beneficial if it is effective in clearing the air passages and removing accumulations of stagnant mucus. It can be harmful if done excessively, because it can exhaust the patient and traumatize the respiratory tissues and thoracic structures. A chronic cough can greatly limit the patient's activities, even eating, because she hesitates to do anything that might trigger a bout of severe coughing.

Effective coughing techniques usually must be taught to the patient. The nurse should explain that deep-breathing and coughing maneuvers are the most effective ways to remove sputum (Patient Teaching 12–1).

Cough medicines are administered either to assist with thinning the sputum so that it can be coughed up and expectorated or to suppress the cough. **Antitussive** agents inhibit the cough reflex in the cough center in the brain. Many sedative cough mixtures contain codeine or other drugs that decrease the desire to cough. The liquefying agents and diluents discussed later in this unit are examples of expectorants. Cough syrups are given to soothe the nerve endings in the upper respiratory mucosa. These medications are given in small doses to coat and protect the throat. **Water should not be taken immediately after a cough syrup.**

In bacterial infections and chronic respiratory diseases, the sputum often is foul smelling, leaving a bad taste in the mouth and offensive breath odor. Frequent oral hygiene is important for patients with this problem. Mouth care is especially needed before meals, when the taste or odor of the sputum may adversely affect appetite. **Frequent mouth care also helps remove pathogenic microorganisms from the oral cavity and thereby diminishes the possibility that they will be aspirated deep into the air passages.**

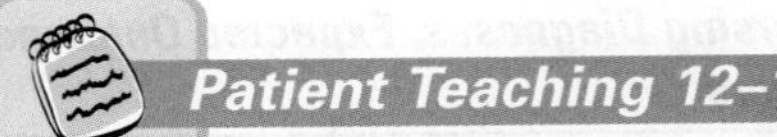

Guidelines for Effective Deep Breathing and Coughing

To instruct the patient in effective deep breathing and coughing, teach these steps.

TO DEEP BREATHE

- Clear the nasal passages.
- Sit with the feet spread about shoulder-width apart.
- Lean forward with the hands or elbows on the knees and the arms and hands completely relaxed.
- Take a deep breath, allowing the diaphragm to drop as you inhale; feel the abdomen expand. Exhale slowly.
- Continue to take several slow, deep breaths.

TO COUGH EFFECTIVELY

- Position tissues or a basin for expectoration.
- While in a sitting position with the feet supported, deep-breathe several times.
- Bend the head forward, and slightly hunch the shoulder forward.
- Take in a deep breath and slowly exhale, coughing three times in succession with exhalation. (The first cough mobilizes secretions and the next two bring secretions up to be expectorated.)
- Repeat the process if secretions are still audible in the lungs.
- Rest in between attempts at coughing.

FOR THE PATIENT WHO WILL NOT EFFECTIVELY COUGH, TEACH THIS METHOD

- After deep breathing, encourage the patient to take a deep breath through the nose and then forcibly exhale through the mouth.
- Repeat the process, producing "huffs" that move secretions upward until they can be expectorated.

Mechanical suctioning of excessive amounts of secretions in the respiratory passages is indicated when the patient cannot clear the airway. Removing secretions from the nose, mouth, and throat (nasopharyngeal suctioning) is a relatively safe and simple procedure. Deep tracheal suctioning, whether through the nose, mouth, or endotracheal tube, however, should only be performed using strict aseptic technique by someone experienced in the correct procedure.

The need for suctioning should be determined on an individual basis when suctioning is ordered as needed. Some patients may require suctioning only once or twice daily to remove deeply situated pools and plugs of mucus that cannot be brought up by coughing. Others require suctioning every 10 to 15 minutes to clear their air passages. It should be remembered that the purpose of suctioning is to facilitate breathing and to allow for an adequate exchange of carbon dioxide and oxygen in the lungs. Even though the procedure may be necessary, the suctioning process removes oxygen, which is the very substance the patient needs to relieve her distress.

Some basic guidelines should be helpful in avoiding the serious consequences of removing oxygen by suctioning:

- Select the proper-size suction catheter; preoxygenate the patient before suctioning by (1) using a manual Ambu (resuscitator) bag attached to 100% oxygen for 2 minutes or (2) using the setting on the ventilator that will briefly hyperoxygenate the patient. Repeat this procedure after suctioning and between repeated sessions of suctioning.
- Suction no longer than 10 to 15 seconds; counting silently while suction is applied is one way to avoid suctioning too long. Apply suction only when withdrawing the catheter.
- The suction gauge pressure should be between 80 and 100 mm Hg when the tubing is unoccluded; no higher pressure should be used.
- If tachycardia or bradycardia develops during suctioning, stop and hyperoxygenate the patient unless the airway is badly occluded by secretions.

See Skill 13–1 on how to suction a tracheostomy in Chapter 13.

INEFFECTIVE BREATHING PATTERNS

Dyspnea or Breathlessness

Mental anxiety is caused by having to struggle for breath or having a sensation of being smothered. Unfortunately, the mental anxiety may only aggravate the situation and increase the distress. Nursing actions that can help relieve dyspnea and its consequences include proper positioning so that the respiratory passages are able to function as best they can, administering oxygen as prescribed, and assuring the patient that everything possible is being done to bring relief.

The position that best facilitates breathing is the high Fowler's position. Proper positioning and support allow the respiratory muscles to function at maximum efficiency. For severe dyspnea, the orthopneic position is most effective. The term **orthopnea** means the ability to breathe only in the upright position (Figure 12–11). The patient should sit upright, lean over the overbed table, which is padded with pillows, and elevate and round the shoulders to allow maximum expansion of the lungs.

Another factor to be considered in caring for the dyspneic patient is that of pressure from organs below or near the lungs and diaphragm. A full stomach can contribute to dyspnea by limiting the amount of space available for expansion of the lungs. For this reason, **small, frequent feedings are preferred to three large meals a day.** Abdominal distention due to a collection of flatus and fecal material also can make breathing more difficult. Pursed-lip and diaphragmatic breathing may lessen dyspnea (see Chapter 14).

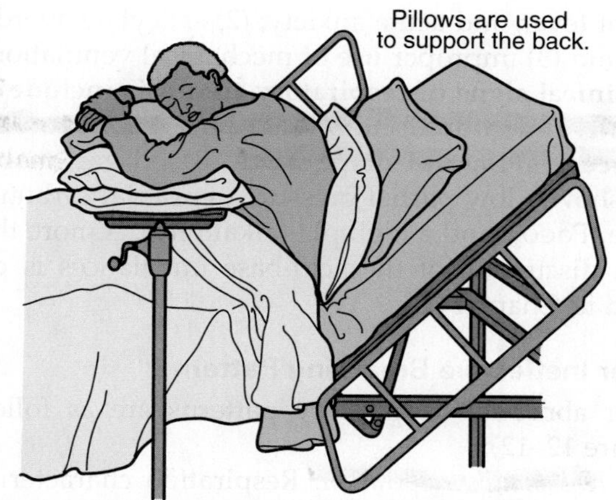

FIGURE **12–11** Orthopneic position.

Hypercapnia

Hyperventilation and hypoventilation were discussed in Chapter 3, as was the effect of either of these abnormal breathing patterns on the acid-base balance of body fluids. **Hypercapnia** (also called *hypercarbia*) is the retention of excessive amounts of carbon dioxide. It is the result of hypoventilation, during which the usual amount of carbon dioxide is not eliminated by exhalation.

Carbon dioxide is a respiratory stimulant; hence the body responds to excessive levels of carbon dioxide by increasing the rate of respirations in an effort to "blow off" larger quantities of the gas. However, if the respiratory centers in the brain are exposed to higher-than-normal levels of carbon dioxide over a long time, they cease to react and a drop in the respiratory rate occurs. The patient then becomes mentally confused, her senses become less acute, and she eventually may fall into a coma. **The heart rate increases to meet the tissues' need for more oxygen. Mental confusion and an increase in pulse and heart rate are indicators of inadequate oxygenation of the blood and tissues.** If the slowing down of respiration is not corrected, the accumulation of carbon dioxide continues, and a vicious cycle begins.

Respiratory failure is defined by arterial blood gases. *It is present when the partial pressure of arterial oxygen (PaO_2) is below 50 mm Hg and the partial pressure of carbon dioxide (PCO_2) is equal to or greater than 50 mm Hg.* The final outcome can be cardiac arrest from respiratory acidosis—a result of respiratory failure.

Hypocapnia

Hypocapnia, which is a deficit of carbon dioxide, occurs as a result of hyperventilation and eventually produces respiratory alkalosis. Conditions associated with hypocapnia include (1) those in which there is an increased metabolic rate, such as thyrotoxicosis, persistent fever, and acute anxiety; (2) salicylate overdosage; and (3) improper use of mechanical ventilation.

Clinical signs of respiratory alkalosis include hyperactive neuromuscular reflexes, tetany, vertigo, blurred vision, and diaphoresis. Blood gas analysis will show a low partial pressure of arterial carbon dioxide ($Paco_2$) and a high pH (alkalinity). A more thorough discussion of the acid-base imbalances is provided in Chapter 3.

Other Ineffective Breathing Patterns

Other abnormal respiratory patterns are as follows (Figure 12–12):

- *Kussmaul's respiration:* Respiration characterized by a distressing difficulty in breathing that occurs as increasing depth and rate of respiration with no expiratory pause. This abnormal breathing pattern is often seen in patients with diabetic acidosis and coma.
- *Biot's respiration:* Respiration that is characterized by irregular periods of apnea alternating with periods in which four or five breaths of identical depth are taken. A respiratory pattern of this kind is seen in patients with increased intracranial pressure.
- *Apneustic respiration (apnea):* Prolonged gasping inhalation, followed by short, ineffective exhalation. The pattern is indicative of damage to the respiratory centers in the brain.
- *Cheyne-Stokes respiration:* Breathing characterized by rhythmic waxing and waning of the depth of respiration, with regularly recurring periods of apnea. This kind of respiration is often seen in patients in coma resulting from a disorder affecting the central nervous system.

Think Critically About . . . Can you name four nursing interventions that can ease breathing for your patient suffering from dyspnea?

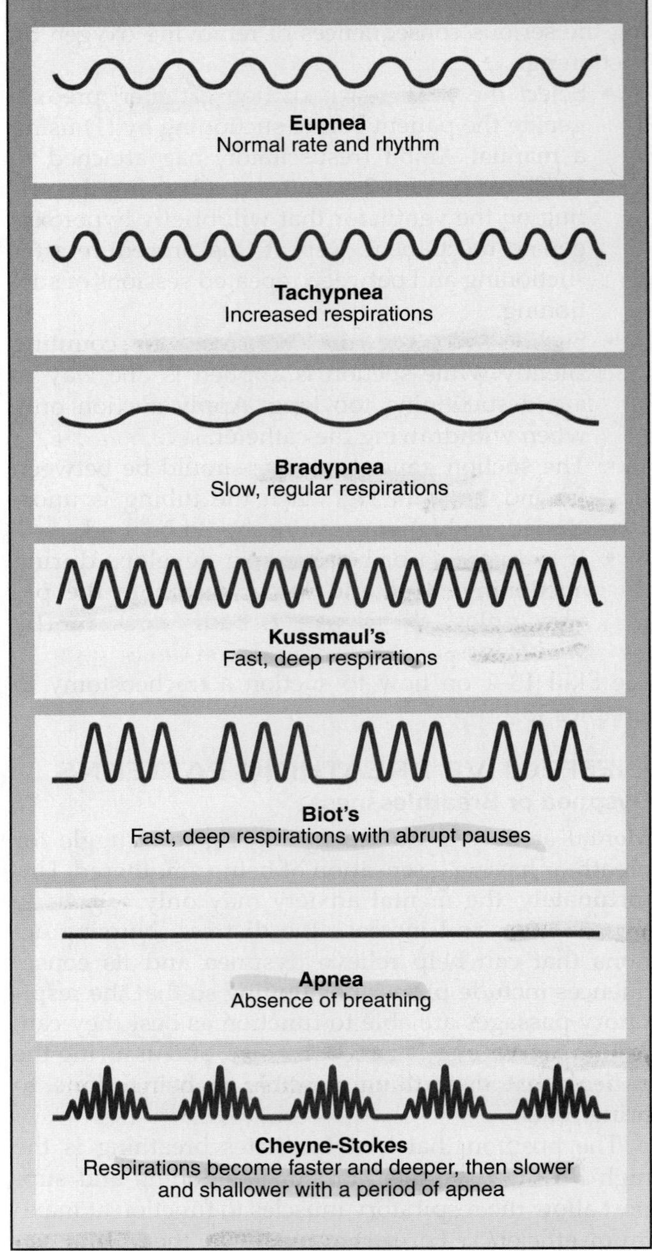

FIGURE 12–12 Respiratory patterns.

RISK OF INFECTION

Many acute URIs are transmitted by droplet infection; that is, the causative organisms are expelled along with the liquid secretions released during coughing and sneezing. Cores of the droplets expelled from the nose or mouth continue to float in the air after the liquid evaporates. These cores are called *droplet nuclei,* and they are teeming with bacteria or viruses when an infection is present.

The patient with a chronic respiratory disorder and the nurse should carefully avoid contamination. Staying out of crowded places where people are coughing and sneezing is advised. Performing hand hygiene frequently, particularly after being out in public places and touching items that are likely to be contaminated, decreases the likelihood of infection. Keeping the hands away from the face and mouth also decreases risk. Patients and family members should be instructed in the proper ways of handling and disposing of secretions. Standing to the side of a person who is coughing and sneezing reduces contamination. **After each contact with a person with a respiratory disorder that produces airborne or droplet secretions, or with articles contaminated by secretions, the hands should be washed thoroughly.**

Most people are not offended by tactfully being told to place a folded tissue over the nose and mouth while sneezing and to turn the head away whenever they are in close contact with another. An alternative is to sneeze or cough into the crook of the elbow so that the hands are not contaminated. Tissues should be disposed of following Standard Precautions, that is, placed in a plastic or waxed paper bag that is sealed before disposal. Gloves should be used when handling used tissues.

ALTERATIONS IN NUTRITION AND HYDRATION

Anorexia and inadequate nutrition are not uncommon in patients with respiratory disorders, particularly when the disorder is chronic in nature. Reasons for this are that:

- The senses of taste and smell may be impaired by nasal congestion.
- The patient might be afraid that chewing and swallowing will bring on an attack of coughing.
- Purulent sputum leaves a bad taste in the mouth and can cause nausea.
- Fatigue can deprive the patient of the will to expend the energy needed to feed herself.

Keep the patient's environment clean, uncluttered, and orderly. Used tissues are disposed of promptly, and sputum cups are kept covered and out of sight.

Frequent oral hygiene and mouth care before meals can help diminish mouth odor and nausea and improve taste. Smaller, more frequent feedings of nutritious liquids and foods are preferable to three large, heavy meals.

Because there is an increased energy expenditure when breathing is difficult, many patients have difficulty maintaining weight even when they do take in normal amounts of calories. Supplements are now available that have an increased fat content and provide more calories in smaller quantities than can be accomplished with carbohydrate substances. Pulmocare is one such supplement. **When a patient is receiving mechanical ventilation, caloric needs rise considerably.** Sometimes total parenteral nutrition or lipid infusions are necessary to prevent malnutrition in a patient with severe chronic airflow limitation (CAL), another term for COPD.

A fluid deficit is likely in patients with respiratory disorders because there is an increased loss of fluid in respiratory secretions. The patient usually breathes through the mouth and exhales large amounts of moisture from the body. Without adequate replacement of these fluids, the patient becomes dehydrated very quickly. Unless contraindicated, an intake of at least 3000 mL of liquid should occur each day. This may include low-sodium bouillon, fruit juices, and other liquids in addition to water.

Humidifying the air breathed by the patient is an effective way to minimize dehydration and liquefy secretions in the air passages. It is especially important to the patient whose secretions are thick and tenacious and difficult to cough up. Humidification of inhaled air is covered under Common Therapeutic Measures in Chapter 14.

FATIGUE

Hypoxia, which is an oxygen deficit in the tissues, produces a loss of energy because it causes a disturbance in cellular metabolism. Patients with respiratory disorders often have hypoxia and, to make matters worse, must use the little energy they have to struggle for breath and cough up secretions.

Patients with respiratory disorders, whether acute or chronic, have some degree of intolerance to physical activity and therefore need periods of rest throughout the day. Treatments and medications should be scheduled so that the patient can rest without interruption. As with any inflammation, repair of damaged tissue is facilitated by resting the affected part. To rest the lungs, the patient should lie down for short periods. Long naps during the day are not recommended, because they interfere with a restful sleep at night. Although rest is needed, the dangers of physical inactivity and the disabilities that can result cannot be ignored. The goal of nursing care, therefore, should be to achieve a satisfactory balance of rest and activity.

Deep-breathing exercises and coughing techniques should be planned whenever the patient is able to do them with or without some assistance. These activities should be followed by good mouth care and a short period of uninterrupted rest.

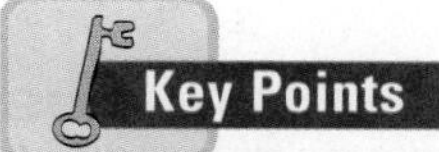

- The best way to prevent URIs is to perform hand hygiene frequently, stay out of crowds, refrain from smoking, and avoid known allergens.
- Immunization against influenza and pneumonia helps prevent respiratory tract infections.
- Causes of respiratory problems include inhalation of infectious organisms and chemical irritants.
- Cardiac disease and other conditions interfere with blood supply to the lungs and distribution of gases.
- There are two major types of ventilatory diseases: restrictive (decreased lung volume) and obstructive (narrowed air passages).
- Restrictive disorders decrease lung capacity. **Scoliosis and kyphosis are restrictive disorders.**
- Obstructive disorders cause problems moving air in and out of the lungs. **Asthma, emphysema, and chronic bronchitis are obstructive disorders.**
- Tumors may cause obstruction of airways and destruction of lung tissue.
- Prevention of respiratory problems includes good health practices: rest, nutrition, and personal hygiene.
- **Stopping smoking decreases the incidence of respiratory ailments.**
- A focused respiratory assessment is essential for the patient with respiratory problems (see Focused Assessment 12–1).
- A thorough lung assessment should be performed when a patient has a respiratory problem.

- A variety of diagnostic tests and procedures are used to diagnose and manage problems of the respiratory system (see Table 12–1).
- Computed tomography and magnetic resonance imaging are performed to locate tumors and other pathologic abnormalities of the larynx and esophagus.
- Appropriate nursing diagnoses depend on the type of problem and the stage of the disorder.
- Expected outcomes are individualized to the patient.
- Interventions are instituted to prevent complications, promote safety, promote nutrition, relieve pain, promote oxygenation, and provide psychosocial support (see Table 12–4).
- Evaluation is performed to determine the effectiveness of the actions and progress toward meeting expected outcomes.
- Effectiveness of interventions and treatment is based on improvements in breathing pattern, arterial blood gas values, and lung sounds.
- Decreased cough, sputum production, wheezing, and dyspnea are other parameters.
- Suctioning may be necessary to remove secretions.
- Positioning in high Fowler's position or sitting with shoulders hunched and arms resting on knees with legs apart eases breathing.
- The orthopneic position is used for severe dyspnea.
- Pursed-lip and diaphragmatic breathing helps relieve dyspnea.
- Hyperventilation or hypoventilation may lead to respiratory failure.
- Signs of respiratory acidosis are excessive P_{CO_2} and rapid respirations.
- Signs of respiratory alkalosis are tetany, vertigo, blurred vision, diaphoresis, and low P_{CO_2} and high pH.
- Other abnormal respiratory patterns are Biot's respirations, Cheyne-Stokes respirations, Kussmaul's respirations, and apneustic respirations.
- Respiratory infections are transmitted by airborne or droplet secretions.
- Anorexia is common in patients with chronic respiratory disease.
- Patient should drink at least 3000 mL/day to help thin secretions.
- Humidification of air can help prevent fluid deficit.
- Hypoxia produces a loss of energy.
- Dyspnea causes an increase in the work of breathing.

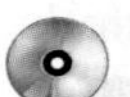
Go to your **Companion CD-ROM** for an Audio Glossary, animations, video clips, and bonus review questions.

evolve Be sure to visit the companion Evolve site at http://evolve.elsevier.com/deWit for interactive NCLEX-PN Exam Style Review Questions, WebLinks, and additional online resources.

NCLEX-PN EXAM STYLE REVIEW QUESTIONS

Choose the best answer(s) for the following questions.

1. Immediately after the physician intubates a patient who is in respiratory arrest, the nurse noted that there were no breath sounds on the left lung fields while hearing breath sounds on the right lung fields. A likely explanation for this clinical finding would be that:

1. the endotracheal tube was placed in the esophagus.
2. the left lung collapsed.
3. the endotracheal tube was inserted too far.
4. there is an underlying pneumothorax.

2. ______________________ is typically heard in children with croup and is caused by partial obstruction of the upper air passages.

3. The respiratory therapist instructs the patient to hold the breath after a maximal inspiration. The volume of gas the lungs can hold at the end of a maximal inspiration is:

1. functional residual capacity.
2. total lung volume.
3. vital capacity.
4. tidal volume.

4. When verifying clinical assessment of the lungs, what is an accurate response by the nurse when asked, "What do you call coarse, low-pitched, rattling lung sounds that are best heard on the anterior lung fields and mid-sternum?"

1. Crackles
2. Rhonchi
3. Pleural friction rub
4. Wheezes

5. On initial assessment of a patient diagnosed with an acute exacerbation of chronic obstructive pulmonary disease (COPD), the nurse is likely to find which of the following signs and symptoms? *(Select all that apply.)*

1. Tensing of the shoulder muscles
2. Unable to tolerate sitting up
3. Flaring of the nostrils
4. Completes sentences with no effort
5. Sternal retraction

6. While taking care of a patient with increased intracranial pressure, the nurse observes irregular apneic episodes with intermittent regular breaths. This characteristic breathing is:

1. Cheyne-Stokes respiration.
2. Kussmaul's breathing.
3. Biot's respirations.
4. apneustic respiration.

7. The nurse attends to the nutritional needs of the patient with chronic respiratory disease by providing oral care. The best rationale for this nursing action would be that:

1. low energy states diminish appetite.
2. respiratory secretions leave a bad taste.
3. chewing is believed to induce coughing spells.
4. nasal congestion reduces the flavor of food.

8. For the nurse taking care of a patient undergoing mechanical ventilation, which of the following nursing interventions would reduce the insensible fluid loss?

1. Suction frequently.
2. Provide humidified air.
3. Increase respiratory rate setting.
4. Reposition every 2 hours.

9. The patient is instructed to take in a deep breath and slowly exhale while coughing three times in succession. The appropriate rationale for these instructions would be that these maneuvers:

1. loosen the respiratory secretions.
2. mobilize secretions and stimulate expectoration.
3. increase the risk for atelectasis.
4. decrease insensible fluid losses.

10. While obtaining sputum for culture and sensitivity, the nurse notes that the specimen was thick, tenacious, and "ropey." A highly probable medical diagnosis would be:

1. pneumococcal pneumonia.
2. pulmonary edema.
3. chronic bronchitis.
4. tuberculosis.

CRITICAL THINKING ACTIVITIES

Read each clinical scenario and discuss the questions with your classmates.

Scenario A

Mr. Kim has undergone diagnostic procedures to confirm suspected cancer of the larynx. He has been admitted to the hospital for a hemilaryngectomy.

1. Describe the teaching plan that would be used for a patient undergoing a direct laryngoscopy.
2. What diagnostic tests would have been done on Mr. Kim?
3. What are the risk factors for cancer of the larynx?
4. How can this type of cancer be potentially prevented?

Scenario B

Ms. Tiber has had frequent bouts of bronchitis. Her physician tells her that this disorder has caused some chronic obstructive pulmonary disease.

1. What measures would you teach her to make breathing easier?
2. Why is it important not to give a COPD patient high-flow oxygen? What would happen?

CHAPTER 13 Care of Patients with Disorders of the Upper Respiratory System

evolve http://evolve.elsevier.com/deWit

Objectives

Upon completing this chapter, you should be able to:

Theory

1. Recognize symptoms of disorders of the sinuses, pharynx, and larynx.
2. Describe the pre- and postoperative care for the patient undergoing a tonsillectomy.
3. Utilize emergency measures for the patient with an airway obstruction.
4. Devise a nursing care plan for the patient who has had a laryngectomy.
5. Describe safety factors to be considered when caring for the patient with a tracheostomy.

Clinical Practice

1. Institute measures to stop epistaxis.
2. Provide tracheostomy care.
3. Devise interventions for the psychosocial care of the patient who has undergone a laryngectomy.

Key Terms

Be sure to check out the bonus material on the Companion CD-ROM, including selected audio pronunciations.

crepitation (KRĔ-Pĭ-tā-shŭn, p. 304)
endotracheal intubation (ĔN-dō-TRĀ-kē-ăl in-tyōō-bā-shŭn, p. 306)
epistaxis (ĕp-ĭ-STĂK-sĭs, p. 301)
follicular pharyngitis (fōl-ik-yĕ-lĕr fĕr-ĭn-jī-tis, p. 301)
laryngectomy (lăr-ĭn-JĔK-tō-mē, p. 305)
laryngitis (lăr-ĭn-JĪ-tĭs, p. 301)
lozenges (p. 302)
obturator (OB-tŭ-ră-tŏr, p. 306)
pharyngitis (fer-ĭn jī-tis, p. 301)
rhinitis (rī-NĪ-tĭs, p. 298)
rhinoplasty (RĪ-nō-plăs-tē, p. 304)
stoma (STŌ-mă, p. 305)
tracheostomy (trā-kē-ŌS-tō-mē, p. 306)

DISORDERS OF THE NOSE AND SINUSES

UPPER RESPIRATORY INFECTION (THE COMMON COLD) AND RHINITIS

The common cold, acute viral **rhinitis,** is an inflammation of the nose and upper respiratory tract. It is the most prevalent infectious disease among people of all ages. Many different strains of viruses can produce the symptoms of a common cold, and that makes total immunity difficult to achieve. Avoiding exposure to those who have a cold and maintaining a state of good health are the only ways one can avoid "catching" a cold.

Etiology and Pathophysiology

Viruses that are spread by airborne droplet sprays from infected people invade the upper respiratory tract. The virus is spread by breathing, speaking, coughing, or sneezing, or by direct hand contact with a contaminated object. Experiencing a chill, fatigue, physical or emotional stress, or a compromised immune status makes one more susceptible to contracting an upper respiratory virus. The inflammation caused by allergic rhinitis also predisposes a person to contracting an upper respiratory virus. The invading organism causes inflammation and swelling of the mucosa.

Signs, Symptoms, and Diagnosis

The common cold usually starts with a mild sore throat or a hot, dry, prickly sensation in the nose and back of the throat. Within hours after the onset of a cold, the nose becomes congested with increased secretions, the eyes begin to water, and sneezing, malaise, and an irritating, nonproductive cough appear. Muscles aches and headache may occur. There usually is no elevation of temperature; if a fever does develop, it is low grade (<101° F. [38.3° C]). The nose becomes more obstructed and the secretions thicken. In most instances, a cold will last 10 to 14 days before all symptoms are gone.

Allergic rhinitis may have many of the symptoms of a cold except there is no fever. It is caused by reaction of the nasal mucosa to an allergen such as pollen or dust. The treatment is symptomatic. Antihistamines, steroids, and sprays that stabilize the mucous cell membranes are often prescribed (Table 13–1). The patient is taught to avoid the offending allergens as much as possible. If the disorder is severe, an allergy evaluation is indicated so that a desensitization program can be started.

Treatment and Nursing Management

There is no cure for the common cold. However, zinc lozenges have proven effective in limiting a cold's duration for many people if started at the first signs of symptoms (Mossad et al., 1996) (Complementary & Alternative Therapies 13–1). A major goal in the care of

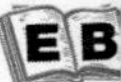

Table 13–1 Commonly Prescribed Drugs for Allergic Rhinitis and Sinusitis

CLASSIFICATION	ACTION	NURSING IMPLICATIONS	PATIENT TEACHING
Antihistamines			
First-generation agents Diphenhydramine (Benadryl) Clemastine (Tavist) Brompheniramine (Dimetane) Chlorpheniramine (Chlor-Trimeton)	Relieve sneezing, excessive secretions, itching, and nasal congestion. Block histamine binding by binding with H_1 receptor sites.	*First-generation agents* tend to cause sedation and slow reaction time. May cause stimulation in some people. May cause GI side effects: anorexia, constipation or diarrhea, or epigastric distress. May cause urinary retention or frequency.	*First-generation agents:* Warn patient not to operate machinery and that driving may be dangerous due to sedation; this usually passes after the first 2 wk of treatment. Ask patient to report changes in heart rate, palpitations, or urinary retention or frequency. Warn that alcohol will have additive depressant effect.
Second-generation agents Loratadine (Claritin) Fexofenadine (Allegra) Cetirizine (Zyrtec)		*Second-generation agents* have limited attachment to H_1 receptors in the brain, do not cause sedation, and have less effect on reflexes. They do not affect bladder function.	*Second-generation agents:* Do not take with alcohol or other CNS-active drug. Do not take with any monoamine oxidase inhibitor. These drugs are more expensive than first-generation drugs.
Corticosteroid Sprays Beclomethasone (Vancenase) Budesonide (Rhinocort) Flunisolide (Nasalide) Fluticasone (Flonase) Triamcinolone (Nasacort)	Inhibit inflammatory response. Have low systemic absorption with normal doses.	Encourage use as directed on a daily basis.	Teach to use on a daily basis rather than PRN. Discontinue if infection occurs. May initially cause some burning in nostrils.
Mast Cell Stabilizer Cromolyn sodium spray (Nasalcrom)	Stabilizes mast cells, preventing inflammatory reaction.	Minimal side effects.	Begin 2 wk before pollen season starts and use throughout pollen season to prevent allergy symptoms. May be used prophylactically for isolated allergy (i.e., cat). Use 10–15 min before exposure.
Decongestants *Oral* Pseudoephedrine (Sudafed) *Nasal spray** Oxymetazoline (Dristan) Phenylephrine (Neo-Synephrine)	Promote vasoconstriction by stimulating adrenergic receptors on blood vessels; reduce nasal edema and rhinorrhea.	May cause insomnia, headache, irritability, dysuria, palpitations, or tachycardia. Can cause rebound nasal congestion.	Some products are contraindicated for those with hypertension, cardiac disease, glaucoma, diabetes, prostatic hypertrophy, or liver or renal disease. Use only 3–4 times a day for no more than 3 days.

Key: *CNS*, central nervous system; *GI*, gastrointestinal; *H_1*, histamine-1; *PRN*, as needed.
*Saline nasal spray is an over-the-counter item. It washes away pollen and dust, thins secretions, and soothes the nasal mucosa.

a common cold is prevention of a secondary bacterial infection. For their own sake as well as that of people around them, individuals with a cold should avoid contact with others so as to avoid picking up a bacterial infection or giving their viral infection to someone else. A person with a cold is contagious for about 3 days after his symptoms first appear.

Colds are spread by droplet infection, and most people realize that coughing and sneezing can send literally millions of viruses into the air. Some are also aware of the danger of spreading a cold by sharing drinking glasses and cups with others. They might not know, however, that a cold can be transmitted by hand. Coughing and sneezing into tissues does limit the viruses' travel by air, but they are also very likely to be on the person's hands, where they can be transferred to anything touched. Turning the head into the crook of the elbow when coughing and sneezing pre-

Complementary & Alternative Therapies 13–1

Alternative Treatment for a URI

A physician in California has discovered that if at the very first signs of a sore throat (burning in the nose or throat) the person takes 400 mg of cimetidine along with 325 mg of acetaminophen, repeats that dose in 6 hours, and then again in another 6 hours, the cold will either be averted or the symptoms greatly reduced.

Alternatively, echinacea, goldenseal, or a combination of herbs, minerals, vitamins, and amino acids such as those contained in the product "Airborne," can be taken at the first sign of a cold or before going into crowded areas during cold season. This product was developed by a schoolteacher and has been effective for many people.

vents contaminating the hands. Hand hygiene is an important part of teaching patients about preventing the spread of a cold to others.

Elder Care Points

- Immune function in the elderly is decreased, and they are therefore more at risk for contracting a cold or upper respiratory infection. They should be encouraged to stay away from people who have such infections.
- If a cold develops, an older person is more likely to develop a secondary infection. Encourage increased fluid intake and lots of rest until the cold symptoms are completely cleared.

The patient should stay indoors, preferably in bed or resting, during the first few days of the illness. Fluid intake should be increased. Fruit juices are recommended, especially citrus juices, because of their vitamin C content.

Aspirin or another mild nonprescription analgesic can help relieve the muscle aches and headache of a cold (Safety Alert 13–1). Decongestant nose drops or sprays containing benzalkonium chloride for the relief of nasal congestion can have a rebound effect, leaving the nose "stuffier" than before if used for more than 3 days (Graf et al., 1995). Frequent use of saline nasal spray decreases congestion without side effects. Antibiotics do not cure a common cold, which is a viral infection.

If a "cold" persists for more than a week to 10 days without improvement, or if the patient begins to feel worse, has a temperature of 101° F (38.3° C), and develops chest pains or coughs up purulent sputum, a bacterial infection that should be treated medically is present.

Think Critically About . . . What are the various ways you can prevent contracting a cold?

Safety Alert 13–1

Caution with Aspirin

Aspirin should not be given to a child under 18 as it has an association with Reye's syndrome, which may result in brain inflammation and possible death. Reye's syndrome occurs after a viral illness. Aspirin should only be given when prescribed by a physician for children under 18 (National Reye's Syndrome Foundation, 2005).

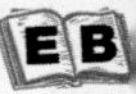

Adults taking anticoagulants or nonsteroidal antiinflammatory drugs should not take aspirin because it will further prolong the clotting time.

SINUSITIS

Sinusitis is an inflammation of the mucosal lining of the sinuses. Causes include infection that has spread from the nasal passages to the sinuses and blockage of normal sinus drainage routes. Pneumococci, streptococci, or *Haemophilus influenzae* is usually the infecting organism. A *deviated septum* or nasal *polyps* can contribute to blockage of the nasal passages. A deviated septum may occur congenitally or from injury to the nose. Polyps occur from repeated inflammation of the nasal mucosa and are tissue growths that obstruct airflow. Sinusitis often occurs after colds or other respiratory infections and during periods of uncontrolled allergic rhinitis. People with a deviated nasal septum or allergy problems tend to have recurrent sinusitis.

As exudate accumulates in the sinuses, pressure builds up causing considerable pain. Symptoms include headache, fever, tenderness over the sinuses, malaise, purulent drainage from the nose, and sometimes a nonproductive cough. The upper teeth may become painful.

Treatment of sinusitis is directed at relieving pain, promoting sinus drainage, controlling infection, and preventing recurrence. Hot, moist packs over the sinus area can be helpful. Inhaling moist steam and increasing fluid intake to thin secretions helps promote drainage. Kits for sinus douche are available at drugstores and seem to help. Medications are prescribed to promote vasoconstriction, reduce swelling, and promote drainage. Decongestants also may be used. Infection may be treated with an antibiotic or anti-infective agent, often for at least 10 days. Rest, reduced stress, a balanced diet, and control of allergies can help prevent recurrence. Analgesics are given for pain. Fluid intake should be increased and dairy product intake lowered to decrease the thickness of secretions.

Think Critically About . . . How would you know if you or a patient has a sinus infection rather than just an ordinary cold?

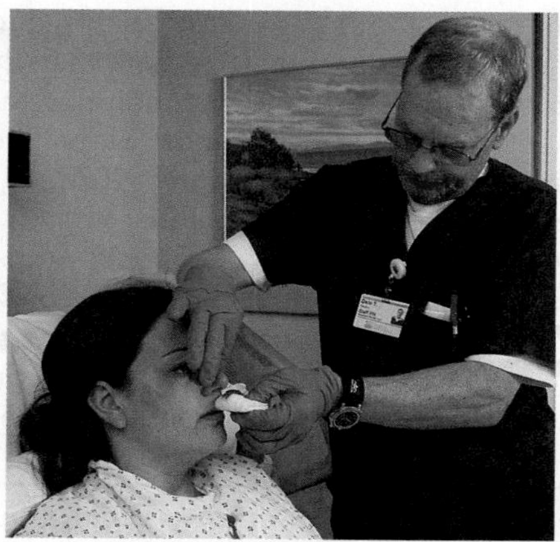

FIGURE 13–1 Stopping a nosebleed by applying pressure to the nose.

Acute or chronic sinus infection should not be ignored because the infection can cause a variety of complications, including septicemia, meningitis, and brain abscess. When sinus infection is chronic, surgery to clean out the sinuses may be necessary. A deviated septum can be surgically repaired, and polyps can be removed by laser treatment.

EPISTAXIS

Epistaxis (nosebleed) is a common occurrence and usually involves minimal blood loss. Nosebleeds may occur for many reasons. Decreased humidity, excessive nose blowing, allergy with inflammation, and nose picking are some causes. Overuse of nasal spray, street drug use (particularly "snorting"), and tumor are other causes. Any condition that prolongs bleeding time or lowers the platelet count may predispose to nosebleeds. They usually result from crusting, cracking, or irritation of the mucous membrane covering the front of the nasal septum and can easily be stopped by the application of pressure. Nosebleeds can also result from trauma, hypertension, and blood disorders such as leukemia. They are common in boys during pubescence.

Bleeding from the nose is the only sign of epistaxis. When epistaxis occurs, the patient should sit forward and apply direct pressure by pinching the soft portion of the nose for 10 to 15 minutes. This is done to avoid having blood run down the back of the throat. Cold compresses or ice, which will constrict the blood vessels, may be applied to the nose, and the patient should suck on ice. If there is still bleeding at the end of a 10- to 15-minute period, a small gauze pad may be inserted into the bleeding nostril and digital pressure applied (Figure 13–1). If the bleeding does not stop, medical attention is needed. If a nosebleed cannot be stopped in this manner, the patient should go to the emergency department, where a physician will cauterize the bleeding vessels or solidly pack the nose, or insert a small balloon device, to stop the bleeding (Figure 13–2). Otherwise the patient will continue to slowly

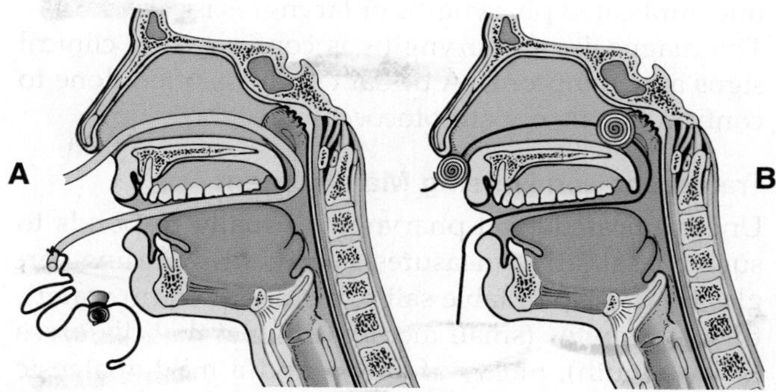

FIGURE 13–2 Placement of nasal packing to stop a nosebleed. **A,** Catheter is passed through the bleeding side of the nose and pulled out through the mouth with a hemostat. Strings are tied to the catheter and the pack is pulled up behind the soft palate and into the nasopharynx. **B,** Nasal pack in position in the posterior nasopharynx. A roll of dental packing placed at the nose helps maintain the packing in the correct position.

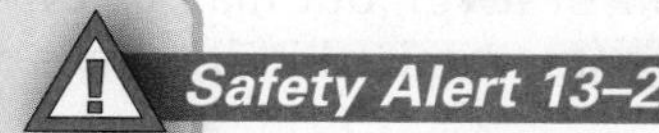

Possible Blood Contact

When attempting to stop a nosebleed, always wear gloves to prevent possible skin or cut contamination by blood.

hemorrhage. Once bleeding stops, the patient should rest quietly for a few hours and be warned not to blow the nose, pick at it, or rub it for 24 hours after the nosebleed has stopped (Safety Alert 13–2).

PHARYNGITIS

Etiology and Pathophysiology

Pharyngitis (inflammation of the pharynx), usually called a *sore throat,* is such a common occurrence that almost everyone has experienced it at one time or another. The inflammation may be caused by a virus, bacteria, or fungus. The majority of cases are viral. Acute **follicular pharyngitis** ("strep throat") is caused by beta-hemolytic streptococcal infection. Fungal pharyngitis occurs with long-term use of antibiotics or inhaled corticosteroids, or in patients with immunosuppression, such as occurs with HIV or AIDS or during cancer treatment. **Laryngitis** (inflammation of the larynx with diminished voice or hoarseness) may occur if the infection progresses into the larynx. If the inflammation extends to the epiglottis, *epiglottitus* occurs. This occurs more commonly in children.

Signs, Symptoms, and Diagnosis

The symptoms include a dry, "scratchy" feeling in the back of the throat, mild fever, headache, and malaise. The throat, tonsils, palate, and uvula may be involved and will be reddened. Dysphagia is also present, with greater discomfort when swallowing one's own saliva than when swallowing food. With laryngitis, the voice may become hoarse or absent. The usual course for uncomplicated pharyngitis or laryngitis is 3 to 10 days. The diagnosis of pharyngitis is confirmed by clinical signs and symptoms. A throat culture is often done to confirm or rule out streptococcal infection.

Treatment and Nursing Management

Uncomplicated viral pharyngitis usually responds to such conservative measures as rest, warm saline gargles (½ to 1 tsp of table salt to a glass of warm water), throat **lozenges** (small medicinal tablet that dissolves in the mouth), plenty of fluids, and a mild analgesic for aches and pains. Antiseptic sprays and lozenges help provide relief from discomfort.

Bacterial pharyngitis requires antibiotic therapy, particularly if the infecting organism is *Streptococcus.* Chronic pharyngitis may require diagnostic procedures to determine the underlying cause, and therapeutic measures such as humidification and filtering of environmental air. Fungal pharyngitis is treated with an agent effective against fungi, but may be difficult to control in immunocompromised individuals.

TONSILLITIS

Etiology and Pathophysiology

An infection with inflammation of the tonsils usually is caused by streptococci, staphylococci, or *H. influenzae* and is different from pharyngitis, even though the symptoms may be somewhat alike. Acute tonsillitis may occur repeatedly, especially in those who have a low resistance to infection. Chronic tonsillitis usually produces an enlargement of tonsillar tissue and adjacent adenoidal tissue as well.

Signs, Symptoms, and Diagnosis

Acute tonsillitis occurs more frequently in young children. There is high fever, sore throat, general malaise, pain referred to the ears, and chills. Inspection of the throat reveals redness and swelling of the tonsils and surrounding tissues with patches of yellow exudate. The white blood cell count becomes elevated.

Chronic infection of the tonsils produces symptoms that may not be as dramatic as those of acute tonsillitis but most certainly are capable of making the person uncomfortable. The child with chronic tonsillitis and enlarged adenoids has frequent colds and appears to be in poor health.

Diagnosis is by physical examination and history. If a streptococcus infection is suspected, a throat culture may be performed, or a quick "strep test" may be done.

Treatment

A throat culture is done before treatment is begun to check for the presence of *Streptococcus,* which can cause rheumatic fever or glomerulonephritis if not treated promptly. Acute tonsillitis is treated with warm saline throat gargles and the administration of specific antibiotics (usually penicillin) to destroy the causative organism. Bed rest, nursing measures to reduce the fever, and a liquid diet to minimize trauma to the tonsils are instituted. After 24 hours on antibiotics, the patient is no longer considered contagious (Mayo Foundation for Medical Education and Research, 2006). EB

Surgery is used to treat tonsillitis when it is recurrent or when enlargement of the tonsils and adenoids obstructs airways. **The physician's rule of thumb is usually to consider surgery if the patient has more than five episodes of tonsillitis per year.** Surgery is performed after the acute infection has cleared.

> *Think Critically About . . .* What would be appropriate foods to offer the patient with pharyngitis or tonsillitis?

Nursing Management

Preoperative Care. These procedures are generally done on an outpatient, same-day surgery basis. Preliminary laboratory testing and patient education begin before the patient is admitted. Physical preparation of the patient involves administration of preoperative medications as ordered and restriction of the patient's diet for 6 to 8 hours prior to surgery. It is especially important that the patient be observed for signs of fever. An elevation of temperature or any signs of an upper respiratory infection (URI) should be reported. Surgery is usually postponed if these signs are present. The patient also has an easier time swallowing postoperatively.

Postoperative Care. Following tonsillectomy or adenoidectomy, the nurse's chief concern is observation for hemorrhage. Although tonsillectomy and adenoidectomy patients usually recover from surgery rapidly and rarely suffer any complications, be vigilant because hemorrhage is a real danger. **Vital signs are checked frequently, and the patient is observed for frequent swallowing, which may indicate bleeding in the throat. Restlessness can be another clue to excessive bleeding.** An ice collar may be placed around the neck to reduce swelling and prevent the oozing of blood from the operative site.

Although it is difficult to keep a child in one position for very long, positioning should be on his side or abdomen as long as there is drainage from the surgical wound. If the child is thrashing about in the bed when recovering from the anesthesia, it is best to collect secretions from the mouth in a large towel rather than use a metal emesis basin, which may cause injury. Older children may sit up in a semi-Fowler's position after they have recovered from the anesthesia and are often more comfortable this way. A younger child usually can be kept calm and quiet by holding and rocking. Preventing crying and agitation helps prevent hemorrhage from the operative site. Providing love and affection gives reassurance during a frightening and uncomfortable experience.

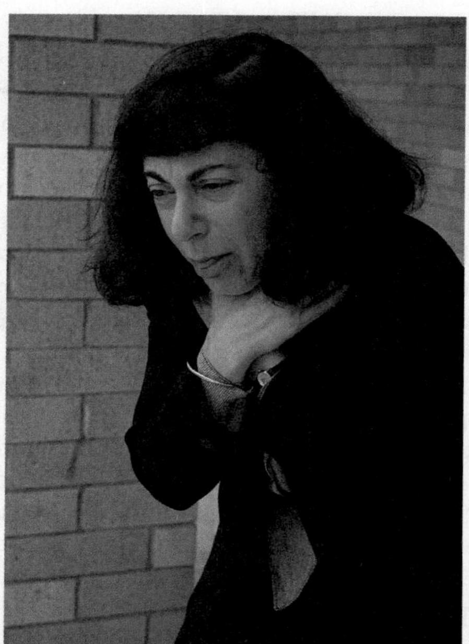

FIGURE 13–3 The hands grasping the throat is the universal signal for choking.

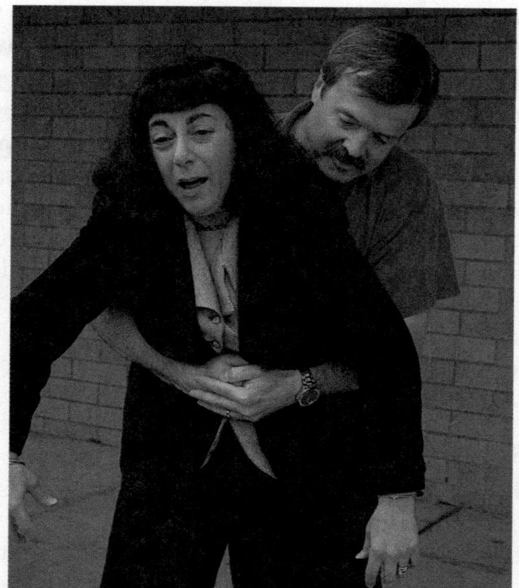

FIGURE 13–4 Heimlich maneuver.

The postoperative diet usually consists of ice-cold liquids, Popsicles, and gelatin (without red coloring), progressing to ice cream, custards, and other semisolid foods for the first 24 hours. Citrus fruits, hot fluids, and rough foods should be avoided until the throat has completely healed. Caution against the use of straws because sucking may cause bleeding. Written instructions are reviewed with the caregiver and sent home when the child is discharged from the same-day surgery unit. Sneezing, coughing, and vomiting are discouraged. The parents are given a phone number to call in case of emergency or if they have questions.

? *Think Critically About . . .* What sign would alert you to the probability that the tonsillectomy patient was experiencing bleeding and that the blood was running down the throat where you cannot see it?

OBSTRUCTION AND TRAUMA

AIRWAY OBSTRUCTION AND RESPIRATORY ARREST

Laryngeal edema from inflammation of an infection or an allergic reaction may obstruct the airway. An injury that crushes the larynx may cause airway obstruction. Sometimes the airway becomes obstructed with a foreign object or food that goes down the airway rather than the esophagus. If the person seems to be choking and cannot breathe or speak, a set pattern of responses should occur. Hopefully the person will make the universal signal for choking, signaling for help by grasping at the throat with the hands (Figure 13–3). In this event, if it seems the breathing is severely restricted, the Heimlich maneuver should be performed. The arms are wrapped around the victim from behind. One hand makes a fist with the thumb inward positioned just above the umbilicus. The other hand wraps around the fist. Five squeeze-thrusts are delivered upward into the abdomen to try to dislodge anything stuck in the airway (Figure 13–4). See Chapter 44 for more information. **In the unconscious adult or child over 1 year of age, the most common cause of airway obstruction is the tongue.** When obstruction is present, an artificial airway may be inserted to prevent hypoxia and assist the patient to breathe (Figure 13–5). The airway may be inserted orally or through the nose.

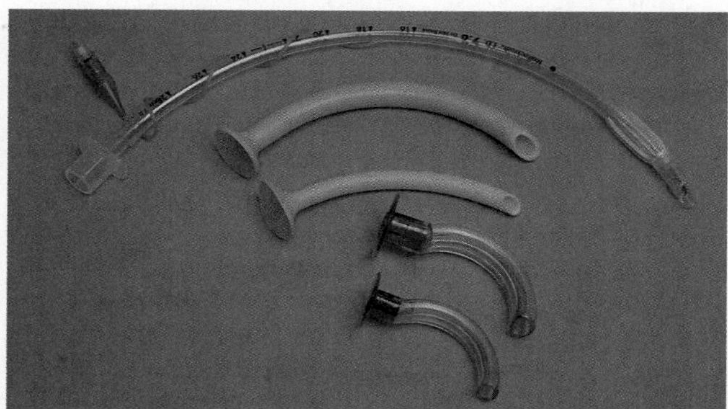

FIGURE 13–5 Types of airways inserted during a respiratory emergency (endotracheal, nasal, oropharyngeal).

If the airway is obstructed for an extended period, the heart may stop due to hypoxia. If the obstruction is cleared, but the victim has no pulse, cardiopulmonary resuscitation must be started (see Chapter 44).

SLEEP APNEA

Sleep apnea is a condition in which the person stops breathing for brief periods during sleep. Obstruction by muscle relaxation at the back of the throat is the most common cause. Breathing stops for 10 seconds or more, until the person reflexively gasps from lack of air. The abrupt intake of air causes the person to awaken. Snoring is frequent with this condition. A sleep study should be performed to determine the specific type of disorder. Sleep apnea is treated with continuous positive airway pressure (CPAP) applied with a mask or nasal prongs. Untreated sleep apnea can contribute to myocardial infarction or stroke. It also causes constant fatigue.

NASAL FRACTURE

Nasal fracture often results from sports injuries, motor vehicle accidents, or physical assault. If the cartilage or bone is not displaced, complications are unlikely and no treatment is needed. Displacement of the cartilage or bone can interfere with airflow, cause deformity of the nose, and become a potential spot for infection.

Diagnosis is by visual inspection for deformity, a change in nasal breathing, and presence of **crepitation** (sound or feel similar to touching small-diameter bubble wrap) upon palpation. If the patient is seen within the first 24 hours after injury, a closed reduction is most often performed using local or general anesthetic. Treatment includes pain relief and the use of ice or cold compresses to reduce swelling.

If the fracture is severe, **rhinoplasty** (surgical reconstruction of the nose) may be done to improve airflow and cosmetic appearance. After surgery, the patient will have packing in both nostrils and a small plaster splint or cast to provide support. A drip pad of folded gauze is secured as a "mustache" dressing beneath the nose.

The patient is observed for frequent swallowing postoperatively, which could indicate posterior nasal bleeding. Vital signs are monitored closely, and the amount of drainage on the dressing is observed. Rest is important, and the patient should be in a semi-Fowler's position. Cool compresses are utilized to decrease nose and facial swelling. Nonsteroidal anti-inflammatory drugs and aspirin are to be avoided as they may cause bleeding to occur in the early postoperative period (Warltier et al., 2003). Forceful coughing and straining at stool (Valsalva maneuver) are to be avoided. A humidifier is used to decrease mucosal drying. After recovery from anesthesia, the patient is usually discharged to recuperate at home. It may take 6 to 12 months before the final result of the surgery is evident.

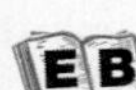

Cosmetic rhinoplasty is often performed for noses to improve physical appearance. Care is the same as for the procedure for a fractured nose.

CANCER OF THE LARYNX

Etiology and Pathophysiology

Airway obstruction may occur from cancer of the larynx. This type of cancer occurs most often in men in their 60s to 80s, but it can strike anyone. It was predicted that there would be 11,300 new cases of cancer of the larynx in 2007 (American Cancer Society, 2007). It is easily cured when diagnosed early, and about 90% of all patients treated by early radiation and/or surgery are cured. Although the cause of cancer of the larynx is unknown, there is some evidence that predisposing factors include cigarette smoking, alcohol abuse, diets rich in spicy foods, infection with human papillomavirus, chronic laryngitis, abuse of the vocal cords, exposure to radiation, and a familial tendency to cancer. Exposure over long periods to environmental pollutants, such as asbestos, diethyl sulfate, mustard gas, sulfuric acid, or wood dust, are other risk factors (Harvard Reports on Cancer Prevention, 1996).

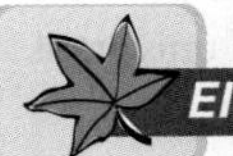

Elder Care Points

Elderly men with a long history of smoking and heavy alcohol use are most likely to develop laryngeal cancer. A thorough assessment should be carried out for these individuals.

The most common malignant tumor of the larynx is squamous cell carcinoma. It grows from the mucous membrane lining the respiratory tract. Metastasis may occur to the lung.

Signs, Symptoms, and Diagnosis

Because the larynx, sometimes called the voice box, is directly involved with the production of vocal sounds, a tumor of the larynx will quickly produce persistent hoarseness that does not respond to usual methods of treatment (Health Promotion Points 13–1).

After the cancer has spread beyond the vocal cords (and is much more difficult to treat), the symptoms may include difficulty in swallowing or breathing,

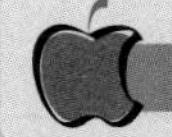

Health Promotion Points 13–1

Signs of Possible Throat Cancer

Tell patients to seek medical attention if the following signs of cancer of the larynx or throat occur:

- Hoarseness lasting more than 3 weeks.
- Sore throat that lasts more than 2 weeks.
- Consistent pain in or around the ear when swallowing.
- Difficulty swallowing.
- Dry, persistent cough for no known reason.
- Blood in phlegm or saliva lasting more than a few days.
- Lumps or knots on the neck indicating enlarged cervical lymph nodes.

halitosis, blood-tinged sputum, fatigue and weakness, a sensation of having a lump in the throat, cough, enlarged lymph nodes in the neck, and pain in the region of the Adam's apple.

Diagnosis is established by visualizing the larynx via a laryngoscope, computed tomography scan of the larynx and throat, magnetic resonance imaging, and microscopic examination of a sample of tissues taken from the site.

Treatment

Once the type of cancer is determined, it is staged so that treatment can be formulated for the best result. Radiation alone is 85% effective in treating early cancer of the larynx. Radiation may be combined with laser cordectomy for certain types of lesions. Brachytherapy along with external-beam irradiation is used for certain types of lesions. Several types of surgical procedures may be performed to treat laryngeal malignant disease. Most often this disorder can be treated on an outpatient basis. If the tumor is large or not restricted to the vocal cords, the surgeon may perform a partial **laryngectomy** in which the thyroid cartilage is split, and only the tumor and involved portion of the larynx and vocal cords are removed. A partial laryngectomy does not permanently eliminate voice sounds. A *tracheostomy* (surgical opening into the trachea) may be done to facilitate breathing temporarily, but the opening made for the stoma eventually is closed, and the patient may resume talking after the affected area is healed completely.

Microlaryngoscopy combined with laser treatment is now the method of choice for removing vocal cord polyps and carcinoma that has not spread. Cure rates for malignancy of the true vocal cords treated by laser are about 90%. Other advantages include the absence of mechanical trauma and swelling when laser is used, which means that the patient returns to normal activities within about 3 days. There is, however, no need for extended voice rest; 2 days is usually sufficient.

A total laryngectomy is performed if the tumor has progressed to the point of paralyzing the vocal cords. The surgeon excises the entire larynx, epiglottis, thyroid cartilage, hyoid bone, cricoid cartilage, and two or more rings of the trachea (Figure 13–6). A newer procedure, near-total laryngectomy, that preserves voice production and swallowing in advanced disease is being performed by some surgeons.

If the tumor has extended to the lymph nodes, a radical neck dissection is performed on the side of the lesion. All the muscle, lymph nodes, and soft tissue from the lower edge of the mandible to the clavicle and from the top of the trapezius muscle to the midline are removed. Range-of-motion exercises are needed postoperatively to restore muscle movement. A tracheostomy is performed at the same time. The trachea is diverted to a surgically constructed opening **(stoma)** in the neck. The patient then has a permanent tracheostomy with no connection between the nose and mouth and the lower respiratory system; the stoma is used for breathing. A laryngectomy tube, which is shorter and wider than a tracheostomy tube,

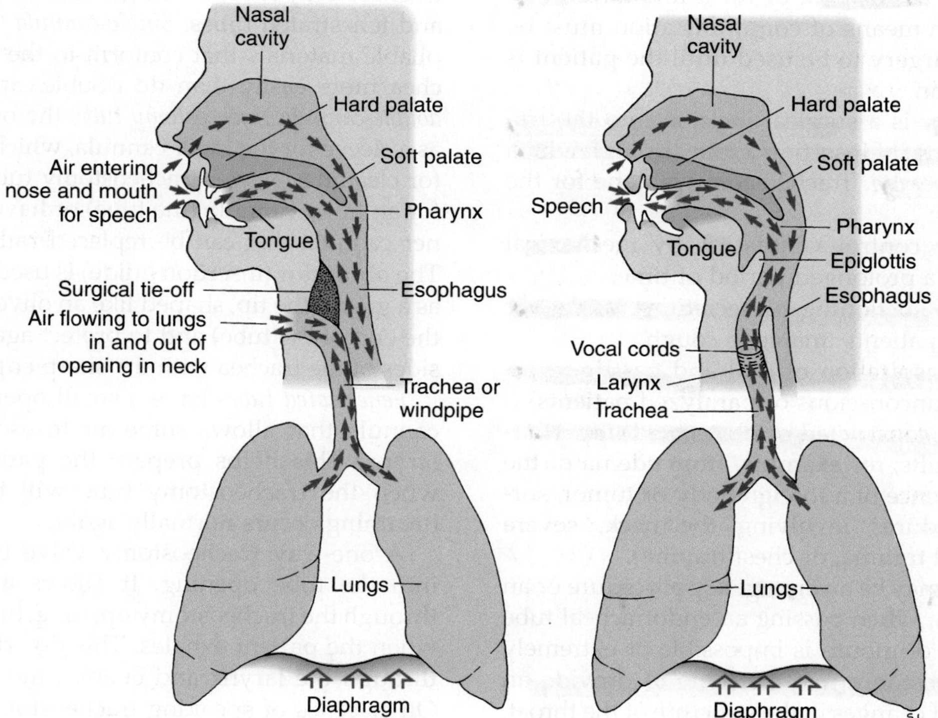

FIGURE **13–6** Airflow after laryngectomy *(left)* and in a normal respiratory tract *(right)*.

is put into place before discharge. After the stoma is completely healed and matured, about 6 weeks after surgery, the tube can be taken out as long as there is no compromise of the airway.

A thin feeding tube is placed during surgery for postoperative use for about 10 to 14 days. The patient has only intravenous fluids initially but then progresses to regular tube feedings. When healing is far enough along that the danger of contamination of the operative site is not a concern, training in eating and swallowing is begun. When the patient is discharged from the hospital, a visiting nurse or clinic nurse will work with the patient on eating skills. Some patients have to rely on a feeding tube if they cannot master the swallowing procedure without aspiration. The indwelling tube may then be replaced with a gastrostomy tube.

? *Think Critically About . . .* How can nurses help decrease the incidence of cancer of the head and neck?

Endotracheal Intubation and Tracheostomy. **Endotracheal intubation** means that an endotracheal tube is inserted into the trachea via the nose or the mouth with the use of a laryngoscope (Figure 13–7). An endotracheal tube is placed for airway protection against aspiration when there is upper airway obstruction and when mechanical ventilation is necessary. Endotracheal tubes are used for short-term respiratory support, such as for immediate relief of airway obstruction, during anesthesia, or for a few days postoperatively. Some means of communication must be devised before surgery to be used until the patient is able to speak again.

A **tracheostomy** is a surgical incision into the trachea for the purpose of inserting a tube through which the patient can breathe. Tracheostomy is done for the following reasons:

- To assist or control ventilation by mechanical means over a prolonged period of time.
- To facilitate suctioning of secretions in the air passages of patients unable to cough.
- To prevent aspiration of oral and gastric secretions (as in unconscious or paralyzed patients).
- To bypass a constricted or obstructed upper airway (as results, for example, from edema of the larynx, presence of a foreign body or tumor, surgical procedures involving the neck, severe burns, facial trauma, or chest trauma).

Tracheostomy may be an emergency procedure or an elective operation. When passing an endotracheal tube through the nose or mouth is impossible or extremely difficult, a tracheostomy may be done to provide an airway. Because of changes in the structure of the throat, some patients will need a tracheostomy tube for the rest of their lives. A tracheostomy tube is inserted when the

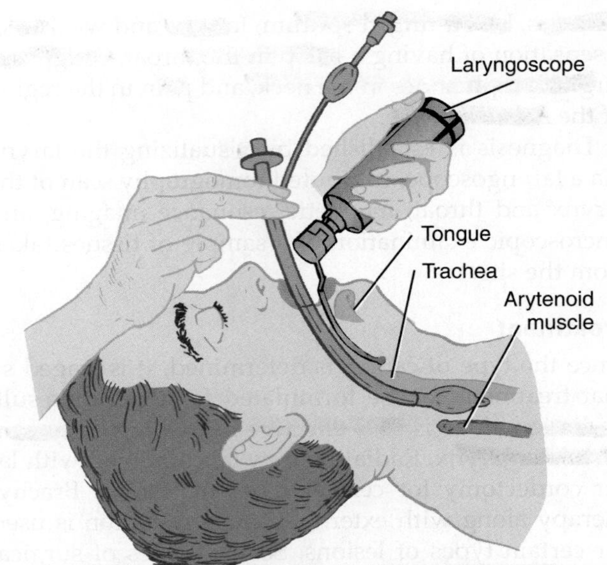

FIGURE **13–7** With the use of a laryngoscope, an endotracheal tube is inserted with the neck extended to align the airway.

patient is expected to need an artificial airway for an extended period, usually longer than 7 to 10 days. In the immediate postoperative period, the patient may need mechanical ventilation and/or oxygen therapy, which are covered in Chapter 14.

Types of Tracheostomy Tubes. Tracheostomy tubes are available in a variety of materials and styles. Most of the models are made of plastic (Figure 13–8). Tubes made of metal alloys are used chiefly for patients who need a permanent tracheostomy. The three styles of tracheostomy tubes are single-cannula, double-cannula, and fenestrated tubes. *Single-cannula tubes* are made of pliable materials that conform to the shape of the trachea more easily than do double-cannula tubes. In a *double-cannula tracheostomy tube,* the outer cannula acts as a sleeve for the inner cannula, which can be removed for cleaning. Newer tracheostomy tubes have no need for an inner cannula (the tube) or have a disposable inner cannula that can be replaced rather than cleaned. The **obturator** (insertion guide) is used during insertion as a guide (the tip, shaped like an olive, extends beyond the end of the tube) and to protect against scraping the sides of the trachea with the sharp edge of the tube.

Fenestrated tubes have a small opening in the outer cannula that allows some air to escape through the larynx. This helps prepare the patient for the time when the tracheostomy tube will be removed and breathing occurs normally again.

A one-way tracheostomy valve box can be fitted into the tube opening. It allows air to be inhaled through the tracheostomy opening, but the valve closes when the patient exhales. This diverts the exhaled air through the larynx and enables the patient to speak. Other types of speaking tracheostomy tubes are now available for the patient who must always have the tracheostomy.

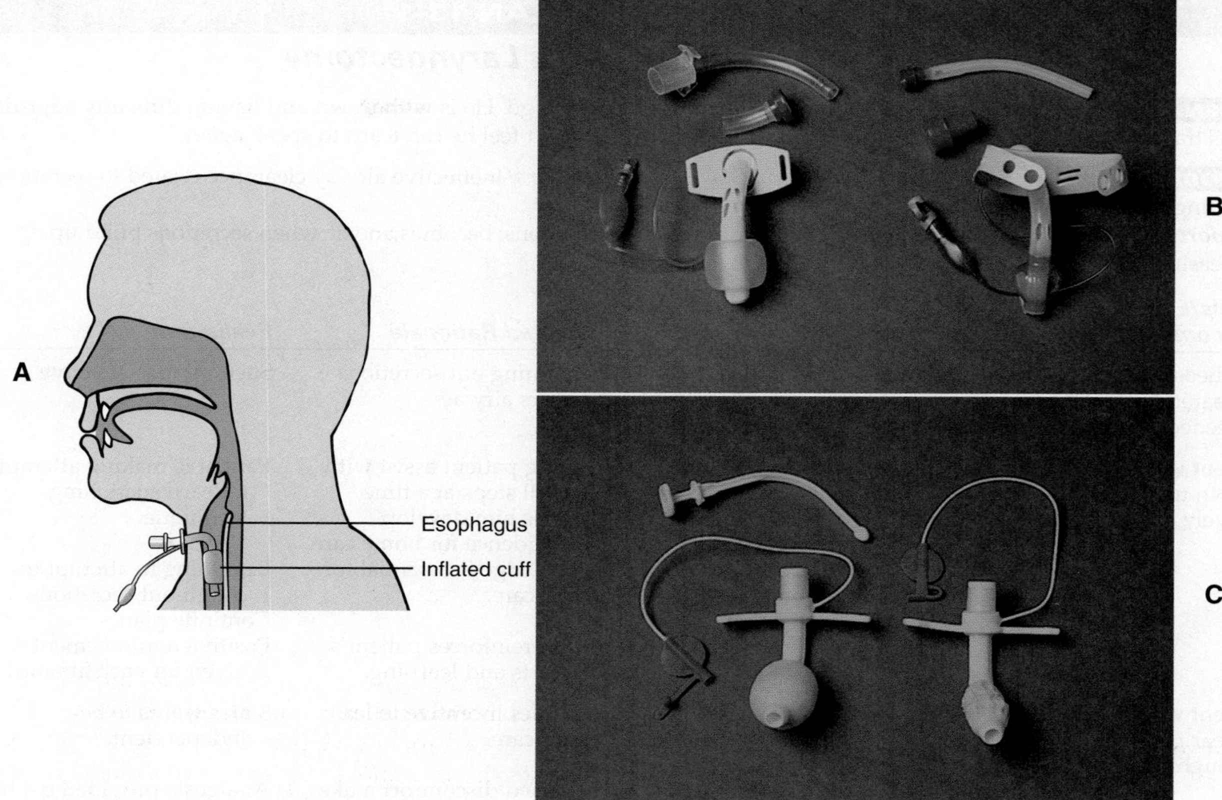

FIGURE **13–8** Types of tracheostomy tubes. **A,** Tracheostomy tube in place with inflated cuff. **B,** Shiley and Portex fenestrated tracheostomy tubes with cuff, inner cannula, decannulation plug, and pilot balloon. **C,** Bivona Fome-Cuf tracheostomy tube with foam cuff and obturator (cuff is deflated on tracheostomy tube).

The *cuffed tracheostomy tube* has a small balloon encircling its tracheal end. It is sometimes called a *balloon tracheostomy tube.* When the balloon is inflated, it fills the space between the outside of the tracheostomy tube and the trachea, thereby providing a seal and preventing the escape of air around the tube. When positive-pressure artificial ventilation is administered, the air passes through the tracheostomy tube *only,* thus providing sufficient pressure to inflate the lungs. **The cuffed tracheostomy tube also reduces the chance of aspiration of mucus and fluids by those patients whose protective reflexes in the larynx and trachea are impaired.**

Foam-cuffed tracheostomy tubes have the cuff bonded to the tube and, of course, do not need to be inflated and deflated. They are disposable and cause minimal tissue necrosis.

Because the lumen of the tube is the only source of air for the patient, watch closely for signs of obstruction of the tube. If the lumen is not suctioned frequently and kept open, the patient will suffocate. To avoid depression of the surface blood vessels in the tracheal wall and resultant necrosis, the cuff must be inflated just enough to seal the trachea without causing extreme pressure against the tracheal wall. Cuff pressure is checked each shift and each time the cuff is reinflated using a manometer.

NURSING MANAGEMENT

Assessment (Data Collection)

A patient with a new tracheostomy requires very specialized nursing care, especially if artificial ventilation through the tube is required. During the first 24 hours, the patient is monitored continuously for signs of respiratory distress. If the patient is unable to cough to remove mucus and drainage, tracheal suctioning is necessary. **A patent airway is the top priority.** However, adequate humidification of the inhaled air helps reduce the need for such frequent suctioning.

The lungs should be auscultated:

- Before suctioning to assess the need
- Afterward to verify that the procedure successfully cleared the airways

Head-to-toe assessment is done as for any surgical patient (see Chapter 5).

Nursing Diagnosis and Planning

Nursing diagnoses are based on the problems identified during assessment. Expected outcomes are written specific to the individual (Nursing Care Plan 13–1).

Implementation

Immediate postoperative care focuses on maintaining a patent airway and observing for hemorrhage. Suctioning is done with a sterile suction catheter, sterile

NURSING CARE PLAN 13–1

Care of the Patient with a Laryngectomy

SCENARIO Mr. Collins had a supraglottic laryngectomy 5 days ago. He is withdrawn and having difficulty adjusting to his tracheostomy, and states, with pencil and paper, that he doesn't feel he can learn to speak again.

PROBLEM/NURSING DIAGNOSIS *Unable to cough up secretions*/Ineffective airway clearance related to secretions resulting from surgery and tracheostomy.

Supporting assessment data *Objective:* Unable to cough out secretions; becomes anoxic when secretions build up, decreasing airflow.

Goals/Expected Outcomes	Nursing Interventions	Selected Rationale	Evaluation
Tracheostomy will be cleared by suctioning as needed.	Suction as needed, at least q 4 hr.	Suctioning out secretions clears airway.	Suctioning is effective.
Patient will learn to suction own tracheostomy effectively by discharge.	Encourage patient to assist with procedure; hold water for moistening catheter, turn on suction.	Having patient assist with small steps at a time helps him develop confidence for home care.	Patient is making attempts to learn suctioning technique.
	Teach to attach catheter to suction tubing; teach to suction self using mirror.	Knowledge is essential for self-care.	Beginning to attempt to cough out secretions. Continue plan.
	Praise for all attempts.	Praise reinforces patient's efforts and learning.	Positive reinforcement given for each attempt.
Patient will learn to clear tracheostomy by coughing effectively.	Point out advantages of not being dependent on others for care of airway.	Provides incentive to learn self-care.	States wants to be independent.
	Medicate for discomfort and encourage patient to cough to remove secretions without suctioning.	Lessened discomfort makes it possible to cough effectively.	Analgesia provided q 4 hr.
	Remind to hold tissues in front of tube rather than the mouth.	Secretions will be coughed out of the tube.	Holding tissues in front of tube when attempts to cough.

PROBLEM/NURSING DIAGNOSIS *Surgical incision*/Impaired skin integrity related to surgical incisions.

Supporting assessment data *Objective:* Supraglottic laryngectomy and tracheostomy.

Goals/Expected Outcomes	Nursing Interventions	Selected Rationale	Evaluation
No infection at incision sites as evidenced by no redness, swelling, or purulent discharge.	Clean incision lines with H_2O_2; apply antibiotic ointment as ordered q shift.	Cleans away bacteria and helps prevent infection.	No evidence of infection. Slight redness around tracheostomy stoma. Continue plan.
	Clean around tracheostomy stoma with acetic acid or normal saline and change gauze pad as needed.		
Skin integrity is intact within 6 wk.	Change tracheostomy ties q 24 hr.		Incision is intact. Continue plan.
	Observe for signs of infection.	Early recognition of infection ensures prompt treatment.	No signs of infection.

NURSING CARE PLAN 13–1

Care of the Patient with a Laryngectomy—cont'd

PROBLEM/NURSING DIAGNOSIS *Unable to speak*/Impaired verbal communication related to loss of larynx.
Supporting assessment data *Subjective:* No verbal communication. *Objective:* Laryngectomy and tracheostomy.

Goals/Expected Outcomes	Nursing Interventions	Selected Rationale	Evaluation
Patient will show interest in learning new style of speech within 6 wk.	Assist him to use Magic Slate or paper and pencil for communication; show patience.	Provides for some means of communication.	Using Magic Slate. Continue plan.
	Obtain order for visit from rehabilitated laryngectomy patient who has mastered some form of speech.	Seeing an example reinforces the possibility of regaining a form of speech.	Visit scheduled.
	Encourage affiliation with community support group for laryngectomy patients.	Support from people with a like problem helps one not to feel so alone and helpless.	Advised about support group. Continue plan.

PROBLEM/NURSING DIAGNOSIS *Chokes when tries to swallow*/Risk for injury related to choking when trying to swallow.
Supporting assessment data *Subjective:* Writes that he doesn't feel he'll be able to swallow or eat by mouth again. *Objective:* Chokes when tries to swallow saliva; tends to aspirate.

Goals/Expected Outcomes	Nursing Interventions	Selected Rationale	Evaluation
Patient will not experience injury from aspiration of food.	Teach to hold his breath and perform the Valsalva maneuver while swallowing.	Valsalva maneuver closes the glottis over the tracheal opening in the throat, preventing food from entering the trachea.	Is still choking when he tries to swallow. Revise plan: Obtain consult with speech therapist for swallowing exercises.
Patient will learn to swallow without aspirating within 6 wk.	Teach to keep the neck relaxed forward when swallowing and forcibly exhale after swallowing.	Exhaling forcibly after swallowing will expel particles that accidentally end up in the trachea.	

? CRITICAL THINKING QUESTIONS

1. What do you think might be psychosocial problems that Mr. Collins could experience?
2. How can you motivate Mr. Collins to participate in suctioning his tracheostomy?

normal saline or sterile water to lubricate the catheter, sterile gloves, and a suction hookup with a drainage container. Sterile technique is important, as the patient with a tracheostomy is very susceptible to respiratory infection. Suctioning technique is presented in Skill 13–1 and is discussed in the section Ineffective Airway Clearance in Chapter 12.

Preventing infection is another nursing responsibility. The incision is an open wound with minimal dressings, is frequently exposed to sputum that is coughed up, and is an ideal entryway for infectious organisms. Tracheostomy care is a sterile procedure until the stoma is well healed.

If the patient is to go home with a tracheostomy, techniques for suctioning and providing the necessary tracheostomy care (Skill 13–2) are taught to both the patient and a family member or caregiver (Patient Teaching 13–1 on p. 314).

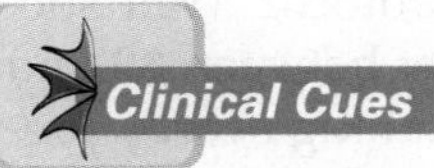

Practicing tracheostomy and endotracheal tube suctioning sufficient times on laboratory mannequins to gain confidence will greatly decrease anxiety when suctioning patients. Considerable skill is necessary to maintain sterile technique while suctioning, yet perform the maneuver quickly and efficiently.

Psychological support of the tracheostomy patient and the family is an essential component of nursing care. The patient has to learn to breathe in a totally dif-

Text continued on p. 314

Skill 13–1 Endotracheal and Tracheostomy Suctioning

Since it is often difficult for a patient to cough out secretions via an endotracheal or tracheostomy tube, the tube must be periodically suctioned. The tracheostomy tube must be kept free of secretions for the patient to breathe or receive oxygen. To determine when suctioning is needed, the lungs are auscultated. A face shield or goggles and mask should be used when suctioning because the patient may spray sputum when coughing. Mouth care should be performed after suctioning the nasopharynx.

■ Supplies

- ✔ Suction source
- ✔ Face shield
- ✔ Sterile normal saline
- ✔ Sterile catheter suction kit
- ✔ Solution container
- ✔ Sterile gloves
- ✔ Sterile suction catheter
- ✔ Resuscitation bag
- ✔ Connecting tubing

Review and carry out the Standard Steps in Appendix 6.

■ Assessment (Data Collection)

1. ***ACTION*** Auscultate the patient's lungs to determine if there are retained secretions present.

   RATIONALE Moist breathe sounds, including gurgles and bubbling, indicate a need for suctioning.

■ Planning

2. ***ACTION*** Be certain all equipment is at hand and think through the procedure before opening sterile supplies.

   RATIONALE Ensures that the procedure will go smoothly.

3. ***ACTION*** Obtain a partner to preoxygenate the patient with the resuscitator bag if possible.

   RATIONALE The patient should be preoxygenated before suctioning so that oxygen is not seriously depleted by suctioning. The procedure is easier to perform with an assistant.

4. ***ACTION*** Attach the connecting tubing to suction source and turn on suction; check the pressure. Place the connecting tubing close at hand.

   RATIONALE Verify that the suction is functioning by occluding end of suction tubing with your thumb and watching pressure on gauge rise. Set pressure according to agency protocol. Wall suction unit pressure is generally set between 80 and 120 mm Hg maximum. Placing tubing nearby prepares tubing to be easily connected to the suction catheter.

■ Implementation

5. ***ACTION*** Perform hand hygiene; open supplies and put on sterile gloves. Set up the water container. Place sterile drape, if available across patient's chest. Pour about 100 mL sterile water into the container with the nondominant hand. With gloved dominant hand holding the catheter, attach the catheter to the connecting tubing. Be careful not to contaminate glove holding the catheter. The hand holding the connecting tubing is no longer sterile.

   RATIONALE Prepares the water for use and maintains sterility of dominant hand. Supplies catheter with suction. Provides sterile field on the chest.

6. ***ACTION*** Have an assistant oxygenate patient by resuscitator bag for 2 minutes with large-volume inspirations while you prepare to suction, or do this yourself. If working alone and the patient is receiving oxygen, increase the concentration to 100% for 2 minutes, keeping hand on oxygen adjustment, or give two or three sigh breaths with the ventilator. Check agency protocol for desired way to preoxygenate the patient.

   RATIONALE Preoxygenation prevents hypoxia during suctioning.

7. ***ACTION*** Moisten the catheter tip in the sterile saline solution and suction up a small bit of the solution to test the system. Disconnect the ventilator

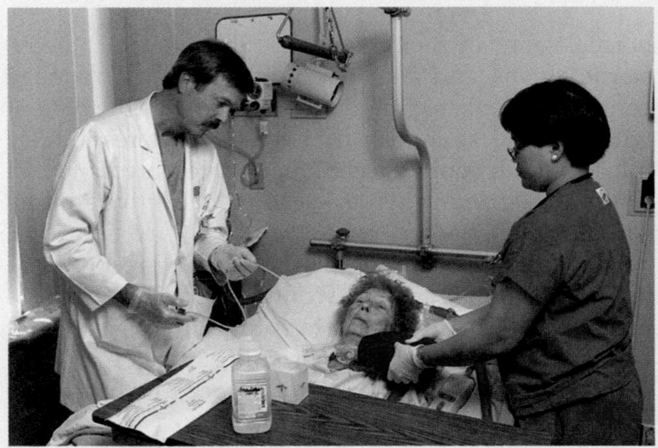

Have assistant oxygenate with resuscitator bag.

From deWit, S.C. (2005). *Fundamental Concepts and Skills for Nursing* (2nd ed.). Philadelphia: Elsevier Saunders.

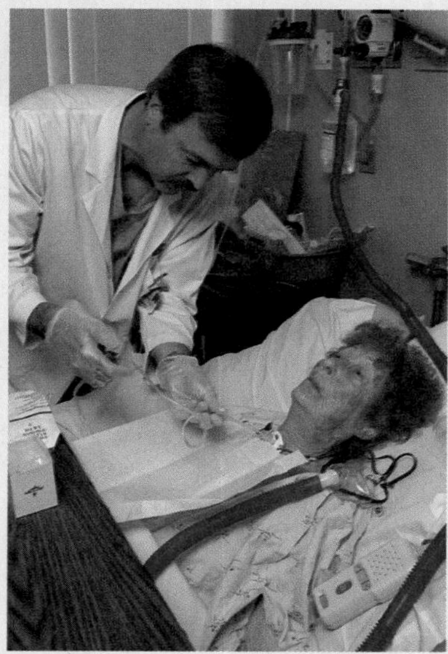
Introduce the suction catheter into the tracheostomy tube.

tubing if ventilator is in use, and immediately introduce the catheter into the endotracheal tube or tracheostomy tube using only sterile gloved hand; *do not* use suction while placing the catheter. Advance the catheter gently until you meet resistance and then pull it back slightly.

RATIONALE Moisture lubricates the catheter and makes it easier to introduce; testing with solution ensures suction is working properly. Suction applied upon entry draws out oxygen. Holding the catheter at a 90-degree angle to the tube to enter it helps prevent contaminating the catheter by touching the patient's face or neck.

8. ***ACTION:*** Apply suction while rotating and withdrawing the catheter. Allow no more than 10 seconds to suction and withdraw the catheter. Counting "1-1000, 2-1000," etc., while suctioning is one way to track the time.

   RATIONALE Suction draws out secretions. Rolling the catheter between your fingers rotates the catheter openings at the tip so that they will suck up secretions around the circumference of the trachea. Suctioning for more than 10 seconds seriously depletes the patient's oxygen.

9. ***ACTION*** Reattach the patient's tube to the oxygen source if one has been in use, and allow a rest period before suctioning again. Hyperoxygenate for 2 minutes or until heart rate and oxygen saturation return to baseline. Keep the catheter sterile while waiting; use the nonsterile hand to reattach the oxygen source. Auscultate the lungs when finished to be certain that secretions have been adequately cleared. Repeat as needed up to three suction passes.

   RATIONALE Suction draws out oxygen as well as secretions and may cause hypoxia. Hyperoxygenation should be done again before each suctioning.

10. ***ACTION*** Suction the nasopharynx if needed.

    RATIONALE Secretions may collect above the cuffed tracheostomy tube and need to be removed.

11. ***ACTION*** Rinse catheter and connecting tubing by suctioning up more solution. Discard the catheter by holding it in your gloved hand and pulling the glove off over it.

    RATIONALE Connecting tubing should be cleared of secretions. A sterile catheter must be used each time tracheobronchial suctioning is performed. Sterile catheters must be kept at the bedside for immediate use. Pulling glove over the used catheter prevents spread of microorganisms.

Suctioning with a Sleeved Catheter

12. ***ACTION*** Open catheter package without disturbing protective sleeve covering the catheter.

    RATIONALE Sleeve maintains sterility of catheter so that it can be reused several times.

13. ***ACTION*** Attach catheter to endotracheal tube or tracheostomy adaptor and to suction tubing.

    RATIONALE Catheter must be connected to suction in order to withdraw secretions.

14. ***ACTION*** As catheter is inserted via endotracheal tube or tracheostomy, sleeve slides back; advance the catheter as far as possible.

    RATIONALE Positions catheter within trachea to carina.

15. ***ACTION*** Apply suction while rotating and withdrawing the catheter. Allow the sleeve to re-cover the catheter as it is withdrawn; pull it back out of the tube opening.

    RATIONALE The sleeve will prevent the catheter from becoming contaminated from environment outside the trachea. Pulling it out of the tube prevents the catheter from occluding the airway.

16. ***ACTION*** Remove gloves and perform hand hygiene. Turn off suction.

    RATIONALE Performing hand hygiene reduces transfer of microorganisms. Suction may remain off between suctioning sessions.

■ Evaluation

17. ***ACTION*** Ask yourself: Did patient tolerate the procedure without drastic changes in heart rate? Are the lungs clear to auscultation? Did suctioning remove secretions? Was sterility maintained?

    RATIONALE Answers provide data to determine if procedure was effective.

Continued

Skill 13–1 Endotracheal and Tracheostomy Suctioning—cont'd

■ Documentation

18. ***ACTION*** Include number of times patient received suctioning, type of technique used, characteristics of secretions, and any problems encountered.

    RATIONALE Documents procedure and any problems encountered.

Documentation Example

5/14 1430 Coughing; gurgling sounds auscultated. Suctioned ×2 with sterile technique and preoxygenation. Moderate white secretions obtained; lungs clear, reattached to ventilator; no signs of dysrhythmia.

____

(Nurse's signature)

■ Special Considerations

- ✔ Some patients can cough secretions out; allow patient to try before suctioning.
- ✔ Holding your breath while you apply suction helps judge the time the patient is without oxygen.
- ✔ Suction container is emptied at the end of each shift or at least every 24 hours; check agency protocol.
- ✔ Do not suction unnecessarily because the procedure is irritating to the tracheal tissues.
- ✔ In the home care situation, suction catheters can be cleaned, sterilized, and reused.
- ✔ The home care patient is taught to perform the suctioning procedure. The teaching plan should be consistently used by all home care nurses working with the patient.

? CRITICAL THINKING QUESTIONS

1. What is one way to hold the suction catheter to introduce it into an endotracheal tube so that it doesn't kink and hit the patient's skin or your hand and become contaminated?
2. What would you need to do before suctioning a patient if you know that this patient frequently forcibly coughs out secretions when being suctioned?

Skill 13–2 Providing Tracheostomy Care

Tracheostomy care is performed every 8 hours. The tracheostomy patient is taught to do this procedure before being sent home with a new tracheostomy. The soiled dressing is removed, the area around the stoma is cleaned, and if needed, the tape or ties holding the tracheostomy tube in place are changed. If there is an inner cannula, it is removed, cleaned, and replaced.

■ Supplies

- ✔ Normal saline
- ✔ Forceps
- ✔ Sterile gloves
- ✔ Hydrogen peroxide
- ✔ Precut tracheostomy dressing
- ✔ Brush or pipe cleaners
- ✔ Tracheostomy tape or tube fastener
- ✔ Scissors
- ✔ Sterile 4 × 4 gauze pad
- ✔ Cotton swabs or Q-Tips
- ✔ Solution containers (2)
- ✔ Discard bag

Review and carry out the Standard Steps in Appendix 7.

■ Assessment (Data Collection)

1. ***ACTION*** Suction as needed before beginning the procedure.

   RATIONALE Clears airway. Movement of the tracheostomy tube during cleaning and care may make patient cough, loosening secretions that could block the airway.

■ Planning

2. ***ACTION*** Set up the equipment on a table close to the patient and plan the order in which to perform the tasks.

   RATIONALE Planning makes work more efficient.

■ Implementation

3. ***ACTION*** Place the patient in a low semi-Fowler's position. Wash your hands, open the supplies, and put on one glove. Separate basins with gloved hand; pour solutions with ungloved hand. Use one part hydrogen peroxide to one part normal saline for the wash solution; normal saline is used to rinse.

   RATIONALE Positioning makes visualization of the tracheostomy site clear; opening supplies prepares them for use. Gloves prevent transfer of microorganisms. Some plastic cannulas are harmed

From deWit, S.C. (2005). *Fundamental Concepts and Skills for Nursing* (2nd ed.). Philadelphia: Elsevier Saunders.

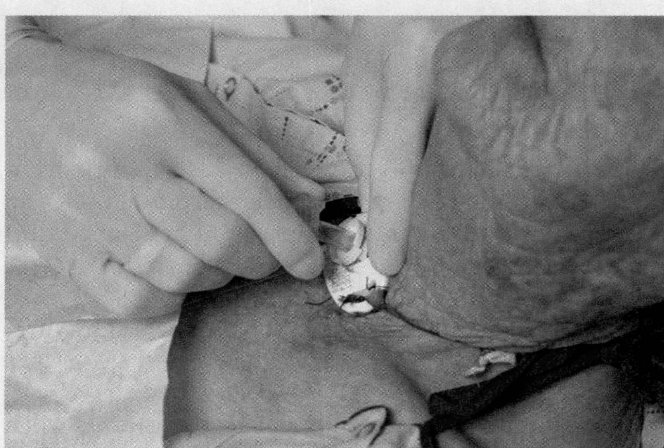
Remove the inner cannula.

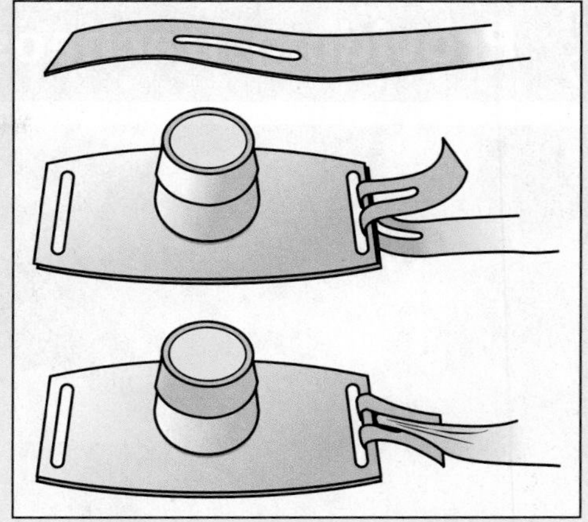
Attach the tracheostomy tube ties.

by hydrogen peroxide; check manufacturer's instructions.

4. ***ACTION*** Put on the second glove. Undo the lock on the outer cannula, stabilizing the tube flange with the index finger and thumb, and remove the inner cannula by gently pulling it out toward you.

   RATIONALE Latch must be unlocked to remove the inner cannula. If tube moves, patient will cough. If difficulty is encountered, obtain assistance.

5. ***ACTION*** Place the reusable inner cannula in the basin of wash solution and clean the lumen thoroughly with pipe cleaners or a small brush. Cleanse the outer surface with the brush. Rinse in the basin of normal saline or sterile water. Place on 4 × 4 gauze pad to drain. Handle silver cannulas carefully because they tend to dent easily.

   RATIONALE Pushing the pipe cleaner all the way through the cannula removes secretions. Some patients will have a second inner cannula available to place into the tracheostomy tube while the one removed is cleaned. In that case, store the removed cannula after cleaning.

6. ***ACTION*** Reinsert the cannula after excessive moisture has been removed. Hold the faceplate of the outer tube securely and, using aseptic technique, insert the inner cannula into the lumen of the outer cannula. Lock in place by turning the latch on the outer cannula one-quarter turn counterclockwise. Check to see that it is properly latched. Many hospitals use disposable inner cannulas that eliminate the need for cleaning.

   RATIONALE Excessive moisture may make the patient cough as the cannula is replaced. Cannula must be firmly locked into place so that it is not coughed out.

7. ***ACTION*** Remove the soiled dressing and dispose of it in the discard bag. Clean around the tube with solution required by agency protocol, using cotton swabs; rinse with saline. Move the tube as little as possible during the cleaning process.

   RATIONALE Soiled tracheostomy dressings are changed as needed. The area around the tube is cleaned every 8 hours or per agency protocol. Moving the tube causes irritation to the trachea and is uncomfortable for the patient. Some agencies require the use of hydrogen peroxide for cleaning; some physicians order acetic acid to be used.

8. ***ACTION*** Replace soiled tracheostomy ties or tube holder. Ask an assistant to help if possible. Punch a hole in the end of the tie with the closed points of the forceps, pass the end through the flange on the side of the tracheostomy tube, and thread the tie through the hole, pulling it taut. Repeat for the other side, and tie the tapes at the side of the neck with a double square knot so that the patient need not lie on the knot. Remove the old ties. The knot should be rotated from one side of the neck to the other with each change. Commercial tracheostomy tube holders may be used in place of tracheostomy tape ties.

   RATIONALE Ties are replaced when soiled or at least once every 24 hours. Ties are easier to replace if done before the new dressing is applied.

9. ***ACTION*** Apply the precut dressing or a "V"-folded gauze. Place it under and around the outer cannula to catch secretions. Forceps may be used to manipulate the dressing into place.

   RATIONALE Cutting a 4 × 4 gauze pad to use as a tracheostomy dressing should not be done because the loose gauze may fall into the tracheostomy tube and be aspirated by the patient.

■ Evaluation

10. ***ACTION*** Ask yourself: Did the procedure go smoothly? Was the tube moved too much, making the patient cough a lot? Are the ties smooth? Is the dressing sitting properly in place?

Continued

Skill 13–2 Providing Tracheostomy Care—cont'd

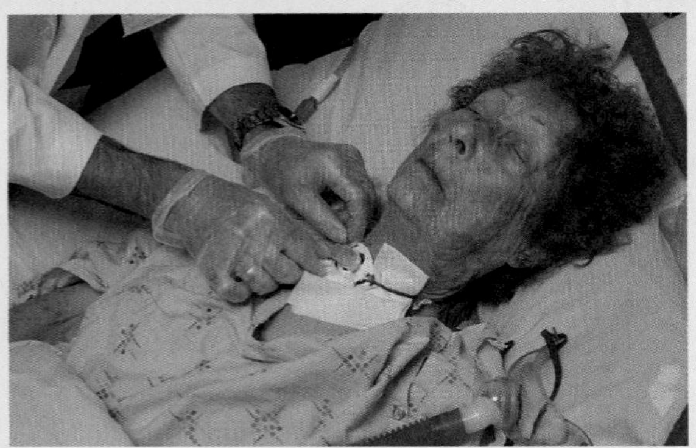

Apply the precut dressing.

RATIONALE Answers to these questions determine if the procedure was done properly and efficiently.

■ Documentation

11. *ACTION* Documentation may be in narrative form or on a flow sheet. Note the care given and the condition of the tracheostomy site.

    RATIONALE Notes that this nursing care was administered.

Documentation Example

6/2 1045 Tracheostomy care given with aseptic technique; reddening 1.5-cm diameter around tube, no complaints of discomfort. Inner cannula cleaned and replaced.

____

(Nurse's signature)

■ Special Considerations

- ✔ For patients with a permanent tracheostomy, teach all steps of tracheostomy care and suctioning. Proceed by explaining the rationale for a step and then demonstrating the step. Teach only a few steps at a time. Have patient demonstrate the procedure with coaching. Obtain a return demonstration of the entire procedure before the patient is discharged.
- ✔ Assess for skin breakdown each time you provide tracheostomy tube care.

?CRITICAL THINKING QUESTIONS

1. What may happen if you do not perform oral suction before deflating an inflatable tracheostomy cuff?
2. Why is it best to prepare the tracheostomy tube ties by cutting a slit in each tie before beginning tracheostomy care?

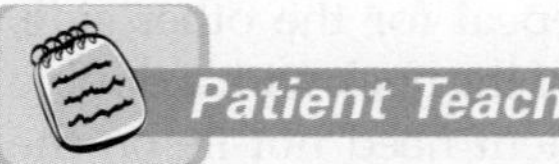

Patient Teaching 13–1

Home Care of a Tracheostomy

The patient and family should be taught the following points:

- Clean the stoma with normal saline, hydrogen peroxide, or acetic acid solution, removing all secretions, on a daily basis.
- Replace the slit gauze pad around the tube as frequently as needed when it becomes soiled.
- It is best to have two people help change the ties, because movement of the tube can easily cause the patient to cough and expel the tube from the stoma.
- Prepare the new ties before loosening the old ones.
- Hold the tube securely in place with thumb and forefinger while the ties are loose.
- Stand to the side of the stoma when providing care because if the patient coughs, mucus may be expelled.

ferent way and cannot speak or call out for help. Continued reassurance is needed both verbally and by actions that show that the nurse is aware of the patient's apprehension and readily available should help be needed. Explanations about what is being done and why are given each time tracheostomy care is provided. Teaching begins as soon as the patient is alert after the tracheostomy tube is placed. The patient who has had a partial laryngectomy will need to be taught how to eat because swallowing without aspirating is difficult (Nutritional Therapies 13–1). With the appropriate encouragement and practice, most patients can master the techniques.

The laryngectomy patient will need to be provided with a means of communication such as a pad and pencil, a Magic Slate, or a picture board device. He will need help and guidance in facing a future in which he will not be able to speak normally. He may be able to use a Passy-Muir speaking tracheostomy valve, or may learn to use esophageal speech (Figure 13–9). External mechanical devices are available to assist with speech. He also may have difficulty eating and swallowing until he masters the technique to avoid the sensations of choking and gagging that frequently occur after a laryngectomy.

Special care must be taken when the ties that hold the tracheostomy tube in place are changed; otherwise the tube may be dislodged by coughing, which movement of the tube tends to cause. Good aseptic technique is a must when caring for the tracheostomy and the neck incisions to prevent infection of the incision areas.

Nutritional Therapies 13–1

Assisting the Partial Laryngectomy Patient with Eating

To assist the patient to eat, practice in swallowing is necessary. The following guidelines are helpful in teaching the patient to swallow, thereby maintaining an adequate nutritional status.

- Explain that swallowing food without choking is possible.
- Obtain a visit from a partial laryngectomy patient who has mastered the procedure.
- Begin practice with soft or semisolid foods.
- Supervise initial practice and explain that someone needs to be with the patient when he eats until swallowing without choking is mastered.
- Teach to swallow by asking the patient to:
  - Take a deep breath and bear down to close the vocal cords.
  - Place a small bite of food in the mouth.
  - Tip the chin toward the chest and swallow.
  - Emit a cough to rid the throat of any food particles.
  - Swallow again.
  - Cough again.
  - Begin breathing normally again.
- Offer encouragement for each effort.

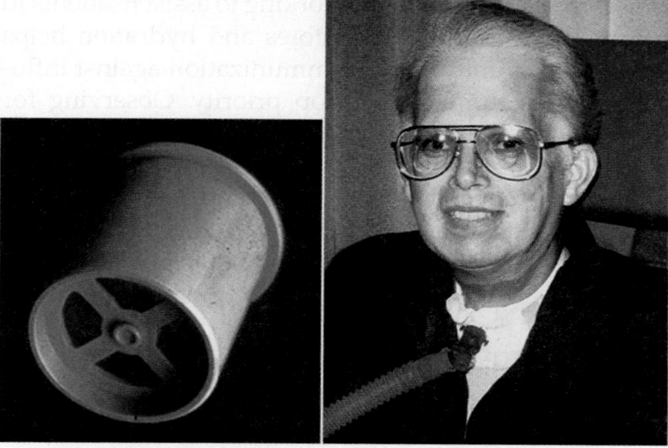

FIGURE **13–9** Passy-Muir speaking tracheostomy valve.

The patient will go through a grief process over losing his natural voice, and perhaps the ability to eat normally, if a total laryngectomy has been done. A radical neck dissection creates further problems with alteration of body image, because the procedure is somewhat disfiguring. Depression is a common problem initially, but contact with others who have had the surgery and are leading full, productive lives may help the patient focus on the benefits of the surgery in saving his own life.

Once the tracheal stoma is healed and well established, protection of the tracheal opening from dust and lint can be accomplished through the use of a simple gauze covering or high-necked clothing. The patient also should be told to avoid swimming and to use care when taking a shower or tub bath so that water is not aspirated through the opening. To protect the patient from inhalation of extremely cold air (he no longer breathes through his nose and mouth, which normally warm the inspired air), the patient may wear a small scarf over the opening during the winter.

Rehabilitation

Proper rehabilitation of the patient plays a very important part in acceptance of surgery and its consequences. The speech therapist works closely with the patient to help with mastery of a new form of speech. Many people are able to learn esophageal speech, in which they first master the art of swallowing air and then moving it forcibly back up through the esophagus. They then learn to coordinate lip and tongue movements with the sound produced by the air passing over vibrating folds of the esophagus. The sounds may be somewhat hoarse, but they can be understood as speech and are more natural than the sounds produced by an artificial larynx. For patients who cannot master esophageal speech in this manner, a tracheoesophageal prosthesis can be implanted. A fistula is created by connecting the esophagus and the trachea. A silicone prosthesis is inserted after healing has taken place. The patient can cover the opening of the prosthesis with a finger or close it with a special valve that diverts air from the lungs up through the trachea into the esophagus and out of the mouth. Speech is formed by the lip and tongue movement as the air is expelled.

A mechanical vibrator device known as an electronic artificial larynx can be used externally when applied to the skin of the esophagus to simulate speech. These are battery powered; they do not produce voicelike speech, but they do provide understandable sounds and make it possible for the patient to communicate (Figure 13–10).

An electronic speech aid with a small tube device inserted into the mouth attached to a pocket-sized power pack can also be used. A button device that can be occluded with a finger can be implanted in the throat, allowing the patient to use diaphragmatic speech.

In various parts of the United States, several groups have been organized for laryngectomy patients who wish to get together for social and rehabilitation purposes. These clubs have names such as Lost Cord, New Speech, New Voice, and Esophageal Speech. Information regarding these clubs and other aspects of postlaryngectomy rehabilitation can be obtained by writing to the American Speech-Language-Hearing Association, 10801 Rockville Pike, Rockville, MD 20852. The e-mail address is actioncenter@asha.org and the website address is www.asha.org/default.htm. Local chapters of the American Cancer Society are also good sources of information and assistance for the laryngectomy patient and his family. Further information regarding care of the laryngectomy patient who has cancer can be found in Chapter 8.

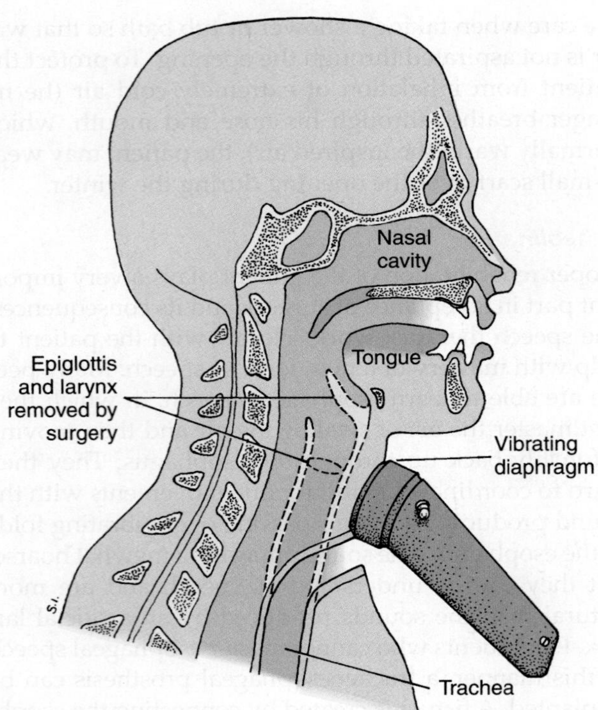

FIGURE 13–10 External electronic larynx. The vibrating cap of the electronic larynx is held against the throat with sufficient pressure to maintain firm contact. Sound vibrations are transmitted into the lower portion of the pharynx and transformed into speech by the normal movements of the tongue, lips, and teeth.

? *Think Critically About . . .* Can you identify all of the health care professionals who would be involved in the collaborative care of the patient undergoing a total laryngectomy and radical neck dissection?

Evaluation

Data are gathered to determine whether the expected outcomes have been met. If not, the nursing interventions are adjusted to better meet the needs of the patient.

COMMUNITY CARE

One of the primary aspects of community care for nurses is to promote immunization for influenza and pneumonia. It also is important to remind the public, now that everyone is so used to having antibiotics to clear up infections, that the best way to prevent infections is through hygiene measures such as frequent handwashing and covering the mouth when coughing or sneezing.

HOME CARE

Home care nurses supervise the follow-up care for the patient recovering from a severe upper respiratory infection (URI). Reviewing the correct methods of deep-breathing and coughing is an important nursing function. **Reminding patients to take every dose of the prescription antibiotic to adequately kill all causative microorganisms is very important in preventing the development of disease-resistant strains of bacteria** (CDC, 2007). 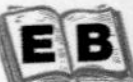 The home care nurse will also be very instrumental in helping the patient with throat cancer recover. Attention to nutritional concerns, wound care, supervision of self-care techniques for care of a tracheostomy, and psychosocial support are the keys to prompt recovery for the laryngectomy patient.

Tracheostomy care in the home setting is a little different from in the hospital. Suction catheters may be used longer and can be disinfected at home for reuse. Once the stoma is healed, the patient learns to adapt supplies to his needs. The patient's economic status may dictate what type of supplies and which type of tracheostomy tube will be best.

EXTENDED CARE

Extended-care facility nurses must be vigilant for signs of URI in residents to prevent the spread of infection to others. Refraining from coming to work with a contagious URI, or diligently wearing a mask and performing hand hygiene, can help prevent introducing URI organisms into the environment. Working to assist residents to maintain adequate protein stores and hydration helps promote immunity. Timely immunization against influenza and pneumonia is a top priority. Observing for early signs of URI and instituting care to attenuate the course of the infection helps prevent pneumonia. Providing for frequent hand hygiene and reminding residents and staff about covering sneezes and coughs decreases the spread of URIs within the facility.

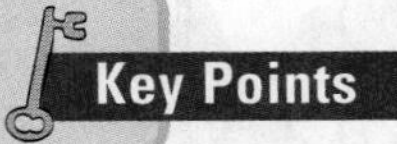

Key Points

- The common cold and rhinitis are caused by many different viruses.
- If a cold persists or high fever develops, the patient should obtain medical attention.
- Rhinitis may be allergic in origin. If it interferes with lifestyle or productivity, desensitization is an option.
- Sinusitis symptoms are headache pain, fever, tenderness over the sinuses, purulent drainage from the nose, painful upper teeth, and malaise. A nonproductive cough may be present.
- Surgery is sometimes necessary to open a drainage tract and clear purulent material.
- Epistaxis is caused by many factors such as irritation from nose blowing, hypertension, trauma, blood dyscrasias, decreased humidity, and nose picking.
- Apply direct pressure to the nose for 10 to 15 minutes to stop bleeding; cold compresses or ice is helpful.
- Pharyngitis is inflammation of the pharynx, or sore throat, that is viral, bacterial, or fungal in origin.

- Treatment for viral pharyngitis is rest, warm saline gargles, throat lozenges, and a mild analgesic.
- A throat culture and antibiotics are usual for bacterial pharyngitis.
- Treatment and nursing interventions for tonsillitis consist of warm saline gargles, throat lozenges, rest, and antibiotics. Surgery may be indicated in some cases.
- After tonsillectomy, check vital signs frequently, keep the patient on his side or abdomen as long as there is drainage from the throat, and limit diet to soft, nonirritating foods until the throat is no longer sensitive.
- Observe for frequent swallowing, which may indicate blood running down the throat.
- Rhinoplasty is performed for severe nasal fracture.
- Cancer of the larynx risk factors are smoking, immoderate alcohol use, chronic laryngitis, and abuse of vocal cords.
- Persistent hoarseness is a first sign of cancer of the larynx; later signs are pain in the throat, coughing, dysphagia, a lump in the throat, or pain in the region of the Adam's apple.
- Surgical treatment for laryngeal tumor is laser treatment, partial or total laryngectomy, and possible radical neck dissection.
- A new speech pattern must be learned by the total laryngectomy patient because there is a permanent opening in the trachea.
- Endotracheal intubation and tracheostomy provide an artificial airway.
- Major concerns of an artificial airway are maintaining an open airway, preventing infection, and maintaining the integrity of skin around the stoma and mucous membranes of the respiratory tract.
- Suctioning of an artificial airway is a sterile procedure (see Skill 13–2).
- Laryngectomy patients are taught self-care for suctioning and tracheostomy care before discharge.
- Prevent respiratory infections in community by promoting immunization for influenza and pneumonia.
- Teach prevention of infection by hygiene measures: proper hand hygiene, and covering the mouth when coughing or sneezing.
- The immune system is less efficient in the elderly, making them more prone to contracting URIs.
- Elderly men with a long history of smoking and heavy alcohol use are most likely to develop throat cancer.
- Elderly people should take care not to be exposed to others with URIs, as immunity is decreased.

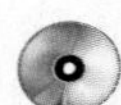

Go to your **Companion CD-ROM** for an Audio Glossary, animations, video clips, and bonus review questions.

evolve Be sure to visit the companion Evolve site at http://evolve.elsevier.com/deWit for interactive NCLEX-PN Exam Style Review Questions, WebLinks, and additional online resources.

NCLEX-PN EXAM STYLE REVIEW QUESTIONS

Choose the best answer(s) for the following questions.

1. On initial assessment, the patient who had recently undergone tonsillectomy and adenoidectomy is found to be restless with noticeable efforts to swallow. The most likely explanation would be:

1. excessive thirst.
1. starvation.
3. bleeding.
4. sore throat.

2. A 45-year-old man eating steak suddenly rises from his seat. His hands are grasping his throat. An immediate action by a bystander would be to:

1. perform finger sweeps when food bolus is seen.
2. wrap the arms around the victim from behind.
3. position the open hand just above the nipple line.
4. deliver three downward squeeze thrusts.

3. Which of the following nursing interventions is appropriate in the immediate postoperative period when caring for a patient who has undergone rhinoplasty? *(Select all that apply.)*

1. Observe for frequent swallowing.
2. Monitor amount of drainage.
3. Position patient flat on the back.
4. Apply warm compresses.
5. Provide humidified oxygen.

4. The spouse of a patient with a tracheostomy asks, "Why did the physician order a fenestrated tracheostomy tube?" An appropriate response by a nurse would be:

1. "It prepares the patient for long-term tracheostomy."
2. "It allows gradual weaning before closure of the tracheostomy."
3. "It prevents aspiration."
4. "It reduces the risk for tracheal wall necrosis."

5. ______________________ is a surgical incision into the trachea for the purpose of inserting a tube through which the patient can breathe.

6. While deciding whether to sign the surgical consent for tracheostomy, the patient's spouse asks, "What is the purpose of this procedure?" Which of the following responses demonstrates nursing knowledge regarding the procedure? *(Select all that apply.)*

1. "The procedure facilitates suctioning of respiratory secretions."
2. "The procedure prevents recurrence of respiratory arrest."
3. "The procedure prevents aspiration of oral secretions in unconscious patients."
4. "The procedure bypasses an obstructed upper airway."
5. "The procedure is a temporary airway for face and neck injuries."

7. A 55-year-old male patient with a new tracheostomy is unable to cough. Breath sounds are diminished. Pulse oximetry is 88% on 100% humidified air. An immediate nursing action would be to:
   1. provide positive ventilation.
   2. suction respiratory secretions.
   3. administer pain medications.
   4. humidify inhaled air.

8. A patient newly diagnosed with a squamous cell carcinoma of the larynx would most likely display which of the following signs and symptoms?
   1. Rhonchi
   2. Hoarseness
   3. Frothy sputum
   4. Drooling

9. The student nurse demonstrates endotracheal suctioning. Which of the following actions indicates a need for further instructions?
   1. Donning sterile gloves prior to suctioning
   2. Lubricating the suction catheter with petroleum jelly
   3. Assessing the need for suctioning
   4. Checking the suction hookup

10. ________________________ is a common occurrence of minimal blood loss that is associated with decreased humidity, excessive nose blowing, allergies, and snorting street drugs.

CRITICAL THINKING ACTIVITIES 

Read each clinical scenario and discuss the questions with your classmates.

Scenario A

Mr. Kim has undergone diagnostic procedures to confirm suspected cancer of the larynx. He has been admitted to the hospital for a hemilaryngectomy.

1. Describe the teaching plan that would be used for a patient undergoing a direct laryngoscopy.
2. What diagnostic tests would have been done on Mr. Kim?
3. Devise a postoperative nursing care plan for Mr. Kim, including interventions for psychosocial problems.
4. What resources in the community could be suggested to help Mr. Kim adjust to his laryngectomy?

Scenario B

Mr. Thomas has undergone a total laryngectomy and radical neck dissection.

1. What structures would have been removed during this surgery and how would his life be affected?
2. When suctioning his tracheostomy, how long would you apply suction?
3. How might you provide for communication with Mr. Thomas during the postoperative period?

CHAPTER

14 Care of Patients with Disorders of the Lower Respiratory System

evolve http://evolve.elsevier.com/deWit

Objectives

Upon completing this chapter, you should be able to:

Theory

1. Compare and contrast commonalities and differences in nursing care for patients with bronchitis, influenza, pneumonia, empyema, and pleurisy.
2. List at least three nursing interventions appropriate for care of patients experiencing the following: persistent cough, increased secretions in the respiratory tract, dyspnea, alteration in nutrition and hydration related to respiratory disorder, and fatigue related to hypoxia.
3. Describe ways a nurse can contribute to prevention and prompt treatment of tuberculosis.
4. Illustrate the pathophysiologic changes that occur during an asthma attack.
5. Identify problems that occur with aging that may cause a restrictive pulmonary disorder.
6. Describe the specifics of nursing care for the patient who has had thoracic surgery and has chest tubes in place.

Clinical Practice

1. Complete a nursing care plan, including home care, for the patient with chronic airflow limitation (CAL).
2. Devise a nursing care plan for the tracheostomy patient on oxygen therapy and on a mechanical ventilator
3. Develop a teaching plan for the patient diagnosed with moderate asthma.
4. Compare emergency nursing care for a patient with a penetrating chest injury with that for the patient with a spontaneous pneumothorax.

Key Terms

Be sure to check out the bonus material on the Companion CD-ROM, including selected audio pronunciations.

aerosol (ĂR-ō-sŏl, p. 349)
asthma (ĂZ-mă, p. 329)
atelectasis (ă-tĕ-LĔK-tă-sĭs, p. 330)
bronchiectasis (brŏng-kē-ĔK-tă-sĭs, p. 328)
bronchodilator (brŏng-kō-DĪ-lā-tĕr, p. 348)
cor pulmonale (kŏr pŭl-mō-NĂ-lē, p. 331)
emphysema (ĕm-fĭ-SĒ-mă, p. 330)
hemoptysis (hē-MŎP-tĭ-sĭs, p. 325)
hemothorax (hē-mō-THŌ-răks, p. 344)
intrathoracic (ĭn-tră-thōr-RĂ-sĭk, p. 346)
leukotriene (lĕw-kō-trī-ēn, p. 349)
nebulizer (NĔ-bū-lī-zĕr, p. 349)
paradoxical respirations (păr-ă-DŎK-sik-ăl rĕs-pĕ-RA-shĕn, p. 342)
pleurisy (PLOOR-ă-sē, p. 329)
pneumonectomy (nū-mō-NĔK-tō-mē, p. 339)
pneumonia (nū-MŌ-nē-ă, p. 321)
pneumothorax (nū-mō-THŌ-răks, p. 343)
polycythemia (pŏl-ē-sī-THĒ-mē-ă, p. 331)
sarcoidosis (săr-koy-DŌ-sĭs, p. 329)
subcutaneous emphysema (sŭb-kū-TĀ-nē-ĕs ĕm-fĭ-SĒ-mă, p. 346)
thoracentesis (thō-ră-sĕn-TĒ-sĭs, p. 329)
thoracotomy (thō-ră-KŎT-ō-mē, p. 346)
thrombolytic (thrŏm-bō-LĬT-ĭk, p. 339)
tuberculosis (too-BĔR-kū-LŌ-sĭs, p. 324)

Please refer to Chapter 12 for a review of anatomy and physiology of the lower respiratory system, along with causes of disorders and ways to prevent them. Information on common problems in caring for people with respiratory disorders, assessment of the respiratory system, and the general nursing management of common respiratory problems is also discussed in Chapter 12.

RESPIRATORY INFECTIOUS DISEASES

ACUTE BRONCHITIS

Acute bronchitis frequently is an extension of an upper respiratory infection involving the trachea *(tracheobronchitis)* and usually is viral in origin. Causes other than infectious agents are physical and chemical agents inhaled in air polluted by dust, automobile exhaust, industrial fumes, and tobacco smoke.

Early symptoms of acute bronchitis are similar to those of the common cold. In acute bronchitis, the symptoms progress to chest pain, fever, and a dry, hacking, and irritating cough. Later the cough becomes more productive of mucopurulent sputum. The fever may be moderate (≤101° F [38.3° C]) and accompanied by chills, muscle soreness, and headache. The physician relies on history and signs and symptoms for diagnosis.

Acute bronchitis is treated conservatively; antibiotics are used only as indicated by sputum that contains specific organisms. Symptomatic treatment includes the use of humidification using either warm or cool moist air, cough mixtures, or bronchodilators to reduce coughing and soothe the irritated tracheal and bronchial mucosa, and bed rest to promote healing. Nutrition and fluid balance should be maintained. Rest is recommended to avoid progression of an acute condition to a chronic one.

INFLUENZA

Etiology

Influenza is an acute, highly infectious disease of the upper and lower respiratory tracts and is caused by any of three major types (A, B, and C) and numerous subtypes of influenzaviruses. It occurs as isolated cases or in epidemics. The most virulent form is type A, which usually affects young adults first and then spreads to the very young and very old in the community (Health Promotion Points 14–1).

Influenza is usually spread by direct and indirect contact with infected people by coughing and sneezing and by virus transferred from contaminated hands to objects. Severe acute respiratory syndrome (SARS) appears to be spread by person-to-person contact, whereas avian flu and West Nile virus are spread by vectors such as certain birds and mosquitoes (CDC, 2001) (Box 14–1).

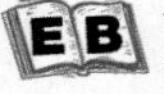

Pathophysiology

The influenzaviruses affect the respiratory mucosa, causing inflammation and necrosis of tissue and shedding of the virus into the secretions. The inflammation may involve the lungs, pharynx, sinuses, and eustachian tubes. The necrosis that occurs provides an environment for the growth of bacteria that cause secondary infection. Bacterial pneumonia is often a consequence of influenza.

Signs and Symptoms

The first symptoms of influenza appear 2 to 3 days after exposure (Safety Alert 14–1). They come on rather suddenly and include headache, fever (often 101° to 103° F [38° to 40° C]) chills, anorexia, and muscle aches. Soon sore throat, hacking cough, runny nose and nasal congestion, and eyes that are light sensitive occur. Children often develop nausea, vomiting, and diarrhea.

Diagnosis

Chest x-ray and auscultation usually show no abnormality. The white cell count is normal or slightly below normal. To actually confirm the diagnosis, viral culture, serology, rapid antigen testing, or polymerase chain reaction and/or immunofluorescence assays must be performed. Diagnosis is usually based on clinical findings.

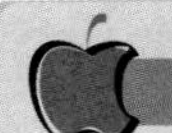

Health Promotion Points 14–1

Protection from Influenza

The Advisory Committee on Immunization Practices (ACIP) recommends annual influenza vaccination for the following groups:

- People at high risk for influenza-related complications and severe disease, including
  - children ages 6 to 59 months
  - pregnant women
  - people >50 years of age
  - people of any age with certain chronic medical conditions
- People who live with or care for persons at high risk, including
  - household contacts who have frequent contact with people at high risk and who can transmit influenza to those individuals
  - health care workers

Treatment and Nursing Management

Uncomplicated influenza usually is managed more effectively by nursing intervention than by drugs or other forms of medical treatment. Rest, increased fluid intake, acetaminophen or ibuprofen, and saline gargles for a sore throat are usually recommended. Antibiotics are given only if there is evidence of bacterial infection secondary to the viral infection.

If a person is known to be at high risk for influenza and has been exposed to type A influenza, the physician may choose to provide prophylaxis with an antiviral agent such as amantadine (Symmetrel), rimantadine (Flumadine), zanamivir (Relenza), or oseltamivir (Tamiflu) (Complementary & Alternative Therapies 14–1). These drugs must be started within 48 hours of the start of symptoms. Aspirin is to be avoided because Reye's syndrome sometimes occurs as a complication and has been linked to aspirin use. Reye's syndrome is more common in children than adults.

Nursing interventions for patients with these problems might include the following:

- Increase oral fluid intake to at least 3000 mL per 24 hours unless contraindicated.
- Encourage patient to take analgesics when discomfort first appears.
- Administer suppressant cough medicine at bedtime and during the night as prescribed.
- Administer cough medicine and analgesics promptly and on a routine basis during the acute phase.
- Perform mouth care at least every 4 hours, before each meal, and more frequently if patient reports bad taste in mouth or has halitosis from sputum.
- Cater to patient's food and drink preferences within limits of dietary restrictions.

Box 14–1 *Emerging Infectious Diseases That May Cause Influenza Symptoms*

AVIAN FLU

A pandemic of *avian influenza* that could kill millions of people is a worldwide fear. Vaccines are under development to try to avert such a problem, but there is no effective vaccine yet. This type of bird flu had been restricted to poultry, but had infected and killed over 100 people as of the summer of 2006. All of these people had been in direct contact with infected poultry or secretions or excretions from poultry. The virus has managed to mutate, infect and sicken humans. Because there is no previous exposure to the virus, and consequently no built-up immunity, it can kill quickly. Symptoms are the same as for common influenza—fever, cough, sore throat, and muscle aches. In some people the disease has progressed to more serious disorders. Complications of pneumonia with acute respiratory distress syndrome have been the cause of death. There have been two probable cases of human-to-human transmission of the virus, and this is the reason for such concern. The drug oseltamivir (Tamiflu) is the only treatment available to decrease the severity of the disease. It is not known how effective this drug would be in a large outbreak.

To prevent the possibility of contracting avian flu when traveling, it is recommended to avoid areas where poultry are raised or kept; to not mingle with wild birds by feeding wild ducks, geese, or swans; and to be certain any poultry eaten is thoroughly cooked. Perform hand hygiene frequently with soap and water or an alcohol-based hand gel. Keep your hands away from your mouth, nose, and eyes.

WEST NILE VIRUS

West Nile virus (WNV) is transmitted by bites from infected mosquitoes. Most WNV infections are mild and inconsequential. The incubation period is 3 to 7 days. West Nile virus may cause flulike symptoms lasting up to 6 days. If infection does occur, it presents as a febrile illness of sudden onset. Symptoms are malaise, anorexia, nausea, vomiting, headache, *myalgia* (muscle ache), eye pain, and lymphadenopathy. A rash may occur. The chances of becoming ill from one mosquito bite are very small. In about 1 in 150 instances of infection, the patient develops severe neurologic disease. This occurs mostly in patients of advanced age. Encephalitis is more frequently the result than meningitis. High fever and changing mental status are the initial signs of neurologic involvement. Treatment of severe disease is supportive, with hospitalization, intravenous fluids, respiratory support, and prevention of secondary infection.

Prevention of WNV is to wear insect repellent containing DEET when outdoors to prevent mosquito bites. Wear a long-sleeved shirt, long pants, and socks with shoes when outside. Clothing should be sprayed too. Avoid being outdoors at dawn and dusk. Keep containers around the yard empty of standing water. Use screens on open windows and doors.

SEVERE ACUTE RESPIRATORY SYNDROME

SARS is caused by a previously unrecognized coronavirus, SARS-associated coronavirus (SARS-CoV). The disease first appeared as a global threat in 2003 and affected people ages 25 to 70. The illness begins with fever >100.4° F. (>38° C) that may be accompanied by chills, headache, malaise, diarrhea, and body aches. Ten percent to 20% of those infected develop diarrhea. After 2 to 7 days respiratory symptoms appear with a dry, nonproductive cough or dyspnea. Hypoxemia requiring mechanical ventilation may develop. Most patients develop pneumonia.

SARS appears to be spread by close person-to-person contact and is thought to be transmitted mostly by respiratory droplets via coughs and sneezes. It is possible that SARS is spread through the air or by other ways not yet known. The severity of SARS ranges from mild illness to death. Supportive treatment and medications used for pneumonia are given. Antiviral agents may be added, but there is no known specific treatment for this disorder.

To prevent the contraction of SARS when in a location in which it exists, use proper hand hygiene, avoid people who have a respiratory infection, and keep your hands away from your eyes, nose, and mouth.

- Give antipyretics and perform sponge bath and other measures to reduce fever.
- Humidify inhaled air.
- Splint chest and abdomen with pillow during coughing attacks.
- Apply emollient to lips and nares as needed.
- Clear nostrils as much as possible to prevent mouth breathing.
- Provide for periods of uninterrupted rest.
- Protect from and monitor for secondary infections such as pneumonia, otitis media, and sinusitis, as the weakened immune system causes greater susceptibility.

People over 65 and those at high risk for influenza should be immunized every year (Gross et al., 1995) (see Health Promotion Points 14–1).

PNEUMONIA

Etiology and Pathophysiology

Pneumonia is an extensive inflammation of the lung with either consolidation of the lung tissue as it fills with exudate or interstitial inflammation and edema. It can affect one or both lungs or only one lobe of a lung (lobar pneumonia). In 2003, 63,241 people died of pneumonia (American Lung Association, 2006b). Pneumonia is classified as community acquired or hospital acquired. Infectious pneumonia may be bacterial or viral. Viral pneumonia tends to be less severe than bacterial pneumonia. Bacterial pneumonia usually produces exudate leading to consolidation. It most commonly affects only one lung. Viral pneumonia does not produce exudate; it causes interstitial inflammation. The most common causative organism of bac-

Precautions When Caring for Patients with Suspected Avian Flu

Follow these safeguards when caring for any patient suspected of having avian flu:

- Place the patient in an airborne isolation room and wear a fit-tested respirator such as a NIOSH-approved N-95 filtering facepiece respirator.
- Use contact precautions for all patient contact, and wear eye protection when within 3 feet of the patient.
- Maintain precautions for 14 days after onset of symptoms or until avian flu has been ruled out.
- Teach the patient about isolation precautions.
- Cover the mouth when coughing or sneezing; instruct the patient in good hand hygiene.

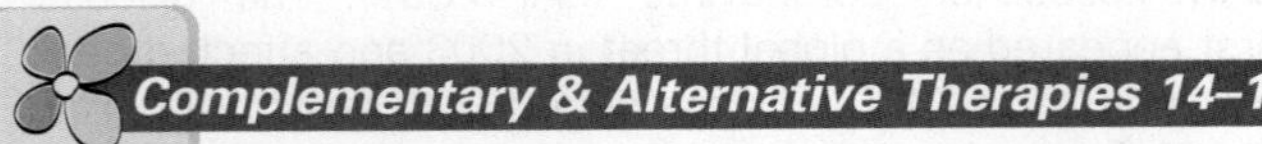

Alternative Therapy for the "Flu"

Elderberry juice has been used for centuries as a treatment to ease symptoms of the flu, colds, and sinus infections. It seems to prevent the influenza virus from latching onto cells. There are antioxidants found in the purple elderberry fruit that have an anti-inflammatory effect comparable to aspirin. This may explain why the juice produces symptom improvement. Elderberry juice is available in health food stores or on line from *www.drugstore.com*. It is said to cut illness time in half.

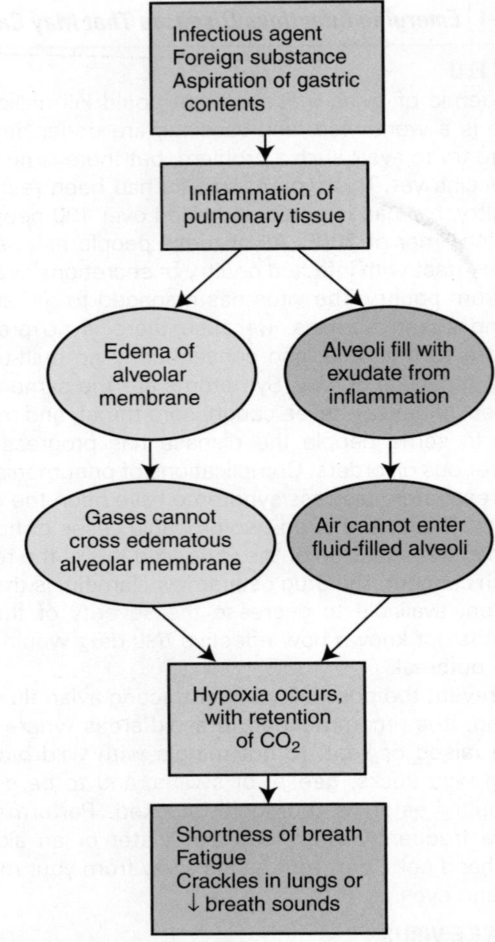

CONCEPT MAP **14–1** Pathophysiology of pneumonia.

terial pneumonia is *Streptococcus pneumoniae*, which also is called *pneumococcus*. Pathogenic microorganisms are always present in the upper respiratory tract and, when resistance is lowered by some other factor, such as chronic disease, alcoholism, physical inactivity, or extremes in age (very young or very old), they may cause pneumonia. It frequently occurs following influenza infection. Concept Map 14–1 presents the pathophysiology of pneumonia.

Pneumonia also can result from inhalation of irritating gases *(chemical pneumonia)* or accidental aspiration of foods or liquids that causes a pneumonitis progressing to pneumonia *(aspiration pneumonia)*. *Hypostatic pneumonia*, which results from lying in bed for extended periods, always is a threat to those with impaired mobility. Lack of physical exercise and inadequate aeration of the lungs are major factors in the development of hypostatic pneumonia, in which retained secretions cause inflammation.

Fungi also may cause opportunistic pneumonia in immunocompromised patients. *Pneumocystis jiroveci* (formerly *Pneumocystis carinii*) pneumonia (PCP) is common in AIDS patients (see Chapter 11).

Prevention

Elderly, weak, debilitated, and immobilized people are all prime candidates for pneumonia, as are those who have some kind of chronic pulmonary disease. People over age 65, and those with chronic respiratory disease, should receive Pneumovax, the pneumococcal pneumonia vaccine. A second dose is needed 6 years after the first dose. This vaccine protects against 23 pneumococcal organisms.

A variety of nursing interventions can help prevent pneumonia. These include:

- Strengthening the patient's natural defenses and avoiding infection.
- Ensuring frequent turning, coughing, and deep breathing for postoperative patients or those who are otherwise unable to ventilate their lungs adequately.
- Carefully watching and properly positioning vomiting patients who are in decreased states of consciousness, such as patients recovering from anesthesia, on their sides.
- Elevating the head of the bed when administering tube feedings and when assisting a patient to

eat, and leaving the head elevated for 30 to 60 minutes after the feeding to prevent aspiration. Check residual before each feeding, or once every 4 hours (Goodwin, 2007).

EB

- Avoiding giving liquids to patients who are prone to aspiration.
- Faithfully following principles of cleanliness and asepsis when caring for debilitated patients and those most susceptible to infection.
- Administering pneumonia vaccine when prescribed for those most at risk for developing the disease .
- Encouraging immunization against influenza.

Nosocomial (hospital-acquired) pneumonia is a major problem that considerably lengthens hospital stays, increasing the cost of health care. Nosocomial pneumonia has a 30% to 50% death rate. Vigilant nurses who provide aggressive respiratory care can greatly decrease the incidence of hospital-acquired pneumonia.

Signs, Symptoms, and Diagnosis

Symptoms of pneumonia vary according to type. In typical infectious pneumonia, there usually is a high fever accompanied by chills, a cough that produces rusty or blood-flecked sputum, sweating, chest pain that is made worse by respiratory movements, and a general feeling of malaise and aching muscles. **Diagnosis is confirmed by chest x-ray, which reveals densities in the affected lung.**

The diagnosis of atypical pneumonia might be missed because of a lack of symptoms usually indicative of pneumonia. Body temperature can be normal or subnormal, breath sounds can be normal with perhaps only occasional crackles and wheezes, and there may be no pleural involvement and therefore no pain, dry cough, or feeling of extreme fatigue. Chest radiography reveals diffuse, patchy areas of density. Cytomegalovirus has become a cause of pneumonia in immunocompromised patients, particularly those with AIDS or transplant patients on immunosuppressive drugs.

Treatment

Typical pneumonia is treated with intravenous (IV) or oral antibiotic agents such as erythromycin or the new macrolides (clarithromycin [Biaxin]), cephalosporins, aminoglycosides, or fluoroquinolones such as ciprofloxacin (Cipro), depending on the type of bacteria responsible and the degree of sensitivity of the causative organism to various antibiotics (Complementary & Alternative Therapies 14–2). Atypical pneumonia caused by *Mycoplasma* usually is treated with either erythromycin or clarithromycin. Viral, atypical pneumonia requires no anti-infective therapy, but antiviral medication may be administered. PCP associated with AIDS is treated with aerosolized and intravenous pentamidine, trimethoprim-sulfamethoxazole (Bactrim), trimetrexate glucuronate (NeuTrexin), dapsone, clindamycin, or atovaquone. Supplemental oxygen is provided as needed. Some patients require mechanical ventilation.

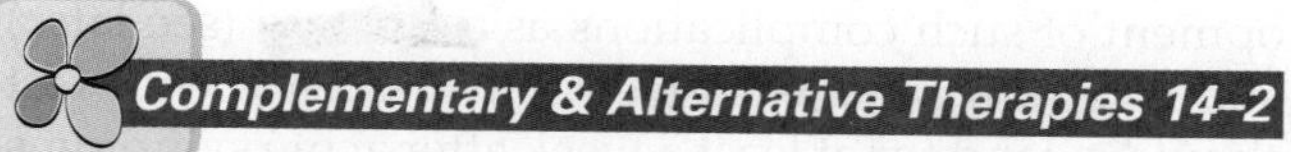

Treatment for Pneumonia

Barberry root bark is used against bacteria, fungi, and viruses as well as other organisms, and is an alternative treatment for pneumonia. It has antimicrobial action against both gram-positive and gram-negative bacteria. It should not be used during pregnancy as it can cause spontaneous abortion.

? *Think Critically About . . .* Can you identify five signs or symptoms found on assessment that might correlate with a diagnosis of pneumonia?

Nursing Management

The nursing care plan for a patient with pneumonia should include interventions to:

- Promote oxygenation
- Control elevated temperature
- Maintain nutritional and fluid intake
- Provide adequate rest
- Monitor vital signs and respiratory status
- Relieve pain and discomfort
- Provide good oral hygiene
- Prevent irritation of the lungs by smoke and other irritants
- Avoid secondary bacterial infections

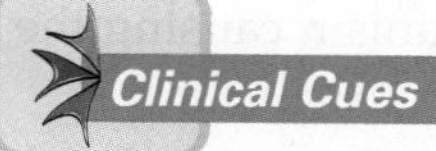

The first signs of decreasing oxygenation may be restlessness or confusion. The patient may want to sit upright to allow for better chest excursion. Respiratory rate will increase and later there will be flaring of the nares, then retraction of respiratory muscles if the condition worsens. Cyanosis is a very late sign.

The patient should deep breathe and cough 5 to 10 times each hour while awake. **It is important that the nurse assess for signs of increasing impairment of gas exchange.**

Fluid intake, unless contraindicated, should be increased to 2500 to 3000 mL/day. Because abdominal distention, nausea, and vomiting also may accompany pneumonia, nursing interventions to deal with these problems may be indicated. Other problems that could be presented by the patient include altered states of consciousness (delirium and confusion) and the development of such complications as empyema (see later) and congestive heart failure. Convalescence with rest should extend for at least a week after acute symptoms subside for the young adult. The older adult needs several weeks to feel able to do usual activities without undue fatigue.

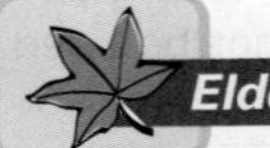

Elder Care Points

A less efficient immune system, decreased action of cilia and other lung protective mechanisms, and less elasticity and muscle tone all cause the elder to be more at risk for influenza and pneumonia.

- Confusion often is the most obvious sign of atypical pneumonia in the elderly.
- It may take 6 to 12 weeks after a bout of pneumonia for the elder to be able to resume normal activities without undue fatigue.
- The very elderly patient may never quite regain the former level of wellness after a serious episode of pneumonia.
- Teach the elderly to seek medical attention quickly if symptoms of pneumonia occur.

EMPYEMA

When the fluid within the pleural cavity becomes infected, the exudate becomes thick and purulent, and the patient is said to have *empyema.* The organisms causing the infection may be staphylococci or streptococci.

Empyema is treated by eliminating the infection through specific antibiotics and by removing excess fluid from the pleural cavity via one or more chest tubes and a closed drainage system. A specimen of the fluid is sent to the laboratory for a culture and sensitivity study. This test determines which exact antibiotic will most effectively destroy the organism causing the infection.

FUNGAL INFECTIONS

PCP has a high incidence in AIDS patients. *Pneumocystis carinii* is now considered a fungus, renamed *Pneumocystis jiroveci.* It is found only in immunocompromised patients and is highly lethal (see Chapter 11).

The incidence of fungal lung disease is increasing in the United States (Box 14–2). These infections are caused by the inhalation of the fungus or spores or by overgrowth of organisms found normally in the body. These infections can cause pneumonia. The most common fungal lung infections are coccidioidomycosis and histoplasmosis.

Coccidioidomycosis occurs in the San Joaquin Valley of California, as well as in Utah, Nevada, New Mexico, Arizona, western Texas, Mexico, and South America. It is contracted by people who engage in desert recreational activities or are working in occupations that require digging in the earth. Most who contract it have only mild respiratory symptoms or are asymptomatic, but 40% of those affected have influenza symptoms with cough, fever, pleuritic chest pain, myalgias, and arthralgias. Sometimes a flat red rash with dark red papules occurs.

Box 14–2 *Fungal Infections of the Lung*

- Histoplasmosis
- Coccidioidomycosis
- Blastomycosis
- Cryptococcosis
- Aspergillosis
- Candidiasis

Histoplasmosis occurs in central and eastern portions of North America, particularly around the Ohio River, Missouri River, and Mississippi River. It also occurs in South and Central America, India, and Cyprus. The fungus lives in moist soil such as that in which mushrooms grow, on the floors of chicken houses and bat caves, and in bird droppings. Clinical signs are fever, fatigue, cough, dyspnea, and weight loss over 1 to 2 months.

The other fungal infections are seen mostly in immunocompromised people. Fungal infections are diagnosed by history, signs and symptoms, and positive skin test reaction to the fungus. Treatment is IV amphotericin B for up to 12 weeks. Cystic fibrosis patients are also susceptible to fungal lung infection.

OCCUPATIONAL LUNG DISORDERS

Coal dust, asbestos, dust from hemp, flax, and cotton processing, and exposure to silica in the air all can cause work-related lung disorders. Asbestos exposure may cause a rare cancer of the chest lining, mesothelioma (Mesothelioma Cancer Research Organization, 2005). It 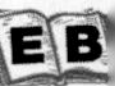

also causes scarring of lung tissue. The other exposures cause obstruction of small airways or scarring and loss of elasticity and compliance. Occupational history should be a part of the respiratory assessment.

TUBERCULOSIS

Etiology

Pulmonary tuberculosis (TB) is an infectious disease of the lung characterized by lesions within the lung tissue. The lesions may continue to degenerate and become necrotic, or they may heal by fibrosis and calcification. The causative organism is the true tubercle bacillus *Mycobacterium tuberculosis.*

Contrary to popular beliefs, tuberculosis is *not* highly contagious. Infection most often occurs after prolonged exposure to the tubercle bacillus, but not everyone contracts the disease, even after close and extensive contact with infected persons (Cultural Cues 14–1).

Tuberculosis still is a major health problem in many countries throughout the world, and in the United States. The increase in the number of immunodeficient people with AIDS and the influx of immigrants who are infected with TB are the two major causes of the increase in the United States. Poor living conditions,

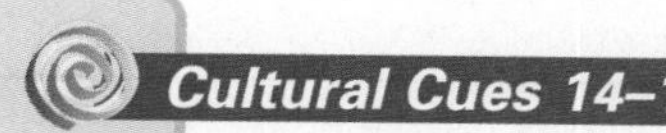

Ethnic Occurrence of Tuberculosis

American Indian, Alaska Natives, Asian/Pacific Islanders, black non-Hispanics, and Hispanics have a high incidence of tuberculosis. The disease is most prevalent in people over 65 years of age in these groups.

New immigrants from areas where tuberculosis is prevalent have incidence rates similar to their former country for the first few years of residence in the United States.

especially in urban areas, and malnutrition increase susceptibility to the tubercle bacillus. The increase in the population of malnourished urban poor is another reason why the disease is spreading.

In countries where there are high rates of tuberculosis, the World Health Organization strongly recommends the widespread use of *bacille Calmette-Guérin* (BCG) vaccine, which is credited with having a favorable impact in reducing the morbidity of tuberculosis. The vaccine's ability to increase resistance is in question, and it is rarely used for this purpose in the United States.

Pathophysiology

Mycobacterium is an acid-fast, aerobic, slow-growing bacillus. When the organism enters the lungs, a local inflammatory reaction occurs, usually in the upper lobe. Bacilli migrate to the lymph nodes and activate a cell-mediated hypersensitivity response. This triggers granuloma formation with influx of macrophages and lymphocytes at the site of inflammation. The bacillus is walled off, forming a *tubercle.* Caseation necrosis, a core of cheeselike material, develops in the center of the tubercle. In a healthy person, the tubercles eventually calcify. In the unhealthy individual, the bacilli spread to other parts of the lung and to other organs. Bacilli may remain viable in a dormant state inside the tubercle for many years. The bacilli are difficult to eradicate when released into the environment because the bacillus is resistant to drying and to many disinfectants.

Signs and Symptoms

The onset of tuberculosis is gradual; a patient may have an active and progressing lesion before symptoms appear. Typical symptoms are cough, low-grade fever in the afternoon, anorexia, loss of weight, fatigue, night sweats, and sometimes **hemoptysis** (blood in sputum). Tight or dull chest pain and mucopurulent sputum may occur as the disease progresses.

Diagnosis

Early detection of tuberculosis is of great importance because:

- The anti-TB drugs are more effective in the early stages of the disease.
- The period of disability is much shorter.
- The complications are fewer.

Tuberculin Skin Testing. Skin testing for tuberculosis is done by the *Mantoux* test. Food handlers, those working with children, and health care workers must be periodically tested. Others who are symptomatic or have been exposed to someone with TB should be tested. The multipuncture test is no longer approved. In this test, 0.1 mL of purified protein derivative (PPD) tuberculin containing 5 tuberculin units is injected intradermally. The test is now referred to as the tuberculin skin test (TST) rather than the PPD test. Skin testing is not used on people who have received BCG vaccine within the previous 10 years. This includes those in whom BCG has been used to treat bladder cancer. The test is *positive* when the swelling at the site of injection is more than 5 mm in diameter 48 to 72 hours after injection in people who have a history of contact with infectious TB or in immunocompromised patients. Induration of more than 10 mm in diameter is *positive* in recent immigrants from countries where TB is prevalent, in medically underserved groups, and the homeless. For those persons at low risk, induration of more than 15 mm is considered positive.

A positive tuberculin test indicates that the person has been infected with the tubercle bacillus at some time. It does not indicate whether the disease is active or inactive at that time, only that the body tissues are sensitive to tuberculin. A positive reaction indicates a need for further evaluation. Once a skin test is positive, the person will always show a positive reaction to the skin test.

A new test, the QuantiFERON-TB Gold, is a blood test and is less likely to produce false-positive readings. It means one visit to the clinic or office for a blood draw, rather than the two required for the TST (the second visit is for reading the result). It is accurate even for people who have had BCG. Both tests cost about the same amount.

X-Rays and Sputum Cultures. An x-ray examination of the chest may or may not reveal tubercular lesions in the lung, but calcified and healed lesions, as well as active lesions, usually can be seen on x-rays. **A diagnosis of active tuberculosis is established when the tubercle bacillus has been found in the sputum or gastric washings.** Because people are quite likely to swallow sputum rather than expectorate it, a sample of stomach contents may be examined if the patient cannot produce an adequate sputum specimen *(gastric analysis).* Sputum cultures are slow growing, and culture results take 1 to 3 weeks to allow identification of the bacillus.

Treatment

Before the advent of anti-TB drugs, patients with pulmonary tuberculosis were treated in sanitoria, where they were isolated to avoid spreading the disease. In the 1960s, the trend was to treat patients with active tuberculosis in general hospitals for a short time and

Table 14–1 ***Drugs Commonly Used in the Treatment of Tuberculosis***

	DOSAGE				
	DAILY	TWICE WEEKLY	MOST COMMON SIDE EFFECTS	TEST FOR SIDE EFFECTS	REMARKS
PRIMARY DRUGS					
Isoniazid (INH)	5–10 mg/kg up to 300 mg PO or IM	15 mg/kg PO or IM	Peripheral neuritis, hypersensitivity, jaundice	AST/ALT (not as a routine)	Bactericidal. Pyridoxine 10 mg as prophylaxis for neuritis; 50–100 mg as treatment.
Ethambutol (Myambutol)	15–25 mg/kg PO	50 mg/kg PO	Optic neuritis (reversible with discontinuation of drug; very rare at 15 mg/kg), skin rash	Red-green color discrimination and visual acuity	Use with caution with renal disease or when eye testing is not feasible.
Rifampin (RMP) (Rifadin)	10–20 mg/kg up to 600 mg PO	Not recommended	Hepatitis, febrile reaction, purpura (rare)	AST/ALT (not as a routine)	Bactericidal. Orange secretion color. Affects action of other drugs.
Streptomycin	15–20 mg/kg up to 1 g IM	25–30 mg/kg IM	VIIIth cranial nerve damage, nephrotoxicity, hypersensitivity	Vestibular function, audiograms; BUN and creatinine	Use with caution in older patients or those with renal disease.
Pyrazinamide	15–30 mg/kg up to 2 g PO	Not recommended	Hyperuricemia, hepatotoxicity	Uric acid, AST/ALT	Under study as first-line drug in short-course regimens.
SECONDARY DRUGS					
Kanamycin (Kantrex)	15–30 mg/kg up to 1 g IM	Secondary drugs are not recommended for twice-weekly dosage	Similar to streptomycin	BUN, creatinine	Increase hydration; evaluate hearing before therapy starts.
Capreomycin (Capastat)	15–30 mg/kg up to 1 g IM		Similar to streptomycin	BUN, creatinine	Periodic hearing evaluation needed.
Cycloserine (Seromycin)	10–20 mg/kg up to 1 g PO		Depression, psychosis, hypersensitivity	Neurologic exam	Warn to avoid alcohol; monitor serum blood levels of drug.
Ethionamide (Trecator)	15–30 mg/kg up to 1 g PO		Peripheral neuritis, GI distress, dermatitis	AST/ALT	Pyridoxine used for neuropathy. Give with meals; avoid alcohol.
Para-aminobenzoic acid (PAS)	150 mcg/kg up to 12 g PO		GI distress, hepatotoxicity, hypersensitivity	AST/ALT	Give with meals; monitor for hepatotoxicity.

Key: *ALT,* alanine aminotransferase; *AST,* aspartate aminotransferase; *BUN,* blood urea nitrogen; *GI,* gastrointestinal; *IM,* intramuscularly; *PO,* orally.
Adapted from Lewis, S.M., Heitkemper, M.M., & Dirksen, S.R. (2007). *Medical-Surgical Nursing: Assessment and Management of Clinical Problems* (7th ed.). St. Louis: Mosby.

then send them home on medication. Now uncomplicated pulmonary tuberculosis is managed in the outpatient setting. People in close contact with the patient have usually been exposed before the disease was diagnosed.

Treatment consists of at least four drugs for an extended period of time (Table 14–1). The MODS test described in Chapter 13 is used to determine the best drugs to employ. The drugs are given in varying combinations on varying numbers of days per week. Noncompliance is an issue because of side effects, the requirement to avoid alcohol, and the long duration of therapy (Complementary & Alternative Therapies 14–3). Two new drug combinations have made compliance easier for patients: Rifamate, containing rifampin and isoniazid, and Rifater, containing rifampin, isoniazid, and pyrazinamide. Close contacts are monitored with skin testing. Effective cure can be obtained within 6 to 9 months for most patients with pulmonary tuberculosis (Legal & Ethical Considerations 14–1).

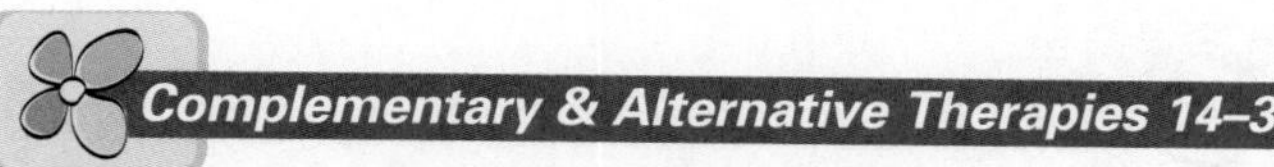

Complementary & Alternative Therapies 14–3

Vitamin D to Prevent Tuberculosis

Vitamin D has been found to be successful in the prevention and treatment of tuberculosis (TB) in two small studies (*Science*, Feb. 23, 2006). White blood cells convert vitamin D into an active form that helps make a protein that kills tuberculosis bacteria. Perhaps this is why moving to a sunny climate and a solarium environment years ago helped people with TB. Indonesian scientists used 10,000 units of vitamin D daily on 70 patients for 9 months and attained a 100% cure rate.

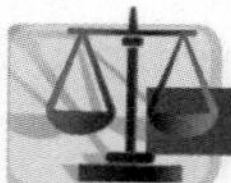

Legal & Ethical Considerations 14–1

Noncompliance with Medication

When someone is found to have tuberculosis and the person is noncompliant with the treatment, is it legal or ethical to compel the person to come for treatment? What will happen if the person is allowed to remain in the community without treatment?

A new drug, PA-824, that is in early stage clinical trials holds promise for shortening the TB treatment regimen (National Institute of Allergy and Infectious Diseases, 2005). It seems to be effective in both actively dividing and slow-growing *M. tuberculosis.* This drug could solve a lot of the problems with compliance with therapy.

There is an increase in the incidence of multidrug-resistant TB, and patients with these infections do not fare so well. For this reason, directly observed therapy is recommended for patients who are known to be at 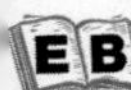 risk of noncompliance with therapy (Munro et al., 2000).This involves the visual observation of the ingestion of each required dose of medication for the entire course of treatment. Often a public health nurse administers the medication at a clinic site. Follow-up visits are necessary for 12 months after completion of therapy to monitor for the presence of resistant strains. Nurses can help the United States to meet the *Healthy People 2010* objectives 22 to 25: *Increase to at least 90% the proportion of all tuberculosis patients who complete curative therapy within 12 months.*

Nursing Management

Assessment is performed by first taking a complete history and looking for possible risk factors for TB. A focused assessment of the respiratory system is performed as described in Chapter 12 (see Focused Assessment 12–1).

Because tuberculosis is an infectious disease, nursing goals are similar to those for other diseases of this type. Nursing objectives concerned with prevention and control of infectious diseases are:

- To control the spread of the infectious agent
- To promote immunity to infectious diseases
- To support and strengthen the capacity for recovery in a patient who has an infectious disease.

Nursing diagnoses for the patient with tuberculosis may include:

- Ineffective breathing pattern related to decreased lung capacity
- Noncompliance related to lack of knowledge of disease process and long-term requirement for treatment
- Activity intolerance related to fatigue, febrile status, and poor nutritional status
- Imbalanced nutrition: less than body requirements related to anorexia, fatigue, and productive cough

Control of Infection. Pulmonary tuberculosis is transmitted principally by way of the respiratory tract. Airborne Infection Isolation in addition to Standard Precautions (see Appendix 5) is recommended for the hospitalized patient who has an active case of tuberculosis and is just beginning drug therapy. The patient is placed in a negative-pressure isolation room with an anteroom, and a high-efficiency particulate arresting (HEPA) respirator mask that tightly fits the face is required for all personnel when caring for the patient. The patient is encouraged to rest because fatigue is common during the active phase of infection and the beginning of medication treatment. The home care patient does not need Airborne Infection Isolation because family members have already been exposed by the time of diagnosis. The patient is taught to cover the mouth when coughing or sneezing, dispose of tissues in plastic bags, practice good hand hygiene, and wear a mask when in contact with crowds until medication effectively suppresses the infection. Sputum examinations are required every 2 to 4 weeks; when three consecutive sputum cultures are negative, the patient is considered no longer infectious and may resume work and other usual social activities. Another aspect of infection control is the identification and prompt treatment of potential and active cases of tuberculosis within the community.

A person with dormant TB may develop active TB later if the immune system is weakened by a serious illness such as HIV, or when the system is less efficient, as with advanced age.

Promotion of Immunity. Fortunately, tuberculosis is one of the most easily avoided of all serious respiratory illnesses. The body's innate immune system cannot work well, however, when a person is malnourished, physically debilitated, and subject to extreme physical and emotional stress. Improvement of living conditions and carrying out sound health practices are essential to maintaining a natural resistance to tuberculosis.

Preventive therapy with isoniazid (INH) has been particularly successful in reducing the transmission of tuberculosis. It is estimated that the drug is 85% effective in reducing the chances of contracting tuberculosis in persons who are most exposed. The drug is given prophylactically once daily for a full year (Weichel, 2000). Those for whom a course of INH therapy is recommended include:

- Those living in the house with or closely associated with a person who is newly diagnosed as having tuberculosis.
- People who have positive skin reactions but normal chest radiographs.
- Positive skin reactors who suffer from a chronic disease (e.g., diabetes mellitus), are taking steroids, or have had a gastrectomy.
- Those who have recently shown a positive skin reaction, but no sign of active disease, and have a history of previous negative reactions.

A new recombinant vaccine, rBCG30, has been developed at the University of California at Los Angeles, and the first clinical trials in humans began in 2004. It is hoped that this vaccine will provide a strong protective immune response against TB.

Support. Even though drug therapy failure occurs in a quite small percentage of patients, many people still dread the disease. When a person first learns that she has tuberculosis, she will need reassurance and continued support in sorting out her feelings and overcoming any fears and misinformation she might have.

In addition, it is important that the patient name all close contacts so that they can be reached and started on preventive therapy. Giving the names of contacts may be very difficult for the patient because of the social stigma that is still attached to tuberculosis in certain cultural groups.

The vast majority of newly diagnosed tuberculosis patients are treated on an outpatient basis. Only those who are extremely debilitated or suffering from another chronic illness are hospitalized. Because much of the responsibility for care probably rests with the patient and possibly with family members, **health education is a major intervention in the management of tuberculosis** (Patient Teaching 14–1).

Evaluation of nursing care requires gathering data to see if expected outcomes and goals have been met.

EXTRAPULMONARY TUBERCULOSIS

It is possible for the tubercle bacillus to attack and damage parts of the body other than the lungs. This is called *extrapulmonary* or *miliary tuberculosis.* The areas most frequently affected are the bones, meninges, urinary system, and reproductive system. Tuberculosis of the spine, called *Pott's disease,* is now quite rare in the United States. The deformity most commonly seen in Pott's disease is *kyphosis,* or "hunchback."

BRONCHIECTASIS

Bronchiectasis is a chronic respiratory disorder in which one or more bronchi are permanently dilated. It is thought to occur as a result of frequent respiratory infections in childhood. It often is classified with chronic airflow limitation (CAL), and its management is similar.

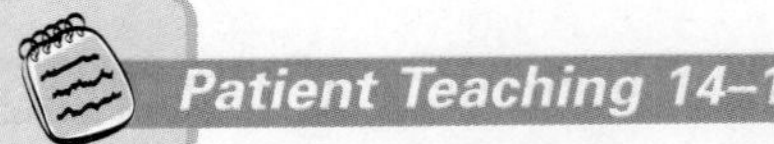

Health Teaching Essential for the Patient with Tuberculosis

Teach the patient to:

- Cover the mouth and nose when coughing or sneezing.
- Place contaminated tissues in a plastic bag.
- Observe sputum and report changes in appearance.
- Take each dose of medication as prescribed at the correct time without fail.
- Wash the hands frequently and correctly.
- Take medication as directed in relation to meals so that food does not interfere with absorption.
- Obtain sufficient, high-quality rest and balance with light activity to promote healing.
- Eat healthy, well-balanced meals that include sufficient vitamin C and protein to promote healing.

Teach the family and close contacts:

- How the disease is transmitted and how it affects the lungs.
- The importance of taking preventive medication continuously and without fail to prevent active infection.
- The importance of maintaining a healthy immune system to avoid active infection.

Cystic Fibrosis

Cystic fibrosis (CF) is a major cause of bronchiectasis. It is a genetic disease in which there is excessive mucus production because of exocrine gland dysfunction. It occurs most often in white children. The lungs, intestines, sinuses, reproductive tract, sweat glands, and pancreas are all affected. It is diagnosed by history, physical examination, and a positive sweat test.

Lung damage occurs in cystic fibrosis patients as a result of excessive secretion of abnormally thick mucus, impairment of ciliary action in the lungs, airway obstruction, and repeated infections, which cause scarring. Cystic fibrosis eventually results in CAL. It was once solely a pediatric disease, because children with cystic fibrosis died before reaching adulthood. Today the median life span is 33 years. A few cystic fibrosis patients live into their 40s because of aggressive respiratory treatment and antibiotics. The drug dornase alfa (Pulmozyme) reduces the frequency of respiratory infections and improves pulmonary function in patients with CF. Breathing exercises and chest physiotherapy are used daily. A handheld device called the flutter valve that looks like a fat pipe aids in loosening and bringing up lung secretions that are blocking airways. It combines positive expiratory pressure with high-frequency oscillations at the airway opening. By exhaling actively into the pipe, the device causes vibrations of the airway walls, loosening secretions so that they can be coughed up. DNase, a recombinant DNA medication, also is used to reduce the number of lung infections and to improve lung function. This may extend the present average life span of the CF patient considerably.

Treatment includes bronchodilators, expectorants, oral pancreatic enzymes, double doses of fat-soluble vitamins, and mucolytics. A high-protein, high-calorie, moderate-fat diet is prescribed. Lung transplantation is a possible lifesaving measure.

Research has finally identified the gene responsible for cystic fibrosis (National Human Genome Research Institute, 2006). Work is continuing on ways to isolate and replace the missing gene to prevent or cure the disease.

INTERSTITIAL PULMONARY DISEASE

Sarcoidosis

Sarcoidosis is a lung disease characterized by granulomas. This disease causes fibrotic changes in the lung tissue over time, and the cause is unknown. It affects other tissues in the body as well. A cellular immune response seems to be responsible for the tissue changes. Sarcoidosis is 10 times more common in blacks than in whites, and most cases occur between ages 20 and 40. The fibrotic changes cause a reduction in function in lung tissue. Although there is no specific treatment for sarcoidosis, occasionally patients recover without treatment.

Pulmonary Fibrosis

Pulmonary fibrosis occurs from severe infection, repeated infection, or inflammation that causes scarring of the lung tissue. The scarring decreases functional lung tissue. Occupational inhalation of lung irritants, smoking, and chronic aspiration are risk factors.

Signs and symptoms are exertional dyspnea, nonproductive cough, and inspiratory crackles, and sometimes clubbed fingers. Diagnosis is by chest x-ray and pulmonary function testing. There is a 30% to 50% survival rate at 5 years after diagnosis. Treatment is with corticosteroids, immunosuppressants, and the antifibrotic agent colchicine. Lung transplantation is an option for those who meet the qualifying criteria.

RESTRICTIVE PULMONARY DISORDERS

Restrictive pulmonary disorders are caused by decreased elasticity or compliance of the lungs or decreased ability of the chest wall to expand. Disorders of the central nervous system or the neuromuscular system can cause a restrictive lung disorder. Myasthenia gravis and arthritis are good examples of extrapulmonary causes of a restrictive disorder. *Kyphosis* of the spine or severe *scoliosis* may also hamper lung expansion, though in these disorders the lung tissue remains normal.

PLEURISY

Pleurisy, an inflammation of the pleura, occurs from several causes. Tuberculosis, pneumonia, neoplasm, and pulmonary infarction all can cause pleurisy. Pleurisy pain is sharp and abrupt in onset and is most evident on inspiration. This causes shallow breathing. A pleural friction rub may sometimes be heard. Treatment is aimed at treating the underlying cause and providing pain relief. Lying on the affected side may provide some relief. The affected side should be splinted during coughing. An intercostal nerve block may be done for severe pain.

PLEURAL EFFUSION

Pleural effusion is a collection of fluid in the pleural space. It is a sign of serious disease. The effusion is termed *transudative* or *exudative* according to the protein content of the fluid. A transudate occurs in noninflammatory conditions and is often a result of congestive heart failure, chronic liver failure, or renal disease. Transudate is a thin fluid containing no protein that passes from cells into interstitial spaces or through a membrane. Exudate is thicker, contains cells and other substances, and is slowly discharged from cells into a body space or to the outside of the body.

Exudative pleural effusion occurs in an area of inflammation due to the increased capillary permeability characteristic of the inflammatory reaction. This type of effusion occurs with lung cancer, pulmonary embolism, pancreatic disease, and pulmonary infections.

When pleurisy is accompanied by effusion of serous fluid, the physician may perform a thoracentesis (removal of fluid from the pleural cavity) for diagnostic tests or symptom relief. It is not uncommon for as much as 500 mL to be removed at one time during a thoracentesis (see Table 12–3 for further information).

OBSTRUCTIVE PULMONARY DISORDERS

Obstructive pulmonary disorders **are characterized by problems moving air into and out of the lungs.** Narrowing of the openings in the tracheobronchial tree increases resistance to the flow of air, making it difficult for oxygen to enter, and contributes to air trapping, as exhalation also is difficult. Asthma is a reactive airways disease causing narrowed airways and mucus production. **Asthma, emphysema, and chronic bronchitis are examples of diseases that cause chronic airflow limitation (CAL).** CAL ranks fourth among the major causes of death in the United States, and the number of its victims is increasing. This represents billions of dollars in economic loss as a result of inability to work and the expense of repeated visits to the physician and hospitalizations. The American Lung Association estimates that about 33.9 million Americans suffer from CAL, and the number is increasing each year (National Center for Health Statistics, 2006). The dramatic increase in the rate of morbidity and mortality due to CAL is attributed to increases in habitual cigarette smoking and rising levels of air pollution. A third factor is genetic susceptibility to the destruction of lung tissue. A serum protein, *alpha$_1$-antitrypsin* (AAT), is deficient in certain people, and the deficiency runs in families. This protein inhibits the activity of the enzyme *elastase,* which tends to break down lung tissue. In the absence of AAT, lung tissue is more easily destroyed by the enzyme. Patients with a deficiency of AAT may develop severe lung disease at an early age.

ATELECTASIS

Atelectasis is an incomplete expansion, or collapse, of alveoli. It may occur from compression of the lungs from outside, a decrease in surfactant, or bronchial obstruction that prevents air from reaching the alveoli. Postoperatively it occurs from retained secretions that accumulated during anesthesia, positioning on the operating room table for an extended period without movement, and hypoventilation related to surgical pain. It usually is a reversible condition. Breath sounds are diminished when the airways are collapsed, and oxygen saturation (Sao_2) will decrease. Treatment consists of ridding the bronchial tree of excess secretions by coughing and providing air to the depths of the lung by deep breathing and use of the incentive spirometer.

CHRONIC OBSTRUCTIVE PULMONARY DISEASE

Chronic obstructive pulmonary disease (COPD) is the term used to describe a condition that includes two diseases, *emphysema* and *chronic bronchitis.* Approximately 16.8 million people in the United States have COPD (National Center for Health Statistics, 2006).

Etiology and Diagnosis of COPD

Smoking and AAT deficiency are the primary causes of emphysema and chronic bronchitis, with air pollution and occupational exposure to irritating fumes and industrial chemicals being contributing factors.

Diagnosis is by history, physical assessment, chest x-ray, pulmonary function testing, arterial blood gas analysis, and, if needed, lung biopsy.

EMPHYSEMA

Pathophysiology

Emphysema is essentially a disease of the *terminal* respiratory units. There is destruction of alveolar and alveolar-capillary walls, as well as narrowed and tortuous small airways. This leads to large, permanently inflated alveolar air spaces. Air that is inhaled becomes trapped, causing the victim to work harder to *exhale* air than to inhale it (Figure 14–1). As emphysema progresses, the patient suffers further loss of lung elasticity. The two major types of emphysema are centrilobular and panlobular. Panlobular emphysema involves destruction of the whole lobule versus the central part of the lobule. Chronic bronchitis is associated with centrilobular emphysema, and this type is more common than the panlobular emphysema.

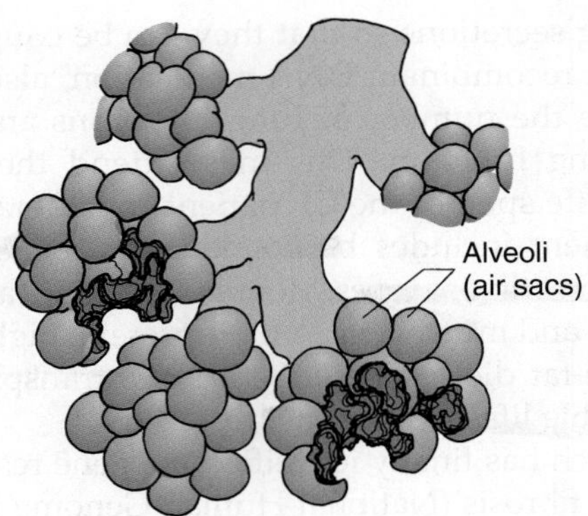

FIGURE **14–1** Alveoli in emphysema.

Signs and Symptoms

Dyspnea is an early symptom of emphysema. There is minimal coughing with small amounts of mucoid sputum. As the disease progresses, dyspnea worsens and eventually interferes with activities of daily living. The diaphragm becomes permanently flattened by overdistention of the lungs, the muscles of the rib cage become rigid, and the ribs flare outward. This produces the "barrel chest" that is typical of many patients with emphysema.

To compensate for the loss of muscular action that normally aids respiration, the patient begins to use other muscles, mainly those of the neck and shoulders. She holds her shoulders high in an attempt to enlarge the space in which her lungs can expand. Her facial expression conveys the anxiety and tension that result from her struggle to get enough air into her lungs. The skin is a pink tone in whites even though hypoxia may be present. Carbon dioxide is usually not retained, and therefore an acid-base imbalance is unlikely.

CHRONIC BRONCHITIS

Pathophysiology

In chronic bronchitis there is excess secretion of mucus that interferes with airflow and inflammatory damage to the bronchial mucosa that causes a productive cough.

Inflammation of the bronchi is considered chronic when the recurrent cough is present for at least 3 months of each year for at least 2 years. Chronic bronchitis can range from a mildly irritating "cigarette" cough in the morning with production of small amounts of sputum to a severe disabling condition. The latter extreme is characterized by increased resistance to airflow, hypoxia, and frequently hypercapnia (excess CO_2) and *cor pulmonale.* Cor pulmonale is a heart condition characterized by pulmonary hypertension and an enlarged right ventricle, both of which are secondary to chronic lung disease. Cor pulmonale places the patient at risk for right-sided heart failure.

Table 14–2 Comparison of Pulmonary Emphysema and Chronic Bronchitis

CLINICAL FEATURE/CHARACTERISTICS	EMPHYSEMA	CHRONIC BRONCHITIS
Age of Onset	40–50	30–40
Pathophysiology	Destruction of alveolar walls. Loss of elasticity, impaired expiration, hyperinflation	Increased mucous secretion, inflammation and infection, obstruction of airways
Health History	Generally healthy	Frequent URI, acute episodes
Smoking	Usually	Usually
Clinical Features		
Barrel chest	Yes	May be present
Weight loss	May be severe in late disease	Infrequent
Shortness of breath	Absent early; pronounced late in disease	Early symptom; especially with activity
Decreased breath sounds	Yes	Variable
Wheezing	Usually absent	Variable
Rhonchi	Absent or minimal	Often present
Sputum	Absent or develops late in disease	Early sign; frequent infections with purulent sputum
Cyanosis	Usually absent; appears late in disease with low Pa_{O_2}	Yes; worsens as disease progresses
Cor pulmonale	Occasional	Common
Polycythemia	May appear in advanced disease	Frequently present
Blood gases	Normal until late in disease	May display hypercapnia Hypoxemia frequent

Key: *Pa_{O_2}*, partial pressure of arterial oxygen; *URI*, upper respiratory infection.

Signs and Symptoms

The primary clinical characteristics of chronic bronchitis include a productive cough due to hyperplasia of the bronchial glands and increased secretion of thick, tenacious mucus that decreases ciliary function. The thick mucus becomes a breeding ground for bacteria, and respiratory infections are frequent.

Airways become edematous and narrowed, and air trapping occurs. Initially the larger airways are affected, and then the smaller airways become obstructed also. The patient suffers from hypoventilation and hypoxemia.

Pulmonary function testing reveals an increased residual volume due to the premature closure of the narrowed airways during exhalation. The patient has a marked increase in her partial pressure of arterial carbon dioxide (Pa_{CO_2}) levels and a marked decrease in partial pressure of arterial oxygen (Pa_{O_2}) levels. **The retention of carbon dioxide and deficiency of oxygen give the skin and/or mucous membranes a reddish blue color.** The reddish color also is due to an increase in the red blood cell count (**polycythemia**). Laboratory tests will show elevated hemoglobin and hematocrit levels. The increase in production of red blood cells is an attempt by the body to compensate for the chronic hypoxia. Table 14–2 presents a comparison of emphysema and chronic bronchitis.

Treatment of COPD

COPD is treated with bronchodilators and anti-inflammatory agents. When bacterial infection is present, antibiotics, and sometimes steroid anti-inflammatories, are used (Table 14–3). In later stages of disease, when hypoxemia is present, oxygen therapy is initiated. Smoking cessation is very important. Respiratory rehabilitation programs can help increase exercise tolerance and improve quality of life.

Nutrition is very important for the patient with COPD. The extra work of breathing for the emphysema patient uses more calories. The tissue damage in both disorders requires protein for repair of tissue. Anorexia may be a problem. It is beneficial to maintain as normal a weight as possible for height and age. Nutritional Therapies 14–1 on p. 334 presents helpful ideas for the COPD patient.

Complications of COPD

Cor Pulmonale. **Cor pulmonale** is enlargement of the right side of the heart as a result of pulmonary hypertension caused by constriction of the pulmonary vessels in response to hypoxia. Constant hypoxia stimulates erythropoiesis with resulting polycythemia and more viscous blood. Eventually right-sided heart failure develops. Right-sided heart failure causes systemic venous congestion. Distended neck veins, right upper quadrant tenderness from an engorged liver, peripheral edema, weight gain, gastrointestinal distress, and ascites may occur.

Treatment is continuous low-flow oxygen and medications to treat the heart failure and fluid volume overload.

Acute Respiratory Failure. An acute respiratory tract infection in a COPD patient who already has compromised respiration is the most common cause of respiratory failure. Indiscriminate use of sedatives and narcotics for surgery in COPD patients may lead to this problem because they depress respiration. Careful monitoring of arterial blood gases (ABGs), treatment

Table 14–3 ***Commonly Prescribed Drugs for COPD and Asthma****

CLASSIFICATION	ACTION	NURSING IMPLICATIONS	PATIENT TEACHING
BRONCHODILATORS			
Beta-Adrenergic Agonists Metoproterenol (Alupent, Metaprel) Albuterol (Proventil, Ventolin) Pirbuterol (Maxair) Terbutaline (Brethine, Brethair) Bitolterol (Tornalate) Salmeterol (Serevent)	Stimulates beta-adrenergic receptors, producing bronchodilation Increases ciliary action and mucus clearance Selectively stimulates beta-adrenergic receptors, producing bronchodilation Long acting	All may be administered by MDI. Some can be administered orally or by nebulizer. Monitor tachycardia, BP changes, nervousness, palpitations, muscle tremors, and dry mouth. May cause nausea, headache, insomnia, and hypokalemia. Acts in 5–10 min and lasts for 3–4 hr.	Should not be used in patients with cardiac disorders or angina. Increase fluid intake; watch for signs of potassium deficit. Wait 5 min before using a glucocorticoid inhaler (anti-inflammatory). Teach to use MDI correctly.
Methylxanthine Derivative Aminophylline (Theo-Dur, Slo-Bid, Uniphyl, Aerolate, Uni-Dur)	Relaxes bronchial smooth muscle, improves diaphragm contractility, increases ciliary action and mucus clearance, stimulates respiration and pulmonary vasodilation, improving exercise tolerance	Administered orally or IV. CNS effects cause nervousness, irritability, headache, and insomnia. Causes tachycardia, BP changes, dysrhythmias, muscle twitching, flushing, anorexia, nausea and vomiting, epigastric pain, and diarrhea. Several drugs may increase theophylline levels. Monitor theophylline levels.	Length of drug action is decreased by smoking. Take with food to decrease GI effects. Lie down if dizziness occurs. Take medication regularly and only as prescribed. Teach to take pulse. Instruct not to use over-the-counter medications without checking with health care provider. Wear an ID bracelet stating asthmatic status. Check interactions with herbal products.
ANTI-INFLAMMATORY AGENTS†			
Beclomethasone (Vanceril, Beclovent) Triamcinolone (Azmacort) Flunisolide (Aerobid) Fluticasone (Flovent) Budesonide (Pulmicort) Cromolyn (Intal) Nedocromil (Tilade)	Provide anti-inflammatory and immunosuppressive effect, decreasing edema in airways Decrease mucous secretion Stabilize cell membranes possibly by inhibiting release of histamine and SRS-A by acting on mast cells	All can be administered by MDI. Cromolyn can be used in a nebulizer. Work synergistically with beta-adrenergic agonists. May affect potassium and glucose levels. Monitor weight. May mask infection. Monitor for edema. May have transient unpleasant taste.	Teach to carry ID indicating is a steroid user. Rinse mouth after each use of inhaler to prevent oral fungal infection. Do not discontinue use abruptly. Wash inhaler with warm water and dry after each use.
Advair diskus	Exact mechanism unknown Contains glucocorticoids and salmeterol Helps keep asthma in check when used daily	Relieves airway constriction and inflammation.	Same as above.
ANTICHOLINERGICS			
Ipratropium (Atrovent)	Causes bronchodilation by blocking action of acetylcholine	Do not mix with cromolyn sodium. Use cautiously in those with narrow-angle glaucoma, prostatic hypertrophy, or bladder neck obstruction.	Do not take more than two puffs at a time. Avoid excessive use of caffeine.
Ipratropium and albuterol (Combivent)	Bronchodilation by stimulating beta-adrenergic receptors, and blocking action of acetylcholine		

Key: *BP,* blood pressure; *CNS,* central nervous system; *GI,* gastrointestinal; *IV,* intravenously; *MDI,* metered-dose inhaler; *OTC,* over the counter; *SRS-A,* slow-reacting substance of anaphylaxis.

*There are many other drugs that are also prescribed for asthma.

†Systemic corticosteroids (hydrocortisone, methylprednisolone, or prednisone) may be administered orally or intravenously when severe or refractory asthma attacks occur.

Table 14–3 **Commonly Prescribed Drugs for COPD and Asthma—cont'd**

CLASSIFICATION	ACTION	NURSING IMPLICATIONS	PATIENT TEACHING
LEUKOTRIENE MODIFIERS			
Zafirlukast (Accolate) Montelukast (Singulair)	Block action of leukotrienes in the lung once they are formed Provide both bronchodilation and anti-inflammatory effects	Administered orally. May cause headache, dizziness, nausea, vomiting, diarrhea, fatigue, or abdominal pain. Not to be used for acute asthma episodes.	Should take drug 1 hr before or 2 hr after meals daily. Increase fluid intake. Do not stop taking other asthma medications.
LEUKOTRIENE INHIBITOR			
Zileuton (Zyflo)	Inhibits the synthesis of leukotrienes, providing bronchodilation and anti-inflammatory effect	Administered orally. Monitor liver enzymes. May cause dizziness insomnia, dyspepsia, and abdominal pain. May interfere with warfarin (Coumadin) therapy and theophylline. Is not used to treat acute asthma attacks.	Check all medications and OTC drugs for ephedrine, which will increase stimulation. Teach to avoid alcohol. Notify health care provider of nausea, vomiting, anxiety, or insomnia. Continue to take even if symptom free.
MUCOLYTIC			
Acetylcysteine (Mucomyst)	Breaks down mucoproteins by enzyme action Decreases viscosity and aids in mobilization of secretions	Administered by nebulizer. Nausea and vomiting may occur. May cause bronchospasm or hemoptysis. Usually combined with bronchodilator. Monitor respirations.	Warn that secretions may become profuse. Teach that unpleasant odor will decrease with use. Discoloration of solution after bottle is opened does not impair its effectiveness.

of the infection, and adjustment of the patient's usual medications, plus aggressive respiratory therapy, may correct the problem. See the section on Respiratory Failure later in this chapter.

Pneumonia. Pneumonia is often a complication of COPD. Purulent sputum is the usual sign. Fever, chills, and an elevated white blood cell count may not be present. Pneumonia is treated as previously discussed.

Peptic Ulcer and Gastroesophageal Reflux Disease. It is thought that peptic ulcer and gastroesophageal reflux disease (GERD) occur as a result of long-term use of the bronchodilators and corticosteroid drugs used to treat COPD. GERD can trigger worse symptoms of the COPD due to the reflux of acid in the esophagus because it stimulates a vagal reflex that causes bronchoconstriction.

Spontaneous Pneumothorax. Pneumothorax may occur due to ruptured alveoli. This can be a repetitive problem.

ASTHMA

Etiology

Asthma is a chronic lung disease characterized by reversible airway obstruction, airway inflammation from edema or swelling, and increased airway sensitivity to a variety of stimuli. The person with asthma has a hypersensitivity of the trachea and bronchi to various kinds of stimuli. Most likely no single cause is responsible for the group of symptoms known as asthma. Among the factors implicated in the occurrence of asthma are allergens, viruses and other infectious agents, occupational and environmental toxins, exercise, perfumes, and emotional stress. Recent studies have indicated a genetic correlation that, along with environmental factors, predisposes to a tendency to develop asthma.

Pathophysiology

Asthma is a chronic lung disease characterized by reversible airway obstruction, airway inflammation from edema or swelling, and increased airway sensitivity to a variety of stimuli. When a precipitating factor is encountered by the person with asthma, a series of physiologic responses occur. Inflammation of the airways is the underlying mechanism that causes bronchospasm. Inflammation of the airways, mucosal edema, and excessive secretion of mucus causes mucous plugging of the small airways. When combined with bronchoconstriction, there is further obstruction and narrowing of the airways, causing airflow limitation (Figure 14–2).

Signs, Symptoms, and Diagnosis

The symptoms of asthma are due to constriction of the bronchi, inflammatory changes in the mucosa, accumulations of secretions in the bronchi, and changes in the elastic recoil of the lungs. The symptoms may be continuous or episodic. Findings include wheezing, cough that is worse at night, difficulty breathing, and chest tightness (Concept Map 14–2).

Nutritional Therapies 14–1

Nutritional Suggestions for the Chronic Obstructive Pulmonary Disease (COPD) Patient

The following tips may prove helpful for the patient with COPD:

- Drink 6 to 8 glasses of noncaffeinated fluids per day to keep mucus thin and easier to cough up. Check with your physician if you are on fluid restrictions.
- Rest before eating.
- Avoid overeating and foods that cause gas or bloating as a distended stomach may make breathing more difficult.
- Eat four to six small meals a day rather than three regular meals to decrease stomach fullness and reduce fatigue.
- Eat a well-balanced diet with adequate protein for your needs.
- Avoid lying down for an hour after eating.
- If you become short of breath while eating or right after meals:
  - Clear the airways 1 hour before eating.
  - Take small bites and chew food slowly.
  - Choose foods that are easy to chew.
  - Drink beverages at the end of the meal rather than during it.
  - Use your oxygen cannula while you eat.
- Take in sufficient calcium via dairy products, vegetables, and supplements—steroid medications put you at risk for osteoporosis; keep your bones strong.
- Cook when feeling most energetic; make extra portions and freeze them for easy, quick, frozen dinners.

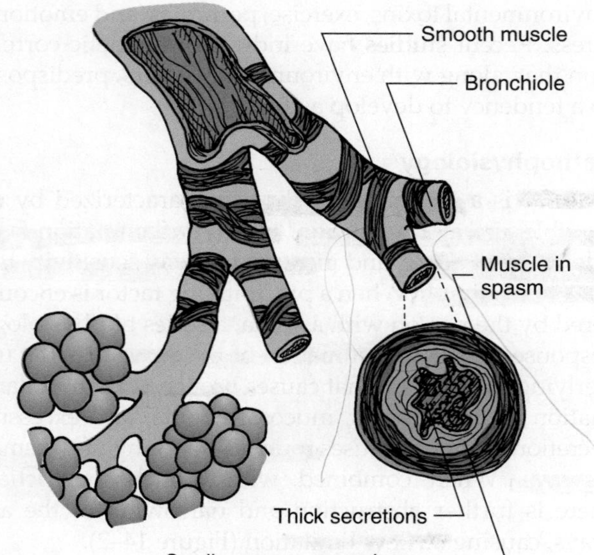

FIGURE 14–2 Bronchial asthma.

Cough usually indicates obstruction of the larger airways. Dyspnea, another common symptom, is indicative of edema or mucus in the smaller airways. **Both patients and nurses need to know that a severe, acute asthma attack can cause death from hypoxia.**

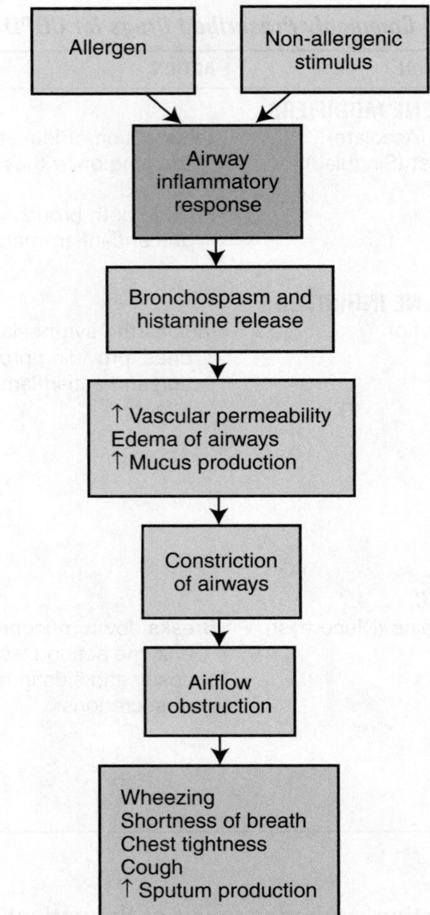

CONCEPT MAP 14–2 Pathophysiology of asthma.

Unrelieved asthma attacks become status asthmaticus and are very serious. Respiratory distress without wheeze is an ominous sign.

Diagnosis is by history, physical, pulmonary function testing, arterial blood gas analysis, and chest x-ray.

Treatment

Asthma is classified by a step system that considers the degree and frequency of symptoms (Table 14–4). Treatment is aimed at managing the underlying symptom for each step. The goals of medical treatment are to:

- Minimize irritation of the air passages and relieve obstruction by secretions, edema, or bronchospasm
- Prevent or control infection and allergy
- Increase the patient's tolerance for activity
- Determine the best drug combination in the least amount that will control symptoms

A *Healthy People 2010* goal is: *Promote respiratory health through better prevention, detection, treatment, and education efforts.* Health Promotion Points 14–2 lists the specific objectives related to asthma.

Bronchodilators in the form of beta-adrenergic agonists, theophyllines, or anticholinergic agents

Table 14–4 Asthma: The Step System of Treatment

CLINICAL MANIFESTATIONS	TREATMENT RECOMMENDATIONS
I. MILD INTERMITTENT • Symptoms or episodes occur twice per week or less. • Client is symptom free between episodes/exacerbations. • Episodes/exacerbations are short, lasting only a few hours. • Symptoms are present at night no more frequently than twice per month. • PFTs are normal between episodes. • During episodes/exacerbations, FEV_1 or PEF is at least 80% of normal. • PEF variability is less than 20%.	• No daily medication needed. • Use of short-acting inhaled beta agonist during episodes (rescue inhaler). • Increased use of rescue inhaler indicates the need to start long-term therapy.
II. MILD PERSISTENT • Symptoms or episodes occur more than twice per week but not daily. • Symptoms are present at night more than twice per month. • During episodes/exacerbations, FEV_1 is at least 80% of normal. • PEF variability is 20%–30%. • Activity is affected during episodes/exacerbations.	• Use of a daily anti-inflammatory. • Inhaled CSC. • Inhaled cromolyn. • Leukotriene antagonist. • Use of a rescue inhaler for relief during episodes.
III. MODERATE PERSISTENT • Symptoms occur daily. • Symptoms or episodes occur more than twice per week and may persist for days. • Patient uses short-acting inhaled bronchodilator daily. • Symptoms are present at night at least once per week.	• Daily use of inhaled CSC (low to moderate dose). • Use of long-acting inhaled beta agonist (bronchodilator). • Use of a rescue inhaler for relief during episodes (daily use means the patient should be evaluated for progression to step IV).
IV. SEVERE PERSISTENT • Symptoms are continuously present. • Episodes/exacerbations are frequent. • During episodes/exacerbations, FEV_1 or PEF is less than 60% of normal. • Physical activity is limited. • Symptoms are frequently present at night. • PEF variability is greater than 30%.	• Daily use of inhaled CSC (high dose). • Daily use of long-acting inhaled bronchodilator. • Frequent courses of systemic CSCs. • May include systemic methylxanthines.

Key: *CSC*, corticosteroid; *FEV_1*, forced expiratory volume in 1 second; *PEF*, peak expiratory flow; *PFTs*, pulmonary function tests.
From Ignatavicius, D.D., & Workman, L. (2006). *Medical-Surgical Nursing: Critical Thinking for Collaborative Care* (5th ed.). Philadelphia: Elsevier Saunders, p. 588.

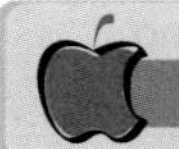

Health Promotion Points 14-2

Healthy People 2010 Asthma

24-1 Reduce asthma deaths.
24-2 Reduce hospitalizations for asthma.
24-3 Reduce hospital emergency department visits for asthma.
24-4 Reduce activity limitations among persons with asthma.
24-5 Reduce the number of school or work days missed by persons with asthma due to asthma.
24-6 Increase the proportion of persons with asthma who receive formal patient education, including information about community and self-help resources, as an essential part of the management of their condition.

such as ipratropium bromide (Atrovent) are used as the main form of therapy (Complementary & Alternative Therapies 14–4). Corticosteroids, mucolytics, antibiotics, and oxygen also may be prescribed (see Table 14–3).

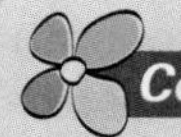

Complementary & Alternative Therapies 14–4

Biofeedback for Asthma

Research has been found that biofeedback may be a way for asthma patients to reduce their symptoms and doses of inhaled steroids. With biofeedback, the patient uses conscious control of body functions through the use of electronic monitoring. A small research study demonstrated that those with asthma significantly reduced the severity of their asthma and lowered their use of inhaled steroids without having a worsening of symptoms after using biofeedback for 10 weekly sessions.

The asthma patient is taught to use a peak flowmeter to determine the drug dosage needed to control the asthma, to predict the effectiveness of therapy, and to detect airflow obstruction buildup before it becomes serious and requires hospitalization (see Figure 12–9). Peak flow monitoring is based on the greatest airflow velocity that can be produced during a forced expira-

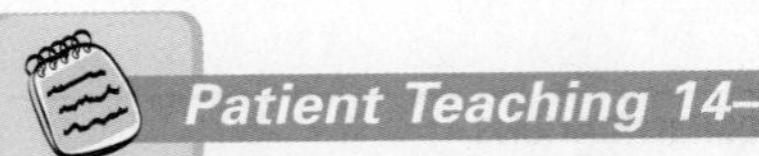

Patient Teaching 14–2

Using a Peak Flowmeter

Peak flow should be monitored daily. Know your "green zone"—when airflow is normal; your "yellow zone"—when usual airflow has decreased and routine medications should be increased; and your "red zone"—when you need to use rescue medications and call your health care provider.

To properly use a peak flowmeter, instruct the patient to:

- Set the pointer to zero.
- While standing, take a deep breath.
- Put the mouthpiece in the mouth and clamp the lips firmly around it for a tight seal.
- Blow out the breath into the meter as hard and fast as possible.
- Record the value and reset the pointer.
- Rest for a couple of breaths.
- Repeat the procedure for a total of three readings.
- Record the highest reading on the peak flow sheet.

tion that starts from fully inflated lungs (Patient Teaching 14–2). It assesses airflow obstruction. Readings are recorded, and, once a baseline for the patient's personal best peak flow is set, readings are compared to it. If a reading is 60% below the patient's best, treatment should be adjusted.

Oxygen is prescribed for moderate and severe hypoxemia. For acute episodes of CAL with hypoxemia, oxygen is given to raise the Sao_2 to 90 mm Hg or greater. Oxygen is used in patients with chronic CAL who have consistent Pao_2 levels less than 55 to 59 mm Hg. Oxygen always is used cautiously in patients with CAL, as they have adjusted to high levels of CO_2, which normally provides the drive to breathe, and are dependent on low oxygen levels to stimulate breathing. **If too much oxygen is given, the patient may cease to breathe and require mechanical ventilation.**

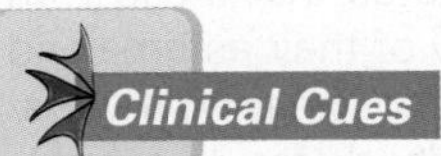

Clinical Cues

When a patient's respiratory disease status is unknown and oxygen has to be applied in an emergency situation, it is best to start it at no more than 2 L a minute by nasal cannula. Once a physician is present and the patient's record has been checked for COPD, the oxygen rate of administration can be changed if appropriate. Oxygen also is prescribed for moderate and severe cases of dyspnea. Patients who continue to experience exertional dyspnea after discharge may be taught to administer their own oxygen at home. A portable oxygen tank can be used to allow the patient to increase her level of activity without triggering severe and frightening episodes of dyspnea.

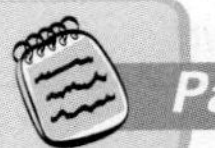

Patient Teaching 14–3

Pursed-Lip Breathing and Diaphragmatic Breathing

Instruct the patient with obstructive lung disease to breathe with pursed lips, to promote better exhalation and decrease air trapping.

PURSED-LIP BREATHING

- Sit up tall and move the back away from the chair; place the feet about shoulder-width apart. Lean forward slightly with hands or elbows on the knees.
- Close the mouth, and breath in through the nose.
- Purse the lips as though to gently whistle or blow out a candle; keep the lips and cheeks relaxed.
- Breath out slowly without puffing out the cheeks; control the flow of exhaled air as if you wanted to cause a candle to flicker but not extinguish.
- Take twice as much time to let the breath out as it did to take it in.
- Tense the abdominal muscles to force as much air from the lungs as possible.
- Use pursed-lip breathing during any physical activity.
- Refrain from holding your breath when lifting objects or performing other physical activities.

ABDOMINAL ("BELLY") OR DIAPHRAGMATIC BREATHING

- Initially practice lying down.
- Lie on the back with the knees bent. Take a deep breath through the nose with the abdomen relaxed and, with the palm of one hand, feel the abdomen rise. Exhale slowly to a count of 4.
- Exhale slowly through pursed lips, tightening the abdominal muscles that push the diaphragm up, forcing more air out of the lungs.
- Once comfortable with the abdominal breathing technique, use it when standing or sitting. This type of controlled breathing will provide more endurance during physical activity.

Nursing Management and Rehabilitation of Patient with Chronic Airflow Limitation

Rehabilitation and education of the patient and family are the chief long-term goals of nursing intervention. With proper home care, the patient with CAL can live longer and have a higher quality of life, reduce the number of hospitalizations and visits to her physician, and have fewer psychosocial problems related to inactivity and a feeling of hopelessness.

It is very important that the family, as well as the patient, be educated so that there is an understanding of the need for appropriate exercise and activity, and of the desire for independence. Families often tend to become very overprotective of the patient because of their fear of episodes of dyspnea. Rehabilitation needs to be a joint effort by the patient and family to help the patient attain as high a quality of life as possible while avoiding the complications of CAL.

The major problem of chronic, diffuse, and irreversible obstruction of the airways must be dealt with in a

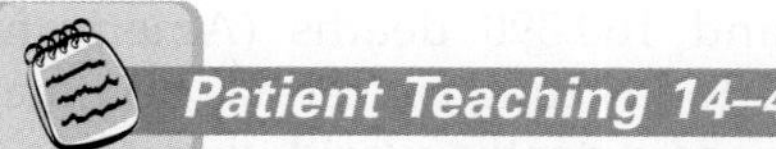

Patient Teaching 14–4

Instructions for the Patient with Chronic Airflow Limitation

- To make mucus more liquid and easier to cough up, drink at least 2 and preferably 3 quarts of liquid every day.
- When you exert yourself, as in lifting something or getting up from your chair, exhale slowly through pursed lips rather than holding your breath. You should do the same thing when you are walking for exercise. It is natural for all of us to hold our breath when we exert ourselves, so you may need practice to get into the habit of exhaling on exertion.
- Eat three or four small, balanced meals rather than one or two large ones each day.
- Practice your breathing exercises every day without fail.
- Try to avoid crowds during the flu and cold seasons.
- Do not take over-the-counter drugs. They can interact with your prescribed drugs, and some may be harmful because of their effects on your breathing. Antihistamines can dry out the mucus even more and make it more difficult for you to clear your air passages.
- Don't smoke or inhale the tobacco smoke of others.

Note: Normal sputum is white and slightly viscous and has no odor or taste.

systematic way. This means working with the patient, identifying specific difficulties she is experiencing, assessing current ability to cope with them, and devising plans to accomplish specific goals for improvement.

To prevent frequent hospitalizations for acute flare-ups of her disease, the patient will need to be taught how to avoid bronchial irritation and infection and prevent such complications as right-sided heart failure (cor pulmonale). Patient Teaching 14–3, 14–4, and 14–5 show some helpful techniques and pointers for the patient with CAL.

Encouragement to quit smoking is of major importance for those with CAL who still smoke. Continued smoking will seriously compromise the extent and quality of life for this patient. The American Lung Association has both literature and community programs directed to assist CAL patients with this problem.

Smoking Cessation. Nicotine is extremely addictive and quitting smoking is not easy, but quitting in the early stages of COPD can slow the progression of the disease. A *Healthy People 2010* goal is *Reduce illness and disability and death related to tobacco use and exposure to second-hand smoke.* Nurses can help achieve that goal by educating patients and offering support.

After quitting, pulmonary function gradually improves and after 10 to 20 years the chance of lung cancer is again equal to that of a nonsmoker. Explain the importance of quitting smoking to the patient and share knowledge of community resources and the various programs designed to help people quit. There are nicotine patches, nicotine gum, nicotine nasal spray, and nicotine inhalers to help the patient wean off the addictive substance. Work with the patient to develop a plan

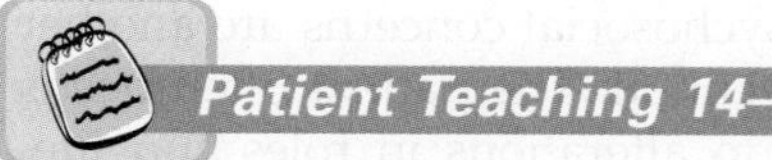

Patient Teaching 14–5

How to Use a Metered-Dose Inhaler (MDI)

When a patient is taking both a corticosteroid and a bronchodilator, teach her to take the bronchodilator first to open the airways so that the corticosteroid will be absorbed.

Instruct the patient to use the following steps:

- Always sit or stand to use the MDI.
- Attach the medication canister by holding the long end of the mouthpiece and inserting the stemmed top of the canister into it.
- Shake the canister several times to mix the medication with the propellant, and remove the mouthpiece cap.
- Breathe out through the mouth, emptying the lungs.
- With the bottom of the canister pointing up, place the mouthpiece 1 to 2 inches (2.5 to 5 cm) in front of the mouth. If using a spacer attachment or an Azmacort or Advair inhaler, place the mouthpiece in the mouth and close the lips around it.
- Breathe in slowly through the mouth. While starting to inhale, press the canister down to release the medication. Keep inhaling slowly until a full breath is taken. Hold the breath for 10 seconds and try not to cough. This allows the medication to penetrate the lung mucosa.
- If a second puff is ordered, wait at least 1 minute by the clock before repeating the procedure. This allows the first dose to be fully absorbed before the second is given.
- If you can't inhale slowly or are unable to depress the canister while inhaling, a spacer or extender can be added to the mouthpiece. The spacer encloses the dose and then delivers it to the lungs when inhalation occurs.
- When using a spacer, place the lips around the mouthpiece of it, completely exhale through the nose, depress the canister to release the medication into the spacer, and then inhale slowly and hold the breath for 10 seconds. Exhale through the nose and take two or three short breaths to obtain the remaining medication in the spacer.
- When using both bronchodilator and corticosteroid inhalers, use the bronchodilator inhaler first. Rinse the mouth and spit out the fluid after using a corticosteroid inhaler.
- Rinse the L-shaped mouthpiece and cap, and the spacer if used, with warm running water at least once a day. Wash them with warm, soapy water at least once a week. Always let them air dry.

Modified from deWit, S.C. (2005). *Fundamental Concepts and Skills for Nursing* (2nd ed.). Philadelphia: Elsevier Saunders, p. 653.

to quit that seems possible to achieve. The drug bupropion (Zyban) is available by prescription and will help decrease nicotine cravings. The FDA has recently released another drug to help with smoking cessation. It is varenicline tartrate (Chantix) and is in tablet form. Chantix is taken for 12 weeks and has been shown by research to be more effective than Zyban (FDA, 2007). Decreasing stress levels and improving coping techniques aid success. Exercise is a good distracter for the urges to use tobacco. A support group can be very helpful. Encouragement and praise for progress are essential components of the treatment program.

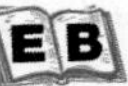

Psychosocial Care. Psychosocial concerns are another area for nursing intervention. The patient often needs help with adjustment to alterations in roles and lifestyle. She may have problems with self-esteem, body image, and sexuality that stem from her chronic disease. A trusting relationship between nurse and patient opens the way for discussing the most personal concerns and provides a means to explore possible solutions or adaptations for problems in these areas. Referral to community support groups also can be beneficial, as the patient then has an opportunity to see and hear how others in her situation have learned to cope and adapt.

Patient and Family Teaching. The teaching plan for the CAL patient is extensive and includes:

- Management of medications and side effects
- Use of respiratory therapy measures and care of equipment
- Management of dyspnea
- Control of the immediate environment and avoidance of allergens
- Maintenance of nutrition
- Balancing exercise and adequate rest
- Signs of complications
- Need for close medical supervision

Education of the patient and family can be overwhelming if it is not planned carefully, allowing enough time for them to gain confidence in one aspect of care before introducing more information.

Most patients with CAL have difficulty getting sufficient rest and sleep because of their dyspnea, anxiety, and decreased mobility. Sedatives and tranquilizers are contraindicated because they tend to depress respiration. Tension and anxiety often can be relieved if the patient is taught some relaxation techniques (Borkovec & Costello, 1993). It should be emphasized that these techniques must be *taught to the patient*. Simply telling her to relax or to stop worrying will not be helpful; she is using almost every muscle in her body to struggle for breath or is extremely tense in anticipation of an attack of breathlessness. Some patients become very agitated and talkative if dyspnea is not too severe. It is best to display a calm attitude, stay with the patient, hold a hand, and state, "Sh-h, we'll talk in a minute. Catch your breath first."

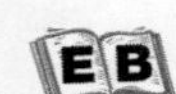

Relaxation exercises can be learned, but it takes a bit of practice to use them whenever relaxation is needed. See Box 7–2 for the script from which the patient can make a "relaxation" tape.

Think Critically About . . . Can you list five nursing interventions that might help your CAL patient avoid episodes of dyspnea?

LUNG CANCER

Etiology

Lung cancer cases have been rising every year. In 2002 there were about 169,500 new cases of lung cancer. In 2006, it was estimated that there would be 213,380 new cases and 160,390 deaths (American Cancer Society, 2007). Today lung cancer has become the leading cause of cancer deaths worldwide. **Cigarette smoking is the primary cause of lung cancer.** A person living with a smoker has twice the risk of lung cancer as someone not regularly exposed to smoke. Other risk factors are increasing air pollution, asbestos exposure, lung diseases such as TB and COPD, and radon exposure. Approximately 85% of lung cancer is thought to be directly linked to cigarette smoking. Lung cancer is found most often in people 40 years of age or older. About 14% of patients diagnosed with lung cancer survive more than 5 years (American Cancer Society, 2006). One of the *Healthy People 2010* objectives is *Reduce the lung cancer death rate.*

Pathophysiology

Most lung tumors begin in the epithelial lining of the bronchi. Tumors arising from the bronchial epithelium are the most common lung malignancy. Squamous cell carcinoma and adenocarcinoma are both seen. Small cell or "oat" cell tumors grow rapidly and are often located near a major bronchus in the central part of the lung. Non–small cell tumors are usually found in the lung periphery and have undifferentiated cells that have slow growth and tend to metastasize.

Chronic irritation of the epithelial tissue in the lung causes changes in cell structure. This makes the tissue more vulnerable to the carcinogens and irritants inhaled when smoking. Dysplasia develops and the tumor grows. Common sites of metastases for cancer of the lung are the brain, bone, and liver.

Signs and Symptoms

There are few symptoms at first, usually only a cough and some wheezing. As the tumor grows larger, the patient may have some pain or discomfort in the chest, exertional dyspnea, and expectoration of blood-streaked sputum. More specific symptoms depend on the location and size of the malignant tumor and the areas to which it has metastasized. If, for example, the malignancy has involved the esophagus, there will be ulceration, bleeding, and dysphagia. Tumors pressing against the trachea can produce hoarseness and paralysis of the vocal cords. Fatigue, anorexia, and weight loss are common because lung cancer is usually advanced when discovered.

Diagnosis

Multiple tests are used to diagnose lung cancer definitively. These include chest x-ray; sputum cytology; low-dose computed tomography (CT); magnetic resonance imaging (MRI); cytology of specimens obtained by mediastinoscopy, bronchoscopy, or thoracentesis; fine needle biopsy of the tumor; and video-assisted thoracoscopic surgery (VATS).

Treatment

Treatment is based on the type of cancer, small cell or non–small cell. The stage of the disease is determined by diagnostic testing. It may be possible to remove the affected area of the lung by surgery if the malignancy is in its earliest stages and is localized. Surgical procedures include wedge resection, in which a small area of the lung is removed; segmental resection, which includes removal of lung tissue and surrounding blood vessels and bronchioles; lobectomy, with removal of an entire lobe of the lung; and **pneumonectomy**, in which an entire lung is removed. Lobectomy is the most common procedure used for small cell lung cancer. Radiation may be used before and after surgery; however, some types of lung cancers are radiation resistant. Small cell tumors respond dramatically to chemotherapy, but if the disease is extensive, the malignancy tends to recur because of metastasis that occurred before diagnosis. Five drugs are used in various combinations to treat small cell tumors: cyclophosphamide, doxorubicin, vincristine, cisplatin, and etoposide.

Non–small cell lung cancer is very aggressive and difficult to treat. Unless it is caught in the very early stages, the prognosis is not good. Combinations of one or two chemotherapy drugs, biotherapy agents, radiotherapy, and photodynamic therapy (PDT) are used depending on the stage of the cancer and the symptoms of the patient. For PDT, the patient is given a drug that is taken up by the tumor cells, making them very sensitive to light and/or heat. The tumor is then exposed to a laser beam that destroys the malignant cells. The laser is introduced into the bronchi via a bronchoscope. Tumors in the main bronchi are particular targets for this type of therapy.

Nursing Management

Care of the patient undergoing thoracotomy for cancer of the lung follows later in the chapter. See Chapter 8 for nursing care of the patient with cancer. Because lung cancer is so lethal, it is a primary function of the nurse to educate the patient about tests and treatments to reduce anxiety and provide hope (Nursing Care Plan 14–1).

PULMONARY VASCULAR DISORDERS

PULMONARY EMBOLISM

Etiology and Pathophysiology

Pulmonary embolism (PE) occurs when a pulmonary vessel is plugged with a mass or clot. Emboli can occur in solid, liquid, or gas forms and can occur from fracture of a long bone (fat embolus), from amniotic fluid during childbirth, from air introduced through a central line, and from clots formed elsewhere in the body, such as from a deep venous thrombosis or thrombi that form in the heart when the patient has dysrhythmias. Regardless of the origin of the embolus, the result is the same: interference with blood flow in the lung distal to the point where the embolus lodges. The obstruction causes shunting to occur at the alveoli that are no longer filling with air. Blood flows past without receiving oxygen or giving up carbon dioxide, and hypoxia results.

The elderly are especially prone to developing deep venous thrombosis when they are immobilized from surgery or for a major illness. **Preventing dehydration in these patients helps prevent thrombus formation** (Gerontological Nursing Center, 2004). Many elderly patients with heart disease suffer cardiac dysrhythmias that predispose to the formation of thrombi in the heart. The dysrhythmia atrial fibrillation, when uncontrolled, is a direct cause of pulmonary emboli. The discovery of a new irregularity of heartbeat upon assessment of the elderly patient should be reported to the physician promptly.

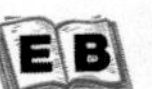

Long airplane flights and sitting for long periods with the legs crossed are other potential causes of venous thrombosis that then may lead to pulmonary embolus.

Signs and Symptoms

Symptoms depend on the size and location of the clot in the lung and whether it is one clot or multiple small clots. **The general symptoms are respiratory distress with dyspnea, chest pain, cough, hemoptysis, and anxiety.** Hypotension and tachycardia may occur. **A sudden onset of dyspnea in a patient at risk of thrombus formation is very suggestive of PE.** The consequences of pulmonary embolism can be minor or life threatening.

Diagnosis

If the data seem to indicate that the cause of symptoms is PE, a ventilation-perfusion scan is performed. If the lung scan is inconclusive, a pulmonary angiogram may be ordered, but it is an expensive procedure that is invasive and not without risk because it involves a right-sided heart catheterization. A spiral CT scan may also be used to diagnose a PE. Plasma D-dimer testing may be recommended when a PE is initially suspected (see Table 12–3).

Diagnosis is made by ruling out other problems, such as heart failure, and by tests to support a diagnosis of pulmonary embolus. A specimen for arterial blood gases is drawn, a 12-lead electrocardiogram and chest x-ray are ordered, and an echocardiogram will most likely be done.

Treatment

Treatment depends on the size and location of the embolus. Intravenous heparin is usually begun and continued for 7 to 10 days. Warfarin (Coumadin) is initiated several days before discharge and is continued at home for up to 1 year. Some physicians are performing trials with **thrombolytic** (dissolves thrombi) therapy using streptokinase, urokinase, or tissue plasminogen activator. There is concern about whether the benefits of decomposing the clot outweigh the risk of bleeding

NURSING CARE PLAN 14–1

Care of the Patient with Lung Cancer

SCENARIO A 62-year-old female smoker with a diagnosis of early lung cancer is scheduled for a right thoracotomy and lobectomy. She has no other medical problems except mild arthritis, for which she occasionally takes aspirin.

PROBLEM/NURSING DIAGNOSIS *Unfamiliar with surgery*/Deficient knowledge related to postoperative care for thoracotomy.

Supporting assessment data *Subjective:* "I've never had surgery before."

Goals/Expected Outcomes	Nursing Interventions	Selected Rationale	Evaluation
Patient will demonstrate leg and arm exercises	Teach deep breathing, coughing, use of incentive spirometer, leg and arm exercises; obtain return demonstration.	Learning the techniques before surgery and sedation will make them easier to perform postoperatively.	Is performing leg and arm exercises, but is hesitant to do the full arm exercise at this point in time. Uses spirometer correctly.
Patient will verbalize understanding of postoperative routine of frequent monitoring of vital signs, chest tube care, and respiratory treatments	Explain kind and purpose of tubes, drainage apparatus, and oxygen equipment. Explain need for early ambulation. Describe methods of pain control.	Being familiar with equipment and what to expect after surgery decreases fear of the unknown.	Verbalizes understanding of what equipment is for. Says will try to ambulate this afternoon. States understands use of PCA pump for pain control. Outcomes met.

POSTOPERATIVE PERIOD

PROBLEM/NURSING DIAGNOSIS *Excision of lobe of lung*/Risk of impaired gas exchange related to surgical removal of portion of lung and possible complications.

Supporting assessment data *Objective:* Thoracotomy and lobectomy.

Goals/Expected Outcomes	Nursing Interventions	Selected Rationale	Evaluation
Patient will display normal respiratory rate and normal blood gas exchange within 36 hours	Position on back or operative side; turn, cough, deep-breathe using incentive spirometer q 2 hr; splint incision with small pillow to minimize pain.	Position allows good lung to fully expand. Incentive spirometer use opens alveoli, promoting better gas exchange and resolving atelectasis	Turned q 2 hr; using spirometer and coughing q 2 hr. Splints incision when coughing.
	Administer humidified oxygen as ordered.		Receiving humidified oxygen.
	Monitor vital signs q 4 hr and respirations frequently; auscultate lung fields q shift; monitor blood gas levels. Pulse oximetry readings q 1 hr × 4; then q 2 hr. Report Sao_2 <90%.	Respiratory rate, lung sounds, blood gas levels, and pulse oximetry readings provide data regarding respiratory status and can indicate decline or improvement.	Vital signs stable; slightly tachypneic. Left lung with normal breath sounds; right lung with diminished sounds in bases and absent over middle lobe area. Sao_2 95% average.
	Encourage use of PCA to promote better cooperation with respiratory therapy, coughing, and deep breathing, but avoid oversedation and respiratory depression.	If pain is minimized, patient is able to more fully expand the lungs.	Using PCA appropriately; pain at 4 on a scale of 1–10.
	Maintain intact, functioning closed chest water-seal drainage system.	Intact system prevents air from entering pleural space and collapsing lung.	Chest drainage system intact with 150 mL drainage.
	Observe for signs of subcutaneous emphysema; assess for signs of pulmonary embolism.		No subcutaneous emphysema; no signs of pulmonary embolism.
	Monitor abdomen for signs of distention or ileus.	Distention can cause pressure on diaphragm, decreasing lung expansion.	Abdomen soft and nondistended.

Key: *CBC*, complete blood count; *IV*, intravenous; *PCA*, patient-controlled analgesia; *Sao_2*, oxygen saturation; *WBC*, white blood cell.

NURSING CARE PLAN 14–1

Care of the Patient with Lung Cancer—cont'd

PROBLEM/NURSING DIAGNOSIS *Surgical incision*/Risk for infection related to surgical incision and chest tubes.

Supporting assessment data *Objective:* Thoracotomy and lobectomy; chest tube in place.

Goals/Expected Outcomes	Nursing Interventions	Selected Rationale	Evaluation
No signs of infection as evidenced by clean incision, temperature in normal range, normal WBC count, and clear breath sounds.	Use aseptic technique for dressing changes and care of chest tube.	Prevents introduction of pathogenic organisms.	Incision clean and dry.
	Assess temperature trends q 24 hr; monitor WBC count.	Provides data that might indicate beginning infection.	Temp 99.4° F, (37.4° C), CBC not back yet.
	Observe wound for signs of infection.		Wound not observed; dressing intact and dry.
	Protect from people with infections; maintain adequate nutrition and fluid intake.	Helps prevent respiratory infection.	Taking clear liquids. IV line patent at 125 mL/hr.
	Auscultate lungs each shift.		Breath sounds clear, but diminished in bases and absent over right middle lobe. Continue plan.

PROBLEM/NURSING DIAGNOSIS *Worry over diagnosis and treatment*/Anxiety related to diagnosis of cancer of the lung, treatment, and prognosis.

Supporting assessment data *Subjective:* "I'm scared. I don't want to die of cancer. Will I have to have chemotherapy? Will there be a lot of pain?" *Objective:* Anxious look on face.

Goals/Expected Outcomes	Nursing Interventions	Selected Rationale	Evaluation
Patient will cope positively with diagnosis of cancer by determined attitude to do whatever she can to fight the cancer by discharge.	Establish trusting relationship; use active listening. Encourage verbalization of fears and concerns, answer questions honestly.	A trusting relationship promotes sharing of feelings and fears.	Attempting to actively listen, but patient is not verbalizing much.
	Establish hope; discuss what patient can do to optimize chances of survival: quit smoking, exercise program, diet, relaxation techniques, stress reduction.	Focuses on hope of what patient can do to help herself.	Reminded that many people have survived for many years after having lung cancer. Discussed aids for quitting smoking. Not willing to try relaxation exercise yet.
	Advise that oncologist will discuss modes of treatment after full pathology report is back.	Type of tumor cells, degree of aggressiveness, and rate of growth dictate treatment.	Advised that oncologist would be in tomorrow morning to talk about options.
	Focus on positives of her life now and for each day in the future; assure her that pain control is possible.		Encouraged to look at what is positive in life. Continue plan.

? CRITICAL THINKING QUESTIONS

1. Why shouldn't this patient be positioned on the unoperative side after surgery?
2. What would you do if you noticed that the amount of drainage in the disposable water-seal chest drainage system was not increasing?

complications. Pulmonary embolectomy is a last resort because the surgery carries a high mortality rate. An intracaval filter may be placed in the vena cava to prevent clots from traveling to the lungs in the future. Oxygen therapy is initiated to decrease hypoxia. The patient is kept on bed rest in semi-Fowler's position initially, but turning, deep breathing, and coughing are important to prevent atelectasis.

Nursing Management

Initial care for the patient who might be experiencing a PE is to stay with the patient, raise the head of the bed to a high Fowler's position, begin low-flow oxygen therapy if there is oxygen in the room, assess vital signs, notify the physician of the patient's symptoms, and administer heparin when it is ordered. If an IV access is not in place, one should be initiated. Prepare the patient for the diagnostic tests and probable treatment. The patient is likely to be very frightened and needs reassurance and a calm attitude from the nurse.

PRIMARY PULMONARY HYPERTENSION

Pulmonary hypertension is elevated pressure in the pulmonary artery. It is rare as a primary disease, but has occurred after taking the appetite suppressant fenfluramine (Fen-Phen). The drug was removed from the market in 1996. There is no cure for primary pulmonary hypertension. The classic symptoms are dyspnea and fatigue. Other symptoms are chest pain with exertion, dizziness, and syncope. The disorder eventually causes right-sided heart enlargement (cor pulmonale), followed by heart failure.

Treatment can improve or relieve symptoms and increase the quality and length of life. Diuretics and anticoagulant therapy are used to reduce right ventricular overload and prevent thrombus formation and thrombosis. Calcium channel blockers may be used for their vasodilating effects to help reduce the load on the heart. Epoprostenol (Flolan) promotes pulmonary vasodilation and reduces the vascular resistance, and its use has contributed to long-term survival. It must be administered through a central IV line and requires extensive education of the patient and family. Bosentan (Tracleer) is an oral form of the drug. An inhaled form is under investigation. A new drug, sildenafil citrate (Revatio), improves exercise ability, but must be used with caution as it can result in myocardial infarction or dysrhythmia.

Lung transplantation is reserved for those who do not respond to epoprostenol and who progress to severe right-sided heart failure.

LUNG TRANSPLANTATION

Lung transplantation is a viable option for a variety of end-stage lung diseases. Options include single lung, bilateral lung, and heart-lung transplantation. Patients must undergo extensive evaluation and psychological counseling, and meet stringent criteria. There must be no history of malignancy within 2 years, no presence of HIV, and no renal or liver impairment. The average wait for a suitable organ is 1 year.

The most common cause of mortality after lung transplantation is infection, with cytomegalovirus being the main organism responsible. Infection often occurs within 4 to 6 weeks.

Immunosuppressive therapy to prevent organ rejection must continue for the life of the patient. After transplantation and stabilization, patients are entered into a rehabilitation program to improve physical endurance.

CHEST INJURIES

Injury to the chest wall and underlying structures can range from minor bruises to major trauma to the pulmonary and cardiovascular systems. Thoracic trauma is a major cause of accidental death, exceeding head and facial injuries. Whenever there is evidence of chest injury, a very real state of emergency exists because the condition of the victim can rapidly deteriorate to death.

The major complications of chest trauma involve either the lungs and air passages or the heart and major blood vessels, or both. Pneumothorax and hemothorax frequently occur as a result of a blunt (nonpenetrating) or penetrating injury to the chest wall. These conditions can cause partial or total collapse of one or both lungs. There also can be contusion of the myocardium, rupture of the aorta, and tracheobronchial or tracheoabdominal injuries. The procedure to correct pneumothorax or hemothorax is to insert a thoracostomy tube (chest tube) (Figure 14–3).

Major concerns in the care of patients with chest injuries are:

- Maintenance of an airway
- Assurance of adequate ventilation
- Treatment of circulatory problems to ensure circulation of oxygenated blood

FRACTURED RIBS

Fractured ribs are very painful as breathing causes movement at the site of injury. The treatment goal is to decrease pain so that the patient can breathe adequately. Intercostal nerve block with local anesthesia may be used to control pain. Narcotic drug therapy is used cautiously since it can depress respirations. Binding the ribs is no longer recommended.

FLAIL CHEST

When a patient experiences severe chest trauma in an automobile accident or fall, often several ribs are broken. When three or more ribs are broken in two or more places, the chest wall becomes unstable. This condition is called *flail chest.* It produces "**paradoxical respirations.**" When the patient breathes in, the fractured portion of the chest is drawn inward instead of

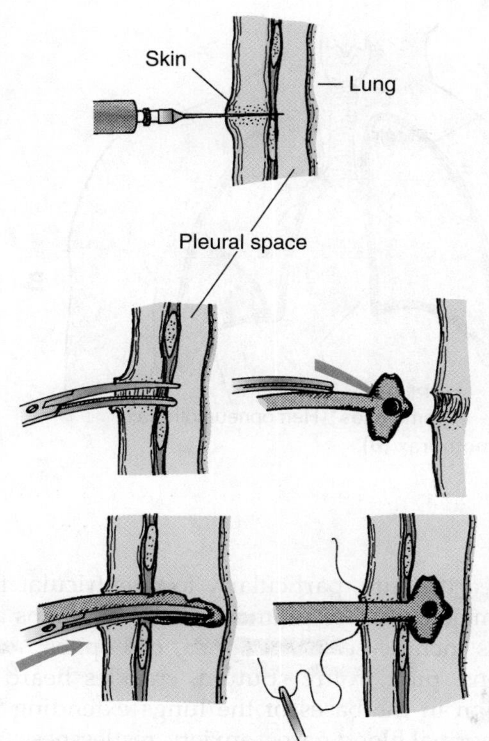

FIGURE 14–3 Insertion of a thoracostomy tube (chest tube).

expanding outward as the rest of the chest does; when she exhales, the flail portion expands outward as the rest of the chest collapses normally. This process interferes with oxygenation, as the lungs cannot expand normally. Emergency treatment consists of turning the patient onto the affected side so that the ground or bed will act as a splint and reduce the pain of breathing. The patient is observed for signs of external and internal bleeding, pneumothorax, and shock. The fractured ribs may cause tissue damage to the lung.

Once the patient is in an emergency facility, flail chest is treated by intubation and mechanical ventilation while the ribs heal. This causes considerable pain, and the patient often has to be given a neuromuscular blocking agent such as pancuronium bromide (Pavulon) to prevent fighting the action of the ventilator. Pain must be controlled as well. Sedation is used to decrease anxiety over being totally paralyzed. The patient should never be left totally alone without a nurse or personnel in sight as the fear of being paralyzed and having something go wrong with the ventilator or tubing connections when totally alone is terrifying.

PENETRATING WOUNDS

Victims of stabbing can have an open chest wound that creates serious respiratory difficulties. An open, or "sucking," chest wound is one in which pneumothorax results from penetration of the pleural cavity, which allows air and gas to accumulate there. Symptoms of pneumothorax include labored, shallow respirations and lack of movement on one side of the chest when the person inhales and exhales. A sucking chest wound should be covered at the end of a forceful expiration with an *occlusive dressing*—that is, one made of plastic wrap, aluminum foil, Vaseline-covered gauze, or any other material that seals the wound and prohibits the flow of air into the pleural cavity. **One corner of the dressing is left unsealed to allow accumulated air to escape.** Place the patient in a semi-Fowler's position if possible.

If a knife or other item is stuck into the chest cavity, do not remove it; instead, stabilize it so that it does not move around and cause more damage as the patient is transported to an emergency facility. The object may be wedged against severed vessels, preventing them from bleeding; removing it may cause hemorrhage.

PNEUMOTHORAX AND HEMOTHORAX

The space within the pleural membranes is an airtight compartment. Pressure within this compartment is less than that of the atmosphere and therefore is called a *negative pressure.* This negative pressure is necessary to allow sufficient space for normal breathing in which the tidal movement of air in and out of the lungs inflates and deflates them. If, however, there is a break in the airtight compartment, either along the surface of the lung or from outside the pleural sac, air rushes in and collapses the lung. The presence of air or gas within the pleural cavity is called **pneumothorax** (Figure 14–4).

Pneumothorax always is a threat in chest injury, as well as in the period following chest surgery. However, the condition also can occur spontaneously when there is a pathologic opening on the surface of the lung that allows a leakage of air from the bronchi into the pleural cavity. This condition is called a *spontaneous pneumothorax.* Treatment for spontaneous pneumothorax may require nothing more than rest and the administration of oxygen to relieve discomfort. If the amount of air in the pleural space is minimal, a large-bore needle may be used to aspirate it. For greater amounts of air or fluid, a chest tube connected to water-seal drainage may be inserted to remove the air and allow reexpansion of the lung.

Tension pneumothorax develops when air enters the pleural space on inspiration but remains trapped there rather than being expelled on expiration. It can occur from trauma, mechanical ventilation, or rib fracture during cardiopulmonary resuscitation. The air in the pleural space increases with each breath, and the pressure within the chest builds, which gradually collapses the lung. If unrelieved, this increasing pressure will cause a *mediastinal shift,* resulting in a decrease in cardiac output and blood pressure. Mediastinal shift means that the structures in the mediastinum—the heart, great vessels, trachea, and esophagus—are all shifted to the unaffected side of the chest. The vena cava can become "kinked" and cause cardiac arrest. In this case, a flutter valve needle or Heimlich valve may be used until a chest tube can be placed to remove the

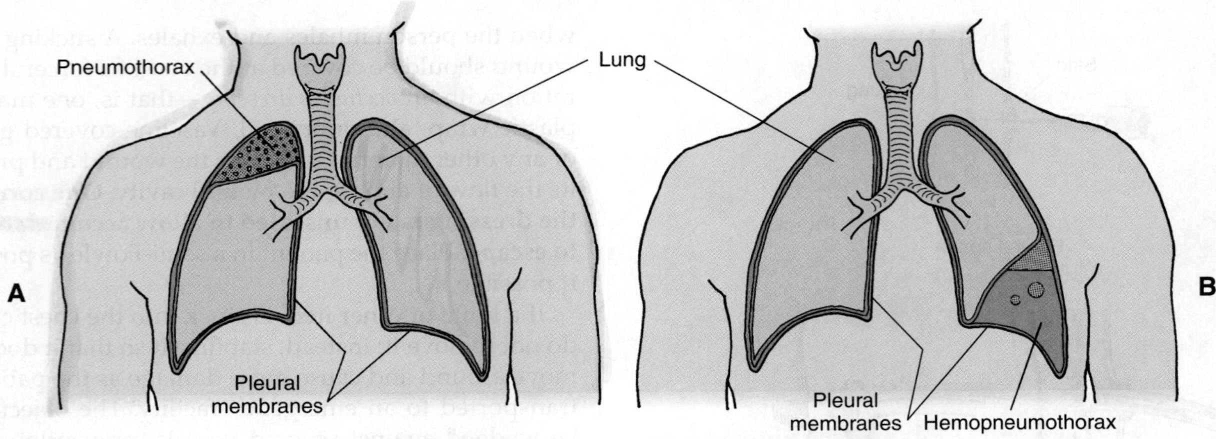

FIGURE **14–4** Pneumothorax **(A)** and hemothorax **(B)**.

air from the pleural cavity. Care of chest tubes and water-seal drainage is discussed in the later section, Common Therapeutic Measures.

Hemothorax is the presence of blood within the pleural cavity. It can occur as a result of laceration of the lung, heart, and blood vessels within the thorax. The accumulation of blood in the pleural cavity can have the same effect as accumulations of gas or air, that is, it fills up space and causes partial or total collapse of the lung. There also is the possibility of mediastinal shift in hemothorax and the likelihood of impaired venous return in the pulmonary blood vessels. The blood is removed by chest drainage.

Assessment of a patient for pneumothorax, hemothorax, or a combination of the two (hemopneumothorax; see Figure 14–4), includes awareness of the patient's history in regard to acute or chronic respiratory disease, accidental injury to the chest, or chest surgery. The condition is suspected when the patient complains of sudden chest pain or a feeling of tightness in the chest. There is an increase in both pulse rate and rate of respirations, a drop in blood pressure, and the absence of normal chest movements and absent or diminished breath sounds on the affected side.

Think Critically About . . . You come upon an automobile accident and stop to assist. You are on your way to work and have your stethoscope with you. Name three assessment criteria that would lead you to believe that the driver of the vehicle has suffered a pneumothorax.

LUNG DISORDERS

PULMONARY EDEMA

Pulmonary edema is an abnormal collection of fluid in the interstitial spaces of the lung and inside the alveoli. Acute pulmonary edema is a medical emergency. Congestive heart failure, particularly left ventricular failure, is a major cause of pulmonary edema. Signs and symptoms include severe dyspnea, orthopnea, noisy respirations, pink frothy sputum, crackles heard on auscultation in the bases of the lungs extending upward, abnormal blood gases, anxiety, restlessness, and possibly confusion. The patient will be very anxious and pale with cold, clammy skin. Diagnosis is based on ruling out other disorders, such as pneumonia, asthma, or pulmonary embolism, and on determining the cause. Treatment depends to some degree on whether the edema is a result of heart problems or from another cause (see the section on Adult [Acute] Respiratory Distress Syndrome below).

Both IV morphine sulfate and furosemide are given for fluid diuresis. The morphine reduces anxiety and the workload on the heart. Oxygen is started immediately, and continuous positive airway pressure (CPAP) may be necessary. Drugs for the underlying heart disorder also are administered.

Nursing care involves placing the patient in high Fowler's position. Sodium and fluids are restricted. Reassurance is provided to the patient to decrease anxiety. Other interventions are to closely monitor fluid intake and output, administer drugs, and perform continuous respiratory and cardiac assessment to evaluate the effectiveness of treatment.

ADULT (ACUTE) RESPIRATORY DISTRESS SYNDROME

Etiology and Pathophysiology

Adult (acute) respiratory distress syndrome (ARDS) is a form of pulmonary edema that is not heart related. It results from pulmonary changes that occur in connection with many disorders, including sepsis, trauma, cardiac or other major surgery, and any critical illness. The alveolar capillary membrane becomes injured and more permeable to intravascular fluid. Alveoli fill with fluid, and oxygen and carbon dioxide cannot cross the alveolar membrane into and out of the capillaries. ARDS is particularly dangerous when a patient has multisystem disorders; the mortality rate in these patients is 50% to 90%.

Signs, Symptoms, and Diagnosis

Dyspnea, tachypnea, cough, and restlessness occur. Auscultation may reveal fine, scattered crackles. Initially there may be mild hypoxemia and respiratory alkalosis from the tachypnea. As ARDS progresses, symptoms worsen because of increased fluid accumulation and decreased lung compliance.

Diagnosis is by physical presentation, history of a disorder or event known to cause ARDS, arterial blood gas determination, and chest x-ray. **The hallmark for diagnosis is a Pa_{O_2} below 70 mm Hg even with 100% oxygen delivery.** Pulmonary edema and lung stiffness occur, resulting in severe hypoxemia. There is diffuse fluid and exudate infiltration that gives a "whiteout" appearance to lung x-rays.

Treatment and Nursing Management

Treatment is ventilatory support with positive end-expiratory pressure (PEEP), treatment of the underlying disorder, careful fluid and electrolyte management, and total care for basic needs. Antibiotics, bronchodilators, and corticosteroids may be administered depending on the situation (Complementary & Alternative Therapies 14–5). Parenteral nutrition may be started to maintain nutritional status. Prone positioning has come back into favor because research showed that the dorsal parts of the lungs are more affected in ARDS and perfusion is greater in the dorsal areas no matter the position. The prone position seems to allow fluid to shift from the dorsal aspects, enabling undamaged alveoli to fill with oxygenated air, thereby decreasing hypoxemia. However, prone positioning is again being questioned as to effectiveness overall.

Partial liquid ventilation may become the favored treatment for ARDS (see the section on Mechanical Ventilation later). A substance called perfluorocarbon is infused into the endotracheal tube. This liquid allows oxygen and carbon dioxide to freely diffuse. It is under investigation, but as yet its use has not decreased mortality. Nursing care is supportive and attempts to prevent other complications.

RESPIRATORY FAILURE

Hyperventilation and hypoventilation were discussed earlier, as was the effect of either of these abnormal breathing patterns on the acid-base balance of body fluids (see Chapter 3). *Hypercapnia* (also called *hypercarbia*) is the retention of excessive amounts of carbon dioxide. It is the result of hypoventilation, during which the usual amount of carbon dioxide is not eliminated by exhalation. Respiratory distress is evident.

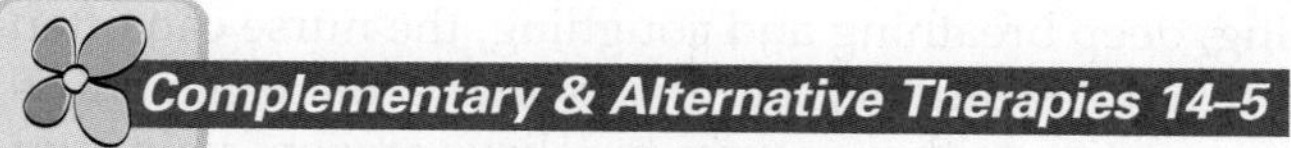

Alternative Therapy for Adult (Acute) Respiratory Distress Syndrome (ARDS)

Anesthesiologists from the Mayo Clinic found that a nutritional supplement composed of borage seed oil, fish oil, protein, carbohydrates, and antioxidants was associated with a 35% reduction in mortality in patients with ARDS. The supplement is administered by enteral tube. Gamma-linolenic acid, a component of the borage seed oil, is thought to reduce inflammation and improve oxygen flow.

Carbon dioxide is a respiratory stimulant; hence the body responds to excessive levels of carbon dioxide by increasing the rate of respirations in an effort to "blow off" larger quantities of the gas. If, however, the respiratory centers in the brain are exposed to higher-than-normal levels of carbon dioxide over a long time, they cease to react and a drop in the respiratory rate occurs. The patient then becomes mentally confused, the senses become less acute, and eventually a coma may ensue. **The heart rate increases to meet the tissues' need for more oxygen. Mental confusion and an increase in pulse and heart rate are indicators of inadequate oxygenation of the blood and tissues.** If the slowing down of respiration is not corrected, the accumulation of carbon dioxide continues, and a vicious cycle begins. The final outcome can be cardiac arrest from respiratory acidosis—a result of respiratory failure.

Signs and symptoms of respiratory failure depend somewhat on the cause. There may be a rapid, shallow breathing pattern or a respiratory rate that is slower than usual. The patient may use pursed-lip breathing and sit upright, bent forward. Inability to speak without pausing for breath occurs. Retraction of respiratory muscles occurs as the work of breathing increases. Breath sounds become abnormal.

Respiratory failure is defined by arterial blood gases. **It has occurred when the Pa_{O_2} is less than 50 mm Hg and the partial pressure of carbon dioxide (P_{CO_2}) is more than 50 mm Hg.**

Blood gas analysis is the best way to determine whether respiratory acidosis is either threatening or already present. Results of the analysis will show a high level of Pa_{CO_2}, a high bicarbonate (HCO_3^-) level, and a low pH (acidosis) if the condition has been present for several days.

Treatment is with oxygen and respiratory therapy, including mechanical ventilation, measures to reduce and remove secretions, drugs to reduce bronchospasm and airway inflammation, correction of acidosis, and treatment of the underlying cause.

By vigilant observation and assessment of patients with respiratory problems and close attention to turning, deep breathing and coughing, the nurse can often prevent respiratory failure. Nursing management is supportive with measures to relieve anxiety, pain, and agitation. Maintenance of adequate nutrition is important, as is monitoring fluid balance.

COMMON THERAPEUTIC MEASURES

INTRATHORACIC SURGERY

Intrathoracic surgery requires opening the chest wall and entering the pleural cavity. For example, in addition to resection of lung tissue and other pulmonary structures, intrathoracic surgery also is necessary to repair the heart and great vessels and to correct defects of the esophagus.

Today, video-assisted thoracoscopic surgery (VATS), is replacing the traditional standard **thoracotomy** (incision with entry into the thorax) (McKenna et al., 2006) for many surgical procedures in the chest cavity. About 70% of thoracic procedures can be performed in this manner, including pulmonary resections, biopsy or resection of mediastinal tumors or masses, and drainage of pleural effusions. An endoscope equipped with a multichip minicamera, along with intense lighting, magnifies the image of the cavity and structures and transmits it to a video monitor. Instruments can be guided through the endoscope to biopsy or remove tissue and to place surgical staples. One to four 1-inch incisions are used to accommodate the endoscope, instruments, and suction.

Preoperative Care

Assessment of the patient's respiratory status prior to chest surgery depends on whether the surgery is elective or in response to accidental trauma. If there is time, a health history as well as subjective and objective assessment data should be obtained prior to the surgery (see Chapter 12 for data collection and assessment).

Preoperatively, efforts are made to improve the respiratory status of the patient as much as possible. Special exercises may be prescribed to strengthen chest and shoulder muscles and accessory muscles of respiration and to remove accumulated secretions from the air passages.

When standard thoracotomy is to be performed, arm and leg exercises are also taught preoperatively to avoid thrombophlebitis in the lower extremities and problems with movement of the arm on the operative side. Movement of the arm may be very painful, because of either the position in which the patient was placed during surgery or the surgical involvement of muscles that control the arm. If the arm is not moved in spite of discomfort, the patient may develop a "frozen" (immobile) shoulder. Patients undergoing VATS do not have this complication.

Preoperative patient education focuses on teaching the patient techniques to use after surgery to improve lung ventilation. Information about chest tubes, suctioning, mechanical ventilation, use of an incentive spirometer, and any other procedures that are anticipated as part of postoperative care is given.

Postoperative Care

During the immediate postoperative period, nursing assessment and intervention focus on special observations (in addition to routine postoperative ones; see later), positioning, routine turning, coughing and deep breathing, and attention to chest tubes and the closed drainage system. In spite of the tubes and machines used postoperatively, the patient with chest surgery usually must ambulate early. An advantage of VATS is that the patient is out of bed and into a chair within 4 to 6 hours of surgery. Because pain is less, the patient is better able to move around and can more quickly resume normal activities. Whereas the standard thoracotomy patient has a 4- to 6-week recovery, the VATS patient resumes activities of daily living in 3 to 4 days and can even return to work within 1 week.

Interpleural analgesia may be used for the postoperative standard thoracotomy patient. An analgesic agent is administered through a catheter that has been placed percutaneously in the interpleural space or is introduced via an injection lumen of the chest tube. Suction is turned off for 15 minutes when medication is instilled. Injections are given every 4 to 6 hours rather than on an as-needed basis. The effect of this type of analgesia is controversial.

Special observations include watching for signs of pneumothorax, hemothorax, or both; observing for symptoms of respiratory distress; and auscultation and palpation of the upper chest and neck for swelling caused by **subcutaneous emphysema,** which is an accumulation of air or gas under the skin. It usually occurs after thoracic surgery when air leaks into the tissues around chest tubes. It could be a sign of malfunctioning of the drainage system and should be reported. Inspecting the drainage system for signs of air leak is essential. Assessing for signs of infection, both respiratory and incisional, is very important.

Gastric distention and paralytic ileus also are possible complications of standard thoracic surgery. **Distention of the stomach and intestines is particularly hazardous for the post-thoracotomy patient, as it can cause these organs to push up on the diaphragm and impair ventilation, which is already severely compromised by the surgery.**

Positioning for comfort, optimal ventilation, and adequate drainage of the operative site is an important aspect of post-thoracotomy care. In most cases the patient is allowed to lie on her back and operative side. Many surgeons do not permit lying on the unaffected side because this position diminishes the expansion of

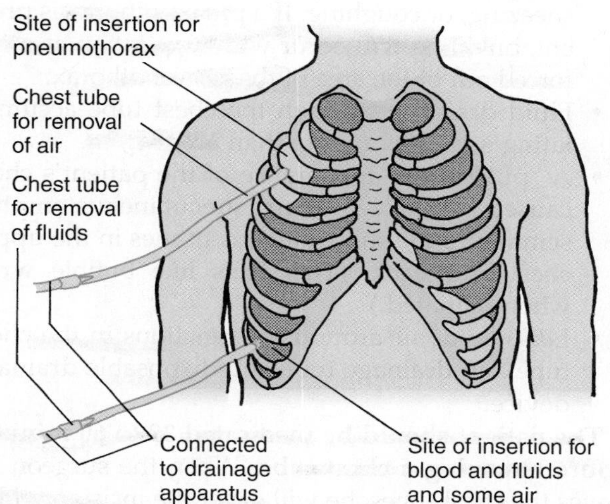

FIGURE 14–5 Location of sites for insertion of chest tubes for drainage of air and fluids.

the good lung. When the patient has a tube inserted for drainage from the operative site, lying on the operative side facilitates the flow of drainage. **Care must be taken when positioning the patient to prevent kinking the chest tubes.**

A pneumonectomy patient is never turned onto her unoperated side, because first, tension pneumothorax and mediastinal shift could occur, and second, the bronchial stump where the lung was removed could leak and the patient could drown in accumulated fluid.

When in doubt about positioning a patient who has had chest surgery, it is always best to check the physician's orders before turning the patient or raising the head of the bed.

Care of Patients with Chest Tubes and Closed Drainage. Of all the special procedures and techniques used to care for a patient who has had chest surgery, the use of tubes and a drainage system to allow reexpansion of the lung is probably the most anxiety-producing for many nurses (Figure 14–5).

Chest tubes inserted during surgery may be attached to any of a variety of drainage systems. Among these are *disposable plastic water-seal drainage systems* and bottle systems with one, two, or three bottles. **Whatever system is used, its purposes are:**

- **To provide for drainage of air and blood from within the pleural cavity**
- **To allow for gradual reexpansion of the lung**

Figure 14–6 shows a disposable system. Note that the water in the left-hand chamber serves as a seal to avoid the return of air to the chest cavity. **The water level will fluctuate as the patient breathes.** There should not be bubbles in this chamber except when the suction is first turned on. The collection chamber, located on the far right of the device, is calibrated for more accurate measurement of drainage from the chest. It also contains float valves, which prevent the

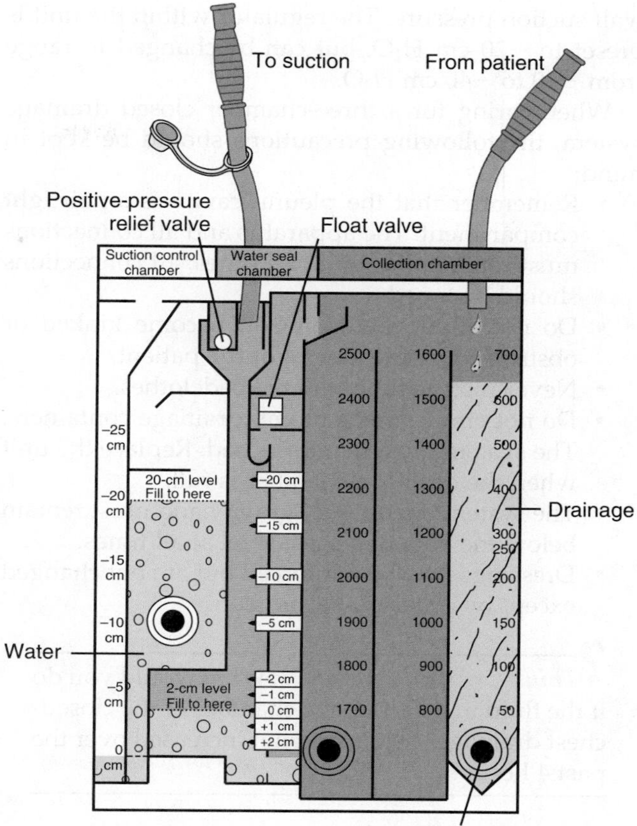

FIGURE 14–6 Disposable water-seal drainage system; note the three chambers.

entry of air or fluid back up into the chest. Suction can be attached to the device to better facilitate removal of air and secretions from the lung. Gentle bubbling in this chamber will be continuous. Specialized chest drainage systems are used to collect the patient's blood from the chest after surgery so that it can be reinfused in an autologous transfusion.

A flutter valve, or Heimlich valve, may be substituted in chest drainage systems. This valve permits the flow of air and fluid from the pleural space into a collection area, but prevents the return flow of air or fluid, and is inserted between the chest tube and the drainage collection apparatus.

Ambulatory patients may be using a small portable chest drainage system that has only one chamber with a dry seal and does not contain water. The collection chamber must be emptied when full. The system is used for certain patients who have less than 500 mL of drainage daily. Two other devices, the Pneumostat and the Pleurx pleural catheter, are available for chest drainage for the home care patient. Each comes with specific care directions.

A dry-suction system is sometimes used in place of water-seal suction. It provides more consistent flow because the suction adjusts automatically to changes in the patient's pleural pressure or to fluctuations in wall suction pressure. The regulator within the unit is preset to −20 cm H_2O, but can be changed to range from −10 to −40 cm H_2O.

When caring for a three-chamber closed drainage system, the following precautions should be kept in mind:

- Remember that the pleural cavity is an airtight compartment. The apparatus and all connections must remain airtight at all times; all connections should be taped.
- Do not allow the tubing to become kinked or obstructed by the weight of the patient.
- Never pin the tubing to the bedclothes.
- Do not empty thoracotomy drainage containers. The system must remain closed. Replace the unit when the drainage chamber is full.
- The system operates by gravity and must remain below the patient's chest level at all times.
- Dressings may be reinforced but are not changed except by order of the surgeon.

Think Critically About . . . What would you do if the fluid in the drainage chamber of the closed-chest drainage system had not increased over the past 4 hours?

Special Aspects of Patient Care

Monitor the patient who has a chest tube regularly and frequently. There are three major areas of assessment:

- The respiratory status of the patient
- The site at which the tube is inserted into the chest and the length of the tube (for kinks)
- The amount and character of the drainage in the collection chamber

The patient is assessed for ease of breathing, pain or discomfort, level of consciousness and orientation, and anxiety and restlessness. The rate and character of respirations are noted, as are breath sounds. The entry site is assessed for unusual drainage, integrity of sutures, and the presence of subcutaneous emphysema.

The drainage tubing must be patent at all times, unless clamped off by the surgeon. If the system becomes disrupted, rather than clamping the tube, place it in a cup of sterile water so that air can escape from the pleural space, but air cannot enter it and cause a tension pneumothorax. The tubing must not be occluded by kinks, compression, or dependent loops; otherwise gas, air, and fluid have no way of escaping from the pleural cavity. It must be airtight; otherwise air will enter the pleural cavity and collapse the lung.

In addition to respiratory distress in the patient, conditions that require immediate attention are:

- Persistent bubbling in the underwater seal, which indicates a leak in the system. Fluid in the chamber *should* fluctuate as the patient breathes air in and out. Occasional bubbles are usual as air escapes from the pleural space with breathing, sneezing, or coughing. If a pneumothorax is present, bubbling will occur with inspiration as air is forced out of the area of the pneumothorax.
- Fluid drainage through the chest tube accumulating at a rate of more than 100 mL/hr.
- A "puffed-up" appearance of the patient's chest caused by leakage of air (subcutaneous emphysema) into the subcutaneous tissues in the upper chest and neck. (This feels like bubble wrap when palpated.)
- Leakage of air around the junctions in the chest tube and drainage tube and disposable drainage device.

The patient should be medicated 30 to 60 minutes before removing a chest tube. When the surgeon removes the chest tubes, he will cover the incision with a dressing containing sterile petroleum jelly to close off the opening so that air does not enter the pleural space. This type of dressing is also applied if a chest tube is accidentally pulled out. Auscultate the lungs after chest tube removal to verify that a pneumothorax has not occurred. Eventually the incision will seal itself. A sample plan with interventions for a patient having thoracic surgery is shown in Nursing Care Plan 14–1.

Think Critically About . . . What would you do if you went to assess your first-day postop standard thoracotomy patient and the water in the closed drainage system was not fluctuating with the patient's breathing?

MEDICATION ADMINISTRATION

A wide variety of drugs are used to treat respiratory disorders. Patients often take several drugs simultaneously, and **it is vitally important that the nurse monitor side effects and drug interactions.** Current drug treatment of lower respiratory system disorders is mainly by inhalation, but some drugs are taken orally.

Bronchodilators are drugs that act directly on the smooth muscle of the bronchi to relax them and thereby relieve bronchospasms. See Box 14–3 for general nursing implications for these drugs. Liquefying agents help to thin the bronchial secretions, making them more liquid and less tenacious. Anti-infectives are helpful in controlling infectious agents in the respiratory tract. These may include the tetracyclines, penicillin, cephalosporins, macrolides (clarithromycin [Biaxin]), fluoroquinolones (ciprofloxacin [Cipro]), and the sulfa drugs.

Corticosteroids are a major part of inhalation therapy for patients with CAL. However, acute respiratory problems are sometimes treated with oral corticosteroids.

When corticosteroids are part of drug therapy, the patient must be closely watched for infection, as steroids may mask signs and symptoms. She must be cautioned to never abruptly to stop taking a steroid drug; it is to be slowly tapered over several days to prevent the serious problems of abrupt steroid with-

Box 14–3 General Nursing Implications for the Administration of Bronchodilators

When giving a bronchodilator drug, you should:

- Check the ID band of the patient before administering each dose to ensure that the right patient receives the drug. Utilize a second means of identification as well.
- Follow the "five rights" of medication administration to prevent errors and injury to the patient.
- Verify allergies and inquire about previous adverse reaction to the drug.
- Auscultate the lungs to ascertain types of lung sounds present.
- Take pulse and count respirations to establish ranges prior to drug administration.
- Use these drugs cautiously in patients with cardiac disease as they affect heart action.
- Consult the physician before administering a bronchodilator to a patient who has a current cardiac dysrhythmia.
- Give the drug with a full glass of water or with meals to decrease the possibility of gastrointestinal upset.
- Give each dose of the drug as close to the ordered time as possible to maintain a steady blood level of the drug.
- When the patient is taking theophylline, check drug serum levels; the therapeutic range is 10 to 20 mcg/mL. Withhold drug if the level is above 20 mcg/mL and notify the physician.
- Warn elderly patients that the drug may cause dizziness and to take precautions when changing positions.
- Monitor the patient for effectiveness of the drug by performing a respiratory assessment.

Regarding possible side effect or adverse effects of the drug, you should:

- Warn the patient about the possibility of paradoxical bronchospasm and advise her to consult the physician if this happens before administering another dose.
- Tell the patient to chew sugarless gum or suck on hard candy to relieve dry mouth.
- Monitor the patient for specific side effects of each drug; general side effects of bronchodilators are dry mouth, insomnia, nervousness, dizziness, palpitations, gastrointestinal upset, and changes in blood pressure.

You should teach the patient taking a bronchodilator drug to:

- Take the drug with a full glass of water; if it causes gastrointestinal upset, take the drug with a meal.
- Take the drug 15 to 60 minutes before exercising (check specific time for individual drug as time depends on form of the drug, i.e., inhalant or oral tablet).
- Follow correct procedure for inhaling the drug: shake the inhaler gently before using, clear the nose and throat, take a deep breath, relax, and completely exhale before inhaling drug.

Adapted from Lewis, S.M., Heitkemper, M.M., Dirksen, S.R. et al. (2007). *Medical-Surgical Nursing: Assessment and Management of Clinical Problems* (7th ed.). St. Louis: Mosby.

drawal. **Potassium loss must be replaced and monitoring for elevated blood glucose performed.**

Antihistamines are used to treat respiratory symptoms of an allergic disorder. They reduce the secretions of the nasal and bronchial mucosa. Decongestants are prescribed for symptoms of the common cold and sinusitis.

Leukotriene inhibitors are the newest addition to the treatment for asthma. They help control symptoms by blocking the activity of these substances that mediate inflammation.

Metered-dose inhalers (MDIs) are used to deliver a variety of drugs to the respiratory patient. The patient should be taught to use a MDI properly (see Patient Teaching 14–5).

Bronchodilators, liquefying agents, and some anti-infectives may be administered directly onto the mucous membranes of the respiratory tract by means of nebulizers and mechanical ventilators.

HUMIDIFICATION

Aerosols are fine suspensions of very small particles of a liquid or solid that constitute a gas. Water is the most important of all aerosols in respiratory therapy. Without adequate humidity, mucous secretions become extremely thick and tenacious, and the mucous membranes become dry, crusted, and irritated. They are then more susceptible to invasion by pathogenic microorganisms. Aerosols other than water include a variety of bronchodilating or mucolytic drugs (see Table 14–3).

The four general purposes of aerosol and humidity therapy are:

- Relief of edema and spasms of the bronchi
- Liquefaction of bronchial secretions
- Delivery of medication
- Humidification of the respiratory mucosa

Aerosols are delivered by a **nebulizer** (device producing a fine spray) via face mask, face tent, or tracheostomy collar. Most aerosols are produced in a jet nebulizer in which a high-velocity gas shatters the liquid into small aerosol particles. Patients may use a handheld nebulizer at home. In the hospital, the nebulizer is attached to oxygen so that hypoxemia can be treated as medication is being administered. Nebulizer treatments are usually 20 to 30 minutes long and are given two, three, or four times a day.

The patient is taught to breathe through the mouth during the treatment. She should sit in a comfortable chair. Halfway through the treatment and after the treatment, deep breathing and coughing are performed to raise loose mucus. Equipment is cleaned and dried before storing.

PULMONARY HYGIENE

Patients with chronic pulmonary disease can benefit from a program of pulmonary hygiene that is designed to remove secretions for more efficient exchange of oxygen and carbon dioxide. This will help them control their breathing so that it is more effective in moving air in and out of the lungs. Pulmonary hygiene programs are achieved by administering prescribed drugs, humidification of the air inhaled, nebulizer and MDI therapy, chest physiotherapy, and breathing exercises. A handheld flutter mucus clearance device may be used to provide positive expiratory pressure.

Chest physiotherapy includes postural drainage when possible and percussion and vibration. *Postural drainage* involves positioning the patient so that the forces of gravity can help remove secretions deep in the bronchi and lungs (Figure 14–7). The nurse who assists a patient with postural drainage should obtain specific directions from the physician or physical ther-

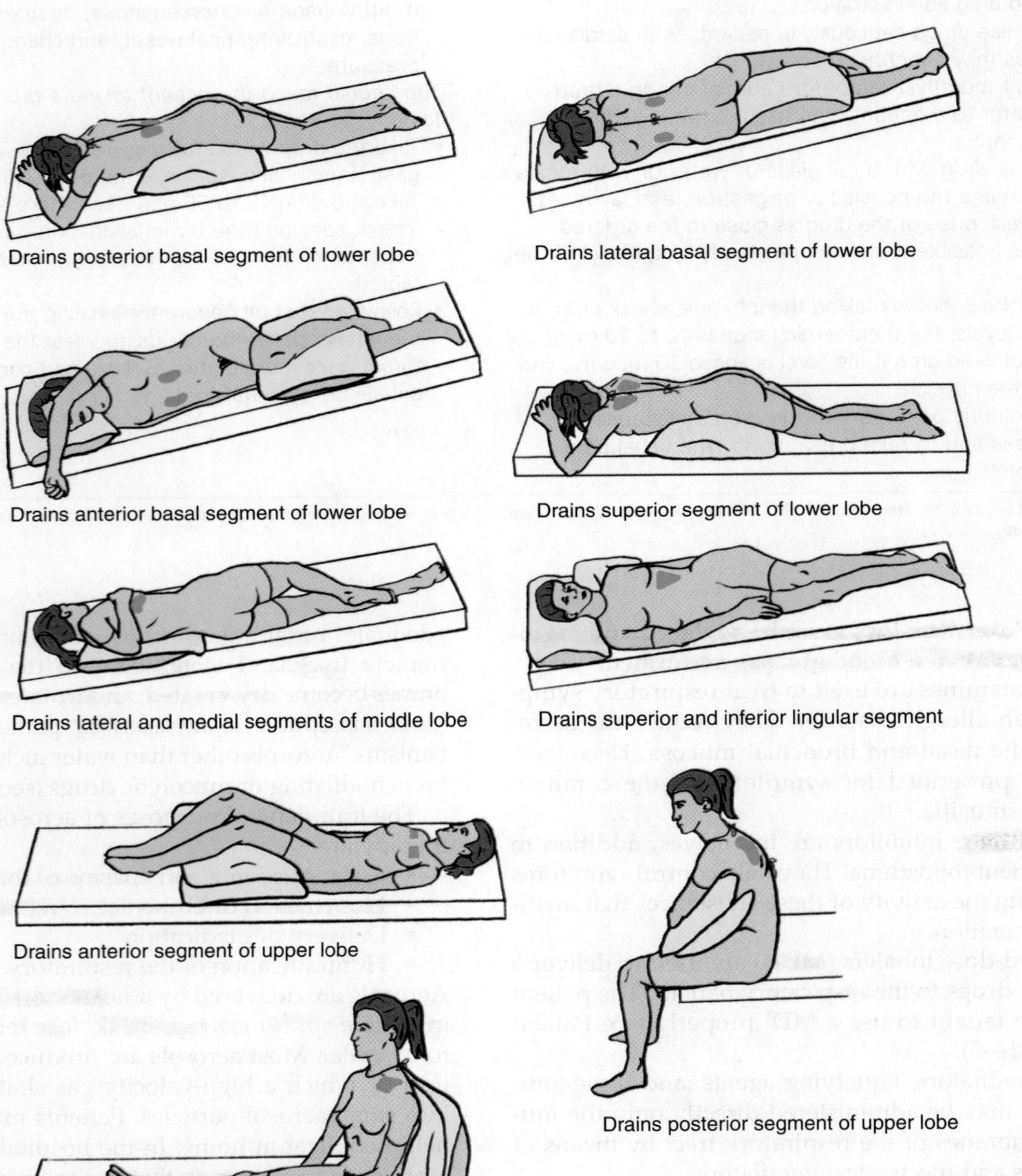

FIGURE 14–7 Positions for postural drainage.

apist so that the patient can be positioned properly. Tapping, clapping, and vibrating techniques sometimes are used during postural drainage. These measures are carried out for the purpose of dislodging mucus plugs so that they can be coughed up more easily (Abboud, 1992). They must be done with precision and only by someone who has received adequate instruction in the proper technique. Family members can be taught the procedures if they are to be continued after the patient goes home.

Because there is likely to be some gagging during coughing episodes that take place during postural drainage, it is best to carry out the procedure before meals, when the stomach is relatively empty and vomiting is less likely.

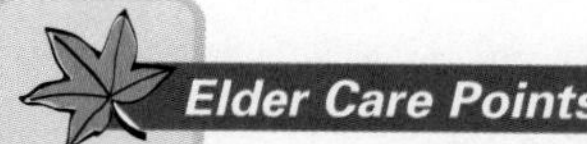

Elder Care Points

Elderly patients with osteoporosis are at risk for fractures of the vertebrae and ribs. Clapping should not be used on these patients. Vibrating techniques are more appropriate.

If the patient is to have postural drainage only once a day, it should be done in the morning when she awakens. At this time, secretions that have accumulated during the night can be removed. After postural drainage is completed, good mouth care, including brushing the teeth and using a refreshing mouthwash, should be given.

The most important aspects of breathing exercises include blowing through relaxed pursed lips, exhaling slowly, and *not* forcing the air out of the lungs (this can bring about the collapse of the airway structures). Breathing through pursed lips is described in Patient Teaching 14–3.

The mechanics of respiration can become less efficient as chronic respiratory disease progresses. The patient suffers a loss of lung elasticity, a flattened diaphragm, and fixation of the rib cage as she becomes more and more dependent on the muscles of her upper chest and neck for breathing. Difficulty in breathing causes respiratory muscle fatigue.

The purpose of breathing exercises is to help correct this situation by strengthening the abdominal muscles so that they can push upward against the diaphragm and assist in the expiration of air from the lungs. These exercises also help overcome rigidity of the thorax so that the lungs can inflate and deflate more easily.

Patients who follow the exercises prescribed for them often find that they can lead more active and useful lives than formerly possible because their exertional dyspnea is less severe (Puhan et al., 2005). This means that they can make better use of all the muscles of their body and are less likely to develop complications that accompany immobility. They are also better able to cough up secretions that would otherwise remain in the lower bronchi and serve as a growth medium for bacteria or a cause of atelectasis. The psychological value of being able to indulge in ordinary activities that once left the patient breathless cannot be overestimated. Abdominal and diaphragmatic breathing are described in Patient Teaching 14–3.

OXYGEN THERAPY

Because oxygen acts as a drug, it must be prescribed and administered in specific doses to avoid oxygen toxicity. The dosage of oxygen is stated in terms of *concentration* and rate of *flow*.

High concentrations (above 50%) may be prescribed to treat acute conditions in which the patient can benefit from prompt treatment of hypoxia, as in cardiovascular failure and pulmonary edema. The rate of flow may be as high as 12 L/min.

Moderate concentrations of oxygen usually are prescribed when increased metabolic rate raises the consumption of oxygen or when there is poor distribution of oxygen because of either congestive heart failure or pulmonary embolism. **The concentrations of oxygen given in a moderate dosage are about 28% to 30% at a rate of flow of 4 to 7 L/min.**

Low concentrations of oxygen of about 24% to 28% delivered at a rate of 1 to 3 L/min are indicated when the patient needs oxygen over an extended period. These percentages and rates of flow are approximate amounts. The exact dosage depends on the method of administration and the patient's individual need for additional oxygen supply. Even though oxygen is essential to life, excessive amounts are toxic and can have serious adverse effects on the tissues of the body. High concentrations of inhaled oxygen can bring about collapse of the alveoli, because the oxygen displaces some of the nitrogen there. Another effect of high oxygen concentration is an interruption in the production of *pulmonary surfactant*, a substance that stabilizes the alveoli and prevents atelectasis.

Short-term oxygen therapy, which is the administration of oxygen to treat hypoxemia, is indicated when:

- There is an inadequate intake of oxygen because of obstruction or restriction of airflow through the air passages.
- Oxygen is not distributed throughout the body because of circulatory failure.
- There is an inadequate supply of hemoglobin to transport the oxygen.
- Carbon dioxide or other gases displace the oxygen in the blood.

Objective criteria for oxygen needs include Pa_{O_2} less than 60 mm Hg or Sa_{O_2} less than 90%.

Outward signs of hypoxia vary in patients and therefore cannot be completely relied on as indications that additional oxygen is needed. Dyspnea and confusion are the most common signs seen. More reliable indicators are the results obtained from blood gas analysis and determination of the blood pH. Not all patients with hypoxia can benefit from oxygen therapy.

Long-term oxygen therapy for patients with CAL is used to:

- Relieve hypoxemia
- Reverse tissue hypoxia and its signs and symptoms
- Allow the patient to function better mentally and physically, thereby allowing greater self-reliance

Home oxygen units and portable units are available for patients who require long-term therapy (Patient Teaching 14–6). The patient with CAL obtains signals to breathe from oxygen levels in the blood. **If this patient is given too much oxygen, it will depress respiration.**

The manner in which additional oxygen is supplied to a patient depends on her particular need for oxygen and her physical condition. Methods of administration are divided into high-flow and low-flow systems (Figure 14–8, Table 14–5).

Nursing Management

The nurse checks the oxygen delivery system at the beginning of the shift and then periodically to verify that the flow is set according to the physician's order. Tubing is checked to see that it is not kinked, blocking the flow of oxygen. This is particularly important whenever the patient is repositioned. Oxygen should be humidified before delivery to the patient, especially if the flow rate is more than 3 L/min. Oxygen is *not* explosive. However, it does support combustion, which means that a spark or flame can cause a major fire in a short time. **Smoking is not allowed when oxygen is used.**

The tubing should be kept off the floor and the connections should be handled aseptically to prevent contamination of the system. Microorganisms grow easily in a warm, moist environment.

When oxygen therapy is discontinued, it is usually done gradually. The patient is "weaned" from dependence on oxygen by reducing the dosage and then alternating periods of breathing room air with periods of breathing low concentrations of oxygen.

? *Think Critically About . . .* Can you describe the assessment points you would cover at the beginning of the shift for a patient who is receiving oxygen therapy? Consider both the patient and the oxygen setup system.

MECHANICAL VENTILATION

Mechanical ventilation is needed when the patient cannot maintain adequate ventilation because of respiratory, neurologic, or neuromuscular problems or trauma. There are two major types of basic ventilators used to give support to patients with ventilatory problems: negative-pressure and positive-pressure ventilators. Negative-pressure ventilators are mainly used for patients with normal vital capacities who have neuromuscular disease, central nervous system disorders (e.g., spinal cord damage), and COPD. Negative-pressure ventilators include the iron lung, cuirass, poncho, and body wrap.

Positive-pressure ventilators are seen far more frequently. There are several types of positive-pressure ventilators and various modes of ventilation. These ventilators work by delivering a positive driving pressure to the patient's airway. The pressure delivered is greater than that within the airway and alveoli; therefore, gas flows into the lungs, either assisting or controlling inhalation. When the pressure is released, exhalation takes place without effort on the

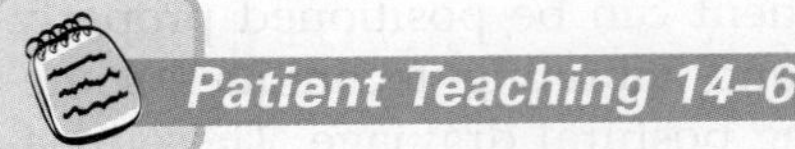

Oxygen Use in the Home

Teach the patient the following points for use of oxygen at home:

GUARD AGAINST FIRE

- Post "No Smoking" signs in the home where both family and visitors will see them.
- Refrain from using electrical appliances (e.g., electric razors, portable radios, electric blankets, electric toothbrushes, electric heating pads) or mineral oils in the area where oxygen is in use.
- Do not allow anyone to smoke in the house.
- Do not use oxygen around a stove or open fire.
- Do not use wool blankets or static-producing clothing in the area.

CANNULA/MASK CARE

- Adjust straps so they are not too tight.
- Pad any pressure points.
- Inspect ears for pressure areas or breakdown.
- Assess oral and nasal mucous membranes two or three times a day.
- Remove the device several times a day and wash and dry the skin where the straps or tubing rubs and stimulates the skin.
- Cleanse the mask or cannula prongs two or three times a day with water.
- Use a water-based lubricant on the lips and nares to decrease dryness.
- Provide humidification via humidifier or nebulizer.

DECREASE RISK FOR INFECTION

- Change disposable equipment frequently.
- Perform oral hygiene several times a day.
- Remove secretions coughed into mask immediately.
- Cleanse skin under mask and inspect for cuts or abrasions; cleanse nares three times a day.

Monitor amount of oxygen remaining in canister and order more ahead of need.

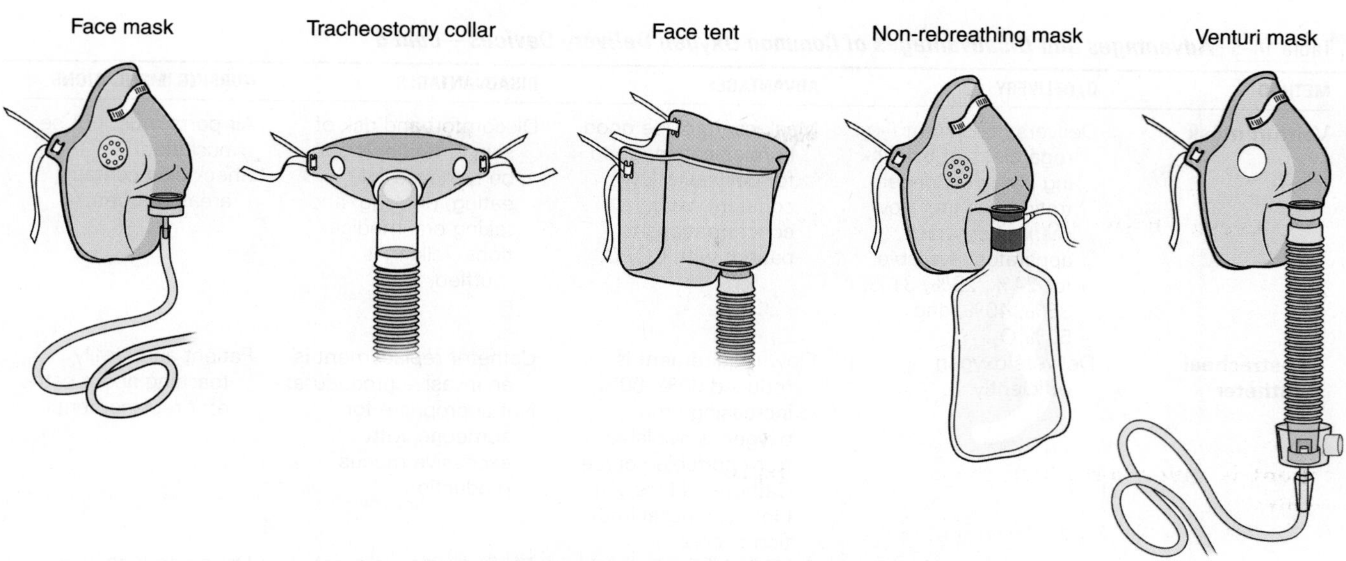

FIGURE **14–8** Various oxygen delivery devices.

Table 14–5 ***Advantages and Disadvantages of Common Oxygen Delivery Devices***

METHOD	O_2 DELIVERY	ADVANTAGES	DISADVANTAGES	NURSING IMPLICATIONS
Nasal cannula (nasal prongs)	Low concentrations; dependent on rate and depth of breathing *Flows:* 1 L = 24% O_2 2 L = 28% O_2 3 L = 32% O_2 4 L = 36% O_2 5 L = 40% O_2 6 L = 44% O_2	Patient can move about, eat, and talk while receiving oxygen. Most COPD patients can tolerate 2 L/min flow.	Restless patients can easily dislodge the prongs. Risk of skin irritation at nares, ears, and cheeks. Flow rate 3 L and above requires humidification as it will dry and irritate nasal mucosa.	Prongs should be facing down toward mouth when inserted in nose; check frequently as patients tend to replace the prongs incorrectly. Clean prongs every few hours.
Simple face mask	Low to medium concentrations; 35%–50% can be achieved with flow rate of 6–12 L/min.	Mask provides adequate humidification; delivers oxygen quickly for short-term therapy.	Discomfort and risk of pressure necrosis caused by tight seal between face and mask. Device must be removed for patient to eat, drink, or take medications. Muffles voice when talking. Requires at least 5-L flow to prevent accumulation of expired air in mask.	Wash and dry under mask and wipe out mask q 1–2 hr. Mask must fit snugly. May need to pad straps at ears to prevent necrosis.
Partial rebreathing mask	Higher concentrations; 40%–60% at flow rates of 6–10 L/min.	Mask is lightweight; reservoir bag traps portion of exhaled breath that is high in oxygen for rebreathing.	Risk of pressure necrosis with long-term use. Cannot be used with high humidity.	Bag should not be allowed to deflate during inspiration. Check skin under straps frequently.
Non-rebreather mask	Highest concentrations; 60%–90% can be achieved.	Delivers high concentration of oxygen accurately.	Cannot be used with high humidity. Flow rate must be sufficient to prevent bag from deflating during inspiration.	Mask should fit snugly; check skin contact areas for pressure necrosis.

Key: *COPD*, chronic obstructive pulmonary disease.

Continued

Table 14–5 Advantages and Disadvantages of Common Oxygen Delivery Devices—cont'd

METHOD	O_2 DELIVERY	ADVANTAGES	DISADVANTAGES	NURSING IMPLICATIONS
Venturi mask	Delivers consistent FIO_2 regardless of breathing pattern. Concentration and liter flow marked on mask apparatus; available for 24%, 28%, 31%, 35%, 40%, and 50% O_2.	Mask can provide good humidification; good for delivering low, constant oxygen concentrations to patient with COPD.	Discomfort and risk of skin irritation. Must be removed for eating, drinking, and taking oral medications. Talking is muffled.	Air ports must not be occluded. Check skin contact areas frequently.
Transtracheal catheter	Delivers oxygen efficiently.	Flow requirement is reduced 60%–80%, increasing time oxygen is available from portable source. Catheter is less visible. Less nasal irritation occurs.	Catheter replacement is an invasive procedure. Not appropriate for someone with excessive mucus production.	Patient and family teaching about catheter replacement.
Tracheostomy collar	Delivers O_2 and humidification via tracheostomy; must be connected to a nebulizer with FIO_2 set at 24%–100%.	Adds humidity to help liquefy secretions. Lose some of O_2 flow since collar is not tight fitting.	Must drain condensation in tubing often. Risk of nosocomial respiratory infection.	Drain condensation from tubing into receptacle, being careful not to allow fluid to go into tracheostomy. Remove and clean collar device and check skin under straps at least q 4 hr.
T-bar (Briggs adapter)	Delivers O_2 and humidification to tracheostomy; must be connected to a nebulizer with FIO_2 set at 24%–100%.	Fits more tightly than tracheostomy collar. Adds humidity to liquefy secretions.	Must drain condensation in tubing often. Risk of nosocomial respiratory infection.	Drain condensation from tubing into receptacle; be careful not to get fluid into tracheostomy. Remove and clean T-bar device q 4 hr.

Key: FIO_2, fraction of inspired oxygen.

part of the machine or the patient. The ventilator patient most often has an endotracheal tube or tracheostomy tube through which ventilation will occur. (See Chapter 13 for care of endotracheal and tracheostomy tubes.)

Time-cycled ventilators deliver air into the lungs for a preset length of time. The volume of gas delivered may vary. The Babybird and the Siemens Servo are examples of this type. These are mainly used for infants and children.

Volume-cycled ventilators deliver a preset volume of gas to the bronchi and lungs. Pressure limits also are set. If the ventilator meets with too much pressure to deliver the selected volume of gas, an alarm sounds to tell the nurse that the patient is not receiving the correct tidal volume. Most commonly this occurs because there is a buildup of secretions in the lungs and the patient needs to be suctioned. Ventilators of this type are most often used in a critical care setting, in which severe chest disease or surgery has severely compromised normal respiratory function. This type of ventilator will deliver adequate tidal volume even when airway resistance is great (e.g., in patients suffering from severe obstructive lung disease).

High-frequency jet ventilation is used to supplement volume ventilation. It provides good ventilation of the patient with the use of relatively small tidal volumes at very high respiratory rates. The oxygenation and ventilation are accomplished by gas diffusion and convection rather than a high flow of gas. Because the intrathoracic pressures needed for this type of ventilation are much lower, there are fewer complications (e.g., barotrauma, hypotension, and pneumothorax) than with other types of ventilation.

Modes of Ventilation

In *controlled-mode* ventilation, the machine is set to deliver a fixed number of breaths per minute, no matter how the patient tries to breathe. This is used during periods of central nervous system depression, such as during anesthesia and drug overdose.

In *assist-mode* ventilation, the frequency of ventilation is determined by the patient. When she takes a breath, the machine is triggered to deliver a set tidal volume. This mode is not used alone in the clinical setting, but is combined with the control function to provide an *assist-control mode.* If the patient's respiratory rate falls, the machine will deliver a set number of breaths per minute; if the patient is breathing within the set rate, the machine assists only by delivering the set tidal volume. This mode considerably decreases the work of breathing for the patient.

Intermittent mandatory ventilation (IMV) and *synchronized intermittent mandatory ventilation* (SIMV) are the most common modes of ventilation found in critical care settings. These allow the patient to breathe spontaneously and yet provide a preset number of ventilator breaths at a preset tidal volume to ensure adequate ventilation without respiratory muscle fatigue.

For example, IMV can "stack" breaths by having the machine deliver a breath at the end of normal inspiration , adding more air to what was normally inspired. SIMV is activated by the patient's own breathing and is therefore synchronized with her breathing pattern. One of the main advantages of these modes is that the respiratory muscles do not become as weak during mechanical ventilation from lack of use, and it is then easier to wean the patient from the ventilator by steadily decreasing the number of mandatory breaths per minute.

Positive end-expiratory pressure (PEEP) also can be delivered by most ventilators. When using PEEP, the pressure in the airways never falls below a certain level (usually between 5 and 15 cm H_2O). This has the effect of holding the smaller air passages open, thus limiting atelectasis. It also holds alveoli in expansion so that there is more time for gas to diffuse across the alveolar membrane and correct hypoxemia. It is used for ARDS and respiratory failure when there is a Pao_2 less than 50 and a Pco_2 greater than 50.

Inverse-ratio ventilation supplies controlled breaths with an inspiratory-to-expiratory duration ratio of 1:2, 1:3, or 1:4. The rationale is that a prolonged inspiratory time will open stiff alveolar units and a shorter exhalation time will not allow them time to recollapse. It is an alternative to PEEP. A disadvantage of this mode is that because it is often uncomfortable for the patient, it requires sedation or the use of a neuromuscular blocking agent. Monitoring the patient requires observing for signs of compromised cardiac function related to the prolonged inspiratory pressures.

Pressure Support Ventilation. Pressure support ventilation (PSV) provides pressure support only during inspiration. The patient controls both the duration and volume of inspiration. It is designed to eliminate the pressure or work required by the patient to draw airflow through the ventilator tubing during spontaneous efforts, preventing tiring. PSV has proven very beneficial during weaning from IMV because it minimizes the workload. Another form of PSV is support ventilation max or PSV_{max}. It also is used during weaning and provides higher pressures to produce tidal breaths equivalent to those on conventional positive-pressure ventilation.

Partial Liquid Ventilation. This mode may be used for treatment of respiratory distress syndrome (RDS) and ARDS. The ventilator mixes air with Perflubron liquid, which is capable of dissolving and carrying large quantities of oxygen. The method gently expands the alveoli and transfers the oxygen into the blood and removes carbon dioxide. Perflubron is a cousin to Teflon and does not trigger any side effects because it does not chemically react with anything in the human body. The method is sometimes used for both premature infants with RDS and patients with ARDS.

Continuous Positive Airway Pressure. Continuous positive airway pressure (CPAP) and bilevel positive airway pressure (BiPAP) can be used for patients who are breathing spontaneously but are showing signs of hypoxemia. It is used for infants with mild RDS and for adults in the early stages of respiratory failure. The patient does not have to be intubated for CPAP to be used. It can be given with nasal prongs. These modes are also used for sleep apnea.

Nursing Management

When caring for a patient on mechanical ventilation, you should:

- Check the physician's order each shift and then the ventilator for the proper settings: mode, F_{IO_2} (fraction of inspired oxygen, or the oxygen concentration that is delivered), respiratory rate, tidal volume, peak inspiratory pressure, and PEEP (Figure 14–9).
- Check alarms to see that they are turned on. Alarms should not be turned off when disconnecting the patient in order to suction as they may not be reactivated.
- Keep tubing clear of pooled water; empty the water into an appropriate receptacle as needed.

The patient is observed for signs of complications, such as gastric distention, pneumothorax, and impaired cardiac output from decreased venous return, and the need for increasingly higher pressures to deliver the set tidal volume, which can indicate stiffening of the lungs (decreased compliance). Providing mouth care with chlorhexidine paste reduces the risk for ventilator-associated pneumonia (Barclay & Vega, 2006). 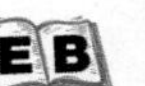 **Auscultate the lung fields to be certain that both lungs are being ventilated.** Arterial blood gas levels are monitored to determine the effectiveness of ventilation treatment (Safety Alert 14–2).

For ventilation to be effective, the lungs must be kept clear of secretions. Many patients can cough up secretions and do not need to be suctioned; others may need suctioning as frequently as every 15 minutes. **Endotracheal and tracheal suctioning must be done with strict aseptic technique.** Mechanical ventilation places the patient at considerably greater risk of respiratory infection because of its invasive nature.

The intubated patient on the ventilator cannot talk and must be given an alternative means of communication such as a Magic Slate, VitalVoice Communication device, or paper and pencil. Being hooked up to a

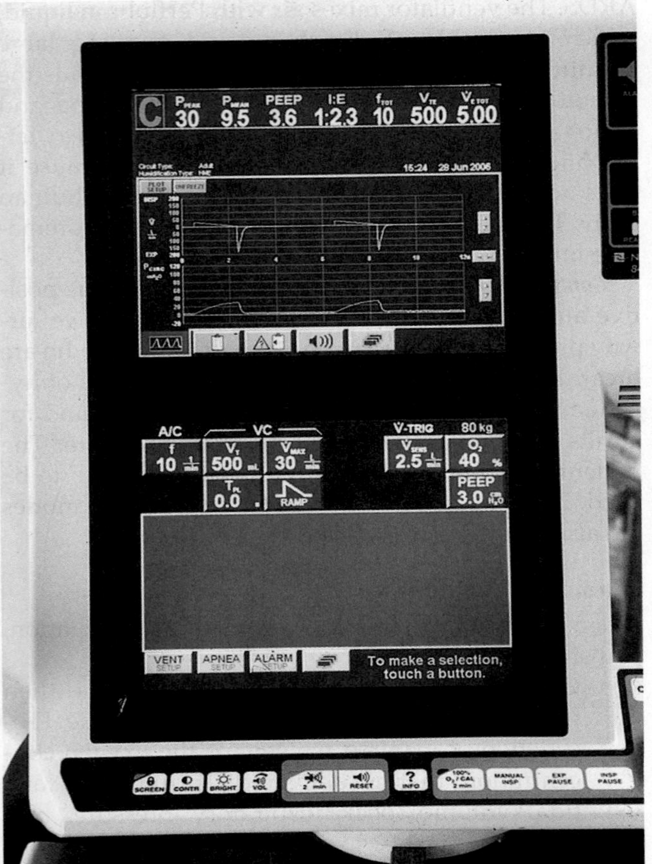

FIGURE **14–9** Check the ventilator settings against the orders each shift.

ventilator is very frightening for most patients, and it is important that the nurse assure the alert patient that she will not be left alone.

Any time a patient is turned or repositioned, the endotracheal or tracheal tube must be checked to be certain that the ventilator tubes are not pulling on it too much.

Attention must be paid to adequate nutrition, as the patient cannot eat by mouth when she is connected to a ventilator. Additional calorie intake is needed just to maintain weight when a ventilator is used. Continuous enteral feeding is the method most often used to prevent malnutrition in these patients, but whatever method is used, the nurse should monitor nutritional parameters to assess whether nutrition is adequate.

If a ventilator alarm sounds and the problem cannot be located quickly, the patient should be disconnected from the machine and ventilated with a manual resuscitator bag and oxygen until the problem is solved. Table 14–6 summarizes the dangers of mechanical ventilation.

Care for a patient who is receiving mechanical ventilation is extremely complex. No one should care for such a patient without extensive training and supervised practice. The patient will require protection from infection, continuous monitoring of vital signs, observation for hypoventilation and hyperventilation, measurement of intake and output, and prevention of the disabilities of inactivity.

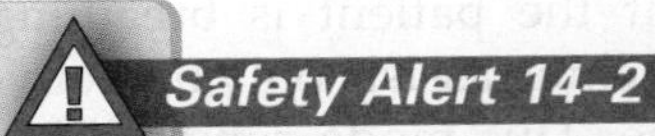

Preventing Ventilator-Acquired Pneumonia

A 2007 National Patient Safety Goal is *Reduce the risk of health-care associated infections.* Ventilator-acquired pneumonia falls into that category. Be certain to use sterile equipment and to maintain sterile technique when suctioning an endotracheal tube or tracheostomy. All respiratory equipment should be cleaned and/or exchanged according to agency policy to help prevent ventilator-acquired pneumonia. Provide mouth care with chlorhexidine paste. Keep people with respiratory infections out of the vicinity of the patient to help prevent nosocomial infection.

Think Critically About . . . You have just assisted another nurse in turning a patient who is attached to a mechanical ventilator. The patient has been positioned on the left side and the ventilator is on the right side of the bed. What all would you check before you leave the bedside?

COMMUNITY CARE

Many patients in long-term care facilities have chronic respiratory disorders. Home care nurses see a large number of respiratory patients, and outpatient clinic nurses frequently see patients with respiratory infections as well as those with chronic respiratory disorders. Home care nurses often monitor patients for signs of pulmonary edema and must become adept at detecting the signs of fluid in the lungs. All nurses must have a solid knowledge of the care required by respiratory patients. Careful assessment techniques can often catch a respiratory problem before it becomes serious.

People who are on gastrointestinal acid-suppressive therapy should be educated that this may make them more susceptible to community-acquired pneumonia (Barclay & Vega, 2004). Normal gastric acid helps prevent pathogens from colonizing the upper GI tract, where they can then be introduced into the respiratory tract. 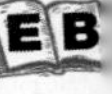

Teaching the techniques to promote better breathing and more effective coughing is a simple measure that can greatly improve the life of the patient with CAL. Working with patients to promote compliance with their exercise and medication regimen is a primary function of the nurse in the community. Teaching use of the peak airflow meter and the MDI can save considerable health care dollars by decreasing serious episodes of acute respiratory dysfunction.

Table 14–6 Dangers of Mechanical Ventilation

DANGER	MANIFESTATIONS
Barotrauma	Sudden increase in peak inspiratory pressure; absent breath sounds over one area of lung; pneumomediastinum; pneumothorax; subcutaneous emphysema; high-pressure alarm goes off frequently.
Oxygen toxicity	Parenchymal damage and absorption atelectasis; alveolar membrane damage; nonproductive cough; decreasing vital capacity; decreased compliance; increased peak inspiratory pressure.
Impaired cardiac output	Decreased blood pressure; poor peripheral perfusion; decreased level of consciousness.
Infection	Change in sputum color, quantity, and consistency; crackles and rhonchi; increased white blood cell count; fever; infiltrate on chest radiograph.
Fluid retention	Increasing body weight; fluid intake more than output; peripheral edema; crackles in lungs or diminished breath sounds.
Gastric distention	Increasing abdominal girth; complaint of distention; tender to palpation.
Gastrointestinal bleeding	Positive stool guaiac; "coffee grounds" aspirate from gastric suction; dropping hemoglobin; black or bloody stool.

Rehabilitation of the chronic respiratory patient is directed at:

- Improving breathing
- Improving activity tolerance
- Decreasing infection
- Preventing acute episodes

Rehabilitation issues are covered in Chapter 9.

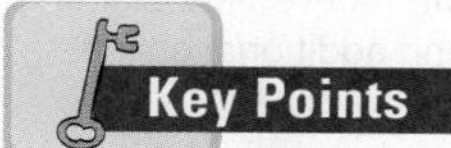

Key Points

- Acute bronchitis is usually a viral disorder.
- Symptoms of influenza are headache, fever, chills, and muscle aches, followed by hacking cough, runny nose and nasal congestion, and eyes that are sensitive to light.
- Hospital-acquired pneumonia can often be prevented by use of aseptic technique and good respiratory care.
- Symptoms of infectious pneumonia are high fever, chills, cough with rusty sputum, chest pain, diaphoresis, malaise, and aching muscles. There will be diminished or abnormal breath sounds.
- Fluid should be increased for patients with respiratory infections.
- The elderly are at considerable risk for pneumonia.
- Treatment of tuberculosis requires multiple medications for a period of 6 to 9 months (see Table 14–1).
- A large percentage of cases of TB occur in immigrant groups.
- Cystic fibrosis is a major cause of bronchiectasis.
- Restrictive lung disorders include pleurisy, pleural effusion, kyphosis, severe scoliosis, and arthritis of the chest wall.
- Chronic obstructive lung disorders include emphysema and chronic bronchitis.
- Emphysema causes destruction of the terminal respiratory units and narrowed, stiff airways with loss of lung elasticity; it causes air trapping and CO_2 retention.
- Chronic bronchitis causes inflammation and excess secretion of mucus with chronic cough with increasing resistance to airflow and hypoxia. Retention of carbon dioxide occurs, and polycythemia develops.
- Asthma causes intermittent, reversible inflammation and obstruction of the airways.
- Treatment of obstructive lung disorders involves a variety of medications (see Table 14–3).
- Smoking cessation is one of the most important measures in the treatment of obstructive lung disease.
- Asthma has many causes and triggers that result in bronchospasm and excessive secretion of mucus with bronchoconstriction, causing airflow limitation and hypoxia.
- A severe asthma attack can kill if not relieved.
- Treatment is with medications in various forms and avoidance of triggers (see Table 14–4); patients are taught to monitor peak flow to avert serious attacks.
- Rehabilitation programs for patients with CAL can improve exercise tolerance and quality of life.
- Patients with COPD often have nutritional problems.
- Lung cancer is primarily caused by cigarette smoking.
- Symptoms of lung cancer are cough, wheezing, chest discomfort, exertional dyspnea, and expectoration of blood-streaked sputum.
- Treatment of lung cancer may include surgery, radiation, chemotherapy, and biotherapy agents. Photodynamic therapy is sometimes used.
- Signs and symptoms of pulmonary embolus are dyspnea, chest pain, cough, hemoptysis, and anxiety.
- Anticoagulant therapy is used when pulmonary embolus occurs.
- Lung transplantation is an option for end-stage lung disease.
- Flail chest occurs when three or more ribs are broken in two or more places; it compromises respirations as the chest wall is unstable.
- Flail chest is treated with intubation and mechanical ventilation.
- Cover a sucking chest wound with an occlusive dressing at the end of an expiration, leaving one corner of the dressing unsealed.
- Do not remove an object stuck in the chest as massive bleeding may occur in the thoracic cavity.
- Pneumothorax and hemothorax decrease lung capacity; they are treated with chest tubes and a closed drainage system.
- Pulmonary edema is a medical emergency.

- Adult respiratory distress syndrome is life threatening and is treated with ventilatory support with PEEP.
- Respiratory failure occurs when Pa_{O_2} is below 50 mm Hg and the P_{CO_2} is over 50 mm Hg.
- Many intrathoracic surgeries are performed by video-assisted thoracoscopic surgery (VATS).
- Preoperative teaching focuses on techniques to improve lung ventilation after surgery.
- The water level in the water chamber of the drainage system should fluctuate with breathing.
- Position the patient according to the surgeon's orders; the usual position is on the back or on the operative side.
- Never allow chest tubes to become kinked.
- Frequent respiratory assessment is essential for the patient with chest tubes.
- Report chest drainage of more than 100 mL/hr.
- Medicate the patient 30 minutes before chest tube removal.
- COPD patients are taught diaphragmatic breathing and pursed-lip breathing techniques to assist aeration of the lungs.
- Postural drainage is used to help drain secretions from various segments of the lungs.
- An incentive spirometer helps open alveoli and prevent atelectasis.
- Oxygen is a medication used to treat hypoxemia and can be toxic.
- There are a variety of types of oxygen delivery devices (see Table 14–5).
- High concentrations of oxygen are not used for COPD patients as it can diminish their drive to breathe; use only low-flow oxygen of 1 to 2 L/min.
- Oxygen delivery equipment must be kept clean and uncontaminated as the respiratory patient is at high risk for infection.
- Mechanical ventilation is necessary after chest surgery and for respiratory failure, ARDS, flail chest, and neuromuscular disorders that interfere with the respiratory muscles.
- Ventilator settings should be carefully checked each shift.
- Never turn off ventilator alarms.
- Auscultate the lungs to be sure both lungs are being ventilated.
- Observe for complications of mechanical ventilation.
- Keep the lungs clear of secretions with suctioning.
- Nutritional needs are increased during mechanical ventilation.
- Residents in long-term care facilities must be continually monitored for respiratory infections and protected from those who are infected.

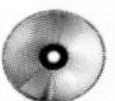
Go to your **Companion CD-ROM** for an Audio Glossary, animations, video clips, and bonus review questions.

evolve Be sure to visit the companion Evolve site at http://evolve.elsevier.com/deWit for interactive NCLEX-PN Exam Style Review Questions, WebLinks, and additional online resources.

NCLEX-PN EXAM STYLE REVIEW QUESTIONS

Choose the best answer(s) for the following questions.

1. The nurse is caring for a patient with signs and symptoms of influenza. Home care of this respiratory condition includes which of the following?

1. Schedule adequate periods of rest and activity.
2. Provide warming measures.
3. Restrict fluid intake.
4. Consider analgesics and antipyretics.

2. During a home visit, the nurse encourages frequent repositioning and sitting to a frail older adult. The nurse understands that immobilization and lying in bed for extended periods of time place the patient at risk for:

1. aspiration pneumonia.
2. hypostatic pneumonia.
3. opportunistic pneumonia.
4. sentinel infections.

3. A 58-year-old male patient is admitted with bacterial pneumonia. He has high fever accompanied by chills, a cough productive of rust-colored sputum, and a general feeling of malaise. The medical diagnosis is confirmed by:

1. blood cultures.
2. chest x-rays.
3. white blood cell count.
4. bronchoscopy.

4. A 37-year-old patient seen in the emergency department for shortness of breath and fatigue is afebrile with occasional crackles and wheezes. The nurse would most likely expect which of the following clinical findings?

1. Diffuse patchy area of density on chest x-ray
2. Productive cough
3. Extreme fatigue
4. Dehydration

5. A frail 40-year-old female patient is admitted with complaints of fever, fatigue, coughing, difficulty of breathing, and weight loss. Which of the following supports the probable medical diagnosis of histoplasmosis?

1. Employment in a paint factory
2. Exposure to bird droppings
3. Recent desert expedition
4. Exposure to asbestos

6. A positive tuberculosis skin test indicates:
   1. exposure to the tubercle bacilli.
   2. active pulmonary tuberculosis.
   3. allergic reaction to tuberculin.
   4. immune deficiency states.

7. The definitive diagnosis of active tuberculosis is confirmed by:
   1. serial chest x-rays.
   2. tuberculin skin tests.
   3. acid-fast bacilli in sputum.
   4. elevated white blood cell count.

8. ______________________ is visual observation of the ingestion of the required medication for the entire course of treatment. It is designed for patients who are known to be at risk of noncompliance.

9. The nurse admits a patient who was diagnosed with active pulmonary tuberculosis. Appropriate nursing interventions to control the spread of the disease include: *(Select all that apply.)*
   1. implementation of airborne isolation.
   2. assigning the patient to a positive-pressure isolation room.
   3. wearing a HEPA respirator mask when providing direct patient care.
   4. explaining the importance of covering the mouth when smiling.
   5. practicing good hand hygiene.

10. A 55-year-old man was admitted for complaints of a recurring irritating "smoker's" cough with small amounts of sputum. If he has emphysema, the most likely clinical finding would be:
    1. blood-streaked sputum.
    2. decreased white blood cells.
    3. pale mucous membranes.
    4. elevated hemoglobin and hematocrit.

CRITICAL THINKING ACTIVITIES

Read each clinical scenario and discuss the questions with your classmates.

Scenario A

You are assigned to take care of Janet Blair, a 26-year-old who has pneumococcal pneumonia. She is receiving oxygen by nasal cannula at 5 L/min. She is on bed rest with bathroom privileges. She is receiving nebulization, chest physiotherapy, and postural drainage treatments from respiratory therapy. She is very weak and runs a temperature of 104.6° F in the afternoons and evenings, which sometimes seems to cause delirium.

1. What would be an appropriate plan of care for Janet?
2. How would you evaluate the effectiveness of the nursing interventions listed on the plan of care?
3. What psychosocial problems might Janet have? How would you help her with these?

Scenario B

Mrs. Wester is 62 years of age. She has suffered from emphysema for several years but has not sought help in coping with the problems it presents. While in the hospital with an acute respiratory infection, she becomes very depressed and says she will never be able to take care of herself again because of her breathlessness. She is not willing to give up smoking and has not been taught any techniques for pulmonary hygiene.

1. What do you think might be the attitude of some health care professionals in regard to Mrs. Wester's problems?
2. Devise a teaching plan to help her with her problem of fatigue and breathlessness.
3. List interventions that would be appropriate in helping with her nutritional and hydration needs.

Scenario C

Mr. Cohen is admitted to the hospital for pneumonectomy. His diagnosis is early lung cancer. He is 56 years old and has worked in a cotton mill since he was 16. He is slightly underweight but is physically strong and has an optimistic outlook about his surgery and chances for recovery.

1. What special preoperative instruction would you expect Mr. Cohen to need?
2. What nursing interventions would you expect to be on his postoperative nursing care plan?
3. How would you help Mr. Cohen deal with the diagnosis of cancer, treatment, and prognosis?

CHAPTER 15 The Hematologic System

evolve http://evolve.elsevier.com/deWit

Objectives

Upon completing this chapter, you should be able to:

Theory

1. Describe the structures and functions of the hematologic system.
2. Differentiate between the various types of blood cells and their functions.
3. Discuss factors that may alter the function of the hematologic system.
4. Identify ways in which the nurse might help prevent blood disorders.
5. List at least five different kinds of information that can be obtained from a complete blood count (CBC).
6. Describe ways to accomplish hemostasis.
7. Apply the nursing process to patients with problems of the hematologic system.

Clinical Practice

1. Explain the procedure and care for a bone marrow aspiration to a patient about to undergo the procedure.
2. Perform a focused assessment on a patient with a problem of the hematologic system.
3. Choose nursing interventions for common problems exhibited by patients with problems of the hematologic system.

Key Terms

Be sure to check out the bonus material on the Companion CD-ROM, including selected audio pronunciations.

agranulocytosis (p. 364)
aplastic anemia (ā-plas-tik ă-NĒ-mē-ă, p. 364)
dyscrasia (dis-KRĀ-zhə, p. 364)
erythropoiesis (ĕ-rĭth-rō-pō-Ē-sĭs, p. 362)
gingivitis (jĭn-jĭ-VĪ-tĭs, p. 369)
hemarthrosis (hē-măr-THRŌ-sĭs, p. 370)
hematocrit (hē-MĂT-ō-krĭt, p. 366)
hemolysis (hē-MŎL-ĭ-sĭs, p. 364)
iatrogenic (ĭ-ă-trō-JĔN-ĭk, p. 364)
jaundice (JĂWN-dĭs, p. 368)
leukopenia (loo-kō-PĒ-nē-ă, p. 364)
melena (MĔL-ĕh-nă, p. 370)
petechiae (pĕ-TĒ-kē-ă, p. 368)
polycythemia (pŏl-ē-sī-THĒ-mē-ă, p. 368)
thrombocytopenia (thrŏm-bō-sīt-ō-PĒ-nē-ă, p. 364)

Blood sustains life for every cell of the body. The cardiovascular system is composed of blood, the heart pump that propels the blood throughout the body, and the veins, arteries, and capillaries that form an interconnecting network for carrying blood to the cells. Any disorder that affects the blood or blood-forming organs interferes with the vital functions the blood performs.

This chapter discusses causes and prevention of blood disorders, diagnostic tests for the hematologic system, and common problems of patients with disorders of this system. The lymphatic system, which drains the fluid from the spaces around each cell and channels it into the circulatory system, was discussed in Chapter 11.

? *Think Critically About . . .* The CBC of your patient shows the following values:
RBCs: 4.8 million/mm^3
WBCs: 6.7 million/mm^3
Hemoglobin: 10.2 g/dL
Platelets: 250,000/mm^3
What abnormalities, if any, do these results indicate?

CAUSES OF HEMATOLOGIC DISORDERS

Several disorders that interfere with normal function of the blood are inherited. Hemophilia, sickle cell disease, and thalassemia types of anemias are examples (Cultural Cues 15–1). Accidental tearing or cutting of the vessels of the cardiovascular system and

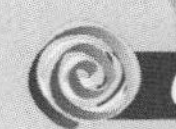

Cultural Cues 15–1

Genetic Hematologic Tendencies

- African Americans have the highest incidence of sickle cell disease.
- Pernicious anemia is more prevalent among those of Scandinavian descent and among African Americans.
- People of Middle-Eastern origin may have a genetic predisposition to thalassemia.

OVERVIEW OF ANATOMY AND PHYSIOLOGY OF THE HEMATOLOGIC SYSTEM

What are the functions of blood?

- **Blood transports water, oxygen, nutrients, hormones, enzymes, and medications to the cells.**
- **Blood transports carbon dioxide and other waste products away from the cells.**
- The 4 to 5 L of blood in the body help regulate fluid volume and electrolyte distribution.
- The blood regulates the pH and acid-base balance by its buffering ability.
- Blood assists in regulating body temperature.
- Blood provides clotting factors for hemostasis

What are the components of blood?

- Blood is composed of formed elements and plasma (Figure 15–1).
- About 45% of the blood is made up of various types of cells—the formed elements—and the remainder of the blood is plasma.
- The formed elements are erythrocytes, neutrophils, lymphocytes, monocytes, eosinophils, basophils, and platelets.
- Plasma contains proteins, water, salts, dissolved gases (such as CO_2), bicarbonate (HCO_3^-), hormones, glucose, and wastes.
- The plasma proteins are albumin, globulins, and fibrinogen.

What are the functions of the plasma proteins?

- Albumin raises osmotic pressure at the capillary membrane, preventing fluid from leaking out into the tissue spaces. (Osmotic pressure is covered in Chapter 3.)
- The alpha and beta globulins work as carriers for drugs and lipids by combining with them and transporting them throughout the body; gamma globulins act as antibodies.

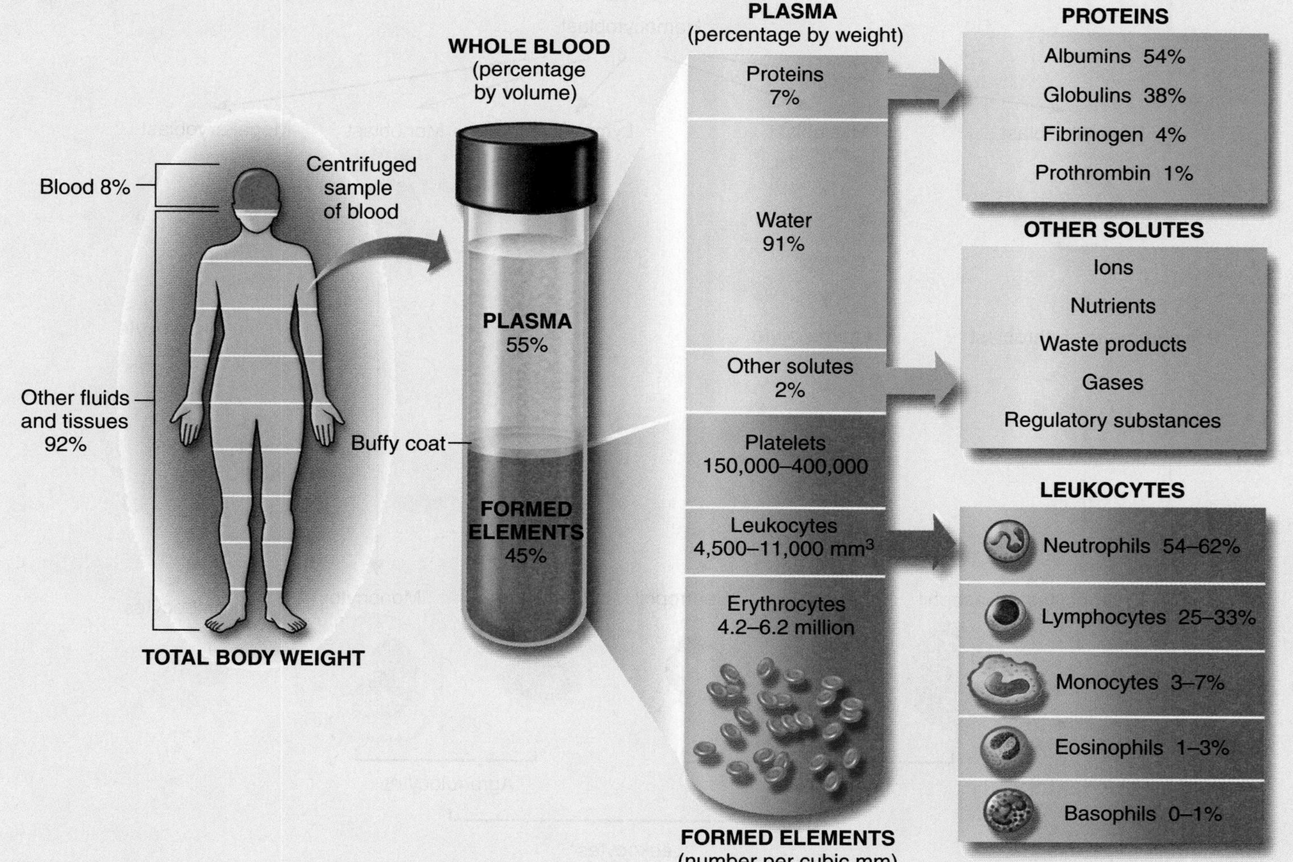

FIGURE **15–1** Components of blood.

Continued

OVERVIEW OF ANATOMY AND PHYSIOLOGY OF THE HEMATOLOGIC SYSTEM—cont'd

- Fibrinogen is essential to the formation of blood clots.

How does the body produce blood cells?

- Blood cells develop from stem cells located in the bone marrow through **erythropoiesis** (Figure 15–2).
- The kidney produces the majority of erythropoietin-stimulating factor, which prompts erythropoietin to be released from the liver for erythrocyte production.
- Erythropoiesis requires iron, vitamins B_{12}, C, and E, folic acid, and amino acids from proteins.

What are the functions of the red blood cells?

- Red blood cells (RBCs or erythrocytes), the most numerous of the blood cells, contain hemoglobin, which carries oxygen to the cells and a portion of carbon dioxide away from the cells.
- Each person has a hereditary blood type based on the antigens on the RBCs.
- **The normal range for adults for RBCs is 4.2 to 6.2 million/mm^3.**
- **The normal range for hemoglobin in adults is 12.0 to 18.0 g/dL.**
- Decreased numbers of RBCs or decreased hemoglobin results in a reduction in the amount of oxygen that can be carried to the cells of the body.

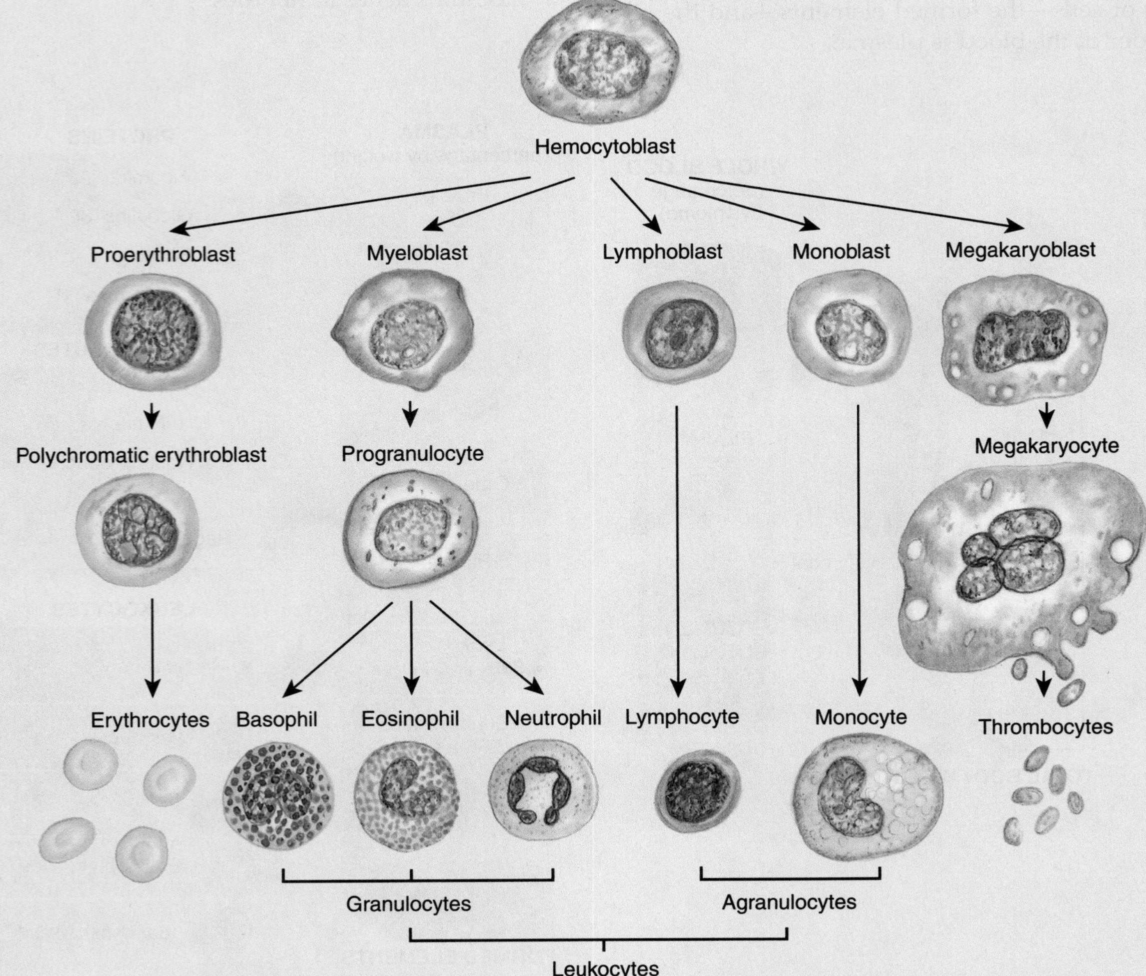

FIGURE 15–2 Development of the formed elements of blood, originating from stem cells in the bone marrow. Erythrocytes (RBCs), leukocytes (WBCs), and thrombocytes (platelets) are the end products.

- RBCs live for approximately 120 days.
- Old, damaged red cells are removed by the spleen and the liver.

What are the functions of the white blood cells?

- White blood cells (WBCs or leukocytes) provide the first line of defense against microbial agents.
- The normal adult range for total leukocytes (WBCs) is 4500 to 11,000/mm^3.
- Leukocytes are divided into granulocytes and agranulocytes, meaning with and without granules in the cell nucleus (see Figure 15–2).
- Leukocytes migrate out into the tissues and are carried by the bloodstream to locations where they are needed (Table 15–1).
- Granulocytes are divided into neutrophils, eosinophils, and basophils and are produced in the red bone marrow.
- Neutrophils make up 50% to 70% of the WBC count and work by engulfing and destroying bacteria by the process of *phagocytosis.*
- An infection in the body stimulates increased production of neutrophils, resulting in a higher-than-normal WBC count, or leukocytosis.
- Eosinophils, which make up 1% to 5% of the total WBCs, help detoxify foreign proteins; they increase in number during allergic reactions and in response to parasitic infections.
- Basophils, which comprise up to 1% of the total WBC, release histamine in response to allergens and help prevent clotting in the small blood vessels.
- Agranulocytes consist of lymphocytes and monocytes.
- Agranulocytes are produced in the red bone marrow and in lymphatic tissue.
- Lymphocytes comprise 25% of the WBCs and occur as B cells and T cells. B cells synthesize antibodies. Some T cells are killer cells and help B cells destroy foreign proteins (see Chapter 11).
- Lymphocytes are produced in the red bone marrow and the lymphatic tissue.
- Monocytes become macrophages when out in the tissues and are active as phagocytes, fighting infection and ridding the body of foreign substances.
- A differential blood cell count gives information about the numbers of different types of leukocytes present in the blood and about the type of inflammatory process that is occurring.

What are platelets and what is their function?

- Platelets, also called thrombocytes, are fragments of megakaryocytes that are produced by the bone marrow.
- Platelets provide the first line of protection, after vasospasm, to prevent bleeding by promoting clotting when the wall of a blood vessel has been damaged.
- Platelets are involved in maintaining hemostasis by a complex process that balances the production of clotting and dissolving factors.
- Fibrin strands derived from the plasma protein fibrinogen attach to aggregated platelets to help form a clot.
- The normal adult platelet count range is 150,000 to 400,000/mm^3; the life span of a platelet is about 10 days.
- Although the body can withstand a substantial drop in the number of platelets, when the platelet count is low, there is risk of spontaneous bleeding into the skin, kidney, brain, and other internal organs.

How does the lymphatic system interact with the vascular system?

- The lymphatic system consists of lymph nodes, lymph channels, the spleen, and the thymus gland (see Chapter 11).
- The spleen, located in the upper left abdominal cavity below the diaphragm and behind the stomach, filters the blood, removing pathogens, old blood cells, and debris, and produces lymphocytes.
- The spleen is a reservoir for extra blood; in response to hemorrhage, it contracts, adding blood to the cardiovascular system.
- If the spleen is removed, its functions are taken over by other lymph tissue and the liver.
- Lymph nodes (bundles of lymphatic tissue) and lymphatic tissues, located along the lymphatic vessels, produce lymphocytes and filter out leukocytes and cell debris from inflammations and infections.

What changes occur with aging?

- Plasma volume decreases after age 60; the older person has less blood volume.
- Bone marrow activity decreases by about 50% as years advance; the marrow becomes infiltrated with fat and fibrotic tissue.

Continued

OVERVIEW OF ANATOMY AND PHYSIOLOGY OF THE HEMATOLOGIC SYSTEM—cont'd

- Immune response is decreased, making the older person more susceptible to infection and autoimmune disease.
- New cells are produced at a slower rate, and correction of anemia is a longer process.
- When blood loss occurs, the elderly patient is at greater risk for hypovolemia and shock.
- Blood is more prone to coagulate because platelets tend to aggregate more with advancing age, and there are alterations in clotting activity. The increased incidence of thrombosis in coronary and cerebral arteries may be related to changes in clotting activity. Daily low-dose aspirin sometimes is prescribed to counteract this phenomenon.

Table 15–1 *Leukocytes and Their Functions*

CELL TYPE AND % OF LEUKOCYTES	FUNCTION
GRANULOCYTES	
Eosinophils (1%–3%)	Detoxify foreign proteins; increase in allergic reactions and in parasitic infections.
Basophils (0%–1%)	Prevent clotting in small vessels; release histamine in response to allergens.
Neutrophils (54%–62%)	Engulf and destroy bacteria via phagocytosis.
AGRANULOCYTES	
Monocytes (3%–7%)	Change into macrophages, move out into tissue, and perform phagocytosis.
Lymphocytes (25%–33%)	Divided into B lymphocytes and T lymphocytes; B lymphocytes change into plasma cells that produce immunoglobulins responsible for the humoral immune response. T lymphocytes fight antigens and are responsible for the cell-mediated immune response.

surgery cause bleeding and loss of blood. Blunt trauma to the spleen, such as might occur in an automobile accident, may cause tearing and massive internal hemorrhage. Chemicals and transfusions of the wrong blood type can cause **hemolysis** (destruction of red blood cells).

Some blood disorders are **iatrogenic**; that is, they are brought on by medical treatment. For example, blood **dyscrasias** (imbalance in numbers of types of cells) or other pathologic conditions of the blood can be induced through at least four kinds of actions:

- Bone marrow suppression, which interferes with the production of blood cells
- Interference with normal cell function
- Destruction of the blood cells by cytotoxic drugs
- Destruction of cells by a transfusion reaction of mismatched blood

Some antineoplastic drugs, for instance, act to depress the bone marrow, which inevitably causes a reduced supply of blood cells. Other drugs, such as phenytoin (Dilantin), primidone (Mysoline), and oral contraceptives, can produce anemia by interfering with the absorption and utilization of folic acid, a substance needed to produce RBCs.

Diuretics such as furosemide (Lasix) and hydrochlorothiazide (HydroDIURIL) sometimes cause **leukopenia** (decreased numbers of white cells), **aplastic anemia** (deficient cell production due to a bone marrow disorder), and abnormally low counts of platelets and granulocytes. Procainamide hydrochloride (Pronestyl) and quinidine, which are used to correct dysrhythmias of the heart, also can cause **thrombocytopenia** (too few platelets), **agranulocytosis** (decrease in granulocyte production), and aplastic anemia. Keep in mind that most drugs are powerful chemicals that are capable of producing undesirable side effects, even though the drugs can be of great value.

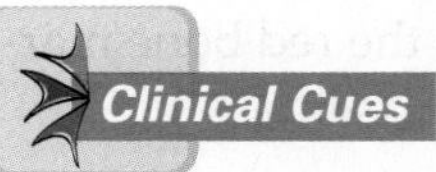

If the patient is showing signs of a blood disorder, review the medications that are being taken and their side effects.

Nutritional deficiencies, such as low protein or lack of vitamin C, can interfere with erythropoiesis and normally functioning blood cells (Nutritional Therapies 15–1). Abnormal red cells are more prone to rapid destruction, which can result in anemia. Bone marrow damage from toxic substances may also interfere with the production of blood cells.

Malignant conditions such as leukemia cause growth of abnormal blood cells and interfere with the production of normal cells. Box 15–1 presents factors that alter hematologic system function.

Nutritional Therapies 15–1

Nutrients Needed for Building Red Blood Cells (Erythropoiesis)

NUTRIENT	ROLE IN ERYTHROPOIESIS	FOOD SOURCES
Cobalamin (vitamin B_{12})	RBC maturation	Red meats, especially liver
Folic acid	RBC maturation	Green leafy vegetables, liver, meat, fish, legumes, whole grains
Iron	Hemoglobin synthesis	Liver and muscle meats, eggs, dried fruits, legumes, dark green leafy vegetables, whole-grain and enriched bread and cereals, potatoes
Vitamin B_6	Hemoglobin synthesis	Meats (especially pork and liver), wheat germ, legumes, potatoes, cornmeal, bananas
Amino acids	Synthesis of nucleoprotein	Eggs, meat, milk and milk products (cheese, ice cream), poultry, fish, legumes, nuts
Vitamin C	Conversion of folic acid to its active forms; aids in iron absorption	Citrus fruits, leafy green vegetables, strawberries, cantaloupe

Key: *RBC,* red blood cell.

PREVENTION OF HEMATOLOGIC DISORDERS

When considerable blood is lost through hemorrhage, the patient becomes anemic. Sometimes excessive blood loss can occur during menstruation. **You can often prevent hemorrhage after surgery or childbirth by vigilantly assessing the amount of blood loss and by instituting measures to stop the loss if it is excessive.**

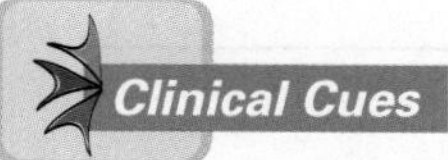

Clinical Cues

The average amount of blood loss via menstruation is less than 80 mL. A better way to estimate that blood loss is to count the number of saturated pads or tampons. Each saturated pad is equal to about 50 mL of blood loss.

You can help prevent anemia by promoting proper nutrition and educating the public about the possibility of nutritional anemia. Nutritional anemia is a particular concern for individuals who subsist mostly on "fast food."

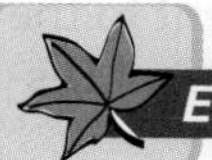

Elder Care Points

- An elderly person, especially one who lives alone, is at high risk of poor nutrition. Problems with arthritis, vision, and chronic diseases make it more difficult to shop and prepare food. An elderly person may substitute cookies, toast, or cereal for a well-balanced meal. It is important to obtain a food intake history.
- Secretion of intrinsic factor from the stomach and absorption of vitamin B_{12} is decreased in the elderly. This can lead to pernicious anemia.

Box 15–1 *Factors that May Alter Function of the Hematologic System*

GENETIC DISORDERS
- Hemophilia
- Sickle cell disease
- Agranulocytosis
- Fanconi syndrome

HEMORRHAGE (ANEMIA)
- Surgical blood loss
- Blood loss from childbirth or spontaneous abortion
- Traumatic blood loss

ANEMIA
- Iron deficiency
- Folic acid deficiency
- Pernicious anemia
- Chronic slow blood loss
- Aplastic anemia

HEMOLYSIS
- Blood transfusion reaction
- Genetic types of anemia

BONE MARROW SUPPRESSION
- Antineoplastic agents used in treatment of cancer
- Radiation treatment used for cancer
- Excessive exposure to ionizing radiation
- Exposure to toxic chemicals that damage bone marrow
- Drugs that suppress the bone marrow

BONE MARROW PROLIFERATION OR ABNORMALITY
- Leukemia

Monitoring patients for drug side effects, and alerting the physician should blood-related side effects occur, can prevent a serious blood disorder from developing (Health Promotion Points 15–1). Carefully monitoring blood transfusions and promptly reporting any untoward reaction may decrease the incidence of hemolysis from a reaction.

Health Promotion Points 15–1

Preventing Blood Disorders

To prevent blood disorders, nurses in the community should:

- Caution the public about the dangers of exposure to ionizing radiation and harmful chemicals to help decrease the incidence of blood disorders related to harmful substances.
- Suggest genetic counseling regarding the possibility of transmitting a genetic blood disorder to offspring to those adults who have such a disorder.
- Inform patients about medications they are taking that can cause blood disorders and remind them to be alert for signs of excessive bruising or easy bleeding. Suggest that CBCs be checked periodically for monitoring purposes.

DIAGNOSTIC TESTS AND PROCEDURES

A surprising amount of information can be obtained from a stained blood film using only a 5-mL sample of uncoagulated blood. Each of the formed elements can be studied for shape, maturity, and number. Other kinds of studies include those done on the plasma to measure the rate at which RBCs settle out from plasma (called the *sedimentation rate*) and to separate and classify various kinds of proteins, including antibodies, in the plasma.

Your responsibility with blood tests is to explain the venipuncture procedure and the purpose of the test to the patient. Many patients have a great fear of needles. Others are concerned about having what seems like a lot of blood withdrawn. A few words of assurance and explanation can do much to relieve anxiety about a needle stick and promote cooperation. If you are to perform the venipuncture, Standard Precautions and aseptic technique must be followed, and the correct tubes for each sample must be used. Latex or impermeable gloves must be worn any time a venipuncture is performed, and equipment must be disposed of according to Standard Precautions (see Appendix 5).

Leukocyte counts provide information about infection and possible immune disorders (see Chapter 11). Data about the number of platelets are valuable in diagnosing a variety of diseases affecting or affected by the clotting of blood.

There are at least 12 different types of hemoglobin in human blood. The types are designated by letters—for example, hemoglobin A is normal adult hemoglobin, hemoglobin F is normal fetal hemoglobin, and hemoglobin S is found in sickle cell disease. A **hematocrit** is a test that measures the volume of blood cells in relation to the volume of plasma. When there has been a loss of body fluids but no loss of cells, as in dehydration, the cell volume is high in proportion to the amount of liquid (plasma) in the bloodstream (i.e., the hematocrit rises). On the other hand, when either hemorrhage or anemia has depleted the supply of cells, the blood is "thinned" and the cell volume is low. Table 15–2 presents the most common diagnostic tests and related nursing care for the hematologic and lymphatic systems.

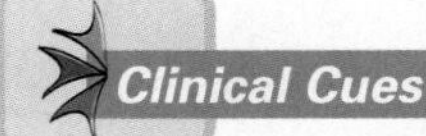

Clinical Cues

- Increased numbers of eosinophils often indicate allergy.
- A viral infection prompts the production of additional lymphocytes.
- Bacterial infection stimulates the production of neutrophils, and segmented neutrophils (segs) increase.
- Ongoing bacterial infections cause immature neutrophils to appear in the blood as *bands* (immature forms of segmented granulocytes). This is referred to as a "shift to the left."
- A "shift to the right" occurs when there are more mature neutrophils than usual; this occurs with anemia from vitamin B_{12} or folic acid deficiency.

Think Critically About . . . When caring for a patient who has been in an automobile accident and has sustained trauma to the trunk of the body, what laboratory values should the nurse check daily?

NURSING MANAGEMENT

Assessment (Data Collection)

History

The nurse assesses patients for signs and symptoms that indicate abnormalities in the blood. Abnormal symptoms result from too little circulating blood or too little hemoglobin, too few platelets, deficiency of normal neutrophils or lymphocytes, and too many abnormal blood cells. **When there is insufficient hemoglobin to carry oxygen to the cells, signs of oxygen deficit occur.** Using the guide for history taking in Focused Assessment 15–1 on p. 369 will provide an appropriate history concerning factors pertinent to the blood and lymphatic system. Inquire about renal disease as this may be a cause of anemia.

Physical Assessment

In addition to the usual initial and ongoing assessment conducted by the nurse caring for a patient, some special observations are relevant for patients with blood disorders (Focused Assessment 15–2, p. 369).

Skin. Although pallor may be a sign of anemia, it is not the most reliable sign. Many other factors can affect

Table 15–2 ***Diagnostic Tests for Disorders of the Hematologic Systems***

TEST AND NORMAL RANGE	PURPOSE	DESCRIPTION	NURSING IMPLICATIONS
Complete blood count (CBC)	Determine whether abnormalities are present in the numbers of blood cells or types of blood cells; assess the amount of hemoglobin present. Useful to diagnose anemia.	Fill a lavender-top tube containing EDTA with a venous sample of blood. Use a site where there is little chance of dilution from intravenous solution. Mix the blood and the EDTA by gently rotating the tube.	Warn the patient that a "stick" is about to occur, but that the pain will be short-lived. Apply pressure directly to the puncture site after withdrawing the needle; at the antecubital space, do **not** have the patient flex the arm as this tends to cause a hematoma.
Erythrocytes Hemoglobin: females: 12.0–16.7 g/dL; males: 13.0–18.0 g/dL Red blood cell (RBC) count: females: 4.2–5.4 million/mm^3; males: 4.6–6.2 million/mm^3 Hematocrit: female: 37%–47%; male: 40%–54% *Leukocytes* White blood cell (WBC) count: 4500–11,000/mm^3 *Differential count* Granulocytes Neutrophils: 54%–62% of WBCs Eosinophils: 1%–3% of WBCs Basophils: 0%–1% of WBCs Agranulocytes Lymphocytes: 25%–33% of WBCs Monocytes: 0%–7% of WBCs Thrombocytes (platelets): 150,000–400,000/mm^3 of blood Mean corpuscular hemoglobin (Hb) (MCH): 26–34 pg/cell Mean corpuscular Hb concentration (MCHC): 32–36 g/dL Mean corpuscular volume (MCV): 80–96 μm^3			
Erythrocyte sedimentation rate (ESR) Wintrobe: Males: 0.5 mm/hr Females: 0–15 mm/hr Westergren: Males: 0–15 mm/hr Females: 0–20 mm/hr	To detect inflammation and infection.	Fill a blue-top tube with venous blood. The laboratory determines the rate at which the RBCs settle.	Explain that this test helps diagnose an inflammatory process but is nonspecific.
Hemoglobin electrophoresis Hemoglobin A_{1c}: 3%–5% Hemoglobin A_2: 1.5%–3% Hemoglobin F: <1% of total	Useful in diagnosing various types of anemia.	Performed on venous sample using lavender-top tube with EDTA.	Same as for CBC.
Tests for anemia Ferritin, serum: 20–200 ng/mL Total iron-binding capacity: 250–410 mcg/dL Saturation 20%–55%	Detect reason for anemia.	Performed on a venous blood sample.	Same as for CBC.
Coagulation tests Prothrombin time (PT): 12–14 sec Activated partial thromboplastin time (APTT): 20–25 sec Bleeding time, Ivy: 2.75–8.0 min	Determine abnormalities of clotting time.	Performed on a venous blood sample; use a blue-top tube	Same as for a CBC; pressure may need to be applied longer than usual if the patient has an abnormal clotting time or is on heparin or warfarin therapy.

Note: Normal values differ between laboratories.

Continued

Table 15–2 ***Diagnostic Tests for Disorders of the Hematologic Systems—cont'd***

TEST AND NORMAL RANGE	PURPOSE	DESCRIPTION	NURSING IMPLICATIONS
D-Dimer Negative: <0.5 mcg/mL	Blood test that provides assay of fibrin degradation to assess thrombin and plasmin activity. Useful for diagnosing pulmonary embolism and disseminated intravascular coagulation (DIC).	Collect blood sample in a blue-top tube.	No fasting is required.
Sickledex 0	Test for the presence of hemoglobin S.	Performed on a venous blood sample; use a lavender-top tube.	Client may be anxious about the result; be sensitive to feelings. Positive result indicates need for genetic counseling.
Bence Jones protein test Presence of Bence Jones proteins in the urine is abnormal	Assist in the diagnosis of multiple myeloma.	Obtain a 10-mL fresh morning specimen of urine in a clean container. Must be refrigerated or tested immediately.	Explain the procedure to the patient.
Schilling test ≥7% excreted within 24 hr	Determine ability to absorb vitamin B_{12}; used to diagnose pernicious anemia.	Radioactive B_{12} is given orally, followed in 2 hr by an intramuscular injection of B_{12}. A 24-hr urine specimen is collected.	Assess kidney function. Requires an 8- to 12-hr fast. No B vitamins for 3 days prior; no laxatives for 24 hr. Subnormal levels of B_{12} in the urine indicate the lack of intrinsic factor, which facilitates absorption of vitamin B_{12}.
Bone marrow aspiration and biopsy Normal cell counts	To help diagnose blood disorders.	Cells are withdrawn by needle from the sternum or iliac crest. Leukocytes, platelets, and erythrocytes are examined in the various stages of development to determine abnormalities. Assists in identifying certain anemias, leukemia, and thrombocytopenia.	Explain that the aspiration is done at the bedside. Seek an order for prebiopsy medication to decrease the discomfort. Explain that there is a feeling of pressure when the needle is inserted and sharp, brief pain when the marrow is aspirated. The area of aspiration is surgically prepped. The patient must hold perfectly still. Pressure is applied to the site afterward to prevent hematoma formation. Posttest, observe for swelling and tenderness indicating continued bleeding or infection.

a person's complexion and skin color, including thickness of the skin, amount of skin pigment, and number and distribution of blood vessels near the surface of the skin. Pale mucous membranes or pale conjunctiva of the eye is a better indicator. A very ruddy complexion with a red, florid appearance is typical of an excessive number of red blood cells **(polycythemia).**

Jaundice, or a yellowing discoloration of the skin and sclera of the eyes, can occur as a result of excessive destruction of red blood cells (hemolysis). When red blood cells are ruptured, bilirubin is released. The pigment eventually finds its way into the bloodstream, where it causes jaundice. If hemolysis is occurring, the urine will often contain bilirubin, giving it a brown tea color.

Bruises and small, red, pinpoint lesions **(petechiae)** are typical of *thrombocytopenic purpura*, a hemorrhagic disease sometimes associated with a decrease in the number of circulating platelets. In dark-skinned people, check the palms of the hands and soles of the feet for petechiae. Bleeding under the skin and formation of bruises in response to the slightest trauma frequently occur in anemias, leukemias, and diseases affecting the bone marrow and spleen. These appear as darker areas on brown-skinned people.

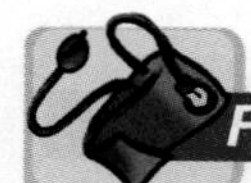

Focused Assessment 15–1

Data Collection for the Hematologic System

Ask the patient the following questions:

- Do you or does anyone in your family have a genetic blood disorder, such as hemophilia, thalassemia, sickle cell trait or disease, aplastic anemia, agranulocytosis, or thrombocytopenia purpura?
- What is your occupation?
- Have you ever been told you had anemia?
- Do you have frequent sore throats or other infections?
- Do you frequently feel as though you have a fever?
- Do you ever have night sweats?
- Are your joints painful? Do they swell?
- Do you bruise easily or develop pinpoint blood spots?
- Do you suffer from itching?
- Do you have any swollen lymph nodes in the groin or armpits?
- Do you ever have tingling or numbness in the extremities?
- Do you have frequent headaches? Palpitations?
- Have you become more irritable than usual?
- Do you get dizzy frequently? Do you suffer fainting spells?
- Do you get short of breath when you walk a short distance or when you climb stairs?
- Do your gums bleed when you brush your teeth? Does your tongue get sore? Do you have frequent mouth sores?
- Do you have any difficulty eating?
- How much alcohol do you drink in a day?
- Do colds or other infections seem to last a very long time for you?
- Do you frequently feel fatigued even when you haven't been doing much?
- Have you been exposed to chemicals, such as pesticides, cleaning agents, or industrial chemicals of any kind?
- Have you ever noticed that you have black, tarry-looking stool or smoky or brown urine?
- Do you have stomach pain or indigestion? Have you ever had an ulcer?
- Are your menstrual periods unusually heavy (if appropriate)?
- What do you usually eat for each meal?
- Are you often cold when others are not?

Elder Care Points

- The elderly bruise more easily because of thinner skin and greater fragility of blood vessel walls.
- Aspirin or other drug therapy also may make the elderly person more prone to bruising.
- Bruising is not necessarily an unusual sign in this agegroup.

Cyanosis, or a bluish tint to the skin, can indicate hypoxia resulting from inadequate numbers of circulating erythrocytes. The gums or the roof of the mouth is the best place to check for a bluish color in dark-skinned people.

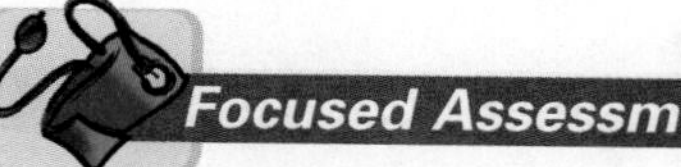

Focused Assessment 15–2

Physical Assessment of the Hematologic System

Gather the following data:

HEAD AND NECK

- Color of conjunctiva and sclera of eye
- Condition of gums and oral mucous membranes; condition of tongue
- Presence of enlarged cervical lymph nodes

SKIN

- Color (pale) (Check conjunctivae, palms of hands, and roof of the mouth in people with dark skin.)
- Condition of fingernails (brittle, spoon-shaped)
- Presence of ecchymoses or petechiae
- Jaundice
- Nasal or gingival bleeding
- Hair (dry, brittle, thinning)

CHEST AND ABDOMEN

- Presence of swollen lymph nodes in armpits or groin
- Rapid respirations; shortness of breath upon exertion
- Rapid pulse rate at rest
- Widened pulse pressure (greater distance between systolic and diastolic pressure)
- Epigastric tenderness
- Abdominal distention

EXTREMITIES

- Presence of swollen or painful joints
- Different lengths of fingers and toes

URINE AND STOOL

- Signs of blood

Mucous Membranes. Nutritional deficiencies contributing to anemia and resultant hypoxia may cause sore and painful gums and tongue. The patient may have difficulty chewing and eating. The tongue may be smooth and beefy red. Bleeding of the gums (**gingivitis**) may occur with tooth brushing when the platelet count is low.

Abdomen. Stomach pain or nausea can be caused by bleeding ulcers, a frequent cause of chronic blood loss. Black, tarry, stools or coffee-ground emesis indicates gastrointestinal (GI) bleeding. Hiatal hernia also can cause a chronic blood loss (Assignment Considerations 15–1).

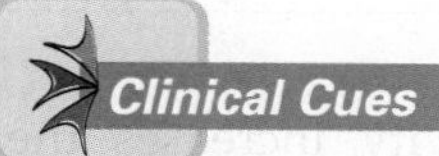

For the patient with thrombocytopenia, abdominal girth should be measured daily to detect internal bleeding. Place marks on the lateral aspects of the abdomen where the measuring tape is placed and measure at the umbilicus. Put the measuring tape in the same place each day.

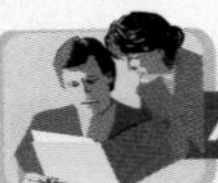

Assignment Considerations 15–1

Observing for Blood

If a nursing assistant will be assisting the patient with toileting, remind that person to check stool for signs of **melena** (dark stool containing blood pigments) and the urine for a smoky color indicating blood.

Swollen and Painful Joints. Bleeding into the joints **(hemarthrosis)** is not uncommon in certain kinds of anemia, such as sickle cell disease, or in hemophilia. This might be evidenced by swelling and slight redness in the area of the joints, or the patient may move more slowly and with obvious discomfort.

Lymph Tissue Involvement. Enlarged lymph nodes occur in a number of different blood disorders as well as in infections and immune disorders. The nodes most often inspected and palpated are those under the arm, in the neck, and in the *inguinal* (groin) region. Lymph node enlargement is often found while bathing a patient or helping him with activities of daily living (ADLs) (Assignment Considerations 15–2).

Enlargement of the spleen, which also accompanies polycythemia and several other blood disorders, might be described by the patient as a feeling of fullness on the left side of the upper abdomen. Palpate the abdomen gently in a patient with a suspected blood disorder. Do not palpate deeply if there is tenderness in the area of the spleen as this could cause rupture of the spleen.

Mental State. Irritability and mental depression are often found in patients with blood disorders. **Irritability, dizziness, difficulty in concentrating, and headache may be caused by a decreased supply of oxygen to the brain.** Depression often accompanies the chronic lack of energy, difficulty in eating and enjoying food, and the many other problems from which patients with blood disorders often suffer.

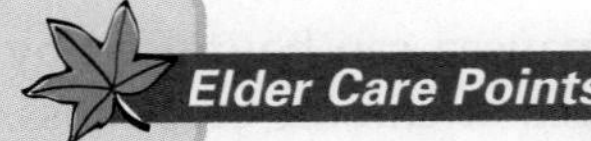

Elder Care Points

An elderly person who has developed pernicious anemia may present with confusion and a loss of mental faculties. This state may be initially thought to be Alzheimer's disease. A blood count is important to establish the diagnosis.

Activity Intolerance. Physical activity increases the demand for oxygen, but if there are not enough circulating RBCs to carry the necessary oxygen, the patient becomes physically weak and unable to engage in physical activity without severe fatigue. Note whether the patient is able to do things for himself or needs help to complete specific ADLs.

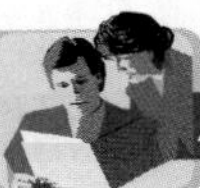

Assignment Considerations 15–2

Changes to Report

When assigning tasks to a certified nursing assistant (CNA) or an unlicensed assistive personnel (UAP), ask the person to report any swellings she notices when assisting with bathing. State that the person may bruise easily and to report any new bruised areas or patient complaints of bleeding of gums or elsewhere.

? *Think Critically About . . .*

- Can you name four signs or symptoms that you might encounter when taking a patient's history that could indicate your patient may be anemic?
- How can the conjunctiva and the sclera of the eye provide information about anemia or jaundice?
- What signs and symptoms might indicate that the patient is suffering a chronic blood loss?

Nursing Diagnosis

Nursing diagnoses for hematologic and lymphatic disorders are based on the problems the disorders cause for the patient. Nursing diagnoses commonly associated with hematologic disorders are listed in Table 15–3. They must be individualized for each patient.

Planning

Nursing care should be planned to provide rest periods for the patient. Planning dietary teaching or consultation with the dietitian is important for patients with anemia. **The patient with a blood abnormality is at higher risk for infection, so using aseptic technique is extremely important.** Such patients should not be exposed to people who are ill with contagious diseases, such as colds or influenza, whether health care workers or visitors. Nursing goals include:

- Prevent infection.
- Conserve patient's energy and prevent undue fatigue.
- Correct nutritional deficiencies.
- Provide treatment to halt or slow disease process.
- Control pain or discomfort.

Specific expected outcomes are written for individualized nursing diagnoses.

Implementation

Nurses should handle patients with blood dyscrasias gently to prevent bruising and hematomas. Care is taken to apply pressure for 5 to 10 minutes after injections or venipuncture (Assignment Considerations 15–3). Good skin care is essential, as the skin acts as a

Table 15–3 Common Nursing Diagnoses, Expected Outcomes, and Interventions for Patients with Blood Disorders

NURSING DIAGNOSIS	GOALS/EXPECTED OUTCOMES	NURSING INTERVENTIONS
Imbalanced nutrition: less than body requirements, related to:	Protein levels will be within normal limits within 6 weeks.	Teach the patient about foods that meet required needs. Obtain dietary consultation as needed Administer iron preparation; if liquid, give through straw.
Iron deficiency from inadequate intake or blood loss	Hemoglobin levels will be within normal range within 3 mo.	Give iron with vitamin C–containing juice or food. Warn that stool may be greenish black.
Vitamin B_{12} deficiency	The patient will administer his own B_{12} injections on a regular schedule.	Administer vitamin B_{12} as ordered; advise that lifetime therapy is needed.
Inflammation of mucous membranes	The patient performs mouth care diligently on schedule. Patient displays normal-appearing mucous membranes. CBC shows increasing RBCs and Hb within 3 wk.	Give gentle mouth care before meals and q 2 hr. Provide bland, easily chewed foods. Monitor CBC count for evidence of increase in RBCs and Hg.
Activity intolerance related to decreased RBCs or HgA	Patient is using oxygen as ordered. Patient alternates activities with rest. Patient seeks assistance with ambulation when dizzy.	Administer oxygen by nasal cannula at 3–6 L/min as ordered for patient with sickle cell crisis. Space activities, allowing rest periods for patient with fatigue. Assist with ADLs to prevent fatigue. Maintain skin integrity. Turn frequently. If dizzy, caution to change position slowly; call for assistance with ambulation.
Pain related to ischemia and swollen joints	Patient verbalizes that pain is controlled by analgesics. Patient verbalizes that pain has decreased within 48 hr.	Elevate swollen joints, and apply hot or cold packs. Encourage high fluid intake. Monitor IV fluid therapy. Teach to avoid strenuous exercise. Use bed cradle to support bed covers. Administer analgesics as ordered PRN.
Risk for injury, related to low platelet count	Platelet count within safe limits after platelet administration. Patient will have no new hematoma formation or other evidence of bleeding.	Assess for signs of internal bleeding (bruises, blood in urine or stool); measure abdominal girth q day. Minimize trauma; handle gently. Apply ice packs and gentle pressure if hematoma seems to be forming. Monitor administration of platelets PRN. Use small-gauge needle for injections; rotate sites. Apply pressure to puncture site for 10 min.
Risk for infection, related to decreased leukocytes	Patient will have no evidence of infection.	Observe for early signs of infection and report. Use strict aseptic technique for wound care and invasive procedures. Use protective isolation as needed. Teach patient good personal hygiene. Maintain integrity of skin and mucosa. Administer anti-infective drugs precisely as ordered.
Deficient knowledge, related to substances that damage bone marrow	Patient verbalizes knowledge of drugs and chemicals that are harmful to the bone marrow within 1 wk.	Assess for exposure to substances that could have damaged the bone marrow. Teach about drugs and chemicals that are harmful to bone marrow and how to prevent damage. Seek feedback to validate understanding of content taught.

Key: *ADLs*, activities of daily living; *CBC*, complete blood count; *Hb*, hemoglobin; *IV*, intravenous; PRN, as needed; *RBCs*, red blood cells.

Continued

Table 15–3 Common Nursing Diagnoses, Expected Outcomes, and Interventions for Patients with Blood Disorders—cont'd

NURSING DIAGNOSIS	GOALS/EXPECTED OUTCOMES	NURSING INTERVENTIONS
Anxiety related to unknown outcome of diagnostic tests and knowledge of disease, treatment, and prognosis	Patient verbalizes purpose and expected experience for each diagnostic test ordered. Patient verbalizes fears regarding disease, treatment, and prognosis.	Provide teaching regarding each diagnostic test. Encourage verbalization of fears. Offer emotional support to patient and family.
Situational low self-esteem, related to inability to perform usual activities	Patient defines ways to cope with physical limitations. Patient verbalizes strengths. Patient discusses possibility of seeking counseling.	Assist to cope with limitations of the illness. Help plan ways to maintain appropriate activity. Help to focus on the things he can still do. Obtain counseling referral if psychological disturbance indicates need.
Risk of disabled family coping, related to expense of treatment and possible death of patient	Patient and family seek assistance from community resources as needed. Patient and family verbalize understanding of disease, treatment modalities, and their implications.	Refer leukemia patient and family to community resources, such as the American Cancer Society, for assistance. Assist family and patient to understand the disease, treatment modalities, and their implications. Encourage attendance for all family members in a support group. Obtain referral to social worker for further assistance. Encourage open communication within family.

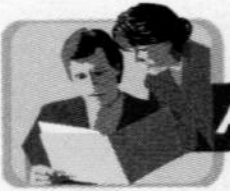

Assignment Considerations 15–3

Report Oozing of Blood

Although the nurse is responsible for checking the patient for signs of bleeding, when a patient with a blood disorder has had blood drawn or an invasive procedure, ask the CNA or UAP to report any oozing noticed at the site or on bandages when she is providing basic care such as feeding or toileting.

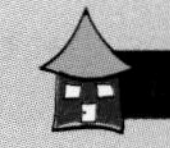

Home Care Considerations 15–1

Evaluating Treatment

It is important that each home care nurse evaluate how closely the patient is following the prescribed treatment plan. Determine whether the treatment is effective, and, if it is not, consult the physician about changing the plan.

protective barrier against infection. Teaching about nutrition and medication administration, prevention of infection, and measures to prevent bleeding is a major part of the nursing care for these patients. Pain control is important for the patient with sickle cell anemia in crisis, the hemophiliac with hemarthrosis, and the advanced leukemia patient.

Specific interventions for patients experiencing blood disorders are listed in Table 15–3. Other interventions are included in the discussion of the various disorders in Chapter 16.

Evaluation

The evaluation process provides data to determine whether the specific outcome criteria are being met for each patient. Monitoring laboratory values for blood counts and determining whether counts are improving is vital to determine if treatment and nursing actions are meeting the patient's needs. Assessing for side effects and evaluating how the patient is tolerating the medication or other treatment for the underlying disorder is important (Home Care Considerations 15–1).

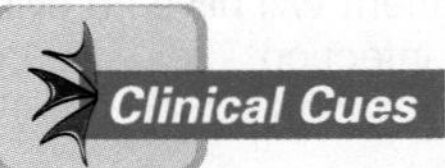

When a patient with leukemia is undergoing chemotherapy, evaluate the blood count results to determine that safe levels of leukocytes and platelets are present before administering another dose of a drug that inhibits their production.

COMMON PROBLEMS RELATED TO DISORDERS OF THE HEMATOLOGIC SYSTEM

EXCESSIVE BLEEDING

When injury has occurred, or spontaneous bleeding happens, you should immediately apply pressure to stop the bleeding (Figure 15–3). Severe bleeding can lead to irreversible hypovolemic shock and circulatory collapse from loss of intravascular fluid. Blood loss

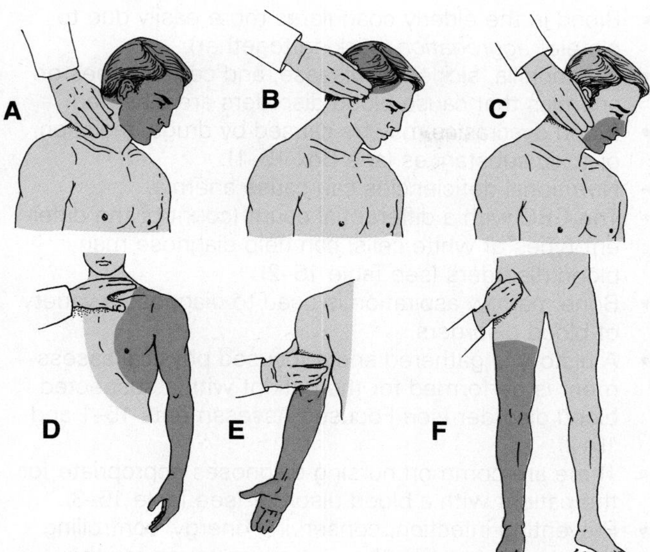

FIGURE 15–3 Locations of commonly used digital pressure points to stop hemorrhage. The screened areas are those within which hemorrhage may be controlled by pressure on a specific artery. **A,** Carotid artery. **B,** Temporal artery. **C,** External maxillary artery. **D,** Subclavian artery. **E,** Brachial artery. **F,** Femoral artery.

from an artery is bright red and will gush forth in spurts at regular intervals as the heart contracts. Blood loss from an artery is more rapid than that from a vein. Blood from a severed or punctured vein leaks slowly and steadily and is dark red. Box 15–2 presents techniques to control bleeding. If bleeding is due to absence of sufficient clotting factors, a transfusion of that factor or platelets will be ordered. See Chapters 3 and 16 for information on transfusions.

Box 15–2 *Techniques to Control Bleeding*

Severe bleeding can lead to irreversible hypovolemic shock from loss of intravascular fluid and to circulatory collapse.

PROCEDURE

- Position the body part that is bleeding over a firm surface and immobilize the part.
- Place a sterile dressing or clean cloth over the wound.
- With the flat palm of the hand or several fingers, apply direct pressure on the wound continuously for 5 minutes.
- Check whether bleeding has stopped after 5 minutes; if bleeding is occurring, apply pressure continuously for another 10 minutes.
- When bleeding has stopped, gently remove hand pressure and apply a pressure dressing over the cloth or dressing by folding another dressing or piece of cloth several times and tying it firmly over the wound.
- Check circulation distal to the wound to be certain that the pressure dressing is not so tight that circulation below the wound is cut off.
- Reinforce the dressing as needed by applying yet another layer of dressing as blood soaks through; do not remove previously applied dressings.
- If direct pressure will not stop the bleeding, and bleeding is considerable, apply pressure over the artery leading to the wound. **(Cut off arterial flow only as a last resort.)**
- Check for adequate pressure over the artery by determining a lack of pulse distal to the wound and patient report of a sensation of tingling and numbness in the wound area.

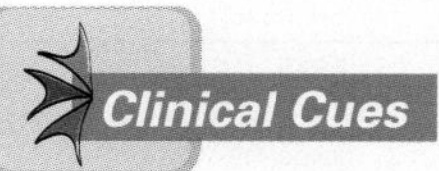

Blood loss from the GI tract from an ulcer, tumor, or hiatal hernia can be in small amounts or in a large enough amount to make stool appear black *(melena)*. Loss of 50 to 75 mL of blood from the upper GI tract is required before melena will appear.

FATIGUE

Spacing activities throughout the day with frequent rest periods will help decrease fatigue. If fatigue is due to anemia, assure the patient that his stamina will improve as his red cell count and hemoglobin rise. Work with the patient and family to decrease chores and expectations while fatigue is being experienced. Fatigue is very common with anemia and affects all

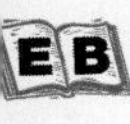

aspects of the patient's life (Ferrell et al., 1996).

ANOREXIA

Serving small, frequent meals is best. Meals should be high in protein, vitamin C, and iron unless contraindicated. Provide mouth care before each meal. Offer foods that are appealing to the patient. Keep the eating environment pleasant and free of odors. Ask family to sit with the patient and offer socialization and encouragement during meals.

PAIN

If the patient is experiencing pain, all comfort measures should be employed. Assess pain level at least every 4 hours and medicate as ordered. Teach relaxation and imagery and assist the patient to perform these techniques (see Chapter 7). Pain may escalate quickly for the sickle cell anemia patient in crisis, so assess pain level at least every 2 hours.

INFECTION

When a patient is moderately to severely anemic, the oxygen-carrying capacity of the blood is considerably decreased. Less than optimal tissue perfusion and tissue hypoxia make it easier for pathogens to invade and cause infection. When WBCs are decreased or abnormal, there are fewer cells to fight infection. Patients with abnormalities of the blood need to be taught how to protect themselves from infection. Good hand hygiene is essential. Staying away from crowds and individuals with infections is necessary. Getting enough sleep and eating a well-balanced diet help keep the immune system as healthy as possible under the circumstances. Prophylactic antibiotics may be given in certain situations. Precautions for the patient who is prone to infection because of neutropenia are located in Chapter 16.

If the patient develops an infection, close monitoring of therapy and symptoms is needed. Rest, plenty of fluids, and sufficient protein and vitamin C are required to help the patient heal.

Key Points

- Blood transports needed substances to the cells and transports waste products away from the cells.
- Blood is composed of RBCs, WBCs, platelets, and plasma.
- Plasma proteins are albumin, globulins, and fibrinogen.
- Plasma proteins raise osmotic pressure and keep fluid from leaking out of the vessels.
- Blood cells develop in the bone marrow.
- When there is a decreased number of RBCs or decreased hemoglobin, there is a reduction in the amount of oxygen that reaches the cells.
- Leukocytes are the first line of defense against microbial agents.
- Neutrophils perform phagocytosis.
- Lymphocytes such as B cells and T cells destroy foreign proteins.
- Platelets are the first line of cell protection to prevent bleeding when trauma has occurred.
- When the platelet count is low, spontaneous bleeding may occur.
- Bone marrow activity decreases by 50% in the elderly.
- Blood in the elderly coagulates more easily due to platelet *aggregation* (sticking together).
- Hemophilia, sickle cell disease, and certain types of anemias that cause blood disorders are inherited.
- Blood dyscrasias may be caused by drugs, radiation, or toxic substances (see Box 15–1).
- Nutritional deficiencies can cause anemia.
- The CBC with a differential count (count of the different types of white cells) can help diagnose many blood disorders (see Table 15–2).
- Bone marrow aspiration is used to diagnose a variety of blood disorders.
- A history is gathered and a focused physical assessment is performed for the patient with a suspected blood disorder (see Focused Assessments 15–1 and 15–2).
- There are common nursing diagnoses appropriate for the patient with a blood disorder (see Table 15–3).
- Preventing infection, conserving energy, controlling pain, and correcting the underlying cause are the goals of care for the patient with a blood disorder.
- Patients with blood disorders must be handled gently.
- Checking serial CBCs is part of the evaluation process.
- Methods to stop bleeding should be taught to patients and families.
- Self-care measures are taught to each patient to prevent infection.

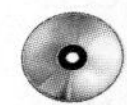

Go to your **Companion CD-ROM** for an Audio Glossary, animations, video clips, and bonus review questions.

evolve Be sure to visit the companion Evolve site at http://evolve.elsevier.com/deWit for interactive NCLEX-PN Exam Style Review Questions, WebLinks, and additional online resources.

NCLEX-PN EXAM STYLE REVIEW QUESTIONS

Choose the best answer(s) for the following questions.

1. For a patient with the clinical finding of leukocytosis, the nurse should:

1. initiate reverse isolation.
2. inspect for signs of active bleeding.
3. anticipate a physician order for antibiotic coverage.
4. schedule periods of rest and activity.

2. For an elderly patient admitted for recent falls, which of the following clinical findings are associated with the aging process? *(Select all that apply.)*

1. Decreased hematocrit
2. Decreased red blood cells
3. Prolonged prothrombin time
4. Increased neutrophils
5. Increased platelets

3. The physician informs the nurse that the patient has a "shift to the right." The nurse understands this to mean that the patient has a(n):

1. bleeding disorder.
2. folic acid deficiency anemia.
3. allergic reaction.
4. emerging infection.

4. To confirm the diagnosis of pernicious anemia, the patient is given an oral dose of radioactive vitamin B_{12}, followed 2 hours later by an intramuscular injection of vitamin B_{12}. A 24-hour urine specimen is also collected. This procedure is referred to as the:

1. Schilling test.
2. Bence Jones protein test.
3. erythrocyte sedimentation rate.
4. total iron-binding capacity.

5. The nurse describes the patient's skin as having a ruddy complexion with a red, florid appearance. The condition is most likely caused by:
   1. increased red blood cells.
   2. decreased platelets.
   3. increased basophils.
   4. decreased neutrophils.
6. The patient diagnosed with thrombocytopenic purpura has characteristic pinpoint lesions referred to as:
   1. ecchymosis.
   2. purpura.
   3. angioma.
   4. petechiae.
7. After removing a peripheral vascular access device, the nurse notes profuse bleeding at the site. An appropriate immediate nursing action would be to:
   1. tape a sterile dressing over the site.
   2. initiate request for blood transfusion.
   3. apply direct pressure.
   4. elevate the extremity.
8. The nurse taking care of an elderly female patient with pernicious anemia demonstrates understanding of the functional implications by:
   1. promoting rest.
   2. actively listening to the patient concerns.
   3. monitoring for bleeding.
   4. administering antibiotics.
9. The nurse initiates neutropenic precautions for a patient who has undergone chemotherapy. Which of the following are considered appropriate nursing actions? *(Select all that apply.)*
   1. Use clean technique for wound care and invasive procedures.
   2. Use protective isolation as needed.
   3. Allow visitors.
   4. Maintain integrity of skin and mucosa.
   5. Provide analgesics, as needed.
10. The nurse formulates the following patient goal statement: "The patient will have no new hematomas or other evidence of bleeding." An appropriate nursing intervention would be to:
    1. suggest the patient use a soft toothbrush.
    2. measure the patient's chest circumference daily.
    3. apply warm packs over hematoma sites.
    4. use a large-gauge needle for injections.

CRITICAL THINKING ACTIVITIES

Read each clinical scenario and discuss the questions with your classmates.

Scenario A

You come upon an automobile accident and stop to help.

1. The first victim has a gash in his thigh and blood is spurting at regular intervals from the wound. What method would you use to stop the bleeding?
2. The second victim has a bleeding wound on the forehead. What method would you use to stop the bleeding?

Scenario B

Mr. Jones has a disorder that has caused leukopenia. He lives alone. To prepare him for discharge home, you would need to provide teaching for him.

1. What would you teach him about preventing infection?
2. What would you suggest regarding visitors who wish to see him?
3. What would you tell him about performing necessary errands?

CHAPTER 16

Care of Patients with Hematologic Disorders

evolve http://evolve.elsevier.com/deWit

Objectives

Upon completing this chapter, you should be able to:

Theory

1. Identify the causes of the various types of anemias.
2. Develop a plan of care for the patient with an anemia.
3. Explain the pathophysiology and care of sickle cell disease.
4. Compare cell abnormalities of polycythemia vera to those of leukemia.
5. Formulate a teaching plan for the patient with leukemia.
6. Consider why multiple myeloma is a disease affecting older people.
7. Discuss the problems and treatments the hemophilia patient faces.

Clinical Practice

1. Considering the goals of care, write expected outcomes for each of the appropriate nursing diagnoses for a patient with a blood disorder.
2. Prepare to provide pre- and postprocedure care for the patient undergoing a bone marrow aspiration.
3. Perform an assessment on a patient with a suspected hematologic disorder.
4. Assist with the development of a plan of care for an adult with leukemia.
5. Assess for signs and symptoms of disseminated intravascular coagulation.

Key Terms

Be sure to check out the bonus material on the Companion CD-ROM, including selected audio pronunciations.

allogeneic (ĂL-ō-JĔN-ĭk, p. 397)
anemia (ă-NĒ-mē-ă, p. 376)
autologous (aw-TŎL-ō-gŭs, p. 393)
disseminated intravascular coagulation (dĭ-SĔM-ĭ-nāt-ĕd ĭn-tră-VĂS-cū-lăr kō-ăg-ū-LĀ-shŭn, p. 393)
ecchymosis (ĕk-ĭ-MŌ-sĭs, p. 390)
hemarthrosis (hē-măr-THRŌ-sĭs, p. 392)
hemoglobinuria (HĒ-mō-glō-bĭn-Ū-rē-ă, p. 395)
hemolysis (hē-MŎL-ĭ-sĭs, p. 377)
hypovolemia (hī-pō-vō-LĒ-mē-ă, p. 376)
leukapheresis (loo-kă-fĕ-RĒ-sĭs, p. 387)
purpura (PŬR-pū-ră, p. 390)
splenomegaly (splē-nō-MĔG-ă-lē, p. 386)
stomatitis (stō-mă-TĪ-tĭs, p. 388)
thrombocytopenia (thrŏm-bō-sīt-ō-PĒ-nē-ă, p. 390)

Disorders of the lymphatic system are presented in Chapter 11 along with the immune disorders since those systems function in conjunction with one another.

DISORDERS OF THE HEMATOLOGIC SYSTEM

ANEMIA

In a healthy person, a balance is maintained between the production of new red blood cells (RBCs) and the disposal of old "worn-out" cells. When something happens to upset this balance or interferes with maturation of cells, anemia results. **Anemia** is a state in which there are insufficient numbers of functioning RBCs, or a lack of hemoglobin, to meet the demands of the tissues for oxygen. When anemia occurs, there **are not enough healthy blood cells to carry sufficient oxygen throughout the body.**

Etiology

There are three major classifications of anemia according to cause:

- Anemia resulting from blood loss
- Anemia resulting from a failure in blood cell production
- Anemia associated with an excessive destruction of red cells

Rapid, severe bleeding leads to anemia from blood loss, **hypovolemia** (decreased volume of circulating blood), and potentially shock. The bleeding may be external, or it may be internal and therefore more difficult to detect. A blood loss that leads to anemia may result from severe trauma to the blood vessels and massive hemorrhage or may be more gradual, as from a small, bleeding peptic ulcer that causes a chronic blood loss.

The amount of blood loss that leads to hypovolemic shock varies depending on the ability of the patient's body to compensate for the lost fluid volume. A blood loss of even 500 mL in an adult who had normal circulating volume may cause hypovolemic shock. See Chapter 44 for the treatment of shock. Table 16–1 shows the amount of blood loss and consequent clinical manifestations.

Table 16–1 Clinical Manifestations of Acute Blood Loss

VOLUME LOST	CLINICAL MANIFESTATIONS
10%	None
20%	At rest, no signs or symptoms; slight postural hypotension when standing; tachycardia with exercise.
30%	Blood pressure and pulse normal when supine; postural hypotension and tachycardia with exercise.
40%	Below-normal blood pressure, central venous pressure, and cardiac output at rest; rapid, thready pulse and cold, clammy skin.
50%	Shock and potential death.

Adapted from Lewis, S.M., Heitkemper, M.M., Dirksen, S.R., et al. (2007). *Medical-Surgical Nursing: Assessment and Management of Clinical Problems* (7th ed.). St. Louis: Mosby, p. 695.

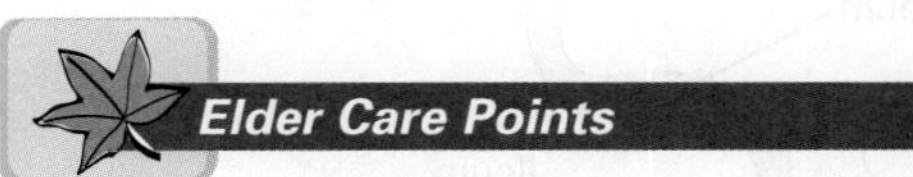

The elderly may develop shock with smaller blood loss because of decreased vascular tone and impaired cardiac function.

Anemia caused by a failure in cell production is the result of either a deficiency of certain substances necessary for the formation of RBCs or abnormal function of bone marrow. Examples of this type of anemia are:

- Nutritional anemia, in which there is an inadequate intake of foods containing proteins, folic acid, and iron
- Anemia resulting from bone marrow suppression by toxic substances
- Pernicious anemia, in which there is faulty absorption of specific nutrients, such as vitamin B_{12}

Iron or folic acid may not be well absorbed in people who have an intestinal malabsorption syndrome.

Hemolytic anemias, in which red cells are destroyed prematurely in the body, have many causes. They can be caused by genetic defects that affect cell structure, causing the cells to disintegrate quickly. Some of the hemolytic anemias, such as *thalassemia,* are inherited, whereas others are caused by exposure of the erythrocytes to poisonous agents, such as chemicals or certain bacterial toxins.

Immune reactions can cause blood cell **hemolysis** (destruction of red cells). The presence of toxins in the blood, infections such as malaria, transfusion reactions, and changes in blood chemistry may cause red cell hemolysis. Blood incompatibility in the newborn *(erythroblastosis fetalis)* is another cause.

Pathophysiology

Iron deficiency anemia occurs when total body iron is insufficient and erythropoiesis is diminished. The lack of iron impedes the formation of hemoglobin (Hb) (Concept Map 16–1).

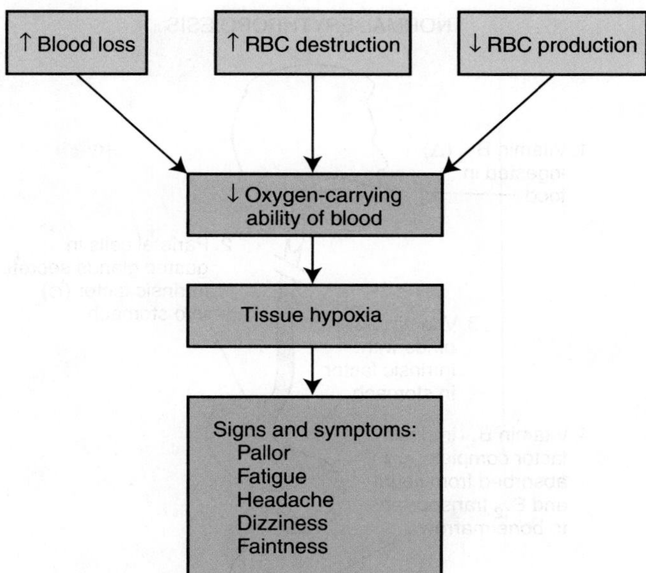

CONCEPT MAP **16–1** Pathophysiology of anemia.

In *pernicious anemia,* the intrinsic factor is missing from the gastric juices, and vitamin B_{12} is not absorbed without it. Vitamin B_{12} acts as a coenzyme in conjunction with folate metabolism and is important in the utilization of iron and protein for the manufacture of RBCs. The result of the missing intrinsic factor is that the red cell production is decreased, and those red cells that are produced are abnormal in structure and function (Figure 16–1). To correct this condition, the physician will order the administration of vitamin B_{12}. A folic acid deficiency also contributes to anemia (British Columbia Ministry of Health, 2006). 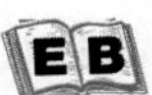

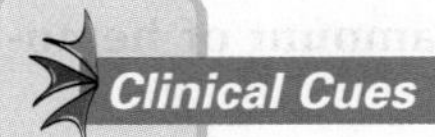

- If your patient has had gastric bypass surgery or a gastrectomy, there is a risk of pernicious anemia as there will be a decrease of available intrinsic factor. Observe for signs of pernicious anemia in this patient.
- Patients who take medications over a long period of time that suppress gastric acid secretion (histamine-2 inhibitors, proton pump inhibitors) must be watched for signs of pernicious anemia. Supplementation with vitamin B_{12} injections or sublingual vitamin B_{12} may help avoid this problem.

Hemolytic anemias associated with excessive destruction of RBCs are quite rare. When red cells are not normal, they break up easily or are destroyed by the body more quickly than normal red cells. This causes the anemia.

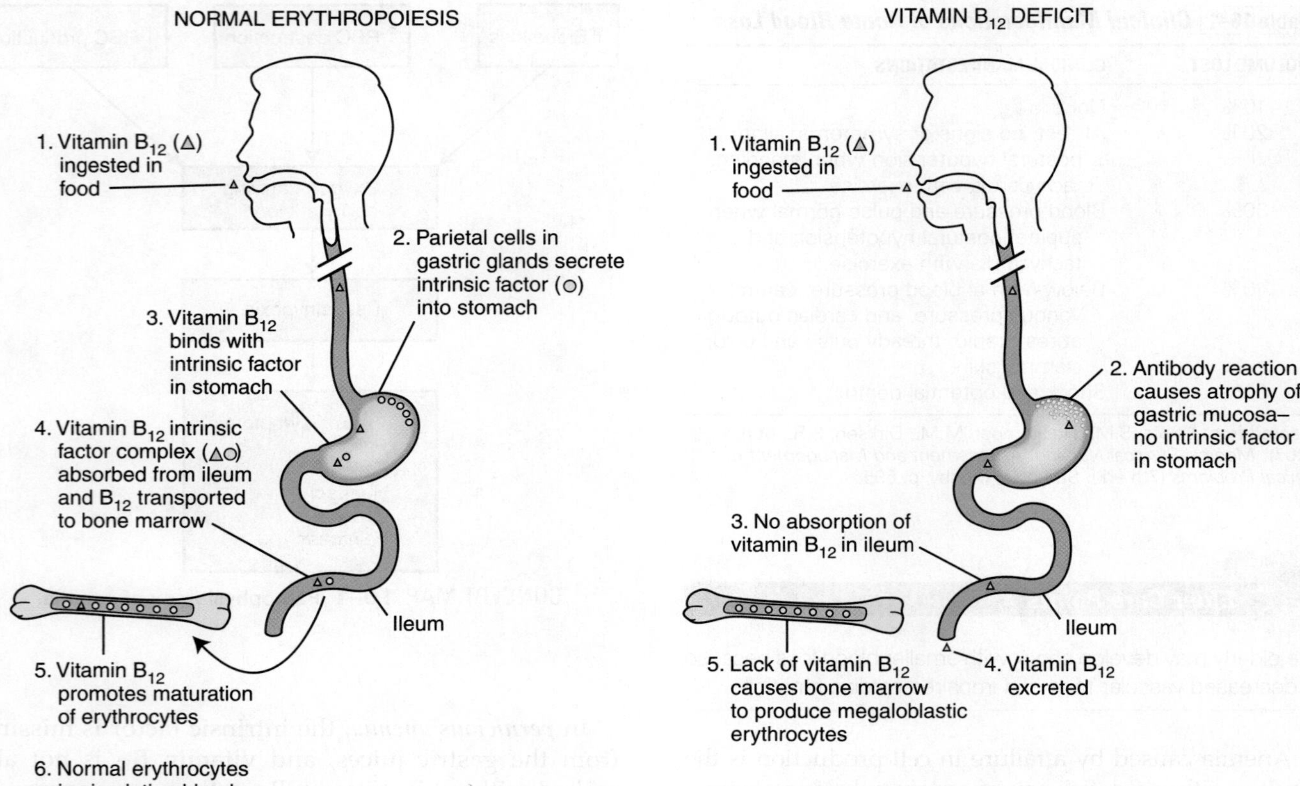

FIGURE 16–1 Development of pernicious anemia.

Anemia occurs in end-stage renal disease patients when there is a deficiency of production of *erythropoietin,* a substance necessary to stimulate the production of RBCs in the bone marrow. This problem is usually corrected by the administration of epoetin alfa (Epogen), which stimulates red cell production (Agency for Healthcare Research and Quality, 2001).

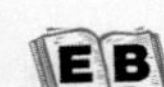

Oxygen transport depends on the number and condition of the red cells and the amount of hemoglobin they contain.

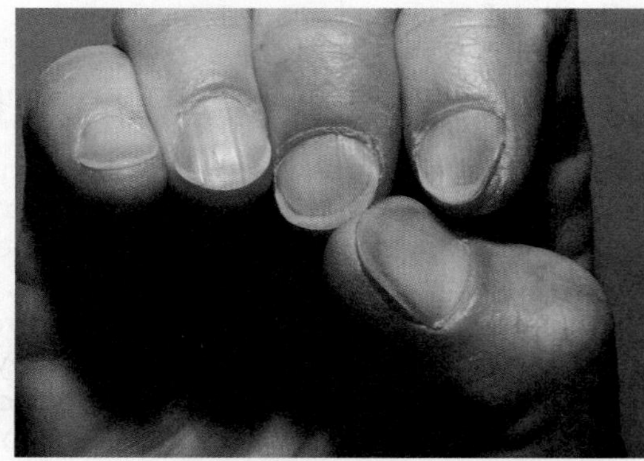

FIGURE 16–2 Thin, concave (spoon-shaped) nails with raised edges may be seen on people with iron deficiency anemia.

Signs and Symptoms

Signs and symptoms of anemias from causes other than rapid bleeding depend on whether the anemia is mild, moderate, or severe (Figure 16–2). Signs and symptoms of mild anemia (Hb 10 to 14 g/dL) are mild headache, palpitations, and dyspnea upon exertion. Moderate anemia (Hb 6 to 10 g/dL) may include pallor, fatigue, headache, and dizziness or faintness. Table 16–2 presents the many signs and symptoms of severe anemia. Tachypnea and tachycardia develop due to the decreased ability of the blood to transport sufficient oxygen to the tissues.

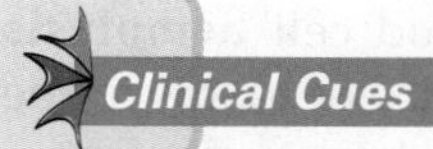

The classic signs and symptoms of hypovolemic shock are falling blood pressure; rapid, weak pulse; cool, damp skin; thirst; decreased urine output; and restlessness progressing to decreased consciousness.

Diagnosis

The microscopic appearance of the red cells on a film of blood that has been spread over a slide (a peripheral smear) gives information about abnormalities in size, shape, and color of erythrocytes circulating in the patient's bloodstream. The complete blood count (CBC) and differential cell count results are diagnostic when anemia is present. Measuring the quantity of hemoglobin tells whether the cells have sufficient amounts to carry adequate oxygen to the body.

Table 16–2 Signs and Symptoms of Severe Anemia

BODY SYSTEM	SIGNS AND SYMPTOMS
General	Sensitivity to cold, lethargy, weight loss
Eyes	Blurred vision, yellowing of conjunctiva and sclera, retinal hemorrhage
Skin	Pallor, pruritus, jaundice
Tongue	Glossitis, smooth tongue
Cardiovascular	Tachycardia, angina, systolic murmur, widened pulse pressure, intermittent claudication, CHF, possible MI
Respiratory	Tachypnea, orthopnea, dyspnea at rest
Gastrointestinal	Anorexia, difficulty swallowing, sore mouth, enlarged liver, enlarged spleen
Musculoskeletal	Bone pain
Neurologic	Headache, dizziness, impaired thinking, irritability, depression, fatigue

Key: *CHF,* congestive heart failure; *MI,* myocardial infarction.

The prefix *normo-* refers to normal, the suffix *-cyte* refers to cell, and the suffix *-chrom* refers to color. Thus a normocytic, normochromic anemia is characterized by cells that are normal in size and color but there is a deficiency in the number of RBCs and a low hematocrit. **This type of anemia usually occurs as a result of sudden blood loss.**

A hypochromic, microcytic anemia is characterized by decreased levels of hemoglobin (not enough color) and small (micro) cells. **This type of anemia is typical of an iron deficiency anemia.**

Treatment

Anemia from chronic, slow blood loss is treated by correcting the underlying problem and then building replacement blood cells. Anemia caused by inadequate iron, folic acid, or protein intake is managed with oral iron supplements, vitamins, and diet adjustment (Nutritional Therapies 16–1). If the anemia is serious, blood transfusions may be given, or iron supplementation may be administered intravenously (IV) with iron dextran (Imferon).

Pernicious anemia is treated by regular injections of vitamin B_{12}, as the deficiency of intrinsic factor prevents adequate absorption of this vitamin from food. There should be sufficient folic acid in the diet or it should be supplemented. Table 16–3 presents the medications most commonly prescribed for hematologic disorders.

For *hemolytic* anemia, the underlying cause is found and corrected if possible, and then the blood volume is rebuilt with added iron and appropriate diet. If the anemia is severe, blood transfusion may be indicated.

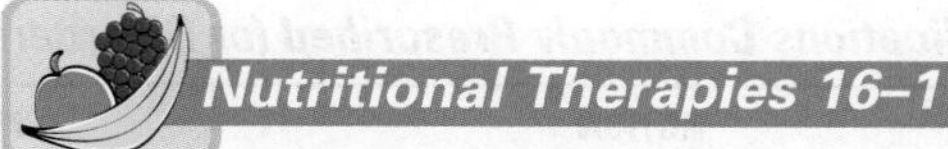

Common Foods High in Iron and Folic Acid

FOODS HIGH IN IRON

- Beef liver
- Blackstrap molasses
- Chicken livers
- Cooked oatmeal
- Cooked prunes
- Cooked shrimp
- Dried apricots
- Egg yolks
- Kidney beans
- Lean beef
- Lima beans
- Whole grains
- Prune juice
- Raisins
- Spinach and green leafy vegetables
- Turkey

Adding raw spinach to dinner salads and snacking on raisins or dried apricots can quickly improve iron intake. Iron-enriched cereals and breads also can be added to the diet.

FOODS HIGH IN FOLIC ACID

- Asparagus
- Beef
- Fish
- Cabbage
- Brussels sprouts
- Broccoli
- Legumes (kidney beans, etc.)
- Liver
- Eggs
- Whole grains

Note: Many of the foods high in iron also are high in folic acid.

? *Think Critically About . . .* Your patient who has suffered a blood loss and is now anemic complains that she is short of breath. Can you explain how blood loss might affect respiration?

NURSING MANAGEMENT

Assessment (Data Collection)

Whenever a patient presents with complaints of fatigue, headaches, or shortness of breath, anemia should always be considered. Besides the CBC results, data regarding physical signs and symptoms are collected (Focused Assessment 16–1, p. 382).

Nursing Diagnosis

Nursing diagnoses are chosen based on the clinical findings and problems identified. Common nursing diagnoses include:

- Activity intolerance related to weakness and fatigue

Table 16–3 Medications Commonly Prescribed for Disorders of the Hematologic System

CLASSIFICATION	ACTION	NURSING IMPLICATIONS	PATIENT TEACHING
MINERAL			
Ferrous sulfate (Feosol, Fer-in-Sol) Ferrous gluconate (Fergon) Ferrous fumarate (Feostat, Ircon) Iron dextran (Imferon)	Increases elemental iron as a component in the formation of hemoglobin. Used to treat iron deficiency anemia.	May cause GI upset: nausea, diarrhea, or constipation; monitor for constipation. Tell patient that oral form will turn stool black. Do not give with milk as it reduces absorption. Dilute elixir in juice and give through a straw to prevent staining of the teeth. Do not crush enteric-coated or sustained-release tablets or capsules. For IM form, give with at least a 3-inch, 19- to 20-gauge needle and use Z-track technique to prevent staining of the skin. Change needles after drawing up the solution. When given IV, monitor closely for anaphylactic reaction. Flush line with 10 mL saline postinfusion.	Take oral form with orange juice or other vitamin C–rich food. Avoid taking iron with milk products. Keep out of reach of children as it is toxic. Have Hb checked according to physician's schedule to check response to medication. Eat foods high in iron. Increase fluids and roughage if constipation occurs.
VITAMINS			
Folic acid (Folvite)	Promotes normal erythropoiesis; used in certain types of anemia.	May interfere with anticonvulsant blood levels. Chloramphenicol interferes with absorption. Increase foods high in folic acid.	Have blood count monitored according to physician's schedule to determine effectiveness of therapy.
Vitamin B_{12} Cyanocobalamin (Rubramin, Anacobin)	Acts as coenzyme for cell replication and hematopoiesis. Used in pernicious anemia, other GI disorders that decrease vitamin B_{12} absorption, and cases of dietary deficiency.	Give Subcut or IM daily for 5–10 days and then once monthly for maintenance. Can cause anaphylactic reaction when given IV. Deficiency more common in strict vegetarians.	Teach importance of maintaining monthly injections for life for prevention of further episodes of pernicious anemia. Encourage increased intake of vitamin B_{12} in diet if deficiency is diet related.
ANTIMETABOLITE			
Hydroxyurea (Hydrea)	Inhibits DNA synthesis. Used to reduce episodes of sickling in sickle cell anemia. Used to eradicate abnormal cells in leukemia, myeloma, and some solid tumors.	Discontinue if WBC count is $<2500/mm^3$ or platelet count is $>100,000/mm^3$. Capsule granules may be mixed with water if taken immediately. May cause GI problems: stomach upset, stomatitis, vomiting, diarrhea.	Use cautiously in presence of renal dysfunction. Radiation therapy increases toxicity. Monitor intake and output. Monitor for infection. Monitor blood counts for neutropenia and thrombocytopenia; bone marrow suppression. Caution to avoid exposure to infection and to report signs or symptoms of infection promptly. Increase fluid intake to maintain adequate hydration. Give mouth care q 4 hr to prevent stomatitis. Report bleeding to the physician.

Key: *BP,* blood pressure; *CBC,* complete blood count; *GI,* gastrointestinal; *Hb,* hemoglobin; *HIV,* human immunodeficiency virus; *IM,* intramuscularly; *IV,* intravenously; *RBCs,* red blood cells; *Subcut,* subcutaneously; *WBCs,* white blood cells.

Table 16–3 ***Medications Commonly Prescribed for Disorders of the Hematologic System—cont'd***

CLASSIFICATION	ACTION	NURSING IMPLICATIONS	PATIENT TEACHING
BIOLOGIC RESPONSE MODIFIERS			
Epoetin alfa; erythropoietin (Epogen, Procrit)	Controls rate of red cell production; a natural hormone produced by recombinant DNA techniques. Stimulates the bone marrow, functioning as a growth factor. Used to combat reduced production of erythropoietin in end-stage renal disease. Used as adjunct therapy in HIV-infected patients with anemia secondary to drug therapy.	Also used for patients with anemia secondary to chemotherapy and in rheumatoid arthritis patients who experience anemia from therapy. May be used to increase RBCs in anticipation of autologous blood transfusion before surgery.	May cause seizures. Monitor blood count closely; dosage may need to be reduced if hematocrit rises too rapidly. Monitor blood pressure closely; may cause rise. May cause pain in limbs and pelvis. Explain the purpose of the injections. Remind that the drug must be refrigerated; discard after 6 hr at room temperature.
Filgrastim (Neupogen)	Stimulates production, maturation, and activation of neutrophils.	CBC with differential before beginning therapy and twice weekly thereafter. Monitor BP as may cause transient increase.	Teach to inform physician if fever, chills, severe bone pain, chest pain, or palpitations occur.
Pegfilgrastim (Neulasta)	Regulates production of neutrophils within bone marrow. Increases phagocytic activity.	CBC and differential before therapy and routinely thereafter. Monitor for allergic reaction (i.e., peripheral edema). Assess muscle strength. Observe mouth for stomatitis, mucositis.	Inform of possible side effects and how to watch for allergic reaction. Remind that regular blood counts are important.
Chemotherapy drugs are presented in Chapter 8.			

- Impaired gas exchange related to decreased hemoglobin
- Imbalanced nutrition: less than body requirements related to poor nutritional intake and anorexia
- Ineffective therapeutic regimen management related to lack of knowledge about appropriate nutrition and medication regimen

Planning

Expected outcomes are written for the specific individual nursing diagnoses chosen to resolve the patient's problems. For the nursing diagnoses listed above, they might include:

- Patient will be able to perform hygiene, dressing, and grooming activities without needing to rest between activities within 1 month.
- Patient will be able to carry out usual daily activities without shortness of breath or fatigue within 2 months.
- Patient will eat three nutritious meals containing sufficient iron, folic acid, vitamin C, and protein daily.
- Patient will verbalize understanding of dietary and medication regimen within 1 week.

Implementation

Intervention begins with an understanding of the particular kind of anemia affecting the patient. Anemia from blood loss presents problems quite different from those related to chronic, and possibly incurable, aplastic or hemolytic anemia.

Actions are directed toward preventing complications for patients with anemias that interfere with clotting and tend to cause bleeding episodes. Assistance with activities of daily living is essential for any patient with anemia severe enough to cause fatigue. Planned rest periods must be provided for these patients.

Administering blood, iron, vitamin B_{12}, and folic acid and monitoring for desired effect are nursing functions. Patient education about needed dietary adjustments also is done. Nutritional Therapies 16–1 provides suggestions for increasing iron and folic acid. **Patients should be taught that iron is absorbed more readily if vitamin C is present in the gastrointestinal (GI) system at the same time.** Taking iron medication with orange juice provides the necessary vitamin C.

Elder Care Points

- Iron supplements should be taken 1 hour before or 2 hours after a meal, as long as they don't cause GI distress.
- Many elderly people have chronic conditions that require daily medication. Antacids and many other drugs interfere with iron absorption.
- Check all drugs a patient is receiving to determine whether drug interactions might interfere with iron absorption.

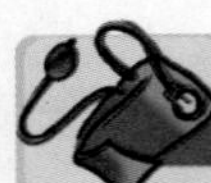

Focused Assessment 16–1

Data Collection When Anemia Is Suspected

Gather the following data:

HEALTH HISTORY

- Have you had any recent blood loss or trauma?
- Do you have chronic liver, endocrine, gastrointestinal, or renal disease?
- What medications, vitamins, supplements, or herbal products do you take?
- What surgeries have you had and when?
- Have you ever had radiation treatments or chemotherapy?
- Is there a history of genetic blood disorders in your family?
- Has your appetite or weight changed?
- Have you noticed any changes in your urine or stool?
- Are you experiencing shortness of breath, weakness, or fatigue?
- Have you noticed any heart palpitations?
- Do you get frequent headaches?
- Have you noticed any changes in vision or dizziness?
- Do you have pain or itching anywhere?
- Do you become cold when others are not?

PHYSICAL ASSESSMENT

Check for the following:

- **Skin:** Pale skin and mucous membranes; pale conjunctiva, yellowing of sclera; cracks in lips; brittle, spoon-shaped fingernails; jaundice; petechiae; ecchymoses; dry, brittle, thinning hair
- **Respiratory:** Tachypnea, orthopnea, dyspnea upon exertion or at rest
- **Cardiac:** Tachycardia, systolic murmur, angina, ankle edema
- **Gastrointestinal:** Sore mouth, stomatitis, beefy red tongue, abdominal distention, enlarged liver or spleen
- **Neurologic:** Headache, dizziness, confusion, irritability, *ataxia* (unsteady gait), paresthesia

PERTINENT LABORATORY VALUES

- CBC, serum iron, ferritin, folate, cobalamin (vitamin B_{12}), stool for guaiac, urinalysis, serum erythropoietin

Analgesia for headache or joint pain is given as ordered, and the patient is monitored for adverse side effects. More nursing diagnoses commonly associated with hematologic problems, including anemia, and lists of appropriate interventions are included in Table 15–3.

Evaluation

Evaluation data are gathered to determine whether expected outcomes are being met. Laboratory values are particularly important when evaluating the care of the patient with anemia. However, data showing that the problems caused by the anemia are resolving are equally important.

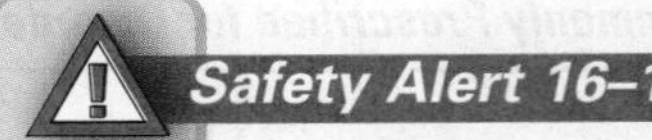

Safety Alert 16–1

Monitor Drug Side Effects

It is your responsibility to monitor blood studies carefully for all patients who are receiving any drug that is potentially damaging to the bone marrow.

APLASTIC ANEMIA

Etiology and Pathophysiology

Aplastic anemia, a rare disorder, may develop after a viral infection, as a reaction to a drug, or because of an inherited tendency. **The disease is characterized by bone marrow depression and is thought to probably be an immune-mediated disease. Red cells, white cells, and platelet levels are decreased.** The toxic effects of certain substances can be responsible for aplastic anemia. Some of these agents include benzene; insecticides; drugs, such as chloramphenicol (Chloromycetin), phenylbutazone (Butazolidin), and sulfonamides; some anticonvulsants; gold compounds used to treat rheumatoid arthritis; and alkylating agents or antimetabolites used in chemotherapy (Safety Alert 16–1). Many other drugs can cause aplastic anemia, but this adverse effect is rare. Radiation exposure is another factor in the development of the disorder.

Impairment or failure of bone marrow function leading to the loss of stem cells is the cause of aplastic anemia (Concept Map 16–2). The bone marrow has decreased cells and increased fatty tissue.

Signs and Symptoms

Signs and symptoms are the same as those of iron deficiency anemia, but also include ecchymosis, petechiae, and hemorrhage related to low platelet count. Infection is frequent and may not cause an inflammatory response because of the very low leukocyte count. There is often frequent bleeding in the mouth.

Diagnosis and Treatment

Diagnosis is by blood count with differential, bone marrow biopsy, and ruling out other disorders. **Aplastic anemia causes an emergency situation.**

Treatment must eliminate any identifiable underlying cause. Packed red cells and platelets are administered. Protective isolation is no longer considered necessary to prevent infection in patients with low leukocyte counts (Mank & Van der Lelie, 2003). Antibiotics are given for identified infection; oxygen is sometimes administered to patients with low erythrocyte counts. Bone marrow transplantation (BMT) is the treatment of choice for those under 45 years of age with severe bone marrow depression, but there must be an identical human leukocyte antigen (HLA) match.

Immunosuppressive therapy with antithymocyte globulin (ATG) and cyclosporine is showing promise

```
Toxic drugs      Toxic chemicals      Radiation
        \              |              /
         Damaged bone marrow
                 |
 Inability to produce adequate normal erythrocytes,
        leukocytes, or platelets
                 |
 Anemia, neutropenia, and thrombocytopenia
                 |
         Infection, bleeding
                 |
               Death
```

CONCEPT MAP **16-2** Pathophysiology of aplastic anemia.

at improving outcomes. ATG contains polyclonal antibodies against human T cells.

Think Critically About . . . What chemical products in your home or garage are capable of causing bone marrow depression? (Read the labels)

Nursing Management

Prevention of hemorrhage and infection is a top priority. Psychological support of the patient and family is important when they are faced with this life-threatening condition. Nursing diagnoses might include:

- Activity intolerance related to fatigue from oxygen deficiency to tissues
- Risk of injury related to potential bleeding
- Deficient knowledge related to the disease process and treatment
- Anxiety related to potential death
- Risk of infection related to low leukocytes
- Ineffective coping related to treatment of the disease

Safety measures are priorities (Health Promotion Points 16–1). Actions for problems of weakness and fatigue are the same as those presented for anemia earlier in the chapter. Other common nursing actions are included in Table 15–3 in Chapter 15. Precautions and actions for the patient with leukopenia/neutropenia are presented in Patient Teaching 16–1 (Shelton, 2003). For

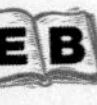

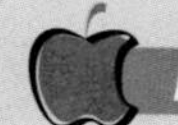

Health Promotion Points 16–1

Dangers of Toxic Agents

All nurses should promote public education about the dangers of toxic agents. It is vitally important that people read and follow the label instructions on all cleaning agents, insecticides, and chemical compounds.

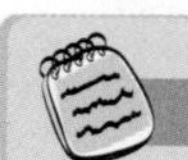

Patient Teaching 16–1

Leukopenia/Neutropenia—Prevention of Infection

Teach the patient the following:

- Perform hand hygiene frequently; use liquid soap or alcohol based hand rub.
- Perform hand hygiene as soon as you return from an outing, after touching a pet, or after shaking hands with someone.
- Dishes should be washed in hot soapy water or put through a dishwasher.
- Do not reuse a dish, cup, utensil, or glass without washing it.
- Drink only water that is fresh or from a fresh bottle.
- Avoid crowds and large gatherings where people might be ill.
- Avoid bacteria-containing foods such as raw milk, salad greens, and raw fruits and vegetables.
- Keep plants and flowers out of the immediate environment because of the bacteria and mold they carry.
- Run cutting boards through the dishwasher after cutting meat or produce that contains bacteria; obtain a bacteria-resistant cutting board.
- Eat meat that has been cooked well-done.
- Use only your own towels and washcloths.
- Bathe daily if possible.
- Clean your toothbrush daily by soaking in a 1:10 solution of bleach and water and then rinsing well, or by running it through the dishwasher.
- Wash the rectal area after each bowel movement with warm water and soap. Pat dry.
- Take your temperature twice a day and record it.
- Report to your physician
  - Elevated temperature greater than 100° F (38° C)
  - Foul-smelling drainage from any body opening or open skin lesion
  - Persistent cough
  - Cloudy or foul-smelling urine or burning upon urination
- Do not work with houseplants or dig in the garden.
- Do not clean the cat's litter box or clean up after any animal.
- Do not let pets lick you or sleep on your bed or chair.
- Do not share personal articles with others (toothbrush, razor, toothpaste, deodorant, hairbrush, bar soap, etc.)
- Obtain sufficient sleep and rest.
- Eat a well-balanced, adequate diet, if possible.
- Take your medications as prescribed.

Patient Teaching 16–2

Thrombocytopenia Safety Measures

Teach the patient to:

- Use a soft toothbrush and brush teeth gently; do not floss teeth.
- Use an electric razor only.
- Apply ice immediately to any bump or scrape.
- Avoid intramuscular injections.
- Observe for blood in the stool or urine; report its presence.
- Measure the abdominal girth daily.
- Avoid chewing on hard foods.
- Be sure dentures fit well.
- Avoid dental work, especially extractions.
- Avoid contact sports.
- Wear shoes with firm soles whenever walking.
- Be careful to avoid injury.
- Promptly report oozing of blood or frank bleeding.

safety measures when thrombocytopenia is present see Patient Teaching 16–2.

SICKLE CELL DISEASE

Etiology

Sickle cell disease is a genetic disorder in which the gene is inherited from both parents (homozygous gene). It is characterized by erythrocytes that contain more hemoglobin S than hemoglobin A. Sickle cell disease is found in less than 1% of African American newborns, but also affects some people whose ancestors were from the Mediterranean region, the Middle East, and India. Approximately 8% of African Americans carry the gene.

Sickle cell trait, in which only about 50% of an individual's total hemoglobin is affected, is present in about 10% of the African American population of the United States. The trait is heterozygous, meaning that the person has an inherited gene for the trait from one parent only. These people are carriers and can transmit the gene to their children even when they don't show signs of the disease. Therefore, genetic counseling and adequate screening for early detection of the disease are considered extremely important to control sickle cell anemia. Approximately 50% of patients with sickle cell disease do not survive beyond age 20, and the rest usually die by age 50.

Pathophysiology

When the patient with sickle cell disease experiences lower oxygenation than normal, the defective S hemoglobin forms clumps in the red cells, causing them to assume a sickle shape, blocking blood vessels, breaking apart, and forming thrombi that cause organ damage (Figure 16–3). Sickle cells are destroyed by the body very quickly, causing anemia.

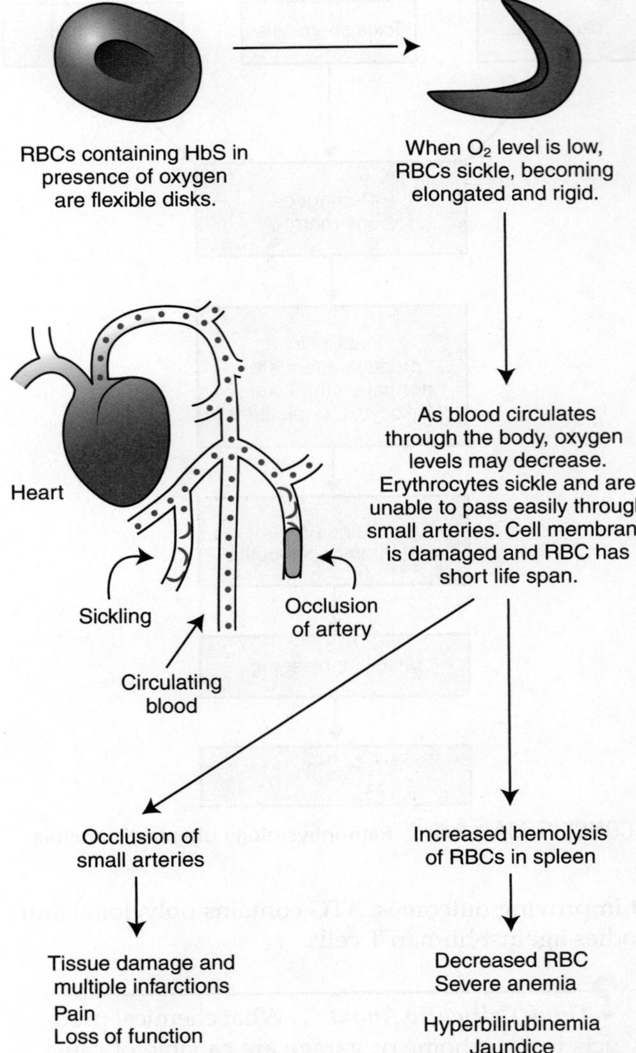

FIGURE **16–3** Sickle cell anemia and the effects of sickling.

Sickle cell trait occurs in people who have only one gene, rather than a pair of genes, for sickle cell anemia. They usually do not have problems with cells assuming a sickle shape unless they experience severe oxygen deficiency. Table 16–4 compares the four major types of anemia in this chapter.

Signs and Symptoms

The signs and symptoms of sickle cell disease are those that indicate lack of oxygen and blood flow, such as pallor, lethargy, and pain. The problems from interrupted normal blood flow affect many organs (Figure 16–4). Painful swelling of the hands and feet related to bone infarction from the sickled cells (hand-foot syndrome) may occur. After sickle cell crisis, signs typical of anemia occur because the abnormally shaped cells are very fragile, break easily, and are destroyed. The RBC and hemoglobin counts can drop very quickly during a crisis.

Table 16–4 Comparison of Four Types of Anemia

ANEMIA	CHARACTERISTIC RBC	ETIOLOGY	ADDITIONAL EFFECTS
Iron deficiency anemia	Microcytic, hypochromic Decreased hemoglobin production	Decreased dietary intake, malabsorption, blood loss	Only effects of anemia
Pernicious anemia	Megaloblasts, immature nucleated cells	Deficit of intrinsic factor due to immune reaction	Neurologic damage Achlorhydria
Aplastic anemia	Often normal cells Pancytopenia	Bone marrow damage or failure	Excessive bleeding and multiple infections
Sickle cell anemia	RBC elongates and hardens in "sickle" shape when O_2 levels are low—short life span	Recessive inheritance	Painful crises with multiple infarctions Hyperbilirubinemia

Key: *RBC*, red blood cell.
From Gould, B.E. (2006). *Pathophysiology for the Health Professions* (3rd ed.). Philadelphia: Saunders.

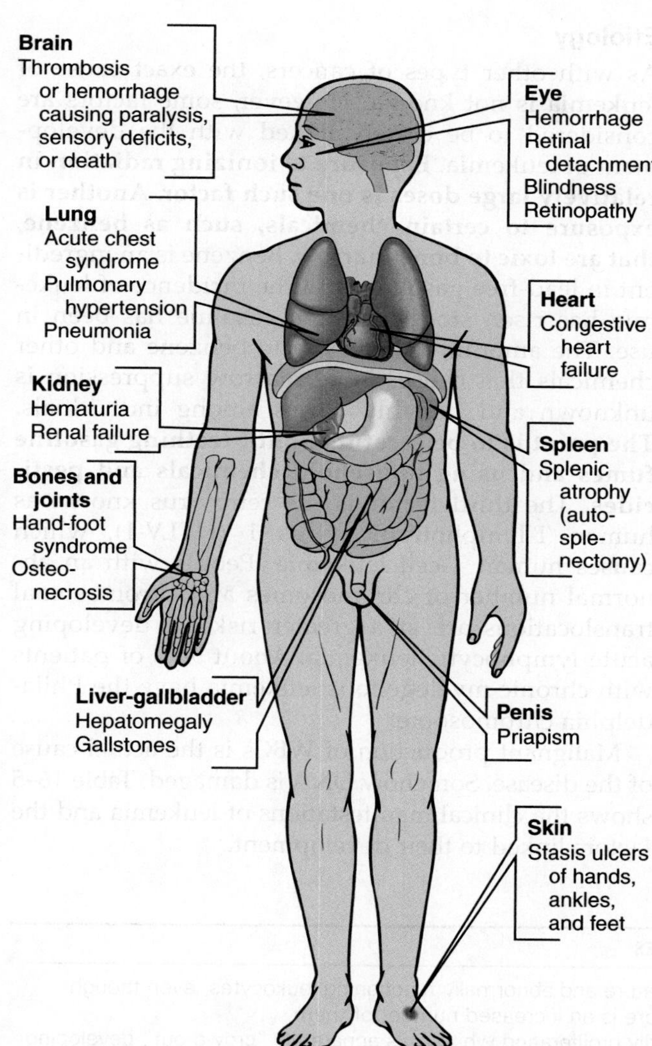

FIGURE **16–4** Clinical manifestations and complications of sickle cell disease.

Diagnosis

A peripheral blood smear can show sickled cells. The sickling test, which exposes RBCs to a deoxygenating agent, is diagnostic. Hemoglobin electrophoresis identifies the presence of abnormal hemoglobin. During crisis, there will be elevations of serum bilirubin because of the hemolysis of the abnormal red cells. Bone and joint abnormalities are revealed by skeletal x-rays.

Treatment

There is no cure or specific treatment for sickle cell anemia; treatment is primarily symptomatic and preventive. Patients should be taking folic acid regularly and eating a diet with sufficient protein to help build red cells. Infection is to be avoided, and the patient should receive all recommended immunizations against influenza, hepatitis A and B, pneumonia, tetanus, and the like. Adequate intake of fluid on a daily basis is important to keep the blood as fluid as possible. Alcohol and recreational drugs are to be avoided. Quick attention for illness should be sought.

The drug hydroxyurea (Hydrea) has been found to reduce the frequency of sickling episodes. Patients on this drug have shown a 50% decrease in the number of hospitalizations for crisis. Should crisis occur, the patient is often treated at home with bed rest, adequate fluid intake, and analgesics. During a crisis, careful attention must be paid to pain control. Narcotic analgesia is administered on a continuous basis, usually by patient-controlled analgesia pump, while the patient is in crisis. If the patient's hemoglobin drops considerably or her condition suddenly deteriorates, she is hospitalized, given oxygen, and transfused with packed red cells. In addition, IV fluids are given. An attempt is made to mobilize the sickled cells and to prevent damage to major organs. Infection is treated with appropriate antibiotics.

There are many complications of sickle cell disease including cholecystitis, stroke, congestive heart failure, and damage to all major organs. One of the most common problems is leg ulcers from impaired circulation to the legs and feet. Protecting the feet and lower legs from injury is important, since small wounds tend to develop into difficult-to-heal ulcers.

BMT is the only available treatment that can cure some patients. The scarcity of donors, the cost, and the risks involved greatly limit the use of this option. Gene therapy is offering hope for future treatment of sickle cell disease.

Nursing Management

Nursing care is aimed at relieving the symptoms from complications of the disease and minimizing organ damage. Patients are taught to avoid high altitudes, vigorous exercise, and iced liquids; to maintain adequate fluid intake; not to smoke; and to obtain treatment for infections promptly. Adequate rest is important as patients with sickle cell anemia experience fatigue. During an acute crisis, the patient will receive continuous IV pain relief. **Assessment for adequate pain relief is a top priority** (American Pain Association, 1999). Intake and output will be monitored to prevent overloading the patient with fluid. Oxygen therapy is instituted if the patient is hypoxic. This helps prevent further cellular damage.

POLYCYTHEMIA VERA

Excessive production of RBCs results in polycythemia vera. White cell numbers also increase, but not to the degree that they do in leukemia. The cause of this disorder is unknown, but it is considered a neoplastic disorder. The blood becomes thick from the increased numbers of cells, blood vessels become distended, and blood flow is sluggish. Because of the sluggish flow, there is a tendency to develop blood clots. Blood pressure is elevated and the heart hypertrophies. Hemorrhage is frequent in areas of distended blood vessels. Signs and symptoms include a reddish face with deep-red purplish lips, fatigue, weakness, dizziness, headache, enlarged spleen **(splenomegaly)**, and congested liver. Minor injury may result in excessive bleeding.

Treatment is aimed at reducing the number of blood cells. Phlebotomy, antineoplastic agents, and radiation therapy are all used. In phlebotomy, a blood vessel is pierced, and blood is drawn off. As much as 500 mL of blood at a time may be withdrawn every 2 to 3 months. Increased fluid intake is essential to decrease blood viscosity, and aspirin is used to decrease platelet clumping and clot formation.

A secondary polycythemia may develop in response to prolonged hypoxia and increased erythropoietin secretion. It does not have the same effects as primary polycythemia.

LEUKEMIA

The word *leukemia*, translated literally, means "white blood." Actually, the white blood cells (WBCs) would have to number 1,000,000/mm^3 before the blood would have a milky white appearance, and, although leukemia is characterized by an increase in the number of leukocytes, their number rarely rises above 500,000/mm^3. In addition to the increase in number, however, **the leukocytes of the patient with leukemia are abnormal cells that do not function as normal white cells do.**

Etiology

As with other types of cancers, the exact cause of leukemia is not known. However, some factors are considered to be closely linked with the development of leukemia. **Exposure to ionizing radiation in relatively large doses is one such factor. Another is exposure to certain chemicals, such as benzene, that are toxic to bone marrow.** Benzene is an ingredient in lead-free gasoline, and the incidence of leukemia has risen since lead-free gasoline has been in use. The amount of exposure to benzene and other chemicals that causes bone marrow suppression is unknown and possibly varies among individuals. **The point is to be careful about breathing gasoline fumes and using household chemicals and pesticides.** The third factor is the retrovirus known as human T-lymphotropic virus 1 (HTLV-1), which causes human T-cell leukemia. People with an abnormal number of chromosomes and chromosomal translocations are at a greater risk for developing acute lymphocytic leukemia. About 90% of patients with chronic myelogenous leukemia have the Philadelphia chromosome.

Malignant production of WBCs is the actual cause of the disease. Somehow DNA is damaged. Table 16–5 shows the clinical manifestations of leukemia and the factors linked to their development.

Table 16–5 *Causes of Clinical Signs of Leukemia*

MANIFESTATIONS	CAUSES
Severe infections	Immature and abnormally functioning leukocytes, even though there is an increased number of them.
Symptoms of anemia	Rapidly proliferating white cells apparently "crowd out" developing red cells and platelets.
Enlarged spleen, liver, and lymph nodes	Excess white cells accumulate within organs, causing distention of tissues.
Weakness, pallor, and weight loss due to elevated metabolic rate	Increased production of white cells requires large amounts of amino acids and vitamins. Increased destruction of cells leads to more metabolic wastes that must be disposed of by the body.
Renal pain, urinary stones and obstruction to flow of urine, and urinary tract infection	Large amounts of uric acid are released when white cells are destroyed by antileukemic drugs.
Headache, disorientation, and other central nervous system symptoms	Abnormal white cells infiltrate the central nervous system.

Pathophysiology

An acute leukemia is one in which there are a large number of primitive cells, called blasts. In chronic leukemia, the predominant cells are more mature. Leukemias are also classified by the origin of the abnormal cells. *Myeloid leukemia* arises from the bone marrow, whereas *lymphoid leukemia* has its origin in the lymphatic system. There are four types of leukemia: acute myelogenous leukemia (AML), chronic myelogenous leukemia (CML), acute lymphocytic leukemia (ALL), and chronic lymphocytic leukemia (CLL).

About 44,240 people will develop leukemia in 2007 and 21,790 people in the United States will have died from it. In acute leukemia there is a sudden, rapid growth of immature blast or stem cells, rapid progression of the disease, and a short survival if the disease is not treated.

Chronic forms of leukemia have a more gradual onset, slower disease progression, and a relatively longer survival time. **CLL is common in men over age 50 and accounts for one third of the new cases of leukemia annually.** CML is most common in young and middle-aged adults. Over time it progresses to the acute form, and eventual death is common.

Leukemia has three major effects:

- Increased numbers of abnormal, immature leukocytes
- Accumulations of these cells within the lymph nodes, spleen, and other organs
- Eventual infiltration of the malignant cells throughout the organs of the body

Signs, Symptoms, and Diagnosis

Patients with chronic leukemias are often asymptomatic, and the disease is detected during a regular physical examination and routine CBC. Signs and symptoms of other leukemias include fever, malaise, frequent infections or infections that won't go away (sore throat, flu, etc.), swollen lymph nodes, enlarged spleen, bone pain, weight loss, and easy bleeding or thrombosis.

Diagnosis is made by history, physical examination, CBC with differential, and bone marrow studies to rule out other disorders.

Treatment

Treatment is aimed at:

- Slowing down the growth of the malignant blood cells
- Maintaining a normal level of red cells, hemoglobin, and platelets
- Managing the symptoms and meeting the special needs of each patient

Acute leukemia treatment consists primarily of chemotherapy with a combination of antineoplastic agents targeted at different phases of the cell cycle. The drug therapy is divided into three phases: induction, consolidation, and maintenance. *Remission induction* therapy is initiated at the time of diagnosis and consists of an intensive combination chemotherapy aimed at achieving a complete remission of symptoms. *Consolidation* therapy is another course of the same agents, or others, at a different dosage level, and the goal is cure. *Maintenance therapy* is usually oral chemotherapy at lesser doses taken for 2 to 5 years to maintain remission.

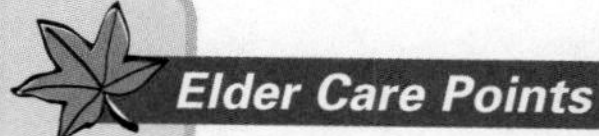

Elder Care Points

Patients over the age of 65 require reduced doses of chemotherapeutic drugs to prevent toxicity because they have decreased kidney and liver function and the drugs are not metabolized as quickly as in a younger person.

Before chemotherapy is started, the patient should be well hydrated and given allopurinol orally to prevent hyperuricemia and kidney stones.

Radiation therapy is used supplementally to increase the success of treatment and to decrease discomfort from enlarged organs (spleen, liver). Cure is sometimes possible, as has been evidenced in children with ALL. Results in adults have not been as good. BMT is a possibility for patients who have had an initial remission with chemotherapy. Eventually it is hoped that monoclonal antibody treatment can be combined with BMT to provide lasting remission (see the section on therapies frequently used in the management of hematologic disorders later in this chapter).

Chronic lymphocytic leukemia (CLL), the most common leukemia in the elderly, is not treated until the patient experiences symptoms. At that time a combination of chemotherapy agents is used.

Chronic myelogenous leukemia (CML) is currently treated with imatinib (Gleevec). Trials using a combination of imatinib with other agents are underway with the hope that the response rate and duration of remission will be enhanced. Recombinant human alpha interferon has been shown to reduce the growth and division of leukemic cells in 55% to 60% of patients. Hydroxurea (Hydrea) may be used as a single chemotherapeutic agent. **Leukapheresis** (separation of white cells) may be done to reduce the massive number of circulating leukocytes that clog organs and cause damage. Blood is drawn and the unwanted white cells are separated out, and the remainder is returned to the patient. A small percentage of patients are likely candidates for BMT.

Transfusions of blood components are prescribed to maintain a near-normal blood picture. Platelet transfusion during or after chemotherapy often is necessary. Antibiotics may be given prophylactically during chemotherapy and are started immediately upon signs of infection because the body's defense mechanisms are seriously compromised.

Box 16–1 lists the chemotherapy agents used to treat the various types of leukemia.

Box 16–1 ***Chemotherapeutic Agents Used to Treat Leukemia***

CHRONIC LYMPHOCYTIC LEUKEMIA
- Chlorambucil
- Fludarabine
- Cyclophosphamide
- Vincristine
- Prednisone

CHRONIC MYELOGENOUS LEUKEMIA
- Imatinib
- Hydroxyurea
- Interferon alfa

ACUTE MYELOGENOUS LEUKEMIA
- Cytosine arabinoside
- Anthracycline

ACUTE LYMPHOCYTIC LEUKEMIA/ACUTE LYMPHOBLASTIC LEUKEMIA
- Daunorubicin
- Vincristine
- Prednisone
- L-Asparaginase
- Cyclophosphamide
- Cytarabine
- 6-Mercaptopurine
- Methotrexate
- Cytosine arabinoside
- Clofarabine
- Nelarabine

Nursing Management

A thorough health assessment is performed and specific problems are identified. Nursing diagnoses for the patient with leukemia include those appropriate for anemia, leukopenia, and thrombocytopenia. Nursing problems to be addressed are:

- Potential for infection
- Abnormal bleeding
- Anemia
- Nutritional alteration with severe anorexia and weight loss
- Increased levels of uric acid in the urine and blood (due to chemotherapy)
- Psychosocial problems related to the effects of the disease as well as the prescribed treatment

Collaboration with the dietitian as well as the pharmacist is a key point in nursing care of the leukemic patient. Nursing Care Plan 16–1 presents care for common problems of the leukemia patient.

Infections from bacteria, viruses, and fungi are the most common cause of death in people with leukemia. Infection is a threat to the patient with leukemia either because of abnormal function of bone marrow that is characteristic of the disease or because of suppression of bone marrow function as a result of therapy. Nursing measures to prevent infection are essential, as is vigilant assessment for early signs. Patient Teaching 16–1 includes measures for the patient at risk for infection due to the effects of chemotherapy or radiation.

Abnormal bleeding as a result of a very low platelet count is the second most common and dangerous complication of leukemia. Observation of the patient, awareness of her current platelet count, and prevention of trauma to body tissues and blood vessels are primary concerns in nursing management. See Patient Teaching 16–2 for guidelines for the patient prone to bleeding.

Elder Care Points

- The elderly patient already has decreased immune system function. When leukemia develops, or is treated, this patient is at very high risk for infection.
- In addition, hemorrhage is not tolerated as well in the elderly and must be carefully guarded against.
- Other conditions also may affect appetite. Emphasis on an appropriate diet, supplements, and good nutritional status can make a marked difference in the quality of life of the elderly leukemia patient.

Anemia and its associated problems of fatigue, hypoxia, GI upsets, and cardiovascular complications affect the patient with leukemia. The anemia can result from the disease itself, from excessive bleeding, or from the therapy administered. Nursing measures previously described for the patient with anemia are appropriate to the care of the patient with leukemia. Colony-stimulating factor drugs sometimes are used to counteract the anemia and neutropenia caused by treatment for leukemia. However, these drugs may stimulate the growth of abnormal cells, making the condition worse, and are used with caution.

Nutritional problems arise from any of a number of conditions. **Extreme weight loss and cachexia are nearly always seen in patients with advanced cancer.** Failure to eat sufficient amounts of nutritious foods is not the only reason this is so. As was explained in Chapter 8, metabolic changes that occur with the proliferation of malignant cells in the body also are responsible for weight loss and emaciation. If nursing measures to alleviate or minimize **stomatitis** (inflammation of the mouth), nausea, and vomiting are not effective, parenteral nutrition may be necessary.

The increased level of uric acid that results from rapid cell destruction during therapy often causes the uric acid crystals to settle out in the kidney structures, causing impaired renal function. Maintaining adequate hydration and administering drugs to decrease the production of uric acid are important nursing measures, as is close observation of fluid intake and urinary output.

The emotional impact of a diagnosis of cancer and the psychosocial needs of the cancer patient and her family are discussed in Chapter 8.

NURSING CARE PLAN 16–1

Care of the Patient with Leukemia

SCENARIO James Cathcart, a 42-year-old man, has acute myelogenous leukemia (AML). He is undergoing outpatient chemotherapy and is being followed at home by a home care agency nurse.

PROBLEM/NURSING DIAGNOSIS *Very low white blood cell count*/Risk for infection related to low WBCs.
Supporting assessment data *Objective:* WBCs 2000/mm^2.

Goals/Expected Outcomes	Nursing Interventions	Selected Rationale	Evaluation
Patient will remain free of infection	Monitor temperature daily. Report elevation >100.4° F (>38° C) that lasts for more than 4 hr.	Temperature elevation may indicate beginning infection.	Temp. remains at 99.2° F (37.3° C).
	Teach patient and family to perform hand hygiene frequently.	Hand hygiene helps prevent infection.	Hand hygiene used consistently.
	Use meticulous hand hygiene when caring for patient.	Helps prevent transmission of microorganisms.	
	Have patient deep-breathe q 2 hr while awake.	Respiratory exercises help prevent respiratory infection from pooled secretions.	Using incentive spirometer regularly.
	Administer transfusion of granulocytes as needed.	Granulocyte transfusion provides WBCs to help fight infection.	Transfusion not ordered yet. Continue plan.

PROBLEM/NURSING DIAGNOSIS *Has no energy*/Fatigue related to chemotherapy side effects.
Supporting assessment data *Subjective:* States has no energy; frequently falls asleep.
Objective: RBCs 3.2 million/mm^3, Hct 33 mL/dL.

Goals/Expected Outcomes	Nursing Interventions	Selected Rationale	Evaluation
Patient will be able to bathe and dress self without assistance	Provide bathing assistance daily.	Conserves patient's energy.	Bathing assistance given daily.
	Encourage resting between care activities.	Prevents undue fatigue.	Is resting between activities.
	Encourage to perform ADLs in small segments.	Preserves energy.	Is combing hair and brushing teeth.

PROBLEM/NURSING DIAGNOSIS *Patient can't work*/Disabled family coping related to loss of patient's income.
Supporting assessment data *Subjective:* Patient too weak to work. Wife seeking full-time employment.

Goals/Expected Outcomes	Nursing Interventions	Selected Rationale	Evaluation
Patient's wife will cope effectively as primary wage earner	Assist wife with defining alternatives for employment.	Helps focus direction for employment.	Wife is considering possible alternatives.
	Arrange consult with social worker to coordinate patient's care when wife returns to work.	Social worker can arrange in-home assistance.	Social Services appointment made.
	Suggest community resources that might help wife find employment.		Wife given list of community resources for employment. Continue plan.

Key: *ADLs*, activities of daily living; *CBC*, complete blood count; *RBCs*, red blood cells; *WBCs*, white blood cells.

Continued

NURSING CARE PLAN 16–1

Care of the Patient with Leukemia—cont'd

PROBLEM/NURSING DIAGNOSIS *Low platelet count*/Risk for injury related to decreased platelets.

Supporting assessment data *Objective:* Platelets 106,000/mm^3.

Goals/Expected Outcomes	Nursing Interventions	Selected Rationale	Evaluation
Patient will not experience episodes of bleeding	Monitor CBC and platelet counts.	Will detect further decrease in platelets.	CBC remaining stable, but platelets down to 104,000/mm^3.
	Instruct to report oozing of blood from the gums.	Alerts to potential for impending bleeding episode.	No oozing of blood.
	Instruct to observe stool and urine for signs of bleeding.		
	Administer stool softener to prevent constipation.	Soft stool will not injure rectal mucosa, causing bleeding.	Stool soft without signs of blood.
	Instruct to use soft toothbrush or toothettes to clean teeth. Instruct to use an electric razor to shave.	Helps prevent small breaks in mucosa or skin that might cause bleeding.	Using soft toothbrush and electric razor. Continue plan.

? CRITICAL THINKING QUESTIONS

1. What measures are necessary for a patient who is immunosuppressed from chemotherapy and is susceptible to infection?
2. How could you help shore up Mr. Cathcart's self-esteem now that he has been forced to give up his role as the family wage earner?

? *Think Critically About* . . . Why is it common for the leukemia patient to have frequent infections? What causes this problem? When caring for a leukemia patient, what would you need to assess to detect early signs of infection?

THROMBOCYTOPENIA

Thrombocytopenia occurs when the platelet count drops to less than 150,000/mm^3. It can be a life-threatening condition. Causes include bone marrow depression from chemotherapy or radiation, autoimmune diseases, bacterial and viral infections, disseminated intravascular coagulation (DIC), and overfunction of the spleen. Certain drugs, such as nonsteroidal anti-inflammatory drugs (NSAIDs) and thiazides, also can result in platelet deficiency.

Immune thrombocytopenic purpura is the most common acquired thrombocytopenia. It is an autoimmune disease in which there is abnormal destruction of circulating platelets. The platelets are covered with antibodies. In the spleen, these platelets are recognized as foreign and are destroyed by macrophages. This disorder commonly occurs in women between 20 and 40 years of age. The chronic form has a gradual onset with transient remissions.

Heparin therapy sometimes causes a type of thrombocytopenia that can be life threatening. Porcine-prepared heparin seems to cause less of this problem than other types of heparin.

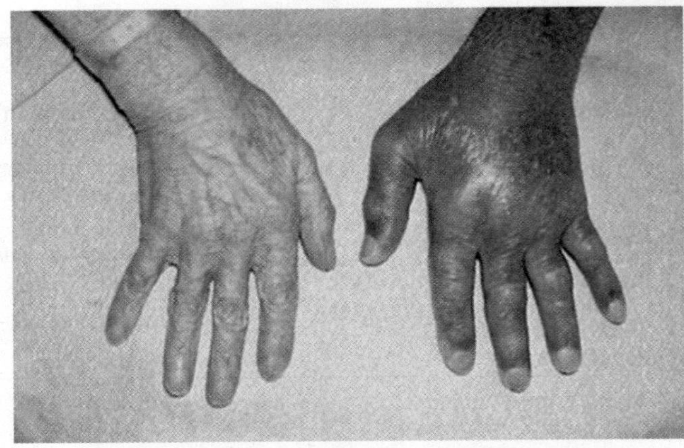

FIGURE **16–5** Ecchymoses of the hand from thrombocytopenia.

Many patients with thrombocytopenia are asymptomatic. Signs and symptoms of thrombocytopenia include **purpura** (small areas of multiple petechiae in the skin and mucous membranes) or large bruised areas caused by hemorrhage that are called **ecchymoses** (Figure 16–5). Bleeding can occur in any part of the body. Hemorrhage is the major danger.

Some patients recover spontaneously. Otherwise, transfusion of platelets is used to control hemorrhage. Splenectomy is done when the cause of the thrombo-

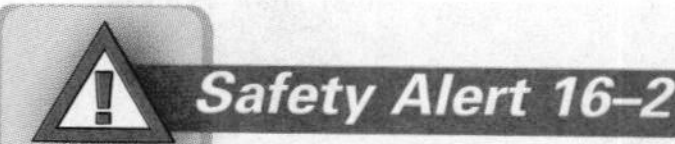

Safety Alert 16–2

Prevent Bleeding

For a patient with a low platelet count, whenever venipuncture is performed, an injection is administered, or an intravenous catheter or needle is discontinued, pressure over the site must be maintained for 10 minutes to prevent continuous oozing.

cytopenia is unknown and the patient does not respond to other therapy, with the hope that this will remove the cause of platelet destruction.

Nursing care is focused on prevention of bleeding by careful handling of the patient, close observation for signs of spontaneous bleeding, and quick intervention (Safety Alert 16–2). Invasive procedures are used only when essential. Patients are taught to avoid activities that might induce bleeding (see Patient Teaching 16–2).

MULTIPLE MYELOMA

Multiple myeloma is a disease in which neoplastic plasma cells infiltrate the bone marrow and destroy bone. It occurs in about 4 in 100,000 people. Men are affected twice as often as women, and the disease occurs in African Americans twice as often as whites. The disease usually occurs after age 40, with the average age at diagnosis being 65 years.

Etiology and Pathophysiology

The cause of multiple myeloma is unknown. Risk factors include a family tendency toward the disease, ionizing radiation, and exposure to herbicides, insecticides, and chemicals (particularly benzene). Genetic factors and viral infections may play a role.

Multiple myeloma is a condition in which abnormal plasma cells multiply out of control in the bone marrow. These abnormal cells produce excessive amounts of abnormal immunoglobulin and cytokines. The accumulation of the abnormal cells in the bone marrow disrupts normal RBC, leukocyte, and platelet production. The disruption of normal cell production leads to anemia, impaired immune response with susceptibility to infection, and bleeding tendencies. The tumors disrupt normal bone marrow function and weaken the bone, predisposing the patient to frequent fractures.

Signs, Symptoms, and Diagnosis

The onset of multiple myeloma is gradual, and symptoms appear when the skeletal system is heavily involved. The patient may experience backache, bone pain that is worse with movement, or pathologic fractures and severe pain. Multiple myeloma is diagnosed by x-ray studies, bone marrow biopsy, and blood and urine tests. The appearance of light chains from the abnormal immunoglobulins in the urine, or Bence Jones proteins, is a diagnostic sign. Because the bone destruction releases calcium, a hypercalcemia occurs that may lead to kidney stone formation and renal impairment. The CBC will show anemia, leukopenia, and thrombocytopenia. Bone marrow studies show large numbers of immature plasma cells.

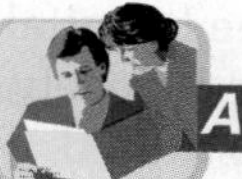

Assignment Considerations 16–1

Assisting Patients with Blood Disorders

When enlisting the assistance of a certified nursing assistant or nursing care aide to help with positioning, moving, or toileting the patient, remind the person that the patient is very prone to bruising, bleeding, or fractures as the case may be. Do not assign ambulation of a patient with multiple myeloma to assistive personnel. Any slight bump or twist of the body may cause a fracture.

Treatment

Chemotherapy or palliative radiation is used to combat the disease. Pain control is a primary concern. Hypercalcemia and osteoporosis often develop, and patients must be monitored and treated for these complications. Measures must be taken to prevent pathologic fractures.

The most common chemotherapy regimen is melphalan and prednisone. It is given orally for 4 to 7 days and repeated at 4- to 6-week intervals. Interferon alfa may be used to prolong a remission. Other chemotherapy agents may be used as needed. Thalidomide (Thalomid), an immune-modulating drug, is being used as an experimental drug for cases that continue to progress despite treatment. Bisphosphonates such as etidronate (Didronel), pamidronate (Aredia), or zoledronic acid (Zometa) inhibit bone breakdown and thereby decrease skeletal pain and hypercalcemia. The drug is given IV once a month. There is no cure for multiple myeloma.

Nursing Management

Supportive care for the many complications of the disease and treatment is provided. Encouraging adequate hydration with an intake of 3 to 4 L of fluid a day to minimize problems from hypercalcemia is a priority. Pain assessment and management are crucial to the quality of life for the patient. Acetaminophen and NSAIDs are used along with narcotic analgesics. Care is taken in moving the patient due to the potential for fractures (Assignment Considerations 16–1). Psychosocial care is essential as the disease has remissions and exacerbations and is eventually fatal. The nursing care for the patient with a neoplastic disorder is covered in Chapter 8, Care of Patients with Cancer.

The patient and family must be taught about the signs and symptoms of hypercalcemia and instructed to report them immediately to the physician. Measures to prevent falls must be instituted both in the hospital and in the home. Mental status is monitored closely, and measures to protect the patient are instituted if confusion arises.

HEMOPHILIA

Etiology

Hemophilia is an inherited X-linked disorder in which there is a deficiency of specific clotting factors. Classic hemophilia, or hemophilia A with a factor VIII deficiency, affects 1 in 5000 male births in the United States. Hemophilia B, or Christmas disease, causes a deficiency of factor IX. Christmas disease affects 1 in 30,000 male births. Both types are characterized by a delayed blood coagulation time that produces a prolonged period of bleeding after injury or surgery. These types of hemophilia almost always occur in males and are genetically transmitted through the female. Although the female does not have the disease herself, she and all her female descendants can transmit classic hemophilia to their offspring. Acquired hemophilia can affect both men and women, but it is rare. Hemophilia can develop as a result of formation of antibody to these clotting factors in blood transfusions, in patients with collagen vascular disease, or after a drug reaction. Idiopathic occurrence may be seen in people older than 50 years of age.

Pathophysiology

The hallmark of hemophilia is bleeding into joints, causing loss of mobility and unequal extremity lengths. In all types of hemophilia, there is a decrease in the amount of activity of one of the 11 different clotting factors normally present in blood and essential to the formation of clots.

Hemophilia A results from a deficiency in factor VIII. Hemophilia B, or Christmas disease, is the result of a deficiency of factor IX. In von Willebrand's disease, there is a decrease in the activity of factor VIII, even though the factor is present in normal amounts in the plasma. The blood of a hemophiliac patient forms a clot immediately after injury, but the clot breaks down and does not effectively stop bleeding.

There are varying degrees of severity in the types of hemophilia, depending on the amount of the factor present and the role of the factor in clot formation. For patients with mild cases, who have 25% to 50% of the deficient factor present in the serum, symptoms may not appear at all until a severe injury or surgery is followed by prolonged bleeding and the hemophilia is thus discovered. In very severe cases, in which less than 1% of the factor is present, the affected individuals may bleed spontaneously without injury, and severe hemorrhage can develop very quickly whenever an injury does occur.

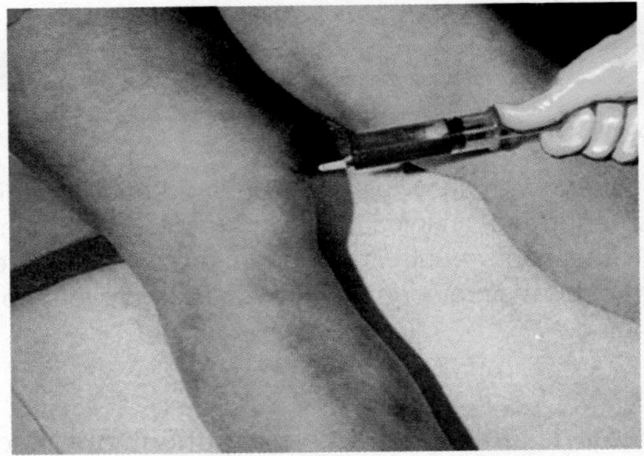

FIGURE **16–6** Aspiration of the knee to relieve the hemarthosis common in hemophilia.

Signs and Symptoms

The most obvious symptom of hemophilia is, of course, bleeding. However, it is not surface bleeding that causes the most serious complications of hemophilia. Bleeding most often occurs internally, with leakage of blood into the joints, the intestinal wall or peritoneal cavity, and the deeper tissues of the body. Hemarthrosis, or bleeding into the joints, produces swelling, pain, warmth, and limitation of movement similar to that suffered by the patient with rheumatoid arthritis (Figure 16–6). This is the primary problem for most hemophiliac patients. If the bleeding occurs in the intracranial spaces and thereby increases intracranial pressure, the patient may experience convulsions and brain damage that can be fatal. Other serious complications from internal bleeding in the person with hemophilia include obstruction of the airway as a result of hemorrhage into the neck or pharynx and intestinal obstruction resulting from bleeding into the intestinal wall or peritoneum.

Diagnosis and Treatment

Diagnosis is by history, physical examination, CBC, and tests for the various clotting factors in the blood.

In the more common types of hemophilia, transfusion of the blood factors is used to replace the missing factors and prevent bleeding. These factor replacements include those needed to treat von Willebrand's disease, factor VIII deficiency (classic hemophilia), and factor IX deficiency (Christmas disease). The availability of these replacement factors has greatly improved the outlook for those with hemophilia and helped them live a more normal life. Recombinant forms of factor VIII and factor IX are now available and decrease the risk of transmission of undetected viruses and prions in the donor blood.

For mild hemophilia A and some subtypes of von Willebrand's disease, desmopressin acetate (DDAVP), which is a synthetic form of vasopressin, may be given to stimulate an increase in factor VIII and von Willebrand factor. Tranexamic acid (Cyklokapron) and aminocaproic acid (Amicar) are administered to inhibit fibrinolysis by increasing clot stability.

Safety Alert 16–3

Avoid Taking Aspirin

Aspirin must never be taken by hemophiliac patients as it increases the bleeding problems. Patients must read labels on every over-the-counter preparation to be certain that it does not contain aspirin or acetylsalicylic acid.

Analgesic drugs and corticosteroids may be used to treat the joint inflammation and pain caused by hemarthrosis and the frequent resultant arthritis. Safe analgesics include acetaminophen, oxycodone, propoxyphene, and pentazocine (Safety Alert 16–3).

Prophylactic factor treatment may be administered prior to dental procedures or other invasive diagnostic tests and unavoidable surgery.

Many patients with hemophilia have been receiving blood products for a number of years. Unfortunately many older patients have been infected with the human immunodeficiency virus (HIV) and/or hepatitis C from contaminated plasma concentrates. Before the invention of an HIV-specific blood test, and screening for hepatitis C, there was no way to tell whether blood donors carried these viruses. This problem has created additional psychological stress for the patient with hemophilia. About 90% of older people with severe hemophilia are HIV positive. Death from AIDS has been common. Fortunately adequate screening is in place now and the problem is resolving.

Hemophilia is a complex disease requiring individual treatment and nursing care based on the needs of each patient. The hemophiliac patient should be encouraged to lead an active life insofar as he is able while avoiding situations that predispose him to injury and illness.

Nursing Management

In addition to administering the necessary clotting factors, interventions include elevating the injured body part, applying cold packs, controlling pain, observing for further bleeding, and providing psychological support for the patient and family. The nurse should also encourage genetic counseling for family members if this has not been done previously.

DISSEMINATED INTRAVASCULAR COAGULATION

Disseminated intravascular coagulation (DIC) is a complicated disorder that usually occurs in conjunction with tissue destruction. It accompanies serious problems, such as severe trauma, gram-negative sepsis, shock, respiratory distress syndrome, malignancy, and abruptio placentae.

Damaged tissue liberates tissue thromboplastin, creating a state of excessive clotting in the microcirculation throughout the body. Hemorrhage follows when the blood's clotting factors are depleted, leading to hypotension or shock. DIC always carries the risk of being life threatening.

The first signs are usually continued bleeding from an injection or IV site, extensive bruising in areas of injury, ecchymoses where there has been no trauma, and petechiae. There may be oral, vaginal, or rectal bleeding. Laboratory studies will reveal a decreased hemoglobin and low platelet count. The prothrombin and activated partial thromboplastin times will be increased. The fibrinogen level is reduced and the fibrin degradation products level is increased. The D-dimer result is elevated.

Treatment consists of correcting the underlying problem (e.g., trauma, infection). Vascular volume is maintained with fluid replacement, vasopressor medications are given to decrease bleeding, and mechanical ventilation is needed for ventilatory support and tissue perfusion. Fresh frozen plasma and packed RBCs are administered to restore blood volume and replenish clotting factors (Levi & ten Cate, 1999). 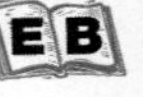

Being alert to the possibility of the development of DIC whenever a patient has a condition that predisposes to it is a nursing priority. Early detection of external bleeding and monitoring sensorium and vital signs for indications of internal bleeding are extremely important.

THERAPIES FREQUENTLY USED IN THE MANAGEMENT OF HEMATOLOGIC DISORDERS

TRANSFUSIONS

A blood transfusion involves the administration of a blood component. To minimize the risks of circulatory overload, HIV, hepatitis, transfusion reaction, and other problems related to the administration of blood, it usually is transfused only when there has been a large blood loss, when the patient has a deficiency of a blood component, or when there must be a total blood exchange in a newborn. Table 16–6 shows some commonly used blood products, the usual amount given per transfusion, and reasons why each is used.

Autologous (originating in one's self) blood transfusion is commonly used when the patient's own blood can be collected and reinfused. Blood either is collected during or after surgery, such as from chest drainage, or is donated by the patient during the weeks prior to surgery for later use. Laboratory procedures that separate the various components by centrifuge or other means allow for the administration of only the particular element of blood needed by a particular patient.

Table 16–6 **Blood Products and Their Use**

COMPONENT	VOLUME	INFUSION TIME	INDICATIONS
Packed red blood cells (PRBCs)	200–250 mL	2–4 hr	Anemia; hemoglobin <6 g/dL, depending on symptoms
Washed red blood cells (WBC-poor PRBCs)	200 mL	2–4 hr	History of allergic transfusion reactions Bone marrow transplantation patients
Platelets			
Pooled	About 300 mL	15–30 min	Thrombocytopenia, platelet count <20,000/mm^3 Patients who are actively bleeding with a platelet count <80,000/mm^3
Single donor	200 mL	30 min	History of febrile or allergic reactions
Fresh frozen plasma	200 mL	15–30 min	Deficiency in plasma coagulation factors Prothrombin or partial thromboplastin time 1.5 times normal
Cryoprecipitate	10–20 mL/unit	15–30 min	Hemophilia A or von Willebrand's disease Fibrinogen levels <100 mg/dL
White blood cells (WBCs)	400 mL	1 hr	Sepsis, neutropenic infection not responding to antibiotic therapy

Adapted from Ignatavicius, D.D., & Workman, M.L. (2006). *Medical-Surgical Nursing: Critical Thinking for Collaborative Care* (5th ed.). Philadelphia: Elsevier Saunders, p. 913.

Legal & Ethical Considerations 16–1

Consent for Blood Administration

The patient must have signed a consent to receive a blood transfusion. If the patient is unable to sign, and the condition is life threatening and no family member is reachable, the physician may make the decision to transfuse the patient.

Dextran, a plasma expander similar to human albumin, is often used to replenish volume quickly while obtaining needed blood products from the blood bank. Several artificial substitutes for human blood that eliminate the need for cross-matching are being tested. So far none has been released for use by the Food and Drug Administration.

Special precautions are always taken when any blood component is given. Blood banks have written procedures and policies for withdrawing and dispensing blood for transfusion (Legal & Ethical Considerations 16–1). Although many reactions and complications cannot be anticipated, carelessness in handling transfusion products cannot be excused.

An LPN who is not qualified to transfuse blood may be asked to assist in checking the blood with the RN and to help *monitor* the patient during the infusion (Figure 16–7; Legal & Ethical Considerations 16–2). All blood bank and agency policies must be strictly followed to decrease the possibility of an adverse reaction or the administration of wrong blood to the wrong patient.

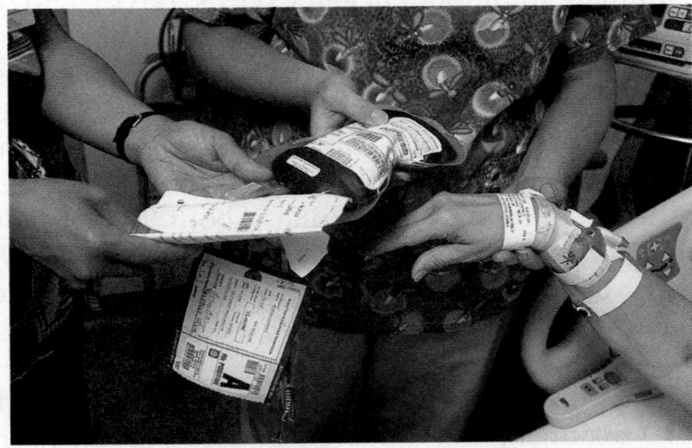

FIGURE **16–7** Two nurses must check the label on the blood product bag, the blood administration form from the blood bank, and the patient's armband and blood bracelet.

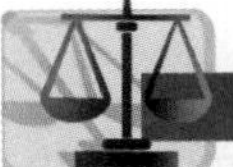

Legal & Ethical Considerations 16–2

Check the LPN/LVN Role

Some states have expanded their LPN practice act to include the administration of blood products. Check your nurse practice act to see if that procedure is within legal practice in your state.

Nursing Management

Determine whether the patient has an IV site already established and what size catheter is in place. It is best to give blood through an 18-gauge or larger catheter.

Blood is normally administered through a Y-type infusion set with 250 mL of 0.9% saline on the other

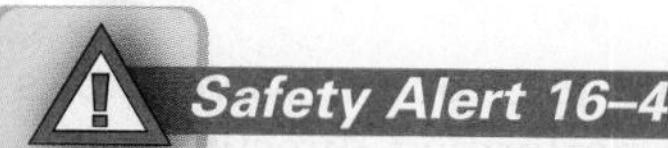

Safety Alert 16–4

Blood Product Safety

Blood bags should never be heated in a microwave oven or placed in hot water. Blood should never be allowed to hang for more than 4 hours as it is an excellent medium for bacterial growth. No other solution or drug is ever administered through the same line or to the same site through which blood is infusing. Destruction of the cells might occur or a precipitate might be formed that could cause emboli.

Elder Care Points

- Vessels in the elderly are fragile. A 22-gauge cannula may be used rather than an 18-gauge for transfusion.
- Blood products should be transfused more slowly to allow the body time to adjust to the added fluid.
- Careful assessment for fluid overload during and after the transfusion is essential.
- A lag period of 2 hours can be observed between each unit transfused to prevent fluid overload.

side of the Y. If a reaction to the blood occurs, the blood can be quickly shut off and the normal saline opened to maintain patency of the IV site. A special blood filter is included in the Y-type infusion set, and the drop factor is different from that of a regular IV tubing set. This infusion system is usually set up before the blood is obtained from the blood bank.

The blood bag should be handled very gently to prevent damage to the cells (Safety Alert 16–4). After obtaining the blood from the blood bank, immediately inform the nurse in charge of the patient that the blood is ready to be infused. The blood must be started within 30 minutes of arrival on the unit and should never be left at room temperature for more than 4 hours; it takes from 1½ to 4 hours for a unit of packed cells to infuse. *(The Skill for blood transfusion is located on the Companion CD-ROM with this book.)*

Think Critically About . . . If there has been carelessness in the proper identification method used to ensure that the right blood is given to the right patient, and the patient has a reaction, could the nurse be sued for negligence?

Transfusion Reaction

The word *reaction,* when used in reference to the transfusion of blood or the infusion of fluids, means sensitivity to the blood itself or to the preservatives or other substances that have been added to a solution. Reactions to RBCs are the result of incompatibility between blood types. There are antigens on the surfaces of RBCs that can bring about a reaction if exposed to blood that is not the same type and is incompatible. The antigen-antibody reaction causes the cells to clump together and obstruct the flow of blood through the capillaries. Common signs and symptoms of a reaction are:

- Chills
- Fever
- Shortness of breath
- Itching or rash
- Apprehension
- A sense of impending doom
- Headache
- Pain in the low back or chest
- Tachycardia
- Tachypnea
- Hypotension
- **Hemoglobinuria** (hemoglobin in the urine)
- Shock

The symptoms of a transfusion reaction may be so mild that they go unnoticed or so severe that death is the eventual outcome (Table 16–7). In milder cases the patient may develop a rash, hives, itching, or facial flushing. In more severe reactions the patient may experience a variety of problems including shock. A delayed reaction due to hepatitis, syphilis, malaria, or other infectious agents might not be evident until 4 to 6 weeks or longer after the blood has been given.

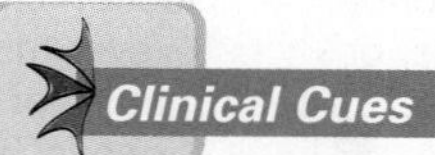

Clinical Cues

If there is **any** sign of reaction, the blood transfusion is stopped immediately, saline is started, vital signs are taken, and the physician and charge nurse are notified.

Diphenhydramine hydrochloride (Benadryl) may be ordered by injection if an allergic reaction is suspected. In severe anaphylactic reactions the treatment is the same as for anaphylaxis due to any extreme hypersensitivity. Should the patient's temperature rise above 100.4° F (38.0° C), the infusion is stopped, the saline started, and the physician notified. Hospitals and other health care facilities in which blood transfusions are administered have written policies and procedures to guide the nursing staff when a patient shows signs of an adverse reaction.

As long as there are no signs of adverse reaction, the patient is assessed and vital signs are taken every 30 to 60 minutes until the transfusion is completed, depending on agency policy.

? *Think Critically About . . .* Your patient is receiving a unit of packed RBCs. When you assess her after the first hour of the transfusion, her pulse rate has increased from 78 to 84, she is slightly restless, and she is complaining of discomfort in her back. Her temperature has risen from 98.4° F to 99° F She has no skin rash and denies nausea. What would you do?

LEUKAPHERESIS

This procedure is performed to clear excessive WBCs from the blood. It may be performed directly on the patient or on separated blood products. The patient is connected to a blood separator machine. Blood is drained a bit at a time from the patient, the WBCs are washed out of the blood, and the red cells and plasma are returned to the patient. This treatment is used to lower the WBC count in CML patients and is some-

Table 16–7 *Acute Transfusion Reactions*

REACTION	CAUSE	CLINICAL MANIFESTATIONS	MANAGEMENT	PREVENTION
Acute hemolytic	Infusion of ABO-incompatible whole blood, RBCs, or components containing 10 mL or more of RBCs. Antibodies in the recipient's plasma attach to antigens on transfused RBCs, causing RBC destruction.	Chills, fever, low back pain, flushing, tachycardia, tachypnea, hypotension, vascular collapse, hemoglobinuria, acute jaundice, dark urine, bleeding, acute renal failure, shock, cardiac arrest, death	Treat shock if present. Draw blood samples for serologic testing slowly to avoid hemolysis from the procedure. Send urine specimen to the laboratory. Maintain BP with IV colloid solutions. Give diuretics as prescribed to maintain urine flow. Insert indwelling urinary catheter or measure voided amounts to monitor hourly urine output. Dialysis may be required if renal failure occurs. Do not transfuse additional RBC-containing components until blood bank has provided newly cross-matched units.	Meticulously verify and document patient identification from sample collection to component infusion.
Febrile, nonhemolytic (most common)	Sensitization to donor WBCs, platelets, or plasma proteins.	Sudden chills and fever (rise in temperature of >1° C), headache, flushing, anxiety, muscle pain	Give antipyretics as prescribed—avoid aspirin in thrombocytopenic patients. *Do not restart transfusion* unless physician orders.	Consider leukocyte-poor blood products (filtered, washed, or frozen) for patients with a history of two or more such reactions.
Mild allergic	Sensitivity to foreign plasma proteins.	Flushing, itching, *urticaria* (hives)	Give antihistamine as directed. If symptoms are mild and transient, transfusion may be restarted slowly. Do *not restart transfusion* if fever or pulmonary symptoms develop.	Treat prophylactically with antihistamines. Consider washed RBCs and platelets.
Anaphylactic and severe allergic	Sensitivity to donor plasma proteins. Infusion of IgA proteins to IgA-deficient recipient who has developed IgA antibody.	Anxiety, urticaria, wheezing, progressing to cyanosis, shock, and possible cardiac arrest	Initiate CPR, if indicated. Have epinephrine ready for injection (0.4 mL of a 1:1000 solution Subcut or 0.1 mL of 1:1000 solution diluted to 10 mL with saline for IV use). *Do not restart transfusion.*	Transfuse extensively washed RBC products, from which all plasma has been removed. Use blood from IgA-deficient donor. Use autologous components.

Key: *BP,* blood pressure; *CPR,* cardiopulmonary resuscitation; *IgA,* immunoglobulin A; *IV,* intravenous; *RBC,* red blood cell; *Subcut,* subcutaneously; *WBC,* white blood cell.

From Lewis, S.M., Heitkemper, M.M., Dirksen, S.R., et al. (2007). *Medical-Surgical Nursing: Assessment and Management of Clinical Problems* (7th ed.). St. Louis: Mosby, p. 733.

Table 16–7 Acute Transfusion Reactions—cont'd

REACTION	CAUSE	CLINICAL MANIFESTATIONS	MANAGEMENT	PREVENTION
Circulatory overload	Fluid administered faster than the circulation can accommodate.	Cough, dyspnea, pulmonary congestion, headache, hypertension, tachycardia, distended neck veins	Place patient upright with feet in dependent position. Administer prescribed diuretics, oxygen, morphine. Phlebotomy may be indicated.	Adjust transfusion volume and flow rate based on patient size and clinical status. Have blood bank divide unit into smaller aliquots for better spacing of fluid input.
Sepsis	Transfusion of bacterially infected blood components.	Rapid onset of chills, high fever, vomiting, diarrhea, marked hypotension, or shock	Obtain culture of patient's blood and send bag with remaining blood and tubing to blood bank for further study. Treat septicemia as directed—antibiotics, IV fluids, vasopressors.	Collect, process, store, and transfuse blood products according to blood banking standards and infuse within 4 hr of starting time.

times used to treat certain immune disorders such as myasthenia gravis.

BIOLOGIC RESPONSE MODIFIERS: COLONY-STIMULATING FACTOR THERAPY

Drug research with DNA-recombinant techniques has developed drugs that stimulate the bone marrow to produce erythrocytes or neutrophils. Erythropoietin (Epogen) is given parenterally to patients who have decreased erythropoietin resulting from end-stage renal disease or who have suppressed bone marrow from the toxicity of chemotherapy given for malignancy, rheumatoid arthritis, or HIV.

Granulocyte colony-stimulating factor (G-CSF; Neupogen, Neulastra) is given parenterally to combat neutropenia. It is used for patients who have bone marrow suppression from chemotherapy, particularly in those with non–blood-related malignancies. Sometimes it is used in leukemia patients, but there is a danger of stimulating the growth of abnormal cells in these patients.

Granulocyte-macrophage colony-stimulating factor (GM-CSF; Leukine), accelerates the recovery of bone marrow after autologous BMT in ALL, Hodgkin's disease, or non-Hodgkin's lymphoma patients who have undergone total destruction of the bone marrow during therapy. Drugs to increase platelet counts are being developed and, one hopes, will be released soon.

BONE MARROW TRANSPLANTATION

Bone marrow transplantation (BMT) is aimed at providing healthy bone marrow when the patient's own bone marrow is faulty or has been destroyed by chemotherapy and/or irradiation in an attempt to rid the body of leukemic or other cancer cells. The bone marrow used for transplantation can be **allogeneic** (from another person) or autologous (from the patient).

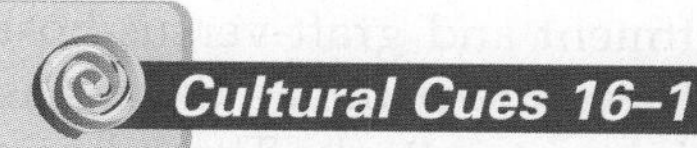

Cultural Cues 16–1

Bone Marrow Donations

Most people willing to donate bone marrow are white. There is a 30% to 40% chance of a human leukocyte antigen (HLA) match for a white patient and donor marrow. Far fewer African Americans have signed up at the bone marrow registry, and the chance for an HLA match for an African American patient is less than 20%. Efforts are being made to encourage African Americans to become bone marrow donors.

Peripheral stem cells or stem cells from umbilical cord blood can also be used if there is a good match with the patient. If the transplant is to be autologous, it is taken from the patient during a period of remission of disease either by bone marrow aspiration or by pheresis for peripheral stem cells. Allogeneic bone marrow is harvested from an HLA-matched person. The HLA match is determined by tissue typing. Finding a good HLA match is difficult, and there is only a 25% chance of matching with the patient's own brother or sister (Cultural Cues 16–1).

Bone marrow harvest is done in the operating room, where multiple aspirations from the iliac crests are performed. About 500 to 1000 mL of marrow is harvested. The marrow is filtered and may be purged to rid autologous marrow of cancer cells or to rid the allogeneic marrow of T cells. Autologous marrow is then frozen. **Nursing care after harvest consists of monitoring the dressings for bleeding and medicating the donor for pain in the hip area. Nonaspirin analgesics often are sufficient to control pain.**

The patient undergoes a conditioning regimen to rid the body of malignancy or to obliterate the diseased bone marrow. This usually takes 5 to 10 days. The process involves intensive high-dose chemotherapy and often includes total body irradiation. The patient experiences all the side effects of these treatments: bone marrow suppression, diarrhea, stomatitis, severe nausea, and vomiting. The patient is at extreme risk for infection. Meticulous supportive and preventive nursing care is essential during and after this phase.

At least 2 days after the end of chemotherapy, the BMT infusion takes place through a central line over approximately 30 minutes. If the bone marrow or stem cells are from an allogeneic donor, the infusion takes place right after harvest. The process of engraftment begins as the cells find their way to the marrow-forming locations in the patient's bones and establish themselves there. Engraftment takes 2 to 5 weeks and is considered successful when the patient's erythrocyte, leukocyte, and platelet counts begin to rise. The patient is at dire risk of infection and hemorrhage until engraftment is complete. Other complications include failure of engraftment and graft-versus-host disease, wherein the cells see the patient's tissues as foreign and mount an immune attack. Thrombosis and phlebitis in the liver also can occur and will cause liver damage if not resolved.

OXYGEN THERAPY

The administration of low concentrations of oxygen may be employed to relieve severe dyspnea and hypoxia during the acute phase of a blood disorder. The treatment is mostly symptomatic, but it does offer some relief if there is sufficient hemoglobin to carry the oxygen to the tissues. In this case it may prevent a myocardial infarction. The care of a patient receiving oxygen therapy and the need for careful monitoring of blood gases are discussed in Chapter 14.

IRON THERAPY

Iron is one of the principal elements in the production and maturation of RBCs. When the body lacks iron, the amount of hemoglobin is decreased in the red cells, making them very small and pale in color. In simple iron deficiency anemia, the condition is relieved by administering iron salts. The iron preparations most often used are ferrous sulfate and ferrous gluconate. Ferrous sulfate is thought to be absorbed the best.

Although iron salts are absorbed better from an empty stomach, they are irritating to the GI tract. There will be fewer gastric upsets if this medication is given in divided doses and immediately after meals. The patient should be warned that taking iron salts by mouth produces greenish black stools and that there is no cause for alarm if this change in the color of stools occurs. Because iron salts may form deposits on the teeth and gums, causing a discoloration, the liquid forms of this medication should be given through a straw. Following administration of each liquid dose, the teeth should be thoroughly cleansed and the mouth well rinsed.

Some patients suffer such severe gastric disturbances from the oral intake of iron salts that the medication must be given by another route. Patients who are anemic because of gastric or intestinal bleeding cannot take iron by mouth because the irritation aggravates their condition. The drug of choice in these cases is iron dextran (Imferon), an iron preparation that is given IV or injected deep into the muscle. Such intramuscular (IM) injections must not exceed 2 mL at each site, and the sites of injection should be rotated to allow for proper absorption and to minimize the hazards of local inflammation. The Z-track technique for IM injection is recommended. Patients receiving an IV infusion of iron dextran must be watched closely for anaphylactic and other adverse reactions.

Vitamin C usually is given with iron because it enhances iron's absorption. If a pharmaceutical preparation of vitamin C is not prescribed, the patient can take the iron salts with orange juice or another juice that is a good source of the vitamin.

? *Think Critically About* . . . What would you teach a home care patient who is complaining that the iron medication is causing a mild nausea, stomach discomfort, and constipation?

VITAMIN B_{12} THERAPY

Vitamin B_{12} has two main functions in the body. First, it is needed for RBCs to develop into mature, normally functioning cells; second, it is necessary for nerve cells to function normally. Another B-group vitamin, folic acid, also is needed for RBC maturation, but it has no effect on the nervous system. Vitamin B_{12} is used to treat pernicious anemia.

Injections of vitamin B_{12} are given daily for the first few weeks and later may be spaced a week apart. As the patient improves, the injections may be necessary only once a month, but must continue for the duration of life.

In addition to administration of supplemental iron and vitamins, the patient with nutritional anemia should eat nutritionally balanced, high-protein meals. Hints for adding protein to the diet are shown in Nutritional Therapies 16–2.

SPLENECTOMY

Indications for surgical removal of the spleen include:

- Severe trauma to and rupture of the spleen
- Splenomegaly due to rapid destruction of blood cells
- Splenomegaly from blood disorders, such as leukemia

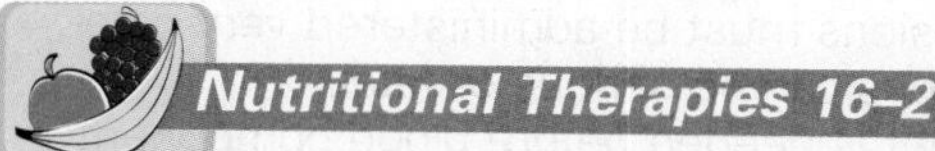

Nutritional Therapies 16–2

Hints for Adding Protein to the Diet

- Mix dry skim milk into the milk called for in recipes.
- Provide between-meal shakes made with commercial protein powder available at the grocery or health food store.
- Add dry skim milk to hot or cold cereal, scrambled eggs, soups, gravies, meal loaf or meatballs, casseroles, and desserts.
- Add diced or ground meat to soups and casseroles.
- Drink commercial canned high-protein drinks (available from pharmacies) between meals, or use instant breakfast drink mix.
- Add cream cheese or peanut butter to breakfast breads.
- Eat peanut butter on crackers, apple, celery, or toast for snacks.
- Mix cooked diced shrimp, tuna, crab, or ham with sliced boiled eggs in cream sauce and serve over cooked rice, pasta, biscuits, or toast.
- Eat desserts made with eggs.
- Eat commercial high-protein bars for snacks, available at the grocery, health food store, or sporting goods store.

Although the known functions of the spleen are important and other functions have not yet been identified, the spleen is not an essential organ. The other organs of the monocyte-macrophage system take over many of its chores once it has been removed. However, those individuals who no longer have a functioning spleen, whether as a result of disease or surgical removal, are at a very high risk to develop life-threatening infections, especially those caused by pneumococci. It is recommended that these persons receive vaccination against 23 strains of pneumococcal bacteria with the Pneumovax vaccine. They are advised to consult a physician and take preventive antibiotics as prescribed when they experience even a seemingly trivial respiratory infection.

The patient with a ruptured or torn spleen is in immediate danger of hemorrhage and shock. Whenever an accidental blow, stab wound, or gunshot wound occurs in the vicinity of the spleen, the patient must be watched closely for signs of internal bleeding such as an expanding abdomen and increased pain. After surgery, the patient is observed for early signs of infection, abdominal distention, and other more general complications of abdominal surgery.

COMMUNITY CARE

Patients with blood disorders are treated in many different places in the community. Patients undergoing chemotherapy may attend an outpatient clinic to receive the doses of the drugs they need. Support groups for patients with the various disorders may meet in hospitals, clinics, churches, or schools, or at other community locations. Patients with sickle cell disease or hemophilia may attend ambulatory clinics.

Patients with blood disorders are frequently treated as home care patients. The elderly patient with pernicious anemia who is home-bound may need a nurse to give her vitamin B_{12} injections and draw laboratory specimens for periodic blood counts. The leukemia patient frequently is followed at home during chemotherapy and recovery periods. The patient with sickle cell problems is more likely to be treated in the home setting after the initial crisis period is over. In some instances blood products are administered at home. Some types of chemotherapy agents are given in the home setting, and the nurse must monitor the patient for all of the adverse effects that such therapy can cause.

The home care nurse must do considerable patient and family teaching about prevention of infection, prevention of and treatment of bleeding episodes, appropriate nutrition, and regulation of medication. The home care nurse manager will coordinate care for the patient with the physician, pharmacist, home infusion company, home health aide, and family.

Key Points

- Anemia results in insufficient oxygen for the body's needs.
- Anemias result from blood loss, failure in blood cell production, or excessive destruction of red cells.
- Hypovolemia from blood loss may result in shock.
- Blood cell production requires protein, folic acid, and iron.
- Pernicious anemia results from lack of intrinsic factor and faulty absorption of vitamin B_{12}.
- There are a variety of causes of hemolytic anemia, some of which are genetic.
- A CBC and differential (peripheral smear) are used for diagnosis of blood disorders.
- Sickle cell disease is a genetic inherited disorder wherein the affected gene is transmitted from both the father and the mother.
- Abnormal hemoglobin causes red cells to sickle when oxygen tension in the blood is lowered.
- There are many signs and symptoms and problems for those with sickle cell disease (see Figure 16–4).
- Nursing care for sickle cell disease and crisis is aimed at relieving the symptoms of complications and minimizing organ damage.
- Treatment of anemia is aimed at curing the underlying disorder and providing nutrients or supplements needed for building red blood cells.
- Aplastic anemia can be life threatening and may require a bone marrow or stem cell transplant.
- Polycythemia vera causes blood to become too thick and predisposes to blood clots.
- Thrombocytopenia affects the platelets and causes bleeding that can be life threatening.

- Nursing care for thrombocytopenia focuses on preventing bleeding.
- There are four major types of leukemia.
- Agents that are toxic to the bone marrow are a key factor in the development of leukemia.
- Leukemia is acute or chronic according to the phase of cell development present and the symptoms.
- The leukemia patient may be asymptomatic or present with fever, malaise, and frequent infections.
- Treatment is aimed at slowing the growth of malignant blood cells and maintaining normal levels of red cells, hemoglobin, and platelets.
- Bone marrow transplantation is one option for certain types of leukemia.
- Infection and hemorrhage are two major complications of leukemia.
- Hemophilia is mostly an inherited disorder affecting the blood's ability to clot.
- Bleeding into the joints is the major problem of hemophilia.
- Blood factor replacement is the treatment for hemophilia.
- Disseminated intravascular coagulation occurs in conjunction with many disorders.
- There is clotting in the microcirculation and bleeding in DIC.
- Blood transfusions must be administered very carefully as reactions can be serious or fatal.
- Patient consent is needed before blood component transfusion.
- There are many signs and symptoms of a blood transfusion reaction (see Table 16–7).
- If there is any sign of a transfusion reaction, the transfusion is stopped immediately.
- Bone marrow transplantation requires an HLA match and is a dangerous procedure.
- Iron, vitamin C, folic acid, and vitamin B_{12} supplementation used to treat anemias.
- Home care patients need teaching for proper care and for prevention of infection and bleeding episodes.

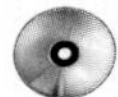

Go to your **Companion CD-ROM** for an Audio Glossary, animations, video clips, and bonus review questions.

evolve Be sure to visit the companion Evolve site at http://evolve.elsevier.com/deWit for interactive NCLEX-PN Exam Style Review Questions, WebLinks, and additional online resources.

NCLEX-PN EXAM STYLE REVIEW QUESTIONS

Choose the best answer(s) for the following questions.

1. While reviewing the laboratory results for a patient who had recent gastric bypass, the nurse notes that the amount of red blood cells has remarkably decreased. The nurse suspects that the anemia is related to:

1. vitamin B_{12} deficiency.
2. chronic renal failure.
3. iron deficiency.
4. bone marrow suppression.

2. An emergency department patient has a suspected gunshot wound to the abdomen. The nurse finds a profusely bleeding abdominal wound. The nurse anticipates which of the following signs and symptoms?

1. Increased blood pressure
2. Rapid, weak pulse
3. Urine output >50 mL/hr
4. Warm, dry skin

3. As part of the discharge instructions, the nurse reminds the patient with iron deficiency anemia to take iron supplements with:

1. meals.
2. orange juice.
3. antacids.
4. vitamin D.

4. ____________________ refers to the painful swelling of the hands and feet related to bone infarction from sickled red blood cells.

5. The physician suspects sickle cell disease in a 20-year-old male patient who presents with pallor, lethargy, and generalized pain. Which of the following diagnostic tests would most definitively confirm the medical diagnosis?

1. Peripheral blood smear
2. Hemoglobin electrophoresis
3. Sickling test
4. Bone and joint deformities on x-rays

6. An elderly female patient was admitted with complaints of fever, malaise, frequent sore throat, swollen lymph nodes, enlarged spleen, bone pain, weight loss, and easy bleeding. The nurse understands that the most likely type of leukemia would be:

1. acute myelogenous leukemia.
2. chronic myelogenous leukemia.
3. acute lymphocytic leukemia.
4. chronic lymphocytic leukemia.

7. The nurse starts a peripheral venous access site on a patient who had multiple traumatic injuries. The nurse notes blood in the urine and the feces. Suspecting disseminated intravascular coagulopathy, the nurse expects which of the following?

1. Increased hematocrit
2. Elevated platelet count
3. Increased activated partial thromboplastin time
4. Decreased D-dimer

8. After the first few minutes of transfusing packed red blood cells, the patient has a temperature of 101.5° F, heart rate 120 per minute, and blood pressure 90/50 mm Hg with complaints of back pain. An important immediate nursing action would be:
   1. flush the line with normal saline.
   2. stop the transfusion.
   3. notify the physician.
   4. administer diphenhydramine (Benadryl).

9. A bone marrow transplant is performed after a cancer patient undergoes chemotherapy and total body irradiation; the patient continues under close observation. Engraftment takes from
   1. 2 to 5 days.
   2. 2 weeks.
   3. 2 months.
   4. 2 to 5 weeks.

10. The nurse is about to administer iron salts to a patient with anemia. An important patient teaching consideration would be to:
    1. take on an empty stomach.
    2. watch for watery stools.
    3. use a straw when taking liquid preparations.
    4. take with vitamin B.

CRITICAL THINKING ACTIVITIES 

Read each clinical scenario and discuss the questions with your classmates.

Scenario A

Mrs. Hutton is a young mother who has three small children. She is admitted to the hospital with a severe anemia. Her hemoglobin is 7.5 g/dL, and her red cell count also is very low. Mrs. Hutton confides in you that she has never eaten as she should, especially when she was a teenager. With the added strain of having the children to care for at home, she doesn't take the time to cook the meals she knows they should have because she is so tired all the time. Her husband makes a fairly good salary, but Mrs. Hutton is under the impression that an adequate diet would cost more than they can afford at present.

1. How can you teach the patient the value of nutritious food and help her with shopping practices that would provide her family with food items that are not expensive?
2. Which foods that are high in iron would you suggest she include in her diet?
3. What practical suggestions could you make to help Mrs. Hutton cope with fatigue?

Scenario B

Mr. Tate is a 24-year-old who has acute lymphocytic leukemia. He is receiving chemotherapy with cyclophosphamide, vincristine, prednisone, and daunorubicin. He is experiencing many of the problems associated with a blood disorder, as well as the problems caused by the side effects of the potent drugs he is receiving.

1. Describe the physiologic problems Mr. Tate is likely to experience as a result of the disease and the therapy.
2. Identify psychosocial concerns that Mr. Tate might have.

Scenario C

Mr. Harris, a 72-year-old white man, has just been diagnosed with chronic myeloid leukemia (CML). He has started chemotherapy with hydroxyurea and imatinib. If this is unsuccessful, he will begin treatment with interferon alfa.

1. What do you need to teach Mr. Harris about the drugs he is taking? Will he be on other drugs to control the side effects of this chemotherapy?
2. His wife asks whether he would be eligible for a bone marrow transplantation. What should you answer?

CHAPTER 17 The Cardiovascular System

evolve http://evolve.elsevier.com/deWit

Objectives

Upon completing this chapter, you should be able to:

Theory

1. Describe the normal anatomy and physiology of the cardiovascular system.
2. Discuss the risk factors and incidence of cardiovascular disease.
3. Explain ways to modify risk factors for the development of cardiovascular disease.
4. State ways in which nurses can contribute to the prevention of cardiovascular disease.
5. Describe the diagnostic tests, specific techniques, and procedures for assessing the cardiovascular system.
6. Identify three likely nursing diagnoses for patients who have common problems of cardiovascular disease and list the expected outcomes and appropriate nursing interventions for each.

Clinical Practice

1. Teach patients about the more common diagnostic tests and procedures to diagnose and evaluate cardiovascular diseases.
2. Assist patients to form plans to modify cardiovascular disease risk factors.

Key Terms

Be sure to check out the bonus material on the Companion CD-ROM, including selected audio pronunciations.

arteriosclerosis (ăr-tē-rē-ō-sklĕ-RŌ-sĭs, p. 408)
cardiomyopathy (kăr-dē-ō-mī-ŎP-ăth-ē, p. 418)
cellulitis (sĕl-ū-LĪ-tĭs, p. 422)
coarctation (kō-ărk-TĀ-shŭn, p. 408)
dysrhythmia (dĭs-RĬTH-mē-ă, p. 407)
endocarditis (ĔN-dō-kăhr-DĪ-tĭs, p. 409)
hypertension (hī-pĕr-TĔN-shŭn, p. 408)
intermittent claudication (ĭn-tĕr-MĬT-ĕnt klaw-dĭ-KĀ-shŭn, p. 418)
ischemia (ĭs-KĒ-mē-ă, p. 408)
oscilloscope (ŏz-ĬL-ō-skōp, p. 411)
palpitation (păl-pĭ-TĀ-shŭn, p. 429)
pericarditis (pĕr-ē-kăhr-DĪ-tĭs, p. 409)
rubor (rōō-bôr, p. 421)
sympathectomy (SĬM-pă-th-ĔK-tō-mē, p. 430)
syncope (SĬN-kō-pē, p. 421)

Cardiovascular disease (CVD) affects one in three people in the United States. The death rate from heart disease has seen a steady decline since 1979, but the rate has begun again to climb. More than 600,000 people die in the United States as a result of cardiovascular problems each year. Preventing and controlling cardiovascular disease are major factors in the attempt to control health care costs. Cardiovascular disease is responsible for the largest portion of Medicare funds spent each year. Each nurse can be instrumental in educating the public regarding prevention and in promoting a heart-healthy lifestyle.

Heart disease in women has been increasing. Nearly 39% of all female deaths in the United States occur from CVD. It is the number one killer of women. Low blood levels of "good" cholesterol (high-density lipoprotein, or HDL) appear to be a stronger predictor of heart disease in women than in men, particularly in the over-65 age group. High blood levels of triglycerides are another particular risk factor in women (Health Promotion Points 17–1 on p. 409). Although it was once thought that hormone replacement therapy (HRT) was heart protective, it was discovered that there were more cardiovascular events in women who were on HRT (Hlatky et al., 2002). EB

To understand the various disorders of the cardiovascular system, it is necessary to recall the structure and normal functions of the heart and blood vessels.

Together with the heart, the vascular system provides the body with nutrients and oxygen needed for life. It also transports metabolic wastes that are excreted by the lungs and the kidneys. When a disorder of the cardiovascular system occurs, homeostasis is upset. Many of the disorders that afflict the cardiovascular system can be prevented or controlled. The public must be educated about the risk factors for the various peripheral vascular and cardiac disorders and about lifestyle changes that may decrease those risks.

The peripheral blood vessels are those situated some distance from the heart. Disorders of the peripheral veins and arteries are almost always chronic, affect people in older age-groups, and are associated with other diseases of the cardiovascular system. For example, atherosclerosis affects both the aorta and the arteries

Text continued on p. 408

OVERVIEW OF ANATOMY AND PHYSIOLOGY OF THE CARDIOVASCULAR SYSTEM

What are the structures of the heart and their functions?

- The heart wall consists of three layers. The epicardium is the outer layer of tissue; the myocardium is the middle layer of muscle fibers that contract to pump blood, and the endocardium is the lining of the inner surface of the heart chambers.
- A membranous sac, the pericardium, surrounds the heart.
- The pericardium is a double-layered sack. It helps provide a barrier to infection and helps prevent overfilling of the heart.
- The pericardial space contains a thin layer of fluid (5 to 20 mL).
- The four chambers of the heart make up two coordinated pumps: The right-side pump is a low-pressure system; the left-side pump is a high-pressure system.
- The right atrium and right ventricle receive deoxygenated blood from the vascular system and pump it through the lungs.
- The left atrium and left ventricle receive oxygenated blood from the lungs and pump it through the systemic circulation.
- A septum separates the right and left sides of the heart.
- The cardiac valves direct the flow of blood through the heart chambers.
- Blood enters the right atrium via the superior and inferior venae cavae and goes to the right ventricle through the tricuspid valve.
- Blood leaves the right ventricle through the pulmonic valve and goes into the pulmonary artery to circulate in the lungs, exchanging carbon dioxide for oxygen. Other arteries in the body carry oxygenated blood.
- The left atrium receives oxygenated blood from the pulmonary veins, and the mitral valve controls the flow from the atrium into the left ventricle. Other veins in the body carry blood containing carbon dioxide.
- The left ventricle ejects the blood through the aortic valve into the aorta and the systemic circulation (Figure 17–1).

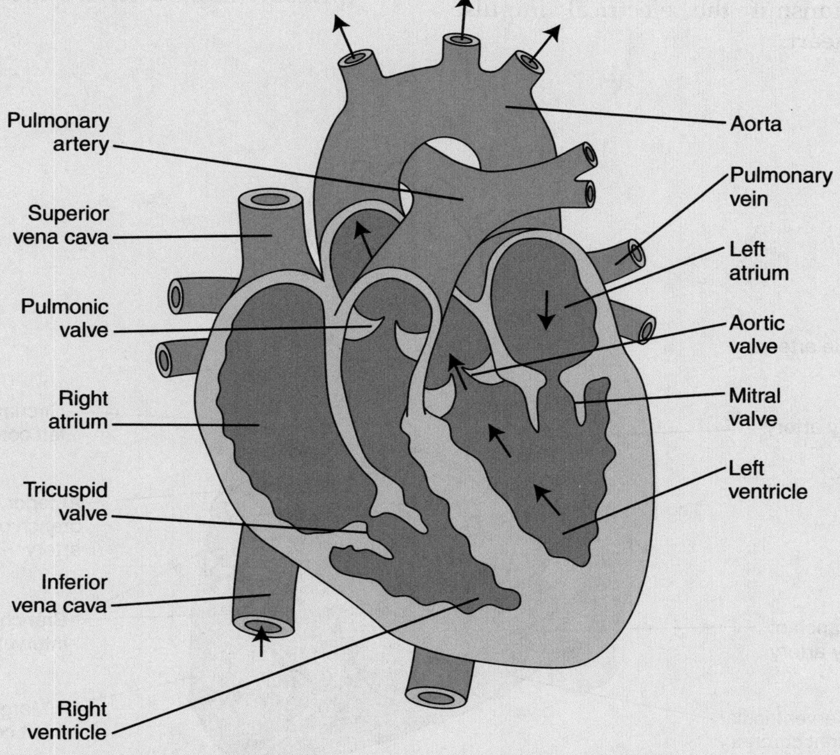

FIGURE **17–1** Heart structures and path of oxygenated blood out of the heart.

Continued

OVERVIEW OF ANATOMY AND PHYSIOLOGY OF THE CARDIOVASCULAR SYSTEM—cont'd

- The coronary arteries branch from the aorta and supply the cardiac muscle with blood.
- The left coronary artery divides into the anterior descending and the circumflex arteries providing blood for the left atrium and the left ventricle.
- The right coronary artery supplies the right atrium, right ventricle, and part of the posterior wall of the left ventricle, as well as the atrioventricular node of the cardiac conduction system (Figure 17–2).
- The heart is located within the mediastinum and is tilted forward and to the left side of the chest.
- The point of maximal impulse (PMI) can normally be felt between the fifth and sixth ribs on a line dividing the left clavicle in half. Listen to the apical heart rate at this location.

What causes the heart to contract and pump blood?

- The heart's pumping action is sparked by specialized pacemaker cells and conduction fibers that initiate spontaneous electrical activity, causing muscle contractions that result in a heartbeat.
- The conduction pathways are located in the myocardium and transmit the electrical impulse throughout the heart.
- The sinoatrial (SA) node is located in the right atrium and is called the "pacemaker" of the heart because it normally initiates the electrical impulses.
- The atrioventricular (AV) node is located in the lower part of the right atrium. It relays the impulse from the SA node to the bundle of His and throughout the ventricles via the Purkinje fibers (Figure 17–3).
- The heart rate and rhythm also are influenced by the autonomic nervous system; factors affecting that system can speed up or slow down the heart rate.

What is the cardiac cycle?

- The cardiac cycle consists of contraction of the muscle (systole) and relaxation of the muscle (diastole).
- The heart pumps out about 5 L of blood every minute (cardiac output).
- The amount of cardiac output depends on the heart rate, the amount of blood returning to the heart (venous return), the strength of contraction, and the resistance to the ejection of the blood (pressure in the arterial system)

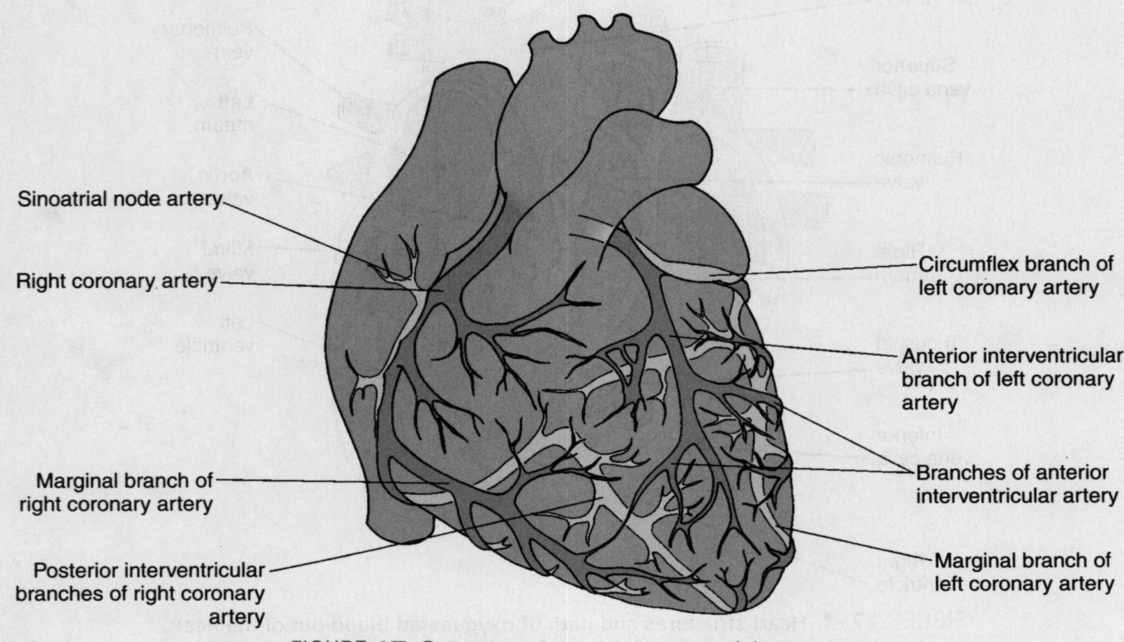

FIGURE 17–2 A view of the coronary arterial system.

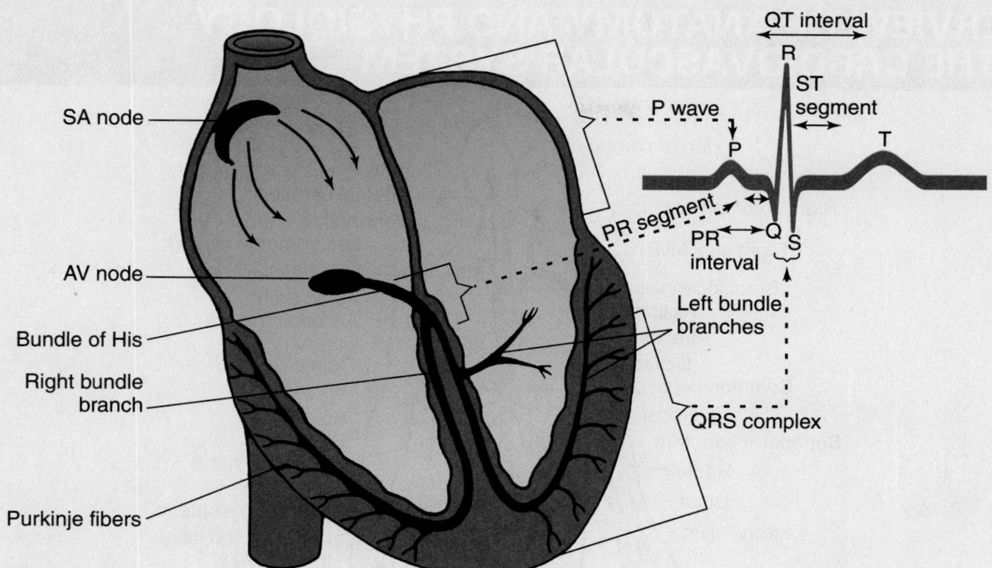

FIGURE 17–3 The cardiac conduction system.

What is the ejection fraction?

- The ejection fraction is the percentage of blood that is ejected from the heart during systole.
- A normal ejection fraction is 50% to 70%.
- As ejection fraction decreases with heart failure, tissue perfusion diminishes.
- A decreased ejection fraction causes backup of blood into the pulmonary vessels.
- Too much blood and the increased pressure in the pulmonary vessels can cause pulmonary edema.
- **Stroke volume** equals the amount of blood pumped out of the heart each minute.
- **Cardiac output** equals stroke volume multiplied by the heart rate for 1 full minute.

How does the vascular system function to carry blood throughout the body?

- Three types of blood vessels make up the vascular system: arteries, veins, and capillaries; these vessels conduct the blood from the heart to the body tissues and back through the lungs to the heart.
- Arteries carry oxygenated blood away from the heart. Veins carry oxygen-depleted blood back to the heart for reoxygenation by the lungs (Figure 17–4). Figure 17–5 depicts the venous system.
- Small veins, *venules*, and small arteries, *arterioles*, are connected by the capillaries.
- The aorta is the largest artery in the body, and it receives blood from the left ventricle.
- The inferior and superior vena cava are the largest veins in the body and empty blood into the right atrium of the heart.
- Arteries are elastic and accommodate changes in blood flow by constricting or dilating.
- Three layers of tissue make up the artery wall; the outer layer, the *tunica adventitia*, is connective tissue; the middle layer, the *tunica media*, is smooth muscle; and the inner layer, the *tunica intima*, consists of endothelial cells.
- Veins have the same three layers but with less smooth muscle and connective tissue. The veins are thinner and less rigid, and for that reason the veins can hold more blood.
- The heart pumps blood through the arterial system with each contraction. Skeletal muscle contraction, respiratory movements that change pressures in the chest, and constriction of the veins propel blood back to the heart.
- Sets of valves in the medium and large veins open and close, keeping blood flowing toward the heart.
- For blood to circulate the arteries must be unobstructed, and they must be able to dilate and constrict as necessary to regulate the blood flow. Veins also must be patent, their valves must function normally, and surrounding muscles must

Continued

OVERVIEW OF ANATOMY AND PHYSIOLOGY OF THE CARDIOVASCULAR SYSTEM—cont'd

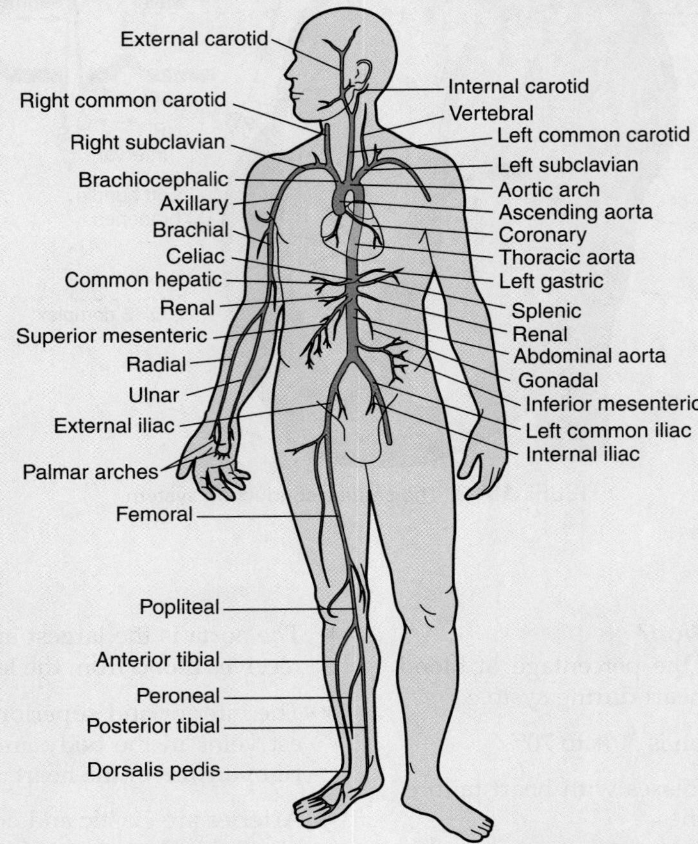

FIGURE **17–4** Major arteries in the body.

contract so that venous blood is continually being moved in the direction of the heart.

What is blood pressure and what affects it?

- Arterial blood pressure is the force that the blood exerts against the walls of the aorta and its branches.
- The blood pressure is greatest during ventricular contraction, *systole,* when blood is ejected into the aorta.
- Diastolic pressure is the pressure when the ventricles are in the relaxation phase, *diastole,* just before the next contraction of the ventricles.
- The difference between the systolic blood pressure and the diastolic blood pressure is called the *pulse pressure.*
- If the caliber of blood vessels becomes smaller because of **atherosclerosis,** blood pressure increases in an effort to force the blood through the smaller opening. Atherosclerosis is the condition in which fibrous plaque with fatty deposits forms in the interior layers of the arteries, causing narrowing.
- If there is an increase in the volume of fluid in the blood vessels, the pressure within the vessels increases, and the heart must work harder to pump the increased volume of fluid through the vessels.
- If blood volume decreases, the kidneys secrete the enzyme renin in the blood (Figure 17–6).
- Renin acts on certain blood proteins to produce angiotensin.
- Angiotensin acts directly on the blood vessels, causing them to constrict, and stimulates the adrenal gland to release aldosterone. Angiotensin increases resistance to blood flow in the peripheral vessels and causes sodium and water retention by the renal tubules through its influence on secretion of aldosterone.

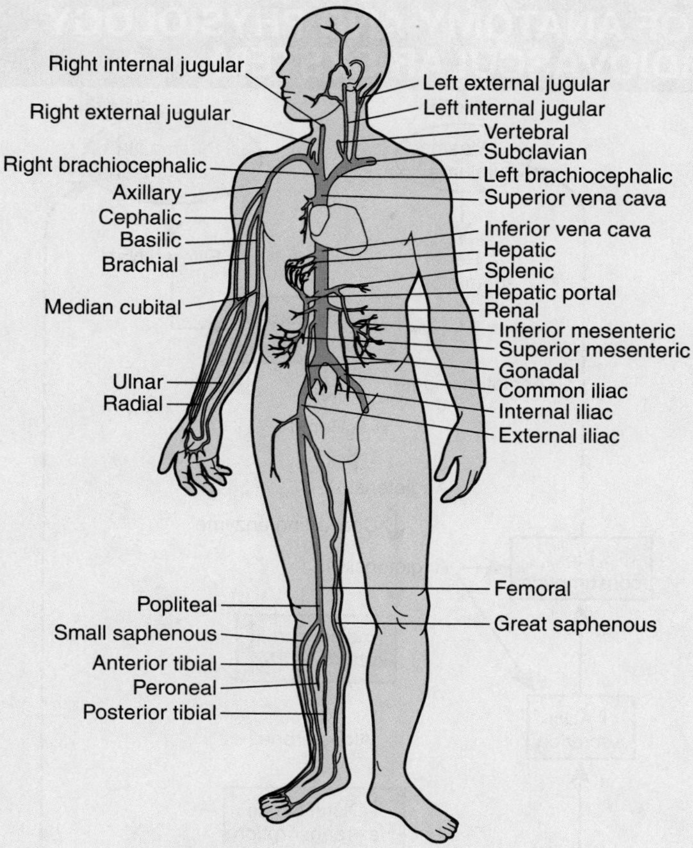

FIGURE **17–5** Major veins in the body.

- The retained sodium and water increase the blood volume, causing increased cardiac output and blood pressure elevation.
- Blood flow is affected by the amount of resistance in the vessels and by the viscosity of the blood.
- Vascular resistance is controlled by the nervous system, hormones, blood pH, and some ions that regulate the diameter of the vessels.
- **When the vessel diameter increases, resistance falls and blood flow increases. When vessel diameter decreases, resistance rises and blood flow decreases.**
- The sympathetic nervous system plays a major role in regulating vessel diameter because it prompts the release of the hormones norepinephrine and epinephrine that cause vasoconstriction.
- Blood viscosity is affected by the hydration status of the body. When dehydration occurs, blood viscosity increases; thicker blood causes an increase in blood pressure.

What changes occur in the cardiovascular system with aging?

- The aging heart becomes stiffer and contractile ability decreases, resulting in decreased stroke volume in the elderly.
- The coronary arteries become tortuous and dilated and have areas of calcification.
- The cardiac valves become thickened, particularly the mitral and aortic valves, which are subject to higher pressures. A systolic murmur is common in those older than age 80.
- The SA node loses about 40% of the pacemaker cells over time predisposing to cardiac **dysrhythmias** or SA node failure.
- The aorta becomes stiffer, contributing to an increase in systolic blood pressure because the left ventricle must pump against greater resistance.
- Atherosclerosis is a natural part of the aging process, and atherotic plaque begins to occur after age 20.

Continued

OVERVIEW OF ANATOMY AND PHYSIOLOGY OF THE CARDIOVASCULAR SYSTEM—cont'd

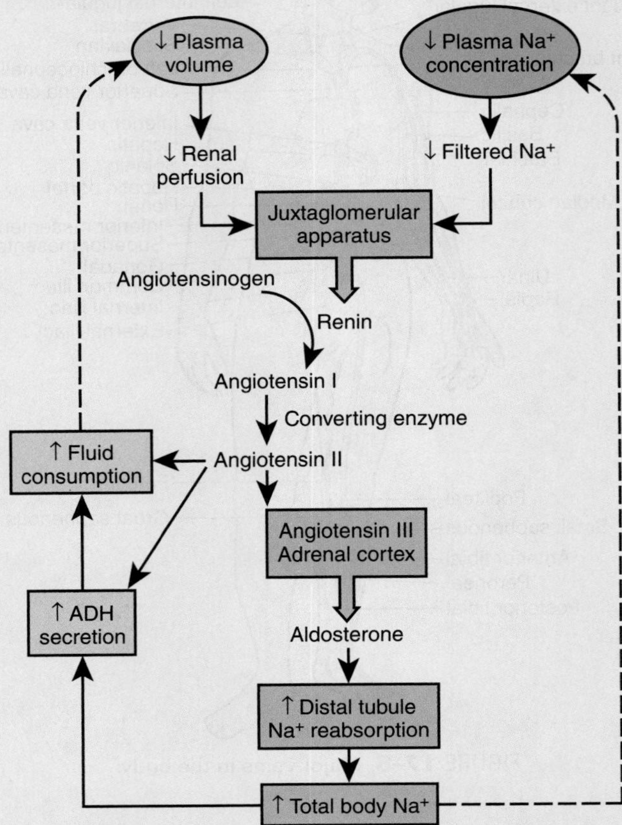

FIGURE **17–6** The renin-angiotensin-aldosterone system.

- The arterial walls thicken and lose elasticity, making them less able to adjust to changes in volume and to comply with sympathetic stimulation.
- Varicose veins develop in the elderly as veins lose their elasticity, valve function lessens, and the leg muscles weaken and atrophy from decreased exercise.
- Platelet aggregation and increased coagulation potential lead to a greater incidence of thrombus formation, deep vein thrombosis, and thrombophlebitis in those of advanced age.
- Chronic health problems and failing eye sight often lead to less activity in the elderly, predisposing to vascular problems.

branching from it. Diseases of the peripheral arteries invariably lead to **ischemia** (localized deficiency of blood) of the tissues. If the ischemia is not relieved, the ultimate outcome is tissue necrosis and gangrene.

Resistance to the flow of blood through the veins leads to increased pressure within the walls of the vessel. When blood is not moved out of the veins of the lower extremities, it accumulates there and provides a medium for the growth of bacteria and may contribute to the formation of leg ulcers.

? *Think Critically About . . .* Can you think of two physiologic reasons why the elderly are more at risk for hypertension?

CAUSES OF CARDIOVASCULAR DISORDERS

Causes of cardiovascular disorders can be congenital or acquired. Narrowing of the aorta **(coarctation)**, holes in the septum, or abnormal formation of a cardiac valve can occur congenitally. Acquired defects include narrowing or hardening of the blood vessels from **arteriosclerosis** or atherosclerosis and aneurysms of the large vessels. Inflammation of the valve structure may cause narrowing (stenosis) or incomplete closure (insufficiency) of the valve. Alteration of the myocardial muscle tissue by extra growth with thickening (hypertrophy) or fibrosis may occur as a result of systemic **hypertension,** pulmonary hypertension, or valve problems. Lack of adequate blood supply

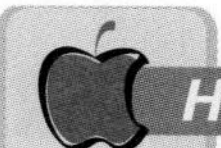

Health Promotion Points 17–1

Preventing Cardiovascular Disease in Women

Public awareness among women needs to be increased concerning the following ways to prevent cardiovascular disease:

- Obtain regular physical activity—at least 30 minutes four or five times a week.*
- Maintain HDL >50 mg/dL, LDL <129, and triglyceride levels <150 mg/dL.
- Refrain from smoking.
- Do not consume more than 1 alcoholic drink per day
- Obtain and maintain a healthy weight as it reduces the chance of type 2 diabetes.* Type 2 diabetes increases the risk of cardiovascular disease.
- Maintain a body mass index (BMI) of <25.
- Discontinue use of estrogen contraception/supplementation as soon as possible.
- Reduce the amount of *trans* fat in the diet.
- If diabetes is present, keep blood sugar <100 mg/dL.
- If hypertension is present, take medication regularly to keep pressure within 130/80 (<115/75 is optimal).
- Incorporate stress reduction techniques into the daily lifestyle, as increased stress is a risk factor for cardiovascular disease.

*These factors play an even larger role in prevention of heart disease in women than in men.

(ischemia) or **infarct** (area of tissue that has died from lack of blood supply) may occur from coronary artery stenosis. Deterioration of the pacemaker cells and conduction fibers related to hypertrophy or inflammation of tissues may cause conduction disorders.

Several disorders involving either the heart or the vessels through which it pumps blood can eventually weaken and damage the heart muscle and lead to pump failure. This condition, called *heart failure,* is a complication of many cardiovascular diseases, as discussed in the following chapters.

Disturbances in any part of the heart's conduction system can result in an increase in heart rate (tachycardia), a slowing down of the heart rate (bradycardia), and disturbances in the rhythm of the heartbeat (dysrhythmias).

Infection and inflammation also can take their toll on the structure and function of the heart. **Endocarditis,** inflammation within the lining and valves of the heart, and **pericarditis,** an inflammation of the sac surrounding the heart, can occur as primary diseases, but they are more often secondary to infection and inflammation elsewhere in the body. An example is rheumatic heart disease, which occurs after a streptococcal infection.

Substances in the blood, such as excess carbon dioxide and certain drugs, can affect the rate and rhythm of the heart through their effect on the autonomic nervous system. The heart also responds to physiologic changes that indicate a need for more or less oxygen.

The arterial walls can be injured by several factors. Hypertension (persistently elevated blood pressure) causes a mechanical injury by applying increased pressure continuously on the arterial walls. For each increment of 20/10 mm Hg above a pressure of 115/75, the risk of CVD doubles (National Heart, Lung, and Blood Institute, 2003). 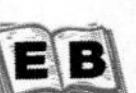 Elevated levels of low-density lipoproteins (LDL) and decreased levels of high-density lipoproteins (HDL) predispose to the deposition of fatty deposits in the arterial walls, causing a narrowing of the vessels. Chemical toxins, such as carbon monoxide, present in the blood when a person smokes, and the toxins caused by renal failure, cause injury to the arterial walls. Physiologic disorders, such as diabetes mellitus, directly cause physical changes in the vessel walls, leading to more rapid arteriosclerosis (loss of elasticity), possibly from elevated blood glucose levels, an increased rate of atherosclerosis, and an earlier onset of hypertension. Some inherited disorders, such as hyperlipidemia, contribute to atherosclerosis.

Obesity, a sedentary lifestyle, and stress are all directly related to the increased incidence of atherosclerosis and hypertension. Smoking, and the changes it causes in the vessel walls, is directly related to arteriosclerosis of the peripheral vessels and decreased circulation in the lower extremities. Long-term hypertension causes arteriosclerosis and is a direct factor in the development of aortic aneurysm in many patients. Essential hypertension cannot be prevented, but it can be managed with diligent therapy and cooperation of the patient. Through the efforts of the American Heart Association and the National Heart, Lung, and Blood Institute, the American public is becoming more aware of the risk factors of hypertension and the need to develop more sensible and wholesome habits of daily living.

PREVENTION OF CARDIOVASCULAR DISEASE

Cardiovascular diseases claimed 871,500 lives in 2004 in the United States (American Heart Association, 2006). Heart disease remains the major cause of death in the United States. Cardiovascular diseases also account for a large percentage of the chronic illnesses that disable, to some degree, a large portion of the U.S. population.

Although the numbers for death and illness from cardiovascular diseases are high, it should be remembered that not all heart problems are either fatal or totally disabling. There are many kinds and degrees of heart disease. Advances in medical science have made it possible either to cure or successfully manage a large number of cardiovascular problems. Reasons for the decline in deaths from heart disease since the mid-1980s include improved emergency treatment of persons experiencing a coronary occlusion or "heart at-

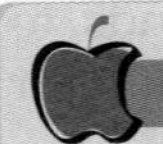

Health Promotion Points 17–2

Know the Signs of a Heart Attack

All patients, family, and friends should be taught the warning signs of a heart attack:

- **Chest discomfort:** A feeling of tightness, pressure, or a crushing or squeezing pain lasting more than a few minutes, or it comes back.
- **Pain or discomfort in other areas of the upper body:** Arms, shoulder, back, neck, jaw, or the top of the stomach.
- **Shortness of breath:** May occur with or without chest discomfort.
- **Breaking out in a cold sweat,** nausea, or lightheadedness with or without chest discomfort.
- **Feeling of impending doom** that doesn't go away.
- **Chest pain** unrelieved by prescribed doses of nitroglycerin.

Call 911 or emergency number immediately—get help!

Table 17–1 ***Risk Factors for Cardiovascular Disease***

UNMODIFIABLE RISK FACTORS	SIGNIFICANCE
Heredity	Children of parents with cardiovascular disease are more likely to develop the same problem.
Race	African Americans experience high blood pressure two to three times more frequently than whites. Consequently the risk of heart disease in this group is higher.
Sex	Males experience more heart attacks than females earlier in life. After age 65, the death rate from heart disease increases in women.
Age	Four out of five people who die of a heart attack are age 65 or older. Increasing age increases risk.
MODIFIABLE RISK FACTORS	**MEANS OF MODIFICATION**
Obesity	Keep weight within normal limits by diet and exercise.
High cholesterol >200 mg/dL	Low-fat diet and exercise; medication.
Hypertension	Encourage blood pressure <120/80.
Diabetes	Good control by keeping blood sugar within normal limits (<110 mg/dL).
Cigarette smoking	Quit smoking.
Sedentary lifestyle	Exercise program of 30-min sessions 3 to 5 times a week.
Excessive stress	Use stress-reduction techniques regularly, such as exercise, relaxation techniques; reduce hostility; maintain a positive support system.
Excessive alcohol intake	Limit alcohol consumption to no more than recommended levels: Men—2 drinks/day; Women—1 drink/day.
Cocaine use	Do not use cocaine.

tack," improved education of the public regarding ways to prevent heart disease, and teaching about the warning signs of a heart attack. Every nurse has a responsibility to assist with public education about heart disease (Health Promotion Points 17–2).

Table 17–1 presents the risk factors for heart disease. Metabolic syndrome is particularly an indicator of cardiovascular risk (Gami et al., 2007). It is diagnosed when three or more of the components in Box 17–1 are present. Modifiable risk factors are the major focus for education to prevent heart disease. Old habits are hard to change, but there is strong evidence that reducing these risk factors can greatly cut down the chance of developing heart disease and thereby improve the quality of an individual's life.

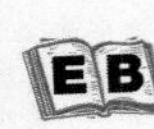

The use of cocaine and methamphetamine has added to the problem of heart disease (National Institute on Drug Abuse, 2007). Cocaine causes vasoconstriction and is thought to speed up the atherosclerosis process. Also, cocaine has been known to cause sudden cardiac death, or stroke, in susceptible individuals. Research is finding that the ingestion of both alcohol and cocaine greatly increases the chance of cardiac death. Methamphetamine increases heart rate, causes vasoconstriction that can lead to hypertension, and

Box 17–1 ***Metabolic Syndrome Components***

When three or more of the following are present, the patient is diagnosed with metabolic syndrome. People with metabolic syndrome are at increased risk of cardiovascular disease. Approximately 50 million Americans have it.

- Elevated waist circumference indicating abdominal obesity; men >40 inches (102 cm), women >35 inches (88 cm)
- Elevated triglycerides >150 mg/dL
- Reduced HDL cholesterol; men <40 mg/dL and women <50 mg/dL
- Elevated blood pressure at or above 130/85 mm Hg
- Elevated fasting glucose indicating insulin resistance; glucose ≥100 mg/dL

speeds up electrical conduction, potentially causing dysrhythmias and myocardial infarction (MI). Cigarette smoking–related health problems are heavy contributors to heart disease, and smoking is a key factor in sudden cardiac death.

Unmodifiable risk factors cannot be prevented by an individual. However, control of diseases such as hypertension and diabetes mellitus, and the reduction of high cholesterol, which are factors in the development of atherosclerosis, are possible and can help prevent the early onset of heart disease. If a person with diabetes can keep the blood sugar consistently below 110 mg/dL, the risk of atherosclerosis is lessened (American Diabetes Association, 2001). Management of hypertension is one of the major tools for heart disease prevention.

> ***Think Critically About . . .*** Can you identify two risk factors you can modify to decrease your risk of heart disease?

A major component in the prevention and control of high blood pressure is education. Nurses can play an important role in teaching others about the disease and supporting their efforts to avoid hypertension and its long-term consequences.

Although systolic blood pressure rises as a natural process of aging because arteries become less elastic, systolic hypertension should be treated in the elderly patient. Hypertension in the elderly is associated with an even higher risk of heart disease, stroke, and death from coronary thrombosis (Brooks, 2007). Hypertension has been associated with more rapid memory loss and loss of cognitive function in some research studies.

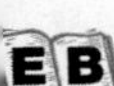

You can contribute to reducing the incidence of the harmful effects of hypertension by participating in community screening programs to detect hypertension in its early stages, confirm its presence, and initiate prompt treatment. In addition, nurses and other health care professionals have an obligation to serve as models for a healthy lifestyle.

DIAGNOSTIC TESTS AND PROCEDURES

In addition to a routine physical examination and medical history, the physician has access to a number of both noninvasive and invasive procedures and tests to help diagnose cardiovascular disease. Because of the hazards and risks of invasive procedures that require entry into the cardiovascular system or the injection of substances into the circulating blood, noninvasive procedures usually are performed first. A chest x-ray is ordered to visualize the size of the heart.

Nuclear imaging often is combined with an exercise ECG—the stress test. Echocardiography also can be done from inside the esophagus using an esophagogastroscope and special transducer. Digital subtraction angiography (DSA) is a form of computer-enhanced angiography that provides a clearer picture of the coronary arteries and their patency. Magnetic resonance arteriography is a new test that may someday replace angiography. Specific cardiovascular diagnostic tests and their nursing implications are listed in Table 17–2. In women, a thallium exercise stress test or electron-beam computed tomography for coronary artery calcium scoring may be better than the standard treadmill test for detecting heart disease. A stress echocardiogram also is helpful (Figure 17–7 on p. 417).

TELEMETRY

Continuous monitoring of cardiac rate and rhythm often is done by telemetry. Disposable electrodes and wire leads from a bedside monitor or battery-operated transmitter unit are applied to the patient. The wave pattern signals are sent to a monitor in a central station, where they are continually observed (Figure 17–8 on p. 417). This allows patients to walk around the nursing unit while being monitored. The wave may also be displayed on a bedside **oscilloscope.** An oscilloscope is a machine that shows a picture of electrical current and its variations. In this instance, the patient's movement is limited by the wire attachments. Modern computerized telemetry monitors can detect specific dysrhythmias (abnormal variations of heart rhythm), automatically store the wave pattern, and alert the nurse to the abnormality with an alarm. Telemetry monitoring is used for patients experiencing an acute cardiac disorder, after cardiac surgery, and after pacemaker insertion. Figure 17–9 on p. 418 shows proper placement for telemetry leads.

SPECIFIC TESTS FOR VASCULAR DISORDERS

Diagnosing a vascular problem begins with a history and physical examination that includes a variety of tests for risk factors for vascular disorders. A complete blood (CBC) count, urinalysis, blood lipid and cholesterol assessment, including high-density lipid (HDL) and low-density lipid (LDL), or sequential multiple analyzer (SMA) panel that screens liver and kidney function, electrolytes, and blood glucose are ordered. If blood pressure is elevated, tests of thyroid, adrenal glands, kidneys, and renal arteries are done to rule out the possibility of another disease that might cause secondary hypertension. Hyperthyroidism, Cushing syndrome, pheochromocytoma, nephrosclerosis, and renal arterial stenosis all elevate blood pressure.

Doppler flow studies are performed to detect a thrombus when one is suspected and to assess the patency of the carotid arteries. Angiography may be performed to determine areas of narrowing in arteries or to detect a lodged embolus. Nuclear medicine scans are performed to detect emboli in the lungs.

The *retrograde filling test* is performed to assess the competency of the valves in the saphenous and communicating veins of the legs. Position the patient supine and raise his leg to 90 degrees to drain the venous blood. Place a tourniquet around the upper thigh to occlude the vessels. If the vein does not fill from below within 35 seconds, the valves are not functioning correctly. Release the tourniquet and observe vein filling. Normal valves slow the filling process; if valves are incompetent, filling occurs immediately.

Text continued on p. 417

Table 17–2 Common Diagnostic Tests for the Vascular System

TEST	PURPOSE	PROCEDURE	NURSING IMPLICATIONS
Electrocardiography 12-lead electrocardiogram	Records electrical impulses of the heart to determine rate, rhythm of heart, site of pacemaker, and presence of injury at rest.	Small electrodes are placed on the chest and extremities, to show conduction patterns in different directions of electrical flow. Figure 17–3 shows a basic ECG tracing.	Inform patient that there is no discomfort with this test. Maintain electrical safety. Normal finding: normal ECG.
Exercise ECG stress test	Records electrical activity of the heart during exercise. Insufficient blood flow and oxygen show up in abnormal waveforms.	Small electrodes are placed on the chest, and a tracing is made while the patient exercises on a treadmill, bicycle, or stairs. The degree of difficulty of the exercise is increased as the test continues to see how the heart reacts to increasing work demands. Vital signs are continuously recorded. May be combined with radionuclide imaging or echocardiograph. Physician is present.	Requires a signed consent form. Have patient wear comfortable clothes and walking shoes. Light meal 2–3 hr prior, then NPO Regular medications are given. Chest is shaved as needed for electrode placement. Inform patient that the test will be stopped if chest pain, severe fatigue, or dyspnea develops.
Ambulatory ECG: Holter monitor	Correlate normal daily activity with electrical function of the heart to determine whether activity causes abnormalities.	Patient wears a small ECG recorder for 6, 12, or 24 hr while going about usual tasks. A diary is kept to show at what time the various activities were performed and any symptoms experienced. The tape is analyzed to correlate any dysrhythmia with the activity at that time.	Remind patient that all activities must be recorded in the diary: brushing teeth, climbing stairs, sexual intercourse, bowel movements, sleeping, etc. Caution patient not to remove the electrodes and not to get the recorder or wires wet. Have patient wear a loose shirt during test.
Echocardiography	Useful in evaluating size, shape, and position of structures and movement within the heart. Test of choice for valve problems.	A metal wand that emits sonar waves is guided over the chest wall while the patient is supine or turned on the left side. Takes 30–60 min. May be done in combination with the exercise (stress) test. Transesophageal echocardiography may be performed with a gastroscope to position the wand.	Inform patient that there is no discomfort, although conduction jelly may feel cool. Normal finding: No abnormalities of size or location of heart structures; normal wall movement. Used for very obese patients or those with a barrel chest. Positioning the gastroscope requires sedation.
Stress echocardiogram	Detect differences in left ventricular wall motion before and after exercise.	Resting echocardiogram images are obtained. The patient exercises, and then within 1 min, postexercise images are obtained.	Explain the procedure and the importance of returning to the examining table immediately after exercising. No heavy meal beforehand, no smoking or caffeine for 6–8 hr before test. Tell patient to wear walking shoes.
Dobutamine echocardiogram	A substitute for an exercise stress test when individual cannot exercise. Detects abnormal heart wall motion.	IV dobutamine, a positive inotropic agent, is infused. The dosage is increased at 5-min intervals during the echocardiogram.	Administer IV dobutamine as ordered. Monitor vital signs; watch for symptoms of distress.
Coronary angiography	Determines patency of coronary arteries and presence of collateral circulation.	Performed by dye injection during cardiac catheterizations. Video recording made during procedure for later review.	Same as for cardiac catheterization.
Intravascular ultrasound	Provide visual information about the interior of a coronary artery.	A flexible catheter with a miniature transducer at the tip is introduced into a peripheral vessel and advanced into a coronary artery. The transducer emits high-frequency sound waves, which create 2- or 3-dimensional image of the vessel lumen.	Consent form required. See cardiac catheterization for posttest care.

Table 17–2 **Common Diagnostic Tests for the Vascular System—cont'd**

TEST	PURPOSE	PROCEDURE	NURSING IMPLICATIONS
Cardiac catheterization	Assesses pumping action of both sides of the heart. Measures pressure within the heart chambers. Measures cardiac output. Calculates differences in oxygen content of arterial and venous blood.	Requires a signed consent form, as it is not without risk. Catheter is inserted into vein or artery, depending on which side of the heart is to be tested. Femoral artery or brachial vein is often used. With local anesthetic and sedation, the catheter is threaded up into the heart, and pressure readings and oxygen saturation determinations are taken. Contrast media may be injected to visualize the size and shape of the chambers and structures. Takes 1½–3 hr. Fluoroscopy is used during the procedure.	Patient is NPO for 6–8 hr prior to test. Assess for allergy to iodine, shellfish, or contrast dye. Have patient void before giving preop medication. Record baseline vital signs and mark location of pedal pulses. Inform patient that procedure involves being strapped to a table that tilts, will have an IV, and patient must lie still during test. ECG leads will be in place during the test. If dye is used, patient will feel a hot flush for a minute after the dye is injected. Patient may be asked to cough during the procedure. He will be constantly monitored and emergency equipment is at hand. Posttest: vital signs q 15 min × 4, q 30 min × 4, then q 1 hr × 4, or until stable. Assess peripheral pulses with vital signs and question patient about numbness or tingling. Inspect insertion site for bleeding or sign of hematoma. Pressure dressing and sandbag weight are left in place for 1–3 hr. If femoral insertion site was used, keep patient flat and leg extended for 6 hr. If brachial site was used, immobilize arm for 3 hr. If dye was used, encourage fluids unless contraindicated. Mark location of distal pulses before the procedure. Postprocedure, prevent hip flexion on affected side.
Electrophysiology studies	Measures and records electrical activity from within the heart to determine the area of origin of the dysrhythmia and the effectiveness of the antidysrhythmic drug for the particular dysrhythmia.	Three to six electrodes are placed in the heart through the venous system. They are attached to an oscilloscope that records the intracardiac and ECG waveforms simultaneously. After baseline tracings are taken, the cardiologist tries to trigger the dysrhythmia that is to be studied by programmed electrical stimulation through the electrodes. Once the dysrhythmia is triggered, an antidysrhythmic drug is administered to determine its effectiveness in stopping the abnormal rhythm. Studies may take from 1½–4 hr; serial studies may be done on different days.	Provide psychologic support for the patient, who is often scared of having dysrhythmias induced. Antidysrhythmic drugs may be stopped 24 hr or more before the test to eliminate them from the patient's system. Assure the patient of constant monitoring and that emergency equipment and staff will be on hand. Keep patient NPO after midnight. Patent IV line is maintained. Electrodes are placed using fluoroscopy. Patient will be supine on an x-ray table. Chest surface electrodes will be placed before the electrodes are threaded into the heart. The femoral vein is most commonly used; the groin is shaved, and local anesthesia is used. Posttest care: much the same as for cardiac catheterization.
Nuclear imaging (thallium perfusion imaging)	Evaluates blood flow in various parts of the heart; determines areas of infarction.	Thallium-201 is injected IV, radioactive uptake is counted over the heart by a gamma scintillation camera. May be done in conjunction with an exercise ECG stress test.	Explain that the radioactivity used is a very small amount and lasts only a few hours. Explain that a camera will be positioned over the heart. ECG electrodes are placed on the chest; scanning is done 10–15 min after injection; can be done as an outpatient procedure. May be done in two parts a few hours apart.

Continued

Table 17–2 **Common Diagnostic Tests for the Vascular System—cont'd**

TEST	PURPOSE	PROCEDURE	NURSING IMPLICATIONS
Dypyridamole (Persantine) stress test	Used for those who cannot exercise for an ECG stress test.	An ECG is done, and IV dypyridamole (Persantine) is given. Blood pressure and pulse are taken and recorded q 15 min while the drug takes effect by diverting blood flow from the coronary arteries, causing cardiac ischemia. Thallium is injected, and scanning images are taken over a period of about 40 min. Repeat scan is done several hours later. The patient is NPO during the test.	Mild nausea or headache may occur. Explain that patient will lie on back for the imaging. If BP drops too low, phenylephrine is given.
Ultrasound Doppler flow studies	Detect clot in vessel; determine degree of narrowing of vessel or detect arterial spasm. Most commonly performed on the lower extremities and the carotid vessels.	A gel is applied to the skin. An ultrasound wand is moved over the skin above the vessel; the skin should be clean and dry with no lotions or powders.	Explain that the test takes about 30 min.
Venogram	To detect thrombosis or narrowing of a vein	Requires a consent form as radiopaque substance is injected into the vessel and radiographs are taken.	Explain that the procedure is somewhat uncomfortable as the dye can be irritating to the vessels, causing a burning sensation.
Venous imaging B-mode	Ultrasound detection of deep vein thrombosis. B/mode shows a two-dimensional image.	Uses real-time duplex scanning. Patient is placed supine in reverse Trendelenburg position; the vessels are scanned. Then patient is placed prone for further vessel examination.	Explain positioning necessary and that the scan head will be moved down the leg to scan each venous segment.
Angiogram (arteriogram)	Determine areas of narrowing or structural changes, such as an aneurysm in an artery. Detect the presence of an embolus. Most frequently performed on vessels in the heart, lungs, or head.	Requires a consent form. A catheter is threaded into an artery and a radiopaque dye is injected. Radiographs are taken. Preoperative preparation is necessary. Postoperative care includes careful monitoring for bleeding from the catheter insertion site, and neurologic signs and vital signs are taken often to monitor for the possibility of embolus or bleeding. Sensation distal to the catheter insertion site also is checked, as internal bleeding can cause a hematoma that presses on nerves.	Preparation is similar to that for surgery. Explain that preoperative medication will be given. Increase fluids if a contrast medium was used to flush the dye through the kidneys. Consent form required.
Impedance plethysmography	Estimates blood flow in a limb based on electrical resistance present before and after inflating a pneumatic cuff placed around the limb. Used to detect deep vein thrombosis.	Measurements of electrical resistance are taken before and after a pneumatic cuff placed around the limb is inflated. Electrodes are placed on opposite sides of the limb.	Instruct to wear loose clothing. Explain that some discomfort may occur during inflation of the cuff. The patient is placed on an examination table and positioned supine in a relaxed comfortable position. The limb is properly positioned, and electrodes and the pneumatic cuff are applied.
Nuclear medicine scan	Detect blood clots, particularly pulmonary emboli.	A radioisotope is injected, and after a waiting period for uptake, a scintillation scanning camera is used to measure the amount of radioactivity present in the area in question.	Determine whether patient has an allergy to the dye. Posttest encourage large fluid intake to flush the dye through the kidneys.

Table 17–2 ***Common Diagnostic Tests for the Vascular System—cont'd***

TEST	PURPOSE	PROCEDURE	NURSING IMPLICATIONS
CT scan	Determine size and condition of aortic aneurysm.	Noninvasive, unless dye contrast used. Patient is positioned on scanning table and moved under the scanner.	Instruct in necessity of holding still during scan.
Carotid duplex examination	Study blood flow in external carotid arteries.	Patient is positioned supine with neck extended. The probe is moved up and down each side of the neck over the external carotid arteries.	Explain that plaque in the arteries can be visualized in this manner. This test assists in determining need for endarterectomy surgery.
Technetium pyrophosphate scan and multiple-gated acquisition (MUGA) scan	Determine area and extent of myocardial infarction. Assess left ventricular function.	Technetium-99m (^{99m}Tc) is injected IV and is taken up by areas of infarction, producing hot spots when scanned. Multiple serial images are obtained. Best results occur when done 1–6 days after a suspected MI.	Inform patient that scan is done 1½ to 2 hr after injection of the ^{99m}Tc. Explain that the test will determine whether any damage occurred from an MI.
Positron emission tomography	Evaluate myocardial perfusion.	IV nitrogen-13-ammonia is injected and a scan performed to show myocardial metabolic function. Then fluoro-18-deoxyglucose is injected and a scan performed. In a normal heart, the scans will match; in an ischemic heart, the scans will differ.	Explain that radioisotopes will be given IV. It will be necessary to lie still while the machine scans the heart. The patient's glucose must be between 60–140 mg/dL. If scan is combined with exercise, patient will need to be NPO and must refrain from tobacco and caffeine for 24 hr before the test.
Magnetic resonance imaging (MRI) **Magnetic resonance arteriography (MRA)**	Evaluate cardiac tissue integrity, detect aneurysms, determine ejection fraction and cardiac output, and determine patency of proximal coronary arteries.	Noninvasive magnetic resonance is used to depict tissue images. IV gadolinium is injected as a contrast medium for the MRA.	Explain about the cylinder within which the patient will be positioned. Warn that there will be loud noises from the machine. Administer antianxiety medication if needed and ordered; provide music if patient desires it.
Electron-beam computed tomography (EBCT)	Assist in predicting whether a patient will develop heart or arterial disease.	Noninvasive 10-min scan is performed to detect calcification within the vessels that indicates plaque.	Helpful for patients with high blood pressure and/or elevated cholesterol to determine cardiovascular event risk.
Hemodynamic monitoring via Swan-Ganz catheter	Determine pressure, flow and oxygenation within the cardiovascular system. *Normal values:* *Preload:* RAP* 2–8 mm Hg PAWP* 6–12 mm Hg PADP 4–12 mm Hg *Afterload:* MAP* 70–105 mm Hg *Oxygenation:* Arterial Hgb O_2 Sat 95%–99% Mixed venous Hgb O_2 Sat 69%–80%	A special catheter, infusion system, and a transducer, and a monitor are prepared and the catheter is placed by the physician in the heart or great vessels.	The system must be calibrated to perform properly. Readings are taken for right atrial, pulmonary artery, and pulmonary wedge pressures. Other data can then be calculated regarding stroke volume, cardiac output, and oxygenation.

Key: *MAP,* mean arterial pressure; *PAWP,* pulmonary artery wedge pressure; *PADP,* pulmonary artery diastolic pressure; *RAP,* right atrial pressure.

Continued

Table 17–2 Common Diagnostic Tests for the Vascular System—cont'd

TEST	PURPOSE	PROCEDURE	NURSING IMPLICATIONS
Laboratory tests			
Cardiac serum enzymes	Measures specific enzyme levels to determine what type of cells have been injured and to what extent.	Creatine kinase (CK) is found in the heart, skeletal muscle, and brain cells. It rises within 6 hr of MI and returns to normal within 48–72 hr. CK-MB is a fraction of the enzyme, or isoenzyme, that is specific to heart muscle cells. Lactic dehydrogenase (LDH) rises following MI but is not specific. LDH_1 and LDH_2 are the isoenzymes contained in heart muscle. If $LDH_1/LDH_2 > 1$, it indicates MI has occurred. Aspartate aminotransferase (AST) rises 6–8 hr after MI, peaks within 24–48 hr, and returns to normal in 4–8 days but is not specific to heart damage. Cardiac enzymes are usually tested q 8 hr × 3.	Explain purpose of laboratory work. Inform patient that blood will be drawn at intervals to check the rise and fall of enzyme levels.
CK	*Normal values:* Female: 5–35 mU/mL Male: 5–50 mU/mL		
CK-MB	<5% total CK		
LDH	15–450 U/mL		
LDH1	17%–27%		
LDH2	27%–37%		
AST	5–40 U/mL		
Serum protein troponin T	Quick test for acute MI	Done by enzyme-linked immunosorbent assay. Provides results in 2 hr. Is very accurate from 10–120 hr after onset of MI symptoms.	Quicker and more accurate than other cardiac enzyme blood tests.
Serum lipids	Determines level	Elevation of cholesterol is a risk factor for atherosclerotic heart disease.	Patient is NPO except for noncaloric liquids for 12 hr.
	Normal values:		
Cholesterol	150–200 mg/dL		
HDL	32–75 mg/dL		
LDL	73–200 mg/dL		
Triglycerides	50–250 mg/dL	Triglycerides contribute to arterial disease. As triglycerides rise, so do low-density lipoproteins, which are a factor in atherosclerosis. The lipoproteins (LDL, VLDL, and HDL) are increased in hyperlipidemia. Lipoprotein fractions are determined by electrophoresis and are used to assign a "risk" factor in cardiovascular disease. High levels for HDL appear to protect against coronary artery disease and MI, whereas increased levels of LDL are associated with increased atherosclerosis and MI.	
Myoglobin	To detect damage to the myocardium from a myocardial infarction. *Normal range:* <90 mcg/L	Requires a blood draw of 5 mL in a red-top tube. Apply pressure to venipuncture site.	Explain procedure. No fasting is required.

The ankle-brachial index (ABI) test evaluates circulatory status in the lower extremities. A regular blood pressure cuff is placed above the malleolus. Another blood pressure cuff is positioned over the brachial artery. A Doppler probe is used to check the systolic end point at the dorsalis pedis and the posterior tibial sites. The brachial blood pressure is measured. The ABI is calculated by dividing the ankle pressure by the brachial pressure. An ABI of 1 or more is considered normal. An abnormal ABI indicates arterial disease and can confirm a vascular cause for ischemic pain at rest and **claudication** (cramping pain in the calves). Table 17–2 presents the diagnostic tests used to detect other problems in the vascular system. Serum cholesterol and lipids are discussed more fully in Chapter 18.

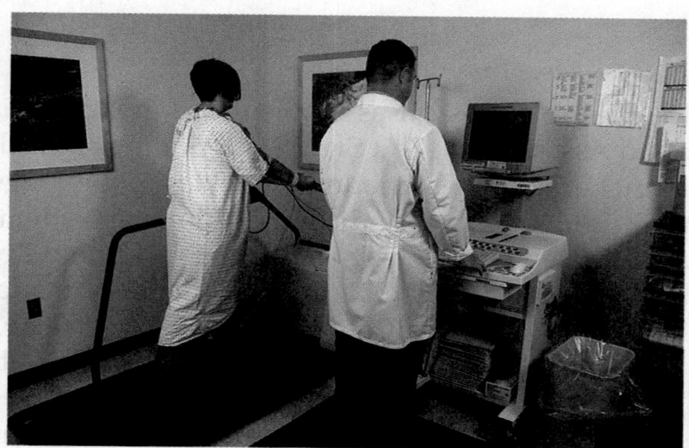

FIGURE **17–7** Cardiac treadmill stress test.

? *Think Critically About . . .* Can you identify four teaching points to be covered for the patient who is to undergo an arteriogram?

NURSING MANAGEMENT

Assessment (Data Collection)

History Taking

It is important to determine whether there are risk factors for cardiovascular disease. Important data include any family history of heart disease, diabetes mellitus, high blood pressure, hyperlipidemia, stroke, gout, or kidney disease. It is helpful, too, to know about the patient's lifestyle, such as smoking, drinking, drug use, and eating habits; weight gains or losses; type and amount of daily exercise; occupation; and sources of stress.

Much of this information is obtained by the physician or nurse practitioner during history-taking and by the admitting nurse during a complete nursing assessment. Some additional information, however, will be gathered in less formal interactions when the patient becomes more relaxed and comfortable with the nurses who care for him.

Information concerning the patient's actual eating habits, such as snacking on "junk" food or daily consumption of several drinks containing caffeine, is more likely to be obtained during nursing care activities than during the initial assessment. Data concerning stressors in the patient's life and his response to them are more easily assessed while interacting over time.

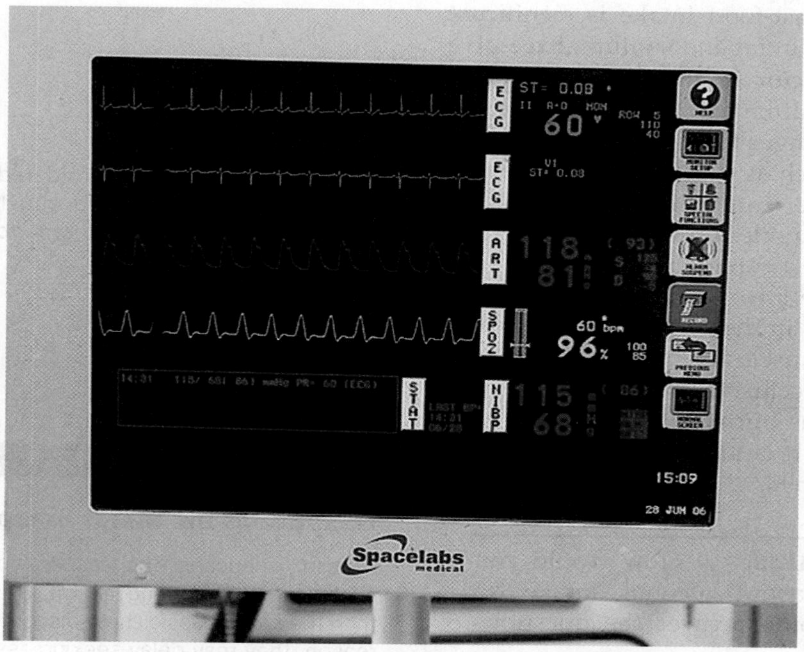

FIGURE **17–8** Telemetry monitor in an intensive care unit.

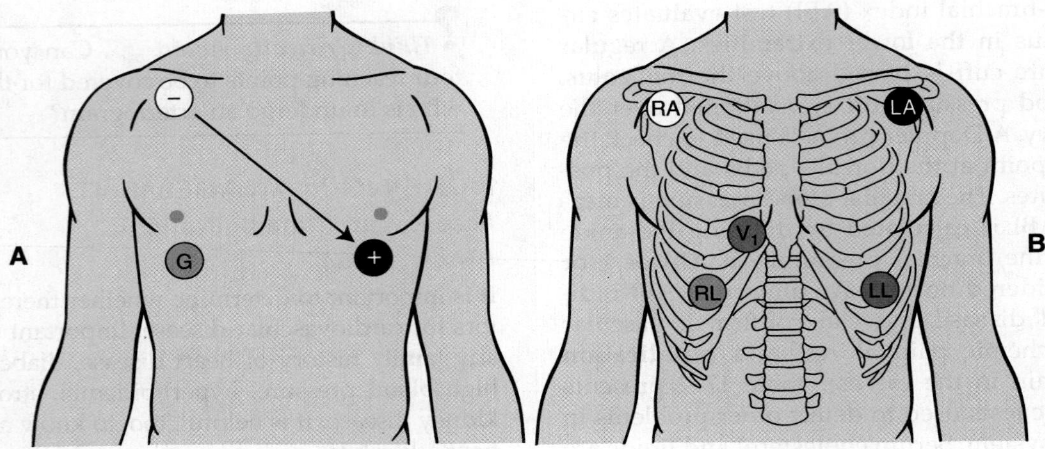

FIGURE 17–9 Placement of the most commonly used telemetry leads. **A,** 2 Lead (three-electrode system); **B,** 5 lead (five-electrode system).

An understanding of the patient's perception of his disorder and overall health are necessary to plan appropriate teaching for him. The effectiveness of your communication with the patient will determine the quality of subjective data obtained. A history-taking guide is in Focused Assessment 17–1.

Other subjective data include questions regarding medications taken regularly, both prescription and nonprescription, as many drugs can cause vasoconstriction and elevate blood pressure. Cold remedies, decongestants, and diet pills are particularly noted for having this effect. Other prescription medications that may affect the heart are bronchodilators, anticoagulants, contraceptives, psychotropic medications, and street drugs. A careful, specific diet history should be gathered. Fast-food intake is significant because it is often high in fat and sodium. **Excessive alcohol intake is a factor in the development of hypertension and** cardiomyopathy. Questions are asked that relate to changes from damage to the cardiovascular system, such as (CHF) heart failure, angina, or kidney failure. **Intermittent claudication,** cramping pain in the muscles brought on by exercise and relieved by rest, is a common symptom of arterial insufficiency to the lower extremities. This pain most frequently occurs in the calves of the legs, but it also can affect the muscles of the thighs and buttocks. Often chronic occlusive arterial disease will cause pain described as burning and tingling, with numbness of the toes. It is most noticeable at night when the patient is in bed.

Think Critically About . . . How would you phrase questions about alcohol intake so that the patient would answer the questions honestly?

Physical Assessment

Guidelines for physical assessment are presented in Focused Assessment 17–1. Significant findings include abnormal or extra heart sounds, crackles in the lungs, or pink frothy sputum indicating pulmonary edema (Cultural Cues 17–1). Chest pain, if present, should be further assessed using the "PQRST" memory device (Table 17–3). Other significant findings might be a bluish cast to skin; pallor or diaphoresis (sweating); clubbing of the fingers; or pitting edema of the feet, ankles, or sacral area. There may be distended jugular veins, an abnormal rate or volume of pulses, or a pulse deficit. A pulse deficit is the difference between the apical and radial pulse rate when they are counted at the same time.

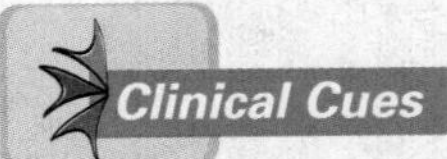

Chest pain should be considered cardiac in origin until such a cause can be ruled out. Many things can cause chest pain, but it is important to always think "cardiac first."

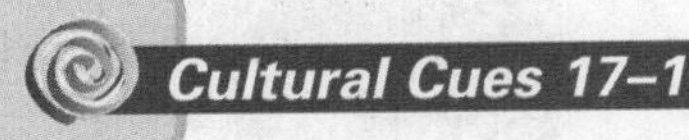

Dyspnea as the Major Symptom

African Americans often experience dyspnea as the most acute symptom during an MI. Dyspnea is more common than the more classic chest discomfort in this group. For this reason, they may delay seeking assistance.

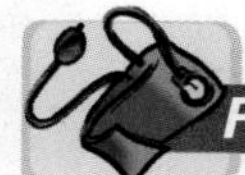

Focused Assessment 17–1

Data Collection for the Cardiovascular System

HISTORY TAKING

When interviewing the patient who has a probable cardiovascular problem, ask the following questions:

- Do you ever have any chest discomfort or pain? What does it feel like? What, if anything, seems to bring it on? What makes it worse? How long does it last? Is it worse when you breathe in deeply? What gives relief? Does the pain radiate (spread) to other parts of the body, for example, down the arm or up into the neck or jaw, or to the upper abdomen? Is it localized, or does it cover a large area? On a scale of 1 to 10, with 10 being the worst and 1 being the least, how do you rate your pain? Do you have numbness, tingling, nausea, diaphoresis, shortness of breath, anxiety, or dizziness when you have chest pain?
- Have you or any member of your family ever been told that you have diabetes mellitus; cardiovascular, thyroid, or renal disease; arteriosclerosis; atherosclerosis; peripheral vascular disease; blood disorder; kidney disease or an immune disorder such as lupus erythematosus?
- Do you become easily fatigued? Dizzy or lightheaded?
- Do you become short of breath? When? Do you sleep on more than one pillow? Is your shortness of breath worse after physical activity? What kind of activity? Walking up steps? Does it occur when you are at rest? Does resting relieve it? Do you wake up at night short of breath or feeling like you are suffocating? Does sitting up on the side of the bed or getting up give you relief?
- Do you have a cough? What kind ? Dry and hacking, or wet and productive? What does the sputum look like? Is there ever any blood in your sputum?
- Do you notice your heart beating very fast or pounding in your chest (palpitations)? Does it skip a beat?
- Have you ever fainted or felt like you were going to faint?
- Do you get up in the night to urinate? How many times do you get up each night?
- Have you noticed any sudden weight gain or swelling in the feet and legs?
- Do you experience pain in your legs when walking?
- Are your feet always cold?
- Have you ever had a bad injury to either leg?
- Have you ever had a deep vein thrombosis (DVT) or thrombophlebitis?
- What medications do you take that are prescribed by your physician? What over-the-counter medications do you take?
- Do you smoke? Have you ever smoked? How much and for how long?
- Do you drink alcohol? What do you usually drink? How many drinks do you have? About how many times a week do you drink something alcoholic?
- What do you usually eat? Can you tell me what you generally eat for breakfast, lunch, and dinner? Do you have a midmorning, midafternoon or evening snack? What do you eat for a snack? Do you eat fast food often? What type? What do you usually drink at meals? Do you drink liquids between meals?
- Do you regularly add salt to your food?
- Do you have leg pain at night?
- Have you ever had a sore on your foot or lower leg that was slow to heal?

PHYSICAL EXAMINATION

When assessing the cardiovascular system, check for:

- Skin color, temperature, and texture
- Facial expression; signs of pain or anxiety
- Vital signs
- Heart sounds; S_1, S_2, abnormal sounds, murmurs
- Apical pulse rate and rhythm; presence of pulse deficit
- Quality of peripheral pulses
- Breath sounds, presence of crackles in lung bases
- Shape of fingers; presence of clubbing
- Appearance of neck veins; presence of venous jugular distention
- Abdomen; presence of distention; abdominal pulsation
- Degree of body tension
- Ankles and feet; presence of edema and degree
- General body appearance; presence of edema
- Weight; gain of 2 lb or more over a few days
- Varicosities in lower extremities

An apical pulse rate should be taken on all patients upon admission. Privacy should be provided before baring the chest and the room should be warm. Heart sounds are auscultated at least every 8 hours on all patients who have a known dysrhythmia or a potential for dysrhythmia, a valve problem, or heart failure (Figure 17–10). The diaphragm of the stethoscope is placed over the bare skin at the mitral area to listen to the apical pulse. S_1 (lub) and S_2 (dub) should be distinguished. S_1 occurs with the closing of the AV valve during systole. S_2 is the closure of the pulmonic and semilunar valves during diastole. Extra sounds or gallops may occur as S_3 sound. Splitting of the S_2 sound may be normal in children and young adults, but may be abnormal in adults. S_4 is usually heard just before S_1 and can indicate various heart diseases.

The bell of the stethoscope is used to listen for heart murmurs. **It must be placed lightly on the skin for the sounds to be heard**. Murmurs usually have a "swooshing" sound from turbulent blood flow. Children may have an innocent murmur that disappears as they grow. Murmurs are commonly from damaged valves, causing abnormal blood flow in the heart. As heart sounds often are very soft, ask the patient to refrain from talking, and turn off the television or radio while listening. (Just remember to turn it back on.) Having the patient roll to the left side or lean forward may make the sounds louder and clearer.

Table 17–3 PQRST for Pain Assessment

This memory device is used to assist in obtaining information from any patient experiencing chest pain or discomfort.

FACTOR	QUESTIONS TO ASK
P Precipitating events	What events or factors precipitated or caused the pain or discomfort?
Q Quality of pain or discomfort	What does the pain or discomfort feel like? Is it aching, dull, sharp, tight, heavy pressure, etc.?
R Radiation of pain	Where is the pain located? Does it radiate to the back, arms, jaw, teeth, shoulder, or elbow?
S Severity of pain	On a scale of 1 to 10, with 10 being the most severe, how do you rate the pain?
T Timing	When did the pain or discomfort begin? Has it changed since it started? Has this type of pain occurred before?

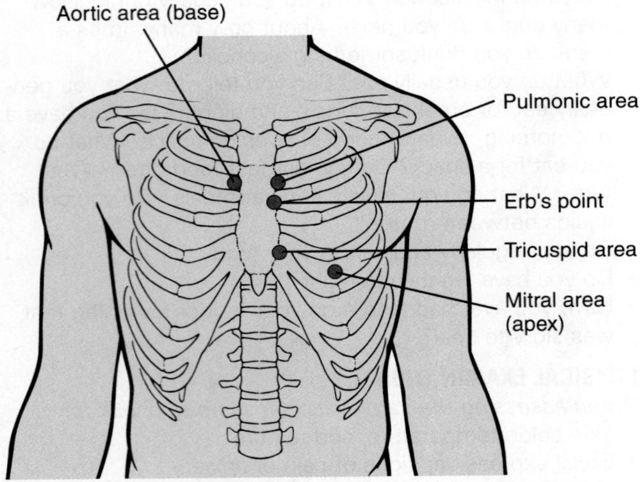

FIGURE 17–10 Sites for auscultation of heart sounds. S_1 is loudest at mitral and tricuspid areas. S_2 is loudest at aortic and pulmonic area. Listen at in the mitral area for S_3 and S_4 sounds.

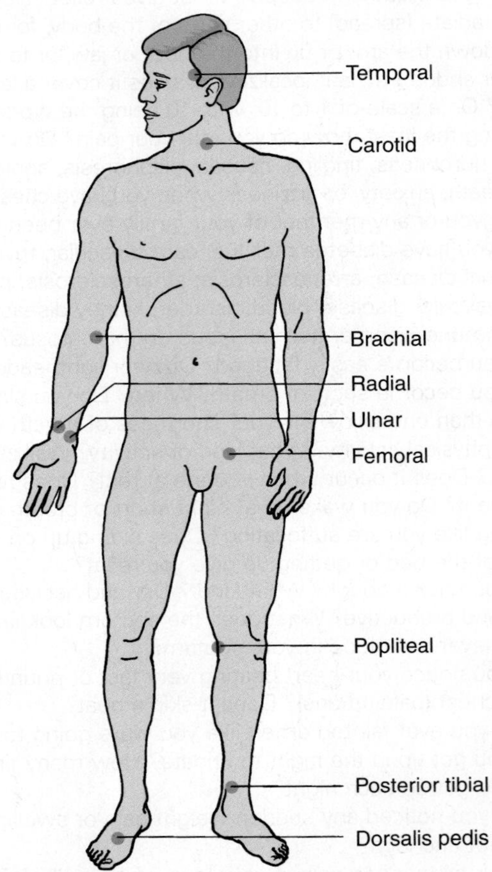

FIGURE 17–11 Palpation sites for arterial pulse.

Box 17–2 Scale for Grading Pulse Quality

0 Absent
1+ Weak, thready
2+ Light volume
3+ Normal volume
4+ Full, bounding

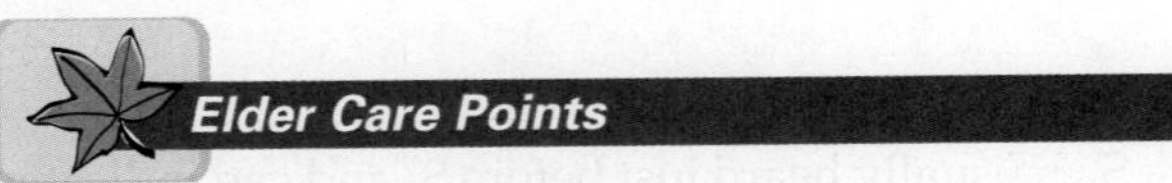

Elder Care Points

The thickening of valve leaflets with age may cause a systolic murmur common in persons older than age 80.

Pulses. Check the arterial pulses and determine the pulse rate, rhythm, and character (force) of the pulse (Box 17–2). When performing a cardiovascular assessment, the radial pulse should be assessed and compared with the apical pulse. **The apical pulse should be counted for a full minute.** The carotid, femoral, popliteal, and pedal pulses should also be palpated and compared bilaterally, noting quality and character. Figure 17–11 indicates the arterial pulse sites. The pulse may be described as *normal* or *absent*, *regular* or *irregular*, *strong*, *weak*, or *thready*.

If pulsations are weak or undetectable, use a Doppler stethoscope to check them. A Doppler stethoscope measures the velocity of blood flow through a vessel with ultrasound waves. It can sense weak pulsations even in severely narrowed arteries (Figure 17–12).

Think Critically About . . . Can you recall the correct way to locate a dorsalis pedis and a posterior tibial pulse? Could you demonstrate the technique to a classmate?

Examine the abdomen with the patient lying supine for a visual abdominal pulsation from the aorta. This sometimes indicates the presence of an aneurysm.

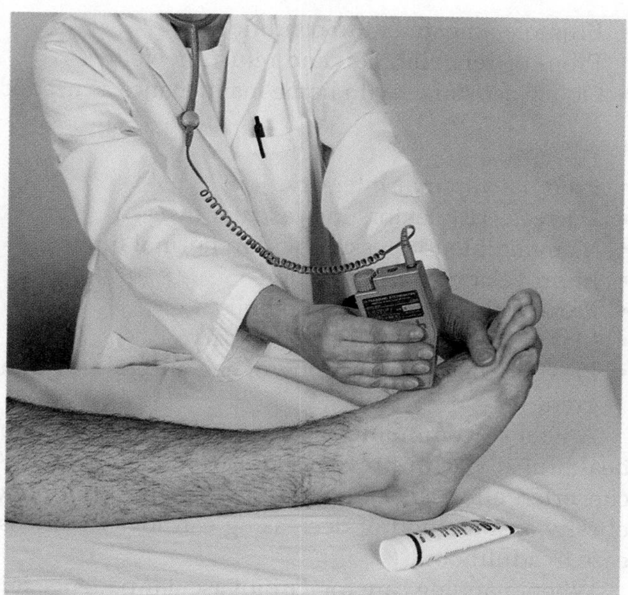

FIGURE **17–12** The Doppler stethoscope is used to detect a faint pulse.

Bruits. A whooshing or purring sound is made when blood passes through a partially obstructed artery. To detect bruits, listen with the bell of the stethoscope applied lightly over the skin of the carotid arteries, abdominal aorta, and femoral arteries. Observe the jugular veins for prominence when the patient is in an upright position; this may indicate CHF.

Blood Pressure. For more accurate readings, be certain the patient has not had a cigarette or any caffeine for the past 30 minutes. Blood pressure should be carefully measured with the correct size cuff. The cuff should fit the upper arm with the lower edge 2.5 cm (1 inch) above the antecubital space. If it is too narrow, the pressure will be falsely elevated. Cuffs are available in child, normal adult, and large adult sizes. The bladder must be centered over the brachial artery, and its length should cover at least 80% of the extremity's circumference when positioned correctly. The pressure should be taken sitting, lying supine, and standing for a thorough assessment. Standing blood pressure measurements also are important when a patient is started on a new medication, particularly an angiotensin-converting enzyme (ACE) inhibitor. Blood pressure should be measured on both arms. The patient's arm on which the cuff is placed should be supported at heart level. The patient should be resting quietly for 5 minutes before the measurement is taken. The equipment used should be calibrated, and the valve should open and close smoothly. The cuff should be deflated slowly and smoothly to obtain a correct diastolic reading.

Orthostatic or postural hypotension occurs when the blood pressure drops with standing. It is a common cause of syncope (fainting) in older patients.

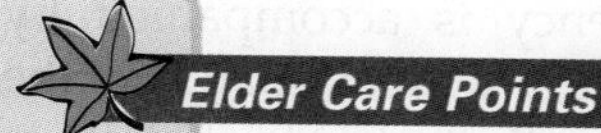

Elder Care Points

The blood pressure of the elderly patient will be lower right after a meal. For accurate readings, assess blood pressure between meals.

Skin. Tissues in light-skinned people that are receiving an adequate supply of oxygenated blood appear pink and rosy, whereas tissues deprived of normal amounts of arterial blood appear pale and mottled. In dark-skinned people, the mucous membranes will be rosy and pink if oxygenation is adequate. However, the environment must be taken into account. Pale and mottled skin also can indicate that the patient is just cold. Reddish blue color can indicate venous insufficiency.

One way to assess arterial blood flow more accurately is by having the patient elevate his feet and legs above the level of the heart for 1 to 3 minutes until pallor occurs. Have the patient lower the legs to a dangling position while sitting. Compare both feet, noting the time necessary for pinkness to return (usually about 10 seconds). Note the time it takes for the veins of the feet and ankles to fill (usually about 15 seconds). For African Americans, inspect the soles of the feet for color change and use a light shining at an angle to visualize vein filling.

Return of color to the lowered feet is delayed in arterial insufficiency. If there is severe ischemia, the dangling feet soon take on a dusky red color (rubor). **This indicates permanent dilation of the vessels; they are no longer able to constrict as they should. In addition to being reddened, the feet and ankles may appear swollen and edematous.**

A cold environment and immobility will cause the extremities to feel cold to the touch. However, when a patient experiences persistent coldness of an extremity in a warm environment, arterial insufficiency should be suspected. When observing a patient for signs of arterial disease, the nurse should note differences in skin temperature in various areas of the same limb, as well as differences between limbs.

Skin that is chronically malnourished because of decreased blood supply has a characteristic appearance: it appears smooth, shiny, and thin, and there is little or no hair on its surface. The nails are thick with deposits of thick, cornlike material under them.

Hair loss is a natural occurrence with aging, as is thickening of fingernails and toenails. These signs are not reliable indicators of vascular problems of the extremities in the elderly.

If there is severe malnutrition of the tissues for several days, the tissues become necrotic. This causes the skin to assume a purple-black color. This is a deep cyanotic condition indicative of gangrene. Gangrene of the toes is not an uncommon complication in the diabetic patient who has poor circulation in the feet.

Chronic venous insufficiency is accompanied by chronic edema. This in turn leads to inflammation of the tissues **(cellulitis)** and eventually to the formation of ulcers. Edema is either present, absent, pitting, or non-pitting. Pitting means that a fingertip pressed into the area for 5 seconds leaves an indentation. Increased pigmentation of the skin, dryness and scaling, and excoriations are objective signs of venous insufficiency.

The capillary refill test has traditionally been used to check peripheral circulation. A fingernail or a toenail is squeezed over the bed of the nail sufficiently to cause blanching; the pressure is removed and an observation of how quickly the color returns is made. Normally the color returns immediately. Although it is a good gross assessment of circulation to the extremity, this test is unreliable as many factors can cause a decrease in time for color to return. This test is most useful for determining whether circulation is occluded by constriction or thrombosis above the area. Review Chapter 3 for assessment and staging of edema.

Homans' sign is tested by having the patient raise the leg with the knee bent, then straightening the leg and dorsiflexing the foot as the leg is lowered to the bed. A positive Homans' sign may indicate a deep venous thrombosis.

Nursing Diagnosis

Table 17–4 presents general nursing diagnoses and nursing interventions for patients experiencing cardiovascular problems. Nursing diagnoses may be added to the care plan for problems secondary to treatments, such as drug therapy or surgery. Additional nursing diagnoses that also may apply include:

- Risk for infection related to inflammation of lining of heart structures
- Anxiety related to life-threatening disease
- Insomnia related to pain in the legs while at rest
- Chronic low self-esteem related to activity intolerance or inability to perform usual roles because of chronic leg ulcers

Planning

General nursing goals for care of patients with cardiovascular disease are:

Cardiac

- Prevent death and complications
- Monitor for complications
- Promote adequate oxygenation
- Alleviate or control pain
- Decrease fear and anxiety
- Balance activity and rest to prevent fatigue and provide adequate tissue perfusion
- Assist with activities of daily living (ADLs) until patient can resume self-care
- Educate regarding disease, surgery, treatments, and self-care
- Promote adjustment to condition
- Promote rehabilitation and return to wellness
- Obtain assistance with home maintenance as needed

Vascular

- Promote vascular integrity
- Decrease risk factors for vascular disease
- Maintain blood pressure within normal limits
- Improve circulatory function
- Prevent thrombosis and embolism
- Maintain or restore tissue integrity
- Prevent the complications of leg ulcers and gangrene

A goal of community nursing is the promotion of healthful living to prevent cardiovascular disease. A concerted effort is being made to decrease childhood obesity as a method of decreasing cardiovascular disease in adulthood.

When planning care for cardiovascular patients, it is important to schedule nursing activities to conserve the strength of the patient and prevent excessive fatigue. Patients undergoing telemetry monitoring should not be disconnected from their monitor for any extended time. Check to see whether it is all right to disconnect the device before having the patient shower. **Reconnect the leads immediately afterward.**

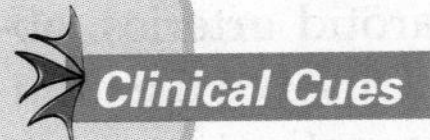

If you detach the cardiac monitor without alerting the person monitoring the telemetry monitors, she may think the patient's heart has stopped beating and call a "code." Always alert the monitor watcher when you remove the patient from telemetry and when you reattach the leads. That way she knows that she needs to watch that screen again.

Planning the timing of medication administration is necessary because many patients prefer to take cardiovascular medications with food in their stomach. If medications are due when a meal is not scheduled, plan to take some juice to the room with the medications. Always check to see that the medication can be taken with food before administering with juice or milk.

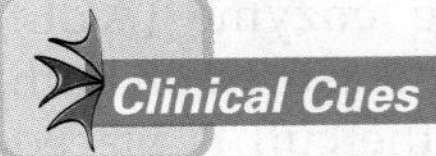

Know what the patient's last blood pressure and pulse measurements were before going to the room with cardiovascular medications. Often you will need to take an apical pulse rate and blood pressure reading before administering certain medications. You need to know what those measurements had been previously in order to evaluate the patient's status properly. Plan time to take these measurements and record them.

Text continued on p. 426

Table 17–4 **Common Nursing Diagnoses and Interventions for Patients with Heart Disorders**

NURSING DIAGNOSIS	GOALS/EXPECTED OUTCOMES	NURSING INTERVENTIONS
CARDIAC DISORDERS		
Activity intolerance related to decreased perfusion	Patient will not experience undue fatigue with activity as evidenced by changes in vital signs.	Space activities of daily living and nursing procedures to prevent undue fatigue. Encourage use of oxygen as ordered. Implement actions to promote rest.
Risk for injury related to dysrhythmia or complications of MI or CHF	Patient will not experience myocardial infarction or congestive heart failure as a result of dysrhythmia. Patient will not experience complications from MI or CHF.	Monitor ECG or telemetry tracings, observing for changes and life-threatening dysrhythmias. Assess for complications: • Monitor lungs for crackles. • Check for jugular venous distention. • Auscultate for changes in heart sounds, extra sounds, changes in rhythm. • Assess respirations for increasing dyspnea. • Assess for signs of inflammation or infection; check temperature trend, WBCs. • Assess for chest pain upon exertion or at rest. • Monitor for central and peripheral edema. • Assess trends in daily weight. • Assess trends in 24-hr intake and output. • Monitor vital signs.
Decreased cardiac output related to dysrhythmia or ineffective cardiac muscle	Patient will demonstrate adequate cardiac output as evidenced by normal pulses, vital signs, skin color, and urine output.	Assess apical pulse q shift. Administer antidysrhythmic and cardiotonic medications, as ordered. Observe for side effects of medications. Assess for adequate perfusion: • Check peripheral pulses. • Assess color of extremities and around mouth. • Assess mentation. • Monitor urine output (related to perfusion of kidneys). • Auscultate lungs for crackles every shift. • Assess level of fatigue. • Treat impaired oxygenation and fluid imbalance.
Impaired gas exchange related to cardiac failure	Patient will not experience impaired oxygenation; Sao_2 will be within normal limits; Po_2 between 80 and 100.	Place in high Fowler's position. Administer oxygen, as ordered. Feed frequent small meals to decrease oxygen demand. Administer diuretics as ordered. Monitor intake and output. Enforce fluid restrictions. Assist with ADLs. Promote relief of anxiety. Give morphine, as ordered, to ease breathing and decrease anxiety. Monitor lung sounds, pulse oximetry, and blood gases. Assist to use incentive spirometer q 2 hr, as ordered. Provide measures to drain pulmonary fluid, as ordered (i.e., postural drainage, suction, nebulizer treatments).
Self-care deficit, bathing/hygiene, toileting, dressing/grooming, related to fatigue, weakness, or dyspnea	Patient will increase performance of own ADLs of 1 to 3 METs within 1 wk. Patient will not experience constipation.	Assist with all ADLs as needed. Plan nursing treatments to provide rest periods. Encourage to do small tasks of ADLs as condition improves. Assist to turn in bed q 2 hr. Assess skin q shift and when turning. Provide mouth care before meals to stimulate appetite. Give stool softeners or laxatives, as ordered, to prevent straining at stool (Valsalva maneuver).

Key: *ADLs*, activities of daily living; *METs*, metabolic equivalent.

Continued

Table 17–4 Common Nursing Diagnoses and Interventions for Patients with Heart Disorders—cont'd

NURSING DIAGNOSIS	GOALS/EXPECTED OUTCOMES	NURSING INTERVENTIONS
CARDIAC DISORDERS—cont'd		
Fear related to life-threatening illness	Patient will verbalize feelings and fears regarding life-threatening condition. Patient will identify own best coping mechanisms.	Perform a spiritual assessment. Determine usual coping style. Support in coping mechanisms. Obtain clergyman if patient desires contact. Provide privacy for prayer and devotions. Assist to ventilate fears to reduce anxiety. Keep informed of what is being done for treatment and what to expect. Inform of positive gains toward wellness. Allow state of denial in acute stage as denial may be protective. Provide time with loved ones. Provide therapeutic touch if patient is accepting. Assess cultural meanings of events to patient. Actively listen to the patient's fears and concerns. Offer realistic reassurance as appropriate.
Impaired home maintenance related to fatigue, dyspnea, and activity intolerance	Appropriate home services will be in place before discharge.	Refer for social services consult. Consider home health care services. Offer information on homemaker aide services. Consult with family regarding ongoing care of patient at home. Collaborate with patient regarding plans for home care.
VASCULAR DISORDERS		
Ineffective tissue perfusion related to: Vascular damage	Patient's blood pressure will be within normal range within 3 mo.	Assess blood pressure; determine effectiveness of therapy. Administer medications to lower blood pressure. Discourage intake of caffeine and excess sodium. Discourage smoking. Teach to arise slowly and stabilize before walking to counteract postural hypotension effect from medication. Teach anxiety- and tension-reduction techniques to decrease blood pressure. Encourage regular rest, relaxation, and exercise program.
Obstructed blood flow	Patient will not develop other deep vein thromboses. Thrombosis will resolve within 10–14 days.	Assess for signs and symptoms of deep vein thrombosis and impaired blood flow. Maintain activity restrictions as ordered. Elevate affected extremity as ordered. Increase fluid intake to 3000 mL/day unless contraindicated. Administer anticoagulants as ordered; monitor for side effects. Teach to prevent future episodes by encouraging not to sit with legs crossed, not to sit for long periods, and not to put pressure on the back of the knees. Apply elastic stockings or sequential pneumatic devices to promote venous return.
Surgical revascularization	Patient will not develop thrombosis.	Check incisions for bleeding q 1–2 hr × 24 hr then q 4 hr × 6, then q shift. Assess for internal hematoma by checking sensation below surgical area. Assess for adequate blood flow by checking pulses distal to incision on same schedule. Assess skin color and temperature above and below incision when checking for bleeding. Reinforce dressing as needed; change dressing per orders, using strict aseptic technique.

Table 17–4 Common Nursing Diagnoses and Interventions for Patients with Heart Disorders—cont'd

NURSING DIAGNOSIS	GOALS/EXPECTED OUTCOMES	NURSING INTERVENTIONS
VASCULAR DISORDERS—cont'd		
Pain related to decreased blood flow and edema	Patient will verbalize adequate pain control attained from analgesics and comfort measures provided.	Assess type and location of pain experienced. Handle gently and avoid jarring the bed. Use a bed cradle or footboard to prevent pressure from bed linens. Administer analgesics and antiinflammatory agents as ordered. Apply heat as ordered; monitor closely to prevent burns. Teach relaxation techniques, imagery, or distraction to decrease pain. Elevate edematous extremity. Apply elastic stockings or sequential pneumatic devices to encourage venous return and decrease edema. Medicate for sleep as ordered if discomfort is interfering with rest.
Activity intolerance related to pain in legs when walking	Patient will develop own activity program within 3 wk. Patient will exercise regularly according to devised program.	Collaborate with physical therapist to encourage prescribed exercises. Assist to plan walking swimming, or cycling program.
Disturbed body image related to: Diagnosis of chronic illness Edema and dilated veins in the legs Loss of limb by amputation Inability to maintain former lifestyle	Patient will verbalize feelings regarding diagnosis, body changes, and needed lifestyle changes. Patient will identify personal strengths and coping mechanisms. Patient will become as independent as possible in tasks of daily living (within 2 mo).	Allow to ventilate feelings about illness and disease process. Assist through the grief process. Assist to identify personal strengths. Reinforce coping mechanisms that have been helpful before. Be with patient for first dressing change. Clarify misconceptions about physical limitations after amputation. Involve patient in care of the wound after initial period of adjustment. Foster independence in tasks of daily living. Assist to explore lifestyle changes. Encourage significant others in their support of the patient. Teach ways to decrease risk of further amputation.
Impaired tissue integrity related to: Ulcer from decreased circulation Surgical wound (Risk for infection may be used here also)	Patient will not develop a wound infection.	Use strict aseptic technique for wound care. Treat and dress wound per physician's orders. Promote adequate nutrition to promote healing. Administer medication, as ordered, to prevent infection.
Risk for impaired tissue integrity related to bed rest and impaired circulation	Patient will not develop impaired tissue integrity.	Position affected limb, as ordered. Maintain correct body alignment. Inspect pressure points q 2 hr. Turn at least q 2 hr. Maintain smooth linens on bed, provide appropriate padding to prevent pressure areas. Keep skin clean and dry. Refrain from raising the knee section of the bed. Encourage foot and ankle exercises q hr while patient is awake. Prevent shearing when patient is moving in bed by using a lift sheet and two people to turn the patient. If skin breakdown occurs, notify physician immediately and provide appropriate wound care.

Continued

Table 17–4 Common Nursing Diagnoses and Interventions for Patients with Heart Disorders—cont'd

NURSING DIAGNOSIS	GOALS/EXPECTED OUTCOMES	NURSING INTERVENTIONS
VASCULAR DISORDERS—cont'd		
Knowledge deficient related to inadequate information about disease process, medications, and self-care	Patient will verbalize knowledge of disease process and ways to prevent further damage. Patient will verbalize how to take medications and side effects to report. Patient will demonstrate self-care techniques.	Explain what is happening in the body to cause the decreased blood flow. Allow time for questions. Instruct in ways to decrease risk factors. Teach self-care methods, including exercises, skin care, foot care, dietary changes, lifestyle changes. Teach about medications, including schedule of administration, action, side effects, what to report to the physician. Encourage regular visits to the physician.
Noncompliance related to refusal to follow treatment regimen	Patient will verbalize frustrations and problems in complying with treatment regimen and lifestyle changes. Patient will demonstrate compliance with treatment regimen.	Reinstruct about disease process. Explore problems with treatment regimen. Allow to express feelings about lifestyle changes. Explore ability to obtain and afford medications. Explore any difficulty in swallowing medications. Explain progression of disease and consequences of poor control; discuss complications and impact on lifestyle. Seek support system for compliance with treatment program. Give praise for each attempt at compliance. Respect the patient's right to make decisions about compliance.
Risk for injury related to: Embolus or bleeding from anticoagulant medication	Coagulation times will remain within safe therapeutic range. Patient will have no signs of bleeding. Patient will have no signs of embolus.	Do not massage affected extremity. Encourage activity restrictions as ordered. Monitor laboratory values: PT or APTT and notify physician when values are outside of accepted therapeutic limits. Assess urine and stool for signs of blood. Assess patient for excessive bruising; bleeding gums, nosebleeds, bleeding at puncture sites. Check injectable anticoagulant dosages and IV admixtures with another nurse before administration to verify correct ordered dosage and rate of infusion.
Circulatory occlusion from embolus		Assess for signs of embolus: chest pain, shortness of breath, change in level of consciousness, sudden headache, or other neurologic signs.

When a patient has a history of thrombosis, the nurse must plan measures to prevent recurrence regardless of what patient problem is currently the focus of treatment. If the patient has arterial insufficiency, the nurse should be alert to prescribed medications that may cause further vasoconstriction.

Appropriate exercise is important to treat vascular disease, and the nurse collaborates with the physical therapist about activity, exercises, and the reinforcement of teaching. Collaboration with the dietitian is vital to the patient who has atherosclerosis and a high cholesterol count. Specific expected outcomes must be written on an individual basis. Examples are included in Table 17–4.

Implementation

A large part of what the nurse does for the patient with a cardiovascular disorder is to monitor the condition and determine whether treatment is effective. Considerable time is spent on teaching patients about the disease, self-care, and medications. Monitoring side effects or adverse effects of medication is very important.

Remember that any patient experiencing fatigue or weakness takes longer to accomplish the tasks of daily living. Space nursing actions appropriately. Place patient in an upright position to administer oral medications. It is especially important that the elderly patient be upright to aid swallowing; have the patient take a sip of water to wet the throat and then give the medication.

Watch the patient receiving cardiac drugs for postural hypotension; have her **hold on to the bedrail and steady herself for a couple of minutes after arising before beginning to walk.** This will help prevent falls.

Appropriate nursing interventions are discussed with the various disorders in the following chapters. Specific nursing interventions for common nursing diagnoses related to cardiovascular conditions also are found in the nursing care plans in those chapters and in Table 17–4.

Collaboration

Cardiovascular patients often are being treated by the physical therapist, dietitian, and respiratory therapist, as well as the physician and nurse. It is important that the nurse consult with the other health professionals involved in the patient's care. Early collaboration with the discharge planner is important to provide continuity of care after discharge. The nurse's work will go more smoothly if it is possible to plan when other health professionals see the patient. Providing others on the health care team with information useful to them promotes a good working relationship.

Evaluation

Evaluation involves both subjective and objective data. This means that good communication skills must be used to ask the right questions and gather the required information from the patient. Ask the patient to describe any "different" feelings she has experienced. Inquire about changes in appetite and bowel movements that could indicate possible medication toxicity. Check laboratory values for therapeutic drug levels before giving doses of medication, and note the latest blood levels of electrolytes. Assess for signs and symptoms of toxicity and fluid or electrolyte imbalance. Ask yourself whether the patient is showing signs indicating that the medication you are giving is effective. The nursing care plan should be checked daily to evaluate whether each nursing action is effective. If an action is ineffective over time, it should be deleted and a new action should be devised to resolve the problem.

It is important to look at serial blood pressure readings to evaluate the effectiveness of treatment and of nursing interventions. Pressures that are consistently higher than normal in between medication doses indicate a need to change either the dosage schedule or the medication.

Carefully evaluating pulses and comparing them bilaterally is an important part of nursing care for patients with problems of the cardiovascular system. Writing a good description of the quality and character of the pulses monitored in the nurse's notes will give coworkers an accurate assessment baseline on which to evaluate changes in the pulse.

It is important to determine if skin color and temperature have changed since the last assessment. Areas of discoloration should be accurately measured and documented in the nurse's notes. Ulcerated areas are monitored closely and are measured to determine whether healing is occurring. The color of the healing tissue and presence of exudate also are evaluated. If the wound is growing or not improving, the nursing actions or treatment must be changed.

Often the nurse must rely on subjective data from the patient to evaluate whether treatment and nursing actions are effective. Increases in peripheral circulation may be evident only by a decrease in pain or an ability to walk further without pain.

COMMON PROBLEMS OF PATIENTS WITH CARDIOVASCULAR DISORDERS

FATIGUE AND DYSPNEA

In the early stages of heart disease, the patient may be only slightly aware of the inability to do as much physical work as she formerly could. If she lets the problem go too long, she will find that physical activities will become increasingly restricted, because she will lack the energy to perform the simplest of tasks and will become short of breath after the slightest exertion.

When the coronary arteries fail to supply adequate oxygen to the cells of the heart muscle, the heart is unable to perform as it should when extra demands are placed on it. The result is a general hypoxia of the tissues throughout the body, which causes fatigue and dyspnea on exertion.

Traditionally, prolonged bed rest was prescribed for every patient with a heart condition. Currently, bed rest with bedside commode privileges is ordered for the first 24 to 72 hours for MI and severe CHF. The patient may feed herself and assist with her sponge bath. She should be cautioned against any isometric activity, such as pushing up in bed. Stool softeners are given to prevent straining at stool (Valsalva maneuver), which causes a sudden increase in cardiac workload (Felker et al., 2006). Straining while coughing or repositioning in bed can cause the Valsalva as well and is to be avoided. Activity progresses to chair sitting, ambulating to the bathroom, and then down the hall. Patients are monitored by telemetry units to watch for dysrhythmias or excessive heart rate changes during ambulation. The amount of energy used in activity is expressed in *metabolic equivalents* (METs). The patient is guided from 1 to 3 METs before discharge. Sitting, eating, washing hands and face, and conversing are 1 to 3 MET activities. Box 17–3 shows the metabolic equivalents for various activities.

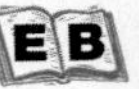

Criteria used to determine whether the patient is tolerating the activity include the following:

- The heart rate does not rise more than 20 beats per minute.
- Systolic blood pressure does not drop.
- There is no complaint of chest pain, dyspnea, or severe fatigue.
- There is no abnormal heart rate or rhythm.

Activity progression often is jointly supervised by a physical therapist and a nurse. More information on cardiac rehabilitation is presented in Chapter 9.

FLUID OVERLOAD: EDEMA

Edema is an accumulation of fluid in the interstitial fluid compartment. It becomes a problem in heart disease when the blood flow into or out of the heart is in-

Box 17–3 ***Energy Expenditure in Metabolic Equivalents***

	CALORIES BURNED
LOW-ENERGY ACTIVITIES (Less Than 3 METs or Less Than 3 cal/min)	
Activities in Hospital	
Resting supine	1.0
Sitting	1.2
Eating	1.4
Conversing	1.4
Washing hands, face	2.5
Activities Outside Hospital	
Sewing by hand	1.4
Sweeping floor	1.7
Painting, sitting	2.5
Driving car	2.8
Assembling a radio	2.7
Sewing by machine	2.9
MODERATE-ENERGY ACTIVITIES (3–6 METs or 3–6 cal/min)	
Activities in Hospital	
Sitting on bedside commode	3.6
Walking at 2.5 mph	3.6
Showering	4.2
Using bedpan	4.7
Walking at 3.75 mph	5.6
Activities Outside Hospital	
Bricklaying	4.0
Tractor plowing	4.2
Ironing, standing	4.2
Mopping floor	4.2
Bowling	4.4
Cycling at 5.5 mph on level ground	4.5
Golfing	5.0
Dancing	5.5
HIGH-ENERGY ACTIVITIES (6–8 METs or 6–8 cal/min)	
Ambulating with braces and crutches	8.0
Performing carpentry	6.8
Mowing lawn by hand	7.7
Playing singles tennis	7.1
Riding on trotting horse	8.0
Walking at 5 mph	6.5
Ascending stairs	7.0

Adapted from Lewis S.M., Heitkemper M.M., Dirksen S.R. et al. (2007). *Medical-Surgical Nursing*, (7th ed.). St Louis, Mosby.

hibited, causing a slowing down of the normal movement of body fluids and their eventual excretion.

Continually assess the fluid balance of a patient with cardiac disease by looking for signs of abnormal collections of fluid in the body tissues. Daily weight change is considered the best indicator of fluid buildup. The feet and ankles of ambulatory patients are checked for signs of dependent edema, and bed rest patients are watched for signs of swelling in the area of the sacrum, buttocks, and thighs. The patient is observed for progressive signs of shortness of breath, and lung fields are auscultated each shift to detect crackles, a sign of beginning pulmonary congestion.

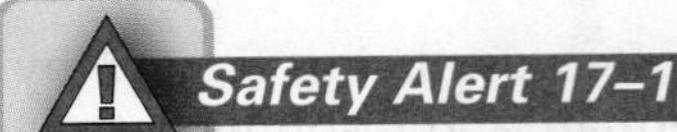

Be Alert for Hypokalemia

Be alert for the following signs of hypokalemia: fatigue, muscle weakness, muscle cramps, drowsiness, confusion, new onset of bradycardia, or postural hypotension. Hypokalemia may cause life-threatening cardiac dysrhythmia.

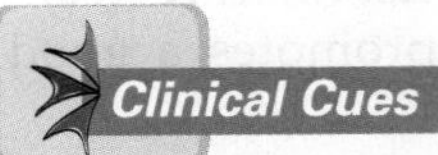

A weight gain of 3 lb or more in a 24-hour period indicates fluid retention.

Nursing responsibilities include recording the patient's weight daily before breakfast, supervising fluid restriction, accurately measuring intake and output, and assessing for signs of both fluid deficit and fluid overload. Elderly patients on fluid restriction and diuretics can easily become dehydrated.

Therapeutic measures to control edema include the administration of diuretics and restriction of sodium and, possibly, fluid. You must observe for adverse effects of medication, such as electrolyte imbalance and postural hypotension. Potassium supplementation may be ordered for the patient who is experiencing hypokalemia (Safety Alert 17–1).

PAIN

Severe pain is most often associated with heart disease of an acute nature (e.g., MI). Anginal pain caused by narrowed coronary arteries can interfere with the patient's lifestyle, as well as cause discomfort. Acute anginal pain is treated with nitroglycerin, oral nitrates, oxygen, reassurance, and careful monitoring for relief. Nitrates and other medications that dilate coronary arteries to promote better blood flow and decrease ischemia are used to control or prevent anginal pain.

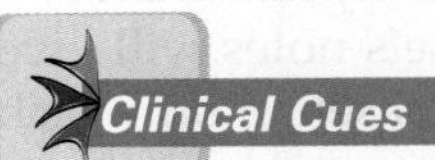

If chest pain is not relieved after administering three nitroglycerin sublingual tablets 5 minutes apart, notify the physician. Institute oxygen therapy according to agency protocol, monitor vital signs, and stay with the patient. The patient may be experiencing an MI. (Do check to make certain that the nitroglycerin causes tingling under the tongue. If not, the tablets are too old and will not work.)

If pain is not relieved, the analgesic drug used most often in an emergency situation is morphine sulfate, as it decreases both anxiety and cardiac workload, as well

EB as alleviates pain (Webb et al., 2000). The drug is given IV initially for quick pain relief. As the acute phase and severe pain subside, these drugs may be replaced with oral dosages or milder sedatives that promote relaxation and freedom from anxiety.

The patient's pain may be increased because of nervousness and anxiety, and you can do much to help relieve pain by providing a restful environment, interacting therapeutically with "active listening," and balancing rest with prescribed physical activity.

Pain can be a symptom of a life-threatening heart event. Each episode of pain is carefully assessed by noting when it started, the location and radiation pattern, degree on a scale, activity prior to onset, associated symptoms such as nausea, diaphoresis, or **palpitations**, and vital signs.

Sleep deprivation and fatigue can increase the pain. Turning, administration of medications, visiting, exercise, and other procedures should be coordinated so that the patient is not disturbed more than necessary.

Determining those factors that seem to trigger an attack can identify stressors that the patient may be able to avoid. Relaxation and other noninvasive techniques to manage pain are discussed in Chapter 7.

ALTERED TISSUE PERFUSION

In peripheral vascular disease, blood flow may be sluggish or altered by constriction of the vessels. The smooth muscles of the arterial walls respond to temperature by constricting in the presence of cold and extreme heat and relaxing in the presence of warmth. Therefore the nurse's care plan should include (1) providing a warm environment for the patient; (2) covering the hospitalized patient with warm blankets; dressing her in warm clothing; and (3) instructing the patient to avoid extremes of cold and heat.

The constricting effect of extreme heat rules out the use of local applications in the form of hot water bottles. In addition to the danger of burning the patient because of decreased sensitivity to extremes of temperature, local heat increases metabolic activity in the tissues to which it is applied and therefore upsets even more the balance of supply and demand for blood flow to all the tissues.

The goal in application of additional warmth is even distribution throughout the body.

? *Think Critically About . . .* What would you recommend to the elderly home care patient to keep his lower extremities warm during the winter? The patient does not have the funds to keep the house heated above 68° F (20° C).

A second consideration is that of *pressure* against the walls of the blood vessels. Constricting clothing is avoided, particularly circular garters and elastic materials in underclothing. Frequent position changes are essential; position must be changed at least every 2 hours.

The patient with poor venous circulation can benefit from periodic elevation of the lower extremities to facilitate venous return of blood to the heart. Elevation above the level of the heart is preferred.

Even, well-distributed support of the vessels near the surface of the body will help improve venous return. To provide this kind of support, the physician may prescribe an elastic bandage or fitted elastic stockings. The stockings or elastic bandage should be applied early in the morning, before the legs are placed in a dependent position, because the blood vessels are less congested after a prolonged rest. Bandages and hose should be applied by beginning at the feet and working upward to avoid trapping blood in the lower leg. The patient should have two pairs of elastic hose and should wash them after each day's wearing. Elastic hose should be replaced every 6 months as they lose their elasticity. When stockings are removed, the heels should be checked for pressure areas. **Elastic stockings are not used for patients with arterial disorders.**

Exercise is especially beneficial to patients with decreased blood flow. Walking is ideal exercise for the ambulatory patient. Bed-ridden patients will need range-of-motion (ROM) exercises and the other kinds of muscular movements described in Chapter 9. Use of a treadmill for patients who cannot exercise by walking outside is very beneficial. An Exercycle is another alternative.

In addition to mechanical factors, certain chemical factors affect the constriction of blood vessels. *Nicotine*, which is inhaled with tobacco smoke, has the effect of producing spasmodic narrowing of the peripheral arteries. Patients with arterial insufficiency are encouraged to stop smoking. Used in conjunction with a community stop smoking support program, the booklet *You Can Quit Smoking*, available from the Agency for Health Care Research and Quality Publications Clearinghouse (540 Gaither Rd., Rockville, MD 20850), can be very helpful.

? *Think Critically About . . .* Can you describe the specific actions you would take to help a patient recognize the need for and to establish a "quit smoking" program?

Alcohol is a mild vasodilator when taken in moderate amounts (Health Promotion Points 17–3). Unless the patient has moral or religious convictions against its use, the physician may approve a daily intake of a specific, small amount of wine or liquor. It is important to find out whether alcohol will interfere with the action of medications being taken.

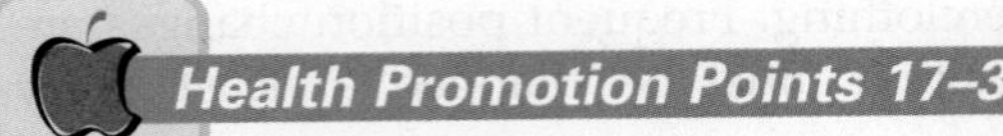

Health Promotion Points 17–3

Drink in Moderation

Promote proper use of alcohol for those who do consume alcoholic beverages. Moderate alcohol intake for a man is two drinks in any one day. For a woman, the appropriate amount is one drink per day. One drink is 1½ ounces of alcohol, 4 ounces of wine, or 12 ounces of beer.

Drugs that are helpful to relieve vasoconstriction and improve blood flow are prescribed. These drugs are of value only when the arteries are still capable of dilating. Severely sclerosed vessels respond very poorly to therapy of this kind. Some think that vasodilators may actually be harmful because they shunt blood away from the zone of ischemia to well-perfused tissues.

Sympathectomy is a surgical technique that may be used to relieve vasoconstriction. Because this procedure severs sympathetic nerve fibers supplying the peripheral vessels, it is of benefit only to those patients who do not have advanced pathologic changes in these vessels.

IMPAIRED TISSUE INTEGRITY

Tissues that have a diminished blood supply are subject to severe and permanent damage from the slightest injury, because the normal processes of healing and repair are impaired. Arterial and venous stasis often lead to chronic leg ulcers.

These ulcers are particularly distressing to the patient because they heal very slowly and many never completely heal. Patients must be taught to avoid conditions that contribute to injury of the extremities and to report any injury, no matter how minor.

Prevention of leg ulcers includes (1) wearing elastic bandages or support hose; (2) proper positioning and exercise; (3) avoiding injury to the feet and legs; and (4) avoiding extremes of heat and cold and other mechanical and chemical factors that contribute to obstruction of blood flow. Information on care of the patient with a venous stasis ulcer is provided in Chapter 18.

Key Points

- Cardiovascular disease is the leading cause of death in the United States.
- Cardiac and vascular disorders cause considerable disability.
- The heart and vessels become stiffer with age and there is less cardiac reserve.
- Atherosclerosis and arteriosclerosis are major contributors to cardiovascular disease.
- Close to a third of the population in the United States has elevated blood pressure.
- Many risk factors for cardiovascular disease are modifiable.
- Control of hypertension and obesity could lower the incidence of cardiovascular disease.
- Understanding diagnostic tests for the cardiovascular system will assist you to prepare and care for patients properly.
- Good interview skills help you to obtain comprehensive data for a cardiovascular assessment.
- Physical data gathering involves a variety of techniques for assessment of the cardiovascular system (see Focused Assessment 17–1).
- Peripheral pulses should be compared bilaterally.
- Blood pressure should be taken, using correct technique, lying, sitting, and standing.
- Skin color and texture can tell much about cardiovascular status.
- Comprehensive nursing care plans should be holistic and may need to include problems secondary to the cardiovascular disease.
- Planning should include time management, as many heart medications need to be given as close to the prescribed time as possible to maintain a steady blood level of the drug.
- Collaboration with other health care team members assists in providing consistent, thorough care for the patient with a cardiovascular disorder.
- Evaluation involves checking blood levels of electrolytes, lab values for cardiac drugs to determine adequate dosing or toxicity, and monitoring blood counts for adequate red cells and hemoglobin to carry sufficient oxygen to the tissues of the body.
- Fatigue and dyspnea occur when the heart cannot pump sufficiently to carry adequate oxygen and nutrients to the tissues.
- Activity during cardiac rehabilitation is measured in metabolic equivalents; activity is started slowly and may progress according to the body's response.
- Heat therapy is applied cautiously to extremities of patients with peripheral vascular disease.
- When blood flow out of the heart is inhibited, there is a slowing of normal movement of body fluids and their excretion, causing edema.
- Daily weight change is the best indicator of fluid buildup.
- Watch patients who have fluid imbalances for accompanying electrolyte imbalances.
- Measures to reduce or prevent edema are often needed for the patient with peripheral vascular disease.
- Pain from an MI is acute in nature.
- Nitroglycerin and morphine are the drugs of choice for myocardial pain.
- Anginal pain is treated with nitroglycerin and other drugs to promote arterial vasodilation.

- Decreasing anxiety and promoting rest may decrease anginal pain.
- It is very important to encourage the patient with cardiovascular disease to quit smoking, as nicotine is a vasoconstrictor.
- Patients with peripheral vascular disease have difficulty healing lower leg and foot wounds.

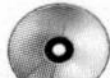

Go to your **Companion CD-ROM** for an Audio Glossary, animations, video clips, and bonus review questions.

evolve Be sure to visit the companion Evolve site at http://evolve.elsevier.com/deWit for interactive NCLEX-PN Exam Style Review Questions, WebLinks, and additional online resources.

NCLEX-PN EXAM STYLE REVIEW QUESTIONS

Choose the best answer(s) for the following questions.

1. Which of the following statements are true regarding drug use and the risk of cardiac disease? *(Select all that apply.)*

1. The vasodilation effects of cocaine hasten atherosclerosis.
2. Sudden cardiac death is associated with cocaine use.
3. Methamphetamine dilates blood vessels.
4. Cigarette smoking contributes heavily to heart disease.
5. Methamphetamine can cause myocardial infarction.

2. The nurse compares the blood pressure taken at the ankle with that taken at the arm to evaluate the circulatory status in the lower extremities. This procedure is known as:

1. retrograde filling test.
2. ankle-brachial test.
3. Doppler flow studies.
4. Allen's test.

3. ______________________________ is a common manifestation of arterial insufficiency to the lower extremities that is described as muscle cramping brought on by exercise and relieved by rest.

4. During initial assessment of an older adult, the nurse found that the skin appears smooth, shiny, and thinned, with little or no hair on the surface. Which is the most appropriate nursing diagnosis?

1. Ineffective tissue perfusion
2. Risk for infection
3. Disturbance in body image
4. Deficient fluid volume

5. When taking care of a patient with cardiac disease, the nurse teaches the importance of decreasing the cardiac workload. Which of the following nursing interventions would reinforce patient instructions?

1. Caution against pushing up in bed with the feet.
2. Prevent straining at stool.
3. Encourage coughing.
4. Promote exercise and progressive activity.

6. The nurse weighs a patient with congestive heart failure and determines that there is a net weight gain of 5 pounds within the last 24 hours. Which of the following nursing interventions is most appropriate?

1. Administering ordered diuretics
2. Restricting of potassium intake
3. Monitoring pulse oximetry
4. Forcing oral fluids

7. The nurse administered two consecutive sublingual nitroglycerin tablets to a patient complaining of moderate chest pain. The patient's blood pressure is 110/70 mm Hg with continued chest pain. An appropriate nursing action would be to:

1. administer morphine sulfate.
2. start a 500-mL fluid challenge.
3. give another sublingual nitroglycerin.
4. provide emotional support.

8. When interviewing a patient complaining of moderate chest pain, an appropriate question would be: *(Select all that apply.)*

1. Who witnessed the pain?
2. What does the pain or discomfort feel like?
3. What relaxation strategies were implemented?
4. Where is the pain located?
5. Where does the pain radiate?

9. The nurse assesses the older adult who complains of easy fatigability with exercise. Which of the following clinical findings is associated with aging?

1. Hypertension
2. Confusion
3. Muscle atrophy
4. Diastolic murmur

10. As the nurse prepares to administer a dose of losartan (Cozaar) the patient asks, "What does this medication do?" An accurate statement by a student nurse would be:

1. "The medication blocks the effect of a potent vasoconstrictor."
2. "The medication stimulates angiotensin secretion."
3. "The medication slows your heart rate."
4. "The medication stimulates the production of red blood cells."

CRITICAL THINKING ACTIVITIES

Read each clinical scenario and discuss the questions with your classmates.

Scenario A

Debra Johnson, a 20-year-old African American college student on your campus, comes to the health center complaining of frequent headaches. The assessment data show that she is 5′ 4″ tall, weighs 149 lb, Temp. 98.8° F, P = 82, R = 14, and BP 138/84. She smokes about half a pack of cigarettes a day. She has a heavy academic schedule and rarely exercises. She eats a lot of "food on the run" at the local fast-food places. Her mother and uncle both have hypertension.

1. Which of her data is abnormal for her age?
2. What risk factors does she have for cardiovascular disease?
3. Which risk factors are modifiable?

Scenario B

Aiko Sukura, a 64-year-old man, comes into the ER after experiencing chest pain and diaphoresis. His ECG is abnormal. He is scheduled for a cardiac catheterization.

1. Is a permit required for this procedure? If so, would he be able to sign it?
2. What questions would you need to ask him when preparing him for this diagnostic test?
3. What would be the priorities of care related to this diagnostic test after the procedure is finished?

CHAPTER

18 Care of Patients with Hypertension and Peripheral Vascular Disorders

evolve http://evolve.elsevier.com/deWit

Objectives

Upon completing this chapter, the student should be able to:

Theory

1. Describe the pathophysiology of hypertension.
2. Describe the complications that can occur as a consequence of hypertension.
3. Briefly describe the treatment program for mild, moderate, and severe hypertension.
4. Discuss the risk factors and incidence of vascular disease.
5. List four factors that contribute to peripheral vascular disease.
6. Describe the pathophysiology of arteriosclerosis and atherosclerosis.
7. Describe the signs, symptoms, and treatment of aneurysm.
8. Compare venous stasis ulcer with arterial leg ulcer.
9. List four nursing interventions for the patient undergoing anticoagulant therapy.
10. List types of surgery performed for problems of the peripheral vascular system.

Clinical Practice

1. Develop and implement a teaching plan for a patient who has hypertension.
2. Describe the points to be included in the teaching plan for the patient who has experienced thrombophlebitis.
3. Differentiate between venous and arterial insufficiency during a physical assessment.
4. Describe nursing interventions for the patient with arterial insufficiency.
5. Identify three likely nursing diagnoses for patients who have common problems of vascular disease and list the expected outcomes and appropriate nursing interventions for each.

Key Terms

Be sure to check out the bonus material on the Companion CD-ROM, including selected audio pronunciations.

bruit (BRŬ-ē, p. 449)
debride (dă-BRĒD, p. 452)
dependent rubor (dĕ-PĔN-dĕnt RŪ-bŏr, p. 442)
embolus (ĔM-bō-lŭs, p. 441)
gangrene (găng-GRĒN, p. 446)
intermittent claudication (ĭn-tĕr-MĬT-ĕnt klăw-dĭ-KĀ-shŭn, p. 442)
scleropathy (sklĕr-ŎP-ă-thē, p. 451)
stent (p. 444)
thrombectomy (thrŏm-BĔK-tō-mē, p. 456)
thrombophlebitis (thrŏm-bō-flĕ-BĪ-tĭs, p. 441)
thrombus (THRŎM-bŭs, p. 444)
varicose veins (VĂR-ĭ-kōs vānz, p. 449)
vascular (VĂS-kū-lăr, p. 436)

Review Chapter 17 for an overview of the vascular system, including anatomy and physiology and diagnostic tests.

HYPERTENSION

Hypertension is defined as persistently high blood pressure. In adults, this means a systolic pressure that is equal to or greater than 140 mm Hg and/or a diastolic pressure equal to or greater than 90 mm Hg. The pressure is taken twice on two different occasions two weeks apart and is averaged before the diagnosis is made. *Prehypertension* is a systolic pressure equal to or greater than 120 mm Hg and a diastolic pressure equal to or greater than 80 mm Hg. Table 18-1 presents ranges for the classification of hypertension. Ideal blood pressure is 115/75 mm Hg.

Hypertensive individuals usually die of long-term damage to the end organs or target organs; that is, the brain, heart, and kidney. More than half the deaths associated with persistent and unrelieved hypertension are caused by myocardial infarction. Immediate causes of death related to high blood pressure include cerebral hemorrhage and heart failure.

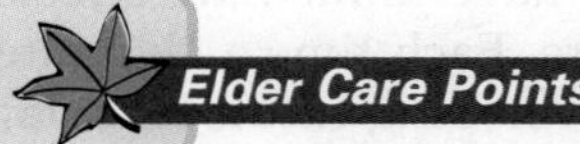

Elder Care Points

Can you think of two physiologic reasons why the elderly are greater risk for hypertension?

Table 18–1 American Heart Association Blood Pressure Recommendations

CLASSIFICATION	SYSTOLIC	DIASTOLIC	PATIENT ACTION
Normal	Less than 120	Less than 80	Continue to monitor if risk factors are present.
Prehypertension	120-139	or 80-89	Make lifestyle changes such as dietary modifications, increase exercise, lose weight, stop smoking.
High			
Stage 1	140-159	or 90-99	May need antihypertensive drugs prescribed. One drug and a diuretic may be prescribed initially.
Stage 2	160 or higher	or 100 or higher	More antihypertensive drugs may be added to the regimen until the patient achieves the desired blood pressure measurements. (Below 140/90, lifestyle modifications must be continued.)

Etiology

Hypertension is a reflection of homeostatic mechanisms that:

- Control the caliber of blood vessels and their responsiveness to various stimuli
- Regulate fluid volume in the intravascular and extravascular compartments
- Control cardiac output

There are two major types of hypertension: essential (primary or idiopathic) and secondary hypertension. About 90% of all cases of hypertension are classified as essential hypertension. The etiology of hypertension is unknown, and the goals of treatment are (1) reduction of high blood pressure and (2) long-term control to decrease the risk of stroke, heart attack, and kidney disease.

In the remaining 10%, the hypertension is actually a symptom of another disorder; that is, the hypertension is secondary to another disease. If the primary disease can be detected and treated successfully, the problem of hypertension is eliminated. Examples of diseases that can produce secondary hypertension include renal vascular disease (e.g., atherosclerosis of the renal artery), dysfunction of the adrenal cortex and medulla, atherosclerosis of the arteries of systemic circulation, and coarctation of the aorta.

Some major factors associated with essential hypertension are age, race, obesity, and sodium intake. Female hormone therapy, nicotine, and caffeine consumption appear to be contributing factors in some people. Persons with a family history of hypertension also are at greater risk for developing essential hypertension.

Obesity is closely associated with hypertension. There is a correlation between an increase in body weight over a period of years and a simultaneous increase in blood pressure. Many times a loss of excess weight alone can return a slightly elevated blood pressure to normal.

Nicotine and caffeine can have immediate effects on the level of blood pressure. Each time a cigarette is smoked, the chances of developing cardiovascular disease increase and blood pressure is elevated significantly.

There is evidence that salt intake also is a factor. Epidemiologic studies have shown that many people who consume large amounts of salt have abnormal blood pressure; others are not affected by a high-sodium diet. A possible explanation is that sodium brings out an inherent susceptibility to hypertension in some people. At any rate, a moderate reduction of salt intake has been effective in lowering the blood pressure of some persons with mild or moderate hypertension.

There is continuing research on the relationship of race, gender, and ethnicity on the incidence and effects of hypertension. African Americans tend to have a higher incidence of hypertension than other minority groups and whites; they also have a higher noncompliance, complication, and mortality rate. Economic issues, access to health care, dietary practices, and weight have been identified as possible reasons for the disparities (*Research Activities*, 2006). Women also tend 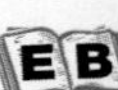 to experience more complications and the inability to properly manage hypertension than the general population. The rising incidence of childhood obesity has resulted in an increase in the incidence of hypertension. Health promotion activities targeting nutrition and exercise habits of children are increasing. Some school districts are changing the types of foods and beverages served in school cafeterias and available in vending machines in an effort to combat the problem of childhood obesity.

Pathophysiology

Blood pressure equals the amount of blood pumped out by the heart (cardiac output) multiplied by the peripheral vascular resistance. If the caliber of blood vessels becomes smaller because of atherosclerosis or vasoconstriction, blood pressure increases in an effort to force the blood through the smaller opening. If there is an increase in the volume or viscosity of fluid in the blood vessels, the pressure within the vessels increases and the heart must work harder to pump the fluid through the vessels. A pathologic response to stress can result in an elevation in blood pressure by stimulating the sympathetic nervous system and causing peripheral vasoconstriction and increased heart rate.

In some instances of hypertension, an excess of renin is secreted by the kidneys. Renin acts on a substance called *angiotensinogen*, converting it to angioten-

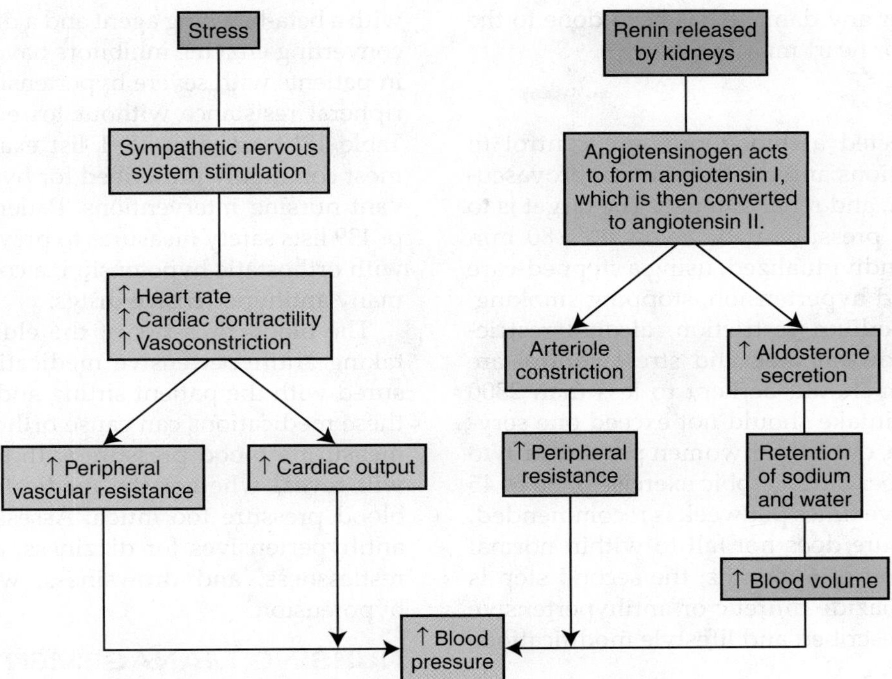

CONCEPT MAP **18–1** Pathophysiology of hypertension.

sin I. Angiotensin I is converted to angiotensin II by another enzyme. Angiotensin II acts directly on the blood vessels, causing them to constrict, and stimulates the adrenal gland to release aldosterone. Angiotensin thereby increases resistance to blood flow in the peripheral vessels and causes retention of sodium and water by the renal tubules through the influence of aldosterone. The retained sodium and water increase the blood volume, causing increased cardiac output and elevation of blood pressure. Concept Map 18–1 shows the pathophysiology of hypertension.

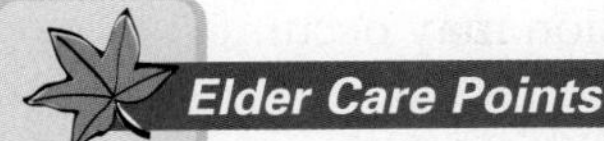

Elder Care Points

The arteriosclerosis that causes blood vessel rigidity is a natural part of aging. Systolic blood pressure may be higher in the elderly person. The baroreceptors that normally help adjust blood pressure become less sensitive with age. The lack of elasticity of the vessels and the decreased sensitivity of the baroreceptors cause the elderly to be at risk for orthostatic (postural) hypotension when changing position.

Signs, Symptoms, and Diagnosis

Hypertension has been called the "silent killer" because in early stages it does not usually cause discomfort or any other subjective signs and symptoms to indicate its presence. About one third of those who have hypertension are not aware of it. Signs may appear only in the later stages when damage has already been done to the target organs—that is, the kidney (renal ischemia), brain (arteriosclerosis and microaneurysms), aorta (aortic aneurysm), and heart (left ventricular hypertrophy and reduced cardiac output). **Patients with symptoms may complain of headache, dizziness, blurred vision, blackouts, irritability, fatigue, or nervousness.**

Hypertensive patients develop coronary heart disease at a rate two to three times greater than that of persons with normal blood pressure. If blood pressure is maintained at or below 120/80, the risk in patients with hypertension does not increase.

Malignant hypertension is a term describing rapidly progressive moderate to severe hypertension that is difficult to control. Diastolic pressure ranges from 140 to 170 mm Hg, and unless effective intervention is found, the patient may suffer heart, kidney, and brain damage.

Hypertensive crisis is a life-threatening emergency in which the patient experiences severe headache, blurred vision, nausea, and possibly confusion. It may occur if a patient has stopped taking antihypertensive medication, or it may be secondary to another disease process. The patient is placed in the intensive care unit and treated with intravenous emergency drugs, such as IV sodium nitroprusside or nitroglycerin, to lower the blood pressure. Short-acting nifedipine (Procardia) may be given orally.

If no underlying disease can be identified as elevating the patient's blood pressure, the patient is said to have *essential hypertension.* Examination of the blood vessels of the retina will reveal any damage to the retinal vessels. This assessment gives an indication about how much damage the high blood pressure has done to vessels throughout the body. If damage has occurred, it is an indication that the person's hypertension is moderate to severe. An electrocardiogram (ECG) and cardiac stress testing may be ordered to determine whether any damage has been done to the coronary arteries or heart muscle.

Treatment

Treatment is directed at blood pressure control to prevent complications and death from cerebrovascular, cardiovascular, and renal damage. The target is to maintain a blood pressure at or below 120/80 mm Hg. Treatment is individualized, using a stepped-care approach. For mild hypertension, stopping smoking, weight control, sodium restriction, alcohol restriction, exercise, a low-fat diet, and stress control are tried first. Sodium should be kept to less than 2300 mg/day. Alcohol intake should not exceed one serving of liquor, wine, or beer for women per day or two servings for men per day. Aerobic exercise of 30 to 45 minutes three to five times per week is recommended. If the blood pressure does not fall to within normal limits over a period of 6 months, the second step is initiated, and a thiazide diuretic or antihypertensive drug is usually prescribed and lifestyle modifications suggested.

Other drugs are added, if needed, to keep the blood pressure consistently within normal limits. Patients with more severe hypertension often require more than two drugs to attain control. The third step is to add such drugs. Other drug possibilities include angiotensin-converting enzyme (ACE) inhibitors, beta-blocking agents, calcium channel–blocking agents, and adrenergic inhibitors or vasodilators. The dose of each drug is increased as needed to achieve the desired blood pressure level unless side effects occur. In this event, another drug is substituted. A common combination used is a diuretic, a vasodilator, and an adrenergic inhibitor. Many of the newer blood pressure medications are very expensive, and there is an ongoing debate as to whether these drugs are really more effective than the older, less expensive medications.

If a potassium-wasting diuretic is prescribed, the patient is taught to increase his or her potassium intake. A potassium supplement is added to treatment, and electrolyte levels are monitored regularly.

Patients often are told to monitor their blood pressure at home and keep records of the readings. Periodic visits to the physician's office for regular examinations are necessary. The better the blood pressure is controlled and kept within normal limits, the less damage there will be to the target organs.

Antihypertensive Therapy. The drugs prescribed to reduce blood pressure work by decreasing blood volume, cardiac output, or peripheral resistance.

Diuretics reduce circulating blood volume. Drugs that decrease both cardiac output and peripheral resistance include the beta-adrenergic inhibitors (beta blockers) and calcium channel blockers. Adrenergic inhibitor medications decrease peripheral resistance. Vasodilators are most commonly used in combination with a beta-blocking agent and a diuretic. Angiotensin-converting enzyme inhibitors have been very effective in patients with severe hypertension. They reduce peripheral resistance without lowering cardiac output. Table 18–2 and Box 18–1 list examples of the drugs most commonly prescribed for hypertension and relevant nursing interventions. Patient Teaching 18–1 on p. 439 lists safety measures to prevent falls for patients with orthostatic hypotension, a common side effect of many antihypertensive drugs.

The blood pressure of the elderly patient who is taking antihypertensive medication should be measured with the patient sitting and standing. Many of these medications can cause orthostatic hypotension; measuring blood pressure with the patient standing will reveal whether the medication is reducing the blood pressure too much. Assess patients receiving antihypertensives for dizziness, confusion, syncope, restlessness, and drowsiness, which may indicate hypotension.

NURSING MANAGEMENT

Assessment (Data Collection)

The patient should be assessed for indications of modifiable and nonmodifiable risk factors for development of cardiac disease. Physical assessment of the cardiac system should also be performed. Assessment of blood pressure and documentation of levels and potential influences on values is an important aspect of nursing care. Accurately assess the patient's blood pressure, as hypertension is a major risk factor in the development of **vascular** disorders. The pressure should be taken sitting, lying supine, and standing for a thorough assessment. Standing blood pressure measurements also are important when a patient is started on a new medication, particularly an ACE inhibitor because orthostatic hypotension may occur.

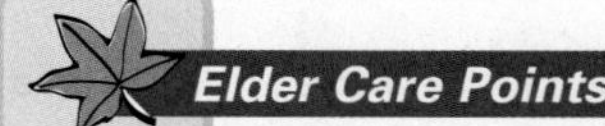

The blood pressure of the elerly patient will be lower immediately after a meal. For accurate readings, assess blood pressure between meals.

Nursing Diagnosis and Planning

Common nursing diagnoses for a patient with hypertension include:

- Excess fluid volume related to impaired regulatory system
- Risk for injury related to complications of hypertension
- Deficient knowledge (disease process, medications), related to new diagnosis of hypertension
- Imbalanced nutrition: more than body requirements, related to high-fat diet
- Anxiety related to potential complications of disease process

Table 18–2 ***Drugs Commonly Used for Patients with Vascular Disorders***

TYPE OF DRUG	ACTION
DIURETICS	
Thiazides and related drugs Hydrochlorothiazide (Esidrix, HydroDIURIL, Dyazide) Metolazone (Diulo, Zaroxolyn) Indapamide (Lozol)	These drugs increase the excretion of water, sodium, potassium, and chloride by blocking the reabsorption of sodium and chloride.
Loop diuretics Bumetanide (Bumex) Furosemide (Lasix) Torsemide (Demadex)	These drugs work in the loop of Henle to block reabsorption of sodium and chloride. This prevents passive reabsorption of water and promotes its excretion. These drugs produce the greatest amount of diuresis.
Potassium-sparing diuretics Spironolactone (Aldactone) Triamterene (Dyrenium)	These drugs block the action of aldosterone in the distal nephron. This prevents the promotion of sodium uptake in exchange for potassium secretion usually caused by aldosterone, and potassium is "spared" (not secreted) and sodium is excreted. These drugs cause very little diuresis.
ANTIHYPERTENSIVES	
Adrenergic Inhibitors	
Beta blockers Atenolol (Tenormin) Propranolol (Inderal) Metoprolol (Lopressor, Toprol XL) Timolol (Apo-timol) Bisoprolol (Zebeta) Carvedilol (Coreg)	It is not certain how these drugs work to reduce blood pressure. Blockade of the $beta_1$ receptors lowers cardiac output by decreasing heart rate and contractility. Action on the $beta_1$ receptors in the kidney decreases the release of renin, which is a factor in rising blood pressure.
Alpha blockers Doxazosin (Cardura) Prazosin (Minipress) Terazosin (Hytrin)	These drugs block $alpha_1$ stimulation on arterioles and veins, preventing sympathetic vasoconstriction. This action results in vasodilation, reducing peripheral vascular resistance and venous return to the heart.
Alpha-beta blocker Labetalol (Normodyne, Trandate)	This drug blocks both $alpha_1$ and $beta_1$ receptors, producing decreased heart rate, contractility, peripheral vascular resistance, and venous return.
ACE inhibitors Benazepril (Lotensin) Captopril (Capoten) Enalapril (Vasotec) Fosinopril (Monopril) Lisinopril (Prinivil) Quinapril (Accupril)	These agents lower blood pressure by inhibiting the conversion of angiotensin I into angiotensin II, thereby preventing vasoconstriction. They also restrict volume expansion mediated by aldosterone.
Calcium channel blockers Diltiazem (Cardizem) Nicardipine (Cardene) Nifedipine (Procardia) Verapamil (Calan, Isoptin)	These drugs reduce blood pressure by causing dilation of arterioles. Calcium channels are blocked, preventing the influx of calcium that promotes contraction.
Central-acting agents Clonidine (Catapres) Guanabenz (Wytensin) Methyldopa (Aldomet)	These agents act within the brainstem to suppress sympathetic impulses to the heart and blood vessels. This action decreases the release of norepinephrine by sympathetic nerves, reducing activation of peripheral adrenergic receptors, and promotes vasodilation. The agents also decrease heart rate and cardiac output.
Peripherally Acting Adrenergic Blockers Guanethidine (Ismelin) Reserpine (Serpaline)	These agents reduce blood pressure by blocking adrenergic receptors in the postganglionic sympathetic neurons and causing decreased sympathetic stimulation of the heart and blood vessels.
Direct-Acting Vasodilators Hydralazine (Apresoline) Minoxidil (Loniten)	These agents reduce blood pressure by promoting arteriole vasodilation.
Direct Renin Inhibitors Aliskiren (Tekturna)	This new class of drugs inhibits renin secretion from the kidney, reducing angiotensin I and angiotensin II, inhibiting vasoconstriction.

Box 18–1 General Nursing Interventions for the Administration of Diuretics and Antihypertensive Drugs

DIURETICS

- Follow the "five rights" of medication administration to prevent errors and injury to the patient: *right* patient, *right* drug, *right* dose, *right* route, *right* time.
- Verify allergies with the patient before administering the drug. Thiazide and thiazide-like diuretics are related to sulfonamides. Patients allergic to sulfas may have adverse reactions.
- Monitor intake and output to determine amount of diuresis and the drug's effectiveness.
- Track the patient's weight to determine the drug's effectiveness.
- Evaluate for decreased edema.
- Check all drugs the patient is receiving for drug interactions with the diuretic drug to prevent toxicity or lack of absorption. Several diuretics are ototoxic, and this adverse effect may be potentiated by other ototoxic drugs.
- If possible, administer dose in the morning, and if a second dose is required, give it midafternoon to avoid sleep interference by need to urinate.
- Provide assistance with urination in a timely manner (answer call bell quickly).
- Assess for signs of dehydration and hypotension; take blood pressure on a set schedule. The elderly are prone to excessive diuresis and can quickly become dehydrated.
- Monitor diabetic patients for increased blood glucose levels when taking loop or thiazide diuretics, as these drugs may cause hyperglycemia.

Regarding possible side effects or adverse effects of the drug, the nurse should:

- Monitor potassium levels frequently if patient is taking a potassium-wasting diuretic; assess for signs of hypokalemia: weakness, tremor, muscle cramps, change in mental status, cardiac dysrhythmia.
- If the patient also is taking digoxin, consult the physician before administering the dose if the potassium level is below 3.5 mEq/L or if the patient exhibits signs of hypokalemia, as hypokalemia increases risk of fatal cardiac dysrhythmia in patients taking digoxin.
- If patient is taking a potassium-sparing diuretic and potassium level is above 5 mEq/L, or if signs of hyperkalemia develop (abnormal cardiac rhythm), consult the physician before administering the dose.
- Monitor blood pressure. If it drops considerably, speak with the physician before giving another dose of the medication.
- Monitor the patient for signs of constipation, as diuresis may cause this problem.
- Monitor patients with a history of DVT for recurrence, as diuretics reduce circulating fluid volume.
- Monitor the patient for side effects or adverse effects of the particular drug taken. The most common general side effects are constipation, electrolyte disturbance, gastric upset, and hypotension. Adverse effects are dehydration, ototoxicity, hyperglycemia, hyperuricemia.
- Monitor the patient for signs of allergic reaction, such as rash or itching.

Teach the patient taking a diuretic to:

- Expect frequent need to urinate and increased volume of urine.
- Report any new heartbeat irregularity.
- Report any signs of ringing of the ears, roaring sounds, a feeling of fullness in the ears, or decreased hearing.
- Eat foods high in potassium, such as bananas, orange juice, cereals, meats, tomatoes, potatoes, and raisins, unless taking a potassium-sparing diuretic.
- If taking a potassium-sparing diuretic, restrict foods high in potassium.
- Take potassium supplement regularly if one is prescribed.
- Increase fiber in the diet if prone to constipation; consult physician if constipation occurs. The elderly patient who is inactive is more prone to constipation.
- Watch for signs of postural hypotension, such as dizziness or light-headedness when changing position. Encourage patient to arise slowly from a supine position and to sit a minute before standing. (The elderly are particularly prone to this side effect.)
- Avoid the sun or take precautions; do not use a sun lamp when taking a loop or thiazide diuretic as the medication may cause photosensitivity.
- Watch for signs of gout (tenderness or swelling of joints) when taking a loop or thiazide diuretic and notify the physician if these occur. Loop diuretics may cause an increase in uric acid levels.
- When taking spironolactone, menstrual irregularities or impotence may occur; report these occurrences to the physician.

ANTIHYPERTENSIVE DRUGS

- Establish that the patient is not hypotensive before giving a dose of an antihypertensive drug. If the patient's blood pressure is below normal levels, consult the physician before giving the dose.
- Monitor the heart rate for bradycardia or tachycardia. Follow specific parameters for administration of the specific drug; some drugs may cause bradycardia, others may cause tachycardia.
- Follow the "five rights" of medication administration, and check the patient's ID band before *each* dose.
- Measure blood pressure standing and sitting to determine whether the patient is experiencing orthostatic hypotension; several antihypertensives may cause orthostatic hypotension.
- Note contraindications and precautions for each specific drug the patient is taking. Angiotensin-converting enzyme (ACE) inhibitors are contraindicated during pregnancy.
- Check all drugs the patient is receiving for drug interactions to prevent toxicity or increased severity of side effects. Many of the antihypertensive drugs have a depressant effect on the heart.
- Monitor blood pressure readings to evaluate effectiveness of the drug.

Box 18–1 ***General Nursing Interventions for the Administration of Diuretics and Antihypertensive Drugs—cont'd***

ANTIHYPERTENSIVE DRUGS—cont'd

Regarding possible side effects or adverse effects of the drug, the nurse should:

- Monitor the patient for the side effects of each drug administered.
- Monitor serum glucose levels in patients with diabetes who are taking a beta-blocker drug, as the drug may mask hypoglycemia.
- Monitor lipid levels for changes in patients taking beta-blocker drugs, as these drugs interfere with lipid metabolism.
- Observe for hypersensitivity reactions such as rash; ACE inhibitors may cause hypersensitivity.
- Monitor patients for signs of congestive heart failure, such as edema; beta blockers, calcium channel blockers, and other drugs that decrease cardiac output may precipitate heart failure in patients with borderline cardiac function.
- Check the skin of the patient using a clonidine patch for signs of irritation, a potential side effect of the patch. Be certain the old patch is removed when applying a new one.
- Give the first dose of an ACE inhibitor at bedtime, as it often causes hypotension.
- Monitor the potassium level of the patient taking an ACE inhibitor. Because it suppresses the release of aldosterone, it increases potassium retention.
- Monitor liver function tests for patients taking centrally acting drugs, such as clonidine, as these drugs may cause liver damage in some patients
- Monitor renal function tests in patients taking hydralazine, as this drug may cause renal impairment.

Teach the patient taking an antihypertensive to:

- Monitor blood pressure regularly and keep a log of the readings.
- Alter lifestyle factors that contribute to hypertension, such as smoking, excess weight, excessive stress, excessive alcohol ingestion, high-salt diet, and lack of exercise.
- Rise slowly from a lying position and stabilize before standing for a couple of minutes.
- Report alteration in sexual response, as some of the antihypertensive drugs may cause impotence.
- Report persistent side effects and any adverse effects of the drug.
- Monitor for weight gain from retention of sodium and water by weighing at least twice a week; report weight gain of more than 2 lb to the physician.
- Report signs of ankle edema, as several of the antihypertensive drugs can precipitate congestive heart failure.
- Be aware that methyldopa may cause dark urine for the first few weeks of therapy.
- Refrain from abruptly discontinuing centrally acting antihypertensives, such as clonidine, as rebound hypertension may occur.
- Check with the physician before taking over-the-counter drugs, as many are contraindicated in hypertension.
- Comply with medication therapy even when blood pressure is normal, as long-term compliance is the key to preventing the organ damage that hypertension can cause.
- Set own goals for lifestyle changes and medication therapy; a patient-directed program has a better chance of success.

Expected outcomes for a patient with hypertension may include:

- The patient will experience a decrease of edema in feet and ankles
- The patient's blood pressure will return to within normal limits
- The patient will verbalize an understanding of teaching related to medications and disease process
- The patient will lose 10% of body weight in a designated period
- The patient will be able to choose low-fat and low-sodium items from a variety of menus

Implementation

Nursing interventions target assisting the patient to make necessary lifestyle changes that will help control her blood pressure and slow further atherosclerosis. Diet changes are often the most difficult for the patient. It is best to work with the patient's current dietary likes and dislikes, modifying methods of food preparation to decrease sodium and fat content

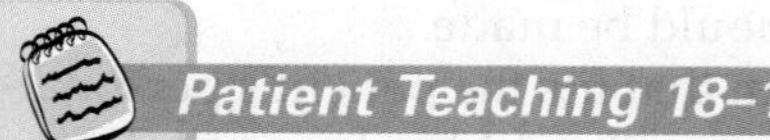

Safety Measures to Prevent Falls for Patients with Orthostatic Hypotension

Teach the patient who experiences the side effect of orthostatic hypotension from medication to:

- Rise slowly from a lying to a sitting position; do not hold your breath as you arise. Sit for 1 minute before standing; stand slowly holding on to a stable object. Stand for 1 minute before walking.
- While seated, flex and rotate the feet several times before attempting to stand; have feet firmly planted on the floor before standing.
- When walking, do not turn your head or body abruptly.
- When feeling unsteady while standing, call for assistance before walking.
- Report lightheadedness or sudden dizziness.
- Use the bathroom before meals and try to avoid getting up for 30 to 60 minutes after meals.

Cultural Cues 18–1

Diet Variations

Working with patients from diverse cultures who have very different diets is a challenge. You should encourage fat and sodium restriction in the cultural diet of the patient. This requires working with the patient to discover food preferences and food preparation patterns inherent in the family

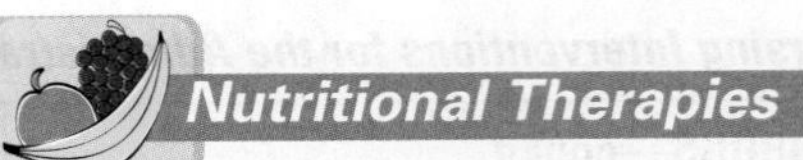

Nutritional Therapies 18–1

Decreasing Sodium in the Diet

For the patient who must reduce the sodium in the diet, instruct to:

- Avoid "convenience" foods: ready-mixed sauces, frozen dinners, cured or smoked meats (including lunch meats), canned soups, and prepared salad dressings, unless the label truly indicates a low sodium content.
- Be aware that regular canned vegetables often contain a large amount of sodium; in some instances rinsing will greatly decrease the sodium content. Use fresh or frozen vegetables or those canned without sodium when possible.
- Check soft drink labels for sodium content; avoid those that contain more than 140 mg of sodium.
- Check cereal box labels for sodium content; switch to a lower-sodium cereal, such as shredded wheat.
- Use one fourth to one half the amount of salt that a recipe calls for.
- Avoid adding salt to food after cooking.
- Make a salt substitute seasoning of: ½ tsp garlic powder, mixed with 1 tsp each of basil, black pepper, marjoram, onion powder, parsley, sage, savory, and thyme; or use a product such as Mrs. Dash or lemon pepper instead of salt.
- When ordering at restaurants, ask which dishes are low in sodium; or ask that the cook refrain from adding salt to your meal.
- Ask fast food restaurants to supply you with a list of their available foods showing sodium content of each item.
- Do not eat preserved or commercially prepared smoked meats, such as bacon, hot dogs, salami, pastrami, ham, smoked turkey, or sausage.
- Read all labels on food containers looking for the words "sodium" or "NaCl."
- Check condiments for amount of sodium. Catsup, soy sauce, steak sauce, and others containing high quantities of sodium.

(Cultural Cues 18–1). Sources of hidden sodium should be learned, and the patient should be taught how to read food labels, looking for the words *salt*, *sodium*, and the letters *NaCl*. Smoked or preserved meats or other products that contain a large amount of sodium should be avoided. Nutritional Therapies 18–1 presents guidelines for decreasing sodium in the diet. Patients who need to increase potassium intake are taught to include citrus fruits and juices, beef and turkey, tomatoes, and potatoes in the diet. The person who does the shopping and food preparation must be included in the diet instruction process. **Weight loss is the most important lifestyle change in obese clients.** The goal is a weight that is within 15% of ideal body weight.

If caffeine restriction is recommended, teach the patient to gradually decrease her caffeine consumption so that she will not experience withdrawal symptoms, such as headache and nervousness. Remind the patient that many types of soft drinks, as well as coffee, tea, and chocolate, contain caffeine. Most of these beverages are available in decaffeinated formulas. Because it produces vasoconstriction, nicotine has a major impact on blood vessels and blood pressure. Stopping smoking can be a difficult task for many patients. Referral to a self-help program should be made.

An exercise program that fits the patient's personality, ability, and preference should be designed. Walking to work from a parking lot a few blocks away, climbing stairs instead of using elevators, and a daily walk in the neighborhood often are sufficient. Other patients might prefer to use a stationary bicycle or treadmill. The object is to work on something that the patient will continue to do for the rest of her life.

Weight loss will begin to occur if the patient is faithful to the prescribed diet and exercise program. As her weight decreases, remind the patient of the direct effect these efforts have had on the blood pressure. Even a moderate weight loss of 7 to 12 lb (3 to 5 kg) can reduce blood pressure. Positive reinforcement should be given for even small amounts of weight loss.

Stress reduction requires an evaluation of lifestyle. Meditation, yoga, leisure activities, or just saying no to extra obligations can all decrease stress. You should help the patient determine where her stressors are and what can practically be done to manage them.

Lifetime compliance with diet, exercise, stress reduction, and medication plans is difficult for most patients. Many do not understand or accept that it is up to them to control their disease. They do well for several months or a few years, but then, because they feel well (while their blood pressure has been controlled), they stop taking their medication and gradually return to previous lifestyle patterns. By teaching them what high blood pressure does to the blood vessels and the heart, brain, eye, and kidneys, you can do much to encourage patients to follow the treatment plan for life. Patient Teaching 18–2 presents guidelines for teaching patients about the complications of uncontrolled hypertension. Each patient needs continuing praise for maintaining blood pressure control.

There are many resources to help hypertensive patients manage their illness more effectively. The American Heart Association, Heart Center Online, the National Institutes of Health, and many others offer educational materials for patients with hypertension. *Healthy People 2010* goals and objectives have been written for hypertension (Health Promotion Points 18–1).

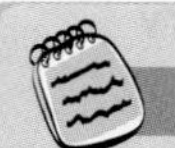

Patient Teaching 18–2

Complications of Uncontrolled Hypertension

The following information should be included in the teaching plan of the patient at risk for noncompliance with treatment of hypertension:

- Hypertension can contribute to and accelerate atherosclerosis, placing an increased workload on the heart. This may cause myocardial infarction, left ventricular hypertrophy, and congestive heart failure.
- Atherosclerosis of the vessels in the brain disrupts circulation and may lead to transient ischemic attacks (TIAs) and stroke,
- Hypertension may cause accelerated atherosclerosis and rigidity of the renal vessels and may lead to kidney failure
- Hypertension damages the arteries of the eye, causing the formation of clots or occurrence of hemorrhage that may lead to blurred vision or blindness.

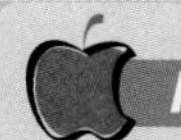

Health Promotion Points 18–1

Healthy People 2010 Management of Hypertension

The patient with hypertension requires intense teaching to assist in achieving health management goals. You must ensure the patient understands the needed lifestyle changes and how to accomplish behavior modification. The patient may be referred to a local support group as a resource in the management of his health. The following *Healthy People 2010* goals are for improving cardiovascular health, particularly in those with hypertension.

OVERALL GOAL

The overall goal is to *improve cardiovascular health and quality of life* through the prevention, detection, and treatment of risk factors; early identification and treatment of patients with heart attacks and strokes; and prevention of recurrent cardiovascular events.

OBJECTIVES: BLOOD PRESSURE

12-9 Reduce the proportion of adults with high blood pressure

12-10 Increase the proportion of adults with high blood pressure whose blood pressure is under control

12-11 Increase the proportion of adults with high blood pressure who are taking action (for example, losing weight, increasing physical activity, or reducing sodium intake) to help control their blood pressure

12-12 Increase the proportion of adults who have had their blood pressure measured within the preceding 2 years and can state whether their blood pressure was normal or high

Evaluation

You must evaluate the effectiveness of medical treatment and lifestyle changes of individuals with hypertension. Consistent maintenance of blood pressure within prescribed limits is a primary indicator of effectiveness of disease management. Evaluate the patient's knowledge of prescribed medications, including use, side effects, and administration. Knowledge of dietary management, exercise activities, stress management, and smoking cessation should be discussed at follow-up sessions. The patient's compliance with the management of hypertension is critical to preventing or minimizing complications of the disease process.

PERIPHERAL VASCULAR DISEASES

Peripheral vascular disease involves loss of function, narrowing, or obstruction of peripheral blood vessels, either arterial or venous. These vessels may be in the arms, neck, abdomen, or lower extremities (Figure 18–1). Diabetes, particularly when uncontrolled contributes to vascular disease.

Other causes of problems include spasm of the smooth muscles in the arterial walls (e.g., Raynaud's disease), structural defects in the arteries (aneurysms), trauma, or **embolus** (blood clot or debris that travels and lodges in a blood vessel) that causes occlusion. Peripheral venous problems are caused by defective valvular function and formation of **venous thrombosis** (blood clots), which may be accompanied by **thrombophlebitis** (inflammation of a vein).

Prevention of peripheral vascular disease is focused on decreasing atherosclerosis and arteriosclerosis, controlling diabetes mellitus, controlling hypertension, and preventing smoking. Prevention of smoking or smoking cessation is important because nicotine causes vasoconstriction resulting in elevation of blood pressure. Maintaining a healthy lifestyle with a low-fat, low-sodium, heart-healthy diet; regular exercise; normal weight; prevention of excessive stress; and control of diabetes mellitus and hypertension can reduce the incidence of peripheral vascular disease.

ARTERIOSCLEROSIS AND ATHEROSCLEROSIS

Arteriosclerosis (hardening of the arteries) is a general term for a variety of arterial changes. It occurs with aging as degenerative changes occur in the small arteries and arterioles. The disorder is characterized by thickening of the artery walls that progresses to hardening as calcium deposits form. Vessel elasticity is lost. The thickening and calcification reduce the diameter of the vessels and cause slowing of blood flow. This may lead to ischemia and necrosis in various tissues. **Atherosclerosis** is a form of arteriosclerosis. Lipids are deposited along the vessel walls and combines with cells, fibrin, and cell debris to form plaques. As the plaque grows and extends into the lumen of the artery, platelets tend to break up and clump at the site and form thrombi. Atheromatous plaque with thrombi form primarily in the larger ar-

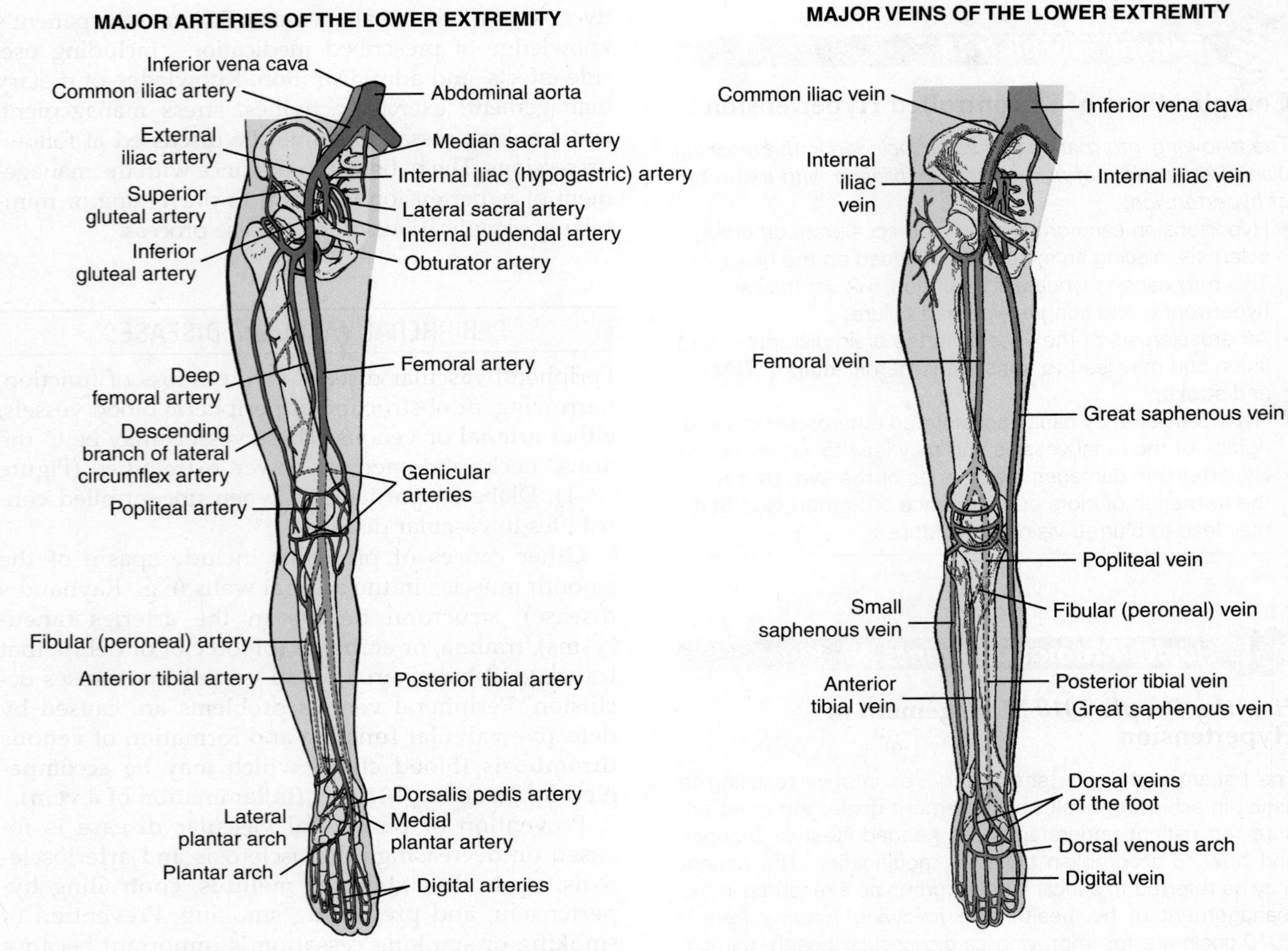

FIGURE 18–1 Diagram of the peripheral vascular system. Veins and arteries of the lower extremities.

teries and the carotid arteries. Diabetes mellitus, particularly when uncontrolled, speeds the development of arteriosclerosis and atherosclerosis. Hypertension is a major factor in arteriosclerosis. The most common etiology of peripheral arterial disorders is atherosclerosis.

PERIPHERAL ARTERIAL DISEASE (PAD) (ARTERIAL INSUFFICIENCY)

Etiology and Pathophysiology

The most common etiology of arterial insufficiency is atherosclerosis. The vessel walls become narrowed or the lumen obstructed, leading to loss of blood flow to the extremity. Hypertension, heart disease, family history, smoking, and improper diet may be contributing factors.

Restriction or cessation of blood flow in the arteries leads to ischemia and tissue death (necrosis). Arterial ulcers may result. Arterial insufficiency may be acute or chronic. Embolism is the most common etiology of acute interruption of arterial blood flow. Arterial insufficiency may occur in the carotid, coronary, and peripheral arteries.

Signs, Symptoms, and Diagnosis

Obtain a complete history and physical examination of the patient. A distinction should be made between signs and symptoms of venous disorders and arterial disorders. Table 18–3 summarizes signs and symptoms of venous and arterial disorders.

Signs and symptoms of peripheral arterial insufficiency of the lower extremities include **intermittent claudication** (pain when walking that diminishes at rest), pain at rest, and ischemic changes. Occlusion in the peripheral system produces the "5 Ps"—pain, pallor, pulselessness, paralysis, and paresthesia. Blood pressure in the affected extremity is lower.

Patients with arterial insufficiency have pallor in the affected extremity when elevated. The skin may appear tight and shiny. Hair is usually absent on the affected extremity. Dark redness **(dependent rubor)** may occur when the extremity is dependent. Pulses are diminished or absent. There also is a temperature change distal to the occlusion. The severity of these symptoms depends on the extent of the lesion, degree of occlusion, and amount of collateral circulation that has been established. If severe ischemia oc-

Table 18–3 Differences in Signs and Symptoms of Arterial and Venous Disease

CHARACTERISTIC	ARTERIAL DISEASE	VENOUS DISEASE
Pulses	Diminished, weak, or absent	Strong and symmetrical; may be difficult to palpate if edema is present
Skin	Pallor, dependent rubor; thin, dry, shiny, cool	Mottling with brown pigmentation at ankles, veins may be visible; legs or feet bluish when dependent; dermatitis; warm at ankle
Edema	Absent or mild	Present, particularly around ankle and in foot
Ulceration	On toes or at pressure points on feet	At bones of ankle
Necrosis and gangrene	Likely	Unlikely
Pain	Intermittent claudication when walking; sharp, stabbing, gnawing; lessens when at rest	Aching, cramping, particularly when dependent; may have nocturnal cramps
Nails	Thick, brittle (normal in elderly)	Normal
Hair	Hair loss distal to area of occlusion (hair loss normal in elderly)	Normal

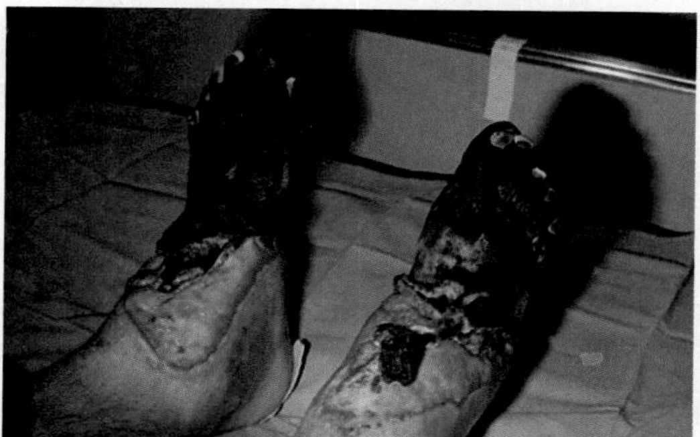

FIGURE **18–2** Patient with gangrene of toes.

curs from occlusion of arterial blood flow, tissue distal to the occlusion blanches, becomes cold, hurts, and eventually becomes numb as necrosis occurs. Eventually the affected part may develop cellulitis, edema, and become gangrenous, necessitating amputation (Figures 18–2 and 18–3). The toes and foot are often affected.

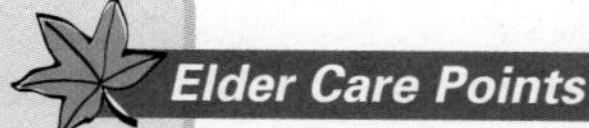

Elder Care Points

Hair loss is a natural occurrence with aging, as is thickening of fingernails and toenails. These signs are not reliable indicators of vascular problems of the extremities in the elderly.

Diagnosis is made using the ankle-brachial index (ABI). The normal value is 1 (i.e., the ABI is the same at the ankle and brachial artery sites). Radiographic and ultrasound procedures also may be performed. Figure 18–4 shows an example of a patient with arterial insufficiency.

Think Critically About . . . Can you recall the correct way to locate a pedal and posterior tibial pulse? Could you demonstrate the technique to a classmate?

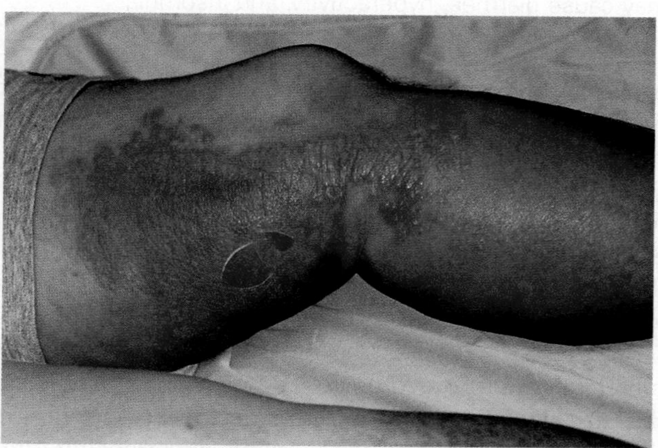

FIGURE **18–3** Patient with cellulitis of the legs.

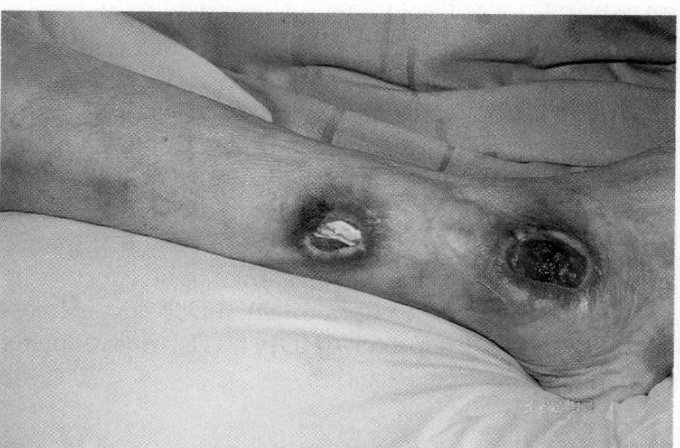

FIGURE **18–4** Patient with arterial insufficiency. Arterial ulcers of the lateral malleolus and distal and lateral portion of the leg. Note round, smooth shape.

Treatment

The best treatment for arterial occlusive disease is regular exercise. Walking vigorously for 20 minutes twice a day will encourage growth of collateral circulation and reduce the severity of claudication in the majority of patients. The exercise program is started slowly, working up to a faster pace and the full 20

Complementary & Alternative Therapies 18–1

L-Carnitine

Several research studies have shown that L-carnitine, a natural substance found in muscle, heart, brain, and nerve cells, may be beneficial in improving the exercise capacity of individuals with peripheral artery disease. L-carnitine, especially in the form of proprinylcarnitine, improves muscle recovery following exercise.

L-carnitine can be found in many foods, with higher concentrations in red meat and dairy products. It is supplied as a dietary supplement in 50- to 500-mg tablets. Recommended dosage for persons with peripheral artery disease is 600 to 1200 mg three times per day or 750 mg twice daily. Side effects are few; however, these dosages in this range may cause diarrhea, hyperactivity, and insomnia.

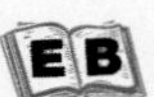

minutes (Johnson, 2006). Some dietary supplements have proven helpful in increasing circulation (Complementary & Alternative Therapies 18–1).

The goal of treatment of arterial insufficiency is directed toward increasing blood flow through the peripheral arteries and decreasing the risk of clot formation in the vessels. Antiplatelet agents, thrombolytics, and platelet inhibitors may be used alone or in combination with other drugs. Aspirin is the most commonly used antiplatelet agent. It prevents the aggregation of platelets in the arteries. Platelet inhibitors, such as clopidogrel (Plavix), may be prescribed. Patients experiencing intermittent claudication may achieve relief of symptoms when prescribed pentoxifylline (Trental) or cilostazol (Pletal). Research has shown cilostazol to be the more effective drug (Zolli, 2004). These drugs increase blood flow by inhibiting clot formation in the vessel. Selected patients may be eligible for thrombolytic therapy. Thrombolytic agents, such as reteplase (Retavase) or alteplase (Activase), are injected directly into the vessel to destroy clots that have accumulated along the vessel wall. Cholesterol-lowering drugs (e.g., atorvastatin [Lipitor], simvastatin [Zocor]) have been shown to be effective by decreasing low-density lipoprotein (LDL) and increasing high-density lipoprotein (HDL) levels, thus reducing plaque deposits in the arteries.

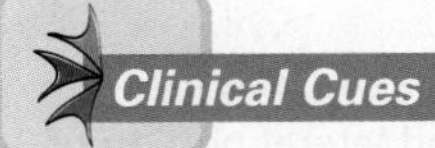

Clinical Cues

Medications to treat arterial insufficiency may cause serious adverse reactions. The major adverse reaction is bleeding. Observe the patient for and report immediately evidence of excessive bruising or bleeding, prolonged clotting after a needle stick, hematuria, changes in vital signs, or changes in neurologic signs.

Surgical treatment of peripheral arterial insufficiency is a palliative measure only. It does not cure the disease or halt the atherosclerotic process. It can, however, relieve ischemic pain, help avoid amputation, and add years to a patient's life. The purpose of vascular surgery is to revascularize and nourish cells in the affected area.

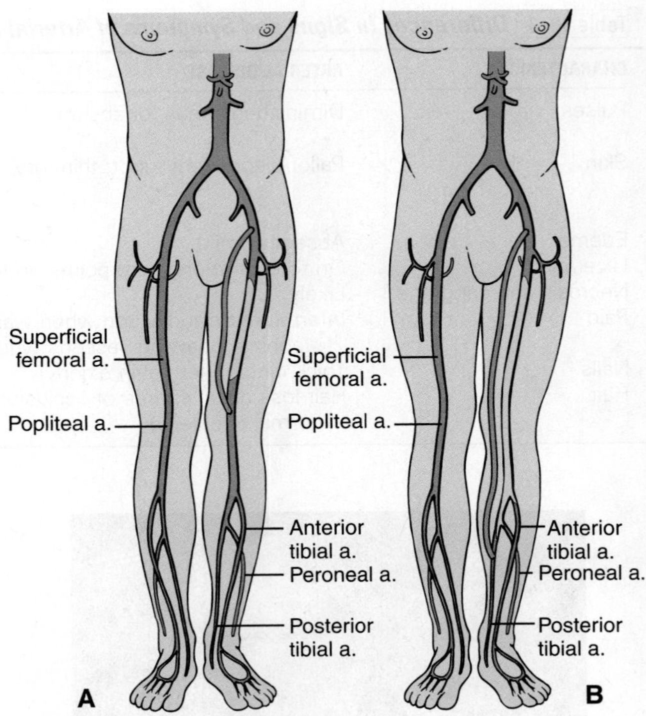

FIGURE 18–5 Femoral popliteal bypass graft. **A,** Femoropopliteal bypass graft around an occluded superficial femoroartery. **B,** Femoropopliteal bypass graft around occluded superficial femoropopliteal and proximal tibial arteries.

Laser angioplasty is now used more commonly to open clogged arteries. This procedure is done in a fashion similar to percutaneous balloon angioplasty. The surgeon enters the artery with a catheter and uses the laser to destroy the plaque buildup that is occluding the artery. Cryotherapy is a new treatment used to open arteries.

Percutaneous transluminal angioplasty (PTA) may be done to open an occluded artery. A catheter is introduced into the artery, and when the proper spot is reached, a balloon is inflated multiple times to dilate the vessel, promoting better blood flow. A metal or mesh **stent** (tubular device to give support to a vessel interior) may be placed to prevent narrowing or closure of the artery (see Chapter 20 for a similar stent illustration).

An aortoiliac bypass or a femoropopliteal bypass is performed to correct arterial occlusion of the leg to prevent the need for amputation. A synthetic graft is placed to divert blood around the obstructed area, or the occluded portion is dissected and replaced by a graft from the patient's saphenous or other vein. Figure 18–5 shows a schematic of a femoropopliteal bypass graft surgery. Postoperative care is the same as for other operative procedures but includes careful assessment of pulses distal to the graft to detect **thrombus** (clot) formation. As with any vascular surgery, extra attention is paid to assessment for signs of bleeding. An aortoiliac bypass requires both an abdominal and a groin incision.

A hyperbaric oxygen chamber is sometimes used for patients with severely compromised circulation to a lower extremity to increase tissue oxygen and avoid amputation.

NURSING MANAGEMENT

Assessment (Data Collection)

You should perform a physical assessment of the patient's affected extremity at least every 4 hours or as required by the facility. Feet should be assessed for warmth, paresthesia, and pulses. All findings must be documented, including any changes. If ulcers are present, assessment and documentation of skin integrity should be included. A major role of the nurse is early detection and prevention of complications. Acute changes in assessment of patients with arterial insufficiency are unlikely; however, you must maintain a record of the patient's condition in the event of development of complications.

Nursing Diagnosis and Planning

The major nursing care goals for patients with peripheral arterial insufficiency are (1) maintaining arterial blood flow to the lower extremities; (2) protecting tissues from further injury from pressure and constriction of blood flow; and (3) preventing wound infection.

Nursing diagnoses may include:

- Impaired skin integrity related to ulcers on lower extremities
- Injury related to loss of peripheral circulation
- Acute pain related to ischemia to lower extremities

Expected outcomes may include:

- The patient will not experience loss of skin integrity.
- Peripheral pulses will remain palpable
- The patient will report reduction in pain level in the lower extremities

Rehabilitation of the patient requires instruction and guidance in special exercises to increase collateral circulation to the legs. See Table 17–4 for common nursing diagnoses and interventions appropriate for patients with peripheral arterial occlusive disease.

Implementation

The nurse can encourage blood flow by keeping the patient and the environment warm. Constricting clothing is to be avoided, and the leg gatch on the bed should never be used, as it puts added pressure on the back of the knees and further occludes blood flow. The nurse should encourage the patient to change her position frequently while awake. The lower extremities should be positioned below heart level to facilitate arterial blood flow. The legs are elevated only if edema is impeding circulation.

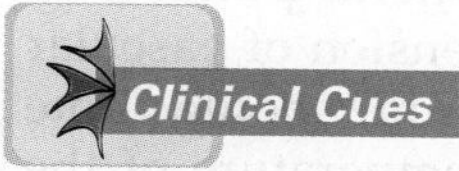

Assess the affected extremity and document and report significant changes in pain level, pulses, sensation, and skin temperature. Additional medical intervention may be needed to prevent complications that could result in amputation of all or part of an extremity.

Encouraging exercise is especially beneficial to patients with decreased blood flow. Walking regularly every day is best for the ambulatory patient. Swimming also is good because it applies light pressure to the surface of the legs and requires muscle action that encourages venous return. Bed rest patients should be encouraged to do foot and leg exercises at least once each hour. You can encourage those who watch television to do the exercises during commercial breaks.

Think Critically About . . . Rhonda, a 63-year-old executive, is experiencing worsening intermittent claudication. Describe how you would interact with her to develop an exercise program that could lessen her symptoms.

Patients should be dressed in warm, nonrestrictive clothing. Blankets or throws may be added for additional warmth. The room temperature should be maintained at the patient's comfort level.

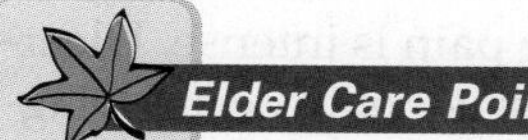

Elderly adults are less tolerant of cold temperatures because of decreased subcutaneous fat tissue as a result of the aging process. Room temperatures must be maintained at the patient's comfort level. Chilling can result in vasoconstriction and contribute to discomfort of patients with vascular disorders.

Tobacco use, especially smoking, contributes to peripheral vascular disease because of the vasoconstriction effect of nicotine. If appropriate, patients should be referred to a smoking-cessation program. Information concerning the effects of alcohol on vascular disorders, surgical interventions, patient teaching, and interventions to prevent leg ulcers can be reviewed in Chapter 17.

Think Critically About . . . Can you describe the specific actions you would take to help a patient recognize the need for, and to establish, a smoking-cessation program?

Evaluation

Evaluation of the effectiveness of the plan of care involves assessing changes in peripheral pulses and skin integrity. Improvement or extension of vascular ulcers should be documented. You should note changes in color, sensation, and temperature of the lower extremities. Patient's perception of pain level should be documented using a scale of 0 to 10. Evaluate the patient's level of compliance with establishing an exercise routine. Include type, frequency, and tolerance of exercise activities. Evaluate the patient's ability to meet established goals and revise the plan as needed.

BUERGER'S DISEASE (THROMBOANGIITIS OBLITERANS)

Etiology and Pathophysiology

Thromboangiitis obliterans, or *Buerger's disease,* involves the small and medium-size arteries. Inflammation, thickening of the arterial walls and occlusion of the vessels in the hands and feet occur. The disease occurs more often in men than women and is commonly found in people from the Middle East, the Far East, India, and Southeast Asia. There is increasing incidence of the disease in women older than age 50. Moderate to heavy cigarette smoking is directly linked to the progression of the disease. It may also be classified as an autoimmune disorder in which the body reacts to properties in nicotine.

Signs, Symptoms, Diagnosis, and Treatment

The signs and symptoms include numbness and tingling of the toes or fingers in cold weather, pain in the feet, and intermittent claudication that progressively becomes more severe. The pain is intense. Ulcerations and **gangrene** (death of tissue) may occur. Diagnosis is made through patient history and symptoms.

Cessation of smoking is the single most important treatment factor. Cigarette smoking must be stopped immediately. Those who do not stop smoking are at great risk for gangrene and amputation of fingers or toes. Exercise may be used to increase circulation in the legs and feet.

NURSING MANAGEMENT

Assessment (Data Collection), Nursing Diagnosis, and Planning

The most important role of the nurse is patient teaching and reinforcement of the need to stop smoking. Assessment of the extremities for skin impairment is essential.

Common nursing diagnoses for a patient with Buerger's disease are as follows:

- Fear related to risk for amputation of fingers
- Risk for infection related to skin impairment
- Risk for injury due to loss of oxygen supply to fingers related to continued cigarette smoking
- Acute pain related to ischemia to extremities

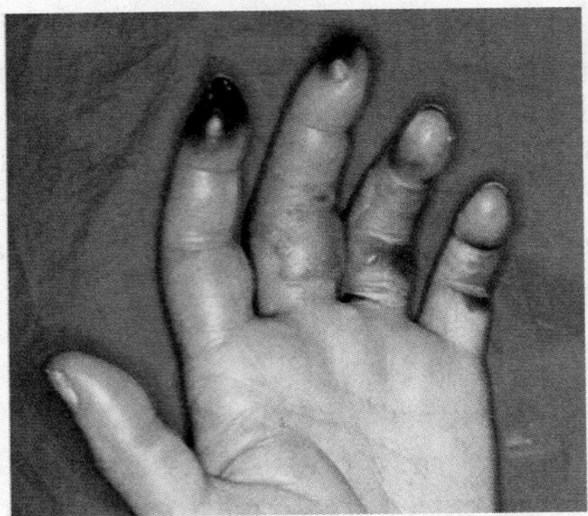

FIGURE 18–6 Raynaud's disease.

Expected outcomes include the following:

- The patient will verbalize reduced anxiety
- The patient will remain free of signs of infection
- The patient will enter a smoking cessation program
- The patient will report a reduction in pain level

Implementation and Evaluation

You should develop a teaching plan to assist the patient to avoid complications of the disease. Priority concerns are protection of extremities from further injury and maintenance of skin integrity. Teach the patient to protect extremities from extremes of heat and cold. The patient should be referred to a smoking cessation program, as this is a priority measure to prevent further complications.

Objective data such as skin integrity, color, and warmth of the extremities should be assessed. The patient's compliance with cessation of smoking should also be determined. Subjective data, including pain, numbness, and loss of sensation, should be included in the evaluation of the effectiveness of treatment. The degree of improvement is measured against the expected outcomes.

RAYNAUD'S DISEASE

Etiology and Pathophysiology

The etiology of Raynaud's disease is unknown. Raynaud's disease is characterized by spasm of the arteries. The body has an exaggerated response to cold and stress, resulting in vasospasm. The disease is seen more often in young women. It mostly affects the fingers and toes. Raynaud's disease can be a primary disorder or may occur secondary to another disease such as lupus erythematosus, rheumatoid arthritis, smoking, repetitive trauma, or scleroderma. In the latter instance it is known as *Raynaud's phenomenon.*

The arterial spasm occurs in response to emotional stress or exposure to cold. Blood vessels normally constrict in cold environments; however, with Raynaud's disease, this process is excessive. The affected body part changes color, ranging from white to blue to red. Figure 18–6 depicts characteristics of Raynaud's disease. When the spasm stops, there often is burning pain and throbbing. In about 10% of those affected, the disease progresses to the point at which ischemia from arterial spasm is so severe that gangrene occurs and amputation is necessary.

Signs and Symptoms

Signs and symptoms of Raynaud's disease include:

- Fingers and toes may display a series of color changes from white to blue to red; these changes are evident on the dorsal surface of the hands and feet
- The patient may experience numbness or a prickly sensation on warming and relief of stress
- There may be decreased sensory perception
- Edema may be present
- Discomfort may occur in the extremity

Diagnosis and Treatment

Diagnosis is usually made by evaluation of patient symptoms. The physician may order laboratory studies such as erythrocyte sedimentation rate (ESR) to determine the presence of autoimmune disorders, or antinuclear antibody test (ANA), which also determines the presence of immune responses. A nail fold capillaroscopy may be performed to detect deformed blood vessels in the nail fold indicative of underlying disease. Medical therapy consists of stress control, avoidance of exposure to cold, and cessation of smoking. Calcium channel blockers may be used to dilate capillaries in the hands and feet. Other drugs such as alpha blockers and vasodilators may be used to achieve vasodilatation in the small blood vessels in the hands.

NURSING MANAGEMENT

Assessment (Data Collection), Nursing Diagnosis, and Planning

Assessment of the extremities and the patient's response to treatment are essential nursing care.

Appropriate nursing diagnoses for a patient with Raynaud's disease are:

- Deficient knowledge related to management of medical condition
- Anxiety related to complications of disease process
- Risk for injury related to effects of cold on extremities
- Relocation stress syndrome related to potential need to relocate residence

Expected outcomes:

- The patient will verbalize understanding of disease process
- The patient will not sustain injury to extremities
- The patient will verbalize a reduction in anxiety related to lifestyle changes needed for disease management
- The patient will consider relocating to a warmer climate if possible

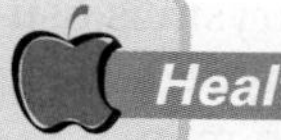

Health Promotion Points 18–2

***Healthy People 2010* Smoking Cessation**

Healthy People 2010 *lists several goals related to tobacco use among Americans. Selected goals include:*

27-1 Reduce tobacco use by adults
27-2 Reduce tobacco use by adolescents
27-3 Reduce the initiation of tobacco use among children and adolescents
27-4 Increase the average age of first use of tobacco products by adolescents and young adults
27-5 Increase smoking cessation attempts by adult smokers
27-6 Increase smoking cessation attempts during pregnancy
27-7 Increase smoking cessation attempts among adolescent smokers
27-8 Increase insurance coverage for evidenced-based treatment of nicotine dependency

You should encourage smokers with vascular disorders to seek smoking cessation programs in their communities. The American Lung Association program "Freedom from Smoking" is offered free of charge online at the American Lung Association website. Other programs such as nicotine replacement therapy are also discussed. Group programs are also offered in many communities, hospitals, American Lung Association affiliates, and community-based health programs.

Implementation and Evaluation

The major nursing intervention is teaching the patient to protect extremities and prevent injury. The patient should be taught to dress warmly when in cold environments. Clothing should be layered and hat and gloves should be worn. Warm socks should be worn to protect feet. The patient should be taught to wear protective gloves when reaching into or removing utensils from ovens, or when handling extremely cold items. Teaching the patient to avoid cold temperatures when possible, manage stress, and stop use of tobacco products should also be provided. If appropriate the patient should be referred to a smoking cessation program (Health Promotion Points 18–2).

You should evaluate the progression of symptoms, including changes in skin color and sensation. Any changes in skin integrity should be noted. The patient's compliance with recommended lifestyle changes should be evaluated and the plan revised as needed to assist the patient to meet established goals.

ANEURYSM

Etiology

Aneurysms occur in a weakened area of a blood vessel, usually the result of plaque formation, genetic predisposition, or hypertension. They may also occur in areas weakened by trauma or surgical procedures. Aneurysms may occur in cerebral vessels (cerebral aneurysms). Aortic aneurysms can occur in the area below the stomach (abdominal aneurysm) or in the chest (thoracic aneurysm). An abdominal aortic aneurysm is usually located below the kidneys. Long-term hypertension and smoking are risk factors, particularly in men.

Congenital malformations predispose to many types of aneurysm. However, atherosclerosis and hypertension are thought to be the major factors in their development. Atherosclerotic plaque weakens the vessel wall, and hypertension puts extra pressure on the weakened walls. Diabetes mellitus and hyperlipidemia are two other conditions that contribute to the development of such vessel problems.

Pathophysiology

An aneurysm can occur along any artery. It is an outpouching of the wall of the artery due to a structural defect in the layers of the arterial wall. Blood flow may become stagnant along the wall of the aneurysm, and clots can form, causing either thrombosis or embolus. Once an aneurysm develops, it continues to grow larger. Aneurysms may eventually rupture if not repaired.

Signs, Symptoms, and Diagnosis

Aneurysm rupture is common in the cerebral vessels, causing intracerebral bleeding and stroke. Aortic aneurysms can occur along either the thoracic or the abdominal portion of the vessel. A ruptured aneurysm often leads to sudden death. Aneurysms often display no obvious symptoms, although patients with cerebral aneurysms may experience headaches, impaired speech, or blurred vision. Patients with an aortic aneurysm may report back pain or a feeling of pressure and may have a visible pulsation of the abdomen. An aortic aneurysm in the thoracic area may cause substernal or tracheal pressure and difficulty with breathing.

Diagnosis of aneurysms is difficult because of lack of symptoms. Physical examination and screening of patients with a family history may be the best means of early detection. The presence of an aneurysm can be verified by chest or abdominal x-ray, ultrasound, magnetic resonance imaging (MRI), or computed tomography (CT) scans. It is recommended that men who have hypertension and a history of smoking undergo ultrasound screening for abdominal aortic aneurysm.

Treatment

If an aortic aneurysm is detected early, it often can be surgically repaired before it ruptures. The size and location of the aneurysm guides the need for surgical intervention. Aneurysms in the ascending aorta are life threatening; therefore, emergency surgery is performed. Those located in the descending thoracic and abdominal aorta may not warrant immediate action. The aneurysm is carefully watched for continued growth. Patients may also be prescribed antihypertensive drugs, such as beta blockers, to reduce the pressure on the arterial walls. If symptoms occur, surgical intervention may be necessary to prevent rupture of the aneurysm.

Surgery involves replacing the area of the vessel wall that is weakened with a graft. The use of a **stent graft** is a minimally invasive procedure. A mesh stent is placed in the area of the aneurysm. It provides support to the vessel wall and allows blood to flow through the stent, thus reducing pressure on the vessel wall. Refer to Figure 20–5 for an illustration of stent graft placement in a coronary vessel. The patient is evaluated every few months with ultrasound tracking of the size of the aneurysm. Surgery may be performed when the aneurysm is about 6 to 8 cm in diameter. Some patients may continue for years without surgery, especially those whose medical condition places them in a high-risk category for surgery.

NURSING MANAGEMENT

Assessment (Data Collection)

Careful physical assessment is needed to detect the presence of an aneurysm. You should immediately report findings of pulsations in the abdomen or other structures in which this is abnormal. Information concerning family history of aneurysm should be gathered during the patient history interview. Assessment of pain patterns, especially changes in intensity and location, is needed to identify progression of the patient's condition that may be life threatening.

Nursing Diagnosis and Planning

The main goal for a patient with an aneurysm is the prevention of rupture. Rupture of an aneurysm is a medical emergency and can lead to death. You should advise the patient to report any change in symptoms, such as pain intensity, apprehension, lightheadedness, or any unusual sensation.

Nursing diagnoses may include:

- Risk for injury from potential rupture of aneurysm
- Acute pain related to pressure of aneurysm on body structures and nerves
- Deficient knowledge related to management of medical condition

Other nursing diagnoses will depend on the location of the aneurysm and whether there is leaking.

Expected outcomes might be:

- The patient will not experience rupture of the aneurysm
- The patient will report absence of pain
- The patient will verbalize understanding of management of medical condition

Implementation

Patient education is important for the presurgical patient. The patient must be taught signs and symptoms that should be reported to the health care provider immediately. Teaching concerning the medical and surgical treatment regimen should be included along with what to expect postoperatively.

Think Critically About . . . You detect a pulsation in the patient's abdomen during physical examination. She states it has been present for several years and the physician is "watching it." List indications that could indicate need for surgical intervention.

Attentive postsurgical care is very important. The surgical procedure and nursing care depend on the location of the aneurysm. Cerebral aneurysm is treated by craniotomy; this is covered in Chapter 23. Aortic aneurysm is treated by thoracotomy or abdominal surgery depending on the location of the aneurysm, and the care is similar to that of other types of thoracic and abdominal surgery. The main difference is that you must also carefully assess pulses and function distal to the repair site. Renal function must be watched closely as blood flow to the kidneys is briefly cut off when the aorta is clamped for surgical repair.

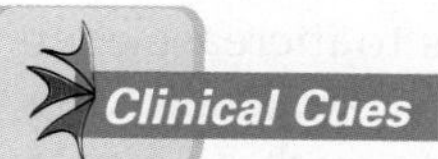

Monitor urinary output at least every 30 minutes in the immediate postoperative period, then every 2 hours. The urinary output should be at least 30 mL/hour. Report falling output immediately.

The patient spends 24 to 48 hours in an intensive care unit postoperatively. A ventilator is used, and thereafter you assist the patient to deep-breathe and cough every 1 to 2 hours. Paralytic ileus occurs for a few days after abdominal surgery and a nasogastric tube will be in place. You should auscultate the abdomen every shift for the return of bowel sounds.

The patient undergoing thoracic aortic aneurysm repair will undergo chest surgery with placement on the cardiopulmonary bypass machine. The care is the same as for other chest surgery patients. Chest tubes will be in place. This patient is especially at risk for atelectasis and pneumonia. Pain management is necessary to promote adequate respiratory effort. You also must monitor for the presence of cardiac dysrhythmias.

Evaluation

Objective data, including vital signs, neurologic status, and respiratory status should be assessed. Subjective data, including pain level and loss of sensation, should also be determined. Evaluation of the patient's understanding of teaching related to disease process, potential complications, follow-up appointments, medications, and recommended lifestyle changes should be assessed and appropriate revisions made to the plan or goals.

CAROTID OCCLUSION

When atherosclerosis has narrowed the carotid arteries leading to the brain, the signs and symptoms include carotid **bruit** (a purring sound heard with a stethoscope), confusion, visual abnormality in one eye, fainting, extremity weakness or paralysis, or other signs of decreased blood flow to the brain. The condition is treated by *carotid endarterectomy,* which surgically removes the atherosclerotic plaque, or bypass surgery, which connects an artery from outside the cranium to an area on the cerebral artery beyond the obstruction. Both procedures are done to prevent the occurrence of stroke (see Chapter 23).

Specific postoperative care for endarterectomy includes assessing for signs of bleeding, for pressure from hematoma on the trachea (evidenced by increasing hoarseness), and for neurologic problems caused by thrombosis or embolus. Neurologic signs are monitored every 2 to 4 hours. If a carotid bypass is done, the patient must have a craniotomy; see Chapter 23 for nursing care of the craniotomy patient.

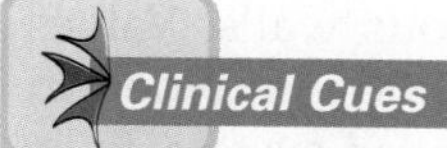

There is risk for cerebrovascular accident (stroke) following carotid endarterectomy. You should assess the patient for signs of disorientation, impaired speech, impaired swallowing, hemiparesis, facial asymmetry, aphasia, and hypertension. These findings should be reported immediately to the surgeon. Because there may be swelling in the neck that may occlude the airway, observe for difficulty breathing.

The patient is taught to maintain adequate hydration, comply with drug therapy for hypertension and diabetes, if applicable. Teaching is provided regarding antiplatelet or anticoagulant drugs. Signs and symptoms of further problems are reviewed and the patient is advised to call 911 for emergency assistance if sensory or motor deficits appear.

VENOUS INSUFFICIENCY AND VARICOSE VEINS

Etiology

Varicose veins are enlarged and tortuous veins that are distorted in shape by accumulations of pooled blood. Veins that develop varicosities have incompetent valves that allow reflux of blood from the deep to the superficial veins. The increased blood flow and resultant pressure on the vein walls cause the vessel to dilate and become tortuous.

The exact etiology of venous insufficiency and varicose veins is unknown. Contributing factors include obesity, family or personal history of atherosclerosis, trauma, hypertension, smoking, pregnancy, long periods of bed rest, and standing for long periods. Individuals who must be on their feet a great deal are encouraged to wear support stockings to encourage venous return. Patients must be taught to avoid wearing excessively constricting clothing; weight reduction is a better alternative than a girdle.

? *Think Critically About . . .* Can you identify two lifestyle changes you could personally make that would decrease your risk of a vascular disorder later in life?

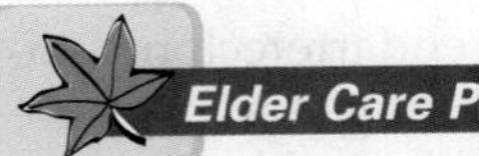

Elder Care Points

Varicose veins develop in the elderly as the veins lose their elasticity and the leg muscles weaken and atrophy from decreased exercise.

Pathophysiology

Venous return is accomplished by the pumping action of the calf muscles against the venous walls. Valves within the veins protect against backflow of blood in the venous system. When the valvular system fails, venous return is compromised, leading to enlargement of superficial and deep veins (varicose veins). As pressure increases in the veins, fluid leaks into the interstitial spaces. As the process progresses, blood also leaks into the spaces, leading to deposits of hemosiderin and discoloration of the skin, usually around the ankles and shins. Venous ulcers may develop because of maceration of skin (Figure 18–7).

Signs, Symptoms, and Diagnosis

Signs and symptoms include dilated, twisted-appearing, superficial vessels on the legs. Swelling of the foot and ankle on the affected leg may occur by the end of the day and is often accompanied by aching. The patient may complain of pain, itching, or both along varicose veins (Figure 18–8). The legs may feel full and heavy during walking or exercise. Patients may tire easily due to decrease in venous return and pooling of blood. An area of inflammation and skin impairment is typical where venous ulcers are present. Figure 18–9 depicts characteristic skin changes in venous insufficiency. Increased pigmentation of the skin, dryness and scaling, and excoriations are objective signs of venous insufficiency (see Figures 18–2 and 18–3).

Diagnosis is made by thorough physical assessment and patient history.

Treatment

Treatment includes the use of elastic support hose, exercising the legs and feet periodically throughout the day, and elevating the legs whenever possible. Prolonged standing, sitting, or crossing the legs is to be avoided. Weight reduction is recommended for obese patients. Exercises such as walking or swimming are beneficial because the muscle contraction encourages venous return to the heart. Treatment of venous insufficiency and varicose veins includes behavior modification to reduce risk factors. You should encourage patients to increase exercise, adhere to a heart-healthy diet, stop smoking, and gain optimal control of diseases such as hypertension and diabetes.

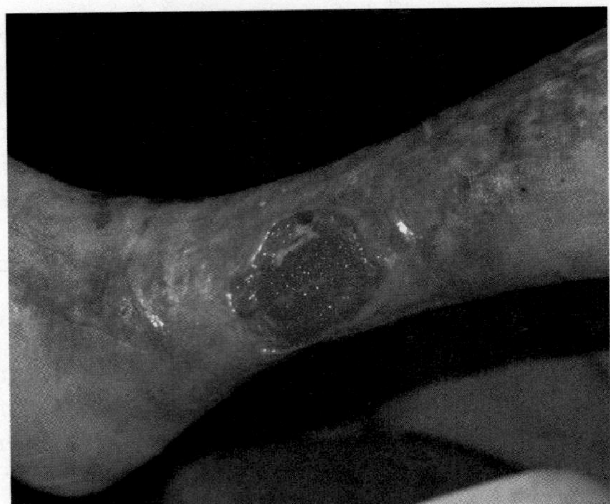

FIGURE **18–7** Venous stasis ulcer.

Constricting clothing should be avoided, particularly circular garters and elastic materials in underclothing. Frequent position changes are essential; position must be changed at least every 2 hours. The patient with poor venous circulation can benefit from periodic elevation of the lower extremities to facilitate venous return of blood to the heart. Elevation above the level of the heart is preferred. Well-distributed support of the vessels near the surface of the body will help improve venous return. To provide this kind of support, the physician may prescribe a compression device or fitted elastic stockings. The stockings or elastic bandage should be applied early in the morning, before the legs are placed in a dependent position, because the blood vessels are less congested after a prolonged rest. Bandages and hose should be applied by beginning at the feet and working upward to avoid trapping blood in the lower leg. The patient should have two pairs of elastic hose and should wash them after each day's wearing. Elastic hose should be replaced every 6 months as they lose their elasticity. When stockings are removed, the heels should be checked for pressure areas.

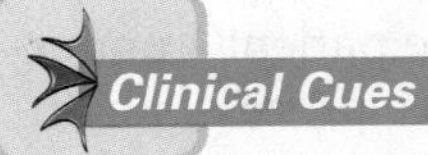

Clinical Cues

Follow directions carefully and measure the patient's calf and legs prior to choosing a pair of elastic stockings. Accurate fit is crucial to effectiveness of treatment.

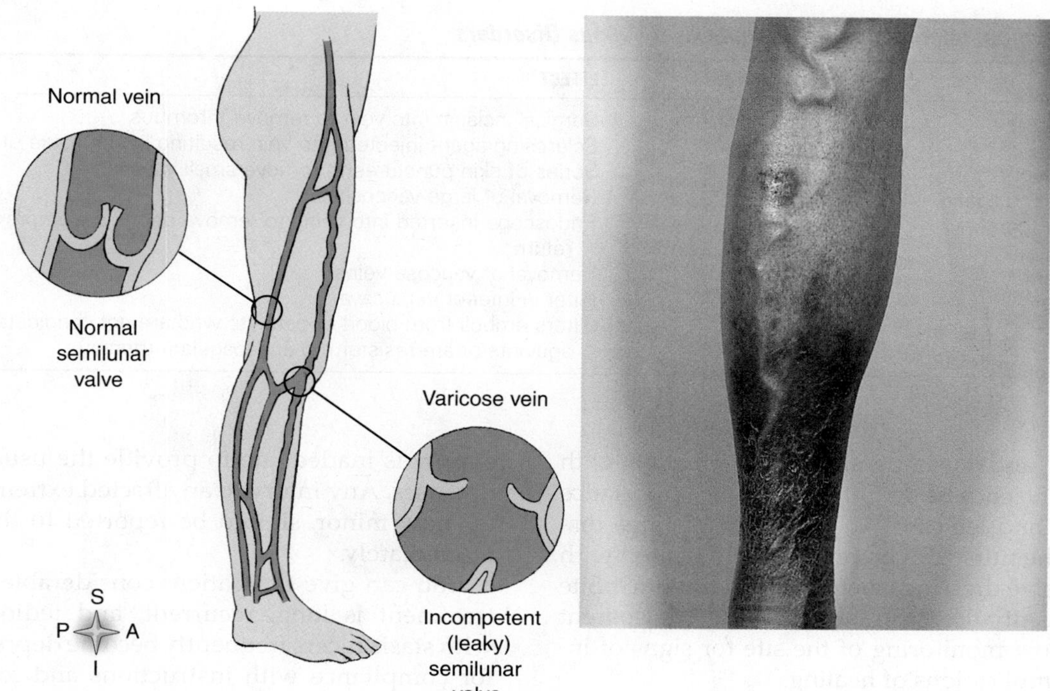

FIGURE 18–8 Varicose veins.

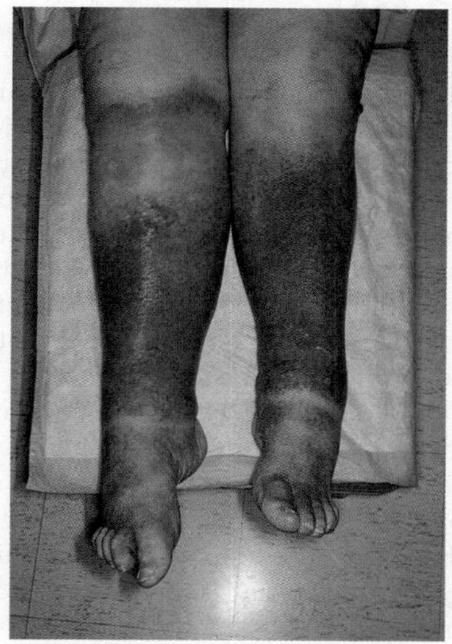

FIGURE 18–9 Characteristic skin changes in the patient with venous insufficiency.

Exercise is especially beneficial to patients with decreased blood flow. Walking is ideal exercise for the ambulatory patient. If a patient is unable to ambulate, you should promote venous return through range-of-motion (ROM) exercises and the other kinds of muscular movements. Use of a treadmill for patients who cannot exercise by walking outside is very beneficial. A stationary exercise bicycle is another alternative.

Medications such as nonsteroidal antiinflammatory drugs (NSAIDs), and if thrombus occurs, thrombolytics or anticoagulants may be prescribed. Surgical procedures may be used when medical treatment is ineffective. Table 18–4 describes surgical interventions for venous disorders.

Small varicosities can be treated by **scleropathy**, which involves injecting an agent that will sclerose the vessel, causing thrombosis, thereby preventing further blood from filling the area. Veins with multiple, severe varicosities (more than 4 mm in diameter) are treated by vein stripping, done as an outpatient procedure. Generally there will be multiple incisions along the leg to ligate and strip out the vein. Newer, less invasive procedures include endovenous occlusion using laser, radiofrequency closure, or transilluminated powered phlebectomy. The legs are wrapped with elastic bandages postoperatively to decrease bleeding and hematoma formation. Bed rest and leg elevation the night after surgery are recommended. ROM exercise of the legs is done every hour to help prevent thrombosis. Prevention of infection after this procedure is essential.

Venous Stasis Ulcers. Chronic venous insufficiency causes chronic skin and tissue lesions on the lower extremities, especially around the ankle (see Figure 18–7). The diabetic patient with venous insufficiency is at high risk for this disorder because of compromised circulation in the extremities and a slow rate of healing. Blood flows into the area, but is not adequately returned to the heart because of valvular problems in the veins. The ulcers may extend deeply into the tissue and are very slow and difficult to heal because of tissue congestion and edema that prevent nutrients from reaching the cells. The ulcer may begin as a small, tender, inflamed area and becomes very painful. With the slightest trauma, the skin breaks and the ulcer grows. Any skin trauma to the lower extremity may cause an

Table 18–4 Surgical Intervention for Patients with Venous Disorders

PROCEDURE	USE	EFFECT
Thrombectomy	Thrombus occlusion	Surgical incision into vein to remove thrombus
Sclerotherapy	Varicose veins	Sclerosing agent injected into vein resulting in shrinkage of vein
Ambulatory phlebectomy	Varicose veins	Series of skin punctures to remove small varicosities
Vein stripping and ligation	Varicose veins	Removal of large varicosities
Endoscopic surgery	Venous ulcers	Endoscope inserted into veins to remove debris and improve venous return
Laser treatment	Varicose veins	Removal of varicose veins
Vena cava filter	Recurring emboli	Filter in inferior vena cava Filters emboli from blood of patients who are not candidates for anticoagulants or are resistant to anticoagulant therapy

ulcer to form, and it is imperative that the patient with venous insufficiency be taught the extreme importance of good foot and leg care. An inflamed skin area discovered by the nurse can be preventively treated with a clear occlusive dressing, such as Tegaderm or OpSite to help prevent ulcer formation. These transparent dressings allow monitoring of the site for signs of infection or complications of healing.

Treatment for the hospitalized patient with an open ulcer consists of leg elevation, a dry or wet-to-dry saline dressing, and hydrotherapy. Dressings are changed several times a day, helping to **debride** (i.e., peel away dead tissue) the area. Often the wound needs a graft to heal completely. Prior to grafting, the ulcer is debrided and varicosities in the area are removed. A split thickness graft or bioengineered skin such as Apligraf or Dermagraft may be used. You should ensure that the patient understands the need to avoid injury to the graft site. Patients are placed on bed rest for several days after grafting to protect the site. Venous stasis ulcers can take weeks to months to heal. Ambulatory patients are treated with compression dressings.

Compression dressings are not used if arterial insufficiency is also present. Compression therapy options include compression stockings, elastic tubular support bandages, intermittent compression devices, a paste bandage such as Unna boot, or placement of two to four layers of compression dressings to the affected area. Each layer is applied differently to accomplish maximal venous return. One layer may be spiral wrapped, the next applied in a figure eight, etc. Venous return is accomplished as the patient moves her leg and achieves pressure on the calf muscles. Compression dressings can be placed over wound dressings. The dressings help to reduce ulcer pain, keep the wound moist, and assist debridement. You should teach the patient with a venous ulcer that compression is a lifelong process because venous injury does not go away. The dressing is changed from every 2 to 3 days to every few weeks, as needed.

You should teach the patient about proper self-care and signs of beginning skin breakdown. The slightest injury to an ischemic area can take a very long time to heal and can easily become infected, as the blood supply is inadequate to provide the usual leukocyte defenses. Any injury to an affected extremity, no matter how minor, should be reported to the physician immediately.

You can give the patient considerable support, as treatment is long, recurrent, and tedious. Patients with stasis ulcers frequently become depressed. Praise for compliance with instructions and for any small gains made toward healing can do much for their morale.

NURSING MANAGEMENT

Assessment (Data Collection)

Subjective information is gathered during history taking. Objective assessment data should include status of the skin, noting color, warmth, and moisture. Venous insufficiency causes a brownish appearance of the skin. Stasis dermatitis may be present and pruritus is common. Edema is a common finding. A description of any stasis ulcer should be included with documentation of size, presence of exudate, color, and odor. Patient statement of pain at the site on a scale of 0 to 10 should be assessed. You should also assess the patient's experience with pain, including intensity, when pain occurs, and how it is relieved. Assess arterial pulses and determine the pulse rate, rhythm, and character (force) of the pulse. Focused Assessment 18–1 is a guide to history taking when assessing a patient with a vascular disease. For diagnostic tests refer to Table 17–3.

Nursing Diagnosis and Planning

Nursing diagnoses are chosen based on the assessment data that indicate problems for the patient. Common nursing diagnoses associated with vascular disorders are listed in Table 17–4. Nursing diagnoses may be added to the care plan for problems secondary to treatments, such as drug therapy or surgery. Other nursing diagnoses sometimes used include:

- Insomnia related to pain in the legs while at rest
- Situational low self-esteem related to inability to perform usual roles because of chronic leg ulcers

The nursing goals for the patient with venous insufficiency are developed to promote circulation and

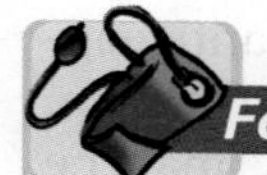

Focused Assessment 18–1

Data Collection for Vascular Disorders

Gather data on the following while interviewing a patient with vascular disorders:

HEALTH HISTORY
- Family history of cardiovascular disease, diabetes mellitus, or peripheral vascular disease
- History of trauma to the lower extremities
- Personal history of peripheral vascular disease
- All medications taken on a regular basis (prescribed and over-the-counter)
- History of tobacco use, especially smoking
- History of alcohol use
- Dietary practices, especially sodium and fat intake
- Current or history of central nervous system occurrences, such as dizziness, headaches, or loss of consciousness
- Occurrence of edema in the legs, feet, or ankles
- Occurrence of leg pain during walking. When? How is it relieved?

HEAD AND NECK
- Color of skin
- Observe for jugular vein distention
- Auscultate carotid arteries for presence of bruit

CHEST
- Auscultate heart sounds and note any abnormalities

ABDOMEN
- Any visible abdominal pulsation over aorta?
- Auscultate over aorta for presence of bruit

EXTREMITIES
- Assess peripheral pulses and compare bilaterally
- Assess blood pressure on both arms, sitting and standing
- Assess skin for temperature, color, appearance, lesions, dryness, presence or absence of hair
- Note presence of varicosities
- Assess capillary refill

prevent complications associated with reduced blood flow. Appropriate exercise is important to treat vascular disease. You should collaborate with the physician and physical therapist about activity, exercises, and 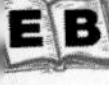 the reinforcement of teaching (Bartley, 2006). Collaboration with the dietitian is vital to the patient who has atherosclerosis and a high cholesterol level. Specific expected outcomes must be written on an individual basis. Examples are included in Table 17–4.

Implementation

A major role of the nurse caring for a patient with venous insufficiency is to monitor the condition and determine whether treatment is effective. Considerable time is spent on teaching patients about the disease, self-care, and medications. Monitoring side effects or adverse effects of medication is very important. Table 17–4 lists helpful interventions for the most common nursing diagnoses associated with problems of the vascular system. Nursing interventions for selected problems in a patient with a venous stasis ulcer are summarized in Table 17–4 and in Nursing Care Plan 18–1.

Evaluation

You must evaluate the patient's response to treatment to determine effectiveness and potential development of complications. Subjective and objective data may be used. Carefully evaluating pulses and comparing them bilaterally is an important part of nursing care for patients with problems of the vascular system. Documenting a good description of the quality and character of the pulses monitored in the nurse's notes will give coworkers an accurate assessment baseline on which to evaluate changes in the pulse.

It is important to determine if skin color and temperature have changed since the last assessment. Areas of discoloration should be accurately measured and documented in the nurse's notes. Ulcerated areas are monitored closely and measured to determine whether healing is occurring. The color of the healing tissue and presence of exudate also are evaluated. Documentation of the characteristics of any exudate should be included. If the wound is enlarging or not improving, the nursing actions or treatment must be changed.

Often you must rely on subjective data from the patient to evaluate whether treatment and nursing actions are effective. Increases in peripheral circulation may be evident only by a decrease in pain or an ability to walk further without pain. The patient should be able to demonstrate understanding of the disease process, preventive measures, medications, signs and symptoms to report to the health care provider, and follow-up care.

THROMBOPHLEBITIS

Etiology, Pathophysiology, Signs, Symptoms, and Diagnosis

Thrombophlebitis is inflammation of a superficial vein caused by a blood clot. It occurs from inactivity, trauma, and irritation to the vein, infection from an IV line, or contaminated IV drug needles.

Trauma to venous walls leads to inflammation and aggregation of blood components at the site of the inflammation. A clot forms at this site, leading to obstruction of blood flow. If not treated, the clot may become an embolus and travel to the lungs, heart, or brain, resulting in pulmonary embolus, myocardial infarction (MI), or cerebrovascular accident (CVA).

Signs and symptoms include swelling, redness, warmth, and considerable tenderness and pain upon touching. Diagnosis is by using ultrasound and venography as a means to detect the clot. Physical examination, patient history, and evaluation of signs and symptoms are important to diagnosing thrombophlebitis.

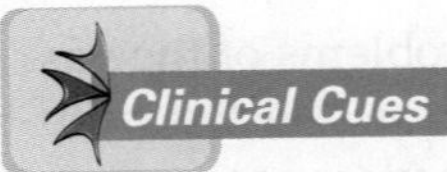

Whenever a patient has a known thrombophlebitis, watch for signs of pulmonary embolus: dyspnea, hemoptysis, tachypnea, tachycardia, chest pain, a feeling of impending doom, cyanosis, and possibly coughing and altered mental status. These signs indicate an emergency situation.

Treatment and Nursing Management

Treatment includes discontinuing the source of irritation; applying warm, moist heat; elevating the extremity; and administering NSAIDs and antibiotics. Patients are encouraged to stay off the feet and elevate the legs.

Nursing management of the patient with thrombophlebitis includes assessment and documentation of the color, warmth, circumference, and pulses of the affected extremity. The patient may be required to remain on complete bed rest or have bathroom privileges. Explain the importance of adhering to the prescribed activity level and potential complications if not in compliance. Make certain that the patient receives medications as prescribed including anticoagulants and medication for pain management. Warm, moist compresses to the affected extremity may be ordered. Emphasize the importance of this treatment. Develop a discharge teaching plan related to the disease process, medications, activity level, home care, and follow-up. Components of teaching may include the following:

- Avoidance of sitting for long periods
- Management of anticoagulants (side effects, signs of complications, follow-up laboratory studies)
- Application of antiembolism stockings, if prescribed
- Activity limits
- Preventive measures

Think Critically About . . . What teaching points would you cover for a 52-year-old female who is being discharged after hospitalization for thrombophlebitis of the right leg? The patient is employed as a waitress.

NURSING CARE PLAN 18–1

Care of the Patient with a Venous Stasis Ulcer

SCENARIO Mrs. Hunter, age 52, with chronic PVD has a large stasis ulcer on the inner aspect of the lower third of her left leg. There is a copious amount of drainage from the ulcer. Her lower right leg is edematous and has dry, scaly skin with brownish discoloration. The ulcer is being treated with calcium alginate dressings, bed rest with bathroom privileges, and elevation of the leg. Patient states she is afraid ulcer will not heal and she will "lose her leg."

PROBLEM/NURSING DIAGNOSIS *Stasis ulcer*/Impaired skin integrity related to decreased peripheral circulation.
Supporting assessment data *Subjective:* Patient verbalizes fear she may need amputation of leg. *Objective:* History of chronic peripheral vascular disease; presence of large stasis ulcer on left leg.

Goals/Expected Outcomes	Nursing Interventions	Selected Rationale	Evaluation
Ulcer will heal completely	Apply and change alginate dressings as prescribed.	Alginate dressing will form a gel and absorb wound drainage.	Dressings changed, less drainage noted; edges less reddened; WBC count; 9500.
	Assess for signs of improvement or worsening of ulcer; purulent drainage, elevated WBC count, increased size of wound.	Elevated temperature, increased WBC, change in character of drainage and wound may indicate infection.	Continue plan.

PROBLEM/NURSING DIAGNOSIS *Cigarette smoking*/Noncompliance related to inability to stop smoking.
Supporting assessment data *Subjective:* States she quit smoking for 3 months; has resumed smoking ½ pack per day.

Goals/Expected Outcomes	Nursing Interventions	Selected Rationale	Evaluation
Patient will join a smoking cessation program in her community within 60 days	Obtain literature on the smoking cessation programs in her community from the American Lung Association (ALA).	Patient more likely to be successful if she has convenient access to a smoking cessation program.	Agreed to join smoking cessation program.
	Reinforce information concerning effects of smoking on peripheral circulation.	Smoking causes vasoconstriction, which further compromises peripheral vascular disease.	Began teaching relaxation exercises; gave ALA literature on quitting smoking; discussed smoking effects on vessels again.
	Teach relaxation exercises.		Continue plan.

NURSING CARE PLAN 18–1

Care of the Patient with a Venous Stasis Ulcer—cont'd

PROBLEM/NURSING DIAGNOSIS *Limited information about disease process*/Deficient knowledge related to care of skin and prevention of ulcers.

Supporting assessment data *Subjective:* States she has not been wearing support hose, obtaining little exercise; cannot verbalize points of proper self-care.

Goals/Expected Outcomes	Nursing Interventions	Selected Rationale	Evaluation
Patient will verbalize six points in proper self-care	Explain how sluggish circulation contributes to breakdown of skin and tissues.	Understanding of effects of disease can help with gaining compliance.	Verbalized understanding of effects of circulation on skin integrity.
	Encourage active exercise: ankle rotation and leg bending while on bed rest; walking when ambulatory.	Promotes venous return.	Performs foot and ankle exercises each day.
	Teach patient and spouse how to apply elastic stocking before she arises in A.M.	Promotes venous return.	Demonstrated proper application of elastic stockings. Continue plan.
	Teach her to inspect feet and legs each day after bath; use lotion bid to ease drying and scaling.	Early detection of skin impairment can prevent extension of problem.	States she inspects feet each day using a mirror for better visualization.
	Teach her to report any sign of reddening or break in skin to physician immediately.		
Patient will not cross legs or ankles when sitting	Teach her not to cross ankles or legs at knee when sitting and to avoid prolonged standing.	Causes vasoconstriction and impedes blood flow.	Observed changing position when realizing legs are crossed while sitting.
	Teach patient to place wedge under foot of mattress at home to raise the legs above the level of the heart	Promotes effective circulation.	States she keeps legs elevated when sitting.
	Teach her to elevate legs when sitting.		
Patient will wear support hose daily			

? CRITICAL THINKING QUESTIONS

1. What are other risk factors that contribute to development of peripheral vascular disease?
2. How would you differentiate between a venous and arterial vascular problem?

Evaluation of patient success in meeting goals would include absence of complications of the disease process or medications and demonstrated evidence of understanding of discharge teaching. Often you must rely on subjective data from the patient to evaluate whether treatment and nursing actions are effective. Increases in peripheral circulation may be evident only by a decrease in pain or an ability to walk further without pain. Nursing interventions for selected problems in a patient with a venous stasis ulcer are summarized in Table 17–4 and in Nursing Care Plan 18–1.

THROMBOSIS AND EMBOLISM

Thrombosis is the formation, development, or presence of a clump of blood elements, particularly platelets and fibrin that form a clot in a blood vessel and diminish or completely obstruct blood flow.

A thrombus can occur or develop as a result of injury to vascular endothelium, sluggish flow of blood (venous insufficiency), or changes in the number of blood elements (for example, an increase in the number of red blood cells or platelets). Immobility is a major factor in the formation of thrombi. Thrombosis can be present in either veins or arteries, but because the flow of blood is slower through the veins than through the arteries, venous thrombosis is more common.

The effects of thrombosis depend on (1) the location and size of the thrombus; (2) whether it completely or only partially blocks blood flow through a vessel; and (3) whether the body is able to establish collateral circulation to prevent ischemia in the area formerly served by the obstructed vessel.

An embolism is the sudden obstruction of an artery by a mass of foreign material that has been brought to the site by the blood current. The embolus usually is a blood clot that has broken off from a thrombus. However, it can be a globule of fat, air bubble, piece of tissue, clump of bacteria, or bolus of liquid that is not dissolved in the blood. The effects of an embolism depend on the site at which it is lodged and its size compared with the caliber of the blood vessel in which it is located.

Arterial thrombosis is treated according to the severity of the symptoms it is causing. If total blockage of an artery is occurring, surgical **thrombectomy** (surgical removal of thrombus) may be necessary. If there is collateral circulation to provide nutrients for the tissues distal to the thrombus, intraarterial enzyme dissolution of the thrombus may be used. A catheter is threaded into the artery and an enzyme substance such as urokinase or streptokinase may be used to dissolve the clot over a 36- to 72-hour period. IV heparin may be used to prevent further clotting, and the patient is closely monitored while the body breaks down the thrombus.

DEEP VEIN THROMBOSIS

Etiology

A clot in a deep vein, or *deep vein thrombosis (DVT)*, most often occurs in the lower leg, although it can occur in any vein in the body. A great many factors contribute to the formation of a DVT. Immobility, trauma, sepsis, clotting problems, surgical procedures, dehydration, obesity, cancer, estrogen hormone therapy, or any condition that causes slowing of venous flow can cause a clot to form. Venous thrombosis occurs fairly often during long plane flights or car trips. Staying well hydrated, exercising the leg and calf muscles frequently during the trip, and walking every 1 to 2 hours helps to prevent clots from occurring. Wearing support hose at work aids venous return and helps prevent thrombosis in those who have varicose veins (Van Wicklin, 2006).

EB

Pathophysiology

A clot in a deep vein may lead to obstruction of venous outflow. If this is not corrected, increased pressure in the vein could result in destruction of venous valves and development of venous insufficiency. **Embolism** may be caused when a portion of a DVT in a leg breaks loose and travels to the lungs, heart, or brain. The embolus lodges in small vessels, especially those in the pulmonary and cardiac systems. Blood flow is interrupted and loss of oxygenation and interruption of blood flow to the myocardium may occur. Cardiac dysrhythmias, such as atrial fibrillation, also cause emboli. Release of fat droplets from a long-bone fracture and amniotic fluid introduced into a vein during the birthing process also can result in the formation of an embolus. The most acute and serious result of DVT is development of an embolus that may lodge in respiratory vessels, causing severe respiratory distress or death

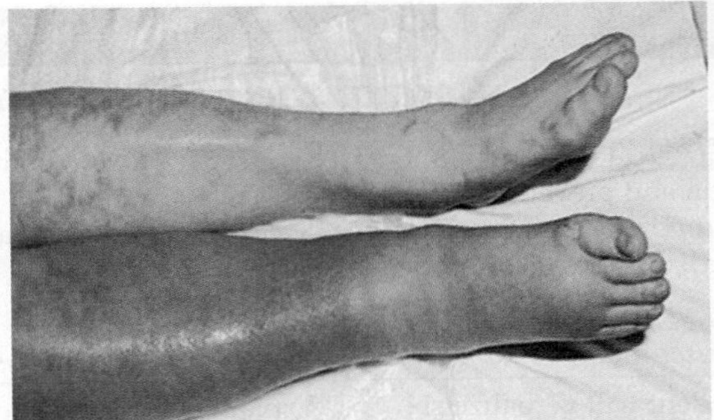

FIGURE 18–10 Patient with DVT.

Although some emboli dissolve on their own, the condition can be life threatening. Treatment may consist of thrombectomy (excision of the clot) or thrombolytic therapy with an enzyme substance.

Signs, Symptoms, and Diagnosis

The main sign of a DVT is edema in one extremity. Figure 18–10 depicts a patient with DVT. There may be pain in the calf of the leg when the foot is dorsiflexed (Homans' sign). The area over the thrombosis may feel warm. You should never rub or vigorously palpate the area, as this can dislodge the clot and send it into the circulation, which can cause severe damage or death. Early ambulation postoperatively helps promote circulation and reduces the risk of clot formation. Encouraging patients on bed rest to perform leg and ankle exercises each hour while awake can do much to decrease the incidence of DVT. Factors that contribute to DVT include venous stasis, changes in the lining of the veins, dehydration, and increased ease of clotting.

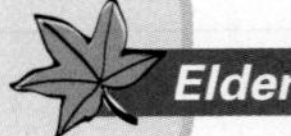

Elder Care Points

Elderly patients who have problems with mobility or stress incontinence tend to drink less fluid so that they do not have to visit the bathroom so often. This can lead to dehydration and more viscous blood, which in turn can predispose to thrombus formation in those susceptible to this disorder. Encourage adequate fluid intake to promote circulation, and provide a means for convenient toileting for these patients. The occurrence of thrombophlebitis increases with advanced age.

The most common method of diagnosing DVT is duplex sonography. Sound waves detect blood flow through the veins and identify areas of abnormality. If sonography is not clear, a venogram may be done to detect DVT. The venogram requires injection of a dye to identify areas of obstruction. You should obtain the patient's allergy history prior to this procedure.

Treatment

Medical treatment usually consists of bed rest and IV heparin and then a low-molecular-weight heparin such as enoxaparin (Lovenox), and oral warfarin sodium (Coumadin) (Agency for Healthcare Research and Quality, 2003). Anticoagulants will not dissolve the clot but will prevent it from growing larger. The body dissolves the clot on its own over time. Thrombolytic therapy may be used to dissolve the thrombus; streptokinase, urokinase, or alteplase (t-PA) are some of the agents used.

EB

There is a high risk of bleeding with these drugs. A thrombolytic agent is followed by a few additional days of heparin while the patient is started on warfarin. Warfarin takes at least 3 days to build to an effective blood level. Elastic stockings may be prescribed for continuous use thereafter.

If a patient is considered at risk for further embolus formation from DVT, a vena caval umbrella may be inserted to prevent damage from emboli. This is a strainer-like device positioned in the vena cava that catches the emboli, preventing them from traveling further. The umbrella is collapsed, and with the use of a special catheter, threaded into the vena cava. The umbrella catches the emboli and the body slowly dissolves and disposes of them.

The outcome of thrombosis or embolus can range from mild local congestion and edema to sudden death from occlusion of a major artery in the brain, lungs, or heart.

NURSING MANAGEMENT

Assessment (Data Collection)

You should assess patients at risk for DVT each shift for signs and symptoms. Homans' sign is a common method of assessment; however, it is not conclusive. The calf pain associated with Homans' sign may be related to factors other than DVT. Assessment should include:

- Observation of the extremity for asymmetric size
- Areas of warmth and redness over a vein
- Calf pain and/or tenderness
- Pitting edema of the affected extremity
- Measurement of calf circumference

Nursing Diagnosis and Planning

Nursing care of the patient with a DVT and thrombophlebitis is presented in Nursing Care Plan 18–2. Information and nursing care for the administration of anticoagulants are presented in Chapter 19.

Nursing diagnoses include:

- Risk for injury related to embolus formation
- Risk for injury related to bleeding associated with anticoagulant therapy
- Deficient knowledge related to medication regimen

Expected outcomes include:

- The patient will avoid complications such as pulmonary embolism
- The patient will verbalize understanding of anticoagulant therapy
- The patient will verbalize understanding of medication regimen

See Nursing Care Plan 18–2 for a more extensive list with outcomes and rationales.

Implementation

Elastic stockings are usually prescribed to prevent recurrence of the thrombus. Support stockings, thromboembolic disease (TED) hose, or Jobst hose should be applied in the morning before the legs have been dependent. Hose must be properly fitted and should be checked and straightened frequently so that they do not bunch up and put pressure on the back of the knee.

Sequential compression devices (SCDs) (see Figure 5–3) often are applied postoperatively to the legs of patients who will be confined to bed and are at risk of deep vein thrombosis. These must be applied properly and checked for positioning frequently. They may be used along with elastic stockings. The SCDs may be removed when ambulating to the bathroom, for personal hygiene care, or as prescribed by the physician.

The patient with thrombosis is taught not to rub the extremity. The nurse encourages increased fluid intake to reduce blood viscosity. Elastic hose are applied correctly, and the procedure for their use is explained to the patient. They must be kept smooth. They are removed only for bathing. You should administer anticoagulant therapy and monitor for adverse side effects, checking for bleeding and monitoring coagulation times. Specifically check for signs of bruising, petechiae, bleeding gums, and blood in the urine or stool. The patient receiving IV heparin should be placed on a Biofoam or similar bed pad before therapy begins to reduce bruising. The patient must be told to move cautiously, to avoid hitting the head or bumping into furniture, doors, or other objects. The IV site should be monitored closely, as heparin can be irritating to the vessel in some people. At the first sign of inflammation, the IV site should be changed. Firm pressure should be applied to any needle stick for at least 5 minutes to prevent hematoma formation. You must be alert for signs of pulmonary embolus (dyspnea, chest pain, hemoptysis, tachypnea, tachycardia).

The patient with DVT is taught to prevent venous stasis by exercising, keeping well hydrated, quitting smoking, avoiding substances that cause the blood to coagulate more easily (e.g., hormones), and avoiding sitting for long periods. The legs should not be crossed to avoid compression of arteries resulting in compromised circulation.

NURSING CARE PLAN 18–2

Care of the Patient with a Deep Vein Thrombosis

SCENARIO Mrs. Hanson, age 72, sustained multiple bruises and a concussion in an automobile accident. She has cardiac dysrhythmia and was admitted 2 days ago for observation and recuperation. She has now developed pain in her right calf, and her lower leg is swollen, with a hot, tender area in the midcalf region. She has been placed on a continuous heparin drip.

PROBLEM/NURSING DIAGNOSIS *Circulatory compromise*/Ineffective tissue perfusion related to presence of clot in vein and inflammation.

Supporting assessment data *Subjective:* "My leg really hurts." Complains of pain in right calf. *Objective:* Thrombus in saphenous vein, right calf. Reddened, warm, tender area on midcalf. Temperature, 101.2° F (38.4° C).

Goals/Expected Outcomes	Nursing Interventions	Selected Rationale	Evaluation
Thrombus will resolve within 2 weeks as evidenced by Doppler flow studies	Maintain on bed rest with bathroom privileges; keep right lower leg elevated.	To avoid further injury from clot.	Heparin drip continuous; IV site without redness or swelling; right leg elevated; active ROM on left leg at 8, 10, 12, and 2; moist heating pad to right calf for 30 minutes each hour; edema decreased slightly; continue plan.
Thrombophlebitis will resolve by discharge as evidenced by normal temperature and no calf tenderness, redness, or swelling	Active ROM of left ankle, knee, and hip.	Maintain venous circulation.	
	Elastic stocking on left leg.	Promote venous return.	
	Warm packs to right leg; handle right leg gently.	Provide comfort, decrease edema.	
	Maintain heparin drip on IV pump at ordered rate; assess IV site q hr for infiltration.	Prevent formation of additional thrombi.	
	Assess legs every shift for status of thrombus and development of other problems.	Heparin can cause bleeding.	
	Auscultate lung sounds every shift; be alert for signs of pulmonary emboli.	Early detection of pulmonary emboli for immediate intervention.	Lung sounds clear to auscultation.
	Monitor level of consciousness (LOC) and neurologic status every shift.	Change in central nervous system status could indicate cerebral embolism.	Alert and oriented × 3.
	Observe for bleeding of gums, excessive bruising, blood in urine or stool, nosebleeds, and abdominal pain and rigidity.	Catches early symptoms of side effects of heparin therapy.	States slight bleeding from gums during oral care.
	Monitor Hb and hematocrit to detect blood loss.	Determines if hidden bleeding is occurring.	No significant changes.
	Begin Coumadin therapy as ordered 3 days before heparin is stopped.	Takes 3 days for Coumadin level to be effective.	Began Coumadin today.
	Handle patient very gently.	Anticoagulant therapy makes patient prone to bruising.	No evidence of bruising; handling gently.

PROBLEM/NURSING DIAGNOSIS *Risk for thrombus formation*/Risk for injury related to heparin drip and to possibility of embolus.

Supporting assessment data *Objective:* Heparin drip 50,000 U in 500 mL at 50 mL/hr. DVT in right leg.

Goals/Expected Outcomes	Nursing Interventions	Selected Rationale	Evaluation
Patient will not experience embolus during hospitalization	Auscultate lung sounds every shift; be alert for signs of pulmonary emboli.	Assists in early detection of pulmonary emboli so immediate intervention can occur.	Lungs clear to auscultation.

NURSING CARE PLAN 18–2

Care of the Patient with a Deep Vein Thrombosis—cont'd

Goals/Expected Outcomes	Nursing Interventions	Selected Rationale	Evaluation
No hemorrhage from heparin as evidenced by no sign of bleeding internally or externally	Monitor LOC and neurologic status every shift.	Change in central nervous system status could indicate cerebral embolism or bleed.	Pupils equal, round and reactive to light and accommodation (PERRLA) without headache, alert and oriented.
	Observe for bleeding of gums, excessive bruising, blood in urine or stool, nosebleeds, and abdominal pain and rigidity.	Catches symptoms of side effects of heparin therapy.	Slight bleeding of gums. Bruising from previous needle sticks; buttocks bruised from bed rest.
	Monitor Hb and hematocrit to detect blood loss Monitor PTT and INR and advise physician immediately if values rise above 2½ times the control value.	May indicate need to change infusion rate or administer antidote.	PTT 2 × control value, INR 2.7; no change in Hb and hematocrit; no evidence of blood in urine or stool; bowel sounds present all four quadrants, abdomen soft.
	Begin Coumadin therapy as ordered 3 days before heparin is stopped. Handle patient very gently.	Anticoagulant therapy will continue when discharged home.	Continue plan.

PROBLEM/NURSING DIAGNOSIS *Lack of knowledge about medication* /Deficient knowledge related to precautions necessary when taking Coumadin.

Supporting assessment data Will go home on Coumadin for at least 6 to 12 months. Has never taken this medication.

Goals/Expected Outcomes	Nursing Interventions	Selected Rationale	Evaluation
Patient will verbalize danger signs to report to physician and proper dosage schedule before discharge	Teach the following: Avoid foods high in vitamin K (give list). Avoid over-the-counter medications and drugs that might extend clotting time or interfere with action of Coumadin (e.g., aspirin, etc.).	Vitamin K interferes with the action of Coumadin. Some over-the-counter drugs have anticoagulant actions that may increase risk of complications of drug therapy.	Began teaching regarding dangers of Coumadin; needs time to absorb information; will continue teaching tomorrow; gave written instruction sheet. Continue plan.
	Move around carefully, trying not to hit head on anything or bump into things.	Injury could cause bruising and hematoma formation.	Slight bruising noted on buttocks. Continue to monitor.
	Observe urine and stool for signs of bleeding.	May indicate elevated PT and INR.	No signs of bleeding in urine or stool.
	Maintain good hydration by drinking at least 10 glasses of fluid a day.	Hydration supports blood flow and reduces risk of additional clot formation.	Oral intake 1500 mL/day.
Patient will verbalize understanding of need for regular medical follow-up and periodic clotting times before discharge	Instruct her to maintain close contact with physician to monitor clotting times.	Monitoring of PT important to evaluate effectiveness of Coumadin therapy.	Verbalizes need to keep appointments for follow-up laboratory studies.
	Explain dosage schedule. Give written instruction sheet.	Provide additional reference for safe administration of drug.	

? CRITICAL THINKING QUESTIONS

1. List the signs and symptoms of pulmonary embolism.
2. What additional assessment data would you expect to find during the physical examination of a patient with deep vein thrombosis?

Patients at risk for embolus should be assessed for signs and symptoms including sudden chest pain, cough, apprehension, and changes in respiratory status. These changes must be reported to the physician immediately.

Evaluation

Evidence that the patient with DVT has met the established outcomes include the absence of respiratory complications and development of pulmonary emboli, absence of complications associated with anticoagulant therapy (i.e., hematuria, bleeding from venipuncture sites), decreased pain and edema in the affected extremity, and patient verbalization of information taught concerning medications and home care.

COMMUNITY CARE

Many patients with vascular disease are treated in outpatient clinics and their homes. Patients who have venous stasis ulcers are often treated by the home health nurse. With early discharge after surgery, many patients receive postoperative care in the home. Patients with arterial bypass may be referred for rehabilitation exercise programs at a rehabilitation center. Your role in these settings is focused on ongoing assessment, coordination of care with other members of the health care team, monitoring progress and compliance with treatment, and patient education. Wound care and dressing changes are a daily function of the home care nurse.

You must include careful monitoring of the blood pressure for the presence of hypertension. Hypertension is a major risk factor in vascular disorders. Patients should be aware of expected blood pressure levels and critical levels to report to the health care provider. You should evaluate the home care patient's understanding of medication, diet, and exercise to accomplish optimal management of hypertension.

Some patients may have the capability of monitoring their coagulation status through home monitoring devices. This is especially important for patients who are taking drugs such as warfarin. The prothrombin time (PT) and international normalized ratio (INR) can be monitored by use of the AccuCoag device. The patient has more information to manage his coagulation status and avoids missed lab appointment. You should be aware of patient use of these devices and ensure the patient is using them correctly.

Key Points

- Hypertension is more prevalent and more severe in African Americans than in other minority groups and whites.
- Treatment of hypertension involves measures to assist the patient to maintain blood pressure at or below 120/80 mm Hg.
- Antihypertensive drugs work by decreasing blood volume, cardiac output, or peripheral resistance.
- Nursing care of patients with hypertension includes counseling and education about lifestyle changes, diet, weight control, stress relief, and exercise.
- Noncompliance with medical regimen for hypertension can result in blindness, stroke, and kidney failure.
- Education, public screening, and encouragement for compliance with treatment can decrease the incidence of damage from hypertension.
- Arterial wall injury may be caused by hypertension, deposit of fatty plaque, chemical toxins, or diabetes mellitus.
- Obesity, stress, and sedentary lifestyle contribute to the incidence of atherosclerosis and hypertension.
- Atherosclerosis is the most common etiology of peripheral vascular disease (PVD).
- Disorders of peripheral arteries invariably lead to ischemia.
- Quitting smoking, following a low-fat diet, controlling diabetes mellitus, and following an exercise program decrease the incidence of PAD.
- Signs and symptoms of PAD include intermittent claudication, pain at rest, and ischemic changes. The "5 Ps" are pain, pallor, pulselessness, paralysis, and paresthesia.
- The best treatment for arterial insufficiency is exercise, specifically walking.
- Nursing goals for management of patients with arterial insufficiency include maintenance of blood flow, protection from injury, encouraging exercise, and prevention of wound infection.
- Buerger's disease affects small and medium-size arteries. Moderate to heavy smoking is directly linked to Buerger's disease.
- The etiology of Raynaud's disease is exaggerated response to cold environment and stress.
- Aneurysms may develop in cerebral vessels and the aorta.
- Long-standing hypertension and atherosclerosis are factors in the development of aneurysms.
- Aneurysms may be repaired by surgical resection and graft.
- An aneurysm rupture frequently causes death.
- Carotid occlusion is signified by a carotid bruit, confusion, blackouts, extremity weakness or paralysis, visual abnormality in one eye, or other neurologic symptoms.
- Treatment includes carotid endarterectomy or bypass surgery.
- Varicose veins are enlarged, tortuous veins engorged with pooled blood.
- The symptoms of varicose veins include fatigue, a feeling of heaviness in the legs after prolonged standing or sitting, pain, and itching along the course of the blood vessel.
- Medical management involves support hose, treatment of obesity, and exercise.
- Surgical treatment may include scleropathy, vein stripping, or ligation.

- Venous stasis ulcers are skin lesions, usually on the lower leg, from venous insufficiency.
- Treatment includes acute debridement and prevention of infection
- A thrombus is the formation of a clot within blood vessels.
- The effects of a thrombus depend on the location and size of the clot and the degree of obstruction to blood flow.
- Thrombophlebitis is the development of a clot and inflammation of a vessel.
- DVT is a clot in a deep vein occluding blood flow.
- The etiology of DVT includes immobility, trauma, surgery, dehydration, and abnormal clotting.
- Treatment of DVT may include IV heparin, subQ enoxaparin, oral warfarin, and hydration; thrombolytic therapy may be used.
- Medical management: elevation of extremity, support hose, warm moist packs, NSAIDs, and sometimes antibiotics. Surgical intervention (thrombectomy) may be required.

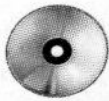
Go to your **Companion CD-ROM** for an Audio Glossary, animations, video clips, and bonus review questions.

evolve Be sure to visit the companion Evolve site at http://evolve.elsevier.com/deWit for interactive NCLEX-PN Exam Style Review Questions, WebLinks, and additional online resources.

NCLEX-PN EXAM STYLE REVIEW QUESTIONS

Choose the best answer(s) for the following questions.

1. A 40-year-old woman complains of leg pains that are associated with fullness during walking. She describes itching on the lower leg over a twisted-appearing swelling in her legs. The nurse would likely suspect:

1. venous stasis ulcers.
2. deep vein thrombosis.
3. arterial insufficiency.
4. varicose veins.

2. The nurse reinforces discharge instructions to a patient who is diagnosed with chronic venous insufficiency. An appropriate nursing statement would be:

1. "You must consider increasing your length of sitting and standing."
2. "Consider swimming and biking."
3. "Wear tight clothing."
4. "Apply elastic stockings in the afternoon."

3. A patient complains of intermittent claudication. The nurse would expect which of the following clinical findings?

1. Strong, symmetrical peripheral pulses
2. Skin mottling
3. Dependent rubor when legs are dependent
4. Ankle edema

4. A patient diagnosed with a venous disorder asks, "What is sclerotherapy?" An accurate explanation would be:

1. "An instrument is inserted into the blood vessel to remove tissues."
2. "An injection of a medication that shrinks the vein."
3. "A surgical procedure that cuts through the vein to remove clots."
4. "An insertion of a filter to prevent the spread of blood clots."

5. A patient is started on antihypertensive medications. Which of the following patient statements indicates effectiveness of teaching?

1. "I will be able to perform sit-ups in the morning."
2. "I need to take the medication when I feel dizzy."
3. "It helps reduce the incidence of a blood clot."
4. "Sudden changes in position may cause dizziness."

6. The nurse is receiving a patient who had femoropopliteal bypass surgery. Initial nursing interventions must include which of the following?

1. Assessing the pulses proximal to the graft
2. Monitoring for signs of bleeding
3. Determining range of motion
4. Checking bowel sounds

7. The nurse is reinforcing the physician's instructions to an elderly woman who is newly diagnosed with hypertension. The patient does not speak the nurse's language and is legally blind. What is an appropriate nursing action?

1. Recruit a translator to provide instructions.
2. Speak slowly.
3. Use a loud voice.
4. Illustrate instructions using stick figures.

8. A 54-year-old man complains of pain and numbness of his lower extremities. Upon examination, the nurse notes that both extremities are pale and cool to touch. An appropriate actual nursing diagnosis would be:

1. Activity intolerance.
2. Ineffective coping.
3. Deficient fluid volume.
4. Risk for injury.

9. A patient with peripheral vascular disease is prescribed a daily dose of aspirin. The nurse accurately explains the prescription by stating:
   1. "Aspirin controls the body temperature to reduce vasoconstriction."
   2. "Aspirin helps prevent formation of clots."
   3. "Aspirin reduces local inflammation."
   4. "Aspirin reduces pain associated with inadequate tissue perfusion."

10. The nurse promotes lifestyle modifications to a 39-year-old male patient who is diagnosed with prehypertension. Recommended lifestyle modifications include which of the following? *(Select all that apply.)*
   1. Smoking cessation
   2. Restrict sodium intake to 5000 mg/day
   3. Aerobic exercise
   4. Alcohol intake of three servings per day.
   5. Low-fat diet

CRITICAL THINKING ACTIVITIES

Read each clinical scenario and discuss the questions with your classmates.

Scenario A

Mrs. Dunn is being discharged from the hospital after being treated for arterial insufficiency in both lower extremities. Her physician requests that Mrs. Dunn receive instruction in the care of her feet and legs prior to discharge.

1. What findings do you expect on physical examination of Mrs. Dunn's legs?
2. What medication and treatment do you expect the physician to prescribe? Why are these prescribed?
3. List five priority teaching points you should establish for Mrs. Dunn.

Scenario B

Ms. Yao, age 27, developed a DVT in her left thigh after surgery to repair a fractured right femur. She is receiving heparin IV and will begin enoxaparin Subcut the following morning.

1. Describe the pathophysiology of DVT. How does Ms. Yao's diagnosis relate to development of DVT?
2. Identify essential information you need to safely administer the medications prescribed.
3. Develop a teaching plan for Ms. Yao.

CHAPTER

19 Care of Patients with Cardiac Disorders

evolve http://evolve.elsevier.com/deWit

Objectives

Upon completing this chapter the student should be able to:

Theory

1. Describe the nursing assessment specific to the patient who is admitted with congestive heart failure.
2. Discuss how nursing interventions for patients with a valvular disorder differ from those for a patient with a cardiac dysrhythmia.
3. State nursing responsibilities in the administration of cardiac drugs.
4. Describe under what circumstances cardiac surgery is appropriate treatment.
5. Discuss the nurse's role in caring for elderly patients with heart disorders in the long-term care facility or the home.
6. Develop a teaching plan with dietary recommendations for heart disease.

Clinical Practice

1. Develop a plan of care for a patient who has heart failure.
2. Perform a basic physical assessment on a patient who has a mitral valve prolapse and dysrhythmia.
3. Use the nursing process to care for assigned patients who have cardiovascular disorders.
4. Safely administer medications for patients with cardiac disorders.
5. Provide support to patients undergoing diagnostic testing and treatment for cardiac disorders.
6. Develop a teaching plan for patients with cardiac disorders.

Key Terms

Be sure to check out the bonus material on the Companion CD-ROM, including selected audio pronunciations.

ablation (ăb-LĀ-shŭn, p. 473)
arrhythmia (ă-RĬTH-mē-a, p. 471)
atrial fibrillation (p. 472)
cardiac tamponade (KĂR-dē-ăk tăm-pŏn-ĀD, p. 479)
cardiomyopathy (kăr-dē-ō-mī-ŎP-ă-thē, p. 480)
cardioversion (kăr-dē-ō-VĔR-zhŭn, p. 478)
dysrhythmia (dĭs-RĬTH-mē-ă, p. 471)
effusion (ĕ-FŪ-zhŭn, p. 480)
endocarditis (ĔN-dō-kăhr-DĪ-tĭs, p. 479)
friction rub (FRĬK-shŭn, p. 481)
infarct (ĭn-făhrkt, p. 471)
orthopneic position (ŏr-thŏp-NĒ-ĭk, p. 468)
palpitation (păl-pĭ-TĀ-shŭn, p. 472)
pericardial effusion (pĕr-ĭ-KĂR-dē-ăl ĕ-FŪ-zhŭn, p. 479)
pericardiocentesis (pĕr-ĭ-KĂR-dē-ō-sĕn-TĒ-sĭs, p. 481)
pericardiotomy (pĕr-ĭ-KĂR-dē-ŏt-ō-mē, p. 481)
pulsus paradoxus (p. 481)

Chapter 17 presented the degree of morbidity and the economic costs of heart disease in the United States. In recent years, heart disease in women has risen considerably. In women, the symptoms of heart attack tend to be more subtle and different than those men experience. Often, diffuse chest pain similar to that of gastroesophageal reflux is the main symptom in a woman (Agency for Healthcare Research and Quality, 2006). 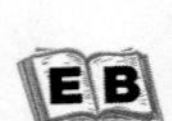 Or there may be some persistent pain in the neck and shoulder or the jaw. Careful assessment of a woman experiencing such a problem, including her risk factors for cardiovascular disease, can save many lives (Sherrod, 2007). 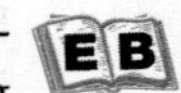 To assist in understanding the following cardiac disorders, review the anatomy and physiology of the heart in Chapter 17. This chapter discusses the various disorders of the heart, how they occur, their diagnosis and treatment, and the nursing care and teaching involved in returning the patient to an optimal level of wellness. Refer to general assessment and data collection for the cardiovascular system in Chapter 17.

DISORDERS OF THE HEART

HEART FAILURE

Heart failure (HF) is a complication of other cardiovascular conditions, rather than a disease in itself. Heart failure can occur any time the muscular strength of the heart weakens, causing it to fail as a pump and a circulator of blood. There are about 5 million Americans with HF, and approximately 550,000 are diagnosed each year. The prevalence is increasing and it is a major chronic condition. Half of patients diagnosed with HF will die within 5 years.

Etiology

Weakness of the heart can be caused by many factors. Infection of the muscle, dilation from blood backup behind stenosed valves, damaged myocardial tissue as a result of myocardial infarction (MI) or long-term

Table 19–1 **Comparison of Left-Sided and Right-Sided Heart Failure**

	RIGHT-SIDED FAILURE	LEFT-SIDED FAILURE
Selected etiology	Pulmonary stenosis, pulmonary hypertension Severe emphysema	Coronary artery disease, MI, valvular disease,
Pathophysiology	The myocardium of the right atrium and ventricle becomes thickened, and contraction strength is reduced	Weakness of the left ventricle resulting in reduced cardiac output and backup of fluid in the pulmonary system
Signs and symptoms	Fatigue Edema in sacrum, legs, feet, ankles Hepatomegaly Abdominal distention as a result of ascites Weight gain Dyspnea	Fatigue Dyspnea Wheezing Orthopnea Sleep apnea Pulmonary edema (pink, frothy sputum) Pallor Clammy skin

alcohol consumption, are common factors. Longstanding hypertension, and aging, may also contribute to heart failure. (Coronary artery disease [CAD] and myocardial infarction [MI] are covered in Chapter 20, along with cardiac surgery.)

Pathophysiology

The key to understanding HF is the word *congestion.* Congestion develops because the heart is unable to move blood as quickly as it should. This may occur because the heart muscle is too weak or because the blood vessels throughout the body are narrowed and constricted (due to atherosclerosis or arteriosclerosis). Therefore, the vessels cannot accommodate a normal supply of blood, causing the heart muscle to become exhausted trying to overcome the resistance. Poorly functioning valves may cause the chambers to dilate from blood backup, causing thinning of the myocardium and decreased pumping ability.

HF may be classified as right-sided HF or left-sided HF. Left-sided failure typically occurs first. Normally, the ventricles of the heart contract, while the atria relax, allowing for the filling and emptying of each chamber. If the muscle wall of the left ventricle cannot contract effectively, some of the blood is left in the ventricle. This prevents part of the blood in the left atrium from progressing into the ventricle. In turn, the blood backs up into the pulmonary vessels, pressure within those vessels increases, and fluid leaks into the lung tissue, producing congestion and, eventually, pulmonary edema. If not corrected, left-sided failure, because of the backup of blood, will soon lead to failure of the right side of the heart. Table 19–1 compares the signs and symptoms of left-sided and right-sided HF.

If the right ventricle does not contract as strongly as it should, it cannot completely empty and becomes engorged with blood. The blood flow is slowed, preventing movement of blood out of the atrium. As it backs up, it prevents normal movement of blood flow out of the vena cava, thus increasing the pressure in the vena cava, the neck veins, and all other veins of the body.

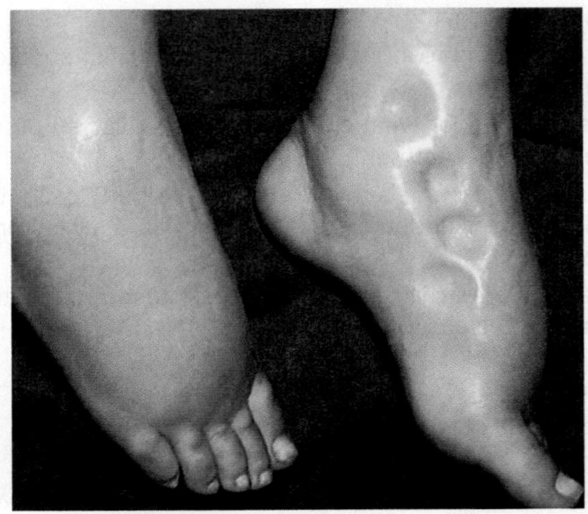

FIGURE **19–1** Dependent/pitting edema.

As the rate of blood flow slows down and pressure in the vessels increases, the fluid from the intravascular fluid compartment begins to leak into the interstitial compartment. This produces retention of fluid and edema. When the right side of the heart fails, the edema is first evident in the lower extremities (*dependent* or *pitting edema*; Figure 19–1). There also is an accumulation of fluid in the liver and abdominal organs, as the portal circulation becomes involved. Congestion of blood flow to and from the kidneys may lead to impaired renal function, preventing normal excretion of urine and causing more accumulation of body fluids. Inadequate circulation to and from the brain may cause mental confusion and irritability, which sometimes progresses to delirium and coma.

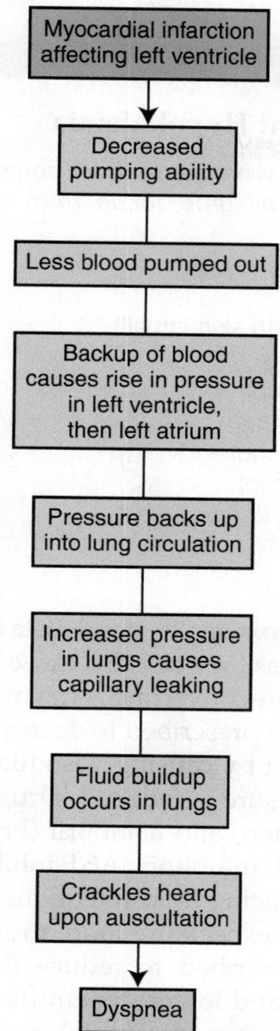

CONCEPT MAP **19–1** Pathophysiology of CHF after an MI.

The systemic backup of blood that occurs in right-sided HF may eventually lead to left-sided heart failure, as the heart will have to pump against increasing pressure in the aorta and systemic circulation. The circulatory system is exactly that: a system. Failure of one component affects the entire system. Concept Map 19–1 shows the pathophysiology of HF resulting from MI.

Think Critically About . . . Can you explain to a patient in simple terms what happens in the body when heart failure occurs?

Signs, Symptoms, and Diagnosis

The diagnosis of HF is based on the patient's history of cardiovascular disease and the symptoms he or she presents. Table 19–1 presents the signs and symptoms of heart failure. Diagnosis is made on the basis of signs and symptoms, chest x-ray, echocardiogram (ECG), and cardiac enzyme levels.

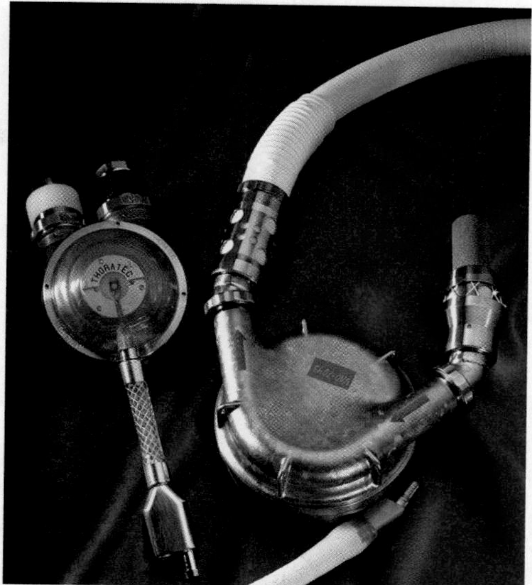

FIGURE **19–2** Heartmate left ventricular assist device.

Think Critically About . . . You auscultate the lung sounds of a patient with HF. You hear crackles. Which side of the heart is failing?

Treatment

Treatment of the underlying cause should be initiated. Surgical correction of valve or septal abnormalities may reverse heart failure. Medical treatment is largely symptomatic. Drugs and other therapies are used to reduce or eliminate the symptoms and complications of HF, but they only control the condition; they do not cure it. Efforts are made to (1) reduce the demand for oxygen and the workload of the heart; (2) strengthen the heart's pumping action; (3) relieve venous congestion in the lungs; and (4) minimize sodium and water retention in the tissues. Other treatments may include:

- Implantable cardioverter-defibrillators (ICD). This device detects shockable dysrhythmias and delivers a shock to convert the rhythm to normal providing more regular pump action.
- Left ventricular assist devices (LVADs) may be used to help with the heart's pumping action. This device is implanted in the patient's abdomen and attached to the heart. These devices have proven to be beneficial to children and adults diagnosed with severe HF. The device may be used while the patient is awaiting transplant and, with continued research, may possibly eliminate the need for transplant in some patients (Figure 19–2).
- Surgery to reduce the size of an enlarged heart (ventricular restoration surgery) may be effective for some patients. This procedure, now in experimental stages, may change the course of

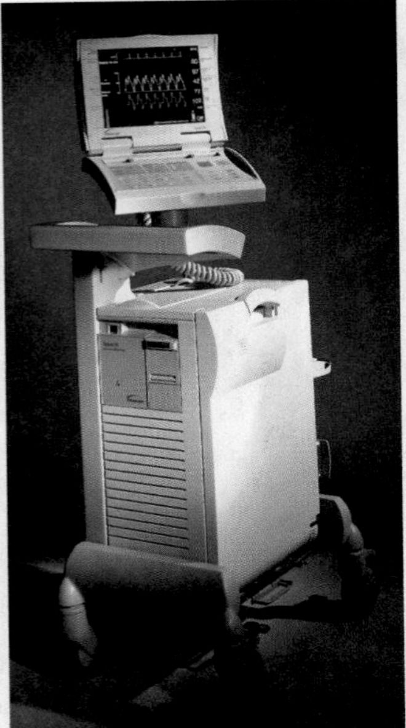

FIGURE 19–3 Intraaortic balloon pump.

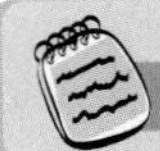

Patient Teaching 19–1

Ways to Prevent Hypokalemia

Teach the patient who is at risk for potassium loss due to medications to consume foods from the following list daily:

- Apricots (3)
- Avocado (½)
- Baked potato with skin (small)
- Banana (1 med)
- Cantaloupe (1 cup)
- Orange juice (½ cup)
- Pinto beans (½ cup)
- Prune juice (½ cup)
- Cooked spinach (½ cup)

treatment for HF. The less effective portions of the left ventricle are removed and the remaining muscle is reattached and shaped to form a more efficient pump.

- Heart transplant may be the only alternative for patients with advanced HF who do not respond to other medical or drug treatment. Heart transplant is discussed in Chapter 20.
- Short-term treatment for HF after an MI or open-heart surgery is accomplished with the intraaortic balloon pump (IABP). The IABP is positioned in the descending aorta. It is designed to increase blood supply to the myocardium and allow it to rest. The balloon pump will inflate and deflate during systole and diastole, thus increasing perfusion to the coronary arteries (Figure 19–3).
- The pumping action of the atria and ventricles may be synchronized for more efficient pumping by use of the *biventricular* pacemaker. This procedure is cardiac resynchronization therapy (CRT), in which wires are placed in the heart to send electrical impulses to the right and left ventricles.

To accomplish the goals of medical intervention, the following may be prescribed:

- Limited physical activity or bed rest in semi-Fowler's or high Fowler's position.
- Reduction of emotional stress.
- Oxygen therapy.
- Beta-adrenergic blockers (e.g., metoprolol [Toprol XL]), are used to slow the heart rate if tachycardia is causing the heart failure, thereby decreasing oxygen demand. Beta blockers are used cautiously as they can also cause heart failure.
- Angiotensin-converting enzyme (ACE) inhibitors may be prescribed to decrease the work load of the heart by causing vasodilation. As a result blood pressure is reduced. Drugs such as captopril (Capoten) and lisinopril (Prinivil) are classified as ACE inhibitors. ACE inhibitors also play a role in reducing fluid retention.
- Diuretics, especially loop diuretics, are commonly prescribed to reduce fluid retention in the lungs and lower extremities. Loop diuretics include furosemide (Lasix), and torsemide (Demadex). Thiazide diuretics such as hydrochlorothiazide (Diuril) may also be prescribed. Measures are taken to prevent electrolyte imbalances from the use of these drugs (Patient Teaching 19–1).
- Digitalis to increase the force of heart contraction (i.e., an inotropic agent) and slow the rate, thereby increasing cardiac output. The most commonly used drug in this category is digoxin (Lanoxin). Several large doses of the drug are given initially, followed by a lower, regular-maintenance dose.
- Venous vasodilators such as isosorbide dinitrate (Isordil) and nitroglycerin (NTG), which relax and dilate blood vessels, allowing them to accommodate larger percentages of the total blood volume (Heidenreich et al., 1999).

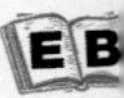

- Morphine is prescribed if pulmonary edema is present to relieve anxiety and make breathing easier.
- Lifestyle modifications, including regular exercise as tolerated, and limitation of sodium intake to 2 to 4 g/day, and in severe cases, restriction of fluid intake (American Heart Association, 2006a) (Nutritional Therapies 19–1; see Table 17–1).

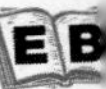

Nutritional Therapies 19–1

Guidelines for a Heart-Healthy Diet

- Limit meat intake to no more than 6 oz of cooked lean meat, fish, and skinless poultry (singly or in combination) per day. Fix main dishes with pasta, rice, beans, or vegetables mixed with small amounts of lean meat, poultry, or fish to create "low-meat" dishes. Restrict intake of organ meats, such as liver, brains, chitterlings, kidney, gizzards, and sweetbreads, as they are very high in cholesterol.
- Eat five to seven servings of fruit and vegetables per day.
- Increase intake of fiber and carbohydrate by eating six or more servings of whole-grain products, such as cereals and breads, per day. Check labels to see that the product really contains *whole* grains.
- Use skim or 1% fat milk and nonfat or low-fat yogurt, cheeses, and ice creams.
- Avoid as much *trans* fat as possible. Read product labels. Limit food high in saturated fat, including tropical oils, and partially hydrogenated vegetable oils.
- Cook using little or no fat; broil, bake, roast, poach, stir fry, microwave, or steam foods rather than frying them.
- Eliminate as much fat as possible by trimming meat and skinning poultry before cooking. After browning meats, drain off all fat. Chill soups, stews, etc. after cooking and skim off fat before reheating to serve.
- Limit consumption of egg yolks to three or four per week, including those in baked or cooked items. Check store packages for listing of eggs or egg yolk as an ingredient.
- Eat less than 6 g of salt (sodium chloride) per day (2400 mg of sodium).
- Have no more than one alcoholic drink per day if you are a woman and no more than two per day if you are a man. Examples of one drink are 12 oz of beer, 4 oz of wine, 1½ oz of 80-proof spirits.

Note: The healthy heart diet is promoted by the American Heart Association.

NURSING MANAGEMENT

Assessment (Data Collection)

The effects of HF can range from very mild to extremely serious. A thorough nursing assessment can help identify specific patient care problems and guide the physician in her evaluation of the patient's response to medical treatment and her decisions to continue or change prescribed drugs and other therapies. The symptoms displayed by a patient with right-sided HF are indications of changes taking place in tissues at some distance from the heart. For example, edema in the lower extremities, and diminished flow of urine reflect involvement of the peripheral circulation, kidneys, and circulation of blood to and from the liver and intestine. It is important to ask the patient if his clothes, rings, or shoes fit tighter than previously. Feelings of breathlessness or having to catch the breath in midsentence may indicate fluid in the lungs and left-sided HF.

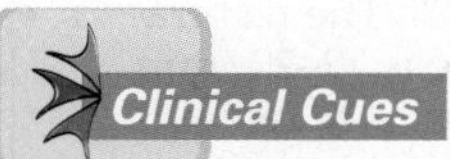

Clinical Cues

Maintain a clinical environment conducive to conserving patient energy. Organize patient activities carefully, keep needed items accessible, and assist as needed. The goal is to reduce cardiac workload.

Significant findings that may indicate heart failure in patients at high risk include the following:

- Increasing fatigue as a result of tissue hypoxia and shortness of breath; this may be caused by left ventricular failure and resultant fluid in the lungs.
- Cough.
- Feeling "bloated" and a loss of appetite due to diminished venous return from abdominal organs, liver enlargement resulting from increased pressure in the portal veins, edema in the intestine, and accumulations of fluid in the abdominal cavity.
- Jugular venous distention; visible jugular vein pulsation more than 4.5 cm above the clavicle when patient is in semi-Fowler's position. These signs are related to right ventricular failure.
- Complaint of feeling "warm" when others are comfortably cool because of vasoconstriction and poor circulation, which prevents removal of body heat.
- Feelings of anxiety, irritability, or depression, and difficulty concentrating and remembering due to diminished blood flow to brain.
- Pale, cool, and dry skin, which are signs of poor peripheral circulation; mottling of skin.

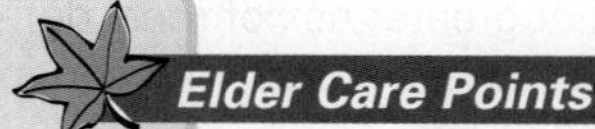

Elder Care Points

Elderly patients who have little cardiac reserve can be placed at risk for CHF by any condition that increases the body's demand for blood or oxygen. Generalized infection, pneumonia, severe trauma, and other conditions that increase the metabolic rate and demand for oxygen can be the precipitating factor. Monitor elderly patients in your care with other conditions for signs of CHF.

- Cyanosis of nail beds, indicating oxygen deficit.
- Dependent, pitting edema (assess feet and ankles in ambulatory patient or one sitting up most of the time. Assess thighs and sacral region in patient confined to bed, due to congestion of the venous system and increased capillary pressure, which forces fluid out of the intravascular fluid compartment and into the tissue spaces).
- Diminished or absent peripheral pulses.
- Gradually increasing heart rate, even when the patient is at rest, this is caused by attempts by the heart to remove blood from a distended ventricle.
- Reduced urinary output, which reflects the kidney's response to poor perfusion by retaining sodium and water.
- Crackles heard on auscultation of the lungs.
- Extra heart sound (S_3).

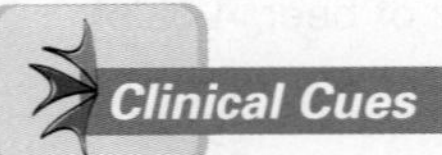

Assess urinary output of elderly patients. Renal function is decreased due to the aging process. Loss of perfusion related to HF will place the patient at greater risk of renal deficiency or failure. Monitor patients who develop infection in any body system closely for signs of HF.

? *Think Critically About . . .* What signs detected during your beginning-of-shift assessment of the patient recovering from an MI might indicate CHF?

Nursing Diagnosis and Planning

See Nursing Care Plan 19–1 for specific nursing diagnoses for the patient with HF. Other nursing diagnoses that might be included on the care plan for the individual patient are in Table 17–4 in Chapter 17.

Plan extra time when caring for the patient with HF. Fatigue, possible lack of mobility, and oxygen deficit cause the patient to move slowly and need more time to accomplish the activities of daily living. Specific outcome criteria are written for each individual's nursing diagnoses and may include:

- The patient will decrease activity to reduce the workload of the heart
- The patient will demonstrate increased ability to complete activities of daily living without fatigue and dyspnea
- The patient will have loss of excess fluid evidenced by decreased respiratory distress and edema.

NURSING CARE PLAN 19–1

Care of the Patient with Heart Failure

SCENARIO Miguel Garcia, age 60, is admitted to the nursing unit with exacerbation of left- and right-sided heart failure. Physical examination reveals 3+ pitting edema of the right lower extremity and 4+ pitting edema of the left lower extremity. He is in acute respiratory distress and is positioned in high Fowler's to facilitate breathing. He has oxygen per simple mask at 10 L/min. T 98° F (36.6° C), P 96, R 28, BP 160/90, O_2 Sat 90%, Wt. 255 (20-lb increase).

PROBLEM/NURSING DIAGNOSIS *Dyspnea*/Impaired gas exchange related to fluid in lung tissue, O_2 Sat 90% on 10 L oxygen.

Supporting assessment data *Subjective:* States he has difficulty breathing while lying down. *Objective:* O_2 Sat. 90%, elevated respiratory rate, uses **orthopneic position** to facilitate breathing.

Goals/Expected Outcomes	*Nursing Interventions*	*Selected Rationale*	*Evaluation*
O_2 Sat 93%–95% on room air	Assess vital signs and O_2 Sat q 2 hr. Report increase in respiratory rate or decrease in oxygen saturation.	Change in vital signs and oxygen saturation may indicate improvement or deterioration of condition.	O_2 Sat remains within 93%–95%. The respiratory rate is 12–22/min. The heart rate remains between 60 and 100.
	Increase oxygen to maintain O_2 Sat at level specified by physician.	Maintain oxygen saturation at levels that indicate effective gas exchange.	O_2 Sat 94%. O_2 at 5 L/min.
	Assess lung sounds at least q 4 hr	Changes in lung sounds indicate positive response to therapy or need to modify treatment plan	Lung sounds clear on right, fine crackles on left
	Maintain high Fowler's position as needed for comfort. Teach patient pursed-lip breathing.	Promotes optimum expansion of thoracic cavity to facilitate breathing and improve gas exchange.	Head of bed at 45 degrees. Continue plan.

NURSING CARE PLAN 19-1

Care of the Patient with Heart Failure—cont'd

PROBLEM/NURSING DIAGNOSIS *Fatigue: unable to complete activities of daily living without assistance*/Activity intolerance related to fluid in lungs, fluid retention lower extremities.

Supporting assessment data *Subjective:* States feet have become more swollen over the past 3 days. *Objective:* Pitting edema both lower extremities, dyspnea on exertion, crackles in bases bilaterally.

Goals/Expected Outcomes	Nursing Interventions	Selected Rationale	Evaluation
Patient will be able to complete activities of daily living and personal hygiene without fatigue	Assess activity tolerance	Guideline for planning care activities.	Able to complete partial bath. Becomes fatigued, requires assistance
	Assist with personal hygiene initially	Conserve patient energy	
	Monitor oxygen saturation		
	Provide frequent rest periods.	Avoid overtiring by scheduling activities to maximize energy use.	Patient remains fatigued.
	Coordinate care with other health care providers to conserve energy.		Continue plan; reassess readiness to meet goals.

PROBLEM/NURSING DIAGNOSIS *Fluid retention lower extremities, crackles in lung fields*/Excess fluid volume related to pulmonary and venous congestion.

Supporting assessment data *Subjective:* Patient reports nonproductive cough. *Objective:* 3–4+ edema both lower extremities. Crackles in lung bases on auscultation.

Goals/Expected Outcomes	Nursing Interventions	Selected Rationale	Evaluation
Lung fields will be clear, pitting edema in lower extremities 0–1+.	Assess lung sounds q 4 hr.	Identifies changes in condition.	Fine crackles on auscultation. Less distress.
	Assess lower extremities each shift.	Identifies effectiveness of drug therapy.	2+ pitting edema bilaterally.
	Administer diuretics as prescribed by the physician.	To reduce fluid retention through diuresis.	Urinary output 2500 mL q 8 hr. Weight 245 lb.
	Maintain accurate intake and output. Daily weights.	Identify positive or negative response to treatment.	Continue plan.

? CRITICAL THINKING QUESTIONS

1. List three additional nursing diagnoses that are appropriate for this patient.
2. List five items to be included in the discharge teaching plan for this patient.
3. What assessment data might indicate a worsening of this patient's condition?
4. What assessment data might indicate improvement of this patient's condition?

- The patient will demonstrate stabilization of vital signs to within normal limits

Implementation

Patients with mild HF may not be hospitalized but do require instruction in self-care. This includes balancing rest with physical activity, limiting sodium intake, and following other dietary restrictions. Self-administration of medications with awareness of adverse side effects that must be reported must be taught, along with the dangers of drug-to-drug interaction when taking nonprescription drugs. Modifying lifestyle as needs indicate (diet, smoking, physical activity) and knowledge of symptoms that should be reported to the physician if they become worse or appear for the first time are other areas for patient education.

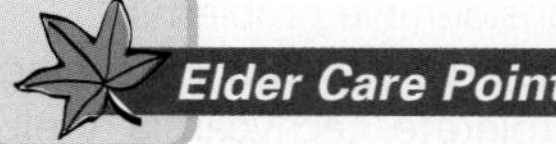

Elder Care Points

The elderly patient who is experiencing CHF often is taking many medications. It is especially important to look for drug interactions and to monitor for signs and symptoms of toxicity.

It is of vital importance to monitor patients with heart failure for electrolyte imbalances, especially imbalance of sodium or potassium. **Electrolyte imbalances may cause serious cardiac dysrhythmias** (MayoClinic.com, 2006).

Patients with chronic HF will need encouragement to follow the prescribed regimen. If treatment does not stop the progress of the disease, the patient may be admitted to the hospital for reevaluation and a change in therapies. Sometimes the patient's heart continues to fail in spite of aggressive therapy, and such complications as pulmonary edema and liver and renal failure occur.

? *Think Critically About . . .* Why does weighing the patient daily help you with evaluating the treatment for HF? How would you know that the treatment is not effective?

Partial or full assistance with activities of daily living will decrease oxygen demand. Scheduling all activities to promote as much rest as possible is a high priority. Activity is alternated with rest throughout the day. Several pillows may be required to achieve a comfortable position. Accurate recording of intake and output is very important. Daily weight is recorded at the same time each day, preferably before breakfast. Careful attention to turning and skin care is essential, as edematous tissue breaks down easily. Particular attention should be given to the sacral area due to pressure points of patient on bed rest. Bed rest causes venous pooling, and active or passive leg exercises should be performed

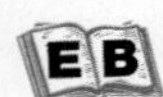

every 1 to 2 hours to help prevent thrombosis (Barclay & Lie, 2004). Elastic stockings or sequential compression devices to prevent venous pooling may be prescribed. Observation for side effects of medications is another major responsibility. Careful ongoing physical assessment is essential. Nursing interventions for selected problems in a patient with HF are summarized in Nursing Care Plan 19–1.

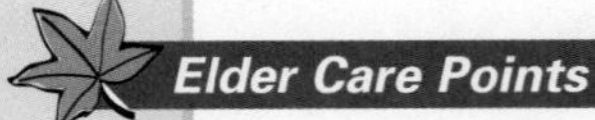

Elder Care Points

Any infection in an elderly patient who has cardiovascular disease may cause HF. An infection increases the metabolic rate, thereby increasing the demand for oxygen by the tissues. The heart that is already having difficulty meeting normal body oxygen demands cannot respond. Carefully assess the lungs for signs of crackles that might indicate beginning HF. Your quick action can save the patient from considerable problems.

Use of oxygen by the heart is less efficient with increasing years, and the heart does not tolerate tachycardia well. Tachycardia brought about by fever and the metabolic demands of infection can give rise to HF rather quickly in the older adult who has heart disease.

Evaluation

The patient with heart failure requires extensive treatment with medication and lifestyle changes. You must evaluate objective and subjective data to determine if patient goals are met. Objective data include the results of lab and hemodynamic studies, assessment of vital signs and body systems., The respiratory and cardiovascular system especially should be monitored for improvement of status. Observation of the patient for the improvement of symptoms including edema, respiratory quality, and activity tolerance will also give indications of patient progress. Note subjective data related to activity tolerance, respiratory status, comfort, and understanding of teaching related to the disease process and self-management. Understanding of the medication regimen is key to determining the patient's progress.

Complications

Acute Pulmonary Edema. Acute pulmonary edema, a complication of HF, is a medical emergency that must be treated promptly. The patient with this condition has severe dyspnea; a cough productive of frothy, pink-tinged sputum; tachycardia; and moist, bubbling respirations with cyanosis.

Nursing interventions for acute pulmonary edema include placing the patient in high Fowler's position to relieve the dyspnea; administering oxygen, diuretics, morphine, and other prescribed drugs; limiting and monitoring activity; and assessing cardiopulmonary status. Provide emotional support during this frightening event.

CARDIAC CONDUCTION DISORDERS

A normal heart is capable of generating tiny electrical impulses that are essential to normal contraction of the heart's ventricles and atria. The impulses originate in the sinoatrial (SA) node and the atrioventricular (AV) node. The SA node is located in the wall of the right atrium between the openings for the inferior and superior vena cava. It stimulates contraction of the atria. The AV node is located in the septum between the atria and transmits impulses via the bundle of His and the Purkinje fibers to the ventricles, causing them to contract (Figure 19–4). The healthy heart beats in normal sinus rhythm (NSR) at 60 to 100 beats per minute (bpm). Figure 19–5 shows the ECG pattern of normal sinus rhythm, and Box 19–1 provides the procedure for evaluating an ECG strip. The goal for the beginning nurse is to be able to determine when the tracing is not normal sinus rhythm.

Etiology

Alterations in the conduction of cardiac electrical impulses that create heart rate and rhythm may occur due to congenital abnormalities, electrolyte disturbances, too much caffeine, and medication side effects.

Valvular disorders, damage to the heart from **infarct**, and neurologic changes may also contribute to conduction disorders.

Pathophysiology

The SA node generates impulses 60 to 100 times per minute. Each impulse travels through the atria to the AV node, which relays the impulse via the bundle of His and the Purkinje fibers to the ventricles, causing them to contract (see Figure 19–4). If the SA node fails to produce an electrical impulse, the AV node will initiate an impulse at 40 to 60 beats per minute. If neither the SA nor the AV node is functioning, the ventricles will initiate an impulse at a slower rate. When there is disruption of the normal electrical conduction in the heart, abnormal heart rhythm occurs. This is called an **arrhythmia** or **dysrhythmia**. A pulse below 60 indi-

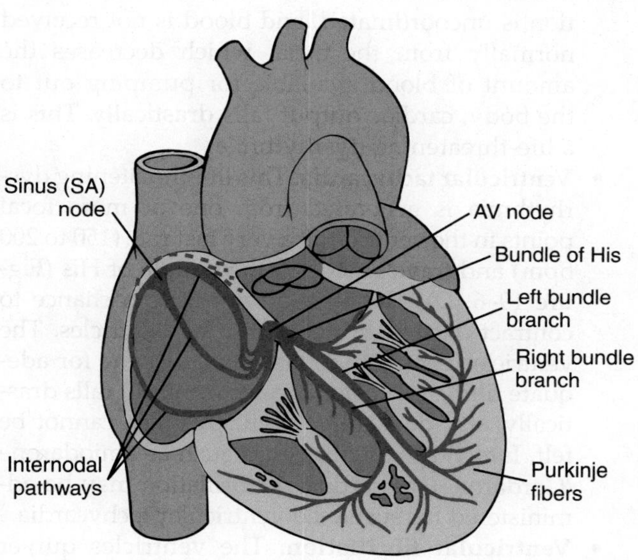

FIGURE **19–4** Cardiac conduction system.

Box 19–1 *Evaluating an ECG Rhythm Strip*

- Obtain a strip with at least 10 large graph squares.
- Calculate the rate. Count the number of 0.2-sec divisions between two consecutive QRS complexes and divide this into 300 to determine the rate. For irregular rhythms, count the number of cycles or complexes in 6 sec and multiply by 10.
- Measure the distance between the P waves. Is the distance the same? If so, the rate is regular. Calculate the atrial rate by counting the number of small boxes between the P waves and dividing that number into 1500. If the atrial rate is irregular, are there premature atrial beats?
- Measure the P-R interval. Is it normal (0.12–0.20 sec)? Does it vary?
- Measure the QRS duration. Is it normal (0.04–0.12 sec)? Measure with calipers from R wave to R wave throughout the tracing to determine whether the rate is regular. Are there premature QRS complexes? Do all the QRS complexes look the same? Calculate the ventricular rate by counting the number of small squares between R waves and dividing that number into 1500. Are the atrial and ventricular rates the same? A rough calculation can be made by counting the number of complexes in a 6-sec tracing and multiplying by 10.

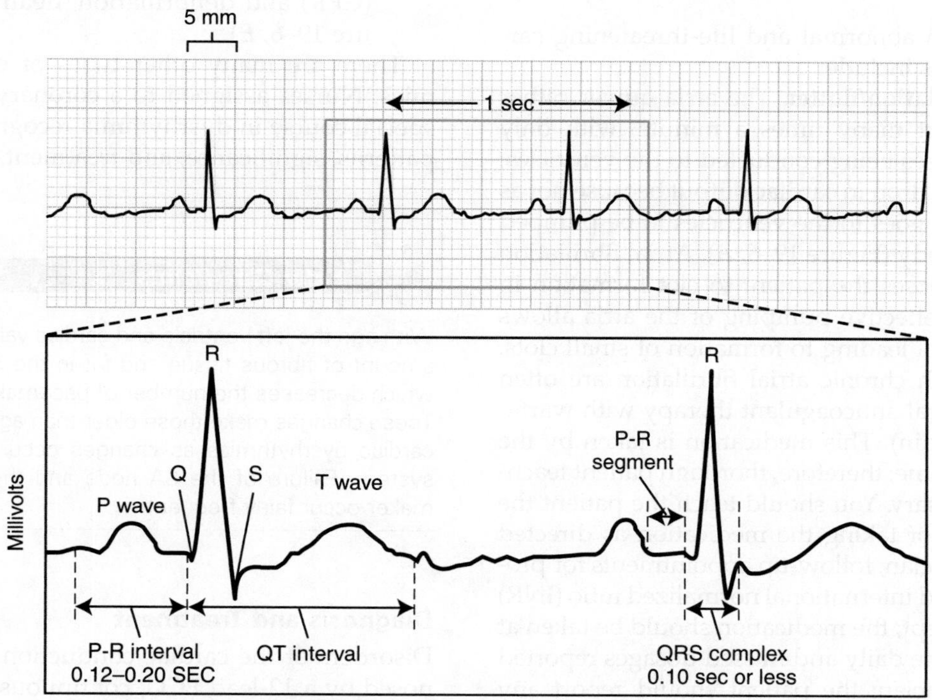

FIGURE **19–5** ECG tracing of normal sinus rhythm.

cates *bradycardia,* one type of dysrhythmia. Bradycardia may drop cardiac output enough to cause the patient to have symptoms of decreased blood flow.

Signs and Symptoms

If the heart rate rises above 100 to 120 bpm, the patient has a dysrhythmia known as *tachycardia*. When the heart beats this fast, the ventricles do not have adequate time to fill with blood and therefore cannot pump effectively. As a result, cardiac output falls.

When the heart's electrical conduction system fails, the normal contractions of the heart that are necessary for its pumping action do not occur, and adequate blood is not pumped out to the body. Symptoms the patient may experience include dizziness, **palpitations** (abnormally rapid throbbing or fluttering of the heart), fatigue, chest pain, loss of consciousness, and possibly death. The severity of the symptoms depends on whether the abnormal rhythm is atrial or ventricular in origin, the amount of cardiac output, and whether the dysrhythmia is persistent.

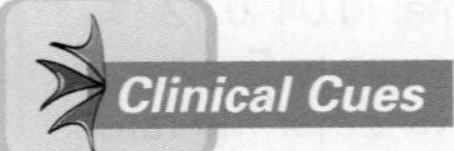

Any time a person notices an irregular or rapid heartbeat, first ask her how much caffeine she is taking in each day. If the caffeine consumption is minimal, ask about medications she is taking, such as decongestants. Inquire about the person's stress levels. Many times caffeine, drugs, or stress can be the benign cause of dysrhythmia. The problem disappears when the precipitating factor is removed or remedied.

Other common abnormal and life-threatening cardiac dysrhythmias include:

- **Atrial fibrillation/flutter.** The atria quiver rather than contract many times a minute, with only some impulses being conducted to the ventricles; this causes a drop in cardiac output because not as much blood goes to the ventricles to be pumped out to the body (Figure 19–6, *A*). Atrial fibrillation also predisposes the patient to clot formation in the atria. Ineffective pumping of the atria allows blood to pool leading to formation of small clots. Patients with chronic atrial fibrillation are often placed on oral anticoagulant therapy with warfarin (Coumadin). This medication is taken by the patient at home; therefore, thorough patient teaching is necessary. You should teach the patient the importance of taking the medication as directed by the physician; follow-up appointments for protime (PT) and international normalized ratio (INR) should be kept; the medication should be taken at the same time daily and missed dosages reported to the physician; the patient should report any unusual bruising or bleeding.
- **Premature ventricular contractions (PVCs).** The ventricular impulse causes ventricular contraction before impulse and contraction of atria are complete (Figure 19–6, *B*). Blood is not received from the atria to be pumped out to body. A few PVCs are not abnormal, but when there are more than six or seven in a minute, cardiac output may fall. This dysrhythmia also makes the heart more likely to develop ventricular tachycardia or ventricular fibrillation.
- **Complete heart block (third-degree heart block)** (Figure 19–6, *C*). Separate impulses cause contraction in the atria and in the ventricles; contraction is uncoordinated, and blood is not received normally from the atria, which decreases the amount of blood available for pumping out to the body; cardiac output falls drastically. This is a life-threatening dysrhythmia.
- **Ventricular tachycardia.** This life-threatening dysrhythmia is generated from one or more focal points in the ventricle at a very fast rate (150 to 200 bpm) and travels through the bundle of His (Figure 19–6, *D*). The atria do not have a chance to contract and push blood into the ventricles. The ventricles contract too fast to allow time for adequate filling with blood; cardiac output falls drastically, and death may occur. A pulse cannot be felt. Intervention with drugs such as amiodarone (Cordarone), or cardiac defibrillation may be administered for sustained ventricular tachycardia.
- **Ventricular fibrillation**. The ventricles quiver rather than contract; there is no cardiac output, and without cardiopulmonary resuscitation (CPR) and defibrillation, death will occur (Figure 19–6, *E*).

There are many other types of cardiac dysrhythmias. Nurses assigned to a coronary care unit take a special course in dysrhythmia recognition to learn the patterns, significance, and treatment of each type.

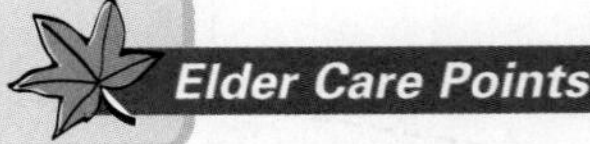

With age the left ventricle and cardiac valves thicken and the amount of fibrous tissue and fat in the SA node increases, which decreases the number of pacemaker cells it contains. These changes make those older than age 75 more prone to cardiac dysrhythmias as changes occur in the conduction system. Failure of the SA node and the need for a pacemaker occur fairly frequently.

Diagnosis and Treatment

Disorders of the cardiac conduction system are diagnosed by a 12-lead ECG, continuous ECG monitoring (Holter monitoring), patient history, and electrophysi-

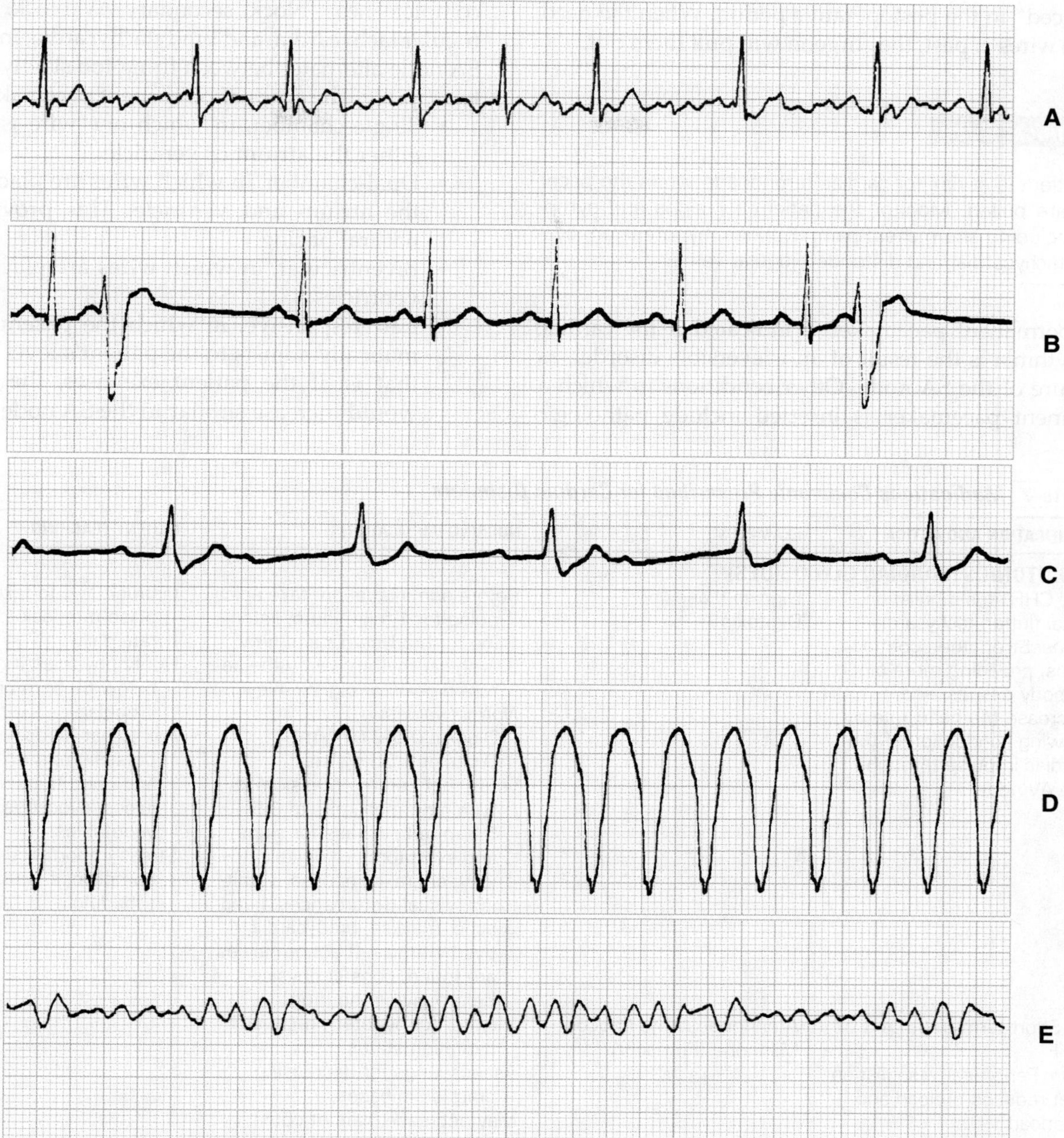

FIGURE 19–6 ECG patterns of abnormal and life-threatening dysrhythmias. **A,** Atrial fibrillation. **B,** Premature ventricular contractions. **C,** Complete (third-degree) heart block. **D,** Ventricular tachycardia. **E,** Ventricular fibrillation.

ology tests, which can be performed during cardiac catheterization (see Chapter 17, Table 17–3.)

Drug therapy is effective in correcting or controlling dysrhythmias in many cases. A variety of antidysrhythmia agents may be used alone or in combination to regulate the heart beat (Table 19–3).

When drug therapy does not control a life-threatening dysrhythmia, surgical destruction **(ablation)** of the tissue initiating the abnormal impulse can sometimes correct the problem if such an area can be located during electrophysiology testing.

Artificial pacemakers may be used to manage chronic and life-threatening dysrhythmias. Pacemakers are commonly used to treat symptomatic bradycardia. Artificial cardiac pacing can be a temporary measure if the problem is an emergent, transient condition, such as drug toxicity. An external pacemaker often is used in the emergency room. A temporary transvenous pacemaker is placed if transient complete heart block (i.e., no impulse travels from the atria to the ventricles) develops after an MI. Pacemaker wires are often placed during cardiac surgery for quick use should the patient need to be "paced" in the postoperative period. When the need for the wires is past, the surgeon will pull them out.

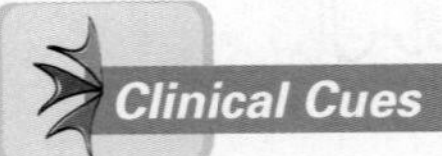

The patient is at risk for cardiac tamponade when the pacer wires are pulled. Monitor the patient for signs and symptoms including sharp chest pain, dyspnea, hypotension, cyanosis, tachycardia, and distended jugular veins.

A permanent pacemaker is indicated if the cardiac dysrhythmia is the result of an irreversible disorder, as in failure of the SA node. Other conditions in which a permanent pacemaker is inserted include pathologic complete heart block, secondary AV block, supraventricular tachycardia, and bradytachycardia, in which the SA node alternates between firing too slowly and firing too rapidly. The types of permanent pacemakers are:

- Single-chamber, in which one wire is placed in either the atrium or ventricle.
- Dual-chamber, in which wires are placed in both the atrium and ventricle. This provides more natural pacing.
- Biventricular, in which wires are placed in both ventricles.
- Rate-responsive, in which the pacemaker automatically adjusts to the patient's level of activity, that is, if the patient exercises, the heart rate would increase similar to the SA node response.

Table 19–3 *Medications Commonly Prescribed for Cardiac Disorders*

CLASSIFICATION AND ACTION	EXAMPLES*	NURSING IMPLICATIONS	PATIENT TEACHING
CARDIOTONICS (CARDIAC GLYCOSIDES)			
Uses: CHF, atrial fibrillation, atrial flutter, tachycardia *Actions:* Strengthen contractions, providing more blood to body tissues, and decrease the heart rate by slowing conduction of the cardiac impulse through the AV node	Digoxin (Lanoxin) Digitoxin	Before administration: take apical pulse for 1 full minute, listening for bradycardia and new irregular rhythm; verify the serum digoxin or digitoxin level. *Normal values:* Digoxin 0.5–2.0 ng/mL Digitoxin <35 ng/mL Verify that serum potassium is within normal limits of 3.5–5.3 mEq/L; assess for signs and symptoms of digitalis toxicity: anorexia, nausea, vomiting, visual disturbances, headache, malaise, bradycardia, dysrhythmias. If abnormalities are found, consult physician before giving the drug.	Instruct how to take own pulse rate; ask to record rate daily. Notify physician if rate is below 60 bpm or newly irregular. Ask to eat foods high in potassium, such as fresh and dried fruits, citrus fruit juices, avocados, and vegetables. Stress importance of compliance with dosage schedule.
Use: Short-term treatment of CHF *Action:* Peripheral vasodilation that reduces preload and afterload	Amrinone lactate (Inocor) Milrinone (Primacor)	Monitor for hypotension; watch hydration status. Assess lungs for decreasing crackles in bases. May decrease platelet count.	
ANTIANGINALS (NITRATES)			
Uses: Angina pectoris, conditions helped by increased blood flow *Actions:* Relaxes and dilates the vessels and lowers cardiac workload by decreasing venous return to the heart	Nitroglycerin (Nitrostat) Nitroprusside (Nipride) Nitro-Bid (Isosorbide dinitrate [Isordil]) Pentaerythritol (Peritrate) Transderm Nitro Nitroglycerin lingual spray (Nitrolingual) Nitroglycerin buccal tablets (Nitroguard) Nitroglycerin transdermal patch (Nitrodur II)	Take baseline blood pressure before administering sublingual form; take blood pressure again at 5 min and at 10 min. If blood pressure continues to rise, call physician. Observe for possible hypotension. Use gloves to apply ointment; wash hands afterward. Check transdermal patch q shift to see that it is intact.	Teach to wet sublingual tablet with saliva and place it under the tongue. Warn it may cause headache. May repeat dose every 5 min, up to three tablets. If pain persists, call emergency number. For patch: remove old patch when applying new one; rotate sites. Take oral tablets on an empty stomach either 30 min before meals or 1–2 hr after meals. Store tablets in cool place in light-proof container. Carry tablets at all times. Replace supply q 3 mo.

*Generic drugs are listed first, followed by brand name(s) in parentheses.

Table 19–3 Medications Commonly Prescribed for Cardiac Disorders—cont'd

CLASSIFICATION AND ACTION	EXAMPLES	NURSING IMPLICATIONS	PATIENT TEACHING
ANTIANGINALS (BETA BLOCKERS)			
Uses: Angina pectoris, MI, some dysrhythmias *Actions:* Slows the heart rate and decreases strength of cardiac contraction, thereby decreasing cardiac workload	Propranolol (Inderal) Atenolol (Tenormin) Metoprolol (Lopressor, Toprol XL) Nadolol (Corgard)	Contraindicated in patients with asthma (may cause bronchoconstriction) or diabetes mellitus (masks signs of hypoglycemia). Check apical pulse rate before administering. Notify anesthesiologist before surgery that patient is taking a beta blocker. Elderly may experience prolonged drug action; watch for toxic effects. Monitor blood pressure and potassium levels regularly. Elderly may experience prolonged drug action.	Take medication with meals. Do not stop taking the drug abruptly. Do not break, crush, or chew this medication. Protect capsules from direct sunlight.
CALCIUM CHANNEL BLOCKERS (ANTAGONIST)			
Uses: Angina pectoris, hypertension, some dysrhythmias, treat vasospasm post-MI *Actions:* Decreases cardiac contractility and may slow pulse, thereby decreasing cardiac workload; dilates coronary arteries	Verapamil (Calan) Nifedipine (Procardia) Diltiazem (Cardizem) Nicardipine (Cardene) Amiodipine (Norvasc) Bepridil (Vascor)	**See information under Class II and Class III antidysrhythmics.** Monitor drug serum level for therapeutic range. Monitor pulse and blood pressure for new dysrhythmia, bradycardia, or hypotension before administering. Assess for side effects: nausea, vomiting, diarrhea, urinary retention, or confusion. Assess for side effects particular to specific drug. Check for drug interactions with other drugs patient is receiving.	Instruct to report side effects and adverse reactions. Stress drug dosage schedule compliance. Advise to avoid caffeine, alcohol, and smoking. Warn about hypotension and encourage to change from lying to sitting position to standing slowly.
CLASS I ANTIDYSRHYTHMICS (ANTIDYSRHYTHMICS)			
Uses: Atrial and ventricular dysrhythmias *Actions:* Slows the sodium channel, prolongs time of depolarization, and increases refractory period	Quinidine sulfate Procainamide (Pronestyl, Procan) Disopyramide (Norpace) Lidocaine (Xylocaine) Phenytoin (Dilantin) Tocainamide (Tonocard)	Quinidine: monitor for cinchonism: tinnitus, headache, nausea, vertigo, and disturbed vision. Observe for changes in ECG pattern. If patient is taking digitalis, monitor for digitalis toxicity as quinidine can double digoxin levels. Cimetidine increases effects of quinidine. Quinidine may enhance action of anticoagulants. Monitor for diarrhea. Monitor drug level. Procainamide: monitor for systemic lupus erythematosus–like syndrome: joint pain; hepatomegaly; unexplained fever; soreness of the mouth, throat, or gums. Discontinue medication if this occurs. Observe for side effects or adverse effects of particular drug administered. Monitor electrolyte levels; watch for postural hypotension, especially if patient is taking antihypertensives.	Instruct to report signs of adverse effects of the drug. Report noticeable changes in cardiac rhythm to the physician. Advise to take quinidine with meals to prevent GI upset. Advise to minimize citrus fruit intake as it changes the urine pH and decreases excretion of quinidine. Procainamide is absorbed best on an empty stomach; if GI upset occurs, take immediately after a meal.

Continued

Table 19–3 Medications Commonly Prescribed for Cardiac Disorders—cont'd

CLASSIFICATION AND ACTION	EXAMPLES	NURSING IMPLICATIONS	PATIENT TEACHING
CLASS II ANTIDYSRHYTHMICS (BETA BLOCKERS)			
Uses: Atrial and ventricular dysrhythmias *Action:* Slows sinoatrial nodal impulses	Propranolol (Inderal) Acebutolol (Sectral) Atenolol (Tenormin) Nadolol (Corgard) Timolol (Apo-Timol) Metoprolol (Lopressor, Toprol XL) Pindolol (Visken) Esmolol (Brevibloc)	Monitor for signs of CHF; monitor pulse and blood pressure, watching for bradycardia and hypotension. Monitor electrolytes. Carefully monitor blood sugar in diabetic patients.	Instruct not to discontinue the drug abruptly. Notify physician if skin rash, confusion, fever, sore throat, or unusual bleeding or bruising occurs. Monitor weight and report gain of >2 lb/wk. Report edema or shortness of breath.
CLASS III ANTIDYSRHYTHMICS			
Uses: Control supraventricular and ventricular dysrhythmias *Actions:* Increases the refractory period and action potential duration	Amiodarone (Cordarone) Bretylium (Bretylol)	Check for drug interactions and for side or adverse effects of specific drug administered. Monitor heart rhythm, blood pressure, and pulse. Monitor renal function.	Instruct to report adverse reactions to specific drug being taken. Advise of need for physician supervision. Report any new heart rhythm irregularities.
CLASS IV ANTIDYSRHYTHMICS (CALCIUM CHANNEL BLOCKERS)			
Use: Paroxysmal supraventricular tachycardia (PSVT) *Action:* Converts PSVT to normal sinus rhythm by slowing conduction time through the nodes	Verapamil (Calan, Isoptin, Verelan)	Monitor heart rate and rhythm; watch for signs of CHF. Observe for hypotension and edema. Use very cautiously with beta blockers.	Instruct to report signs of edema, shortness of breath, or weight gain of >2 lb in 1 wk. Notify physician of new changes in heart rhythm.
DIURETICS: THIAZIDES AND RELATED DRUGS			
Uses: Edema and hypertension *Actions:* Block tubular reabsorption of water, sodium, and chloride; promote excretion of potassium	Chlorothiazide (Diuril) Chlorthalidone (Hygroton) Hydrochlorothiazide (Esidrix) Indapamide (Lozol) Metolazone (Zaroxolyn)	Observe for side effects of thiazide diuretics: electrolyte imbalances, elevated blood sugar, and elevated uric acid levels. Hyperlipidemia also may occur. Potassium supplementation is frequently necessary. Patients also should be monitored for constipation.	Ask patient to monitor weight to determine effectiveness of diuretic. Instruct to eat foods high in potassium or take prescribed potassium supplement as ordered. Increase fiber intake and exercise to decrease potential for constipation.
DIURETICS (LOOP DIURETICS)			
Uses: Edema, hypertension, CHF *Actions:* Inhibits reabsorption of sodium in the loop of Henle; promotes water and sodium excretion; potassium also is excreted	Ethacrynic acid (Edecrin) Furosemide (Lasix) Bumetanide (Bumex)j Torsemide (Demadex)	Patients with a history of thrombophlebitis who are taking a diuretic should be monitored closely for recurrence. Given in once a day doses in the a.m. to promote diuresis before bedtime. Loop diuretics are potent drugs. Side effects and nursing implications are much the same as for the thiazide diuretics except that loop diuretics promote calcium excretion and can be ototoxic (hearing loss). Monitor for changes.	Instruct in the signs of hypokalemia and the importance of taking in sufficient potassium while taking a loop diuretic. Ask to keep a daily weight chart and report any weight gain of >2 lb/wk without any alteration in diet or exercise.

Table 19–3 Medications Commonly Prescribed for Cardiac Disorders—cont'd

CLASSIFICATION AND ACTION	EXAMPLES	NURSING IMPLICATIONS	PATIENT TEACHING
POTASSIUM-SPARING DIURETICS			
Uses: Edema, hypertension *Actions:* Acts on distal renal tubules, promoting water and sodium excretion and inhibiting potassium excretion	Spironolactone (Aldactone) Amiloride (Moduretic) Triamterene (Dyazide, Maxide)	Potassium intake should not be increased. Observe for signs of sodium depletion. Electrolyte levels should be checked periodically for all patients receiving daily diuretics.	Patient receiving diuretics must be taught: (1) the purpose and desired effects of the drug; (2) the importance of taking the drug exactly as prescribed; (3) that signs of side effects and toxicity should be reported to the physician; (4) symptoms of potassium and sodium depletion.
ANTICOAGULANTS			
Uses: Prevents clot extension, new clots, and emboli formation *Actions:* Heparin blocks the conversion of prothrombin to thrombin and fibrinogen to fibrin. Warfarin sodium inhibits the synthesis of vitamin K needed to form clotting factors	Heparin Warfarin sodium (Coumadin) Dicumarol Enoxaparin (Lovenox) Dalteparin (Fragmin)	Observe for signs of abnormal bleed by periodically checking vital signs; monitoring urine and stool for signs of internal bleeding; inspect skin for bruises and petechiae; ask about bleeding of gums with toothbrushing. For patients on IV heparin drips, place extra foam mattress on bed to prevent bruising of thighs and buttocks. Monitor for interactions with other drugs the patient is receiving as drug interactions can enhance or counteract the effect of coumarin. Aspirin and other salicylates are contraindicated when the patient is receiving an anticoagulant. Patients on oral anticoagulants may experience fatigue. Monitor clotting times. For heparin: APPT or PPT should be 1½ to 2 times the control value. Consult physician if APPT or PT is approaching 70 sec. For coumadin: PT should be 2 to 2½ times the control or, if reported as international normalized ratio (INR), should be between 1.5 and 3.0; hold the medication and report values greater than this to the physician immediately.	Explain the rationale for the administration of heparin. For patients receiving oral anticoagulants, instruct about the drug being given; the hazards of hemorrhage; the reason for frequent blood tests, safety precautions, foods that affect clotting, and not to take over-the-counter medications without consulting the physician as they may alter the drug's effect. Warn specifically not to take aspirin or other salicylates.

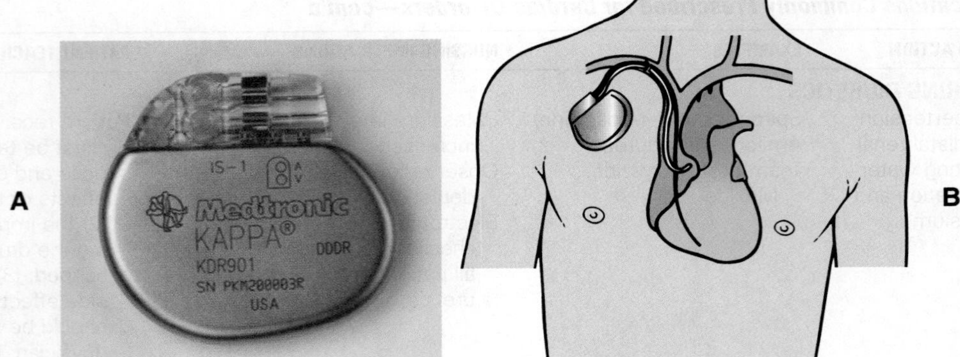

FIGURE **19–7** Thoracic placement of permanent pacemaker and transvenous catheter. **A,** Pacemaker. **B,** Placement of pacemaker and wires.

Transvenous pacemakers are inserted by fluoroscopy with local anesthesia. Patient consent is required, and a sedative is given to the patient before the procedure. A permanent pacemaker is inserted in the operating room or cardiac catheterization laboratory to ensure an aseptic environment, even though the procedure is relatively minor (Figure 19–7). Set-rate pacemakers are still used in patients with atrial fibrillation, as sensors have a problem interpreting the chaotic electrical activity of the atrium.

Patients who experience supraventricular tachycardia or atrial fibrillation that does not respond to drug therapy may be treated with **cardioversion.** A mild electrical shock is delivered to the heart at a specific time in the cardiac cycle to interrupt the abnormal rhythm and begin a new, normal rhythm of electrical impulse and contraction. The patient is given a sedative before the procedure. Signed consent is required. The procedure may be performed in the cardiac catheterization laboratory or the emergency department by the physician. Resuscitation equipment must be at hand. The patient must be monitored for response to treatment, including heart rate, rhythm, and blood pressure.

Automatic implantable cardiac defibrillators (AICD) are used for patients who have repeated episodes of life-threatening ventricular fibrillation or cardiac asystole (arrest). The defibrillator is implanted in the operating room. This device monitors the heartbeat and provides an electrical shock similar to that delivered in cardiac defibrillation when a life-threatening rhythm is detected. The patient is warned not to go through airport metal detecting systems, as the defibrillator is turned on and off by a magnet. The patient should carry a letter from the physician with this information when traveling. Not all pacemakers are affected by these systems, but patients with susceptible devices should avoid the scanning wand used for screening passengers. Alternative methods of screening can be done.

Nursing Management

If inserting a pacemaker is not an emergency procedure, you will have opportunities to assess the patient's knowledge of and feelings about having a pacemaker regulate his heart rate. Although the physician is responsible for explaining the purpose of the pacemaker and its benefits to the patient, these explanations can raise more questions and possibly create fears and anxiety. You should assess the patient's learning needs and seek to identify the source of his fear and the level of his anxiety.

Both the American Heart Association and the manufacturers of pacemakers provide illustrated booklets to help patients learn more about their cardiac pacers. You can go over these booklets with the patient and perhaps show him a demonstration model and explain how it works to his advantage.

Care of the patient who has a temporary pacemaker includes checking the connections of the lead wires to the pulse generator, keeping the device and wires dry, checking the control settings, and protecting the patient from electrical shock and infection. For protection, the pulse generator and exposed wires are placed in a rubber glove, and contact is avoided with all electrical apparatus (e.g., unplug bed; do not use an electric razor). Other care is identical to that for the patient receiving a permanent pacemaker.

Postoperative nursing care for the permanent pacemaker patient includes continuous monitoring of heart rate and rhythm, dressing changes, and care of the insertion site according to the protocol of the nursing care unit. Vital signs, peripheral pulses distal to the insertion site, and level of consciousness are checked frequently during the immediate postoperative period.

Discharge instructions for the patient with a permanent pacemaker should include the amount of physical activity allowed until healing occurs and the electrode is securely in place. This usually takes no more than 6 weeks, after which time the patient can be as physically active as he wishes, although he is warned not to engage in contact sports or other activities that may result in injury to the chest.

Although the newer pacemakers have a shield to protect them from electromagnetic signals from machinery, the patient should be cautioned not to expose his pacemaker unnecessarily to high-voltage equipment. Faulty microwave ovens, lawn mower motors, and other sources of electromagnetic signals can "confuse" a pacemaker with impulses that could cause it to malfunction. Should this occur, function will return to normal as soon as the patient moves away from the source of electromagnetic signals. A cell phone or cordless telephone should be placed on the ear opposite where the pacemaker battery is placed. The battery in a pacemaker should last 6 to 9 years, depending on the type, but it could weaken prematurely. Weakening results in a drop in pulse rate, which should be reported to the physician immediately.

The patient will need to know how to take his pulse so that he can regularly evaluate the performance of his pacemaker. He should take his pulse for 1 full minute every day while he is in a resting position.

A patient with a pacemaker should wear medical identification, such as a bracelet or necklace at all times and carry an identification card stating that he has a pacemaker. Follow-up care is essential for every person with a pacemaker. The patient must understand the importance of periodic evaluations of his condition for the rest of his life. Some pacemakers have a telephone monitoring device that allows the patient to call a monitoring station and have the pacemaker checked. Instructions for the use of the pacemaker and monitoring device are included in the owner's manual.

Because of the sensors implanted in the chambers of the heart, the patient is at risk for infection of the lining of the heart **(endocarditis).** He should be given prophylactic antibiotics before any invasive medical or dental procedure (Safety Alert 19–1).

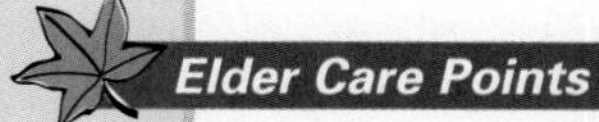

Elder Care Points

Older patients who have SA node disease and resulting cardiac dysrhythmias can achieve a far better quality of life with an implanted pacemaker. Many patients are fearful of the surgery required and can benefit from talking to another patient who has had a successful pacemaker implantation.

Think Critically About . . . What would you include in a teaching plan for the patient who has received a pacemaker? How would the teaching differ for a temporary pacemaker versus a permanent pacemaker?

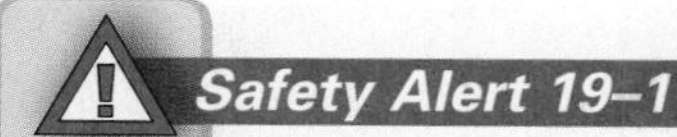

Safety Alert 19–1

Infective Endocarditis

Streptococcus viridans, a bacteria found in the mouth, is responsible for about 50% of cases of infective endocarditis. The patient must provide the health care provider of his medical history so that appropriate prophylactic treatment can be provided. Children with congenital heart conditions and adults with heart-valve disorders are usually started on antibiotic therapy prior to dental and other invasive procedures.

INFLAMMATORY DISEASES OF THE HEART

Etiology

The tissues of the heart are subject to the same inflammatory conditions that affect other parts of the body. The inflammation may be present in the inner lining (endocarditis), the heart muscle (myocarditis), or the sac surrounding the heart (pericarditis). The process also may involve the valves between the heart chambers or those located at the base of the major vessels leading from the heart. The inflammation of acute pericarditis may occur after MI, rheumatic fever, systemic lupus erythematosus, or a viral infection. Cancer and its treatment, renal failure, or trauma can also cause pericardial inflammation. Pericarditis can be bacterial or viral in origin or can result from inflammation in tissue damaged from MI. If the inflammation causes an excessive amount of fluid in the pericardial sac, a **pericardial effusion** occurs. Should the fluid become excessive, **cardiac tamponade** may occur as the fluid restricts the filling and pumping of the heart. If unresolved, cardiac tamponade is soon fatal, because the heart cannot supply the body with needed oxygen and nutrients.

Infection of the heart can result from an acute infection elsewhere in the body. The infection may be caused by staphylococci, pneumococci, gonococci, bacilli, or fungi. This condition is called *infective endocarditis* (IE), *bacterial endocarditis* (BE), or *subacute bacterial endocarditis* (SBE), depending on the cause. In adults the introduction of bacteria during dental or invasive diagnostic procedures is a frequent cause of endocarditis. Subacute bacterial endocarditis occurs most frequently in people who have a congenitally damaged heart or a prosthetic valve. Intravenous drug injection with unclean needles is another cause of endocarditis.

Although antibiotics, particularly penicillin, have decreased the incidence of rheumatic fever, the danger is still present. Today, untreated strep throat is the most common cause of cardiac inflammation in children who do not have congenital cardiac abnormalities. Strep throat is a common disease of childhood

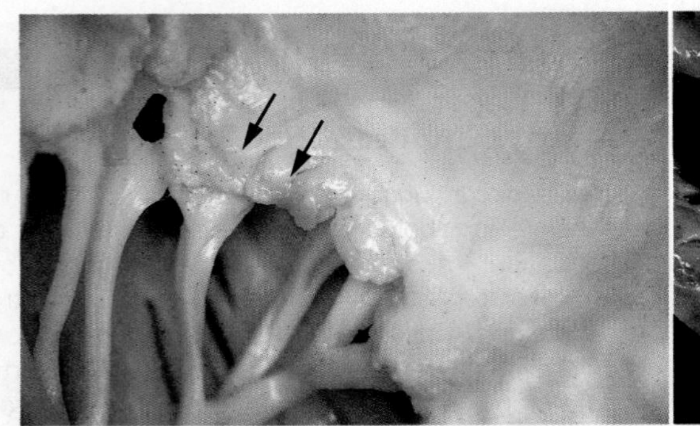

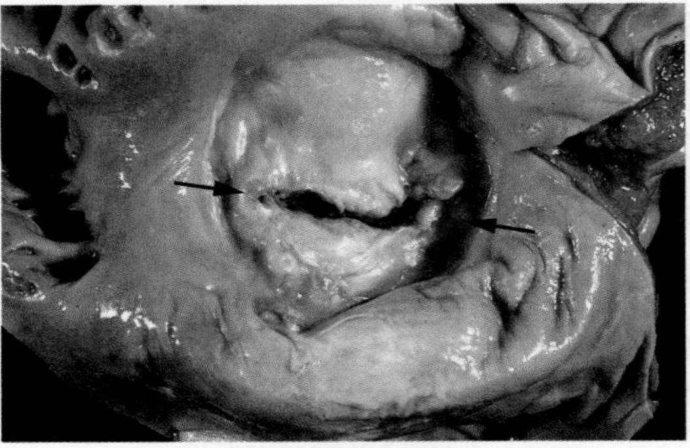

FIGURE **19–8** **A,** Thickening and valve leaflet distortion from infection and inflammation of the endocardium. **B,** Mitral stenosis.

caused by group A streptococcus. Throat culture should be performed any time there is a question that beta *Streptococcus* A is the organism responsible for a strep throat. If the streptococcal infection is treated early with antibiotics, inflammation in the heart may be avoided. Rheumatic fever is much less common in adults. In adults circulating microorganisms in the bloodstream may attack the endocardium.

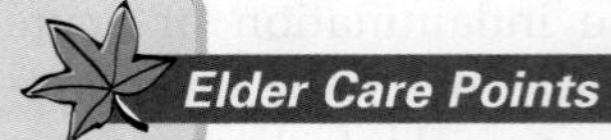
Elder Care Points

In the elderly, systemic infections of the respiratory, urinary, or gastrointestinal tract, or skin often are the causes of endocarditis. Diagnosis is difficult because symptoms are frequently vague. The aortic valve is most often affected.

Pathophysiology

The inflamed tissues of the heart become rough and swollen. The serous fluids that typically are produced by inflammation may cause an **effusion** (accumulated fluid) in the pericardium. If the effusion becomes large, it can affect the filling of the heart and the cardiac output.

Invading microorganisms may attack the heart valves or areas of the endocardium that are congenitally abnormal, causing small deposits on the valve called *vegetation.* Vegetation decreases the effectiveness of the valve and is frequently the reason for valve replacement. The mitral valve is the most frequent location of infection (Figure 19–8).

A viral infection can cause myocarditis and **cardiomyopathy**. The virus attacks the muscle tissue, causing inflammation and resultant fibrosis. Cardiomyopathy is a term for cardiac degeneration from a source other than CAD, hypertension, cardiac structural disorders, or pulmonary disease. The heart enlarges and becomes an inefficient pump. Other causes of cardiomyopathy include alcoholism, drug toxicity, crack cocaine use, pregnancy, immune disorders, and

Box 19–2 ***Types of Cardiomyopathy***

There are several types of cardiomyopathy including:

- **Ischemic** Usually related to myocardial infarction
- **Idiopathic** Related to unknown cause
- **Dilated** Usually idiopathic, characterized by extensive enlargement of the left ventricle
- **Hypertropic** Increased growth of left ventricle muscle. May be hereditary
- **Alcoholic** Follows chronic alcohol abuse
- **Peripartum** Occurs during last trimester of pregnancy or after childbirth
- **Restrictive** Heart cannot relax adequately after systole, affecting ventricular filling

nutritional deficiencies (Box 19–2). The major problems exhibited by patients with cardiomyopathy are HF and dysrhythmias.

Think Critically About . . . How many medical conditions or procedures that might cause a pericardial effusion or tamponade can you name?

Signs, Symptoms, and Diagnosis

The signs and symptoms of IE vary considerably. The sedimentation rate and leukocyte count are elevated, and signs of low-grade intermittent fever are evident. The spleen becomes enlarged. Splinter hemorrhages (thin black lines) can occur under the nails, and there may be petechiae inside the mouth. Cardiac inflammation (endocarditis) may be recurring. Each instance of endocarditis further damages the heart valves. The scar tissue that occurs as the inflammation subsides may cause the valve to leak, resulting in insufficiency (lack of closure), or the valve leaflets may become thickened and calcified, causing narrowing or stenosis. An existing cardiac murmur may worsen, or a new murmur may appear as a valve is damaged. The mitral and aortic valves are most often affected. When mitral or aortic stenosis or insufficiency causes symptoms sufficient to interfere with the patient's usual lifestyle, surgery becomes necessary (see section on cardiac surgery in Chapter 20). Stenosis and insufficiency of cardiac valves may eventually cause HF.

Symptoms of pericarditis include tachycardia, chest pain eased by sitting up and leaning forward, dyspnea, and a pericardial **friction rub.** The rub is a high-pitched scratchy sound heard with the diaphragm of the stethoscope placed at the lower left sternal border of the chest. The ECG will show changes.

If effusion is present, there may be malaise and fatigue related to decreased cardiac output and perfusion of the tissues with oxygen. When the effusion grows and seriously compromises the ability of the heart to function, cardiac tamponade (compression of the heart) occurs (Figure 19–9). This is a life-threatening occurrence. Watch for muffled heart sounds, tachycardia, restlessness, anxiety and confusion, distended neck veins, and **pulsus paradoxus**—a drop in systolic BP greater than 10 mm Hg upon inspiration.

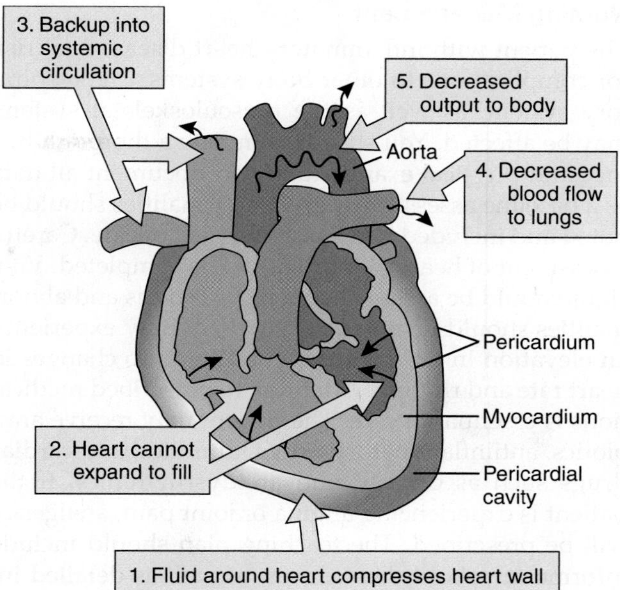

FIGURE 19–9 Effects of pericardial effusion.

Diagnosis is made by history and physical and confirmed by echocardiogram and blood cultures. Inflammatory conditions are primarily treated with rest of the affected part, and the same is true of inflammatory diseases of the heart. Treatment consists of measures intended to decrease the workload of the heart. The patient is placed on bed rest with bathroom privileges during the acute stage of the infection.

Signs and symptoms of cardiomyopathy include dyspnea, activity intolerance, angina, dizziness, hypertension, and palpitations. Diagnosis is made through history plus chest x-ray, cardiac catheterization, echocardiography, ECG, or MRI/CT scans.

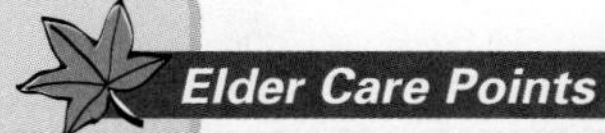

Elder Care Points

The valve leaflets thicken with age; this gives rise to the common systolic murmur heard in persons over age 80.

Treatment

Medications. Specific medications for the treatment of inflammatory conditions of the heart include the antiinflammatory agents used for pericarditis and antiinflammatory agents plus antiinfective drugs used for infective endocarditis. Choice of drug is determined by blood culture for the particular organism responsible for the infection and sensitivity testing for the drug that destroys the organism quickly. Generally a combination of at least two antibiotics is given IV through a central line for 4 to 6 weeks, with further oral therapy thereafter. Hearing must be tested frequently during therapy because some antibiotics may cause hearing loss. After the initiation of therapy and stabilization, the patient often is discharged home, usually within 7 to 10 days, and the medications are administered by home health nurses, the patient, or the family.

Medical treatment for cardiomyopathy includes drugs to increase contractility, such as digoxin, antihypertensive drugs, diuretic, antidysrhythmia drugs, and anticoagulants. Severe cardiomyopathy can be rapidly fatal. These patients are possible candidates for a heart transplant.

Surgical Treatment. Pericarditis may be surgically treated by **pericardiotomy** (opening of the pericardium) or **pericardiocentesis** (opening of the pericardium and removal of fluid). Repair of congenital cardiac problems, such as atrial or ventricular septal defect, may be done. Balloon valvuloplasty is a procedure sometimes used to open stenosed valves. It is performed with a balloon-tipped catheter much like the one used for cardiac angioplasty. However, it is questionable whether the valve will just close again with time. Valve replacement is an open-heart surgical procedure in which the valve is replaced with a porcine (pork), bovine (beef), or synthetic valve (see Chapter 20). When a synthetic valve is used, the patient must be on anticoagulant therapy for the rest of his life, as the synthetic material tends to cause breakup of blood cells and clumping of platelets, which in turn cause clots and emboli. Prophylactic antibiotics are necessary before any invasive procedure (dental, endoscopy, etc.) for any patient who has had an inflammatory cardiac disorder.

Nursing Management

The patient with inflammatory heart disease is at risk for complications to other body systems. The respiratory system, as well as the musculoskeletal system, may be affected. You should complete a thorough history and physical examination and document all data as a baseline assessment. Any abnormalities should be noted and included in the nursing plan of care. Careful assessment of heart sounds should be completed. Vital signs should be assessed on a regular basis and abnormalities should be noted. The patient may experience an elevation in temperature in addition to changes in heart rate and rhythm. Attention to prescribed medications is essential to care. The patient may receive antibiotics, antiinflammatory drugs, diuretics, and cardiac drugs such as digoxin and antidysrhythmics. If the patient is experiencing angina or joint pain, analgesics will be prescribed. The teaching plan should include information about these drugs, as well as detailed information about the specific disease process. Some patients may require complete bed rest. You should make the patient as comfortable as possible and reinforce the rationale for this activity level. Oxygen administration may be required, and the importance of this treatment should be discussed with the patient. Discharge planning should include evaluation of the patient's physical status, assessment of the patient's understanding of the home care requirements, and teaching related to medications and treatment.

> *Think Critically About* . . . Can you list four diagnostic procedures prior to which a patient with an artificial or defective heart valve should take prophylactic antibiotics?

CARDIAC VALVE DISORDERS

Besides congenital abnormalities, rheumatic fever, and BE, long-term hypertension also can cause cardiac valve disorders. Problems most commonly occur in the mitral valve between the left atrium and ventricle. The aortic valve is the second most commonly diseased valve.

Etiology and Pathophysiology

Valve disorders are of two types: stenosis or insufficiency. In valvular stenosis, a narrowing of the valve opening occurs and causes an obstruction to normal blood flow. When stenosis occurs, the chamber that pumps the blood through the valve must do more work to force blood through. With valvular insufficiency (also called *incompetency* or *regurgitation*), the diseased valve is unable to close properly and blood flows back into the chamber after contraction, causing an overfilling.

Mitral stenosis causes the left atrium to work harder to pump blood through the narrowed valve into the left ventricle. *Mitral insufficiency* results in blood flow back into the left atrium with every contraction of the left ventricle. This makes more work for the left atrium. With both conditions, the left atrium dilates and thickens in response to the increased workload. The increasing pressure of the extra blood in the left atrium causes a backward increase in pressure in the pulmonary circulation and the eventual development of HF. As the atrial tissue dilates, the conduction system may be disrupted and dysrhythmias, particularly atrial fibrillation, may occur.

When atrial fibrillation occurs, clots may form in the atria and be pumped out into the circulation as emboli, lodging in the coronary vessels, the brain, or elsewhere in the body. An MI or stroke may result.

Aortic stenosis causes the left ventricle to work harder to force blood through the valve into the aorta. *Aortic insufficiency* allows blood to backflow into the ventricle after it is pumped into the aorta. With these conditions, the left ventricle dilates and thickens in an effort to handle the extra pressure and volume of blood in the ventricle. Eventually, left ventricular failure occurs.

Signs, Symptoms, and Diagnosis

Signs and symptoms of mitral valve disorders include a cardiac murmur, progressive fatigue, exertional dyspnea, irregular heart rate, and the gradual onset of HF. Confirmation of a suspected valve disorder is made by echocardiogram or cardiac catheterization.

Signs and symptoms of aortic valve disorders include cardiac murmur, syncope, angina, dysrhythmia, dyspnea, and signs of HF. Aortic insufficiency causes a widened pulse pressure. Diagnosis is by echocardiogram or cardiac catheterization.

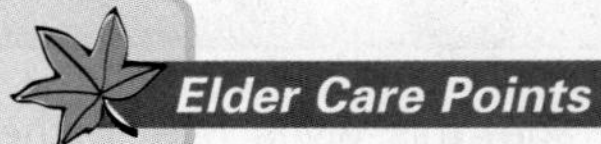

Elder Care Points

Elderly people with long-term hypertension are at risk for aortic stenosis because of increased arteriosclerosis and stiffening of the aorta. Carefully assess aortic valve sounds of the elderly patient, especially if hypertension is not well controlled.

Treatment

Treatment for mitral valve disorders is aimed at controlling atrial fibrillation and HF with digitalis, diuretics, and antidysrhythmic medications, and prophylactic anticoagulants to prevent clot formation and emboli. Valve surgery is performed on the dysfunctional valve when the person's lifestyle is restricted by cardiac failure (see Chapter 20).

Treatment for aortic valve disorders is essentially the same as for mitral valve disorders, except that different antidysrhythmic medication is used for ventricular dysrhythmia. There is a greater danger of sudden death with aortic stenosis due to decreased blood flow to the coronary arteries. For all types of valve disorders, the patient is encouraged to attain and maintain a normal weight to minimize the workload of the heart.

Nursing Management

The primary nursing goals for patients with cardiac valve disease are to maintain homeostasis, control dysrhythmias, and prevent or control HF. Careful assessment of the patient for signs of developing heart failure, teaching the patient about prescribed medications, and preparing the patient for surgical procedures should be included in the nursing plan of care. See Chapter 17 for common nursing diagnoses and interventions for problems related to valve problems.

CARDIAC TRAUMA

Blunt chest trauma often causes myocardial contusion, but it also can cause tears in the great vessels and massive bleeding. Contusion may result in cardiac dysrhythmia; therefore, the patient's cardiac rhythm is monitored closely when such trauma has occurred. Penetrating trauma usually causes a hemothorax. Cardiac tamponade can occur from either type of wound if bleeding into the pericardial sac occurs. The fluid compresses the heart and restricts blood flow in and out of the ventricles. Cardiac output falls and venous pressure rises; the arterial blood pressure falls and there is a narrowing of pulse pressure accompanied by tachycardia. Shock and death will result if the bleeding is not stopped and the fluid removed. Pericardiocentesis may be performed to remove the fluid from the pericardial sac. Every effort is made to restore normal cardiac output.

CARDIOGENIC SHOCK

Cardiogenic shock may occur as a result of hypovolemia or cardiac tamponade caused by trauma. It also may occur from serious dysrhythmias, cardiac arrest, myocardial degeneration, and as a complication of MI or cardiac surgery. It results from circulatory failure due to the failure of the heart to pump sufficient blood.

Signs and symptoms are those that accompany decreased cardiac output, such as confusion; restlessness; diaphoresis; rapid, thready pulse; increased respiratory rate; cold, clammy skin; and diminishing urinary output to less than 20 mL/hour. If cardiogenic shock is stemming from a mechanical defect, use of the intraaortic balloon pump until surgical repair can correct the defect may stabilize the patient. The best position for the patient is with the head of the bed elevated to 45 degrees to help breathing and oxygenation. The patient is cared for in the intensive care unit, where a variety of drugs aimed at improving cardiac output may be administered. See Chapter 44 for further information on shock.

COMMON THERAPIES AND THEIR NURSING IMPLICATIONS

The medical treatments most commonly used to manage heart disease include (1) oxygen therapy (2) pharmacologic agents, and (3) dietary controls. Patient education and rehabilitation of the cardiac patient also must be included.

Surgical treatment of cardiac conditions most often is used to correct structural defects of the heart and great vessels.

OXYGEN THERAPY

The administration of supplemental oxygen to relieve the dyspnea and hypoxemia of a cardiac patient is a routine therapeutic measure. Any patient experiencing chest pain is started on low-dose oxygen. Your responsibilities regarding oxygen therapy for a cardiac patient are primarily concerned with observation to determine a patient's need for supplemental oxygen, maintenance of the ordered flow rate, and the response to therapy once it has been initiated.

It is important that you be alert for signs of changing oxygen needs, such as increased pulse rate and symptoms of cerebral anoxia, including irritability, confusion, and disorientation.

The patient's oxygen saturation can be monitored by pulse oximetry or blood gas analysis.

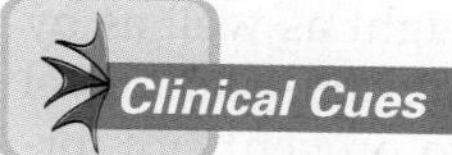

The patient's oxygen saturation should be maintained between 90% and 100%. Patients with history of pulmonary disease such as emphysema may exhibit an oxygen saturation between 85% and 90%.

PHARMACOLOGIC AGENTS

Many types of drugs are used to treat heart disorders. The most commonly administered drugs are listed in Table 19–3. Digitalis in its various forms is a widely prescribed drug. However, it is a potent drug that can produce serious toxicity. See Table 19–3 for signs and symptoms of digitalis toxicity. It can be very effective in treating certain kinds of cardiac disorders, but its therapeutic range is quite narrow. A therapeutic dose is only about one third less than the dose that will induce toxicity. Moreover, physiologic changes resulting from age, electrolyte imbalances (particularly hypokalemia or hypercalcemia), renal impairment, metabolic disturbances, and certain heart conditions can predispose a patient to digitalis toxicity. Other drugs given simultaneously, including erythromycin, also can alter the effects of digitalis and make it more toxic. When the pulse rate is less than 60 bpm, you should consider the other drugs the patient is taking. Both beta blockers and calcium channel blockers will lower the heart rate. Learn each physician's guidelines regarding a pulse rate lower than 60 bpm and check the nursing unit protocols.

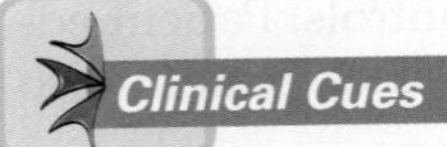

Remember that digitoxin has a slower and more prolonged action and is 10 times more potent than digoxin. **For this reason, digitoxin and digoxin are not interchangeable.**

Some physicians may not want you to hold a dose of digitalis if the patient's pulse rate is below 60 bpm, as long as there are no signs of digitalis toxicity. Check the physician's order sheet before administering the medication if the pulse rate is less than 60.

When life-threatening complications arise from digitalis toxicity, Digoxin Immune Fab is given to counteract the excess digitalis. This drug is used cautiously, as side effects include hypotension, hypokalemia, worsening of HF, and rapid ventricular rates if the patient is experiencing atrial fibrillation.

Anticoagulants are prescribed to inhibit the formation of clots within blood vessels. Anticoagulants do not dissolve clots that have already formed, but they can prevent existing ones from growing larger and can interfere with the development of new clots. Heparin, in some institutions, is beginning to be administered in doses calculated by the patient's weight as well as by clotting times, which provides a more consistent level of the heparin in the right amount to prevent clot formation.

? *Think Critically About . . .* Can you list four signs and symptoms that might indicate your patient is experiencing digitalis toxicity?

DIETARY CONTROL

Contrary to popular opinion, obesity itself is not a direct cause of heart disease. However, the National Heart, Lung and Blood Institute lists obesity as a risk factor for cardiac disorders. When obesity is present in conjunction with other factors, such as hypertension, diabetes mellitus, smoking, and family history of heart disease, the likelihood of cardiovascular problems is increased.

To prevent heart disease and decrease the factors that predispose one to cardiovascular disease, the American Heart Association recommends the measures listed in (Health Promotion Points 19–1).

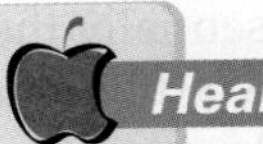

Health Promotion Points 19–1

American Heart Association Diet and Lifestyle Recommendations

- Use up as many calories as you take in
- Eat a variety of nutritious foods from all food groups
- Eat less nutrient-poor foods
- Decrease saturated fat
- Choose lean meat, poultry without skin, fish
- Choose fat-free, 1%, or low-fat dairy products
- Reduce consumption of foods with *trans* fats
- Decrease intake of high-cholesterol foods
- Decrease intake of beverages and foods with added sugars
- Refrain from adding salt to foods. Make low-sodium food choices
- Avoid smoking tobacco and avoid tobacco smoke

From American Heart Association 2006 Diet and Lifestyle Recommendations. Reprinted with permission. www.americanheart.org.

One Harvard study has indicated the great benefit of adding fiber to the diet to cut cholesterol levels. Increased fiber will lower cholesterol even without cutting down on dietary fat. Adults should consume about 35 g of fiber per day; the national average consumption is about 12 g. Increasing fiber in the diet also lowers the risk of cancer.

Another study indicates that regular cube margarine may be as harmful as butter in raising cholesterol levels because of the *trans*-fatty acids it contains. Foods containing *trans* fats increase the cholesterol level, especially low-density lipoprotein. A tub, soft-style margarine that lists water or liquid vegetable oil as its first ingredient contains less *trans*-fatty acids than other types (American Dietetic Association, 2006). Patients should be taught to read food labels for the presence of *trans* fat. Manufacturers are now required to list the amount of *trans* fats on the food labels. 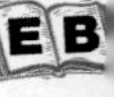

There are excellent resources for information and support for patients who have a cardiovascular disease and are attempting to follow a dietary regimen as part of their overall treatment plan. Many community hospitals sponsor weight management programs. Local chapters of the American Heart Association provide pamphlets and other sources of information about diet.

Although some persons are more susceptible to hypertension than others, such as the obese person, a high intake of sodium is thought to contribute to the development of high blood pressure in susceptible individuals. Limiting sodium intake is an important part of preventing and treating hypertension. Teaching efforts should recognize the patient's willingness to change his or her eating habits and the support and encouragement received from the family. Several cookbooks that make low-sodium, low-cholesterol meals easier to plan and prepare are sponsored by the American Heart Association and others. The fact that the tendency to develop cardiovascular disease is familial gives the patient and the family good reason to develop good eating habits and to change to more heart-healthy foods.

Many health professionals consider the self-help groups to be most successful in assisting people to lose pounds and then to keep their weight within normal range once the excess is lost. These groups include Weight Watchers, TOPS (Take Off Pounds Sensibly), and Overeaters Anonymous. Results of studies have shown that the behavior-modification techniques these groups use are very successful.

Restriction of sodium, prescribed because of sodium's association with retention of water in the tissues, is discussed in Chapter 3. Patients who are on sodium-restricted diets require special encouragement and instruction in methods to avoid an intake of sodium that would be harmful. Nutritional Therapies 18–1 suggests ways to decrease sodium in the diet.

Traditionally iced drinks, hot drinks, and those containing caffeine were denied to the MI patient. Today post-MI patients can safely drink some coffee or iced beverages if there are no changes in heart rate, rhythm, or blood pressure after drinking them.

Dietary programs to reverse coronary heart disease have been introduced by many proponents of severe restriction of saturated fat in the diet. These programs (e.g., the Pritikin Diet, Dr. Dean Ornish Diet) claim that arteriosclerosis and other factors that lead to heart disease can be reversed if a diet high in complex carbohydrates, fiber, and limited fat is followed. In addition, consistent exercise, weight management, managing emotional stress, and maintaining positive relationships are emphasized to reduce modifiable risk factors. These programs take considerable personal motivation. The entire family and support system must be involved to achieve optimum success.

Think Critically About . . . How could you specifically change your eating habits in a way that would help you follow a more heart-healthy diet?

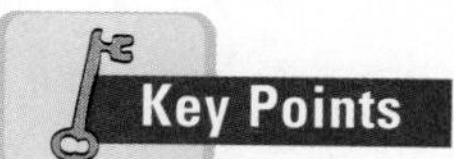

Key Points

- HF is the inability of the heart to pump as it should, and flow of blood becomes sluggish, backing up into lungs and systemic circulation.
- Left-sided symptoms of HF: dyspnea, cough, decreased urinary output, weight gain.
- Right-sided symptoms of HF: pitting peripheral edema, abdominal distention, weight gain.
- Medical treatment of HF includes limited activity initially; oxygen therapy; medications such as digoxin, loop diuretics, antihypertensive drugs; restricted sodium intake, smoking cessation.
- Careful, thorough, ongoing assessment is vital to assess the patient's response to therapy or development of complications.
- Record daily weight and accurate intake and output.
- Maintain fluid restrictions as required every 24 hours.
- The heart's conduction system is controlled by the SA node at the rate of 60 to 100 bpm. The SA node is the heart's natural pacemaker.
- Disruption of normal SA node conduction leads to dysrhythmias; lack of normal regular myocardial contraction decreases cardiac output.
- Life-threatening dysrhythmias include ventricular tachycardia, ventricular fibrillation, and asystole.
- Dysrhythmias causing decreased cardiac output include severe bradycardia, atrial fibrillation, complete heart block, and frequent PVCs.
- Dysrhythmias are diagnosed using 12-lead ECG, continuous ECG monitoring, patient history, and electrophysiologic testing.
- Failure of the heart's natural pacemaker may result in replacement by an artificial pacemaker.
- Artificial pacing can be temporary or permanent, external, transvenous, or internal.
- AICDs may be used in patients with repeated episodes of ventricular tachycardia, ventricular fibrillation, or asystole.
- Inflammation of the heart may occur as endocarditis, myocarditis, or pericarditis.
- Medical treatment includes rest to reduce workload of heart; antiinfective drugs to control infection; surgery to replace or repair valves damaged by the inflammatory process. Severe cardiomyopathy is treated by heart transplant.
- Cardiac valve disorders are caused by congenital defect, rheumatic fever, endocarditis, or long-term hypertension.
- Types of valvular disorders include stenosis and insufficiency. Changes in pressures cause the heart chamber to dilate and thicken.
- HF is the final consequence of progressive, untreated valve disease.

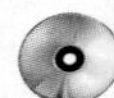

Go to your **Companion CD-ROM** for an Audio Glossary, animations, video clips, and bonus review questions.

evolve Be sure to visit the companion Evolve site at http://evolve.elsevier.com/deWit for interactive NCLEX-PN Exam Style Review Questions, WebLinks, and additional online resources.

NCLEX-PN EXAM STYLE REVIEW QUESTIONS

Choose the best answer(s) for the following questions.

1. The nurse is about to administer the first dose of torsemide (Demedex) to a patient diagnosed with congestive heart disease. Common drug reactions include which of the following? *(Select all that apply.)*
   1. Hypocalcemia
   2. Ototoxicity
   3. Hypoglycemia
   4. Light-headedness
   5. Hypertension

2. After careful discussion of treatment options, the patient consents to have an implantable cardioverter-defibrillator (ICD). Upon seeing the nurse, the patient asks, "What exactly does this procedure do for me?" An appropriate response is:
   1. "You sound anxious. Everything will be fine."
   2. "Do you want to talk to your physician?"
   3. "You consented to the implantation of a device that detects and treats shockable dysrhythmias."
   4. "Do you want to review your procedure consent?"

3. ________________ is the delivery of a mild electrical shock at a specific time of the cardiac cycle to interrupt an abnormal rhythm and to possibly initiate a normal rhythm.

4. Immediate postoperative nursing care of a patient who has had a permanent pacemaker inserted includes which of the following?
   1. Encouraging active range-of-motion exercises.
   2. Monitoring cardiac rate and rhythm.
   3. Checking bowel sounds.
   4. Determining optimal level of function.

5. A 48-year-old patient is admitted for tachycardia, chest pain eased by sitting up and leaning forward, and difficulty in breathing. The nurse auscultates a high-pitched scratchy sound at the lower left sternal border of the chest. The patient most likely has:
   1. heart failure.
   2. pericarditis.
   3. pneumonia.
   4. pulmonary stenosis.

6. The 60-year-old patient complains of shortness of breath and fatigue on exertion. The nurse determines that the patient would not be able to fully manage the day-to-day functioning in a home setting and formulates the nursing diagnosis "Self-care deficit related to low energy states and tiredness." An appropriate patient expected outcome would be that:
   1. the patient will have clear lung fields and reduced peripheral edema at the end of the shift.
   2. the patient will be able to optimally participate in activities of daily living and personal hygiene at the time of discharge.
   3. the patient will be able to verbalize concerns and issues during hospital stay.
   4. the patient will be able to demonstrate effective coping strategies at the time of discharge.

7. Which of the following patient statements regarding healthy food choices demonstrates a need for further teaching?
   1. "I can have egg yolks up to three or four times per week."
   2. "I need to skim all the fat off soups and stews."
   3. "Regular milk is a great source of protein."
   4. "Organ meats are high sources of cholesterol."

8. The nurse explains the importance of reducing salt in the diet to a Mexican American man who was recently diagnosed with heart disease. The nurse realizes that the relatives are at the bedside with the patient. An appropriate nursing action would be to:
   1. involve the youngest male in the family to translate.
   2. ensure patient privacy by directing the relatives out of the patient room.
   3. determine who does the cooking in the family.
   4. include all the relatives in the diet teaching.

9. In discussing heart failure with a patient, the physician explains that the underlying weakness of the left ventricle results in reduced cardiac output and back-up of fluid in the pulmonary system. The nurse anticipates which of the following signs/symptoms?
   1. Edema in sacrum, legs, feet, ankles
   2. Hepatomegaly
   3. Frothy pink sputum
   4. Ascites

10. The patient asks, "Why am I taking digoxin (Lanoxin)?" An accurate statement by the nurse would be:
    1. "The medication increases the force of contraction of the heart."
    2. "The medication increases the heart rate."
    3. "The medication causes vasodilation."
    4. "The medication reduces the amount of fluid going to the heart."

CRITICAL THINKING ACTIVITIES

Read each clinical scenario and discuss the questions with your classmates.

Scenario A

Mr. Jenkins, age 56, is admitted to the telemetry unit with a diagnosis of atrial fibrillation. Physical assessment reveals a restless, apprehensive male with a heart rate of 96 and irregular, dyspnea.

1. Describe the rhythm you expect to note on the telemetry monitor
2. What medications do you expect the physician to prescribe for Mr. Jenkins?
3. List five priority teaching points you should establish for Mr. Jenkins.

Scenario B

Mr. Zulic, age 76, received a permanent pacemaker to correct complete heart block. He is 3 days postoperative and preparing for discharge home.

1. What are indications for a pacemaker?
2. Describe the types of pacemakers and indications for their use.
3. Describe preoperative and postoperative nursing interventions when caring for a patient receiving a pacemaker.

CHAPTER 20

Care of Patients with Coronary Artery Disease and Cardiac Surgery

evolve http://evolve.elsevier.com/deWit

Objectives

Upon completion of this chapter the student should be able to:

Theory

1. Discuss the causes of coronary artery disease.
2. Describe the pathophysiology of coronary artery disease.
3. Compare and contrast the different types of angina.
4. Outline nursing interventions to care for a patient experiencing angina, including medication administration and patient teaching.
5. Discuss the pathophysiology of myocardial infarction.
6. Develop a nursing care plan for a patient experiencing a myocardial infarction.
7. Describe the nursing care of a patient undergoing cardiac surgery.
8. List five complications of cardiac surgery.

Clinical Practice

1. Identify signs and symptoms that indicate a patient may be experiencing a myocardial infarct.
2. Administer medications to patients experiencing cardiac disorders within the scope of practice.
3. Develop a teaching plan for a patient with coronary artery disease.
4. Collaborate with other health care providers to care for patients after cardiac surgery
5. Contribute to discharge planning for a patient after cardiac surgery.

Key Terms

Be sure to check out the bonus material on the Companion CD-ROM, including selected audio pronunciations.

angina pectoris (ăn-JĪ-nă PĔK-tŏr-ĭs, p. 492)
atherosclerosis (ăth-ĕr-ō-sklĕ-RŌ-sĭs, p. 488)
CABG (KĂ-bĭdg, p. 498)
cardiomyoplasty (kăr-dē-ō-mī-ō-plăs-tē, p. 504)
coronary insufficiency (KŎR-ō-nĕr-ē ĭn-să-FĬSH-ăn-sē, p. 488)
drug-eluting stent (stĕnt, p. 498)
infarction (ĭn-FĂRK-shŭn, p. 493)
MET (p. 500)
myocardial infarction (mī-ō-KĂR-dē-ăl ĭn-FĂRK-shŭn, p. 488)
necrosis (nē-KRŌ-sĭs, p. 489)
valvuloplasty (văl-vū-LŌ-plăs-tē, p. 504)

CORONARY ARTERY DISEASE

Coronary artery disease (CAD) is a progressive disease leading to narrowing or occlusion of the coronary arteries. The coronary arteries are responsible for supplying oxygen and nutrition to the myocardium (Figure 20–1). As the vessel narrows, the patient may experience symptoms of ischemia, such as chest tightness and angina. When a sudden obstruction to blood flow through one or more major coronary arteries occurs, cutting off oxygen and nutrients to the cardiac cells, a **myocardial infarction** (MI) occurs.

Obstruction of blood flow usually is caused by **atherosclerosis** and thrombus formation but can also result from embolus or arterial spasm.

Etiology

A major factor in the development of CAD is atherosclerosis, in which plaque-containing cholesterol is laid down inside the arteries. It can affect the cerebral vessels, the aorta, and arteries other than the coronaries. It is one form of arteriosclerosis. *Arteriosclerosis* is a general term for disorders that cause thickening and loss of elasticity of the arteries.

The process of atherosclerosis begins during childhood, when streaks or islands of fatty material are laid down on the inner walls of the arteries. Low-density lipoprotein (LDL) is the major contributing factor to the formation of this fatty material. Deposits accumulate, particularly where there has been irritation or inflammation of the vessel. Later, fibrous plaques are formed as a result of inflammation and healing. The plaque area protrudes into the artery, decreasing the vessel's size, and platelets begin to adhere to the plaque (Figure 20–2). The plaque areas eventually rupture, causing platelet clumping and clotting (thrombosis). Over time, the plaque begins to calcify, causing rigidity of the vessel wall. Narrowing of the coronary arteries causes **coronary insufficiency** (decreased or insufficient blood flow). Obstruction occurs from this process and from thrombosis. Spasm of the artery may contribute to occlusion and consequent heart muscle damage.

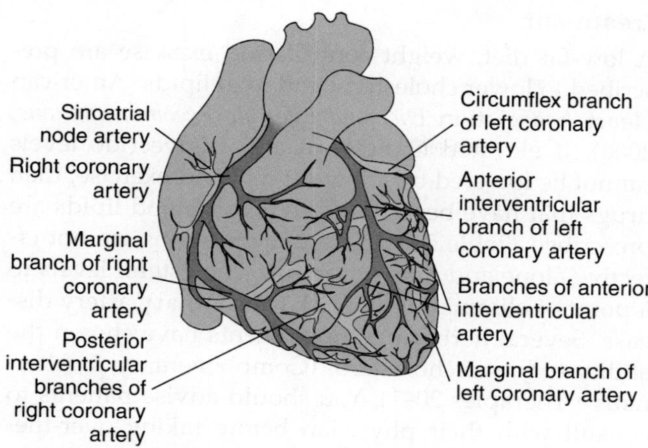

FIGURE **20–1** View of coronary artery circulation.

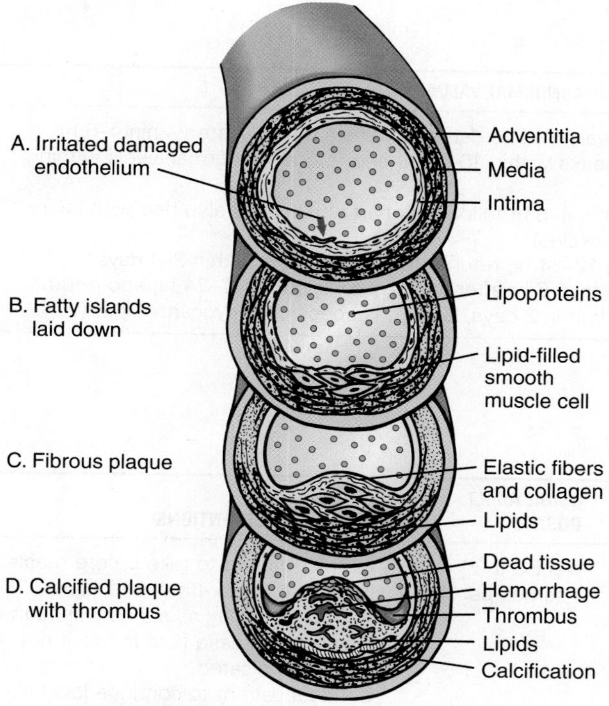

FIGURE **20–2** Progression of atherosclerosis.

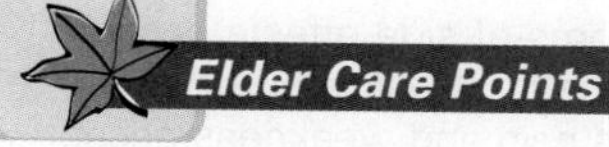

Elder Care Points

Coronary blood flow in a 60-year-old is decreased in relationship to the amount of flow in a 25-year-old. Elderly people have less *cardiac reserve,* meaning that added oxygen demands may compromise the coronary circulation and the heart's ability to pump properly.

There is a proven link between high serum cholesterol or high levels of LDL and atherosclerosis. Cigarette smoking and a history of hypertension and diabetes mellitus also are factors that lead to a higher incidence of atherosclerosis.

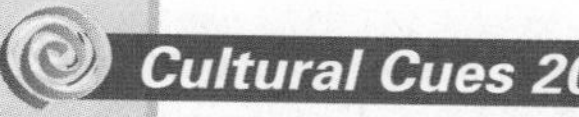

Cultural Cues 20–1

Ethnicity and Coronary Artery Disease

The incidence of coronary artery disease is disproportionately higher in African Americans, especially African American males. Research continues to determine the etiology of this finding and approaches to decrease the incidence. Ethnicity-based treatment of heart disease is also explored, as research has demonstrated that some classifications of medications are more effective for persons of diverse ethnicity

Factors such as age (>age 40), gender, and race (risk higher in African Americans) contribute to the disease; however, these cannot be modified (Cultural Cues 20–1). Those who have had one or more immediate family members die of coronary artery disease during their middle years are considered to be at high risk for the disorder. Postmenopausal women, and women who use oral contraceptives or estrogen replacement therapy, are at greater risk.

Pathophysiology

As coronary artery disease progresses, the coronary vessels become more narrow, decreasing blood supply to the myocardium. This lack of blood supply leads to ischemia and eventually **necrosis** (cell death) of the myocardium. If loss of muscle tissue occurs (MI), the heart muscle is unable to pump effectively and cardiac output is reduced. Cardiac dysrhythmias and death may occur if medical intervention is not obtained.

Signs and Symptoms

Signs and symptoms of coronary artery disease are related to the lack of oxygen supply to the myocardium and inability of the heart to pump blood effectively to oxygenate tissues and cells. Angina pectoris, acute coronary syndrome (ACS), or sudden cardiac death may occur. When the oxygen supply can be improved with medication and lifestyle changes, the condition is called *stable angina.* Signs and symptoms may include:

- Chest discomfort, including feeling of tightness, aching, burning
- Chest pain (angina pectoris) radiating to the arm, jaw, or back
- Dyspnea (shortness of breath)
- Palpitations or tachycardia
- Nausea and vomiting
- Weakness and inability to complete usual activities without chest pain or dyspnea

Acute coronary syndrome presents as either unstable angina, MI with non–ST-segment elevation, or MI with ST-segment elevation on the echocardiogram (ECG).

Diagnosis

Diagnosis of coronary artery disease is accomplished through serum lab tests, such as cardiac enzymes and lipid levels, cardiac angiography (cardiac catheterization), and electron beam computed tomography. The most common cardiac enzymes are troponin (I and T), creatine phosphokinase (CPK), and creatine kinase (CK)-MB. These enzymes are found in the body in low levels, but when myocardial damage occurs their blood levels increase. Troponin and CK-MB levels are more specific for cardiac tissue damage. CPK levels may increase when damage to other body tissues occurs. An elevation of troponin levels is most significant in diagnosing damage to the myocardium. Table 20–1 summarizes the cardiac enzymes and their significance.

Treatment

A low-fat diet, weight control, and exercise are prescribed to lower cholesterol and total lipids (American Heart Association *Diet and Lifestyle Recommendations,* 2006). If elevated cholesterol and triglyceride levels cannot be lowered by a low-fat diet and exercise, then drugs that have been found to lower blood lipids are prescribed (Table 20–2) These medications are not effective alone and may not reduce cholesterol levels to a point of eliminating the risk for coronary artery disease. Several herbs and supplements have shown the ability to lower cholesterol (Complementary & Alternative Therapies 20–1). You should advise patients to consult with their physician before taking over-the-counter medications.

Table 20–1 *Cardiac Enzymes*

ENZYME	NORMAL VALUE	SIGNIFICANCE OF ABNORMAL VALUE
Troponin I (TnI) Troponin T (TnT)	<0.3 mcg/L <0.1 mcg/L	Specific to heart muscle damage. Levels may elevate within 4–6 hr after MI, peaks within 10–24 hr and returns to normal levels within 10 days.
CPK (creatine phosphokinase)	Men: 55–170 IU/L Women: 30–135 IU/L	Elevated within 4–8 hr following heart attack (may also rise with injury to other muscles). Peaks within 12–24 hr, returns to normal levels within 3–4 days.
CK-MB	<3 ng/mL	Elevates within 2–6 hr after an MI, peaks within 12–24 hr, and returns to normal within 3 days. CK-MB is specific to myocardial injury.

Table 20–2 *Commonly Used Drugs to Treat Hypercholesterolemia*

DRUG	ACTION	COMMON SIDE EFFECTS	USUAL ADULT DOSAGE	NURSING INTERVENTIONS
Bile acid sequestrants Cholestyramine, (Questran) Colestipol (Colestid) Colesevelam (Welchol)	Bind bile acid in the GI tract, resulting in decreased absorption of cholesterol	Abdominal pain, constipation, nausea	4 g PO 1–2 times per day	Instruct patient to take before meals Instruct to mix with 4–6 oz liquid. Advise drug may cause constipation and to increase fluid intake if not contraindicated. Counsel patient to continue low-fat diet and exercise.
Fibric acid derivatives Gemfibrozil (Lopid) Clofibrate (Atromid) Fenofibrate (Tricor)	Reduces triglyceride production by the liver	Abdominal pain, diarrhea, epigastric pain	600 mg PO bid	Encourage to keep appointments for follow-up lab studies. Encourage to notify physician if symptoms of side effects occur.
HMG-CoA reductase inhibitors (statins) Atorvastatin (Lipitor) Lovastatin (Mevacor) Simvastatin (Zocor) Rosuvastatin (Crestor)	Inhibits the enzyme HMG-CoA reductase, which is responsible for synthesis of cholesterol	Abdominal pain, constipation, diarrhea, flatus, heartburn, rash	Individual drug dependent	Teach to notify physician if severe muscle pain and weakness occur. Encourage to keep follow-up appointments and have periodic lab work performed. Pregnancy category X. Advise female patients to notify physician immediately if pregnancy is suspected. Notify physician of alcohol intake. May be at risk for liver disease.
Cholesterol absorption inhibitor Ezetimibe (Zetia)	Inhibits intestinal absorption of cholesterol	Possible headache and mild GI distress; infrequent	10 mg daily	Can be used along with other antilipemics. Do not use for those with active liver disease. Take bile acid sequestrant 2 hr before or 4 hr after this drug. Obtain periodic lipid levels and liver function enzymes.

Nursing Management

Patients should be encouraged to adopt a healthy lifestyle, including exercise and a diet low in saturated fat (Nutritional Therapies 20–1). Obtain a referral to a dietitian and assist the patient by reinforcing the need for changes in dietary habits. Help the patient choose an exercise regimen that she can manage on a long-term basis. Emphasize the importance of maintaining a normal body weight.

If the patient is on a statin drug to lower cholesterol, remind her that she needs to have blood work drawn to determine if the drug is effective and to monitor for serious side effects of the drug (Health Promotion Points 20–1).

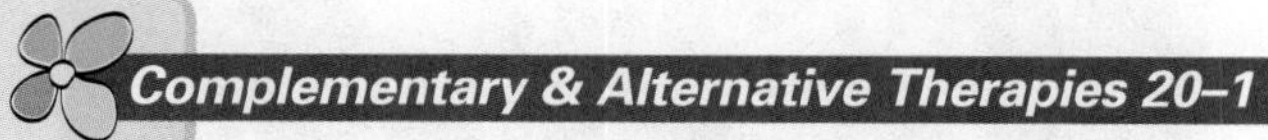

Complementary & Alternative Therapies 20–1

Herbs and Supplements that Naturally Lower Cholesterol

The following have been found to lower cholesterol in patients with hyperlipidemia.

- Garlic
- Niacin (nicotinic acid)
- Omega-3 fatty acids
- Red rice yeast
- Milk thistle
- Fiber
- Phytosterols
- Soy
- Coenzyme Q_{10}

Patients who choose to use these substances should check for interactions with other medications they are taking. Some of the substances just lower cholesterol and LDL; others raise HDL.

Nutritional Therapies 20–1

Ways to Lower Fat and Cholesterol in the Diet

When trying to lower your total cholesterol, LDL, and triglyceride levels, the following actions will help.

- Avoid all fried foods; trim fat from meat and stick to 3-oz portions of meat per meal (a piece the size of a deck of cards). Remove skin from poultry.
- Eat fish with omega-3 fatty acids at least twice a week (salmon, mackerel, tuna).
- Use egg whites or Egg Beaters as cholesterol-free egg substitutes, both for breakfast cooking and in recipes.
- Decrease or eliminate all commercial baked goods containing *trans* fat, saturated fat, or high levels of fat. Check the labels. Pies, doughnuts, croissants, and pastries are very high in fat.
- Use unsaturated fats for home baking and cooking. Avoid palm oil, coconut oil, kernel oil, lard, bacon fat, and hydrogenated vegetable shortening. Use olive oil whenever possible in salad dressings and for cooking. Do not use cube margarine as it contains *trans* fats.
- Microwave bacon on paper towels to decrease the amount of fat; use turkey bacon rather than regular bacon.
- Check the amount of fat in cheeses and choose the lower-fat varieties. Eat only small amounts of cheese.
- Drink nonfat milk and use a nondairy, no-cholesterol creamer if you must have creamer in your coffee.
- Decrease the use of all dairy products and use only the low-fat or nonfat varieties.
- Eat more high-fiber whole grains and vegetables.

Clinical Cues

- Because statins can injure muscle tissue and are toxic to the liver in some patients, blood should be drawn for levels of CK, an enzyme released from damaged muscle, and for liver enzymes. Elevated liver enzymes may indicate toxic damage to the liver.
- Patients should be told to report any unexplained muscle tenderness or pain persisting for more than a few days. Baseline blood values should be obtained before therapy when a statin drug is begun. Repeat laboratory tests for liver enzymes are recommended every 1 to 2 months for the first 18 months of therapy.
- Grapefruit juice should not be consumed when taking a statin drug. Grapefruit juice interferes with the metabolism of the drug, which can lead to increased serum levels and risk of toxicity (Skidmore, 2007).

Health Promotion Points 20–1

Healthy People 2010 Cardiovascular Health

Healthy People 2010 *is a government initiative to encourage positive health practices and outcomes among American citizens. Selected objectives related to cardiovascular health include:*

12.1	Decrease coronary heart disease deaths
12.2	Increase proportion of adults age 20 years or older who are aware of the early warning signs of heart attack and the importance of accessing rapid emergency care by calling 911
12.6	Decrease hospitalization of older adults with congestive heart failure as a primary diagnosis
12.9	Decrease proportion of adults with hypertension
12.13	Decrease mean total blood cholesterol levels among adults
12.15	Increase proportion of adults who had their cholesterol levels checked in the past 5 years
12.16	Increase proportion of adults with coronary artery disease with LDL level <100 mg/dL www.healthypeople.gov
22.1	Decrease proportion of adults who engage in no leisure-time physical activity
22.2	Increase proportion of adults who engage regularly, preferably daily, in moderate physical activity for at least 20 minutes per day

ANGINA PECTORIS

Etiology and Pathophysiology

Angina pectoris (chest pain) occurs when blood supply to the heart is decreased or totally obstructed. The ischemia of the heart tissue causes pain. Angina may be caused by atherosclerosis or arterial spasm.

The decreased blood flow that occurs when the coronary arteries are partially or totally obstructed causes pain due to ischemia of the myocardial tissue. The resulting chest pain is known as *angina pectoris.* Decreased blood flow is caused by atherosclerotic plaque narrowing the artery or by arterial spasm. Any activity that increases the heart's workload increases its need for oxygen. When the occluded coronary arteries cannot deliver adequate amounts of blood to meet these needs, the patient experiences an angina attack. Attacks can be precipitated by physical exertion, emotional excitement, eating a heavy meal, exposure to cold, infection, or any disorder or activity that increases the oxygen demand and consumption or decreases the availability of oxygen to the myocardial tissue.

When the patient's angina is no longer adequately controlled by medication and her attacks become more frequent or severe, surgery may be indicated to prevent a life-threatening MI.

Signs, Symptoms, and Diagnosis

The type of pain or discomfort may vary in individuals, but in most cases it is described as a dull pain or tightness under the sternum or pain that radiates to the neck or jaw. The pain may also radiate down one or both arms. It most commonly radiates down the left arm. The patient may experience dyspnea, pallor or flushing of the face, profuse perspiration, apprehension, and nausea and vomiting. Angina is most often described as a dull ache and is seldom sharp or stabbing. There are three types of angina:

- **Stable or exertional angina:** Triggered by physical activity or stress, and is related to atherosclerosis. Goal of therapy is to reduce intensity and frequency of attacks.
- **Variant or vasospastic angina:** Caused by coronary artery spasms that restrict the blood flow to the myocardium. The goal of treatment is to reduce the number and severity of attacks.
- **Unstable angina:** Medical emergency. Usually caused by occlusion of coronary arteries. May not respond to drug therapy. Morphine sulfate often used for the pain.

Medical diagnosis is established on the basis of history, clinical signs and symptoms, and whether rest and nitroglycerin provide relief during an acute attack. Response of the heart muscle to increased oxygen demands can be determined by exercise stress testing. Cardiac catheterization with coronary angiography may be performed (Figure 20–3). Echocardiography may be ordered to rule out a valve disorder or to evaluate left ventricular function. Laboratory levels of blood lipids will be ordered, and cardiac enzymes may be ordered to rule out an MI. An electrocardiogram is a standard diagnostic procedure.

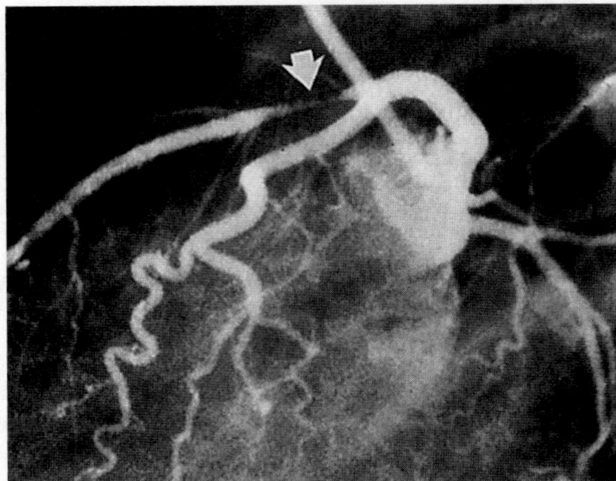

FIGURE 20–3 Stenosis *(arrow)* of the left anterior descending coronary artery.

Treatment

The treatment of angina pectoris is mostly symptomatic, with emphasis on eliminating those factors that are known to precipitate an attack in the individual patient. With guidance and teaching, the patient may soon be able to correlate certain activities with an attack and thereby learn to avoid one whenever possible. Medications commonly used for patients with angina are presented in Table 19–3. Nitroglycerin, nitrates, calcium antagonists, and beta blockers are used in combination with drugs to lower cholesterol and prevent platelet aggregation. A low daily dose of aspirin (81 mg or 325 mg) may be prescribed for the treatment of CAD. Aspirin helps prevent clotting and may prevent a thrombus that could cause an MI (*ACP Journal Club 88,* Nov/Dec., 2001). If the patient is allergic to aspirin, clopidogrel (Plavix) is prescribed. Nitroglycerin administered sublingually is the most common drug for treatment of angina. An aerosol spray and a buccal form of the drug are also available.

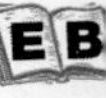

Nursing Management

You should assess thoroughly a patient experiencing chest pain to collect data that assist in determining the type of angina the patient is experiencing. Patients with a history of angina may experience increased episodes when exposed to very cold environments. Externally cold temperatures result in vasoconstriction. The patient should be instructed to wear warm clothing when exposed to cold and may consider remaining indoors when the weather is extremely cold. See Patient Teaching 20–1 for teaching guidelines for patients who experience angina. Nursing interventions for selected problems related to angina pectoris are summarized in Nursing Care Plan 20–1.

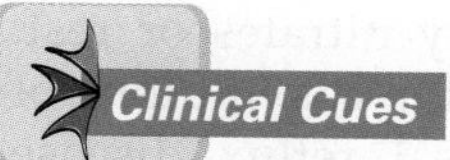

Sublingual nitroglycerin is the standard treatment for an anginal attack. The tablets should be kept in a cool, dark place and should be carried by the patient at all times. If the mouth is dry, a sip of water should be taken before placing the tablet under the tongue. If possible, the patient should lie down when using nitroglycerin. In the hospital, a baseline blood pressure should be measured, a tablet given, and then the pressure should be checked again in 5 minutes. If the pain has not eased or the pressure has risen, another tablet is placed under the tongue. Check the blood pressure again in 5 minutes. The blood pressure should decrease. If it has not or if the pain is still present, administer a third sublingual tablet at the end of 15 minutes from the first tablet. Notify the physician immediately if the pain worsens or does not resolve after the three tablets. If oxygen is available, administer it according to hospital policy while waiting for communication from the physician.

ACUTE MYOCARDIAL INFARCTION

About 1,300,000 Americans suffer an MI annually. Although male victims outnumber females almost 2 to 1, females die more frequently after an MI. According to the American Heart Association, heart disease is the leading cause of death among American women, claiming about 500,000 lives each year. The incidence of heart disease, including MI, continues to rise among women. Women are more likely to experience heart attacks after reaching menopause; however, poor dietary habits, sedentary lifestyle, and increased levels of stress contribute to development of cardiovascular disease earlier in life for an increasing number of women.

Etiology and Pathophysiology

An MI may be caused by thrombosis due to atherosclerosis, embolus from somewhere else in the body that blocks a coronary artery, or sustained arterial spasm in a coronary artery. An embolus may result from atrial fibrillation or valvular disease. Whatever the cause, blood flow is stopped to a portion of the myocardium. MI occurs most often in those older than age 45.

An **infarction** is an area of necrosis in tissue caused by an obstruction to the flow of blood to that area for a prolonged period (Figure 20–4). *Myocardial* means "pertaining to the heart muscle." In an MI, there is an area of necrosis (cell death) in the heart muscle. That portion of the heart muscle cannot contract normally to help pump blood out of the heart. Dead tissue does not return to normal and scar tissue forms and interferes with the normal functions of pumping and electrical conduction. Obstruction of blood flow in the coronary arteries may be caused by thrombosis, embolus, or severe arterial spasm. Most cases are related to obstruction from atherosclerosis.

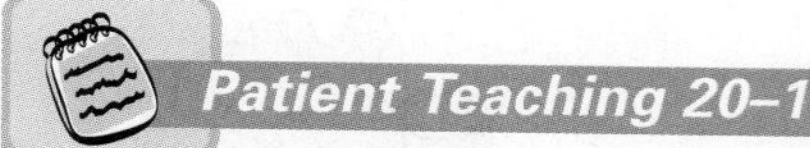

Guidelines for the Patient with Angina

Patients who experience anginal attacks are taught to:
- Avoid eating heavy meals.
- Avoid physical activity for an hour after meals to prevent excessive oxygen demands.
- Take nitroglycerin before heavy physical activity that is known to cause an attack, such as intercourse or sports activities.
- Avoid exposure to cold; do not walk into a cold wind.
- Decrease controllable risk factors, such as lifestyle stress, obesity, hypertension, and improper diet.
- Adopt a graduated exercise program.
- Stop smoking.
- Learn meditation or other deep relaxation techniques.
- Take a sublingual nitroglycerin tablet and lie down at the beginning of an anginal attack. Make certain that the tablet produces a tingling sensation where it contacts mucous membrane. Nitroglycerin may be repeated twice more at 5-minute intervals for a total of three tablets if the pain persists. If the pain has not eased within 15 minutes, call 911, and notify the physician.
- Check pulse rate once daily if taking a calcium channel blocker or a beta-adrenergic blocker. These drugs should never be stopped abruptly; call physician if heart rate drops below 60 beats per minute.
- Rise slowly from a supine or sitting position because of potential postural hypotension.
- Cleanse area of previous application of nitroglycerin paste when applying a new dose.
- Keep appointments for regular checkups.
- Obtain sufficient rest daily.
- Avoid high environmental temperatures and high humidity; stay in air-conditioned areas when such conditions occur as they increase cardiac workload.
- Nitrates may initially cause a headache and hypotension.

The prognosis of the patient who suffers an acute MI depends on the size of the artery obstructed, the location, and the amount of heart tissue that is damaged. If a large area of the heart is affected, instant death may occur. Smaller ischemic areas may heal if treated promptly and effectively. Patients whose bodies have a strong compensatory mechanism may have a well-developed collateral circulation that delays or prevents the occurrence of MI over time. As the coronary vessels narrow, small blood vessels are formed that supply oxygen to the myocardium. A patient with a well-established collateral circulation may experience milder heart attacks with fewer complications. Most MIs occur in the left ventricle, the main "pump."

Signs and Symptoms

The clinical picture presented by the patient with an acute MI is one that most people recognize as a "heart attack." There is a sudden, severe pain in the chest, usually described as tightness, pressure, squeezing,

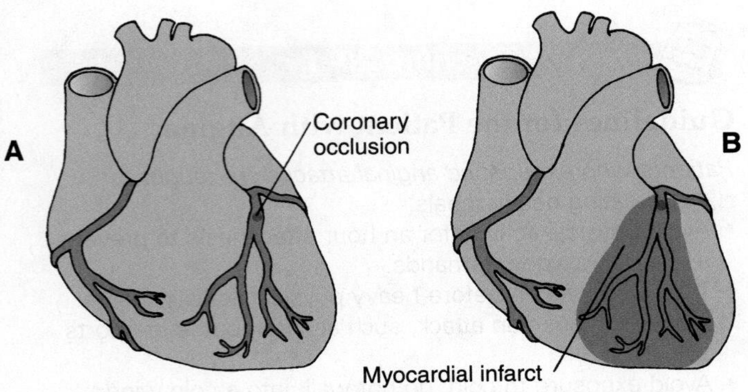

FIGURE **20–4** Occlusion of a major coronary artery **(A)** leads to area of infarct, **(B)** resulting from ischemia.

or crushing that is not relieved by nitrates or rest. Sometimes the pain is mistaken for a symptom of acute indigestion, gastroesophageal reflux disease (GERD), or anginal pain the patient has experienced before. The patient also shows symptoms of dyspnea, nausea with or without vomiting, or wheezing. Signs of shock, with pallor, profuse sweating, and anxiety may occur. The heart rate may be very fast (tachycardia) or very slow (bradycardia), or the pulse may be irregular. In older adults, the attack may present as fatigue, syncope, or weakness. Women often complain of recent episodes of extreme fatigue, with inability to complete daily activities without prolonged

NURSING CARE PLAN 20–1

Care of the Patient with Angina

SCENARIO Mrs. Ralston, age 63, is admitted to the telemetry unit. She has a history of chest pain and dyspnea precipitated by physical or emotional exertion. Her BMI is 30, and she has a history of smoking two packs of cigarettes per day for 40 years. She is admitted for control of chest pain and evaluation of cardiac status. Cardiac enzymes are negative for MI.

PROBLEM/NURSING DIAGNOSIS *Chest pain unrelieved by sublingual nitroglycerin*/Acute pain related to cardiac ischemia.

Supporting assessment data *Subjective:* States she took five nitroglycerin tablets before admission with no relief of chest pain. *Objective:* BP 100/70, HR 90, R. 26. O_2 Sat 92% on 5 L oxygen via nasal cannula.

Goals/Expected Outcomes	*Nursing Interventions*	*Selected Rationale*	*Evaluation*
Pain will be relieved within 15 min by sublingual nitroglycerin	Assess level and duration of angina.	Determines severity of pain and need for additional intervention.	Pain relieved after two nitroglycerin tablets 5 min apart.
	Teach to notify nurse and lie down and rest when pain occurs.	Early intervention for pain relief and assessment of change in condition.	Blood pressure maintained within 4 mm Hg of beginning of episode.
	Assess vital signs during episodes of angina and medication administration.	Recognize side effects, such as hypotension and patient's response to treatment.	Continue plan.

PROBLEM/NURSING DIAGNOSIS *Apprehensive concerning upcoming tests and possible change in condition*/Anxiety related to diagnostic tests and recurrent chest pain.

Supporting assessment data *Subjective:* Asks, "Are you sure I didn't have a heart attack this time?" *Objective:* Scheduled for cardiac catheterization in the A.M.

Goals/Expected Outcomes	*Nursing Interventions*	*Selected Rationale*	*Evaluation*
Patient will verbalize that anxiety has decreased within 12 hr	Assess level of anxiety. Administer medication if appropriate.	Increased anxiety can precipitate episodes of angina.	Required Valium 5 mg PO for anxiety.
	Allow patient opportunity to express concerns.	Active listening will help to reduce patient's anxiety.	Patient verbalized fear of dying from heart attack or complications of procedures.
Patient will verbalize understanding of cardiac catheterization	Provide information related to cardiac catheterization.	Adults desire straightforward information concerning their medical status.	Verbalized understanding of procedure. Some anxiety.
	Answer questions or refer to appropriate health care provider as needed.	Provides level of control for decision making.	Reevaluate and continue plan.

NURSING CARE PLAN 20-1

Care of the Patient with Angina—cont'd

PROBLEM/NURSING DIAGNOSIS *BMI 30, cholesterol level 235*/Deficient knowledge related to lack of understanding impact of diet on medical condition or methods to improve cardiac health.

Supporting assessment data *Subjective:* "I just can't exercise, and I don't understand how to choose and cook foods without salt or frying." *Objective:* Wt. 195 lb, elevated cholesterol, resting HR 98.

Goals/Expected Outcomes	Nursing Interventions	Selected Rationale	Evaluation
Within 2 days, patient will be able to verbalize how to choose and prepare foods that are low in fat and sodium	Assess current knowledge of food content and reading food levels.	Provides starting point for teaching.	Patient able to choose low-fat and low-sodium foods from a menu list.
	Refer to dietitian and reinforce teaching.	Expert knowledge of dietitian needed to determine caloric needs and develop nutrition plan.	Still voices concern these foods will not be enjoyable and remainder of family will not eat them.
	Determine if patient is candidate for cardiac rehabilitation program. Make referral after collaboration with physician.	Provide structured, monitored exercise program that also includes dietary and emotional counseling.	States she will consider participation in a cardiac rehab program if funds are available. Reevaluate plan, refer to social services for assistance with financial concerns. Collaborate with patient and physician about evaluation of emotional status that may interfere with ability to remain compliant.

PROBLEM/NURSING DIAGNOSIS *Has not quit smoking and has recurrent episodes of angina*/Risk for injury related to continued cigarette smoking.

Supporting assessment data *Subjective:* "I have tried to quit smoking but it just doesn't work."

Goals/Expected Outcomes	Nursing Interventions	Selected Rationale	Evaluation
Patient will agree to enter a community smoking cessation program	Assess willingness to reduce amount of or stop smoking.	Patient must be internally motivated for optimal success.	Patient states she had tried many times to stop smoking with limited success.
	Teach complications related to heart disease and smoking.	Provide understanding of role of smoking and vasoconstriction that lead to episodes of angina.	States she understands need to quit smoking and the impact smoking has on her health.
	Refer to social services for community programs available.	Social services personnel are aware of community resources that can benefit patient care.	Identified smoking cessation program within patient's neighborhood in nearby church. Patient states she will contact program before discharge. Continue plan.

? CRITICAL THINKING QUESTIONS

1. What are five risk factors for coronary artery disease? What are complications?
2. List the three types of angina. Which category would you place Mrs. Ralston? Why?
3. Provide a teaching plan for a patient with angina. Include commonly used medication administration and side effects.
4. What is the most commonly used medication for angina/chest pain? How should it be administered?

rest periods. These episodes may be accompanied by chest pressure, followed by eventual return to full energy state. Feelings of "indigestion" are common. **A woman may never experience typical chest pain during an MI.** Denial is a real factor in seeking treatment (Rosenfeld, 2005).

Think Critically About . . . A patient experiences chest pain. The physician orders lab studies. Which results may indicate MI versus an episode of angina?

Although these symptoms are usually present in an acute MI, they are not always severe, and in some cases patients have described their pain as mild. Sometimes the patient only experiences pain in the left arm, jaw, or back.

Diagnosis

The ECG may or may not show evidence of an MI initially. For this reason ECGs are repeated serially every 8 to 12 hours for three times or on a daily basis for 3 days. Changes slowly evolve and will occur in the QRS complex, ST segment, and T wave when ischemia or damaged tissue occurs. The severity of the symptoms will depend on the size of the area of ischemia or infarction. When there is necrotic tissue anywhere in the body, the white cell count increases and the sedimentation rate rises. Within 24 hours of an acute attack, the temperature of the patient with MI rises slightly, and mild leukocytosis appears.

In addition to the clinical manifestations, ECG changes, and other diagnostic tests, laboratory determinations of specific enzymes are used to establish a diagnosis of MI and evaluate the extent of damage done to the heart muscle. Troponin levels are the preferred biomarker for diagnosis. Serum troponin T and troponin I are also accurate within a few hours. Troponin is found only in cardiac tissue. CK isoenzymes, lactic dehydrogenase (LDH), and LDH isoenzyme levels are observed over a 72-hour period. The CK is fractionalized into CK-MB, an enzyme that is only found in heart muscle. They are 100% accurate from 10 to 120 hours after symptom onset. The level of CK-MB rises in 4 to 8 hours and begins to decline in 12 to 24 hours; LDH level increases 24 to 48 hours after an MI and stays high for up to 2 weeks. The most significant lab finding for diagnosis of MI is an elevated troponin level, especially if accompanied by an elevated CK-MB.

The albumin cobalt-binding (ACB) test is new. Albumin structures change when an MI occurs. The test measures how much cobalt is bound to albumin. The test is used in conjunction with the ECG and troponin testing.

Safety Alert 20–1

Contrast Dye

When your patient has received a contrast dye for a diagnostic test, promote good hydration either by oral or IV fluids. Keeping the patient hydrated will increase the rate of urine flow, dilute the urine, and help prevent kidney damage as the dye is excreted.

Think Critically About . . . How would you prepare the patient who has experienced a probable MI for the diagnostic tests she will most likely undergo? What teaching is required?

Cardiac catheterization and angiography may be done soon after the patient is admitted to the emergency room if MI is the probable diagnosis. This provides immediate, definitive diagnosis and treatment for occluded vessels. The nurse must thoroughly assess the status of the patient after cardiac catheterization. The patient must remain flat for 4 to 8 hours after the procedure and avoid flexing the hip joint on the access leg (usually the right leg). Distal pulses on the affected leg must be assessed frequently and the groin area must be assessed for presence of hemorrhage or a hematoma. Renal function should be monitored because of potential adverse effects of contrast dyes used during the procedure (Safety Alert 20-1).

After the patient is stabilized, further testing will be done. Chest x-ray, magnetic resonance imaging (MRI), echocardiography, and a technetium-99m sestamibi scan may be performed to determine the full extent of the infarction.

Treatment

In many large cities and some rural areas of the United States, there are specially designed and equipped mobile units staffed with trained personnel to give immediate care to the patient who has had a heart attack. Chewing an aspirin when signs of an MI occur has been adopted as part of the emergency treatment protocol to decrease or prevent heart damage by decreasing platelet aggregation (American Heart Association, 2002).

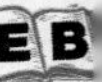

Outside the hospital a trained emergency response team should be called immediately. If the patient shows signs of cardiac or respiratory arrest, help should be called and cardiopulmonary resuscitation (CPR) with defibrillation, if indicated, should be started immediately. Many public areas, such as airports and shopping malls, have automated external defibrillators (AED) available. These can be used by individuals trained in CPR to detect and treat shockable rhythms until emergency personnel are on the scene.

As soon as a patient with an acute MI is brought to the emergency room, measures are taken to relieve pain, decrease ischemia, and prevent further circulatory collapse and shock. Patients who present to the emergency room with symptoms of heart attack are triaged and treated immediately. The MONA (morphine, oxygen, nitrates, aspirin) regimen is initiated (Bull & Willcox, 2002). Oxygen via nasal cannula or mask is started, intravenous (IV) access is obtained for administration of fluids and emergency drugs, and the patient is placed on a cardiac monitor. Pain medication is given along with an aspirin of 160 to 325 mg to chew. A thorough cardiac history is obtained. Emergency care and CPR are of critical importance in preventing death from an MI.

Sublingual nitroglycerin is given unless contraindicated. Drugs administered to control pain in a patient with acute MI are morphine sulfate, or hydromorphone hydrochloride (Dilaudid). One of these is given IV to provide immediate relief; morphine is the drug of choice because of its vasodilation property. A nitrate infusion also may be started. Antidysrhythmia drugs are given as indicated by ECG-abnormal rhythms. Antianxiety agents, such as lorazepam (Ativan), are administered to relieve anxiety.

Close assessment of respiration is essential, as the drugs for pain can depress respiration at a time when the heart's oxygen demand is increased. Pulse oximetry is instituted quickly to measure oxygen saturation. **Pain medication given IV has a shorter duration, and doses must be repeated more frequently to keep the patient comfortable.**

If the patient sought immediate medical attention upon experiencing the symptoms of MI, she may be given thrombolytic agents in an attempt to dissolve a clot obstructing the coronary artery. Thrombolytic therapy must be started within 12 hours to prevent necrosis of the myocardium and is indicated when the ECG shows ST-segment elevation. Agents used IV to dissolve the clot include alteplase (t-PA, Activase), streptokinase, tenecteplase (TNKase), and reteplase (Retavase). These drugs are contraindicated in patients who have severe, uncontrolled hypertension or a history of a hemorrhagic stroke, gastrointestinal (GI) bleed, intracranial or intraspinal surgery within the past 2 months, a brain tumor, arteriovenous malformation, or aneurysm. After one of these agents is infused, a heparin drip may be started to prevent reocclusion. Heparin is continued for 3 to 4 days until the patient is stabilized on warfarin sodium (Coumadin), an oral anticoagulant. When a patient is not a candidate for thrombolytic therapy, heparin and low-dose aspirin may be administered to prevent further thrombosis.

If there is ST-segment elevation and the clinical picture indicates that there is complete occlusion of a coronary artery, the patient may immediately undergo cardiac catheterization and balloon angioplasty with placement of stents to restore blood flow.

Acute Care. If myocardial damage is less extensive, the patient may be admitted to a telemetry unit. If damage is considered extensive, admission to the intensive care unit (ICU) or coronary care unit (CCU) is the rule. Generally the patient is kept in the ICU/CCU for 1 to 2 days, then on a step-down telemetry unit for 2 to 4 days unless damage is very extensive and the patient is unstable. The patient is placed in bed and kept on bed rest with bedside commode privileges for 12 to 24 hours. Physical activity is gradually increased according to the patient's individual condition and response to therapy. An IV line or a saline lock is inserted to provide a route for administration of emergency drugs to control blood pressure and dysrhythmias.

Vital signs are continuously monitored by electronic means and are assessed every 15 minutes to 2 hours. Blood pressure, heart rate, mean arterial pressure, and oxygen saturation are also monitored electronically. Continuous ECG (cardiac telemetry monitoring) is essential to provide an accurate evaluation of the status of the heart. Death occurs most frequently within the first 2 hours and is due to ventricular fibrillation. Many complications can occur, and you must be vigilant for the onset of their signs and symptoms.

While in ICU/CCU, a pulmonary artery flow-directed catheter (Swan-Ganz type) may be inserted to read central venous pressure (CVP), pulmonary artery pressure (PAP), and pulmonary capillary wedge pressure (PCWP), which give a better picture of the injured heart's ability to pump. The patient may be placed NPO or on a liquid diet for the first 24 hours. Then a low-sodium, low-fat diet is ordered when the patient's vital signs have stabilized. A stool softener is given to decrease the risk of bradycardia, which can be caused by straining to have a bowel movement. Potassium and magnesium are monitored closely as imbalances can cause dysrhythmias. Medication to correct dysrhythmia is ordered as needed. Measures to correct acid-base imbalance are begun. A beta-adrenergic blocker, such as metoprolol (Toprol XL, Lopressor), may be ordered to decrease the heart's workload. An angiotensin-converting enzyme (ACE) inhibitor such as captopril (Capoten) may also be prescribed. Continuous oxygen via mask or nasal cannula is begun at a rate of 2 to 5 L/minute. Various IV drugs may be used to regulate blood pressure or to control dysrhythmias; these include sodium nitroprusside (Nitropressin) to lower blood pressure and dobutamine (Dobutrex) to raise blood pressure.

A temporary pacemaker may be inserted if the patient's heart rate drops below 40 and remains there, or if she experiences complete heart block where the electrical impulse does not go through the atrioventricular (AV) node to the ventricles and the ventricles are not signaled to contract (see Chapter 19).

If only a few areas of stenosis are identified, the patient may have a percutaneous transluminal coronary angioplasty (PTCA) rather than coronary artery bypass graft surgery (CABG) to improve blood flow. PTCA is a nonsurgical technique to open blocked coronary arteries. It is performed in the cardiac catheterization laboratory using fluoroscopy. A catheter with a balloon attachment is threaded into the blocked artery, and when the narrowed area is reached, the balloon is inflated, flattening the plaque and widening the interior of the artery. A **drug-eluting stent** (continually releases an anticoagulant/antiplatelet drug) may be left in place to help maintain the opening (Figure 20–5). A stent is made of stainless steel and acts as a brace for the artery wall. Research had shown that the drug-eluting stents may reduce the need to restent the vessels over time because of cellular hyperplasia as the body adjusts to the foreign body. Newer research is questioning this assertion. As the tissue surrounding the traditional stent increases, reocclusion occurs. Some stents are coated with paclitaxel, a drug that interferes with the process of cellular proliferation, thus reducing the risk of the stent becoming occluded. Concerns have been expressed concerning the safety of drug-eluting stents because of increased incidence of thrombus, MI, and death following the procedure. Additional research has been inconclusive related to effectiveness and safety (Stone et al., 2007). Abciximab (ReoPro), tirofiban (Aggrastat), or eptifibatide (Integrilin) is given to reduce platelet aggregation for up to 48 hours after stent placement to prevent cardiac ischemia. When a stent is placed, the patient must take antiplatelet agents, such as aspirin, or clopidogrel (Plavix) for up to 1 year following placement. Another procedure, called *rotoablation,* uses a similar catheter and a rotating device that shaves away plaque and extracts it to clear the artery. This is sometimes used when a patient has reocclusion after CABG and PTCA. CABG surgery is covered in the section on cardiac surgery.

Studies are ongoing to determine whether a regimen consisting of a very–low-fat diet, regular exercise, reduction of stress, and practice of relaxation techniques can reverse CAD without surgery. These methods have been effective in people who can maintain the discipline to stick to the program.

If the left ventricle is badly damaged, cardiogenic shock may occur and the intraaortic balloon pump (IABP) may be used to ease the heart's workload while it begins to heal. This device uses a balloon catheter positioned in the aorta that inflates during diastole and deflates during systole, effectively decreasing the workload of the heart and increasing blood flow through the coronary arteries. This procedure is done while the patient is in ICU/CCU. Only registered nurses who are certified in the care of the patient on an IABP are assigned to care for these patients.

Nursing Management

All patients with heart disease should be taught the signs of MI and advised that the best survival rate is directly related to obtaining medical attention as early as possible.

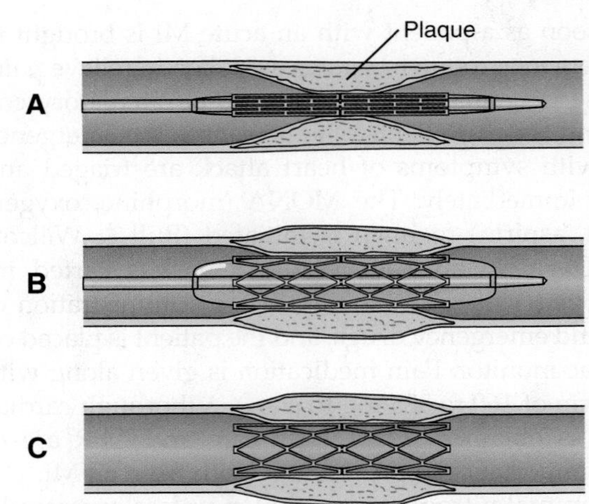

FIGURE 20–5 Placement of coronary artery stent. **A,** The stent is positioned at the site of stenotic lesion. **B,** The balloon is inflated, expanding the stent. The balloon is then deflated and removed. **C,** The implanted stent is left in place.

Nursing care is directed toward:

- Promoting rest.
- Administering ordered medical therapy and observing for side effects.
- Assisting with activities of daily living (ADLs) and ambulation.
- Monitoring physical status by performing a thorough cardiovascular assessment every 4 to 8 hours, and monitoring vital signs every 2 to 4 hours.
- Recording daily weight and comparing with previous weight. Intake and output are accurately recorded and compared with previous amounts and urine output is closely monitored.
- Maintaining a patent IV access at all times.
- Limiting visitors and monitoring the heart rate closely during visits.
- Monitoring for signs of complications of MI, such as dysrhythmia, congestive heart failure (CHF), pulmonary edema, pericarditis, cardiogenic shock, or cardiac arrest (Table 20–3). Quick identification and treatment of complications is life-saving and greatly reduces the cost of treatment during recovery.
- Decreasing anxiety and stress for the patient. It is helpful to explain the function of all equipment and tests in simple terms. Explain also the routine of frequent assessment and tests so the patient will know what to expect. You will need to help decrease the family's anxiety by reinforcing what the physician has told them about the patient's condition and treatment.

Through its local chapters, the American Heart Association provides an abundance of written material designed for the person recovering from an MI. Patients and their families should know about this valuable source of information and support as they work toward the goal of rehabilitation.

Intermediate Care. As the patient recovers from the acute phase of her illness, she is quickly weaned

Table 20–3 Signs and Symptoms of Complications after Myocardial Infarction

COMPLICATION	SIGNS AND SYMPTOMS
Dysrhythmia	Irregular pulse; abnormal ECG pattern. Report more than three PVCs per minute, heart rate of <120 or >40 bpm.
CHF	Dyspnea; pedal edema; sacral edema; crackles in lung bases; distended neck veins; enlarged, tender liver; weight gain of more than 2 lb in 24 hr.
Pulmonary edema	Crackles throughout lungs; severe dyspnea and orthopnea; frothy sputum; high anxiety; feelings of impending doom.
Cardiogenic shock	Significant drop in systolic blood pressure (>20 points); diaphoresis; rapid pulse; cold, clammy skin; gray skin; restlessness.
Pericarditis	Pericardial friction rub upon auscultation; chest pain aggravated by movement and lessened by sitting up and leaning forward.

away from intensive care. When very frequent assessment and monitoring are no longer essential and the patient is able to participate in her personal hygiene activities without detrimental effects on the healing heart tissues, she is transferred out of ICU/CCU into a telemetry, or "step-down," medical unit. For some patients, this move is frightening because they know they will no longer have a nurse giving constant attention. Every effort is made to assure the patient that she is making progress toward recovery and no longer needs intensive care. While the patient is on the telemetry unit, physical activities are gradually increased according to ability to tolerate exercise, as evidenced by stable heart rate, blood pressure, and respiratory rate. There is close monitoring for subjective and objective symptoms of excessive strain on the heart, such as dysrhythmia or dyspnea, or the development of complications.

These measures may minimize damage from an MI, but the patient still has CAD, requires treatment, and must attend to lowering her risk factors.

Rehabilitation

As the patient gains an understanding of her illness and ways in which she can help herself toward recovery, she should become more confident and optimistic about her condition. Realization that one has suffered a serious heart attack is frightening. You will see a variety of emotional and behavioral responses (Box 20–1). The patient and her family will need much help and support as they work to make the necessary adjustments.

Many hospitals offer an outpatient cardiac rehabilitation program to help the patient make lifestyle changes to reduce future risk of cardiac problems. The program provides counseling on dietary changes for a heart-healthy diet; stress-reduction techniques; reduction of risk factors, such as avoiding tobacco use; controlling hypertension and diabetes; and a supervised exercise program with continuous ECG monitoring for 4 to 6 weeks. Progressive, supervised exercise is continued for an additional 6 to 8 weeks, and then a maintenance program is devised that the patient can do independently. Research has shown that women and ethnic minorities are less likely to access or complete cardiac

Box 20–1 Emotional and Behavioral Responses to Acute Myocardial Infarction

DENIAL
- May have history of ignoring symptoms related to heart disease
- Minimizes severity of medical condition
- Ignores activity restrictions
- Avoids discussing MI or its significance

ANGER
- Is commonly expressed as, "Why did this happen to me?"
- May be directed at family, staff, or medical regimen

ANXIETY AND FEAR
- Fears death and long-term disability
- Overtly manifests apprehension, restlessness, insomnia, tachycardia
- Less overtly manifests increased verbalization, projection of feelings to others, hypochondriasis
- Fears activity, recurrent heart attacks, and sudden death

DEPENDENCY
- Is totally reliant on staff
- Is unwilling to perform tasks or activities unless approved by heath care provider
- Wants to be monitored by ECG at all times
- Is hesitant to leave ICU or hospital

DEPRESSION
- Experiences mourning period concerning loss of health, altered body function, and changes in lifestyle
- Realizes seriousness of situation
- Begins to worry about future implications of health problem
- Shows manifestations of withdrawal, crying, anorexia, apathy
- May be more evident after discharge

REALISTIC ACCEPTANCE
- Focuses on optimum rehabilitation
- Plans changes compatible with altered cardiac function

Key: *ECG,* electrocardiogram; *ICU,* intensive care unit; *MI,* myocardial infarction.

From Lewis S.M., Heitkemper M.M., Dirksen S.R., et al. (2007). *Medical-Surgical Nursing: Assessment and Management of Clinical Problems,* (7th ed.). St Louis, Mosby.

rehabilitation programs. There has been no clear explanation for this other than income and accessibility.

One area of major concern is sexuality. The patient may be fearful of resuming intercourse, thinking that it may cause a heart attack. The spouse/partner, too, often has these fears. Both partners need reassurance that resumption of normal sexual activities will be possible. The patient may need to take a more passive role during intercourse, at least for a while, using alternate positions that cause less strain and less oxygen demand. The patient should be told that the workload of intercourse with a known partner is equal to climbing a flight of stairs. If she can climb a flight of stairs without much change in heart rate, respirations, or blood pressure, intercourse should not cause harm. The physician should discuss this area with the patient and her spouse/partner, but if she does not, you should see that the proper information is given. Sexual dysfunction may occur at first, but with patience on the part of both partners, it usually passes.

Patients should be taught to plan sexual activity for times when they are well rested and to avoid an environment that is too hot or too cold. It is best to space such activity at least 2 hours after eating a meal or drinking any alcohol. Nitroglycerin should be used prophylactically if intercourse causes angina symptoms. If angina does occur, the patient should cease activity, place a nitroglycerin tablet under her tongue, lie down, and rest. Intercourse may be resumed 3 to 6 weeks after an MI and 4 to 6 weeks after open heart surgery, depending on the patient's exercise tolerance as determined by stress testing. The target heart rate for exercise is aimed at 70% of that which the patient could safely achieve during graded exercise testing without an ischemic heart response (angina) or significant dysrhythmia.

Levels of physical activity are designated through metabolic equivalent (MET) units. One MET is the amount of oxygen needed by the body at rest. The patient's rehabilitation program slowly progresses stepwise to higher energy expenditures over a period of months. See Chapter 17, Box 17–3 for examples of activities and their MET expenditures.

Rehabilitation involves three major aspects: (1) a program of increasing activity based on the patient's individual progress and needs; (2) instruction of the patient and family about the nature of the illness and the rationale for every aspect of its management; and (3) assistance to the patient and family as they work toward the goal of accepting the limitations imposed and the changes in lifestyle that may be required.

In spite of all efforts to educate the post-MI patient about her illness and the need to continue her exercise program and modify her lifestyle, long-term continued compliance with the prescribed regimen is not as high as desired. The main purpose of instruction is to provide the patient with the information she needs to avoid the problems and complications that can occur once she leaves the structured program.

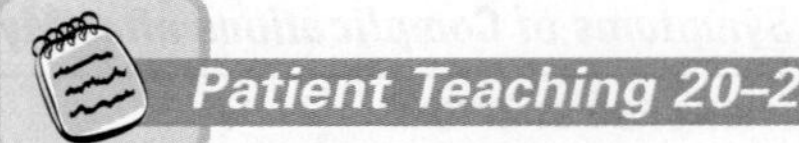

Patient Teaching 20–2

Guidelines for Recovery from an MI

Teach the patient to:

- Recognize the signs of recurrent MI and to seek immediate medical attention should they occur. These are chest pain, diaphoresis, nausea, and anxiety.
- Adopt a lifetime regular, graduated exercise program.
- Alter controllable risk factors: reach and maintain a normal weight; cease smoking; keep alcohol consumption at a moderate level (no more than 1.5 oz per day); keep cholesterol within normal limits; control hypertension.
- Reduce stress and learn relaxation techniques.
- Observe for complications, such as irregular pulse rate, dyspnea and fatigue, chest pain, and fever.
- Continue on a low-fat, low-sodium diet individualized to taste.
- Take medications as ordered and monitor for side effects.

The patient's perception of her own situation greatly influences whether she will comply with the instructions she has received for continued treatment and preventive therapy. She may not follow instructions if she does not see herself as particularly susceptible to a condition—that is, if she does not think she is at risk for complications or further damage. She must also understand the rationale for the therapy and necessary lifestyle changes (Patient Teaching 20–2).

It is important to stress to the patient that she has control over her rehabilitation and prognosis. She and her physician and other health professionals are partners in fighting the disease that has caused her problem. She alone has full control over her lifestyle changes and the treatment program. She needs to know that she is the master of her own destiny. When the patient feels that she, rather than the physician, is in control, she is much more likely to remain on the treatment program.

CARDIAC SURGERY

Until the 1950s, little could be done in the way of surgical procedures involving the heart itself because prolonged interruption of circulation meant certain death for the patient. However, with the introduction of the cardiopulmonary bypass machine and hypothermic techniques, surgeons can now repair or replace damaged valves, correct many congenital heart defects, and bypass clogged coronary arteries.

The heart-lung machine, which has many variations in design and appearance, functions as an artificial heart (pump) and lung (oxygenator). For this reason, it is sometimes called a *pump-oxygenator.* Because all this is done outside the patient's body, the procedure is called *extracorporeal circulation.* The surgeon inserts large tubes in the vena cava and reroutes the unoxygenated

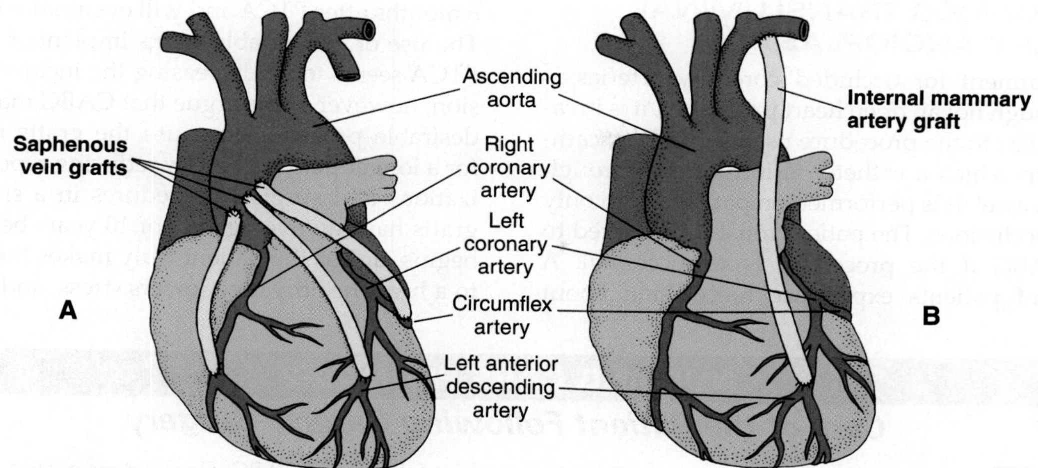

FIGURE 20–6 Two methods of coronary artery bypass grafting. **A,** Saphenous vein grafts. **B,** Internal mammary artery graft.

venous blood through the heart-lung machine. There, the blood is exposed to an atmosphere of oxygen in which an exchange of gases takes place (carbon dioxide is released and oxygen is taken up), and the oxygenated blood is returned to the patient via the femoral artery. The blood may be cooled so that the patient's body temperature is lowered (hypothermia), thereby reducing the body's metabolic needs during surgery.

Open heart surgery is performed by extracorporeal circulation or off pump and hypothermia. Congenital heart defects, valve replacements, bypass of clogged coronary arteries, and heart transplant are accomplished by open chest techniques.

CORONARY ARTERY BYPASS SURGERY

CABG is performed when angina cannot be controlled medically or to prevent more occlusions and consequent MI. The surgery bypasses the artery that is blocked, replacing it with sections of a vein or artery taken from another part of the patient's body. Usually the mammary artery or sections of saphenous vein are grafted. An end of the mammary artery is dissected and attached to beyond the stricture in a coronary artery. A saphenous graft is attached to the aorta and then to the distal portion of a coronary artery. Although the heart is not "opened," its activity often is stopped for the procedure. The patient will have a midsternal incision and, if saphenous veins were used for the grafts, will have leg incisions as well. Figure 20–6 shows CABG procedures using vein grafts or the internal mammary artery.

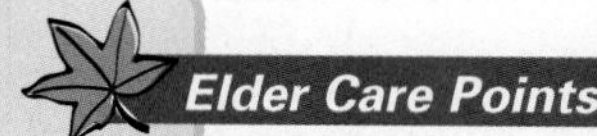

Elder Care Points

Elderly patients tolerate coronary artery bypass graft surgery well, but the recovery period is longer because of the slower healing rate and lessened ability of the body to handle this degree of physical stress.

Other techniques for CABG procedures, minimally invasive direct coronary artery bypass (MIDCAB) or off-pump coronary artery bypass (OPCAB), do not require stopping the heart's activity and therefore do not require using the heart-lung machine. These procedures are done on about 25% of patients who undergo coronary artery bypass. The procedure requires only a 3-inch incision, is performed with the use of drugs to slow or stop the heart briefly, and special instruments, and takes approximately one third the time to complete as traditional CABG. Patients may be discharged home in less than 36 hours. It is also only one third the cost of CABG. However, only patients with one or two lesions in an easily accessible area of a major coronary artery are candidates for this simplified procedure. The main advantage of this procedure is to the patient in the areas of cost, time spent in the hospital, recovery time, and avoidance of large surgical incisions. Studies have not shown that there is significant difference in outcome or prognosis between the different procedures (Plomondon et al., 2005). EB

Coronary bypass surgery is expensive, averaging $21,000 to $30,000 for surgery, anesthesia, and in-hospital care. Less invasive approaches average $3000 to $5000 less. Anginal chest pain disappears in about 65% of patients, and another 25% show improvement. There is an average of a 10-year patency rate for CABG using the left internal mammary artery and even greater success rates when the right internal mammary artery is used. Some physicians still question the benefits of such surgery compared with the cost and effectiveness of more conservative medical therapies. At present, many of those patients who had a coronary artery bypass in the past 10 years are returning for a second operation because the new arteries have become occluded. A greater emphasis is being placed on the need for dietary and exercise therapy after the procedure. Nursing Care Plan 20–2 summarizes care of the patient following cardiac surgery.

PERCUTANEOUS TRANSLUMINAL CORONARY ANGIOPLASTY

Another treatment for occluded coronary arteries is PTCA. Although not an open heart procedure, it is invasive and similar to the procedure used for cardiac catheterization, in which a catheter is introduced through the femoral vessel. It is performed on patients with only one or two occlusions. The patient must be prepared to undergo CABG if the procedure is unsuccessful. A percentage of patients experience reocclusion about 6 months after PTCA and will eventually need a CABG. The use of expandable stents implanted at the time of PTCA seems to be decreasing the incidence of reocclusion; however, some argue that CABG may be the more desirable procedure because the grafts remain patent for a longer period, thereby reducing repeated hospitalizations and surgical procedures in a short time. The grafts have an average life of 10 years before occlusion begins, unless the patient truly makes the commitment to a heart-healthy diet, lowers stress, and exercises reg-

NURSING CARE PLAN 20–2

Care of the Patient Following Cardiac Surgery

SCENARIO Mr. Jacobi, age 57, is admitted to the telemetry unit following a CABG. He is 2 days postop. Mr. Jacobi is married with three teenaged children. He plans to return to his job as a truck driver after surgical recovery.

PROBLEM/NURSING DIAGNOSIS *Unable to ambulate 50′ in the hallway without complaints of dizziness and dyspnea/* Activity intolerance related to postsurgical hemodynamic changes.

Supporting assessment data *Subjective:* States, "I'm feeling faint and short of breath" after ambulating 30′. *Objective:* RR 32, O_2 Sat. 90% after ambulating short distance. O_2 Sat. increases to 95% to 100% when returned to chair, RR decreased to 24.

Goals/Expected Outcomes	*Nursing Intervention*	*Selected Rationale*	*Evaluation*
Patient will be able to ambulate 50′ in hallway without complaints of dizziness and dyspnea	Assess O_2 Sat. and vital signs before and after ambulation.	Provides baseline values for evaluation.	O_2 Sat. 96%, no complaints of dizziness by third postop day.
	Provide safety during ambulation (e.g., follow with wheelchair, use gait belt, instruct to use handrails).	Prevent falls if hemodynamic changes occur.	Patient did not sustain fall.
	Provide rest periods every 15′.	Improve success of ambulation.	Patient able to ambulate 100′ without rest period by third postop day.
	Gradually increase distance of ambulation as condition stabilizes.	Decrease workload on heart and facilitate patient recovery.	Patient ambulated 100′ tid without complaints of dizziness and dyspnea by third postop day. Continue plan.

PROBLEM/NURSING DIAGNOSIS *Midsternal and left lower leg surgical incision*/Impaired skin integrity related to thoracotomy and saphenous vein graft.

Supporting assessment data *Subjective:* Patient asks about care of wounds to chest and left lower leg. *Objective:* Incisions to midsternum and left lower leg. Both incisions intact, no areas of redness noted.

Goals/Expected Outcomes	*Nursing Intervention*	*Selected Rationale*	*Evaluation*
Surgical incisions will remain intact and free of signs of infection	Assess and document status of incision at the beginning of each shift.	Determine changes in status of wound, such as development of redness, edema, opening of suture lines.	Midsternal incision intact, no signs of infection. Incision to left lower leg slightly edematous, ½-inch opening of wound on fourth postop day. Document and report. Continue to monitor.
	Assess vital signs, especially temperature and heart rate.	Elevated temperature and heart rate may indicate beginning of wound infection.	HR 72, T 100° F (37.8° C). Continue to monitor.
	Include wound management in discharge teaching plan.	Provides knowledge to prevent and recognize complications associated with wound healing.	Demonstrated appropriate wound care. Verbalized signs and symptoms of infection.

NURSING CARE PLAN 20–2

Care of the Patient Following Cardiac Surgery—cont'd

PROBLEM/NURSING DIAGNOSIS *Complains of incisional pain during deep-breathing exercises and use of incentive spirometer*/Acute pain related to midsternal surgical incision.

Supporting assessment data *Subjective:* States, "It hurts too much to do these breathing exercises." *Objective:* Unable to reach incentive spirometer goals. O_2 Sat 91%.

Goals/Expected Outcomes	Nursing Intervention	Selected Rationale	Evaluation
Patient will verbalize decreased pain during deep-breathing exercises	Assess pain level before deep-breathing exercises and use of incentive spirometer. Provide pain medication as needed. Teach to splint incision during respiratory exercises.	Patient will be more likely to complete exercises if he is pain free.	Completes breathing exercises without pain medication by third postop day.
Patient will reach incentive spirometer goals within 24 hr	Encourage patient to use incentive spirometer at least q 2 hr. Gradually increase goal.	Prevent postoperative respiratory complications.	Reaches 90% of incentive spirometry goal by third postop day.
O_2 Sat will remain above 95%	Monitor O_2 Sat before and after use of incentive spirometer.	Baseline values to determine effectiveness of treatment.	O_2 Sat 95% before and after use of incentive spirometer. Continue plan.

PROBLEM/NURSING DIAGNOSIS *Patient expresses concern about home care management*/Deficient knowledge related to postoperative care after discharge from hospital.

Supporting assessment data *Subjective:* States, "I don't know how I can manage all this at home. When can I return to work?" *Objective:* Patient anxious, irritable during discussion of discharge planning.

Goals/Expected Outcomes	Nursing Intervention	Selected Rationale	Evaluation
Patient will demonstrate knowledge of home care instructions including: wound management, medications, exercise, diet, ADLs, when to return to work	Assess level of understanding of discharge instructions.	Baseline for developing discharge plan.	Verbalized understanding of discharge instructions.
	Provide opportunity to verbalize concerns.	Reduces patient anxiety.	Verbalized concerns openly, stated some anxiety relieved.
	Provide instructions concerning medications, wound care, ADLs.		Demonstrated understanding of instructions.
	Refer to dietitian/nutritionist for dietary requirements.	Knowledge of expectations increases confidence and reduces anxiety.	States understands diet instructions and will attempt to follow them.
	Collaborate with physician concerning additional instructions, such as return to work and cardiac rehab recommendations.	Expert knowledge may be needed to provide appropriate information. Reinforce information as provided by physician.	Verbalized disappointment that he will be unable to return to work for at least 8 wk. May require part-time basis for longer period. Continue plan.

? CRITICAL THINKING QUESTIONS

1. List five additional nursing diagnoses that are appropriate for a patient after cardiac surgery.
2. List five additional priority assessments you should complete for this patient.

ularly. Recent research suggests patients in stable condition with minimal cardiac disease demonstrate results similar to angioplasty with conservative medical treatment alone. Patients managed medically did not experience higher incidence of MI, stroke, or other complications (Boden et al., 2007).

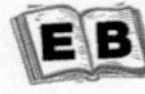

TRANSMYOCARDIAL LASER REVASCULARIZATION

Patients who are critically ill are not candidates for PTCA or CABG, but transmyocardial laser revascularization (TMR) is an option. This procedure may be available to patients with severe chest pain that limits their ability to perform ADLs, who have a history of CABG and no other treatment options. A carbon dioxide laser is used to drill tiny holes in the heart's left ventricle. These channels heal on the outside of the heart, but remain open on the inside, allowing blood to flow into the myocardium, where it was previously diminished because of blocked coronary arteries.

CARDIOMYOPLASTY

Some patients with severe CHF who are not candidates for a heart transplant are undergoing dynamic **cardiomyoplasty** using the latissimus dorsi muscle. Part of the muscle is detached from its natural position and brought around to the front of the body. It is wrapped around the heart and a pacemaker is connected to the heart and the back muscle and implanted in the abdominal wall. The pacemaker makes the muscle contract in conjunction with the normal action of the heart and thereby boosts the heart's pumping power.

VALVULOPLASTY AND VALVE REPLACEMENT

For valve stenosis, balloon **valvuloplasty** may be performed in some cases. A balloon catheter is threaded via the circulatory system through the heart and into the valve and the balloon is inflated to break open the stenosed valve. Valve replacement surgery is more commonly done although valve repair may be performed. Valve replacement can be with a mechanical or biologic device. If a biologic device is used, it may be an autologous graft, an allograft, or a xenograft (Figure 20–7). Patients who receive biologic valve replacement must remain on anticoagulants, such as warfarin (Coumadin), for about 6 months. If a mechanical device is used, anticoagulant therapy is lifelong. Mitral or aortic valve replacement is scheduled when the patient's condition prevents her from going about her usual daily activities, whether the problem is stenosis or insufficiency. Replacement is done as an open heart procedure using extracorporeal circulation with the heart-lung bypass machine and hypothermia. Valve replacements are usually performed as an open heart procedure; however, minimally invasive approaches may be an option for some patients. Mitral valve repair or replacement, and tricuspid valve replacement may be performed through a minithoracotomy. A 2-inch incision is made between the ribs to access the heart and valves. The aortic valve may be replaced through a hemisternotomy procedure. A small incision (4 to 5 inches) is made through the sternum. There is also robotic cardiac surgery. Three small incisions are made in the chest wall and instruments and cameras are placed in the cavity. The surgeon guides the robotic mechanism to perform such procedures as mitral valve repair. Preoperative and postoperative care is much the same as for CABG patients.

Open heart surgeries usually take between 3 and 6 hours, depending on the amount of repair or replacement necessary. The patient returns to the cardiac surgical intensive care unit and remains on a ventilator for 8 to 24 hours. Patient care requires highly skilled nurses, as there are multiple tubes and lines for monitoring physiologic status and for delivering drugs to control blood pressure and dysrhythmias. If the patient's recovery is uncomplicated, she will be transferred to a step-down telemetry unit 1 to 2 days after

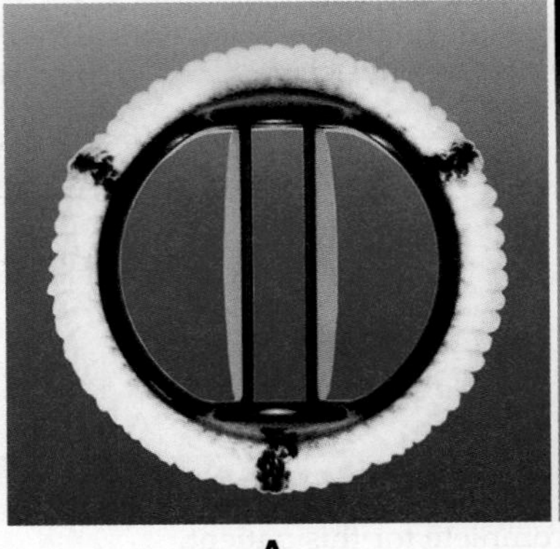

A

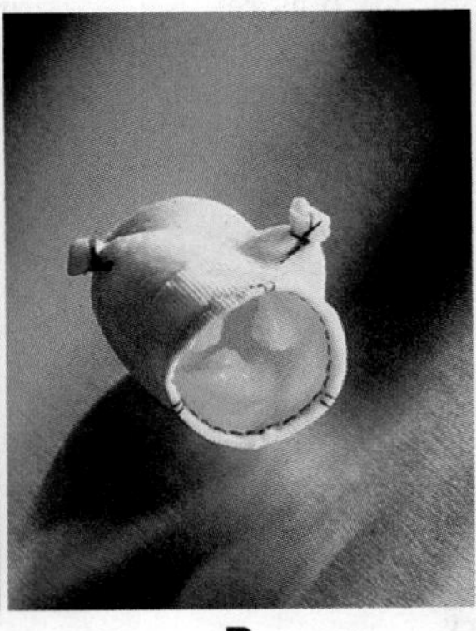

B

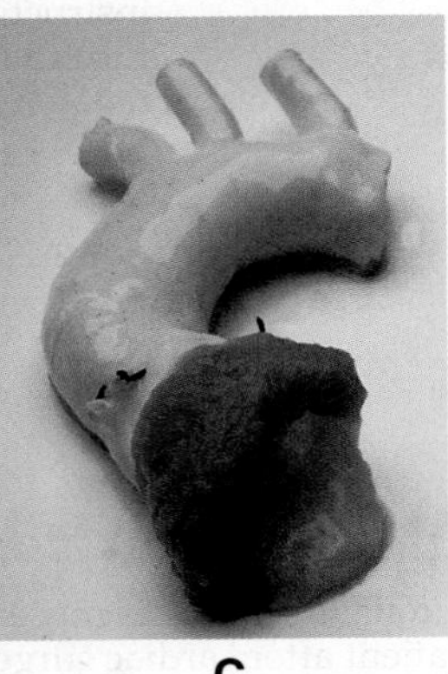

C

FIGURE **20–7** Examples of mechanical and biologic tissue valves for valve replacement. **A,** Bi-leaflet mechanical valve. **B,** Porcine heterograft. **C,** Carpentier-Edwards aortic pericardial valve.

surgery. Ventricular aneurysm resulting from an MI or trauma may be surgically repaired also.

HEART TRANSPLANT

Heart transplants are performed for selected patients who have end-stage left ventricular failure resulting from cardiomyopathy (primary myocardial disease). Ideally, candidates must be younger than age 65, have end-stage cardiac disease with predicted survival of less than 6 months, no other systemic disease, have good renal function, and be psychologically stable. Some patients may fall outside of these parameters because of other health conditions and considerations. There is some flexibility with the age requirements. Other requirements are that the patient be within 20% of ideal weight and not an active tobacco user or alcohol abuser. A history of diabetes beginning more than 10 years before or accompanying complications, or organ damage, is another contraindication. A good tissue match is essential for a transplant.

Candidates for heart transplant undergo an extensive psychological evaluation and thorough physical assessment. Patients must also be evaluated for the ability to remain in compliance with health care instructions and the ability to obtain and administer antirejection medications. Transplant patients must take immunosuppressants and other medications for the remainder of their lives. These drugs can be very expensive. Those without insurance coverage are especially at risk if unable to obtain needed medications. Very few donor hearts are available, and the waiting lists are long. A heart transplant operation takes 5 to 8 hours (Figure 20–8).

Patients who receive a heart transplant face considerable financial cost, a life of taking immunosuppressive drugs that have many serious side effects, including risk for infection, and the constant threat of organ rejection. However, the benefits are considerable with a 1-year survival rate of 80% to 90% and a 3-year survival time of about 70%. A significant number of heart transplant patients are surviving beyond 10 years.

Patients must adhere to strict dietary and exercise regimens to prevent the new heart from becoming affected with problems that led to the original heart failure. Heart transplants are performed in highly specialized medical centers. Patients who are too unstable for care in the home may remain in the hospital for an extended period until a heart is available. Other patients may be given a special pager for notification of an available heart. These patients must be available for immediate admission to the hospital. Patients awaiting a heart transplant are placed on a waiting list. A heart may be available within 24 hours or may be months away. Unfortunately, some patients die before a suitable heart is available. There is ongoing investigation of use of artificial hearts. There has been limited success with use of xenograft and mechanical artificial hearts. The left ventricular assist device has been of benefit to providing needed perfusion for patients awaiting transplant surgery.

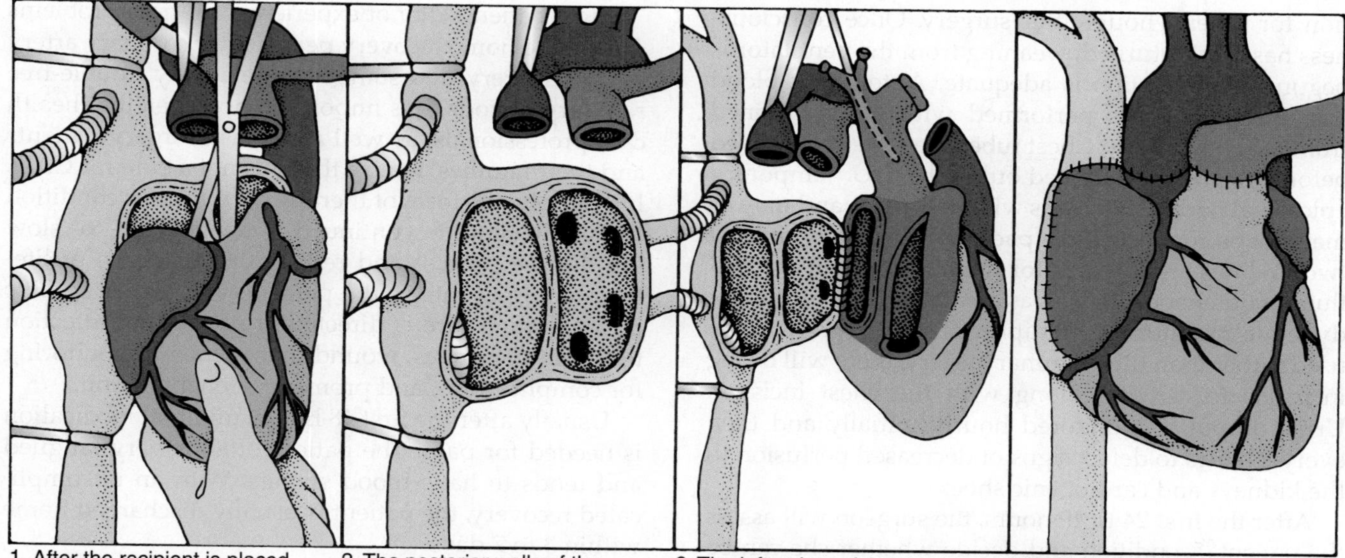

1. After the recipient is placed on cardiopulmonary bypass, the heart is removed.

2. The posterior walls of the recipient's left and right atria are left intact.

3. The left atrium of the donor heart is anastomosed to the recipient's residual posterior atrial walls, and the other atrial walls, the atrial septum, and the great vessels are joined.

POSTOPERATIVE RESULT

FIGURE 20–8 Heart transplantation.

NURSING CARE OF THE PATIENT HAVING CARDIAC SURGERY

PREOPERATIVE CARE

Before cardiac surgery, the patient undergoes a series of diagnostic tests and examinations, mostly on an outpatient basis. Once a decision is made to undergo surgery, measures are taken to ensure that she is in the best possible health. All teaching and psychological preparation is done on an outpatient basis whenever possible. The teaching plan should include expectations during the preoperative and postoperative periods. These are mostly the responsibilities of a nurse. There is considerable apprehension on the part of the patient and the family faced with open heart surgery.

The patient is given information about the procedure, explaining what she can expect and the kind of equipment she will see. She is admitted early the morning of surgery for a scheduled procedure. If she has been on an oral antiplatelet agent (aspirin, Plavix), she is switched to heparin by injection at least 1 day prior to surgery. If time permits, the antiplatelet agent is stopped 4 to 5 days preoperatively. See Nursing Care Plan 20–2 for care of the patient following cardiac surgery.

POSTOPERATIVE CARE

During the early postoperative period, the patient remains in an ICU, where specialized cardiac monitoring equipment is used and highly skilled personnel are in constant attendance. Cardiac rate and rhythm are monitored closely. Chest tubes for drainage and proper reexpansion of the lungs need special attention. The patient often continues to receive mechanical ventilation for several hours after surgery. Once consciousness has fully returned, weaning from the ventilator is begun if oxygenation is adequate. Autologous blood transfusion often is performed with blood drained from the chest cavity. Chest tubes are usually removed before the patient is moved out of the ICU. Temporary epicardial pacemaker leads will be in place and may or may not be connected to a pacemaker. Usually, at least two IV lines are in place for medication delivery and fluid maintenance, as well as an arterial line for hemodynamic monitoring. If saphenous vein grafts were used rather than the mammary artery, there will be leg incisions to care for along with the chest incision. Urine output is monitored hourly initially and then every 2 hours to detect signs of decreased perfusion to the kidneys and cardiogenic shock.

After the first 24 to 48 hours, the surgeon will assess the patient's condition and decide whether she can be transferred to a step-down or general surgical unit. The patient will continue to need very special nursing care. Her vital signs must be taken and recorded at frequent intervals. Her urinary output must be measured and recorded hourly at first, then every 2 to 8 hours, and her fluid intake may be restricted for a period. Daily weight is monitored to assess fluid balance.

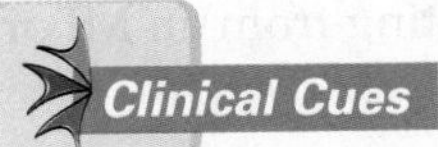

Priorities for care of the postsurgical patient must be established. Plan on frequent assessment of respiratory and cardiac status, care of invasive lines and chest tubes, wound assessment and care, fluid and electrolyte balance, pain management, and assessment of emotional status.

Coronary artery bypass surgery can produce many special problems related to physical and emotional disability and rehabilitation of the patient. Among the physiologic symptoms that can persist into the home recovery period are fatigue and weakness, incisional discomfort, edema in the donor leg, dysrhythmias, loss of appetite, depression, and unusual physical sensations. There also is the possibility of closure of the graft and the reappearance of original symptoms. Sometimes the patient develops Dressler syndrome, a type of pericarditis, which is treated with nonsteroidal antiinflammatory drugs (NSAIDs).

Cardiac transplant patients are threatened by organ rejection, infection, development of CAD in the new heart, and development of a malignant tumor as a result of immunosuppressive therapy to prevent transplant rejection. Heart biopsies are performed regularly.

Depression for weeks to months is not uncommon after heart surgery. Patients should be alerted to this possibility and referred for assistance if this occurs. Women are more likely than men to experience depression following surgery and the cases are more severe.

Most patients do not experience all these problems during the home recovery period after coronary artery bypass surgery, and some have relatively trouble-free recovery periods. It is important, however, that health care professionals, as well as bypass surgery patients and their families, realize that it is not a cure for CAD. It is simply one form of therapy for a chronic condition that will require continued management to slow the disease process and reduce the incidence of life-threatening events in the person's life. Other specific postoperative care is directed at preventing infection to the surgical sites, wound management, monitoring for complications, and promoting rehabilitation.

Usually after the first 48 hours, minimal medication is needed for pain. The patient often is very fatigued and tends to have mood swings. With an uncomplicated recovery, the patient is usually discharged home within 3 to 7 days.

COMMUNITY CARE

With early discharge from the hospital after surgery, many patients have continuing care from home health nurses. Patients recovering from cardiac surgery, MI, atherosclerotic heart disease, angina, or valvular heart disease all may be referred to a cardiac rehabilitation program. The goal of such programs is to reduce risk of further heart problems or death. The program is directed toward restoring and maintaining optimal physiologic function. Improving psychological outlook, maintaining ability to work, and social well-being are other components of the program. A supervised exercise program with cardiac monitoring for 6 to 8 weeks is combined with dietary counseling, classes on stress reduction, and the development of an individual action plan to reduce cardiac risk factors. A support group consisting of other individuals who have the same condition or have had similar surgery often is available. Most insurance coverage will pay for the program, as it has been highly successful in helping people to develop and maintain a healthier lifestyle and to reduce risk factors.

Home care nurses have many patients diagnosed with heart disease. The goal of home care is to monitor the patient's condition and to prevent complications, such as life-threatening dysrhythmias, MI, and CHF. Nurses supervise the medication regimen, monitor weight gain, draw blood for laboratory tests to determine drug levels and electrolyte status, and assess for beginning signs of complications. By detecting complications early, patients can be treated at home rather than at the hospital, thereby decreasing costs of care.

While working in long-term care facilities you will encounter cardiac patients daily because many older adults have a history of cardiac disorders. Assessing changes in condition is a high priority. If changes can be found quickly, the severity of a complication can be reduced.

Key Points

- High levels of cholesterol (LDL) contribute to development of atherosclerosis, a major factor in occlusion of coronary vessels.
- Ischemia occurs as blood supply is lost to the myocardium.
- A cardinal sign of myocardial ischemia is angina pectoris (chest pain).
- Angina may be classified as stable, variant, or unstable.
- Nitrates (nitroglycerin) are the most commonly used drugs to treat angina.
- Patients should be monitored for hypotension and development of a throbbing headache while taking nitroglycerin.
- When a coronary artery becomes completely obstructed, necrosis of myocardial tissue occurs (MI).
- Necrotic myocardial tissue cannot perform its function of pumping.
- Diagnosis of MI is made by patient history, ECG, and serum cardiac enzyme levels.
- A patient may be given an aspirin tablet to chew if a MI is suspected. Aspirin helps prevent clot formation.
- Emergency care for a patient suspected of experiencing an MI includes oxygen; IV access; cardiac monitoring; pain management, usually morphine sulfate IV; ECG; and management of dysrhythmias.
- Medications following MI may include nitrates, antihypertensive drugs, anticoagulants, beta blocker, ACE inhibitor, and antidysrhythmic drugs.
- Cardiac catheterization is likely to be performed on a patient experiencing an MI.
- Nursing care after cardiac catheterization includes cardiac monitoring, maintaining the patient in a supine position with the legs straight, monitoring the femoral area for hematoma formation, assessing peripheral pulses frequently, and monitoring urinary output.
- Stents may be placed to maintain patency of coronary vessels in an attempt to avoid CABG. Stents may be placed during PTCA.
- CABG may be needed when a patient's angina cannot be controlled by medical means or when there is myocardial damage due to occlusion of one or more coronary vessels.
- Alternatives to CABG include OPCAB and MIDCAB.
- A heart transplant may be needed for a patient with end-stage cardiomyopathy.
- Patients must receive extensive physical and psychological assessment before acceptance into a cardiac transplant program. Family counseling is also advisable.
- Donor hearts are not readily available; therefore patients must be carefully screened to determine the most appropriate candidate.
- Patients must be advised of potential complications, the need to follow through on dietary and exercise recommendations, and the need to continue medications, such as immunosuppressants and drugs to treat other cardiac conditions, for the remainder of their lives.
- Nursing care of patients after heart transplant includes intense monitoring in the CCU or ICU; assessing for signs of complications; wound management; administration of emergency, antirejection, and appropriate cardiac drugs; pain management, assessment of respiratory function; and initial return to physical activity such as out of bed to chair.
- Discharge planning should prepare the patient for return to her home and the beginning of care in the community.
- A home health nurse may visit the patient in the home.
- Monitoring the patient's understanding of and compliance with prescribed medications is an important responsibility of the home health nurse.

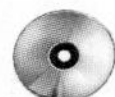

Go to your **Companion CD-ROM** for an Audio Glossary, animations, video clips, and bonus review questions.

evolve Be sure to visit the companion Evolve site at http://evolve.elsevier.com/deWit for interactive NCLEX-PN Exam Style Review Questions, WebLinks, and additional online resources.

NCLEX-PN EXAM STYLE REVIEW QUESTIONS

Choose the best answer(s) for the following questions.

1. After reviewing risk factors for cardiac disease, the patient is prescribed atorvastatin (Lipitor) to reduce cholesterol levels. The nurse must include which of the following instructions? *(Select all that apply.)*

1. Report any muscle weakness.
2. Avoid exposure to sunlight.
3. Schedule for renal function tests.
4. Drink grapefruit juice.
5. Maintain a low-protein diet.

2. The patient asks, "What causes angina pectoris?" An accurate response by a nurse would be:

1. "It is caused by the decreased blood flow to the coronary arteries due to shunting of the blood."
2. "It is caused by a decreased blood flow to the myocardium due to partial obstruction of the coronary arteries."
3. "It is caused by poor oxygenation of the coronary arteries due to poor gas exchange across the alveolar basement membrane."
4. "It is caused by the inflammation of the sternal cartilage."

3. A patient is diagnosed as having attacks of angina pectoris. As part of the discharge instructions, the patient is instructed on the appropriate storage and use of sublingual nitroglycerin. Which of the following patient statements indicates a need for further instructions?

1. "The tablets should be kept in a cool, dark place."
2. "I need to lie down after I take the medication."
3. "I can take the tablet every 15 minutes for angina pains."
4. "I can check my blood pressure between sublingual doses."

4. A 44-year-old patient is admitted with a sudden, severe chest tightness unrelieved by rest or nitroglycerin, and profuse sweating. The nurse would expect the physician to order which of the following tests?

1. Serum troponin
2. Blood urea nitrogen
3. Arterial blood gases
4. Prothrombin time

5. Immediate therapeutic measures given to a patient with an acute myocardial infarction includes which of the following? *(Select all that apply.)*

1. Morphine sulfate
2. Oxygen therapy
3. Furosemide
4. Nitroglycerin
5. Aspirin

6. Which of the following foods have been found to reduce cholesterol levels?

1. Garlic
2. Onion
3. Ginger
4. Nutmeg

7. The physician explains the treatment options to a Hmong female patient diagnosed with occlusion of multiple coronary vessels. Prior to signing an informed consent, the patient is most likely to defer her health care decisions to her:

1. oldest adult son.
2. oldest adult daughter.
3. brother-in-law.
4. husband.

8. The patient with angina pectoris has accompanying some ST-segment elevation on the ECG. An appropriate nursing diagnosis would be:

1. Deficient fluid volume.
2. Ineffective coping.
3. Ineffective tissue perfusion.
4. Activity intolerance.

9. Immediate postoperative nursing care of a patient who has undergone an open heart surgery includes which of the following? *(Select all that apply.)*

1. Assessing cardiac rate and rhythm
2. Checking chest tubes for drainage
3. Monitoring liver enzymes
4. Assessing bowel sounds
5. Managing pain

10. After discussing treatment options with a patient who suffered an MI, the patient asks, "What is percutaneous transluminal coronary angioplasty?" The nurse explains that:

1. "It is a surgical technique to open occluded coronary arteries."
2. "It is an insertion of a balloon catheter to widen narrowed vessels."
3. "It is a systemic injection of thrombolytic agents."
4. "It is a replacement of heart valves."

CRITICAL THINKING ACTIVITIES 

Read each clinical scenario and discuss the questions with your classmates.

Scenario A

Mrs. Yee, a 50-year-old woman, presents to the emergency room complaining of a burning, squeezing sensation in her chest, and a feeling of nausea. She is diaphoretic and apprehensive.

1. Compare and contrast the symptoms of heart attack between men and women.
2. Describe the probable emergency treatment of Mrs. Yee in the emergency room.
3. What lab tests may be ordered to evaluate for possible MI? What is a significant ECG finding indicating MI?

Scenario B

Ms. O'Hare, a 45-year-old, is on the list for a heart transplant. She has a left ventricular assist device and is waiting at home.

1. What are the criteria for heart transplant? List contraindications.
2. Describe the purpose of the left ventricular assist device.
3. Develop a discharge teaching plan for Ms. O'Hare after transplant.

CHAPTER 21 The Neurologic System

evolve http://evolve.elsevier.com/deWit

Objectives

Upon completing this chapter, you should be able to:

Theory

1. Define the vocabulary particular to problems of the nervous system.
2. Discuss the differences in the action of sympathetic and parasympathetic nervous systems.
3. Identify four specific ways in which a nurse can contribute to preventing neurologic disorders.
4. State the appropriate preparation and postprocedure care for patients undergoing lumbar puncture (spinal tap), electroencephalogram (EEG), and radiologic studies of the brain and cerebral vessels.
5. Become familiar with the techniques used for assessment of the nervous system.
6. Compare and contrast the various signs and symptoms of the common problems experienced by patients with nervous system disorders.

Clinical Practice

1. Gather a pertinent history for a patient with a nervous system problem.
2. Demonstrate a "neuro check."
3. Score the neurologic status of a patient with a nervous system disorder according to the Glasgow Coma Scale.

Key Terms

Be sure to check out the bonus material on the Companion CD-ROM, including selected audio pronunciations.

accommodation (p. 526)
aphasia (ă-FĀ-zhă, p. 535)
Babinski's reflex (p. 522)
calculi (KĂL-kŭ-lī, p. 533)
caloric testing (kăl-Ō-rĭk, p. 523)
clonus (KLŌ-nus, p. 522)
decerebrate posturing (dē-SĔR-ē-brāt, p. 525)
decorticate posturing (dē-KŎR-tĭ-kāt, p. 525)
delirium (dĕ-LĬR-ē–ŭm, p. 534)
dysphagia (dĭs-FĀ-jē-ă, p. 533)
hemiparesis (hĕm-ē-pă-RĒ-sĭs, p. 529)
hemiplegia (hĕm-ĭ-PLĒ-jă, p. 529)
nystagmus (nĭs-TĂG-mŭs, p. 525)
quadriplegic (kwŏd-rĭ-PLĒ-jĭk, p. 529)
tetraplegia (TĔT-ră-PLĒ-jă, p. 529)

The nervous system is the communication system of the body. It coordinates all sensory and motor activities by receiving, interpreting, and relaying messages that are vital to the proper performance of all the body's activities. Respiratory, circulatory, digestive, and endocrine functions all depend on an intact and normally functioning autonomic nervous system.

If anything happens to impair the ability of certain nerve cells to receive and conduct impulses, the tissues controlled by those nerve cells cease to function normally. One example of this is severe spinal cord injury. All parts of the body below the level of injury would be paralyzed and have no sensation of heat, cold, pressure, or pain if the spinal cord had been severed and the flow of impulses interrupted. A basic knowledge of the anatomy of the nervous system and how it works is essential to understanding how various disorders affect it. A brief review is provided here as a refresher.

CAUSATIVE FACTORS INVOLVED IN NEUROLOGIC DISORDERS

Many factors can affect neurologic function including genetic and acquired developmental disorders. Infections and inflammation, benign and malignant tumors, vascular or neuromuscular degeneration, and metabolic and endocrine disorders all can cause damage to or interfere with normal function of the nervous system. Chemical or physical trauma often causes permanent damage to the brain or spinal cord. Box 21–1 lists by category the most common neurologic disorders in the adult.

PREVENTION OF NEUROLOGIC DISORDERS

Nurses can help prevent neurologic problems in many ways. The goals for *Healthy People 2010: National Health Promotion and Disease Prevention Objectives* encourage health protection through education about safety and responsible self-care (Health Promotion Points 21–1).

Text continues on p. 518

Box 21–1 Classification of Common Neurologic Disorders

GENETIC/DEVELOPMENTAL DISORDERS
- Cerebral palsy
- Muscular dystrophy
- Huntington's disease (chorea)

TRAUMA
- Head injury
- Penetrating brain injury
- Spinal cord injury
- Ruptured intervertebral disk

CEREBROVASCULAR
- Cerebrovascular accident
  - Ruptured aneurysm
- Arteriovenous malformation
- Migraine, cluster headache

TUMOR
- Brain tumor
- Spinal cord tumor

INFECTION
- Meningitis
- Encephalitis
- Brain abscess
- Poliomyelitis
- Guillain-Barré syndrome

NEUROMUSCULAR DISORDERS
- Multiple sclerosis
- Myasthenia gravis
- Amyotrophic lateral sclerosis

DEGENERATIVE DISORDERS
- Parkinson's disease
- Alzheimer's disease

CRANIAL NERVE DISORDERS
- Bell's palsy
- Trigeminal neuralgia

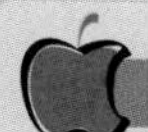

Health Promotion Points 21–1

Protecting the Nervous System

- Encourage people to wear helmets when biking, in-line skating, skateboarding, or riding motorcycles, and when involved in other sports activities that may lead to head injury.
- Remind people that wearing safety hats or helmets when in a workplace where head injury is a danger does reduce the number of injuries.
- Review safety precautions when diving and swimming. Never diving into water of unknown depth helps prevent spinal cord injury.
- Encourage people to fasten their seat belts before putting the car into gear.
- Be certain that children are fastened into appropriate restraints.
- Wear mask, gloves, long pants, and long-sleeved shirt when spraying with insecticide; wash up immediately afterward and change clothes.
- Refrain from using recreational drugs, because they can affect the cardiovascular system and can cause a stroke.

OVERVIEW OF ANATOMY AND PHYSIOLOGY OF THE NEUROLOGIC SYSTEM

How is the nervous system organized?

- The functional unit of the nervous system is the neuron, which consists of a cell body, dendrites, and an axon. Neurons react to stimuli, conduct impulses, and influence other neurons (Figure 21–1). There are afferent and efferent neurons.
- The nervous system consists of the central nervous system (CNS) and the peripheral nervous system (PNS).
- The CNS is made up of the brain and spinal cord (Figure 21–2).
- The brain is divided into the cerebrum, diencephalon, cerebellum, and brainstem, which each perform various functions (see Figure 21–2). Table 21–1 (p. 516) lists the functions of the various divisions of the brain.
- The brainstem consists of the midbrain, pons, and medulla.
- The different parts of the brain control various functions (Figure 21–3).
- The PNS is composed of the sensory organs—eyes, ears, taste buds, olfactory receptors, and touch receptors—12 pairs of cranial nerves, and 31 pairs of spinal nerves and ganglia that link the sensory organs, muscles, and other parts of the body to the brain and spinal cord (Figure 21–4). The distribution pathways of the spinal nerves are called *dermatomes.*
- There are 12 pairs of cranial nerves, some of which are sensory nerves and others of which are motor nerves (Table 21–2, p. 516).

Continued

OVERVIEW OF ANATOMY AND PHYSIOLOGY OF THE NEUROLOGIC SYSTEM—cont'd

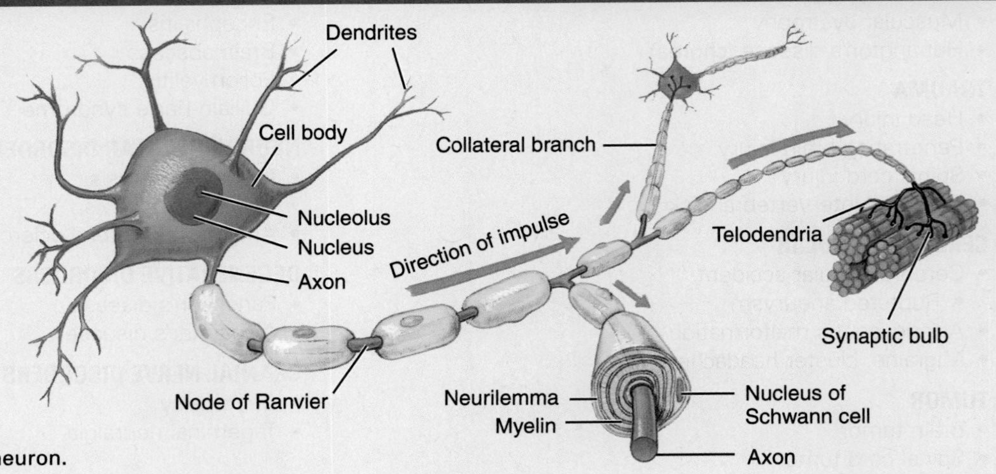

FIGURE **21–1** Structure of a neuron.

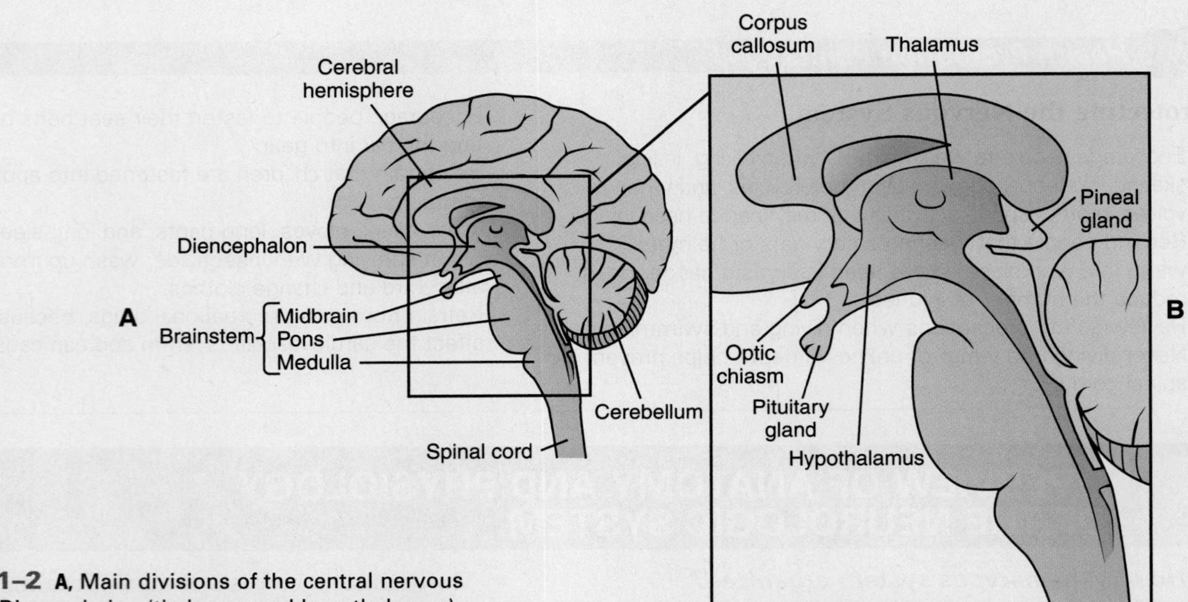

FIGURE **21–2** **A,** Main divisions of the central nervous system **B,** Diencephalon (thalamus and hypothalamus).

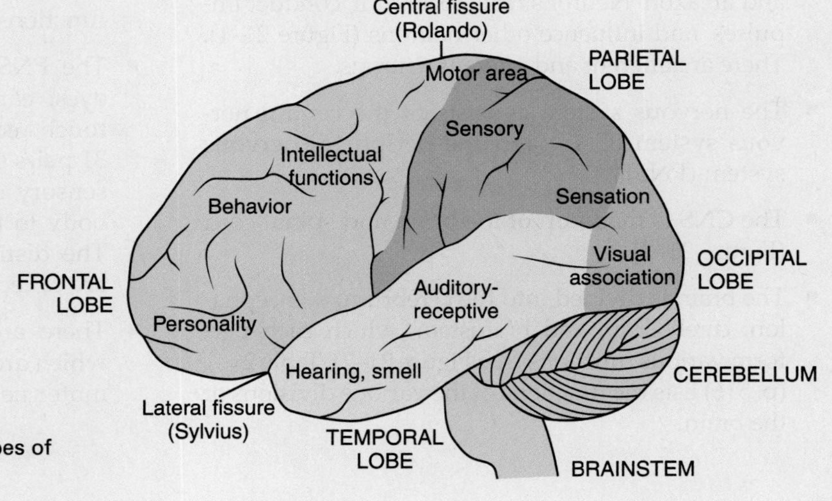

FIGURE **21–3** Specialized functions of the lobes of the cerebrum.

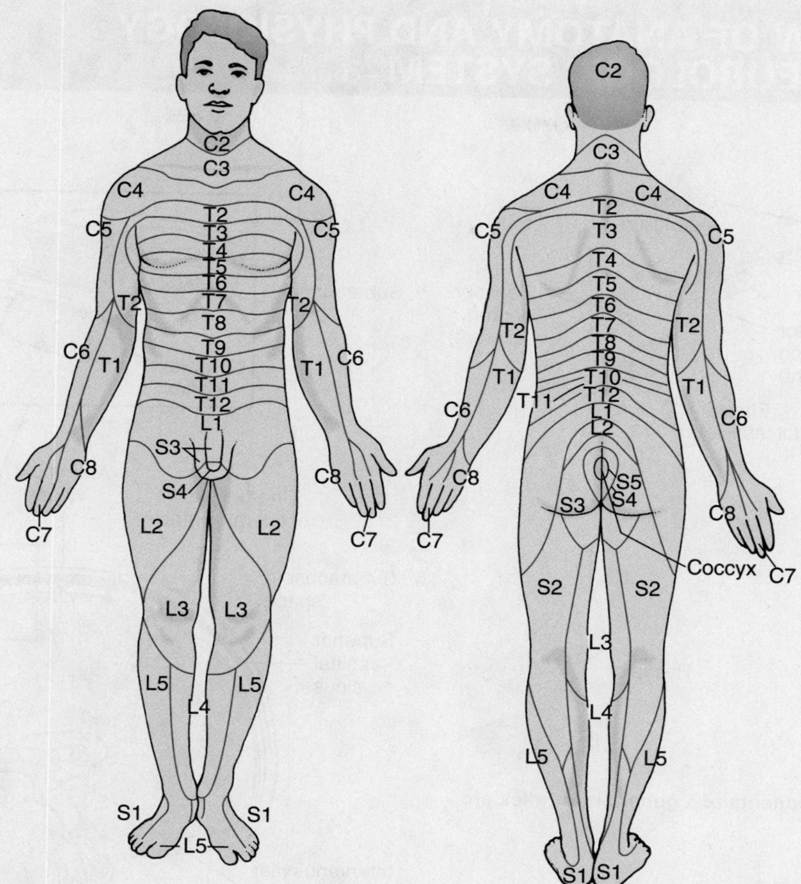

FIGURE 21–4 Dermatomes (cutaneous innervation of spinal nerves). Stimulation of the skin in the depicted area for each nerve causes reflex activity. (Key: *C*, cervical spinal nerves; *T*, thoracic spinal nerves; *L*, lumbar spinal nerves; *S*, sacral spinal nerves.)

- The spinal cord extends from the medulla to the level of the first lumbar vertebra.
- The spinal cord is a conduction pathway for impulses going to and from the brain and also serves as a reflex center for nerve impulse transmission. Sensory impulses travel to the brain on ascending conduction pathway tracts; motor impulses travel on descending tracts.
- Pyramidal tracts are conduction pathways that begin in the cerebral cortex and end in the spinal cord. These tracts control skeletal muscle movement. All other conduction pathways are extrapyramidal tracts, and they control muscle movements associated with posture and balance.

How does the peripheral nervous system interact with the central nervous system?

- The PNS is subdivided into an afferent division and an efferent division. The afferent division carries impulses to the CNS; the efferent division carries impulses away from the CNS.
- The reflex arc is a simple conduction pathway that utilizes a receptor (a sensory neuron centered in the spinal cord) and a motor neuron located in an effector (skeletal muscle). A stimulus travels from the sensory receptor through the spinal cord and back to the effector, causing action (Figure 21–5).
- Reflex arcs are important to most functions of the body, including maintaining an upright position.
- The cranial and spinal nerves are part of the somatic subsystem and respond to changes in the outside world. Because these nerves initiate voluntary action, the somatic system often is called the *voluntary system.*
- The autonomic system of the PNS is active in maintaining internal body balance *(homeostasis)* and is automatic (involuntary) in its actions.
- The autonomic system is divided into the sympathetic nerves, which mobilize energy to initiate changes aimed at maintaining or restoring homeostasis, and the parasympathetic nerves,

Continued

OVERVIEW OF ANATOMY AND PHYSIOLOGY OF THE NEUROLOGIC SYSTEM—cont'd

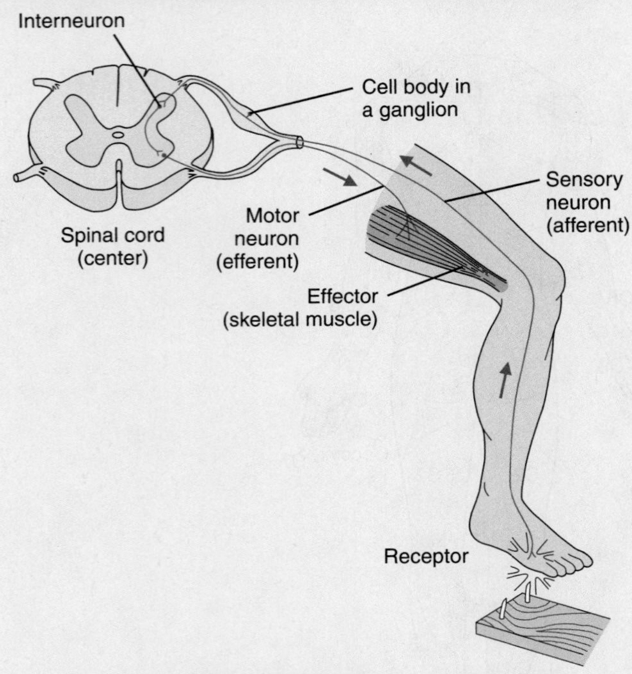

FIGURE 21–5 Components of a generalized reflex arc.

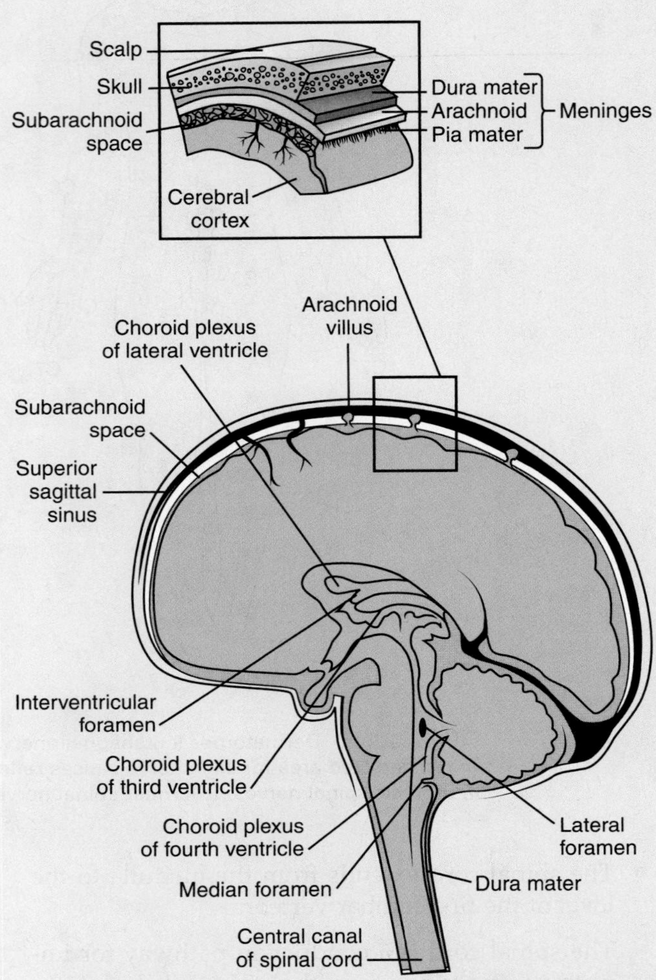

FIGURE 21–6 Flow of the cerebrospinal fluid. *Inset,* Meninges covering the brain.

which conserve and restore energy that has been used to maintain homeostasis.

- **Sympathetic and parasympathetic nerves have opposite effects on many organs** (Table 21–3, p. 517).

How is the central nervous system protected?

- The bones of the skull and the vertebral column form the outer layer of protection for the brain and the spinal cord.
- The meninges are protective membranes that cover the brain and are continuous with the membranes covering the spinal cord. The meninges consist of the pia mater, which covers the brain; the arachnoid, which encases the entire CNS; and the dura mater, which is a tough membrane protecting the brain and spinal cord (Figure 21–6).
- The subarachnoid space is located between the pia mater and the arachnoid membrane and is where the cerebrospinal (CSF) fluid circulates.
- CSF serves to cushion and protect the brain and spinal cord. It is formed continuously as a filtrate from the blood in specialized capillary networks in the choroid plexus, located in the ventricles of the brain. It is reabsorbed by the arachnoid villi of the arachnoid membrane at the same rate at which it is formed. The volume of CSF normally stays constant (see Figure 21–6).
- **Normal CSF pressure is 70 to 125 cm water pressure (cm H_2O).** When there is an excess of fluid in the subarachnoid space, the pressure rises above normal.

How do nerves conduct impulses?

- The axons of many neurons, bundled together and wrapped in connective tissue, make up a nerve. Ganglia are collections of nerve cell bodies outside the CNS.
- When in a state of polarization, neurons have the capacity to become excited (stimulated). They also have the ability to conduct that stimulus along the nerve pathways.

- A stimulus is a physical, chemical, or electrical event that changes the cell membrane and initiates conduction of the stimulus as an electrical impulse along the nerve pathway.
- The stimulus travels from one neuron to another across a *synapse* (the space between two neurons).
- A neurotransmitter secreted by the neuron is necessary for transmission of an impulse across the synapse (Table 21–4, p. 518). Acetylcholine, dopamine, and norepinephrine are the major neurotransmitters.
- Neurotransmitter substances are secreted at the synapse, and these diffuse across the synapse to stimulate the postsynaptic membrane on the next neuron. **When the neurotransmitter is absent or decreased at the synaptic junction, the stimulus cannot travel along the nerve pathways normally.**
- Impulses either travel in a reflex arc, going to the spinal cord and traveling back to an effector site, or they travel along nerve pathways to the brain to be interpreted.
- After impulse interpretation, a message may be sent out from the brain via the spinal cord or cranial nerves (PNS) for appropriate action to be taken. In other words, a stimulus produces a response.
- Many axons are surrounded by a myelin sheath that is a white, fatty covering. The myelin sheath is an excellent electrical insulator and it speeds the conduction of nerve impulses. **When myelin is destroyed, as in multiple sclerosis, impulse transmission is slowed or stopped.**

What are the special characteristics of the nervous system?

- Although some cells in the PNS have an outer membrane called the *neurolemma* that may regenerate after damage, cells of the CNS do not have this capability. **Once destroyed, cells in the brain cannot be replaced.**
- In the PNS, the Schwann cells can regenerate. The Schwann cells form myelin sheaths that wrap around the axons in the PNS.
- Neurons are very sensitive to oxygen and die quickly when deprived of oxygen. **The brain's neurons cannot survive anoxia for more than 4 to 6 minutes.**

What changes occur in the nervous system with aging?

- There is a loss of neurons with aging, and brain weight may drop considerably after age 70; there is no loss of intellectual function attributable to this loss of neurons.
- The number of functioning dendrites decreases with aging. This decrease causes slower impulse transmission and resultant slower reaction time in the older person.
- Blood flow to the brain is decreased with advanced age; this makes the elderly more susceptible to permanent damage if blood flow to the brain is further compromised.
- Loss of neurons and slower nerve conduction cause a decrease in efficiency of the autonomic nervous system in advanced age.
- Body homeostasis is more difficult to maintain or regain in the elderly. Exposure to prolonged cold or to excessive heat may cause death. Adaptation to physiologic stress takes much longer, and recovery often is incomplete.
- Recent, short-term memory is affected by the aging process, but long-term, distant memory is often not affected. The ability to learn is not affected by aging, but the learning process is slower. It takes longer to process new information. Abstract reasoning ability slowly diminishes with advancing age, and perception may become impaired.
- Decreases in secretion of the neurotransmitters norepinephrine and dopamine occur, and there is an increase in monoamine oxidase, which can affect cognitive function, gait, and balance.
- The number of posterior root nerve fibers and sympathetic nerve fibers of the autonomic nervous system declines with aging of the spinal cord. In the PNS, the motor nerve fibers and the myelin sheath degenerate with advancing age; reflexes may become diminished or absent with advanced age.
- Utilizing the brain and keeping it active promotes continued intellectual function in the healthy elderly.

The student is referred to an anatomy and physiology text for a thorough review of the complex nervous system.

Table 21–1 *Functions of the Divisions of the Brain*

DIVISION	FUNCTION
Cerebrum	Center of intellect and consciousness. Receives and interprets sensory information; controls voluntary movements and certain types of involuntary movements; responsible for thinking, learning, language capability, judgment, and personality; stores memories.
Cerebellum	Responsible for coordination of movement, posture, and muscle tone that are the mechanisms of balance.
Diencephalon	Consists of two parts.
Thalamus	Relay center between spinal cord and cerebrum.
Hypothalamus	Controls body temperature, appetite, and water balance; links nervous and endocrine systems.
Brainstem	Consists of three parts.
Midbrain	Mediates visual and auditory reflexes; controls cranial nerves III and IV and certain eye movements.
Pons	Links connecting various parts of the brain; helps regulate respiration.
Medulla oblongata	Contains reticular formation that regulates heartbeat, respiration, and blood pressure; controls center for swallowing, coughing, sneezing, and vomiting; relays messages to other parts of the brain.

Table 21–2 *The Cranial Nerves and Their Functions*

	CRANIAL NERVE (CN)*	TYPE AND FUNCTION
O	Olfactory (CN I)	*Sensory:* smell
O	Optic (CN II)	*Sensory:* visual acuity, field of vision, pupillary response (afferent impulse)
O	Oculomotor (CN III)	*Motor:* eyelid elevation, extraocular eye movement, pupil size, convergence, pupillary constriction (efferent impulse)
T	Trochlear (CN IV)	*Motor:* extraocular eye movement (inferior and lateral)
T	Trigeminal (CN V)	*Sensory:* corneal reflex *Motor:* facial sensation; chewing, biting, lateral jaw movement
A	Abducens (CN VI)	*Motor:* extraocular eye movement (lateral)
F	Facial (CN VII)	*Sensory:* taste *Motor:* facial muscle movement, including muscles of expression; lacrimal gland and salivary gland control
A	Acoustic (CN VIII)	*Sensory:* hearing, sense of balance
G	Glossopharyngeal (CN IX)	*Sensory:* sensations of the throat, taste (posterior tongue) *Motor:* gagging and swallowing movements
V	Vagus (CN X)	*Sensory:* sensations of posterior tongue, throat, larynx; impulses from heart, lungs, bronchi, and gastrointestinal tract
S	Spinal accessory (CN XI)	*Motor:* shoulder movement and head rotation
H	Hypoglossal (CN XII)	*Motor:* tongue movement, articulation of speech

*Initials for mnemonic for names of the cranial nerves (see Clinical Cues box, p. 518).

Teaching the dangers of recreational drug use, such as the possibility of stroke from the use of "crack" cocaine and the potential for accidents caused by being under the influence of some drugs, are other areas for public education. Informing the public about the damaging effect of too much alcohol on brain cells, as well as the increased incidence of alcohol-induced accidents, is another area for education.

Promoting immunizations to protect from tetanus, poliomyelitis, and infectious diseases that may cause high fever and resultant brain damage is an area in which nurses can be effective. **Working to decrease the incidence of hypertension and to provide control for those afflicted with this disorder can readily reduce the number of strokes and the damage they cause.** Teaching people to recognize the symptoms of stroke and to seek early treatment may prevent permanent disability. Promoting the benefits of a low-fat diet to decrease plaque buildup from atherosclerosis can help reduce the incidence of stroke as well as help prevent heart disease. These are some of the ways nurses can be effective agents for preventing neurologic disorders.

Pesticides and various chemicals in household and work environments can cause neurologic toxicity and damage. Parkinson's disease has been particularly more prevalent in farm workers and others who handle pesticides or work in areas in which they are frequently used (Miller, 2006). 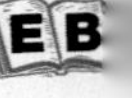 Information on containers of those substances should be read carefully and precautions taken. Long-sleeved clothing and gloves should be used when spraying with pesticides in the garden. Spraying should be done in quiet, nonwindy conditions. Hands and exposed skin should be washed with soap and water afterward, and clothing should be changed and the clothing worn should be laundered.

EVALUATION OF NEUROLOGIC STATUS

The complete neurologic examination performed by the physician, physician's assistant, or advanced practice RN systematically measures the ability of the body to perform its myriad motor and sensory functions. Mental acuity, memory, and emotional stability also are assessed. The physical examination to identify problems of motor and sensory function is a very long procedure and may be performed in stages over sev-

Table 21–3 ***Autonomic Effects on Various Organs of the Body***

ORGAN	EFFECT OF SYMPATHETIC STIMULATION	EFFECT OF PARASYMPATHETIC STIMULATION
Eye		
Pupil	Dilated	Constricted
Ciliary muscle	Slight relaxation (far vision)	Constricted (near vision)
Glands	Vasoconstriction and slight secretion	Stimulation of copious secretion (containing many enzymes for enzyme-secreting glands)
Nasal		
Lacrimal		
Parotid		
Submandibular		
Gastric		
Pancreatic		
Sweat glands	Copious sweating (cholinergic)	Sweating on palms of hands
Apocrine glands	Thick, odoriferous secretion	None
Blood vessels	Most often constricted	Most often little or no effect
Heart		
Muscle	Increased rate Increased force of contraction	Slowed rate Decreased force of contraction (especially of atria)
Coronaries	Dilated (β_2); constricted (α)	Dilated
Lungs		
Bronchi	Dilated	Constricted
Blood vessels	Mildly constricted	Dilated
Gut		
Lumen	Decreased peristalsis and tone	Increased peristalsis and tone
Sphincter	Increased tone (most times)	Relaxed (most times)
Liver	Glucose released	Slight glucose synthesis
Gallbladder and bile ducts	Relaxed	Contracted
Kidney	Decreased output and renin secretion	None
Bladder		
Detrusor	Relaxed (slight)	Contracted
Trigone	Contracted	Relaxed
Penis	Ejaculation	Erection
Systemic arterioles		
Abdominal viscera	Constricted	None
Muscle	Constricted (α-adrenergic) Dilated (β-adrenergic) Dilated (cholinergic)	None
Skin	Constricted	None
Blood		None
Coagulation	Increased	None
Glucose	Increased	None
Lipids	Increased	None
Basal metabolism	Increased up to 100%	None
Adrenal medullary secretion	Increased	None
Mental activity	Increased	None
Piloerector muscles	Contracted	None
Skeletal muscle	Increased glycogenolysis Increased strength	None
Fat cells	Lipolysis	None

From Guyton, A.C., & Hall, J.E. (2006). *Textbook of Medical Physiology with Student Consult Access* (11th ed.). Philadelphia: Elsevier Saunders, p. 754.

eral days. However, gross assessment of the cranial nerves, coordination and balance, muscle strength, and reflexes is standard for every patient with a neurologic complaint. Often the physician or nurse practitioner carries out a thorough assessment, but if not, the nurse should check cranial nerve function.

CRANIAL NERVES

The 12 cranial nerves (designated as CN I through CN XII) control both sensory and motor activities within various parts of the body. The patient may be tested for the sense of smell (CN I), sight and pupil constriction (CN II and III), and hearing and balance (CN VIII). The ability to change facial expression (CN V, VII, and XII), gag reflex and swallowing (CN IX and X), ability to move the eyes (CN IV and VI), and head and shoulder movement (CN XI) also are evaluated. Table 21–2 presents the cranial nerves and their functions. Table 21–5 tells how to perform a basic assessment of cranial nerve function.

Table 21–4 Neurotransmitters that Affect Transmission of Nerve Impulses

NEUROTRANSMITTER	LOCATION	FUNCTION	COMMENTS
Acetylcholine	CNS and PNS	Generally excitatory but is inhibitory to some visceral effectors	Found in skeletal neuromuscular junctions and in many ANS synapses
Norepinephrine	CNS and PNS	May be excitatory or inhibitory depending on the receptors	Found in visceral and cardiac muscle neuromuscular junctions; cocaine and amphetamines exaggerate the effects
Epinephrine	CNS and PNS	May be excitatory or inhibitory depending on the receptors	Found in pathways concerned with behavior and mood
Dopamine	CNS and PNS	Generally excitatory	Found in pathways that regulate emotional responses; decreased levels in Parkinson's disease
Serotonin	CNS	Generally inhibitory	Found in pathways that regulate temperature, sensory perception, mood, onset of sleep
Gamma-aminobutyric acid (GABA)	CNS	Generally inhibitory	Inhibits excessive discharge of neurons
Endorphins and enkephalins	CNS	Generally inhibitory	Inhibit release of sensory pain neurotransmitters; opiates mimic the effects of these peptides

Key: *ANS,* autonomic nervous system; *CNS,* central nervous system; *PNS,* peripheral nervous system.
From Applegate, E. (2006). *The Anatomy and Physiology Learning System* (3rd ed.). Philadelphia: Elsevier Saunders, p. 161.

Table 21–5 Quick Gross Assessment of Major Cranial Nerves

CRANIAL NERVE TESTED	QUICK METHOD OF TESTING
Olfactory	Have patient smell a sample of ground coffee, perfume, and pickle juice.
Optic	Test visual acuity with a Snellen eye chart. Test visual fields by asking patient to hold the head still and identify items on various areas of a chart.
Oculomotor, trochlear, and abducens	Assess pupil size, direct and consensual constriction and accommodation. Assess the cardinal fields/directions of gaze.
Trigeminal	Ask patient to clamp jaw shut, open the mouth against resistance, open the mouth widely, move the jaw from side to side, and make chewing motions. Test sensation by placing a hot and then a cold item on various portions of the face. Ask whether item is warm or cold.
Facial	Observe the face for symmetry; ask patient to smile, frown, raise the eyebrows, tightly close the eyes, whistle, show the teeth, and puff out the cheeks.
Vestibulocochlear (or acoustic)	Whisper from varying distances and locations behind the patient and ask what was said. Test equilibrium with Romberg's test: ask patient to stand with feet only slightly apart and eyes closed. See if there is swaying of the body.
Glossopharyngeal and vagus	Ask patient to open mouth wide and say "Ah." Place tongue depressor on first third of tongue to flatten it and observe movement of the uvula and palate. They should rise symmetrically with the uvula at midline. Assess gag reflex by touching each side of the pharynx; there should be a brisk response. Have patient swallow a bit of water.
Spinal accessory	Ask patient to elevate the shoulders with and without resistance, turn the head to each side, resist attempts to pull the chin back toward the midline, and push the head forward against resistance.
Hypoglossal	Ask patient to open mouth wide, stick out tongue, and rapidly move it from side to side and in and out. Watch for deviation from midline. Apply pressure to cheek and ask patient to push tongue against hand to check for strength.

*These maneuvers do not check for every function of these cranial nerves, but will provide data indicating whether a more thorough assessment is needed.

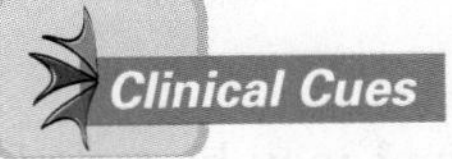

A mnemonic for remembering the cranial nerve names is as follows:

"**O**n **O**ld **Ol**ympus's **T**owering **T**op **A** **F**inn **A**nd **G**erman **V**iewed **S**ome **H**ops" (Olfactory, Optic, Oculomotor, Trochlear, Trigeminal, Abducens, Facial, Acoustic, Glossopharyngeal, Vagus, Spinal accessory, Hypoglossal).

COORDINATION AND BALANCE

This portion of the neurologic examination evaluates functions controlled by the higher centers of the brain, the cerebrum and cerebellum. During the examination, the patient is asked to stand with the feet together and to close the eyes (Romberg's test). If the sense of balance is normal, a steady posture will be maintained and there will not be swaying from side to side. Next ask the patient to walk across the room, and assess the gait. Next the examiner stands in front of the patient, holds up a finger, and asks the patient to touch the finger and then his own nose; the examiner moves the finger to different locations in front of the patient. This tests both the ability to follow directions and coordination.

NEUROMUSCULAR FUNCTION TESTING

Groups of large muscles are tested for strength and coordination. The physician may evaluate the patient's gait while walking, the hand grip strength, and arm and leg strength as the patient pushes against resistance. If this has not been done, then the nurse evaluates muscle function. More sophisticated tests include electromyography (Table 21–6).

REFLEXES

A reflex is an action or movement that is built into the nervous system and does not need the intervention of conscious thought to take place. In other words, it is an automatic response. The knee jerk is an example of the simplest type of reflex. When the knee is tapped, the nerve that receives this stimulus sends an impulse to the spinal cord, where it is relayed to a motor nerve. This causes the quadriceps muscle at the front of the

Text continues on p. 523

Table 21–6 *Diagnostic Tests for Neurologic Disorders*

TEST	PURPOSE	DESCRIPTION	NURSING IMPLICATIONS
Skull and spine x-rays	Detect fractures, bone loss, and other bony abnormalities.	X-rays are taken of the desired area from various angles.	Explain that the test is noninvasive. Advise that various positions will need to be assumed.
Lumbar puncture (spinal tap)	To determine if CSF pressure is elevated; to determine if there is a blockage to the flow of CSF; to inject medications; to obtain fluid for chemical analysis and culture.	Physician performs a sterile puncture into the arachnoid space, using local anesthetic, between L3 and L4 or L4 and L5; opening pressure is obtained; fluid is aspirated and placed in sterile test tubes labeled 1, 2, and 3. Fluid is analyzed for color, pH, cell count, protein, chloride, and glucose; a culture is usually done. Local anesthetic is used.	Obtain signature on consent form. Obtain sterile lumbar puncture tray, local anesthetic, sterile gloves, and tape. Assist patient into position with back bowed, head flexed on chest, and knees drawn up to the abdomen. Patient may be lying or sitting. Assist him to maintain position and to hold still during procedure. Reassure patient and provide emotional support. *Posttest:* Appropriately label tubes with patient data afterward and transport them to the laboratory immediately. Keep patient flat in bed to reduce headache for 1 hr or longer after procedure and encourage fluid intake unless contraindicated. Observe the site for signs of drainage and inflammation.
Electroencephalography (EEG)	To detect abnormal brain wave patterns that are indicative of specific diseases, such as seizure disorder, brain tumor, CVA, head trauma, and infection; to determine cerebral death.	May be performed while patient is asleep, drowsy, or undergoing stimulation such as hyperventilation or rhythmic bright light. Test may be done at the bedside or in the EEG lab. Tracing is taken with patient in reclining chair or lying down. Electrodes are applied to the scalp with an electrode paste. Test takes 45 min–2 hr.	Explain purpose of test to the patient; assure him he will not receive an electric shock, the test is not painful, and that the machine does not determine intelligence or read his mind. Hair should be clean and dry. No sleeping pills or sedatives the night before test; check with physician regarding other drugs to be held; restrict coffee, tea, caffeine, and alcohol for 24–48 hr. If a sleep EEG is ordered, patient may need to be kept up most or all of the night prior to the test; do not keep NPO, as hypoglycemia can affect the test. *Posttest:* Wash hair to remove the electrode paste.
Electromyography (EMG)	To measure electrical activity of skeletal muscle at rest and during voluntary activity to determine abnormalities in muscular contraction. Helpful in diagnosing neuromuscular, peripheral nerve, and muscular disorders.	With the patient sitting in a chair or lying on a table, needle electrodes are inserted in selected muscles. Tracings of electrical activity are taken with the muscles at rest, then with various voluntary activities that produce muscle contraction. The test takes 1–2 hr depending on how many muscles are tested.	Obtain signed informed consent. Explain the procedure to the patient; tell him that there is discomfort when the electrodes are placed. Check with physician regarding medications to be withheld; muscle relaxants, cholinergics, and anticholinergics can influence test result. There is no food or fluid restriction. If serum enzymes are ordered, they should be drawn before the EMG.

Key: *CSF,* cerebrospinal fluid; *CVA,* cerebrovascular accident; *NPO,* nothing by mouth.

Continued

Table 21–6 ***Diagnostic Tests for Neurologic Disorders—cont'd***

TEST	PURPOSE	DESCRIPTION	NURSING IMPLICATIONS
Myelography	To detect spinal lesions, intervertebral disk problems, tumors, or cysts.	Contrast medium is injected into the spinal canal, and fluoroscopic examination and radiographs are made. The study is contraindicated if the patient has increased ICP. The patient is placed prone and strapped to the x-ray table for the spinal puncture; as the contrast medium is injected, the table is tilted. After the test, if oil-based medium was used, it is withdrawn. The patient is kept in bed with head of bed elevated 60 degrees or flat depending on the contrast medium used. Procedure takes 1 hr. Rarely performed.	Requires a signed consent. Explain what to expect. Patient may feel a warm flush when contrast medium is injected. Bowel evacuation regimen may be ordered the night before. Keep NPO for 4–8 hr prior to procedure. Check for medications to be withheld before and for 48 hr posttest. Assess for allergy to iodine or shellfish. Dress in myelogram pajamas; administer preoperative sedative or analgesic if ordered. *Posttest:* Monitor VS q 30 min × 2 hr, then q 1 hr × 4 hr. Assess pulses and sensation in extremities; monitor urinary output; catheterize as ordered if patient cannot void in 8 hr; encourage increased fluid intake. Observe for signs of meningitis.
Computed axial tomography (CAT or CT scan)	To examine the brain from many different angles, obtaining a series of cross-sectional images that provide views from three dimensions. To identify hematomas, tumors, cysts, hydrocephalus, cerebral atrophy, obstruction to CSF flow, and cerebral edema.	May be done with or without contrast dye enhancement. Patient lies on a narrow table with his head cradled and is moved so that his head is inside the circular opening of the machine. A security strap is wrapped snuggly around him. CT scanner produces a narrow x-ray beam. Various clicking and whirring noises are heard as the machine rotates the scanner for different views. The test takes 45 min–1½ hr.	A consent form is required. Explain the procedure and what he will see, hear, and feel. If contrast dye is used, the patient will feel a warm flush and have a metallic taste in his mouth as it is injected. If contrast dye is used, patient should be NPO for 3–4 hr prior to test to prevent vomiting. Assess for allergy to iodine or shellfish. Remove all hairpins, jewelry, and metal from the head and neck. Patient may need to be sedated if he is prone to claustrophobia; the table can be uncomfortable for those with arthritis or back problems. He will be able to communicate with the machine's operator.
Cerebral angiography	To visualize the structure of the cerebral arteries to determine the presence of stricture, tumor, aneurysm, thrombus, or hematoma.	Radiopaque liquid is injected through a catheter inserted into the common carotid artery, and a series of radiographs is taken. Fluoroscopy is used during the procedure. Digital subtraction angiography (DSA) is done by utilizing a computer along with the angiography procedure. Test takes 1–2 hr.	Consent form is required. Assess for allergy to iodine and shellfish. Explain procedure; patient will be supine on x-ray table; local anesthetic will be used to introduce the catheter; an IV line will be started in case of need for emergency drugs; patient will feel a flush as the dye is injected. Patient should be NPO 8–12 hr prior to test; anticoagulants are discontinued beforehand. May be given preprocedure sedative, antihistamine, or steroid to decrease possibility of allergic reaction to dye. *Postprocedure:* Assess for bleeding at catheter site; assess distal pulses; perform neurologic checks; monitor VS q 15 min × 2 hr, then q 1 hr × 4 hr or until stable. Assess for dysphagia and respiratory distress that could indicate internal bleeding in the neck. Activities are restricted for 24 hr.

Key: *CSF,* cerebrospinal fluid; *ICP,* intracranial pressure; *IV,* intravenous; *NPO,* nothing by mouth, *VS,* vital signs.

Table 21–6 ***Diagnostic Tests for Neurologic Disorders—cont'd***

TEST	PURPOSE	DESCRIPTION	NURSING IMPLICATIONS
Radionuclide imaging (brain scan)	To detect an intracranial mass: tumor, abscess, hematoma, or aneurysm.	A radioisotope is administered IV. Abnormal tissue usually absorbs more of the isotope than normal tissue. After a 1- to 3-hr waiting period for absorption, a scintillation scanner is used to image the brain. The test takes 30 min–1 hr.	Explain the procedure; patient will sit or lie on a table; the scanner makes clicking noises; the amount of radioactivity is very low and is not dangerous to the patient or others. Patient will need to lie or sit still during the scanning. A drug may be given the night before to block uptake of the radioactive element by the thyroid and salivary glands. There is no food or fluid restriction; no special aftercare.
Magnetic resonance imaging (MRI)	To visualize soft tissue without the use of contrast media or ionizing radiation; provides excellent images of soft tissue, eliminating bone; can visualize lesions undetected by CT scan. To detect white matter areas in nervous system that represent demyelination, as in multiple sclerosis.	An electromagnet is used to detect radiofrequency pulses produced by alignment of hydrogen protons in the magnetic field. Computer produces tomographic images with high contrast of area studied. Cannot be used in the presence of metal. Is quite expensive. A contrast agent often is used for better visualization and definition of specific structures.	Inform patient that the test is painless; no dietary restrictions. Remove all metal objects before test. Screen the patient for hidden sources of metal, such as bullet fragments, iron filings, aneurysm clips. MRI is contraindicated for patients with pacemakers. Patient must be still during test. Explain that body part to be imaged is moved inside large machine; some patients become claustrophobic. He will be able to communicate with the machine operator. Requires a signed consent for use of contrast media.
Magnetic resonance angiography (MRA)	Evaluates intracranial and extracranial blood vessels. Useful for diagnosing cerebrovascular disease. Is rapidly replacing cerebral angiography.	Similar to MRI. Uses differing signals of flowing blood to collect data. May be enhanced with use of contrast media.	Explain the need for lying completely still for 1 hr. May require sedation. Screen patient for any metal on body before test. Requires a signed consent for use of contrast media.
Magnetic resonance spectroscopy (MRS)	Used to determine loss of neurons with markers of neuronal integrity (e.g., *N*-acetyl aspartate) and to study brain diseases.	Uses MRI to gather information about chemical composition of brain tissue.	Same as for MRI.
Positron emission tomography (PET)	Assesses for cell death, damage in brain tissue.	Radioactive material is given and provides differing color in areas of cellular activity.	Requires signed consent. Explain that two IV lines will be inserted. Patient is to avoid sedatives or tranquilizers before test. Ask to empty bladder before test. Patient may be asked to perform various activities during the test.
Single-photon emission computed tomography (SPECT)	Used to visualize glucose or oxygen metabolism in the brain and to visualize blood flow.	Radiolabeled compounds are injected and their single-photon emissions are scanned. Images are made of the accumulated radiolabeled compounds.	Same as for PET.
Ultrasound arteriography (Doppler flow studies)	To study flow and determine areas of constriction or obstruction in cerebral arteries. To detect arterial spasm.	Noninvasive test. Doppler image scanning device is used with computer to visualize anatomy of major cerebral arteries.	Tell patient that the test is noninvasive and painless. A small Doppler wand is positioned over particular "window" areas on the skull (temples), and with the computer, sound waves are directed so as to produce an image of the interior arteries and their blood flow. No special preparation or aftercare.
Carotid duplex Doppler studies	Determine if blood flow in carotid arteries is decreased or blocked.	Sound waves graph a picture of blood flow in the carotid arteries.	Explain that the test is noninvasive and painless. Patient will lie flat with head turned to one side and then the other.

Continued

Table 21–6 **Diagnostic Tests for Neurologic Disorders—cont'd**

TEST	PURPOSE	DESCRIPTION	NURSING IMPLICATIONS
Evoked potential studies	To measure response of the CNS to visual, auditory, or sensory stimulus. Helpful in detecting tumor of CN VIII, blindness in infants, or brainstem lesions. Also useful in diagnosing multiple sclerosis.	May be done in conjunction with EEG. Electrodes are used to pick up and transmit impulses to a computer while a stimulus is delivered to the patient. Signals are displayed on an oscilloscope, and data are stored for later interpretation.	Explain the procedure to the patient. Visual-evoked potentials: stimulus may be a bright flashing light or checkerboard patterns. Somatosensory-evoked potentials require stimulation of a peripheral sensory nerve with a mild electric shock. Auditory brainstem-evoked potentials utilize various noises or tone bursts through earphones. Discomfort is minimal. Test takes 30–60 min.
Cerebrospinal fluid analysis and culture	To detect abnormalities that are indicative of specific neurologic problems and determine which organism is responsible for infection.	CSF is obtained by lumbar puncture. It is analyzed for color, cell count, protein, chloride, and glucose. The fluid is cultured to detect the presence of organisms; if present, an antibiotic sensitivity test is done to determine which drug will best kill the organism. CSF pressure also is measured. Normal CSF values for the adult are: Color: clear Cell count (WBCs): 0–8 mm^3 Protein: 14–45 mg/dL Chloride: 118–132 mEq/L Glucose: 40–80 mg/dL Pressure: 75–175 cm H_2O	Follow lumbar puncture procedure. Label the test tubes as 1, 2, and 3 and be certain they are filled with at least 3 mL of CSF in this order. Do not refrigerate the tubes; transport to the lab immediately. Maintain Standard Precautions.
PLAC (lipoprotein-associated phospholipase A_2; Lp-PLA_2)	Inflammatory enzyme marker for increased ischemic stroke risk.	This substance is thought to be partly responsible for atherosclerosis formation.	Explain that this is a simple blood test. Results take 7–10 days.

Key: *CN,* cranial nerve; *CNS,* central nervous system; *CSF,* cerebrospinal fluid; *WBCs,* white blood cells.

thigh to contract and to move the leg upward. This reflex, or simple reflex arc, involves only two nerves and one synapse. The leg begins to jerk up while the brain is just becoming aware of the tap on the knee (see Figure 21–5).

The knee jerk, or patellar reflex, tests nerve pathways to and from the spinal cord at the level of the second through fourth lumbar nerves. In addition to testing the patellar reflex, a neurologic examination might include testing the biceps reflex (pathways for the fifth and sixth cervical nerves), triceps reflex (seventh and eighth cervical nerves), brachioradialis reflex (fifth and sixth cervical nerves), and Achilles tendon reflex (first and second sacral nerves). Reflexes are graded as follows: 0/5 = absent; 1/5 = weak response; 2/5 = normal; 3/5 = exaggerated response; and 4/5 = hyperreflexia with clonus. **Clonus** is a continued rhythmic contraction of the muscle while there is continuous application of the stimulus.

Another reflex action widely used as a diagnostic aid in CNS disorders is **Babinski's reflex,** which is elicited by scraping an object such as a key along the sole of the foot. In a normal response to this stimulus, the toes will bend downward. In a *positive* Babinski reflex, the great toe bends backward (upward) and the smaller toes fan outward. A positive Babinski reflex in the adult not under the influence of chemical substances indicates an abnormality in the motor control pathways leading from the cerebral cortex (Figure 21–7).

In the unconscious person, the physician may perform tests to determine brainstem function. After ruling out spinal cord injury, the oculocephalic ("doll's eye") and oculovestibular reflexes are assessed. For the doll's eye reflex, the examiner places a hand on each side of the patient's head, using the thumbs to gently hold open the eyelids. While watching the patient's eyes, the head is rotated briskly to one side and eye movement is observed in relation to head movement. If the brainstem pathways are intact, the eyes appear to move in a direction opposite to that of the head movement; that is, if the head is rotated to the right, the eyes appear to move to the left. After assuring the tympanic membrane is intact, the oculovestib-

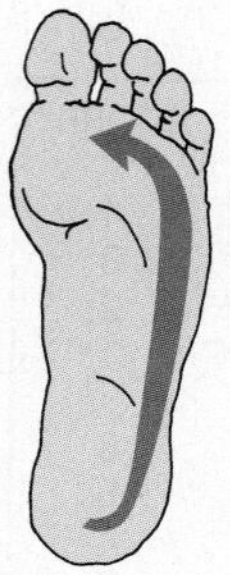

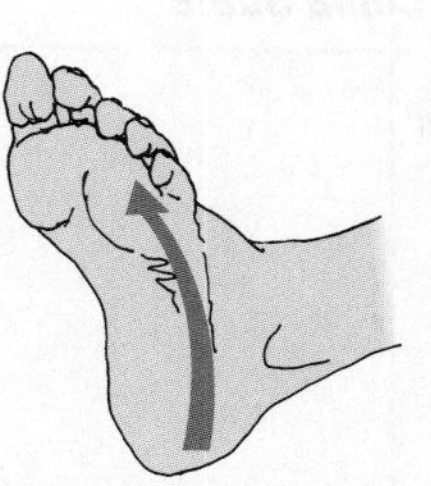

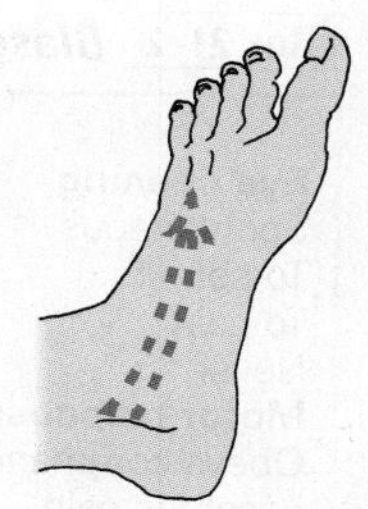

FIGURE **21–7** Normal and Babinski's reflexes.

ular reflex is assessed by **caloric testing**. With the patient's head elevated at least 30 degrees, 20 to 200 mL of cold or ice water is instilled into the ear with a catheter-tipped syringe. While the external ear canal is irrigated, the patient's eye movements are observed. Normally the eyes will show nystagmus, darting away from the irrigated ear. Absence of eye movement may indicate a brainstem lesion.

NURSING MANAGEMENT

Assessment (Data Collection)

Neurologic nursing requires special training and experience in observation, critical judgment, and specific skills to help patients cope with a myriad of problems. The nurse not only must be aware of subtle changes in the patient's condition but also must recognize the *significance* of these changes and act promptly when medical attention is needed. The LPN/LVN assists the RN with the gathering of data for the neurologic assessment (Assignment Considerations 21–1).

Patient History

Because neurologic disorders can be present in conjunction with or in addition to disorders of other body systems, the nurse should always include questions about neurologic status in the initial and ongoing assessments of all patients. For example, a surgical patient could have had a previous stroke, or could have a history of seizures or an existing neuromuscular disease such as multiple sclerosis. Although these may not be the primary reason for admission to a hospital, they will certainly influence the course of the illness or injury for which admission occurred.

Questions that should be asked when assessing a patient with an actual or possible neurologic problem are presented in Focused Assessment 21–1.

Physical Assessment

A basic nursing assessment of neurologic function is performed on any patient who is suspected of experiencing a neurologic problem. Nurses often need to assess for the occurrence of cerebrovascular accident (CVA, or stroke) or of a neurologic deficit after a surgical procedure. Basic neurologic assessment includes assessment of the following areas.

Vital Signs. Assessing and recording temperature, pulse, respirations, and blood pressure are essential. The patient's temperature is important and may be elevated for a number of reasons. Infection or damage to the temperature control mechanisms within the brain from increasing intracranial pressure (ICP) may be present.

Changes in blood pressure, particularly a rise in systolic pressure and a widening pulse pressure, may indicate an ICP increase. The pulse may become slow and bounding, and breathing may become irregular and labored as ICP rises. Changes in breathing pattern often indicate a problem with neurologic control of respiration. Any identified change must be reported to the physician promptly.

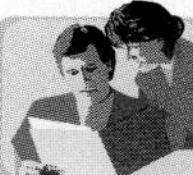

Assignment Considerations 21–1

Reporting Observations

If a patient with a neurologic problem that may affect level of consciousness is assigned to a certified nursing assistant (CNA) for bathing and morning care, remember to remind the assistant to report to you any change in wakefulness, irritability, speech, eye appearance, gait, or balance. It is best not to assign a patient who has already shown some signs of deteriorating level of consciousness to a CNA.

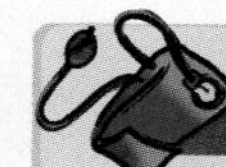

Focused Assessment 21–1

Data Collection for the Neurologic System

When gathering a history for a patient who may have a neurologic problem, ask the following questions.

- Do you or does any member of your family have any genetic disorder of the nervous system?
- Have you ever had a seizure or been told you have epilepsy?
- Have you ever had difficulty in speaking, concentrating, remembering, or expressing thoughts? Have you noticed any changes in these functions?
- Have you had any changes in muscle strength or coordination?
- Have you ever injured your head?
- Have you ever had a really high fever?
- Have you had any severe sinus, ear, tooth, or facial skin infection?
- Do you recall any episodes of tremors, muscle spasms, fainting, dizziness, ringing in the ears, or blurred vision?
- Have you had any "blackout" spells?
- Have you noticed any changes in taste or smell?
- Do you have any numbness or tingling in the extremities?

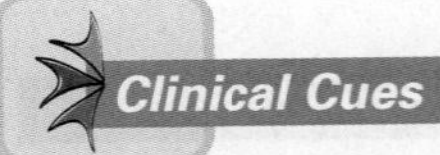

Clinical Cues

When the systolic and diastolic pressure readings are farther apart, a widening pulse pressure has occurred. For example, if the blood pressure was 128/78 earlier and is now 136/64, there is a widened pulse pressure.

Current vital signs should be compared to those from the previous several days to determine any changes or trends. Look for changes in blood pressure, pulse rate and quality, respiratory pattern, and for rising temperature.

Think Critically About . . . If your patient's blood pressure was 138/84 and is now 146/76, what is happening? Is the ICP probably increasing or decreasing?

Mental Function and Level of Consciousness. Patients experience varying levels of consciousness (LOC) and ability to respond. It is necessary to determine where the patient is in relation to level of consciousness, the extremes being alert wakefulness and deep coma (no responsiveness at all).

When observing a patient to determine LOC, the best assessment is based on established criteria or standards that are understood by the observer as well as by others who will be reading the results of the observations. The Glasgow Coma Scale is a tool that is universally used in one form or another for this purpose (Box 21–2). The patient's LOC is scored in three different categories. The first category is eye opening, the second is best motor response, and the third is best verbal response. A number is assigned for each category depending on what the assessment reveals. Assessment in the first and last category determines whether the patient can respond to voice commands or to pain or doesn't respond at all. Verbal responses are evaluated according to whether the patient is oriented and "making sense," confused, making inappropriate remarks, incomprehensible, or silent. **The score in each area is added together, with the optimal score being 15, which indicates a fully alert patient. A score of 3 indicates a totally comatose patient.** Coma level is indicated by a score of 8 or less. Some of the criteria for assessing LOC include: Does the patient awaken easily? Is he oriented to person (himself as well as others), place, and time? Is he able to follow commands? Does he fail to respond to any stimulus, even physically painful ones? Is he restless? Combative? Does he respond to pain with abnormal posturing?

The FOUR (Full Outline of UnResponsiveness) score developed by Dr. Eelco Wijdicks, a neurologist at

Box 21–2 ***Glasgow Coma Scale***

	SCORE*
Eye opening	
Spontaneous	4
To sound	3
To pain	2
Never	1
Motor response	
Obeys commands	6
Localizes pain	5
Normal flexion (withdrawal)	4
Abnormal flexion posturing	3
Extension posturing	2
None	1
Verbal response	
Oriented	5
Confused conversation	4
Inappropriate words	3
Incomprehensible sounds	2
None	1

*A score of 8 or less indicates coma. The highest possible score is 15.

the Mayo Clinic, is becoming preferred for comatose or intubated patients who cannot speak. A score of 0 to 4 is assigned in each of four categories: eye, motor, brainstem, and respiratory function. A score of 0 indicates no function and a score of 4 indicates normal function (Wijdicks et al., 2005). 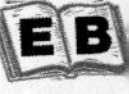

In the alert patient, note changes in mental function by asking questions to determine orientation to person, place, and time: "What day is today? What month is it? Where are you now?" Assessing memory lapses may be done by asking when the patient was born, what state he resides in, what the last major holiday was, and so on. Thinking can be evaluated by asking the patient to add three numbers together; to count by 6s; or to solve a simple puzzle, such as "If a man goes to the store and purchases four oranges at 40¢ each, two apples at 60¢ each, and two bananas for 46¢, how much did he spend?" (Allow pencil and paper to be used.) If the patient can read English, hand him a card with a command written on it, such as "walk to the sink" or "turn on your right side" (assuming he is physically capable of performing such a task).

Judgment can be grossly tested by assessing whether the patient has been making rational choices in his day-to-day life and by asking him what he would do in a particular situation. Asking specifically what he would do should there be a fire in the trash can will provide information about his judgment.

Neurologic and Neuromuscular Status. Basic assessment of cranial nerves and motor function can be performed by watching the patient perform morning activities of daily living (ADLs). Assess the following: Does the face move symmetrically when he smiles? Is speech clear when he answers questions? Does he move left and right extremities without noticeable problems? Is there anything abnormal about his gait as he moves across the room or down the hall? Does he have difficulty eating or swallowing? Observe the pupils of the eye for size and

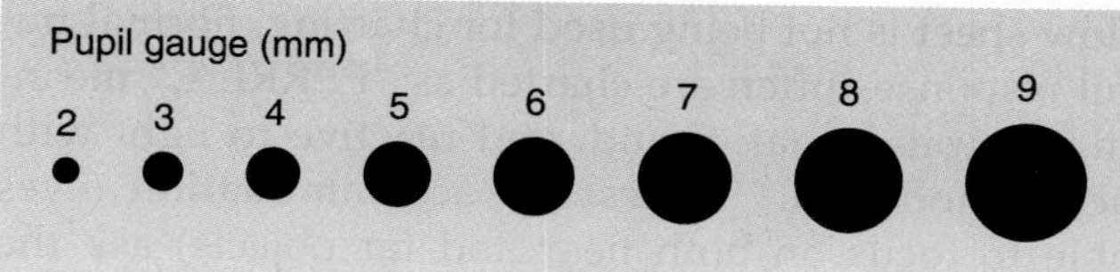

FIGURE 21–8 Pupil gauge (mm).

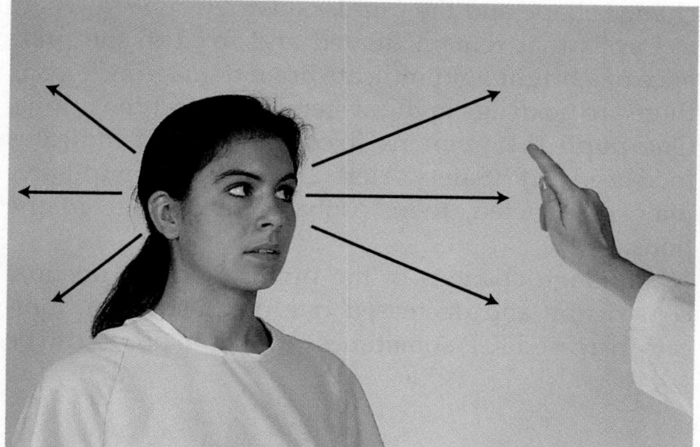

FIGURE 21–9 Checking the cardinal positions of eye movement.

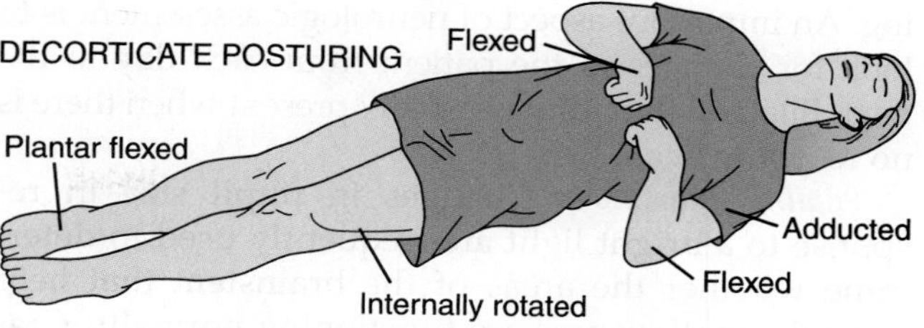

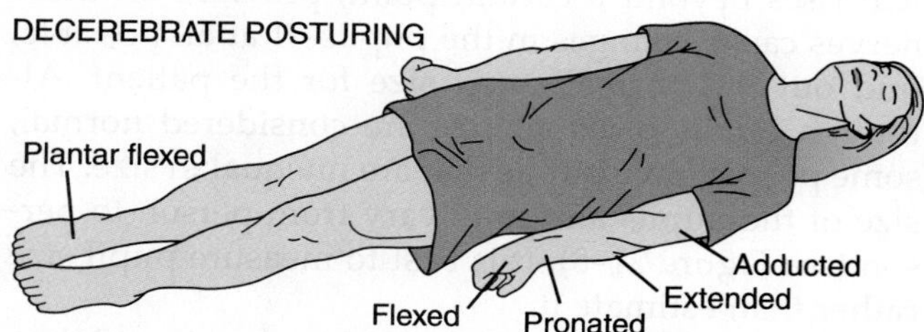

FIGURE 21–10 Decorticate and decerebrate posturing indicating brainstem injury.

equality. Pupils should be equal size and should constrict and dilate readily when the environmental light changes (Figure 21–8). Can he hear you if you speak to him when his back is turned? Does he seem as alert as usual? Is he having any trouble with balance?

Extraocular muscle movements are also evaluated. Ask the patient to follow your finger while you move it through the cardinal positions of gaze (Figure 21–9). Note whether both eyes move together (conjugate) or one deviates. If there is deviation, it is important to note the direction of the deviation. It should be noted if there is any quick back-and-forth oscillation (nystagmus) of the eye at the end points of each direction. Nystagmus can indicate abnormality, such as multiple sclerosis, or can be a side effect of medication, such as phenytoin (Dilantin).

Neuromuscular assessment is concerned with the function of the motor pathways. Each of the upper and lower extremities is tested. Ask the patient to follow verbal commands such as "raise your left leg," "bend your right knee," "touch your left elbow with your right hand," and "touch your face with your left hand." Have him push against the palms of your hands first with one foot and then the other to test the strength of the leg muscles. Have the patient extend his arms in front of him, and press down on each arm one at a time, while asking him to try to raise his arm, to test muscle strength.

If the patient has an extremity that is not responding, another stimulus may be necessary to test it. If the patient does not respond to voice commands at all, and deafness is not an issue, the degree of unconsciousness is tested. First use a louder voice to try to arouse the patient; then, if he doesn't respond, gently shake him as you would to awaken a child. If that is not successful, painful stimuli are applied for 20 to 30 seconds. First try applying pressure above the eye by placing a thumb under the orbital rim beneath the middle of the eyebrow and pushing upward. If there is no response, pinch the trapezius muscle at the angle of the shoulder and neck; twist the fingers slightly. If there is no response, apply pressure to the angle of the mandible with the index and middle fingers. If there is still no response, the sternum is rubbed with the knuckles in the form of a fist; a twisting motion is used. **The sternal rub is performed on subsequent assessments only if there is good reason to believe that the patient's comatose status is changing, as it causes bruising.**

The levels of response are:

- Purposefully withdrawing from the stimulus or an attempt to push it away
- Nonpurposeful response, in which the patient may frown or move his arm or leg in a random fashion
- Failure to respond at all

Nonpurposeful responses to pain occur in two ways. Decorticate (flexor) posturing, which is the extension of the legs and internal rotation and adduction of the arms with the elbows bent upward, occurs with damage to the cortex. In decerebrate (extensor) posturing, the arms are stiffly extended and held close to the body, and the wrists are flexed outward. This response means there is damage to the midbrain or brainstem, which indicates a very serious injury (Figure 21–10). The response may be "lateralization," wherein one side of the body shows typical decorticate or decerebrate posturing. An important aspect of neurologic assessment is to look for changes in the patient from each day to the next. Bilateral flaccidity is usually present when there is no response at all.

Pupillary Reactions. Changes in pupil size in response to a bright light are frequently used to determine whether the areas of the brainstem that help control consciousness are functioning normally. Cranial nerves II and III control pupil movement. When ICP rises beyond a certain point, pressure on these nerves cause changes in the pupils. If at all possible, find out the normal pupil size for the patient. Although pupils of equal size are considered normal, some people have pupils that are unequal in size. The size of the pupils also may vary from person to person (see Figure 21–8). It is best to measure pupil size rather than estimate it.

The pupils should be examined in a room with low light, when the pupils would usually be dilated. A bright light is then directed into each eye from the side while the other eye is covered. One should observe whether the pupil into which the light is shone constricts and whether it does so briskly or sluggishly *(direct reflex)*. Finally, the light is shone into each eye while watching to see if the pupil constricts in the other eye *(consensual reflex)*. Table 21–7 shows pupil abnormalities and the possible causes. **When pupils have been previously reactive, changes in pupil size or reactivity may signal an emergency, and the physician must be notified immediately.** If a flow sheet is not being used for charting, normal pupil responses often are charted as "PERRLA," meaning "pupils equal, round, and reactive to light with accommodation." To test for **accommodation** (eyes able to focus on both near and far objects) ask the patient to look at an object across the room away from the light source, and then to look at your fingers held about 6 inches from the eyes. The lenses should change shape and the pupils constrict.

Pupils that remain dilated and fixed in the presence of a bright light indicate brain damage as long as there are no drugs in the system that affect the pupils. One pupil that remains fixed and dilated indicates increased ICP (Safety Alert 21–1). If both pupils remain constricted, there probably is damage to the pons.

Although changes in the pupils, such as unequal constriction and decreased rate of constriction, indicate increased ICP, sometimes changes in pupils can be

Safety Alert 21–1

Report Changes Immediately

If changes in data indicate a rise in ICP or a decrease in LOC, it is important to alert the charge nurse and physician. This is even more important when possible intracranial bleeding is suspected as it may indicate an emergency situation.

Table 21–7 *Pupillary Abnormalities and Possible Causes*

ASSESSMENT DATA	APPEARANCE	POSSIBLE CAUSES
Unilateral, fixed, dilated pupil. Unreactive to light. May be accompanied by ptosis and deviation to side and downward.		Damage to oculomotor nerve related to increased intraocular pressure, compression of oculomotor nerve, head trauma with epidural or subdural hematoma
Bilateral dilated and fixed pupils that do not react to light.		Hypoxia associated with cardiopulmonary arrest Pressure on midbrain Severe CNS disorder Anticholinergic drug overdose
Bilateral small, fixed pupils that do not react to light. Accompanied by motor deficits, drowsiness, confusion, headache, vomiting, incontinence when due to damage to diencephalon.		Side effect of opiates such as morphine Miotic eye drops Hemorrhage into the pons Damage to the diencephalon
Unequal pupil size; both pupils react to light unless there is underlying pathology.		Ocular inflammation Congenital aberration Adhesion, as of iris to cornea or lens Disturbance of neural pathways

Key: *CNS*, central nervous system.

caused by medications. For example, atropine and scopolamine can produce dilated pupils, and opiates, miotics, and street drugs can cause constriction (see Table 21–7).

The "Neuro" Check. Monitoring the neurologic status of a patient with a known neurologic disorder includes a "neuro" check on a set schedule. It is performed to determine whether increased ICP is present or ICP is rising. For example, monitoring is necessary after a traumatic head injury, after ingestion of an overdose of a drug or other chemical, when a stroke has occurred or is suspected, or for any other condition in which the patient has lost or may lose consciousness. A neurologic assessment flow sheet is used to chart assessment data so that the trend in function of each area can be quickly identified (Figure 21–11). Four areas are monitored: vital signs, LOC, pupil reaction, and motor function (Assignment Considerations 21–2).

"Neuro" checks may be ordered as frequently as every 15 minutes or at intervals from 2 to 8 hours. The findings are recorded on the neurologic flow sheet.

> ? *Think Critically About . . .* You arrive at the home of an elderly lady who has severe heart disease and is very weak. Her spouse says she is confused and lethargic and that she wouldn't try to eat breakfast. He is worried. As her nurse, what specific assessments would you perform in an attempt to determine whether she has suffered a CVA?

Diagnostic Tests. The major diagnostic tests most commonly used to evaluate the neurologic system are presented in Table 21–6. Basic physiologic testing is also done to rule out disease in some other system that might be affecting the condition of the patient. A chest radiograph, electrocardiogram, complete blood cell count, urinalysis, and basic tests for electrolytes, liver function, kidney function, nutritional parameters, and lipid metabolism (such as are included on a sequential multiple analyzer [SMA] profile) are performed. A nerve or muscle biopsy may be done to determine pathologic changes in these tissues. Figure 21–12 shows the technique used for lumbar puncture.

Nursing Diagnosis

The most common nursing diagnoses for patients with neurologic disorders are listed in Table 21–8. Each nursing diagnosis chosen for the patient should be individualized to fit the situation. Nursing diagnoses in a care plan vary according to whether the patient is in the acute stage, recovery stage, or rehabilitative stage of the disorder. Goals and general expected outcomes for each nursing diagnosis are presented in Table 21–8 along with appropriate interventions.

Planning

Overall goals for patients with neurologic disorders depend on whether there is a physiologic possibility that full function may be regained or not. When permanent neurologic deficit occurs, as may occur with some spinal cord injuries, the ultimate goal is for the patient to function at the highest physiologic level. This requires adjusting to limitations imposed by neurologic deficit so that the patient may live his life in a meaningful way. A goal for all patients with neurologic disorders is to prevent injury, whether from complications of immobility, accidents related to lack of sensation, aspiration from difficulty in swallowing, or any of the other problems that the neurologic deficit may cause.

Caring for patients with neurologic deficits can be very time consuming and requires considerable patience and understanding. If the patient has any weakness, paralysis, or decreased sensation in the extremities, or is confused, disoriented, aphasic, or otherwise incapacitated, providing care will take more time than usual. Extended time must be included in the daily work plan. When a patient is comatose or paralyzed, it is best to team up with another helper to provide care and to turn or reposition the patient. By working together, care is smoother and less taxing.

Implementation

Interventions for each nursing diagnosis concerning common problems of neurologic disorders are listed in Table 21–8. Patients should be given information about the disorder and taught about diagnostic tests, and self-care. Positive coping skills should be reinforced and ongoing support offered. Interventions are discussed in the following sections on common care problems and with the specific neurologic disorders in the next chapters.

Evaluation

Evaluation of interventions is performed to determine whether goals are being met. Are the interventions chosen helping to meet the specific expected outcomes written? If not, the plan needs to be changed. Progress often is slow in the patient experiencing a neurologic deficit. It may take a considerable time for improvement to be noted. Long-term goals of a realistic nature are appropriate. Keep in mind that certain types of neurologic deficits, such as those caused by spinal cord severance, may not improve.

SOUTHWEST WASHINGTON MEDICAL CENTER
VANCOUVER, WASHINGTON

ADULT/PEDIATRIC NEURO FLOW RECORD

PATIENT IMPRINT

DATE:		TIME:
1. EYE OPENING	4. Spontaneous 3. To speech 2. To pain 1. No response	
2. ADULT/PEDIATRIC **BEST VERBAL RESPONSE**	5. Oriented 4. Confused 3. Inappropriate 2. Incomprehensible 1. No response	
OR		
3. AGE <2 YR	5. Social smile, orients to sound, follows objects 4. Cries, consolable 3. Inappropriate, persistent cry 2. Agitated/restless 1. No response	
4. BEST MOTOR RESPONSE	6. Spontaneous 5. Localizes pain 4. Withdraws to pain 3. Flexion to pain 2. Extension to pain 1. No response	
5. LEVEL OF CONSCIOUSNESS	5. Alert/oriented 4. Confused/disoriented 3. Drowsy/responding 2. Reacting 1. Unconscious	
6. PULSES	4. Strong 3. Weak 2. Present with Doppler 1. Absent	RT DP/PT LEFT DP/PT Radial pulse
7. DRESSINGS	4. Dry 3. Slight amount 2. Moderate amount 1. Saturated	
8. SWELLING OF POSTOP	4. Absent 3. Slight amount 2. Moderate amount 1. Vast amount	
9. GRIPS AND MOVEMENT	5. Strong 4. Medium strong 3. Weak 2. Minimal 1. Absent	R. Hand grip R. Arm movement R. Leg movement R. Leg pushes L. Hand grip L. Arm movement L. Leg movement L. Leg pushes
10. RESPIRATORY	5. Normal/deep 4. Tachypneic 3. Bradypneic 2. Cheyne-Stokes 1. Respirator assist	
11. PUPILS Size in mm REACTION 3. Normal 2. Sluggish 1. Nonreactive	SIZE 1-Pinpoint ○-2 ○-3 ○-4 ○-5 ○-6 ○-7 ○-8 ○-9	R. Pupil size L. Pupil size R. Pupil reaction L. Pupil reaction
12. INITIALS		

FIGURE 21–11 Neurologic assessment flow sheet.

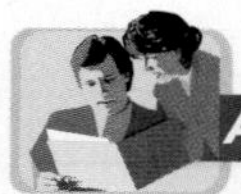

Assignment Considerations 21–2

The "Neuro" Check

Although the measuring of vital signs can be assigned to assistive personnel, the gathering of data for the "neuro check" should not be delegated. It is important to compare current data with previous data and to carefully assess neuromuscular and pupillary response.

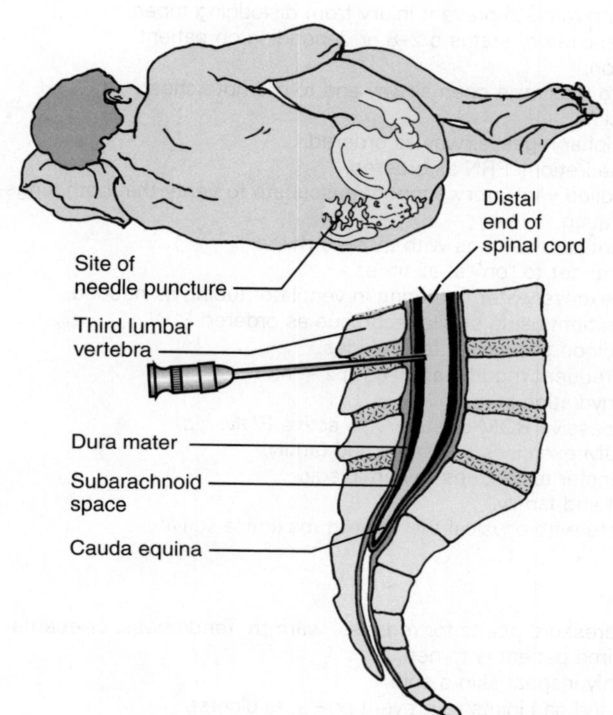

FIGURE **21–12** Lumbar puncture technique.

COMMON NEUROLOGIC PATIENT CARE PROBLEMS

Neurologic disorders and illnesses cause many of the same problems. Whether the patient has encephalitis, has a head injury, is recovering from cranial surgery, has suffered a stroke, or has multiple sclerosis or Parkinson's disease, he may need nursing intervention in one or more of the following areas.

INEFFECTIVE BREATHING PATTERN

Weakness of the diaphragm, respiratory muscles, or interruption of normal brain function may occur with a variety of neurologic disorders. The nurse must monitor the adequacy of respiratory effort and promote a patent airway and chest expansion. Elevating the head of the bed 30 degrees allows the diaphragm to drop more easily and promotes chest expansion. This is only done when there is no spinal injury. When consciousness is depressed, the tongue may be flaccid and fall back, blocking the airway. Positioning the patient on the side allows the tongue to fall to the side and opens the airway. Insertion of an oropharyngeal tube or oral airway also is helpful.

Assisting the patient with deep breathing and the use of an incentive spirometer can help prevent atelectasis and improve ventilation (Agency for Healthcare Research and Quality, 2001). Respiratory assessment is performed every shift and includes auscultating the lungs for signs of atelectasis or retained secretions and judging the quality of respiratory effort. If respiratory efforts are considerably impaired, the patient may need intubation and mechanical ventilation. Interventions for the patient undergoing mechanical ventilation are presented in Chapter 14.

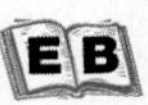

IMPAIRED MOBILITY

The nurse, the physical therapist, and the patient work together to help the patient cope with muscle weakness or paralysis. Activities such as proper positioning and range-of-motion (ROM) exercises are started immediately to preserve proper alignment of joints and limbs and prevent contractures and muscle atrophy. Assistive devices, such as splints and slings, may be used. The patient who suffers **hemiplegia** (paralysis and loss of sensation in an extremity) is taught to become aware of arm or leg placement when he turns or transfers to a chair to avoid injury to the affected extremity.

For example, the patient with left hemiplegia from a CVA may neglect his paralyzed side. He must therefore be taught to attend to the affected side of his body by scanning it frequently. To prevent discomfort in the shoulder and arm on the affected side and to prevent dislocation of the shoulder, care is taken not to pull on the affected arm or shoulder during transfers or ambulation. The affected arm should be supported with pillows or an armrest to keep it from dangling when the patient is seated. Using a sling for comfort and to promote better balance when ambulating and transferring is desirable.

The patient with hemiplegia is taught step by step the safest way to transfer from the bed to a wheelchair and back, and how to use assistance from others. He is also taught how to care for and protect his skin in areas of decreased sensation.

The patient who has **hemiparesis** (one-sided weakness) is taught how to strengthen his muscles and use assistive devices, such as walkers, crutches, or canes, to walk. He is taught the best ways to get out of bed and into and out of a chair. The **quadriplegic** patient (four limbs paralyzed) is helped in learning to cope with this drastic alteration in his life and how he might direct his energies toward different, but attainable, goals. A newer term for quadriplegia is **tetraplegia.**

All patients who have suffered an impairment of mobility need assistance with the grieving process,

Table 21–8 ***Common Nursing Diagnoses, Expected Outcomes, and Nursing Interventions for Patients with Neurologic Disorders***

NURSING DIAGNOSIS	GOALS/EXPECTED OUTCOMES	NURSING INTERVENTIONS
Risk for injury related to decreased level of consciousness; paralysis or decreased sensation	Patient will have no evidence of injury or trauma.	Side rails up at all times patient is unattended. Bed in low position when patient is unattended. Pad side rails if seizure activity or restlessness indicates need. Provide eye care for unconscious patient and if corneal (blink) reflex is absent; lubrication and eye patch or shield as needed. Position carefully, protecting extremities from contact with side rails. Maintain correct body alignment. Administer anticonvulsants as ordered to prevent seizure activity. Protect from thermal injury. Utilize hand mitts to prevent injury from dislodging tubes.
Ineffective breathing pattern related to neurologic disruption of respiration	Maintain a patent airway. Maintain a Po_2 of 80–100 mm Hg. Patient will have no evidence of pulmonary infection.	Assess respiratory status q 2–8 hr depending on patient condition. Position to maximize open airway and to promote chest expansion. Insert oropharyngeal airway as ordered. Suction secretions PRN as ordered. For controlled ventilatory support: auscultate to verify that both lungs are inflating. Check ventilator settings with those ordered. Keep alarm set to "on" at all times. Remove excess water gathering in ventilator tubing as needed. Suction patient using sterile technique as ordered PRN. Monitor blood gas values for changes. Provide frequent mouth care (i.e., q 2–4 hr). Monitor hydration status.
Impaired physical mobility related to CNS deficit, weakness, paralysis, or fatigue	Maintains mobility of all joints. Patient will have no evidence of contractures. Patient will regain optimal physical mobility neurologically possible.	Perform passive ROM or supervise active ROM qid. Teach ROM exercises to patient and family. Teach transfer techniques to hemiplegic patient and family. Collaborate with physical therapist to maximize activity.
Risk for impaired skin integrity related to impaired mobility, decreased sensory awareness, or decreased sensation	Patient's skin will remain intact.	Inspect pressure points for redness, warmth, tenderness, or edema each time patient is turned. Thoroughly inspect skin q shift. Position and pad joints to prevent pressure ulcers. Formulate regular turning/repositioning schedule and stick to it. Use special mattress or special bed to enhance skin protection. Teach patients in wheelchairs to shift weight q 15 min. Teach patient and family to inspect pressure areas and skin for beginning signs of breakdown.
Self-care deficit related to neurologic impairment: paresis, paralysis, decreased LOC, or confusion	Patient will meet self-care needs of hygiene, toileting, feeding, and grooming. Patient will resume self-care at level physiologically and neurologically possible.	Assist with hygiene, toileting, feeding, and grooming as needed. Assist patient to set small, attainable goals for self-care. Explain and demonstrate specific ADL in small, one-task segments. Obtain and demonstrate adaptive devices to assist with ADLs. Offer patience, support, and encouragement for each attempt at self-care. Maintain chart of self-care improvement to track achievement so that patient can see progress.

Key: *ADLs,* activities of daily living; *CNS,* central nervous system; *LOC,* level of consciousness; Po_2, partial pressure of oxygen; *PRN,* as needed; *ROM,* range of motion.

Table 21–8 ***Common Nursing Diagnoses, Expected Outcomes, and Nursing Interventions for Patients with Neurologic Disorders—cont'd***

NURSING DIAGNOSIS	GOALS/EXPECTED OUTCOMES	NURSING INTERVENTIONS
Imbalanced nutrition: less than body requirements related to inability to swallow or danger of aspiration	Patient's nutritional status will remain adequate as evidenced by normal weight and adequate levels of serum protein.	Institute tube feeding as needed. Check tube placement before initiating each feeding; aspirate stomach contents; test acidity if there is doubt about origins of aspirated fluid. Check residual before each intermittent feeding or every 4 hr for continuous feedings; if greater than 150 mL or more than ½ of previous feeding, replace and delay next feeding for 1–2 hr. Position patient with head of bed up at least 30 degrees when feeding and for 30–60 min after feeding. Monitor for adverse side effects such as diarrhea. Flush tube with 30–60 mL water after each feeding. Instill water between feedings to maintain hydration. Monitor glucose levels after initiation of feedings until blood glucose is stable. Weight at least twice a week. Monitor intake and output. **For patient with dysphagia who can take oral feedings:** Serve semisoft foods. Provide six small meals per day; provide non-stressful atmosphere with few distractions for mealtime. Teach to sit upright with head slightly forward and neck flexed; encourage to place food on strongest side of mouth and tongue; encourage to take small bites at a time. Remain with patient to decrease fear of choking; keep suction at hand and turned on during meal. Ensure privacy for meal to decrease embarrassment about drooling, dropping food, or choking. Provide appropriate tube care (see Chapter 23).
Constipation/diarrhea/ bowel incontinence related to decreased level of consciousness, neurogenic impairment, or side effects of medications	Patient will have normal bowel movements as evidenced by soft, formed stool. Patient will attain bowel continence.	Monitor bowel movements and evaluate regularity based on nutritional intake. Administer stool softeners, rectal suppository, or enemas as ordered for constipation. Check for and remove fecal impaction if it occurs, guarding against spinal dysreflexia in the paralyzed patient. Institute bowel training program if needed (see Chapter 23). If diarrhea occurs, determine cause and alleviate if possible. Administer antidiarrheal if ordered. Keep rectal area clean and dry; protect rectal mucosa. Monitor hydration status; evaluate intake and output.
Disturbed sensory perception related to decreased level of consciousness	Patient will respond to family interaction as evidenced by movement, hand squeezing, eye opening, or speech. Patient will return to alert state as evidenced by proper orientation to person, time, and place.	Speak of current events or daily happenings while providing care. Encourage family members and friends to speak to patient of day's occurrences or fun times in past. Play music on the radio that is to the patient's taste. Play videotapes on topics of interest to the patient. Turn on the patient's favorite television shows. Ask questions and patiently listen for a response. With a tape recorder, introduce sounds from the patient's home and work environment.
Social isolation related to immobility and intellectual limits imposed by neurologic impairment	Patient will have social interaction with visiting friends. Patient will maintain relationships with family members and loved ones. Patient will make new friends among support group members.	Encourage friends and family to visit. Instruct friends and family on how to interact with the patient. Encourage patient to discuss his feelings regarding social contact. Encourage participation in an appropriate support group. Encourage development of a social network. Encourage participation in church, civic, volunteer, and social groups in community. Provide referrals to community job retraining resources if patient is unable to resume former employment or lifestyle.

Continued

Table 21–8 *Common Nursing Diagnoses, Expected Outcomes, and Nursing Interventions for Patients with Neurologic Disorders—cont'd*

NURSING DIAGNOSIS	GOALS/EXPECTED OUTCOMES	NURSING INTERVENTIONS
Interrupted family processes related to role changes, uncertainty of the future, and financial constraints	Each family member will demonstrate appropriate coping methods. Each family member will regain an optimistic outlook. Each family member will accept the patient in his changed state. Each family member will use referrals to support groups and community resources.	Assess strengths of each family member; look for signs of stress. Provide opportunity for verbalization of fears and concerns; feelings about patient's changed condition. Refer to social worker and community resources for support services. Arrange for psychological counseling or family therapy as needed. Encourage contact with appropriate support group. Initiate interaction and honest communication between patient and family members when patient and each member is ready. Teach problem-solving methods if coping skills are weak.

help in establishing healthy and effective coping patterns, and assistance with depression.

Attention to pain relief and muscle spasm is necessary for the patient to achieve the highest level of rehabilitation possible. Paralyzed extremities are susceptible to edema and should be elevated when the patient is at rest to decrease this problem. The patient needs to be turned frequently to prevent complications from pressure and sluggish circulation.

Elderly patients may suffer joint stiffness from arthritis. Assess joints for tenderness and pain before performing ROM, and be gentle and considerate when turning and repositioning.

Measures to promote skin integrity are instituted. The patient is placed on a special bed or protective mattress cover or pad, pressure points are inspected frequently, and the skin is kept clean and dry. Chapter 9 discusses the effects of immobility on each body system, along with the nursing activities necessary to avoid disabilities resulting from inactivity. The principles and practices presented in that chapter are relevant to the nursing care of a patient with a neurologic disorder that produces some type of paresis or paralysis, and for the patient who is unconscious.

SELF-CARE DEFICIT

Neuromuscular impairment may interfere with the patient's ability to perform hygiene activities or other ADLs. He may need assistance with bathing, grooming, oral hygiene, dressing, eating, and toileting. Work with the patient as his condition dictates, assisting with techniques to perform self-care in spite of disability when possible, offering encouragement, and praising any effort at accomplishing a self-care task.

Inability to carry out the most basic of self-care activities can erode a person's sense of independence and self-esteem. The ability to feed, clothe, and take care of functions of elimination is an important part of independence. Regaining some level of self-care in these areas is of particular concern to the adult who, because of neurologic dysfunction, may have to relearn ways to perform the simplest of daily activities.

If the patient is unconscious, the mouth must be kept clean to avoid infection of the parotid gland. The lips, tongue, and gums are cleansed and lubricated at frequent intervals as mouth breathing makes them excessively dry. This cleansing may be done by turning the patient to the side, turning on suction to the oral suction device, and, with a toothbrush or a tongue depressor with gauze taped to it, wiping the oral surfaces. A solution of 50% water/50% mouthwash, or water with a small amount of hydrogen peroxide, may be used to moisten the gauze. Too much hydrogen peroxide will cause excessive foaming. Using an irrigation syringe filled with water in one hand and the oral suction device in the other allows rinsing of the mouth while preventing aspiration of the liquid. It is easiest for two caregivers to work together to rinse and suction the mouth. Each time the mouth is cleansed, the patient should be positioned on the opposite side to ensure thorough cleansing of each side of the mouth. Oral suction should be available and turned on any time mouth care is given to a patient who has a weakened gag reflex, cannot swallow normally, or has weakness of the facial muscles. Studies show that tooth and tongue brushing decreases iatrogenic infection significantly.

When the patient cannot shut his eyes, the nurse or caregiver must provide care to prevent keratitis or corneal ulceration. The eyelids are cleansed with warm sterile water or normal saline every few hours to remove discharge and debris. Artificial tears or a lubricant is instilled as prescribed to prevent dryness. If the corneal reflex is absent, an eye shield or patch is placed over the eye. The eyelid is closed before a patch is applied. The eyes are examined each day for signs of inflammation.

The ability of significant others to learn how to care for the patient and their willingness to do so is an important part of assessing and planning for rehabilitation.

Goals for rehabilitation must be realistic and mutually agreed on by the patient, his family, and the nurse.

There are many assistive devices to help patients with neurologic deficits feed and dress themselves. Occupational therapists can help the patient relearn how to perform elementary tasks necessary to daily living. Patients are retaught how to feed themselves, how to get in and out of bed or a chair, how to select and put on clothes and fasten them, and how to bathe, brush their teeth, and comb their hair.

Provide assistance when the patient cannot do a task completely, and, most of all, provide encouragement and praise for efforts made. **When pursuing self-help rehabilitation, the nurse needs to remember that the patient tires easily and tasks must be spaced apart so that energy is available to achieve them.** Pushing the patient to try another task when he is too tired only sets him up for failure and frustration.

DYSPHAGIA

Every patient who has suffered a neurologic insult from head injury, stroke, or intracranial surgery should have the swallowing reflex assessed by trying to sip plain water before attempting to eat food. Checking periodically that the patient automatically swallows saliva should be done before offering water. Patients who have paresis from a stroke or who suffer from myasthenia gravis or other neurologic disorders often have difficulty swallowing **(dysphagia)**. Those patients who have difficulty eating are at risk for nutritional disorders and aspiration pneumonia. Patients with dysphagia should be sitting upright or in a high Fowler's position to eat. The position should be maintained for at least 30 minutes after a meal (Suiter, 2007). A nonstressful meal environment without distractions is best as stress makes dysphagia worse. Patient teaching for dysphagia is located in Chapter 23.

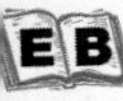

When swallowing without choking or aspiration is not possible, tube feeding is necessary. When the patient is receiving nutrients by tube, the caloric intake should be assessed frequently. The patient is weighed twice a week and intake and output are recorded and evaluated. Interventions for the patient receiving tube feedings are outlined in Chapter 28.

INCONTINENCE

Many patients with CNS disorders experience temporary or permanent urinary or fecal incontinence. Some patients experience constipation. The patient must be kept clean and dry. A condom catheter for the male patient or incontinence briefs or pads are used for urinary incontinence.

Perhaps the first step in planning and implementing either a bladder or a bowel training program is to convince the nursing staff and the patient and his family that something can be done to improve, if not completely relieve, the situation. A negative attitude and lack of persistence can doom a program to failure before it is started. Be content with small successes at first, setting short-term goals that will eventually lead to a satisfactory resolution of the problem.

Bladder Training Program

This is a program designed to help a patient with some degree of loss of normal bladder function and a resulting disturbance of voiding and bladder control. Loss of control can occur in a variety of neurologic disorders, including stroke, spinal cord injury, and tumors and lesions of the spinal cord.

The purposes of a bladder reconditioning program are to prevent urinary complications such as infection and **calculi** (stones) and to allow the patient freedom from fear of embarrassment and loss of self-esteem. Calculi are less likely to develop when there is a high fluid intake and frequent, complete emptying of the bladder.

Bladder function is assessed to determine the optimal neural and muscular control that can be realistically expected in view of the physiologic cause of loss of control and the patient's mental and emotional ability to cooperate and take an active part in carrying out the program.

The cause of urinary incontinence must be known, and the specific symptoms manifested by the patient must be clearly defined. Significant data include information about:

- Difficulty in starting to void
- Any methods the patient uses to initiate voiding (e.g., pressure on the bladder)
- Degree of awareness of the need to void
- Ability to empty the bladder completely and amount of residual urine
- Signs of bladder distention and dribbling or overflow
- Nighttime incontinence
- Stress incontinence
- Usual times for voiding

Spinal cord injuries and lesions produce what is known as a *cord bladder* or *neurogenic bladder.* Patients with disorders of this type are not aware of the need to void and must be trained in techniques to initiate voiding and emptying the bladder.

The second step in a bladder training program is to keep an accurate record of actual voiding times for a 2- to 3-day period. **Some problems of incontinence can be corrected by a simple scheduling of voiding times.** Offering a bedpan or getting the patient up to the bathroom one-half hour before times he is usually incontinent may remedy the problem.

A bladder training program usually begins with a 2-hour schedule for toileting. The patient should attempt to drink 2000 to 3000 mL of fluid between waking up and 6 P.M. Coffee, tea, alcoholic beverages, and soda with caffeine should be avoided after dinner, because they have a diuretic effect. The patient is toileted before retiring for the night. The maintenance of an accurate training record is essential. A trial of 6 weeks is necessary before determining whether the training is successful. Various drugs that affect the voiding process, such as oxybutynin chloride (Ditropan), flavoxate hydrochloride (Urispas), or solifenacin (VESIcare) may be helpful for certain types of patients. The nurse assesses whether the medication is beneficial.

Patients who have nerve damage and paralysis are trained in specific techniques to empty the bladder (Bodner, 2006). Credé's maneuver, in which the open hand is pressed over the bladder area and directed toward the suprapubic area, can facilitate emptying a flaccid bladder. Self-catheterization is taught to paraplegic patients so that they are not dependent on an indwelling catheter or on other people for their urinary elimination (see Chapter 34).

Some patients are candidates for the implantation of an artificial sphincter to control bladder release of urine. More and more types of successful devices are developed each year, but these are primarily for the patient who has no neurologic control over the bladder.

Every patient undertaking a bladder retraining program needs a great deal of understanding and encouragement and a positive attitude to be successful. Praise for each small achievement should be given. Accidents should be expected and not looked on as "failures." Achieving total continence takes considerable time and effort, but is possible for many patients.

Bowel Training Program

Bowel training for the neurologic patient is done to correct incontinence or prevent constipation and impaction. The bowel training program begins with an assessment of the specific patterns of elimination. It also helps to know the patient's former bowel pattern before illness or injury. Did he regularly rely on the use of enemas or laxatives? Has he been prone to constipation? Next, the nurse needs to establish whether the patient is aware of the urge to defecate or has any warning of evacuation.

Bowel training for either constipation or incontinence should incorporate an exercise program that is within the patient's ability, a high-fiber diet, and adequate liquid intake during the day. **An accurate recording of bowel movements correlated with times of oral intake over a 2- to 3-day period will help establish the most opportune times to try to stimulate evacuation and thus establish a habit.** If incontinence occurs at specific times after eating, then toileting 30 minutes sooner and using a rectal suppository or a gloved finger to stimulate the urge to defecate may alter the pattern. Gradually the use of the suppository is discontinued.

For the patient who is prone to constipation and incontinence, increasing liquid intake and administering a stool softener can be effective. If this does not work, a planned regimen of suppository or enema use may be necessary to assist with evacuation at a desired time, thus preventing incontinence.

All patients need to be comfortable when attempting to evacuate the bowel. A raised, padded toilet seat, handrails, and perhaps a footstool can provide enough comfort to allow the patient to relax so that evacuation can occur naturally. Privacy is essential. Remember to provide privacy for the bedridden patient. Most of all, a positive attitude is needed by staff members. Many times, if the nurse and the patient are optimistic and patient, success can be achieved.

PAIN

Many patients with neurologic disorders experience pain. The pain often is chronic in nature. The nurse must work with the patient to identify the characteristics of the pain, its location and spread, its intensity, and how it is affecting the patient's life. When the patient has suffered a head injury or is experiencing increasing ICP, narcotic analgesics may not be given, as they mask the signs of rising ICP. Other methods of analgesia must be employed.

Pain often causes difficulty sleeping. A trusting relationship between the patient and the nurse is necessary for teaching to be assimilated. Teaching the patient about pain and its relief, the adverse effect of stress, anxiety, and unpleasant stimuli, and the benefits of distraction from the pain become part of the plan. Pharmacologic agents and alternative methods for pain control are used (see Chapter 7).

? *Think Critically About . . .* How would you determine if a patient who has a decreased level of consciousness is experiencing pain?

Depression often occurs with chronic pain and lack of sleep. The combination of an antidepressant and pain medication often is more effective for chronic pain control than either type of drug used alone.

CONFUSION

Patients with brain tumors, head injuries, and strokes, as well as degenerative diseases, may experience confusion and deficits in memory, intellectual ability, or judgment. Confusion may be acute and short term, or it may be a permanent state. Confusion also may be mild or severe and may be accompanied by anxiety, agitation, and refusal to cooperate. The person is in a state of disorientation, and until the symptoms subside, he cannot behave rationally. He must be supported and protected, or he may injure himself. In states of severe (acute) confusion **(delirium)** the patient may experience hallucinations, delusions, and severe agitation. This is usually an acute, short-term state caused by fever or metabolic imbalance. Patients who experience confusion after a head injury often become combative as their ICP rises. It is not advisable to restrain these patients; be very careful to stay out of range of flailing arms.

The nurse should be alert to signs of confusion in any patient with a CNS problem. Subjective and objective assessment data include:

- Loss of orientation to person, place, or time
- Inability to cooperate fully with simple tasks and requests, such as eating and bathing
- Inappropriate statements or inappropriate answers to questions
- Restlessness and agitation
- Hostility and anxiety
- Hallucinations or delusions
- Other signs of inability to maintain control over thought processes and behavior

The patient who is confused needs above all else a stable and calm environment. His thought processes are, in a sense, "fractured" and somewhat beyond his control. Stimuli entering his brain are frightening and threatening to him, and he simply cannot make sense out of most of what is going on around him. A calm, consistent, and orderly approach combined with a set daily routine is most helpful.

Attention to safety of the patient is a priority. Family members must be taught measures to protect the patient who wanders, is disoriented, or lacks judgment (see Chapter 48).

These patients need a stable, dependable environment and a consistent schedule. If agitation or confusion causes undesirable behavior, the use of distraction can be beneficial. Handing the patient an item, leading him from the area, or decreasing environmental stimuli (turning off the television or radio) can calm the patient.

The patient with memory loss who can read benefits from written instructions and a posting of the day's schedule of activities. Measures to protect the patient and deal with confusion are presented in Chapter 47.

APHASIA

Aphasia is a defect in the ability to express oneself in speech or writing, or an inability to comprehend spoken or written language. It is caused by disease or injury of the brain centers controlling language comprehension and expression, located in Wernicke's area of the left cerebral hemisphere.

Aphasia may be *receptive, expressive*, or *global*. **The person with receptive aphasia has difficulty interpreting communications to him in either spoken or written form. In expressive aphasia, the person has difficulty expressing himself in speech or writing. Global aphasia is when the person has a combination of receptive and expressive aphasia. Aphasias vary in degree and in type of deficit.** For example, a person may be able to write a message but cannot form the words to say it.

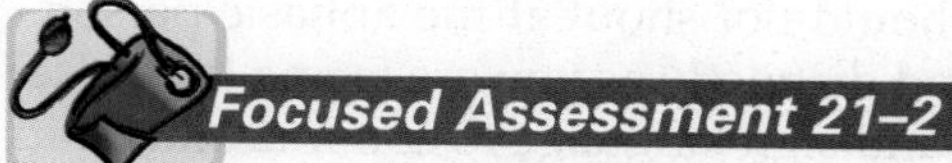

Determining Type of Aphasia Problem

Questions to ask when evaluating the type and degree of aphasia a patient is experiencing include:

- Can he understand yes/no questions? Are his responses of "yes" and "no" reliable (does that seem to be what he means)?
- Can he point to or look toward objects you have named that are in his line of vision?
- Can he name the objects?
- Is he able to follow simple directions (e.g., "Turn your head")?
- Can he repeat simple words? Complex words?
- Can he repeat sentences?
- Can he follow simple written requests?
- Can he write answers to questions?
- Can he write requests?
- Can he read questions or directions?

A comprehensive assessment of the patient who has some type of aphasia usually is a team effort carried out under the leadership of a specially trained speech therapist. Nurses and others responsible for the care of the aphasic patient can assist by noting specific abilities or inabilities of the patient to communicate with them. Some important questions the nurse may ask while observing and assessing the status of a patient who has difficulty communicating because of a neurologic disorder are provided in Focused Assessment 21–2.

The patient who suddenly has a problem speaking or understanding words or signs is likely to suffer from isolation and experience extreme frustration unless an effort is made to establish some means of communicating with him as quickly as possible. Once the patient's specific problem is identified, which could be relatively simple or extremely complex, measures are taken to help the patient communicate as fully as his condition will allow.

Goals for the care of the aphasic patient are focused on stimulating communication without undue frustration and gradually guiding him to appropriate responses and requests. Reaching these goals may take weeks or months, but there are helpful principles and techniques that can be used by all members of the health team and by family members and friends.

Perhaps the most important rule of all is to avoid talking to the aphasic person as if he were mentally incompetent. His inability to communicate does not mean a lack of intelligence. He should be spoken to, not spoken about as if he cannot hear and understand what others are saying in his presence.

Caregivers should not shout at the aphasic person. Speak slowly and distinctly as you are facing him. Use body language and sign language to communicate if it seems to help the patient. Your facial expressions, posture, and gestures can often say more than the words you are saying.

Give the aphasic patient time to respond to questions. Do not ask more than one question at a time. It takes longer for an aphasic person to process what is being said. If you need to repeat a statement or question, use **exactly** the same words. He may have comprehended only half of the sentence the first time. Only one person should speak at a time. Be certain to establish eye contact with the patient before speaking.

It is especially important that the aphasic patient be in an orderly and relaxed environment that is relatively free from distractions that make it difficult to concentrate on communicating.

The speech therapist will plan the patient's speech therapy program and will share with the nurse the details of how best to work with each individual patient. Some general guidelines include:

- Give praise for attempts at communication and for each correctly expressed word or sentence.
- Do not correct the patient's pronunciation, as he is liable to become too frustrated and give up speaking.
- Be very patient.

Problems with aphasia sometimes resolve spontaneously in 3 or 4 months after a CVA. Total speech rehabilitation can take many months and may never reach the prestroke level.

? *Think Critically About . . .* Can you identify three specific techniques you might use to assist a patient with expressive aphasia to communicate his needs?

Among the techniques used to stimulate communication and help the patient deal with his problem of aphasia are self-talk, parallel talk, expansion, and modeling. *Self-talk* helps the aphasic person associate activities with specific words and phrases. The nurse or caregiver talks about what she is doing while performing a task (e.g., making the bed). Self-talk is done in the presence of the patient so he can make connection between what is being said and what he sees being done (Royal-Evans & Marcus, 2004).

EB

Parallel talk describes for the patient what he is doing while he is performing some activity. In *expansion*, the person communicating with the patient completes the patient's sentences when he is able to verbalize but cannot yet speak in complete sentences. No new information is added during expansion. In *modeling*, the patient's sentences are completed, and new information is added.

All of these techniques are helpful in improving communication. They are forms of therapy, however, and are used only in a planned program that has been designed to meet a patient's individual needs. Whatever techniques are chosen, they should not be used in a condescending manner; the adult patient should always be treated respectfully.

The plan of care for the aphasic patient should not neglect the physical condition of his mouth and tongue. Good oral hygiene is needed to keep the oral mucosa clean and moist and in optimal condition so that it is easier for the patient to form words.

SEXUAL DYSFUNCTION

Sexual dysfunction from a lesion in neural pathways should be dealt with by allowing expression of the patient's concerns, beliefs, and feelings. Sexual counseling by someone skilled in working with patients with neurologic deficits should be initiated. Alternate techniques for meeting sexual needs must be explored. Many patients can, with teaching, lead a sexually satisfying life.

PSYCHOSOCIAL CONCERNS

The multiple stresses, alteration in roles, and changes in body image and self-esteem that result from a chronic neurologic disorder can be overwhelming. The patient will need time and assistance in adapting to an altered body image. The nurse must be accepting of the patient's expression of anxiety, anger, denial, regression, and depression. Work to support the patient emotionally, attempting to establish realistic hope for quality of life. Exploring the patient's previous methods of coping with adversity, as well as his support systems, talents, and desires, helps to provide clues on how best to help him. Jointly establishing small, accomplishable goals can do much to rebuild self-esteem.

Collaboration with the social worker concerning referral to support groups and interaction with others with similar disabilities who are coping well can prove most beneficial. Contact with community agencies that offer support services and job retraining, if pertinent, is essential. The patient needs a way to be a productive member of society and to contribute to the welfare of his family.

Reentry into the community and a normal social life are other areas for intervention. Often the patient has been out of touch with his normal social circles for many months during his illness and recovery process. Plans should be made before discharge for social contact to be reinstated. The county or state office of vocational rehabilitation may help with funding.

INEFFECTIVE FAMILY COPING

A chronic neurologic disorder that disrupts normal function for the patient also disrupts normal roles within the family. Family lifestyle is altered, and changes in roles may lead to family conflict. Family members often feel powerless, ambivalent toward the patient, angry, and guilty for having angry feelings. Family members need to be included when educating the patient about his disorder, the possibility of remissions and exacerbations, and the self-care measures necessary. Everyone needs time to adjust to the situation. Referrals to counseling and support groups can be very helpful.

Key Points

- The CNS is made up of the brain and spinal cord.
- The peripheral nervous system is composed of the sensory organs, the cranial nerves, the spinal nerves, and ganglia.
- The cerebrum, diencephalon, cerebellum, and brainstem comprise the brain.
- There are pyramidal tracts and extrapyramidal tracts that are conduction pathways between the brain, the spinal cord, and the skeletal muscles.
- Meninges consisting of the pia mater, the arachnoid membrane, and the dura mater cover the brain and spinal cord inside the bony structures.
- Cerebrospinal fluid cushions and protects the brain and spinal cord and circulates between the pia mater and arachnoid membrane in the subarachnoid space.
- Nerve impulses travel via the neuron axons and dendrites when a stimulus is received.
- A neurotransmitter is necessary for impulse transmission across a synapse from one neuron to another.
- When nerve conduction is normal, a stimulus produces a response. The myelin sheath of the axon speeds the impulse conduction.
- Impulses either travel through a reflex arc or are transmitted to the brain, where they are interpreted and a response is sent out.
- The somatic system, consisting of the cranial and spinal nerves, responds to changes in the environment and initiates voluntary actions.
- The autonomic system of the PNS actively maintains homeostasis and is involuntary in its actions.
- Sympathetic and parasympathetic nerves have opposite effects on many organs (see Table 21–3).
- When deprived of oxygen, neurons die quickly.
- Many changes occur with aging, and after age 70 the brain atrophies somewhat.
- Reflexes diminish or are lost as age advances.
- Preventing accidents and head injuries by teaching safety practices reduces the number of neurologic injuries.
- Discouraging recreational drug use helps prevent neurologic damage.
- Teaching patients how to reduce risk factors for stroke can prevent the devastation that a stroke can inflict.
- Nurses routinely perform gross assessment of the cranial nerves, coordination and balance, muscle strength, and reflexes.
- Vital signs, mental function, neuromuscular status, papillary reactions, and level of consciousness are parts of the physical assessment and are always performed as part of the "neuro check."
- Observing for subtle changes is part of the LPN/LVN's data gathering.
- A thorough history is gathered focusing on areas of neurologic function (see Focused Assessment 21–1).
- Many nursing diagnoses are appropriate for patients with neurologic disorders (see Table 21–8).
- Nursing care is individualized, with outcome objectives and interventions chosen to alleviate the various problems.
- Every effort is made to maintain effective breathing for the neurologic patient.
- Many neurologic patients experience impaired mobility, and nurses attempt to prevent the associated potential problems .
- Assisting with ADLs when patients have self-care deficits is a major part of nursing care for patients with neurologic disorders.
- Specific techniques are needed for the patient who experiences dysphagia to prevent aspiration.
- Many patients with bowel or bladder incontinence can regain continence through bowel and bladder retraining programs.
- Pain control can be a difficult issue because most pain medications dull the sensorium and will interfere with accurate neurologic assessment and signs of decreasing level of consciousness.
- Many patients with neurologic disorders become confused, and there are special techniques nurses use to assist these patients.
- Learning to work with an aphasic patient is essential to providing care for him (see Focused Assessment 21–2).
- When appropriate, neurologic patients should be referred for appropriate sexual counseling.
- When a family member has a neurologic deficit, it affects the whole family and can disrupt normal family functioning; families need help to learn to cope.

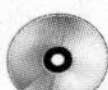

Go to your **Companion CD-ROM** for an Audio Glossary, animations, video clips, and bonus review questions.

evolve Be sure to visit the companion Evolve site at http://evolve.elsevier.com/deWit for interactive NCLEX-PN Exam Style Review Questions, WebLinks, and additional online resources.

NCLEX-PN EXAM STYLE REVIEW QUESTIONS

Choose the best answer(s) for the following questions.

1. While performing an initial assessment, the nurse notes that the patient provides inappropriate responses to verbal communication. This clinical finding is referred as:
   1. dysphasia.
   2. aphasia.
   3. dysarthria.
   4. dysphagia.
2. Regarding the care of a patient with global aphasia, which behavior demonstrated by the nursing assistant warrants immediate attention by the nurse?
   1. The nursing assistant speaks slowly and distinctly.
   2. The nursing assistant waits for the patient's response.
   3. The nursing assistant uses a loud, commanding voice.
   4. The nursing assistant uses simple words.
3. While assisting the patient with feeding, the nurse describes every step in meal preparation in simple language. This is referred to as:
   1. parallel talk.
   2. self-talk.
   3. expansion.
   4. modeling.
4. The nurse is providing discharge instructions to an elderly Iranian man who experienced a stroke. The nurse notices that the patient seems indifferent to teaching. The nurse must consider:
   1. talking to the wife or daughter.
   2. involving the entire family in the care of the patient.
   3. sending the patient to a long-term care facility.
   4. stopping and trying again later.
5. With an open hand, the nurse presses over the flaccid bladder of a patient. When questioned regarding the nursing action, an appropriate response would be:
   1. "The technique increases the muscle tone of the bladder."
   2. "The maneuver facilitates removal of urinary sediments."
   3. "The technique assists with complete bladder emptying."
   4. "The technique reduces the incidence of bladder irritation."
6. The nurse shines a light on the right eye and inspects the left eye. The nurse is assessing:
   1. accommodation.
   2. consensual reflex.
   3. direct reflex.
   4. blink reflex.
7. The nurse uses the Glasgow Coma Scale to evaluate the neurologic responses of a patient. The patient opens eyes to pain, makes incomprehensible verbal sounds, and extends extremities with pain. The score would suggest:
   1. locked-in syndrome.
   2. brain death.
   3. comatose.
   4. lethargy.
8. The nurse demonstrates understanding of the physiologic changes in the nervous system associated with aging by:
   1. providing reminders to optimize level of daily functioning.
   2. performing all the activities of daily living.
   3. anticipating ready responses to open-ended questions.
   4. communicating slowly and loudly with high-pitched tones.
9. The nurse scrapes an object along the sole of the patient's foot and notes that the great toe bends upward and the smaller toes fan outward. The clinical finding is suggestive of:
   1. sensory abnormality of the cortex.
   2. motor abnormality of the cortex.
   3. cerebellar tissue destruction.
   4. a normal finding.
10. Which of the following nursing interventions are appropriate when providing care for a patient with right hemiplegia from a stroke? *(Select all that apply.)*
    1. Reminding the patient to pay attention to the left side.
    2. Protecting extremities during transfers.
    3. Supporting unaffected arm with pillows.
    4. Using slings on the affected arm to promote better balance.
    5. Initiating range-of-motion exercises.

CRITICAL THINKING ACTIVITIES

Read each clinical scenario and discuss the questions with your classmates.

Scenario

Mr. Lawson is to have several diagnostic tests done to determine the cause of his neurologic symptoms, which include headache, visual disturbance, muscular weakness, and personality change.

1. How would you explain an electroencephalogram to Mr. Lawson? A computed tomography scan? Magnetic resonance imaging?
2. If you are to assess Mr. Lawson's "neuro signs" and he is using eyedrops for glaucoma that constrict the pupils, how would you evaluate his pupillary responses?
3. Should Mr. Lawson end up needing a lumbar puncture to obtain cerebrospinal fluid for studies, how would you position him? What would you tell him about the procedure?

CHAPTER 22

Care of Patients with Head and Spinal Cord Injuries

evolve http://evolve.elsevier.com/deWit

Objectives

Upon completion of this chapter you should be able to:

Theory

1. Describe the types of injuries that result from head trauma.
2. Compare and contrast the signs and symptoms of subdural hematoma and epidural hematoma.
3. Explain why an epidural hematoma causes an emergency situation.
4. Discuss the type of procedure performed to relieve a subdural hematoma.
5. Illustrate the pathophysiology of increasing intracranial pressure in a patient who has experienced a severe head injury.
6. Identify the reasons why an elderly person is more at risk for an intracranial bleed from a head injury.
7. Explain the possible ramifications of spinal cord injury.
8. List appropriate nursing interventions necessary to provide comprehensive care for a patient who has suffered a C5 spinal cord injury.
9. Analyze the symptoms of low back pain and correlate them with their cause.

Clinical Practice

1. Teach a family member how to properly assess and care for a patient who has suffered a concussion.
2. Perform a neurologic check on a patient who has suffered head trauma.
3. Participate in a collaborative care planning conference for a patient who has sustained a spinal cord injury.
4. Prepare a plan for teaching self-care measures to a patient who suffers from low back pain.

Key Terms

Be sure to check out the bonus material on the Companion CD-ROM, including selected audio pronunciations.

concussion (cŏn-KŬ-shŭn, p. 540)
contralateral (kŏn-tră-LĂT-ĕr-ăl, p. 542)
contusion (kŏn-TŪ-zhŭn, p. 541)
coup-contrecoup injury (koo kôtre-koo, p. 541)
epidural hematoma (Ĕ-pĭ-DŬ-rŭl hē-mă-TŌ-mă, p. 541)
hydrocephalus (hī-drō-SĔF-ă-lăs, p. 548)
intracerebral hematoma (ĭn-trăh-sĕ-RĒ-brăl, p. 541)
ipsilateral (ĭp-sĭ-LĂT-ĕr-ăl, p. 542)
quadriplegia (kwŏd-rĭ-PLĒ-jă, p. 551)
subdural hematoma (sŭb-DŬ-rŭl, p. 541)
subluxation (sŭb-lŭk-SĀ-shŭn, p. 550)

HEAD INJURIES

Head injuries are a frequent cause of death. About 1.5 million people sustain head and brain injury in the United States each year. Approximately 50,000 die and 1.1 million are treated for traumatic brain injury and released. Those who survive initial head injury require meticulous observation and care so that damage to the brain cells can be kept at a minimum and death averted. There are about 5.3 million people in the United States who have need of lifelong help with activities of daily living due to residual disabilities from brain injury (Brain Injury Association of America, 2007).

Etiology

A blow to the head may cause a laceration of the skin or scalp and fracture of the skull, or may only cause a minor contusion. The injury may cause movement of the brain within the skull, tearing blood vessels. Accidents are the most common cause of head injury, with motor vehicle accidents being the leading cause.

Pathophysiology

When a depressed skull fracture occurs, there is bruising, contusion, or laceration of the underlying brain tissue with the inflammatory changes that occur with any wound. A minor head injury may cause concussion. **Concussion** is the term used to describe a closed head injury in which there is a brief disruption in level of consciousness (LOC), amnesia regarding the occurrence, and headache. Skull fractures are described as:

- Linear or depressed
- Simple, comminuted, or compound
- Closed or open

A *closed* injury is one in which the scalp and skull remain intact, but the underlying brain tissue is damaged. There may be contused areas or hematoma. In an *open* injury there is laceration of the scalp and fracture of the skull with damage to brain tissue.

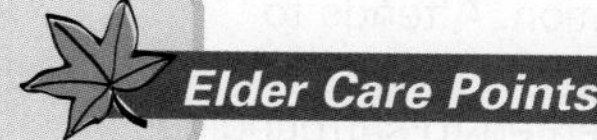

Elder Care Points

The brain atrophies with age and does not take up as much space in the cranial vault. This allows for more movement and more potential for torn vessels and contusions on the brain when an accident occurs that involves a head injury.

In a **contusion**, the brain tissue is bruised, blood from broken vessels accumulates, and edema develops causing increased intracranial pressure (ICP).

A **coup-contrecoup injury**, or an *acceleration-deceleration injury*, occurs when the head is moving rapidly and hits a stationary object, such as a windshield. The contents within the cranium hit the inside of the skull (coup) and then bounce back and hit the bony area opposite the site of impact, causing a second injury (contrecoup) (Figure 22–1).

Subdural hematoma is a common result of head injury. It often happens in the elderly as a result of a fall. Anticoagulant therapy puts a patient at greater risk for a subdural hematoma after even a minor blow to the head. A hematoma is a blood-filled swelling. When a blow is delivered to the head, it may rupture the blood vessels that lie between the delicate arachnoid membrane covering the brain and the tough, fibrous dura mater. As the blood leaks under the dura mater (subdural), the hematoma grows in size, pressing against the softer arachnoid and the brain tissue it is covering (Figure 22–2).

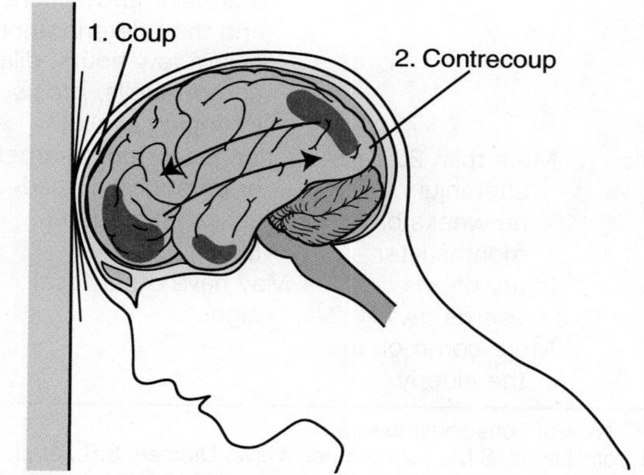

FIGURE 22–1 Coup-contrecoup (acceleration-deceleration) injury.

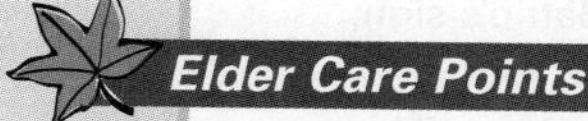

Elder Care Points

Because the brain of the older person tends to move more in the cranial vault when head trauma occurs, small vessels may be torn and the patient is more at risk for a slow developing subdural hematoma. The person should be watched for several months for signs of personality change, decreasing LOC, increased irritability, and other signs of increased ICP.

An **epidural hematoma** occurs more rarely, but when it does, it is caused by rapid leakage of blood from the middle meningeal artery, which quickly elevates ICP (see Figure 22–2). This constitutes a medical emergency. A craniotomy is needed to repair the damaged vessel and relieve the rapidly rising pressure before death occurs from the increased ICP (see Chapter 23 for a discussion of the craniotomy procedure). An **intracerebral hematoma** may occur within the brain.

Signs and Symptoms

The severity of brain damage from a head injury is best judged by the symptoms presented by the patient, a neurologic assessment, the history of the type of blow received, and whether the victim lost consciousness and for how long. The outward symptoms of head injury are fairly obvious; these include bruising,

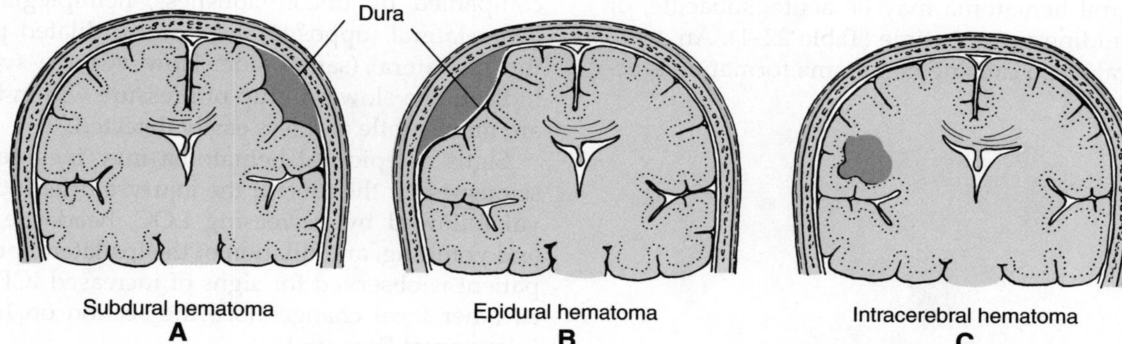

FIGURE 22–2 **A,** Subdural hematoma. As a result of trauma to the head, small ruptured blood vessels leak blood into the space under the dura mater (slower than an epidural bleed). **B,** Epidural hematoma, the result of a head injury that tears a large meningeal artery, causing a rapid bleed with a large amount of blood above the dura mater. If not relieved, subdural and epidural hematomas can be fatal. **C,** Intracerebral hematoma. Small vessels within the brain have torn and bled.

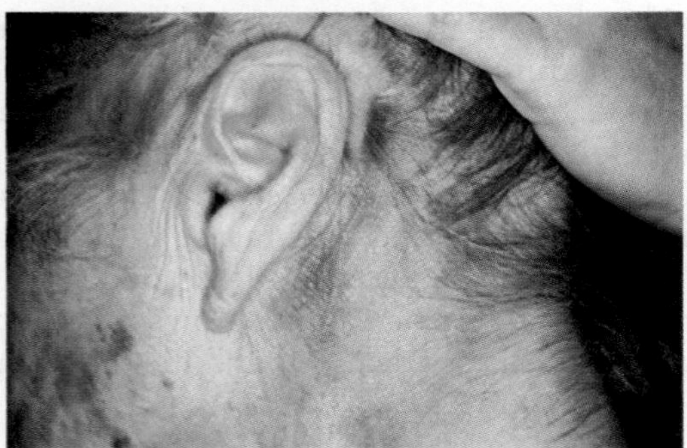

FIGURE **22–3** Battle's sign.

swelling, lacerations, and bleeding. There may be periorbital fractures with *ecchymoses* (raccoon eyes), or ecchymoses behind the ear (Battle's sign) (Figure 22–3). *Otorrhea* (fluid from the ear), *rhinorrhea* (fluid from the nose), tinnitus or hearing difficulty, facial paralysis, and conjugate deviation of gaze wherein both eyes deviate to one side may be present. Otorrhea and rhinorrhea should be tested to determine if there is a cerebrospinal fluid (CSF) leak. If the fluid is clear, it can be tested with a Dextrostix or Tes Tape to see if glucose is present.

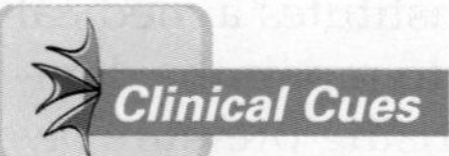

If the fluid from the ear or nose is tinged with blood, a Dextrostix or Tes Tape will not give accurate results. Collect about a teaspoon of the fluid on a white gauze pad. Within a few minutes blood will move to the center and a yellow ring (halo) will form around it if the fluid is CSF (Figure 22–4).

A concussion can cause a brief disruption of the normal LOC, amnesia regarding the event, and headache. A contusion can cause an alteration in LOC and may cause seizures. Box 22–1 shows the downward progression of decreased LOC.

A subdural hematoma may be acute, subacute, or chronic, building up over time (Table 22–1). An acute intracerebral bleed causing hematoma formation is accompanied by unconsciousness, hemiplegia on the **contralateral** (opposite) side, and a dilated pupil on the **ipsilateral** (same) side. However, the symptoms indicating a slow buildup of pressure within the skull are more subtle and less easily detected.

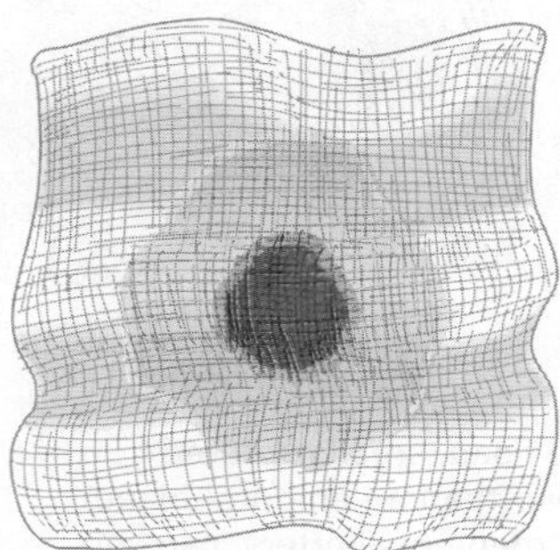

FIGURE **22–4** Assessing for the halo sign on fluid from the nose or ear after a head injury. The blood will draw together in the middle of the gauze pad, leaving a yellow ring (halo) around the blood, indicating the presence of cerebrospinal fluid.

Box 22–1 ***Decreasing Levels of Consciousness (LOC)***

- **Alert:** Responds appropriately to questions and commands with little stimulation. Attends to surroundings.
- **Confused:** Somewhat disoriented to surroundings, time, or people. Judgment may be impaired. Needs to be cued to respond to commands.
- **Lethargic:** Drowsy, but easily aroused; needs gentle touch or verbal stimulation to attend to commands.
- **Obtunded:** More difficult to arouse and responds slowly to stimulation. Needs repeated stimulation to maintain attention and to respond to the environment.
- **Stuporous:** Responds to vigorous stimulation only slightly; may only moan or mutter in response.
- **Comatose:** No observable response to stimulation.

Table 22–1 ***Types of Subdural Hematomas***

TYPE	OCCURRENCE AFTER INJURY	PROGRESSION OF SYMPTOMS
Acute	Within 24–48 hr	Quick; immediate deterioration
Subacute	48 hr–2 wk	Initial unconsciousness, gradual improvement and then deterioration over a few hours, dilation of pupils, *ptosis* (drooping eyelid)
Chronic	More than 20 days after injury; may be weeks or months later	Changes in temperament or personality, headaches, alteration in LOC
	Injury often seems trivial	May have other focal signs
	More common in the elderly	

Key: *LOC,* level of consciousness.
Adapted from Lewis, S.M., Heitkemper, M.M., Dirksen, S.R., et al. (2007). *Medical-Surgical Nursing: Assessment and Management of Clinical Problems* (7th ed.). St. Louis: Mosby.

Signs of epidural hematoma may include unconsciousness at the time of the injury, a brief lucid interval followed by decreasing LOC, headache, nausea and vomiting, and dilation of the ipsilateral pupil. The patient is observed for signs of increased ICP, as well as other focal changes (see the section on Increased Intracranial Pressure).

Diagnosis

The diagnostic tests and examinations commonly used to determine the extent of head injury include a radiograph of the skull, a computed tomography (CT) scan, magnetic resonance imaging (MRI) with contrast, pos-

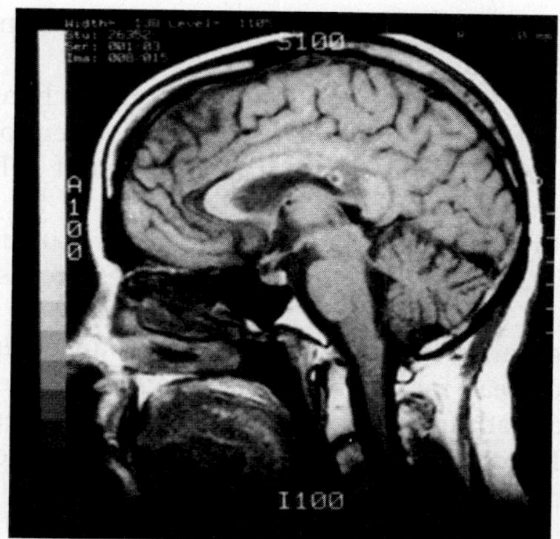

FIGURE **22–5** MRI: midline sagittal view of the brain.

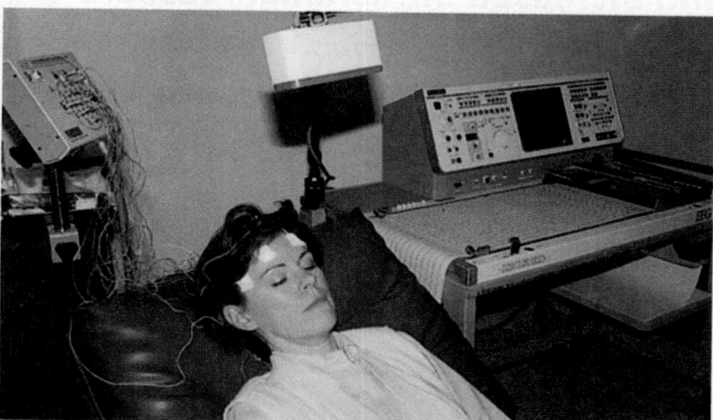

FIGURE **22–6** Electroencephalogram (EEG).

itron emission tomography, evoked potentials, and electroencephalography (Figures 22–5 and 22–6) (see Chapter 21, Table 21–6).

> *Think Critically About . . .* Why should every patient who has sustained a head injury be assessed closely for 24 to 48 hours?

Treatment

The patient with a head injury usually is treated conservatively at first. If the injury causes an increase in ICP, or if the injury is a compound fracture of the skull, then surgical debridement of the wound and removal of splintered bone from the brain tissues or elevation of the skull fragment is performed. All measures to keep ICP from rising are instituted for serious head injuries.

A patent airway must be secured, and the head raised 30 to 45 degrees with the body in correct alignment. Elevation helps reduce ICP. Neurologic signs are monitored closely. An intravenous (IV) line is inserted for access for diuretic drugs if needed and for administration of fluid. Intravenous fluids are infused very slowly so that there is no fluid overload that increases the ICP. Diuretics are used to decrease vascular volume and keep ICP as low as possible.

> *Think Critically About . . .* Why would a nurse check for a patent airway before performing a neurologic assessment on a patient with a head injury?

Surgical Intervention. Subdural hematoma is removed surgically either via burr holes or by craniotomy incision. The hematoma is evacuated by suction or surgical instruments. Epidural hematoma necessitates immediate, emergency craniotomy for access to the brain to stop the bleeding and evacuate the hematoma to prevent death from increased ICP. The craniotomy procedure is described in Chapter 23 along with surgeries of the brain.

Preoperative Period. The patient with a hematoma is quickly prepared for surgery. The operative site usually is not shaved until the patient is under anesthesia in the operating room. For planned surgery, a shampoo may be ordered the evening before surgery. Preoperative preparation is the same as for other surgeries. Any scalp lesions or other unusual conditions that are noted at this time should be reported. Usually the entire head is not shaved, only the operative area, and, if the patient has long hair, any hair that is cut off may be saved to be used as a hairpiece until the patient's hair grows back.

Postoperative Period. During the immediate postoperative period, the patient who underwent a craniotomy is in the intensive care unit for continuous monitoring. Essentially, care will be the same as that for any patient in danger of increasing ICP. Additional specific points in the postoperative care of the patient who has undergone intracranial surgery are as follows:

- Position the patient according to written orders from the attending surgeon. *Make no exceptions.* Positioning is important to prevent added increases in ICP.
- Keep the neck in midline and prevent excessive hip flexion to promote venous drainage from the head and keep ICP from rising (American Association of Neuroscience Nurses, 2007). 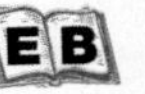
- Use nasal suctioning *only* if there is a written order allowing this as there may be a fracture that allows a pathway to the brain tissue.
- Watch carefully for signs of leakage of CSF from the nose, ear, and operative site, and report evidence of leakage immediately. Use aseptic technique in applying dressings to catch the drainage and prevent microorganisms from easily entering.
- Provide a quiet, nonstimulating environment.
- Administer only those treatments, comfort measures, and medications for which there are specific written orders.
- Report promptly any changes in the neurologic status of the patient.

Nursing Management

If it has been determined that there is indeed leakage of spinal fluid through the nose, ear, or an open head wound, special precautions must be taken to prevent infection and the physician must be notified. These precautions include the following:

- Keep the patient on absolute bed rest with the head of the bed elevated 30 to 45 degrees to promote venous drainage from the head.
- Cover a draining ear with a sterile gauze pad, changing it periodically to look for drainage.
- Instruct the patient *not* to blow her nose or pick at it; blowing may increase ICP, and picking may allow entry of microorganisms.
- Do not plug the nose or ear if there is drainage of CSF as this may increase ICP.
- Remind the patient that she is not to change her position in any way unless she has been told it is all right to do so, in order to prevent ICP from rising.

Continued neurologic assessments are an integral part of care. Specific nursing diagnoses are listed in Nursing Care Plan 22–1.

Observation of a patient treated in an emergency room for head injury and released to go home requires specific instructions (Legal & Ethical Considerations 22–1). Patient Teaching 22–1 includes instructions for the patient's family.

NURSING CARE PLAN 22–1

Care of the Patient with a Head Injury and Increased Intracranial Pressure

SCENARIO A 16-year-old boy who suffered a head injury in an automobile accident is groggy, but arousable.

PROBLEM/NURSING DIAGNOSIS *Blow to skull*/Ineffective cerebral tissue perfusion related to increased intracranial pressure from head injury.

Supporting assessment data *Subjective:* Hit right side of head on dashboard. *Objective:* Nondepressed skull fracture, alteration in LOC, confused as to where he is, what day it is; somewhat combative.

Goals/Expected Outcomes	Nursing Interventions	Selected Rationale	Evaluation
Patient will not display further increase in ICP	Monitor neurologic status q 1 hr using Glasgow Coma Scale (GCS); notify physician of any pupil changes or signs of increasing ICP, such as widening pulse pressure, change in respiratory pattern, slowing of pulse, increase in temperature, or decrease in LOC.	GCS provides good estimate of neurologic status.	GCS maintaining at 11.
	Monitor for seizure activity; institute seizure precautions.	Increased pressure on brain tissue may cause cellular irritability and seizure activity.	No sign of seizure activity. Precautions in place; padded tongue blade at bedside.
	Keep head of bed (HOB) at 30 degrees and body in correct alignment; turn side to side q 2 hr if condition warrants.	Keeping head slightly elevated and in proper alignment helps promote venous drainage from the head.	HOB at 30 degrees; positioned in correct alignment with neck midline. Turned q 2 hr.
	Maintain IV infusion at 50 mL/hr.	Decreasing IV rate helps prevent increased ICP and maintains IV access.	IV infusion at 50 mL/hr; patent without redness or swelling at site.
	Administer diuretic as ordered.	Diuretic decreases vascular volume and intracranial volume, lowering ICP.	No diuretic ordered at this time.
	Keep room calm and softly lit; do not disturb more than necessary; talk to patient while giving care; allow rest periods between any invasive procedures; monitor intake and output; reorient patient frequently.	Invasive procedures raise intracranial pressure.	Room is tidy and softly lit; care procedures grouped at intervals allowing rest; I = 400 mL, O = 375 mL.

Key: *ADLs*, activities of daily living; *I*, input; *ICP*, intracranial pressure; *IV*, intravenous; *LOC*, level of consciousness; *O*, output.

NURSING CARE PLAN 22–1

Care of the Patient with a Head Injury and Increased Intracranial Pressure—cont'd

PROBLEM/NURSING DIAGNOSIS *Unable to bathe and dress self*/Self-care deficit related to confusion, grogginess, and increased ICP.

Supporting assessment data *Objective:* Falls asleep during attempts at bath, etc.; is confused about how to use ordinary objects such as toothbrush.

Goals/Expected Outcomes	Nursing Interventions	Selected Rationale	Evaluation
Patient will have adequate assistance with hygiene and dressing	Provide assistance with all ADLs.		Assisted with morning care.
	Inspect skin when turning; place foam pad on bed.	Pressure-relieving devices helps prevent pressure ulcer formation.	No signs of reddened areas on skin. Foam pad on bed.
Patient will resume self-care by discharge	Encourage self-care as LOC improves.		Continue plan. Not ready for self-care yet.

PROBLEM/NURSING DIAGNOSIS *Mother is very anxious*/Disabled family coping related to patient's decreased LOC and hospitalization.

Supporting assessment data *Subjective:* Mother states she is afraid son is going to die. *Objective:* Mother keeps trying to rouse the patient when she is in the room.

Goals/Expected Outcomes	Nursing Interventions	Selected Rationale	Evaluation
Mother's anxiety will decrease as she gains information about her son's condition and prognosis	Explain to family that confusion and grogginess are usual after head injury.	Knowledge decreases fear of the unknown.	Explained patient's condition to family and measures to keep ICP down. Mother seems less anxious. Discussed need for calm and positive talk in room. Continue plan.
	Explain that the danger is if the ICP keeps increasing; tell what measures are being done to minimize increasing ICP; explain all procedures; explain that calm, rest, and positive talk in the room will help.	Knowing the treatment plan decreases anxiety.	
	Call hospital chaplain or own minister if family desires.	Presence of spiritual advisor can decrease anxiety.	
	Keep family informed of changes in patient's condition.		

? CRITICAL THINKING QUESTIONS

1. Why do you think that it is contraindicated for this patient to strain to have a bowel movement?
2. Why is it important to decrease stimuli and provide a calm, soothing environment for this patient? (Be specific.)

? *Think Critically About . . .* Why is the patient with a head injury positioned with the head of the bed at 30 to 45 degrees' elevation?

The long-term outcome for patients who have suffered a *severe* head injury are unpredictable. Recovery is a long process, and improvement may occur over many months for some patients. Disabilities may be lifelong.

INCREASED INTRACRANIAL PRESSURE

Etiology and Pathophysiology

Because the skull is a closed bony structure in the adult, it is unable to expand. **Any lesion or fluid accumulation that begins to take up space within the cranial cavity causes an increase in the pressure within the cavity.** Therefore, any swelling of the brain tissue from injury or surgery, leakage of blood from ruptured cerebral vessels, or tumors, abscesses, or any

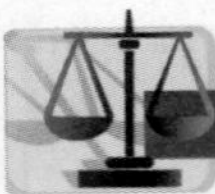

Legal & Ethical Considerations 22–1

Documenting Patient Teaching

Because there are legal ramifications of inadequate patient/family teaching, document all teaching in the medical record and send home clearly written instructions. It is best to have the patient or family sign a form for the record that indicates that teaching and written instructions have been received.

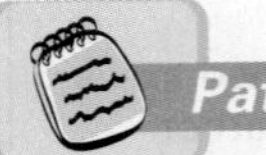

Patient Teaching 22–1

Instructions for Care of a Patient with a Head Injury

Teach the family or significant other to do the following:

- For the first 24 hours, awaken the person every 2 hours to be certain he/she can be easily aroused.
- Question the person about where he/she is, who you are, what happened, and so on, to check orientation.
- Check the pupils to see that they are equal in size and that they will constrict; use a flashlight.
- Avoid strenuous activity for 24 hours.
- Apply icebag to areas of swelling—continue for 24 hours.

For 48 hours, watch for the following signs and report them to the physician or Emergency Medical Services if they occur:

- Change in level of consciousness (e.g., becoming more groggy, difficult to awaken, confused)
- Projectile vomiting (vomit travels a distance) without nausea
- Unusual dizziness, sleepiness, loss of balance, or fall
- Change in vision (i.e., seeing double, blurred vision)
- Jerking movements of the eyes
- An increasing headache that feels worse when moving around
- Any twitching movements of arms or legs that cannot be controlled (seizures)
- A change in speech or ability to find words or converse
- Behavior that is odd for the individual

other space-occupying lesion within the skull presents an increased ICP risk. Pressure against cerebral veins and arteries interferes with the flow of blood, producing a local ischemia and hypoxia. Pressure against the cells themselves can interfere with their vital functions. If it rises very high and remains high for very long, ICP can cause death from inadequate cerebral perfusion or cerebral herniation. Brainstem injuries or pressure on the brainstem from increased ICP causes respiratory depression from pressure on the medulla oblongata. Carbon dioxide accumulates, causing vasodilation and further increases in ICP. Normal ICP is 0 to 15 mm Hg. Concept Map 22–1 shows the relationship between the causes and the pathologic occurrences of increased ICP.

Signs, Symptoms, and Diagnosis

When the body can no longer compensate for the increase in volume in the cranial vault, decompensation begins and clinical signs of increasing ICP become apparent.

The earliest sign of increasing ICP is lethargy and decreasing consciousness, accompanied by a slowing of speech and delay in response to verbal cues.

When ICP rises, it affects the oxygenated blood perfusion of the brain and hypoxia occurs. Nerve cells are particularly sensitive to hypoxia and cannot be replaced once they have been destroyed. Extended periods of hypoxia cause brain cell death. The body tries to compensate by raising blood pressure to force more oxygenated blood through the brain tissue. If ICP continues to rise, the brain tissue will herniate through the tentorial notch at the midline of the foramen magnum. This herniation results in pressure on the vital structures of the midbrain, pons, and medulla and causes changes in the vital signs and pupil reactions characteristic of increased ICP.

As brain tissue swells or fluid volume increases in the cranium, pressure is placed on the optic nerve. Pupils begin to react slowly; pupil size becomes unequal, progressing to dilation, and then the pupil size becomes fixed as reflexes disappear.

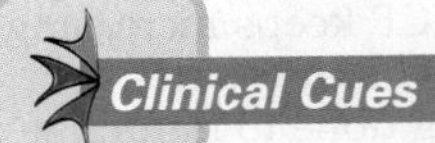

Clinical Cues

Abnormal pupillary responses can reverse to normal if the cause of increased ICP can be resolved in time.

The classic signs of increased ICP, with the first three called *Cushing's triad,* are:

- Rising systolic blood pressure
- Widening pulse pressure
- Bradycardia with a full, bounding pulse
- Rapid or irregular respirations (Figure 22–7)

These tend to be late signs, as are pupil changes, and signal a severe emergency and the need for immediate action to try to prevent the patient's death.

? *Think Critically About . . .* Why does increasing intracranial edema cause a double threat to the brain?

Treatment

The patient with greatly increased ICP is usually placed in an intensive care unit. Increased ICP is treated with supportive care to keep the pressure from rising further and with interventions to decrease the cranial blood or CSF volume. Osmotic diuretics (mannitol, glycerol, urea) are administered to remove fluid from the body, thereby reducing fluid in the brain.

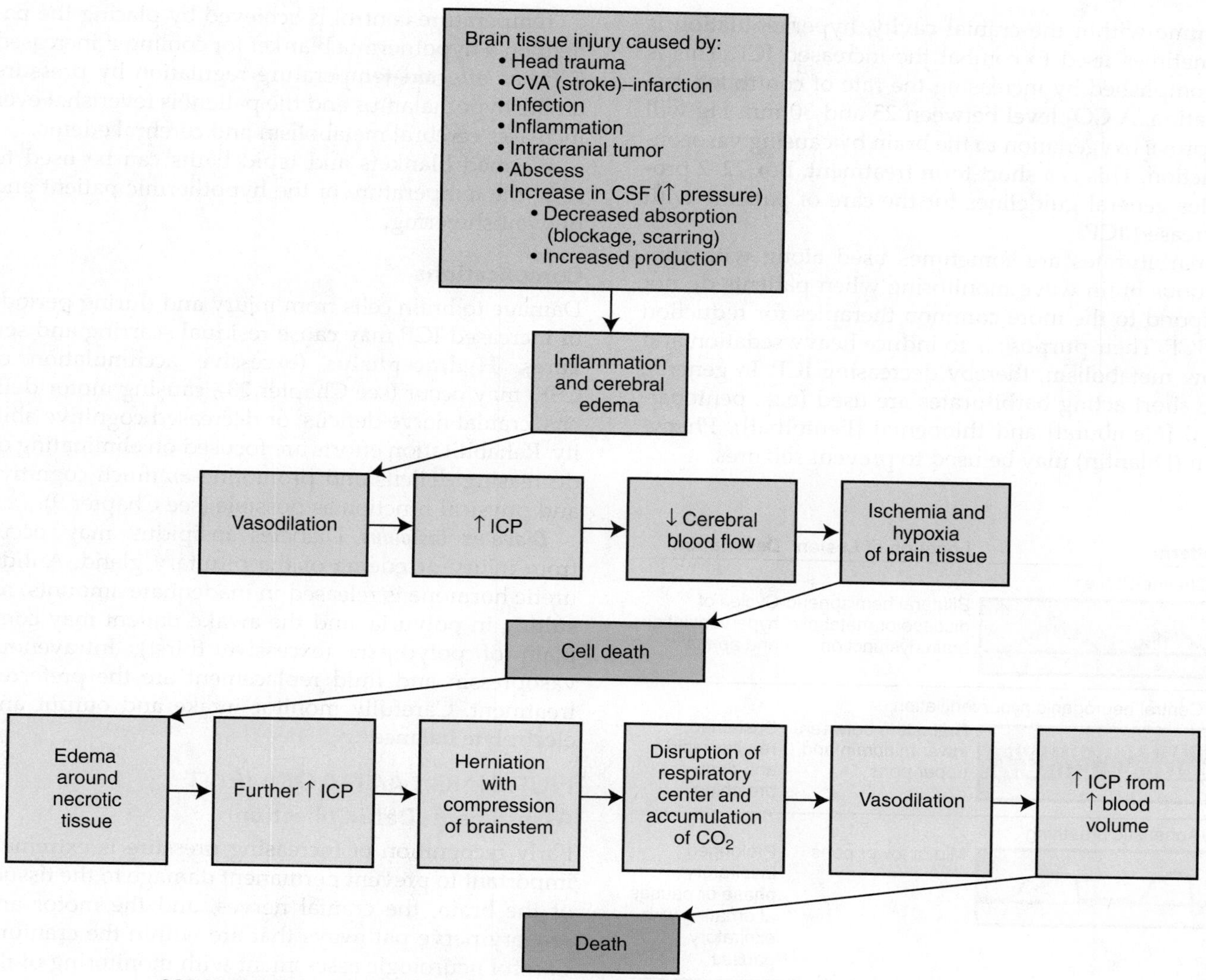

CONCEPT MAP 22–1 Pathophysiologic changes from a brain injury that increase intracranial pressure (ICP) and can lead to death.

Systemic diuretics, such as furosemide (Lasix), also may be given. Dosage is determined by body weight, and electrolytes are monitored every 6 hours, as mannitol and diuretic action can cause electrolyte imbalances. An indwelling urinary catheter is inserted to monitor output. Electrolytes and fluid balance are watched closely.

Dexamethasone (Decadron) may be given to decrease the inflammatory response and cerebral edema if the ICP is caused by a brain tumor or abscess (Meaney & Grady, 2005). Histamine (H_2)-receptor blockers or proton pump inhibitors are administered to protect the gastric mucosa. The patient is positioned with the head of the bed at 30 to 45 degrees to promote venous drainage from the head. The head and neck must be kept positioned midline so that venous drainage into the body is not restricted. Hip flexion should be less than 90 degrees. Rolled washcloths, towels, or trochanter rolls can be used for positioning.

If ICP is dangerously high as indicated by a Glasgow Coma Scale score of 8 or less and an abnormal CT scan, the surgeon may insert an intraventricular catheter into the lateral ventricle, through which CSF can be drained in small amounts to relieve the pressure. A probe can also be positioned in the subarachnoid or epidural area to monitor the pressure. Cerebral perfusion pressure (CPP) must be kept above 60 mm Hg to ensure oxygenation of the brain tissue (CPP = mean arterial pressure − intracranial pressure). Normal CPP is 70 to 100 mm Hg. A monitoring device connected to the inserted probe may be used to measure cerebral blood flow. There are some new devices used to monitor cerebral oxygenation and blood flow (Table 22–2).

If the patient is on a ventilator and is extremely agitated, pancuronium bromide (Pavulon) to paralyze skeletal muscles, in combination with sedation, may be used to prevent further increases in ICP. Because carbon dioxide is a vasodilator and can increase blood volume within the cranial cavity, hyperventilation is sometimes used to combat the increased ICP. This is accomplished by increasing the rate of controlled respiration. A CO_2 level between 25 and 30 mm Hg will improve oxygenation to the brain by causing vasoconstriction. This is a short-term treatment. Box 22–2 provides general guidelines for the care of patients with increased ICP.

Barbiturates are sometimes used along with continuous brain wave monitoring when patients do not respond to the more common therapies for reduction of ICP. Their purpose is to induce heavy sedation and slow metabolism, thereby decreasing ICP. In general, the short-acting barbiturates are used (e.g., pentobarbital [Nembutal] and thiopental [Pentothal]). Phenytoin (Dilantin) may be used to prevent seizures.

Pattern	Location of Lesion	Description
1. Cheyne-Stokes 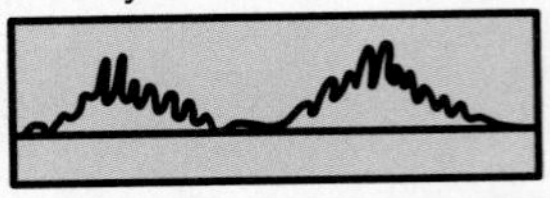	Bilateral hemispheric disease or metabolic brain dysfunction	Cycles of hyperventilation and apnea
2. Central neurogenic hyperventilation 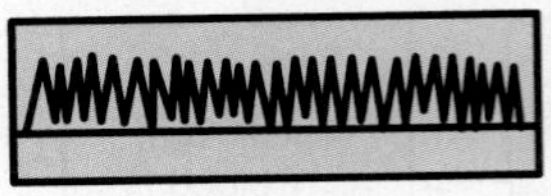	Brainstem between lower midbrain and upper pons	Sustained, regular rapid and deep breathing
3. Apneustic breathing 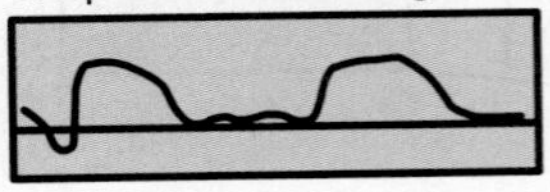	Mid or lower pons	Prolonged inspiratory phase or pauses alternating with expiratory pauses
4. Cluster breathing 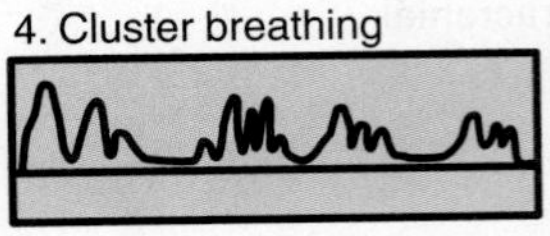	Medulla or lower pons	Clusters of breaths follow each other with irregular pauses between
5. Ataxic breathing 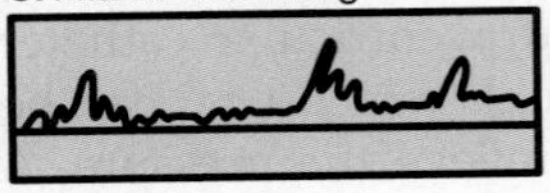	Reticular formation of the medulla	Completely irregular with some breaths deep and some shallow. Random, irregular pauses, slow rate

FIGURE **22–7** Common abnormal respiratory patterns associated with coma.

Temperature control is achieved by placing the patient on a hypothermia blanket for cooling if increased ICP has affected temperature regulation by pressure on the hypothalamus and the patient is feverish. Fever increases cerebral metabolism and cerebral edema.

Warmed blankets and tepid baths can be used to raise the temperature of the hypothermic patient and prevent shivering.

Complications

Damage to brain cells from injury and during periods of increased ICP may cause residual scarring and seizures. **Hydrocephalus** (excessive accumulation of CSF) may occur (see Chapter 23), causing motor deficits, cranial nerve deficits, or decreased cognitive ability. Rehabilitation efforts are focused on eliminating or decreasing deficits and promoting as much cognitive and physical function as possible (see Chapter 9).

Diabetes Insipidus. Diabetes insipidus may occur from injury or edema of the pituitary gland. Antidiuretic hormone is released in inadequate amounts, resulting in polyuria, and the awake patient may complain of polydipsia (excessive thirst). Intravenous vasopressin and fluid replacement are the preferred treatment. Carefully monitor intake and output and electrolyte balance.

NURSING MANAGEMENT

Assessment (Data Collection)

Early recognition of increasing pressure is extremely important to prevent permanent damage to the tissues of the brain, the cranial nerves, and the motor and sensory nerve pathways that are within the cranium. Careful neurologic assessment with monitoring of the patient's LOC, pupillary reactions, level of neuromuscular activity, and vital signs is essential to accurately evaluate the patient's progress. "Neuro checks" are performed every 15 minutes to every 2 hours for the acute patient (see Chapter 21). The following indications that ICP may be rising should be reported immediately:

- Extreme restlessness or excitability following a period of apparent calm
- Deepening stupor and decreasing LOC
- Headache that is unrelenting and increasing in intensity
- Vomiting, especially persistent, projectile vomiting

Table 22–2 ***Noninvasive Devices for Monitoring Cerebral Oxygen and Carbon Dioxide***

DEVICE	PARAMETER MEASURED	MECHANISM OF ACTION
INVOS Cerebral Oximeter	Oxygen saturation in the brain tissue	Sensors are placed on both sides of the forehead and infrared light passes through the skull and tissue to measure cerebral oxygenation
Capnometer	Expired end-tidal carbon dioxide ($EtCO_2$)	Measures the CO_2 in expired volume of breath

- Unequal size of pupils and other abnormal pupillary reactions
- Leakage of CSF from the nose or ear
- Changes in the patient's blood pressure, pulse, or respiration; widening pulse pressure; a slow, bounding pulse

Think Critically About . . . Why do you think an elderly person is at greater risk when a head injury or other cause of increased ICP occurs?

Nursing Diagnosis, Planning, and Implementation

The appropriate nursing diagnosis is "Ineffective cerebral tissue perfusion related to effects of increasing intracranial pressure." Goals of nursing care are:

- Maintain cerebral perfusion
- Reduce ICP
- Maintain adequate respiration
- Protect from injury
- Maintain normal body functions
- Prevent complications

The expected outcome would be "Patient will not experience brain damage from increased intracranial pressure."

Maintaining an open airway and adequate respiration may require suctioning and possibly intubation with mechanical ventilation. (If the patient has sustained a head injury, x-rays to rule out a basilar fracture are necessary before suctioning the nonintubated patient to prevent the possibility of the suction catheter entering the cranial vault.) The patient whose consciousness level is decreased and whose gag and swallowing reflexes are impaired is in danger of aspirating blood, vomitus, mucus, and other material into the air passages.

Position the patient on her side and ask her to exhale as you turn her to prevent a Valsalva maneuver, which could raise ICP. Instruct her not to grip the side rails or push with her feet or elbows against the mattress during repositioning for the same reason. Plan uninterrupted rest periods between activities that cause an increase in ICP, preferably 1 hour at a time. Provide a soothing environment free of noxious odors and noise. Keep the room temperature adjusted to normalize the patient's temperature; prevent shivering (American Association of Neuroscience Nurses, 2007).

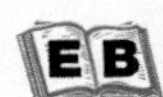

Nutrition supplied early improves outcomes after brain injury and increased ICP as it promotes healing (Yanagawa et al., 2005). If the patient is unable to take food orally, supplementation is begun within 3 days after injury. Full nutritional supplementation should be in place by day 7. Nutrition is planned according to determined metabolic needs and fluid and electrolyte status. Metabolic needs are calculated based on age, weight, and height.

Unless the patient has a tracheostomy or an oral airway in place, she should be positioned on her side, not on her back, as the tongue may occlude the airway, and mucus cannot drain naturally. **The unconscious patient requires care for all basic needs.** See Table 21–8 and the section on common care problems for specific interventions in Chapter 21.

Box 22–2 *Guidelines for Patients with Increased Intracranial Pressure (ICP)*

DO

- Conduct neurologic checks at least once every hour unless more frequent monitoring is indicated.
- Report changes immediately.
- Maintain a patent airway and adequate ventilation to ensure proper oxygen and carbon dioxide exchange.
- Elevate the head of the bed 15 to 30 degrees to facilitate return of blood from the cerebral veins.
- Use measures to maintain normal body temperature. Elevations of temperature raise blood pressure and cerebral blood flow. Shivering also can increase ICP.
- Monitor intake and output. Restrict or encourage fluids according to physician's order.
- Give passive range-of-motion exercises.
- Space activities apart.

DO NOT

- Allow patient to become constipated or perform Valsalva maneuver.
- Hyperextend, flex, or rotate the patient's head.
- Flex the patient's hips (as in female catheterization).
- Place patient in Trendelenburg's position for any reason.
- Allow patient to perform isometric exercises.

Evaluation

Data are gathered regarding the success of the nursing interventions. If the interventions are not helping the patient meet the expected outcomes, the interventions should be changed.

INJURIES OF THE SPINE AND SPINAL CORD

Etiology

A person may suffer from injury to the spinal cord in a number of ways. Injury in the cervical and lumbar areas is more frequent because these segments are more mobile. Automobile accidents, gunshot wounds, diving accidents, and other forms of trauma often inflict severe damage to the spinal cord, but tumors, degenerative disease, and infections also can impair the functions of the spinal cord and its branches. Generally speaking, spinal cord injuries are classified according to their anatomic location; that is, cervical, thoracic, lumbar, or sacral (Figure 22–8). Whatever the cause of spinal cord injury, motor and sensory losses may occur. The amount of loss of function and sensa-

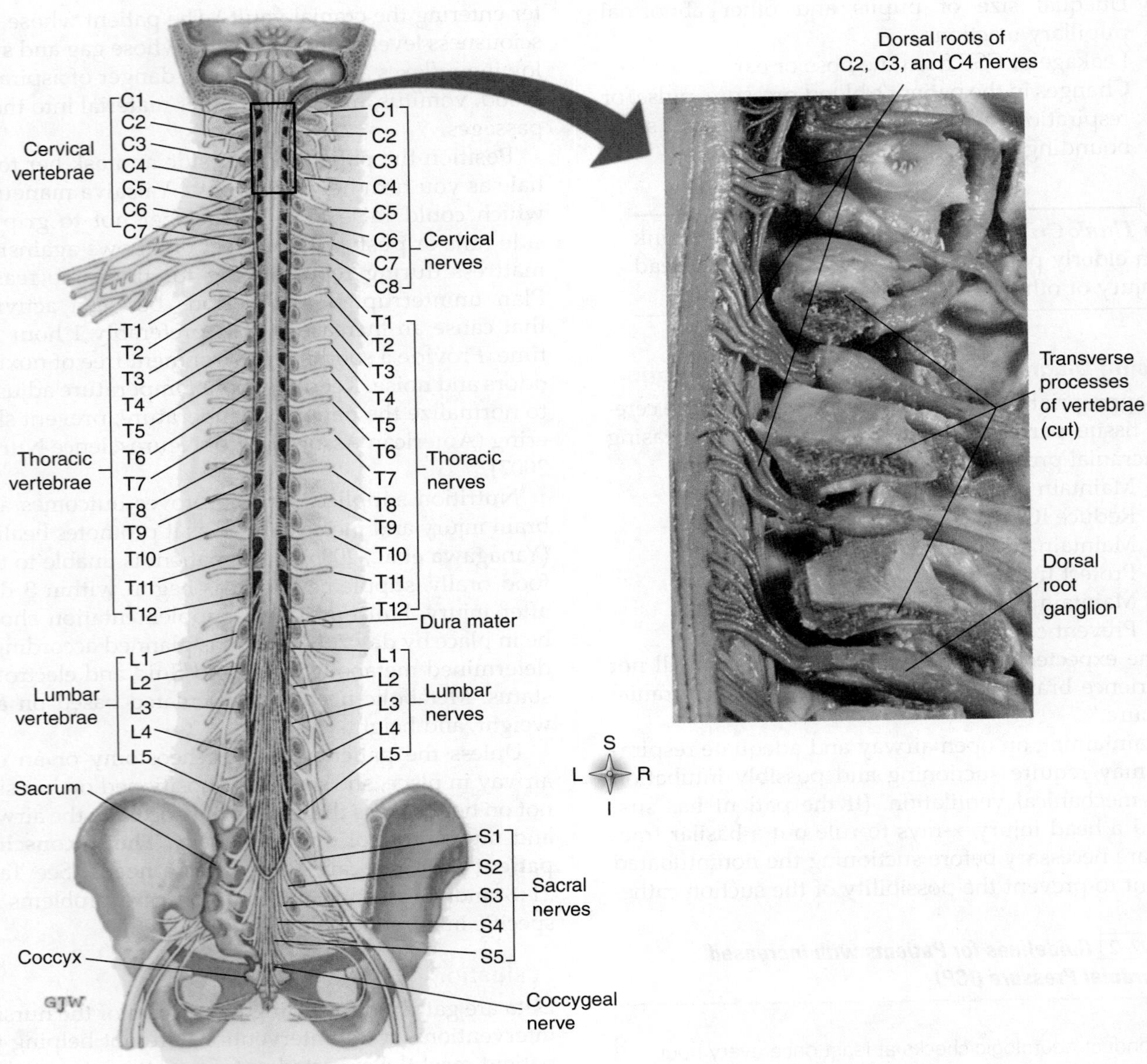

FIGURE 22–8 Divisions of the spinal column and designations of spinal nerves.

tion depends on the level and extent of injury to the spinal cord.

Pathophysiology

Fracture, dislocation, or **subluxation** (partial dislocation) of the vertebral column often results in spinal cord damage. Cord injury is caused by compression, pulling and twisting, or tearing of the cord, with four types of injuries occurring. Penetrating trauma from gunshot or knife wounds or other types of accidents may cause severance, compression, or contusion of the spinal cord. Extreme flexion or hyperextension of the neck, or falling on the buttocks, which causes flexion of the lower thoracic and lumbar spine, all may cause spinal cord damage (Figure 22–9). Tumor growth may compress or destroy spinal cord tissue. Whatever the cause of injury to the spinal cord, nerve transmission to the brain or from the brain may no longer occur below the level of the damage, resulting in paralysis.

Microscopic bleeding occurs in the gray matter immediately after spinal cord injury. Irritation of the cells causes edema to develop and spread along the next one or two cord segments. The edema peaks in 2 to 3 days and subsides in about 7 days after injury. The edema causes temporary loss of function and sensation. Hemodynamic instability with drops in blood pressure may cause decreased blood flow and hypoxia in the cord that increases the initial damage. The inflammatory process may injure the myelin covering the axons, and the chemical and electrolyte changes interrupt nerve impulse transmission.

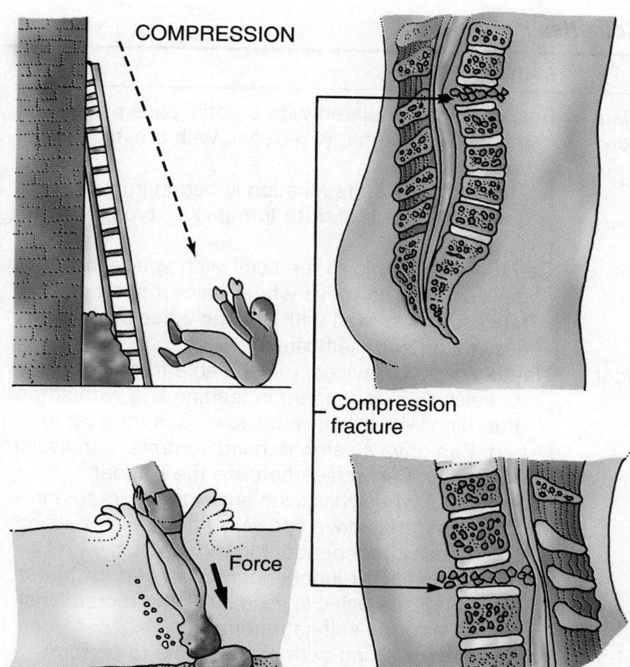

FIGURE 22–9 Accidents can cause vertical compression on the cervical or lumbar spine.

Box 22–3 American Spinal Injury Association (ASIA) Impairment Scale

A = **Complete:** No motor or sensory function is preserved in the sacral segments S4-S5.

B = **Incomplete:** Sensory but not motor function is preserved below the neurologic level and includes the sacral segments S4-S5.

C = **Incomplete:** Motor function is preserved below the neurologic level, and more than half of key muscles below the neurologic level have a muscle grade less than 3.

D = **Incomplete:** Motor function is preserved below the neurologic level, and at least half of key muscles below the neurologic level have a muscle grade of 3 or more.

E = **Normal:** Motor and sensory function are intact.

From American Spinal Injury Association, Atlanta, Ga.

Signs, Symptoms, and Diagnosis

A complete severance, or damage to the entire thickness, of the cord results in a total loss of sensation and control in the parts of the body below the point of injury. If the cord is damaged in the cervical region, the paralysis and loss of sensory perception may include both arms and both legs (tetraplegia), also called **quadriplegia.** Severe injury to the cord above the level of the fifth cervical vertebra often is fatal if emergency care is not immediate because the phrenic nerves that innervate the diaphragm originate in the third, fourth, and fifth cervical segments. Branches of these nerves play a major role in the control of respiration, and when they are severed, respiration must be maintained by artificial means. If the damage is only partial (incomplete) there will be some losses, but not all motor and sensory innervation is lost (Box 22–3).

Interruption of the thoracic spinal cord through L1 and L2 causes paraplegia (paralysis of both legs). Table 22–3 presents activities possible at varying levels of cord injury.

Injury to the spinal cord that does not involve complete severance of the cord may result in a temporary paralysis, which may subside as the spinal cord recovers from the swelling and initial shock of the injury.

Diagnosis is by made by physical examination and testing of reflexes. CT scan or MRI may be performed to determine the extent of the damage and to see whether the cord is completely *transected* (severed). This helps determine if neurologic deficits are likely to be permanent. A myelogram may be performed when other tests do not reveal sufficient information.

Treatment

There are four main objectives in the treatment and nursing care of the patient with an injury of the spinal cord:

- To save the victim's life
- To prevent further injury to the cord by careful handling of the patient
- To repair as much of the damage to the cord as possible
- To establish a routine of care that will improve and maintain the patient's state of health and prevent complications, so that eventual physical, mental, and social rehabilitation is possible

As soon as an injury to the spinal cord occurs, the patient must be handled with extreme care (Safety Alert 22–1). Because a nurse or physician may not be at the scene of the accident to supervise the moving of the victim, laypersons should learn the proper emergency care of such injuries. When an accident victim complains of neck or back pain, or cannot move the legs or has no feeling in them, treat the victim as if she has a spinal cord injury. **To avoid flexion of the neck, *no pillow or other kind of support is placed under the head. Do not move the victim unless life-threatening conditions require it.***

Transfer of the patient to the hospital should be done only by trained emergency medical technicians or others qualified to administer first aid and immobilize the spine. In the emergency department of the hospital, the patient's condition is stabilized and a thorough examination is conducted to establish the extent of her injuries. A large dose of methylprednisolone, a corticosteroid, may be given as soon as the examination and diagnosis of cord injury are made. If given within 8 hours of injury, it is thought to mini-

Table 22–3 Level of Spinal Cord Damage, Function Present, and Activities Possible

LEVEL OF INJURY	FUNCTION PRESENT/NEUROLOGIC DEFICIT	ACTIVITY POSSIBLE
C1-C3	No respiratory function; usually fatal unless immediate emergency help is available to establish respiration Quadriplegia	Respirations stimulated with phrenic pacemaker. Can manipulate electric wheelchair with breath, chin, or voice control.
C4	Loss of diaphragm movement; breathe with assistance Quadriplegia	May live if assisted respiration is begun immediately. Can use a mouthstick to turn pages, type, or write.
C5	Partial shoulder movement; partial elbow movement	Can turn head. Able to feed self with special adaptive devices. Able to move wheelchair for short distances, moves well with electric wheelchair. Can assist a bit with self-care.
C6	Retains gross motor function of arms; partial shoulder, elbow, and wrist movement possible Paraplegia	Needs adaptive devices; may be able to propel wheelchair. Independent in feeding and with some grooming with adaptive devices. Can roll over in bed. Can drive a car with hand controls. Can assist in transfer. Can self-catheterize the bladder.
C7	Shoulder, elbow, wrist, hand partial movements possible Paraplegia	Manipulates wheelchair with arms; transfers to and from chair; may drive specially fitted car. Excellent bed mobility. Independent in most ADLs.
C8	Normal arm movement; hand weakness Paraplegia	Bed and wheelchair independent. Can perform most ADLs and may achieve vocational and recreational goals. Performs self-catheterization.
T1-T10	Normal arm movement and strength; loss of bowel, bladder, and sexual function	May achieve walking with braces. Able to perform ADLs and achieve vocational and recreational goals.
T11 and below	Loss of bowel, bladder, and sexual function	Wheelchair not essential. Able to perform ADLs, work, and recreation activities.

Key: *ADLs,* activities of daily living.

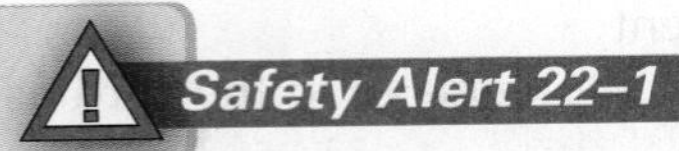

Prevent Further Spinal Injury

Anyone with a head injury is treated as if she has also suffered a spine injury until proven otherwise. The neck must be stabilized to prevent any movement. When no cervical collar is available, use a shirt, towel, coat, or other material rolled and placed around the neck as a collar to keep the neck as straight as possible, preventing it from flexing or hyperextending. If the victim must be moved to safety, she should be rolled like a log, as one straight piece, onto a flat surface, such as a piece of plywood or a door removed from its hinges. She is rolled as one piece onto her side, the flat surface placed beside her, and then she is carefully rolled back onto the board. This is done slowly and carefully to avoid twisting or bending the spinal column. The victim is kept still.

mize further damage and improve the return of both motor function and sensation (National Institutes of Health, 2006). Use of a corticosteroid is controversial due to recent research about the lack of evidence of benefit versus the many side effects of the drug.

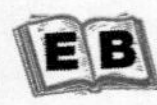

Normal saline is used for fluid replacement, and drugs such as dopamine (Intropin) may be given to sustain a sufficient blood pressure to prevent cord hypoxia. Pulmonary edema, and increased ICP if a head injury is present, are potential problems, and fluid balance is watched carefully.

Respiratory Management. Intubation and mechanical ventilation are often required to sustain life in patients with an injury at C5 or above. Patients with intact phrenic nerve innervation may receive a phrenic nerve stimulator that assists them to breathe by stimulating action of the diaphragm. Patients who can breathe when they first arrive at the hospital may be intubated because as cord edema progresses, respiration may become impaired. Mechanical ventilation relieves the muscle work of breathing and conserves the patient's energy during the emergent phase of the injury. An oral airway may be placed if a tracheostomy is unnecessary.

Immobilization and Surgery. Surgery on the spine with removal of bone fragments is performed to relieve pressure, provide stabilization, and prevent further injury. **Cervical spinal cord injury is usually treated with traction to immobilize the affected vertebrae and maintain alignment.** Traction can be accomplished by a head halter; skeletal traction using Crutchfield or Gardner-Wells tongs with ropes, pulleys, and weights (Figure 22–10); or a halo ring and fixation pins (Figure 22–11). The halo is often used for cord injury not requiring surgery and allows for early ambulation.

Selecting the type of bed to be used for a patient with spinal cord injury depends on many factors. Some physicians and nurses prefer placing the patient in a special lateral rotation bed designed to prevent the problems of immobility while maintaining traction (Figure 22–12). If halo traction is used and the patient

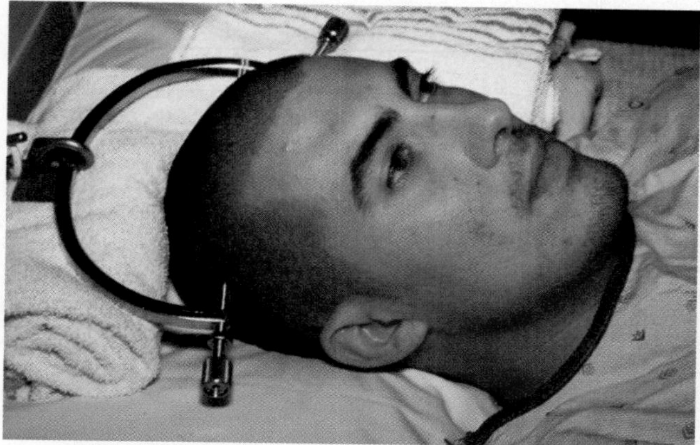

FIGURE 22–10 Crutchfield tongs for cervical traction.

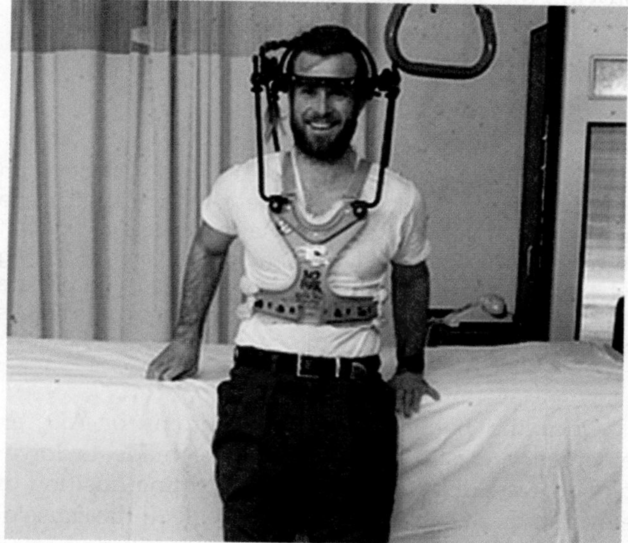

FIGURE 22–11 Halo traction vest for cervical stabilization. Note the rigid shoulder straps and encompassing vest. Various vest sizes are available prefabricated. The halo ring superstructure and the vest are magnetic resonance imaging (MRI) compatible.

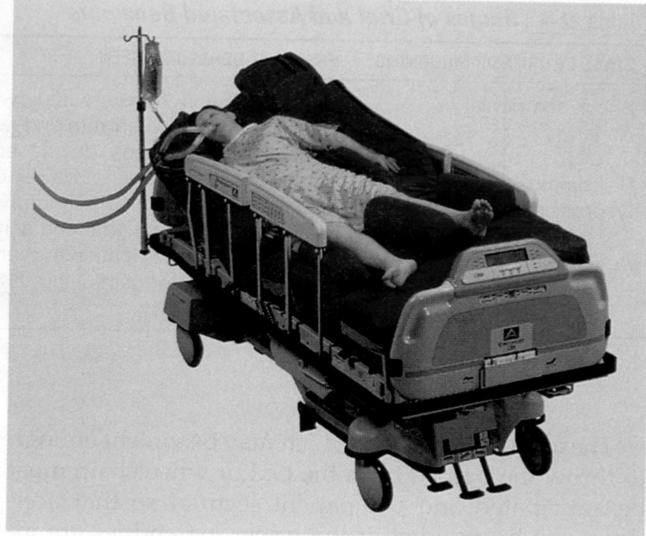

FIGURE 22–12 The Roto-Rest oscillating bed.

has an incomplete spinal cord injury, a standard orthopedic bed may be used. All measures to prevent the problems of immobility are instituted (see Chapter 9).

Urinary Management. An indwelling urinary catheter is inserted to prevent bladder distention and protect the skin from reflex bladder emptying. After the first week, a bladder management program will be initiated (see Chapter 21).

Psychological Care. The short-term and long-term psychological changes brought about by spinal cord injury and paralysis are difficult, if not impossible, to measure. Adjustment to such a drastic change in one's lifestyle is a continuous process that may well last a lifetime (see Chapter 9).

Grief and Mourning Response. Sustaining a spinal cord injury that causes permanent neurologic deficit brings with it many losses. Most patients experience grief and mourning of the losses experienced and the changes that such losses bring to their roles and lifestyle. Table 22–4 presents a review of the stages of grief and the behaviors that might be seen. Use active listening, be supportive, and help the patient to focus on positive strengths and possibilities for the future.

Sexual Concerns. One area of concern to the patient and her family members that sometimes receives inadequate attention is that of sexual function and sexuality following spinal cord injury. Discussions of sexual conduct and the larger concept of human sexuality are not easily approached and participated in by many individuals. The nurse who wishes to help a patient deal with problems of sexuality must first come to terms with his own feelings and attitudes and clarify his own values. He should not be critical or judgmental in his discussions about the patient's sexuality. The patient and her partner must be encouraged to verbalize their concerns and questions and should be given guidance in alternative ways to express sexuality and meet sexual needs.

Complications

Spinal Shock (Neurogenic Shock). The disruption in the nerve communication pathways between upper motor neurons and lower motor neurons immediately causes spinal shock. It is characterized by flaccid paralysis, loss of reflex activity below the level of the damage, bradycardia, hypotension, and occasionally paralytic ileus. Vital signs become labile. Treatment is aimed at maintaining adequate blood pressure and heart rate.

Muscle Spasms. Immediately after a cord injury, the patient will usually have a flaccid type of paralysis. Later, as the cord adjusts to the injury, the paralysis will become spastic, and there will be strong, involuntary contractions of the skeletal muscles.

Table 22–4 *Stages of Grief and Associated Behaviors*

STAGE OF GRIEF OR MOURNING	FREQUENT BEHAVIORS SEEN
Shock and denial	Complete dependence, withdrawal, excessive sleep, struggle for survival, unrealistic expectations.
Anger	Hostility toward caregivers and family, manipulative behavior, abusive language, refusal to discuss paralysis and losses, decreased self-esteem.
Bargaining	Bargaining with a higher power or fate: "If you'll let me walk again, I'll pray every day."
Depression	Sadness, "blue" mood, withdrawal, insomnia, agitation, refusal to participate in education for self-care, suicidal thoughts and comments.
Adjustment	Begins active participation in therapy and education for self-care, planning for future, expresses hope for future functioning, finds meaning in whole experience of injury and therapy, return of usual personality.

These muscle spasms, which may be violent enough to throw the patient from the bed or wheelchair, must be anticipated and the patient secured so that accidents can be avoided. If the upper extremities are involved, she is likely to tip over glasses, water pitchers, or anything within reach of her arms when seized with uncontrollable muscle spasms.

The patient and family may interpret these spasms as a return of voluntary function of the limbs and will have false hopes of complete recovery. The nurse or the physician must explain to them that these spasms are frequently seen in patients with spinal cord injuries.

To avoid stimulating the muscles when moving the patient and thereby precipitating a spasm of the muscles, avoid grasping the muscle itself. The palms of the hands are used to support the joints above and below the affected muscles. The administration of antispasmodic medications such as baclofen (Lioresal) may decrease the severity of the spasms (Table 22–5).

Autonomic Dysreflexia (Hyperreflexia). Autonomic dysreflexia (AD) is an uninhibited and exaggerated reflex response of the autonomic nervous system to some form of stimulation. It is a response that occurs in 85% of all patients who have spinal cord injury at or above the level of the sixth thoracic vertebra (T6). The response is potentially dangerous to the patient, because it can produce vasoconstriction of the arterioles with an immediate elevation of blood pressure. The sudden hypertension can, in turn, cause a seizure, retinal hemorrhage, or a stroke. Less serious effects include severe headache, changes in pulse rate, sweating and flushing above the level of the spinal cord lesion, and pallor and "goose bumps" below the level of injury.

It is important for nurses and others participating in the care of a patient with quadriplegia and other kinds of spinal cord disorders at or above the T6 level to be aware of the circumstances that can trigger AD, its manifestations, and the correct measures to take if it happens. The problem can occur any time after a spinal cord injury; in some cases it has first appeared as late as 6 years after the injury.

There are many kinds of stimulation that can precipitate AD. Most are related to the bladder, bowel, and skin of the patient. For example, catheter changes, a distended bladder, the insertion of rectal suppositories, enemas, and sudden changing of position can provide the stimulation that results in AD (National Spinal Cord Injury Association, 2006). 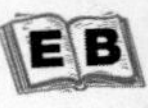

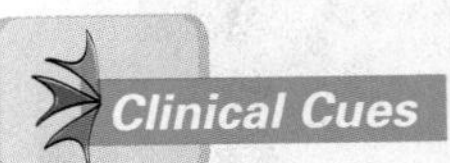

Careful attention must be paid to keeping the bladder from becoming overdistended. Check the catheter and drainage tubing for the indwelling catheter every couple of hours if the patient is on bed rest. Monitor output and time of voiding for the patient without an indwelling catheter and palpate the bladder for distention every few hours when voiding has not occurred.

Once the patient exhibits symptoms of AD, an emergency exists. Efforts should be made to lower blood pressure by placing her in a sitting position or elevating her head to a 45-degree angle. If the cause of the stimulation is known—for example, an impacted bowel, overdistended bladder, or pressure against the skin—the stimulus should be removed as gently and quickly as possible. The physician should be notified immediately so that the appropriate medications can be prescribed and administered. Patients who experience repeated attacks of AD may require surgery to sever the nerves responsible for the exaggerated response to stimulation (Agency for Healthcare Research and Quality, 2007). 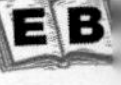

Orthostatic Hypotension. Vasoconstriction is impaired after spinal cord injury, and the lack of muscle function in the legs causes pooling of blood in the lower extremities. Sudden change in position from supine to sitting or sitting to standing may cause dizziness and fainting. Compression stockings, moving slowly, and a reclining wheelchair may help prevent this problem.

Deep Venous Thrombosis. Decreased blood pressure combined with lack of muscle movement slows venous return to the heart. Thrombosis may occur. Compression stockings, sequential compression devices, and/or heparin injections may be needed to prevent deep venous thrombosis.

Table 22–5 Medications Commonly Used for Patients with Head and Spinal Cord Injury

CLASSIFICATION	ACTION	NURSING IMPLICATIONS	PATIENT TEACHING
CORTICOSTEROID			
Methylprednisolone (Solu-Medrol)	Decreases inflammation by suppression of leukocyte migration to injury site; decreases capillary permeability.	Give as IV bolus. May cause insomnia, increased susceptibility to infection, and GI distress. May delay wound healing. Monitor electrolyte levels. H_2 receptor blocker or proton pump inhibitor often given concurrently to prevent stress ulcer.	Advise to report heartburn or stomach pain.
SKELETAL MUSCLE RELAXANT			
Baclofen (Lioresal)	Inhibits synaptic responses in CNS by decreasing GABA, thereby decreasing frequency and severity of muscle spasms.	Monitor for seizure activity. Observe for muscle weakness and fatigue. Assess for allergic symptoms: rash, fever, respiratory distress.	Advise not to drink alcohol as it increases CNS depression. Do not discontinue medication quickly or abruptly.
ADRENERGIC ACTION VASOCONSTRICTOR			
Dopamine (Intropin)	Acts on alpha receptors causing vasoconstriction in blood vessels, thereby raising blood pressure.	Monitor vital signs closely; assess for chest pain. Monitor I&O. Place patient on a cardiac monitor during therapy. May cause nausea, vomiting, or diarrhea. Be certain that IV access is patent as drug will cause necrosis if extravasation into the tissue occurs.	Explain purpose of drug is to raise blood pressure so that brain has adequate perfusion and oxygen. May cause headache.
OSMOTIC DIURETIC			
Mannitol	Increases osmotic pressure of glomerular filtrate; promotes diuresis.	Monitor vital signs closely. Track I&O, assess skin turgor and mucous membranes for signs of dehydration. Monitor electrolytes. Observe for nausea, backache, hives, and chest pain.	Explain that the drug will cause increased urine output and that this is its intended action.
NEUROMUSCULAR BLOCKING (PARALYZING) AGENT			
Pancuronium (Pavulon)	Inhibits transmission of nerve impulses, producing skeletal muscle relaxation for surgery, endotracheal intubation, and mechanical ventilation when patient is fighting the ventilator.	Be certain that alarms are properly set on the ventilator. Observe patient frequently. Keep Ambu bag at bedside. Monitor electrolytes and I&O. Observe for urinary retention. Observe for allergic reaction: rash, fever, pruritus. Protect the eyes with artificial tears and keep lids closed.	Explain that patient will be paralyzed and unable to move. Assure that she will be monitored at all times and that there are backup measures in place in case of power outage when ventilator wouldn't work.

Key: *CNS,* central nervous system; *GABA,* gamma-aminobutyric acid; *GI,* gastrointestinal; *H_2,* histamine$_2$; *I&O,* intake and output; *IV,* intravenous.

Infection. Impaired respiratory muscles with decreased cough and shallow respirations predisposes the patient with spinal cord injury to respiratory infection. Mechanical ventilation with intubation provides an avenue for microorganisms to enter the lungs and is a risk factor for infection. Urinary catheterization for loss of bladder control is a risk factor for infection as well.

Skin Breakdown. Lack of sensation and inability to move for repositioning places the patient at great risk for skin breakdown and pressure ulcers. Pressure-relieving devices, meticulous skin care with regular inspection, and manual repositioning are essential to prevent this problem.

Renal Complications. Urinary reflux from the bladder to the kidney often occurs due to impaired bladder function. Catheterization and immobility predispose to bladder infection, which may travel up the ureters to the kidneys. Permanent damage may eventually occur from the infections.

? *Think Critically About . . .* Can you name three care interventions that might trigger an episode of AD? How could you possibly avoid causing this reaction?

NURSING MANAGEMENT

There often is a tendency to treat a physically disabled patient as if she were less than a "whole" person with the same desires, hopes, and anxieties that all humans share. The nurse can serve patients by reacting to and interacting with them in an open and honest manner. When the nurse feels unprepared to handle a certain problem, there is no reason not to readily admit embarrassment, confusion, or lack of information and seek assistance from other members of the health care team. Rehabilitation of patients with spinal cord injuries is discussed in detail in Chapter 9.

Assessment (Data Collection)

Continued assessment for signs of decreased oxygenation, blood pressure instability, infection, skin breakdown, gastrointestinal or nutrition problems, and urinary problems is essential. A daily review of systems and collection of data regarding physical status is performed. Assessment of a tracheostomy tube, traction devices and pins, correct placement and use of sequential compression devices or compression stockings, indwelling catheter, IV cannula, feeding tube, and the like is essential each shift.

Nursing Diagnosis

Nursing diagnoses appropriate for the patient with a spinal cord injury may include:

- Impaired gas exchange related to paralysis, diaphragm fatigue, or retained secretions
- Impaired physical mobility related to vertebral column instability, disruption of the spinal cord, and traction
- Decreased cardiac output related to hypotension and decreased muscle action causing venous pooling
- Imbalanced nutrition: less than body requirements related to increased metabolic demand from healing injuries, slowed gastrointestinal motility, and inability to feed self
- Impaired urinary elimination related to decreased innervation of the bladder
- Constipation related to loss of nerve stimulation to the bowel and immobility
- Risk for autonomic dysreflexia related to reflex stimulation of sympathetic nervous system
- Risk for impaired skin integrity related to immobility and loss of sensation
- Risk for ineffective coping related to loss of control over bodily functions and altered lifestyle secondary to paralysis
- Disturbed body image related to paralysis and loss of control over bodily functions
- Interrupted family processes related to change in role within the family because of neurologic deficits
- Grieving related to neurologic deficits and changes in roles and lifestyle

Planning, Implementation, and Evaluation

Specific, individual expected outcomes are written for each nursing diagnosis supported by data gathered. Long-term goals are considered, and planning for rehabilitation begins with hospitalization. The patient will often be transferred to a rehabilitation facility for intensive rehabilitation and retraining in activities of daily living.

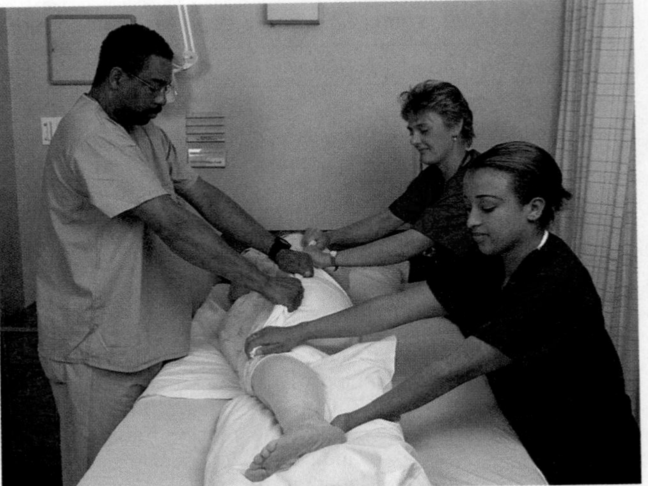

FIGURE 22–13 Log-rolling procedure using a lift sheet and three people.

Care for the patient with a spinal cord injury can be very complex depending on the level of the injury. Often a head injury accompanies the trauma to the spinal cord. When a stabilization device is in place on the head, assessment and care of the pin sites are performed every shift initially and then twice a day. Sterile technique is used and is performed according to agency policy. Solutions such as sterile normal saline, hydrogen peroxide, or ointments such as povidone-iodine or bacitracin may be used. Weights used for cervical traction must be kept hanging free to be effective. Traction pull should never be interrupted. If the patient is wearing a halo fixation device, skin care must be given frequently and the skin checked to see that the jacket or cast is not causing pressure ulcers. One finger should be able to slip easily beneath the cast or jacket to be sure it is not too tight. The patient is never moved or turned by holding or pulling on the halo device. **The halo jacket is never unfastened unless the patient is supine as head movement will immediately occur.** Moving the patient as a unit, or "log rolling," must be done with extreme care to avoid twisting the vertebral column and further damaging the spinal cord (Figure 22–13; Assignment Considerations 22–1).

All the nursing measures designed to prevent the disabilities that may result from immobility, to promote healing, and to avoid complications are used to help the patient achieve the goals of rehabilitation. Bladder and bowel training programs, as well as instruction in moving from bed to chair and other aspects of self-care, may be necessary. Realistic goals should be set for the patient and every effort made to achieve them.

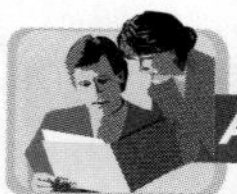

Assignment Considerations 22–1

Inappropriate Delegation

Although many tasks may be delegated to the certified nursing assistant (CNA) or UAP, moving or positioning the patient with neurologic injury or surgery should *not* be delegated. If given proper, complete instructions, the CNA or UAP may help log roll the patient with the nurse's help and supervision.

Implementation of actions requires encouraging the patient to do whatever she can for herself as soon as feasible. The overall goal is to promote as much independence as possible. A great deal of encouragement and praise are required. You can be a pillar of support for the patient.

Evaluation is ongoing to see if the interventions have been successful in achieving the expected outcomes. If they have not been successful, the plan is rewritten.

Rehabilitation

A full team of professionals will be involved in the care and rehabilitation of the patient with a spinal cord injury. The physical therapist, occupational therapist, psychologist, physician, respiratory therapist, pharmacist, and ancillary personnel will collaboratively plan the patient's care. The patient and family are often invited to participate in the planning process.

The use of robotics and computers is providing hope for some patients to walk again (Barker, 2005). A system called functional electrical stimulation (FES) is used to generate neural activity and overcome lost function. The system stimulates muscles to make walking motions. The patient is suspended in a harness to support body weight and is retrained to walk using a treadmill. Research is underway on a neuroprosthetic microchip implant that would help certain patients to walk again. A pacemaker for the bladder is under study for the treatment of urinary incontinence.

Communication between team members is crucial to the success of the individual plan. When the patient is discharged, all plans and specifics required for her care must be shared with home caregivers and home care nurses who will be involved in her care. Her primary physician must be fully briefed.

BACK PAIN AND RUPTURED INTERVERTEBRAL DISK ("SLIPPED DISK")

Etiology

Back pain is surpassed only by headache pain. Emergency physicians treat more than 6 million cases of back pain annually. In people under age 45, it is the most common cause of work absence and is the most costly health condition for employers. Carelessness and incorrect methods of lifting contribute to a large percentage of back problems. On-the-job accidents and resultant trauma to the spine are another cause. Obesity and lack of exercise, and poor lifting and moving techniques, contribute to the stress placed on the back muscles and to the occurrence of injury or the severity and duration of pain. Exercise promotes good muscle tone. Other risk factors include lack of exercise causing poor muscle tone, poor posture, cigarette smoking that decreases oxygenation to the disks and predisposes to degenerative disease, and stress. Repetitive heavy lifting also may cause back pain. This is often a factor for health care workers. Causes of musculoskeletal back pain include:

- Acute lumbosacral strain
- Instability of lumbosacral spine
- Osteoarthritis of the spine
- Intervertebral disk degeneration and spinal stenosis
- Herniation of the intervertebral disk

Preventing back pain and disorders begins with proper posture and the use of correct lifting techniques. Maintaining one's weight within normal limits also helps decrease back strain. Sufficient physical exercise that maintains the condition of the back muscles and specific exercises to strengthen the abdominal and back muscles can greatly decrease the repeated incidence of back pain.

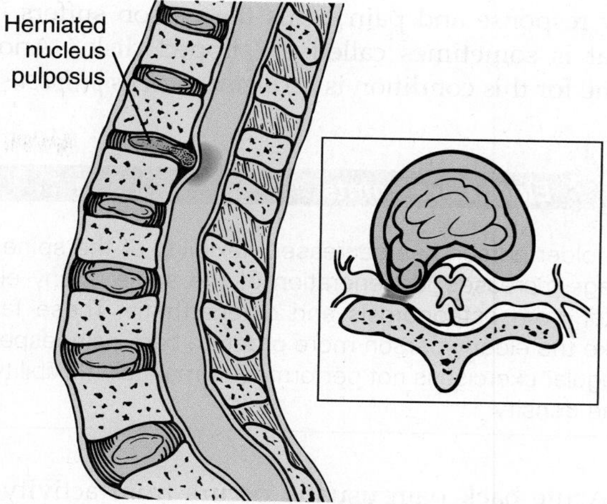

FIGURE 22–14 Herniated disk (nucleus pulposus) with compression of spinal cord.

Pathophysiology

The bodies of the vertebrae lie flat on one another like a stack of coins. Between the vertebral bodies there is a disk of fibrous cartilage filled with gelatinous substance (in the nucleus) that acts as a cushion to absorb shocks to the spinal column. This disk may be ruptured by an injury, such as strain caused by lifting a heavy object or wrenching or falling on the back. When the disk ruptures, part of the contents squeeze out from between the vertebrae and disk fragments may lodge in the spinal canal. The disk compression on the adjacent nerve root causes the pain (Figure 22–14). When protein from the disk contents leaks out into the canal, the body perceives it as a foreign substance, causing an inflammatory response and pain. Thus the person suffers from what is sometimes called a "slipped disk." Another name for this condition is *herniated nucleus pulposus.*

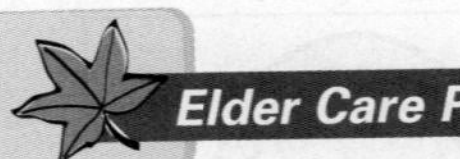

Elder Care Points

The older person has decreased flexibility of the spine and, as age increases, degeneration of the spine. Many elderly suffer from osteoporosis and osteoarthritis. These factors make the elderly person more prone to back pain, especially if regular exercise is not performed to maintain flexibility and bone density.

Acute back pain usually occurs from activity that puts stress (hyperflexion) on the tissues of the lower back. Back pain that is a result of muscle spasm is usually self-limiting and often resolves within 4 weeks. Chronic back pain is pain that lasts for more than 3 months or is a repeat episode. It may be due to degenerative disk disease or osteoarthritis, but lack of exercise, prior injury, and obesity are frequent factors.

The most common sites of disk rupture are L4-L5 and L5-S1. Herniation may also occur at C5-C6 or C6-C7.

Signs, Symptoms, and Diagnosis

Sometimes a lumbar herniated disk causes pain radiating down the sciatic nerve into the buttock and below the knee. Muscle weakness and paresthesias may occur. Cervical herniated disk causes pain in the neck and shoulder, radiating down the arm with numbness and tingling in the hand. Muscle tightening and spasm in the area of injury are common.

Diagnosis requires a history and physical examination. The straight-leg-raising test is often used for low back pain. While supine, the leg is raised off the bed or examination table and the foot is flexed. The test confirms a disk problem if there is pain in the low back. Reflexes may be decreased or absent. The patient may experience muscle weakness or paresthesias in the legs or feet.

If conservative therapy does not relieve the pain, diagnostic x-rays, MRI, or CT scanning is performed. An electromyogram may be ordered to determine the degree of nerve irritation and to rule out other pathologic conditions.

Treatment

In most instances, the physician will treat back pain initially with conservative measures in the hope that surgical correction will not be necessary. If there is no sciatic pain, bed rest is not recommended as the research has shown that walking provides a quicker recovery. When sciatic pain is present, bed rest for 2 to 3 days is helpful. During this period, the patient is encouraged to get up and walk around every 2 to 3 hours while awake even if this causes pain (Hilde et al., 2005). Ice packs are applied for 5 to 10 minutes at a

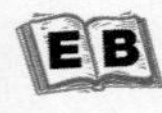

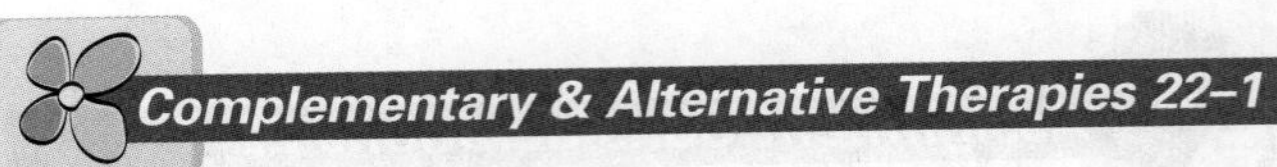

Complementary & Alternative Therapies 22–1

Help for Pain

Acupuncture, acupressure, and massage therapy have all proven beneficial for back pain. Research from the National Institutes of Health has proven that acupuncture is effective for back pain. For those with chronic back pain, it certainly is worth trying. Massage and acupressure help relieve muscle spasm, especially when heat is applied to the affected muscles first.

time each hour for the first 48 hours to reduce muscle spasm in the back. After 48 hours, heat may be more helpful as it relaxes strained muscles. Ultrasound treatments are often helpful. Heating pads, hot packs, and hot showers work well to relax the muscles (Complementary & Alternative Therapies 22–1). A study done at Johns Hopkins showed that wearing a portable heat wrap for 8 hours on 3 consecutive days decreased pain by 60% in a group of patients with back pain. Transcutaneous electrical nerve stimulation may help relieve the patient's pain. Back strengthening exercises are prescribed as soon as acute symptoms subside and are initially supervised by a physical therapist. The exercises are encouraged for a lifetime as muscles need to be toned to prevent back strain. Specially designed corsets or back braces are sometimes used to maintain proper alignment of the spine when the patient is allowed out of bed. The patient is cautioned not to lift anything heavier than 2 to 5 lb and not to twist when reaching for things. The patient should be up moving about frequently rather than sitting for long periods. High heels should be avoided.

Swimming or walking for short distances frequently is very beneficial. Standing for long periods is to be avoided, and when standing, the patient should shift weight from one foot to the other frequently. Adjustments and treatments by a chiropractor may also help relieve pain, although chiropractic treatment is not appropriate for all types of back injuries. Chiropractic help seems most effective if the pain has been present less than 16 days and the pain is all above the knee.

If pain continues beyond 3 to 4 weeks, there is evidence of neurologic deficit, or pain is worsening, surgery may be indicated.

Gentle yoga movements have been more successful in relieving pain than prescribed back exercises for many patients. For others, core body stretching and muscle strengthening works well.

Surgical Procedures. For those patients who cannot find relief through conservative measures, surgical removal of the damaged disk may be the only alternative. A diskectomy often is performed to decompress the nerve root. This is a microsurgical technique that utilizes a very small incision through which the herniated intervertebral disk material is dissected and extracted. If the area cannot be handled with microsurgery, an open incision diskectomy or laminectomy, which involves removal of the posterior arch of the vertebra along with the disk, is done. A laminectomy may be done in conjunction with spinal fusion.

A percutaneous laser diskectomy is an outpatient procedure. A tube is passed through the retroperitoneal soft tissues to the disk's lateral border. Local anesthesia and fluoroscopy are used during the procedure. A laser is utilized to cut away and destroy the herniated portion of the disk. Small stab wounds are used, there is minimal blood loss, and rehabilitation time is shorter.

A spinal fusion is necessary in some patients to stabilize the spine. In a spinal fusion, a piece or pieces of bone from the iliac crest or cadaver bone are grafted onto the vertebrae to strengthen them. Fixation with metal rods and screws may be employed to decrease spinal motion and irritability. A new device, the InFuse Bone Graft/LT-CAGE, is being used to avoid the need to use bone from the patient for grafting (Perina, 2006). Genetically engineered protein contained in the device stimulates new bone growth at the site.

A laminectomy may be done for conditions other than a ruptured disk—for example, for such degenerative diseases of the spine as Pott's disease (tuberculosis of the spine), for fractures of the spine, and for spinal dislocation. Once a laminectomy with a fusion has healed, the fused vertebrae are immobile.

Nursing Management

Preoperatively, a baseline neurologic assessment is performed and documented (Focused Assessment 22–1). Other preoperative care is the same as for other types of general surgery. The major concern after spinal fusion, laminectomy, or diskectomy is to keep the spinal column in alignment so that healing can take place and no further injury occurs to the spinal cord. Pillows are placed under the thighs when the patient is on her back and between the legs when on the side to maintain correct spinal alignment and decrease the pressure to the back. If the surgeon allows the patient to be turned to the side, log rolling is used to avoid twisting the spine (see Figure 22–13). Sometimes the surgeon will allow the patient to be positioned only on the back or sometimes the abdomen. Whenever the patient's position is changed, there should be ample people to help move her. The patient who has had cervical spine surgery is placed in a cervical collar and continues to wear a collar for several weeks.

When the laminectomy or spinal fusion patient is allowed out of bed, the physician sometimes orders a back brace or corset to support the spinal column until complete healing has occurred. The patient is not allowed to sit for any length of time for several weeks. She must walk or lie down. Standing for long periods is discouraged. The microdiskectomy patient is usually up and about the day after surgery. However, weeks to many months of exercises and physical therapy are necessary before recovery is complete.

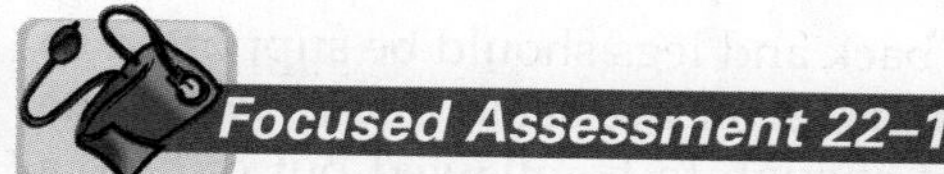

Focused Assessment 22–1

Data Collection Following Spinal Surgery

Immediately postoperatively, assess every 15 to 30 minutes; after first 4 hours, assess every 2 to 4 hours postoperatively. Assess the following areas and compare findings with preoperative data:

SENSATION
- Check extremities for numbness and tingling.
- Check all anatomical surfaces of forearms and hands, upper and lower legs, and feet.

MOVEMENT
- Check for ability to move shoulders, arms, hands, legs, and feet.

MUSCLE STRENGTH
- Check each extremity for weakness by having the patient push against your hands while you apply downward pressure to the extremity.

WOUND
- Assess surgical (and donor) site for drainage, noting amount, color, and characteristics.
- Check carefully for signs of CSF leak at surgical site.
- Determine adequacy of analgesia.

PAIN
- Assess for site of pain, characteristics of the pain, and degree of pain on a scale of 1 to 10, with 10 being the worst pain.
- Reevaluate pain after administering analgesia for effectiveness.
- Monitor respirations and vital signs.

SKIN PRESSURE POINTS
- Check for reddened areas on bony prominences when turning patient.

Key: *CSF,* cerebrospinal fluid.

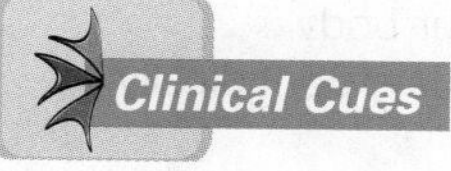

Clinical Cues

At the time of discharge, the instructions about not sitting or standing for any length of time should be reinforced. Patients tend to overdo when they get home and become very fatigued, have more pain, and become discouraged.

An IV opioid may be ordered for pain control the first 24 to 48 hours after surgery. It is usually administered by patient-controlled analgesia pump. Additional boluses for adequate pain control may be needed. Assess frequently for effectiveness of the pain medication. Once fluids are being taken, oral analgesia is started with acetaminophen with codeine, hydrocodone (Vicodin), or oxycodone (Percocet). Muscle relaxers may be given as well.

After spinal surgery a small fracture bedpan is used for toileting if the patient is not to be allowed up. The patient's back is firmly supported while she is resting on the pan. The back and legs should be supported so that all of her body is on the same plane. When the patient is steady enough to be allowed out of bed, a bedside commode, or for the male patient, standing at the bedside is encouraged to promote complete bladder emptying. Provide privacy for toileting activity. If difficulty with voiding occurs, intermittent catheterization or an indwelling catheter will be required.

Interference with bowel function and paralytic ileus may occur after laminectomy or spinal fusion. Observe for nausea, abdominal distention, return of bowel sounds, and constipation. Stool softeners are used to help prevent constipation. Incontinence or difficulty with bowel evacuation may indicate nerve damage and should be reported to the surgeon.

Activity allowed varies according to the underlying pathology and the patient's progress. Be clear about activity orders, whether a brace or corset is to be worn, and whether such is to be put on while lying down, sitting, or standing.

If a bone graft has been performed, the donor site must be assessed regularly and care provided. Pain is usually greater at the donor site than at the spinal fusion site. If the fibula is the donor site, neurovascular assessments of the limb must be performed on a regular schedule as edema can occur.

Depending on the type of spinal surgery performed, many weeks to months are needed for complete recovery. The patient must learn to perform activities without twisting the spine (Patient Teaching 22–2).

Patient Teaching 22–2

Guidelines for the Patient with Low Back Pain or Spinal Surgery

DO

- Bend knees, with back straight, and crouch to lift an item off the floor.
- Carry items close to the center of your body.
- Perform your back exercises twice a day; periodically review the correct way to do them.
- Maintain appropriate body weight; lose weight if overweight.
- Use a lumbar pillow or roll when sitting and particularly when driving for long distances.
- Stop and walk around at least every 2 hours when on long trips.
- Consider how to safely perform a task before starting to do it.

DO NOT

- Lean over without bending the knees.
- Reach to lift items; lift heavy items higher than level of the elbows.
- Stand for long periods.
- Sleep with legs out straight without pillow cushioning under the thighs or between the legs when on the side.
- Bend from the waist to pick up an item.
- Twist to the side to lift things (e.g., groceries or things in the car or trunk).

Key Points

- Head injuries are open or closed and result in concussion, contusion, acceleration-deceleration injury, skull fracture, or tearing of cranial vessels.
- Subdural or epidural hematoma may result from a head injury; epidural hemorrhage is a life-threatening event.
- A significant head injury causes disruption in normal LOC.
- Drainage from the ear or nose should be evaluated to determine the presence of CSF.
- Symptoms of increasing ICP may be subtle or acute. Changes in LOC, in pupil size and action, and in vital signs are some of the signs and symptoms that occur.
- X-rays, CT scans, and MRI are the most common diagnostic tests for initially determining the extent of a head injury.
- Any lesion or extra fluid that begins to take up space in the cranial vault causes an increase in ICP.
- The earliest sign of increased ICP is decreasing LOC.
- Treatment of increased ICP includes maintaining a patent airway, administering diuretic agents to decrease edema, monitoring neurologic signs for increased ICP, regulating temperature, maintaining adequate blood pressure, and instituting nursing measures to prevent further increases in ICP (see Table 21–8, Nursing Care Plan 22–1).
- Neurologic assessment is performed every 15 minutes to 2 hours for the acute patient with injury or surgery to the brain.
- For maintenance of a patent airway, intubation or a tracheostomy and mechanical ventilation may be necessary.
- Early nutritional support is very important for both head injury and spinal cord injury patients.
- The unconscious patient requires care for all basic needs; the eyes must be protected from injury since the blink reflex may be absent.
- Complications of head injury and increased ICP include hydrocephalus and diabetes insipidus.
- The extent of permanent cord damage often cannot be assessed until many days after injury because of edema and resulting pressure on the cord that it causes.
- The degree of neurologic impairment and activities that the patient will still be able to perform depend on the level and extent of the injury (see Table 22–3).
- Autonomic dysreflexia is potentially very dangerous to the patient as it can severely elevate blood pressure.
- Traction provided by Crutchfield or Gardner-Wells tongs, or a halo ring and fixation pins, immobilizes the spine while healing takes place.
- The patient is included in establishing the long-term care plan, and the goal is to promote as much independence as possible.
- Back pain can be caused by muscle strain or herniated or ruptured intervertebral disk.

- Two controllable factors that contribute to back pain for many people include lack of exercise with poor muscle tone and obesity.
- Back pain should be treated conservatively before surgery is considered.
- A herniated lumbar disk can sometimes cause sciatic nerve pain that runs from the buttock down the leg to below the knee.
- Straight-leg raising is a test for a ruptured lumbar disk.
- Treatment depends on whether or not a disk rupture is present and on the severity of the pain and disability.
- Conservative treatment includes rest, gentle exercise, ice or heat, analgesics, and muscle relaxants.
- Surgical procedures include microdiskectomy, laminectomy with or without fusion, percutaneous laser diskectomy, and spinal fusion.
- Postoperative care depends on the type of procedure performed.
- Patients are taught measures to prevent future episodes of back pain.

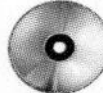

Go to your **Companion CD-ROM** for an Audio Glossary, animations, video clips, and bonus review questions.

evolve Be sure to visit the companion Evolve site at http://evolve.elsevier.com/deWit for interactive NCLEX-PN Exam Style Review Questions, WebLinks, and additional online resources.

NCLEX-PN EXAM STYLE REVIEW QUESTIONS

Choose the best answer(s) for the following questions.

1. A 75-year-old patient is admitted for apparent personality changes, decreased level of consciousness, and irritability. The physician suspects a possible subdural hematoma. A family member asks about the condition. An accurate explanation would be:

1. "It is the presence of bleeding in the brain parenchyma."
2. "Bleeding occurs between the skull and the dura mater."
3. "It is the collection of blood between the brain and the inner surface of the dura mater."
4. "It is the intermittent blockage of circulation in various areas of the brain."

2. The nurse is admitting a patient with a possible periorbital fracture. Which of the following clinical findings would likely confirm the diagnosis? *(Select all that apply.)*

1. Battle's sign
2. Partial blindness
3. Otorrhea
4. Rhinorrhea
5. Swallowing difficulty

3. An appropriate nursing intervention to prevent further increases in intracranial pressure for a patient with head injury would be:

1. securing a patent airway.
2. positioning flat in bed.
3. performing passive range-of-motion exercises.
4. administering large amounts of fluids.

4. The nurse keeps the postcraniotomy patient's neck in midline position and ensures that there is no excessive hip flexion. The rationale for the nurse's action would be:

1. "This position helps restore neutral position of the joints."
2. "This position improves adequate venous drainage."
3. "This position promotes comfort and rest."
4. "This position prevents the formation of blood clots."

5. The nursing assistant is attending to the needs of a patient with head injury who is lethargic and has increased intracranial pressure. Which of the following actions by the nursing assistant indicates a need for further teaching?

1. Stopping the patient from blowing her nose
2. Monitoring blood pressure
3. Dangling the patient on the side of the bed
4. Reporting soaking of the dressings

6. ______________________ refers to the classic signs of increased intracranial pressure, including rising systolic blood pressure, widening pulse pressure, and a full, bounding, slow pulse.

7. The surgeon inserts an intraventricular catheter into the lateral ventricle of a patient with increased intracranial pressure. When asked by a relative regarding the procedure, an accurate response by the nurse would be:

1. "The catheter allows direct visualization of the brain tissue."
2. "The catheter is used to monitor brain waves."
3. "The catheter is used to remove excess fluid inside the brain."
4. "The catheter is used to infuse fluids and medications into the brain."

8. A 40-year-old man with a T4 spinal cord injury suddenly complains of severe headache, increased pulse rate, sweating, and flushing above the level of the spinal cord lesion, and "goose bumps" below the level of injury. Immediate nursing actions should include which of the following? *(Select all that apply.)*

1. Place flat in bed.
2. Identify cause of stimulation.
3. Administer antihypertensives.
4. Provide measures to facilitate bowel movement.
5. Clamp indwelling catheter.

9. Which of the following nursing interventions promotes a soothing environment for optimum care of the patient with increased intracranial pressure?
   1. Provide continual background music.
   2. Provide periods of uninterrupted rest.
   3. Apply cooling blankets.
   4. Maintain constant cool airflow in the room.

10. A 30-year-old male patient is admitted to the emergency department after a motor vehicle accident. On examination, the patient is diagnosed with a T6 spinal cord injury. He has flaccid paralysis, slowed heart rate, low blood pressure, and no bowel sounds. The patient must be developing:
    1. autonomic dysreflexia.
    2. muscle spasms.
    3. spinal shock.
    4. diabetes insipidus.

CRITICAL THINKING ACTIVITIES  *Read each clinical scenario and discuss the questions with your classmates.*

Scenario A

Mary is a 22-year-old college student who has suffered a head injury in an automobile accident. She was healthy prior to her accident. The Emergency Medical Services team brought her to the emergency room. She is stabilized in the ER, cervical spine injury is ruled out, and she is admitted to the neurologic intensive care unit. She is confused and groggy and has leakage of cerebrospinal fluid (CSF) from one ear and irregular respirations.

1. What assessments would you perform?
2. What specific nursing measures would you include in your care plan concerning the leaking CSF?
3. What measures would you take to provide appropriate respiratory care?

Scenario B

Gus Berrini is a 40-year-old truck driver who received a severe spinal injury when he was shot in the back by a hitchhiker. The bullet severed the spinal cord at the sixth thoracic vertebra.

1. What kinds of activities should Mr. Berrini eventually be able to perform?
2. How would you plan his care during the acute stage of his illness so that efforts at rehabilitation might be successful?
3. What other members of the health care team might participate in his care and rehabilitation?

CHAPTER

23 Care of Patients with Disorders of the Brain

evolve http://evolve.elsevier.com/deWit

Objectives

Upon completion of this chapter you should be able to:

Theory

1. Describe the appropriate nursing actions and observations to be carried out for a patient experiencing a seizure.
2. Explain why seizure may be a consequence of a stroke, tumor, or infection in the brain.
3. Compare the subjective and objective findings of thrombotic stroke and intercerebral bleed.
4. Devise a nursing care plan for the patient who has suffered a cerebrovascular accident (CVA, stroke).
5. Discuss nursing actions to assist the patient who has developed a complication after a cerebrovascular accident.
6. Describe subjective and objective findings indicative of a brain tumor.
7. Explain the pathophysiology behind the symptoms of a brain tumor.
8. Diagram the mechanism by which infection in the brain may cause increased intracranial pressure.
9. Recall the signs of increasing intracranial pressure from early to late signs.
10. Compare and contrast symptoms of meningitis and encephalitis.
11. Explain the assessment data that differentiate migraine headaches from cluster headaches.
12. Compare the signs, symptoms, and treatment of trigeminal neuralgia and Bell's palsy.

Clinical Practice

1. Teach a teenage patient recently diagnosed with epilepsy what he needs to know about his disorder and care.
2. Perform neurologic checks on a patient who is admitted with a suspected CVA.
3. Assist with the care of a patient who has had intracranial surgery.
4. Devise a teaching plan for the patient who has suffered a CVA and has right-sided hemiplegia.

Key Terms

Be sure to check out the bonus material on the Companion CD-ROM, including selected audio pronunciations.

agnosia (ăg-NŌ-zhă, p. 572)
aneurysm (ĂN-ūr-ĭ-zĭm, p. 569)
aphasia (ă-FĀ-zhă, p. 572)
apraxia (ă-PRĂK-sē-ă, p. 572)
ataxia (ă-TĂK-sē-ă, p. 588)
aura (ĂW-ră, p. 564)
automatisms (ăw-TŌM-ă-tĭsmz, p. 564)
dysarthria (dĭs-ĂHR-thrē-ă, p. 572)
dysphasia (dĭs-FĀ-zhă, p. 572)
embolus (EM-bō-lus, p. 569)
epilepsy (Ĕ-pĭ-lĕp-sē, p. 563)
homonymous hemianopsia (hō-MŎN-ĭ-mŭs hĕ-mē-ă-NŎP-sē-ă, p. 572)
hydrocephalus (hī-drō-SĔF-ă-lăs, p. 582)
infarct (ĭn-fährkt, p. 568)
nuchal rigidity (NOO-kăl, p. 582)
postictal (PŌST-ĭk-tĕl, p. 565)
ptosis (TŌ-sĭs, p. 587)
scotoma (skō-TŌ-mă, p. 586)
status epilepticus (STĂ-tŭs ĕp-ĭ-LĔP-tĭ-kŭs, p. 565)

SEIZURE DISORDERS AND EPILEPSY

Etiology

Seizures can be symptomatic of a large number of disorders. Brain injury from a stroke, pressure from a brain tumor, infectious diseases with high fever, end-stage renal disease with uremia, toxicity (such as that occurring in eclampsia during pregnancy or in drug poisoning), epilepsy, and tetanus are but a few examples of seizure-producing disorders. **Seizures also can occur any time the brain is deprived of oxygen.**

Seizures may be symptoms of an underlying illness. Metabolic disturbances such as acidosis, electrolyte imbalances, hypoglycemia, hypoxia, and water intoxication may cause seizures. Alcohol or barbiturate withdrawal can cause seizures. In children, a high temperature is a frequent cause of seizures. There are at least 40 types of seizure disorders linked to genetic defects. Epilepsy is present when correcting the metabolic problem does not stop the seizures. Epilepsy affects up to 10 in 1000 people in the United States.

Pathophysiology

Epilepsy is a chronic disturbance of the nervous system characterized by recurrent seizures that are the result of abnormal electrical activity of the brain. Epilepsy is characterized by spontaneous recurring seizures. It is thought that a group of abnormal neurons fire spontaneously. Some unknown stimulus causes the cell membranes to depolarize. The depolarization of the neurons causes abnormal sensory or motor activity and may cause unconsciousness. The neurons involved have a low threshold for excitation. The excitation spreads to surrounding cells, spreading the activity to a small area or throughout the brain. Seizures are classified as *partial* or *generalized* (Box 23–1). Each seizure lasts a few seconds or a few minutes. The abnormal electrical activity generated can be captured by an electroencephalogram (EEG).

Signs and Symptoms

Partial Seizures. Partial seizures are further divided into three subgroups: simple partial seizures, in which consciousness is not impaired but there are other motor, sensory, autonomic, or psychological symptoms; complex partial seizures, in which there is some impairment of consciousness with or without **automatisms** (repetitive, automatic actions such as lip smacking); and partial seizures that become generalized as the seizure continues.

Partial seizures also are called simple or focal seizures and result from an abnormal localized cortical discharge. Partial seizures with complex symptomatology, also called psychomotor or temporal lobe seizures, usually, but not always, originate in the temporal lobe of the brain. Partial seizures can be unilateral, with involvement on only one side of the brain and activity only on one side of the body.

Generalized Seizures. Generalized seizures are bilaterally symmetrical (affecting both sides of the body equally) and do not have a local onset; that is, they do not typically begin in one part of the body. Generalized seizures have symptoms or activity that is bilaterally symmetrical and include absence, myoclonic, clonic, tonic, tonic-clonic, and atonic seizures and infantile spasms (usually caused by increased temperature).

Generalized seizures are characterized by bilateral synchronous electrical discharges in the brain. The whole brain is affected and there is no warning or **aura** (preceding sensation). The patient usually quickly loses consciousness lasting for a few seconds up to several minutes.

The manifestations of epilepsy depend on the area of the brain where the abnormal firing occurs. **Absence or petit mal seizures last only a few seconds. The onset is sudden, with no aura or warning and no postictal symptoms.** Seizures of this type tend to affect children between 5 and 12 years of age and disappear during puberty. There usually is a twitching about the eyes and mouth. The person remains standing or sitting and appears to have had no more than a lapse of attention or a moment of absentmindedness.

Box 23–1 ***International Classification of Epileptic Seizures***

I. Partial seizures
- A. Simple partial seizures
  - 1. With motor signs
    - a. Focal motor without march
    - b. Focal motor with march (jacksonian)
    - c. Versive
    - d. Postural
    - e. Phonatory
  - 2. With somatosensory or special-sensory symptoms
    - a. Somatosensory
    - b. Visual
    - c. Auditory
    - d. Olfactory
    - e. Gustatory
    - f. Vertiginous
  - 3. With autonomic symptoms or signs
  - 4. With psychic symptoms
    - a. Dysphasia
    - b. Dysmnesic
    - c. Cognitive
    - d. Affective
    - e. Illusions
    - f. Structured illusions
- B. Complex partial seizures
  - 1. Simple partial seizures at onset, followed by impairment of consciousness
    - a. With simple partial features
    - b. With automatisms
  - 2. With impairment of consciousness at onset
    - a. With impairment of consciousness only
    - b. With automatisms
- C. Partial seizures evolving to secondarily generalized seizures
  - 1. Simple partial seizures evolving to generalized seizures
  - 2. Complex partial seizures evolving to generalized seizures
  - 3. Simple partial seizures evolving to complex partial seizures evolving to generalized seizures

II. Generalized seizures
- A. Absence seizures
  - 1. Typical absence seizures
    - a. Impairment of consciousness only
    - b. With mild clonic components
    - c. With atonic components
    - d. With tonic components
    - e. With automatisms
    - f. With autonomic components
  - 2. Atypical absence seizures
- B. Myoclonic seizures
- C. Clonic seizures
- D. Tonic seizures
- E. Tonic-clonic seizures
- F. Atonic seizures

Adapted from Holmes, G.L. (1997). Classification of seizures and the epilepsies. In Schachter, S.C. & Schomer, D.L. (Eds.): *The Comprehensive Evaluation and Treatment of Epilepsy.* San Diego, CA: Academic Press. With permission from Elsevier (www.elsevier.com).

With tonic convulsions, there is continued contraction of all muscles and the body becomes rigid. Grand mal or tonic-clonic seizures usually begin with bilateral jerks of the extremities or focal seizure activity. There is loss of consciousness with both tonic and clonic convulsions. The patient may be incontinent during the attack, and there is danger of biting the tongue. In the **postictal** (after a seizure) phase, the person is confused and drowsy.

Atonic or akinetic seizures are characterized by loss of body muscle tone that results in nodding of the head, weakness of the knees, or total collapse and falling ("drop attacks"). The person usually remains conscious during the attack.

The third major group, unclassified seizures, simply means that not enough data have been obtained to determine which type of seizure the patient is experiencing.

The fourth designation, status epilepticus, indicates prolonged partial or generalized seizure without recovery between attacks. **Status epilepticus** is a grave condition in which there is a rapid, unrelenting series of convulsive seizures without intervening periods of consciousness, and an absence of respiration. **Irreversible brain damage can occur if the seizures are not controlled.**

In classifying epileptic seizures on the basis of origin, seizures are grouped as either idiopathic or symptomatic. Idiopathic epilepsy has no known cause. Symptomatic epilepsy has a known physical cause (e.g., brain tumor, injury to the head at birth, a wound or blow to the head, toxicity, or an endocrine disorder).

Diagnosis

Diagnosis of epilepsy is based on the history and the actual signs and symptoms observed during a seizure. A thorough physical examination and tests for underlying disease are ordered based on the history and physical findings. Confirmation of the diagnosis is by EEG and magnetic resonance imaging (MRI). These tests help locate the site, or locus, and possibly the cause of the seizures.

Treatment

When the cause of seizures is known, as in cases of high fever or drug toxicity, medical treatment is aimed at controlling or eliminating whatever is responsible for the seizures. However, when there are recurrent seizures, as in epilepsy, the condition usually is managed with anticonvulsant drug therapy.

The major antiepileptic drugs are presented in Box 23–2. Patient education is extremely important, be-

Box 23–2 *Medications Commonly Used for Seizure Control*

DRUGS FOR GENERALIZED TONIC-CLONIC AND PARTIAL SEIZURES

- Phenytoin (Dilantin)
- Fosphenytoin (Cerebyx)
- Carbamazepine (Tegretol)
- Primidone (Mysoline)
- Lamotrigine (Lamictal)
- Phenobarbital
- Felbamate (Felbatol)
- Gabapentin (Neurontin)
- Levetiracetam (Keppra)
- Oxcarbazepine (Trileptal)
- Tiagabine (Gabitril)
- Topiramate (Topamax)
- Valproic acid (Depakene)
- Zonisamide (Zonegran)
- Vigabatrin (Sabril)

DRUGS FOR ABSENCE, AKINETIC, AND MYOCLONIC SEIZURES

- Valproic acid (Depakene)
- Ethosuximide (Zarontin)
- Clonazepam (Klonopin)
- Divalproex (Depakote)
- Phenobarbital

GENERAL NURSING IMPLICATIONS

- Educate patient about the importance of taking the drug exactly as it is prescribed.
- All these drugs cause some degree of sedation, drowsiness, and lethargy. Warn about driving or operating machinery when these effects are significant. Advise not to drink alcohol or use other central nervous system depressants.
- The patient should not stop taking an anticonvulsant abruptly without consulting the physician.
- Check interactions with other drugs before administering any of these drugs. Interaction with anticoagulants, oral contraceptives, digoxin, aspirin, certain antibiotics, antacids, folic acid, and other drugs are significant. Some anticonvulsant drugs interact with each other (e.g., phenobarbital).
- Periodic blood work, every 1 to 3 months, should be done when taking an anticonvulsant.
- Dosages of each drug are based on therapeutic blood level of the drug.
- Anticonvulsants have a narrow therapeutic range; toxicity occurs if too much of the drug is taken.
- Patient should be under the close supervision of the health care provider.
- All of the anticonvulsant drugs can produce some unpleasant side effects, such as fever and leukopenia and, in the case of phenytoin, gingival hyperplasia and rash.
- Physical dependence can become a problem for patients taking either phenobarbital or primidone, which is largely converted to phenobarbital in the bloodstream.
- Toxic side effects such as ataxia, drowsiness, nausea, sedation, and dizziness are not uncommon.

cause the patient will need to report any untoward effects to the physician or nurse clinician so the dosage can be adjusted or the drug changed. Most anticonvulsant drugs cause some grogginess and fatigue.

Surgical Treatment. Surgical treatment of epilepsy is an alternative for some persons who have the disorder. The procedures involve removing the epileptic focus or preventing the spread of epileptic activity by sectioning the corpus callosum. A temporal lobe resection may eliminate seizures in more than 70% of patients with temporal lobe seizures. For patients with extensive damage in one side of the brain that causes intractable seizures, a hemispherectomy may be performed. Surgeries are not without danger and are reserved for those patients whose seizures cannot be managed by medical treatment and in whom the focus of the seizures is accessible.

A NeuroCybernetic Prosthesis (vagal nerve stimulator) can be implanted in the chest with a wire tunneled to stimulate the vagus nerve. It acts similar to a pacemaker and provides a tiny stimulus every 5 minutes that stimulates the brain to interrupt seizures (Rielo, 2006).

Biofeedback techniques are geared to teaching the patient to maintain a certain brain-wave frequency that isn't susceptible to seizure activity.

Treatment of status epilepticus depends on its cause. Many times patients who are known to have epilepsy arrive in the emergency room with status epilepticus because, for one reason or another, they stopped taking the medication that controls their seizures. Treatment in this instance would involve administering diazepam, phenytoin, or phenobarbital in a dose sufficiently high to stop the seizures. Rectal diazepam has been approved by the Food and Drug Administration (FDA) in a system called Diastat AcuDial. It can be used at home by nonprofessional caregivers, and clinical studies have shown that the system resolved seizures in 85% of patients (Waknine, 2005).

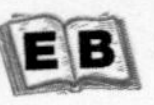

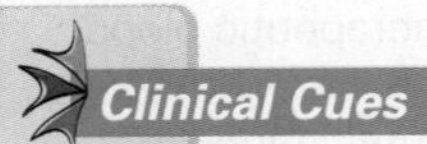

When phenytoin is ordered to be administered intravenously (IV), mix it in 0.9% saline solution and flush the line before and after administration if a glucose IV solution is running. Glucose is incompatible with phenytoin. Never administer IV phenytoin faster than 50 mg/min because of the risk of cardiac dysrhythmia. For patients with a history of heart problems, administer the solution no faster than 25 mg/min.

Uncontrolled seizures secondary to hypoglycemia (as in improperly controlled diabetes mellitus) can be relieved by IV administration of 50% dextrose. If the unrelenting seizures are caused by chronic alcoholism or withdrawal, treatment consists of IV administration of thiamine. Although these kinds of seizures are known as status epilepticus, they should not be confused with chronic epileptic seizures.

NURSING MANAGEMENT

Assessment (Data Collection)

Patients with a known seizure problem usually are treated on an outpatient basis. However, these patients also are seen in hospitals or long-term care facilities and must be assessed carefully to provide optimal safety and care. Significant history information includes the kind of seizures they experience, whether they have any sensation just before the appearance of clinically observable signs, what medications they are taking, and what measures are known to be helpful either to prevent a seizure or to assist while they are having a seizure and afterward. Assessment should include any factors that could have triggered the seizure (e.g., hyperventilation, bright lights [photosensitivity], alcohol and other drugs, fluid and electrolyte imbalances, lack of sleep, and emotional stress). Focused Assessment 23–1 lists signs to be observed during a seizure.

When caring for a patient who is likely to experience a seizure during an acute illness, periodically observe the patient for tremors, unexplained sensory

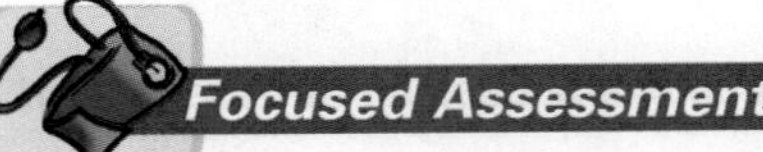

Observations to Make During a Seizure

Observe as much of the following as possible and document your findings.

- Time the seizure began and the time it ended
- What the patient was doing just before the seizure (was the patient picking at clothing?)
- Where in the body the seizure began, what parts of the body are involved
- Which way eyes are moving, whether they constrict or dilate, deviate to the right or the left, or roll upward
- Which side the head turns toward
- Whether the patient cries out or screams as the seizure begins
- Whether there is evidence of repetitive movements: lip smacking, chewing, grimacing, tapping, or "pill rolling"
- Whether movements are bilateral and symmetrical
- Incontinence of urine or stool, vomiting, frothing at the mouth, or bleeding
- Whether the patient becomes apneic or cyanotic
- Changes in skin color or profuse perspiration

Postictal assessment, after a patent airway is ensured, includes determining:

- Length of time before regaining awareness
- Presence of lethargy or confusion
- Presence of headache
- Presence of speech impairment
- Presence of muscle soreness
- Whether there was an aura before the seizure began
- Effects of the seizure on the patient's vital signs

or motor changes, mental changes that indicate confusion or disorientation, and restless or agitated behavior. **In many cases, a change in the neurologic status of a patient can signal the possibility that a seizure might occur.**

Nursing Diagnosis, Planning, and Implementation

The main nursing diagnosis for the patient who experiences seizures is "Risk for injury related to seizure activity." Expected outcomes are written for the individual patient and the type of seizure disorder, its possible triggers, and its manifestations.

Nursing care of patients with epileptic seizures is concerned with immediate care during and after a seizure and long-term management and control of seizures and their psychosocial implications. Witnessing a seizure for the first time can be a frightening experience. The nurse's first responsibility is to stay calm, remain with the patient, and call for assistance.

The environment of a patient at risk for seizure should be made as safe as possible. If the patient is very likely to have seizures, the side rails and headboard of the bed are padded. Never try to pry open the patient's mouth or insert something into it once the jaw is clamping down as teeth may be broken and the airway may be obstructed.

If a seizure comes on without warning and the patient drops to the ground, leave him wherever he is lying. If he is on a hard surface, his head should be protected from injury by placing a rolled blanket or coat under it. The head should be turned to the side, if possible, to prevent aspiration. Do not attempt to restrain the patient's movements or to move him to a bed or chair during the seizure. If supplemental oxygen is near, it should be administered if possible. Call for help and provide privacy if possible. When the seizure is over, turn the patient to the side, and suction the airway if needed. Check oxygen saturation with a pulse oximeter. Check the glucose level, if possible, and assess for injuries. Stay with him until he is completely conscious. When consciousness is regained, reorient and reassure him. The patient should be allowed to rest or sleep after the seizure. Thoroughly document the event in the medical record with time, duration of the seizure, and observations of the seizure activity and any aura that occurred prior to its start.

The long-term management of epileptic seizures is primarily focused on providing the patient with the information and support he needs to care for himself and avoid recurring and debilitating seizures. Psychosocial support is necessary to encourage the patient to talk about his fears and concerns. Lifestyle changes will have to be made if he is not permitted to drive. Most states allow resumption of driving when a patient has been seizure free for 1 year. A referral to the local epilepsy society for connection with a support group can be very helpful for both the patient and his family.

Most individuals who suffer from epileptic seizures are perfectly normal between seizures; they are not mentally retarded and are quite capable of becoming contributing members of our society if only they are given the chance to prove their worth.

Patient Education

Self-care for the epileptic patient requires that he understand the nature of his disorder, the purpose of his prescribed medications, their side effects, and the signs of toxicity that should be reported to the physician. He must understand the necessity for compliance with the prescribed regimen to avoid recurrent seizures. He will need assistance in developing coping mechanisms to deal with the psychosocial impact of having epilepsy.

The teaching plan should also include information about possible seizure-triggering mechanisms and the importance of avoiding them whenever possible. Alcohol is especially contraindicated for the patient with seizures, as it interferes with the effectiveness of the medications, causes excessive sedation, and may trigger seizures. Fatigue also can make the patient more prone to seizure activity. He must be helped to plan for adequate rest each day.

The patient is taught not to swim or participate alone in activities that could have dangerous effects if he had a seizure and was alone. Women need to know that menstruation puts additional stress on the body, and they are more prone to seizures during this period each month. People with epilepsy should wear a Medic Alert bracelet or necklace and carry a list of the medications they are taking and names and phone numbers of their physician and others to be notified in an emergency.

? *Think Critically About . . .* What would you teach a 22-year-old man who has just been diagnosed with grand mal seizures regarding safety?

Evaluation

Evaluation is based on whether the expected outcomes are being achieved. This probably will include whether the patient is seizure free, or whether the number of seizures has decreased. Patient compliance with the medication regimen and avoidance of triggers for seizure activity is evaluated as well. Patient teaching may need to be reinforced. If progress toward the achievement of outcomes is not occurring, the plan must be revised.

TRANSIENT ISCHEMIC ATTACK

Many patients with a narrowing of the lumen of the arteries supplying the brain experience what are called *transient ischemic attacks* (TIAs). TIAs can be caused by small emboli or a brain blood vessel rupture. Recreational drugs that constrict vessels are another cause of TIAs. Although they usually are not recognized as such, TIAs often are warnings that a more serious neurologic event may occur. During the attack, the person may feel a sudden weakness or numbness on one side of the body, slurring of speech or inability to talk, visual disturbances such as blindness or double vision, confusion, diminished coordination or ability to balance, and a headache. Symptoms are similar to those of a stroke. **These symptoms last from a few minutes to 24 hours and completely resolve without residual deficits.** Unless the person knows the signs of a TIA and their importance, he will not seek medical treatment and will not further investigate the cause. About 30% of those individuals who experience a TIA will have a complete stroke within a year.

If the patient seeks medical assistance, a thorough history of the event, how it began, the symptoms experienced, and how long it lasted is essential. If carotid obstruction is suspected, carotid duplex ultrasound studies are done to determine if obstruction in the carotid arteries is preventing normal blood flow from reaching the brain. Multiple tests may be performed if carotid occlusion is ruled out, including blood tests, MRI, and EEG. If there is greater than 60% occlusion, either an angioplasty procedure with stent implantation or a carotid endarterectomy is considered. If occlusion from plaque obstruction is less than 60%, medical treatment with diet and lifestyle modification and medication to prevent platelet aggregation (i.e., aspirin, clopidogrel [Plavix], dipyridamole [Persantine]) is prescribed.

CEREBROVASCULAR ACCIDENT (STROKE, BRAIN ATTACK)

Etiology

There are more than 700,000 first and repeat strokes in the United States each year. Stroke is the leading cause of disability and the third leading cause of death. The incidence is about 19% higher in males than in females. About 25% of cases occur in people younger than age 65 (American Heart Association, 2007). An increase in public education about the risk factors and signs of stroke could result in lessened disability and death from stroke (Cultural Cues 23–1). Health Promotion Points 23–1 lists the risk factors for stroke.

Control of high blood pressure, quitting cigarette smoking, decreasing intake of cholesterol and controlling blood lipids, maintaining a normal blood sugar level, avoiding excessive alcohol intake, getting sufficient exercise, avoiding obesity, and living a lifestyle that helps prevent heart disease can help reduce the risk of stroke. Atherosclerosis is a major cause of stroke as it can predispose to thrombus formation in the brain vessels or plaque in other arteries that can break off and become emboli.

Pathophysiology

A cerebrovascular accident (CVA) is the result of an interruption of blood flow to a specific area of the brain (i.e., *cerebral ischemia*) (Health Promotion Points 23–2). Ischemia of cells directly causes cellular *necrosis* (death) and **infarct** (area of tissue that has become necrotic from lack of blood supply). Ischemia can be caused by:

- Cerebral thrombosis (formation of a blood clot in a cerebral artery)

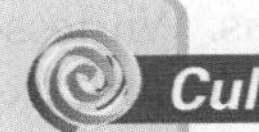

Cultural Cues 23–1

Greater Incidence of Stroke in African Americans and Hispanic Americans

It is known that African Americans have about a 60% greater incidence of stroke than whites. A study at the University of Michigan found that Hispanic Americans have a far greater chance of suffering a stroke than non-Hispanic whites. It is thought that untreated hypertension may be the risk factor involved (Morgenstern et al., 2004).

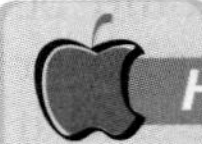

Health Promotion Points 23–1

Risk Factors for Stroke

Educate all patients about the risk factors for stroke and encourage measures to alter those factors that can be changed.

RISK FACTORS THAT CAN BE TREATED

- Cigarette smoking
- Using cocaine or other recreational drugs
- Drinking more than TWO drinks per day
- Heart disease (especially atrial fibrillation)
- Diabetes
- High blood pressure
- High cholesterol
- Sedentary lifestyle
- High red blood cell count (polycythemia)
- Transient ischemic attacks (TIAs)
- Use of oral contraceptives or hormone replacement therapy

RISK FACTORS THAT CANNOT BE CHANGED

- Age over 65
- Asymptomatic carotid bruit (indicates atherosclerosis, which increases stroke risk; a bruit is a swishing sound in an artery)
- Diabetes mellitus
- Heredity (family history of stroke increases individual risk)
- Prior stroke
- Race (African Americans have a 60% higher risk rate)
- Sex (incidence is 30% higher in men)

- An **embolus** (a traveling clot, fat, bacteria, or tissue debris that lodges in a vessel, occluding it)
- Intercerebral hemorrhage (the blood vessel ruptures and leaks blood into brain tissue or an aneurysm or arteriovenous malformation in the brain leaks or ruptures)
- Pressure on a blood vessel

Figure 23–1 shows the events causing stroke (CVA).

The carotid arteries supply a major portion of the blood that goes to the brain (Figure 23–2). **If plaque forms in these arteries as a result of atherosclerosis, the person is at risk for a stroke as blood supply to the brain is diminished or stopped.** Less common causes of stroke are arterial spasms, compression of cerebral vessels by a tumor, local edema, rupture of a cerebral aneurysm, or another disorder.

Think Critically About . . . How many risk factors for stroke are present for each member of your family?

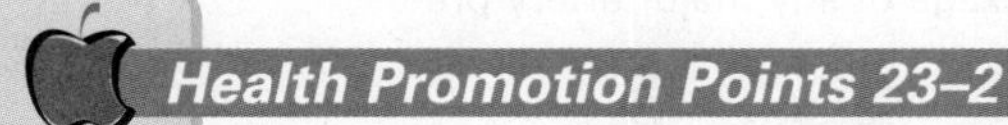

Health Promotion Points 23–2

Dangers of Cocaine or Methamphetamine Use

Caution people about the dangers of using cocaine or methamphetamine. Both of these drugs can cause vasoconstriction and brain ischemia. Cocaine may also cause hemorrhage. Using these drugs causes a fivefold increase in the incidence of stroke. The incidence of this type of stroke has greatly increased in young adults (Vega, 2007).

EB

Cerebral Aneurysm and Arteriovenous Malformation. Structures that can cause an intercerebral hemorrhage are an aneurysm and an arteriovenous malformation. An **aneurysm** is an abnormal ballooning of an artery wall (Figure 23–3). It may be congenital or caused by a weakening of the artery wall from chronic hypertension. Rupture of a brain aneurysm causes bleeding into the subarachnoid space or into the ventricles. An arteriovenous malformation (AVM) is a congenital abnormality and is a tangled mass of malformed, thin-walled, dilated vessels that form an abnormal communication between the arterial and venous systems. An AVM can leak, causing an intracerebral hemorrhage. Vasospasm often occurs after intercerebral bleeding, leading to further ischemia of the brain tissue and more neurologic impairment. Resultant deficits are the same as for other kinds of strokes.

Subarachnoid hemorrhage, which refers to bleeding in the brain below the arachnoid, often causes rapid onset of neurologic deficit and loss of consciousness. A leaking cerebral aneurysm may cause a severe headache. However, sometimes bleeding is slower, producing a more gradual progression of headache, neck stiffness, and other neurologic signs, such as blurred vision.

Stroke Prevention

Many strokes can be prevented by either surgical procedures or medical management of diseases that predispose a person to a CVA. **Surgery for the prevention of a major stroke is reserved for carotid arteries that are 70% to 99% occluded and involves the removal of plaque deposited on the inner wall of the carotid ar-**

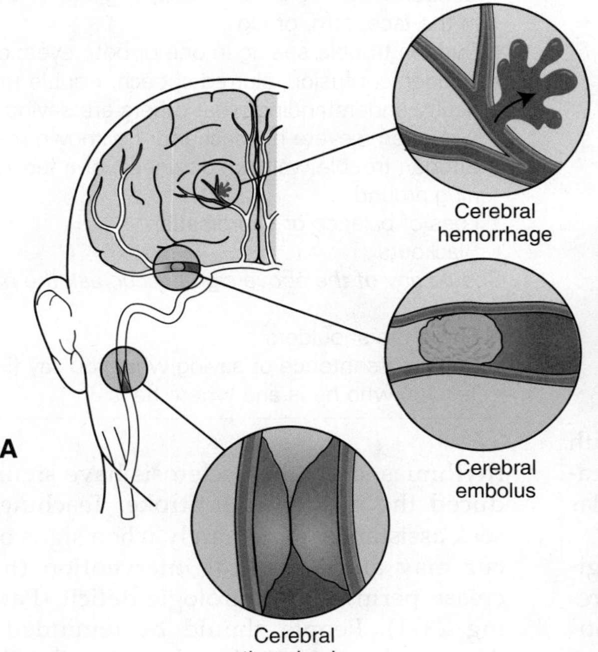

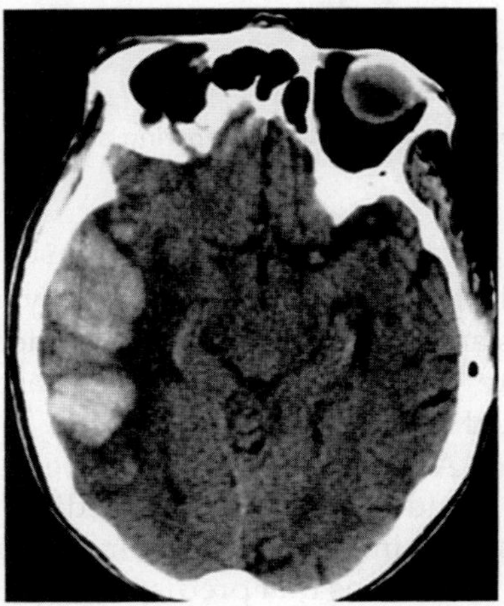

FIGURE **23–1** **A,** Events causing stroke. **B,** Magnetic resonance imaging showing hemorrhagic stroke in the left cerebrum.

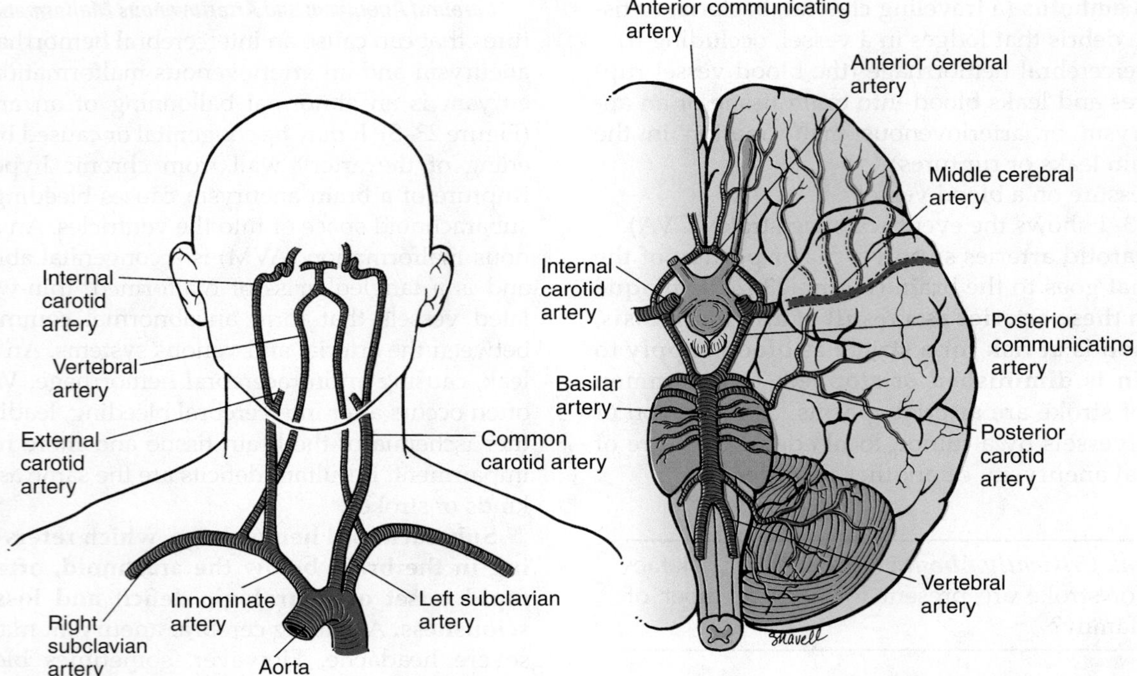

FIGURE 23–2 Major arteries supplying blood to the brain. Blockage of any major artery precipitates a cerebrovascular accident (CVA).

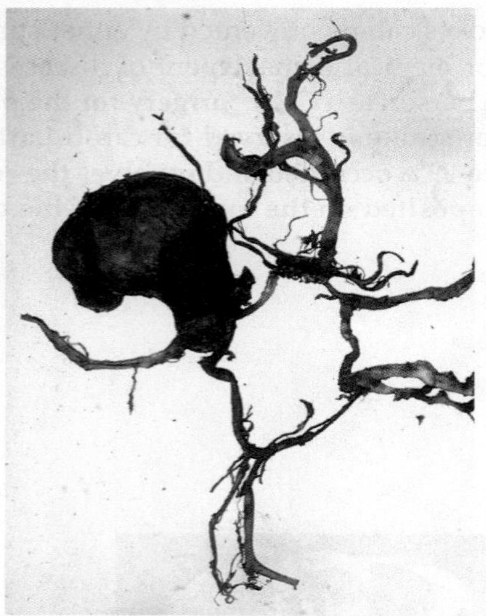

FIGURE 23–3 Dissected circle of Willis showing a large cerebral aneurysm.

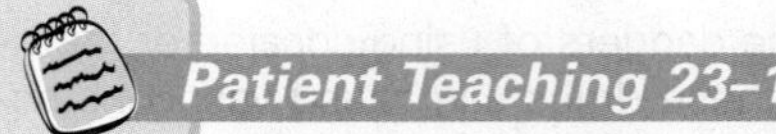

Patient Teaching 23–1

Warning Signs of Stroke

Teach people to seek immediate medical attention in an emergency room if any of the following warning signs of stroke appears:

- Sudden weakness, numbness, tingling, or loss of feeling in the face, arm, or leg
- Sudden trouble seeing in one or both eyes; double vision
- Sudden confusion, slurred speech, trouble talking, or difficulty understanding what others are saying
- A sudden, severe headache for no known reason
- Sudden trouble walking, dizziness, or a feeling of spinning around
- Loss of balance or coordination
- Blackouts

Should any of the above signs occur, ask the person to:

- Smile
- Shrug the shoulders
- Repeat a sentence or saying what you say first
- Tell you who he is and where he is

tery (carotid endarterectomy). An angioplasty with stent placement is an option for opening occluded carotid arteries. Care for patients undergoing vascular surgery is presented in Chapter 20.

Aneurysms and AVMs can sometimes be surgically corrected if found before rupture. Medical preventive measures are aimed at eliminating or managing some of the conditions that predispose a person to stroke. Control of hypertension and the effective treatment of rheumatic heart disease, cardiac dysrhythmias, and atherosclerosis have significantly reduced the incidence of stroke. Teaching people to seek assistance immediately when signs of stroke occur may allow medical intervention that will decrease permanent neurologic deficit (Patient Teaching 23–1). People should be reminded about the danger of cocaine-induced stroke. Cocaine use can greatly increase blood pressure, causing a brain vessel to rupture.

Table 23–1 Medications Commonly Used for Patients after a CVA

DRUG	ACTION	NURSING IMPLICATIONS	PATIENT TEACHING
t-PA (alteplase; tissue plasminogen activator)	Converts fibrin to plasminogen, causing lysis of thrombus or embolus of CVA	Frequent VS; monitor for dysrhythmias; frequent neurologic checks; assess for bleeding until 24 hr after infusion. Monitor for hypersensitivity; monitor clotting/bleeding studies. Do not give concurrently with anticoagulants, antiplatelet aggregation drugs, or NSAIDs.	Explain that the intermittent IV infusion is for the purpose of breaking up the clot stopping blood flow to part of the brain.
Dipyridamole (Persantine; Aggrenox with aspirin)	Decreases platelet aggregation by inhibiting the enzyme phosphodiesterase	Monitor VS and for orthostatic hypotension.	Must be taken continuously in evenly spaced doses as directed. Report dizziness; rise slowly from a supine or seated position and stand for a couple of minutes before walking. Do not use alcohol or OTC medications without prescriber's knowledge.
Clopidogrel (Plavix)	Inhibits platelet aggregation	Monitor blood studies: CBC, PT, and cholesterol. Watch for signs of leukopenia. Administer with food. Stop drug 3–7 days before surgery. Drug is very expensive ($3+ a tablet)	Ask to report diarrhea, skin rash, bleeding, excessive bruising, chills, fever, sore throat. Advise all health care workers that drug is being taken.
Aspirin (Ecotrin)	Decreases platelet aggregation	Administer with food; observe for signs of intestinal bleeding, tinnitus. Monitor blood count and liver enzymes.	Instruct to take with a full glass of water and when in an upright position. Ask to report any blood in stool, bleeding gums, nose bleeds, or excessive bruising. Report ringing in the ears or skin rash. Caution not to crush the pill. Do not take OTC products containing aspirin or salicylic acid.
Phenytoin (Dilantin)	Alters ion transport, inhibiting spread of seizure activity to motor cortex	Assess for skin rash; monitor drug levels, CBC; observe for respiratory depression. Shake suspension well; dilute before giving via feeding tube. Flush IV line with NS before and after administering slowly by IV piggyback. May cause Stevens-Johnson syndrome.	Teach that PO doses should be taken with meals; urine may turn pink; not to stop taking drug abruptly; take as directed; brush teeth and floss thoroughly and regularly, and visit dentist every 3–6 mo; do not use alcohol. Do not use antacids within 2 hr of the drug. Adjust to drug before operating machinery or performing hazardous activities.
Nimodipine (Nimotop)	Inhibits calcium ion flux across cellular membrane; decreases or prevents cerebral vasospasm	Frequent neurologic assessment and VS; monitor liver enzymes; assess BP and apical pulse immediately prior to administration. Hold if systolic BP is <90 mm Hg. Monitor for hypotension.	Advise that the drug may cause hypotension and dizziness with movement.

Key: *BP,* blood pressure; *CBC,* complete blood count; *CVA,* cerebrovascular accident; *IV,* intravenous; *NS,* normal saline; *NSAIDs,* nonsteroidal anti-inflammatory drugs; *OTC,* over the counter; *PO,* oral; *PT,* prothrombin time; *t-PA,* tissue plasminogen activator; *VS,* vital signs.
See Chapter 20 for information on warfarin (Coumadin) given when atrial fibrillation is present.

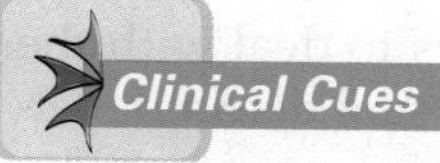

Valve disorders and arrhythmias such as atrial fibrillation predispose to stroke from emboli. Emboli form in the chambers of the heart when blood flow is abnormal and can be ejected into the cerebral circulation.

Medications that reduce platelet aggregation and decrease the chance of thrombosis often are used. Low-dose enteric-coated aspirin, dipyridamole (Persantine), clopidogrel (Plavix), or ticlopidine (Ticlid) is prescribed for patients who have TIAs or to prevent the recurrence of stroke from thrombosis (Table 23–1).

A combination of two inflammatory marker blood tests is showing promise in predicting which middle-aged people are at risk of a stroke. Researchers reported that C-reactive protein and lipoprotein-associated phospholipase A_2 (LP PLA_2) were higher in those who later had an ischemic stroke than in those who did not have a stroke (Baldwin, 2006).

Cerebral ischemia caused by thrombosis causes signs that progress slowly. Thrombosis develops in an area of the vessel where there is atherosclerotic plaque.

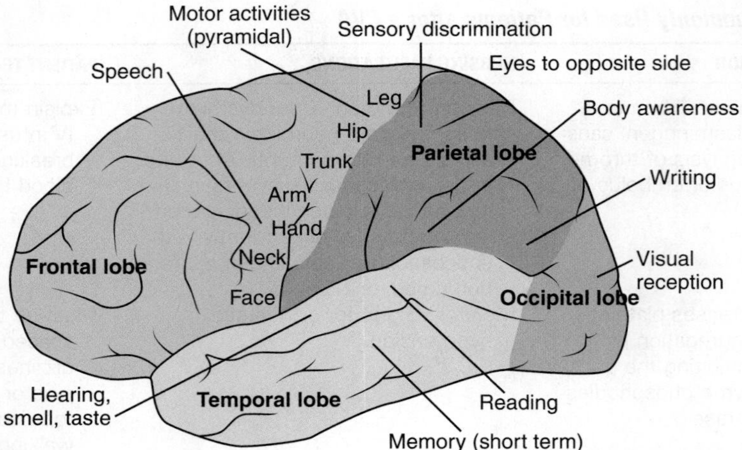

FIGURE **23–4** Each area of the brain controls a particular activity.

Lodging of an embolus in a major cerebral vessel causes sudden neurologic deficit. Emboli most often are the result of heart disease and resultant atrial fibrillation, a cardiac dysrhythmia.

Signs and Symptoms

The neurologic effects of stroke can range from mild motor disturbances to profound coma. Figure 23–4 shows selected control zones of the brain and motor and sensory functions likely to be affected by a stroke.

Signs and symptoms will depend on the type of event that has caused the stroke and the location of the clot or bleed. There may be weakness **(hemiparesis),** inability to speak or understand **(aphasia),** difficulty with vision, loss of balance or poor coordination, decreased level of consciousness, and confusion. Incontinence may occur. Bleeding into the brain or edema around necrotic tissue causes intracranial pressure (ICP) to increase (see Chapter 22 regarding increasing ICP).

Motor function deficits affect mobility, respiratory function, swallowing and speech, gag reflex, and self-care abilities. Because the pyramidal pathways cross at the level of the medulla, injury to brain cells in the right hemisphere affects the left side of the body and damage to cells in the left hemisphere affects the right side of the body. There may be **hemiplegia** (one-sided paralysis) or hemiparesis. Muscle tone is usually flaccid at first, and then there may be spasticity and hyperreflexia. Keeping the body parts in good alignment to prevent contractures is very important.

Language disorders involve expression and comprehension of both written and spoken words. Aphasia or **dysphasia** (minimal speech activity) or a mixed type of aphasia may occur (see Chapter 21). Many stroke patients experience **dysarthria** (difficulty in speaking) due to lack of muscular control of the tongue. A speech therapist works with the patient to improve speech capability. There are computer software programs for rehabilitation of the aphasic patient that have been beneficial to many.

Emotional responses may be exaggerated after a stroke, and may be unpredictable. Many stroke patients tend to cry easily, and they find this embarrassing. The frustration of trying to perform a function that has always been easy before the stroke may cause the patient to cry. Alternatively, the patient may display an angry emotional outburst, and sometimes foul language.

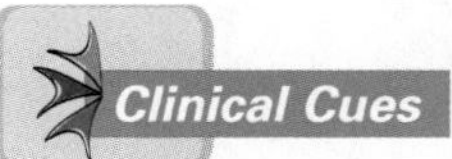

Because of the insult to the nervous tissue, fatigue is another problem for the stroke patient. When working with the patient to relearn walking, dressing, or other activities, keep the session short and allow for adequate rest periods between activities.

Memory and judgment may be affected by the stroke. The ability to learn may be affected, which makes relearning activities to promote independence slow. A great deal of patience and encouragement is needed from the staff working with the patient.

Spatial-perceptual deficits may cause the patient to totally neglect input from the affected side of the body. He must be taught to attend to the body parts on that side of the body in order to protect them from injury. **Homonymous hemianopsia** (blindness in part of the visual field of both eyes) adds to the spatial-perceptual problems by making it difficult to judge distances (Figure 23–5). The patient is taught ways to deal with the problems of the particular type of visual defect developed. **Agnosia** (inability to recognize an object by sight, touch, or hearing) makes it difficult to do ordinary tasks. **Apraxia** (the inability to carry out learned sequential movements on command) adds to the difficulty in regaining independence.

Bladder and bowel incontinence are often temporary after a stroke. Constipation does occur because of immobility, weakened abdominal muscles, dehydration, and diminished response to the defecation reflex. The inability to express needs and difficulty in managing clothing

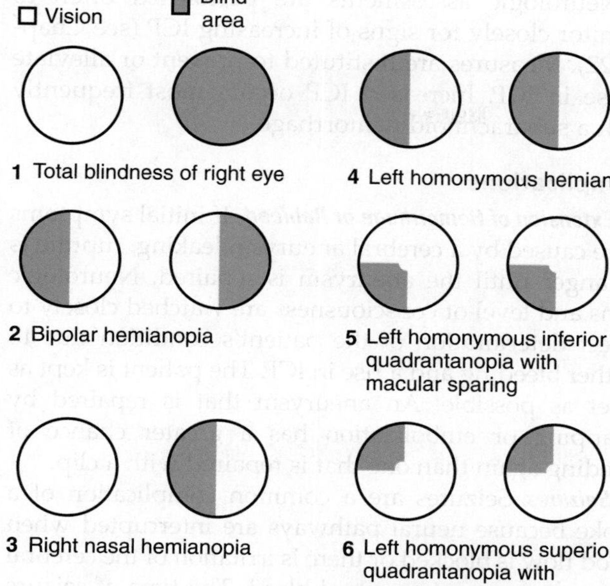

FIGURE 23–5 Homonymous hemianopia: visual field defects that can occur after a stroke.

contributes to bladder and bowel incontinence and constipation. With time, these problems can be overcome.

Diagnosis

In addition to a complete physical and neurologic examination, the physician may order a computed tomography (CT) scan, a cerebral angiogram, or MRI to determine the specific cause of the stroke and rule out a different neurologic problem. An EEG is performed; brain scans or transcranial Doppler flow studies and carotid artery Doppler studies may be ordered. Testing for blood levels of glutamate, which will increase and damage brain tissue during a progressive ischemic stroke, may alert physicians to patients whose condition is likely to rapidly deteriorate.

Treatment

Immediately after a person is suspected of having suffered a stroke, it is especially important to maintain an open airway. If breathing difficulty is present, all constricting clothing around his neck should be removed, and the patient should be turned to one side to prevent aspiration of saliva and obstruction of the air passages. When outside of the hospital, no attempt should be made to move the person until an ambulance has arrived. Reassure the patient regardless of whether or not he is able to respond. If he is conscious, elevate the head slightly to reduce ICP.

Once under medical care, if breathing is impaired or the patient is comatose, an artificial airway is inserted to maintain a patent airway, and the patient may be mechanically ventilated. Hypovolemia is treated with fluids, and hypertension of greater than 220/130 mm Hg will be treated. Vital signs may be unstable. Two IV lines for drug and fluid access are inserted, and nor-

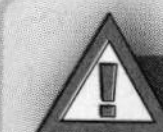

Safety Alert 23–1

Cranberry Juice Interaction

The consumption of cranberry juice while taking warfarin (Coumadin) can produce an interaction that increases the serum level of the drug, extending clotting time. Patients who drink cranberry juice should consult their physicians. Off-and-on intake of cranberry juice will affect the prothrombin time and INR.

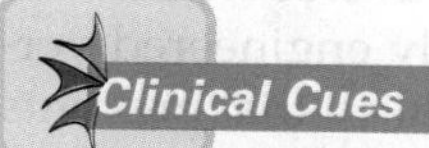

Clinical Cues

There is a fine line between keeping blood pressure high enough to perfuse the brain when an obstruction is present and keeping it low enough to prevent vessel rupture or increased bleeding from a rupture that has occurred.

mal saline is administered. Electrolytes are assessed frequently to prevent imbalances. If the temperature is elevated and rising, a hypothermia blanket may be used to keep the temperature down.

Once the specific cause of the stroke has been determined, the physician is able to plan a more effective regimen of care. Systemic tissue plasminogen activator (t-PA) is used to dissolve clots and emboli in nonhemorrhagic stroke. It must be administered within 3 hours of the onset of symptoms, with the greatest effect occurring if it is administered within 90 minutes (Hacke et al., 2004). The drug is effective in about 1 of 8 patients treated with it. A procedure undergoing clinical trial administers t-PA directly to the clot via a catheter positioned during angiography. Results have been promising. Platelet inhibitors and anticoagulants may be given to prevent further clot formation. If t-PA has been given, no anticoagulants or antiplatelet aggregation drugs are given for 24 hours (Safety Alert 23–1). **The drug is *not* administered to anyone with a known risk of bleeding or who has had an intercerebral bleed.** Heparin infusion is no longer used for thrombotic stroke as it has not proven to be very effective and can cause dangerous bleeding. Antihypertensive drugs are ordered as appropriate. Nimodipine or nifedipine may be given to decrease arterial spasm if the stroke is from subarachnoid hemorrhage. Testing of new drugs continues in an effort to find a way to decrease the resultant damage from a stroke. Another neuroprotective drug being tested—citicoline, which appears to limit the size of the stroke, speed recovery, and improve the victim's mental functioning—is showing promise (Castillo, 2007).

EB

A study at the University of California at Los Angeles (UCLA) is using "Fast-Mag," a twice-normal amount of magnesium sulfate, in the blood via infusion. It is believed that the chemical can slow the process that kills cells after a stroke. So far the study is showing success when administered within 2 hours of onset of symptoms (UCLA Stroke Center, 2005). A recombinant human interleukin-1 receptor antagonist has been shown to be effective in patients with acute stroke symptoms in reducing the amount of injury and residual deficits. Research is continuing to see if these results can be reproduced in larger studies. Use of a natural growth factor, neuregulin-1, that protects brain cells from the damage caused by stroke is also under study. The biggest benefit of neuregulin-1 is that its therapeutic window is much longer than t-PA and it can be administered up to 13 hours after the onset of the stroke. This drug has shown no adverse side effects to date. Desmoteplase is a genetically engineered version of a protein in a vampire bat's saliva that prevents clotting. The drug can break down a clot without affecting the coagulation system, thereby decreasing the risk of intracerebral bleeding. It works when given within 9 hours of a stroke and has been given fast-track status by the FDA. Researchers are also studying recombinant activated factor VII. It slowed hematoma growth and reduced mortality among 400 patients who suffered an intercerebral hemorrhage (Reddrop et al., 2005). Further studies are in progress.

Surgical Procedures. About one third of all strokes can be traced to obstruction of any one of the four arteries in the neck that supply blood to the brain. These arteries are generally accessible, so the surgeon can open the artery and remove the obstruction, which is usually from plaque buildup. The vessel wall is then sutured or a Dacron patch is sewn at the incision, leaving the vessel larger than before.

A procedure using a mechanical device to remove an embolus or thrombus was approved by the FDA in 2004. The Mechanical Embolus Removal in Cerebral Ischemia (MERCI) Retriever can be used up to 8 hours after the onset of an ischemic stroke to remove a thrombus. A catheter is threaded up through the femoral artery to the brain and a wire device is guided through the catheter to the brain. The end of the wire resembles a corkscrew and ensnares the clot, which is

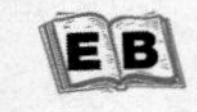

pulled out through the catheter (Becker & Trott, 2005). The interventional radiologist performs this procedure during angiography. If successful, blood flow can be restored to the brain within 20 minutes.

A cerebral aneurysm may be repaired during a craniotomy by placing a clip around the stalk of the aneurysm. The aneurysm may be wrapped with a material that prevents the wall from rupturing if it cannot be clipped or resected. A radiologic procedure wherein a small platinum wire is guided carefully into the aneurysm is another option. Coils of wire are curled into the aneurysm sac, filling it (Figure 23–6). Electricity is sent down the wire to break the wire off and leave the coils in the aneurysm. Thrombosis completes the solidification of the aneurysm, effectively eliminating it. AVMs are treated in much the same way, but may be eliminated using radiosurgery. More than one type of intervention may be used.

Neurologic assessments are performed often to monitor closely for signs of increasing ICP (see Chapter 22). Measures are instituted to prevent or alleviate a rise in ICP. Increased ICP occurs most frequently with a subarachnoid hemorrhage.

Complications

Extension of Hemorrhage or Rebleed. If initial symptoms were caused by a cerebral aneurysm leaking, rupture is a danger until the aneurysm is repaired. Neurologic signs and level of consciousness are watched closely to detect deterioration of the patient's condition due to further bleeding and a rise in ICP. The patient is kept as quiet as possible. An aneurysm that is repaired by wrapping or embolization has a greater chance of bleeding again than one that is repaired with a clip.

Seizures. Seizures are a common complication of a stroke because neural pathways are interrupted when blood flow is blocked or there is irritation of the cerebral cortex from an intercerebral bleed. The type of seizure depends on the area of the brain involved and the extent of the intercerebral bleed or blockage of blood flow. Generalized seizures may occur. The patient may be started on an anticonvulsant to prevent seizure occurrence. The tensing of muscles during a generalized seizure increases ICP. Anticonvulsant therapy may be continued for many months to 2 years after the last seizure occurs.

Hydrocephalus. If blood has leaked into the ventricular system, it interferes with the resorption of cerebrospinal fluid (CSF), causing hydrocephalus. This is more common when a subarachnoid hemorrhage has

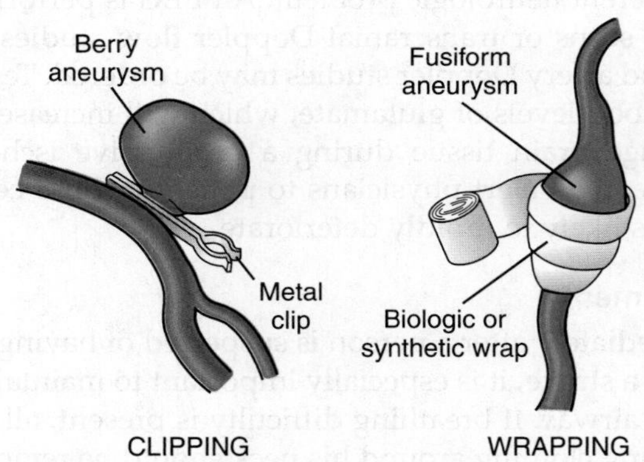

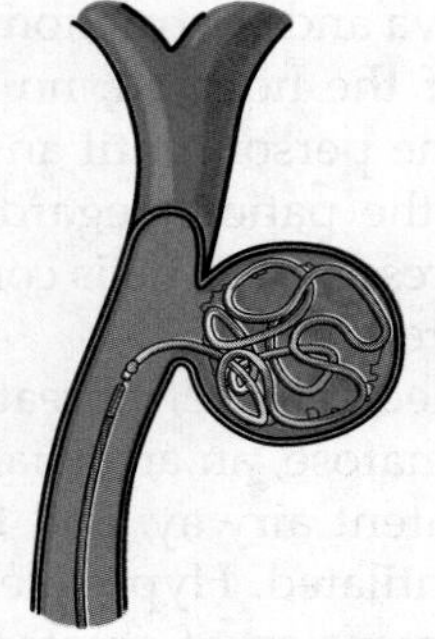

FIGURE 23–6 Techniques used for aneurysm repair.

occurred. A catheter placed into the lateral ventricle and then tunneled down to the right atrium or the peritoneal cavity may be necessary to prevent increased ICP by shunting the fluid out of the brain.

NURSING MANAGEMENT

When the stroke patient is first admitted to the hospital, the general state of health is assessed as well as effects of the stroke *(see TIA/Acute Ischemic Stroke Admission Form on the **companion CD-ROM** accompanying this text).* EB The Agency for Healthcare Research and Quality (1995) has issued clinical practice guidelines for post-stroke rehabilitation. Standardized, validated assessment tools are used to determine deficits and to measure progress toward recovery.

Care of the stroke patient can be divided into three phases: *phase 1,* or initial care; *phase 2,* which is concerned with rehabilitation efforts; and *phase 3,* during which plans are made for continuity of care once the patient returns home. These are not phases in the sense that one begins only after another is finished. There is overlapping of activities in each phase. Because about 80% of all stroke victims survive the first or initial phase of their illness, rehabilitation and plans for self-care are of the utmost importance. Chapter 9 discusses concepts of rehabilitation.

PHASE 1

Assessment (Data Collection)

Immediate assessment of breathing and respiratory rate is essential. Level of consciousness (LOC) is assessed next. Initial care of the stroke patient includes careful assessment to determine the extent to which neurologic functions have been affected. Complete hemiplegia is a common effect of stroke. **Paralysis on the left side indicates focal damage to the right side of the brain because the motor pathways cross to the opposite side before extending down to the spinal cord. Aphasia often indicates ischemia of the brain cells on the left side of the brain and is usually accompanied by right-sided hemiplegia.** Figure 23–7 illustrates deficits often experienced by damage to the left or right side of the brain.

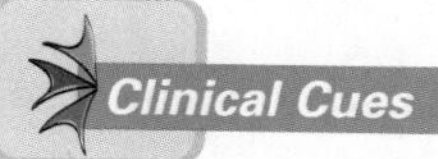

If any change in the patient's thought processes or level of consciousness appears, or the patient becomes more restless, notify the physician immediately as these may be early signs of increasing intracranial pressure. Treatment to decrease intracranial pressure may prevent disability and may prevent death from herniation of the brain.

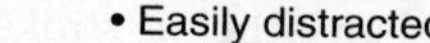

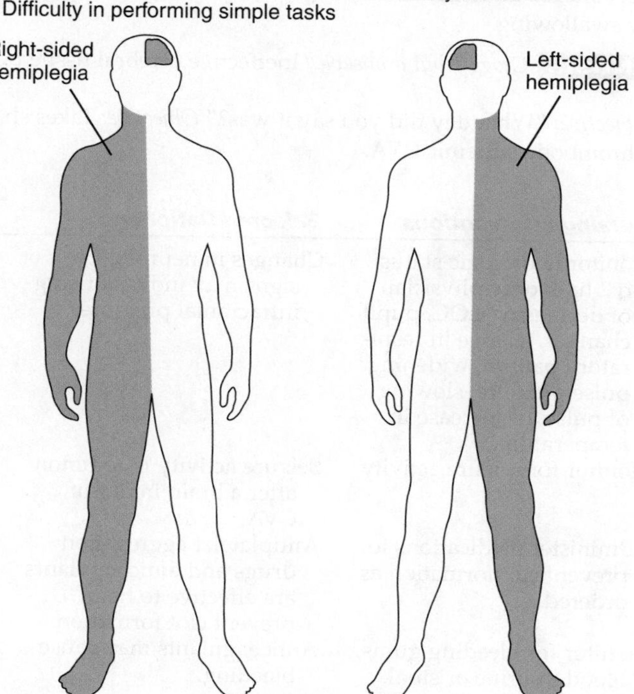

FIGURE **23–7** Comparison of deficits and behavior related to damage to the left and right sides of the brain.

After the acute stage of the stroke has passed and there is physiologic stability, an assessment of functional abilities is performed so that rehabilitation goals and plans can be devised. Assessment of and nursing intervention for the patient with problems of immobility, incontinence of urine and feces, aphasia, delirium or confusion, and altered LOC are discussed in the section on Common Neurologic Patient Care Problems in Chapter 21. Because the patient who has suffered a stroke is at risk for a second occurrence, assessment for new signs of neurologic impairment is ongoing.

Nursing Diagnosis and Planning

Nursing diagnoses for the patient who has experienced a CVA commonly include:

- Risk for injury related to weakness, paralysis, confusion, decreased consciousness, or unilateral neglect
- Impaired physical mobility related to weakness or paralysis
- Imbalanced nutrition: less than body requirements related to impaired swallowing and hemiparesis or hemiplegia
- Self-care deficit related to inability to perform activities of daily living (ADLs; feeding, bathing, grooming) without assistance
- Functional urinary incontinence, related to neurologic deficits
- Bowel incontinence, related to impaired mobility and neurologic impairment
- Risk for impaired skin integrity related to decreased mobility, paresis, or paralysis
- Impaired verbal communication related to inability to clearly verbalize or inability to comprehend communication
- Disturbed body image related to neurologic damage and hemiplegia
- Disturbed sensory perception: visual, related to loss of vision in parts of visual field; kinesthetic, related to decreased sense of touch on one side of the body
- Situational low self-esteem related to alteration in body image and dependence on others
- Ineffective coping related to loss of usual lifestyle, neurologic deficits, and dependence on others

Planning for specific goals must take into account the individual patient's previous lifestyle, age, general health or illness status, and specific problems of care (Nursing Care Plan 23–1). The 80-year-old retired person will not have the same goals for rehabilitation and recovery as the 47-year-old mother of three who had been working full time as a schoolteacher before her attack. *(Refer to Plan of Care form for TIA/Acute Ischemic Stroke Clinical Path on the Companion CD-ROM.)*

Major nursing goals during the first phase are to:

- Maintain an adequate airway

NURSING CARE PLAN 23–1

Care of the Patient Who Has Experienced a Stroke

SCENARIO Mr. Lewis, age 68, suffered an ischemic stroke (CVA) 4 days ago. He is experiencing left-sided paresis, decreased alertness, and difficulty swallowing.

PROBLEM/NURSING DIAGNOSIS *Groggy, but arousable*/ Ineffective cerebral tissue perfusion related to obstruction from a thrombus.

Supporting assessment data *Subjective:* "What day did you say it was?" *Objective:* Takes shaking his shoulder and calling his name to arouse him. Thrombotic ischemic CVA.

Goals/Expected Outcomes	Nursing Interventions	Selected Rationale	Evaluation
Patient will show no further decrease in LOC	Monitor neurologic status q 2 hr. Notify physician of decreasing LOC, pupil changes, change in respiratory pattern, widening pulse pressure, slowing of pulse, or increase in temperature.	Changes in neurologic signs may indicate rising intracranial pressure.	No changes in neurologic signs. Difficult to arouse, but orients quickly.
	Monitor for seizure activity.	Seizure activity is common after a brain injury or CVA.	No signs of seizure activity.
	Administer medications to prevent clot formation as ordered.	Antiplatelet aggregation drugs and anticoagulants are effective to help prevent clot formation.	First dose of Coumadin administered. Managed to swallow the tablet.
	Monitor for bleeding gums, blood in urine or stool.	Anticoagulants may cause bleeding.	No signs of blood in urine or stool; gums not bleeding.

Key: *CVA*, cerebrovascular accident; *LOC*, level of consciousness; *ROM*, range of motion.

NURSING CARE PLAN 23–1

Care of the Patient Who Has Experienced a Stroke—cont'd

PROBLEM/NURSING DIAGNOSIS *Trouble swallowing food and large pill*/Impaired swallowing related to weakness of swallowing muscles.

Supporting assessment data *Subjective:* "I almost choked on that capsule." *Objective:* Coughing when trying to swallow capsule.

Goals/Expected Outcomes	Nursing Interventions	Selected Rationale	Evaluation
Patient will not aspirate food	Place in high Fowler's position for meals, snacks, and oral medication administration.	Gravity will assist swallowing in this position.	Raised to high Fowler's for oral intake.
	Instruct to tilt head and neck forward when attempting to swallow.	Facilitates elevation of the larynx and posterior movement of the tongue allowing food to go into esophagus rather than trachea.	Is tilting head and neck forward when swallowing.
	Have swallow a sip of water before eating or taking an oral medication.		Swallows sip of water without much difficulty now.
	Assist to choose foods for meals that are easily swallowed.	Custard, eggs, canned fruit, mashed potatoes, and other soft foods are more easily swallowed.	Choosing soft foods for tomorrow's meals.
	Encourage to take small bites of food.	Small amounts are more easily swallowed than large amounts.	Is taking small bites of food.
	Use a thickening agent in liquids if they are particularly hard to swallow.	Thickening makes liquids easier to swallow without aspirating.	Thickening agent not needed.
	Avoid putting foods of different texture in the mouth at the same time.		Is eating one type of food at a time.
	Reinforce swallowing techniques/exercises recommended by speech therapist.	Muscle strengthening exercises may improve swallowing if done regularly.	Is practicing techniques suggested by speech therapist to improve swallowing.

PROBLEM/NURSING DIAGNOSIS *Left arm and leg weakness*/Risk for injury related to muscle weakness in left extremities.

Supporting assessment data *Subjective:* "I can't put full weight on my left leg." *Objective:* Left leg unable to push much against resistance; when trying to stand, left leg won't support full weight.

Goals/Expected Outcomes	Nursing Interventions	Selected Rationale	Evaluation
Patient will not fall or sustain injury before or after discharge	Assist to stand and walk to the bathroom.	Assistance prevents falling.	Using gait belt and cane to walk to bathroom.
	Instructed not to get up without assistance.		Asking for assistance to go to the bathroom.
	Place call bell within reach each time he is repositioned.	Allows patient to call for help when wishing to arise.	
	Encourage ROM exercises and strengthening exercises taught by physical therapist.	Working the muscles may improve muscle tone.	Performing ROM and strengthening exercises 3 times/day.

Continued

NURSING CARE PLAN 23–1

Care of the Patient Who Has Experienced a Stroke—cont'd

PROBLEM/NURSING DIAGNOSIS *Is left-handed and cannot shave himself or comb his hair well*/Self-care deficit related to weakness and fatigue.

Supporting assessment data *Subjective:* I'm too weak to hold the razor properly to shave. *Objective:* Hand shakes when trying to grip razor and shave.

Goals/Expected Outcomes	Nursing Interventions	Selected Rationale	Evaluation
Patient will resume some self-grooming by discharge	Assist with bathing, dressing, and grooming.	Assistance prevents undue fatigue. Assistance helps accomplish daily hygiene activities.	Assistance with bathing, dressing, and grooming provided.
	Encourage patient to attempt to comb hair and brush teeth.	Small accomplishments provide hope of independence.	Attempted to comb hair with right hand; praise given.
	Praise for every successful attempt at self-care.	Praise reinforces desired behavior.	
	Help to practice shaving with electric razor using right hand.	New skills improve with practice.	Wife will bring in an electric razor for him tomorrow. Continue plan.

PROBLEM/NURSING DIAGNOSIS *Left extremity weakness, difficulty in remembering things*/Ineffective coping related to memory impairment, difficulty swallowing, and paresis of left extremities.

Supporting assessment data *Subjective:* "I don't want to be a burden to my wife." *Objective:* Tends to forget what wife or nurses have told him. Eyes filled with tears at times.

Goals/Expected Outcomes	Nursing Interventions	Selected Rationale	Evaluation
Patient will express hope of full recovery before discharge	Assure that it is too early to tell if there will be any permanent disability from the stroke.	Validates that the future is not known at this time.	Assurance given during bathing discussion.
	Help patient explore his fears and anxieties about his condition and his future.	Expressing fears decreases anxiety.	Spoke about fear of being dependent upon wife for daily care.
	Actively listen with patience when patient shares his thoughts.	Actively listening establishes trust and provides emotional support.	Sat with patient, established eye contact, and listened to his concerns.
	Do not express negative thoughts or opinions about his condition or progress in his or his wife's presence.	Negative thoughts can destroy hope.	No negative comments made.
	Point out each small bit of progress in self-care, eating, and mobility.	Acknowledging progress toward recovery helps dispel fear of permanent dependence.	Acknowledged improvement in swallowing at noon meal. Continue plan.

? CRITICAL THINKING QUESTIONS

1. How would you incorporate Ms. Lewis into the care of her husband?
2. What might be accomplished with a social service consult for this patient?
3. How could a social service consult be helpful for this patient and his wife?

- Establish baseline data regarding vital signs, LOC, neuromuscular function, and neurologic status
- Preserve joint and muscle function
- Prevent complications that may interfere with rehabilitation

Specific individual expected outcomes are written for each identified problem or nursing diagnosis.

Implementation

The amount of activity permitted a stroke patient during the initial acute stage of his illness depends on the cause of the stroke. If there is danger of continued hemorrhage from a ruptured artery and resultant increase in ICP, physical activity will necessarily be limited, and the patient care challenges will not be the same as for a patient with stroke from another cause. When there is no danger of further damage to his brain, the patient usually is encouraged to become active as soon as his condition has stabilized.

Many patients have dysphagia (difficulty swallowing) as a result of the stroke. The speech therapist should be called to do a swallowing study and to devise a plan to improve swallowing. Be certain the patient has a gag reflex by having him sip a small amount of water before feeding orally. Nutritional Therapies 23–1 provides suggestions for working with the dysphagic patient.

Measures to prevent complications, such as subcutaneous low-molecular-weight heparin injections and elastic stockings to prevent deep venous thrombosis, skin care to minimize the risk of skin breakdown, physical therapy and splinting to prevent contractures and spasticity, and measures to prevent falls, are included in the plan of care. To reduce the possibility of recurrence of a stroke, risk factors are identified and teaching is begun to modify them.

Evaluation

Evaluation is based on whether the interventions are effective in achieving the expected outcomes. Assess whether the overall goals have been met. If the outcomes are not being met, the care plan must be revised.

PHASE 2

Rehabilitation

Plans for rehabilitation should begin the moment the patient is admitted. This means maintenance of an adequate airway and aeration of the lungs, proper positioning, range-of-motion exercises for affected limbs, adequate nutrition and fluid intake and output, prevention of pressure ulcers, use of devices to keep extremities in anatomical position, and all other nursing measures directed toward maintaining normal body functions until the patient is able to maintain them on his own. *(An Interdisciplinary Care Plan for Ischemic Stroke is located on the **companion CD-ROM** accompanying this text.)*

If the patient suffers from homonymous hemianopsia, he has a visual defect affecting the same half of the visual field in each eye. He will not be able to see past the midline toward the side opposite the lesion and must turn the head to scan that side (see Figure 23–5). The problem may cause accidents when ambulating. The patient must be taught ways to deal with this visual problem.

If disabilities from inactivity are avoided, rehabilitation has a much better chance of success. During phase 2, various members of the health care team collaborate with the patient and his family to help resolve both psychosocial and physical problems. Among the team members helping the stroke victim may be the physical therapist, speech pathologist, social worker, psychologist, and occupational therapist. The patient usually is transferred from the hospital to a rehabilitation facility.

During phase 2, the patient is encouraged with physical therapy to strengthen his muscles as well as his resolve to help himself. He will need to exercise his muscles actively and retrain them.

There are many ways to encourage the patient. Instead of feeding him every item on his tray, let him hold bread and other "finger foods," suggesting that he feed himself these things. Chewing may be slow at

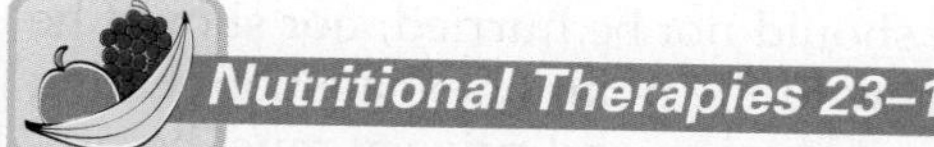

Nutritional Therapies 23–1

The Patient Who Has Dysphagia

The patient with dysphagia is in danger of aspiration. To help prevent aspiration, teach the patient to:

- Sit up straight to eat, and tilt your head slightly forward.
- Place only one teaspoon of food in your mouth at a time.
- If you have paresis from a stroke, the food should be placed on the unaffected side of your mouth.
- Place your chin on your chest and swallow; wait a few seconds and swallow again.
- Refrain from taking liquids and solids at the same time.
- Sip from the cup or glass rather than use a straw.
- Remain in an upright position for 45 to 60 minutes after a meal.

Interventions to assist the patient to eat without aspirating include:

- Plan a 30-minute rest and relaxation period before each meal.
- Allow plenty of time for a relaxed meal.
- Serve food cold or well-warmed; lukewarm foods are more difficult to swallow.
- Serve foods in the consistency ordered; some patients find semi-solid food easier to swallow.
- Avoid serving peanut butter, syrup, and bananas because they are sticky and difficult to swallow.
- Avoid serving dry foods such as rice, popcorn, toast, or crackers as they tend to be more difficult to swallow and can stick in the throat.
- Keep the container for liquids less than two-thirds full so that the patient does not have to tilt the head back too far to drink. Tilting the head back tends to cause fluid to go into the trachea.

first; the patient should not be hurried, nor should he be allowed to chew to the point of exhaustion. Eating often is difficult and messy, and privacy must be provided. If hemiplegia is causing the patient to "pocket" food in the folds of the mouth, the mouth should be checked after meals.

Combing and brushing the hair is good exercise for the arm and shoulder, as are brushing the teeth and washing the face and hands. The patient may not be able to carry all these procedures through to completion at first, but with occupational therapy encouragement he can gradually improve until he is able to perform much of his own personal care. **The patient who has suffered brain injury becomes fatigued very quickly, and this must be kept in mind when performing self-care activities.** Encouragement and praise for the smallest accomplishment can help the patient's tattered self-esteem.

The stroke patient can be prone to rapid mood swings and spontaneous weeping. All health care workers must be patient and accepting, and an explanation to the patient and family that this is very common after a stroke can ease his embarrassment.

Various rehabilitation techniques are undergoing trials to see if more function can be regained in the extremities. Thermal stimulation, in which heat and then cold are applied to the affected upper extremity in 10 cycles 5 days a week for 6 weeks, brought improvement in grasping strength and wrist extension (Jia-Ching, 2005). Another technique is called constraint-induced movement therapy (CIMT). It emphasizes use of the disabled extremity. The unaffected extremity is restrained and the patient works with a therapist to slowly learn to use the affected limb again. The therapy is thought to take advantage of brain plasticity—its ability to adapt and reorganize. The therapy only succeeds if patients work at it 6 hours a day, 5 days a week for

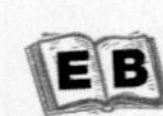

2 to 3 weeks (Barker, 2005). Further information on rehabilitation programs is located in Chapter 9.

PHASE 3

In phase 3, plans are made for discharge and referral to individuals and agencies outside the hospital that will help the patient and his family adjust to his new way of life. A visiting nurse often is assigned for a period of time to coordinate rehabilitation efforts, assist with teaching, and assess the patient's status. The patient continues rehabilitation as an outpatient under the physician's supervision.

BRAIN TUMOR

Etiology and Pathophysiology

About 200,000 new brain tumors are discovered each year in the United States. About 40,000 of those are primary tumors and the rest are metastatic tumors from a different site of origin (Table 23–2). It is not known how brain tumors begin, and there are over 120 different types. Low-grade astrocytomas are more common in young people than in older adults. High-grade gliomas are more prevalent in the elderly. Cerebellar tumors are more common in children.

Table 23–2 *Different Types of Brain Tumors**

TUMOR	TYPE OF TISSUE
Gliomas (malignant)	
Glioblastoma multiforme	Primitive stem cells (glioblasts)
Astrocytoma	Astrocytes and glial cells
Medulloblastoma	Primitive neuroectodermal cells
Oligodendroglioma	Oligodendrocytes
Ependymoma	Ependymal epithelium
Pituitary adenoma (usually benign)	Pituitary gland cells
Acoustic neuroma (usually benign)	Myelin sheath cells of the VIIIth cranial nerve
Meningioma (most often benign)	Cells of the meninges
Hemangioblastoma (benign)	Cells from blood vessels in the brain
Metastatic tumors (malignant)	Mostly from lung, breast, kidney, thyroid, and prostate carcinomas

*Primary brain tumors are classified by the type of tissue from which they derive.

Neoplasms within the confines of the skull are space-occupying lesions, and thus create problems of increasing ICP by compressing adjacent tissues. If the tumor arises from brain cells, the cranial nerves, or the pituitary gland, the neoplastic cells can infiltrate and destroy these structures, although other types of tumor can destroy tissue through pressure. Many brain tumors are benign, such as a meningioma or acoustic neuroma. However, because of the increased ICP tumors cause and the way they can invade brain tissue, a benign tumor also presents a serious condition.

Intracranial tumors may begin in the brain itself, or they may begin in the meninges, cranial nerves, or pituitary gland. Primary malignant brain tumors rarely metastasize outside the brain, but an intracranial tumor may be secondary to malignant lesions outside the skull, such as a malignancy of the breast, lung, or melanoma of the skin.

Signs, Symptoms, and Diagnosis

There can be as many symptoms of intracranial tumors as there are functions of the structures within the skull. The symptoms depend on location and may appear gradually, or, if the tumor is a highly malignant, fast-growing type, they may appear suddenly. In a slow-growing type of tumor, the patient may first show personality changes, disturbances in judgment and memory, loss of muscular strength and coordination, or difficulty in speaking clearly. Headache awakening the patient is a key sign. Vomiting, visual problems, and other signs of increased ICP also may occur. Approximately 20% to 50% of adults with brain tumors develop seizure activity.

Diagnostic procedures to identify the site and extent of intracranial tumors include MRI, arteriography, and CT scan.

Treatment

The three modes of therapy for intracranial tumors are the same as those for neoplastic diseases elsewhere in the body: surgery, radiation therapy, and chemotherapy. Radiation is usually given 5 days a week for 6 weeks. With brachytherapy, tiny radioactive particles are inserted into the tumor tissue via an implanted catheter. This treatment extends over about 5 days. Radiation precautions are needed during this period. If the tumor is found while it is still very small, a stereotactic Cyberknife or gamma knife procedure may destroy it. Gamma knife procedures use a steel frame attached to the head with ports through which radiation is directed from several angles. Cyberknife procedures use a molded head mask or body mask to keep the patient from moving during treatment. Measurements are calculated by a computer to precisely locate the tumor, and the radiation is delivered only to the tumor, which spares surrounding tissue. These procedures also can be used for small recurrent tumor growth (see Figure 8–4).

Most chemotherapy drugs cannot cross the blood-brain barrier. To get the drugs into the brain circulation, an Ommaya reservoir may be implanted between the scalp and the skull. It consists of a port attached to a catheter that is placed in the lateral ventricle of the brain (Figure 23–8). Chemotherapy drugs can be injected into the port and instilled into the CSF in the ventricle. In this way the chemotherapy drug is carried to the tumor cells in greater quantity than can be achieved by infusion of the drugs into the bloodstream. In patients for whom chemotherapy and radiation have previously failed, implantation of carmustine (BiCNU; Gliadel) wafers into a glial cell tumor slows growth. The drug is inserted into brain tissue after removal of the glioma to fight the malignancy and slow or prevent regrowth. Temozolomide (Temodar) is an oral chemotherapeutic drug that does cross the blood-brain barrier. Trials with local hyperthermia are underway, as are trials of biologic therapy. Treatments are discussed more thoroughly in Chapter 8. If there are signs of increased ICP, measures are instituted to try to lower the ICP and to provide supportive care (see Chapter 22).

Surgery. Whenever possible, intracranial tumors are removed surgically, and the other modes of treatment are used to destroy remaining cells. Sometimes, however, the tumor has infiltrated vital parts of the brain that must not be traumatized by surgical procedures. If the tumor is located in the cerebrum, an operation called a *craniotomy* is done. A "window flap" of scalp and bone is cut and pulled down, the dura is opened, and the tumor is removed. Tumors in or near the *cerebellum* are removed through an incision under the occipital bone. If all of the tumor cannot be removed, a portion of the tumor may be removed to relieve compression of the brain against the skull. This procedure is only a temporary measure to relieve the patient's symptoms. Care of the patient after brain surgery is presented in Chapter 22.

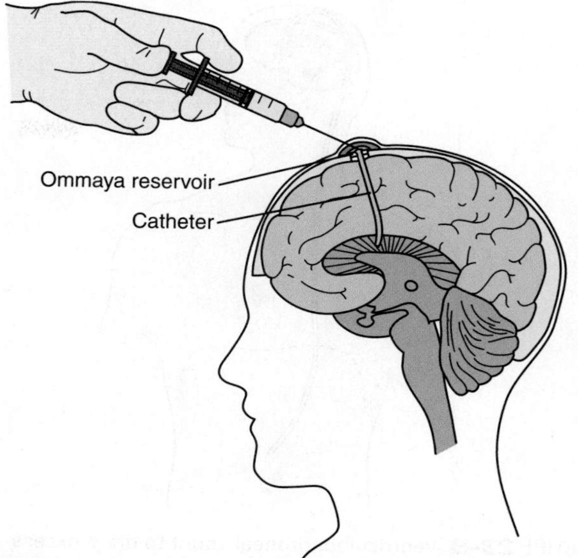

FIGURE 23–8 Implantation of an Ommaya reservoir for chemotherapy of a brain tumor.

Nursing Management

Routine neurologic assessments are performed as well as assessment of ability to perform ADLs. Pain assessment and control are important. Helping the patient and family to communicate fears and cope with the situation should be part of the care plan.

Nursing diagnoses commonly used for the patient with a brain tumor are:

- Ineffective tissue perfusion related to tumor pressure and cerebral edema
- Pain related to cerebral edema and increased ICP
- Self-care deficit related to altered neuromuscular function, sensory deficits, or decreased LOC
- Anxiety or fear related to diagnosis and prognosis
- Risk for injury related to seizure activity caused by the tumor
- Risk for injury related to increasing ICP from tumor growth
- Impaired memory related to damaged cells from pressure
- Impaired home maintenance related to physical impairments
- Disturbed personal identity related to inability to work

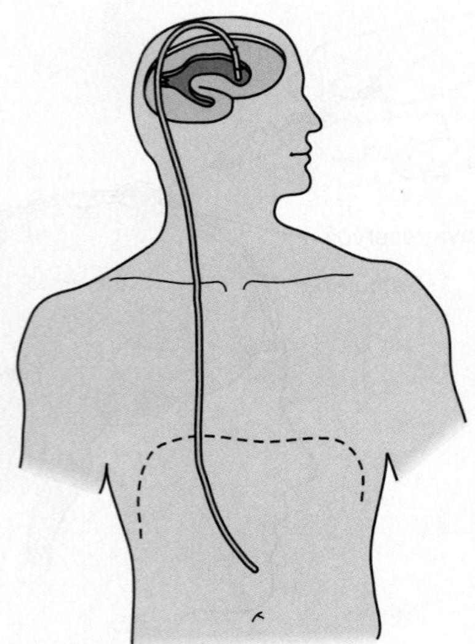

FIGURE **23–9** Ventriculoperitoneal shunt to drain excess cerebrospinal fluid into the peritoneal cavity, where it is absorbed through the mucosa.

Specific outcomes appropriate for the individual are written and interventions planned to help the patient meet the outcomes. Evaluation is based on data that indicate the outcomes are being met. (See Chapter 21 for care for common problems and interventions for various nursing diagnoses related to neurologic problems; see Nursing Care Plan 22–1 and the section on Increased Intracranial Pressure in Chapter 22 for further interventions.)

Complications

Hydrocephalus. Obstruction of CSF flow may require placing a shunt to reduce CSF pressure and prevent increased ICP. A shunt is a tube attached to a small manual pump that moves excess CSF fluid from the ventricles to the peritoneal cavity or into the atrium of the heart, from where it is absorbed (Figure 23–9).

Intercerebral Hemorrhage. Bleeding in the brain may occur as the tumor erodes blood vessels. Depending on the condition of the patient, the size of the tumor, and prognosis, various measures to stop the bleeding and reduce ICP will be employed.

INFECTIOUS AND INFLAMMATORY DISORDERS OF THE NERVOUS SYSTEM

BACTERIAL MENINGITIS

Etiology and Pathophysiology

Meningitis is an inflammation of the membranes covering the brain and spinal cord and is caused by an infectious agent. The membranes can become infected in a number of ways, because infectious agents can be carried through the bloodstream to the membranes, or brain tissue can become affected as an infection in a particular area of the brain spreads. Infection can spread from the spinal cord and sinuses to the brain. Two examples of how infectious organisms may enter the cranial vault are:

- Through an opening in the skull in a head injury or from surgery
- By accidental introduction of infectious agents into the spinal canal during spinal puncture

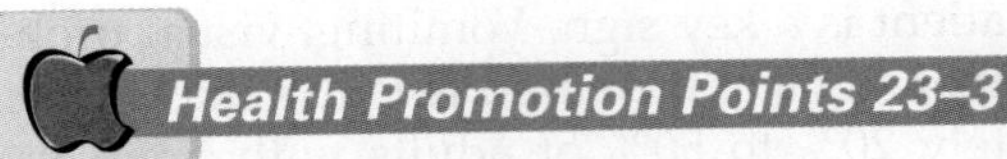

Health Promotion Points 23–3

Meningitis Immunization

Meningitis vaccine is available and is required for all students entering college. It should be encouraged for adults living in a communal situation. Meningitis can spread quickly when people are in proximity, such as in classrooms or dormitory rooms.

Many different strains of bacteria can cause meningitis, but the causative organisms are usually the bacteria *Streptococcus pneumoniae* and *Neisseria meningitidis.* In children the causative organism may be *Haemophilus influenzae* type B. Bacterial meningitis frequently follows an upper respiratory infection. Immunization against *H. influenzae* type B has been recommended for all infants for many years (Health Promotion Points 23–3).

A consequence of bacterial meningitis can be an increase in circulating CSF due to obstruction of normal mechanisms of CSF absorption. Bacteria, white blood cells, and debris block the arachnoid villi, resulting in an obstructive **hydrocephalus** (increased CSF in the ventricles of the brain) that increases intracranial pressure (ICP). Meningitis can cause permanent neurologic damage and may cause severe vasoconstriction that requires amputation of part of a limb.

Signs and Symptoms

The most outstanding symptom of meningitis is the **sudden onset of fever and a severe and persistent headache that is greatly aggravated by moving the head.** Other signs of meningeal irritation include pain and stiffness of the neck when the head is bent forward, flexing the neck **(nuchal rigidity),** as well as exaggerated deep tendon reflexes, irritability, photophobia, and hypersensitivity of the skin. A positive Brudzinski's sign can be elicited by placing a hand behind the patient's head and, with the other hand on the chest, gently flexing his neck forward by moving his chin toward his chest. If there is flexion of the knees and hips when you try to flex the neck, Brudzinski's sign is positive and indicates meningeal irritation. For Kernig's sign, have the patient supine and with the hip and knee flexed at 90-degree angles, and slowly extend the knee (Figure 23–10). If there is pain, not just discomfort, behind the knee, Kernig's sign is positive, indicating meningeal irritation. **Meningococ-**

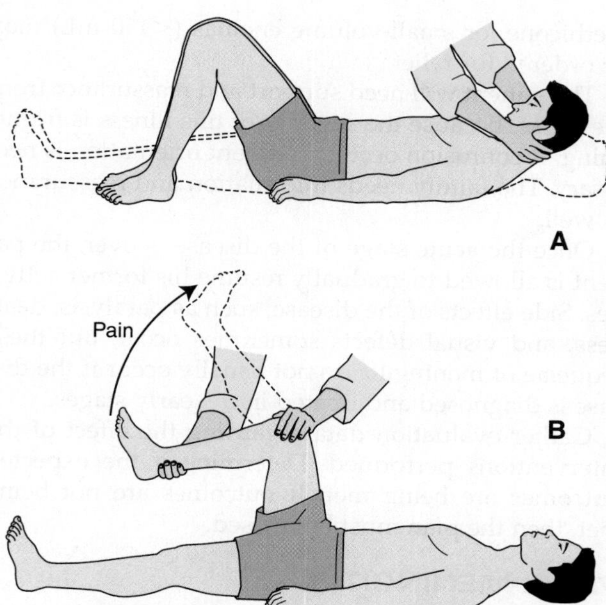

FIGURE **23–10** **A,** Positive Brudzinski's sign: Passive flexion of the head and neck causes flexion of the thighs and legs. **B,** Positive Kernig's sign: Inability to extend the leg from a position of 90-degree flexion at the hip due to pain and spasms in the hamstring muscle.

cal meningitis often is accompanied by a petechial rash covering the chest and extremities. Seizures frequently occur, as well as nausea and vomiting, in the patient with meningitis.

Diagnosis

When meningitis is suspected, a spinal tap is performed, and the CSF is examined for the number and type of organisms present. The CSF pressure is elevated (see Chapter 21). A Gram stain identifies the causative organism. Blood tests may be performed to rule out other disorders that can mimic meningitis.

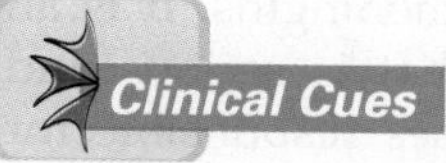

When meningitis is present, the spinal fluid may appear milky as a result of the increased number of white cells suspended in the fluid. Other abnormal findings in the CSF include the presence of protein and decreased amounts of glucose.

Treatment

Successful treatment of meningitis and prevention of permanent disability depend on early recognition and prompt treatment. Antibiotics are started immediately for bacterial meningitis, and when the causative organism has been identified, specific antibiotics to which the organism is sensitive are administered. A combination of two antibiotics is common. The disease usually responds well to IV antibiotic therapy followed by oral doses given for a total of 10 days. Dexamethasone has proven beneficial to decrease inflammation for many patients and may be continued for 4 days. Anticonvulsive drugs are administered to control seizures, and ibuprofen, aspirin, or acetaminophen is given for headache.

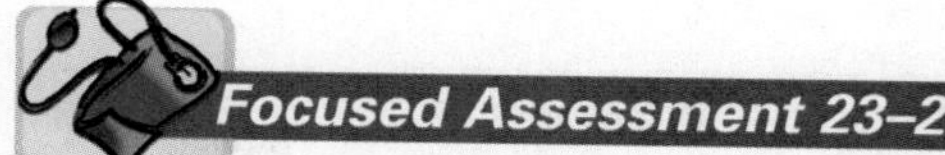

Assessment of the Patient with Brain Infection

An assessment (data collection) should be performed each shift for the following areas:

- Neurologic check for increasing intracranial pressure
- Stiff neck or paralysis
- Temperature and monitoring of temperature trend
- Assessment for electrolyte and fluid imbalance; skin turgor, mucous membranes, condition of lips; intake and output
- Gastrointestinal assessment: bowel sounds, distention, constipation, diarrhea, nausea, vomiting
- Intravenous access site
- Skin condition
- Psychosocial concerns

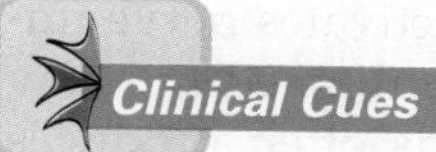

Narcotics are rarely used for pain control in patients with increased ICP, as they cause sedation and prevent accurate neurologic assessment.

Prophylactic antibiotics are usually given to those in close contact with the patient to prevent the spread of the disease. Mortality occurs in about 20% of cases.

NURSING MANAGEMENT

Assessment (Data Collection) and Nursing Diagnosis

In addition to noting the specific signs and symptoms of meningitis, assess the patient for subjective and objective data relevant to each of the patient care problems that might accompany the disease. Examples include convulsive seizures, elevated body temperature, nausea and vomiting, delirium, pain, increased ICP, and fluid and electrolyte imbalances. Ongoing, vigilant neurologic assessment is a high priority in monitoring for signs of increasing ICP, changes in condition, and response to treatment. An ongoing assessment should be done each shift (Focused Assessment 23–2).

Nursing diagnoses are written for the specific problems identified via data collection (see Table 21–8, Nursing Care Plan 22–1, and Nursing Care Plan 23–1).

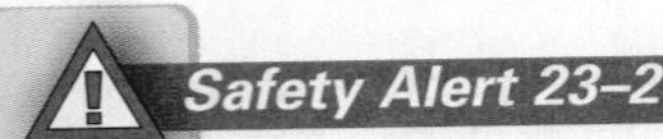

Factors that Can Raise ICP

Large-volume enemas should not be given because they may increase intracranial pressure (ICP) by being absorbed into the body's fluid compartment and causing fluid overload or by initiating the Valsalva maneuver for defecation. Performance of the Valsalva maneuver stimulates the vagus nerve, causing hypotension.

Administration of corticosteroids, mineralocorticoids, estrogens, and progesterones can increase ICP because they cause fluid retention.

Planning, Implementation, and Evaluation

Expected outcomes are written for the nursing diagnoses chosen. Specific nursing interventions in the care of the patient with meningitis are primarily concerned with measures to:

- Conserve the strength of the patient
- Prevent seizures
- Promote healing

Preventing the spread of infection includes use of Standard Precautions and droplet precautions.

The patient's room should be quiet and dimly lit. Sudden noises or bright flashes of light can cause a seizure because the sensory input activates nerve impulses. Care and treatments are coordinated to allow as much rest as possible. Meningitis often produces mental confusion and delirium, as well as the possibility of seizures. Herpes simplex (fever blisters) frequently accompanies meningitis.

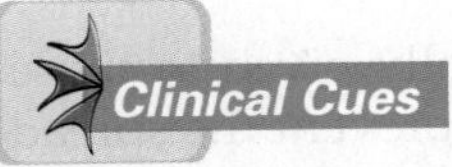

The presence of herpes lesions, plus drying of the lips and mouth from fever and dehydration, requires special mouth care. Using Standard Precautions (see Appendix 6), the lips and mouth should be cleansed and lubricated at least every 2 hours during the acute stage of the disease.

Fluid volume deficit is often a problem. Monitor the patient's intake and output and prevent dehydration. Excessive vomiting or outward signs of early dehydration should be reported promptly so that IV fluids may be given to correct fluid volume deficits (Safety Alert 23–2).

Irritation of the neural centers in the brain may cause a decrease in the peristaltic action of the intestines in the patient with meningitis and can lead to an accumulation of flatus and fecal material with severe abdominal distention. Check the patient's abdomen for distention, and note bowel sounds and record them in the medical record. Rectal tubes, suppositories, simethicone, or small-volume enemas (<150 mL) may be ordered for relief.

The patient will need support and reassurance from the nurse, because the severity of this illness is frightening. If confusion occurs, frequent orientation is necessary. The family needs information and reassurance as well.

Once the acute stage of the disease is over, the patient is allowed to gradually resume his former activities. Side effects of the disease, such as paralysis, deafness, and visual defects sometimes occur, but these sequelae of meningitis do not usually occur if the disease is diagnosed and treated in the early stages.

Gather evaluation data regarding the effect of the interventions performed. Determine if the expected outcomes are being met. If outcomes are not being met, then the plan must be revised.

VIRAL MENINGITIS

Several viruses can cause meningitis, and the most common ones are enteroviruses, arboviruses, HIV, and herpes simplex virus. Viral meningitis tends to be milder than bacterial meningitis. The presenting signs and symptoms include a headache, fever, photophobia, and stiff neck. Brain involvement symptoms are not usually present.

Examination of the CSF is performed to confirm the diagnosis. A complete blood count will show increased lymphocytes *(lymphocytosis)*. A polymerase chain reaction (PRC) test to detect virus-specific DNA or RNA can diagnose central nervous system (CNS) viral infection.

The disease is self-limiting and is managed symptomatically. Full recovery of the patient is usual within 7 to 10 days. Sometimes residual effects such as persistent headaches, mild mental impairment, and incoordination occur.

ENCEPHALITIS

Etiology and Pathophysiology

Encephalitis is less common than meningitis. It is an acute inflammation of the brain that is serious and sometimes fatal. Some of the viruses responsible for encephalitis are associated with particular seasons of the year or with geographic locations. Ticks and mosquitoes are the vectors that transmit the disease (Health Promotion Points 23–4). Examples of viruses in the United States that cause encephalitis are eastern equine encephalomyelitis, western equine encephalomyelitis, La Crosse encephalitis, St. Louis encephalitis, and West Nile viruses. Encephalitis may occur as a complication of the viral diseases chickenpox, measles, and mumps. Postviral encephalitis is an immune-mediated disorder and follows the end of the viral infection by 2 to 12 days. Herpes simplex virus 1 (human herpesvirus 1) is frequently the cause of non–vector-transmitted encephalitis. Cytomegalovirus encephalitis is a complication in patients with AIDS.

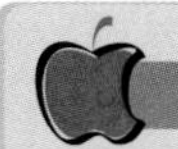

Health Promotion Points 23–4

Protect Against Mosquitoes and Ticks

During mosquito season, wear insect repellent and protective clothing. Prevent water from standing in containers around the home and property to discourage the breeding of mosquitoes. Avoid being out of doors for recreational purposes at dusk and at night, when mosquitoes are more likely to be about. Use insect repellent and protective clothing when out in wooded areas. Skin should be inspected for ticks after the outing.

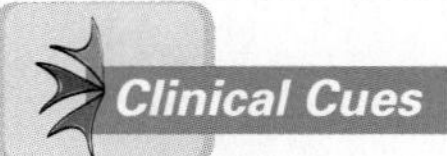

Clinical Cues

Whenever a patient is admitted with symptoms of a brain infection, check the skin thoroughly and question the patient about a recent history of herpes lesions. If you find any herpes lesions, or are told that they were present within the past several days, notify the physician immediately. Herpes encephalitis can be fatal if not treated early.

Once the virus crosses the blood-brain barrier and enters neural cells, disrupting normal neural function, hemorrhage and an inflammatory response occur in the gray matter.

The severity of the illness may be mild or fatal. The most common type of viral encephalitis in the United States is that caused by herpes simplex virus 1. West Nile virus has emerged as a cause of encephalitis since 1999.

Neurologic impairment is caused by direct infection of neural cells. Western equine encephalomyelitis is spread by the mosquito and occurs most frequently  between April and September (Nandalur, 2005). Herpes simplex encephalitis spreads from neural tissue to the CNS. It can be a primary or secondary infection and can occur from reactivation of latent virus. **If treatment for the herpes simplex is not started before coma occurs, death is almost certain.**

Signs, Symptoms, and Diagnosis

The onset of encephalitis may be either sudden or insidious. There may be behavioral and personality changes and a decreased LOC. **Stiff neck, photophobia, and lethargy are classic symptoms of encephalitis. Seizures, acute confusion, and flaccid paralysis may occur.** CNS signs usually appear 1 to 4 hours after the onset of other symptoms. Lethargy may progress to coma. The patient with herpes simplex encephalitis may exhibit flulike symptoms that rapidly progress. West Nile virus should be considered if an adult over age 50 develops encephalitis in the summer or early fall.

Encephalitis symptoms differ from those of meningitis in that with encephalitis there is altered mental status, motor or sensory deficits, and speech or movement disorders.

Diagnosis is confirmed by the presence of the virus in the CSF or bloodstream. The CSF in herpes simplex encephalitis will show a slightly elevated white blood cell count, a small increase in protein, and normal glucose levels. PCR tests for herpes simplex virus DNA and RNA levels in CSF allow for early diagnosis. MRI, positron emission tomography scanning, and an EEG may be performed to demonstrate inflammation and the disruption of normal neural impulses. A brain biopsy may be required to verify the responsible organism so proper treatment can begin.

Treatment and Nursing Management

The treatment of encephalitis is primarily symptomatic, with general supportive measures to maintain cardiac and respiratory function, maintain the patient's strength, promote healing, and prevent complications. Herpes simplex type 1 encephalitis is treated with antiviral IV acyclovir or fascine.

Specific nursing measures are essentially the same as for any patient who is subject to seizures, high fever, delirium, or altered LOC. See Table 21–9 for appropriate nursing diagnoses, expected outcomes, and nursing interventions. The nursing care plan must be individualized to the patient's needs.

Complications

Permanent neurologic disabilities may occur, such as problems with walking, paralysis, cognition, memory, and self-care. About 65% of survivors of encephalitis have long-term problems.

BRAIN ABSCESS

A brain abscess is a collection of purulent material in a cavity within the brain. A bacterial infection that has traveled from the gums or teeth, sinus, ear, or mastoid region to the brain usually is the cause. An abscess can form from bacteria introduced at the time of any type of head injury or cranial surgery. **Signs and symptoms are headache, fever, and progression to lethargy and confusion.** If the abscess is not treated, ICP will rise as the size of the abscess increases. Teach patients who experience sinus infections with purulent drainage to seek treatment if symptoms last for more than a few days.

HEADACHES

Headaches are the most common complaint of pain in people. Headaches are commonly caused by allergy and related sinus problems, or by tension, or are vascular in origin. Arthritis, cervical spondylitis, and temporomandibular joint syndrome may also cause headaches. The pain of a headache may be minor or

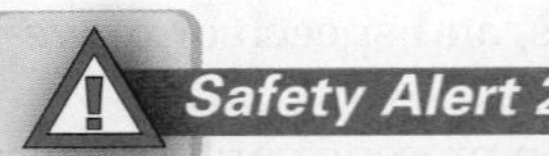

Safety Alert 23–3

Triptans and Antidepressant Use

Patients who are taking triptans migraine medication should not also take antidepressant/mood disorder medications that are selective serotonin reuptake inhibitors (SSRIs) or selective serotonin/norepinephrine reuptake inhibitors (SNRIs). There is a greater risk of increased serotonin levels occurring if triptans are combined with SSRIs or SNRIs, and the resulting serotonin syndrome can be life threatening. Signs and symptoms of serotonin syndrome include restlessness, hallucinations, loss of coordination, tachycardia, rapid changes in blood pressure, hyperthermia, overactive reflexes, nausea, vomiting, and diarrhea. Consult with the physician rather than abruptly stopping the SSRI or SNRI medication.

severe. Persistent headache requires testing to rule out organic problems such as anemia, brain tumor, or cerebral aneurysm.

Treatment for severe, recurrent headaches begins with determining the cause, if possible, and identifying factors that seem to precipitate the headache. Mild headaches usually are relieved by rest and a mild analgesic.

MIGRAINE HEADACHES

Approximately 23 million Americans have at least one migraine headache a year. Women experience them more than men. It is thought that constriction and subsequent dilation of cerebral arteries cause migraine headaches. Attacks usually occur irregularly and may begin with a prodromal period of visual disturbances such as "spots before the eyes" **(scotoma).** The visual aura preceding the attack may take other forms and often occurs up to an hour before the onset of pain. Pain usually begins on one side of the head and is described as throbbing in character. A migraine headache is often accompanied by nausea and vomiting. Symptoms may last for several hours or a day or more. Light causes irritation and sensitivity, and for some sufferers, certain types of light set off the headache. Frequent migraine headaches are very debilitating (Safety Alert 23–3).

Lying in a darkened, quiet room that is odor free with the eyes closed decreases the symptoms. Sometimes doing this at the very beginning of symptoms can prevent a full-blown migraine headache. Metoclopramide (Reglan) is often prescribed for the nausea that accompanies a migraine. Various behavioral treatments such as biofeedback and relaxation therapy, combined with physical treatments seem to offer the best result (McCrory, 2000).

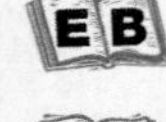

Treatment consists of using one or more of the agents listed in Box 23–3 (Silberstein, 2000). A cold compress to the temple, eye, and occiput areas is helpful. For some people, compression of the temporal artery on the affected side is beneficial. Identifying food or other substances that seem to trigger an attack is very important (Nutritional Therapies 23–2). If migraine headache tends to occur around the time of menses, taking a prescribed diuretic for 3 to 5 days before onset of menstruation may be effective in preventing the headache (Complementary & Alternative Therapies 23–1).

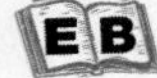

Occipital nerve stimulation is under study at Rush University Medical Center to control migraine and other headache pain. Two nerve stimulator electrodes are implanted under the skin at the base of the head at

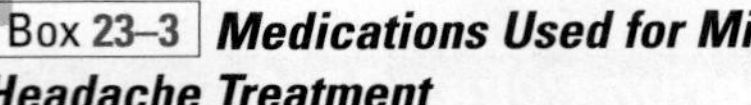

Box 23–3 Medications Used for Migraine Headache Treatment

DRUGS THAT ABORT MIGRAINE SYMPTOMS
- Sumatriptan (Imitrex, Imigran)
- Zolmitriptan (Zomig, Zomig ZMT)
- Naratriptan (Amerge, Naramig)
- Rizatriptan (Maxalt, Maxalt MLT)
- Almotriptan (Axert)
- Frovatriptan (Frova)
- Eletriptan (Relpax)
- Ergotamine tartrate (Cafergot)
- Methysergide (Sansert)
- Acetaminophen-isometheptene-dichloralphenazone (Midrin)
- Dihydroergotamine (D.H.E. 45 injections, Migranal Nasal Spray)

PREVENTIVE DRUGS (TAKEN DAILY)
- Valproic acid (Depakote)
- Topiramate (Topamax)
- Amitriptyline (Elavil)
- Nortriptyline (Pamelor)
- Propranolol (Inderal) and other beta blockers
- Timolol (Blocadren)
- Verapamil (Covera) and other calcium channel blockers
- Cyproheptadine (Periactin)

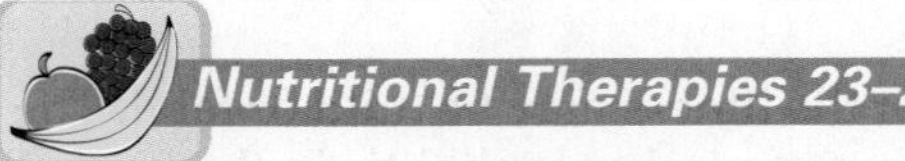

Nutritional Therapies 23–2

Finding Foods that Trigger a Migraine Headache

Ask patients who suffer from migraine headaches to keep a food diary and see if any of the following foods or additives are triggering the attacks:
- Alcohol
- Caffeine
- Chocolate
- Artificial sweeteners (aspartame, sucralose, saccharin)
- Monosodium glutamate (MSG)
- Citrus fruits
- Meats with nitrites (bacon, salami, etc.)
- Salt
- Foods containing tyramines: peanuts, raisins, vinegars, soy sauce, aged cheese, yogurt, sour cream, chicken livers, sausages, bananas, avocados, pickled herring, freshly baked breads, pork, beans

Complementary & Alternative Therapies 23–1

Vitamin B_6, Herbs, and Vitamin B_2

If taking a diuretic drug is contraindicated for some reason, taking time-release vitamin B_6 tablets for 3 to 5 days before the start of menses will often cause enough diuresis of fluid buildup to be helpful. Vitamin B_6 should not be taken continuously as toxic levels can occur that cause neuropathy.

All herbs should be approved by the health care provider as they may interfere with other medications the patient is taking. Herbs that have been found to help prevent or alleviate migraine headache are:

- Feverfew
- Willow
- Bay
- Ginger
- Lemon balm
- Purslane
- Red pepper

A supplement that is beneficial for some patients in preventing migraine headaches is vitamin B_2 400 mg/day.

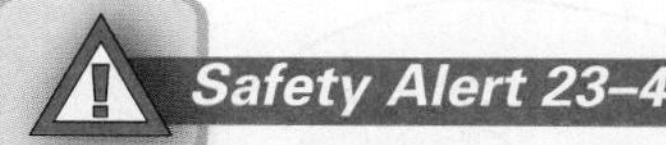

Safety Alert 23–4

Caution When Taking Analgesics

Fiorinal should be avoided for long-term use as it contains a barbiturate and is habit forming. Drugs containing acetaminophen should be used within the dosage guidelines and not used daily as this drug can cause liver failure and impaired renal function. The guidelines are to refrain from taking more than 4 g of acetaminophen per 24 hours. Remind patients who take acetaminophen not to combine it with alcohol as doing so can cause liver damage in some people.

Those taking aspirin, ibuprofen, or a drug containing either should monitor themselves for peptic ulcer and gastric bleeding. Signs and symptoms to report are epigastric pain, dyspepsia, black stool, or vomiting of blood. Fatigue, headache, and dizziness may indicate anemia from a slow gastric bleed.

the back of the neck. The neurostimulator control is implanted on one side in the lowest part of the back. The stimulator impulse can be adjusted depending on the level of stimulation that blocks pain. It is hoped that the device will diminish pain perception and the person will be able to function normally again (Rush University, 2006).

CLUSTER HEADACHES

Cluster headaches occur more frequently in men, and are not as common as migraine headaches. A cluster headache causes the most severe headache pain. The pain is abrupt in onset and usually lasts 30 to 90 minutes. It may start during sleep. The headache may recur several times a day, and the clusters usually last 2 to 3 months. The cause and pathophysiology are not clearly known, but the trigeminal nerve is implicated. Vasodilation occurs, causing the headache. It is thought that the disorder may be caused by dysfunction of the biologic clock mechanisms of the hypothalamus. Alcohol can trigger this type of headache.

Signs and symptoms include severe unilateral orbital, supraorbital, or temporal pain along with one of the following: redness of the conjunctiva of the eye, tearing, nasal congestion, dripping nose, facial swelling, pupil constriction, or **ptosis** (drooping) of the eyelid. The person becomes restless and often paces the floor, and is sensitive to touch.

History usually is sufficient to diagnose a cluster headache, but CT scan, MRI, or magnetic resonance angiography may be performed to rule out tumor, aneurysm, or infection.

Treatment for cluster headache includes a combination of analgesic and 100% oxygen by face mask, sumatriptan succinate (Imitrex) and other triptans, internasal lidocaine 4% aqueous solution, transdermal clonidine, or dihydroergotamine mesylate (D.H.E. 45). Opiates are to be avoided as they can cause rebound headache (Safety Alert 23–4).

TENSION HEADACHES

Tension headaches are quite common, but are not as severe as migraine or cluster headaches. This type of headache usually involves the head along with neck stiffness and limitation of range of motion of the neck. Analgesic medication, muscle relaxants, tension-reducing medication or relaxation techniques, massage, yoga, and biofeedback are often helpful. Biofeedback can be very effective in preventing or averting headaches for many people.

CRANIAL NERVE DISORDERS

TRIGEMINAL NEURALGIA (TIC DOULOUREUX)

Etiology and Pathophysiology

Trigeminal neuralgia is a relatively rare facial pain syndrome. The cause of trigeminal neuralgia is not known, although it can be related to pressure on the nerve root by a tumor, or to a lesion of the blood vessels. Multiple sclerosis can be a factor. Often, no cause can be found and the disorder is considered idiopathic. This disorder most commonly affects people over age 60.

This disorder involves one or more branches of the fifth cranial (trigeminal) nerve. The three branches of this nerve are the ophthalmic, the mandibular, and the maxillary (Figure 23–11). In most cases of trigeminal neuralgia, the ophthalmic nerve is not involved. The mechanism of pain production is controversial. It may be due to increased afferent firing in the nerve or failure of inhibitory mechanisms.

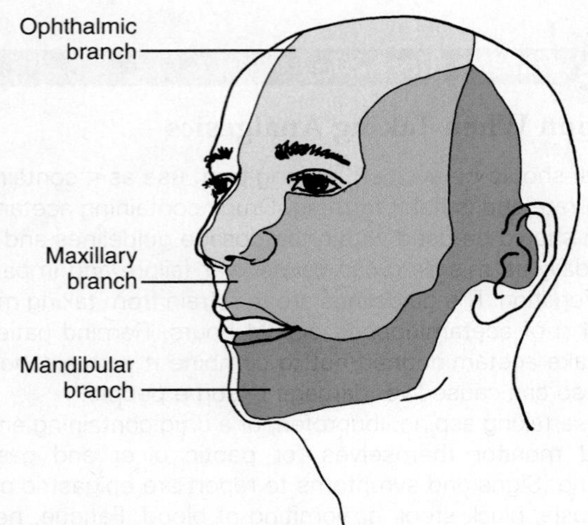

FIGURE 23–11 Areas of innervation by each of the three branches of the trigeminal nerve.

Signs, Symptoms, and Diagnosis

The most notable symptom of trigeminal neuralgia is severe facial pain, which is described as sharp and intense, lasting for 1 to 2 minutes, and located along the pathway of one of the branches of the trigeminal nerve. The pain is localized on one side of the face, rarely affecting both sides. It can extend from the midline of the face across the cheek and jaw to the ear.

Attacks are usually triggered by exposure to drafts, light touch or vibration, drinking cold or very hot liquids, chewing, brushing the hair, shaving, or washing the face. The pain causes a brief muscle spasm of the facial muscles—the tic. Between acute flare-ups the patient may experience no pain, or may report a dull ache. The pain during the acute phase is so severe that many patients live in constant fear they will do something to provoke an attack.

Diagnosis is based on the patient's history and chief complaint and tests to rule out a cerebellopontine angle tumor that is affecting the nerve. There is no test to confirm the diagnosis, and there are no observable pathologic changes.

Treatment

Medical management usually is preferred to surgical intervention, because the latter involves dissection of nerve rootlets with resultant loss of motor and sensory function.

The drugs most frequently prescribed to prevent or relieve spasmodic pain are the anticonvulsants carbamazepine (Tegretol) and phenytoin (Dilantin) and the muscle relaxant baclofen (Lioresal). Other anticonvulsants are effective in some patients. Relief of severe pain usually can be obtained by injecting glycerol into the terminal branch of the trigeminal nerve (glycerol rhizotomy).

NURSING MANAGEMENT

Assessment (Data Collection) and Nursing Diagnosis

Observing the patient between acute attacks can help identify clues to affirm the presence of trigeminal neuralgia. The patient may not want to wash his face or shave, and he will guard his face or hold it immobile to avoid an attack. He is very sensitive to any contact with his face and will indicate the area of pain by pointing to, but never touching, it.

The universal nursing diagnosis for patients with trigeminal neuralgia is, of course, pain. Because chewing can provoke an attack of pain, the patient may be susceptible to nutritional deficit. Small, frequent feedings consisting of food that is moderately warm can help provide adequate nutrition and at the same time avoid precipitating an acute attack.

Planning, Implementation, and Evaluation

Specific expected outcomes are written for the patient regarding the control of pain and its triggers. Nursing intervention for the patient who is being treated medically includes instruction about the expected actions and adverse side effects of the drug he is taking. Phenytoin can produce **ataxia,** skin eruptions, overgrowth of the gums, nystagmus, and Stevens-Johnson syndrome (a serious immune reaction). Carbamazepine can damage the bone marrow and produce such hematologic reactions as leukopenia, aplastic anemia, and decreased platelet count. Skin eruptions also can occur as a reaction to carbamazepine or baclofen. The patient's blood count and liver function must be closely monitored to detect early signs of drug toxicity. Baclofen may cause transient drowsiness, nausea, weakness, or fatigue.

Surgical treatment of trigeminal neuralgia brings about problems related to potential for damage to the cornea when the ophthalmic branch is dissected. The patient must be taught to avoid rubbing his eyes or exposing them to foreign objects because the normal protective corneal reflex is no longer functional. He should get into the habit of wearing protective goggles when there is the possibility of getting dust and debris in his eyes, and should try to blink his eyes often to cleanse their surfaces.

Dissection of the second or third branches of the trigeminal nerve produces problems of potential damage to the oral mucosa and teeth. The patient cannot feel hot liquids and foods and could be burned, could bite the inside of the mouth without realizing it, or may have dental caries that will not cause pain. Good oral hygiene and periodic dental examinations are particularly important when the body's natural warning system is not operative.

Evaluation data are gathered to see if the specific expected outcomes are being met.

BELL'S PALSY

Bell's palsy is weakness or paralysis of the muscles supplied by the facial nerve. It usually affects only one side of the face, and usually occurs in people over age 30. The disorder affects about 23 per 100,000 people and affects the right side of the face most often. The etiology of Bell's palsy is controversial. It is thought to be caused by edema and ischemia that compresses the facial nerve. The herpes simplex virus is thought to be a cause. Stress can be a factor also. Exposure to cold is a risk factor. Sometimes the disorder occurs during pregnancy, most often in the third trimester. **Signs and symptoms are numbness and partial or total paralysis of the facial muscles suddenly or over a few days.** There may be taste disturbances. The eyelid on the affected side loses its blink reflex and the mouth droops, causing problems with drooling.

Diagnosis is by history and exclusion of other neurologic or muscular disorders, and Lyme disease. If the patient is asked to raise the eyebrows, the eyebrow on the affected side will not move. When asked to smile, the face becomes distorted as the affected side of the mouth and face will not move normally.

Treatment consists of closing and patching the eye if it loses the blink reflex. Artificial tear eyedrops also are used to prevent dryness of the cornea. Corticosteroids are given if they can be started right after the beginning of symptoms. They are ineffective if delayed more than 7 days. Acyclovir may be prescribed as well, since herpesvirus may a causative organism (Grogan, 2001). Recovery is individual; some patients with total paralysis may not achieve full recovery but will improve as inflammation declines. Eighty percent to 90% of patients recover completely within 6 weeks to 3 months. Bell's palsy recurs in 10% to 15% of patients.

EB

Key Points

- Many conditions can cause a seizure. Epilepsy is a chronic condition in which abnormal electrical activity is triggered in the brain without an underlying metabolic cause.
- Seizures are classified as generalized or partial (see Box 23–1).
- Signs of seizure depend on the type and location of the seizure in the brain.
- Irreversible brain damage can occur if seizures are unrelenting and uncontrolled.
- Treatment of epilepsy is by drugs and/or surgery (see Box 23–2).
- Close observation of a seizure with documentation by the nurse is very helpful (see Focused Assessment 23–1).
- Patient education is extremely important for safety and for the prevention of recurrent seizures.
- A cerebrovascular accident is caused by a thrombus, embolus, or an intracranial hemorrhage that interrupts circulation to an area of the brain.
- Risk factors for stroke are high blood pressure, atherosclerosis, cigarette smoking, excessive alcohol intake, insufficient exercise, high cholesterol, obesity, and diabetes.
- t-PA must be given within 3 hours of the onset of symptoms to be effective for thrombotic stroke.
- Cerebral aneurysms and arteriovenous malformations may leak or burst and cause a stroke.
- Subarachnoid hemorrhage is a medical emergency.
- People should be encouraged to seek medical help immediately if signs of a stroke are experienced.
- A thrombosis causes cerebral ischemia that progresses slowly; an embolus causes sudden neurologic deficits.
- Homonymous hemianopsia, hemiplegia or hemiparesis, agnosia, apraxia, aphasia, and dysphagia are some of the problems caused by a CVA.
- Fatigue and emotional lability with crying or outburst may be common after a stroke or other injury to the brain, depending on the area of the brain involved.
- Hydrocephalus may be a complication of several disorders of the brain; a shunt can be placed to divert the excess CSF to the peritoneal cavity (see Figure 23–9).
- Rehabilitation for the stroke patient is extremely important and takes extensive work.
- Brain tumors may be benign or malignant; many are metastatic from a different malignant site (see Table 23–2).
- Brain tumors compress adjacent tissue, causing problems and increased ICP.
- Some common signs of brain tumors are personality change, disturbance in judgment and memory, loss of muscular strength and coordination, and difficulty speaking clearly. Headache, projectile vomiting, visual problems, and signs of increased ICP may be present.
- Depending on the site and type of brain tumor, treatment is by surgery, radiation, and/or chemotherapy.
- Viral and bacterial infections cause the inflammation of the membranes covering the brain and spinal cord in meningitis.
- Severe and persistent headache with nuchal rigidity are classic signs of meningitis, but a spinal tap is needed for diagnosis.
- Meningitis causes an increase in ICP.
- Encephalitis is most often the result of a viral infection or the toxins produced by viral organisms such as measles, chickenpox, and mumps.
- West Nile virus is a cause of encephalitis and is spread by mosquitoes
- Stiff neck, photophobia, and lethargy are classic symptoms of encephalitis.
- Nursing care is geared toward the problems of seizures, high fever, and delirium of altered LOC (see Table 21–9).
- A brain abscess can develop from a severe sinus, ear, or tooth or gum infection.
- Headaches are very common, and approximately 23 million Americans suffer from migraine headaches.

- Tracking triggers for migraine, avoiding them, and taking medication helps prevent migraine attacks (see Nutritional Therapies 23–2, Box 23–3).
- Migraine headaches most often cause pain on one side of the head.
- Migraine is often preceded by an aura.
- Cluster headaches cause severe pain and tend to be periodic in nature.
- Trigeminal neuralgia is a painful disorder affecting the fifth cranial nerve and the muscles of the face. Only one side of the face is usually affected.
- The patient is taught to avoid pain triggers in trigeminal neuralgia.
- Bell's palsy is thought to be caused by edema and ischemia that compress the facial nerve. It causes weakness or paralysis of the muscles supplied by the nerve.
- Numbness and partial or total paralysis of the facial muscles, usually on one side, occurs with Bell's palsy.
- Corticosteroids and acyclovir are the drugs used to treat Bell's palsy.

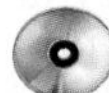

Go to your **Companion CD-ROM** for an Audio Glossary, animations, video clips, and bonus review questions.

evolve Be sure to visit the companion Evolve site at http://evolve.elsevier.com/deWit for interactive NCLEX-PN Exam Style Review Questions, WebLinks, and additional online resources.

NCLEX-PN EXAM STYLE REVIEW QUESTIONS

Choose the best answer(s) for the following questions.

1. A 25 year-old patient is admitted for "drop attacks" characterized by the loss of muscle tone. The patient recalls nodding, feeling weakness in the knees, and falling. A likely condition would be:

1. malingering.
2. atonic seizure.
3. tonic-clonic seizure
4. petit mal seizure.

2. The nurse determines that the appropriate nursing diagnosis for a patient with status epilepticus would be "Risk for injury related to seizure activity." An appropriate expected outcome would be:

1. everyone will stay calm during the episodes.
2. the caregiver will stay with the patient during the episodes.
3. the patient will be free from any injuries associated with the seizures.
4. standing orders will be obtained to medicate acute seizure episodes.

3. Nursing care of a patient who just had a seizure includes which of the following nursing interventions? *(Select all that apply.)*

1. Assess for injuries.
2. Check the glucose level.
3. Reassure and reorient patient.
4. Provide uninterrupted periods of sleep and rest.
5. Provide a 24-hour sitter.

4. Which of the following patient statements indicates a need for further teaching regarding the prevention of injuries associated with seizures?

1. "I need to avoid situations that could potentially trigger a seizure."
2. "Alcohol can counter the effects of my seizure medications."
3. "I must carefully evaluate my work schedule and social obligations."
4. "I am less likely to have seizures during menstruation."

5. The ________________ is a tangled mass of malformed, thin-walled, dilated blood vessels that form a connection between arterial and venous systems.

6. The nurse assesses the readiness for transfer to another level of care of a patient who had a cerebrovascular accident. The patient continues to have agnosia and apraxia. These clinical findings indicate that the patient would:

1. require assistance with undertaking activities of daily living.
2. demonstrate independence in performing ordinary tasks.
3. prompt self to complete sequential tasks.
4. understand verbal communication.

7. An appropriate nursing intervention for a patient with homonymous hemianopsia includes which of the following:

1. consider bold print editions.
2. turn the head to scan both sides.
3. avoid bright lights.
4. wear prescription glasses.

8. A 21-year-old male patient complains of a sudden onset of fever, severe headache, and stiffness of the neck. The nurse notes a petechial rash over the chest and extremities. The following nursing actions are appropriate *except for:*

1. instituting Standard Precautions and droplet precautions.
2. administering antibiotics.
3. maintaining a quite and dimly lit patient room.
4. encouraging increased physical activity.

9. A patient is admitted to the urgent care center for complaints of an abrupt onset of severe headache. Clinical history indicates that symptoms started during sleep and recurred several times during the day. These symptoms suggest:

1. hangover.
2. migraine.
3. cluster headaches.
4. tension headaches.

10. The nurse providing care to a 60-year-old Chinese patient with trigeminal neuralgia identifies that pain is the priority nursing diagnosis. Effective pain management would be:

1. assessing the level of pain based on facial expressions.
2. initiating patient-controlled analgesia.
3. place warm cloth on face.
4. anticipating request for pain medications.

CRITICAL THINKING ACTIVITIES

Read each clinical scenario and discuss the questions with your classmates.

Scenario A

Jack Thompson, age 36, suffered a seizure while walking down the hall at work. He fell to the ground and demonstrated jerking motions of his body.

1. What type of seizure is this most likely to be?
2. What observations should be made if he has another seizure?
3. How would you care for Mr. Thompson after the seizure is over?
4. If Mr. Thompson is diagnosed with epilepsy, what patient teaching will he need?

Scenario B

Mr. Foster is a 77-year-old retired teacher who complained of a severe headache during dinner and then slumped over the table, unconscious. He was rushed to the hospital, and a tentative diagnosis of cardiovascular accident (CVA) was made.

1. What diagnostic tests might be appropriate for Mr. Foster?
2. What emergency care could you have given Mr. Foster if you had been present at dinner?

Mr. Foster's diagnostic tests indicate a subarachnoid hemorrhage from a ruptured aneurysm. He is comatose; his pupils are equal and reactive to light; and he responds to pain with decorticate posturing, opens his eyes at random, and seems to be paralyzed on the right side.

3. What are the priorities of care for Mr. Foster?
4. If Mr. Foster survives, what potential complications might he experience if he has had an intracerebral hemorrhage?

Scenario C

Janice Pringle, age 19, has been experiencing headaches more frequently over the past 6 months. She comes to the student health center on her college campus to seek help. This headache is really bad and she is nauseated.

1. What subjective and objective assessment data would you gather regarding this young lady and her headaches?
2. What are your priorities of care for Janice?
3. What interventions would you suggest at this time?

CHAPTER 24

Care of Patients with Degenerative Neurologic Disorders

evolve http://evolve.elsevier.com/deWit

Objectives

Upon completion of this chapter you should be able to:

Theory

1. Compare and contrast the pathophysiology of Parkinson's disease and myasthenia gravis.
2. Discuss treatments for Parkinson's disease.
3. Describe the nursing care needed for the patient with Parkinson's disease.
4. Explain why multiple sclerosis might be difficult to diagnose.
5. Devise a home care plan for the patient with multiple sclerosis.
6. Compile a nursing care plan for the patient with Guillain-Barré syndrome.
7. Identify the differences between Huntington's disease and amyotrophic lateral sclerosis.
8. Illustrate the signs and symptoms of myasthenia gravis.
9. Compare and contrast the complications of Parkinson's disease with those of myasthenia gravis.

Clinical Practice

1. Teach a newly diagnosed patient about the medications for Parkinson's disease.
2. Teach a patient about the diagnostic tests that might be ordered if multiple sclerosis is suspected.
3. Write a nursing care plan for the myasthenia gravis patient who is hospitalized with a respiratory infection.

Key Terms

Be sure to check out the bonus material on the Companion CD-ROM, including selected audio pronunciations.

bradykinesia (brā-dē-kĭ-NĒ-zē-ă, p. 593)
chorea (kă-RĒ-ă, p. 605)
demyelination (dē-MĪ-ē-lĭ-nā-shŭn, p. 598)
diplopia (dĭ-PLŌ-pē-ă, p. 605)
hyperesthesia (hī-pĕr-ĕs-THĒ-zē-ă, p. 603)
Lhermitte's sign (lăr-mētz sīn, p. 599)

PARKINSON'S DISEASE

Parkinson's disease (PD) is named after James Parkinson, who first described the syndrome in 1871. It is a degenerative disorder with symptoms that are neurologic in nature and become progressively more incapacitating. It has sometimes been called "shaking palsy," because the outstanding manifestation is a tremor or involuntary motion of the muscles.

PD is considered a major health problem because of its crippling effects. It is a progressive disorder, beginning rapidly at first and then advancing more slowly. It affects more men than women and occurs most frequently after age 60. One million people in the United States are affected with PD, and 1 in every 100 people over age 60 has this disease.

Etiology

The specific cause of PD is unknown, but it involves degeneration of the dopamine-producing neurons in the substantia nigra of the midbrain. Genetic susceptibility and environmental toxins appear to play a role. The most common type of PD is *idiopathic*, that is, the primary or specific cause is not known. The syndrome can be drug induced, especially by reserpine-type antihypertensives such as methyldopa, phenothiazines, some tranquilizers such as the butyrophenones (e.g., haloperidol [Haldol]), some antiemetics, methamphetamine, and a few other drugs. These drugs block the uptake of dopamine at the receptors in the brain cells. Pesticide exposure is also implicated as a cause of PD.

Pathophysiology

PD is a disorder of the extrapyramidal system, in particular the motor structures in the basal ganglia. This is the part of the brain that controls balance and coordination. The basal ganglia are gray matter that is scattered throughout the white matter of the cerebrum beneath the cerebral cortex. Stimulation of the basal ganglia causes muscle tone in the body to be inhibited and promotes refined voluntary movements. Two neurotransmitters accomplish this action: dopamine and acetylcholine (ACh) (see Table 21–4 for the action of the common neurotransmitters). ACh-producing neurons transmit

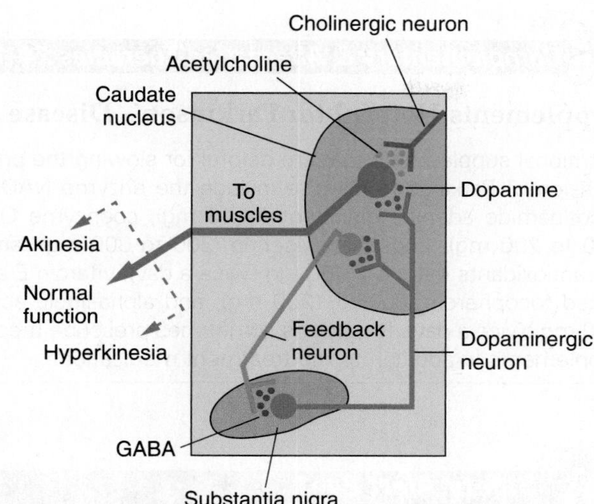

FIGURE **24–1** Dopaminergic synaptic activity is mediated by dopamine. Cholinergic synaptic activity is mediated by acetylcholine. A balance between the two kinds of activity produces normal motor function. A relative excess of cholinergic activity produces akinesia and rigidity. A relative excess of dopaminergic activity produces involuntary movements.

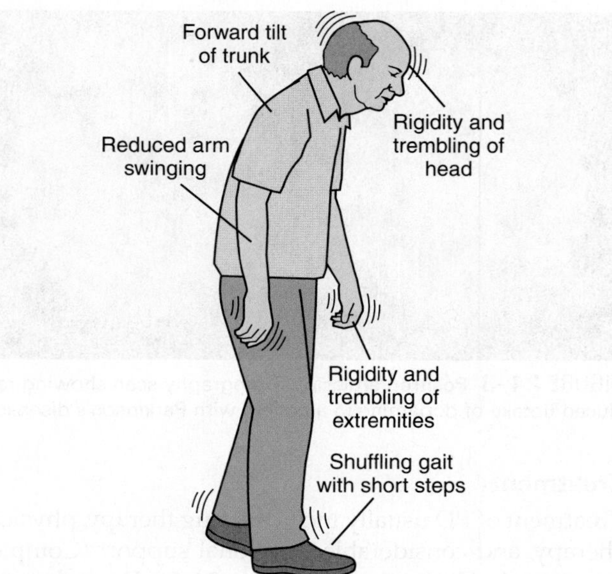

FIGURE **24–2** Parkinson's disease causes abnormalities of movement. Movements are jerky in nature.

excitatory messages throughout the basal ganglia. Dopamine inhibits the function of these neurons so that there can be control of voluntary movement (Figure 24–1). There is usually a balance between these neurotransmitters. The degenerative changes in the basal ganglia lead to a decrease in dopamine. The ACh-secreting neurons remain active, creating an imbalance between excitatory and inhibitory neuronal activity. The excessive excitation of neurons prevents a person from controlling or initiating voluntary movements.

Signs and Symptoms

The onset is gradual and may involve only one side of the body initially. A triad of symptoms are characteristic of PD: tremor, bradykinesia, and rigidity. The first, *tremor,* occurs when the body is at rest, decreases when there is voluntary movement, and is absent when the patient is asleep. The tremor is most often a "pill-rolling" motion of the thumb against the fingers. This is when there is a circular rubbing of a finger or two as if rolling a piece of string or fuzz into a "pill." If the patient suffers stress and emotional tension, the tremor becomes more pronounced.

Bradykinesia (condition exhibiting slow movement and speech) produces poor body balance, a characteristic gait, and difficulty initiating movement. The gait is shuffling, with short steps that become quicker (Figure 24–2). There is decreased swinging of the arms when walking. A foot may drag or may be stiff, producing a limp. In advanced stages there is a stiff, bent-forward posture when walking. Earlier in the disease process, the patient may lean slightly to one side, propel forward uncontrollably, or fall backward.

The third symptom is *rigidity* affecting the skeletal muscles and contributing to postural changes and difficulty in movement. Postural changes affect coordination and balance. The face becomes blank or masklike in appearance with little or no expression. Speech becomes low in tone, monotonous sounding, and slow; enunciation becomes difficult due to the decreased dopamine and the excitatory response from the increased acetylcholine. Drooling may occur. The patient may experience decreased tearing, constipation, incontinence, excessive perspiration, heat intolerance, and decreased sexual ability. PD does not usually affect intellect; however, a percentage of patients do develop a dementia similar to that of Alzheimer's disease. Mood disturbance does occur, and depression is a problem. Stress tends to make symptoms worse.

? *Think Critically About . . .* A patient comes into the clinic complaining about hand tremors and "stiffness" of the joints that started recently, excessive sweating, and some urinary incontinence. You notice that her gait is abnormal. What would be a priority question you would ask her as you start history taking?

Diagnosis

The characteristic symptoms of the disease are used to diagnose the disorder. Laboratory tests usually reveal findings within normal ranges. However, magnetic resonance imaging (MRI) scans of the brain may be performed to rule out other neurologic disorders. Positron emission tomography can display the reduced uptake of dopamine (Figure 24–3).

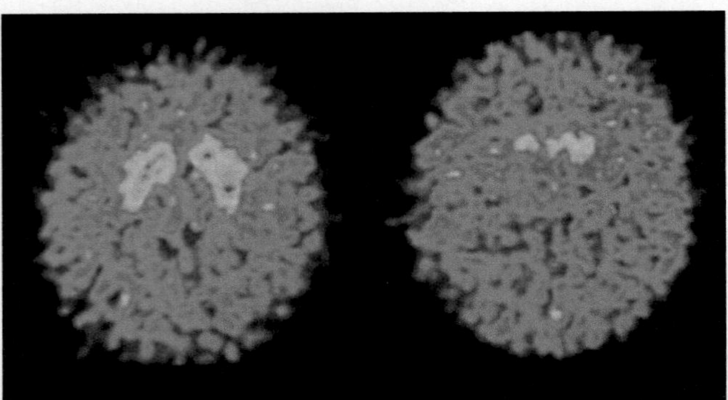

FIGURE **24–3** Positron emission tomography scan showing reduced uptake of dopamine in a patient with Parkinson's disease.

Treatment

Treatment of PD usually includes drug therapy, physical therapy, and considerable emotional support (Complementary & Alternative Therapies 24–1). Drug therapy aims to provide dopamine to the basal ganglia and thus reduce symptoms. Anticholinergics, dopamine agonists, and monoamine oxidase inhibitor (MAOI) drugs are used to control symptoms. MAOIs block the metabolism of dopamine. In the early stages of the disease when disability is not evident, selegiline (Eldepryl), a drug that increases dopamine's action, may be given (Safety Alert 24–1). When disability is present, L-dioxyphenylalanine (L-dopa, or levodopa) or a combination of levodopa and carbidopa (Sinemet) is given. Sinemet is given in increasing doses until control of the symptoms is achieved. It is not without side effects, however. Other drugs used either along with L-dopa or sometimes alone to treat early stages of PD or to minimize the side effects of L-dopa are presented in Table 24–1. The antihistamine diphenhydramine (Benadryl) may be added for its anticholinergic effects and may help with insomnia.

Think Critically About . . . What would be appropriate nursing interventions for the patient who is beginning to experience dysphagia?

Surgical Treatment. Stereotactic neurosurgery may be done if the drug therapy fails. In one such procedure the area in the thalamus that is causing the involuntary movements is destroyed. Microsurgical procedures such as pallidotomy improve rigidity and bradykinesia (Agency for Healthcare Research and Quality, 2003).

Other procedures with some success in relieving symptoms include transplanting tissue from the adrenal medulla into the brain, or implanting fetal tissue or stem cells. Fetal substantia nigra tissue is transplanted into the caudate nucleus of the brain. This is still experimental, but the procedure has shown substantial clinical improvements in motor function (National Institutes of Health, 2006). Stem cell implantation done in various ways has shown some promising results. There is much controversy about using stem cells because of the issues related to abortions and stored human embryos from which fetal stem cells can be obtained.

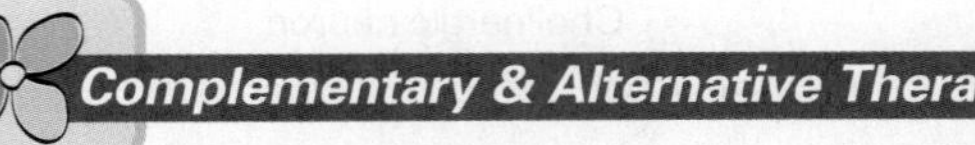

Supplements Helpful for Parkinson's Disease

Nutritional supplements that are helpful for slowing the progression of Parkinson's disease include the enzyme NADH (nicotinamide adenine dinucleotide; 10 mg), coenzyme Q_{10} (100 to 200 mg), phosphatidylserine (200 to 300 mg), and the antioxidants ester-C (1000 mg twice a day), vitamin E as mixed tocopherols (800 to 1200 mg), and alpha-lipoic acid (100 mg twice a day). Physicians sometimes prescribe these supplements in addition to the treatment medications.

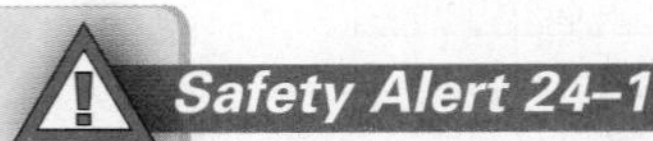

Caution When Administering MAOIs

When a patient with Parkinson's disease has been prescribed selegiline, a monoamine oxidase inhibitor (MAOI), caution her against eating foods containing tyramine such as aged cheeses, anything fermented, smoked fish or meat, yeast extract, some imported beers, Chianti wine, dietary protein supplements, and soy sauce. Giving meperidine to someone taking an MAOI can cause *hyperpyrexia* (excessive elevation of temperature) and possible death. Many drugs interact adversely with MAOIs, and the health care provider or pharmacist should be consulted before taking any other drug with an MAOI.

Deep brain stimulation (DBS) uses electrode implants that control tremors by constant electrical shocks that block them. The device can be adjusted as the patient's symptoms change or worsen (National Institute of Neurological Diseases and Stroke, 2007). There has been considerable success with DBS, but it is expensive at $10,000 for the unit and another $8000 every few years for battery replacement.

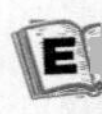

Depression is frequent in Parkinson's patients, but most respond well to a selective serotonin reuptake inhibitor (SSRI) antidepressant.

Complications

Swallowing may become difficult, and dysphagia develops (Assignment Considerations 24–1). Mobility becomes severely limited as the disease progresses. Problems of immobility occur (see Chapter 9). Constipation, urinary incontinence, and insomnia may develop.

NURSING MANAGEMENT

Assessment (Data Collection) and Nursing Diagnosis

A thorough history is gathered and a physical examination is performed for the patient who has or is thought to possibly have PD. Focused Assessment 24–1 presents the points to cover.

Table 24–1 Drugs Commonly Used for Patients with Parkinson's Disease

DRUG CLASSIFICATION	USE
ANTIPARKINSONIAN/ADRENERGICS	
Levodopa (L-dopa) Levodopa-carbidopa (Sinemet) Bromocriptine mesylate (Parlodel) Pergolide (Permax) Pramipexole (Mirapex) Ropinirole (Requip) Apomorphine (Apokyn)	Decrease presence of tremor, rigidity, and bradykinesia and improve motor function.
ANTIVIRAL	
Amantadine (Symmetrel)	Decrease presence of rigidity, bradykinesia.
ANTICHOLINERGICS	
Trihexyphenidyl (Artane) Biperiden (Akineton) Benztropine (Cogentin)	Decrease tremor.
MONOAMINE OXIDASE INHIBITOR	
Selegiline (Eldepryl, Carbex) Rasagiline (Azilect)	Decrease presence of tremor, rigidity, and bradykinesia, and improve motor function.
CATECHOL-*O*-METHYLTRANSFERASE (COMT) INHIBITOR	
Tolcapone (Tasmar) Entacapone (Comtan)	Slow the breakdown of dopamine, thereby prolonging the action of levodopa.

MAJOR NURSING IMPLICATIONS

When giving a drug for Parkinson's disease:

- Pay close attention to dosage amount as therapy is individualized to each patient.
- Check other medications patient is receiving to see if there may be interactions with the antiparkinsonian drug, contraindicating administration of the drug.
- Administer the drugs as close to the time ordered as possible to maintain a consistent blood level of each drug.
- Carbidopa-levodopa may cause many neurologic disturbances, including psychiatric problems; discuss any onset of new symptoms that occur with the physician.
- Administer anticholinergic medications with meals to decrease gastrointestinal irritation.
- Selegiline may increase the side effects of carbidopa-levodopa. If this occurs, seek an order to decrease the dosage.
- Monitor for effectiveness of each drug by observing for a decrease in Parkinson's symptoms, such as tremor, rigidity, or drooling; assess for decrease in side effects of carbidopa-levodopa when anticholinergic drugs are given for that purpose.
- Continually assess the patient for worsening of symptoms that may be due to disease progression, side effects of medication, or failure of medication.

Regarding possible side/adverse effects of the drug:

- Monitor patients taking carbidopa-levodopa, amantadine, bromocriptine, or pergolide for orthostatic hypotension and urinary retention.
- Assess patients who are taking carbidopa-levodopa for excessive or inappropriate sexual behavior.
- Bromocriptine may cause changes in mental status; report observed changes.
- Amantadine and pergolide may cause insomnia and should not be administered at bedtime.
- Many of these drugs can cause nausea, dyspepsia, and abdominal pain.
- Anticholinergics are contraindicated in patients with acute narrow angle glaucoma.
- Anticholinergics cause dry mouth and constipation; increase fluids to 3000 mL/day; treat constipation as needed per orders; add fiber to diet.
- Monitor blood pressure and pulse during initiation and adjustment of anticholinergic medication; report tachycardia.
- Consult pharmacology book or drug insert for specific side effects of each particular drug.

Teach the patient taking antiparkinsonian drugs:

- Selegiline may cause dizziness; warn patient to move cautiously during initiation of therapy.
- Orthostatic hypotension causes dizziness and can precipitate falls; it is important to allow the blood pressure to stabilize in a sitting position before standing, to rise slowly and stabilize while holding on to something when standing before walking.
- Carbidopa-levodopa will turn the urine dark.
- Ropinirole (Requip) may cause drowsiness; advise patient not to operate machinery or drive until adjusted to the drug.
- When taking a COMT inhibitor, it is important to have liver function checked regularly.
- Constipation is a problem with the anticholinergic drugs; increases in dietary fiber, plenty of fluid, and exercise can help control constipation; bowel movement frequency should be monitored to prevent impaction.
- Adjustment of dosages and combination of medications that will control symptoms with the fewest of side effects may take weeks or months to accomplish.

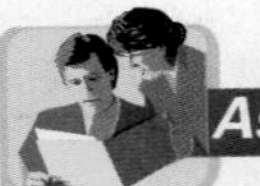

Assignment Considerations 24–1

Feeding the Dysphagic Patient

Unlicensed assistive personnel (UAPs) should not be assigned to feed the dysphagic patient if at all possible. If an aide must be used to help feed a patient with dysphagia, be certain that suction is turned on and at hand and that the aide has been trained in helping a dysphagic patient to eat. Remind the UAP that the patient should be positioned as upright as possible, to give small bites, to wait for that bite to be swallowed before offering another one, and not to rush the patient. Coaching the patient to drop the chin when swallowing helps prevent choking.

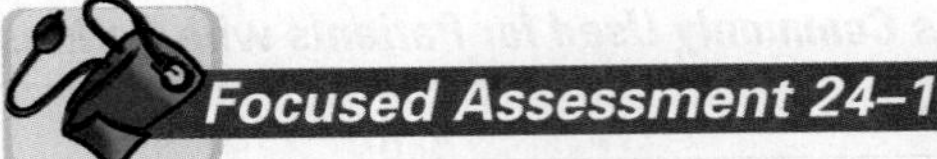

Focused Assessment 24–1

Data Collection for the Patient with Parkinson's Symptoms

Gather subjective data regarding history by asking the following questions:

- Have you ever had a head injury, meningitis, encephalitis, or cerebrovascular disorder?
- Have you ever been exposed to metals, pesticides, or carbon monoxide for extended periods?
- What medications do you take? (Particularly important are major tranquilizers such as haloperidol [Haldol], phenothiazines, reserpine, methyldopa, and amphetamines.)
- Do you have a problem with fatigue?
- Have you noticed excessive salivation and problems handling secretions?
- Do you have any trouble swallowing?
- Have you been steadily losing weight?
- Do you suffer with constipation or urinary incontinence?
- Do you sweat excessively?
- Do you have difficulty initiating walking or other movements? Do you fall frequently?
- Has your dexterity decreased? Has your handwriting deteriorated?
- Do you have insomnia?
- Do you experience pain or cramping?
- Do you have mood swings? Are you depressed? Do you have hallucinations?

Points to cover with physical examination:

- Presence of drooling
- Ability to swallow
- Facial expression or lack thereof
- Presence of ankle edema
- Evidence of postural hypotension
- Presence of tremor at rest; pill-rolling movements
- Rigidity of body and jerky movements of extremities
- Slow start, then quick short steps when ambulating; shuffling gait with bent-forward posture
- Difficulty stopping once ambulating

Nursing Care Plan 24–1 contains the common nursing diagnoses, expected outcomes, and specific interventions for the patient with PD.

Planning, Implementation, and Evaluation

Nursing care focuses on preventing complications of PD, drug therapy, enhancing voluntary movement, and safety. Constipation is a problem and requires the addition of fiber to the diet and an increase in fluids to at least 3000 mL per 24 hours. Grasping coins or other objects may help decrease tremors because it is an intentional action. Walking may be improved by having the patient think about imaginary lines across the pathway on which to walk. Imagining stepping over something helps prevent "freezing" when walking (Patient Teaching 24–1, p. 599). An exercise program is instituted by the physical therapist to maintain muscle function and promote joint mobility. Teach the patient to consciously assume correct posture. Not using a pillow when resting helps prevent flexion of the spine. Learning to sleep prone also is beneficial for posture correction.

Remember that the PD patient needs extra time to finish tasks. A warming tray can be used to keep food hot during meals so that the patient can take rest periods while eating. Considerable patience and understanding are necessary to help the patient deal with the frustration of deteriorating body control and inability to do things that she formerly could easily do. Degeneration of cognitive skills occurs in the late stages of PD.

Falls are common, and safety is a major factor. Using a cane or walker will increase stability and decrease the incidence of falls. Leg braces or foot braces often are helpful to maintain balance. Loose carpets should be removed from the home, and grab bars in the shower and tub, and a raised toilet seat should be installed. Patients with tremor must be cautioned against carrying hot liquids as spills may cause burns. The section on Common Care Problems in Chapter 21 discusses measures to help with the problems typical of many neurologic disorders. Patient and family teaching is an important part of nursing care for patients with PD.

Evaluation includes gathering data about the results of the interventions implemented. Next, determine if the expected outcomes are being met. If progress toward the outcomes is not occurring, then the plan needs to be revised.

MULTIPLE SCLEROSIS

Etiology

Multiple sclerosis (MS) is a chronic inflammatory disease causing demyelination in the central nervous system. The most common type of MS is characterized by periods of remission and exacerbation. Another type is progressive without remission periods. The cause of MS is not known, but it is thought that an environmental factor (bacteria, virus, or chemical) combined with a genetic predisposition for the disease is responsible.

NURSING CARE PLAN 24–1

Care of the Patient with Parkinson's Disease

SCENARIO A 63-year-old man is admitted to your unit because of increasing incidence of falling. He is diagnosed with Parkinson's disease. He is beginning to have trouble swallowing and his speech has slowed. Has slight tremor in left hand and upper extremity.

PROBLEM/NURSING DIAGNOSIS *Has trouble swallowing*/Imbalanced nutrition: less than body requirements related to dysphagia.

Supporting assessment data *Subjective:* "I can't chew and swallow very well." *Objective:* Difficulty chewing; difficulty getting food to go down.

Goals/Expected Outcomes	Nursing Interventions	Selected Rationale	Evaluation
Patient will not aspirate food Patient will maintain satisfactory body weight	Monitor swallowing during drug administration and meals to assess degree of swallowing difficulty.	Allows assessment of swallowing ability.	Swallowing pills one by one without problem. No choking or difficulty during meal as long as eats slowly.
	Keep suction equipment at hand to remove pooled secretions and prevent aspiration; turn on before meal.	Readies suction and allows removal of secretions.	Suction on and at hand during meals.
	Maintain upright position for drug administration and meals.	Gravity helps food go down to the stomach, and helps prevent aspiration.	Sitting fully upright for medications and meals.
	Provide semisoft and thickened liquids for diet.	Semisoft foods and thickened liquids are easier to swallow.	Has a semisoft diet. Thickener used for liquids.
	Consult speech therapist about swallowing difficulties.	Speech therapist can evaluate swallowing ability and make recommendations.	Speech therapy consult ordered.
	Consult dietitian for dietary recommendations.	Dietitian can design a diet that provides sufficient calories and is easy for the patient to eat.	Dietitian consulted with patient.

PROBLEM/NURSING DIAGNOSIS *Repeated falls*/Impaired physical mobility related to abnormal posture, rigidity, bradykinesia, and difficulty in initiating movements.

Supporting assessment data *Subjective:* "I seem to have trouble with balance. I've fallen four times this month." *Objective:* Rigidity of joints, jerky movements, shuffling gait, stooped posture.

Goals/Expected Outcomes	Nursing Interventions	Selected Rationale	Evaluation
Patient will ambulate safely Patient will maintain joint mobility and muscle strength	Physical therapist to work with patient on joint mobility, muscle strengthening, and ambulation.	Physical therapy helps to decrease rigidity and muscle weakness.	Physical therapist is working with the patient. Patient is performing prescribed exercises with spouse's help.
	Administer antiparkinsonian medication as ordered. Monitor for side effects and effectiveness of medication.	Decreases tremor, rigidity, and bradykinesia.	Receiving ordered medications with no signs of side effects as yet. Rigidity slightly improved.
	Cane or walker provided if necessary.	Assistive device promotes safety.	Using walker when ambulating.
	Teach to perform active ROM exercises bid.	Techniques improve gait and movement.	Performing ROM exercises bid.
	Teach to walk as if over an imaginary line and to rock back and forth to initiate movement.		Physical therapist is coaching the patient in how to walk.

Key: *bid*, twice daily; *ROM*, range-of-motion.

Continued

NURSING CARE PLAN 24–1

Care of the Patient with Parkinson's Disease—cont'd

PROBLEM/NURSING DIAGNOSIS *Having difficulty with swallowing; decreased appetite*/Risk for imbalanced nutrition related to eating difficulties.

Supporting assessment data *Subjective:* "I haven't had much appetite lately and I've choked on food a few times." *Objective:* Slight drooling, weight down 4 lb this month.

Goals/Expected Outcomes	Nursing Interventions	Selected Rationale	Evaluation
Patient will not aspirate food	Obtain consult with speech therapist for swallowing studies.	Detects dysphagia.	Consult with the speech therapist is ordered.
Patient will maintain present weight	Reinforce teaching regarding methods to be used for swallowing.	Various maneuvers can assist with correct swallowing and prevent choking.	Teaching plan is in place and teaching is ongoing.
	Offer six small meals per day.		Offering between-meal small snacks.
	Serve hot meals on warming tray and do not rush patient with eating.	Keeps food warm while patient rests during meal.	Reheating food as needed during meal.
	Offer nutritional supplements between meals if needed.		Taking a protein shake in the afternoon.
	Administer anticholinergic medication as ordered.	Decreases drooling.	Medication is showing effect in decreased drooling.
	Monitor for side effects and effectiveness of medication; observe for urinary retention.	Identifies side effects patient experiences.	No urinary retention or other side effect as yet.
	Increase fiber intake and increase fluids to 3000 mL/day to prevent constipation.		Drank 2800 mL today. Fiber in diet increased.

? CRITICAL THINKING QUESTIONS

1. What are the side effects of Sinemet?
2. What would you suggest be done around the house to help prevent falls?

There are four clinical progressions of MS: (1) relapsing-remitting, (2) primary progressive, (3) secondary progressive, and (4) relapsing-progressive (Table 24–2). There is no cure. The disease appears mostly in people of northern European ancestry. It affects females more frequently than males. Symptoms most often appear between 15 and 50 years of age, but can occur at any age. A genetic factor may be involved as the disease is sometimes seen in more than one family member. There are about 350,000 people in the United States with MS, and every year approximately 10,000 people are diagnosed.

Pathophysiology

Currently it is thought that a viral illness causes an autoimmune reaction that produces antibodies against central nervous system myelin. T cells become reactive to a single myelin protein. Myelin, the protective sheath around the axons that transmits electrical impulses from one neuron to the next, acts as a thick, protective insulator allowing impulse transmission along the nerves. Plaques form along the myelin sheath, causing inflammation. When myelin is eroded by inflammation and replaced by scar tissue **(demyelination),** nerve impulses cannot travel along the damaged neurons (Figure 24–4). Thus the muscles served by the affected nerves do not receive the impulses they need to perform in a well-coordinated and useful manner. When inflammation subsides, some remyelination occurs, but it is often incomplete and nerve transmission is not normal.

Signs and Symptoms

Clinical signs and symptoms reflect the pathologic changes that occur as a result of inflammation and subsequent scarring of myelin covering the nerves. The disorder typically follows a course of unpredictable flare-ups that are followed by periods of partial or complete remission. The very nature of the disease affects a patient's life in terms of ability to make a living, maintain satisfying interpersonal relationships with family and friends, and maintain a positive self-image.

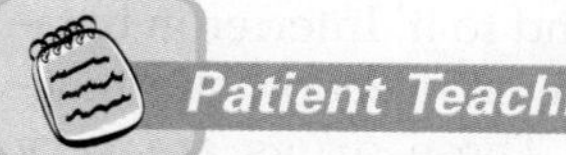

Patient Teaching 24–1

Parkinson's Disease

The following points should be covered in teaching the patient with Parkinson's disease how to cope with the illness. Keep teaching lessons short to prevent excessive fatigue.

MEDICATIONS

- How to take them per a written schedule.
- Purpose of each medication.
- What side effects to expect and what reactions to report.

DIET AND EATING

- Eat smaller, frequent meals.
- How to keep food warm while eating.
- Add more fiber to the diet to prevent constipation.
- Increase fluids to help prevent constipation.
- When attempting to swallow, keep lips closed and teeth together; put food on the tongue, lift the tongue up and back, and then swallow.
- Eat slowly and take small bites.

MOVEMENT AND EXERCISE

- Exercise and stretch regularly to prevent rigidity and contractures.
- Exercise in the morning when energy levels are higher.
- Wear good, sturdy shoes.
- Avoid soft, deep chairs; to get up from a chair, bend over slowly so that your head is over your toes.
- If bradykinesia is present, rock back and forth to begin walking.
- Use a cane or walker if balance is unsteady.
- Concentrate on standing upright.
- Imagine that you are stepping over a series of imaginary lines when walking.
- Count to yourself while walking.
- Visualize your intended movement.
- To calm tremor of the hands, hold change in your pocket or squeeze a small rubber ball.

FOR EXCESSIVE SALIVATION

- Make a conscious effort to swallow saliva frequently.
- Keep the head in an upright position so saliva will collect in the back of the throat and stimulate the swallowing reflex.
- Swallow excess saliva before speaking.

Adapted from Black, J.M., & Hawks, J.H. (2005). *Medical-Surgical Nursing: Clinical Management for Positive Outcomes* (7th ed.). Philadelphia: Elsevier Saunders, p. 2174.

Table 24–2 ***The Four Clinical Progressions of Multiple Sclerosis***

TYPE OF PROGRESSION	CHARACTERISTICS AND CLINICAL COURSE
Relapsing-remitting (most common type)	Clearly defined relapses of acute worsening neurologic function. Partial or complete recovery occurs in remission period.
Primary progressive	Slow but almost continuous worsening with occasional plateaus and temporary minor improvements.
Secondary progressive	Initial period of relapsing-remitting disease followed by a steadily worsening course. May or may not have occasional relapses, minor remissions, or plateaus.
Relapsing-progressive	Disease steadily worsens from onset, but there are clear acute relapses with or without recovery. Disease progresses between relapses.

The more common manifestations of MS are as follows:

- *Motor dysfunction* can include weakness or paralysis of limbs, trunk, and neck; diplopia caused by oculomotor weakness; and spasticity of the muscles.
- *Sensory dysfunction* may include numbness, tingling, burning, and painful sensations; patchy or total blindness or blurring of vision in one or both eyes; dizziness; ringing in the ears and hearing loss; and **Lhermitte's sign** (a sensation like an electric shock down the spine when the neck is flexed).
- *Problems of coordination* include ataxia, intention tremor of limbs and eyes, slurring of speech, and dysphagia.
- *Mental changes* usually are limited to depression and cognitive problems such as impaired judgment, decreased ability to solve problems, and memory loss.
- *Fatigue* is a characteristic of MS and is worsened by heat (e.g., a hot shower or hot weather).
- Other problems that occur late in the disease are related to urinary and bowel incontinence and altered sexual function: loss of male and female self-esteem, physical impotence in the male, and diminished sensation in the female.

The neuromuscular dysfunctions characteristic of MS are unique to each person and can vary greatly from time to time in the same person.

Diagnosis

No laboratory test will definitively establish a diagnosis of MS, although most patients have elevated immunoglobulin G (IgG) levels in their cerebrospinal fluid (CSF), with the presence of oligoclonal bands

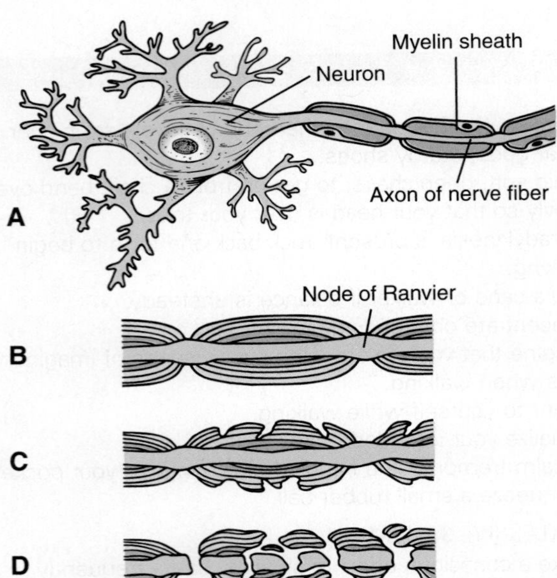

FIGURE 24–4 Effects of multiple sclerosis. **A,** Normal nerve cell with myelin sheath. **B,** Normal axon. **C,** Myelin breakdown. **D,** Myelin totally disrupted; axon not functioning.

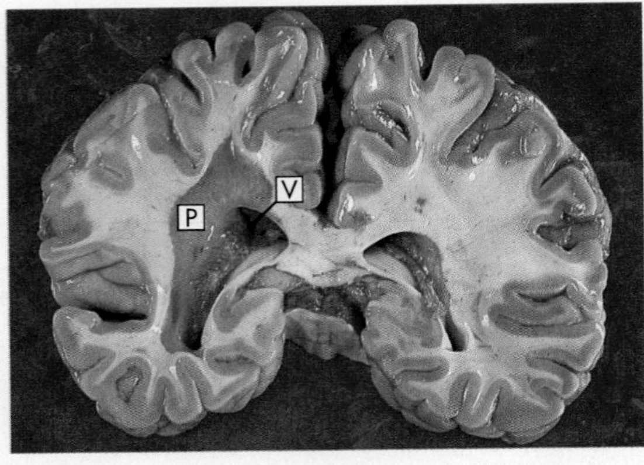

FIGURE 24–5 Chronic multiple sclerosis. Demyelination plaque *(P)* at gray-white matter junction and adjacent partially remyelinated shadow plaque *(V)*.

(bands of IgG produced by electrophoresis of the CSF). An MRI study usually shows characteristic white matter lesions scattered through the spinal cord and/or brain, which confirms the diagnosis of MS (Figure 24–5). However, the clinical signs and symptoms presented by a patient usually are sufficiently characteristic of the disorder to allow the neurologist to make a diagnosis that the patient possibly or probably has MS. The clinical manifestations of the disease reflect the extent to which inflammation and scarring of the myelin have occurred.

Treatment

One of the biologic response modifier drugs, such as interferon beta-1b (Betaseron), is effective for many ambulatory patients with relapsing-remitting MS. It is given by injection. It reduces MS attacks by one third and decreases the number of severe attacks. It is not a cure, and not all patients respond to it. Interferon beta-1a (Avonex, Biogen) causes fewer injection site reactions than interferon beta-1b. These drugs are very expensive and are used for preventive treatment. Acute attacks are treated with intravenous (IV) methylprednisolone for 5 days followed by oral prednisone in tapering doses. Adrenocorticotropic hormone (ACTH) may be given for its ability to suppress immune system activity (Table 24–3). Most therapeutic efforts are centered on supportive measures to maintain resistance to infection, reduce muscle spasticity, and manage specific symptoms, such as diplopia, speech disorders, muscle weakness, fatigue, and depression. The drug regimen is geared to each patient's symptoms.

An exercise program is very beneficial for the MS patient to relieve spasticity and improve coordination (Rietbert, 2005). Swimming provides considerable benefits as exercising in water is less fatiguing than exercising out of water. Because of fatigue, it is often difficult to convince MS patients to exercise.

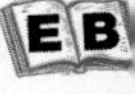

In addition, the patient should be provided the support and physical and psychological means necessary to develop a positive and hopeful outlook. A positive and affirming mental attitude can have beneficial physiologic and biologic effects on the MS patient. There is an understandable tendency to become depressed and pessimistic about the future when confronted with the realities of muscle weakness, incontinence, sexual impotence, and any combination of disabilities likely to be experienced during the course of MS.

NURSING MANAGEMENT

Assessment (Data Collection), Nursing Diagnosis, and Planning

A careful history can provide many clues to the possibility that the patient has MS. Testing extremity strength, looking for visual problems, and checking reflexes are part of the physical examination.

Nursing diagnoses are based on the assessment findings and may include:

- Fatigue related to improper transmission of neural impulses
- Impaired physical mobility related to muscle weakness, spasticity, or paresthesias
- Self-care deficit related to muscle spasticity and neuromuscular deficits
- Reflex urinary incontinence related to sensory motor deficits
- Sexual dysfunction related to neuromuscular deficits
- Risk for impaired skin integrity related to immobility
- Interrupted family processes related to potential financial problems, changing roles, and fluctuating physical abilities
- Ineffective coping related to loss of usual abilities and roles

Table 24–3 Drugs Commonly Used for Patients with Multiple Sclerosis

DRUG	SYMPTOMS RELIEVED	SIDE EFFECTS AND PRECAUTIONS	PATIENT TEACHING
CORTICOSTEROIDS			
ACTH, prednisone, methylprednisolone	Exacerbations	Edema, mental changes (euphoria), weight gain, redistribution of body fat*; widespread effects on many metabolic processes; few adverse effects with use for less than 1 mo at a time	Restrict salt intake. Do not abruptly stop therapy. Know drug interactions.
IMMUNOMODULATORS			
Interferon beta (Betaseron, Avonex, Rebif)	Exacerbations	Flulike symptoms, local skin reactions, depression; monitor CBC, blood chemistries, and liver function tests every 3 mo	Perform self-injection techniques. Report side effects.
Glatiramer acetate (Copaxone)	Exacerbations	Local skin reactions; chest pain, weakness; no laboratory monitoring required	Perform self-injection techniques. Report side effects.
IMMUNOSUPPRESSANTS			
Mitoxantrone (Novantrone)	Exacerbations	Nausea, vomiting, diarrhea, mucositis, alopecia, hepatotoxicity, myelosuppression, cardiovascular disease; lifetime dose limit because of cardiotoxicity; monitor CBC and liver function every month	Receive regular monitoring and follow-up. Consult health care provider before getting immunizations. Be aware that urine may turn a blue-green color initially. Maintain adequate fluid intake.
MONOCLONAL ANTIBODY			
Natalizumab (Tysabri)	Lessens complications, slows vision loss	Arthralgia, UTI, diarrhea, depression, fatigue, headache and progressive multifocal leukoencephalopathy	Observe for side effects regularly. May increase risk of infection in combination with corticosteroids and other immunosuppressants.
CHOLINERGICS			
Bethanechol (Urecholine) Neostigmine (Prostigmin)	Urinary retention (flaccid bladder)	Hypotension, diarrhea, diaphoresis, muscle weakness; history of cardiac dysfunction, hypotension, allergies, peptic ulcer disease, asthma	Consult with health care provider before using other drugs, including over-the-counter drugs.
ANTICHOLINERGICS			
Propantheline (Pro-Banthine) Oxybutynin (Ditropan)	Urinary frequency† and urgency (spastic bladder)	Dry mouth, blurred vision, constipation, hypertension, flushing, urinary retention (too high a dose); contraindicated with history of glaucoma, prostatic hyperplasia, cardiac dysfunction, intestinal obstruction	Consult health care provider before using other drugs, especially sleeping aids, or antihistamines (possibly leading to potentiated effect).
MUSCLE RELAXANTS			
Diazepam (Valium)	Spasticity	Drowsiness, ataxia, fatigue; contraindicated with history of narrow-angle glaucoma	Avoid driving and similar activities because of CNS depressant effects. Be aware of additive potential. Avoid long-term use. Avoid concomitant use of barbiturates, MAO inhibitors, or antidepressants.
Baclofen (Lioresal)	Spasticity	Drowsiness, weakness; use cautiously with a history of hypersensitivity and renal damage; possible exacerbation of seizures in patients with seizure disorders	Do not abruptly stop therapy (possibility of hallucinations). Avoid driving and similar activities because of sedative effects. Avoid use of other CNS depressants. Take with food or milk.

Key: *ACTH,* adrenocorticotropic hormone; *CBC,* complete blood count; *CNS,* central nervous system; *MAO,* monoamine oxidase; *UTI,* urinary tract infection.
*See Chapter 36 for effects of long-term corticosteroid therapy.
†Urodynamic studies must be done before initiation of therapy because patients with multiple sclerosis have multiple lesions, and type of bladder dysfunction cannot be diagnosed from symptoms alone.
Adapted from Lewis, S.M., Heitkemper, M.M., Dirksen, S.R., et al. (2007). *Medical-Surgical Nursing: Assessment and Management of Clinical Problems* (7th ed.). St. Louis: Mosby, pp. 1544–1545.

Continued

Table 24–3 Drugs Commonly Used for Patients with Multiple Sclerosis—cont'd

DRUG	SYMPTOMS RELIEVED	SIDE EFFECTS AND PRECAUTIONS	PATIENT TEACHING
MUSCLE RELAXANTS—cont'd			
Dantrolene (Dantrium)	Spasticity	Drowsiness, dizziness, malaise, fatigue, diarrhea; used cautiously in patients with a history of respiratory or cardiac dysfunction; risk of hepatotoxicity	Avoid driving when drug is used. Avoid use with tranquilizers and alcohol (possibly causing photosensitivity). Obtain baseline liver function tests.
Tizanidine (Zanaflex)	Spasticity	Drowsiness, dry mouth, fatigue, nausea; use cautiously in patients with history of hypersensitivity, liver or renal disease, hypotension, or bradycardia	Avoid driving when drug is given. Avoid use with tranquilizers and alcohol (possibly causing photosensitivity). Eat small, frequent meals to reduce nausea. Change position slowly when going from lying or sitting position to standing.

Expected outcomes are written for each nursing diagnosis specific to the individual's problems.

Implementation and Evaluation

Appropriate care for the patient with MS depends on the severity of the disease and the symptoms. Care is individualized for each patient. During the diagnostic phase, the patient and family need a great deal of emotional support, as most patients realize that there is no cure.

Ongoing care focuses on safety, prevention of complications, assistance with physical therapy, and emotional support. The patient should not be exposed to excessive heat or hot baths, as this causes weakness to become much worse (Multiple Sclerosis Association of America, 2007). Care of the common problems of the neurologic patient is covered in Chapter 21. The importance of proper nutrition with adequate fluids and fiber in the diet should be stressed to maintain proper bowel function and decrease the likelihood of urinary tract infections. Calcium and vitamin D should be included in the diet to help prevent osteoporosis that may result from the IV steroid treatments. Medications to decrease stomach acid and prevent ulceration from the steroids are administered (histamine [H_2]-receptor blockers or proton pump inhibitors).

Help the patient and family establish a consistent daily routine that will promote optimum levels of functioning for the patient. The routine should include daily physical exercise balanced by rest periods to prevent fatigue.

Patient teaching involves:

- Education about the unpredictability of the disease and the need to avoid stress, infections, and fatigue to maintain independence as long as possible
- Referral to the National Multiple Sclerosis Society and local support groups. (Additional information and local sources of help for the patient with MS and the family can be obtained from the Internet at www.nmss.org or by writing to the National Multiple Sclerosis Society, 733 Third Avenue, New York, NY 10017.)

Evaluation of care is based on whether the expected outcomes are being achieved. If they are not, then the plan is revised.

ALZHEIMER'S DISEASE

Alzheimer's disease, a form of dementia due to pathologic changes in the brain tissue of the patient, is covered in Chapter 47. Unfortunately the specific diagnostic changes can be detected only at autopsy. The cause of Alzheimer's disease is unknown, and considerable research is in progress to better define this disease. It can occur during middle age or during the later decades of life and causes devastation to the patient and family. The disease has a slow onset, progresses at varying rates of speed through several stages, and is eventually fatal.

AMYOTROPHIC LATERAL SCLEROSIS

Etiology and Pathophysiology

Amyotrophic lateral sclerosis (ALS), also called *Lou Gehrig's disease,* is a progressive neuromuscular disease characterized by degeneration of the gray matter in the anterior horns of the spinal cord and the lower cranial nerves. Electrical and chemical messages generated in the brain cannot reach the muscles to activate them. Approximately 5 per 100,000 people have ALS. It most often occurs in people between the ages of 40 and 70 years and equally affects men and women. Although some people with ALS can survive for many years, the disease usually progresses rapidly, producing a prognosis of death within about 3 years of the onset of symptoms.

Signs and Symptoms

One of the first clinical manifestations of ALS is weakness of the voluntary muscles, especially of the distal muscles of the extremities. Some patients may notice difficulty swallowing and speaking clearly because of oropharyngeal weakness. As the disease progresses, there is atrophy of the muscles. Until atrophy is complete, however, there may be spontaneous contractions or spasticity of the muscles and abnormal sensations *(paresthesias)*, such as tingling or prickling. The patient also may report pain, which is probably caused by undue strain on weakened muscles.

Only the motor neurons are affected in ALS; therefore, the patient remains mentally alert and does not have sensory impairment. Mental depression is relatively common as a result of the unrelenting progression of muscle weakness and atrophy. Death is usually due to respiratory infection and dysfunction as weakness and atrophy of the respiratory muscles impede normal respiration and mechanisms to clear bacteria and secretions from the lungs.

Diagnosis and Treatment

There is no laboratory test to confirm a diagnosis of ALS; electromyelography in combination with muscle biopsy provide data for positive diagnosis. Other neuromuscular disorders such as MS, myasthenia gravis, and progressive muscular dystrophy must be ruled out.

There is no cure for ALS. Eventually the muscle paralysis renders the patient totally dependent because of inability to move, swallow, speak, and, ultimately, breathe. The drug riluzole (Rilutek), a glutamate antagonist, has been shown to slow the progression in patients in whom nerve degeneration began in the medulla (National Institute of Neurological Diseases and Stroke, 2006). Eventually impaired breathing requires a tracheostomy and mechanical ventilation.

Nursing Management

During the first contact with the ALS patient, conduct a thorough neurologic assessment. As the disease progresses, periodic assessments can identify specific needs. Nursing diagnoses likely to be associated with ALS are those related to difficulty with respiration, all problems of immobility, dysphagia, impaired ability to communicate, pain, ineffective coping, and depression.

In the latter stages of ALS, the patient and family will need more assistance and guidance to maintain some level of independence and comfort for the patient. Rehabilitation includes obtaining equipment and devices such as a walker, wheelchair, hospital bed, suction machine, and nasogastric or gastrostomy tube feeding supplies.

Because of the nature of the disease, issues related to terminal illness, death, and the grieving process are likely to be present (see Chapter 8). The services of a visiting nurse or a hospice program can provide appropriate instruction and physical and emotional support.

GUILLAIN-BARRÉ SYNDROME

Etiology and Pathophysiology

Guillain-Barré syndrome (GBS) is a relatively rare disease that affects the peripheral nervous system, especially the spinal nerves outside the spinal cord. It also can affect the cranial nerves. The cause of GBS is not known, but it usually follows a viral respiratory infection or gastroenteritis in adults within 10 to 21 days. There have been a few cases of Guillain-Barré syndrome in recipients of meningococcal conjugate vaccine (Centers for Disease Control and Prevention, 2006). Authorities believe that the disease is a cell-mediated immunologic response preceded by stimulation from a viral infection, trauma, surgery, viral immunizations, HIV, or neoplasm of the lymphatic system. Cytomegalovirus and Epstein-Barr virus are two viruses that have been linked to GBS.

Pathologic changes include demyelination, inflammation, edema, and nerve root compression. These changes bring about the paresthesia, pain, and progressive, ascending paralysis typical of the syndrome. Autonomic nervous system dysfunction with alterations in both sympathetic and parasympathetic systems may occur, causing orthostatic hypotension, hypertension, abnormal vagal responses, bowel and bladder dysfunctions, facial flushing, and diaphoresis. When the lower brainstem becomes involved, the cranial nerves are affected.

Signs and Symptoms

Objective and subjective symptoms of GBS include mild sensations of numbness and tingling in the feet and hands, followed by muscle pain, tenderness, and aching, especially in the shoulder, pelvis, and thighs. There is progressive muscle weakness, usually starting in the lower extremities and moving upward over 24 to 72 hours. However, it also can affect the cranial nerves and facial muscles first and move downward. Symptoms peak in about 14 days. Sensory loss can also occur, but is not as common as motor loss. If respiratory function is affected, ventilatory support may be needed.

Pain is common and may be evidenced as paresthesias, muscular aches and cramps, and **hyperesthesia** (abnormal sensitivity to stimuli). Pain often is worse at night when there is less distraction in the environment.

Diagnosis

Diagnosing GBS is difficult because its characteristic signs and symptoms are similar to those of several other diseases. Analysis of the CSF is helpful. Typically there is an elevated CSF protein content that tends to rise as the disease progresses, peaking in 4 to 6 weeks. The number of leukocytes remains within normal limits, as does CSF pressure. Electromyelography and nerve conduction studies show reduced conduction velocity. For the most part, the physician must depend on the clinical picture presented by the patient to diagnose GBS.

Treatment

Medical treatment is mainly supportive. Within the first 2 weeks, plasmapheresis, in which the patient's plasma is removed and "washed" to remove antibodies, hastens recovery in some patients and decreases the time ventilatory support is needed (see Chapter 16). The use of IV immune globulin to hasten recovery is also effective (Hughes, 2007).

Nutritional support via tube feedings may be required due to dysphagia. If paralytic ileus occurs, parenteral nutrition will be necessary.

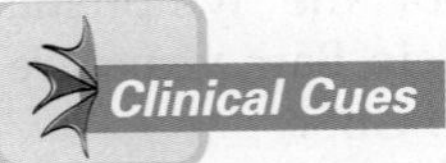

Signs and symptoms of paralytic ileus are absence of bowel sounds, abdominal pain, and considerable abdominal bloating with lack of passage of stool.

NURSING MANAGEMENT

Assessment (Data Collection), Nursing Diagnosis, and Planning

Assessment is the most important aspect of care during the acute stage. Monitor progression of ascending paralysis, assess respiratory function carefully, and assess gag, corneal, and swallowing reflexes closely. Monitor arterial blood gases and oxygen saturation. Observing vital sign trends and watching for orthostatic hypotension and cardiac dysrhythmia can indicate the degree of autonomic nervous system dysfunction.

Nursing diagnoses depend on the degree of nervous system involvement, but may include:

- Impaired spontaneous ventilation related to disease progression affecting respiratory nerves
- Impaired physical mobility related to paralysis of muscles by disease progression
- Risk for aspiration related to dysphagia
- Imbalanced nutrition: less than body requirements related to dysphagia and inability to feed self
- Acute pain related to paresthesias, muscle aches and cramps, and hyperesthesias
- Self-care deficit related to inability to use muscles to accomplish activities of daily living
- Fear related to seriousness of disease and unknown outcome
- Impaired verbal communication related to paralysis of speech muscles or intubation

Expected outcomes must be written for each nursing diagnosis. Overall goals of care are:

- Maintain adequate ventilation.
- Control pain adequately.
- Prevent damage from aspiration.
- Maintain communication.
- Maintain adequate nutritional status.
- Return patient to normal function.

Implementation and Evaluation

There are three phases of GBS: the acute phase, the static phase, and rehabilitation phase. Each demands different kinds of monitoring and intervention. During the *acute* phase, the goals are to sustain life, prevent complications related to immobility, and promote rest and comfort. Respiratory problems are particularly troublesome and may require suctioning, tracheostomy care, artificial ventilation, and other life-support measures.

Vital signs must be checked frequently. Alterations in the autonomic nervous system can cause drastic changes in blood pressure, particularly hypotension. Cardiac arrhythmias also frequently occur, and the patient is continuously monitored.

The paralysis and loss of control that take place with GBS come on so suddenly and are so overwhelming that the patient becomes very frightened. Because the course of the disease usually extends for months with a very slow recovery, the patient begins to have feelings of hopelessness, despair, and isolation. If the respiratory muscles are affected, the patient will be intubated and placed on mechanical ventilation.

The *static* phase is a kind of plateau the patient reaches 1 to 3 weeks after the onset of the illness. During this time the motor loss and paresthesias no longer progress, and the patient's condition becomes somewhat stabilized; she gets no better or no worse. This phase can last from a few days to months.

***Think Critically About* . . .** What problems requiring specific nursing interventions would you expect to encounter for the patient with Guillain-Barré syndrome who is now stable but has paralysis of the lower extremities and paresis of the upper extremities?

During the static phase, nursing care is concentrated on preventing complications of immobility and helping the patient deal with her feelings of anger, depression, and anxiety. Exercises are usually begun, but are limited to passive and gentle range-of-motion and stretching exercises. There must be a balance of rest and exercise and no sudden changes in posture or position, in case blood pressure suddenly drops.

Meticulous skin care is essential because of immobility. Monitoring for thrombophlebitis is important, as this is a frequent complication. Elastic stockings or sequential compression devices are applied to the legs, along with anticoagulant therapy, to try to prevent thrombophlebitis.

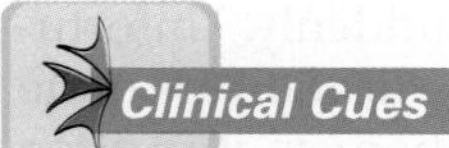

Signs of thrombophlebitis are warmth, swelling, and pain in the extremity and a positive Homans' sign. Temperature may be elevated.

The final phase, *rehabilitation,* is one of gradual recovery. The patient may become elated over the change in her condition and must be prevented from overexertion, which can lead to a relapse. As muscle function returns, the level of exercise and activity is slowly increased (Carroll et al., 2003). It may take up to 2 years for maximal improvement with return to normal functioning. Approximately 80% to 90% of patients have little residual deficit.

POLIOMYELITIS AND POSTPOLIO SYNDROME

Poliomyelitis destroys the motor cells of the anterior horn of the spinal cord, the brainstem, and the motor strip located in the frontal lobe. It is caused by a virus and can be prevented by immunization with the Salk (killed-virus) or Sabin (attenuated live-virus) polio vaccine. It is rare in the United States as immunization is given in childhood, but outbreaks still occur in other parts of the world. *It is mentioned here because some people who had poliomyelitis have developed postpolio sequelae or postpolio syndrome.* A new onset of weakness, pain, and fatigue occurs in people who had the disease over 30 years ago. Disability may be temporary or permanent. Treatment is geared toward making lifestyle modifications to preserve energy and physiologic function. Swimming in warm water has been found to promote comfort and help maintain flexibility.

HUNTINGTON'S DISEASE

Huntington's disease or Huntington's chorea is a rare genetically transmitted degenerative neurologic disorder characterized by abnormal movements **(chorea).** It is accompanied by a decline in intellectual capacity and emotional disturbances. Signs of Huntington's disease usually become evident during the fourth or fifth decade of life, but may occur earlier. Women and men are equally affected. The disorder is progressive and causes disability and then death within 15 to 20 years after signs appear. Death is from neurologic degeneration affecting all body systems. Genetic transmission is by an abnormal gene on the short arm of chromosome 4. It is an autosomal dominant disorder, meaning that 50% of the children of a person who has the disease will inherit it. If a child does not inherit the disease, the gene is not passed on to the next generation.

The person progresses from being fidgety and restless to a state of constant movement. There is no specific test for the disease, and there is no known treatment to alter its course. Voluntary movement deteriorates until the patient is totally helpless. Intellectual decline causes depression, suspiciousness, and eventual dementia.

MYASTHENIA GRAVIS

Etiology and Pathophysiology

The words *myasthenia gravis* literally mean "grave muscle weakness." The disease is a chronic disorder manifested by fatigue and exhaustion that are aggravated by activity and relieved by rest. The muscular weakness can be so mild that it causes a minor inconvenience or so severe that it is life-threatening because of its effect on the muscles used for breathing and swallowing.

Myasthenia gravis is an autoimmune disease in which circulating autoantibody is directed against the postsynaptic acetylcholine (ACh) receptors at the neuromuscular junction (the point at which nerve impulses are transmitted to muscle tissue). The antibody reduces the number of functional receptor sites, restricts the neuron uptake of ACh, and thereby interferes with total neural stimulation of the muscle, which in turn produces muscle weakness.

Signs and Symptoms

Symptoms of myasthenia gravis include **diplopia** (double vision), difficulty chewing and swallowing, and ptosis (Figure 24–6). The patient's voice tends to be hoarse or nasal in quality, and volume decreases toward the end of a sentence. **Severe muscle weakness that improves with rest is the outstanding symptom of the disorder.** Any of the skeletal muscles might be involved; intestine, bladder, and heart muscles are not affected.

Ocular myasthenia may occur first and be demonstrated by diplopia and ptosis. In a small percentage of patients the disease progresses no further. If cranial nerves become more involved, bulbar myasthenia occurs with facial and oropharyngeal muscle weakness causing a blank facial expression and a smile resembling a snarl. Swallowing and speaking become difficult. Further progression to generalized myasthenia involves the muscles of the neck, shoulders, limbs,

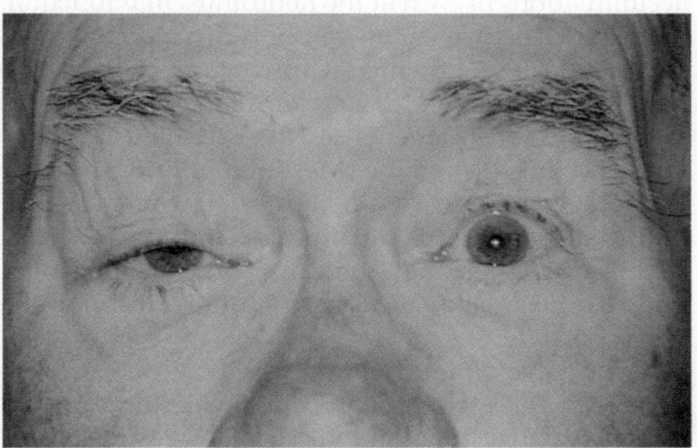

FIGURE 24–6 Ptosis (drooping upper lid) characteristic of the muscle weakness of myasthenia gravis.

hands, diaphragm, and abdomen. The disease does not affect the level of consciousness. Muscles are strongest in the morning and become weaker with activity. Respiratory muscle weakness may require mechanical ventilation.

Diagnosis

Diagnosis is established by history and physical. A Tensilon test may be ordered to confirm the diagnosis. Two divided injections of edrophonium (Tensilon) are administered; a marked increase in muscular strength is noted within 1 minute of the second injection if the patient has myasthenia gravis. The first injection is a test dose to see if the patient will have an adverse reaction to the medication. Atropine is kept on hand to reverse the effects of the Tensilon if necessary. A blood test for antibodies to ACh receptors may also be ordered.

Treatment

There are two main modes of therapy, the choice depending on the severity of the symptoms. In milder cases the physician may manage the disease by dealing with the specific symptoms, rather than trying to induce a remission of the disease. In more severe cases, efforts are made to manage the underlying cause of the symptoms by inducing remission.

Because 80% to 90% of myasthenia gravis patients have autoantibodies against ACh receptors, plasmapheresis can be an effective treatment for the patient in crisis. It is particularly helpful in restoring muscle function when the patient is dependent on a ventilator. The purpose of the plasma exchange is to remove the circulating autoantibodies from the patient's blood (see Chapter 16). This mode of therapy may bring clinical improvement in some patients, but it is not a cure for myasthenia gravis.

Anticholinesterase therapy is the earliest form of treatment for myasthenia gravis. Acetylcholine must be present at the point where nerve impulses are transmitted to muscle for sustained repetitive muscle contraction to occur. Anticholinesterase agents inactivate acetylcholinesterase, a substance that prevents accumulations of ACh at the neuromuscular junction. Anticholinesterase agents temporarily increase muscle strength by allowing ACh to work, but they do not cure the problem. Two drugs commonly used as anticholinesterase agents are neostigmine (Prostigmin) and pyridostigmine (Mestinon). Pyridostigmine is more commonly used because it can be taken orally. Corticosteroids and immunosuppressant drugs such as azathioprine (Imuran) and cyclophosphamide (Cytoxan) may be used to suppress the immune response.

The dosage of anticholinesterase drugs is precisely calculated for each patient. The aim is to achieve a delicate balance between too much and too little ACh at the neuromuscular junction. Stress can quickly alter a patient's need for ACh; hence overmedication or undermedication can occur rather suddenly. Unfortunately, the symptoms of too much medication are quite similar to those of too little medication, so it is often difficult to adjust the dosage correctly.

Another method of treatment is to remove the thymus gland, which decreases the antibody production (Kaiser, 2006). Treatment with IV immune globulin (IVIG) for 5 days may produce a favorable response for 30 to 60 days. 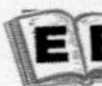

NURSING MANAGEMENT

Assessment (Data Collection), Nursing Diagnosis, and Planning

The severity of myasthenia gravis is assessed by asking about the degree of fatigue, what body parts are affected, and how severe the problem is. Knowledge of the disorder should be determined, and the patient's coping abilities assessed. Assessment of respiratory function is a top priority. Assess muscle strength of the face, swallowing, speech volume and clarity, and cough and gag reflexes. Check the strength of the shoulder muscles and of the limbs.

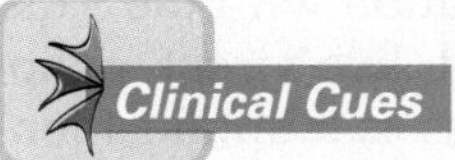

When assessing status of a myasthenia gravis patient, have the patient look up at the ceiling. Watch to see if the eyelids start to move downward. This is often an early sign of the disease or that the medication is insufficient.

Nursing diagnoses will depend on the severity of the disease and may include:

- Ineffective breathing pattern related to diaphragm and intercostal muscle weakness
- Ineffective airway clearance related to weakness of intercostal muscles, and impaired cough and gag reflexes
- Disturbed visual sensory perception related to ptosis and diplopia
- Imbalanced nutrition: less than body requirements related to impaired swallowing ability
- Activity intolerance related to fatigue and muscle weakness
- Impaired verbal communication related to intubation or weakness of larynx, mouth, and pharynx muscles
- Ineffective coping related to inability to maintain usual roles and lifestyle

Expected outcomes are written for each nursing diagnosis based on the specific problem the patient is experiencing.

Implementation and Evaluation

Infection, surgery, and other physical and emotional stresses can precipitate a myasthenic crisis and cause hospitalization. During the crisis, frequent monitor-

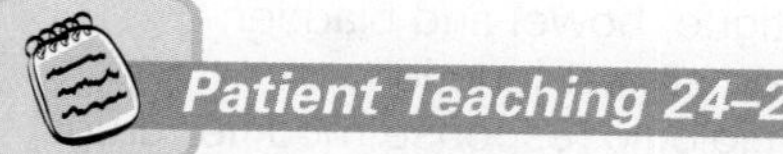

Patient Teaching 24–2

Teaching for the Patient with Myasthenia Gravis

- Use your anticholinesterase medication correctly:
  - Take the drug with food or fluid.
  - Take the drug 30 minutes before meals to permit maximum effect for chewing and swallowing.
  - Adjust drug dosage and times of administration as instructed according to your individual pattern of weakness and daily activities.
  - Do not take over-the-counter or other prescribed medications without the approval of your health care provider or pharmacist.
  - Report signs of cholinergic crisis to the health care provider quickly.
- Modify the diet for ease of chewing and swallowing; soft foods are easier to consume.
- Eat slowly in a calm environment and take small bites.
- Balance rest and activity throughout the day.
  - Figure out ways of doing usual activities that conserve energy.
  - Compensate with extra rest during periods of extra stress, illness, hormone swings during menstruation, and environmental temperature extremes.
- Wear a Medic Alert bracelet or necklace at all times; carry a card in your wallet stating that you have myasthenia gravis and list contact numbers for next of kin or significant other.
- Be aware of the signs and symptoms of myasthenic crisis and report them immediately.

ing is essential. The patient's ability to swallow and breathe on her own can be seriously compromised. Suctioning, tracheostomy, and artificial ventilation may be necessary to maintain life until the crisis is over.

Education of the patient and her family must include instruction about the nature of the illness and the adverse effects of emotional upsets, respiratory infections, and similar stresses (Patient Teaching 24–2). Care focuses on the neurologic deficits and their effect on daily activities. Rehabilitation goals include education and support for the patient and family so that the patient remains as independent as possible.

Because she can become critically ill and need immediate medical attention at any time, the patient with myasthenia gravis should at all times wear a Medic Alert emblem that identifies her as having the disease. The patient, as well as members of the family and the nurses who care for her in the hospital or at home, should know the symptoms of overdosage of anticholinesterase medication. The symptoms of myasthenic crisis caused by underdosage of anticholinesterase agents, a precipitating illness, or stress factors are equally important to know (Box 24–1). If any of these symptoms occurs, the physician should be notified immediately.

Box 24–1 *Signs and Symptoms of Cholinergic Crisis and Myasthenic Crisis*

The nurse, patient, and family should know these signs and symptoms:

SIGNS AND SYMPTOMS OF CHOLINERGIC CRISIS
- Generalized weakness within 1 hour of the dose
- Dyspnea and increased bronchial secretions
- Poor tongue control producing difficulty in chewing
- Difficulty swallowing and excessive salivation
- Restlessness, anxiety, and irritability
- Diaphoresis
- Abdominal cramps, nausea or vomiting, diarrhea

SIGNS AND SYMPTOMS OF MYASTHENIC CRISIS
- Increase in myasthenia gravis symptoms after failure to take drug as prescribed or following a precipitating illness or increased stress:
  - More difficulty swallowing
  - Diplopia
  - Ptosis
  - Dyspnea

Notify the physician immediately if these signs and symptoms appear.

Think Critically About . . . What immediate action would you take if you found your patient in cholinergic crisis?

In addition to being affected by problems arising from the anticholinesterase drugs, the myasthenic patient also can suffer from exaggerated and bizarre effects from a variety of drugs. These include the steroids and thyroid compounds; sedatives and respiratory depressants, such as morphine; tranquilizers, such as the phenothiazines; the mycin antibiotics; and some cardiac drugs, such as quinine and quinidine. Because so many drugs are potentially dangerous to a patient with myasthenia gravis, it is imperative that the nurse check with the physician ordering a medication to be sure there is awareness that the patient has myasthenia gravis. **Always check each drug the patient is to receive for interactions and contraindications.**

COMMUNITY CARE

After leaving the hospital, patients with neurologic problems often are cared for in long-term care facilities, rehabilitation programs, outpatient clinics, and the home. Nurses who work in long-term care facilities must be confident in caring for patients with PD, as a large percentage of residents in these facilities have this disorder. Because elderly patients often have more than one chronic illness, it is essential that you be knowledgeable about medication interactions and side effects. Each patient's medications must be continually assessed for possible adverse effects and side effects as well as for data indicating that each medication is producing a sufficient therapeutic effect to warrant continued administration. A close working relationship with the pharmacist can assist the nurse in judging these matters. Collaborative care between the pharmacist, nurse, nurse aides, physical therapist, social worker, and others who interact with the patient is needed to provide the best plan of care for these patients who require complex care.

The nurse who works with patients who have neurologic deficits that cause some degree of immobility must constantly try to prevent the complications of immobility and to achieve as high a level of function for the patient as possible. The home care nurse interacts with the entire family and needs to continually offer support as the difficulties of learning to live with someone who has a neurologic deficit are met. Family roles often are altered and strained, and the period of adjustment for the patient and family is lengthy. It often is difficult for the family to cope with the personality changes that occur in the patient who has a degenerative neurologic disorder. Referral to community support groups is often helpful for both the patient and the family members. The following agencies can provide materials, information, and support for patients with neurologic disorders. The local library or the Internet can provide current addresses and phone numbers of both national and local offices:

- American Parkinson Disease Association
- Guillain-Barré Syndrome International Foundation
- Myasthenia Gravis Foundation
- National Multiple Sclerosis Society
- National Parkinson Foundation

Key Points

- Parkinson's disease (PD) is a degenerative neurologic disorder affecting a million people in the United States.
- The characteristic triad of symptoms of PD is tremor, bradykinesia, and rigidity.
- Dysphagia is a complication of PD.
- Treatment of PD is with drug therapy, physical therapy, and emotional support (see Table 24–1).
- When drug therapy for PD fails, surgical treatment may be warranted.
- Multiple sclerosis (MS) is a chronic inflammatory disease causing demyelination of the myelin sheath in the central nervous system.
- Four types of clinical progression are seen in multiple sclerosis (see Table 24–2).
- Common manifestations of MS are motor dysfunction, sensory dysfunction, problems of coordination, mental changes, fatigue, bowel and bladder problems, and altered sexual function.
- MS is treated with biologic response modifier drugs and drugs to treat the problems caused by the disease.
- Alzheimer's disease is a form of dementia and is covered in Chapter 47.
- Amyotrophic lateral sclerosis (ALS) is a rare, but devastating disease that usually results in death within 3 years after diagnosis.
- ALS affects the motor neurons and causes weakness of the voluntary muscles.
- Nursing care for the ALS patient focuses on preventing complications and dealing with the problems the disease has caused, particularly immobility, dysphagia, inability to communicate, pain, and depression.
- Guillain-Barré syndrome (GBS) affects the peripheral nervous system and the cranial nerves.
- GBS is a cell-mediated immunologic response to a stimulus from a viral infection, trauma, surgery, viral immunization, HIV, or neoplasm of the lymphatic system.
- GBS usually causes an ascending paralysis and considerable pain.
- Nursing care for GBS is directed at maintaining adequate ventilation, nutrition, and supportive care for immobility and activities of daily living.
- Postpolio syndrome is the reappearance of polio symptoms 30 years after the initial polio illness.
- Huntington's disease (HD) is a genetic disease characterized by chorea.
- HD causes a decline in intellectual capacity, emotional disturbances, and total dependence, with death occurring in 15 to 20 years.
- Myasthenia gravis (MG) is an autoimmune disease affecting the neuromuscular junction.
- MG is chronic and is manifested by fatigue and muscular weakness that improves with rest.
- Ptosis, diplopia, a weak nasal-quality voice, a blank expression, and a smile resembling a snarl are signs and symptoms of MG.
- MG may affect the intercostal muscles and the diaphragm, causing inadequate respiration.
- Anticholinesterase therapy is the common treatment for MG.
- Many environmental situations and illnesses can cause the MG patient's condition to worsen.
- Nurses must know the signs of overdosage of anticholinesterase drugs.

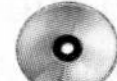
Go to your **Companion CD-ROM** for an Audio Glossary, animations, video clips, and bonus review questions.

evolve Be sure to visit the companion Evolve site at http://evolve.elsevier.com/deWit for interactive NCLEX-PN Exam Style Review Questions, WebLinks, and additional online resources.

NCLEX-PN EXAM STYLE REVIEW QUESTIONS

Choose the best answer(s) for the following questions.

1. During a neurologic examination, the patient demonstrates difficulty initiating movement. The steps are short with quick cadence. Arm swings are decreased with subsequent steps. The clinical findings are referred to as:
   1. ataxia.
   2. bradykinesia.
   3. rigidity.
   4. tremors.

2. A 46-year-old patient complains of weakness of the voluntary muscles of the lower extremities and abnormal tingling and prickling sensations. On initial assessment, the patient is alert, oriented, and coherent. The nurse would likely suspect which of the following?
   1. Multiple sclerosis
   2. Parkinson's disease
   3. Alzheimer's disease
   4. Amyotrophic lateral sclerosis

3. The physician discusses the treatment options with a patient newly diagnosed with Parkinson's disease. The patient asks, "Am I going to die?" An appropriate response would be:
   1. "You seem worried. Let's talk about your concerns."
   2. "Your physician can fully explain your condition."
   3. "You will be all right."
   4. "We all eventually get there."

4. A 45-year-old patient newly diagnosed with multiple sclerosis asks about the nature of the illness. An accurate statement by the nurse would be:
   1. "The condition is a progressive degeneration of the gray matter in the anterior horns of the spinal cord and the lower cranial nerves."
   2. "The condition can only be diagnosed during an autopsy."
   3. "The condition affects the spinal nerves outside the spinal cord and usually follows a viral infection."
   4. "The condition is a chronic demyelinization of the central nervous system with periods of remissions and exacerbations."

5. A 48-year-old female patient is admitted for an acute episode of myasthenic crisis. The nurse would most likely find which of the following signs and symptoms?
   1. Tingling in the extremities
   2. Ptosis
   3. Poor tongue control
   4. Drooling

6. The nurse observes a nursing assistant feed a dysphagic patient. Which of the following actions by the nursing assistant indicates a need for further instruction and guidance?
   1. The wall suction is turned on and readily available for use.
   2. The patient is propped up with one pillow.
   3. The food is cut into small, bite-sized pieces.
   4. The nursing assistant coaches the patient to drop the chin.

7. The nurse reinforces pharmacy instructions regarding safe use of pyridostigmine (Mestinon), an anticholinesterase, by a patient newly diagnosed with myasthenia gravis. Which of the following patient statements indicates effective patient understanding?
   1. "I need to take the medication after meals."
   2. "I can adjust the drug dosage and times depending on daily activities."
   3. "There is no danger in taking over-the-counter medications."
   4. "I must expect some difficulty in swallowing and breathing."

8. Thirty seconds after the administration of edrophonium (Tensilon), the patient is observed to have slowed heart rate, sweating, and cramping. An appropriate nursing action would be to:
   1. start chest compressions.
   2. notify the physician.
   3. administer atropine.
   4. give pyridostigmine (Mestinon).

9. The priority nursing assessment of a patient with myasthenia gravis would be to:
   1. determine the degree of fatigue.
   2. assess the level of knowledge regarding the disease.
   3. monitor the adequacy of respiratory function.
   4. check the patient's swallowing, speech, and protective reflexes.

10. The nurse determines that Risk for injury is the priority nursing diagnosis for a patient diagnosed with Parkinson's disease. Which of the following nursing interventions help prevent any occurrence of falls? *(Select all that apply.)*
    1. Encourage use of wheelchair.
    2. Apply leg braces.
    3. Remove loose carpets or throw rugs.
    4. Install grab bars in the shower and tub.
    5. Install low toilet seats.

CRITICAL THINKING ACTIVITIES 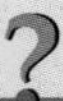 *Read each clinical scenario and discuss the questions with your classmates.*

Scenario A

Your patient had a bout of the "flu" about a week ago. Today he noticed he was having trouble walking. When he got home from an errand, he had trouble pulling his sweater over his head. His wife brought him to the emergency room.

1. Which neurologic problem within this chapter do you think he might have?
2. What might be done to establish a diagnosis?
3. What would be a top priority in his care at this time?
4. What further problems do you think could occur?

Scenario B

Mrs. Jones seems less animated than she has been over the past several months. Her husband tells you she has fallen three times since her last office visit. You notice that she seems more stooped over and her movements are "jerky." The physician examines her and after a thorough history and physical tells the couple that he thinks Mrs. Jones has Parkinson's disease. He prescribes Sinemet for her.

1. What can you anticipate that Mr. and Mrs. Jones will need to be taught?
2. What are the potential complications of Parkinson's disease?

Scenario C

A fellow student in your clinical group confides that she has myasthenia gravis. She takes Mestinon for control of the disease.

1. What factors could cause her symptoms to worsen?
2. What might happen if she forgets to take her medication before reporting for her clinical rotation?

CHAPTER 25

The Sensory System: Eye and Ear

evolve http://evolve.elsevier.com/deWit

Objectives

Upon completing this chapter, you should be able to:

Theory

1. Identify ways in which nurses can help patients preserve their sight and hearing.
2. Identify signs and symptoms of eye problems.
3. Discuss tests and examinations used to diagnose eye and ear disorders.
4. Describe nursing activities associated with assessing the eye and ear.
5. Utilize the nursing process for patients with disorders of the eye or ear.

Clinical Practice

1. Provide teaching for a patient who is to undergo tests for a vision problem.
2. Perform focused assessments for disorders of the eyes and ears.
3. Assist visually impaired patients to find resources to maximize their vision.
4. Instruct a spouse in ways to effectively communicate with a hearing-impaired partner.

Key Terms

Be sure to check out the bonus material on the Companion CD-ROM, including selected audio pronunciations.

cerumen (sĕ-RŪ-mĕn, p. 625)
ectropion (ĕk-TRŌ-pē-ŏn, p. 614)
entropion (ĕn-TRŌ-pē-ŏn, p. 620)
exophthalmos (ĕk-sŏf-THĂL-mŏs, p. 621)
keratitis (kĕr-ă-TĪ-tĭs, p. 614)
nystagmus (nĭs-TĂG-mŭs, p. 628)
otorrhea (ō-tō-RĒ-a, p. 630)
photophobia (fō-tō-FŌ-bē-ă, p. 621)
presbycusis (prĕz-bē-KŪ-sĭs, p. 634)
presbyopia (prĕz-bē-Ō-pē-ă, p. 614)
ptosis (TŌ-sĭs, p. 614)
refraction (rē-FRĂK-shŭn, p. 613)
sensorineural (sĕn-sŏ-rē-NŪ-răl, p. 624)
strabismus (stră-BĬZ-mŭs, p. 615)
xanthelasma (zăn-thĕ-lăz-mă, p. 621)

The loss of vision or hearing may greatly affect the quality of life of an individual. Vision loss is one of the most profound and dreaded of physical disabilities. When a sighted person is no longer able to see, the world changes, and many adjustments must be made. There are two general kinds of patients with impaired vision: those who were born blind, and those who develop some degree of visual impairment later in life. This chapter focuses on the latter type of visually handicapped patient.

Hearing loss is a problem for the patient and for those with whom he lives. Hearing loss can lead to misunderstandings. Social withdrawal is not unusual when hearing becomes severely impaired. The earlier hearing loss is treated, the better. The brain adjusts more readily to a hearing aid if hearing has not been impaired for a long time.

THE EYE

To understand the causes of eye problems, and their effects, it is necessary to recall the anatomy and functions of the structures of the eye (see p. 612).

CAUSES OF EYE DISORDERS

Eye disorders are caused by injury or disease, or are a disorder for which there is a genetic predisposition. Diabetes mellitus and hypertension contribute greatly to visual loss in the United States. Untreated glaucoma causes blindness. Macular degeneration is another major cause of impaired vision. It is now known that smoking has a direct link to the incidence of macular degeneration just as it does to lung cancer. Cataracts eventually cause blindness if they are not removed.

There are approximately 10 million visually impaired or blind people in the United States. Of those, 5.5 million are over 65 years of age. About 7000 Americans use seeing-eye guide dogs (American Foundation for the Blind, 2007).

There have been many new developments in the treatment of a number of potentially blinding diseases. These new surgical techniques and medical treatments offer hope for eyesight preservation to increasing num-

Text continued on p. 615

OVERVIEW OF ANATOMY AND PHYSIOLOGY OF THE EYE

What are the structures of the eye?

- The eyeball is spherical in shape and 2 to 3 cm in diameter (Figure 25–1).
- The sclera, which is part of the wall of the eyeball, is opaque white and covers the posterior ⅚ of the eyeball.
- The transparent cornea is part of the wall of the eyeball and covers the anterior ⅙ of the eyeball.
- The choroid is part of the middle layer of the eyeball. It is a highly vascular layer containing brown pigment located between the sclera and the retina.
- The ciliary body is part of the middle layer of the eyeball and contains finger-like ciliary processes that produce aqueous humor. The ciliary body helps change eye shape for near and far vision.
- The iris is the third part of the middle layer of the eyeball; it is the colored portion of the eye and is a doughnut-shaped diaphragm with the pupil as the central opening. The iris contains two groups of smooth muscles that constrict and dilate the pupil to regulate the entrance of light.
- The biconvex, transparent lens, together with the suspensory ligaments and the ciliary body, forms a partition that divides the interior of the eyeball into two chambers. The anterior chamber between the lens and the cornea is filled with aqueous humor. The posterior chamber, between the lens and the retina, contains vitreous humor.
- The suspensory ligaments connect the ciliary body to the lens.
- The retina is the inner coat of the eyeball and is found in the posterior portion of it. The retina contains several layers. The layer with rods and cones acts as the receptor for light images.
- The optic nerve carries messages from the nerve cells in the retina to the brain.
- The optic disc is formed by the axons of the ganglion cells of the retina.
- The macula lutea is a yellow spot just lateral to the optic disc that allows for visual detail.
- The fovea centralis is the area of the retina that produces the sharpest image.
- The eyelids are composed of skin, connective tissue, and conjunctiva. The conjunctiva is a thin mucous membrane that lines the eyelid and covers the anterior portion of the eyeball except for the cornea.
- Eyelashes line the edge of the eyelid.
- Sebaceous glands are situated with the eyelashes.
- The lacrimal glands are located in the upper outer area above the eyes. The lacrimal ducts and canals carry tears from the eye to the nose.
- Six muscles attach to the eyeball and allow for movement. The muscles come from the bones of the orbit and insert on the outer layer of the eyeball.

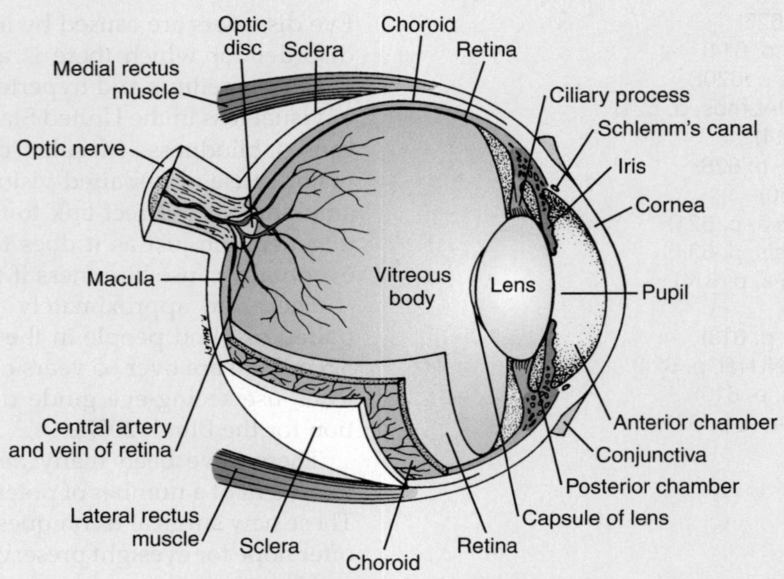

FIGURE **25–1** Structures of the eye.

What are the functions of the eye structures?

- The bony orbit protects the eyeball.
- The eyelashes help trap foreign particles, keeping them from landing on the eyeball.
- The eyelids protect the eyes from foreign matter and help distribute moisture on the eye surface.
- The sebaceous glands secrete an oily fluid that lubricates the lids.
- Blinking of the eyelid 6 to 30 times a minute stimulates the lacrimal glands to produce tears.
- The lacrimal gland secretes tears that moisten, lubricate, and cleanse the surface of the eye. Tears contain an enzyme that helps destroy bacteria and prevent infections.
- The transparent cornea allows light to hit the lens. It assists with the bending of light rays **(refraction),** so that the rays will hit the retina in the right location for images to be transmitted to the brain.
- The choroid's brown pigment absorbs excess light rays that could interfere with vision.
- The ciliary processes secrete aqueous humor that helps maintain the shape of the anterior chamber; it also nourishes the structures in this part of the eye. The aqueous humor assists with refraction of light onto the retina. **The amount of aqueous humor present determines the internal pressure of the eye.** The aqueous humor is reabsorbed by the blood vessels located at the junction of the sclera and the cornea.
- Muscles in the iris control dilation and constriction of the pupil.
- The suspensory ligaments connected to the ciliary body and lens allow light to focus on the lens and retina, which is necessary for close vision.
- The retina's rods and cones are photoreceptors for light and color. The nerves of the retina transmit the images perceived to the brain.
- The optic nerve conducts nerve impulses from the retina to the brain.
- Visualization of the optic disc provides information about the pressure within the eye and within the skull. When intracranial pressure gets higher, the optic disc appears "swollen" or "choked."
- Visual impulses travel along the optic nerve to the optic chiasma just anterior to the pituitary gland; at this point some of the axons cross over to the other side. Images from the medial portion of the left eye and the lateral portion of the right eye are carried by the right optic tract. Images from the medial portion of the right eye and the lateral portion of the left eye are carried by the left optic tract (Figure 25–2). Images are conducted to the visual cortex in the occipital lobe of the brain.
- Six muscles control movement of the eyeball. Table 25–1 lists these muscles and the nerves that control them.

What changes occur in the eye with aging?

- Subcutaneous fat and tissue elasticity decrease and the eyes appear to be sunken.
- *Arcus senilis,* an opaque ring outlining the cornea, sometimes results from the deposition of fatty globules (Figure 25–3).
- The cornea flattens and develops an irregular curvature after age 65, causing astigmatism or making an existing astigmatism worse; vision becomes blurred. Cornea transparency also decreases.
- The sclera develops a yellowish tinge due to fatty deposits; thinning of the sclera may cause a bluish tinge.
- The ability of the iris to dilate decreases, causing difficulty for the older person in going from a bright area into a darkened area.

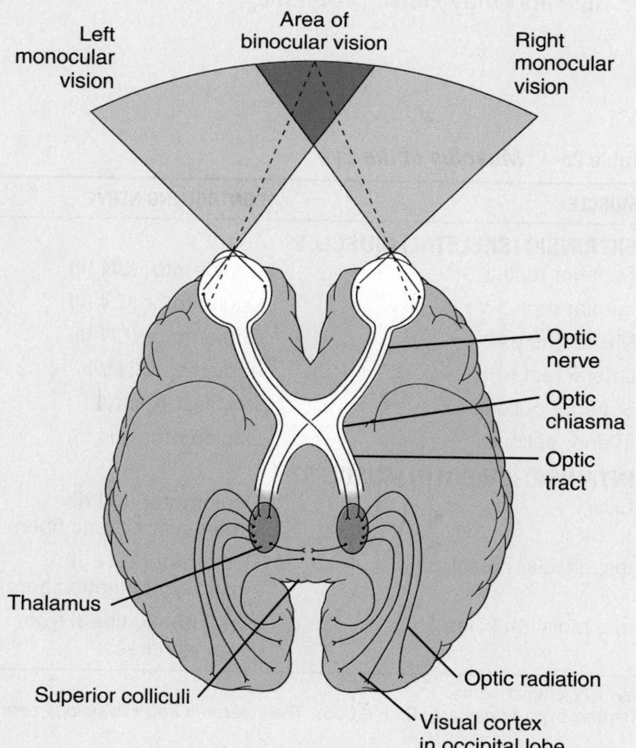

FIGURE **25–2** Visual pathway.

Continued

OVERVIEW OF ANATOMY AND PHYSIOLOGY OF THE EYE—cont'd

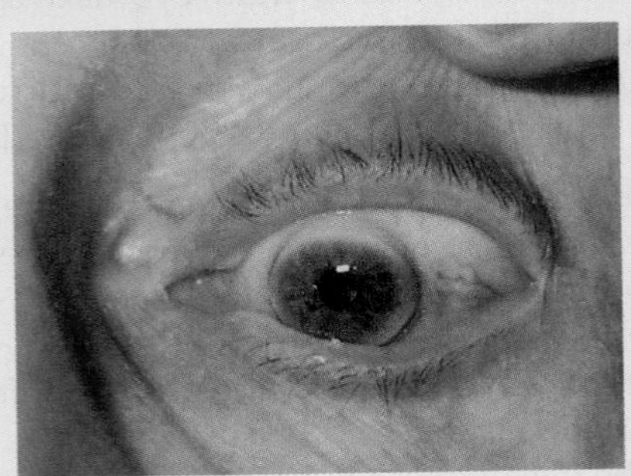

FIGURE 25–3 Arcus senilis, a white ring around the cornea.

- The lens of the eye changes after age 40, gradually losing water and becoming harder. Cataracts may form.
- The ciliary muscle has less ability to allow the eye to accommodate, a process responsible for the gradual extension of distance from the eyes at which an item to be read is held **(presbyopia).** This change begins around age 40.
- The farthest point at which an object can be identified decreases, and the older person has a narrower visual field.
- Color discrimination decreases with advancing age and may cause problems.

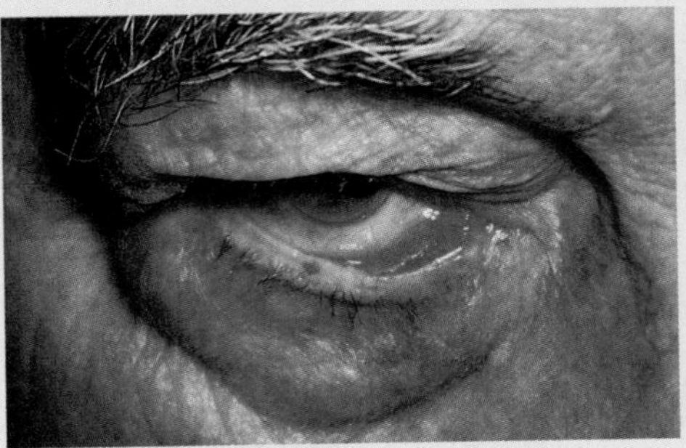

FIGURE 25–4 Ectropion.

- Moisture secretion decreases during the senior years, placing the eyes at greater risk for irritation and infection. This is especially common after age 70. Repeated episodes of **keratitis** (inflammation of the cornea) may seriously compromise vision and can lead to loss of independence for an elderly person.
- Eversion of the lower lid **(ectropion)** occurs because of loss of muscle tone and elasticity (Figure 25–4).
- Decreased muscle tone and decreased elasticity may cause drooping of the upper lid to a point where it interferes with vision **(ptosis).**

Table 25–1 ***Muscles of the Eye***

MUSCLE	CONTROLLING NERVE	FUNCTION
EXTRINSIC (SKELETAL) MUSCLES		
Superior rectus	Oculomotor (CN III)	Elevates eye or rolls it superiorly and toward the midline.
Inferior rectus	Oculomotor (CN III)	Depresses eye or rolls it inferiorly and toward the midline.
Medial rectus	Oculomotor (CN III)	Moves eye medially, toward the midline.
Lateral rectus	Abducens (CN VI)	Moves eye laterally, away from the midline.
Superior oblique	Trochlear (CN IV)	Depresses eye and turns it laterally, away from the midline.
Inferior oblique	Oculomotor (CN III)	Elevates eye and turns it laterally, away from the midline.
INTRINSIC (SMOOTH) MUSCLES		
Ciliary	Oculomotor (CN III): parasympathetic fibers	Causes suspensory ligament to relax, so lens becomes more convex for close vision.
Iris, circular muscles	Oculomotor (CN III): parasympathetic fibers	Decreases the size of the pupil to allow less light to enter the eye.
Iris, radial muscles	Sympathetic fibers from spinal nerves	Increases the size of the pupil to allow more light to enter the eye.

Key: *CN*, cranial nerve.
Adapted from Applegate, E. J. (2006). *The Anatomy and Physiology Learning System* (3rd ed.). Philadelphia: Saunders, p. 189.

bers of people. Efforts also have been made to educate the public about eye care, prevention of eye disease, and periodic examinations to detect eye disorders in their earliest and treatable stages.

Acquired immunodeficiency syndrome (AIDS) is causing blindness as a result of opportunistic infections that the AIDS patient contracts. Ocular problems of the AIDS patient are discussed in Chapter 11.

PREVENTION OF EYE DISORDERS

As health care providers, nurses share responsibility for maintaining good eyesight and for preserving vision throughout the patient's life span. Three major nursing goals to promote good vision are:

- Health education to inform the general public about basic eye care
- Prevention of accidental injury to the eye
- Prevention of visual loss

Healthy People 2010 national goals contains 10 objectives related to preventing vision loss and improving vision for the American public (Health Promotion Points 25–1).

BASIC EYE CARE

The term *eyestrain* has often been used as a catchall to explain various visual defects and diseases of the eye. It is actually very difficult to strain the eye. Inadequate lighting or prolonged use of the eyes for close work can overwork the eye muscles, but this will not damage the eyes any more than straining to hear a distant sound can damage the ears. One should rest the eye muscles periodically when working at the computer, watching television, doing needlework, or performing any activity that demands intensive visual effort. If the eyes tire easily or if there is headache or burning, itching, or redness of the eyes, this is not eyestrain. These are symptoms of a visual problem and are an indication that the person's eyes should be examined. Good nutrition is important to eye health, and certain nutrients such as lutein and zeaxanthin are especially beneficial to vision (Nutritional Therapies 25–1).

Normal eyes do not require irrigations or periodic "washing out" with over-the-counter eye solutions. Normal secretions of the conjunctiva and tear glands should be sufficient to lubricate the eye and wash away small particles of dust that may collect in the eye. **Accumulations of purulent material or excessive tearing usually indicate the need for an eye examination.** Dry eye syndrome that occurs in persons younger than 60 years of age could be symptomatic of an underlying disease.

Health Promotion Points 25–1

***Healthy People 2010* Vision**

28.1 (Developmental) Increase the proportion of persons who have a dilated eye examination at appropriate intervals.

28.2 (Developmental) Increase the proportion of preschool children age 5 years and under who receive vision screening.

28.3 (Developmental) Reduce uncorrected visual impairment due to refractive errors.

28.4 (Developmental) Reduce blindness and visual impairment in children and adolescents age 17 years and under.

28.5 (Developmental) Reduce visual impairment due to diabetic retinopathy.

28.6 (Developmental)Reduce visual impairment due to glaucoma.

28.7 (Developmental)Reduce visual impairment due to cataract.

28.8 (Developmental)Reduce occupational eye injury.

28.9 (Developmental) Increase the use of appropriate personal protective eyewear in recreational activities and hazardous situations around the home.

28.10 (Developmental) Increase vision rehabilitation.

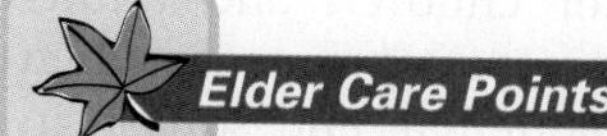

Older persons sometimes suffer from "dry eyes." This is due to decreased production of tears and is treated by instilling "replacement tears," which are commercial preparations or prescriptions of solutions similar in composition to real tears.

Children do not outgrow crossed eyes **(strabismus).** Until a baby reaches the age of 6 to 9 months, he may have some difficulty focusing his eyes, but this problem should not persist. Neglect of strabismus can result in serious loss of vision. It is generally agreed by

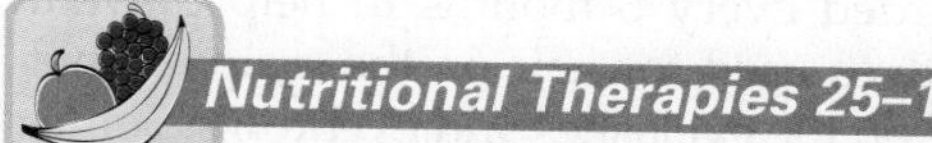

Vitamins and Antioxidants Beneficial to Vision

Vitamin A protects against night blindness, slow adaptation to darkness, and glare blindness. The carotenoids are the precursors for vitamin A and are found in green leafy and yellow vegetables. Carrots, greens, spinach, orange juice, sweet potatoes, and cantaloupe are rich sources of the carotenoids (Barclay & Lie, 2006).

Lutein and zeaxanthin, both antioxidants, may help prevent macular degeneration and cataracts. They are found in yellow fruits and vegetables, red and purple fruits, and greens. Lutein is particularly high in tomatoes, carrots, broccoli, kale, spinach, and romaine lettuce. Corn, cornmeal, kale, Japanese persimmons, and turnip greens have large quantities of zeaxanthin, with corn containing the highest amount. Many vitamin supplements have added lutein to their formulation (National Eye Institute, 2001).

Yet another reason to eat more fruits and vegetables!

ophthalmologists that the sooner treatment is begun, the better the chance of correcting the condition and preserving the child's eyesight.

EB **Every person over the age of 40 should have eye examinations every 2 to 3 years** (Agency for Healthcare Research and Quality, 2005). It is particularly important that a test for glaucoma be made at the time of the examination, because this disease usually is asymptomatic until damage to vision has occurred. People with a family history of glaucoma should be especially careful to have their eyes tested frequently for increased pressure within the eyeball, as this is the basic pathology of glaucoma and the disorder tends to be familial.

PREVENTION OF EYE INJURY

Accidental injury to the eye is a major cause of diminished or total loss of vision, especially in young children. Parents and teachers should be encouraged to teach children the danger of sharp pencils, paper wads, small stones, lawn darts, fireworks, and other small objects children may be tempted to hurl at one another while playing. Older children and adults should be cautioned to wear protective eyewear when engaging in sports such as raquetball and squash in which small balls travel at high speeds. Protective eyewear should be worn when using machinery that might cause debris to fly into the eye, such as lawn mowers, weedeaters, sanders, or power saws.

The rate of occupational accidents has gone down since the establishment and enforcement of rules on wearing goggles and other protective devices for people working in a hazardous environment. The National Institute of Occupational Safety and Health (NIOSH) in Rockville, Maryland, provides information about eye safety and hazards in the workplace.

Cosmetics for the eyelids, eyelashes, and eyebrows can be a source of infection and allergy. Eye makeup should be discarded every 6 months to help prevent infection. Most dyes used for hair on the scalp are not intended for use on the eyelashes and eyebrows. Sometimes it is not the cosmetic but the way in which it is applied that causes eye disease. Saliva should not be used to moisten eye pencils, eye shadow, or mascara, as it may contain organisms that can cause eye infection. When eye cosmetics are being applied, it is important to have a steady hand to avoid accidentally scratching the cornea and eyelids. Cosmetics should never be shared, as this can transmit organisms. To promote prompt treatment of eye disease in its earliest stages, the National Society for the Prevention of Blindness has a list of danger signals (Health Promotion Points 25–2).

PREVENTION OF VISUAL LOSS

Diabetes mellitus and hypertension are chronic diseases that when uncontrolled may cause visual loss. Patients with these disorders are more susceptible to retinopathy (Cultural Cues 25–1). Helping patients gain good control over these disorders can prevent or control visual loss.

Encouraging people who experience an accident causing a corneal abrasion to seek medical attention quickly helps prevent infections that might cause corneal scarring and loss of vision. Promptly seeking medical attention when the eye is inflamed, secreting purulent discharge, or sore assists in treatment of infection that may cause a residual visual loss.

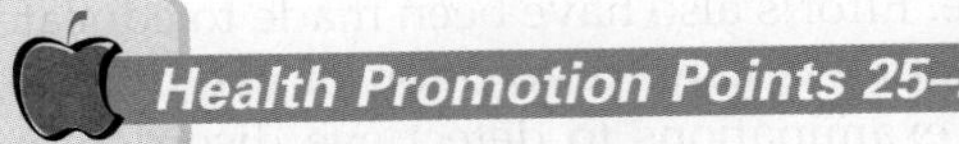

Health Promotion Points 25–2

Danger Signals of Eye Disease

- *Persistent redness of the eye.* Infections and inflammations of the structures of the eye that are not treated may leave scars that can produce loss of vision.
- *Continuing pain or discomfort about the eye, especially following injury.*
- *Disturbance of vision.* Although these symptoms may simply indicate a need for eyeglasses, blurred vision, loss of side vision, double vision, and sudden development of many floating spots in the field of vision may be symptomatic of more serious systemic diseases.
- *Colored light flashes, or a feeling that a curtain has been pulled across the line of vision or a shade has been pulled down.* This can indicate a retinal detachment and requires prompt attention.
- *Crossing of the eyes, especially in children.*
- *Growths on the eye or eyelids or opacities visible in the normally transparent portion of the eye.*
- *Continuing discharge, crusting, or tearing of the eyes.*
- *Pupil irregularities,* either unequal size of the two pupils or distorted shape.

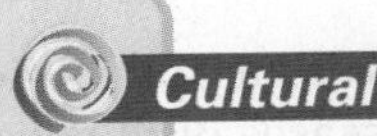

Cultural Cues 25–1

Latinos and Eye Disease

The Los Angeles Latino Eye Study found that Latinos had high rates of diabetic retinopathy and of open-angle glaucoma. The study interviewed and examined 6300 Latinos age 40 and older from the Los Angeles area. Many of those Latinos involved in the study were found to have previously undiagnosed diabetes. Almost half of the individuals in the study who had diabetes had diabetic retinopathy. Seventy-five percent of Latinos with glaucoma were undiagnosed before participating in the study (National Institutes of Health, 2004).

? ***Think Critically About . . .*** Can you identify four specific ways in which you might help prevent eye disorders among your relatives and patients?

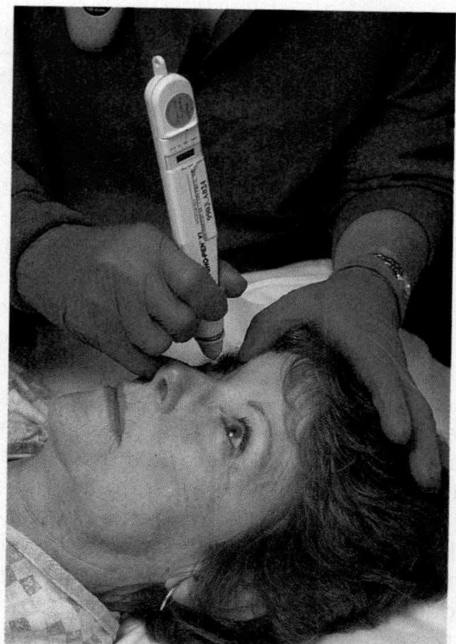

FIGURE 25–5 The Tono-Pen is used to check intraocular pressure.

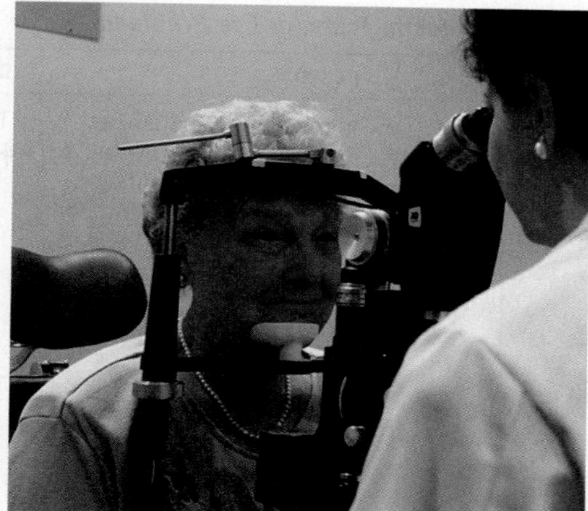

FIGURE 25–6 Slit-lamp ocular examination.

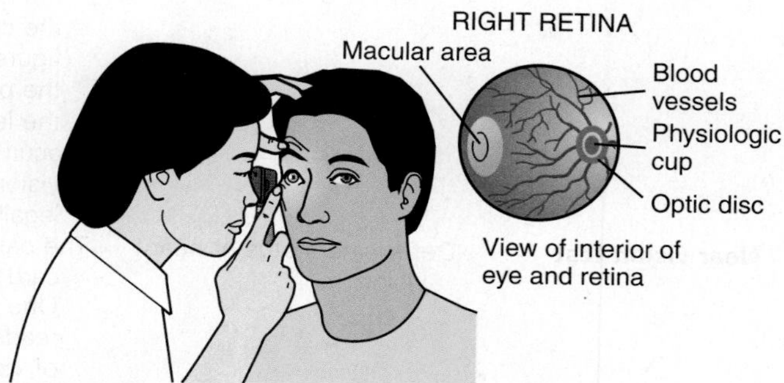

FIGURE 25–7 Examination of the eye with an ophthalmoscope.

Assessing patients for the presence of cataracts and recommending regular periodic eye examinations should be a part of every nurse's practice. Cataract removal can greatly improve vision. Screening for glaucoma reduces the incidence of blindness from that condition. Free screening clinics often are available in most communities. Nurses can inform patients of when and where such screenings are available. The Tono-Pen is often used for such screenings. It is also used in the emergency room when a patient complains of symptoms that might be from increased intraocular pressure (Figure 25–5).

Nurses must be aware that there are many types of visual loss. Some may affect only one area of the field of vision in one eye, whereas others affect parts of the field of vision in both eyes. The degree of visual impairment varies greatly.

DIAGNOSTIC TESTS AND EXAMINATIONS

Diagnostic tests are performed to test visual acuity, prescribe prescription lenses, inspect the interior of the eye, check intraocular pressure and assess the health of the retinal blood vessels (Figure 25–6). Computed tomography, optical coherence tomography, and magnetic resonance imaging may also be used to diagnose eye disorders. Table 25–2 provides further information about diagnostic tests.

NURSING MANAGEMENT

The nursing care of patients with severe visual handicaps demands a special awareness of the unique problems encountered by someone who has either a partial or a total loss of vision. You must be sensitive to these patients' special needs. Patient education is especially important to these patients' acceptance of their visual disorder, their participation in diagnostic and therapeutic measures, and their adjustment to their new surroundings when they are hospitalized or admitted to a long-term care facility.

Assessment (Data Collection)

All nurses should be able to perform a basic eye examination, inspecting the eye for signs of redness or discharge, and checking visual acuity with a Snellen eye chart. Only nurses who have had special training in ophthalmic nursing are qualified to conduct a complete eye assessment (Figure 25–7). Significant data can be obtained by nurses without such specialized education by taking an adequate history.

History Taking

Many systemic diseases, including AIDS, hypertension, and diabetes mellitus, secondarily affect the eye and its functions. In the general assessment of any patient, you should be aware of the more obvious indications of an ophthalmic pathology, whether it be primary or secondary.

Table 25–2 ***Diagnostic Tests for Eye Problems***

TEST	PURPOSE	DESCRIPTION	NURSING IMPLICATIONS
Ophthalmoscopy (retinoscopy)	Inspect the fundus (back portion) of the eyeball to detect abnormalities of the retina, macula, optic disc, and retinal vessels	The examiner uses an ophthalmoscope (see Figure 25–7) to focus light through the pupil onto the fundus.	The room is darkened before the examiner approaches the patient with the ophthalmoscope. Drops may be placed in the eye before this examination to dilate the eye and offer a wider area through which to view the fundus.
Visual acuity	Determine status of vision	The Snellen eye chart is used. It is placed 20 feet from the patient, and first one eye is occluded and then the other eye is occluded. The person begins reading lines of letters that decrease in size. Visual acuity is expressed as a fraction for each eye. The numerator (first) figure indicates the distance between the patient and the chart. The denominator (second) figure expresses the distance at which the person could read at least half of the letters in the line correctly. Visual acuity of 20/20 in each eye is normal; vision of 20/200 (with correction) is legally defined as blindness.	Explain the procedure to the patient. Have the patient hold the occluding card close to the nose so that the entire eye is covered. Start with the third line. If the patient cannot read that, progress upward; if the line is correctly read, go to the next line down; etc. Test the other eye. Record the findings.
Near vision test	Determine status of near vision	The patient is given a Jaeger's Test Type card with different sizes of type on it. One eye is occluded while the patient reads the lines of type. Determination of vision status is made on the basis of what a person with normal vision can read.	Explain that this is a simple test of vision to determine whether there are any problems that might require further testing.
Visual fields test (confrontation test)	Examine the patient's visual fields, detecting problems with peripheral vision	The examiner faces the patient and asks him to look directly into her eyes. The examiner covers her right eye, and the patient covers his left eye. Then the examiner's finger is moved from an area outside of the peripheral vision into the line of vision. The patient should detect the finger about the same time as the examiner. The test is repeated with the other eye covered.	Explain the test to the patient and remind him to keep looking directly into your eyes.
Extraocular muscle function test	Test the function of the extraocular muscles	Ask the patient to hold his head still and to move the eyes to follow a small object such as a pen to each of the six cardinal points: right; upward and right; down and right; left; upward and left; down and left.	Observe for parallel eye movements and any deviation of movement. Nystagmus is a normal finding for the far lateral gaze. Record your findings.
Color vision test	Determine if the patient has any color blindness	Use the Ishihara chart book, which shows numbers composed of dots of one color within an area of dots of a different color. Ask the patient what he sees on the page for each chart. Test each eye separately. Reading the numbers correctly indicates normal color vision.	Explain the purpose of the test. Tell the patient to tell you what number appears on the chart. Record your findings.
Refraction	Determine amount of lens correction necessary to restore person's vision to as near normal as possible with glasses	A series of glass lenses are placed in front of the patient's eyes to determine which lens provides the best vision correction. Each eye is tested separately.	A prescription for glasses will be written depending on the findings of the refraction test. The test may be performed for both near and far vision.

Key: *IV,* intravenous.

Table 25–2 ***Diagnostic Tests for Eye Problems—cont'd***

TEST	PURPOSE	DESCRIPTION	NURSING IMPLICATIONS
Intraocular pressure test	Determine the amount of pressure within the eye; aid in diagnosis of glaucoma	A tonometer is used to measure the pressure. This may be a handheld instrument, but it usually is a device that measures pressure by taking a reading while air is directed at the eye by a pneumotonometer. Another type of tonometer is the applanation tonometer. Normal intraocular pressure is 15–21 mm Hg.	Explain that this is a test to determine whether a patient might have glaucoma. More than one reading on different days is necessary to confirm a diagnosis of glaucoma. If a diagnosis of glaucoma is made, medication can be prescribed to help control the intraocular pressure and preserve vision.
Slit-lamp biomicroscopic examination	Examine the surface of the eye	A beam of light is reduced to a narrow slit that illuminates only a small section of the eye, allowing examination of a thin section of the eye structures at a time.	Explain that this device helps detect "floaters" in the vitreous humor, and abnormalities of the cornea and other structures of the eye. The eyes may be dilated with mydriatic drops for this test.
Topical dye (corneal staining)	To detect abrasions of the cornea or the presence of a foreign body on the cornea	Fluorescein dye drops are administered to the affected eye. The dye remains on the injured tissue or surrounds a foreign body. Such areas usually appear as green spots.	Explain the procedure and the rationale for the test. Warn that the drops may sting slightly for a few minutes. Give the patient a tissue to absorb the excess drops as they may stain clothing.
Fluorescein angiography (retinal angiography)	To detect tumors of the interior of the eye and to help diagnose and measure the extent of retinopathy	An IV injection of sodium fluorescein is given. A short time later photographs of the fundus are taken with a special camera.	An IV injection is necessary. A signed consent form is required to perform the procedure.
Electroretinography	Test the functional integrity of the retina; evaluates degeneration of the photoreceptor cells	Electrodes embedded into a contact lens are placed directly on the anesthetized eye. A light stimulus is introduced. The change in electrical potential of the eye caused by the flash of light is measured.	Instruct the patient that he must fixate on the target and not move the eyes during the test.
Optical coherence tomography (OCT)	Record images of retinal structures Differentiate the anatomical layers within the retina and allows measurement of retinal thickness Detect macular holes, epiretinal membranes, cystoid macular edema, and other pathologies	Focused beams of light are directed into the eye that scan the structural features of the retina. A cross-sectional image similar to a topographic map is produced.	The patient's eyes must be dilated. Tell the patient that he will be looking into a machine. The test takes from 10 to 20 minutes.
Amsler grid test	Detect macular degeneration	Using a handheld card printed with a grid of black lines similar to graph paper, the patient fixates on a center dot and records abnormalities of the grid lines.	Test should be performed every week or two. Instruct the patient to record seeing wavy or missing lines, or distorted areas.
Ultrasonography	Evaluate the characteristics of a lesion, and its size and growth over time, or to determine the presence of a foreign body	A probe is placed directly on the eyeball. Sound waves are transmitted into the eye, bounce back off the various tissues, and are collected by a receiver and amplified on an oscilloscope screen.	Explain the procedure to the patient.

Normal vision depends in part on:

- Adequately functioning nerve cells, including those in the retina as well as the optic nerve
- Adequate circulation of blood to the retinal cells
- Intact and functioning structures of the eyeball itself

A history of neurologic disorders should be noted. Neuromuscular diseases are especially likely to cause diplopia, blurred vision, or inability to move the eyes. Endocrine disorders that secondarily affect the eyes include thyroid disease and diabetes mellitus. Acute hyperglycemia can alter the shape of the lens and temporarily cause blurred vision. **Prolonged hyperglycemia can adversely affect the blood vessels of the retina, causing bleeding and leading to loss of vision.** Liver and kidney failure can produce pathologic changes in both neural and vascular structures within the eye. Retinal changes also can be caused by hypertension and atherosclerosis.

Some drugs are capable of producing either transient or permanent ocular changes that lead to disturbances in color vision and visual acuity and the formation of cataracts, retinopathy, and glaucoma. Among common drugs that have possible ocular side effects are digitalis leaf, corticosteroids, indomethacin (Indocin), and sulfisoxazole (Gantrisin).

A family history of eye disorders can be significant because disorders such as strabismus, retinitis pigmentosa, glaucoma, and cataracts tend to run in families or follow a pattern of inheritance (Focused Assessment 25–1).

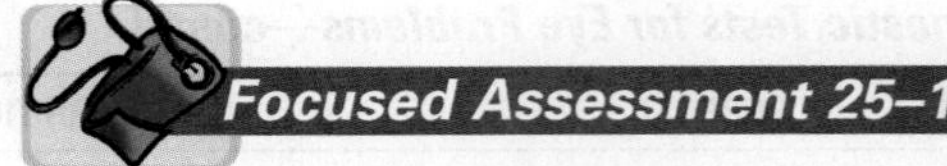

Focused Assessment 25–1

Data Collection for Eye Disorders

The following questions should be asked when gathering history regarding an eye disorder:

- Have you noticed a change in your vision?
- Do you have any pain or discomfort in the eyes? Itching? Burning? Stinging? Excessive tearing or watering?
- Have you had any episodes of blurred vision? Double vision? A loss in the field of vision? Blind spots? Floating spots?
- Do you have difficulty with vision at night?
- Is there any pain in the eyes when you are in bright light?
- Do you have headaches in the brow area?
- Do you see halos around lights?
- Have you ever injured an eye in any way?
- Do you experience frequent reddening of the eye *(conjunctivitis)?*
- Do you ever experience discharge or sticky matter in the eye?
- Do you find that your lids are crusty when you awaken?
- Do your eyes feel dry? Do you frequently use eyedrops?
- Do you wear contact lenses? Use glasses?
- What medications do you take regularly?
- Is there any history of glaucoma in your family?
- Have you ever been told you have diabetes? Hypertension?
- When did you have your last eye examination?
- *For those patients who have a previous visual loss:* How do you cope with your loss of vision?

Table 25–3 *Abnormalities of Lid Position*

ABNORMALITY	CAUSES	SYMPTOMS	TREATMENT
Entropion: Inversion of lid margin; eyelids are turned inward toward eyeball so that lashes rub against eyeball	Scarring and contraction of skin near eyelid (cicatricial entropion); or aging of skin with laxness of tissues supporting the lid and contraction of orbicularis muscle (spastic entropion)	Pain, tearing, redness, and corneal ulceration due to lid margin and eyelashes rubbing against cornea	Splinting the lid, using a pressure patch, or taping lid into everted position Surgical correction by tightening musculature and everting lid margin
Ectropion: Eversion or outward turning of the lower lid	Aging and laxness of skin and muscle tissues, facial paralysis, edema of conjunctiva lining the lid, or contraction of scar tissue	Irritation of palpebral conjunctiva, spilling of tears down the cheeks due to blocked outlet, irritation of skin of cheeks, symptoms of conjunctivitis	Usually responds to patching of the eye Surgical correction necessary if paralysis of orbicularis muscle is permanent or if there is severe scarring and contraction of skin near the lid
Ptosis: Drooping of the eyelid so that it partially or completely covers the cornea	Congenital weakness of the levator superioris muscle or long-term presence of foreign body; one of first signs of myasthenia gravis	Obvious drooping of eyelid If not corrected in infants, can lead to blindness because light rays cannot enter and stimulate development of the eye Patient may be observed tilting head back or raising eyebrows in an effort to see from under eyelids	Surgical correction Removal of foreign body, if that is the cause

Sometimes patients are not aware of gradual changes in vision, but have noticed that they have had more minor accidents lately, seem to be more easily fatigued, or are less interested in doing things that once gave them pleasure, such as sewing or some other hobby.

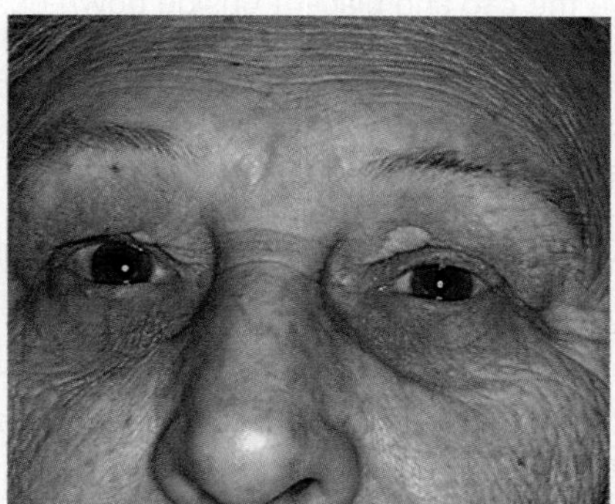

FIGURE **25–8** Xanthelasma.

Physical Examination

Observe the patient's eyes and eye area for redness of the conjunctiva, swelling of the eyelids or in the periorbital space, excessive tearing, change in visual acuity, secretions and encrustations on the eyelids, abnormal position of the eyelid, and **exophthalmos** (protrusion of the eyeball). Abnormalities of lid position are described in Table 25–3. **Xanthelasma,** or soft, raised, yellow areas, sometimes appear on the eyelid after age 50 (Figure 25–8). Signs and symptoms of selected eye diseases are listed in Table 25–4. In addition to the more obvious signs of eye disease, visual impairment also can be assessed by noting the patient's head, hand, and eye movements. Tilting the head to one side to improve vision could mean that the patient has double vision or that one eye is much stronger than the other. Squinting could mean poor vision. Shading the eyes with the hands may indicate an increased sensitivity to light **(photophobia).**

Table 25–4 ***Clinical Signs and Symptoms of Selected Eye Diseases, Medical Treatment, and Nursing Interventions***

DISEASE	SIGNS AND SYMPTOMS	MEDICAL TREATMENT AND NURSING INTERVENTIONS
Blepharitis: Infection of glands and lash follicles along lid margin	Itching, burning, sensitivity to light Mucus discharge and scaling; eyelids crusted, glued shut, especially on awakening Loss of eyelashes	Warm compresses to soften secretions; scrub eyelids with baby shampoo; stroke sideways to remove exudate and scales Antibiotic eyedrops; systemic and topical antibiotics if skin is infected
Chalazion: Internal stye; infection of meibomian gland	Astigmatism or distorted vision, depending on size and location of chalazion Small, hard tumor on eyelid	Chalazion may require surgical excision and antibiotics to avoid chronic state and cyst formation
Hordeolum: External stye. Infected swelling near the lid margin on inside	Sharp pain that becomes dull and throbbing Rupture and drainage of pus bring relief Localized redness and swelling of lid	Hordeolum usually resolves spontaneously Warm compresses qid for 10–15 min to bring stye to a head and hasten rupture Caution patient never to squeeze swelling, as this could spread infection; poor health status can predispose a person to recurrence of styes
Conjunctivitis: Inflammation of the conjunctiva; "pink eye" is a specific type caused by chemical irritants, bacteria, or virus	Varying degrees of pain and discomfort Increased tearing and mucus production Itching; sensation of a foreign body in the eye	Depends on type of infecting organism; antibiotic eyedrops and ointments Special care when handling infective material
Keratitis: Inflammation of the cornea	Varying degrees of pain and discomfort Photophobia; blurred vision if center of cornea is affected	Depends on specific causes; could be allergy, microbes, ischemia, or decreased lacrimation. Most superficial lesions are self-healing. Antibiotic eyedrops or ointment used for bacterial infections. Steroids can reduce inflammation and discomfort; however, herpes infection can rapidly worsen keratitis unless an antiviral agent is given simultaneously Patient is encouraged to use good personal hygiene, frequent hand washing
Corneal abrasion or ulceration	Moderate to severe pain and discomfort aggravated by blinking History of trauma, contact lens wear	Change or discontinue use of contact lens Teach patient proper way to insert, remove, and care for contact lens Caution patient not to moisten lens with saliva

Observation of the patient's ability to move the eyebrows and eyes can be helpful in diagnosing nerve damage. Inability to raise the eyebrows indicates damage to the facial nerve. Movement of the eyeball to direct the gaze is controlled by no less than six muscles, which are themselves under the control of three cranial nerves: the oculomotor nerve (third cranial), the trochlear nerve (fourth cranial), and the abducens nerve (sixth cranial) (see Table 25–1).

Nursing Diagnosis

Nursing diagnoses are based on the data obtained from assessment. The LPN/LVN collaborates with the RN in formulating the nursing care plan and selecting the nursing diagnoses. Some of the nursing diagnoses most frequently encountered in the care of patients with eye disease include:

- Disturbed sensory perception related to decreased visual acuity
- Risk for injury related to decreased visual field
- Fear of blindness related to consequences of diabetic retinopathy
- Impaired home maintenance management related to impaired or lost vision
- Deficient diversional activity related to visual limitation
- Deficient knowledge related to proper method and schedule of instillation of eyedrops

Planning

Expected outcomes for the above nursing diagnosis might be:

- Patient will compensate for decreased visual acuity and not suffer sensory deprivation.
- Patient will not experience injury.
- Patient will verbalize decreased fear as treatment begins to help condition.
- Patient will seek assistance with home maintenance within 7 days.
- Patient will explore other means of diversion than reading and watching television.
- Patient will demonstrate proper installation of eyedrops and will verbalize the schedule for the eyedrops.

When a patient is visually impaired, the nurse must plan extra time to assist with personal care to allow the patient to perform as much self-care as possible. The instillation of preoperative eyedrops is a very time-consuming nursing task (Box 25–1). The nurse must plan for this when creating the work plan for the shift. Hands must be washed before and after instilling eyedrops. Often an eyepatch must be removed, and then a new one placed, after instilling eye medication. Planning also must be done to incorporate patient teaching on the administration of medication, self-care instructions for the patient with glaucoma, and postoperative instructions.

Box 25–1 *Instillation of Eyedrops and Eye Ointment*

Check the label of the medication and be certain which eye is to receive the medication. Follow the Five Rights of medication administration. Wash the hands and apply gloves.

FOR EYEDROPS

- Remove the cap and place it upside down on the table.
- With the patient sitting or reclining, ask the patient to look up at the ceiling and tilt the head slightly toward the eye receiving the drop.
- With a tissue beneath the fingers, retract the lower lid downward, exposing the conjunctival sac.
- Stabilize the eyedrop container above the eye and drop the designated number of drops directly into the conjunctival sac. Do not place drops on the cornea. Block the entrance to the lacrimal gland by placing a finger over it.
- Carefully replace the cap on the container without contaminating the dropper tip.
- Ask the patient to close the eyelids gently and move the eyes from side to side under the lids to distribute the medication.

FOR EYE OINTMENT

- Remove the cap from the tube and set it down on the table upside down.
- Expose the conjunctival sac.
- Apply a thin ribbon of ointment along the entire length of the conjunctival sac.
- To end the ribbon, twist the tube with a lateral movement of the wrist without touching the eye.
- Recap the tube.
- Ask the patient to gently close the eyelids and roll the eyes around under the lids to distribute the medication.

Implementation

Nursing Interventions for the Visually Impaired Patient

Considerable adjustments must be made by those who are deprived of optimum sight. A sense of hopelessness and despair may be experienced by people who have lost their eyesight. The patient goes through stages of grief in much the same way the dying person does. A different lifestyle must be learned, but it is not necessarily less meaningful.

Remember that the person has a vision impairment, he is not deaf. Speak normally. Speak to the person and identify yourself as you enter the room, and do not touch him until after you have spoken to him. This prevents startling or frightening him when he may not have heard you enter the room. Be certain that he is oriented to the room and can easily locate the call bell.

Prevention of accidents is an important part of the care of a blind person. Aside from the physical effects of bumping into objects or falling over them, the visually impaired person also suffers from a loss of self-confidence and security if movement is not safe and independent. **Doors should be kept closed or completely open. They must never be left ajar.** Always return things to their places when working in the room. If it is necessary to move any object in the room, ask for consent and state its new location. *When you leave the room, tell the visually impaired person that you are going.* This will prevent him from becoming frustrated by resuming a conversation only to find that no one is there. When ambulating with the patient, lead with the patient holding your arm as he follows.

Pity is neither expected nor appreciated by the visually impaired. They only want to be treated as normal people and would prefer to ask for your help when they need it rather than have you do everything for them. If you are assigned to the care of a visually impaired person, determine the amount of assistance the patient needs and wants by asking. Do not assume that the person is helpless, but avoid neglect when help is needed.

When a visually impaired patient is admitted, he will require special orientation to the room and surroundings. If there is total blindness, describe the size of the room and the placement of furniture, using the bed as the focal point. An ambulatory patient can be walked around the room and to the bathroom to develop familiarity with the location of the commode, bath, and sink. As with any patient, show how to locate and use the call system, the radio, and the telephone if there is one at the bedside.

Most patients prefer to feed themselves if at all possible. However, it usually is necessary to set up the meal tray of the visually impaired patient, using the "clock" method for placement of food on the plate. The patient is told what food is in which area (i.e., "The potatoes are at 2 o'clock"). Setting up the meal tray includes opening containers of milk and juice, pouring coffee or tea, and cutting meat into bite-sized pieces, unless the patient is accustomed to doing these things (Assignment Considerations 25–1).

Do not give a visually impaired person a straw or drinking tube unless you are asked to, because it may be awkward to use. If you must feed the patient all of a meal, work slowly and calmly. Indicate about hot and cold foods on the tray, and alternate dishes rather than feeding all of one thing before offering another. Avoid talking too much, thus forcing the patient to either stop eating or answer you with a mouth full of food. Whenever possible, help the patient select finger foods such as sandwiches and raw fruit or vegetables from the menu. The goal is to help the patient maintain dignity and self-respect while meeting his personal needs.

If a guide dog is present, don't interfere with it or pet it as it is working. Don't feed the dog; let the patient feed at the appropriate time. Be sure the dog is near the bed on its own mat. Ask if the mat may be on the side of the bed that the staff are less likely to use.

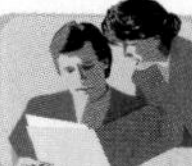

Assignment Considerations 25–1

Assisting the Visually Impaired Patient

If a certified nursing assistant (CNA) or unlicensed assistive personnel (UAP) is assigned to help feed, ambulate, or care for a visually impaired patient, be certain that the person understands what the visual impairment is and whether one or both eyes are affected. Ask that the aide announce her presence with a knock on the door and to speak before touching the patient. Review how to feed the blind patient and how to assist with ambulation. Gently remind the CNA or UAP that the patient is blind and not deaf, unless deafness is also a patient problem.

? *Think Critically About . . .* Can you think of three specific ways in which you can assist a blind patient who is admitted to the hospital to maintain as much independence in this setting as possible?

Evaluation

Evaluation is based on reassessing data and determining whether expected outcomes have been met. This is an ongoing process. Some questions to be asked when gathering data for evaluation include: Is the patient compliant with the use of eye medications? Is an infection resolving? Is vision improving? If interventions have not been effective in helping the patient achieve expected outcomes, the plan of care should be altered.

COMMUNITY CARE

Nurses in all settings should be conscious of eye safety for themselves and those around them. Public education about using sunhats, visors, and dark glasses when out of doors to protect the eyes from ultraviolet UVA and UVB rays is another function of all nurses. School nurses also should institute "case finding" methods with the teachers or faculty to identify students who may have vision problems that have not been identified.

Nurses working in home care often find patients who have not had eye care in many years; prescriptions have not been changed, and their quality of vision has decreased. Arranging for referral to an appropriate agency to set up an eye examination should be done when the patient cannot afford an eye exam from a provider in the community. Glaucoma testing should be encouraged every 2 to 3 years for all adults over the age of 40.

THE EAR

Approximately 28 million people in the United States have a significant loss of hearing (National Institute on Deafness and Other Communication Disorders, 2005). The number has risen dramatically in the last three decades. About 40% of the hearing impaired are under the age of 65. The inability to hear causes difficulty with communication (Health Promotion Points 25–3). Approximately 2 in 1000 babies born in the United States have some form of congenital hearing problem. After age 75, about half of the population has some degree of hearing loss. Almost 90% of people over age 80 have a hearing loss. It is thought that the trend of playing very loud music, causing damage to the acoustic nerve, will result in considerably more hearing loss in the coming decades.

There are two types of hearing loss related to problems in the ear, *sensorineural* and *conductive*. About 80% of hearing loss is due to a disorder of the hearing nerve **(sensorineural)**. Conductive hearing loss is caused by a problem of sound impulse transmission through the auditory canal, the tympanic membrane, or the bones of the middle ear. Hearing impairment is the nation's number one disability, affecting 1 in every 15 people. Causes of sensorineural and conductive hearing impairment are listed in Table 25–5.

Arteriosclerosis can cause decreased blood flow to the otic nerve (eighth cranial nerve), resulting in sensorineural hearing loss. This often contributes to hearing loss in the elderly.

A loss of hearing, like a loss of sight, burdens its victims with physical, emotional, psychosocial, and financial problems. Hearing allows for communication with others in everyday conversations, in the classroom, and in business transactions. Without the ability to hear, one can be deprived of many of the joys and pleasures of life: music, drama, exchange of ideas, and the thousands of sounds in one's environment. Because hearing warns one of danger, an inability to hear can cause anxiety and fear. Adults who have a hearing deficiency might lose their job and alienate friends because of their communication handicap. Nurses must learn ways to help prevent hearing loss and to assist patients who already have such a loss.

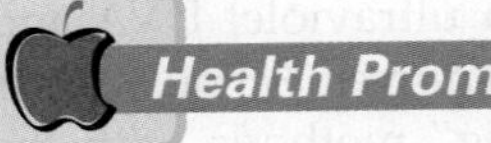

Health Promotion Points 25–3

Coping with Hearing Loss

The sooner the person with a hearing loss obtains and learns to use a hearing aid, the greater the hearing improvement. The brain does better at integrating the hearing aid transmissions when hearing has not been gone for a very long time. Encourage those individuals with any hearing loss to be tested and to try a hearing aid if one is recommended. The person should be told that there is an adjustment curve with new hearing aid use, and it often takes several trips back to the hearing aid center for minor adjustments to the instrument to be made. It also takes practice in using the aid to achieve better hearing.

Inner ear disorders can cause problems with balance. Dizziness, vertigo, and ataxia can greatly interfere with an individual's ability to work or to perform usual activities of daily living. Accidental injury and fractures from falls may occur. To understand the problems affecting the ear, it is necessary to recall its normal structure and functions (Overview of Anatomy and Physiology of the Ear).

CAUSES AND PREVENTION OF HEARING LOSS

A glance at the causes of hearing loss listed in Table 25–5 will help identify some of the ways the nurse can help prevent hearing loss. Not all cases of hearing disability can be prevented, but education of the general public about causes of hearing loss can reduce its incidence. *Healthy People 2010* includes eight objectives to prevent hearing loss and improve hearing in the American public (Health Promotion Points 25–4). **Adequate treatment of severe ear infections helps preserve hearing.** Research is questioning whether antibiotics should be used for the average case of otitis media in childhood as most cases will resolve on their own. Loud noise is a major cause of sensorineural hearing loss, and the use of headphones contributes considerably (Table 25–6, p. 627) (Grant, 2005). 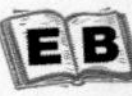

Hairpins, the ends of pencils, and other assorted objects should never be used to relieve tickling or itching in the ear, or to remove cerumen. Earwax normally moves on its own out of the ear canal to the outer ear, where it can be removed without danger of damaging the delicate lining of the ear canal or the tympanic membrane (eardrum). Obstructing cerumen should be removed by using drops that dissolve it or by a physician or nurse skilled in removing impacted cerumen. Foreign objects, such as beans, peas, and other organic substances, also should be removed by someone who is experienced and aware of the potential for ear damage.

Table 25–5 Common Causes of Sensorineural and Conductive Hearing Loss

CONDUCTIVE LOSS	SENSORINEURAL LOSS
• Obstruction by impacted cerumen • Infection with labyrinthitis • Otosclerosis • Trauma and scarring of the tympanic membrane • Congenital malformation of the outer or middle ear	• Presbycusis • Heredity with congenital loss • Ototoxic drugs • Loud noise exposure • Tumor (acoustic neuroma) • Ménière's disease • Severe infection such as measles, mumps, meningitis • Rubella in utero

OVERVIEW OF ANATOMY AND PHYSIOLOGY OF THE EAR

What are the structures of the ear?

- The external ear consists of the pinna (auricle) and the canal (auditory meatus). The pinna is the fleshy part of the ear situated on the side of the head (Figure 25–9).
- The auditory meatus is a tube about 2.5 cm long extending from the pinna to the tympanic membrane.
- The meatus is lined with numerous hairs and glands that secrete a waxy substance called **cerumen** (earwax).
- The middle ear contains the auditory bones (ossicles) and opens into the eustachian tube.
- The auditory ossicles are three small bones: the malleus (hammer), the incus (anvil), and the stapes (stirrup).
- The malleus attaches to the tympanic membrane.
- The stapes attaches to the oval window.
- The incus links the malleus and the stapes.
- The tympanic membrane (eardrum) separates the middle ear from the external ear.
- The eustachian tube connects the middle ear with the throat.
- The oval window and the round window connect the middle ear to the inner ear.
- The inner ear is divided into the vestibule, the semicircular canals, and the cochlea.
- The inner ear contains a bony labyrinth with a membranous labyrinth lining and is located in the temporal bone of the skull.
- A clear fluid, endolymph, fills the membranous labyrinth.
- The cochlea contains the organ of Corti, which is composed of sound receptors.

What are the functions of the ear structures?

- The pinna collects sound waves and channels them into the auditory meatus.
- The hairs and cerumen in the canal help prevent foreign objects from reaching the tympanic membrane.
- The tympanic membrane vibrates when sound waves hit it; the sound vibrations are conducted to the malleus.
- The bones of the middle ear transmit the sound vibrations to the inner ear. The malleus transmits them to the incus and the incus transmits them to

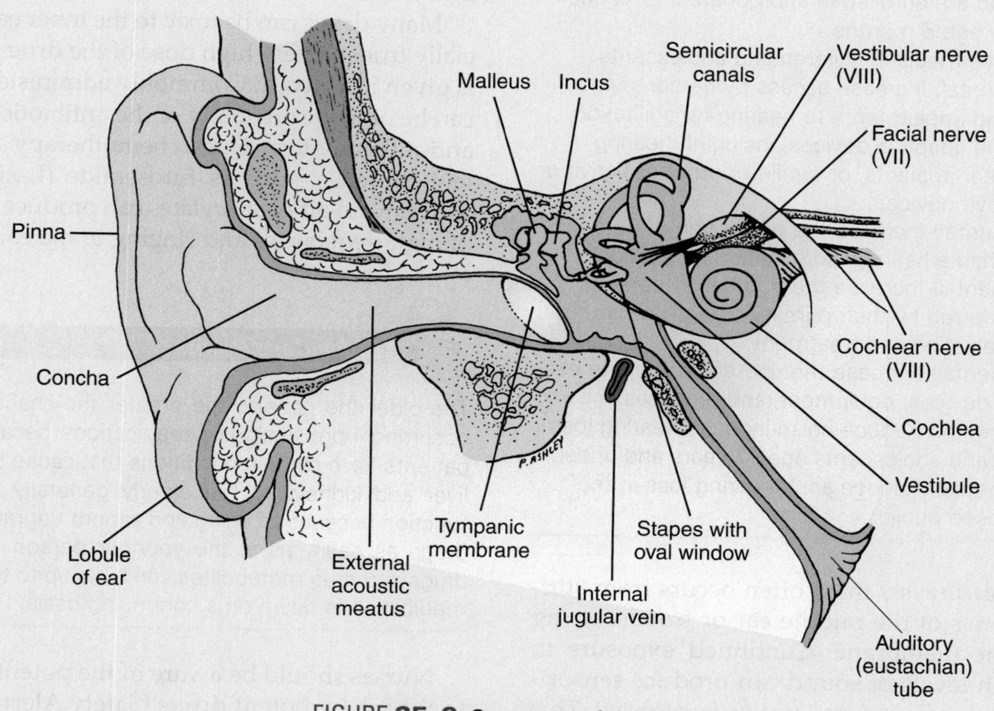

FIGURE **25–9** Structures of the ear.

Continued

OVERVIEW OF ANATOMY AND PHYSIOLOGY OF THE EAR—cont'd

the stapes. The stapes transmits the sound vibrations to the oval window, which transfers the motion to the fluid in the inner ear.

- Fluid motion in the inner ear stimulates the sound receptors in the cochlea and the organ of Corti.
- The organ of Corti transmits impulses to the cochlear branch of the vestibulocochlear nerve (cranial nerve VIII). This nerve carries the impulses to the medulla oblongata, the thalamus, and then to the temporal lobe of the brain that contains the auditory cortex.
- The eustachian tube helps equalize pressure in the middle ear.
- Receptors responsible for equilibrium (balance) are located in the inner ear within the bony vestibule and at the base of the semicircular canals.
- Impulses from the equilibrium receptors are transmitted to the brain via the vestibular branch of the vestibulocochlear nerve (cranial nerve VIII). The cerebellum is important in mediating the sense of equilibrium and balance.

What changes occur in the ear with aging?

- Cerumen becomes harder, containing less moisture, and its buildup within the ear may contribute to a hearing loss in the low-frequency range.
- The tympanic membrane loses elasticity.
- The joints between the auditory bones become stiffer, which interferes with the transmission of sound waves, but this is not clinically significant by itself.
- There is a gradual loss of the receptor cells in the organ of Corti after age 40.
- With increasing age, the number of nerve fibers in the vestibulocochlear nerve decrease, contributing to hearing loss and sometimes affecting balance and equilibrium.

Health Promotion Points 25–4

Healthy People 2010 Hearing

28.11 (Developmental) Increase the proportion of newborns who are screened for hearing loss by age 1 month, have audiologic evaluation by age 3 months, and are enrolled in appropriate intervention services by age 6 months.
28.12 Reduce otitis media in children and adolescents.
28.13 (Developmental) Increase access by persons who have hearing impairments to hearing rehabilitation services and adaptive devices, including hearing aids, cochlear implants, or tactile or other assistive or augmentative devices.
28.14 (Developmental) Increase the proportion of persons who have had a hearing examination on schedule.
28.15 (Developmental) Increase the number of persons who are referred by their primary care physician for hearing evaluation and treatment.
28.16 (Developmental) Increase the use of appropriate ear protection devices, equipment, and practices.
28.17 (Developmental) Reduce noise-induced hearing loss in children and adolescents age 17 years and under.
28.18 (Developmental) Reduce adult hearing loss in the noise-exposed public.

Conductive hearing loss most often occurs from stiffening of the bones of the middle ear or from scarring of the tympanic membrane. Continued exposure to excessively high levels of sound can produce sensorineural loss called *noise-induced hearing impairment.* This condition is particularly likely to occur in industrial settings where machinery operation creates loud noise. The standards of the Occupational Safety and Health Administration (OSHA) require the wearing of ear protectors in such settings.

A more recent phenomenon is the potential damage to the inner ear caused by amplified music. **Authorities recommend that continual exposure to music amplified to more than 104 to 111 decibels be avoided.**

Many drugs can be toxic to the inner ear. This is especially true if a very high dose of the drug is given or if it is given incorrectly. Commonly administered drugs that can be ototoxic are many of the antibiotics, nonsteroidal anti-inflammatory drugs, chemotherapy agents, and potent diuretics, such as furosemide (Lasix) (Box 25–2). Aspirin and other salicylates can produce loss of hearing of high frequencies and ringing in the ears *(tinnitus).*

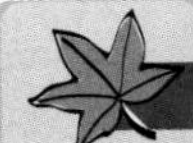

Elder Care Points

The older the patient, the greater the chance of ototoxicity occurring from analgesic medications because many older patients have chronic conditions that cause chronic pain. The liver and kidneys in the elderly generally have decreased function because of aging and cannot degrade and eliminate drugs as easily as in the younger person. For that reason drugs and drug metabolites can build up to toxic levels when medication is taken on a continuing basis.

Nurses should be aware of the potential for damage to the ear by potent drugs (Safety Alert 25–1). Nonsteroidal anti-inflammatory drugs are more toxic in

Table 25–6 Range of Sounds Audible and Hazardous to the Ear

LEVEL IN DECIBELS (dB)	EXAMPLE
0	Lowest sound audible to the human ear
30	Quiet library, soft whisper
40	Living room, quiet office, bedroom away from traffic
50	Light traffic at a distance, refrigerator, gentle breeze
60	Air conditioner at 20 ft, conversation, sewing machine
70	Busy traffic, noisy restaurant; at this decibel level, noise may begin to affect hearing if exposure is constant
HAZARDOUS ZONE FOR HEARING LOSS	
80	Subway, heavy city traffic, alarm clock at 2 ft, factory noise; these noises are dangerous if exposure to them lasts for >8 hr
90	Truck traffic, noisy home appliances, shop tools, lawn mower; as loudness increases, the "safe" time exposure decreases; damage can occur in <8 hr
100	Chain saw, stereo headphones, pneumatic drill; even 2 hr of exposure can be dangerous at this decibel level; with each 5-dB increase, the safe time is cut in half
120	Rock band concert in front of speakers, sandblasting, thunderclap; the danger is immediate; exposure of 120 dB can injure ears
140	Gunshot blast, jet plane; any length of exposure time is dangerous; noise at this level may cause actual pain in the ear
160	Rocket launching pad; without ear protection, noise at this level causes irreversible damage; hearing loss is inevitable

Adapted from Lewis, S.M., Heitkemper, M.M., Dirksen, S.R., et al, (2007). *Medical-Surgical Nursing: Assessment and Management of Clinical Problem* (7th ed.). St. Louis: Mosby.

elderly and when used at maximum dosages over an extended period of time.

DIAGNOSTIC TESTS AND EXAMINATIONS

VISUAL EXAMINATION OF THE EAR

The two instruments most commonly used to examine the ear canal and tympanic membrane are the otoscope and the aural speculum. The otoscope is fitted with a light and a magnifying lens to facilitate inspection (Figure 25–10). The aural speculum is used with a special circular, slightly concave head mirror that has a hole in its middle. The head mirror is positioned so that the central hole lies in front of one eye of the examiner. A source of light, such as a lamp, is placed behind the examiner so that it shines on the head mirror and is reflected into the ear.

The simple speculum can be modified by attaching a special tube and inflatable bag (pneumatic otoscope),

Box 25–2 Ototoxic Drugs and Environmental Chemicals

Ototoxicity (ear poisoning) is due to drugs or chemicals that damage the inner ear or the vestibulocochlear nerve. The vestibulocochlear nerve sends balance and hearing information from the inner ear to the brain. Ototoxicity may result in temporary or permanent disturbances of hearing, balance, or both. Environmental chemicals can be toxic from inhalation of fumes or powder residue or from skin contamination.

DRUGS THAT MAY CAUSE OTOTOXICITY

Antibiotics

- Tobramycin
- Gentamicin
- Streptomycin
- Kanamycin
- Amikacin
- Neomycin
- Netilmicin
- Dihydrostreptomycin
- Erythromycin (IV)
- Vancomycin
- Chloramphenicol
- Minocycline
- Capreomycin
- Dibekacin
- Etiomycin

Antineoplastic Drugs

- Cisplatin
- Carboplatin
- Bleomycin
- Nitrogen mustard

Loop Diuretics (IV)

- Furosemide
- Torsemide
- Bumetanide
- Ethacrynic acid

Salicylates

- Aspirin

Nonsteroidal Anti-inflammatory Drugs

- Ibuprofen
- Naproxen sodium

Quinidine Derivatives

- Quinidex
- Atabrine
- Plaquenil
- Quinine sulfate
- Mefloquine
- Chloroquine

ENVIRONMENTAL CHEMICALS

- Metals (lead, mercury, gold, arsenic)
- Aniline dyes
- Toluene
- Carbon monoxide
- Trichloroethylene
- Xylene
- Povidone-iodine
- Nicotine
- Potassium bromate

Key: *IV*, intravenous.

Safety Alert 25–1

Dangers of Ototoxic Drugs

Know the toxic effects of the drugs you administer. Patients should be assessed frequently while receiving a potentially ototoxic drug. Any signs of ototoxicity, such as ringing in the ears, subtle changes in hearing ability, and difficulty in hearing, should be reported immediately. Many times ototoxicity occurs because patients are taking more than one drug that can be toxic to the ear. Teach patients who are taking daily doses of aspirin or nonsteroidal anti-inflammatory drugs for arthritis or other chronic pain conditions to immediately report the signs of ototoxicity.

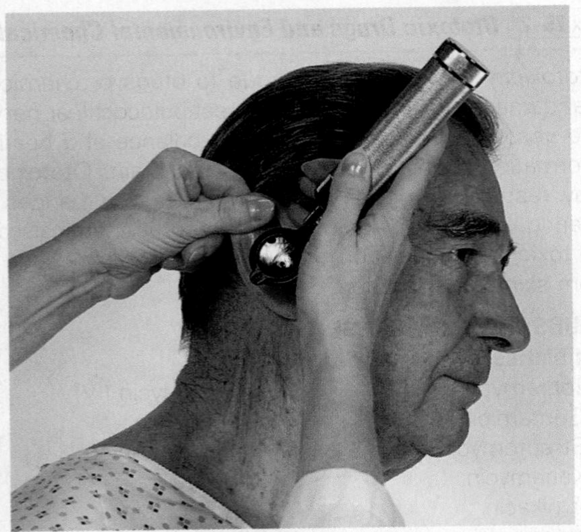

FIGURE **25–10** Examination of the ear with an otoscope.

thereby creating an airtight system. This allows the examiner to determine whether the tympanic membrane responds to positive and negative pressure. The normal eardrum moves in response to pressure. Healed perforations and scars on the eardrum can be seen when the tympanic membrane is moved.

A simple hearing test is the *whisper test.* The examiner stands behind the patient and whispers a question to the patient. If the patient hears the question, an answer is forthcoming. The examiner backs up a step and whispers another question, and so on.

TUNING FORK TESTS

Tuning forks measure hearing by air conduction or by bone conduction (Weber's test and Rinne test). A tuning fork is activated by holding it by the stem and striking the tines softly on the back of your hand (Table 25–7).

TEST FOR NYSTAGMUS

To test for **nystagmus** (involuntary rhythmic jerking of the eyes), the nurse holds a finger directly in front of the patient at eye level. The patient is asked to follow the finger without moving the head. The nurse moves the finger slowly from the midline toward the right ear about 30 degrees. Then the finger is moved back to the midline and then slowly toward the left ear about 30 degrees. The patient's eyes are watched for any jerking movements. Nystagmus other than at the extremes of lateral gaze is abnormal and may indicate an inner ear problem, an intracranial tumor, or paralysis of an eye muscle.

THE ROMBERG TEST

This is a test of equilibrium. The patient stands with the feet together, the arms out to the sides, and the eyes open. The nurse notes ability to maintain an upright posture without swaying. The patient is then asked to close the eyes and posture is observed again. If the patient loses balance, it may indicate a problem with the inner ear or the cerebellum. Table 25–7 lists other diagnostic tests for the ear.

NURSING MANAGEMENT

Assessment (Data Collection)

Patients over the age of 60 should always be assessed for hearing loss. If a patient has a known hearing impairment, the nurse should assess how the patient is coping with it. Hearing and balance are subjective problems and require a good history from the patient. Focused Assessment 25–2 presents guidelines for history taking. Diagnosis of infection requires an otoscopic examination. It should be noted that the color, texture, and amount of cerumen varies among individuals. In whites and African Americans it tends to be moist and rust-brown colored. Native Americans and Asians have cerumen that is lighter in color and drier. Normally, the top of each pinna is aligned with the corner of the eye on each side of the head. Lesions on the pinna may indicate skin cancer, particularly in the elderly patient. There should be no secretions other than cerumen from the ear. Ear pain may be referred from other parts of the head and neck and may occur from sinusitis, dental problems, or temporomandibular joint syndrome. Focused Assessment 25–3 presents a guide to systematic physical examination of the ear.

The ears of elderly in long-term care facilities should be checked with an otoscope at regular intervals for cerumen. Many long-term care residents have a correctable hearing loss related to impacted cerumen. Cerumen can be removed by using cerumen softener drops and then irrigating the external ear canal (Figure 25–11).

Nursing Diagnosis

Nursing diagnoses are chosen based on the data provided during the assessment. Table 25–8 presents the most commonly encountered nursing diagnoses for patients with ear problems, along with the expected outcomes and nursing interventions.

Planning

General goals for the patient with problems of the ear or hearing are:

- Promote knowledge to protect hearing
- Prevent infection and injury
- Promote effective communication
- Promote coping with hearing loss

Expected outcomes are written for each nursing diagnosis chosen for the patient's care plan. Writing the outcomes should be done in collaboration with the patient and other health team members. In addition to the nurse and physician, an audiologist, hearing aid specialist, and speech therapist may be involved in the patient's care. Both long- and short-term goals for the patient should be considered.

Table 25–7 ***Diagnostic Tests for Ear Problems***

TEST	PURPOSE	DESCRIPTION	NURSING IMPLICATIONS
Weber's test	Determines loss of hearing in one ear or both	Tuning fork is struck, and then the handle is placed on the patient's forehead. Normal hearing or equal loss in both ears is demonstrated by hearing the sound in the middle of the head.	Explain purpose and procedure to patient.
Rinne test	Determines whether hearing loss is sensorineural or conductive	Tuning fork is struck, and then the handle is placed on the mastoid bone; the fork is removed and struck again and held beside the ear. The patient is asked in which position he heard the sound better or longer.	Explain procedure to patient.
Audiometry	Determines degree of hearing loss in each ear	Earphones are placed on the patient's ears and, with the use of an audiometry machine, the audiologist channels sounds of different decibels and pitch into one ear and then the other of the patient. The patient signals when he hears the tone.	Explain procedure to patient.
Caloric test	Checks for alteration in vestibular function in each ear	With patient in a seated or supine position, each ear is separately irrigated with a cold and then a warm solution to determine vestibular response. Normal response is nystagmus, vertigo, nausea, vomiting, falling; decreased response indicates abnormality.	Explain procedure to patient; tell him he may experience nystagmus, vertigo, nausea, and vomiting, but these will indicate a normal response.
Electronystagmography (ENG)	Assesses for disease of vestibular system	Electrodes are placed near the patient's eyes. Caloric test is performed; movement of the eyes is recorded on a graph. Decreased response is abnormal.	Explain procedure and equipment to patient. Tell him that nausea, vertigo, etc., indicate a normal response.
Evoked-response audiometry (ERA); auditory brainstem response (ABR)	Determines abnormality of nerve pathways between eighth cranial nerve and brainstem	Electrodes are attached to the client's head in a darkened room; similar to EEG. Auditory stimuli are directed to the patient, and a computer is used to track and separate the auditory electrical activity of the brain from other brain waves.	Explain procedure and equipment to patient. Tell him the room will be darkened.
Magnetic resonance imaging (MRI)	Detects tumor of the eighth cranial nerve, acoustic neuroma	Huge electromagnet is used to detect radiofrequency pulses from the alignment of hydrogen protons in the magnetic field. A computer translates the pulses into cross-sectional images. Provides high-contrast views of soft tissue.	Explain to patient that his head will be placed in a machine that looks like a large tube. He will need to lie very still during the test; all metal must be removed before the test.
FTA-ABS blood test	Blood test for syphilis	Blood is drawn and sent to the lab for determination of presence of syphilis. Syphilis can cause problems with nerve transmission from the ear.	Explain that a blood sample is needed.

Key: *EEG,* electroencephalography; *FTA-ABS,* fluorescent treponemal antibody absorption.

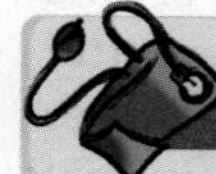

Focused Assessment 25–2

Data Collection for Ear Disorders

Ask the following questions:

- Have you had any pain in the ear?
- Have you had a recent temperature elevation?
- Do you suffer from allergies?
- Do you have frequent upper respiratory infections?
- Have you ever been exposed to very loud noise? Do you work in an area that is noisy? Do you listen to loud music?
- Have you ever had a head injury?
- Do you scuba dive, hunt or shoot skeet, or fly in small airplanes?
- Do you ever have ringing, buzzing, or odd sounds in the ears?
- Do you feel your hearing ability has decreased? Do people you live with think that you do not hear as well as you used to hear? Do you frequently have to ask people to repeat things that have been said to you?
- Is there a history of hearing loss in your family?
- Have you ever had a really high fever?
- What medications are you taking regularly? Are there other medications that you have taken for an extended period in the past? Do you take aspirin?
- How do you clean your ears?
- Do you ever suffer with dizziness, vertigo, or loss of balance?

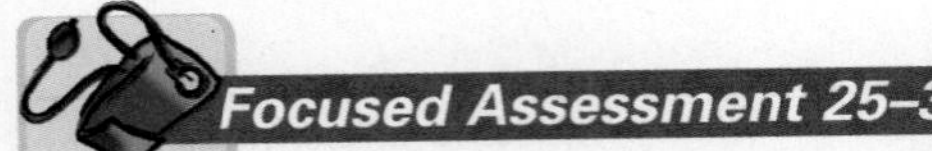

Physical Assessment of the Ear

- Compare the pinna from one side to the other for symmetry and placement.
- Palpate the pinna for the presence of nodules.
- Observe for the presence of lesions on the pinna.
- Check for drainage **(otorrhea)** from the ear; note color and odor.
- Observe the gait to detect any problem with balance.
- Observe for wavering when arising from a supine or seated position that might indicate dizziness or equilibrium problems.
- Observe for signs of bruising on the body from falls that may indicate problems with balance.
- Observe to see whether the person speaks in a voice louder than necessary.
- Observe to see whether facial expression indicates difficulty in understanding what is being said.
- Determine whether responses to statements are inappropriate.

Note: Someone qualified and experienced in using an otoscope should inspect the auditory meatus and the tympanic membrane.

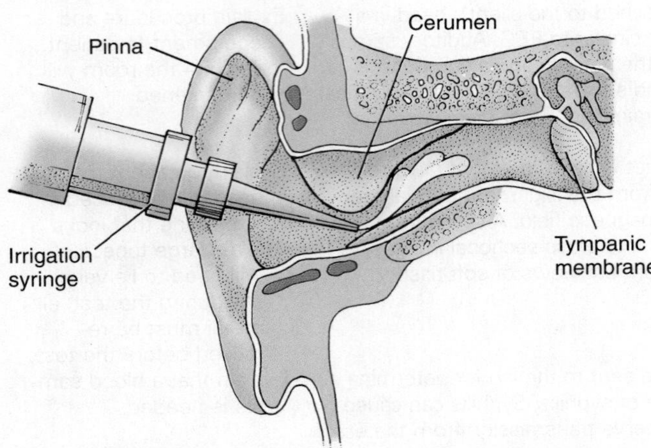

FIGURE **25–11** Irrigating the external ear canal. Warm water is used to remove cerumen and debris from the canal. Aim the stream of water above or below the impaction to allow back pressure to push it out rather than farther down the canal.

When a patient is severely hearing impaired, communication with the patient for treatments and activities of daily living may take longer than with normally hearing patients. The nurse should take this into consideration when creating the daily work plan. If the patient does not have adequate aids for hearing, the nurse must devise an acceptable method of two-way communication with the patient.

Implementation

Interventions for the patient with a hearing or balance problem are geared toward patient education, treatment of infection, pre- and postoperative care and instructions, measures for communication, and referral to resources (Box 25–3). The hearing aid must be cared for properly (Box 25–4).

Instillation of Ear Medication

Eardrops may be ordered to dissolve cerumen, relieve pain, or combat infection in the auditory meatus. The patient should be positioned in a supine lateral position so that the affected ear is uppermost. The medication should be at room temperature. Cold eardrops may cause discomfort or dizziness. For the adult, the ear canal is straightened by drawing the pinna upward and toward the back of the head (Figure 25–12). For a child under age 3, the pinna is pulled down and back. Following the "Five Rights" of medication administration, draw up the correct amount of medication. Insert the tip of the dropper into the external ear canal and instill the medication (Box 25–5). Place cotton in the external meatus to prevent the medication from escaping. Have the patient remain in the lateral position for 5 to 10 minutes.

Interventions for Communication with the Hearing Impaired Patient

The patient who is hearing impaired has unique problems of communication when in the hospital or long-term care facility. If he cannot hear well and misunderstands or misinterprets the voices and sounds in the unfamiliar surroundings, he is likely to be frustrated, fearful, and anxious. Unless a special effort is made to have frequent contact with the patient, social isolation may occur.

When speaking to a hearing-impaired patient, sit at eye level facing the patient. Gain eye contact and speak slowly and enunciate clearly. When trying to communicate with a person who is hearing impaired, bear in mind that attempts to answer questions without fully understanding what is asked may occur. Past experience has taught many hearing-impaired persons that to ask for repetition of questions irritates people and causes them to think the person is stupid. **For this reason, many people who cannot hear well frequently smile and say "Yes," when such an answer is either incorrect or inappropriate.** Another problem is that the individual may fill in parts of sentences with similar-sounding words. For example the words "Knott's Berry Farm" may be interpreted as "not very far." Some guidelines to help the hearing-impaired patient and improve the nurse's ability to communicate are given in Box 25–3.

? ***Think Critically About . . .*** What three techniques of communication with a hearing-impaired patient do you think would be the most helpful?

Table 25–8 ***Nursing Diagnoses, Expected Outcomes, and Nursing Interventions for Patients with Ear Disorders***

NURSING DIAGNOSIS	GOALS/EXPECTED OUTCOMES	NURSING INTERVENTIONS
Disturbed sensory perception related to damage from infection or obstruction	Patient will verbalize ways to prevent further hearing loss. Patient will be free of ear infection within 10 days.	If cerumen is obstructing the auditory canal, irrigate as ordered; warm the irrigation solution to body temperature. If infection is present, instruct regarding antibiotic medication and encourage to take entire prescription. Instruct in use of hearing aid if one is prescribed. Advise of ways to prevent further hearing loss: avoid loud noise or wear ear protectors; seek treatment immediately for signs of ear infection.
Pain related to inflammation in the ear	Pain will be controlled with analgesia within 8 hr. Pain will be resolved within 7 days.	Administer analgesics as ordered as needed. Warm analgesic eardrops to room temperature before administration. Have patient rest head on heating pad turned on "low" setting if this seems to decrease pain.
Impaired verbal communication related to inability to receive messages or to decode and interpret them	Patient will assist in choice of methods to improve ability to communicate. Patient will try hearing aid for 2 wk if there is an indication that this device would help hearing.	Plan with patient the best way to communicate so that instructions and information are comprehended; explore tone of voice, level of volume, distance from patient when speaking, writing out communication, etc. Refer for evaluation by audiologist. Encourage daily use of hearing aid if one is prescribed. Explain that time and adjustments are necessary to obtain the optimum result. Give praise for efforts to use hearing aid.
Anxiety related to inability to hear warnings, perform at work, or communicate in social settings	Patient will explore methods of maintaining safety within 2 wk. Patient will verbalize ways in which assisted hearing devices might assist in performance in the work environment.	Encourage verbalization of fears. Utilize means to enhance communication. Advise of assisted-hearing devices, hearing aids, and availability of "hearing ear" dogs. Introduce means of learning alternative communication methods, such as sign language and speech reading. Explore methods of enhancing attention to visual cues of dangers in the environment (i.e., close attention to signal lights, or observing others at street crossings). Discuss problems of communication in social settings and explore possible solutions (i.e., masking devices for use in crowds, having interaction with only one or two people at a time, avoiding noisy restaurants, or using hearing aid).
Risk of injury related to impaired equilibrium	Patient will verbalize methods to ensure safety within 3 days. Patient will not experience a fall or injury.	Administer medication for vertigo as ordered. Encourage a low-sodium diet. Instruct to change positions very slowly. Encourage to hold on to something solid or to someone when rising from a sitting to a standing position. If vertigo is present, do not ambulate without assistance. Teach or reinforce vestibular/balance exercises as prescribed. Assist to identify any aura (presence of symptoms that precede an attack). Instruct to lie down and keep the eyes open and focused straight ahead when experiencing vertigo.
Deficient knowledge related to the nature of disability, self-care, and availability of community resources for the hearing impaired	Patient will verbalize ways to enhance safe self-care within 2 wk.	Explain nature of hearing loss or vertigo and possible causes. Describe measures to assist the hard-of-hearing person to adapt; refer to support groups and sources for information. Refer to community agencies and resources for the hearing impaired.
Social isolation related to difficulty in communicating	Patient will establish an adequate social network within 2 mo.	Assist patient to consider possibilities for social contact despite hearing problems. Help patient obtain a telephone for the hearing-impaired person. Encourage the use of computer email for contact with friends and family and social interaction with others.

Box 25–3 Communicating with the Hearing-Impaired Person

- If the person uses a hearing aid, encourage its use and see that it is situated, turned on, and adjusted before beginning speaking.
- Be certain you have the person's attention before beginning speaking.
- Sit facing the person with the light on your face rather than from behind you.
- Ask permission to turn down the volume or turn off the television or radio.
- The best distance for speaking to a hearing-impaired person is 2½ to 4 feet. Place yourself on eye level with the person. Do not speak directly into the person's ear as this prevents the person from obtaining visual cues while you are speaking.
- Do not smile, chew gum, or cover the mouth while speaking.
- Use short, simple sentences. If the patient does not appear to understand or responds inappropriately, state the message again using different words. Try to limit each sentence to one subject and one verb.
- Give the person time to respond to questions.
- Ask for oral or written feedback to make certain your message is understood.
- Avoid using the intercom system as it may distort sound.

Box 25–4 Caring for a Hearing Aid

When a hearing aid does not work:

- Check that the switch is "on."
- Examine the ear mold for attached wax or dirt; clean the sound hole.
- Check the battery to see that it is inserted correctly.
- Check the connection between the ear mold and the receiver.
- Replace the battery. Batteries last an average of 12 to 14 days depending on type of aid.
- Check placement of the ear mold in the ear; it should fit snugly.
- Adjust the volume.
- If all else fails, take the hearing aid to an authorized service center for repair.

To clean the hearing aid:

- Turn the hearing aid off.
- Wash the ear mold with mild soap and warm water; do not submerge in water.
- Use a pipe cleaner or toothpick to gently cleanse the opening or short tube that fits into the ear.
- Dry the mold completely before turning on the aid or before reattaching it to the hearing aid (if it is separate).

A piece of tape or sign of some kind should be placed over the terminal on the intercom system that designates the room of a hearing-impaired patient. This serves to remind the person answering the light to go to the patient's room rather than try to talk over the intercom system.

Box 25–5 Instilling Otic Medication

Follow the Five Rights of medication administration. Read the order carefully to determine which ear is to receive the medication.

- Position the patient supine and in the lateral position so that the affected ear is uppermost.
- Draw medication into the medicine dropper by depressing the bulb and letting it go.
- Straighten the ear canal by drawing the pinna upward and toward the back of the head. For children younger than 3 years, draw the earlobe slightly down and back.
- Insert the tip of the medicine dropper into the external ear canal and depress the bulb to dispense the medication. Withdraw the dropper.
- Place cotton in the external meatus to prevent the medication from escaping.
- Have the patient remain in the lateral position for 5 to 10 minutes.

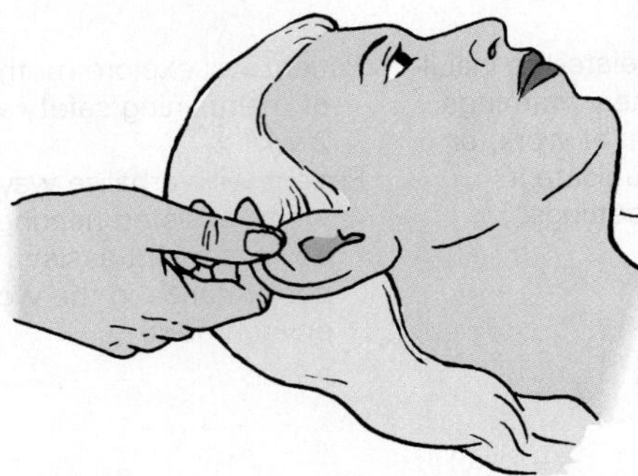

FIGURE **25–12** Straightening the ear canal to instill eardrops.

Evaluation

Evaluation involves reassessment to determine whether the expected outcomes are being met. Determining whether hearing has improved is the criterion by which effectiveness of treatment is evaluated. Improvement is verified by audiometry. Fading or resolution of dizziness and vertigo indicate that actions and treatments for these problems have been effective. Resolution of infection is determined by the appearance of the eardrum, absence of pain, and normal temperature.

COMMON PROBLEMS OF PATIENTS WITH EAR DISORDERS

HEARING IMPAIRMENT

Hearing impairment ranges from difficulty in hearing certain ranges of tones or in understanding certain words to total deafness (Assignment Considerations 25–2). Persons with sensorineural hearing loss typically have more difficulty hearing high-pitched tones than low-pitched ones; thus they frequently can un-

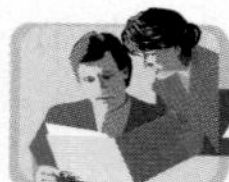

Assignment Considerations 25–2

Caring for the Hearing Impaired

When assigning tasks for a hearing-impaired patient to UAPs and CNAs, remind the person how to effectively communicate with the patient: face the patient and obtain the patient's attention before speaking; speak slowly and enunciate clearly in a normal voice. If the patient wears a hearing aid, it should be in the ear and the patient should be reminded to turn it on before communication begins.

derstand the speech of men better than that of women. Another characteristic of sensorineural hearing loss is difficulty hearing softly spoken and poorly enunciated words. Speaking slightly louder to the person with sensorineural hearing loss may help, but it is especially important to speak slowly and clearly and to face the person when communicating with him. Because people with sensorineural hearing loss do not hear their own voices as well as a person with normal hearing, they tend to speak louder than necessary.

Hearing aids help some people with sensorineural hearing loss. Aids designed to amplify some pitches and block out others that do not need amplification are most helpful. Hearing aids are not always the answer to a problem of hearing loss, and for some people the most effective therapy is focused on rehabilitation to facilitate acceptance of the loss and learning of new ways to communicate in spite of some degree of deafness.

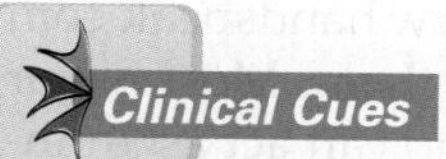

Clinical Cues

The earlier a hearing-impaired person who can benefit from a hearing aid obtains and uses one, the better his brain will adjust and the better the quality of hearing that can be achieved (Ross, 2005). EB

Most hearing aid professionals and companies will offer a 30-day money-back guarantee on any hearing aid so that the patient can try it. The patient will benefit from knowing beforehand that it may take several visits to the hearing aid center for small adjustments before just the right settings are achieved for the hearing aid for the individual.

Central hearing loss occurs in the brain as a result of some pathologic condition above the junction of the eighth cranial nerve and the brainstem. Central hearing loss can be due to a problem of transmission of stimuli in the brain, an inability to decode and sort signals received from one or both ears, or a failure in the transmission of sounds from one hemisphere of the brain to the other. Causes include brain tumors, vascular changes that suddenly deprive the middle ear of its blood supply, and cerebrovascular accident.

Many people have a combination of two or more types of hearing impairment. Often there is a combination of sensorineural and conductive loss.

It should be noted that when a person is fitted with a hearing aid, it takes considerable time of working with the audiologist on adjustments to the device to obtain the best result. Too many people give up on a hearing aid because they have not taken the time to work through the adjustment process.

? ***Think Critically About . . .*** How would you go about working with a hearing-impaired patient who is a candidate for a hearing aid, but adamantly refuses to consider trying out one?

DIZZINESS AND VERTIGO

The sense of balance and equilibrium is governed by the vestibular system in the inner ear. Increases in fluid pressure in the inner ear, inflammations, and vascular disorders that interrupt blood supply to the cochlea can produce dizziness, loss of balance, and nausea and vomiting. These symptoms can range from mildly annoying to completely incapacitating and should always be assessed whenever a person has an ear disorder and loss of hearing. Meniere's disease and labyrinthitis may cause vertigo.

The patient who experiences dizziness and positional vertigo should be cautioned to avoid suddenly turning his head or making other movements that aggravate the vertigo. He should be told to call for assistance whenever he needs to move from his bed or chair. When helping the patient to his feet, move slowly and give him time to stand for a moment before beginning to walk. **Typically, patients with this kind of vertigo feel that the room is spinning around during an attack, and any motion makes the sensation even worse.** While the patient is having an attack of vertigo, he should lie in bed and remain as motionless as possible. Stabilizing his head with a pillow on either side may encourage immobility. Attacks can last from a few minutes to hours.

Medications to reduce motion sickness and nausea should be given precisely as ordered. These are usually given every 3 to 4 hours or on a preventive basis *before* the patient's symptoms become severe.

When increased fluid pressure in the inner ear is suspected as the cause of dizziness, the physician may order a low-sodium diet and limit fluid intake. Patients with recurrent attacks of vertigo are encouraged to stop smoking if they are habitual tobacco smokers. Alcohol is contraindicated as well; in particular, red wine and beer should be avoided. **Stress may affect the frequency of attacks of vertigo in patients with inner ear disorders.** Teaching the patient effective coping mechanisms to handle stress or adding rest periods into the work schedule may be helpful.

TINNITUS

Ringing, buzzing, or other continuous noise in the ear *(tinnitus)* can be mildly annoying or so severe that it interferes with activities of daily living and prevents the patient from getting sufficient sleep and rest. Common causes of tinnitus include **presbycusis** (hearing loss associated with aging), constant exposure to loud environmental noise, inflammation and infection in the ear, otosclerosis, Meniere's disease, and labyrinthitis. Systemic disorders such as hypertension and other cardiovascular disorders, neurologic disease (including head injury), and hyper- and hypothyroidism also can cause ringing in the ears. Tinnitus frequently may be one of the first symptoms produced by an ototoxic drug. Symptoms of tinnitus are subjective, and diagnosis is by patient history.

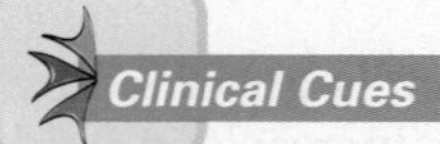

The patient with tinnitus will become more fatigued than others when in a noisy location such as a social gathering, a restaurant, or the like. Family and friends should be informed of this situation. It happens because of the overload of sensory input to the brain.

Medical treatment begins with efforts to determine the underlying cause and treat it. When the cause cannot be found, symptomatic relief is tried. However, some cases of intractable tinnitus resist all modes of conventional therapy. Less traditional measures that have varying degrees of success include biofeedback training and "masking." Sometimes substances that increase circulation are helpful. The benzodiazepines, such as diazepam (Valium) or chlordiazepoxide (Librium), seem to help some people.

Biofeedback training is especially helpful in those cases in which emotional stress and anxiety are thought to be the underlying causes of tinnitus. Through visual or auditory signals, the person learns to relax and exert some degree of control over his autonomic nervous system. This can lower blood pressure and pulse rate and relax muscles that are very tense.

Masking simply provides a low-level noise to block out, or "mask," the head noise heard by the person complaining of tinnitus. Some examples include playing soft music or a tape of sounds of nature, such as a waterfall, while the person is resting or sleeping, providing "white noise" in the working environment, using a hearing aid to amplify sound from the outside and overcome head noise, and wearing a special tinnitus instrument, which is a combination hearing aid and tinnitus masker for people who have both hearing loss and tinnitus. The therapeutic effect of masking is highly individualized. Some people find instant relief, some partial abatement of the head noise, and some do not benefit from any attempts to mask the sounds of tinnitus. Earplugs or ear protection should be worn when noise exposure cannot be avoided.

REHABILITATION FOR HEARING LOSS

Specific measures to rehabilitate a patient with hearing loss depend on the age and aptitude of the patient. Adults who have acquired the skills of speech and language before their loss of hearing occurred are better able than children to pick up language cues and understand what is being said to them, and therefore should have fewer problems with communication by language.

LIPREADING (SPEECH READING)

Instruction in reading lips is one mode of therapy for the hearing impaired, but it is not a remedy for all difficulties. Only about 60% of the sounds in the English language can be identified by watching the lips. Most experienced lip-readers do not catch more than half of the words spoken to them. Communication by lipreading is enhanced by other nonverbal clues, such as facial expressions and hand gestures.

Learning to lip read is difficult. It requires at least average intelligence, exceptional language skills, excellent eyesight, and much persistence and patience.

SIGN LANGUAGE

Many deaf people learn to communicate with sign language. American Sign Language (ASL) is the third most commonly used language in the United States. There are on-line dictionaries for ASL and several websites that provide tutorials: www.handspeak.com and www.deafsign.com are two of them. Most major hospitals have someone on staff who can act as an interpreter for ASL.

HEARING AIDS

An evaluation by a reputable audiologist should be completed before purchasing a hearing aid. In this way a prescription for a hearing aid designed to provide the best possible improvement of hearing is obtained.

The hearing aids produced today can improve hearing for a variety of types of hearing loss. For the person who does not have a defect in the middle ear, a hearing aid can transmit amplified sound from the receiver through the eardrum to the inner ear. This is accomplished by amplifying sound waves transmitted by air conduction and bone conduction.

The design of a hearing aid varies. Some are worn in the ear, others behind the ear, and still others are built into the frame of eyeglasses. Persons with binaural hearing loss (both ears are affected) must wear a hearing aid in each ear. Regardless of the type of hearing aid, it will have a microphone, an amplifier, a receiver, and a battery (Figure 25–13).

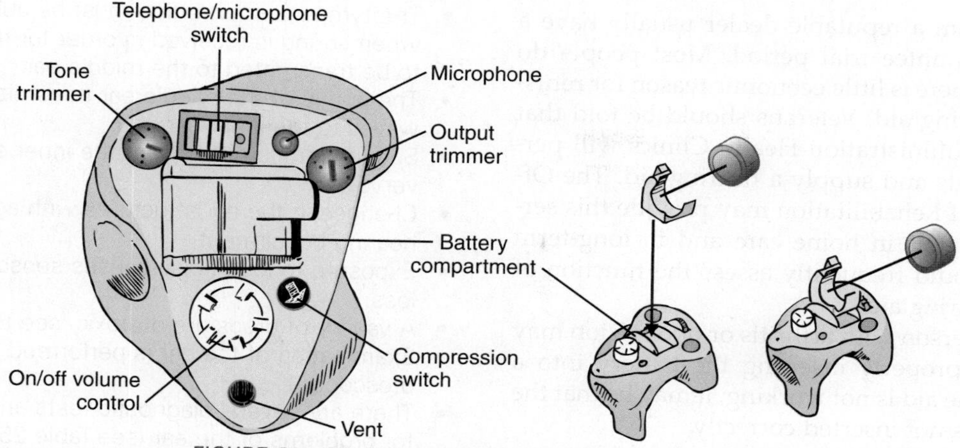

FIGURE 25–13 Parts of a typical in-the-ear hearing aid.

The hearing aid should not be handled roughly or dropped. The ear mold can be cleaned with soap and water, but the other parts of the aid should not get wet (see Box 25–4). Hair spray can damage the microphone of a hearing aid. Regular servicing by a dealer can keep the aid in good working order. When an incapacitated patient has a hearing aid, the nurse is responsible for the security of the hearing aid.

There are many types of hearing aids on the market. Newer digital types can amplify the tones needed while masking other levels of noise. It takes time to adapt to the use of a hearing aid, and the audiologist must make repeated adjustments to the device to achieve optimum function.

COCHLEAR IMPLANT

Cochlear implants are now available for the patient who has no hearing at all. The device is a small computer that changes spoken words into electrical impulses that are transmitted via an implanted coil to the nerve endings in the cochlea. Success with the surgical implant varies considerably from one person to the next. Bone hearing devices and semi-implanted devices are under development (Figure 25–14). A speech therapist works with the patient once the cochlear implant is in place.

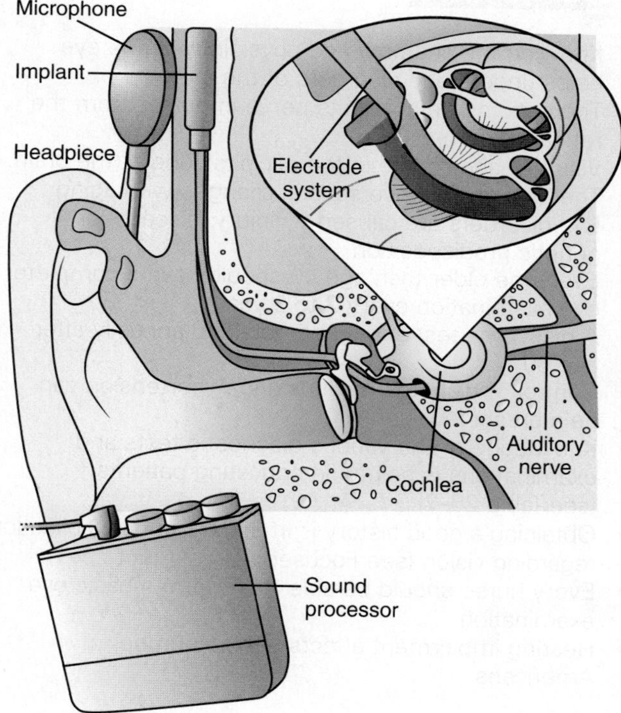

FIGURE 25–14 Cochlear implant.

HEARING-ASSISTIVE DEVICES

Many devices on the market use hearing aid technology. These devices assist people to hear telephone conversations, television, and sound systems, such as those in church or the theater. A telecommunication device for the deaf (TDD) is available. It is a combination typewriter and telephone and can be used to communicate with someone else who has a TDD, or can be used to call a relay center that then communicates the message to the intended person. There are alarm clocks that activate a flashing light, smoke detectors that flash light, and doorbells and telephones that flash a light when a sound is produced. "Hearing ear" dogs are trained to alert their owners to particular sounds and to keep their owners safe when around traffic.

COMMUNITY CARE

Public education about the dangers of loud noise and music could do much to prevent thousands of people from becoming hearing impaired. Teaching people to seek medical attention for symptoms of otitis media quickly prevents damage to the tympanic membrane and preserves hearing ability.

Encouraging those with hearing impairment to have a thorough evaluation and to try a hearing aid could do much to improve the quality of their lives.

Hearing aids from a reputable dealer usually have a money-back guarantee trial period. Most people do not know this. There is little economic reason for refusing to *try* a hearing aid. Veterans should be told that the Veteran's Administration Health Clinics will perform hearing tests and supply a hearing aid. The Office of Vocational Rehabilitation may provide this service as well. Nurses in home care and in long-term care settings should frequently assess the function of the patient's hearing aid.

The elderly person with arthritis or poor vision may have difficulty properly inserting the battery into a hearing aid. If the aid is not working, it may be that the battery simply is not inserted correctly.

Key Points

- Knowing the anatomy and physiology of the eye helps understand disorders of the eye.
- The optic nerve conducts nerve impulses from the retina to the brain.
- Visual images arrive in the occipital lobe of the brain.
- The eyes experience several changes with aging.
- Eye disorders are caused by injury, disease, or genetic predisposition.
- Everyone older than age 40 should have a complete eye examination every 2 to 3 years.
- A glaucoma test should be obtained annually after age 50.
- Control of diabetes mellitus and hypertension can help preserve vision.
- Knowledge of the various diagnostic tests and examinations is helpful in educating patients (see Table 25–2).
- Obtaining a good history is important to data collection regarding vision (see Focused Assessment 25–1).
- Every nurse should be able to perform a basic eye examination.
- Hearing impairment affects a large number of Americans.
- The tympanic membrane must be able to vibrate when sound is received in order for the sound waves to be transmitted to the middle ear.
- The bones of the middle ear transmit the sound waves to the inner ear.
- Sound is transmitted from the inner ear to cranial verve VIII.
- Changes in the ear structures with aging may cause hearing impairment.
- Exposure to loud noise causes sensorineural hearing loss.
- A variety of drugs are ototoxic (see Box 25–2).
- Examination of the ear is performed visually with the otoscope.
- There are several diagnostic tests and examinations for problems of the ear (see Table 25–7).
- Learning to communicate with the hearing-impaired person is important for nurses (see Box 25–3).
- Labyrinthitis and Ménière's disease cause dizziness and vertigo.
- Decreasing stress often decreases dizziness and vertigo.
- Tinnitus is common with a variety of ear disorders.
- A variety of treatments are available to help the patient with tinnitus; biofeedback and masking help many people.
- Lipreading or speech reading is helpful to the hearing-impaired person but is difficult to learn.
- Various types of hearing aids are available, but using one takes practice.
- Cochlear implants are available for the patient who is totally deaf.
- Nurses should actively educate in the community about ways to prevent hearing loss.

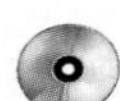

Go to your **Companion CD-ROM** for an Audio Glossary, animations, video clips, and bonus review questions.

evolve Be sure to visit the companion Evolve site at http://evolve.elsevier.com/deWit for interactaive NCLEX Exam Style Review Questions, WebLinks, and additional online resources.

NCLEX-PN EXAM STYLE REVIEW QUESTIONS

Choose or insert the best answer(s) for the following questions.

1. ______________________ is an opaque ring outlining the cornea that sometimes results from the deposition of fatty globules.

2. The proper instillation of ear drops to an adult patient would be to:
   1. draw the pinna upward and toward the front of the head.
   2. draw the pinna upward and toward the back of the head.
   3. pull the pinna downward and toward the front of the head.
   4. pull the pinna downward and toward the back of the head.

3. When communicating with a hearing-impaired patient, the nurse must consider which of the following strategies? *(Select all that apply.)*
   1. Sit at eye level facing the patient.
   2. Chew gum.
   3. Enunciate clearly.
   4. Speak directly into the patient's ear.
   5. Use simple sentences.

4. The nurse evaluates the visual acuity of the patient using the Snellen chart. Which of the following statements is true regarding the use of the Snellen chart?
   1. The chart is placed 40 feet away from the patient.
   2. The patient reads the letters using one eye at a time.
   3. The numerator indicates the smallest line that the patient could read.
   4. The denominator (bottom) refers to the patient's distance from the chart.

5. While looking at a card with a geometric grid of identical squares, the patient is asked to focus on a central dot and to describe any distortions of the surrounding boxes. Which of the following patient statements indicates a need for further diagnostic testing?
   1. "I get dizzy staring at these boxes for so long."
   2. "I am beginning to see color differences in the squares."
   3. "I can see all the boxes surrounding the dot."
   4. "There are wavy lines around the central dot."

6. During a physician visit, a 65-year-old man complains of pain in his right eye associated with excessive tearing. The nurse notes that the eye is red with lashes rubbing against the cornea. A likely condition would be:
   1. ptosis.
   2. ectropion.
   3. hordeolum.
   4. entropion.

7. The nurse applies a vibrating tuning fork to the middle of the patient's forehead. The patient reports hearing the sound in the middle of the head. The patient's response indicates:
   1. sensorineural hearing loss.
   2. conduction hearing loss.
   3. normal hearing.
   4. inconclusive findings.

8. The nurse observes as a patient self-administers eyedrops. Which of the following patient actions indicates a need for further instructions?
   1. The cap is placed upside down after removal.
   2. While reclining, the patient looks up to the ceiling while tilting the head slightly toward the eye receiving a drop.
   3. Eyedrops are placed on the cornea.
   4. The eyes are gently moved side to side to distribute the medication.

9. While ambulating, the patient with Ménière's disease complains of dizziness and vertigo. An immediate nursing action would be to:
   1. provide oxygen.
   2. assist patient to lying position.
   3. administer medications.
   4. notify physician.

10. Which of the following nursing actions demonstrate appropriate care of a visually impaired patient? *(Select all that apply.)*
    1. Introduce self prior to touching.
    2. Speak slowly with a loud voice.
    3. Keep the door ajar.
    4. Ensure ready access to the call button for assistance.
    5. Assist with feeding using the clock method.

CRITICAL THINKING ACTIVITIES

Read each clinical scenario and discuss the questions with your classmates.

Scenario A

Mr. Hartman comes to the ambulatory clinic because he "got something in my eye" while using the weedeater.

1. What type of examinations would you expect the health care provider to perform?
2. What would you teach Mr. Hartman about eye safety before he leaves?
3. What questions would you ask him about basic eye care while you are interviewing him before the physician sees him?

Scenario B

Mrs. Como is admitted to the hospital for management of her hypertension. She has had sensorineural deafness for several years, and it is much worse in her left ear than in her right. Her inability to hear well causes additional stress for Mrs. Como, and she is especially anxious about being in the hospital among strangers. Mrs. Como also suffers from tinnitus, which adds to her stress and inability to relax and rest. This and the stress of not being able to hear adversely affect Mrs. Como's hypertension.

1. What evidence would you expect to find that would indicate that Mrs. Como has a hearing impairment?
2. What can the nurses do to improve communication with Mrs. Como and help allay her anxiety about being in the hospital?
3. Why could her hearing problem make her blood pressure rise?

CHAPTER

26 Care of Patients with Disorders of the Eyes and Ears

evolve http://evolve.elsevier.com/deWit

Objectives

Upon completion of this chapter, you should be able to:

Theory

1. Discuss errors of refraction and their treatment.
2. Consider the nursing care for the patient who is undergoing a corneal transplant.
3. Compare measures used to provide assistance after a chemical eye burn and those for an eye injury with a foreign object.
4. Describe the signs and symptoms of selected disorders of the eye and appropriate medical treatment and nursing interventions for each.
5. Discuss nursing interventions to care for the patient after a scleral buckle or a cataract extraction.
6. Identify aids and resources for people with vision loss.
7. Explore the impact of hearing or vision loss on an individual and her family.
8. List the signs and symptoms of selected disorders of the ear, appropriate medical or surgical treatment, and nursing interventions for each.
9. Teach the patient with tinnitus or vertigo measures that may decrease the symptoms.
10. Discuss aids and resources for people with impaired hearing or tinnitus.

Clinical Practice

1. Provide appropriate care for a patient who is preoperative for eye surgery.
2. Properly administer eye medications.
3. Teach a patient to properly administer ear medication.
4. Provide appropriate care for a postoperative ear surgery patient.

Key Terms

Be sure to check out the bonus material on the Companion CD-ROM, including selected audio pronunciations.

accommodation (ă-kŏm-ō-DĀ-shŭn, p. 638)
astigmatism (ă-STĬG-mă-tĭsm, p. 639)
drusen (drū-zĕn, p. 653)
enucleation (ē-nū-klē-Ā-shŭn, p. 641)
exophthalmos (ĕk-sŏf-THĂL-mŏs, p. 639)
hyperopia (hī-pĕr-Ō-pē-ă, p. 638)
myopia (mī-Ō-pē-ă, p. 638)
nystagmus (nĭs-TĂG-mŭs, p. 657)
photodynamic therapy (fō-tō-dī-NĂM-ĭk, p. 653)
photophobia (fō-tō-FŌ-bē-ă, p. 642)
presbyopia (prĕz-bē-Ō-pē-ă, p. 639)
tympanoplasty (tĭm-pă-nō-PLĂS-tē, p. 657)

COMMON DISORDERS OF THE EYE

There are many disorders of the eye, including infection, irritation, injury, and structural abnormalities. Patients must be taught the eye danger signals indicating the need for a physician's attention (see Health Promotion Points 25–2).

ERRORS OF REFRACTION

The most common visual defects are those of refraction. This means that light rays entering the eye are not "refracted," or bent, at the correct angle and therefore do not focus on the retina. Errors of refraction may be caused by a number of structural defects within the eyeball itself. For example, if the eyeball is constructed so that the distance between the lens and retina is too short, the light rays focus behind the retina. This causes difficulty in seeing objects close at hand and is called farsightedness **(hyperopia)** (Figure 26–1).

If the opposite is true, and the eyeball is too elongated, the light rays will converge and focus in front of the retina. The individual then has difficulty seeing objects at a distance and is referred to as being nearsighted. Nearsightedness is called **myopia** (see Figure 26–1).

Light rays from distant objects do not enter the eye at the same angle as light rays from near objects. When looking off into the distance and then quickly looking down at a book, the eyes must make an adjustment to the difference in the light rays entering the eye. This adjustment, which is called **accommodation,** is accomplished by ciliary muscles and ligaments that change the shape of the lens, making it more rounded or flatter, thereby allowing light rays to fall on the retina (Figure 26–2).

With age, the ciliary muscles become less elastic and cannot readily accommodate the needs of distant and

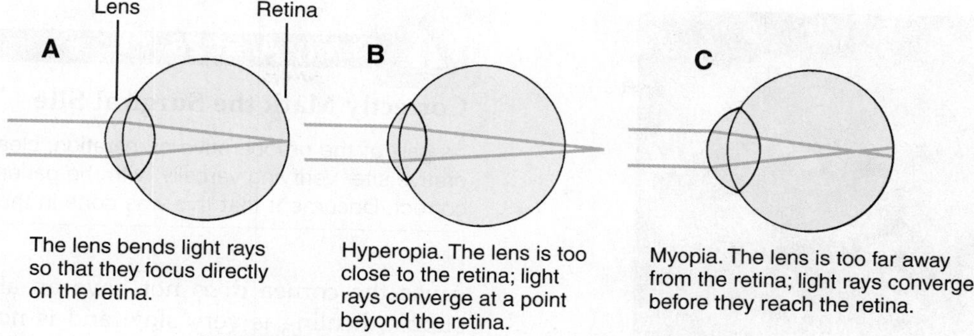

FIGURE 26–1 **A,** Normal vision. **B,** Hyperopia. **C,** Myopia.

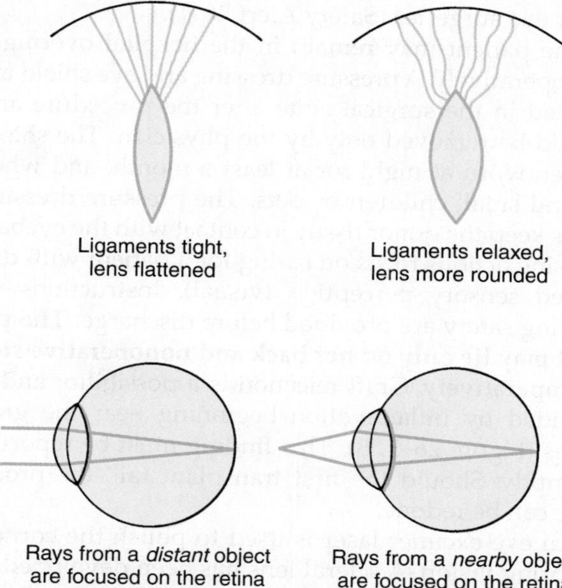

FIGURE 26–2 Flattening and rounding of the lens during accommodation.

near vision. Hardening of the ciliary muscles occurs in many people over 40 years of age and is known as **presbyopia.** Bifocal glasses are usually prescribed for this condition because they allow for two sets of lenses in one pair of glasses, one for viewing distant objects and one for seeing close objects.

Astigmatism is a visual defect resulting from a warped lens or an irregular curvature of the cornea, either of which will prevent the horizontal and vertical rays from focusing at the same point on the retina. Actually, very few people have perfectly shaped eyeballs, and thus there are very few who do not have some degree of astigmatism. If the astigmatism is very slight, the eye can accommodate for its imperfection by changing the shape of the lens. If there is a serious error of refraction, the eyes will tire very easily or the person will have defective vision because the eyes cannot change the shape of the lens enough to compensate for the abnormality.

Serious errors of refraction are treated with prescription artificial lenses and either eyeglasses or contact lenses that are fitted so that the light rays are brought into proper focus on the retina. In recent years, advances have been made in refractive surgery that permit correction of refraction problems for some people. Those who are nearsighted (myopic) can undergo one of three procedures. In *photorefractive keratectomy (PRK)*, an excimer laser is used to remove a thin layer of tissue from the cornea. This corrects the excessive curvature of the cornea that is interfering with the proper focus of light rays through the lens. The preparation takes 30 minutes and the actual procedure takes less than a minute to perform; visual improvement is apparent within 3 to 5 days. *LASIK* (laser in situ keratomileusis) is the most common procedure for nearsightedness in the United States. The middle layer of the cornea is reshaped with a laser after a very thin outer layer of the cornea is peeled back. The outer layer is replaced. Postoperative recovery is very rapid with little discomfort. The procedure takes about 10 to 15 minutes per eye and is done as an outpatient procedure.

Radial keratotomy is used to correct both nearsightedness and astigmatism. Tiny cuts are made in the cornea that flatten it. It is another outpatient procedure. LASIK and PRK have mostly replaced this procedure.

CORNEAL DISORDERS

Keratitis

Keratitis is an inflammation of the cornea caused by irritation or infection. Patients who have had a stroke may develop irritation of the cornea because the eyelid does not close normally. Keratitis may occur in a comatose patient who is not receiving proper eye care. Some people with **exophthalmos** (protruding eyeballs) develop this disorder. Infection caused by bacteria, fungi, or protozoa also is a frequent cause of keratitis. **Such an infection is not uncommon in those who wear contact lenses.** The infecting agent may be in home-prepared saline solution used for cleaning the lenses. The eye becomes reddened, and there may be tearing along with a feeling of grittiness or pain. Discharge from the eye may occur. Treatment of irritation is instillation of

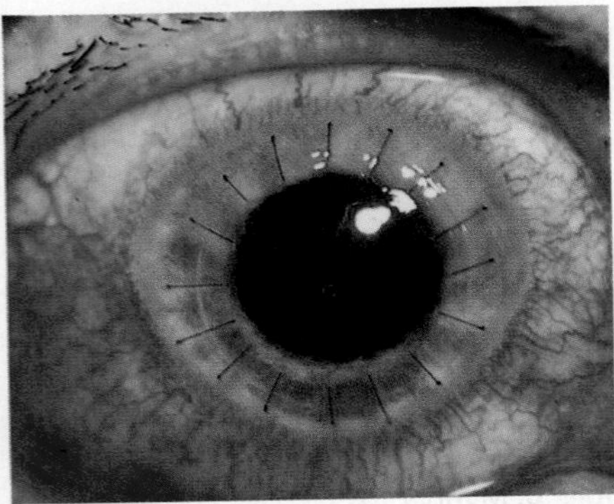

A

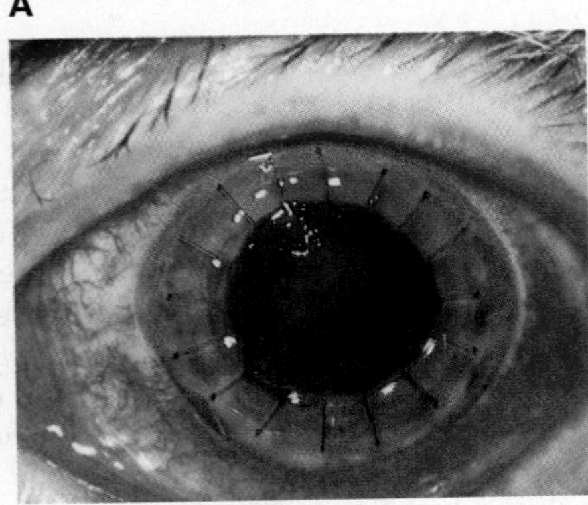

B

FIGURE 26–3 **A,** Keratoplasty (corneal transplant). **B,** Acute transplant rejection.

artificial tears. Infection is treated by a medication to kill the organism. Drugs may be given topically, subconjunctivally, or by intravenous (IV) infusion.

Corneal Ulcer

A corneal ulcer may occur from irritation, infection, or injury. The ulcer is cultured to determine whether there is a causative organism. If so, appropriate medication is supplied. Scarring from corneal ulcers or severe infection is treated by keratoplasty.

Corneal Transplantation (Keratoplasty)

Corneal transplants replace corneas that have been damaged by genetic disorders, trauma, ulcers, or disease, such as *keratitis* (inflammation of the cornea), and help restore corneal clarity. Two types of procedures are done: a full-thickness keratoplasty (corneal transplant), or a lamellar keratoplasty, which replaces only a superficial layer of corneal tissue. The full-thickness keratoplasty restores vision in about 95% of patients (Figure 26–3, *A*). Corneas for transplantation are harvested from cadavers soon after death. The transplantation is performed with regional anesthesia.

The patient must be "on call" to come for the transplantation, as it is unpredictable as to when a matching donor cornea will become available. The patient must realize beforehand that it takes 1 to 2 weeks before any improvement in vision is noticeable and that improvement will continue for several months. Because the cornea does not have an abundant blood supply, healing is very slow and is not complete for about 1 year. **Prevention of infection is extremely important.** Preoperative care is much the same as for other eye surgeries (Safety Alert 26–1).

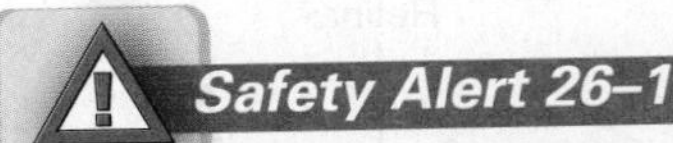

Safety Alert 26–1

Correctly Mark the Surgical Site

As part of the preoperative preparation, clearly mark the operative site, verifying verbally with the patient that the site is correct. Document that this was done in the medical record.

The patient may remain in the hospital overnight postoperatively. A pressure dressing and eye shield are applied in the surgical suite after the procedure and should be removed only by the physician. The shield is then worn at night for at least a month, and when around small children or pets. The pressure dressing helps keep the donor tissue in contact with the eyeball. Nursing actions focus on caring for a patient with disturbed sensory perception (visual). Instructions regarding safety are provided before discharge. **The patient may lie only on her back and nonoperative side postoperatively.** Graft rejection is a possibility and is heralded by inflammation beginning near the graft edges (Figure 26–3, *B*). This finding must be reported promptly. Should the first transplant fail, the procedure can be redone.

An eye excimer laser is used to polish the cornea, restoring vision. A scleral lens has been developed. It is like an oversized contact lens that arches over the cornea. The space between the lens and the cornea is filled with artificial tears, providing lubrication, and thus the scleral lens fulfills the optical functions of the damaged cornea. These innovations may eventually make corneal transplants unnecessary for many people.

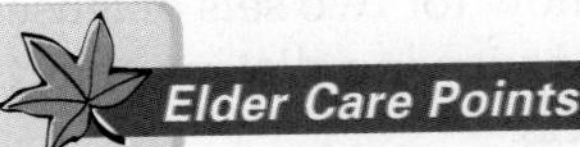

Elder Care Points

The elderly patient who is visually impaired temporarily or permanently may experience a loss of independence and a change in self-perception. This patient will need specific suggestions on ways to maintain independence. After an eye surgery, which is often done on an outpatient basis, the person will need someone to help at home for a few days at least.

EYE TRAUMA

Eye trauma occurs from accidents and from debris in the air. Not using safety goggles or glasses when sanding or operating weedeaters and various types of power equipment accounts for most incidents of foreign bodies landing in the eyes.

Removal of Foreign Bodies from the Eye

If the foreign body is not deeply embedded in the tissues of the eye, it can easily be removed by irrigation. Irrigation with clear, lukewarm water or sterile water or saline is used to remove a foreign body sticking to the cornea. Continuous irrigation can be done with small tubing, and a bottle of solution or an irrigating syringe or bottle can be used. The nurse must be very careful not to touch the eye with the tip of the irrigating device. Sometimes a speck of foreign matter on the cornea can be removed with a moistened, sterile cotton swab. Have the patient tilt the head back and move the eyes away from the site of the particle. Hold the eyelids open to prevent blinking.

If a foreign body is sticking out of the eye, no attempt to remove it should be made. Both eyes should be patched to prevent further eye movement, and the patient should be transported to the emergency room or to an ophthalmologist.

If the patient continues to complain of a sensation that a foreign body is still in the eye after it appears to have been removed by irrigation, or complains of continuing pain, refer to a physician immediately, as there may be a corneal abrasion.

The physician will apply a stain to the eye to assess whether the cornea is abraded. If there is an abrasion, medicated ointment will be prescribed, and the eye will be patched. The patient must be given instructions on how to instill the ointment (see Box 25–1). A thin line of eye ointment is applied from the inner canthus to the outer canthus along the lower eyelid inside the conjunctival sac (Figure 26–4). The patient closes the eyelid and moves the eyeball around in the socket to distribute the ointment. Excess medication is gently wiped away with a tissue, moving from the inner to the outer canthus. If an eyepatch is not applied, the patient is warned that the ointment may blur vision for a while. A corneal abrasion is painful; a nonsteroidal anti-inflammatory drug may be used for discomfort.

Chemical Burns

Chemical burns should be treated by lengthy, continuous irrigation. An IV bag of normal saline is the preferred solution; otherwise, tap water will do. Place the patient supine with her head turned to the affected side. With gloves on, direct the stream of fluid to the inner canthus so that the stream flows across the cornea to the outer canthus, holding the lids apart with your thumb and index finger. At intervals, stop and have the patient close her eyes to move secretions and particles from the upper eye to the lower conjunctival sac; then begin again. The patient should be seen by a physician as soon as possible. All commercial businesses where exposure to chemicals is a possibility must comply with Occupational Safety and Health Administration (OSHA) standards and have an eyewash station within the facility as close as possible to the area where chemicals are likely to be used.

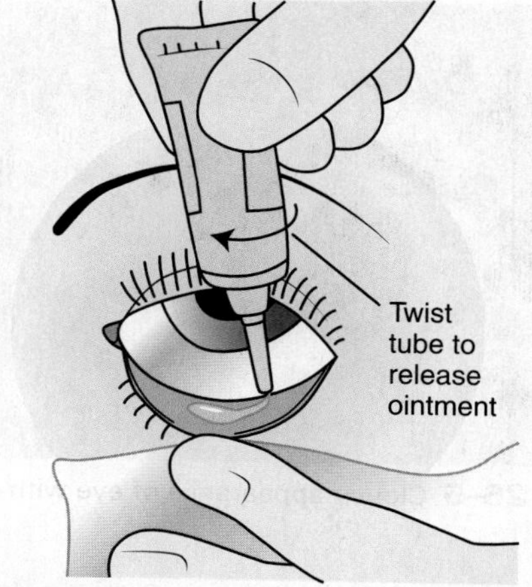

FIGURE **26–4** Applying eye ointment.

Enucleation

If the eye is too damaged by trauma to be salvaged, or is irreparably damaged by disease or tumor, **enucleation** (removal of the eye) is performed. An implant is created to maintain the orbital anatomy while a matching artificial eye is created. The implant is sutured to the muscle structures. When the artificial eye is placed, the muscle attachments allow for coordinated eye movement.

Postoperatively, observe for signs of complications such as excessive bleeding, swelling, increased pain, elevated temperature, or displacement of the implant. Losing an eye is a devastating experience even when there has been a long period of painful blindness preoperatively. Understanding of the emotional impact and support of the patient are prime nursing responsibilities. The permanent prosthesis is placed about 6 weeks after the surgery.

Care of an Artificial Eye. The procedure for cleansing and caring for an artificial eye is similar in many ways to the care of dentures. Both require basic principles of cleanliness, careful handling, and proper storage. An artificial eye is very expensive and must be handled very carefully.

The artificial eye is cleansed with gentle soap and water, unless the patient, her family, or the physician directs otherwise. Keep it in a safe place to avoid damage. When the eye is to be reinserted, it should be cleansed again with soap and water. When inserting or removing the prosthesis, have the head over a padded surface. The patient's upper lid is lifted, and the eye is inserted with the notched end toward the nose. After the prosthesis is placed as far as possible under the upper lid, the lower lid is depressed allowing the eye to slip into place.

CATARACT

The word *cataract* literally means waterfall. It is used to designate an opacity of the lens that produces an effect similar to one a person would get when looking through a sheet of falling water (Figure 26–5). **A cataract causes a blurring of vision because the lens,**

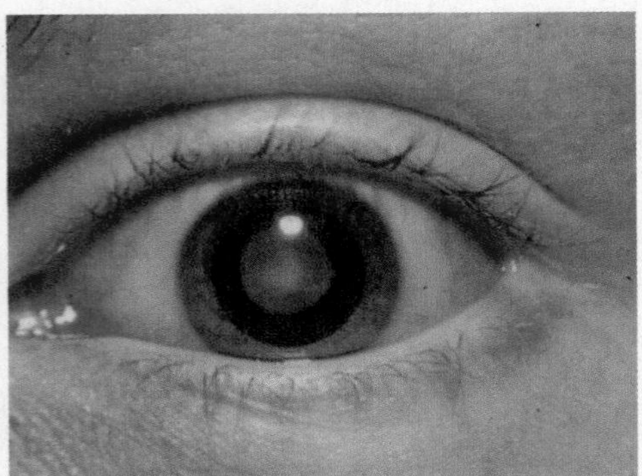

FIGURE 26–5 Cloudy appearance of eye with cataract.

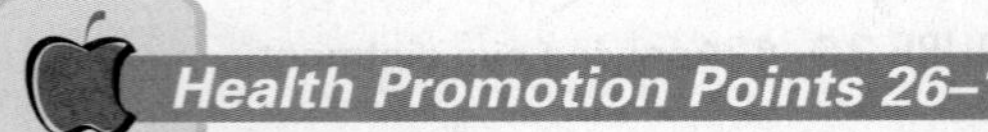

Health Promotion Points 26–1

Cataract Prevention

Encouraging the habit of wearing of sunglasses that protect from ultraviolet light and a hat when outdoors can help prevent the development of cataracts. Cumulative exposure to ultraviolet light is the greatest risk factor for cataracts.

which is normally transparent, becomes cloudy and opaque.

Etiology and Pathophysiology

Cataracts are sometimes present at birth *(congenital cataracts),* but they most often occur as a result of aging and are found in people over the age of 50 *(adult-onset [senile] cataracts).*

Traumatic cataracts may occur from a physical blow or exposure to sunlight, heat, or chemical toxins (Health Promotion Points 26–1). **Cigarette smoking increases the risk of developing cataracts. Heavy drinking also is implicated.** Repeated exposure to lead is implicated in the development of cataracts. Sometimes cataracts occur again after surgery if the lens capsule is left intact during original cataract surgery. Chronic use of corticosteroids predisposes to the development of cataracts.

? *Think Critically About . . .* What would you teach the person with rheumatoid arthritis who is on corticosteroids most of the time about eye care?

Congenital cataracts are most often due to maternal infection with rubella or *Toxoplasma gondii.* Traumatic cataracts occur from disruption of the lens' normal placement and contour. Aging sometimes causes degeneration of the lens and the structures that support it.

Signs, Symptoms, and Diagnosis

In addition to the blurred vision that is typical of opacity of the lens, there may be distortion of vision when looking at distant objects. Vision may be better in low light when the pupil is dilated because more light is transmitted around the opacity. Uncomplicated cataracts are usually painless, but the patient may have **photophobia** (intolerance of light). Assessment may reveal the following symptoms:

- Hazy, blurred, or double vision *(diplopia)*
- Increasing complaints about glare
- Increasing nearsightedness
- Complaints that colors are faded or appear yellowish or brownish
- Desire for increased light by which to read
- Difficulty with night vision
- Frequent need for eyeglass prescription change

The loss of vision associated with cataracts is progressive and sometimes is partially due to secondary glaucoma. As an untreated cataract progresses, the lens of the eye becomes cloudy or milky white, then may turn yellow, and eventually become brown or black (see Figure 26–5). The patient may have difficulty discriminating colors.

Diagnosis of a cataract is confirmed by examining the dilated pupil with a slit lamp, which enables the examiner to see opacities more clearly. Glaucoma should first be ruled out as a possible cause of the symptoms. Tonometry is used to determine intraocular pressure (IOP). For screening purposes, the Tono-Pen may be used (see Figure 25–5).

Treatment

Cataract surgery is performed when the loss of vision greatly affects the quality of the person's life. The only effective method of treating cataracts is surgical removal of the affected lens; cataract surgery is the most commonly performed surgical procedure in the United States. Surgical techniques are (1) *extracapsular extraction,* in which the lens is removed along with the anterior portion of the lens capsule; and (2) *intracapsular extraction,* in which both the capsule and the lens are removed. Extracapsular extraction is most frequently performed because it allows an intraocular lens to be inserted inside the remaining capsule. Lenses are now available that allow for multifocal vision rather than monovision where vision is good at one distance without glasses. There have been some later problems with this type of lens, but other types are being developed. One type of lens is hinged to the ciliary muscle allowing for accommodation of vision for various distances (Claoue, 2004). If a monovision lens is chosen, vision is corrected for nearsightedness or farsightedness by the lens implant and further correction of vision is achieved with regular eyeglasses or contact lenses. Vision is usually fully recovered within 3 months of surgery (Nursing Care Plan 26–1).

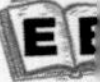

One technique for intracapsular cataract extraction (ICCE) utilizes *cryosurgery,* in which the lens is frozen by a super-cooled probe and then removed. *Phacoemulsification,* in which the tissue is pulverized and the debris is removed by suction, is often used for extracap-

NURSING CARE PLAN 26–1

Care of the Patient Undergoing a Cataract Extraction

SCENARIO Mrs. Fort, age 79, is admitted to the outpatient surgery unit for extraction of a cataract of the left eye with lens implant. The vision in her right eye also is affected by a cataract, but the visual loss is not as severe in that eye. Mrs. Fort suffers from a crippling osteoarthritis of the hands, but her general health is good. She is well oriented, outgoing, and physically active. She lives alone in an apartment building for retired senior citizens. Her daughter and son-in-law live nearby and are in daily contact with her. Mrs. Fort has only been in the hospital once in her life for pneumonia and is concerned about what to expect pre- and postoperatively.

PROBLEM/NURSING DIAGNOSIS *Lack of knowledge*/Deficient knowledge regarding pre- and postoperative procedures and care.

Supporting assessment data *Subjective:* "I have never had surgery before."

Goals/Expected Outcomes	Nursing Interventions	Selected Rationale	Evaluation
Patient will verbalize preoperative routine activities and postoperative procedures and expectations	Teach patient and daughter about eye medications to be used at home and how to instill them; how to dress and shield eye properly, how to remove bandage without contaminating eye.	In order to comply with instructions, teaching must occur on how to instill drops and how to dress and shield the eye and perform care needed.	Provided teaching for patient and daughter. Will ask for return demonstration before discharge. Left printed instructions.

PROBLEM/NURSING DIAGNOSIS *Potential postoperative complications*/Risk for injury related to postoperative complications such as hemorrhage and increased intraocular pressure.

Supporting assessment data *Objective:* Undergoing cataract extraction; hemorrhage and increased intraocular pressure are potential complications.

Goals/Expected Outcomes	Nursing Interventions	Selected Rationale	Evaluation
Intraocular hemorrhage will not occur, and there will not be an increase in intraocular pressure	Teach signs and symptoms of complications that are to be reported to physician immediately: increasing eye pain, purulent discharge, decreasing vision, fever or chills, increasing brow headache.	Patient must know what to look for in order to report complications.	Gave instructions and left printed list. Will ask for feedback before discharge.
	Instruct to refrain from straining at stool; encourage to use milk of magnesia or stool softener to prevent straining as needed.	Preventing the Valsalva maneuver will help prevent an increase in intraocular pressure.	Verbalizes the ways to prevent raising intraocular pressure.
	Wash hands thoroughly before instilling eye medications or changing dressing; teach patient and daughter to wash hands before approaching eye area.	Aseptic techniques help prevent infection. Maintaining asepsis aids in protecting the surgical site from infection and prevents complications.	Patient and daughter state that they understand handwashing and aseptic techniques for postoperative eye care.
	Demonstrate how to put on eye shield for sleep.		
	Instruct patient to avoid rapid or sudden movements and bending from the waist.	Bending from the waist increases intraocular pressure.	Instructed to crouch rather than bend at the waist and to avoid sudden movements.
	Instruct patient to take medication immediately for nausea and vomiting.	Quickly medicating for nausea may avert vomiting.	Instructions given and a written instruction sheet at bedside.
	Remind patient not to lie on affected side.		
	Encourage patient to seek assistance with ambulation while vision is blurred.		

Continued

NURSING CARE PLAN 26–1

Care of the Patient Undergoing a Cataract Extraction—cont'd

PROBLEM/NURSING DIAGNOSIS *Limited use of hands*/Self-care deficit related to disabilities imposed by osteoarthritis.

Supporting assessment data *Objective:* Has severe osteoarthritis of the hands with limited dexterity.

Goals/Expected Outcomes	Nursing Interventions	Selected Rationale	Evaluation
Assistance with administration of postoperative eye medications and eye care will be given by daughter	Teach daughter techniques needed for postoperative eye care and give her a written schedule for that care.	Written instructions and a schedule reinforce the teaching and help care to occur on time.	Daughter observed care and administration of eye medications today; will demonstrate postoperative eye care when meds are next due.

? CRITICAL THINKING QUESTIONS

1. Why should one wait 5 minutes between instilling one type of eyedrop and the next type of eyedrop?
2. What is one of the most important things to teach someone who is to instill eyedrops or ointment postoperatively?

sular cataract extraction (ECCE). These outpatient surgical procedures are performed under procedural sedation and local anesthesia. An intraocular lens implant is placed after extracapsular extraction.

Nursing Management

The patient must be told that there is a period of visual adjustment after cataract surgery. Postoperative care of the patient following implantation of an intraocular lens does not differ greatly from that of a patient with simple cataract extraction. (See the section Nursing Care of the Patient Having Eye Surgery later in the chapter.) The surgeon may prescribe miotic eyedrops after surgery to constrict the pupil and lessen the danger of lens dislocation. **Patient adherence to the schedule for postoperative medications is critical to preventing complications and promoting healing.** Teaching points for home care after cataract extraction are presented in Patient Teaching 26–1.

? *Think Critically About . . .* Can you identify patients who should be carefully assessed for signs and symptoms of cataract?

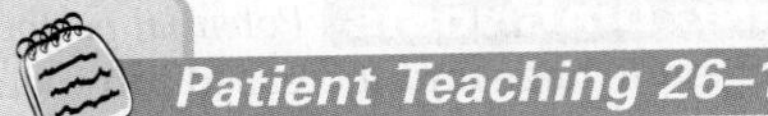

Patient Teaching 26–1

General Care After Eye Surgery

Instructions for the patient and/or family caregiver:

- Always wash the hands before instilling medication. Be careful to check the label of the container of the medication to be certain it is the right medication. Do not contaminate the applicator tip of the medication.
- Instill only the number of drops ordered; apply pressure at the inner canthus to prevent systemic absorption; close the eye gently (do not squeeze the eye shut).
- Change the eye patch dressing at least once a day; change as needed to keep the area clean.
- Follow the medication schedule prescribed by the physician exactly. (Send home a written schedule.)
- Maintain designated head position and activity restrictions.
- Report signs of complications: sudden, increasing pain in the eye, which can indicate hemorrhage; purulent drainage; decreasing vision; signs of increased intraocular pressure, such as brow headache.
- Keep the follow-up appointment with the surgeon.
- Use caution to prevent water in the eye when showering or washing hair.
- Protect the eye during the day with glasses; use sunglasses for outside wear; wear a protective eye shield at night.

GLAUCOMA

Etiology

The term *glaucoma* comprises a complex group of disorders that involve many different pathologic changes and symptoms, but have in common an increased IOP that damages the optic disk, causing atrophy and loss of peripheral vision. Glaucoma may come on slowly and cause irreversible visual loss without presenting any other noticeable symptoms, or it may appear abruptly and produce blindness in a matter of hours. Glaucoma can be present at birth or can develop at any age. It can result from genetic predisposition, trauma, or another disorder of the eye. Glaucoma frequently is a manifestation of diseases and pathologies in other body systems. The amount of increased pressure that causes damage differs from one person's eye to another. **Blindness is preventable if the disorder is treated early.**

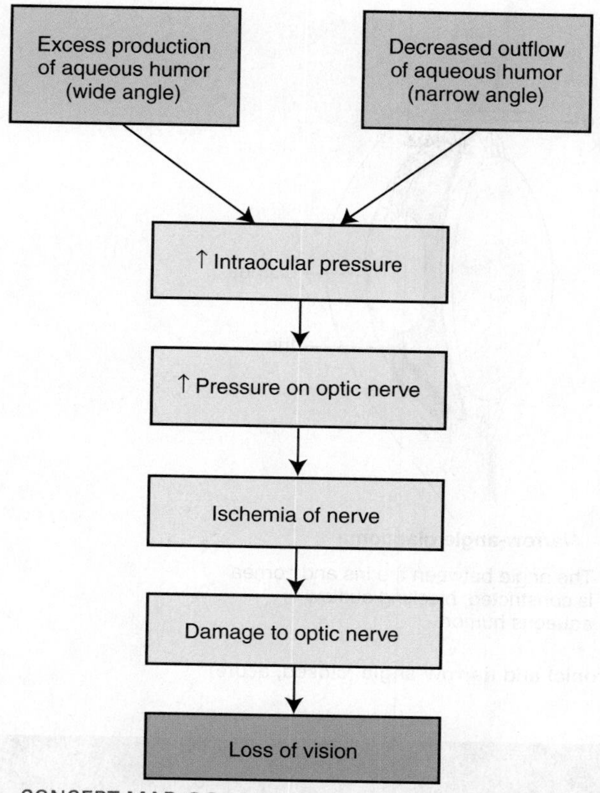

CONCEPT MAP **26–1** Pathophysiology of glaucoma.

Think Critically About . . . How can you include asking about family history or predisposing risk factors for glaucoma into your patient care?

Pathophysiology

The IOP is determined by the rate of *aqueous humor* production and the outflow of the aqueous humor from the eye. Aqueous humor is produced in the ciliary body and flows out of the eye through the canal of Schlemm into the venous system (Concept Map 26–1). An imbalance may occur from overproduction by the ciliary body or by obstruction of outflow. Increased IOP greater than 22 mm Hg requires thorough evaluation. Increased IOP restricts the blood flow to the optic nerve and the retina. Ischemia causes these structures to lose their function gradually. **The vision impairment from damage to the optic nerve or retina is irreversible; it is permanent.**

There are two major types of glaucoma: narrow-angle or angle-closure (acute) glaucoma, and open-angle (chronic) glaucoma (Figure 26–6). The terms *narrow angle* (angle closure) and *open angle* refer to the angle width between the cornea and the iris. *Acute* and *chronic* refer to either the onset or duration of the problem. These two major types differ in their clinical signs and symptoms, treatment, and effects on vision.

NARROW-ANGLE (ANGLE-CLOSURE) GLAUCOMA

Signs, Symptoms, and Diagnosis

Narrow-angle, or acute, glaucoma is a medical emergency in which there is severe pain in the eye accompanied by the appearance of colored halos around lights, blurred vision, and pain in and around the eye. Nausea and vomiting may occur. The cause of narrow-angle glaucoma is the position of the iris, which lies too close to the drainage canal and bulges forward against the cornea, blocking the drainage of aqueous humor (see Figure 26–6). The IOP rises suddenly, sometimes reaching a pressure of 50 to 70 mm Hg. Relief of the situation must be prompt, or damage to the optic nerve will cause blindness in the affected eye.

Diagnosis is by history, testing of IOP, and dilated eye examination.

Treatment and Nursing Management

Emergency treatment in narrow-angle glaucoma consists of measures to reduce IOP as quickly as possible. During the attack, drugs such as pilocarpine, topical epinephrine, and IV acetazolamide are used. Surgery is performed as soon as inflammation subsides to relieve pressure against the optic nerve endings. *Trabeculectomy, laser trabeculoplasty,* or other procedures that allow filtering of the aqueous humor from the anterior chamber into the subconjunctival space are performed. If these procedures fail, sometimes *cyclocryotherapy* (the application of a freezing tip) may be used on the ciliary body to decrease the aqueous production.

Nursing management is the same as for other eye surgeries: teaching about activity precautions during healing, schedule for eyedrops, symptoms to report to the surgeon, and aseptic handling of the eyedrops and eye shield.

OPEN-ANGLE GLAUCOMA

Signs and Symptoms

Open-angle, or chronic, glaucoma, in which there is no angle closure, is much more insidious and more common, occurring in about 90% of people with glaucoma. It often is an inherited disorder that causes degenerative changes in the aqueous humor outflow tracts. It usually is bilateral and can progress to complete blindness without ever producing an acute attack. Its symptoms are relatively mild, and many patients are not aware that anything is wrong until vision has been seriously impaired (Health Promotion Points 26–2).

Diagnosis

People at high risk for glaucoma are:

- Diabetics
- African Americans (at least four times as many African Americans as non–African Americans have glaucoma-related blindness)
- Individuals with a family history of glaucoma

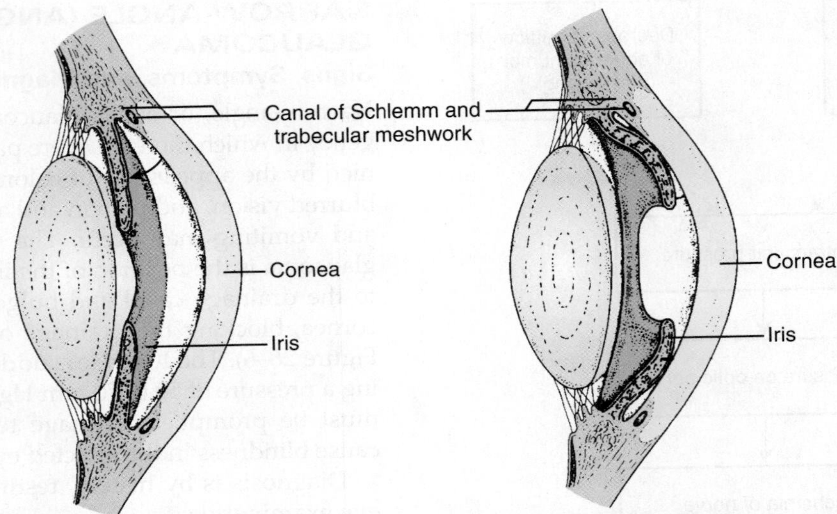

FIGURE **26–6** Comparison of open-angle (wide, chronic) and narrow-angle (closed, acute) glaucoma.

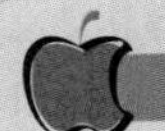

Health Promotion Points 26–2

Danger Signals of Glaucoma

The National Society for the Prevention of Blindness lists the following symptoms as danger signals of open-angle glaucoma:

- Glasses, even new ones, that don't seem to clarify vision
- Blurred or hazy vision that clears up after a while
- Trouble in getting used to darkened rooms, such as in movie theaters
- Seeing rainbow-colored rings around lights
- Narrowing of vision at the sides of one or both eyes

Encourage a complete eye examination if any of these signs is present.

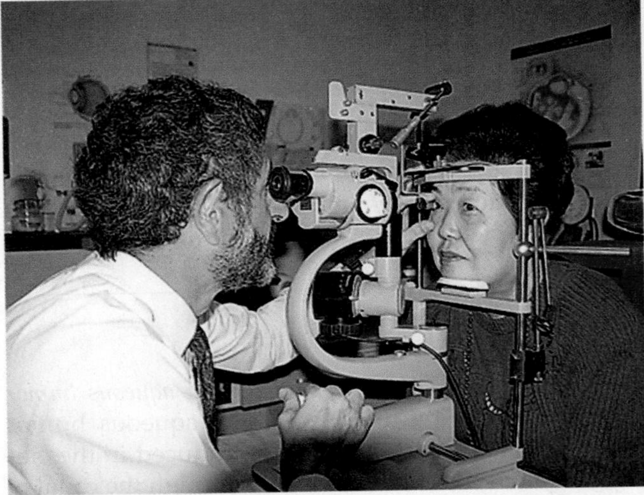

FIGURE **26–7** Applanation tonometer.

A commonly used screening technique for early detection of glaucoma is to measure IOP with an air tonometer. A puff of air is directed at the cornea, which causes a momentary indentation while a pressure reading is taken (Fleming, 2005). The test is painless, and nothing but the air touches the eye. Verification of the diagnosis of glaucoma may require the use of a more complex instrument called an *applanation tonometer* (Figure 26–7). The cornea is flattened and pressure is measured with a slit-lamp biomicroscope.

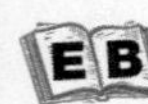

Treatment

The initial treatment of choice for chronic (open-angle) glaucoma is medication rather than surgery (Table 26–1). If drugs are not effective or if they produce worrisome side effects, surgery is performed.

Drugs prescribed are intended to enhance aqueous humor outflow, decrease its production, or both (see Table 26–1). They do this by constricting the pupil (miotics) or by inhibiting the formation of aqueous humor. A commonly used miotic is pilocarpine hydrochloride (Isopto Carpine, Pilocar, Akarpine). Miotics cause blurred vision for 1 to 2 hours after use. Adjustment to dark rooms is difficult because of pupil constriction. Pilocarpine is available in an eye medication disk that resembles a contact lens. The disk is inserted into the conjunctival sac in a patient's lower eyelid, where it can remain for up to 7 days. The medication is slowly released. Use of the disk does not prevent the wearing of contact lenses. Drugs that decrease the formation of aqueous humor are beta-adrenergic blocking agents, such as latanoprost (Xalatan), timolol (Timoptic), and levobunolol (Betagan). Carbonic anhy-

Table 26–1 ***Pharmacologic Management of Eye Disorders***

CLASSIFICATION	EXAMPLES	ACTION/NURSING IMPLICATIONS
GLAUCOMA		
Miotics	*Cholinergics:* pilocarpine hydrochloride (Isopto Carpine), pilocarpine nitrate (Ocusert Pilo-20, Ocusert Pilo-40), carbachol (Pilostat)	Constrict the pupil, promote outflow of aqueous humor, and reduce intraocular pressure. Reduce visual acuity in dim light; advise patient to avoid driving at night. Ocusert is placed in conjunctival sac and replaced weekly.
	Cholinesterase inhibitors: Echothiophate iodide (Phospholine Iodide) demecarium bromide (Humorsol)	Produce miosis, increase aqueous humor outflow, and decrease intraocular pressure. Avoid touching tip of bottle to eye; moisture may interfere with drug potency.
	Beta-adrenergic blockers: timolol maleate (Timoptic), betaxolol (Betoptic), levobunolol (Betagan), metipranolol (OptiPranolol), carteolol (Ocupress)	Reduce production of aqueous humor, thereby reducing intraocular pressure. Betoptic reduces intraocular hypertension. Monitor pulse and blood pressure during initiation of therapy. Blurred vision decreases with continued use. Use beta blockers cautiously in patients with a history of asthma.
Carbonic anhydrase inhibitors	Latanaprost (Xalatan), acetazolamide (Diamox), dichlorphenamide (Daranide), methazolamide (Neptazane), dorzolamide (Trusopt)	Interfere with carbonic acid production, thereby decreasing aqueous humor formation and decreasing intraocular pressure. Taken orally or as eyedrops (TruSopt). When taken orally, these drugs have a diuretic action; observe for dehydration and postural hypotension. Monitor electrolytes. Confusion may occur in the elderly. Check interaction with other drugs patient is receiving.
Sympathomimetics	Epinephrine (Epifrin), dipivefrin (Propine), apraclonidine (Lopidine)	Reduce intraocular pressure by increasing aqueous outflow. May cause brow headache, headache, eye irritation, and blurred vision. Used for open-angle glaucoma only. May cause tachycardia and rise in blood pressure.
Alpha$_2$ adrenergic agonist	Brimonidine tartrate (Alphagan)	Acts on alpha receptors in the blood vessels, decreasing the production of aqueous humor. Do not use with soft contact lenses. Contraindicated in heart disease.
Anti-inflammatories	*Corticosteroids:* Pred Forte, Ocu-Pred, Ophtho-Tate	Decrease inflammation and swelling; reduce miosis. Interact with contact lens materials.
	NSAIDs: ketorolac (Acular), flurbiprofen (Ocufen)	
	Prostaglandin analogue: Lantanoprost	
DRUGS USED TO FACILITATE DIAGNOSIS AND SURGERY OF THE EYE		
Cycloplegics and mydriatics anticholinergic agents	Atropine (Atropisol), cyclopentolate (Cyclogyl), homatropine (Isopto Homatropine), scopolamine (Isopto Hyoscine), tropicamide (Mydriacyl)	Dilate the pupils and paralyze the muscles of accommodation, causing mydriasis and cycloplegia. Mydriasis facilitates observation of the eye's interior during an examination. Cycloplegia prevents movement of the lens during assessment of the eye.
Adrenergic agonist	Phenylephrine (Ocu Phrin)	Induces mydriasis by action on the muscle of the iris. Causes blurred vision. Photophobia may be eased by using dark glasses.
Staining solution	Fluorescein sodium	Turns corneal scratches bright green; a green ring surrounds foreign bodies. Dye will filter through the lacrimal duct into the nasal secretions.
Topical anesthetics	Proparacaine HCl: Alcaine, AK-Taine Tetracaine HCl: Pontocaine	Anesthetize the eye. Caution patient not to rub the eye while it is anesthetized. Patch eye when patient leaves the office if medication is still in effect.
ANTI-INFECTIVE OPTIC MEDICATIONS		
Antibiotics	Gentamicin sulfate (Garamycin Ophthalmic), erythromycin (Ilotycin), polymyxin B sulfate, neomycin sulfate, bacitracin, sulfonamides (Sodium Sulamyd, Gantrisin) ciprofloxacin (Ciloxan), chlortetracycline (Aureomycin), ofloxacin (Ocuflox)	Used to treat infection or for prophylaxis. Caution patient to use a clean washcloth and towel on the face each time to prevent reinfection.
Antifungal	Natamycin (Natacyn Ophthalmic)	To treat *Fusarium.* Caution as above.
Antivirals	Idoxuridine (IDV, Stoxil, Herplex) Trifluradine (Viroptic)	Store in refrigerator. Do not use with boric acid. If no improvement, discontinue after 1 wk.
	Vidarabine (Vira-A Ophthalmic)	Effective against DNA viruses; used for keratoconjunctivitis.

Continued

Table 26–1 Pharmacologic Management of Eye Disorders—cont'd

GENERAL GUIDELINES FOR ADMINISTERING EYEDROPS

- Wash hands before administering eyedrops, and explain the procedure.
- Position the patient supine or with head tilted back, looking up at the ceiling.
- Provide a tissue for the patient to hold to blot excess fluid gently and keep if from running down the face.
- Verify the medication against the order one last time, and consciously review which eye the drops are intended for. Verify correct identification of the patient.
- Put on gloves.
- Remove the eye patch, if one is in place, and gently cleanse the closed eye with cotton and gauze moistened with irrigating solution or water if exudate is present.
- Remove gloves and rewash the hands.
- Remove the cap of the container, and place it upside down so that the inside of the cap does not become contaminated.
- Pull the lower lid of the eye downward to expose the conjunctival sac.
- Place the drops in the conjunctival sac.
- Remind to close the eye gently so that the drops are not displaced.

drase inhibitors also reduce aqueous humor production and include acetazolamide (Daranide, Diamox), dorzolamide (Trusopt) and methazolamide (Neptazane). Epinephrine (0.5% to 2.0%) and latanoprost (Xalatan) also decrease aqueous humor production. Diuretics may be prescribed to reduce the production of aqueous humor fluid. Not all diuretics reduce IOP, and a substitute should not be used for the specific drug prescribed.

Whenever glaucoma is being managed by medication, the patient must continue the eyedrops and oral medications on an uninterrupted basis. Patients admitted to the hospital for disorders other than glaucoma often are allowed to keep their glaucoma medication at the bedside if they are able to administer it themselves.

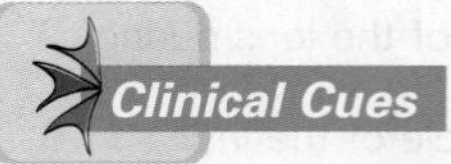

When admitting a patient with a history of glaucoma, check to see that she has her eye medication with her and that there is an order on the chart for leaving it at the bedside. Otherwise, verify that there is an order on the chart for her usual glaucoma medications. If there is no order, call the physician for one.

When drugs do not control glaucoma and increased IOP persists, surgery is an alternative. The goal is to create openings so that excess fluid can escape. A laser is used to create evenly spaced openings in the collecting meshwork (trabeculoplasty) to facilitate aqueous humor drainage in open-angle or chronic glaucoma. Filtering procedures such as *trephination, sclerectomy,* or *sclerostomy* create outflow channels from the anterior chamber to the subconjunctival space. Because scarring closes the openings in about 25% of patients, an antimetabolite such as 5-fluorouracil may be injected subconjunctivally to inhibit fibroblast growth and decrease scarring. If all other surgical procedures fail, the ciliary body may be treated by applying a freezing probe tip *(cyclocryotherapy)*. This permanently damages cells in the ciliary body and decreases the production of aqueous humor.

Laser surgery is performed with procedural sedation. The patient may experience a mild headache and blurring of vision during the first 24 hours. There is a possibility that IOP may increase because of an inflammatory response. **Increasing pain in the eye should be reported to the ophthalmologist immediately.** The patient should be instructed to prevent increasing the venous pressure in the head, neck, and eyes by avoiding the Valsalva maneuver (straining with a closed glottis), not bending over, keeping the head up, and not making any sudden movements. A stool softener is given to prevent constipation. Strenuous exercise is to be avoided for 3 weeks. The head of the bed should be elevated 15 to 20 degrees to decrease pressure within the eyes during sleep. Elevated IOP will persist for a week or so in some patients. Glaucoma medications are continued to meet the patient's individual needs. The patient must understand the importance of frequent checkups and the necessity of consistently following instructions. In other words, the surgical procedure may relieve the immediate problem of greatly increased IOP, but does not always eliminate the need for medication.

Nursing Management

Education of the patient and her family is a major aspect of care, because 90% of all cases of glaucoma are chronic conditions for which there usually is no permanent cure. Failure to follow the prescribed treatment regimen to control glaucoma and neglecting to maintain regular contact with the physician can result in progressive loss of vision and eventual blindness (Figure 26–8).

The patient who has glaucoma needs to be fully informed about the nature of this disorder, how it can affect vision, the treatments available, and the expected result of those treatments. An analogy that can be used

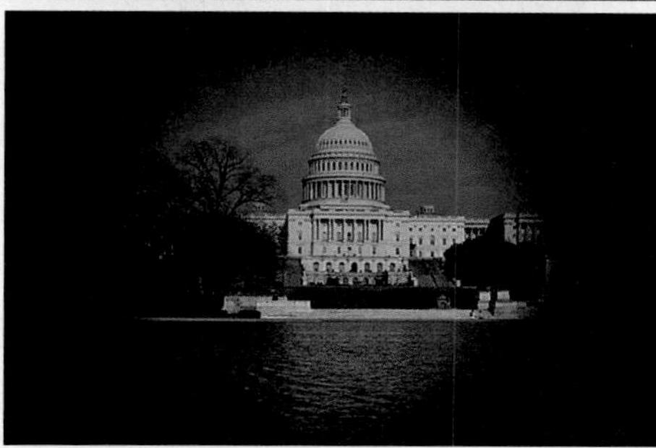
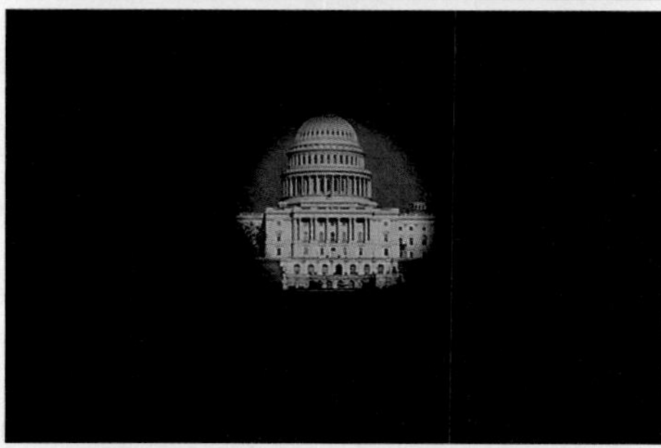
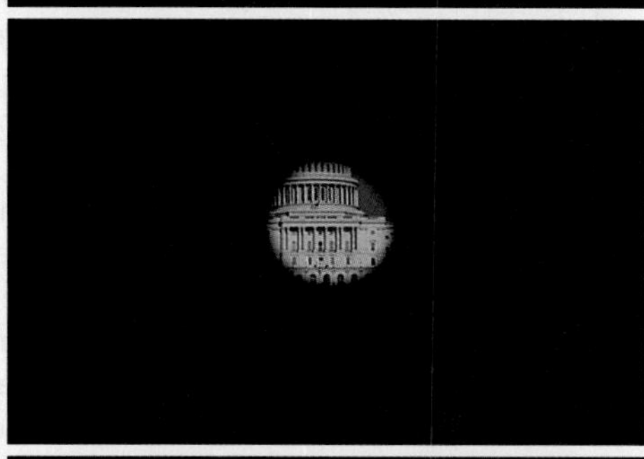

FIGURE 26–8 Glaucoma causes a progressive loss of peripheral vision.

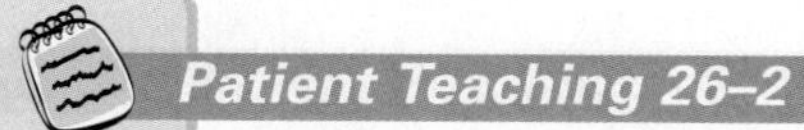

Points to Cover in the Glaucoma Teaching Plan

- Signs of IOP: pain in eye, redness, tearing, blurred vision, halos around lights, frequent need for change in eyeglasses.
- Measures to prevent increase in IOP: low-sodium diet, little caffeine, prevent constipation and Valsalva maneuver, decrease stress.
- Need to take prescribed medications and refrain from taking over-the-counter or other medications without physician's knowledge. Glaucoma medication must be taken regularly for life.
- Use good aseptic technique when instilling eye medication.
- Wear ID tag or bracelet stating "Glaucoma" and carry card in wallet that states what medications are being taken.
- Keep extra bottle of eye medication on hand. Carry eyedrops.
- Maintain close medical follow-up with physician.
- Practice safety habits; avoid night driving if possible.

Key: *ID,* identification; *IOP,* intraocular pressure.

to explain the nature of the disorder is to compare the eye to a sink with an open faucet (the ciliary processes), a drain (angle), and pipes (trabecular structures). As long as water flows into and out of the sink at the same rate, there is no problem. If something blocks the drain or the pipes, the water will fill the sink beyond its holding capacity. Treatment with miotics helps keep the pipes open so that drainage is possible; beta blockers and diuretics can slow down the rate at which water flows from the tap. If the medications do not work or the sink suddenly is blocked by a clogged pipe, it may be necessary for the surgeon to clear the drainage system so that the water can drain from the sink.

In addition to learning about the nature of glaucoma and the expected results of prescribed treatments, the patient also must be made aware of the possibility of vision loss if the condition is not managed. **Teaching should emphasize that glaucoma medications prevent further vision loss but cannot restore vision.** This must be done with tact and sensitivity for the patient's feelings. The information should never be presented in such a way that the patient feels threatened or becomes so fearful that she is unable to participate in the management of her disorder. Patient Teaching 26–2 summarizes a teaching plan for patients with glaucoma.

A new class of drug called glial cell–line derived neurotrophic factor (GDNF) is showing promise in preventing or repairing the damage to the optic nerve by the increased pressure present with glaucoma. Research is ongoing to determine if the drug will be safe to use for this purpose.

RETINAL DETACHMENT

Etiology

Retinal detachments often are classified as either primary or secondary. Primary retinal detachment is the result of spontaneous or degenerative changes in the

Cultural Cues 26–1

Incidence of Retinal Detachment in People of Jewish Descent

Retinal detachment is seen more frequently in people of Jewish ethnicity. The condition is relatively infrequent in African Americans. The reason may be that the Jewish population has more incidence of myopia, and that condition tends to be inherited. Severe myopia is a risk factor for retinal detachment.

retina or the vitreous humor. Secondary retinal detachment is associated with mechanical trauma, inflammation within the eye, or some other ophthalmic disorder, such as diabetic or hypertensive retinopathy. Retinal detachments frequently occur in people with a high degree of myopia (Cultural Cues 26–1). The incidence of retinal detachment increases dramatically after 40 years of age and is most common between the ages of 40 and 70. Fifteen percent of people with retinal detachment in one eye develop detachment in the other eye.

Pathophysiology

Retinal detachment is actually not a detachment of the whole retina but a separation of the sensory layers of the retina from the pigmented epithelial layer, the choroid. Retinal detachment can cause vitreous fluid to leak under the retina, separating a portion of it from the vascular wall and thereby depriving it of its blood supply (Figure 26–9).

Signs, Symptoms, and Diagnosis

Onset can be either gradual or sudden, depending on the cause and extent of the detachment and location of the area involved. The patient may see flashes of colored light accompanied by showers of floaters. Later, cloudy vision or loss of central vision is noticed. In severe cases, there may be complete loss of vision.

> *Think Critically About . . .* What would you say to your friend if you are having a meal together in a restaurant and she comments that she is seeing flashes of colored light in her left eye? What would you tell her to do?

Diagnosis of detached retina can be made with a direct ophthalmoscope, but it is greatly simplified by a stereoscopic indirect ophthalmoscope. This instrument permits visualization of the entire retina and produces an image of the retina with less magnification and distortion than the direct ophthalmoscope. Ultrasound can be used to detect retinal detachment when the eye is clouded by opacity from cataract or hemorrhage.

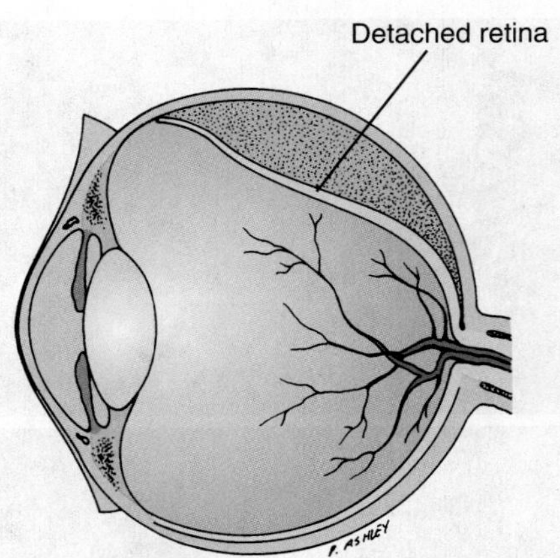

FIGURE **26–9** Retinal detachment.

Treatment

Retinal holes and tears sometimes can be repaired on an outpatient basis with laser therapy that creates an inflammatory reaction, causing the layers to adhere during healing. Those located in the posterior fundus can be coagulated and sealed with a laser beam or photocoagulator. Peripheral retinal holes through which no fluid has leaked can be closed by applying a freezing probe tip (cryotherapy). The frozen area scars over in a few days, and the hole is thus sealed. A third procedure, called *scleral buckling,* requires more extensive surgery. In effect, it places the retinal breaks in contact with the pigmented epithelial layer. Adhesions are formed that bind the sensory and epithelial layers and the choroid together. Prior to the procedure, air or gas is injected into the eye to apply pressure on the retina from the interior of the eye. This helps hold the layers together during healing.

In some instances when hemorrhage into the vitreous obstructs vision, the surgeon may perform a closed vitrectomy during retinal repair. The purpose of this procedure is to remove the cloudy vitreous humor and stabilize the retina against the choroid. Inert gas or air is used to fill the space until aqueous humor eventually refills the area.

Nursing Management

Positioning of the patient and the level of activity allowed after surgery are prescribed by the surgeon. The head is positioned so that the area repaired is dependent, preventing the pull of gravity from disrupting the surgical site. The designated position for the head also is calculated to position the air or gas bubble, if one was used, in the best place to apply pressure to the retina. This requires a supine and lateral position for at least 16 out of 24 hours a day. IOP is monitored closely for at least 24 hours. Vision does not return immediately because of postoperative swelling and the effects of the dilating drops. Vision improves on a gradual basis over several weeks to months. The eyes may both be patched, or just the operative one. Eye patches are changed at least once a day (Box 26–1). A shield is

Box 26–1 *Applying an Eye Patch*

Wash your hands, and cleanse the skin of the patient's forehead and cheek with a skin prep solution or pad.

- Prepare strips of nonallergenic paper or other tape to secure the patch.
- Ask the patient to close both eyes and position the pad over the lid of the eye to be patched.
- Secure the patch by placing strips of tape diagonally over the patch from the cheek to the forehead. Use several strips of tape to ensure adhesiveness.

FOR A PRESSURE PATCH

- Use two eye patches. Fold the first one in half; place it over the closed lid and then place the other patch on top of the folded one. Apply tape as above.

FOR SLEEPING

- A plastic or metal eye shield may be placed over the eye and secured to further protect the eye. Often, the patch can be left off when the shield is placed for sleeping.
- After surgery, the shield is used for 2 to 6 weeks, depending on the surgeon's instructions.

worn when napping and at night. Several types of eyedrops may be ordered for postoperative use, as well as an antibiotic ointment. Strict asepsis is observed when instilling eyedrops and ointment.

There usually is some degree of pain after all types of retinal surgery. Acetaminophen with codeine often is prescribed for this. If the patient is allergic to codeine, extra-strength Tylenol may be sufficient to control the pain.

Flashing lights are common after retinal surgery for the first few weeks. These decrease over 2 to 6 months; if they worsen within several weeks of surgery, the physician should be notified. Light sensitivity is common in both eyes after surgery and may cause tearing. This gradually lessens over a period of 4 to 6 weeks. Wearing dark sunglasses when outdoors helps eliminate this problem. A moderate amount of discharge from the eye is not unusual; it should be yellowish or pink-tinged. If the amount of discharge increases markedly or is accompanied by severe pain, or if it has a foul smell or a greenish tinge, infection may be present; notify the surgeon. Cleanse the eyelid with a gauze pad or cotton ball moistened with irrigating solution or tap water. Wipe from the inner to the outer area of the eye. A separate clean pad or cotton ball should be used for each eye.

The patient is allowed to sponge-bathe, brush the teeth, shave, and comb the hair as long as care is taken not to get water in the affected eye. See the section Nursing Care of the Patient Having Eye Surgery later in this chapter.

At discharge, the patient is cautioned to avoid heavy lifting, straining at stool, and vigorous activity for several weeks. Eyeglasses are worn during the day for protection, and the eye shield is worn at night after an eye patch is no longer necessary. Instructions for care are listed in Home Care Considerations 26–1.

? ***Think Critically About . . .*** How do the signs and symptoms of glaucoma and cataract differ?

RETINOPATHY

Etiology

The two major causes of retinopathy are diabetes mellitus and hypertension. Years of elevated blood pressure cause retinal vasospasm, which damages and narrows the retinal arterioles, thereby decreasing the blood supply to the retina. Contributing factors are excessive use of nicotine and caffeine, and high stress levels.

Pathophysiology

Diabetic patients experience two different forms of retinopathy: proliferative and nonproliferative retinopathy. In the nonproliferative type of retinopathy, microaneurysms develop on the retinal blood vessels. These eventually swell and rupture, causing hemorrhage into the vitreous humor, which interferes with vision. The proliferative form of retinopathy occurs later in the course of diabetes. New blood vessels grow from the existing retinal vessels in a process called *neovascularization*. The new vessels are thinner and rupture more easily, causing hemorrhage. The blood from the hemorrhage causes scarring, which also interferes with vision.

Signs, Symptoms, and Diagnosis

It is important that diabetic patients have regular, frequent eye examinations since, in the early stages of retinopathy, there are no symptoms. As the retinopathy progresses, there are alterations in vision such as blurring, missing areas in the field of vision, and seeing red or black lines or spots. These signs can be observed on ophthalmologic examination of the retina and by fluorescein angiography. When the macula is involved, there is a loss of vision that may progress to blindness. Retinal detachment may occur as a result of proliferative retinopathy.

Treatment

Tight control of blood glucose levels (100 to 115 mg/dL) is very important to prevent excessive diabetic retinopathy. There is no other known way to halt the process. The microaneurysms and the neovascularized vessels are treated with laser photocoagulation therapy to prevent hemorrhage and the consequent scarring and loss of vision. Vitrectomy also can be done if hemorrhage has caused serious impairment of vision.

Research is underway to determine whether a deficiency of insulin-like growth factor (IGF), a hormone that helps maintain nerve function, rather than

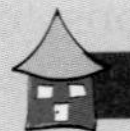

Home Care Considerations 26–1

Home Care Instructions for Retinal Surgery or Vitrectomy

Instructions will vary if the patient has a gas bubble that was injected intraocularly. Positioning and activity are more restricted in this instance.

ACTIVITY

- Restrict activity according to physician's instructions. Bed rest with bathroom privileges for the first few days is usual. The head may need to be positioned to the left or right most of the time. A head-down or semiprone position to the right or left will be required for the majority of the time if a gas bubble was injected into the eye.
- The following activities are allowed immediately after discharge unless a gas bubble has been injected into the eye as part of the procedure:
  - Watching television from a distance of at least 10 feet.
  - Tub bath or shower, using extreme care not to get soap or water into the eyes. Take care not to fall.
  - Walking outdoors with the guidance of a companion.
  - Reading for brief periods.
  - Gentle shampooing of hair with head tilted backward and care not to get soap or water into the eyes
  - Riding in a car as a passenger

EYE CARE

- The operated eye is to be patched at all times and protected by an eye shield or glasses until you are told you may leave the eye uncovered. A patch or shield may still be recommended for use while sleeping. The eye patch is removed only to administer eyedrops or ointment. The eyelid may be cleansed with cotton or gauze moistened with irrigating solution. Each time the patch is changed, check the movement of the eyeballs under the lids. Gently retract the upper lid, and look down as far as possible. Next, look up while retracting the lower lid. This helps break adhesions of the eyeball to the lids.
- The following are expected and should not cause alarm: tearing, a small amount of blood on the eye patch, a scratchy sensation, blurred vision, unusual visual images, a few light flashes, and floaters. Do call the physician if these symptoms *significantly* increase after discharge.
- Have someone else administer the eye medications. Assume a reclining position for eyedrop or eye ointment placement. Pull down the lower lid and, with the patient looking up, place the correct number of drops into the center of the conjunctival sac. Let the lid gently close. The patient should try not to squeeze the eye shut or blink excessively. Wait 3 to 5 minutes between types of eyedrops so that they do not wash each other out and dilute the intended effect. Patch the eye after each set of drops or ointment is administered. If a shield is to be used, it is placed on top of the taped-down eye pad.

COMFORT

- Take a prescribed analgesic or extra-strength acetaminophen to relieve pain. A cool washcloth or ice pack to the forehead may provide comfort. Report pain that grows markedly worse or is accompanied by nausea and vomiting.

PRECAUTIONS

- In case of cough, take cough syrup. Do not try to hold back sneezes. Do not strain at stool; take a stool softener or milk of magnesia if needed to prevent this.

RESTRICTIONS

- Avoid driving a car until visual acuity is 20/40 or better; your physician will tell you when you may resume driving.
- Avoid lifting heavy objects (those over 20 lb) for at least 4 months.
- Refrain from work for 2 to 6 weeks (depending on type of work); your physician will tell you when you may return to work. Light housework that does not require bending over or vigorous scrubbing may be resumed within 1 to 2 weeks depending on the type of surgery performed.
- Avoid vigorous or strenuous activity for 4 months.
- Do not bend with your head down; keep the head upright, and bend at the knees.
- Avoid sports for 3 to 4 months.

---

uncontrolled glucose levels is the cause of diabetic retinopathy. If so, IGF injections may prevent the problem.

Nursing Management

Since within 15 years of becoming diabetic, nearly all patients with type 1 diabetes and 80% of patients with type 2 diabetes develop some retinopathy, the nurse can be instrumental in promoting glucose control and regular eye examinations. Nurses must encourage glucose testing in patients who have a family history of diabetes, or who are in a high-risk category, so that the disease may be discovered early before vascular effects have occurred.

? *Think Critically About* . . . What would you teach your diabetic patient about the prevention of retinopathy? What factors enter into the development of retinopathy?

MACULAR DEGENERATION

Etiology

The macular region of the retina gives us color vision, acute vision, and central vision. Macular degeneration (also called age-related macular degeneration [AMD]) occurs with aging and is the most common cause of visual loss in the elderly. Research is in progress to

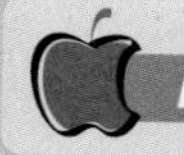

Health Promotion Points 26–3

Tobacco and Alcohol and AMD

Teaching people to quit smoking and to abstain from immoderate drinking (four or more alcoholic drinks a day), can decrease the incidence of age-related macular degeneration (AMD). Smoking is thought to double the risk of AMD. In Britain there is a movement to add the warning about the risk of vision loss to the other warnings on cigarette packages.

determine factors that seem to predispose to this disorder. Inflammation may be a factor as the presence of *Chlamydia pneumoniae* has been found in the eye tissue of some people with the wet form of AMD. Studies showing that both statin drug users and aspirin users may have less incidence of macular degeneration point to inflammation being a factor in its development (*Ophthalmology*, 2005). There is a genetic tendency for the disease, and diabetes and hypertension are associated risk factors (Health Promotion Points 26–3).

Wearing sunglasses regularly when outdoors may help protect against AMD. Certain vitamins, minerals, and antioxidants seem to help prevent or slow AMD (Complementary & Alternative Therapies 26–1).

Pathophysiology

There are two types of macular degeneration: dry (atrophic) and wet (exudative). In the dry form the problem lies with photoreceptors in the macula of the retina that fail to function and are not replaced because of advancing age. This form accounts for 85% to 90% of cases. In the wet form, abnormal vessels develop in or near the macula. The fragile vessel network grows into the subretinal space and may bleed into the macular region, causing central visual impairment.

Signs and Symptoms

The problem usually is bilateral and progressive. Early symptoms may be an inability to see the vividness of colors or to see details. Blurred vision, presence of scotomas, or distortion of vision gradually occurs. Objects may appear to be the wrong size or shape, or straight lines may appear crooked or wavy. As central vision deteriorates, there may be a large dark spot or empty place over the center of what is viewed. The patient retains peripheral vision and can walk, dress, cook, and sometimes even drive if impairment is minimal, but cannot read when the disorder becomes severe.

Diagnosis

Ophthalmologic examination of the retina and macula is the first step in diagnosis. Yellow exudates called **drusen** are found beneath the retinal pigment epithelium. Drusen represent extracellular debris. Patients at risk for macular degeneration, or extension of the

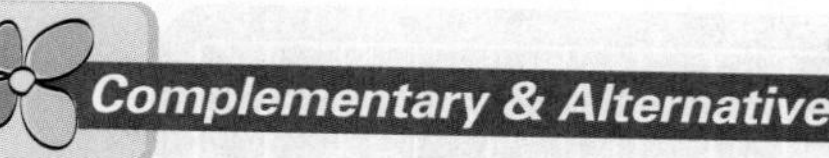

Complementary & Alternative Therapies 26–1

Antioxidants May Help Prevent AMD

The antioxidants acetyl-L-carnitine, concentrated omega-3, and coenzyme Q_{10} have been shown to improve vision in age-related macular degeneration (AMD) patients in a recent Italian study (*Ophthalmology*, 2005). The combination is available in Europe in a supplement called Phototrop.

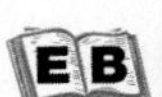

problem, are taught to use an Amsler grid (a small card with lines in a grid formation) at home to assess for progression of the disorder (Figure 26–10). If macular degeneration is occurring, the lines appear wavy. Fluorescein angiography or optical coherence tomography shows the specific areas of the retina involved.

Treatment

Prompt laser treatment to destroy the fragile blood vessels can sometimes be done to prevent further bleeding and visual deterioration. **Photodynamic therapy** using verteporfin (Visudyne) intravenously followed by a low-light-level laser that destroys only the cells that absorbed the dye is a new therapy. This destroys abnormal blood vessels without permanent damage to the photoreceptor cells and the retinal pigment epithelium. Because direct exposure to sunlight or other intense forms of light can activate the dye in the cells, the patient must avoid those forms of light for 5 days, after which the remaining dye will have been fully excreted.

Pegaptanib sodium injection (Macugen) has received Food and Drug Administration (FDA) approval for the treatment of wet AMD. It is injected into the eye, under local anesthesia, once every 6 weeks. This drug, during clinical studies, has limited the progression to legal blindness by 50% compared to the controls.

A newly developed derivative of bevacizumab (Avastin) has been used "off label" and has shown promise in improving wet macular degeneration. There are clinical trials underway. The drug is injected intravenously and is effective within 1 week. Long-term studies are needed to determine if the benefits outweigh the risks. Ranibizumab (Lucentis) has been approved by the FDA for AMD, but it is very expensive at $1950 per treatment. Some patients have experienced a stroke after the treatment. Anecortave acetate (Retaane) is another drug undergoing review by the FDA for the treatment of AMD. It inhibits the abnormal growth of blood vessels in the back of the eye. It is administered onto the outer surface of the back of the eye at 6-month intervals.

A technique under investigation is transplantation of healthy cells of retinal pigment epithelium to replace or enhance degenerating epithelium. It is hoped that transplantation of such cells before vision has greatly deteriorated will slow or eliminate the progression of AMD.

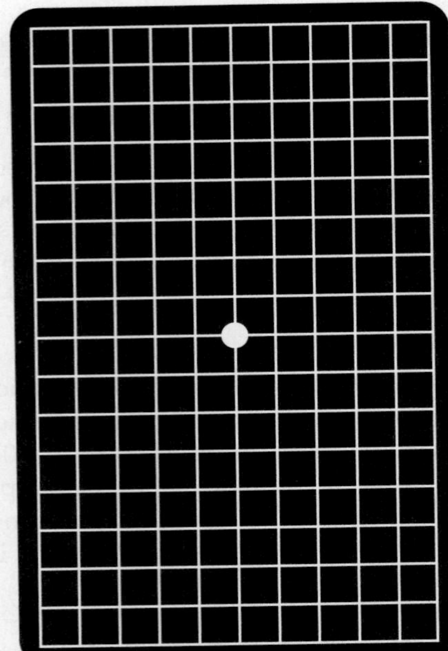

FIGURE **26–10** Amsler grid used to check for macular degeneration.

Nursing Management

The nurse helps patients with permanent vision loss learn to use low-vision aids. A referral to a low-vision device specialist and low-vision support groups often is needed. Devices are available to light and magnify reading material. Books with large print are easier to read. Learning to turn the head and move the eyeballs to work around the central scotoma may help. A closed-circuit television system that magnifies a printed page on screen can be used for reading or doing crossword puzzles. Telescopic lenses can help for watching movies, attending the theater, reading street signs, and seeing traffic lights. A head-mounted low-vision enhancement system provides both distance and close-up enhancement. Easy-to-read watches with large numerals, television screen magnifiers, and guides that fit over checks to assist with writing on them are some of the less expensive low-vision aids that are available.

NURSING CARE OF THE PATIENT HAVING EYE SURGERY

PREOPERATIVE CARE

Most eye surgery procedures are done on an outpatient basis unless the patient has other serious disorders such as cardiac dysrhythmias, severe diabetes, or a chronic disability. Therefore, a large part of nursing care is directed at discharge teaching for home care. One surgery that is performed as an inpatient procedure is a scleral buckle for retinal detachment (see the section on Retinal Detachment).

Stool softeners may be started a day or two before surgery to prevent constipation and the Valsalva maneuver postoperatively. The Valsalva maneuver can increase IOP. Some physicians direct the patient to wash her face with surgical soap several times the evening and morning before surgery. The patient may be given instructions on the administration of eyedrops the night before and the morning of surgery.

After admission, the patient is fully oriented to the outpatient surgery unit and given instructions about the layout of the room and area and the ways in which the nurse can be summoned. Side rails are usually necessary to prevent falls, and the patient should be cautioned against getting up without assistance. Preoperative eyedrops and medications are instilled by the nurses in the outpatient surgery center the morning of surgery. Drugs must be given with extreme care and accuracy, especially if only one eye is affected. **Be sure that the medication is applied to the correct eye.**

Preoperative dilating *(mydriatic)* eyedrops often are administered every 5 minutes for six doses. Other eyedrops may be administered in between these doses. An IV infusion is started shortly before surgery.

Because the great majority of patients undergoing eye operations are elderly and therefore are most likely to be suffering from some additional chronic disease, the nurse must remember to apply the principles of geriatric nursing in administering care. Fear, anxiety over surgery, and confusion about the expected results of the surgery are all factors to be considered when preparing the patient for the operation. Instructions and information should be given both verbally and in writing. Measures to ensure patient safety are very important both pre- and postoperatively since vision is impaired (Safety Alert 26–2).

POSTOPERATIVE CARE

In caring for a patient undergoing any type of eye surgery, the key word is *gentleness*. The patient's head should not be jarred when transferring from the oper-

Safety Alert 26–2

Prevent Falls from Impaired Vision

The elderly person who has an eye patched, or who has low vision, and is in a strange environment is subject to falls. The patient may need to be reoriented to place, time, and surroundings frequently to decrease confusion and agitation.

ating table or stretcher to the bed. Remember to speak before touching a patient who is blind or wearing bandages over the eyes.

Patients are usually kept in the recovery area of the outpatient surgery department for 2 to 3 hours postoperatively. Nausea and subsequent vomiting can wreak havoc with delicate suture lines in the eye. **If the patient becomes nauseated, antiemetic medication should be administered immediately and all food and liquids withheld.**

An eye patch is usually placed over the eye that was operated on (Figure 26–11). If it is necessary to restrict movement of the eyes, then both eyes are patched.

Instructions regarding postoperative medications and how they are to be instilled are given before discharge. The patient or significant other is taught to wash the hands thoroughly, pull the lower lid of the eye downward while the patient is looking up (with the head tilted slightly upward), and squeeze the correct number of drops into the conjunctival sac without touching the tip of the medication container on the eye or lashes (Figure 26–12). The eyelids must be closed gently so as not to squeeze all the medication out of the sac. Different types of eyedrop medications come with color-coded tops for easy identification. Eyedrop bottles also can be "labeled" by wrapping one, two, or three rubber bands around them so that the vision-impaired patient can differentiate one type of drop from another.

Should the patient need to stay in the hospital because of other problems, the nurse must be thoroughly familiar with her individual care needs. It should be known whether the patient can be turned on one or both sides or must remain flat on the back, whether pillows are allowed under the head, and how high the head of the bed may be raised. For certain types of retinal surgery, the head may need to be raised and positioned toward a particular side. If a gas bubble has been injected intraocularly, the patient is positioned supine toward one side or the other according to orders. If the patient is allowed out of bed, care must be taken not to jar the head or move too suddenly.

Sexual activity can usually be resumed in 1 to 8 weeks postoperatively, depending on the procedure performed. The surgeon will explain this to the patient. Make certain that the patient understands the time of the next appointment with the ophthalmologist. The patient and family should be encouraged to follow the physician's directions faithfully during the healing period at home so that nothing will jeopardize the success of the surgery.

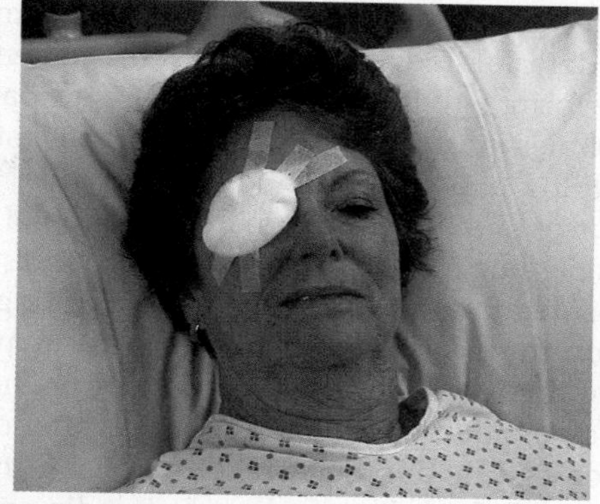

FIGURE 26–11 Patient with eye patch to protect surgical site and prevent eye movement. The head is kept elevated in the immediate postoperative period.

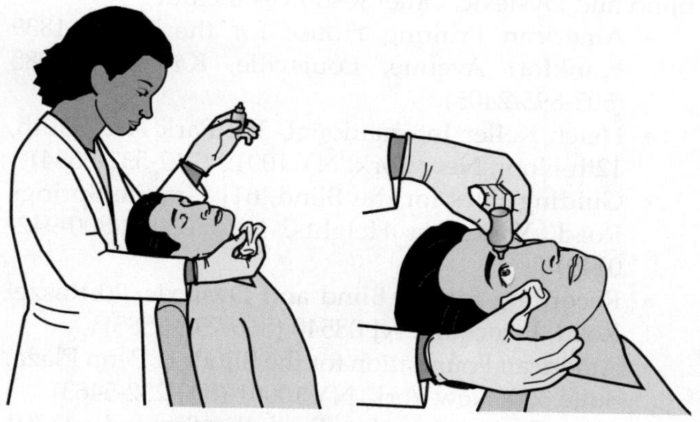

FIGURE 26–12 Instilling eyedrops.

Discharge planning for the patient having surgery from the outpatient department or the hospital is of utmost importance. Refer to Home Care Considerations 26–1 for home care of the patient following retinal surgery or vitrectomy.

COMMUNITY CARE

RESOURCES FOR THE VISION IMPAIRED

Loss of vision need not be devastating for a person if she is given support and encouragement for coping with her impairment. There are resources to help the visually impaired person learn to care for herself, find employment, and enjoy educational and recreational activities. Many colleges provide special funds to enable blind students to hire readers and tape recorders to help them with their studies.

Both home care nurses and those working in long-term care should be alert to signs of progressing macular degeneration. The Amsler grid can assist in identifying this problem. Patients with known eye disorders should be periodically assessed to see how much vision has deteriorated and how much the patient's ability to perform activities of daily living and partake in usual hobbies is affected. Nurses should be instrumental in helping patients obtain low-vision aids.

All nurses should encourage the donation of corneas at death. Signing a donor card for organ harvest should be a consideration for all, as well as indicating "tissue donor" on the driver's license. The nurse may be the person to approach the terminal patient or the family about the possibility of donating corneas after death . . . the gift of sight to another. The Library of Congress in Washington, DC, lends records and recording machines without charge to the blind and maintains a wide selection of recordings. Recordings of required textbooks may be obtained free of charge from Recording for the Blind and Dyslexic. Other resources include:

- American Printing House for the Blind, 1839 Frankfort Avenue, Louisville, KY 40206-0085 (502-895-2405)
- Helen Keller International, 352 Park Ave South, 12th Floor, New York, NY 10010 (212-532-0544)
- Guiding Eyes for the Blind, 611 Granite Springs Road, Yorktown Heights, NY 10598 (800-942-0149)
- Recording for the Blind and Dyslexic, 20 Roszel Road, Princeton, NJ 08540 (866-732-3585)
- American Foundation for the Blind, 11 Penn Plaza, Suite 300, New York, NY 10001 (800-232-5463)
- The Center for the Partially Sighted, 12301 Wilshire Boulevard, Suite 600, Los Angeles, CA 90025 (310-458-3501)
- National Association for Visually Handicapped, 22 West 21st Street, 6th Floor, New York, NY 10010 (212-889-3141)
- National Eye Institute Information Office, National Institutes of Health, 31 Center Drive MSC 2510, Bethesda, MD 20892-2510 (301-496-5248)

COMMON DISORDERS OF THE EAR

EXTERNAL OTITIS

Etiology and Pathophysiology

Infection of the external ear is common and often occurs in the ears of swimmers. It is caused by either bacterial or fungal pathogens, with staphylococci being the most frequent cause. Other infections of the skin may affect the external ear (see Chapter 42). A moist environment, or disruption of the skin from trauma, provides a place for pathogens to grow.

Signs and Symptoms

Pain occurs with the infection. An early sign may be pulling at the pinna or itching in the canal. If swelling occurs in the ear canal, hearing may be impaired as sound waves cannot reach the tympanic membrane.

Diagnosis, Treatment, and Nursing Management

Redness is evident on otoscopic examination, and there may be drainage. A culture of the drainage may be performed. Antibiotic or fungal eardrops and ointments are the usual treatment. A severe infection may require oral antibiotics as well.

Teaching patients to use drops of an alcohol solution in the ears after drying them helps to prevent external otitis. A mild analgesic may help decrease the discomfort during healing.

IMPACTED CERUMEN AND FOREIGN BODIES

Normally the ear canal is self-cleaning, but in certain individuals cerumen may become impacted. Foreign objects such as insects or organic matter may obstruct the canal. In children, small toy parts or beans or peas may become stuck in the ear canal. A feeling of fullness in the ear combined with a hearing loss can indicate that obstruction has blocked the canal, preventing sound waves from reaching the tympanic membrane.

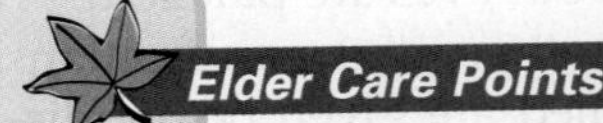

Elder Care Points

With age, the auditory canal narrows and the hairs become coarser and stiffer. The cerumen glands atrophy, causing cerumen to be drier. This combination may result in impaction of cerumen that causes a conductive hearing loss and tinnitus. Elders with this problem should be taught to use cerumen softening drops and an ear syringe to wash out the cerumen periodically. Those who are unable to cleanse the ears themselves should have regular ear checks by their health care provider.

If otoscopic examination reveals hardened cerumen blocking the canal, irrigation of the canal is performed to remove it.

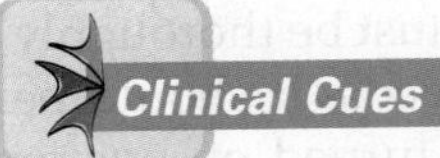

Clinical Cues

When irrigating an ear canal, the water should be tepid. Cold water and too much irrigation pressure can cause dizziness and nausea as well as pain. Check the temperature of the water each time the syringe or irrigation container is refilled. Drape the patient so that the clothing does not become wet.

OTITIS MEDIA

Etiology

This condition is an inflammation of the middle ear caused by various types of bacteria or viruses. Although it is mostly seen in infants and young children, it does occur in adults. It results in the accumulation of fluid behind the eardrum and some temporary impairment of hearing.

Pathophysiology

The inflammation of otitis media usually follows an upper respiratory tract infection or trauma to the ear. It is usually viral in origin, but may be complicated by bacteria. Obstruction of the eustachian tube usually precedes the disorder and is caused by an upper respiratory infection or allergy. Middle ear inflammation occurs when the eustachian tubes that usually drain that area become blocked. The obstruction changes the pressure within the middle ear. The inflammation may provide an environment for *Streptococcus pneumoniae, Haemophilus influenzae, Moraxella catarrhalis,* and *Streptococcus pyogenes,* or other pathogens to invade the tissue.

When the infection is sudden in onset and of short duration, it is termed *acute otitis media.* The eardrum is retracted inward because of negative pressure due to a closed eustachian tube. The pain can be very severe. When the infection is repeated, often causing perforation of the eardrum and drainage, it is called *chronic otitis media.*

Otitis media sometimes is accompanied by an allergy and may be aggravated by enlarged adenoids. Fluid may build up in the middle ear. This disorder is called *serous otitis media.*

Signs, Symptoms, and Diagnosis

Symptoms may be mild and may consist only of a feeling of fullness in the ear and evidence of impaired hearing and tinnitus. There may be pain in the infected ear, headache, fever, and fussing and pulling on the ear in an infant or toddler. Nausea and vomiting may occur with severe infection. If the fluid remains over an extended time, it causes tympanic membrane contraction and can permanently impair its movement.

Depending on the stage of infection, otoscopic examination may show retraction of the eardrum, redness and bulging, or pus behind the eardrum. Perforation may occur with drainage of the pus. This type is termed *suppurative otitis media.*

Treatment

There is great controversy about using antimicrobials for otitis media because so many strains of pathogens are becoming antimicrobial resistant. If there is otitis media with fluid behind the eardrum, and no acute systemic or local evidence of severe infection, antimicrobials are withheld. The condition is treated conservatively with antihistamines and decongestants.

For repeated episodes of otitis with fluid, or when the fluid will not resorb, a *myringotomy* (incision into the eardrum) is done, and a ventilating tube is inserted to drain the excess fluid in the middle ear and to equalize pressure while the eustachian tube is blocked. The tympanic membrane is anesthetized locally. The procedure is painless and takes about 15 minutes. The incision heals within 24 to 72 hours unless a tube is placed in the opening. Tubes remain in place for 6 to 18 months before they are naturally expelled. The hole then heals. If allergy is thought to be responsible for the fluid buildup, antihistamines are prescribed.

Acute otitis media occurs when pus-producing bacteria infect the middle ear. It usually is associated with an upper respiratory tract infection, most often when organisms from the nasopharynx find their way into the middle ear. Treatment consists of systemic therapy with antibiotics for at least 10 days, topical therapy with eardrops, and oral analgesics to reduce pain and fever. With repeated episodes, **tympanoplasty** to repair a ruptured eardrum and damaged ossicles, and, sometimes, mastoidectomy may be needed to eliminate all sources of infection and prevent further degeneration of bone.

Nursing Management

Keeping the patient comfortable at home, encouraging compliance with the medication regimen, and returning for an examination when medication is finished, or when told to return by the health care provider, are usual nursing actions. Show a family member how to instill eardrops properly (see Box 25–5). Temperature should be taken each day during the course of acute otitis media to track improvement.

Infections in the middle ear always have the potential for spreading to the meninges and causing meningitis, or to the mastoid bone, causing mastoiditis. With the advent of antibiotics, surgery to scrape and clean infected mastoid bone is performed far less frequently than it was previously. Although otitis media is a fairly common occurrence, it should always be treated immediately.

LABYRINTHITIS

Etiology and Pathophysiology

Labyrinthitis is an inflammation involving the vestibular portion of the labyrinth in the inner ear. It most commonly occurs as a complication of bacterial meningitis or chronic otitis media, or from a viral infection such as influenza, mumps, or measles. It may occur with a viral upper respiratory infection.

Signs, Symptoms, and Diagnosis

The symptoms include sensorineural hearing loss in the affected ear, tinnitus, severe dizziness with nausea and vomiting, and **nystagmus** (abnormal jerking movements of the eyes). If the disorder is viral, there usually is no tinnitus and resolution occurs within 7 to 10 days. Diagnosis is made from the symptoms and by ruling out tumor or other disease.

Treatment and Nursing Management

Treatment is aimed at removing the source of infection and controlling symptoms. Antibiotics may be given in massive doses to control a bacterial infection. Meclizine (Antivert, Bonine) or another antihistamine that assists in decreasing vertigo and its associated nausea and vomiting also is used. Scopolamine patches behind the ear can be used after the acute phase to control vertigo.

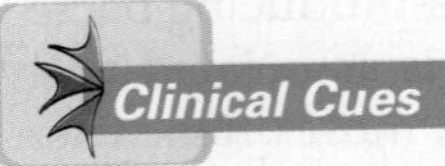

Remind the patient to wash the hands again after applying the scopolamine patch. If the eye is touched after touching the patch, severe eye irritation may occur.

Initially the patient is kept on bed rest to prevent falls and injury. The family is cautioned not to let the patient get out of bed without assistance. If the source of the problem is chronic mastoiditis that won't respond to medical treatment, a mastoidectomy may be done.

Nursing management consists of safety measures to prevent falling and instructions about the medications. Attention to hydration is important if the patient is nauseated to the point of repeated vomiting.

MENIERE'S DISEASE (MENIERE'S SYNDROME)

Etiology and Pathophysiology

The exact cause is unknown, but Meniere's disease occurs most often in people who have had chronic ear disorders and allergic symptoms involving the upper respiratory tract. There is a genetic link, and about 50% of those with the disorder have family members who are also afflicted.

An increase of fluid within the spaces of the labyrinths, with swelling and congestion of the mucous membranes of the cochlea, occurs. Resultant pressure in the labyrinth of the inner ear results in permanent damage to both the cochlear and vestibular structures. The disorder is usually unilateral.

Signs, Symptoms, and Diagnosis

The symptoms include attacks of dizziness, ringing in the ear (tinnitus), poor coordination that makes walking difficult or impossible, and sensorineural hearing loss. **Any sudden movement of the head or eyes during an attack usually produces severe nausea and vomiting.** Diagnosing Meniere's disease usually is not difficult, but because these symptoms could indicate a tumor of the auditory mechanism, a *caloric test* (electronystagmogram [ENG]) may be performed, which involves instilling very warm or cold fluid into the auditory canal. A patient with Meniere's disease will experience a severe attack; a normal person will complain of only slight dizziness. A person with a tumor of the auditory mechanism will have no reaction at all. Tympanometry and audiometry are ordered, and a brainstem-evoked response (BSER) test is performed to rule out an acoustic neuroma or problem in the brain.

Treatment

Treatment of Meniere's disease focuses on relieving symptoms; there is no cure for this condition, although it does disappear spontaneously in some cases. For an acute attack with disabling vertigo, atropine may be given subcutaneously, followed by diazepam (Valium), dimenhydrinate (Dramamine), meclizine (Antivert), or other drugs for motion sickness. To control edema and reduce pressure in the inner ear, the patient may be placed on a low-sodium diet, her fluid intake may be restricted, and diuretics may be ordered. Anticholinergic drugs, such as propantheline (Pro-Banthine) or glycopyrrolate (Robinul), may be given to help control the vertigo and nausea. To improve circulation in the ear, papaverine (Vasospan) or niacin may be prescribed. Some patients find that *Ginkgo biloba,* which acts as a vasodilator, helps. The patient is kept quiet and in bed to avoid aggravating her symptoms. She may be very irritable and withdrawn and may refuse to eat or drink because of fear of vomiting. Care should be taken to avoid increasing her irritation by jarring the bed, turning on bright overhead lights, or making loud noises.

If attacks continue and are very severe despite medical treatment, the endolymph sac from the inner ear can be removed with microsurgical techniques. When hearing loss is total on the affected side, surgical destruction of the eighth cranial nerve may be done to resolve the symptoms. Although this produces permanent deafness in the affected ear, the severe attacks are eliminated. In most persistent cases of Meniere's disease, the patient will eventually suffer a serious or even total loss of hearing regardless of the treatment used.

For those with dizziness and unsteadiness who do not wish to undergo surgery, vestibular rehabilitation therapy may decrease the dizziness and balance problems resulting from inner ear damage (Duke Health, 2005). 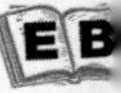

Nursing Management

If the patient uses nicotine products, encourage her to quit as nicotine constricts blood vessels and will decrease inner ear circulation as well. If allergy seems to be a factor in the onset of attacks, encourage consultation with an allergist to obtain control of allergens. Decreasing stress is a helpful intervention when there has been a pattern of attacks after particularly stressful times in the patient's life.

OTOSCLEROSIS

Etiology and Pathophysiology

Otosclerosis is a hereditary degeneration of bone in the inner ear. It occurs twice as often in females and begins in the late teens or early 20s. It may become worse during pregnancy.

The sense of hearing depends in part on the vibration of very small bones of the inner ear. The *stapes,* or stirrup, is particularly important, because it conducts sound waves to the fluid in the semicircular canals in the inner ear. Otosclerosis is a disease process that causes the formation of excess bone. This causes the footplate of the stapes to be fixed so that it no longer vibrates to transmit sound waves.

Signs, Symptoms, and Diagnosis

The patient often complains of difficulty hearing the voices of others, yet her own voice sounds unusually loud. In response to this, she may lower her voice to the point that she can scarcely be heard by others. Diagnosis is by otoscopic examination, Rinne and Weber's tests, and audiogram.

Treatment

The hearing loss of otosclerosis can sometimes be corrected by using a hearing aid. Microsurgical intervention can restore air-conductive hearing by providing a new movable pathway for the sound waves. During the operation, called a *stapedectomy,* the stapes is removed and is replaced with a prosthetic device. This device may be a steel wire and fat implant, a wire and a segment of vein, or a vein graft with polyethylene tubing. In any case, the prosthesis is attached to one end of the *incus* (anvil of the middle ear) so that sound can be transmitted to the inner ear. The surgical procedure is extremely delicate and would not be possible without the dissecting binocular microscope and other modern surgical instruments that allow visualization and manipulation of the very small structures of the middle ear. Care for a hearing aid is presented in Box 25–4 in the previous chapter.

Tympanoplasty is now the more common procedure. Tympanoplasty involves the surgical reconstruction of the tympanic membrane and ossicles to restore middle-ear function. There are five different types of procedures ranging from simple closing of a tympanic membrane perforation to extensive repair of the middle-ear structures. The procedure is performed with an operating microscope via the external auditory canal or through a postauricular incision. Although performed as an outpatient procedure, tympanoplasty requires general anesthesia.

Nursing Management

Postoperative care involves keeping the patient quiet and flat in bed for several hours. The head is turned so that the affected ear is uppermost. When the patient is allowed to move about, she must be warned that dizziness is likely to occur, especially if she turns her head suddenly. Position changes should be accomplished slowly. Coughing and sneezing should be avoided, or if unavoidable, should be accomplished with the mouth open to decrease pressure in the ear (Nursing Care Plan 26–2). See the section on Postoperative Care later in this chapter.

NURSING CARE PLAN 26–2

Care of the Patient Having a Tympanoplasty

SCENARIO Miss Cook, age 38, is a high school teacher who has had progressive hearing impairment as a result of recurrent otitis media of the right ear. She is admitted to outpatient surgery for tympanoplasty. During her initial assessment, the nurse found Miss Cook to be well informed about the nature of her disorder but somewhat anxious about the outcome of surgery. Her physical health status is good; her only previous hospitalization was for an appendectomy when she was 19 years old. Care is for the postoperative period.

PROBLEM/NURSING DIAGNOSIS *Possible disruption of graft*/Risk for injury related to graft displacement.

Supporting assessment data *Objective:* Tympanoplasty.

Goals/Expected Outcomes	Nursing Interventions	Selected Rationale	Evaluation
Graft will be successful as evidenced by restored hearing in affected ear	Position patient side-lying on nonoperative side.	Prevents collection of fluid behind graft and reduces pressure.	Positioned on nonoperative side or back with HOB raised 30 degrees.
	Reinforce preoperative instructions to remain in bed for 4 hr, avoid sudden movements, blowing nose, or sneezing.	These measures help prevent graft disruption.	Compliant with instructions. Continue plan.
	Check vital signs, for evidence of infection bid.	Elevation in temperature may indicate beginning infection.	Temperature within normal range. No sign of infection.
	Give analgesic/sedative as ordered.	Analgesic/sedative will promote rest.	Patient resting comfortably; pain at 2/10.
	Provide quiet environment.		

Key: *bid,* twice daily; *HOB,* head of bed.

Continued

NURSING CARE PLAN 26–2

Care of the Patient Having a Tympanoplasty—cont'd

PROBLEM/NURSING DIAGNOSIS *May experience vertigo and dizziness*/Risk for activity intolerance related to vertigo and instability.

Supporting assessment data *Subjective:* After tympanoplasty, states is very dizzy and nauseated.

Goals/Expected Outcomes	Nursing Interventions	Selected Rationale	Evaluation
Falls and head trauma will be avoided	Up with assistance only. Repeat explanation for safety precautions.	Helps to prevent falls.	Asking for assistance when needs to get up.
	Caution patient to change positions and turn her head very slowly.	Abrupt changes in position are likely to cause vertigo and nausea.	Compliant with instructions.
	Provide well-lighted room when ambulating.	Good lighting prevents tripping over obstacles when ambulating.	Room lighting is adequate.
	Administer medication prescribed for vertigo.	Medication can help control vertigo.	Medication for vertigo is effective.

PROBLEM/NURSING DIAGNOSIS *Lack of knowledge about postoperative care*/Deficient knowledge about postoperative care.

Supporting assessment data *Subjective:* Asks about restrictions and self-care. *Objective:* Cannot verbalize knowledge of medications.

Goals/Expected Outcomes	Nursing Interventions	Selected Rationale	Evaluation
Patient will verbalize knowledge of home self-care before discharge	Instruct to avoid loud noises and pressure changes for 6 mo, especially avoiding flying and diving.	Loud noise and pressure changes can disrupt the graft.	Instructions given gone over verbally and printed instructions left with patient.
	Stress importance of not blowing her nose for at least 1 wk, to avoid an upper respiratory infection; if at all possible, protect her ear against cold; and refrain from any activity that might provoke dizziness or disturb the graft (e.g., straining at stool, bending, and heavy lifting).	Preventing pressure changes helps protect the integrity of the graft.	Provided correct feedback on postoperative precautions.
Patient will demonstrate dressing change correctly before discharge	Teach patient how to change dressing on the external ear.	Will prepare patient for self-care.	Patient has not changed bandage as yet. Continue plan.
	Reiterate importance of taking full course of prescribed antibiotic and reporting to surgeon at scheduled times.	Taking the full course of antibiotics correctly will help prevent infection.	Acknowledges importance of taking antibiotics as directed.
	Reassure patient that because of swelling of tissues and presence of surgical pack, it may be several weeks before she can fully evaluate effectiveness of the surgery.	Inflammation at the surgical site will cause swelling that interferes with hearing initially.	Reassurance given. Yes, but continue plan. States she understands that it may be a while before hearing is as good as it will get.

? CRITICAL THINKING QUESTIONS

1. Why can dizziness and vertigo occur after a tympanoplasty?
2. What level of noise would be considered "too loud"?

NURSING CARE OF THE PATIENT HAVING EAR SURGERY

Most ear surgeries are performed as outpatient procedures. Nursing care is focused on the immediate preoperative and recovery periods and on instructions for home care.

PREOPERATIVE CARE

Nursing care of the patient during the preoperative period usually is rather routine except for the administration of eardrops or other special medications. Physical preparation for ear surgery may or may not involve removing some of the hair from the scalp. Male patients should be clean shaven the morning of surgery. The external ear and surrounding skin should be thoroughly cleansed, preferably with a surgical soap. Female patients with long hair should have it braided or pinned back securely so that it will not become soiled by drainage from the ear or serve as a source of infection at the operative site.

POSTOPERATIVE CARE

The patient will often return from major ear surgery with an ear dressing (Figure 26–13). Positioning of the patient after ear surgery depends on specific instructions from the physician. Often the patient is placed flat in bed, and her head is supported so that she does not turn it from side to side. In addition to noting the vital signs, the nurse should watch for signs of injury to the facial nerve, including inability of the patient to close her eyes, wrinkle her forehead, or pucker her lips. The patient and family are advised to report such symptoms to the surgeon. If they appear later than 12 hours after surgery, they may be due to edema, and the physician may order a loosening of the dressings.

Safety precautions, such as raising side rails, should be taken to avoid injury due to dizziness and loss of balance during the recovery period. Balance is temporarily affected as a result of disturbance to the mechanism that maintains equilibrium. When the patient is allowed to get up and move about, assistance should be provided to prevent falls. The patient should arise slowly to a sitting position and sit for a few minutes. Then the patient stands while holding on to something or being supported by another. Dizziness must pass before the patient attempts walking.

Because the ear is so near the brain, a special effort must be made to avoid contamination of the surgical site. Dressings may be reinforced to keep them dry, but excessive drainage must be reported to the surgeon.

The patient should be instructed beforehand about what is to be expected from the surgery. Hearing is usually slightly impaired immediately after surgery because of edema or bandages, but is expected to improve in time. See Home Care Considerations 26–2 for care after discharge.

Myringotomy (incision of the eardrum) with placement of tubes is a lesser procedure and the only dressing may be a cotton ball in the ear. There is less occurrence of dizziness or nausea with this surgery.

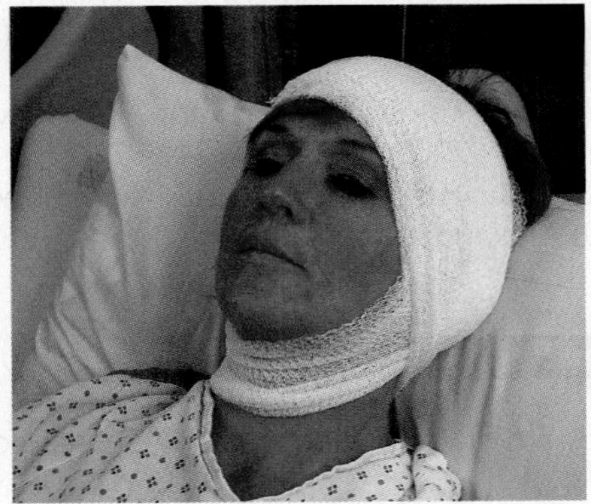

FIGURE 26–13 An ear surgery dressing. The patient is positioned with the head elevated or side-lying on the unaffected side.

Home Care Considerations 26–2

Instructions After Ear Surgery

The following instructions are given to the patient after ear surgery at the time of discharge:

- Sneezing, coughing, and nose blowing are all ways in which the operative site may be disturbed. If necessary, blow the nose gently one side at a time. Cough or sneeze with the mouth open. Continue this for 1 week after surgery.
- Do not drink through a straw for 2 to 3 weeks. Avoid drinking directly from the mouth of a plastic bottle as negative pressure occurs if the bottle opening is sealed.
- Limit physical activity for 1 week after surgery. Refrain from exercising and sports for 3 weeks or until the surgeon discharges you.
- Avoid heavy lifting for 3 weeks. Avoid bending over from the waist or moving the head rapidly for 3 weeks.
- Keep the ear dry for 4 to 6 weeks after surgery by placing a cotton ball covered with petroleum jelly (such as Vaseline) in the ear canal; refrain from shampooing hair with water for 1 week after surgery.
- After the initial dressing is removed, keep a cotton ball in the ear to protect it; change the cotton ball daily.
- Avoid people with colds.
- Do not fly until the surgeon allows it.
- Wear ear protectors when exposed to a loud environment.
- A return to work is usual after 3 to 7 days; strenuous work may not be resumed for 3 weeks.

Note: The surgeon will explain the specific time limitations for each activity based on the type.

COMMUNITY CARE

Cautioning people about the dangers of listening to loud music through earpieces can help curb hearing loss. Teaching adults to seek medical attention for symptoms of otitis media quickly prevents damage to the tympanic membrane and preserves hearing ability.

A hearing assessment should be part of any thorough health assessment. Encouraging those who have any difficulty with hearing to have a thorough evaluation and to try a hearing aid, if the need is indicated, could help improve the quality of their lives. Nurses in home and long-term care settings should frequently assess the function of the patient's hearing aid.

RESOURCES FOR THE HEARING IMPAIRED

Various accommodations can be found to help the hearing impaired. There are even assistance dogs to help keep the hearing-impaired person safe both in the home and on the streets.

Organizations for the Hearing Impaired

- Hearing Loss Association, 7910 Woodmont Avenue, Suite 1200, Bethesda, MD 20814 (301-657-2248)
- American Tinnitus Association, P.O. Box 5, Portland, OR 97207-0005 (800-634-8978)
- Better Hearing Institute, 515 King Street, Suite 420, Alexandria, VA 22314 (703-684-3391)

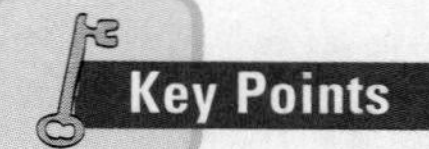

- A problem with refraction is the most common eye disorder.
- Cataracts cause a blurring or loss of vision and usually occur slowly.
- Cataract surgery with lens implant usually restores vision.
- The increase in intraocular pressure, unless treated, will eventually cause blindness.
- Glaucoma medication most often must be used for the rest of the patient's life.
- Acute narrow-angle glaucoma is a medical emergency.
- Retinal detachment symptoms are flashing colored lights followed by the appearance of "floaters."
- Unless treated quickly and successfully, retinal detachment causes vision loss.
- Positioning and restriction of amount of movement are crucial after eye surgery.
- Retinopathy is a disorder that occurs most frequently with diabetes or hypertension.
- Tight glucose control helps prevent diabetic retinopathy.
- Retinopathy is frequently treated by laser.
- Injury and infection cause other eye disorders.
- Keratoplasty may be performed for damaged corneas.
- Macular degeneration is a frequent problem in the elderly, but can occur at an earlier age.
- There is presently no cure for macular degeneration, but new drugs may be able to slow it or reverse some of the vision loss.
- There are many low-vision aids to help the vision-impaired person.
- Eye trauma should be treated by a health care provider promptly.
- Eyedrops must be instilled correctly and accurately both before and after surgery.
- Keep the eye surgery patient quiet and treat nausea immediately.
- External otitis is often a problem for swimmers.
- Otitis media is a common malady and may be induced by allergy or upper respiratory infection.
- Impacted cerumen or foreign bodies in the ear interfere with hearing.
- Otosclerosis is generally hereditary.
- Tympanoplasty may be performed for otosclerosis or for tympanic membrane dysfunction.
- Labyrinthitis and Meniere's disease cause vertigo and tinnitus.
- It is very important that the patient follow postoperative instructions after ear surgery.

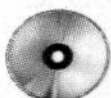
Go to your **Companion CD-ROM** for an Audio Glossary, animations, video clips, and bonus review questions.

evolve Be sure to visit the companion Evolve site at http://evolve.elsevier.com/deWit for interactive NCLEX-PN Exam Style Questions, WebLinks, and additional online resources.

NCLEX-PN EXAM STYLE REVIEW QUESTIONS

Choose the best answer(s) for the following questions.

1. A male patient was informed that he would need to wear a pair of corrective lenses for astigmatism. When asked about the condition, the patient demonstrates understanding when he states that:

1. "Astigmatism is hardening of the ciliary muscles."
2. "Astigmatism is an irregular curvature of the cornea."
3. "Astigmatism enables focusing of light in front of the retina."
4. "Astigmatism is an increased opacity of the lens."

2. Which of the following must be included in the discharge instructions of a patient who has undergone corneal transplant?

1. Increase physical activity.
2. Wear an eye shield when in close contact with children or pets.
3. Remove pressure dressing as needed.
4. Lie only on the operative side.

3. The nurse is providing care of an artificial eye. Which of the following is considered an appropriate nursing action?

1. Clean with soap and water unless directed otherwise.
2. Use a denture cup for safekeeping.
3. Lift the lower lid to insert the prosthesis.
4. Insert the notched end of the artificial eye toward the ear.

4. An elderly patient is admitted for cataract extraction. The nurse anticipates which of the following signs and symptoms associated with the condition?

1. Increased tearing
2. Increasing complaints about glare
3. Increasing farsightedness
4. Bluish discolorations

5. ________________ is a condition of increased intraocular pressure that damages the optic disk, leading to the loss of peripheral vision.

6. Following eye surgery, the patient is instructed to avoid movements that increase the venous pressure in the head, neck, and eyes. Which of these movements increase venous pressure? *(Select all that apply.)*

1. Straining
2. Bending over
3. Keeping the head up
4. Sudden head movements
5. Strenuous exercises

7. Prior to eye surgery, the patient is instructed to take stool softeners. When asked about the rationale for taking the stool softener, the nurse appropriately responds:

1. "The medication reduces the possibility of straining at stool postoperatively."
2. "The medication prevents constipation caused by anesthetic agents."
3. "The medication cleanses the gastrointestinal tract."
4. "The medication enhances surgical recovery."

8. Older adults are more prone to conductive hearing loss and tinnitus because of:

1. hypertrophy of the cerumen glands.
2. hardened cerumen.
3. widening of the auditory canal.
4. hair loss in the auditory canal.

9. The nurse emphasizes safety precautions to a 60-year-old Latin American female patient with Meniere's disease. An appropriate nursing approach would be to:

1. use first name when addressing the patient.
2. include female family members.
3. address decision making to the patient.
4. set specific schedule for providing instructions.

10. Which of the following are appropriate postoperative instructions to a patient who has had ear surgery? *(Select all that apply.)*

1. Cough or sneeze with the mouth open
2. Resume routine exercises
3. Avoid bending or heavy lifting
4. Keep ear dry by plugging with cotton covered with petroleum jelly
5. Drink with a straw

CRITICAL THINKING ACTIVITIES

Read each clinical scenario and discuss the questions with your classmates.

Scenario A

Mr. Lavant, age 52, and his wife, who has diabetes, have heard about a glaucoma screening clinic being held in their community. They are interested in attending the clinic but are very apprehensive about the kind of tests that will be done. They ask you about the tests and whether you think they should go to the screening clinic when they have no symptoms of glaucoma or any other eye disease.

1. How would you explain a test with a tonometer?
2. How would you explain glaucoma in terms Mr. and Mrs. Lavant could understand?
3. Who are among the people at high risk for glaucoma?
4. What is the usual treatment for chronic, open-angle glaucoma?

Scenario B

Mr. Wilson, age 78, is scheduled for a right cataract extraction and intraocular lens implant. He has bilateral cataracts that have made him legally blind for years. He did not consult a physician until recently, because he had always heard that cataracts had to be "ripe" before they could be treated, and he felt he could not afford frequent trips to a physician when nothing could be done for his condition.

Mr. Wilson enters the outpatient surgery area, and you are assigned as his nurse.

1. How would you approach and orient Mr. Wilson to his surroundings?
2. What would you tell Mr. Wilson about the preoperative routine and medications at this time?
3. What nursing diagnoses would be appropriate for Mr. Wilson at this time?
4. What are the advantages of intraocular lens implants over cataract glasses and/or contact lenses?

Scenario C

Mr. Thompson is suffering from a severe attack of Meniere's disease and vertigo. He is severely nauseated, and his vertigo prevents him from getting out of bed.

1. What nursing actions would be appropriate for him?
2. How would you explain this disorder to Mr. Thompson?

The physician wants to rule out the possibility of tumor as a cause of Mr. Thompson's vertigo, and so he is scheduled for an electronystagmogram (ENG) with a caloric test and a magnetic resonance imaging (MRI) scan.

3. How would you explain these tests to Mr. Thompson?

CHAPTER 27 The Gastrointestinal System

evolve http://evolve.elsevier.com/deWit

Objectives

Upon completing this chapter, you should be able to:

Theory

1. Identify three major causative factors in the development of disorders of the gastrointestinal system.
2. Explain three measures to prevent development of disorders of the gastrointestinal system.
3. List nursing responsibilities in the pre- and post-test care of patients undergoing diagnostic tests for disorders of the gastrointestinal system.
4. Describe the assessment of a patient with a possible gastrointestinal disorder.
5. State the care needed for the patient who is having a liver biopsy.

Clinical Practice

1. Perform an assessment of gastrointestinal status.
2. Provide pre- and post-test care of patients undergoing tests of the liver, gallbladder, and pancreas.
3. Provide care for a patient who is experiencing diarrhea.
4. Teach a patient experiencing constipation ways to alleviate the problem.

Key Terms

Be sure to check out the bonus material on the Companion CD-ROM, including selected audio pronunciations.

absorption (ăb-sŏrp-shŭn, p. 664)
adhesion (ăd-HĒ-shŭn, p. 668)
anabolism (ă-NĂB-ŏ-lĭzm, p. 664)
anorexia (ăn-ŏ-RĔK-sē-ă, p. 679)
ascites (ă-SĪ-tēz, p. 676)
catabolism (kă-TĂB-ō-lĭzm, p. 664)
chyme (KĪM, p. 666)
flatus (FLĀ-tŭs, p. 680)
mastication (măs-Tĭ-KĀ-shŭn, p. 665)
metabolism (mĕ-TĂ-bō-lĭzm, p. 664)
pancreatitis (păn-krē-Ă-TĪ-tĭs, p. 669)
peristalsis (pĕr-ēs-TĂL-sĭs, p. 664)

The central role of the intestinal tract and accessory organs of digestion is the intake, absorption, and assimilation of food to provide nourishment for the body. The transfer of nutrients from the intestine into the blood is referred to as **absorption.** Food substances are moved along the intestinal tract by wavelike motions of involuntary muscles within the walls of the organs. This rhythmic squeezing action is called **peristalsis. Metabolism** is the sum of many physical and chemical processes concerned with the disposition of the absorbed nutrients. Metabolic activities involve the synthesis of substances needed to build, maintain, and repair body tissues **(anabolism).** Metabolism is also responsible for the breakdown of larger molecules into smaller molecules so that energy is available **(catabolism).**

The gallbladder, liver, and pancreas are considered the accessory organs of the digestive system. These organs lie outside the gastrointestinal (GI) tract but are directly concerned with digestion. Although the gallbladder can be removed without harm to the individual, the liver is essential to life. If the pancreas is removed or nonfunctional, the patient must take many enzymes and insulin for life. To understand the disorders of the accessory organs, the structure and location of the organs as well as their functions must be clear.

Disorders that affect the GI system may lead to malnutrition and a weakening of the immune system. If sufficient nutrients are not available, manufacture of disease-fighting cells is inadequate. Insufficient nutrition accompanying any other disease or disorder brings a greater degree of illness and a higher mortality. To understand the various problems of the GI system, recollection of the normal anatomy and functions of the system is necessary.

CAUSES OF GASTROINTESTINAL DISORDERS

CAUSES OF GASTROINTESTINAL TRACT DISORDERS

As with all tissues of the body, those of the gastrointestinal tract are subject to infection, inflammation, physical and chemical trauma, and structural defects. Factors that contribute to these pathologic conditions

Text continued on p. 668

OVERVIEW OF ANATOMY AND PHYSIOLOGY OF THE GASTROINTESTINAL SYSTEM

What are the organs and structures of the gastrointestinal system?

- Organs of the gastrointestinal (GI) system are the mouth, pharynx, esophagus, stomach, small intestine, large intestine, rectum, and anus (Figure 27–1).
- The accessory organs are the liver, gallbladder, and pancreas (Figure 27–2).
- The gastroesophageal sphincter (cardiac sphincter) controls the opening from the esophagus into the stomach; it prevents reflux from the stomach into the esophagus.
- The stomach lies in the upper left portion of the abdominal cavity (Figure 27–1).
- The pyloric sphincter controls release of food substances into the small intestine (Figure 27–3).
- The small intestine is divided into the duodenum, jejunum, and ileum and is about 6 m long.
- The ileocecal valve controls the progress of substances into the large intestine.
- The large intestine is divided into the cecum, colon, rectum, and anal canal; the colon is about 1.5 m long.
- The colon has four portions: the ascending, transverse, descending, and sigmoid colon.
- The appendix is attached to the cecum and has no known function in the digestive process.
- The walls of the digestive tract have four layers: mucosa, submucosa, muscular layer, and a serous layer called serosa.
- The peritoneum is a serous sac that lines the abdominal cavity and encloses the intestines, stomach, liver, and spleen and partially encloses the uterus and uterine tubes.

What are the functions of the gastrointestinal system?

- The teeth and tongue are instrumental in the chewing **(mastication)** process, and they help break down food into smaller pieces that can be acted upon by various enzymes.
- Food moves from the mouth through the pharynx down the esophagus to the stomach, where mixing movements occur.

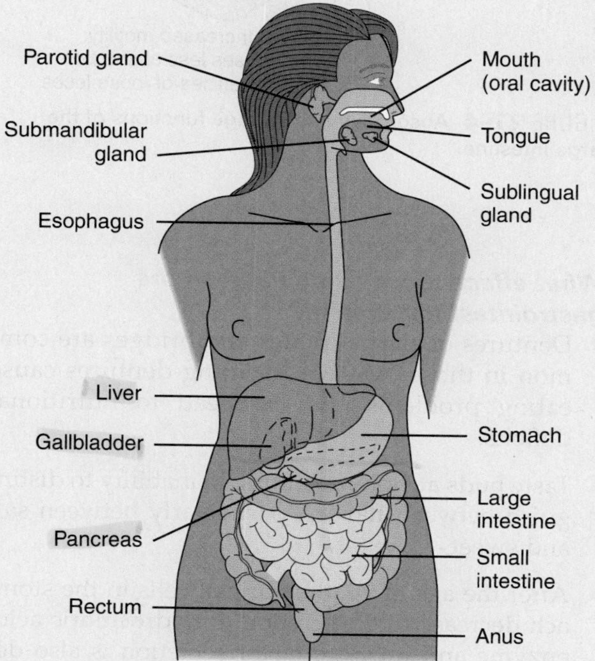

FIGURE 27–1 Organs of the digestive system.

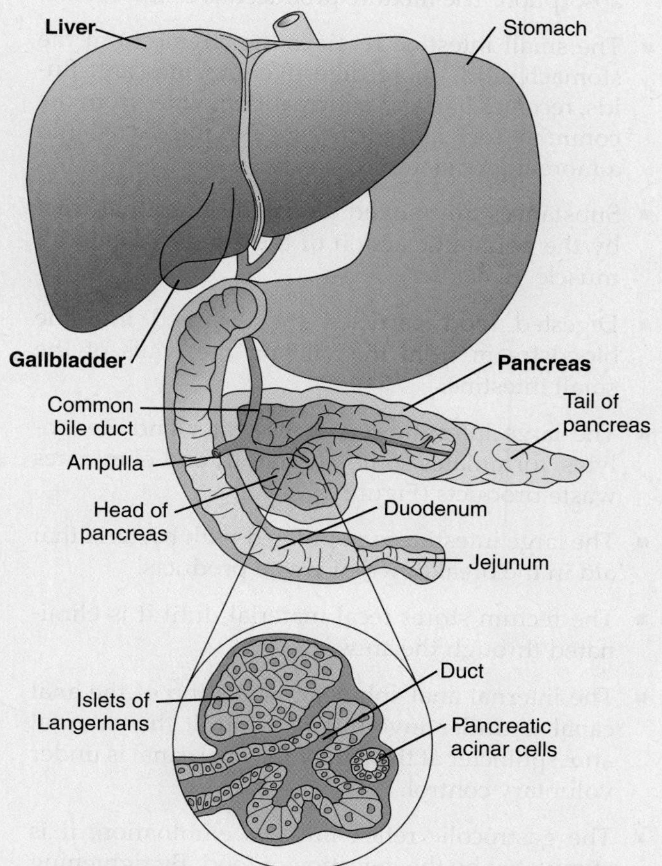

FIGURE 27–2 Accessory organs of the digestive system.

Continued

OVERVIEW OF ANATOMY AND PHYSIOLOGY OF THE GASTROINTESTINAL SYSTEM

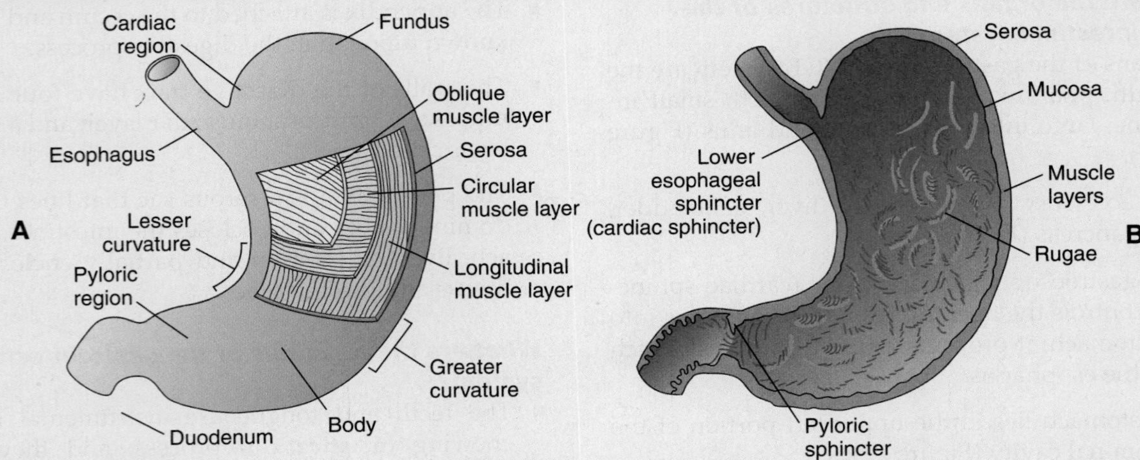

FIGURE 27–3 The stomach. **A,** External view. **B,** Internal view.

- Mucus, hydrochloric acid (HCl), intrinsic factor, pepsinogen, and gastrin are secreted into the stomach from cells within its walls and are mixed into the food to break down further the particles for absorption. The mixture produced is called **chyme.**
- The small intestine receives the chyme from the stomach, adds more digestive enzymes and fluids, receives bile and pancreatic enzymes from the common duct, and further digests the chyme into a more liquid state.
- Substances are moved along the intestinal tract by the peristaltic action of the intestinal smooth muscle.
- Digested food particles are absorbed into the bloodstream from the villi on the walls of the small intestine.
- The large intestine reabsorbs water and electrolytes, formulates some vitamin K, and eliminates waste products (Figure 27–4).
- The large intestine is populated with bacteria that aid in the breakdown of waste products.
- The rectum stores fecal material until it is eliminated through the anus.
- The internal anal sphincter at the top of the anal canal is under involuntary control; the external anal sphincter at the end of the anal canal is under voluntary control.
- The gastrocolic reflex initiates elimination; it is stimulated by the ingestion of food. By tightening the voluntary anal sphincter, the reflex emptying of the rectum can be stopped.

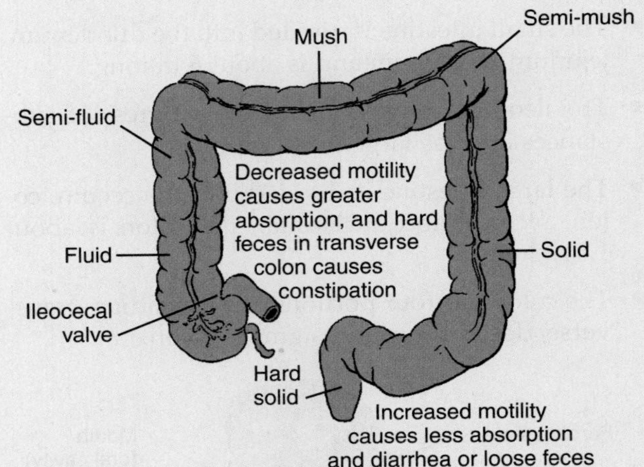

FIGURE 27–4 Absorptive and storage functions of the large intestine.

What effects does aging have on the gastrointestinal system?

- Dentures or partial plates and bridges are common in those over 65. Ill-fitting dentures cause eating problems and can lead to nutritional deficits.
- Taste buds atrophy, resulting in inability to distinguish between flavors, particularly between salt and sweet.
- After the age of 70, the parietal cells in the stomach decrease their secretion of hydrochloric acid; enzyme and intrinsic factor secretion is also decreased. The lack of intrinsic factor may cause pernicious anemia.

- The mucosa of the small intestine becomes less absorptive, and the large intestine may develop diminished motility.

What are the structures and locations of the accessory organs?

- The *gallbladder* is a small sac attached to the lower portion of the liver.
- The *liver* is a large reddish brown organ located in the upper right quadrant of the abdominal cavity under the diaphragm and is protected by the rib cage.
- The portal vein transports venous blood and nutrients absorbed from the small intestine to the liver.
- The *pancreas* is an elongated, flat organ that sits behind the stomach and consists of a "head" and a "tail" (see Figure 27–2).
- The gallbladder connects to the common bile duct that leads from the liver to the duodenum.
- The pancreatic duct extends the length of the pancreas and connects with the common bile duct, conducting its secretions into the duodenum.

What are the functions of the gallbladder, liver, and pancreas?

- The gallbladder stores bile produced in the liver and delivers it as needed to the small intestine; it can store up to 50 mL of bile.
- The liver manufactures and secretes bile and bile salts necessary to digest fat.
- The liver synthesizes albumin, fibrinogen, globulins, and clotting factors.
- The liver is a storage area for glucose (in the form of glycogen); vitamins A, D, E, K, and B_{12}; and iron.
- The liver receives blood directly from the digestive tract via the hepatic portal vein. All nutrients and oral medications pass through the liver before being distributed to other parts of the body.
- The liver is responsible for how drugs are metabolized.
- The liver detoxifies and breaks down many compounds and drugs, preparing them for excretion; it alters ammonia, a by-product of protein metabolism, so that it does not harm the body.
- The liver helps break down and excrete hormones, drugs, cholesterol, and hemoglobin from worn-out red blood cells.
- The liver plays a major role in glucose metabolism, removing excess glucose from the blood, converting it to glycogen, and then, as glucose is needed, converting glycogen back to glucose.
- The liver plays key roles in lipid metabolism, breaking down fatty acids and synthesizing cholesterol and phospholipids, and in converting excess carbohydrates and proteins into fats.
- The liver is instrumental in protein metabolism, converting certain amino acids into different ones as needed for protein synthesis.
- The liver is a large filter containing phagocytic Kupffer cells that remove bacteria, damaged red blood cells, and other toxic materials from the blood.
- The liver may store between 200 and 400 mL of blood.
- The liver synthesizes the prothrombin needed for normal blood clotting.
- The pancreas islets of Langerhans secrete the hormones insulin and glucagon into the blood; insulin is essential to the metabolism of carbohydrates.
- The pancreatic acinar cells secrete digestive enzymes into ducts that connect with the pancreatic duct.
- The major pancreatic enzymes are amylase, protease, trypsin, and lipase; these enzymes are essential to the digestion and absorption of nutrients from the small intestine.
- Secretion of pancreatic enzymes is controlled by secretin and cholecystokinin, two substances secreted by the intestinal mucosa.

How does aging effect the accessory organs of digestion?

- Gallstone incidence is higher in the older person, possibly due to an increase in biliary cholesterol related to diet and to a tendency toward dehydration.
- Secretion of lipase from the pancreas decreases, altering fat digestion, and may contribute to a depressed nutritional state in the elderly.

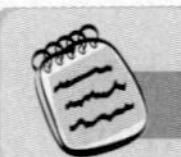

Patient Teaching 27–1

Foods that May Contribute to Colon Cancer

The patient should be taught that the following foods may contribute to the development of colon cancer.

NITRATES AND NITRITES

- Hot dogs
- Bologna and other luncheon meats
- Bacon
- Ham
- Smoked fish
- Some imported cheeses (check labels)

Nitrates and nitrites are used extensively as food preservatives. Check labels on "deli" products. Charred grilled foods or meat cooked at high temperatures also contain substances that are potentially cancer-causing.

include obvious physical ones, such as exposure to infectious agents (as in food poisoning), and less apparent psychosocial factors.

An intestinal tract problem may occur due to blockage of movement of food through the intestine (intestinal obstruction). Postoperative **adhesions** sometimes cause intestinal obstruction. Adhesions are bands of scar tissue that bind two anatomical surfaces together that are normally separate. Tumor may cause intestinal obstruction also. Intestinal disorders may occur from interference with flow of digestive juices and enzymes needed for digestion. Obstruction of this type may occur in the bile or pancreatic ducts. Continued irritation and inflammation of the GI mucosa can lead to intestinal bleeding and to increased peristalsis causing inadequate absorption of nutrients.

Psychological and emotional stresses greatly influence appetite and motility of the stomach and intestines. The secretion of digestive juices in amounts sufficient for the breakdown of food is regulated in part by the emotions. Excessive stimulation of digestive acid and enzymes can cause a breakdown in the integrity of the mucous membrane lining the digestive tract. The damage to the mucous membrane can result in gastric or duodenal ulcers and chronic colitis.

Some disorders, such as Crohn's disease and ulcerative colitis, are correlated with a genetic predisposition. Both disorders also have an ethnic correlation as they are more common among the Jewish population. Certain forms of colon cancer have been identified as having a genetic link. There is a familial tendency for the occurrence of colon cancer. Esophageal and stomach cancer are linked to consumption of charred foods and those containing nitrites (Patient Teaching 27–1). Cigarette smoking is a known link for stomach cancer.

Autoimmune diseases often affect the GI system, causing inflammation or fibrosis of organs. Treatments such as drug and radiation therapy may cause GI problems as a side effect. Some people who have undergone chemotherapy for cancer develop a mechanical form of sprue, a malabsorption problem, that remains even after chemotherapy is complete. Lactose intolerance, which is not uncommon in the older adult, may cause continuous diarrhea and malabsorption.

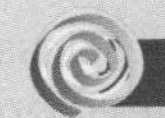

Cultural Cues 27–1

Genetic Gallstone Risk

Native Americans and people of Mexican American ancestry develop gallstones more frequently than the general population. Native Americans secrete high levels of cholesterol in bile. A majority of Native American men have gallstones by age 60, and 70% of the women of the Pima Indians in Arizona have gallstones by age 30. Mexican Americans of both sexes and all ages also have high rates of gallstones (National Digestive Diseases Information Clearinghouse, 2005).

? *Think Critically About* . . . Can you identify any GI problems that seem to run in your family? What measures can family members take to prevent such problems?

CAUSES OF GALLBLADDER DISORDERS

The formation of stones within the gallbladder can cause irritation and create areas susceptible to inflammation and infection. Stones can lodge in the common duct, causing obstruction to the flow of bile. Many people who have used liquid weight loss diets, or who have very rapidly lost weight, have developed gallstones. Women develop gallstones more frequently than men, and the incidence increases with age. Obesity and having several children are risk factors (Cultural Cues 27–1). People who have diabetes mellitus or Crohn's disease are at higher risk for the disorder.

CAUSES OF LIVER DISORDERS

The liver filters out many toxic substances and is constantly exposed to any infectious organisms circulating in the bloodstream. Many parasites migrate to the liver and can cause problems when cysts or abscesses develop. The hepatitis virus in particular attacks the liver, causing inflammation and damage to the tissue. Hepatitis B and C are implicated in liver cancer (Pellegrino, 2006).

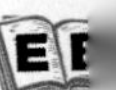

Cancer can affect any of the accessory organs, but is more prevalent in the liver. Cancer in the liver may be primary, or may be secondary to metastasis from a site elsewhere in the intestinal tract.

Many drugs and chemicals are toxic to the liver, and the nurse should always be aware of the drugs a patient is taking that may cause liver damage. Alcohol and other toxic substances are major factors in the development of cirrhosis of the liver (Lehrer, 2006).

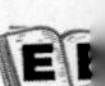

Box 27–1 Drugs and Substances Toxic or Harmful to the Liver

TOXIC DRUGS AND SUBSTANCES

- Acetaminophen (Tylenol)
- Carbon tetrachloride
- Ethyl alcohol
- Mushroom: *Amanita phalloides*
- Polychlorinated biphenyls (PCBs)
- Toluene
- Trichloroethylene
- Yellow phosphorus
- Many pesticides

DRUGS AND SUBSTANCES THAT MAY BE DAMAGING TO THE LIVER

Drugs

- Acetylsalicylic acid (aspirin)
- Amiodarone
- Amitriptyline
- Amoxicillin-clavulinic acid
- Chloroform
- Chlorpromazine (Thorazine)
- Diazepam (Valium)
- Erythromycin
- Ethambutol
- Fluconazole
- Gold compounds
- Halothane (Fluothane) anesthetic agent
- Ibuprofen
- Imipramine
- Indomethacin
- Isoniazid (INH)
- Ketoconazole
- 6-Mercaptopurine
- Methotrexate
- Methyldopa (Aldomet)
- Nifedipine (Verapamil)
- Nitrofurantoin
- Oral contraceptives
- Phenobarbital
- Phenytoin (Dilantin)
- Propylthiouracil
- Rezulin
- Rifampin
- Serzone
- Statin drugs
- Thiazide diuretics
- Tricyclic antidepressants

Chemical Substances

- Acetaldehyde
- Aerosolized paint
- Cadmium
- Ethylene oxide
- Mercury
- Nitrosamines
- Paint thinner
- Many cleaning solvents

Box 27–1 lists the most common drugs and chemicals that can cause liver problems.

Trauma to the liver is not uncommon because of automobile accidents. Liver lacerations may cause massive internal hemorrhage. However, the liver is a resilient organ and, if repair is performed quickly and part of the liver is functional, it will regenerate.

Parasites may cause cirrhosis, but this is not a usual cause of the disorder in the North American continent. Most parasites that damage the liver enter the body when people wade or swim in contaminated water in tropical countries, or eat contaminated food.

CAUSES OF PANCREATIC DISORDERS

Pancreatitis (inflammation of the pancreas) is associated with alcoholism, obstructive cholelithiasis, peptic ulcer, hyperlipidemia, and trauma. Pancreatic cancer incidence rises steadily with age. Although the cause of pancreatic cancer is not known, the incidence is higher in cigarette smokers. Obesity, chronic pancreatitis, and diabetes mellitus are also risk factors for this cancer. (See Chapter 37 for information on diabetes mellitus.)

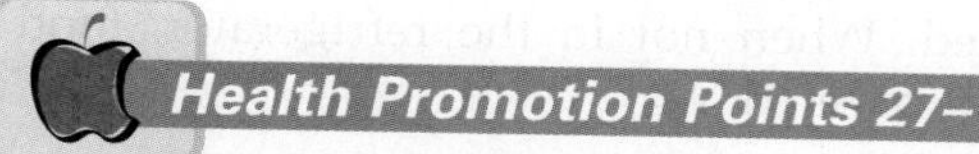

Maintaining Abdominal Tone

Obtaining sufficient daily exercise maintains abdominal muscle tone and contributes to peristalsis and the ability to defecate normally. Defecating at more or less the same time each day aids the defecation process and helps promote continued ability to control defecation.

PREVENTION OF DISORDERS OF THE GASTROINTESTINAL SYSTEM

PREVENTION OF GASTROINTESTINAL TRACT DISORDERS

There are many ways to help prevent GI problems. Eating a normal, well-balanced diet aids digestion. Maintaining good oral health is important to the health of the rest of the body (Gluch & Giorgio, 2006). Consuming sufficient bulk in the diet helps maintain a healthy colon by enhancing the timely passage of waste. A diet lacking in fiber is one factor in the development of diverticulosis, in which pockets form along the colon where waste material can lodge. Drinking at least eight glasses of fluid a day prevents constipation by helping to keep the stool moist.

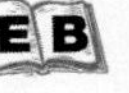

Heeding the need to defecate promptly aids in keeping the gastrocolic reflex functioning well and prevents constipation and hemorrhoids. Straining at stool contributes to hemorrhoids. When defecation must be initiated by straining, intra-abdominal pressure rises, causing the hemorrhoidal vessels to engorge (Health Promotion Points 27–1). Mobility and exercise greatly influence digestion. Decreased mobility in the elderly patient often leads to digestive problems. Increasing mobility in any way possible helps the digestive process.

Maintaining one's body weight within normal limits helps prevent hiatal hernia and esophageal reflux. Developing healthy coping mechanisms and keeping stress within acceptable limits may prevent ulcers and chronic irritability of the bowel.

Mechanical and chemical irritants that produce inflammation often can be identified by elimination diets to determine the foods that cause GI upsets. Once the offending foods are identified, efforts are made to help the patient avoid the foods and to maintain adequate nutrition.

Preventing infections of the intestinal tract is similar to preventing infections elsewhere in the body. Washing the hands before eating and proper cleaning of cooking and eating utensils are prudent. Following general rules of good hygiene and sanitation can prevent many infectious GI upsets. Food poisoning can be prevented by adequate refrigeration and proper canning, freezing, and food-handling methods. Meats and foods containing mayonnaise or dairy products should be kept chilled. When not in the refrigerator, food should be kept covered.

? *Think Critically About . . .* Can you teach your family and friends about ways to decrease the risk of colon cancer? What would you recommend to your parents regarding screening for colorectal cancer?

PREVENTION OF GALLBLADDER DISORDERS

Maintaining a normal body weight, eating a low-fat, low-cholesterol diet, avoiding rapid weight loss diets, and maintaining an active lifestyle help prevent gallstones. Having the gallbladder removed quickly when gallstones are irritating it might help prevent cancer formation.

PREVENTION OF LIVER DISORDERS

Obtaining immunization against hepatitis A and hepatitis B prevents these viral diseases. A vaccine against hepatitis C is under study at present. Using Standard Precautions (see Appendix 5) when handling body fluids, particularly blood, greatly reduces the risk of infection with hepatitis B and C. Hepatitis C can be transmitted via saliva as well as by blood. Hepatitis D and E are usually found in conjunction with hepatitis B or C. Avoiding contraction of hepatitis B and C helps decrease the chance of developing liver cancer (Health Promotion Points 27–2). Refraining from consuming excessive amounts of alcohol decreases the risk of developing cirrhosis of the liver. Avoiding exposure to known toxic or carcinogenic chemicals helps prevent liver damage and liver cancer.

PREVENTION OF PANCREATIC DISORDERS

Avoiding consuming large quantities of alcohol may prevent pancreatitis. Attending to removal of a gallbladder that has gallstones can help prevent obstruction of the pancreatic duct with stones. This prevents backup of pancreatic enzymes that are thought to be a cause of pancreatitis. Compliance with therapy for a peptic ulcer helps prevent irritation of the pancreas and resultant pancreatitis. Avoiding smoking cigarettes decreases the risk of pancreatic cancer.

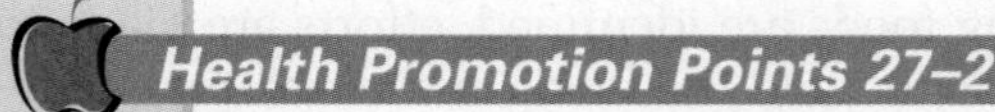

Health Promotion Points 27–2

Avoiding Contraction of Hepatitis

Practicing good hygiene and avoiding contact with substances that transmit the hepatitis virus are preventive measures. Refraining from eating raw oysters and shellfish from contaminated waters may prevent infection with hepatitis A. Avoiding unprotected sex with people who are drug users, or those known to be carriers of hepatitis B or C, helps prevent the contraction of both types of hepatitis.

DIAGNOSTIC TESTS, PROCEDURES, AND NURSING IMPLICATIONS

Diagnostic tests for disorders of the intestinal tract and accessory organs consist of x-rays, computed tomography (CT) scans, nuclear medicine scans, magnetic resonance imaging, ultrasound studies, endoscopy, biopsy, laboratory tests, tests of gastric secretions, and stool and urine studies (Table 27–1).

The patient often is scheduled for a series of tests, some of which use a contrast medium. Check patient's allergies to make certain that a particular contrast medium or injectable marker is not contraindicated. It is important that GI tests be done in the correct order so that the contrast media do not interfere with other tests. For example, if the patient is scheduled for an upper GI series, a gallbladder sonogram, and a barium enema, he should have them done in this order: sonogram, barium enema, and then the upper GI series.

A relatively new test, virtual colonoscopy, is available for colon cancer screening. The procedure combines images from a high-tech spiral CT scan to create a computer-generated three-dimensional picture of the colon. The procedure is less costly than standard colonoscopy and requires no sedation. However, if a polyp or suspicious area is seen, the patient must undergo a regular colonoscopy for tissue specimens to be obtained.

Include instructions to promote comfort when teaching about the preparation phase for a diagnostic test. Many of the studies require cleansing of the GI tract. When laxatives are administered in liquid form, the patient can drink them more easily if they are chilled or poured over ice (Assignment Considerations 27–1).

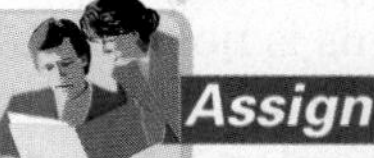

Assignment Considerations 27–1

Assisting with a Bowel Prep

When a UAP or CNA is assigned to care for a patient who is undergoing a bowel prep for a diagnostic test, ask the person to be prompt in answering a call bell for assistance to the bathroom. The need to defecate may be urgent. When a patient is consuming large quantities of fluid, such as with GoLYTELY, ask that any degree of confusion, shortness of breath, extra weakness, or muscle cramping be reported to you immediately. The person may suffer from dehydration, fluid overload, or electrolyte imbalance from the bowel prep routine.

Text continued on p. 674

Table 27–1 **Diagnostic Tests for Gastrointestinal (GI) Disorders**

TEST	PURPOSE	DESCRIPTION	NURSING IMPLICATIONS
RADIOLOGIC EXAMINATIONS			
Upper GI series (UGI)	Radiographic examination with fluoroscopy to locate obstruction, ulceration, or growths in the esophagus, stomach, and duodenum	Patient drinks a contrast medium and is placed in various positions on the x-ray table.	Keep patient NPO for 8–12 hr before the test. Explain what happens during test. After radiographs, increase fluids and give ordered laxatives to clear GI tract of contrast medium and prevent impaction. Stool may be white up to 3 days after test.
Barium enema (BE)	Radiographic examination of the colon using fluoroscopy to locate tumors, obstruction, and ulceration	A radiopaque substance is instilled into the colon by enema. After evacuation of this substance, air may be instilled for contrast studies.	Keep patient NPO for 8 hr before test. Give ordered laxatives and enemas. Bowel must be clear of stool. Explain what will happen during the test. Post-test care is same as for upper GI series.
Computed tomography (CT)	Visualizes soft tissue and density changes when sonography is inconclusive Detects tumors, abscesses, trauma, cysts, inflammation, and bleeding	Radiography is combined with computer techniques to provide a series of sectional pictures of the gallbladder.	Patient is kept NPO for 4 hr when oral contrast is to be used. May require a consent form. Assess for allergy to iodine or shellfish. Explain to patient that he will be positioned supine on a special, narrow table and his body will be in the circular opening of the scanner. He will have a strap over his waist to secure him to the table. Clicking noises will be heard from the machine. The test takes about 30 min. An IV contrast agent that causes a transitory warm feeling may be given to enhance images. He will be asked to hold his breath at certain points in the test. The machine uses narrow x-ray beams.
Virtual colonoscopy	Noninvasive method of determining if there are polyps or abnormalities in the colon Does not allow for biopsy of suspicious areas	Helical CT scan of the colon is performed. An oral contrast agent may be given 1 day before the scan.	Patient must lie still during the procedure. Remove all metal from the body surface. Usually takes about 30 min. Encourage large quantities of fluid postprocedure if barium contrast material was swallowed.
Ultrasonography	Obtains images of soft tissue that indicate density changes Used to diagnose gallstones, tumor, cysts, abscess, etc.	Sonograms are produced with high-frequency sound waves that pass through the body. Echoes vary with tissue density.	Patient is kept NPO after midnight. Explain procedure: will be supine on table, lubricant will be applied to the skin surface, and a handheld metal probe is passed back and forth with light pressure. Test takes about 30 min. Patient needs to remain still.
Magnetic resonance imaging (MRI)	Evaluates abnormalities in the liver	Places the patient in a magnetic field. Uses radiofrequency signals to determine how hydrogen atoms behave in the magnetic field. Provides better contrast than CT between normal tissue and pathologic tissue.	Explain that there is no exposure to radiation. Antianxiety medication may be administered to those patients who are claustrophobic. There are no food or fluid restrictions before the test. The test takes 30–90 min. Remove all metal objects from the body, including dental bridges. Inform patient that he will be required to remain motionless during this study. A thumping sound will be heard during the test. There may be a tingling sensation in metal fillings. A contrast medium may be injected into a vein.

Key: *IM*, intramuscular; *INR*, international normalized ratio; *IV*, intravenous; *NG*, nasogastric; *NPO*, nothing by mouth.

Continued

Table 27–1 ***Diagnostic Tests for Gastrointestinal (GI) Disorders—cont'd***

TEST	PURPOSE	DESCRIPTION	NURSING IMPLICATIONS
NUCLEAR IMAGING SCANS (SCINTIGRAPHY)			
Hepatobiliary scintigraphy (hepatoiminodiacetic acid [HIDA] scan)	Determines blood flow distribution in the liver, biliary tree, gallbladder, and proximal small bowel Confirms cirrhosis, neoplasm, and acute cholecystitis	^{99m}Tc is injected. Patient is positioned under imaging camera and images are taken as radioactive material is distributed.	Only traces of radioactivity are administered and there is little radioactivity danger. Patient will lie flat during scanning.
GI scintigraphy	Determine site of active GI bleeding	Radioactive tracer is administered IV and attaches to red blood cells. Images of the abdomen are obtained at intermittent intervals.	Same as for hepatobiliary scan.
ENDOSCOPIC STUDIES			
Esophagogastroduodenoscopy	Visualizes the esophagus, stomach, and duodenum with a lighted tube (endoscope) to detect tumor, ulceration or obstruction Separate study of esophagus, stomach, or stomach and duodenum may be done	Patient is given preoperative sedation. IV sedation may be given for the test. A local spray or gargle may be used to anesthetize the throat. The patient lies on a table with head extended, and the endoscope is introduced through the mouth.	Keep patient NPO for 8 hr. Obtain signed consent. Explain what he will experience during the test. Give preoperative medication. After procedure, keep patient NPO until gag reflex has returned. Take vital signs q 15–30 min as ordered. Watch for signs of perforation: rising temperature, pain, changes in vital signs.
Endoscopic retrograde cholangiopancreatography (ERCP)	Performed when common radiologic studies do not reveal the cause of the problem Used to identify obstruction and other pathologic conditions in the biliary and common ducts	An endoscope is passed through the mouth into the duodenum with the use of fluoroscopy. A cannula is positioned in the common bile duct, and a contrast medium is injected. Radiographs are then taken.	Obtain a signed consent for procedure. Patient is kept NPO after midnight. Explain the procedure to the patient (same as for esophagogastroendoscopy). A pretest sedative may be ordered. Postprocedure care is same as for esophagogastroendoscopy.
Proctoscopy	Examination of the lining of the rectum and sigmoid colon to detect polyps, tumor, obstruction, or ulceration	The patient is placed in the knee-chest position, often on a special table. A sigmoidoscope is introduced through the anus. Biopsies can be taken from areas of suspect tissue; polyps can be removed. The patient will experience some cramping during the procedure.	Give laxatives and enemas the evening before as ordered. Give clear liquids for dinner the night before, then keep patient NPO until after examination. Explain what he will experience. Encourage use of deep breathing and relaxation techniques to decrease cramping. Observe for rectal bleeding after biopsy or polyp removal.
Colonoscopy	Direct visualization of the lining of the colon with a flexible endoscope	Patient is moderately sedated for this procedure, which takes about 1½–2 hr. Polyps can be removed or biopsies taken.	Give clear liquid diet 1–3 days before test. Patient is kept NPO for 8 hr before test. Give laxatives for 1–3 days before test and enemas the night before. Explain procedure and what he will experience. Obtain signed consent. Give preoperative sedation. After procedure, observe for rectal bleeding and signs of perforation: abdominal distention, pain, elevated temperature.

Table 27–1 ***Diagnostic Tests for Gastrointestinal (GI) Disorders—cont'd***

TEST	PURPOSE	DESCRIPTION	NURSING IMPLICATIONS
ENDOSCOPIC STUDIES—cont'd			
Gastric analysis	Determines the rate of secretion of gastric juices and degree of acidity	A nasogastric tube is inserted, and the stomach contents are aspirated. A substance may be given to stimulate the flow of gastric secretions, and another sample is aspirated in 30 min. Increased secretion can indicate peptic ulcer or pancreatic tumor. A low degree of acidity may indicate gastric ulcer. An absence of acid can accompany cancer of the stomach or pernicious anemia.	Withhold drugs affecting gastric secretion for 24–48 hr before test. No smoking the morning of test (nicotine stimulates secretions). Keep patient NPO for 8 hr before test. Explain use of NG tube and procedure.
Liver biopsy	Removal of a tissue sample for microscopic examination and diagnosis of various liver disorders	Under local or general anesthesia, a special biopsy needle is inserted through the abdominal wall into the desired area of the liver, and a tissue sample is aspirated.	Obtain an informed consent. Patient must be kept NPO 4–8 hr before procedure. Place patient in supine or left lateral position. He will need to hold very still if performed under local anesthesia. The needle is introduced during sustained exhalation. He will feel pain similar to a punch in the shoulder lasting only a minute or so. Procedure takes about 15 min. Take baseline vital signs. Assess for allergy to local anesthetic. Have patient empty the bladder before the procedure. Check coagulation studies for abnormalities. After biopsy, place a small dressing over puncture site; position patient on right side with support to provide pressure over biopsy site for 1–2 hr. Observe for bleeding. Monitor vital signs q 15 min for 1 hr; then q 30 min for 4 hr; then q 4 hr for 24 hr. Assess for tenderness at biopsy site. Observe for respiratory problems, such as dyspnea, cyanosis, or restlessness, that might indicate pneumothorax. Instruct patient to avoid coughing or straining that might increase intra-abdominal pressure. He should refrain from heavy lifting or strenuous activities for 1–2 wk.
Tubeless gastric analysis	Determination of presence or absence of hydrochloric acid in the stomach secretions	The patient is given special granules in 240 mL of water. Urine specimens are collected at specific intervals. If HCl is present in the stomach, the urine will be blue; if none is present, the urine will be normal color.	Explain test and procedure to patient.

Continued

Table 27–1 *Diagnostic Tests for Gastrointestinal (GI) Disorders—cont'd*

TEST	PURPOSE	DESCRIPTION	NURSING IMPLICATIONS
LABORATORY TESTS			
Fecal analysis (stool examination)	Analysis for presence of mucus, elevated fat content, blood (guaiac), bacteria, or parasites	Stool specimen is obtained in bedpan or container in commode. Small smear is made on special paper and tested with special solution for guaiac or with Hemoccult test. Specimen is placed in container and sent to laboratory for testing.	Explain test to patient. Provide means for collection of stool. Promptly retrieve stool, obtain sample for guaiac test, place specimen in laboratory container, and dispatch to laboratory immediately (bacteria will multiply if specimen is left at room temperature for extended period; parasites may disintegrate). Patient must have red meat–free diet for at least 3 days before a stool guaiac test can be considered accurate.
Serum bilirubin *Normal values:* Total: 0.1–1.2 mg/dL Indirect: 0.2–0.8 mg/dL Direct: 0.1–0.3 mg/dL	Detect abnormal bilirubin metabolism Jaundice is present when bilirubin >2.5 mg/dL	Collect 5–7 mL of venous blood. Protect sample from bright light.	Explain that a blood sample will be taken. Some laboratories require an 8-hr fast.
Alanine aminotransferase (ALT) *Normal value:* 1–45 IU/L	An enzyme used to detect liver disease With viral hepatitis, ALT/AST ratio is >1.0 With other liver disease, ALT/AST ratio is <1	Collect 7–10 mL of venous blood in a red-top tube. Injury of liver cells causes release of this enzyme.	Explain that a blood sample will be collected. No fasting is required.
Aspartate aminotransferase (AST) *Normal range:* 1–36 units/L	An enzyme found in heart, liver, and muscle tissue Used to detect acute hepatitis or biliary obstruction	Collect 7–10 mL of venous blood in a red-top tube. Diseases affecting hepatocytes cause this enzyme to rise in the blood.	Explain that a blood sample will be drawn. Avoid hemolysis of sample. IM injection will affect level.
Alkaline phosphatase (ALP) *Normal range:* 35–150 units/L	Enzyme found in bone, liver, and placenta Used to detect liver tumor in conjunction with other clinical findings Rises when there is obstruction of biliary tree	Collect 5–7 mL venous blood in a red-top tube.	No fasting is required.
Ammonia *Normal range:* 10–80 mcg/dL	Is a product of protein metabolism Used to support diagnosis of severe liver disease with encephalopathy	Collect 4–7 mL venous blood in a green-top tube. May need to ice the specimen.	No fasting is required.

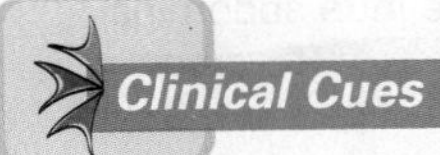

If a patient has trouble with nausea, sucking on an ice cube first and then using a straw to drink the solution for a colon "prep" helps as it decreases taste sensation.

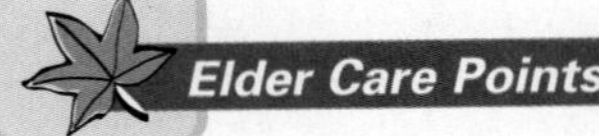

The older patient is especially at risk for problems of electrolyte imbalance and dehydration when undergoing preparation for diagnostic tests that require a fasting state and/or bowel cleansing. Frequent assessment for these problems is essential.

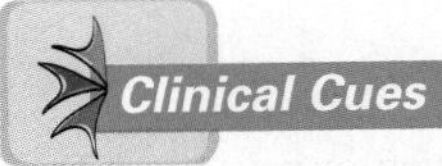

Frequent, loose bowel movements cause rectal irritation. Instructing the patient to apply a lubricant such as A&D ointment, Desitin ointment, or petroleum jelly before the laxatives act can protect this area and make the patient more comfortable.

For many GI tests, the patient is kept on nothing by mouth (NPO) status the night before. In the hospital, mouth care should be offered in the morning, and the door of the room should be kept closed so that food odors do not enter and increase hunger. A food tray should be obtained immediately upon return to the floor, as long as NPO status is no longer in effect.

Table 27–1 ***Diagnostic Tests for Gastrointestinal (GI) Disorders—cont'd***

TEST	PURPOSE	DESCRIPTION	NURSING IMPLICATIONS
LABORATORY TESTS—cont'd			
Gamma-glutamyl transpeptidase (GGT) *Normal range:* 5–10 g/dL	Detects liver cell dysfunction, biliary obstruction, cholangitis, or cholecystitis	Collect 7–10 mL venous blood in a red-top tube.	Explain that a blood sample will be taken. Drugs that affect this test are alcohol, phenytoin, phenobarbital, clofibrate, and oral contraceptives.
Protein *Normal range:* 6.0–8.0 g/dL **Albumin** *Normal range:* 3.5–5.5 g/dL	Detect altered protein metabolism Decreased in liver failure	Collect 5–7 mL venous blood in a red-top tube.	Explain that a blood sample will be drawn. No fasting is required.
Prothrombin time (PT) *Normal range:* 12.0–14.0 sec	Protein produced by the liver and used in blood clotting Depends on adequate intake and absorption of vitamin K Reduced in patients with liver disease, causing a prolonged clotting time	Collect 5–7 mL of venous blood in a blue-top tube.	No fasting is required. Apply pressure to venipuncture site. INR used to determine therapeutic level of anticoagulant medication.
Partial thromboplastin time (PTT) *Normal PTT:* 60–70 sec **Activated PTT (APTT)** *Normal APTT:* 20–35 sec	Detect deficiencies of stage II clotting mechanisms Prolonged in liver disease	Collect 5–14 mL venous blood in one or two blue-top tubes.	No fasting is required. Apply pressure to venipuncture site.
***Helicobacter pylori* antibody test** *Normal:* none present	Detects antibodies to *H. pylori* bacterium in the stomach *H. pylori* is a risk factor for gastric and duodenal ulcers, chronic gastritis, or ulcerative esophagitis	Collect a sample of venous blood according to the laboratory's instructions.	Explain to patient that a blood sample will be drawn. No fasting is required.

You can provide juices and coffee or tea while waiting for the meal tray to be delivered. Frequent assessment for signs of dehydration is necessary. Cleansing enemas and lack of oral intake can quickly dehydrate a patient who has already been ill with nausea, vomiting, or diarrhea.

> ***Think Critically About*** . . . How would you assess an elderly patient for signs of fluid and electrolyte problems resulting from diagnostic tests on the GI system?

Psychological care of the patient should not be overlooked. What seems to be a routine test to the nurse can have very different meaning to the patient. It is best to assess what fears the patient might have before beginning teaching about the test. The purpose, description, and nursing implications for the diagnostic tests of the GI system and accessory organs are listed in Table 27–1.

> ***Think Critically About*** . . . How and what would you teach a patient who is scheduled to have an endoscopic retrograde cholangiopancreatography (ERCP)?

NURSING MANAGEMENT

Assessment (Data Collection)

A focused assessment of the GI system includes the collection of both objective and subjective data. Although assessment for particular problems is covered later, a general guide for history taking is presented in Focused Assessment 27–1.

Assessment for problems of the accessory organs of the digestive system begins during history taking.

Focused Assessment 27–1

Data Collection for the Gastrointestinal System and Accessory Organs

When obtaining a GI history, ask the following questions:

- Have you gained or lost weight recently?
- Do you have any difficulty chewing or swallowing?
- When did you have your last dental examination?
- Do you ever experience indigestion? Do certain foods disagree with you? Do you have known food intolerances?
- Do you drink alcohol? About how often do you drink? How many drinks do you average?
- Has your appetite changed in any way?
- Have you been experiencing any abdominal pain or nausea and vomiting? Do you experience any regurgitation or reflux?
- Can you describe your usual diet? How much of each item do you eat? (Ask about what is eaten at each meal typically, and then ask about between-meal snacks and drinks.)
- What drugs do you take on a regular basis? (aspirin, NSAIDs, and corticosteroids are particularly important)
- Are you able to shop and prepare meals? Is there any problem with obtaining sufficient food (if patient is known to have economic constraints)?
- Do you have any cultural preferences for food?
- How do you handle stress? Blow off steam?
- How do you relax?

Additional questions pertinent to the accessory organs:

- Does eating fatty or fried food give you pain or diarrhea?
- Does your blood take a long time to clot when you hurt yourself?
- Have you had any rapid weight loss from dieting?
- Have you been immobile for a long period of time?
- Have you been exposed to chemical toxins such as cleaning agents, pesticides, or industrial chemicals?
- Have you had hepatitis B and/or hepatitis A immunizations?
- Have you ever had a blood transfusion?
- Have you had any surgeries? If so, what year were they?
- Do you use recreational drugs?
- Do you have any tattoos or body piercings?
- Do you smoke? If so, how much do you smoke? How many years have you smoked?
- Have you experienced any abdominal trauma?
- Do you have a sexual partner? Are you monogamous? Has any sexual partner been a carrier of hepatitis B or hepatitis C?

Key: *NSAIDs,* nonsteroidal anti-inflammatory drugs.

Questions regarding family history, diet, dietary intolerances, presence of pain, and problems with blood clotting are asked. Immunization status is verified. Because of the many functions of the liver, assessment of the patient with liver disease must include all systems of the body. A comprehensive history of illnesses and exposure to toxic agents, both chemical and infectious, is part of a thorough evaluation.

Physical Assessment

Physical assessment includes inspection, auscultation of bowel sounds, palpation, and percussion. The teeth, gums, and oral mucosa are inspected for obvious problems. The skin is inspected for color and lesions, and any discolorations on the abdomen are noted. The presence of edema and **ascites** (fluid in the abdominal cavity) is checked by observing for marked abdominal distention and taut, glistening skin. The contour of the abdomen is checked, and any outpouchings indicating a hernia are noted.

Auscultation of bowel sounds is performed for each quadrant of the abdomen using the diaphragm of the stethoscope (Figure 27–5). **Bowel sounds are caused by air and fluid moving through the intestinal tract and are heard as soft gurgles and clicks every 5 to 15 seconds.** The normal frequency for these sounds is about 5 to 30 in 1 minute. Both the character and frequency of sounds are noted. Loud, frequent sounds occur when there is excessive motility in the bowel. **Auscultation is done before palpation or percussion because palpation may cause peristaltic movement that otherwise would not have occurred.**

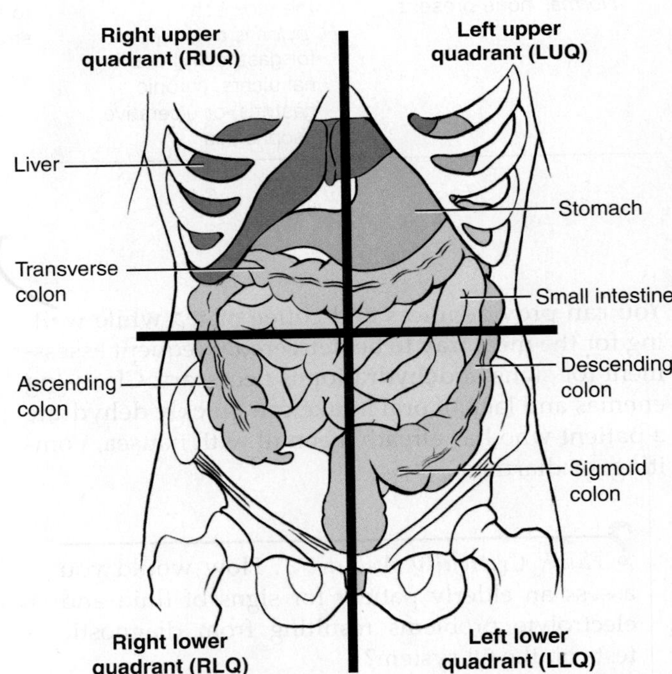

FIGURE 27–5 Auscultate bowel sounds in all four quadrants.

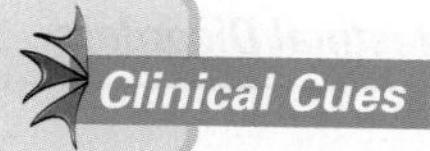

For bowel sounds to be considered absent, it is necessary to verify that no sounds are heard after listening in each of the four quadrants for 5 minutes. Hypoactive bowel sounds can be noted in the medical record when no sounds are heard after listening in each of the four quadrants for 30 seconds.

If hyperactive, high-pitched sounds are heard in one quadrant and another quadrant has decreased sounds, assess for nausea and vomiting as the patient may have an intestinal obstruction.

Light palpation is performed over each quadrant of the abdomen to detect areas of tenderness and any masses that might be present. It is important to watch the patient's face during palpation to detect signs of discomfort.

Percussion is performed by placing the middle finger of one hand on the abdomen and striking the finger lightly below the knuckle and listening for the pitch of sound produced. A resonant sound is heard over areas filled with air and a dull, thudding sound is heard over solid organs. **Percussion detects excessive air in the intestinal tract, which occurs with irritation and inflammation.**

If there is a question of whether ascites is present, abdominal girth is measured. A tape measure is placed around the fullest part of the abdomen, usually at the umbilicus. Small ink marks are placed at the sides of the tape on the axillary lines so that future measurements may be taken at the same place for comparison. If ascites is present and continuing to be produced, the abdominal girth will increase with subsequent measurements.

Ascites can be assessed for by placing the patient supine and exposing the abdomen. With the patient's arms at the sides and knees flexed, observe for *bulging flanks* indicating fluid accumulation. Percuss from the umbilicus to the flanks to detect shifting dullness caused by air rising and fluid shifting to the dependent areas.

Check the laboratory values and diagnostic test results (see Table 27–1). Evaluate the urine for presence of bilirubin, which makes the urine dark or the brown color of tea. Inspect stool for the presence of fat and urobilinogen. If undigested fat is present, the stool will float in the toilet bowl. If bile is not reaching the intestine, the stool appears clay-colored or whitish. Focused Assessment 27–2 presents an outline guide for physical assessment.

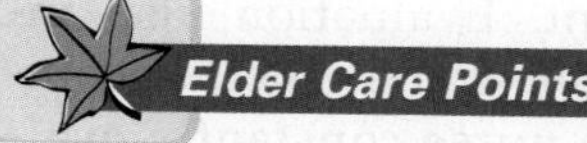

Recording all the medications the elderly patient is taking, both prescription and over-the-counter drugs, is very important when assessing the digestive system. Many drugs affect digestion, bowel motility, and appetite in these patients and can cause constipation or diarrhea.

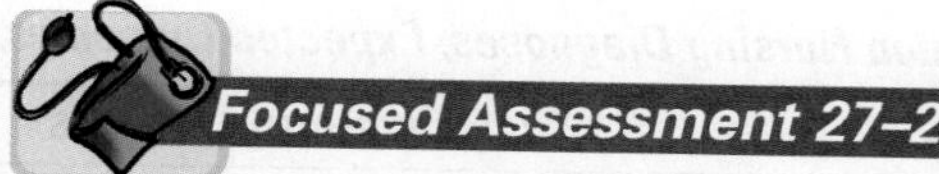

Physical Assessment of the Gastrointestinal System and Accessory Organs

Assess the following:

- Inspect the mouth for condition of teeth, gums, and mucous membranes.
- Inspect swallowing ability.
- Inspect the skin for color, areas of discoloration, and presence of surface vessels and easy bruising.
- Inspect the sclera and mucous membranes for signs of icterus.
- Inspect the contour of the abdomen.
- Auscultate for bowel sounds in all four quadrants.
- Lightly palpate each quadrant of the abdomen.
- Percuss each quadrant of the abdomen if there seems to be a problem with intestinal irritation or inflammation.
- If there is evidence of ascites, measure abdominal girth.
- Inspect stool, if available, for characteristics; test for occult blood if need is indicated.
- Inspect color of urine.
- Inspect anus for presence of external hemorrhoids.
- If vomiting has occurred, inspect vomitus for characteristics; test vomitus for blood if data gathered indicate need.

Nursing Diagnosis and Planning

Nursing diagnoses commonly used for problems of the GI tract are located in Table 27–2.

The planning of nursing care is based on problems determined from data collection. Care is planned in collaboration with the patient and other health team members. More time is often needed to care for a patient who has diarrhea or is incontinent of feces. It is important to consider the time it takes for toileting and cleaning up after loose bowel movements. A bowel retraining program takes patience and time. Administering enemas can be quite time-consuming as well. Measures needed for each patient should be worked into the time plan for the shift.

Desired outcomes are written for individual nursing diagnoses pertinent to the patient's problems. Standard Precautions must be followed whenever a patient has hepatitis. Diapered or incontinent patients may need to be treated using Transmission-Based Precautions. Expected outcomes for common nursing diagnoses for problems of the GI system are provided in Table 27–2.

Implementation

Nursing interventions to control and eliminate pain, maintain fluid and electrolyte balance, promote adequate nutrition, rest, and healing, and prevent complications are instituted. Common nursing interventions for problems of the GI system are located in Table 27–2.

All nurses must ask each patient each day about bowel movements to prevent constipation and possible impaction in ill or hospitalized patients. Nursing actions for patients with various GI disorders are dis-

Table 27–2 Common Nursing Diagnoses, Expected Outcomes, and Interventions for Patients with Gastrointestinal Disorders

NURSING DIAGNOSIS	GOALS/EXPECTED OUTCOMES	NURSING INTERVENTIONS
Deficient fluid volume related to nausea and vomiting or diarrhea	Vomiting will be controlled within 24 hr; diarrhea will be controlled within 24 hr. Fluid volume will be within normal limits within 48 hr as evidenced by adequate skin turgor and urine output >50 mL/hr.	Assess urine output for signs of fluid deficit. Provide mouth care after vomiting to decrease nausea. Medicate for nausea and vomiting as ordered. Provide quiet environment and rest. Medicate for diarrhea as ordered; keep patient clean and dry. Give only small sips of clear liquids by mouth until vomiting subsides. Continue clear-liquid diet until diarrhea is controlled.
Imbalanced nutrition: less than body requirements, related to anorexia, nausea, and vomiting	Patient will ingest at least 1200 calories per day within 7 days after vomiting subsides.	Offer mouth care before meals. Provide six small meals a day plus small, high-calorie snacks between meals. Weigh q 3 days and record. Keep room odor free. Provide company and quiet atmosphere for mealtime.
Diarrhea related to intestinal infection or inflammation	Infection or inflammation episode will resolve within 72 hr. Diarrhea will be controlled to prevent fluid imbalance within 24 hr.	Medicate with antibiotics, anti-inflammatories, and antidiarrheals as ordered. Rest bowel with clear-liquid diet or bland diet as ordered. Protect anal mucosa with barrier ointment. Keep anal area clean and dry. Provide warm sitz bath to soothe anal tissues as needed. Medicate for discomfort from abdominal cramping as ordered. Provide restful environment.
Constipation related to side effects of medication, loss of ability to initiate defecation, or other cause	Patient will have normal bowel movements regularly within 2 wk.	Increase fluid intake to 2500 mL/day unless contraindicated. Add fruit juices to diet. Increase fiber in diet; add slowly to prevent excessive gas formation. Increase exercise on a daily basis. Encourage patient to heed gastrocolic reflex and not delay defecation. Administer stool softener or bulk laxative as ordered. Monitor for fecal impaction.
Bowel incontinence related to lack of sphincter control	Patient will use bowel training program. Continence will be achieved within 2 mo.	Institute bowel training program. Provide toileting opportunity after each meal. Provide privacy and comfort for attempts at defecation. Adjust diet to provide optimal fiber in diet. Keep patient clean, dry, and odor free.
Ineffective coping related to inability to handle excessive stress	Patient will identify desired ways of coping within 3 wk. Patient will learn new coping techniques within 2 mo.	Assist to identify present coping mechanisms. Assist to identify stressors. Instruct in ways to develop more effective coping mechanisms, such as relaxation techniques, alterations in perspective, exercise, or imagery. Refer for counseling as needed.

cussed in the chapters that follow. Specific nursing actions are presented in the nursing care plans, and in the section on specific problems related to ingestion, digestion, and bowel elimination.

Evaluation

Evaluation involves reassessment to determine the effectiveness of nursing interventions, medical treatment, and progress toward desired outcomes. Laboratory values are analyzed to see whether problems are resolving with treatment. Evaluation also involves considering data to determine whether complications are occurring. **The nurse constantly evaluates whether the patient is experiencing adverse side effects of therapy.** When evaluation indicates that desired outcomes are not being met, the plan of care is revised and different nursing measures are tried.

COMMON PROBLEMS RELATED TO THE GASTROINTESTINAL SYSTEM

ANOREXIA

Anorexia is the absence of appetite. Enjoying food partially depends on having an appetite. Physical causes for a diminished interest in eating include poorly fitting dentures, stomatitis, decaying teeth, halitosis, and a bad taste in the mouth. Pain or nausea related to surgical procedures or the presence of a mouth or GI infection or irritation decreases appetite.

Psychosocial factors have a significant impact on one's desire for food. Appetite depends on complex mental processes having to do with memory and mental associations that can be pleasant or extremely unpleasant. Appetite is stimulated by the sight, smell, and thought of food. It is influenced by the physical and social environment in which a person is eating. The enjoyment of eating can be inhibited by unattractive or unfamiliar food, surroundings, or company, and by emotional states such as anxiety, anger, and fear. Mental depression also may cause anorexia.

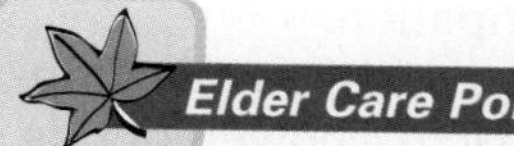

Elder Care Points

Both taste and smell sensation diminish with age. Sometimes this is due to a zinc deficiency. Teeth may be lost because of gingival or dental disease, making eating more difficult. Dental plates may not fit correctly, making eating painful. Many elderly patients take a variety of medications for various conditions. The combination of these medications may greatly affect appetite and digestion. *Polypharmacy* (taking many medications) is a frequent cause of anorexia in the elderly patient.

Because of the complex nature of anorexia, it may be necessary for the nurse to talk with the patient, family, and significant others to learn why appetite has been lost. Consulting the patient's chart may reveal some physiologic, social, or psychological reason why a patient does not eat normally. Once the apparent cause of anorexia is discovered, nursing intervention is aimed at minimizing or alleviating those factors that inhibit appetite.

Nursing Management

Loss of appetite is to be expected when a person becomes ill. However, persistent anorexia must be dealt with to avoid the consequences of inadequate nutrition. Nursing interventions include mouth care before each meal to eliminate or minimize oral causes of poor appetite. Laboratory results regarding albumin and electrolyte levels should be monitored. The percentage of each meal eaten should be noted and documented.

If psychosocial factors are involved, the nurse might try offering preferred foods whenever this is possible and not detrimental to health. Meals that are planned to include a variety of colors, textures, and tastes are more appealing and enjoyable than those that are monotonous and bland. The patient should be given ample time to eat and be encouraged to eat slowly and enjoy the meal. If it is necessary to feed the patient, this should be done cheerfully and in a manner in which you would eat a meal.

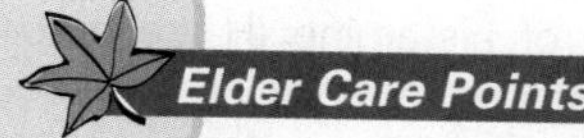

Elder Care Points

If weight loss and loss of appetite occur in an elderly patient without evidence of any specific cause, the possibility of depression should be investigated. The depressed elderly patient may give up hope and just stop eating much.

Eating is a social event, and very few people get as much pleasure eating alone as they would in the company of someone else. The nurse, a family member, or a friend can provide companionship while a patient eats. If there is a patient cafeteria or gathering place for patients to eat together, and the patient is able to go there for meals, this can sometimes alleviate or minimize a problem of anorexia.

Many elderly patients have dental problems that interfere with eating. This possibility should be explored. Some people may be embarrassed by physical limitations that cause them to be awkward with eating and will eat very little in the company of others. Others who have difficulty swallowing and are afraid of choking are afraid to eat alone but embarrassed when eating with others. It is essential to explore the causes of anorexia and feelings about eating for each patient.

Food from home often is a welcome addition to institutional fare. The person bringing the meal will need to be advised of any restrictions on the patient's dietary intake and the importance of adhering to dietary limitations.

NAUSEA AND VOMITING

Interference with comfort and nutrition occurs when nausea and vomiting are persistent. Nausea and vomiting may be related to illness, anesthesia, pain, effects of cancer treatment, or stress. A transient problem is not treated, but when the disorder persists, medication with antiemetics, GI intubation, and administration of intravenous fluids are necessary (Complementary & Alternative Therapies 27–1). Nursing interventions for the patient with nausea and vomiting are discussed in Chapter 3.

ACCUMULATION OF FLATUS (GAS)

Surgical intervention, mechanical obstruction, and accidental injury to the intestinal tract can cause disturbances in the passage of material through it. Whenever ingested material cannot pass through the intestinal tract as it should, it accumulates in the stomach and the intestines. Pressure and distention occur when

Complementary & Alternative Therapies 27–1

Ginger for Nausea

Ginger has been used for centuries in Asia to combat nausea and vomiting, motion sickness, and dyspepsia. It is available candied in capsules, fluid extract, and tablets, and tincture or as fresh gingerroot that can be grated and used to make tea. Ginger may decrease the action of histamine (H_2)-receptor antagonists and proton pump inhibitors and may increase absorption of medications taken orally. Ginger may decrease the effect of antidiabetic medications. It should not be used during pregnancy or lactation.

peristalsis is decreased or the flow of chyme is inhibited by an obstruction. **Flatus** (gas) is formed by the action of digestive juices and bacteria on the ingested material, resulting in bloating.

Nursing Management

Assisting the patient to walk a lot has traditionally been the nursing intervention for sluggish peristalsis or bloating. This works for some patients, but others continue to have discomfort. If the physician will permit it, a slight Trendelenburg position can be useful in speeding the expulsion of gas. Placing the buttocks and legs higher than the trunk and head causes gas to rise toward the rectum, making it easier to expel flatus. For patients who do not have abdominal incisions, massaging the abdomen gently is helpful. Work up the right side, across, and down over the left colon to move gas toward the rectum. Use both hands, placing the left hand behind the right after moving the gas along the bowel before lifting the right hand. This helps prevent gas from moving backward. Patient Teaching 27–2 presents another method for relieving gas.

Advise the patient to avoid chilled or hot drinks as these may create more gas. Antiflatulent medications that contain simethicone, such as Phazyme, are helpful if the patient is not NPO. The physician may order the insertion of a rectal tube or a rectal suppository to help the patient move the gas out of the intestine.

? *Think Critically About . . .* Can you teach a patient three ways to prevent the occurrence of excessive gas postoperatively?

CONSTIPATION

When constipation occurs, the stool is hard, dry, and difficult to pass. There may be a bloated feeling, and pain may be experienced when the patient attempts to defecate. Consistency of stool is greatly influenced by the type of food eaten and the quantity of liquid consumed. A diet low in fiber predisposes to constipation, as does inadequate fluid intake. Physical inactivity,

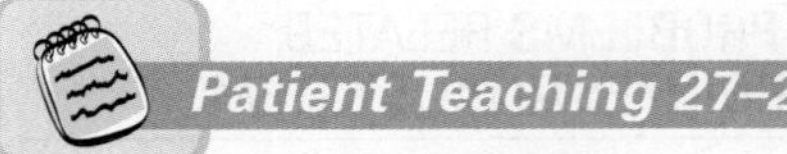

Patient Teaching 27–2

An Exercise to Reduce Gas and Bloating

Teach the patient who is experiencing bloating and excessive gas the following exercise unless contraindicated.

- Lie on your back with your legs extended and a pillow under your knees.
- Slowly raise your right leg, bend the knee, and bring the leg down toward the abdomen.
- Hold this position for a count of 10, then slowly lower your leg back down to the bed.
- Take three slow deep breaths and repeat the exercise with the left leg.
- When you feel the need to expel gas, do so; don't hold back.
- Repeat the exercise three or four times with each leg. Perform the exercise several times a day with rest periods between the exercise periods.

ignoring the gastrocolic reflex, stress, and some neurologic disorders affecting the nerves in the intestinal tract also may contribute to constipation.

Besides not passing stool regularly, signs and symptoms of constipation include hypoactive bowel sounds, abdominal distention, a firm abdomen, and abdominal discomfort or pain.

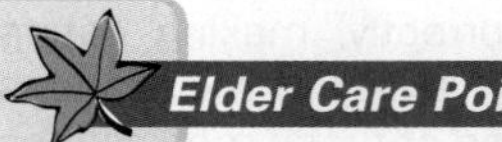

Elder Care Points

Constipation is a problem among many people over age 60. Decreased GI motility, lack of exercise, limited fluid intake, and constipating medications taken for various conditions all contribute. In the very elderly, difficulty getting to the bathroom and suppression of the defecation urge may contribute to the problem. Reliance on laxatives is common among the elderly and is to be discouraged. Counsel with individual patients about ways to increase fiber in the diet that are to their liking, and encourage fluid intake of at least 2500 mL/day if not contraindicated by the presence of cardiac or renal disease.

Nursing Management

The first step is to identify the cause of constipation. Initial treatment may include a rectal suppository or enema to induce evacuation, or the administration of a laxative. A stool softener may be prescribed. Fiber and liquids are increased in the diet. If this does not resolve the problem, the patient is placed on one of the bulk-forming laxatives to be used daily, such as Metamucil. If the patient has become impacted with stool, digital extraction may be needed. In this event, the nurse applies a lubricant, such as K-Y jelly or the anesthetic lubricant xylocaine jelly, into the rectum and around the anus and, using a gloved finger, breaks up and removes the feces. An oil retention enema usually is given prior to this procedure. The patient may be medicated with a mild analgesic 30 to 60 minutes prior to impaction removal to decrease the discomfort of the procedure.

Counsel the patient to add lots of raw fruits and vegetables to the diet, to eat more whole-grain cereals and breads, add bran to the diet, and drink lots of fluids. Fruit juices are particularly helpful as they contain fructose, which is a natural laxative. Help the patient to design an acceptable exercise program, such as walking, biking, running, swimming, or active sports participation. Advise him to heed the urge to defecate quickly and not to put it off.

? *Think Critically About . . .* Can you list six foods high in fiber that a patient might add to the diet to combat constipation?

DIARRHEA

The frequent passage of liquid or semiliquid stool is called diarrhea. It occurs with a variety of illnesses, food poisoning, excessive stress, and inflammation of the bowel. Mild diarrhea is not treated. If diarrhea persists for more than 24 to 48 hours or the number of stools is so excessive that great quantities of fluid are lost, treatment should begin. Signs and symptoms include multiple liquid or semiliquid bowel movements, hyperactive bowel sounds, and abdominal cramping.

Antidiarrheal agents such as diphenoxylate hydrochloride (Lomotil), loperamide hydrochloride (Imodium), tincture of opium (Paregoric), or a combination product, such as Kaopectate, are administered (see Table 29–1). If the diarrhea is severe, nothing is given by mouth until it subsides. If it is moderate, only clear liquids are permitted by mouth. Severe, long-term diarrhea may require the use of total parenteral nutrition. Because diarrhea depletes the natural bacterial flora in the intestine, taking tablets, capsules, or granules containing *Lactobacillus acidophilus* helps replace the flora. When diarrhea is caused by infection, antibiotics are prescribed. Stool cultures may be necessary. As the condition improves, the diet is advanced.

Nursing Management

Monitor intake and output and assess the amount of fluid lost in the stool, measuring it if needed. Administer ordered medications and replace lost fluids. Monitor the patient for electrolyte imbalances and watch for signs of dehydration, such as decreased skin turgor, thick oral secretions, and decreased urine output. Taking small amounts of an electrolyte replacement solution, or Gatorade, helps prevent imbalances. Avoiding coffee or tea helps as caffeine is a gastric stimulant and increases peristalsis. Thorough handwashing is essential when caring for the patient, and Standard Precautions are followed. When infection is the cause of the diarrhea, Contact Precautions to prevent spread of the infection are followed.

The anus and rectal mucosa must be protected from excoriation. The use of barrier ointment or cream helps protect the area. Warm sitz baths may relieve soreness and discomfort in the tissues as well as help cleanse the area without excessive wiping. Keeping the patient clean and dry is a high priority. Relieving odor in the room may be done with a deodorizing spray and by emptying and cleaning bedpans and commodes quickly.

BOWEL INCONTINENCE

Severe illness, trauma, neurologic damage, or prolonged bed rest may bring about bowel incontinence. This is very embarrassing for the alert patient. The nurse must be kind and gentle and must make every effort to keep the patient clean and dry. Tracking the time of incontinent movements and offering toileting after each meal may help eliminate the problem. Should incontinence be persistent, the cause should be identified and then a bowel training program instituted. See Chapter 29 for information on the bowel training program.

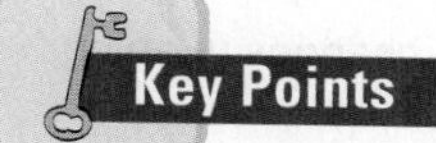

- The role of the gastrointestinal system and accessory organs is to provide nourishment for the body.
- Peristalsis moves food through the GI tract.
- The process by which the nutrients are utilized in the body after digestion and absorption is called metabolism.
- Anabolism is the building of body tissues from the nutrients.
- Catabolism is the breakdown of larger molecules into smaller molecules so that energy is available.
- The gallbladder stores bile and can be removed without harm to the body.
- The pancreas provides enzymes for digestion and insulin, and daily replacement of these substances must occur if the pancreas is removed.
- The secretion of lipase from the pancreas decreases with age, altering fat digestion.
- Problems of the GI system include infection, inflammation, trauma, and structural defects.
- Continued irritation and inflammation of the GI mucosa can lead to intestinal bleeding and increased peristalsis with inadequate absorption of nutrients.
- Consuming adequate fluid and fiber promotes proper bowel function.
- Hygienic practices and proper care of food and food-handling utensils helps prevent infection of the intestinal tract.
- Immunization for hepatitis A and B prevents liver disease.
- Hepatitis B and C are risk factors for liver cancer.
- Controlling alcohol consumption helps prevent cirrhosis of the liver and pancreatitis.

- If damage to the liver is halted before all tissue is affected, the liver can regenerate.
- Not smoking cuts the incidence of pancreatic cancer by 50%.
- Diagnostic tests are performed to determine problems of the GI system (see Table 27–1).
- A focused assessment should be performed on each patient with a problem of the GI system or accessory organs (see Focused Assessment 27–1, Focused Assessment 27–2).
- Check urine and stool for signs that bile ducts are blocked.
- Medications can affect appetite and digestion.
- Taste and smell diminish with age and may decrease appetite. Poor dentition may make eating difficult for the elderly person.
- Eating is a social event, and company at mealtime improves appetite and intake.
- Nausea and vomiting interfere with nutrition and should be treated promptly.
- Ambulation and oral simethicone are helpful in reducing gas.
- Severe diarrhea can cause fluid and electrolyte imbalances and dehydration. Treat diarrhea early.
- Increasing fiber, fluids, and exercise helps prevent or relieve constipation.

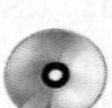
Go to your **Companion CD-ROM** for an Audio Glossary, animations, video clips, and bonus review questions.

evolve Be sure to visit the companion Evolve site at http://evolve.elsevier.com/deWit for interactive NCLEX-PN Exam Style Review Questions, WebLinks, and additional online resources.

NCLEX-PN EXAM STYLE REVIEW QUESTIONS

Choose the best answer(s) for the following questions.

1. In the liver, ______________________ are phagocytic cells that remove bacteria, damaged red blood cells, and other toxic materials from the blood.

2. Which of the following physiologic changes in aging predisposes the older adult to anemia?
   1. Decreased ability to discriminate salt and sweet
   2. Decreased lipase production
   3. Decreased secretion of intrinsic factor
   4. Increased biliary cholesterol

3. The nurse discusses disease prevention measures with a group of older adults during a senior seminar. The nurse provides accurate information when she includes which of the following? *(Select all that apply.)*
   1. Consume sufficient fiber.
   2. Eat a normal, well-balanced diet.
   3. Exercise regularly.
   4. Drink at least three glasses of fluids.
   5. Take laxatives regularly.

4. The nurse is preparing a patient for a gastrointestinal diagnostic procedure. Which of the following nursing interventions promotes psychological well-being of the patient?
   1. Applying skin barrier ointments to prevent breakdown
   2. Attending to patient's fears and anxiety
   3. Providing oral care
   4. Assessing for dehydration and electrolyte imbalance

5. During abdominal assessment, the nurse is observed to auscultate prior to palpation or percussion. An accurate explanation would be:
   1. "The sequence prevents abdominal guarding."
   2. "The sequence provides a more accurate assessment of the presence of peristalsis."
   3. "The sequence reduces patient anxiety during the examination."
   4. "The sequence relieves abdominal tenderness."

6. An elderly female patient of Puerto Rican descent is admitted for persistent anorexia and dehydration. With no apparent organic underlying cause for loss of appetite, which of the following would be culturally appropriate? *(Select all that apply.)*
   1. Determine food preferences.
   2. Encourage family visits.
   3. Provide small amounts of food and fluid frequently.
   4. Consider parenteral nutrition.
   5. Consult dietitian and speech therapy.

7. A patient is consuming large quantities of laxative fluid as part of the bowel preparation for a diagnostic procedure. The nurse must watch for which of the following side effects?
   1. Constipation
   2. Rashes
   3. Dehydration
   4. Chest pains

8. A 30-year-old female was admitted with complaints of severe nausea and vomiting for a couple of days. On admission she was hypotensive and extremely weak. The nurse determines that a priority nursing diagnosis would be:
   1. Ineffective breathing pattern
   2. Activity intolerance
   3. Deficient fluid volume
   4. Decreased cardiac output

9. The nurse is caring for an 18-year-old patient who was diagnosed with anorexia nervosa. The nurse identifies that Imbalanced nutrition: less than body requirements is a priority nursing diagnosis. An appropriate expected outcome would be:
   1. the patient will be able to eat 35% or more of her meals.
   2. the patient will be able to develop improved eating behaviors.
   3. the patient will be able to verbalize the importance of eating.
   4. the patient will be able to identify barriers to eating.

10. The nurse emphasizes the importance of eating natural sources of fiber to a patient who has frequent constipation. Which of the following patient statements indicates effective health teaching?
   1. "I will consider white bread."
   2. "Laxatives would keep me regular."
   3. "I will add more milk to my morning cereal."
   4. "I will eat more fruits and vegetables."

CRITICAL THINKING ACTIVITIES

Read each clinical scenario and discuss the questions with your classmates.

Scenario A

Mr. Bruns, 66-years old, was admitted with jaundice, abdominal distention, abdominal pain, and malaise. He is to undergo an ERCP. He is apprehensive and frightened about what may be wrong with him.

1. What is involved in an ERCP procedure? What is the pretest care? Post-test care?
2. What would you do to try to alleviate Mr. Bruns' apprehension and fear?
3. What could be possible causes of his jaundice?

Scenario B

Ms. O'Malley is a resident in your extended care facility. She has been losing weight, has no appetite, and is becoming more withdrawn. Her daughter has a new job and isn't able to visit as many times a week as she had been.

1. What assessments would you think appropriate for Ms. O'Malley at this time?
2. What nursing interventions could you institute that might improve her nutritional status?
3. What could you do to help her loneliness now that her daughter cannot visit as often?

CHAPTER 28

Care of Patients with Disorders of the Upper Gastrointestinal System

evolve http://evolve.elsevier.com/deWit

Objectives

Upon completing this chapter, you should be able to:

Theory

1. Discuss obesity and its management, including bariatric surgery.
2. Compare the signs and symptoms of oral, esophageal, and stomach cancer.
3. Illustrate the cause of gastroesophageal reflux disease (GERD).
4. Explain the etiology and prognosis for Barrett's esophagus.
5. Describe the pathophysiology, means of medical diagnosis, and treatment for gastritis.
6. Compare and contrast the treatment and nursing care of the patient with GERD and a patient with a peptic ulcer.
7. Devise a nursing care plan for the patient with a gastrointestinal disorder.
8. Review the difference in the care of the patient with a nasogastric tube for decompression and a feeding tube.

Clinical Practice

1. Prepare a teaching plan for a patient who has GERD.
2. Plan postoperative care for a patient having gastric surgery.
3. Demonstrate proper care of the patient with a Salem sump tube for gastric decompression.
4. Manage a tube feeding for the patient receiving formula via a feeding pump.
5. Compare the care for a patient receiving total parenteral nutrition with care of the patient receiving enteral feedings.

Key Terms

Be sure to check out the bonus material on the Companion CD-ROM, including selected audio pronunciations.

achlorhydria (ă-chlŏr-HĪ-drē-ă, p. 702)
anastomosis (ă-năs-tō-MŌ-sĭs, p. 699)
anorexia nervosa (ăn-ō-RĔK-sē-ă nĕr-VŌ-să, p. 687)
bariatric (BĀ-rē-ĂT-rĭk, p. 684)
bulimia nervosa (bū-LĒ-mē-ă nĕr-VŌ-să, p. 688)
dyspepsia (dĭs-PĔP-sē-ă, p. 691)
dysphagia (dĭs-FĀ-jē-ă, p. 688)
Helicobacter pylori (p. 694)
hematemesis (hē-mă-TĔM-ĕ-sĭs, p. 696)
melena (mĕ-LĒ-nă, p. 698)
roux-en-Y (roo-ĕn-WY, p. 687)
stomatitis (stō-mă-TĪ-tĭs, p. 688)
vagotomy (vă-GŎT-ō-mē, p. 699)

A common problem that interferes with ingestion is poor dentition or ill-fitting dentures. Pain or difficulty with eating interferes with nutritional intake. Any time a patient is continuously not eating well, the oral cavity should be examined and a history of dental care taken.

EATING DISORDERS

OBESITY

Obesity is a worldwide problem, and is particularly prevalent in industrialized nations. In the United States, obesity causes approximately 300,000 premature deaths per year. There is an ongoing search to see if there is a genetic predisposition to this disorder. Children are showing a trend for increasing obesity, and community teaching to prevent this problem is a goal of the Healthy People Initiative (Health Promotion Points 28–1). Obesity is contributing to considerable morbidity from high blood pressure and cardiac disease. **Bariatrics** is the specialty that deals with treatment and control of obesity.

Etiology and Pathophysiology

Several factors must interact for obesity to occur, including genetics, eating foods high in calories and fat, lack of exercise, and overconsumption of food. Some medications increase appetite. The readily available high-calorie prepackaged and high-fat fast food, plus growing portion sizes, are known contributors to obesity.

People overeat for a variety of reasons. For some it is a reaction to stress; for others it is a substitute for absent pleasures. There are many theories about why more fat is developed in certain individuals. Some obese people seem to metabolize nutrients differently than others. The way a person develops fat cells and deposits fat is another factor. Genetic predisposition is most likely a factor since obesity seems to occur in several members of a family.

Signs and Symptoms

A person is considered obese if she weighs more than 20% above the ideal weight for her height, age, and body type. Over half of Americans are overweight and 40 million are obese; 3 million Americans are morbidly obese (100% over ideal body weight, or a body mass index over 40).

Obese patients should be counseled to lose weight to avoid developing one or more of the many diseases in which obesity is a contributing factor. Complications of obesity include:

- Diabetes mellitus
- Hypertension
- Hyperlipidemia
- Coronary artery disease
- Obstructive sleep apnea
- Cholelithiasis
- Arthritis with back and/or knee problems

The obese person is more susceptible to infectious disease and has decreased wound healing. A general health assessment should be conducted before a patient is placed on a weight reduction diet.

> ? ***Think Critically About . . .*** How much do you think the intake of bottled and canned soda pop and juice drinks has contributed to obesity? What do they contain and how many calories are in each? (Check the label.)

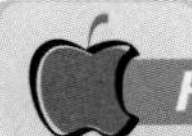

Health Promotion Points 28–1

Healthy People 2010 Obesity

Objectives regarding weight and obesity are:

19-1 Increase the proportion of adults who are at a healthy weight.

19-2 Reduce the proportion of adults who are obese.

19-3 Reduce the proportion of children and adolescents who are overweight or obese.

Diagnosis

To determine whether a patient is obese, use the following measurements:

- Height and weight chart. If more than 20% above ideal body weight for age and body build, the patient is considered obese.
- Measure the waist and then the hip circumference. Calculate the waist-to-hip ratio (waist measurement divided by the hip measurement). If the ratio is more than 1.0 in men or 0.8 in women, it indicates that the person is overweight. This is a more accurate indicator for obesity in the elderly.
- A body mass index (BMI) of more than 30 indicates obesity (Table 28–1).

$$\text{BMI} = \frac{\text{Weight (kg)}}{\text{Height (m}^2\text{)}}$$

Thyroid function should be determined to ascertain that hypothyroidism is not a cause of the weight gain.

Table 28–1 *Body Mass Index (BMI)*

BMI	19	20	21	22	23	24	25	26	27	28	29	30	31	32	33	34	35
HEIGHT	**WEIGHT (IN POUNDS)**																
4′10″ (58″)	91	96	100	105	110	115	119	124	129	134	138	143	148	153	158	162	167
4′11″ (59″)	94	99	104	109	114	119	124	128	133	138	143	178	153	158	163	168	173
5′ (60″)	97	102	107	112	118	123	128	133	138	143	148	153	158	163	168	174	179
5′1″ (61″)	100	106	111	116	122	127	132	137	143	148	153	158	164	169	174	180	185
5′2″ (62″)	104	109	115	120	126	131	136	142	147	153	158	164	169	175	180	186	191
5′3″ (63″)	107	113	118	124	130	135	141	146	152	158	163	169	175	180	186	191	197
5′4″ (64″)	110	116	122	128	134	140	145	151	157	163	169	174	180	186	192	197	204
5′5″ (65″)	114	120	126	132	138	144	150	156	162	168	174	180	186	192	198	204	210
5′6″ (66″)	118	124	130	136	142	148	155	161	167	173	179	186	192	198	204	210	216
5′7″ (67″)	121	127	134	140	146	153	159	166	172	178	185	191	198	204	211	217	223
5′8″ (68″)	125	131	138	144	151	158	164	171	177	184	190	197	203	210	216	223	230
5′9″ (69″)	128	135	142	149	155	162	169	176	182	189	196	203	209	216	223	230	236
5′10″ (70″)	132	139	146	153	160	167	174	181	188	195	202	209	216	222	229	236	243
5′11″ (71″)	136	143	150	157	165	172	179	186	193	200	208	215	222	229	236	243	250
6′(72″)	140	147	154	162	169	177	184	191	199	206	213	221	228	235	242	250	258
6′1″ (73″)	144	151	159	166	174	182	189	197	204	212	219	227	235	242	250	257	265
6′2″(74″)	148	155	163	171	179	186	194	202	210	218	225	233	241	249	256	264	272
6′3″ (75″)	152	160	168	176	184	192	200	208	216	224	232	240	248	256	264	272	279

From National Heart, Lung, and Blood Institute. (1998). *Evidence Report of Clinical Guidelines on the Identification, Evaluation, and Treatment of Overweight and Obesity in Adults.* Bethesda, MD: National Institutes of Health.

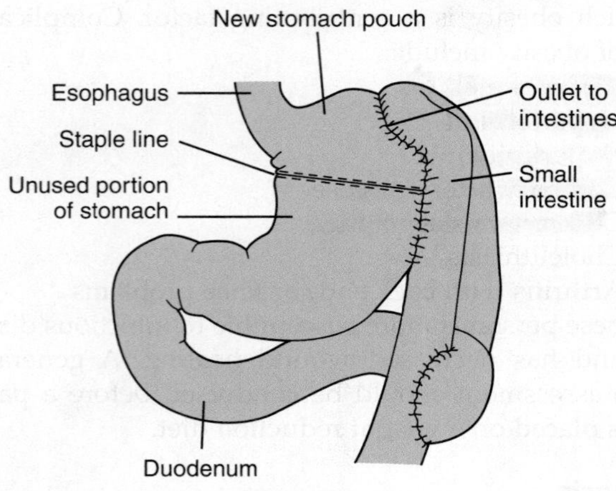

Gastric bypass

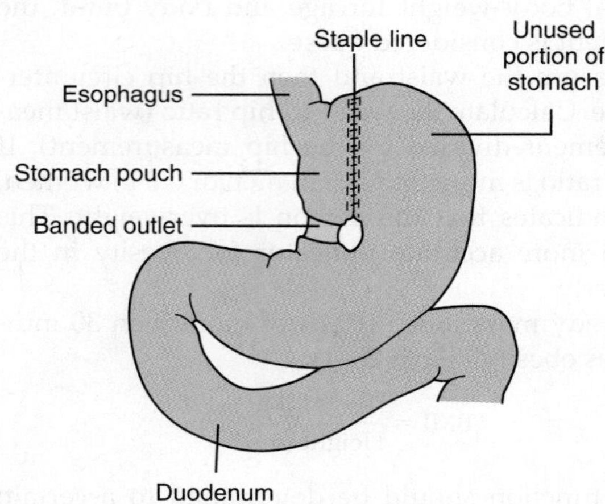

Vertical banded gastroplasty

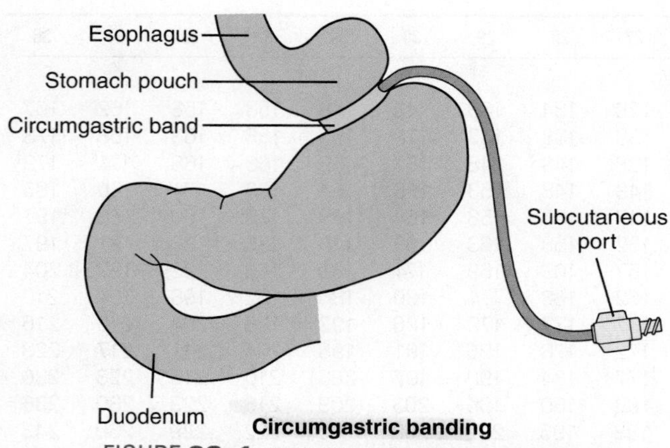

Circumgastric banding

FIGURE **28–1** Bariatric surgical procedures.

Treatment

Physician supervision is the best and safest way to treat obesity. Usually a lower calorie diet and exercise are prescribed. The patient is taught ways to change her thinking about food and her weight. Those with a BMI over 40 may have surgery to achieve weight reduction if they meet established criteria. Participation in a support group and behavior modification with some sort of reward for weight loss are part of the total treatment plan. Teaching stress reduction and alternate ways of coping are essential to success. Medications that suppress appetite or block fat absorption may be used on a short-term basis. Sibutramine (Meridia) is the commonly used appetite suppressant. It is a selective serotonin reuptake inhibitor, which enhances the feeling of fullness when eating, combined with norepinephrine, which increases the metabolic rate, thereby burning more calories. Side effects include dry mouth, insomnia, and constipation. Orlistat (Xenical) inhibits lipase, causing fats to remain partially undigested and unabsorbed. It decreases calorie intake. Gastrointestinal side effects include diarrhea (sometimes uncontrolled), abdominal cramping, and nausea.

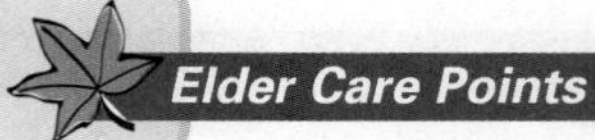

Elder Care Points

The elderly may become obese due to decreased mobility from arthritis or other joint disorders. Cooking and eating are less appealing if the person is living alone. Snacking on junk food may take the place of some meals. Metabolic rate slows with age, and a decreased calorie intake is needed to maintain a normal weight. It is essential to assess for the underlying reason for obesity in an elderly person.

Bariatric Surgery. Bariatric surgery creates reduction of gastric capacity. The patient undergoes extensive counseling and assessment. The patient must agree to modify her lifestyle and follow the stringent regimen required to lose weight and keep it off. Three common types of bariatric surgery are gastric restrictive, malabsorptive, and gastric restrictive combined with malabsorptive surgery. Preoperative care is the same as for any patient undergoing abdominal surgery. There is greater risk of pulmonary and thrombus formation, as well as death, for the obese patient.

Restrictive Procedures. *Circumgastric banding* is performed by placing an inflatable band around the fundus of the stomach. This procedure may be performed laparoscopically. The band is inflated and deflated via a subcutaneous port to change the size of the stomach as the patient loses weight.

For *vertical banded gastroplasty,* the surgeon creates a small stomach pouch by placing a vertical line of staples. A band is placed to provide an outlet to the small intestine (Figure 28–1).

Malabsorptive and Combination Procedures. The total *gastric bypass* procedure causes severe nutritional deficiencies and is no longer recommended. The **roux-en-Y** *gastric bypass (RYGB)* limits the stomach size, and the duodenum and part of the jejunum are bypassed. This limits the absorption of calories.

Think Critically About . . . What impact on nutritional status might a roux-en-Y bypass have on an individual? Why? What might be the physical long-term consequences?

Complications

With the RYGB procedure, there is danger of leakage of stomach contents into the abdomen in the early postoperative period. Later, gastric stretching may cause the staple line to break and a leak to occur. Signs and symptoms are tachycardia, dyspnea, or restlessness. An upper gastrointestinal (GI) series or computed tomography scan can diagnose the problem. The band in the vertical banding procedure may erode into the stomach over time and cause leakage. Other complications of major surgery may occur in the respiratory and cardiovascular systems (see Chapter 5 for complications of surgery). About a third of patients who undergo bariatric surgery develop gallstones. Taking 600 mg of ursodiol daily for 6 months postoperatively greatly decreases gallstone formation (Smith, 2005).

EB

All bariatric surgery patients are at risk of nutritional deficiencies. Those with the RYGB procedure are most likely to develop deficiencies of iron, vitamin B_{12}, calcium, and folate. Supplements must be taken for life.

NURSING MANAGEMENT

Assessment (Data Collection)

Data collection includes establishing whether there is a family history of obesity, determining contributing factors, and obtaining an accurate record of eating patterns for a 7-day period. Physical assessment includes measuring weight and height, figuring BMI, and taking a skinfold thickness measurement. A general health assessment is performed.

Nursing Diagnosis and Planning

Refer to Table 27–2 for many nursing diagnoses pertinent for the obese patient. Two specific nursing diagnoses are:

- Disturbed body image related to excess weight
- Chronic low self-esteem related to excess weight

Goals should be long-term, and expected outcomes might include:

- Patient will make positive statements about decreasing body size.
- Patient will verbalize feelings of self-worth.
- Patient will maintain relationships with significant others.

Implementation

A diet should be chosen with input from the patient. An exercise plan should be designed according to the patient's lifestyle and preferences. Encourage the patient to keep an eating and exercise diary. Weekly meetings for counseling and evaluation are important to provide guidance and support. Offer support by being available to talk about the positive aspects and frustrations of staying on the diet. Discourage fad diets and emphasize the importance of a well-balanced, nutritious, low-calorie diet. Commercial programs are available to assist patients with weight reduction. Weight Watchers and TOPS (Take Off Pounds Sensibly) are two commercial programs that have shown good long-term results with maintenance of normal weight.

Postoperative care for the bariatric surgery patient depends on the type of surgical procedure performed and is generally the same as for any patient having abdominal or abdominal laparoscopic surgery. Because of the weight and size of the client, lifting apparatus must be available as well as an extra-wide bed and chair. Hospitalization may be for 1 to 5 days depending on the procedure and the patient. If a nasogastric (NG) tube is in place, do not reposition it as you might disrupt the suture line. Feedings begin with 1 ounce of clear liquid at a time, advancing to pureed foods, juice, thinned soups, and milk. The diet is increased in 1-ounce increments taken over 5 minutes until the patient's appetite is satisfied. The diet is maintained for 6 weeks and then progressed to regular foods. Nausea, vomiting, and discomfort may occur, especially if too many liquids are ingested. The patient remains under medical supervision to ensure that vitamin deficiency or malnutrition does not occur.

Evaluation

Evaluation data must be gathered to determine whether the nursing actions have been effective in helping the patient meet the expected outcomes for the nursing diagnoses chosen for the care plan. The patient's diet and exercise diary should be evaluated each week if possible. Weight is tracked on a graph to show progress in weight loss. If the outcomes are not being met, the plan's interventions must be reconsidered.

ANOREXIA NERVOSA

Anorexia nervosa is presented in Chapter 45 as it is classified as a psychological disorder. Anorexia nervosa does have serious nutritional consequences. In North America, the emphasis on a slim body has influenced young women's body image. The patient refuses to eat adequate quantities of food, and is in danger of literally starving to death. Although it is a psychiatric disorder, the patient may be admitted to the medical floor for treatment of malnutrition by parenteral therapy. Behavior modification is combined with nutritional treatment.

Anorexia nervosa patients develop intricate food rituals and excessive exercise routines as a means of staying thin. The criteria listed for confirming the psychiatric diagnosis of anorexia nervosa versus malnutrition from another source are:

- Refusal to maintain body weight at or above a minimally normal weight for age and height (body weight less than 85% of that expected).
- Intense fear of gaining weight or becoming fat, even though underweight.
- Disturbance in the way in which one's body weight or shape is experienced or denial of the problem.
- Absence of at least three consecutive menstrual cycles after onset of menstruation in the female.

Diagnosis requires extensive interviewing.

BULIMIA NERVOSA

Bulimia nervosa is another psychological disorder and is covered in Chapter 45. The patient consumes large quantities of food and then induces vomiting to get rid of it so that weight is not gained. Laxatives may be taken to purge the system after an eating binge. Some patients with anorexia nervosa also are bulimic.

Some individuals practice bulimia occasionally without harm. When it is practiced frequently, it can lead to severe fluid and electrolyte imbalances, starvation, and death. Treatment of bulimia includes psychotherapy, antidepressant medication, and behavior modification. Both bulimia nervosa and anorexia nervosa are difficult to cure. Many patients with bulimia are young women.

STOMATITIS

Stomatitis is a generalized inflammation of the mucous membranes of the mouth. Causes include trauma from ill-fitting dentures or malocclusions of the teeth, poor oral hygiene, and nutritional deficiencies. Excessive smoking, excessive drinking of alcohol, pathogenic microorganisms, radiation therapy, and drugs (especially those used in chemotherapy for malignancies and anticonvulsants) are other contributors to the problem.

Common symptoms of stomatitis include pain and swelling of the oral mucosa, increased salivation or excessive dryness, severe halitosis, and sometimes fever. Small crater-like aphthous ulcers may appear in the mouth, commonly called "canker sores" (Complementary & Alternative Therapies 28–1).

Treatment of stomatitis is chiefly symptomatic, unless a specific infectious causative agent is identified. Nursing measures to control the symptoms of stomatitis, including special mouth care, artificial saliva, and diet, are discussed in Chapter 8.

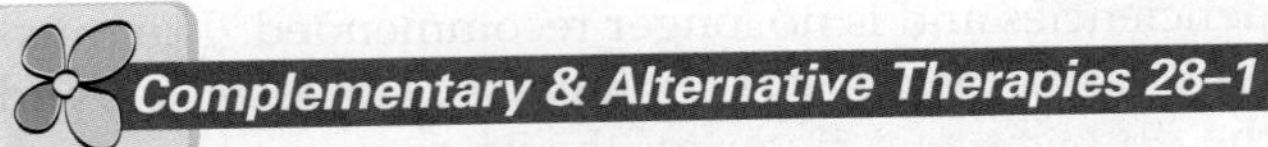

Lysine for Mouth Sores

Many people who develop "canker sores" from food sensitivities or stomach upset often can heal them more quickly by taking the dietary supplement lysine three or four times a day. This often helps cut the time of a "fever blister" on the lips as well (Tabereaux, 2005).

DYSPHAGIA

Dysphagia means difficulty in swallowing. It is the most common symptom of disorders of the esophagus and varies from a mild sensation that something is sticking in the throat to complete inability to swallow solids or liquids. Tumors, esophageal diverticula, inflammation, or motility disorders from a neurologic disorder may cause swallowing problems. If the patient is experiencing choking or difficulty with swallowing, she is kept on nothing by mouth (NPO) status. A modified barium swallow test is ordered to determine the specific cause. Videofluoroscopy is used during the test to visualize the swallowing process. A speech pathologist then can choose the most effective therapy for the patient.

Observe carefully the kinds of food the patient can tolerate and the conditions under which difficulties are experienced. Knowing the consistency and temperature of the foods most easily ingested by the patient is helpful. Some patients may strangle on liquids, tolerate soft and semisolid foods, and have the feeling that high-fiber foods are not moving past a certain point in the esophagus.

Treatment and Nursing Management

Have the patient take some "practice swallows" before beginning the meal. Watch to see that the larynx rises with each swallow. Measures that may be helpful in relieving dysphagia include instructing the patient to chew the food more thoroughly or to eat semisoft or pureed foods. Drinking liquids throughout the meal (if liquids do not cause choking) may help. Sitting upright with the head forward and the neck flexed with the chin slightly tucked aids in swallowing (Suiter, 2007). Head 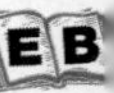 position may be altered depending on the particular type of problem present. Thickening may be added to liquids to assist in swallowing them. An electrical stimulation treatment called VitalStim is approved by the Food and Drug Administration for use with swallowing disorders. It assists in strengthening the muscles involved in swallowing (Chetney and Waro, 2004). Exercise therapy is used along with the electrical stimulation. Meals should be served in a relaxing atmosphere, with pleasant surroundings and relief from emotional stress. Further discussion of dysphagia is found in Chapters 21 and 23 with the neurologic disorders.

Nursing diagnoses for patient with swallowing problems are:

- Impaired swallowing
- Risk for imbalanced nutrition: less than body requirements
- Risk for aspiration

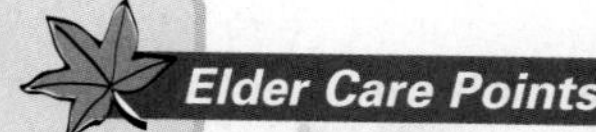

Elder Care Points

With advanced age, the muscles used for swallowing may become weaker. The older patient may have experienced a stroke that has impaired swallowing ability. Difficulty with swallowing pills is frequent in this age-group. Instruct the patient to take a drink of water, swallow, place the pill on the back of the tongue, take another drink of water, tuck the chin down slightly and swallow; follow by drinking at least 6 to 8 ounces of water.

Patients with chronic dysphagia are subject to respiratory problems resulting from the aspiration of food into the respiratory tree. Both acute and chronic dysphagia are likely to produce nutritional deficiencies and electrolyte imbalances. If the dysphagia is such that the patient cannot swallow sufficient amounts of food for adequate nutrition, tube feeding may be indicated. This sometimes is necessary when the dysphagia is the result of cerebral damage, as in cerebrovascular accident.

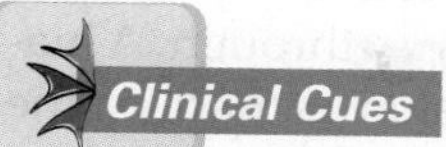

Clinical Cues

Oral suction should always be on and at hand when the patient with a swallowing problem is eating. Aspiration of food can occur quickly. The patient and family, when appropriate, are taught how to quickly use the suction apparatus.

If the patient cannot swallow anything because of a neurologic condition, or if the esophagus is obstructed and cannot be corrected surgically, then the patient must have a gastrostomy. An opening in the wall of the stomach is created, and a permanent feeding tube is sutured in place.

Nursing interventions for the patient with a gastrostomy tube include aspirating for residual contents before each feeding, keeping the skin clean and dry around the tube, flushing the tube after each feeding, and changing the dressing every 24 hours or as needed until the site is healed. Adding a feeding when there is too much residual from the last feeding may cause regurgitation and aspiration.

UPPER GASTROINTESTINAL DISORDERS

CANCER OF THE ORAL CAVITY

Etiology, Pathophysiology, and Signs and Symptoms

There will be an estimated 30,990 cases of oral cancer in the United States in 2007 (American Cancer Society, 2007). Although the specific cause is unknown, oral or throat cancer is curable if discovered early. Oral and pharyngeal cancer risks are cigarette smoking, use of smokeless tobacco, pipe smoking, and heavy alcohol use. The human papillomavirus is another risk factor. Leukoplakia, a precancerous lesion, may occur on the tongue or mucosa. Dental examinations should include inspection for this lesion. Sores or discolorations on the lips or in the mouth that do not heal within 2 weeks should be checked by a physician. Cell mutation occurs until an area of cells becomes neoplastic. A genetic factor is most likely present.

? ***Think Critically About . . .*** Smokeless tobacco is very popular among young men. What could be done to decrease the incidence of its use in your community?

Diagnosis and Treatment

Diagnosis is made by physical examination and biopsy. Oral cancer treatment varies depending on the structures involved. Radiation, chemotherapy, and surgery are treatment options. *Mandibulectomy* (removal of the mandible), *hemiglossectomy* (removal of half of the tongue), or *glossectomy* (removal of the tongue) with resection of other parts of the mouth may be necessary. If the cancer has spread to the cervical lymph nodes, radical or modified neck dissection is performed. This surgery involves wide excision of the primary tumor with removal of the regional lymph nodes, the deep cervical lymph nodes, and lymph channels. A tracheostomy accompanies these procedures to protect the airway (see Chapter 13). A drain is placed to prevent fluid accumulation. Tube feedings are used as long as swallowing is difficult.

Nursing Management

Postoperative care includes close monitoring of respiratory status, airway, and oxygenation. Cold packs and elevation of the head are used to prevent excessive swelling in the neck that might compress the airway, circulation, and nerves. Aseptic wound care and tracheostomy care are provided. Psychological care is very important with these surgeries. The threat of death from cancer, and the disfigurement from the surgery, have a huge impact on the patient's body image and well-being. Nutritional support is an ongoing concern and is very important in the healing process. Many of these patients are malnourished before surgery. See Chapter 8 for the specific care of the cancer patient undergoing radiation and/or chemotherapy.

CANCER OF THE ESOPHAGUS

Etiology and Pathophysiology

Although the cause of esophageal cancer is unknown, it is associated with alcohol ingestion or the use of tobacco (Health Promotion Points 28–2). The cancer is usually well advanced when discovered. It is the second most common cancer in China, but is seen less in

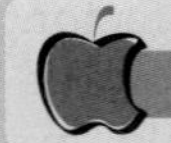

Health Promotion Points 28–2

Cigarettes and Esophageal Cancer

Cigarette smoking is a major cause of esophageal cancer in the United States. When combined with heavy alcohol consumption, the risk for esophageal cancer greatly increases. Both substances are irritants to the mucosa of the esophagus. Cigarettes and smokeless tobacco are responsible for 12,300 deaths from esophageal cancer annually (American Cancer Society, 2007).

North America. The tumor is either adenocarcinoma or squamous cell cancer.

Gastroesophageal reflux disease (GERD) is a cause of Barrett's esophagus, which is a precancerous condition (Stoltey et al., 2007). The cellular changes caused by irritation of the stomach fluids may eventually become malignant.

Signs, Symptoms, and Diagnosis

Signs and symptoms may include progressive dysphagia, a feeling of fullness in the throat, regurgitation of foods, or foul breath. At first the dysphagia only occurs with meat, but then with soft foods and eventually even with liquids. Pain occurs late in the disease and is substernal, epigastric, or in the back and occurs with swallowing. Weight loss is typical.

Barium swallow with fluoroscopy may show a narrowed esophagus. Definitive diagnosis is by esophagogastroduodenoscopy (EGD) and biopsy.

Treatment

Care of the patient with Barrett's esophagus is focused on encouraging measures to prevent GERD and on regular checkups. Patients should be encouraged not to use tobacco products and not to indulge in heavy alcohol use.

Think Critically About . . . If a patient who smokes is awaiting surgery for esophageal cancer, is it appropriate to prevent her from smoking?

Surgery, radiation, and chemotherapy in various combinations are used in treatment. Surgical procedures may include replacement of part of the esophagus with a section of colon, or with a Dacron tube insert. Only part of the esophagus may be removed with anastomosis of the remaining portion to the stomach. Sometimes an esophagoenterostomy is performed. This procedure involves removal of a portion of the esophagus with anastomosis of a segment of the colon. There is a poor prognosis because the disease is usually well advanced when discovered. Surgery may be thoracic or both thoracic and abdominal.

Nursing Management

Postoperative care is the same as for any patient having thoracic or abdominal surgery. Maintaining a patent airway is the top priority. Nutrition is supplied by parenteral fluids initially. When bowel sounds return, small amounts of water are given orally every hour. Gradual progression to small, frequent, bland meals is the next step. The patient should be upright when eating to prevent regurgitation. Monitor for leakage of the feeding into the mediastinum. Pain, increased temperature, and dyspnea indicate leakage. Intolerance of food is evidenced by vomiting and abdominal distention. The patient may need a feeding tube for several weeks or a gastrostomy tube to sustain nutrition.

HIATAL HERNIA (DIAPHRAGMATIC HERNIA)

Etiology and Pathophysiology

Loss of muscle strength and tone, factors that cause increased intra-abdominal pressure (such as obesity or multiple pregnancies), and congenital defects contribute to the formation of a hiatal hernia.

Hiatal hernia is the result of a defect in the wall of the diaphragm where the esophagus passes through. A hiatal hernia is formed by the protrusion of part of the stomach or the lower part of the esophagus up into the thoracic cavity; it is found in 50% of patients over the age of 50. More women than men are affected.

Signs and Symptoms

Signs and symptoms include indigestion, belching, and substernal or epigastric pain or feelings of pressure after eating caused by reflux of gastric fluid into the esophagus. The symptoms are more severe when the patient lies down. The problem is diagnosed by an upper GI series.

Treatment

Treatment includes weight reduction, avoidance of tight-fitting clothes around the abdomen, administration of antacids and histamine (H_2)-receptor antagonists, and elevation of the head of the bed on 6- to 8-inch blocks. If esophagitis is present, proton pump inhibitors are used. The patient is instructed not to eat within several hours of going to bed. Intake of alcohol, chocolate, caffeine, and fatty food is limited, and smoking should be avoided. Ingestion of fats relaxes the sphincter, allowing reflux.

Occasionally a patient with reflux esophagitis, which is caused by the hernia, may bleed extensively. If bleeding or discomfort cannot be controlled, surgical correction of the hernia is required.

Nursing Management

Nursing care is directed at reinforcing the teaching of ways to prevent pain and reflux. Encourage weight reduction if weight is above normal. Remind the patient to stay upright for 2 hours after eating and not to eat for 3 hours before bedtime (Fujiwara et al., 2005).

Lifting and moving heavy items are to be avoided. If the head of the bed cannot be raised, a wedge pillow should be used to elevate the upper body. This position helps prevent reflux and assists gravity in maintaining the stomach in the abdominal cavity. Prescribed H_2 or proton pump inhibitors should be taken at bedtime to prevent reflux and damage from acid entering the esophagus. The patient should avoid foods that cause bloating, which increases abdominal pressure. Increased abdominal pressure may push the stomach upward through the diaphragmatic defect.

GASTROESOPHAGEAL REFLUX DISEASE

Etiology and Pathophysiology

GERD is a syndrome, not a disease. Ninety percent of patients with GERD have a hiatal hernia. GERD occurs equally in men and women. It is caused by transient relaxation of the lower esophageal sphincter. The relaxation allows fluids or food to reflux into the esophagus from the stomach. Delayed stomach emptying is another factor. Certain foods and medications contribute to this mechanical problem. Being overweight is common among patients with GERD. GERD may contribute to bronchoconstriction and asthma symptoms due to irritation of the upper airway by gastric secretions. About 75% of patients with asthma have GERD (Patti et al., 2005).

Signs and Symptoms

Heartburn (**dyspepsia**) and reflux are the most common symptoms of GERD. Other symptoms may include chest pain, coughing, dysphagia, belching, flatulence, and bloating after eating. Some patients do not experience symptoms. In those who do, the symptoms are aggravated by lying down.

Diagnosis

The disorder is diagnosed by EGD and sometimes barium esophagram. Occasionally other tests such as an esophageal manometry or ambulatory 24-hour pH monitoring, or radionuclide measurement of gastric emptying, are performed. Esophageal manometry measures pressures in the esophagus; they will be increased during episodes of reflux. For 24-hour pH monitoring, a tiny tube with a transducer is introduced into the esophagus to take measurements of the esophageal pH.

Treatment and Nursing Management

Diet therapy, lifestyle changes, drug therapy, and education are the mainstays of GERD treatment. The diet should exclude foods that cause sphincter relaxation (Patient Teaching 28–1). Drug therapy may include antacids, H_2-receptor antagonists, proton pump inhibitors (Safety Alert 28–1), and prokinetic drugs. Table 28–2 provides information about these drugs.

Check for drug interactions with other drugs the patient is taking. Verify that the patient can afford the drugs prescribed as some are very expensive.

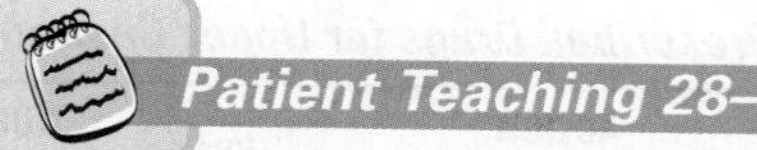

Patient Teaching 28–1

Measures to Decrease the Symptoms of GERD

Teach the patient to:

DIETARY ALTERATIONS

- Avoid any food in the diet that increases gastric acid and causes pain.
- Avoid high-fat and spicy foods, including garlic.
- Do not eat a large meal; rather eat 4 to 6 small meals a day.
- Eat slowly and chew food thoroughly, and avoid using a straw for liquids to decrease belching and reflux.
- Avoid carbonated beverages as they increase bloating.
- Eliminate or limit alcohol, tomato-based products, caffeine, citrus juice, raw onions, chocolate, peppermint, and spearmint from the diet. These foods either relax the esophageal sphincter or increase acid production.

LIFESTYLE ALTERATIONS

- Wait 2 to 3 hours after eating before lying down.
- Do not wear clothes that constrict around the middle of the body.
- If overweight, lose the extra pounds; a 10% weight loss can decrease symptoms considerably.
- Sleep with the head of the bed elevated 4 to 6 inches with blocks or a foam bolster pillow.
- Take medications as directed in relationship to meals and bedtime.
- Stop smoking as it may stimulate gastric acid secretion.
- Participate in regular stress-reducing activities such as exercise, meditation, deep breathing, and laughter.

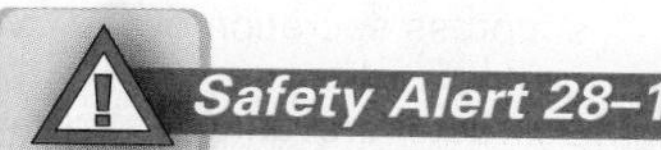

Safety Alert 28–1

Proton Pump Inhibitors and Cardiac Problems

The FDA has issued a warning that long-term use of the proton pump inhibitors esomeprazole (Nexium) or omeprazole (Prilosec) may increase the risk of heart problems. Patients taking these drugs should consult their health care provider.

If the above therapies do not control the problem, endoscopic noninvasive therapies often are effective. Laparoscopic surgical **fundoplication**, wherein the fundus of the stomach is wrapped around the esophagus to create a new valve junction (Figure 28–2), is effective in 92% of patients (Patti et al., 2005). This is the same procedure used to correct a hiatal hernia.

? *Think Critically About . . .* Many patients with GERD and hiatal hernia do not really modify their diet and lifestyle over the long term. They tend to rely on the medications to decrease their symptoms. This adds to the cost of health care in our country and is expensive for the patient. What measures could you use to show patients that lifestyle changes may control symptoms without medication?

Table 28–2 **Commonly Prescribed Drugs for Upper Gastrointestinal Disorders**

CLASSIFICATION*	ACTION	NURSING IMPLICATIONS	PATIENT TEACHING
ANTACIDS			
Gelusil, Maalox, Mylanta-II, Riopan, Di-Gel, etc. There are four antacid families consisting of compounds of aluminum, magnesium, calcium, and sodium.	Neutralize stomach acid	Aluminum hydroxide compounds promote constipation, whereas magnesium hydroxide compounds promote diarrhea. Sodium compounds may adversely affect hypertension and heart failure. All antacids may adversely affect the dissolution and absorption of other drugs. One hour should be allowed between antacid administration and administration of another drug. Magnesium compounds are used cautiously in patients with renal insufficiency.	Antacids for treatment of peptic ulcer should be taken seven times a day: 1 hr and 3 hr after meals, and at bedtime. Separate from other drug administration by 2 hr. Shake liquid preparations well before pouring from container. Chew antacid tablets thoroughly, and follow with a glass of water or milk. Report problems of constipation or diarrhea to the physician. Take even after pain has disappeared; consult physician.
HISTAMINE (H_2)-RECEPTOR ANTAGONIST			
Cimetidine (Tagamet) Famotidine (Pepcid) Nizatidine (Axid) Ranitidine (Zantac)	Suppress acid secretion by blocking H_2 receptors on parietal cells	Cimetidine may interact with many other drugs; check drug interactions for other drugs patient is receiving. Cimetidine may cause confusion and other CNS effects. Separate administration of these drugs and antacids by 1 hr. Monitor for decreased abdominal pain and ulcer symptoms.	These drugs should be taken with meals and at bedtime. Once-a-day dose should be taken at bedtime. Advise patient to avoid cigarettes, aspirin, and other NSAIDs. Advise to avoid alcohol or only consume it in moderation and only in conjunction with food. Advise to utilize stress reduction techniques.
PROTON PUMP INHIBITORS			
Omeprazole (Prilosec) Lansoprazole (Prevacid)	Proton pump inhibitors suppress secretion of gastric acid	May cause headache, nausea, vomiting, or diarrhea. Use is preferably limited to 4–8 wk.	Follow regimen of diet and stress reduction for ulcer healing.
Misoprostol (Cytotec)	Misoprostol prevents gastric ulcers caused by long-term therapy with NSAIDs	May cause diarrhea or abdominal pain. Not safe during pregnancy.	
Rabeprazole (Aciphex)		Do not crush delayed-release tablets.	This is a slow-release preparation that acts throughout the day. Teach patient to wear sunscreen as drug may cause sun sensitivity.
Pantoprazole (Protonix)		Do not crush tablets.	Another slow-release preparation.
Esomeprazole (Nexium)		Do not administer with digoxin, rabeprazole, or iron salts.	May affect absorption of digoxin, rabeprazole, and iron salts.
MISCELLANEOUS MEDICATIONS			
Sucralfate (Carafate)	Sucralfate provides protective coating barrier over ulcer crater	Monitor for constipation.	Take only as directed. Wait 30 min before taking any other drug.

Key: *CBC,* complete blood count; *CNS,* central nervous system; *GI,* gastrointestinal; *NSAIDs,* nonsteroidal anti-inflammatory drugs.
*Names of generic drugs are listed first, followed by the brand names of drugs in parentheses.

Table 28–2 Commonly Prescribed Drugs for Upper Gastrointestinal Disorders—cont'd

CLASSIFICATION	ACTION	NURSING IMPLICATIONS	PATIENT TEACHING
ANTIMICROBIALS			
Clarithromycin (Biaxin)	Suppresses protein synthesis in bacteria Used to kill *Helicobacter pylori*	Assess for drug allergy. Report hematuria or oliguria. Administer q 12 hr to maintain serum levels. Do not crush tablets. Monitor for diarrhea, abdominal pain, or signs of jaundice.	May cause diarrhea, anorexia, or nausea. Must be taken at regular intervals to be effective. Take the entire prescription. Taking acidophilus between doses may alleviate diarrhea. Increase fluid intake if diarrhea occurs.
Amoxicillin (Amoxil)	Causes cell wall of bacteria to swell and burst, preventing replication	Assess for drug sensitivity. Assess for side effects. Monitor renal function. Monitor for blood in stool and abdominal pain.	Take on an empty stomach with a full glass of water. Take at regular intervals around the clock to sustain blood levels. Take entire prescription.
Tetracycline	Bacteriostatic Inhibits protein synthesis in microorganisms	Assess for drug sensitivity. Monitor CBC, liver, and kidney functions. Increases effect of warfarin and digoxin. Decreases effect of penicillin and oral contraceptives.	Do not take with dairy products or antacids; separate by 2 hr. Avoid sun exposure. Avoid using Clinistix, Diastix, or Tes-Tape for diabetic urine testing.
Metronidazole (Flagyl)	Kills amebas and *Trichomonas;* degrades DNA in organism	Do not give during second and third trimesters of pregnancy. Increases action of anticoagulants. Decreases action of phenobarbital and phenytoin. May cause toxicity if administered with cimetidine or lithium. Patient should have vision examination before and after therapy. Monitor for neurotoxicity. Discontinue if fever, chills, rash, or itching occurs.	Do not drink alcohol during or for 48 hr after therapy has ended. May cause severe vomiting and prostration. Urine may turn dark brown. Notify physician of numbness or tingling. Dizziness may occur; avoid hazardous activities. May cause dry mouth; chew sugarless gum or sip water frequently.
ANTISPASMODICS			
Dicyclomine hydrochloride (Bentyl, Antispas) Propantheline bromide (Pro-Banthine)	Block acetylcholine, thereby decreasing smooth-muscle spasm and GI motility and inhibiting gastric acid secretion	These drugs interact with many other drugs; check each drug patient is taking for interactions. Most of theses drugs are contraindicated in glaucoma, prostatic hypertrophy, myasthenia gravis, and other conditions; consult information on each drug individually. May predispose to drug-induced heat stroke. Monitor vital signs and urine output carefully.	Take 30–60 min before meal. Patient can suck on hard candy to relieve mouth dryness unless contraindicated. Drink 2500–3000 mL of fluid to prevent constipation. Avoid driving and hazardous activities if drug causes dizziness, sleepiness, or blurred vision. Report rash or skin eruption to physician.
Metoclopramide (Reglan)	Hastens gastric emptying and relaxes pyloric and duodenal segments of GI tract	Assess for neurologic or psychotropic side effects such as restlessness, anxiety, ataxia, or hallucinations. Not for long-term use.	Take before meals.

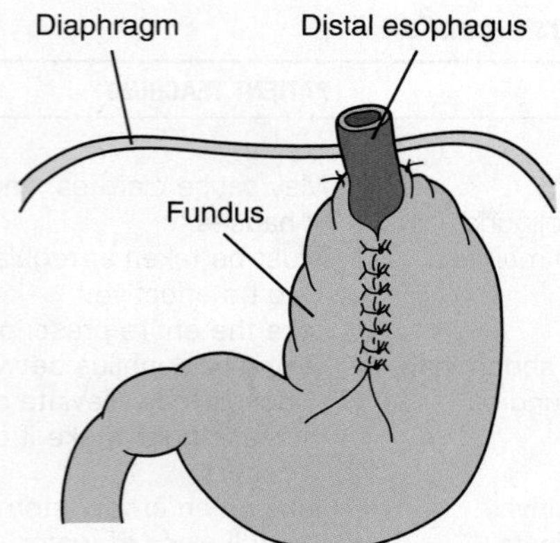

FIGURE 28–2 Nissen fundoplication surgery for hiatal hernia or to treat gastroesophageal reflux disease.

Complications

Continuous reflux into the esophagus of stomach contents containing hydrochloric acid, pepsin, and other enzymes causes irritation. Constant irritation may cause cellular changes such as those in Barrett's esophagus. Barrett's esophagus is a condition in which there are areas of precancerous lesions in the esophageal tissue. Five percent of patients with Barrett's esophagus 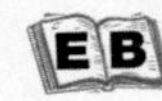 eventually develop esophageal cancer (Patti et al., 2005). Reflux is also a risk factor for aspiration of stomach contents and pneumonitis. Acid reflux into the mouth over time may cause dental caries.

GASTROENTERITIS

Gastroenteritis is inflammation of the stomach and small intestine. It is caused by intake of food or water contaminated with a virus, a pathogenic bacteria, or parasites. The Norwalk virus is a common cause, as are *Giardia* and *Shigella.* Signs and symptoms include vomiting, diarrhea, abdominal cramping, and distention. Fever, elevated white blood cell count, and blood or mucus in the stool may occur. In healthy adults the disorder is self-limiting and does not require hospitalization. The young child, the elderly, and the chronically ill may need intravenous (IV) therapy to take in enough fluid to compensate for the fluid loss.

The patient should be kept NPO until vomiting has stopped. When tolerated, fluids containing glucose and electrolytes should be started (Pedialyte, Gatorade) (Nutritional Therapies 28–1). If diarrhea continues beyond 3 or 4 days, stool studies for the causative organism should be performed. Therapy to eradicate the causative agent can then be started. Rest is important during the course of the vomiting and diarrhea. After 24 to 48 hours, medication may be prescribed for the vomiting, abdominal cramping, and diarrhea.

GASTRITIS

Etiology

The main cause of gastritis is ***Helicobacter pylori*** bacteria. Other contributors to acute gastritis are drinking excessive amounts of alcohol, infection from eating

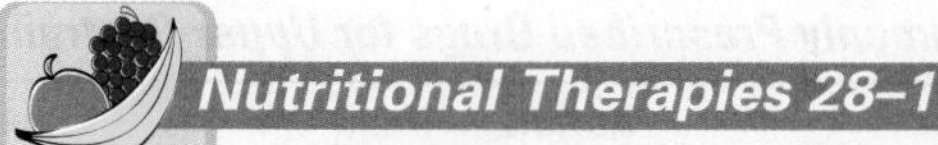

Dietary Guidelines for the Patient with Vomiting

- Stick to a liquid diet for 12 to 24 hours. Avoid milk, ice cream, pudding, cheese, yogurt, citrus juice, and cream soups. Frequent small amounts of clear liquids are best.
- Foods allowed on the liquid diet are electrolyte solutions, carbonated beverages, bouillon, unflavored gelatin, apple juice, peach or pear juice, plain hard candy, sugar, honey, sugar substitutes, and frozen Popsicles.

When nausea and vomiting stop:

- Add some of the following foods for the next 12 to 24 hours: soda crackers, toast and jelly without butter, tea, rice, pretzels, bananas, applesauce, cooked cream of wheat or cream of rice, and fruit or vegetable juice (BRATT diet: banana, rice, applesauce, tea, and toast).
- If above diet is tolerated without further symptoms, add the following foods for the next 12 to 24 hours: potatoes (not fried), soups, soft eggs, custards, puddings, white turkey meat or white chicken meat, and cottage cheese.
- If no further symptoms occur, resume a regular diet but avoid highly seasoned foods, greasy or fried foods, heavy fatty foods, excessively hot or cold foods, raw vegetables, coffee, colas, and other milk products. Avoid those foods for 1 week after symptoms have stopped.

contaminated food, and ingestion of drugs, such as aspirin, ibuprofen, corticosteroids, or nonsteroidal anti-inflammatory agents (NSAIDs).

Pathophysiology

Gastritis is an inflammation of the mucous membrane lining the stomach rather than a disease. Gastritis may be acute or chronic in nature. *Atrophic* gastritis involves all layers of the stomach. It is seen in association with gastric ulcer and malignancies of the stomach. Gastritis associated with uremia is common in the patient with kidney failure. The excessive urea that builds up from the kidney failure causes gastric irritation. Untreated chronic gastritis may progress to ulcer formation and upper GI hemorrhage.

Signs, Symptoms, and Diagnosis

In both acute and chronic gastritis, the main symptoms are anorexia, nausea, vomiting, pain and tenderness in the stomach region, hiccoughs, and sometimes diarrhea. The patient with chronic gastritis may have no symptoms and may suddenly experience massive hemorrhage from the stomach. Diagnosis is by history, physical examination, and endoscopic examination.

Treatment and Nursing Management

Acute gastritis usually is of very short duration. Treatment consists of withholding all foods by mouth and administering drugs that slow down the peristaltic action of the GI tract. If severe dehydration or nausea and vomiting occur, fluids may be given IV.

Elder Care Points

If an elderly patient experiences vomiting and is unable to retain fluids for 12 hours, a trip to the emergency department for intravenous fluids may be needed to prevent severe dehydration.

The patient with gastritis must be watched closely for signs of fluid and electrolyte imbalance.

Chronic gastritis is not as easily treated as acute gastritis. Diet therapy is of primary importance in chronic gastritis because the patient frequently admits to indiscretion in her dietary and drinking habits and finds it difficult to change. The diet for these patients is devoid of spicy or acidic foods. Use tact and patience in encouraging the patient to follow the prescribed diet faithfully.

Treatment consists of antispasmodics to decrease the pain of stomach spasms, antacids, an H_2-receptor antagonist such as ranitidine to decrease acid secretions and change pH, or a proton pump inhibitor to decrease the secretion of hydrochloric acid. If *H. pylori* is present, antibiotic therapy is administered.

PEPTIC ULCER

Etiology

It was thought that the usual cause of peptic ulcer was the presence of too much gastric juice in relation to the secretion of mucus and other substances that neutralize gastric acid. Normally, all areas exposed to the hydrochloric acid and pepsin in gastric juices have an ample supply of mucous glands that secrete a protective alkaline mucus. However, the chief cause is really the bacterium *Helicobacter pylori.*

Theories about genetic and environmental causes of peptic ulcer abound. Both gastric and duodenal ulcers tend to occur in families. Relatives of people with gastric or duodenal ulcers have three times the expected rate for ulcer formation. A genetic link has been found.

Neither hot spicy foods nor caffeine has been proven to be a risk factor for ulcers, but these substances make symptoms worse in many people. Gastric ulcers do occur in those who are poorly nourished because of poverty or because of poor eating habits. Despite the stereotype of the hard-driving executive suffering from an ulcer and gulping antacid tablets, there is a greater incidence of ulcers in blue-collar workers and in laborers.

Stress does have a bearing on the progression of peptic ulcer, however. Tension, anxiety, and prolonged stress do alter gastric function. Prolonged physiologic stress produces what is known as a *physiologic stress ulcer,* which is believed to be the result of unrelieved stimulation of the vagus nerves and decreased perfusion to the stomach. A stress ulcer is pathologically

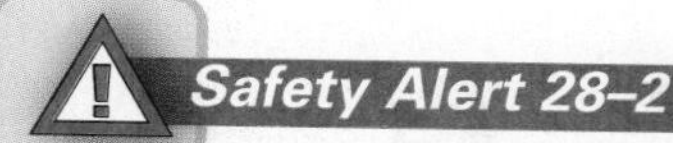

Safety Alert 28–2

Monitor NSAID Use and Acetaminophen

There is an increased risk of peptic ulcer in individuals taking regular OTC doses of NSAIDs such as ibuprofen and naproxen. When combined with more than 2 g of acetaminophen per day, the risk increases. Daily doses of acetaminophen over 2 g along with other NSAIDs increase the risk of upper GI bleeding by twofold. Encourage patients who regularly take an NSAID to check the labels on pain, sleep, and cold medications to monitor acetaminophen intake (Neafsey, 2004).

Key: *GI,* gastrointestinal; *NSAIDs,* nonsteroidal anti-inflammatory drugs; *OTC,* over-the-counter.

and clinically different from a chronic peptic ulcer. It is more acute and more likely to produce hemorrhage. Perforation occurs occasionally, and pain is rare. Stress ulcers are a hazard for patients who are severely ill and in intensive care units for prolonged periods. Patients with multiple trauma, burns, or multiple system disorders are subject to physiologic stress ulcers. Such patients often receive medication to prevent ulcer formation.

Drug-induced ulcers are most often caused by aspirin, NSAIDs, alcohol, and glucocorticoids (Yuan et al., 2006) (Safety Alert 28–2). Cigarette smoking is known to be a causative factor in peptic ulcer, particularly if over one-half pack a day is smoked (Yuan et al., 2006).

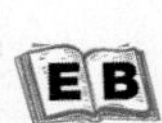

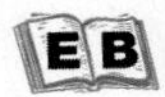

Pathophysiology

Ulcers develop when the mucosa cannot protect itself from corrosive substances, such as gastric acid, pepsinogen, alcohol, bile salts, and irritating food substances. Normally, the upper GI mucosa can resist corrosion. When gastric substances are out of balance, problems arise. A peptic ulcer is an ulceration with loss of tissue of the upper GI tract. The term includes both duodenal and gastric ulcers (Figure 28–3). The most common site for development of a peptic ulcer is in the first few centimeters of the duodenum, just beyond the pyloric muscle. About 25 million people in the United States have experienced a peptic ulcer. *Helicobacter pylori* is rich in an enzyme that may cause corrosion of the upper GI mucosa by damaging its mucous coating, making it more susceptible to damage from gastric acid and pepsinogen.

Duodenal ulcers and some prepyloric ulcers are associated with an increased amount or hyperacidity of the gastric juices, and are 70% associated with *H. pylori.* Gastric ulcers, in contrast, are characterized by normal or abnormally low levels of hydrochloric acid, but 90% have been associated with *H. pylori. Helicobacter pylori* is implicated in the development of gastric cancer as well (Yuan et al., 2006).

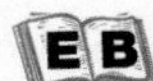

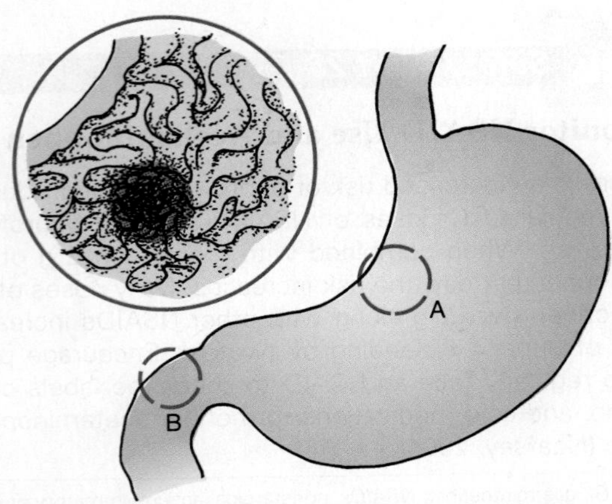

FIGURE 28–3 Peptic ulcers: **A,** Gastric; **B,** duodenal.

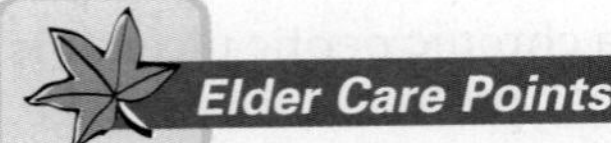

Elder Care Points

By age 60, approximately 60% of the population in the United States is infected with the *H. pylori* bacterium. However, most people never have symptoms of gastritis, and few develop ulcers.

Signs and Symptoms

Subjective symptoms of uncomplicated ulcer include epigastric pain that might be described as burning, gnawing, cramping, or aching and usually comes in waves that last several minutes. The daily pattern of pain is associated with the secretion of gastric juices in relation to the presence of food, which can act as a buffer. **For example, with a gastric ulcer the pain is diminished in the morning when secretion is low and after meals when food is in the stomach, and is most severe before meals and at bedtime.** Discomfort often appears for several days or weeks and then subsides, only to reappear weeks or months later. Other subjective symptoms include nausea, loss of appetite, and sometimes weight loss. Spontaneous vomiting accompanies duodenal ulcer more often than gastric ulcer.

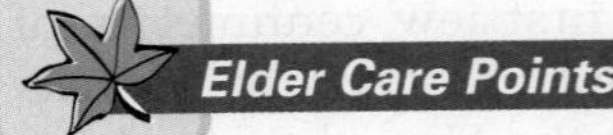

Elder Care Points

The elderly patient may not display the typical symptoms. Pain is less typical and may be poorly localized, or it may be described as lower chest discomfort or left-sided pain. Anorexia, weight loss, general weakness, anemia, nausea, and painless vomiting may occur; peptic ulcer is difficult to diagnose in this population.

Gastrointestinal Bleeding. Subjective signs of acute GI bleeding include complaints of weakness and feeling faint, nausea and vomiting, restlessness, thirst, and mental confusion. Objective signs include the presence of bright red blood in emesis. The appearance of the blood in emesis is similar to coffee grounds and is termed **hematemesis.** Diarrhea, decreased blood pressure, rapid pulse, and other signs of hypovolemic shock may occur. Blood in the GI tract acts as a cathartic and causes diarrhea. If bleeding from the upper GI system is profuse, maroon or bright red blood may appear in stool because of the rapid transit of the blood through the intestinal tract. Black stools almost always indicate the presence of digested blood, which means that the source of bleeding is in the upper GI tract.

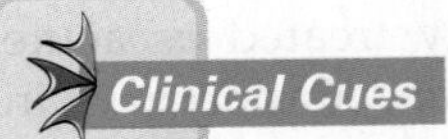

Clinical Cues

Remember that iron salts can cause the stool to be black and that the ingestion of beets can cause the stool to be bright red.

Estimates of blood loss from the GI tract are based in part on blood pressure readings and pulse rates. Blood pressure and pulse rate should be monitored every 15 to 30 minutes when there is evidence of extensive GI hemorrhage. Central venous pressure readings also are helpful in determining the amount of blood lost, especially in hypertensive patients, whose blood pressure may not reflect hypovolemia.

Changes in the vital signs that signal hypovolemic shock do not appear until after the patient has lost 20% or more of the blood volume.

Additional data useful in determining the status of patients with GI bleeding include hematocrit and hemoglobin levels. These levels can be normal or even slightly elevated at the beginning of a bleeding episode. It takes 4 to 6 hours for the body to shift fluids from other compartments to the intravascular compartment. The shift of fluid changes the ratio of formed elements to fluids in the blood. The white cell count may be elevated in massive GI bleeding, probably because of the body's response to injury or hypovolemia. An elevated level of blood urea nitrogen can indicate digestion of large amounts of blood.

Diagnosis

The technique most commonly used to diagnose peptic ulcer is an upper GI series. Endoscopy can help locate the site of ulceration and bleeding and differentiate between benign and malignant ulcerations and between esophageal ulcer and a *diverticulum* (pouching of the intestinal wall).

A gastric analysis to measure the level of hydrochloric acid in gastric juices may be helpful in some cases, but there is a good bit of variation in gastric acid levels among patients with peptic ulcer. Serum tests for *H. pylori* detect antibodies indicating active or recent infection. The urea breath test involves the measurement of gas released in the breath following ingestion of a radiolabeled urea isotope. When *H. pylori* is present, the test is positive.

Think Critically About . . . How do the symptoms of a gastric ulcer differ from those of a hiatal hernia?

When the patient is experiencing extensive GI bleeding, the patient's condition is stabilized and diagnostic procedures are done to locate the source of bleeding. These procedures include endoscopic examination of the esophagus, stomach, and small intestine. Barium studies may be ordered.

Treatment

Peptic ulcer is treated conservatively at first to avoid surgery. Medications to relieve pain from local irritation of the intestinal mucosa include the antacids, which reduce the pain of ulcer by neutralizing gastric acid. Examples of antacids include aluminum hydroxide (Amphojel), aluminum hydroxide–magnesium trisilicate (Gaviscon), and aluminum hydroxide–magnesium hydroxide–simethicone (Gelusil). Antacids effective for antiflatulence include aluminum hydroxide–magnesium hydroxide–simethicone (Gelusil-M, Maalox Plus, and Mylanta).

Treatment of gastric bleeding is begun by inserting a large-bore NG tube and using a normal saline lavage to monitor the quantity of bleeding and evacuate the blood, clots, and stomach contents. This allows the stomach to constrict, halting the blood flow. Antacids are given via the tube to neutralize pepsin and help stop the bleeding. An H_2-receptor antagonist, such as cimetidine (Tagamet), ranitidine (Zantac), or famotidine (Pepcid), is given IV to decrease stomach acid secretion. Proton pump inhibitors such as lansoprazole (Prevacid) or esomeprazole (Nexium) are used to stop acid secretion (see Table 28–1). Eighty percent of GI bleeding will stop with these treatments.

If there is major blood loss, transfusions of whole blood, packed cells, or fresh frozen plasma may be necessary. Normal saline, Plasmanate (plasma protein fraction), and Ringer's solution may be administered until blood is available. Maintenance of fluid balance is of extreme importance. Intake and output must be measured and recorded accurately. Oxygen therapy is started to maximize tissue oxygenation.

If the presence of *H. pylori* has been determined, treatment consists of the administration of clarithromycin (Biaxin) plus another antibiotic, an H_2 inhibitor, and a proton pump inhibitor. Sucralfate (Carafate) tablets may be used for short-term (up to 8 weeks) treatment of duodenal ulcer (Safety Alert 28–3). It has negligible acid-neutralizing capacity. The action of this drug is local. Its benefits probably derive from its adherence to the ulcer site, providing protection from further damage by gastric juices. Misoprostol (Cytotec) is used to replace gastric prostaglandins depleted by NSAID therapy. Misoprostol helps prevent ulcer formation caused by NSAIDs. Sedatives are sometimes prescribed for the peptic ulcer patient to help reduce anxiety and relieve tension.

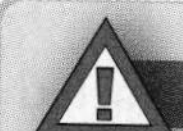

Safety Alert 28–3

Proton Pump Inhibitor Drug Interactions

Because proton pump inhibitors slow the liver's ability to metabolize and clear some drugs from the bloodstream, they should be used with caution in patients taking diazepam (Valium), phenytoin (Dilantin), and warfarin (Coumadin). Patients taking a proton pump inhibitor along with any of these three drugs should be watched closely for signs of toxicity.

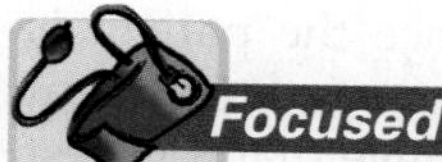

Focused Assessment 28–1

Data Collection for Peptic Ulcer

Assess the following areas:

HISTORY
- Pain: characteristics, what affects pain, what relieves it; when pain began
- Nausea or vomiting; presence of "coffee-ground" emesis
- Dark "tarry" stool, or maroon-colored stool
- Anorexia, weight loss

PHYSICAL ASSESSMENT
- Vital signs and changes from baseline
- Presence of restlessness, confusion, or thirst
- Skin tone
- Appearance of emesis
- Stool color, characteristics, frequency
- Abdominal tenderness, rigidity, guarding, bloating
- Bowel sounds

LABORATORY DATA
- Complete blood count (CBC)
- Blood urea nitrogen (BUN)

NURSING MANAGEMENT

Assessment (Data Collection)

Gather data regarding signs and symptoms using the guide in Focused Assessment 28–1.

Nursing Diagnosis

Common nursing diagnoses for the patient with a peptic ulcer are found in Table 27–2. Specific diagnoses might be:

- Pain related to interruption of the gastric or duodenal mucosa
- Risk for injury related to potential for perforation

If GI bleeding is present, nursing diagnoses would include:

- Deficient fluid volume related to loss of blood
- Risk for ineffective tissue perfusion related to GI bleeding

Planning

Expected outcomes are listed in Table 27–2. Expected outcomes for the previous nursing diagnoses might be:

- Pain will be controlled with medication before discharge.
- Patient will not experience ulcer perforation.
- Fluid volume will be restored prior to discharge.
- Patient will not experience ineffective tissue perfusion.

Implementation

Diet counseling is a top priority once the patient is stable. In the past, diet was a major part of treatment of ulcers. Today, most authorities believe that it is best to restrict only those foods that the patient identifies with the onset of symptoms. A suitable diet is established for the patient. Alcohol and caffeine should be excluded. It is generally agreed that the kind of food eaten by an ulcer patient is not as important as when the food is eaten. The patient is instructed to eat at frequent and regular intervals throughout the day, rather than in two or three large meals. Meals should not be skipped. The patient should try to keep some food in the stomach at all times.

The medication schedule should be reviewed and the purpose of each medication and its potential side effects discussed. Compliance is better if the patient thoroughly understands why each medication is important.

Nursing intervention for GI bleeding must include consideration for the patient's fear and anxiety. Many times these patients are afraid they are going to die. The sight of so much blood loss is frightening to the patient, to whom it usually appears more profuse than it actually is. Whatever procedures are used, the patient and family deserve an explanation and reassurance that everything is being done to control the hemorrhage.

During the time the patient is experiencing GI bleeding and **melena** (black, tarry stool with digested blood), the room must be kept as free of odor as possible. Melena stools cause considerable odor.

After the bleeding has apparently stopped and the patient's vital signs have stabilized, there must be continuous monitoring for signs of persistent or renewed bleeding. Blood pressure and pulse rate are measured regularly. Observe skin color, for diaphoresis or thirst, and for other signs of continued blood loss such as restlessness. Watch for impending hypovolemic shock. Measure intake and output and note the character of vomitus, aspirated gastric fluid, and stools. Measure and record the patient's daily weight.

Before a peptic ulcer can be successfully controlled, the patient must understand how and why the ulcer developed in the first place. Once the predisposing factors are understood, it is easier to avoid them. Unless the patient can cooperate fully, there is a strong possibility that ulcers will develop again despite medical or even surgical treatment (Patient Teaching 28–2). Use tact and patience in encouraging the patient to follow the prescribed diet faithfully. Nursing interventions for selected problems in a patient with a bleeding peptic ulcer are summarized in Nursing Care Plan 28–1.

Evaluation

Data are gathered to determine whether the expected outcomes are being met. If they are not, then the plan of care must be revised.

Complications

The three major complications of peptic ulcer are **hemorrhage, perforation, and obstruction.** Hemorrhage occurs when the ulcer erodes vessels, causing bleeding into the stomach. Signs of hemorrhage include the vomiting of blood. If the hemorrhage is unchecked, hypovolemic shock may occur. Perforation is erosion of the ulcer through all walls of the intestine. A spilling

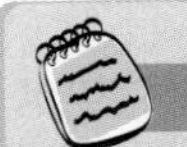

Patient Teaching 28–2

Healing a Peptic Ulcer

Teach the patient to:

- Regulate the types of foods eaten and the schedule for eating. Mealtimes should be unhurried, relaxed, and spaced at regular intervals.
- Control stress and develop healthy coping techniques; avoid extremely stressful situations; fit regular relaxation into the lifestyle.
- Drink a lot of water. Because water dilutes the gastric juices and thereby makes them less corrosive, develop the habit of taking several swallows of water at least every hour during the day.
- Refrain from smoking. If unable to discontinue smoking altogether, moderate smoking habits.
- Cooperate with the physician and remain under medical supervision for as long as the physician deems advisable. Report regularly for periodic assessment to determine progress.
- Report side effects of antacids should they occur, such as constipation or diarrhea, flatulence, and signs of edema resulting from sodium retention.
- Check with the pharmacist about possible drug interactions among all the drugs being taken.
- Unless otherwise ordered, take antacids 1 hour after meals. If antacid tablets are used in preference to liquid preparations, the tablet must be chewed thoroughly and followed by a full glass of water.
- Avoid aspirin and NSAIDs. There are more than 300 prescription and nonprescription medications that contain aspirin. The patient should develop the habit of reading carefully the labels of any medication before taking it. Tell all health care professionals involved in care that aspirin is contraindicated.

Key: *NSAIDs*, nonsteroidal anti-inflammatory drugs.

of the contents of the GI tract into the peritoneal cavity ensues. It constitutes a surgical emergency because of the danger of hemorrhage and peritonitis.

Perforation is characterized by a sudden and severe pain in the upper abdomen that persists and increases in intensity and sometimes is referred to the shoulders. The abdomen is rigid and boardlike and extremely tender. In a short time the patient shows signs of shock. Obstruction occurs as a result of scarring and loss of musculature at the pylorus, narrowing the stomach outlet. It is manifested chiefly by persistent vomiting.

Surgical Treatment of Peptic Ulcer. Surgical treatment becomes necessary when a chronic ulcer fails to respond to medical treatment; when complications such as perforation, obstruction, or hemorrhage occur; or when malignancy is present.

In *pyloroplasty with truncal or proximal gastric vagotomy,* the pylorus, which has been narrowed by scarring, is widened. The branches of the vagus (Xth cranial) nerve that stimulate acid secretion in the stomach are selectively severed **(vagotomy)** so that the stomach does not receive impulses from the brain and therefore does not secrete hydrochloric acid. A vagotomy is often done at the same time a gastric resection is performed.

Subtotal gastrectomy (gastric resection) consists of removing a part of the stomach and then joining the remaining portion to the small intestine by anastomosis. **Anastomosis** is the joining of two hollow organs by suturing the open ends together so that they become one continuous tube. An *antrectomy,* in which the gastrin-producing portion of the stomach (the antrum) is removed, may be done in conjunction with a truncal

NURSING CARE PLAN 28–1

Care of the Patient with a Bleeding Peptic Ulcer

SCENARIO Mr. Lee is a 47-year-old long-distance truck driver admitted to the hospital with a tentative diagnosis of bleeding peptic ulcer. He has had recurrent bouts of epigastric pain that is more pronounced before meals and at bedtime. Mr. Lee states that he eats "whenever I can grab a bite." He eats mostly fried and spicy foods and he smokes two packs of cigarettes a day. He went to the physician because of fatigue and discomfort that seemed to be getting progressively worse in spite of antacid use. He also admits to having some vomiting episodes with blood in the secretions. Mr. Lee is the sole support of his wife and four children and is very concerned about the expense of hospitalization and the time away from work. He is scheduled for an endoscopic examination of the esophagus, stomach, and duodenum.

PROBLEM/NURSING DIAGNOSIS *Worried about costs of hospitalization*/Anxiety related to expenses, time off work, and worry about what is wrong with him.

Supporting assessment data *Subjective:* "I'm the only one working"; expresses worry over hospital expenses; worried about blood in vomitus. *Objective:* Scheduled for endoscopic examinations.

Goals/Expected Outcomes	Nursing Interventions	Selected Rationale	Evaluation
Patient will verbalize reduction in anxiety before discharge	Encourage verbalization of concerns and fears.	Verbalizing fears may decrease their intensity.	Verbalizing specific concerns and fears.
Patient will devise plan to cover hospital expenses so as to decrease anxiety	Ask for financial consultant collaboration regarding handling of hospital expenses.	A plan for meeting financial obligation will somewhat decrease anxiety.	Appointment with social worker to discuss financial situation.
Patient will verbalize understanding of diagnosis and treatment of his condition	Explain all diagnostic procedures and medications.	Decreases the fear of the unknown and lowers anxiety.	Endoscopic procedures and test for *H. pylori* explained; told purpose of each medication.
	Assess usual coping techniques and teach new ways to cope as necessary.	Establishes usual coping methods and provides data for other coping methods to be taught.	Uses smoking and television as relaxation.
	Reinforce wife's assurances that they can manage expenses at home.	Reinforcement of information helps patient remember.	Wife says he tends to be a "worry wart"; reinforced information about her ability to cope with expenses. Continue plan.
	Encourage relaxation techniques.	Relaxation techniques help decrease anxious feelings.	Taught relaxation exercise and encouraged to practice it.

Key: *ac,* before meals; *BP,* blood pressure; *CBC,* complete blood count; *GI,* gastrointestinal; *Hct,* hematocrit; *Hgb,* hemoglobin; *hs,* at bedtime; *pc,* after meals; *PO,* orally.

Continued

NURSING CARE PLAN 28–1

Care of the Patient with a Bleeding Peptic Ulcer—cont'd

PROBLEM/NURSING DIAGNOSIS *Abdominal pain and discomfort*/Pain related to irritation and possible ulceration of gastric mucosa.

Supporting assessment data *Subjective:* Recurrent bouts of epigastric pain more pronounced before meals. *Objective:* Blood-tinged vomitus and blood in stool (positive guaiac test).

Goals/Expected Outcomes	Nursing Interventions	Selected Rationale	Evaluation
Patient will verbalize relief of pain	Assess location and severity of pain q shift.	Provides data regarding condition and need for medication.	Pain is epigastric at 3/10; now occurring between meals.
Patient will verbalize ways to prevent gastric pain	Administer ordered antacids, antispasmodics, and H_2 inhibitors.	Medications neutralize stomach acid or decrease acid production.	Taking meds as ordered.
	Give caffeine-free diet.	Caffeine causes more stomach acid production.	No caffeine drinks; bland diet.
	Encourage him to quit smoking.	Smoking constricts blood vessels, decreasing perfusion to stomach. Decreased perfusion makes the stomach more susceptible to inflammation.	Encouraged him to quit smoking; said he would think about it. Provided community resource information for stopping smoking. Continue plan.
	Give frequent feedings to neutralize gastric acid.	Keeping food in the stomach helps neutralize acid.	Eating a snack every 2 hr between meals.
	Provide quiet, relaxed environment.		

PROBLEM/NURSING DIAGNOSIS *Vomiting episodes with blood*/Ineffective tissue perfusion related to loss of blood from gastric mucosa.

Supporting assessment data *Subjective:* States has experienced blood-streaked vomitus; history suggestive of peptic ulcer; increasing fatigue. *Objective:* Pale conjunctiva; epigastric tenderness, below-normal Hgb and Hct.

Goals/Expected Outcomes	Nursing Interventions	Selected Rationale	Evaluation
Patient will have no signs of intestinal blood loss by discharge	Monitor CBC count for evidence of continued bleeding.	CBC may indicate if bleeding is occurring.	Hgb 11.9 g/dL and Hct 32.
Hemoglobin and hematocrit will be within normal levels within 30 days	Assess vomitus for blood.	Blood in vomitus indicates bleeding is still occurring.	No vomitus this shift.
	Check stool for occult blood as ordered.	Blood in stool indicates GI bleeding.	Stool positive for occult blood × 2.
	Monitor vital signs and assess for continued or rapid blood loss as ordered.	Active bleeding will be reflected by vital signs.	Pulse 92 and BP 138/86.
	Teach about foods high in iron content to correct anemia.	Eating foods high in iron helps correct anemia.	Taught about foods high in iron.
	Administer iron supplements as ordered.	Iron supplementation helps correct anemia.	Iron supplement not ordered yet. Continue plan.

Mr. Lee's physician found a duodenal ulcer on endoscopic examination. He has prescribed sucralfate (Carafate), 1 g PO qid 1 hr ac and hs; ranitidine (Zantac), 300 mg hs; and Mylanta II, 30 mL 30 min pc, in hopes of healing the ulcer and preventing surgery.

PROBLEM/NURSING DIAGNOSIS *No knowledge of risk factors for peptic ulcer*/Deficient knowledge related to factors that contribute to peptic ulcer and information about medications.

Supporting assessment data *Subjective:* States was unaware that cigarette smoking contributed to ulcers; never has heard of the medications prescribed for him, except for the antacid.

NURSING CARE PLAN 28–1

Care of the Patient with a Bleeding Peptic Ulcer—cont'd

Goals/Expected Outcomes	Nursing Interventions	Selected Rationale	Evaluation
Patient will verbalize factors that contribute to ulcer formation	Instruct in contributing factors of ulcer formation.	Knowledge of risk factors helps patient refrain from risky behaviors.	Discussed factors that can contribute to peptic ulcer. States that he will quit eating foods that cause pain (i.e., spicy foods); has cut smoking down to ½ pack per day, states he will try to quit; verbalizes side effects of medications and proper dosage schedule; will begin exercise program for stress reduction.
Patient will attempt to quit smoking within 2 wk			
	Assist him to learn new ways to cope with stress.	Practicing relaxation and deep breathing helps decrease stress.	Taught deep breathing exercise.
	Instruct him in food substances to avoid, including caffeine and alcohol.	Knowing what foods he should avoid helps him make good food selections.	Instructed in what food and beverages contain caffeine. Discussed abstaining from alcohol.
	Discuss ways to manage proper eating when on the road.	Knowing good food choices for his situation can help him eat properly when on the road.	Discussed food places that have appropriate choices and what are appropriate choices.
Patient will verbalize reason for each medication, dosage schedule, and side effects	Teach action, dosage, and side effects of each medication. Obtain feedback for material taught.	Understanding how to take medications and what to expect, or report, helps with compliance and prevents toxic reactions.	Went over each medication and gave list with dosages. Discussed possible side effects and what to report to the physician.

? CRITICAL THINKING QUESTIONS

1. How would you interact with this patient to try to help him quit smoking?
2. What does he need to know about taking an antacid if he is taking other medications?
3. Considering he is a truck driver and on the road a lot, what can you do to help him change his diet?

vagotomy. When the fundus of the stomach is anastomosed to the duodenum, the procedure is known as a *Billroth I.* In the *Billroth II* procedure, the duodenum is closed and the fundus of the stomach is anastamosed to the jejunum. *Total gastrectomy* is the surgical removal of all of the stomach. The esophagus is anastomosed to the small intestine (Figure 28–4).

Nursing Care of the Patient Undergoing Gastric Surgery

Preoperative Care. The diet of the patient is restricted to liquids during the day before surgery. The patient is kept NPO, a nasogastric tube is inserted, and gastric suction is begun to remove all stomach contents before surgery.

The patient receives routine preparations necessary for all major abdominal surgery. These include enemas so that the colon is emptied of fecal material. If the patient has had a barium enema, the nurse should look for and report returns that contain whitish material. This is barium, and it will become hardened if left in the colon, thus presenting the possibility of a fecal impaction later on.

Postoperative Care. Care of the patient having gastric surgery is routine, with the following exceptions. Following surgery in which part of the stomach has been removed, care must be taken in handling the NG tube to avoid injury to the sutures and prevent introduction of infectious agents. The surgeon will have written specific orders about irrigating fluids allowed and movement of the gastric tube.

After the tube is removed, the patient is given small amounts of liquid to determine tolerance. These liquids are gradually increased. The patient's ability to take them without nausea, vomiting, or abdominal distress is assessed. If the liquids are well tolerated, the patient progresses to small, frequent feedings. Within 6 months, most patients are able to take three regular meals a day. The remaining portion of the stomach stretches to accommodate more and more food. Pa-

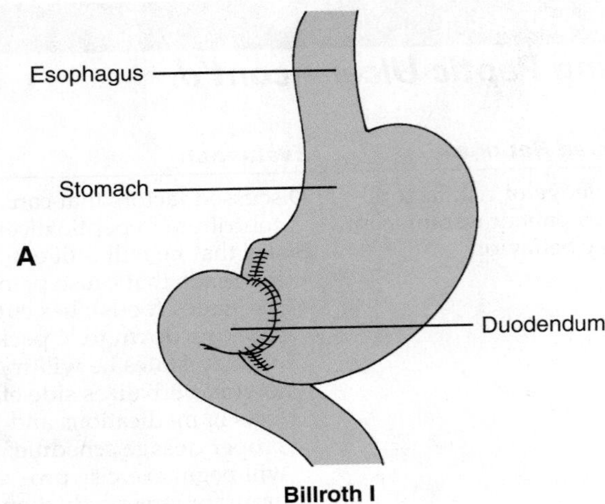

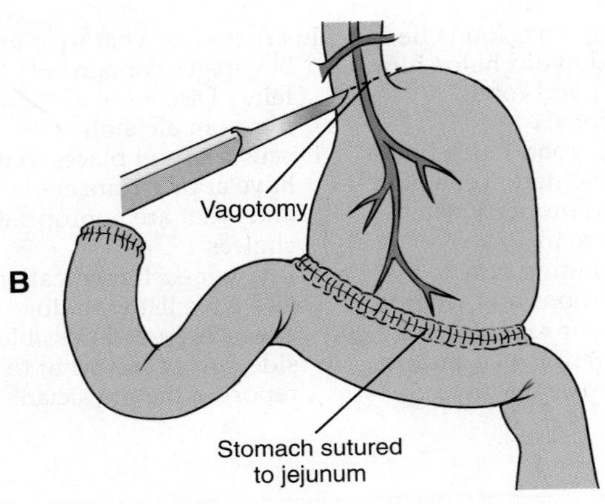

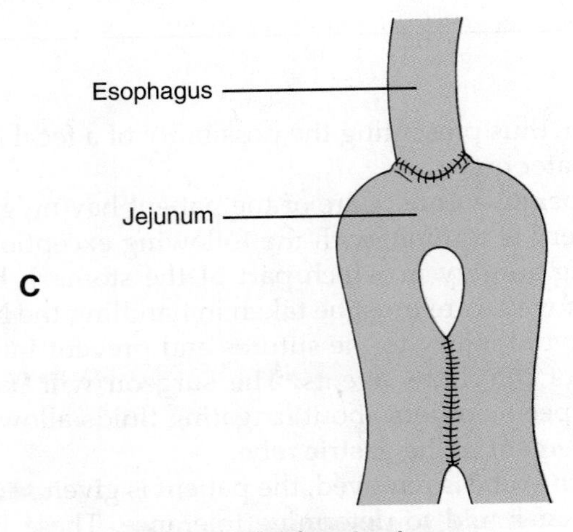

FIGURE **28–4** Stomach surgical procedures. **A,** Billroth I. **B,** Billroth II. **C,** Total gastrectomy.

tients who have had a *total* gastrectomy have restricted diets. They are usually restricted to small, frequent feedings of easily digested semisolids for the rest of their lives. Before discharge, the hospital dietitian usually is called to help the patient and her family learn about the special diet needed after undergoing gastric surgery.

Dumping Syndrome. Some patients who have had a gastrectomy experience a complication known as the "dumping syndrome." **The patient has nausea, weakness, abdominal pain, and diarrhea and may feel faint and perspire profusely or experience palpitations after eating.** These sensations are caused by the rapid passage of large amounts of food and liquid into the jejunum. This occurs because part or all of the stomach and duodenum has been surgically removed. The progress of the ingested foods and fluids is not slowed by passing through the upper portion of the GI tract. When a patient experiences dumping syndrome, instruction is given to avoid eating large meals and to drink a minimum of fluids during the meal. Fluids may be taken in small amounts later, between meals. If sweet foods and liquids seem to aggravate the condition—and they sometimes do—the patient should try to avoid them. It also may be helpful for the patient to lie down flat for 30 minutes after a meal.

GASTRIC CANCER

Adenocarcinoma of the stomach wall is not common, but it is projected that it will cause 13,779 deaths in 2007 in the United States (American Cancer Society, 2007) It is usually discovered very late. The 5-year survival rate is 75% if the disease is caught fairly early and only 30% in those with advanced disease. Metastasis to surrounding organs is common.

Etiology

The cause of gastric cancer is unknown, but pernicious anemia and **achlorhydria** (absence of hydrochloric acid) are often present. It is believed that a diet high in smoked, highly salted, or spiced foods may be a contributor (Nutritional Therapies 28–2). Food preservatives such as nitrates or nitrites increase the risk. The presence of *H. pylori,* particularly if present from an early age, is a definite factor. Genetic influence plays a role as the risk is increased in family members and in those with blood group A (Cultural Cues 28–1).

Pathophysiology

Gastric cancer grows primarily from the mucous glands. Most tumors arise in the antrum or pyloric area. The lesion begins as an ulcerative crater with an irregular border and a raised margin. The tumor eventually spreads through the layers of the stomach and spreads to the lymph nodes, the liver, and the ovaries in women.

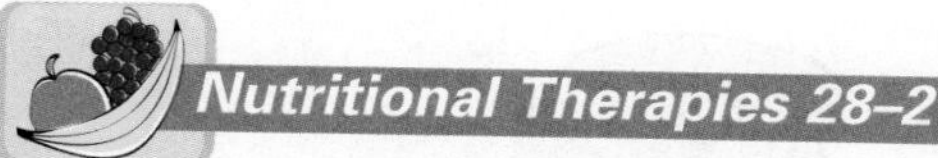

Nutritional Therapies 28–2

Prevention of Gastric Cancer

Refraining from eating a diet high in smoked and salted foods, or pickled vegetables helps prevent gastric cancer. Eating a diet high in fruits and vegetables, particularly those high in beta-carotene and vitamin C, decreases stomach cancer risk. People who eat a lot of red meat each week have double the risk of gastric cancer. Foods such as bacon and many "lunch meats" are high in nitrites, which are carcinogenic. When eating those foods, drinking orange juice reduces the quantity of nitrites. It is the ascorbic acid in the orange juice that counteracts the nitrite concentration.

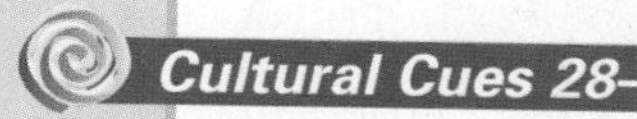

Cultural Cues 28–1

Stomach Cancer Incidence

Stomach cancer is almost double in incidence in African American individuals as in non-Hispanic whites. Native Americans and Hispanic Americans are also at an increased risk for stomach cancer. *Helicobacter pylori* is more common in Hispanic and African American individuals. Research with minority populations is underway to determine how *H. pylori* is transmitted in these populations in an effort to decrease stomach cancer incidence.

Signs and Symptoms

Signs and symptoms are similar to those of peptic ulcer, but may be just intermittent abdominal distress. Belching and the use of antacids may relieve the distress. The patient may become pale and weak and complain of fatigue, weakness, dizziness, and sometimes shortness of breath. Anemia is the underlying cause of those symptoms. There is often blood in the stool.

Diagnosis

Diagnosis is by upper GI series and endoscopic examination of the stomach with biopsy. Anemia, verified with a complete blood count, is usually present. Tumor markers such as carcinoembryonic antigen and carbohydrate antigen (CA) 19-9 are useful in determining the degree of invasion of the tumor, and liver metastasis.

Treatment and Nursing Management

Surgical intervention may relieve symptoms such as obstruction or debulk the tumor. The same surgical procedures are used as for peptic ulcer. There is only a 40% 5-year cure rate with surgery. Adjuvant therapy of radiation and/or chemotherapy may be employed. Radiation has proved to be of value only for palliation. 5-Fluorouracil (5-FU) and cisplatin or 5-FU with epirubicin and cisplatin are the preferred chemotherapy protocols today. A British study recently showed that three cycles of chemotherapy before surgery and three cycles after surgery reduced metastasis and prolonged survival (American Cancer Society, 2006). Cancer therapy and nursing care are discussed in Chapter 8. Nursing care after surgery is the same as for the patient who underwent surgery for a peptic ulcer but with excision of involved lymph nodes.

COMMON THERAPIES FOR DISORDERS OF THE GASTROINTESTINAL SYSTEM

GASTROINTESTINAL DECOMPRESSION

Abdominal distention with increased pressure within the abdominal cavity is very uncomfortable. Excess fluids and gases also interfere with ventilation of the lungs and normal function of other nearby organs.

Measures to relieve distention include inserting an NG tube to remove fluids and gas from the stomach. Gastrointestinal tubes vary in length, design, and purpose. The Levin tube and gastric sump tube are shorter because they are intended to reach only as far as the stomach. The Miller-Abbott, Cantor, and Harris tubes are longer tubes that are directed past the stomach and into the small intestine. Intestinal tubes are described in Chapter 29.

Nursing Management

During GI decompression the patient is observed for continuing signs of abdominal distention, which would indicate that excess fluids and gases are not being removed as intended. **Nausea, vomiting, complaints of feeling full or bloated, increasing shortness of breath, and increase in the girth of the abdomen are signs that the stomach and intestines are not being decompressed adequately.**

Applying too much suction can pull the gastric mucosa into the drainage openings, or "eyes," of the tube, causing damage to the mucosa and traumatic ulceration. Using a gastric sump tube (Salem, ventral) that has an air vent can help prevent this problem. Sump tubes are usually attached to continuous "low" suction; Levin tubes function best with intermittent suction.

Unless ordered otherwise, the low setting is used for suction. The tubing and pigtail should be kept above the level of the stomach. The connecting tubing leading to the suction machine works best if it is kept above the height of entry into the drainage container (Assignment Considerations 28–1).

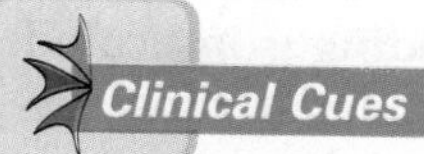

Clinical Cues

The blue pigtail on the Salem sump tube must be kept above the level of the stomach or it will leak stomach secretions. The pigtail can be cleared by instilling a few milliliters of air, and nothing but air should be instilled through it.

Assignment Considerations 28–1

Caring for a Patient with a Salem Sump Tube

When assigning assisted ambulation of the patient with a Salem sump tube, remind the CNA or UAP to keep the tube above the level of the stomach to prevent leaking of stomach contents from the pigtail. The main tube should be plugged for ambulation. When reattaching the tube to suction, suction will resume effectively more quickly if the suction tubing is coiled and placed above the level of the suction machine if it is a portable machine.

Irrigations with normal saline are usually ordered to keep the tube patent. The amount instilled should be added to the patient's intake count, and the amount of drainage is recorded as output for each shift. If the patient has had surgery on the intestinal tract, the irrigation procedure should be done with aseptic technique rather than clean technique.

The characteristics of the drainage are charted each shift. **If coffee ground–like material is noticed in the tube, the drainage should be tested for presence of blood. Blood that has been in contact with gastric juices looks like coffee grounds.** A Hemastix strip dipped into the secretions will reveal the presence of blood. If blood unexpectedly appears in the drainage, the physician should be notified. Fluid and electrolyte imbalance problems that can be caused by continuous suction and irrigation are discussed in Chapter 3.

An NG tube is uncomfortable for the patient. The naris must be checked for signs of pressure, and the tube may need to be repositioned to relieve the problem. Common complaints are sore throat, dry mouth, earache (from congestion of the eustachian tube), and dry lips and nasal mucosa. Frequent mouth care and application of a lubricant to the lips and nares will help. A room humidifier can also be helpful, but this requires a physician's order. The physician may allow the patient to have limited amounts of ice chips, hard candy, or chewing gum to decrease the problem of dry mouth.

After the tube is removed, the patient is monitored for nausea, vomiting, and abdominal distention. Sometimes it is necessary to insert the tube again.

ENTERAL NUTRITION

If a patient has long-term difficulty taking in food orally, as when in a coma, enteral feeding is indicated. Current practice calls for a nasoduodenal tube, frequently the Dobbhoff or similar weighted-tip tube (Figure 28–5). The tube delivers special-formula liquid feedings into the duodenum.

These tubes are inserted by the physician or a registered nurse, and placement in the duodenum is confirmed by x-ray before feedings are started. The feedings can be given at specified times throughout the day or on a continuous basis. If continuous tube feedings are ordered, they frequently are administered with a feeding pump.

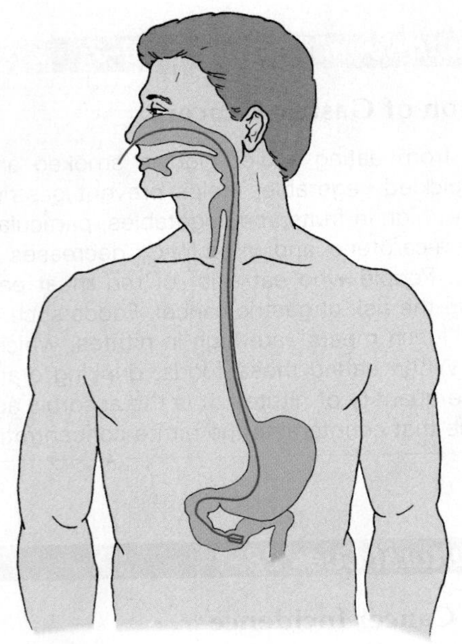

FIGURE 28–5 Small-bore feeding tube placement.

The patient requiring long-term nutritional support for problems such as inability to swallow may undergo percutaneous endoscopic gastrostomy (PEG). A feeding gastrostomy tube is placed endoscopically through the abdominal wall (Figure 28–6). The patient then receives enteral feedings via the gastrostomy tube. The tube is marked with indelible ink at the point of exit so that correct placement can be checked daily. The area is observed for signs of infection and cleansed daily with soap and water until healing is complete. A 4 × 4 gauze dressing is used over the outside bumper until healing has taken place. Change the dressing as needed. Box 28–1 presents nursing interventions for the patient receiving tube feedings.

Sometimes the feeding tube is placed in the jejunum via a jejunostomy. If this is the case, the tube is sutured in place, and the spot where the tube enters the abdominal skin is marked. The mark and suture are checked before beginning a feeding to make certain that the tube has not been dislodged. It is difficult to aspirate anything from a jejunostomy (Safety Alert 28–4).

TOTAL PARENTERAL NUTRITION

Total parenteral nutrition (TPN) is indicated when the patient cannot ingest or digest foods normally or has a problem with malabsorption. If a patient has continued weight loss and a negative nitrogen balance, TPN is indicated. Conditions that could warrant TPN include

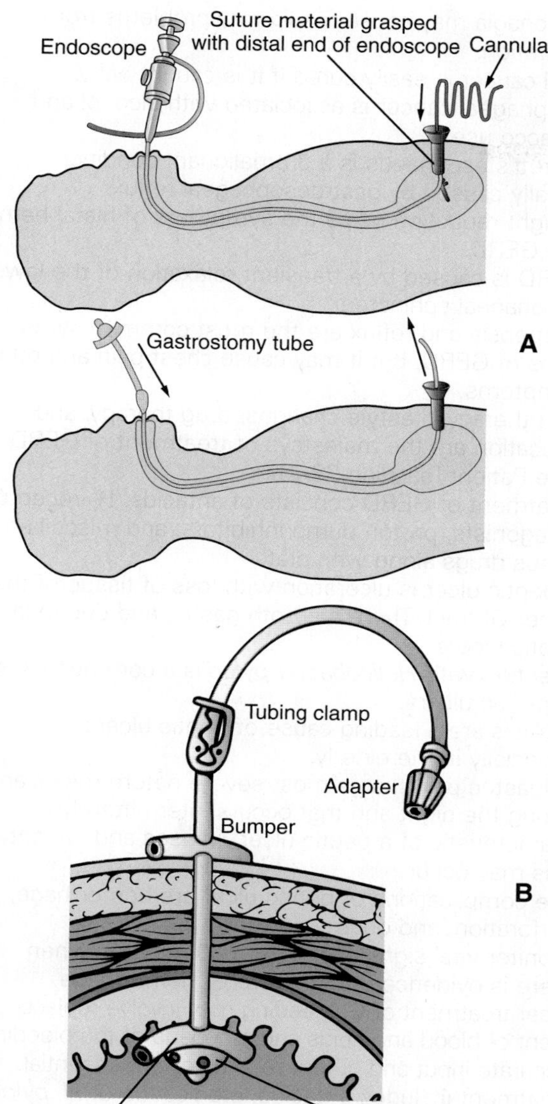

FIGURE 28–6 Percutaneous endoscopic gastrostomy. **A,** Gastrostomy tube placement via percutaneous endoscopy. The gastrostomy tube is inserted through the esophagus into the stomach and pulled through a stab wound made in the abdominal wall. **B,** A retention disk on the inside of the stomach and a bumper disk on the outside secure the tube.

severe trauma to the intestinal tract, as with a gunshot wound, and chronic inflammatory conditions. Regional ileitis that prevents absorption of nutrients is such an inflammatory condition. Other conditions not related to the intestinal tract but nevertheless capable of seriously interfering with normal nutrition over time include prolonged sepsis, fever, extensive burns, and cancer.

TPN is essentially a form of IV feeding. However, because the amounts and kinds of nutrients needed for long-term nutritional maintenance usually cannot be handled as well by peripheral veins, the nutrient mix is given into a larger central vein such as the

Box 28–1 *Nursing Interventions for the Patient Receiving Enteral (Tube) Feedings*

- Be certain tube placement has been checked by x-ray and is correct.
- Check and record the residual volume every 4 hours or as ordered and record it.
- Verify the drip rate for the feeding on the order sheet.
- Assess the feeding pump to be certain it is set up correctly and that the drip setting is accurate. Be certain the formula being instilled is what was ordered.
- Change the feeding bag and tubing every 24 hours. Change the irrigation set every 24 hours also.
- When continuous feeding is ordered, add only 4 hours of formula to the bag at a time to prevent bacterial growth; a closed system may be used for 24 hours.
- Do not use food dye in the formula as it does not prevent aspiration and can cause complications.
- Keep the head of the bed elevated at least 30 degrees during the feeding and for 1 hour after an intermittent or bolus feeding. For continuous feeding, keep the patient in a semi-Fowler's position.
- Monitor laboratory values: blood urea nitrogen, electrolytes, hematocrit, prealbumin, and glucose.
- Monitor for diarrhea or excessive gas.
- Monitor and record input and output.
- Monitor and record the patient's weight at least weekly.
- Flush the tube with 30 to 60 mL of water every 4 hours during continuous feeding, and before and after each intermittent feeding.
- Flush with 30 mL of warm water before and after each individual medication; do not mix medications together or with the feeding formula. Use liquid medications whenever possible.
- If tube becomes clogged, flush with 30 mL of water in a 50-mL piston syringe; use gentle pressure.
- Provide mouth care every 4 hours.
- Clean the nares and around the tube in the naris each shift or twice a day. Inspect the naris for pressure areas.
- Change the tape securing the tube to the nose if it becomes loose or soiled.

FOR GASTROSTOMY TUBE

- Assess the insertion site for signs of infection or excoriation.
- Rotate the tube 360 degrees every day and check for ¼-inch play in and out. If tube cannot be moved, report this to the physician as the retention disk may have become embedded in the tissue.
- Change the dressing once a day, applying a dry sterile dressing.

FOR JEJUNOSTOMY TUBE

- Be certain that the suture holding the tube is in place and that the mark on the tube is at the skin surface before starting or adding to a feeding. If it is not, stop the feeding and notify the physician.
- Do not attempt to aspirate a jejunostomy tube as it will just collapse due to its small interior diameter.
- Inspect the insertion site and change the dressing once a day.

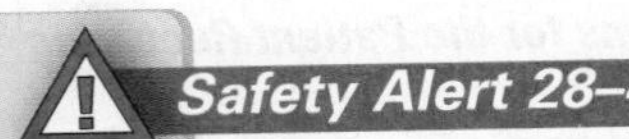

Jejunostomy Tube Displacement

If a jejunostomy tube has moved or the suture is broken, no feeding should be given. Peritonitis may occur if feeding formula spills into the peritoneal cavity. The tube must be replaced by the physician. Always document that placement was checked and whether the suture is intact and the mark is at the skin. If displacement has occurred, document what action was taken.

superior vena cava. To accomplish this, the physician may choose a direct central line into the vena cava or jugular vein. A peripherally inserted central catheter (PICC) line may be inserted and threaded into the vena cava instead. Lipids may be given via a peripheral vein. Further information about TPN and the principles for administration are found in Chapter 3.

Care of the patient must be a team effort on the part of physicians, pharmacists, dietitians, and nurses. Nursing care includes assisting with the insertion of the IV central line or PICC line, changing the tubing with each new bag or bottle, changing the dressing, and removing the tubing when TPN therapy is discontinued. Some institutions have specially prepared TPN nurses to give direct care to these patients. They also supervise TPN care given by general-duty nurses. However, day-to-day care includes monitoring vital signs, glucose levels, and fluid and electrolyte balance. The patient is weighed daily and provided frequent mouth care. Dressing changes with observation of the insertion site are the responsibility of the staff nurse to whom the patient has been assigned. The rate of TPN is slowly decreased to gradually lower the dextrose load before TPN is discontinued.

Key Points

- Poor dentition is a common problem affecting ingestion.
- A calorie reduction diet combined with exercise and behavior modification are the initial treatments for obesity.
- Bariatric surgery may be considered for the obese person with a BMI over 40.
- In anorexia nervosa the patient refuses to maintain a normal body weight. There is disturbance of body image and an extreme fear of becoming fat.
- Bulemia is the practice of induced vomiting after binge eating. Laxatives may be used to help purge the system.
- Stomatitis is generalized inflammation of the mucous membranes of the mouth and has many causes.
- Dysphagia may cause respiratory problems from aspiration.
- Oral cancer is easily cured if it is caught early.
- Esophageal cancer is associated with alcohol and tobacco use.
- Barrett's esophagus is a premalignant condition usually caused by gastroesophageal reflux.
- Weight reduction helps the symptoms of hiatal hernia and GERD.
- GERD is caused by a transient relaxation of the lower esophageal sphincter.
- Dyspepsia and reflux are the most common symptoms of GERD, but it may cause chest pain and other symptoms.
- Diet therapy, lifestyle changes, drug therapy, and education are the mainstays of treatment of GERD (see Patient Teaching 28–1).
- Treatment of GERD consists of antacids, H_2-receptor antagonists, proton pump inhibitors, and miscellaneous drugs along with diet.
- A peptic ulcer is ulceration with loss of tissue of the upper GI tract. There are both gastric and duodenal peptic ulcers.
- Infection with *Helicobacter pylori* is a common cause of peptic ulcers.
- NSAIDs are a leading cause of peptic ulcers, especially in the elderly.
- Epigastric pain that is most severe before meals and during the night and that occurs intermittently is characteristic of a peptic ulcer. Nausea and weight loss may occur.
- The complications of peptic ulcer are hemorrhage, perforation, and obstruction.
- Monitor vital signs every 15 to 30 minutes when there is evidence of extensive GI hemorrhage.
- Ulcer treatment of GI bleeding may involve replacement of blood and fluids and stoppage of the bleeding. Accurate input and output recordings are essential.
- Treatment includes antacids, eradication of *H. pylori* if it is present, an H_2-receptor antagonist, and a proton pump inhibitor.
- Surgical procedures for peptic ulcer include pyloroplasty with vagotomy, subtotal gastrectomy, antrectomy, or total gastrectomy (see Figure 28–4).
- Gastric cancer has often metastasized by the time of diagnosis.
- *Helicobacter pylori*, pernicious anemia, and achlorhydria are all implicated in the development of gastric cancer.
- Symptoms of dumping syndrome are nausea, weakness, abdominal pain, diarrhea, faintness, palpitations, and diaphoresis.
- A nasogastric tube is used for gastric decompression; a nasoduodenal tube is used for enteral feeding.
- After NG tube removal, the patient is monitored for abdominal distention, nausea, and vomiting.
- If long-term enteral feeding is needed, a PEG tube may be inserted.
- A jejunostomy tube is sutured in place; check the integrity of the sutures before feedings.
- When a patient cannot ingest foods and liquids normally, total parenteral nutrition may be required.

- Total parenteral nutrition formula must enter into a vessel with high-volume blood flow.
- TPN solution should not be speeded up beyond the rate ordered.
- The TPN solution must be kept sterile, and the dressing over the catheter site must be changed using sterile technique.

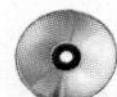
Go to your **Companion CD-ROM** for an Audio Glossary, animations, video clips, and bonus review questions.

evolve Be sure to visit the companion Evolve site at http://evolve.elsevier.com/deWit for interactive NCLEX-PN Exam Style Review Questions, WebLinks, and additional online resources.

NCLEX-PN EXAM STYLE REVIEW QUESTIONS

Choose the best answer(s) for the following questions.

1. After an exhaustive discussion of surgical options, the patient consents to undergo circumgastric banding. When asked about the procedure, the nurse accurately responds:

1. "It removes certain segments of the small intestines."
2. "An inflatable band is placed around the stomach to change the size of the stomach as the patient loses weight."
3. "It bypasses parts of the small intestine and limits the stomach size."
4. "A small stomach is created by placing a vertical line of staples."

2. The nurse determines that an important nursing diagnosis for a female patient who is undergoing elective bariatric surgery would be Disturbed body image related to excess weight. An appropriate patient expected outcome would be:

1. Patient will be able to make positive statements about her body.
2. Patient will be able to develop new social relationships.
3. Patient will be able to meet caloric requirements.
4. Patient will be able to demonstrate happiness.

3. The nurse interviews a 21-year-old woman who was admitted for severe weight loss. The patient denies having any problems and indicates a strong desire to look better. The most likely diagnosis would be:

1. failure to thrive.
2. chronic gastritis.
3. anorexia nervosa.
4. depression.

4. When screening for the presence of risk factors for oral and pharyngeal cancers, the nurse asks which of the following questions? *(Select all that apply.)*

1. How much alcohol do you consume?
2. Have you had any oral lesions?
3. Do you have family members who have cancer?
4. What do you smoke?
5. Have you been exposed to hepatitis virus?

5. ____________________ is considered a precancerous lesion of the oral cavity.

6. The nurse is taking care of a patient who had a modified radical neck dissection surgery. The patient's spouse asks, "Why do you have to apply cold packs and to elevate my husband's head?" The appropriate response by the nurse is:

1. "These interventions facilitate rapid recovery."
2. "These interventions reduce neck swelling."
3. "These interventions promote faster healing."
4. "These interventions reduce the incidence of postoperative fever."

7. A 76-year-old Chinese man complains of progressive difficulty swallowing and fullness of the throat. When making clinical decisions, an effective approach would be to:

1. determine the decision maker of the family.
2. talk privately with the patient.
3. use a family member as an interpreter.
4. schedule a family conference.

8. While obtaining a clinical history, the patient with a known history of peptic ulcers suddenly complains of a severe upper abdominal pain of increasing intensity that spread to the shoulders. The abdomen has board-like rigidity. The nurse anticipates which of the following signs and symptoms? *(Select all that apply.)*

1. Slow deep respirations
2. Increased blood pressure
3. Increased pulse
4. Warm dry skin

9. The nurse reinforces diet recommendations to a patient with gastroesophageal reflux disease (GERD). Which of the following patient statements indicates a need for further teaching?

1. "I should avoid spicy Italian sauces."
2. "Clothes should be loose."
3. "I need to wait 30 minutes after eating before lying down."
4. "I need to consider removing caffeine from my diet."

10. Regarding the nursing care of enteral feeding tubes, which nursing behaviors demonstrate appropriate nursing care? *(Select all that apply.)*
    1. Aspirating intestinal contents of a jejunostomy tube
    2. Gentle flushing of a clogged enteral tube with 30 mL of water
    3. Checking for 1 inch of play on a gastrostomy tube
    4. Monitoring laboratory values such as blood urea nitrogen, prealbumin, hematocrit, electrolytes, and glucose
    5. Rotating the jejunostomy tube 360 degrees every day

CRITICAL THINKING ACTIVITIES 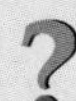 *Read each clinical scenario and discuss the questions with your classmates.*

Scenario A

Ms. Sutton, age 52, is experiencing a lot of abdominal discomfort and reflux. She visits her physician, who believes she has GERD.

1. What measures would be recommended to decrease the symptoms of GERD?
2. What specific instruction would you give Ms. Sutton regarding her diet?
3. Why would losing some weight help her problem? (She is 5′3½″ tall and weighs 158 lb).

Scenario B

Mr. Post, age 47, is admitted to the hospital because he has epigastric pain, is vomiting blood, and has a suspected gastric ulcer.

1. What tests might be done to establish a diagnosis for Mr. Post?
2. What kind of information will help Mr. Post avoid difficulty with his diet after he is discharged?
3. What would Mr. Post need to know to keep his ulcer under control and eventually cure it?

CHAPTER

29 Care of Patients with Disorders of the Lower Gastrointestinal System

evolve http://evolve.elsevier.com/deWit

Objectives

Upon completion of this chapter, you should be able to:

Theory

1. Describe the etiology and signs and symptoms of various types of hernias.
2. Discuss the characteristics of irritable bowel syndrome.
3. Explain how diverticulitis occurs.
4. Illustrate how the two types of intestinal obstruction occur and their danger.
5. Describe the pathophysiology, methods of diagnosis, and treatment for ulcerative colitis and Crohn's disease.
6. List nursing interventions for the patient with inflammatory bowel disease.
7. Differentiate the signs and symptoms of appendicitis from those of peritonitis.
8. Compare the characteristics of hemorrhoids, pilonidal sinus, and anorectal fistula.
9. Create a teaching plan for the prevention of colorectal cancer.
10. Identify nursing interventions for the patient having surgery of the lower intestine and rectum.

Clinical Practice

1. Write a nursing care plan for the patient with cancer of the colon and intestinal obstruction.
2. Formulate a nursing care plan for a patient undergoing colostomy, considering the type of stoma and the effluent it produces.
3. Prepare to provide care for a patient with an ileostomy.
4. List four interventions for helping the patient psychologically adjust to his ostomy.

Key Terms

Be sure to check out the bonus material on the Companion CD-ROM, including selected audio pronunciations.

anastomosis (ă-năs-tō-MŌ-sĭs, p. 723)
colectomy (kŏ-LĔK-tō-mē, p. 723)
colostomy (kŏ-LŎS-tō-mē, p. 723)
cryotherapy (krī-ō-THĔR-ă-pē, p. 721)
diverticulitis (dī-vĕr-tĭk-ū-LĪ-tĭs, p. 714)
diverticulosis (dī-vĕr-tĭk-ū-LŌ-sĭs, p. 714)
diverticulum (dī-vĕr-TĬK-ū-lŭm, p. 714)
hemicolectomy (hĕ-mē-kŏ-LĔK-tō-mē, p. 723)
hemorrhoid (HĔM-rŏyd, p. 721)
hemorrhoidectomy (HĔM-rŏyd-ĔK-tō-mē, p. 721)
hernia (HĔR-nē-ăh, p. 710)
hernioplasty (hĕr-nē-Ō-PLĂS-tē, p. 710)
herniorrhaphy (hĕr-nē-ŎR-ĕ-fē, p. 710)
ileostomy (ĭl-ē-ŎS-tō-mē, p. 728)
intussusception (ĭn-tŭs-sŭs-SĔP-shŭn, p. 715)
lyse (līz, p. 716)
mucorrhea (mū-kō-RĒ-ă, p. 711)
photocoagulation (fō-tō-kō-ăg-ū-LĀ-shŭn, p. 721)
pilonidal (pī-lō-NĪ-dăl, p. 722)
scleropathy (sklĕr-ō-pă-thē, p. 721)
volvulus (VŎL-vū-lŭs, p. 715)

THE LOWER GASTROINTESTINAL SYSTEM

Some disorders, such as Crohn's disease and ulcerative colitis, are correlated with a genetic predisposition. Both disorders also have an ethnic correlation as they are more common among the Jewish population. Certain forms of colon cancer have been identified as having a genetic link and definitely show a familial tendency for occurrence. Autoimmune diseases often affect the gastrointestinal (GI) system, causing inflammation or fibrosis of organs.

Treatments such as drug and radiation therapy may cause GI problems as a side effect. Some people who have undergone chemotherapy for cancer develop a mechanical form of sprue, a malabsorption problem, which remains even after chemotherapy is complete. Lactose intolerance, which is not uncommon in the older adult, may cause continuous diarrhea and malabsorption.

Alleviating the effect of stress on intestinal disorders is difficult as emotions are not always easy to control. Teaching patients ways to relax and to cope with undue stress can be helpful, but it does not guarantee freedom from disorders that usually have multiple causes.

DISORDERS OF THE ABDOMEN AND LOWER GASTROINTESTINAL SYSTEM

ABDOMINAL AND INGUINAL HERNIA

Etiology and Pathophysiology

The internal organs of the body are contained within their respective cavities by the outside walls of the cavity. In the abdomen, the wall is *muscular.* If there is a defect in this muscular wall, the intestine may break through the defect. This protrusion is called a **hernia** or a *rupture.*

The most common locations for a hernia are in areas where the abdominal wall is normally weaker and more likely to allow a segment of intestine to protrude (Figure 29–1). These include the center of the abdomen at the site of the umbilicus and the lower abdomen at the points where the inguinal ring and the femoral canal begin. **The most common contributing factors in the development of a hernia are straining to lift heavy objects, chronic cough, straining to void, straining at stool, and ascites.** Inguinal hernias are more common in men. A hernia may form at an old abdominal surgical incision.

Hernias are classified as *reducible,* which means the protruding organ can be returned to its proper place by pressing on the organ, and *irreducible,* which means that the protruding part of the organ is tightly wedged outside the cavity and cannot be pushed back through the opening. Another name for an irreducible hernia is *incarcerated* hernia. If the protruding part of the organ is not replaced and its blood supply is cut off, the hernia is said to be *strangulated.* An *indirect* hernia protrudes through the inguinal ring. A *direct* hernia protrudes through the posterior inguinal wall.

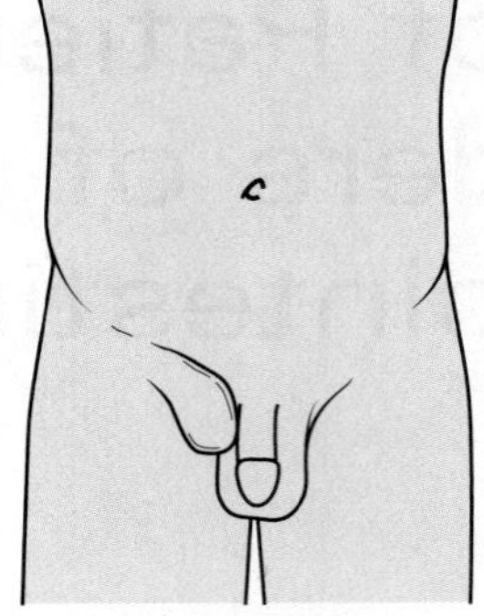
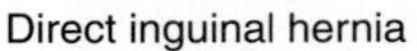

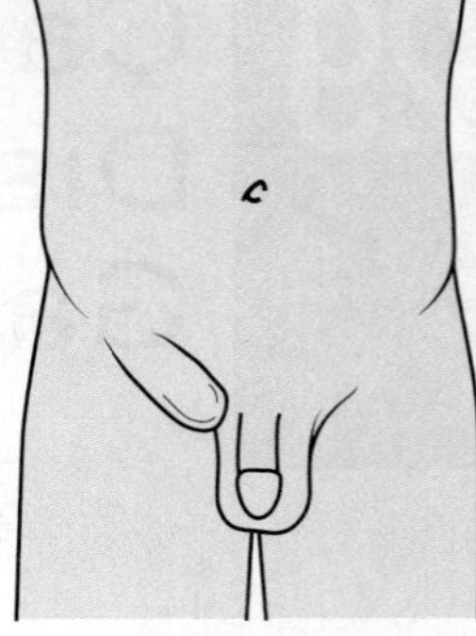

A

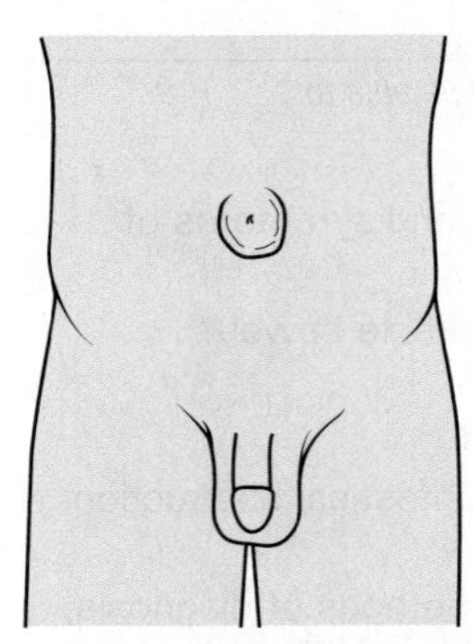

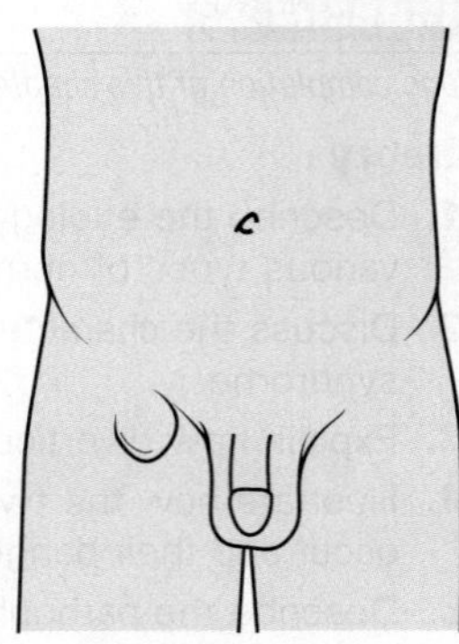

B

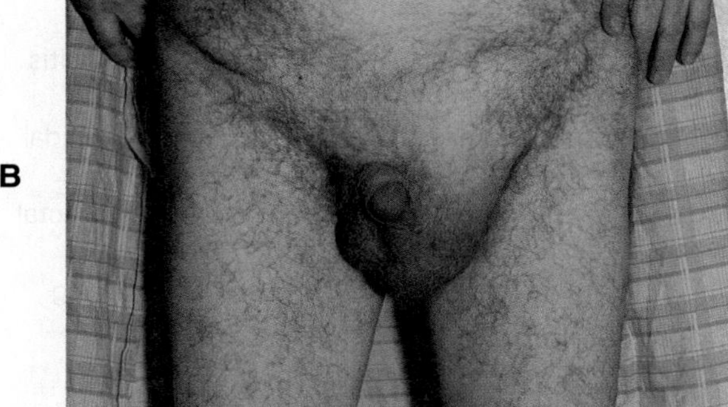

FIGURE **29–1** **A,** Types of hernias. **B,** Indirect inguinal hernia.

Signs and Symptoms

If the hernia is not incarcerated, there will just be an abnormal pouching out from the abdominal wall or in the groin area (inguinal hernia). Some discomfort may accompany the hernia. Pain occurs when the peritoneum becomes irritated or when the hernia is incarcerated or strangulated. **The flow of intestinal contents becomes blocked by an incarcerated hernia, and the patient has symptoms of intestinal obstruction. This is an emergency because when the blood supply is restricted, part of the bowel may die.**

Diagnosis and Treatment

There is a "lump" or local swelling at the site of the hernia. When pressure on the abdominal wall is removed by lying down, the swelling disappears. Lifting of heavy objects, coughing, or any activity that puts a strain on the abdominal muscles may force the organ back through the opening, and the swelling reappears.

Hernias are best treated by surgery. If surgery is not possible because of age or poor surgical risk, the patient may be fitted with an appliance called a *truss.* The truss is put on each morning before the patient gets out of bed, because the hernia is more likely to be reduced at that time. A truss simply reinforces the weakened cavity wall and prevents protrusion of the intestines. It is only a symptomatic measure and does not cure the hernia.

Herniorrhaphy. The surgical procedure used in the treatment of a hernia is called a **herniorrhaphy,** which means a surgical repair of a hernia. The defect is closed with sutures. If the area of weakness is very large, a **hernioplasty** is done. In this procedure, some type of strong synthetic material is sewn over the defect to reinforce the area. The procedure is now most often done on an outpatient basis.

Careful discharge instructions are given to the patient to prevent respiratory problems because the patient should not cough in the immediate postoperative period. Guidelines on signs and symptoms of complications are sent home with the patient, along with a written list of activities to avoid until healing is complete.

Nursing Management

When a hernia is found on assessment, the patient is encouraged to seek repair. Care after hernia repair is directed at pain control and preventing recurrence of the hernia. The patient is cautioned not to do heavy lifting, pulling, or pushing that increases intra-abdominal pressure considerably. Postoperative care is much the same as for other surgical patients (see Chapter 5).

Think Critically About . . . What would you say to a family member who mentions to you that he has a swelling in the groin area and thinks he may have a hernia?

IRRITABLE BOWEL SYNDROME

Irritable bowel syndrome (IBS) is a functional disorder of gastrointestinal motility. In the United States more people suffer with IBS than with diabetes or asthma.

Etiology

The cause of IBS is unknown, but it is thought to be due to a hypersensitivity of the bowel wall leading to disruption of the normal function of the intestinal muscles. In North America, IBS is far more common in women than in men. The disorder often causes the patient considerable pain and discomfort. IBS is a major reason people miss work.

Pathophysiology

An altered bowel pattern and abdominal pain with bloating are caused by altered motility of the small and large intestines. It is thought that there is an abnormality of nerve function in the intestine. A chemical mediator, 5-hydroxytryptamine (5-HT) or serotonin, plays a role in bowel motility and visceral sensitivity. 5-HT may be implicated in the pain that occurs with IBS. There is a familial predisposition. Stress, caffeine, and certain foods such as dairy and wheat products seem to be triggers for IBS in some people. Food sensitivity seems to be a contributing factor, as is stress.

Signs and Symptoms

IBS is a group of symptoms that together represent the most common disorder presented by patients who consult gastroenterologists. The three characteristics typical of this disorder are (1) alteration in bowel elimination, either constipation or diarrhea or both; (2) abdominal pain and bloating; and (3) the absence of detectable organic disease. Although the pattern of bowel dysfunction varies from case to case, each patient seems to have a unique pattern.

Diagnosis

Diagnosis is based on clinical manifestations and ruling out the presence of organic bowel disease. Diagnostic criteria include:

- Abdominal pain or discomfort characterized by the following:
- Relieved by defecation
- Associated with a change in stool frequency
- Associated with a change in stool consistency

Other symptoms that support the diagnosis include:

- **Mucorrhea** (mucus in the stool)
- Abdominal bloating

Treatment

Treatment of IBS is inevitably long and, because of the stress factors involved, often includes such modes of therapy as psychotherapy, biofeedback training, and instruction in relaxation techniques. It is important to reassure the patient that there is no relationship between his disorder and a malignancy of the bowel.

Medications are prescribed according to each patient's need. Drugs that have been used include bulk-forming agents, antidiarrheals, antispasmodics, antidepressants, anticholinergics/sedatives, and mild analgesics to relieve discomfort (Table 29–1). A diet high in fiber also may be prescribed. Metamucil or other bulk stool softeners are recommended.

Gas-forming foods such as legumes and those in the cabbage family should be avoided. Avoiding onions, potatoes, cucumbers, coffee, tea, carbonated beverages, and alcohol can be helpful. In some patients, the intake of milk is restricted if they have shown evidence of intolerance to it. Lactase tablets may be used but may not help if there is sensitivity to dairy products rather than a lactase deficiency (Complementary & Alternative Therapies 29–1).

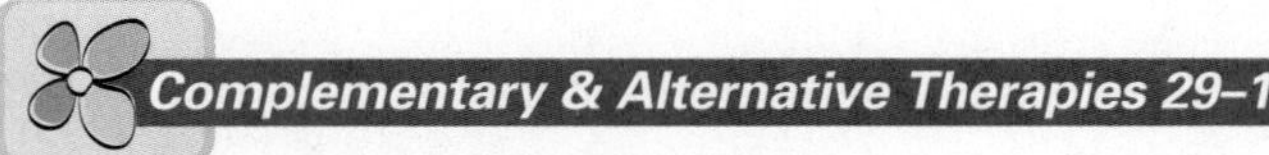

Digestive Enzymes and Probiotics

Digestive enzymes seem to be helpful for some people. Probiotics often temper the symptoms of IBS. A 2- to 4-week trial of regular intake of enzymes and probiotics should tell whether they will be helpful in decreasing symptoms of IBS (*Clinical Nutrition Updates*, 2006). EB

Simethicone caplets seem to be effective to help reduce the gas and bloating associated with episodes of IBS. It prevents formation of gas pockets in the GI tract.

Key: *GI*, gastrointestinal; *IBS*, irritable bowel syndrome.

Table 29–1 ***Commonly Prescribed Drugs for Gastrointestinal Disorders***

CLASSIFICATION	ACTION	NURSING IMPLICATIONS	PATIENT TEACHING
ANTIDIARRHEALS			
Diphenoxylate hydrochloride (Lomotil) Loperamide (Imodium) Opium tincture (Paregoric)	Decrease motility, propulsion, and secretions	Observe for effectiveness; should be effective within 48 hr. Observe for signs of constipation. Use cautiously in patients with prostatic enlargement as may cause urinary retention. Warn that Pepto-Bismol will make stool black.	Warn that medication will cause dry mouth. Instruct not to take more than recommended dosage as toxicity can occur. With Lomotil, warn not to operate machinery until effect on central nervous system is known. Advise to contact physician if acute diarrhea does not abate within 2 days.
Kaolin-pectin combinations (Kaopectate)	Decrease fluid in stool		
Bismuth subsalicylate (Pepto-Bismol)	Binds water; coats mucosa, absorbs toxins		
ANTIFLATULENTS			
Simethicone (Phazyme, Mylicon, Di-Gel)	Defoaming action disperses gas	Warn that the drug does not prevent gas formation, but will decrease bloating and discomfort. Gas is expelled via belching or flatus.	Instruct to chew tablets before swallowing.
LAXATIVES			
Bulk-forming Methylcellulose (Citracel) Psyllium (Metamucil, Konsyl)	Act like fiber, absorbing water in the bowel and hastening transit time through the bowel	None specific; monitor effectiveness.	Instruct to take with an 8-oz. glass of water to prevent esophageal or bowel obstruction.
Surfactants Docusate sodium (Surfak, Colace) Docusate potassium (Dialose)	Facilitate absorption of water by stool by decreasing the surface tension Enhance secretion of fluid and electrolytes in the bowel	Contraindicated for patients with signs of intestinal obstruction. Act in 24–48 hr. Used to prevent constipation rather than treat it.	Instruct to take with a full glass of water. Not to be used for more than 1 wk without physician's knowledge.
Contact laxatives Bisacodyl (Dulcolax) Phenolphthalein (Feen-a-Mint, Ex-Lax, Modane) Cascara sagradra and senna (Senokot, Fletcher's Castoria) Castor oil	Act on intestinal wall to increase secretion of fluid and electrolytes into the intestine	Most act within 6–12 hr to produce a semi-fluid stool. Bisacodyl is available as a rectal suppository as well as an oral tablet. Phenolphthalein may turn the urine pink. Cascara sagradra and senna may cause a brownish yellow or pink tinge to the urine. Castor oil acts within 2–6 hr. Castor oil should not be used routinely to treat constipation. The unpleasant taste of castor oil can be decreased by chilling or pouring over ice or mixing in chilled fruit juice.	Contact laxatives should be used only for occasional treatment of constipation. They are habit-forming, decreasing the natural mechanisms for evacuation. Tablets should not be chewed. Take tablets with a full glass of water. Do not exceed recommended dosage. Take bisacodyl 1 hr after taking antacids or milk. Suppository form may cause burning sensation in the rectum.

Key: *5-ASA,* 5-aminosalicylic acid; *GI,* gastrointestinal; *5-HT$_4$,* 5-hydroxytryptamine$_4$; *IV,* intravenously.

Table 29–1 ***Commonly Prescribed Drugs for Gastrointestinal Disorders—cont'd***

CLASSIFICATION	ACTION	NURSING IMPLICATIONS	PATIENT TEACHING
DRUGS FOR INFLAMMATORY BOWEL DISEASE (IBD)			
Sulfasalazine (Azulfidine) Mesalamine (5-ASA) Olsalazine (Dipentum)	Sulfasalazine is a sulfonamide antibiotic Mesalamine is the active agent in sulfasalazine Olsalazine contains two molecules of 5-ASA These drugs reduce inflammation in the bowel by suppressing prostaglandin synthesis and the migration of inflammatory cells into the affected area	May cause muscle aches, nausea, fever, or rash. Complete blood counts needed periodically as the drugs can cause agranulocytosis and anemia. Determine whether allergy to sulfonamides exists before administration.	Caution patient to avoid direct sunlight and ultraviolet light to prevent photosensitivity reaction. Advise to use form of contraception other than oral contraceptives as these drugs interfere with their effectiveness. Warn that when used with oral hypoglycemics, an increased hypoglycemic effect may occur. Advise that urine may be tinted orange. GI upset may be minimized by taking drug after meals. Instruct to report rash or sensitivity reaction to physician promptly.
Infliximab (Remicade)	Monoclonal antibody that neutralizes the activity of tumor necrosis factor alpha found in Crohn's disease; decreases infiltration of inflammatory cells	Given IV over at least 2 hr. Dose repeated at 2 wk and then q 6 wk from first dose. Observe for anaphylactic reaction.	May initially cause increased diarrhea. Report nausea, vomiting, abdominal pain, itching, or rash to physician. Need periodic blood counts. Do not breast-feed while taking this drug.
ANTISPASMODICS			
Dicyclomine hydrochloride (Bentyl, Antispas) Propantheline bromide (Pro-Banthine) Oxyphencyclamine hydrochloride (Daricon)	Block acetylcholine, thereby decreasing smooth-muscle spasm and GI motility and inhibiting gastric acid secretion	These drugs interact with many other drugs; check each drug patient is taking for interactions. Most of these drugs are contraindicated in glaucoma, prostatic hypertrophy, myasthenia gravis, and other conditions; consult information on each drug individually. May predispose to drug-induced heat stroke. Monitor vital signs and urine output carefully.	Take 30–60 min before meal. Patient can suck on hard candy to relieve mouth dryness unless contraindicated. Have patient drink 2500–3000 mL of fluid to prevent constipation. Avoid driving or hazardous activities if drug causes dizziness, sleepiness, or blurred vision. Report rash or skin eruption to physician.
Hyoscyamine (Levsin)	Inhibits action of acetylcholine at postganglionic receptor sites, decreasing spasm and abdominal pain	May decrease absorption of antacids and antidiarrheals. May increase effects of anticholinergics. May cause urinary retention. Assess for dehydration; encourage adequate fluid intake.	May cause dry mouth. Inform physician of rash, eye pain, difficulty in urinating, or constipation. Avoid hot baths and saunas. May initially cause dizziness or faintness; do not operate machinery until response is known.

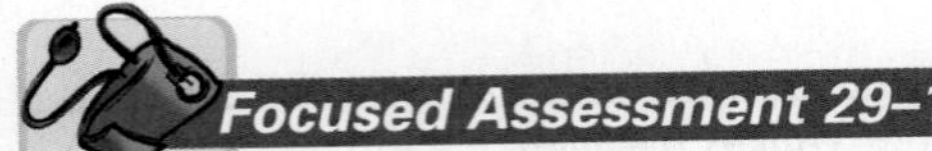

Focused Assessment 29–1

Data Collection for the Patient with Suspected IBS

For the patient with symptoms suggesting IBS, gather the following data.

HISTORY

- When symptoms first began
- Stool pattern: frequency, character of stool
- Presence of bloating and flatus
- Incidence of pain or cramping; location, duration, character
- Pain that awakens the patient at night
- Precipitating factors for cramping or diarrhea
- Known food intolerances
- Methods of self-treatment
- Known stressors
- Methods of coping with stress

PHYSICAL EXAMINATION

- Presence and character of bowel sounds
- Degree of firmness and tenderness of abdomen
- Location of tenderness
- Appearance of stool

Key: *IBS*, irritable bowel syndrome.

NURSING MANAGEMENT

Assessment (Data Collection)

A general health assessment is conducted along with a focused assessment (Focused Assessment 29–1).

Nursing Diagnosis and Planning

The more common nursing diagnoses and interventions for patients with IBS are essentially the same as for any patient with alteration in bowel elimination, either diarrhea or constipation (see Table 27–2). Instructing the patient about the nature of his disease can help diminish unwarranted fears.

Implementation

Ineffective coping patterns in response to stress may be present in these patients. Teaching relaxation techniques is helpful. Consultation with a psychiatric nursing specialist can help the staff nurse develop more realistic goals and effective nursing interventions to improve the patient's coping skills. Instruction is given about the medications and diet therapy. Encourage wearing loose clothing if bloating and increased abdominal pressure are problematic.

Evaluation

Gather data regarding the actions performed. Ask, "Are the actions meeting the stated expected outcomes?" If the outcomes are not being met, the plan must be revised.

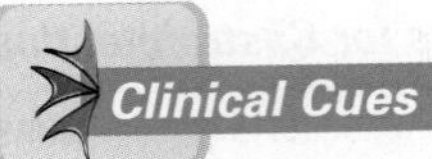

Clinical Cues

Having the patient keep a food diary can be very helpful in identifying foods that cause a reaction with bloating and inflammation. If the diary is kept over a period of weeks, a pattern may be established. Food intolerance symptoms may not show up for up to 4 days after the food is eaten. Sometimes it is one food that greatly increases the symptoms and that food can be simply left out of the diet.

DIVERTICULA

The term **diverticulum** refers to a small, blind pouch resulting from a protrusion of the mucous membranes of a hollow organ through weakened areas of the organ's muscular wall. Diverticula occur most often in the intestinal tract, especially in the esophagus and colon. They are most prevalent in the older individual. When they are present, the patient is said to have **diverticulosis**. If the diverticula become inflamed or infected, the condition is referred to as **diverticulitis**.

Etiology of Diverticulosis and Diverticulitis

Increases in intra-abdominal pressure from constipation and straining to defecate are thought to be factors in the development of colon diverticula. Muscle of the colon hypertrophies, thickens, and becomes rigid. The increased intra-abdominal pressure causes herniation of the mucosa and submucosa through the colon wall. Diverticulitis occurs when food caught in the diverticulum mixes with bacteria. The intestinal wall becomes irritated and infected, and if it is not treated, perforation and peritonitis may occur. Diverticulitis affects one third of adults over age 60.

Esophageal diverticula occur when there is herniation of esophageal mucosa and submucosa into surrounding tissue. The disorder is more common in older patients.

Pathophysiology

Diverticula tend to develop in people over age 50 who have chronic constipation and/or eat a low-fiber diet. Diverticulitis occurs when the diverticula become inflamed or infected. Waste accumulates in the diverticula and can irritate the mucosal wall. Seeds from berries, tomatoes, and items such as popcorn hulls are thought to be especially prone to cause inflammation in the diverticula.

Signs, Symptoms, and Diagnosis

A person may have diverticulosis and remain unaware of his condition for quite a while because it often presents no symptoms. Eventually, however, the diverticula may fill with some material passing through the intestinal tract and become inflamed or infected, causing symptoms. For bowel diverticula, there is usually a history of constipation. There may be rectal bleeding. **Diverticulitis of the intestine produces symptoms of diar-**

Nutritional Therapies 29–1

Diet for Diverticular Disease

A high-fiber diet is encouraged for the patient with diverticular disease. Eating whole-grain cereals and breads, as well as fruits such as apples, seedless berries, peaches, and pears adds fiber. High-fiber vegetables—squash, broccoli, cabbage, and spinach—and legumes, including dried beans, peas, and lentils provides bulk that decreases constipation and speeds the transit time in the intestine. Drinking plenty of fluids and water helps considerably. This diet combined with exercise to prevent constipation can usually control diverticular disease.

Patients who have recurrent diverticulitis are asked to avoid foods with husks, such as peanuts, sunflower seeds, berries with seeds, tomatoes, and popcorn, as a precautionary measure. It is thought that the husks may get into the diverticulum and irritate it, causing inflammation and eventual diverticulitis.

rhea or constipation, left lower abdominal pain, fever, and rectal bleeding. The condition may be complicated by intestinal obstruction or by peritonitis if the intestinal wall ruptures. If bleeding is massive, there will be hypotension and dehydration and eventual shock.

Esophageal diverticula produce complaints of dysphagia, regurgitation, nocturnal cough, and *halitosis* (bad breath). There is a risk of esophageal perforation. Diagnosis of diverticula is by GI series and by endoscopy.

? *Think Critically About* . . . What is the difference in the signs and symptoms of diverticulitis and those of irritable bowel syndrome?

Treatment and Nursing Management

Treatment of diverticulitis consists of parenteral antibiotics, withholding solid food, and providing hydration with intravenous (IV) fluids as necessary. Recurrent episodes of diverticulitis, or perforation and peritonitis, require surgical removal of the part of the colon that is involved.

The symptoms of diverticulosis and diverticulitis will to some extent govern the treatment necessary. Diverticulosis often can be managed conservatively. A high-fiber diet, increased fluids and bulk laxatives, or stool softeners to control constipation may be all that are needed. Diverticulitis may need antidiarrheal medication. The role of the LPN/LVN is in reinforcing education about the diet, fluid intake, and exercise. Mild pain medication may be used for abdominal discomfort in the ambulatory patient (Nutritional Therapies 29–1).

INTESTINAL OBSTRUCTION

Intestinal obstruction is a blockage of the intestinal tract that prevents the normal passage of GI contents

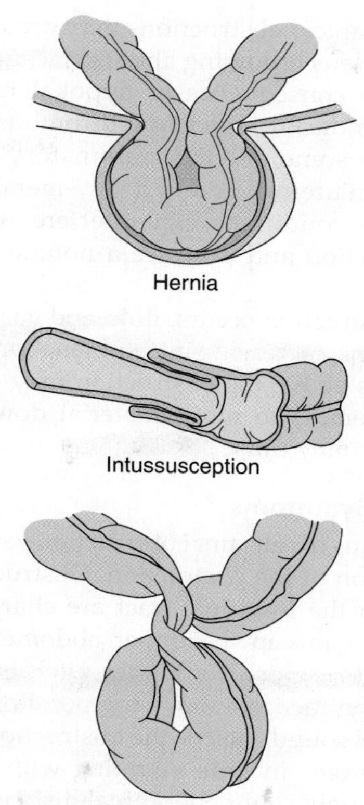

FIGURE **29–2** Mechanical causes of intestinal obstruction.

through the intestines. The condition may occur suddenly or progress gradually.

Etiology and Pathophysiology

Obstruction of the bowel may be mechanical or nonmechanical. Mechanical obstruction results in blockage of the lumen of the bowel. Nonmechanical obstruction results from the absence of peristalsis. Movement of contents through the bowel stops. Mechanical obstructions include tumors, adhesions, strangulated hernia, twisting of the bowel **(volvulus)**, telescoping of one part of the bowel into another **(intussusception)**, gallstones, barium impaction, and intestinal parasites (Figure 29–2). Abdominal adhesions are a common cause of intestinal obstruction. Adhesions form when inflammation from abdominal trauma or surgery has occurred and fibrous bands of scar tissue hold together two segments of bowel that are normally separated.

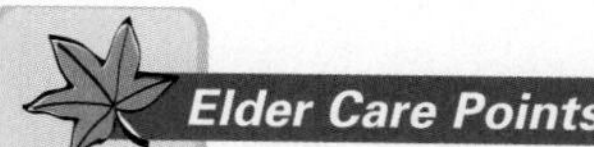

Elder Care Points

The elderly are more prone to the occurrence of volvulus and consequent intestinal obstruction, partially because of decreased muscle tone. Suspect this disorder when the patient complains of sudden abdominal pain with vomiting, has abdominal distention with a palpable mass, has increased bowel sounds on auscultation, and exhibits signs of dehydration.

Nonmechanical obstructions may occur as a result of paralytic ileus following abdominal surgery, infection, or as a consequence of hypokalemia, or they may be secondary to intestinal thrombus. Infections can occur in some pelvic inflammatory diseases or peritonitis, in uremia, and in heavy-metal poisoning. All of these conditions can interfere with normal peristaltic action and produce a nonmechanical obstruction.

When obstruction occurs, fluid and gas accumulate in the intestine, increasing intralumenal pressure. Peristaltic waves above the obstruction may occur as the intestine attempts to move material down the tract. These waves may cause severe pain.

Signs and Symptoms

The symptoms of intestinal obstruction vary according to the location of the obstruction. Obstructions occurring high in the intestinal tract are characterized by sharp, brief pains in the upper abdomen. More frequent bowel sounds of a higher pitch in the area of peristaltic contractions above the point of obstruction occur. Bowel sounds below the obstruction are absent. Other symptoms include vomiting with rapid dehydration and only slight abdominal distention.

Obstructions of the colon are characterized by a more gradual onset with marked abdominal distention as the bowel fills, infrequent vomiting (which occurs late in the process if at all), and **pains that last several minutes or longer and correspond to peristaltic waves.** Bowel sounds are high in pitch above the point of obstruction and are absent below the obstruction.

Diagnosis and Treatment

Diagnostic x-rays will be ordered to determine where the obstruction is located. Surgery is indicated for obstruction caused by adhesions, volvulus, hernia, or tumor.

The physician may first try to relieve the obstruction by using an intestinal tube, which is a long tube inserted via the nose (Figure 29–3). The tube decompresses the intestine above the obstruction. In some patients this treatment can resolve the problem without the trauma of surgery. If surgery is performed, the procedure depends on the type of obstruction encountered. Adhesions are **lysed** (broken apart), a volvulus is untwisted, or a colectomy may be necessary if tumor is involved.

Nursing Management

The patient with acute intestinal obstruction is very seriously ill. He often has respiratory difficulty because of the pressure of the distended abdomen against the diaphragm. Placing the patient in Fowler's position helps relieve this pressure and also aids in removing gas and intestinal contents through the intestinal tube. Fluid and electrolyte status must be monitored closely. Pain is considerable, and prompt attention to pain control is essential. If the obstruction cannot be resolved, surgical correction must be done. Measure abdominal girth every 2 to 4 hours, placing the tape at the same location on the abdomen each time. If unresolved, intestinal obstruction can lead to rupture of the intestine, peritonitis, shock, and death. Postoperative care is the same as for other abdominal surgery patients (see Chapter 5 and the Nursing Care Plans in this chapter).

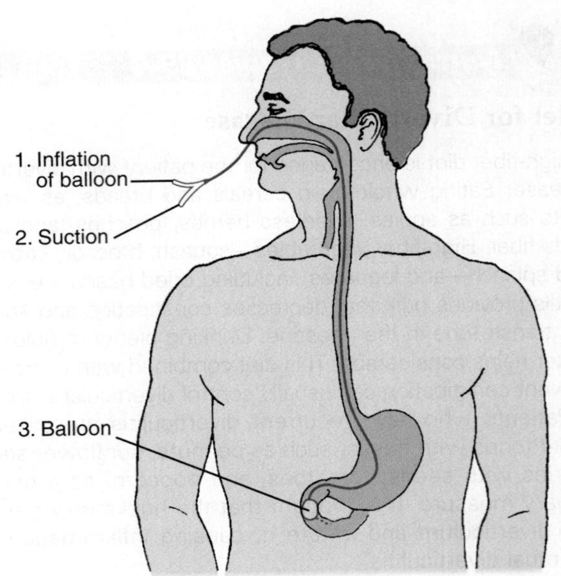

Miller-Abbott tube in place. It is advanced through the intestines to the prescribed point. The Miller-Abbott tube has a double lumen and is weighted with tungsten. *1*, Portion of the metal tip leading to the balloon. *2*, Portion of the metal tip leading to the lumen that can be suctioned. *3*, Balloom inflated with air.

FIGURE **29–3** Miller-Abbott double-lumen intestinal tube used for decompression.

INFLAMMATORY BOWEL DISEASE

ULCERATIVE COLITIS AND CROHN'S DISEASE

Ulcerative colitis is an inflammation, with the formation of ulcers, of the mucosa of the colon. It often is a chronic disease, and the patient usually is free from symptoms between acute flare-ups. Crohn's disease can involve any part of the GI tract, but most commonly affects the small intestine. The onset of inflammatory bowel disease (IBD) is commonly between the ages of 15 and 35.

Etiology

The causes of ulcerative colitis and Crohn's disease are not known. A genetic factor may well be present as there is increased familial incidence. Immunologic activity is thought to be involved as well because anticolon antibodies are often present in the blood. With ulcerative colitis, infections and emotional tension frequently bring about acute attacks. It is more common among those of Jewish descent, and people with the disorder have a 40% higher incidence of some type of arthritis than the general public.

Pathophysiology

The pathophysiology of IBD is being investigated. The end result of the disorders is inflammation of the mucosal lining of the intestinal tract, causing ulceration, edema, bleeding, and fluid and electrolyte loss. Ulcerative colitis and Crohn's disease (regional ileitis) share many of the same characteristics (Table 29–2). One difference is that the inflammatory changes in ulcerative colitis are nonspecific, whereas those in Crohn's disease are granulomatous. Another very important difference is that the patient with long-standing chronic ulcerative colitis is at 10 to 20 times greater risk for developing cancer of the colon than the patient with Crohn's disease. The constant inflammation disrupts normal cell function, and cellular mutations may occur. Crohn's disease can affect any area of the intestine, although it more frequently affects the ascending colon and can affect the small intestine (Figure 29–4). Ulcerative colitis most often affects the rectosigmoid and left colon. Ulcerative colitis changes tend to be continuous along the affected portion of the bowel, whereas those of Crohn's disease are segmental, leaving healthy sections of bowel in between diseased portions ("skip lesions"). On radiograph, there is a cobblestone appearance to the mucosa.

There is a growing tendency to include both disorders under the title of inflammatory bowel disease (IBD). It is suspected that ulcerative colitis and Crohn's disease are immunologic responses to the same as-yet-unknown etiologic agent.

Signs and Symptoms

The patient with IBD suffers from attacks of diarrhea that may be bloody and contain mucus, abdominal pain with cramping, malaise, fever, and weight loss. The color of blood in the stool depends on the degree and rapidity of the bleed. Slow bleeding and oozing will show up as black, tarry stool. If diarrhea is frequent, the blood may be more reddish. The color is also dependent on where in the intestine the bleeding is occurring. Blood tends to be redder when the bleeding location is lower in the intestine.

Table 29–2 *Comparison of Ulcerative Colitis and Crohn's Disease*

	ULCERATIVE COLITIS	CROHN'S DISEASE
Area affected	Mucosa only; usually involves rectum and proceeds up the colon	Full thickness of the intestine; most common in small intestine
Characteristics	Mucosa is red, intestinal wall is edematous and friable, bleeding easily; pseudopolyps are present	Edematous bowel wall, inflammatory cells, mucosal ulcerations, granulomas, and "skip" lesions (normal areas)
Signs and symptoms	Diarrhea, frequently bloody; abdominal cramping relieved by defecation; rectal bleeding	Fever, malaise, fatigue, weight loss, intermittent diarrhea, cramping or steady right lower quadrant or periumbilical pain, postprandial bloating
Complications	Massive hemorrhage; hypovolemia, toxic megacolon, cancer of the colon	Fistulas, anal fissures, perianal disease, bowel obstruction or perforation

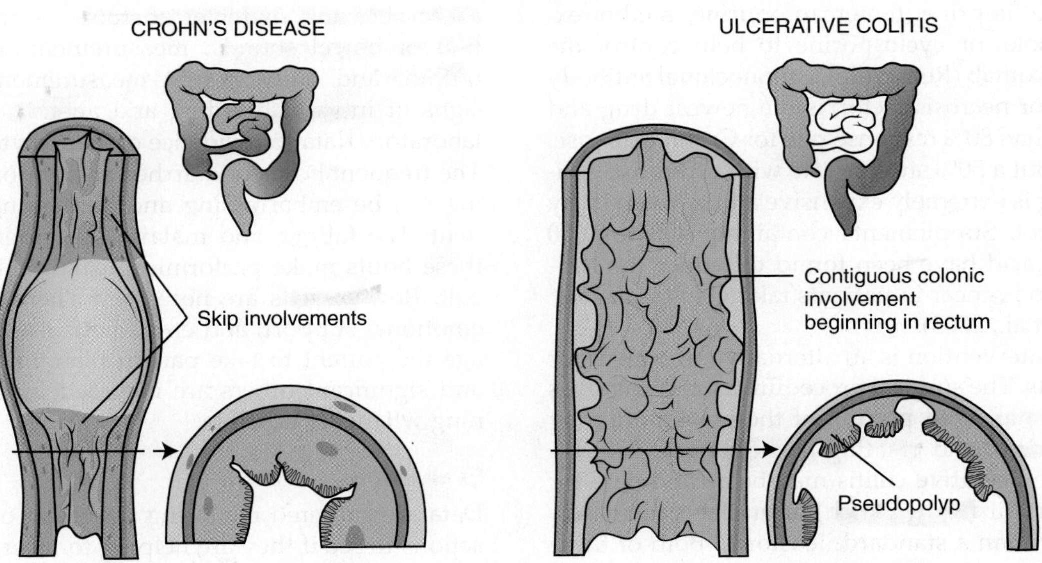

FIGURE **29–4** Comparison of the distribution of disease and characteristics of lesions of Crohn's disease and ulcerative colitis.

The bouts often are precipitated by events that cause undue physical or emotional stress. An acute attack can last for days, weeks, or even months, followed by periods of remission extending from a few weeks to several decades. A few patients experience only one attack and then remain free of symptoms for the rest of their lives. Others suffer such profound disturbances during the first attack that their lives are in danger if they do not receive prompt treatment to stop intestinal hemorrhage and correct fluid and electrolyte imbalances.

Diagnosis

Medical diagnosis usually is based on the patient's medical history and presenting symptoms. Colonoscopy, endoscopy with biopsy, barium enema, and stool analysis may be used to confirm the diagnosis.

Treatment

Treatment for either ulcerative colitis or Crohn's disease varies according to severity of symptoms and whether the condition becomes chronic. Conservative approaches to medical treatment include administration of antidiarrheal drugs, long-term sulfasalazine therapy, and medications to relieve abdominal cramps. A diet of low-fat, low-fiber foods that have a high protein and caloric content is instituted. Small frequent feedings are best. Lactose avoidance helps some patients. Corticosteroids are used for moderate to severe cases to decrease the inflammation. During acute attacks, fluid replacement may be necessary. Blood transfusions are given when anemia is present. Oral 5-aminosalicylic acid (5-ASA) derivatives, such as olsalazine sodium (Dipentum), have recently been found to be useful for those patients who cannot tolerate sulfasalazine (see Table 29–1). Budesonide (Entocort) is used to help control disease in the ileum. Patients with advanced disease who are not surgical candidates may be given azathioprine, 6-mercaptopurine, methotrexate, levamisole, or cyclosporine to help control the disease. Infliximab (Remicade), a monoclonal antibody against tumor necrosis factor, is the newest drug and has greater than 80% response rate for Crohn's disease, but only about a 50% success rate with ulcerative colitis. The drug is extremely expensive and is given IV by a set protocol. Supplements containing 400 to 1000 mcg of folic acid have been found to reduce the incidence of colon cancer in patients taking sulfasalazine
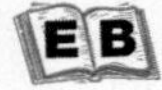
(Diculescu et al., 2003).

Surgical intervention is an alternative treatment for some patients. The surgical procedure usually involves removing the affected portion of the bowel, often by proctocolectomy, and creating an ileostomy. Today a patient with ulcerative colitis may be a candidate for an ileal reservoir (Kock pouch) or an ileoanal anastomosis rather than a standard ileostomy. Both of these new procedures allow the patient control over the discharge of wastes from the reservoir, and consequently a collection pouch is not necessary. The patient uses a catheter to empty the reservoir after the Kock procedure. With an ileoanal anastomosis, the patient retains control over the anal sphincter with voluntary defecation. These procedures are not performed often for Crohn's disease because as the disease progresses, the area of the reservoir is involved.

NURSING MANAGEMENT

Assessment (Data Collection)

A complete health assessment is performed with particular attention to pain, nutritional, and fluid and electrolyte status. A thorough abdominal assessment is performed.

Nursing Diagnosis and Planning

Nursing diagnoses might include:

- Pain related to intestinal inflammation
- Deficient fluid volume related to diarrhea fluid loss
- Diarrhea

Other common nursing diagnoses are listed in Table 27–2.

Expected outcomes might include:

- Patient's pain will be controlled with analgesia within 8 hours.
- Patient will regain fluid balance within 36 hours.
- Patient will experience decreased number of diarrhea bowel movements within 24 hours.

Long-term goals may be concerned with helping the patient adhere to the prescribed regimen, encouraging effective coping mechanisms, and instruction and encouragement in relaxation techniques.

Implementation

The nursing care plan for a patient experiencing an acute attack of IBD should include such observations as number and character of stools, periodic auscultation of bowel sounds, measurement of intake and output, and daily weight measurement. Check for signs of internal bleeding and anemia, and monitor laboratory data for evidence of electrolyte imbalances. The frequent bouts of diarrhea and abdominal cramping can be embarrassing and depressing for the patient. The fatigue and malaise that often accompany these bouts make performing usual daily tasks difficult. Rest periods are necessary. There is a need for emotional support, and empathetic listening. Encourage the patient to take part in planning care. Family and significant others are included in the care planning whenever possible.

Evaluation

Data are gathered regarding the result of the nursing actions to see if they are helping to meet the expected outcomes. If progress is not being made, then the nursing care plan must be revised.

? *Think Critically About . . .* Can you describe three key differences between Crohn's disease and ulcerative colitis?

APPENDICITIS

Etiology and Pathophysiology

Appendicitis is an inflammation of the vermiform appendix (called *vermiform* because it is wormlike and *appendix* because it is an appendage of the cecum). The appendix is a blind pouch and is therefore easily infected by bacteria passing through the intestinal tract.

Signs, Symptoms, and Diagnosis

Pain in the lower right side, halfway between the umbilicus and the crest of the ileum, at McBurney's point is the best-known symptom of appendicitis. It is usually accompanied by muscle guarding. However, the location of the pain may, and often does, vary among individuals. The patient may rest with the right thigh drawn up. Extending the leg causes pain. **A slight temperature elevation (1°), nausea and vomiting, and an increase in the white cell count also are characteristic of appendicitis.**

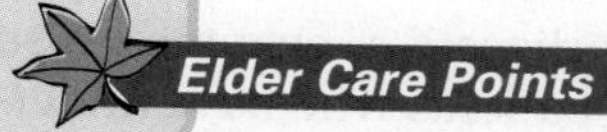

Elder Care Points

Peritoneal inflammation does not necessarily cause abdominal rigidity in the elderly patient. These patients often present with only diffuse abdominal pain, malaise, and weakness. Confusion may be present.

A specific type of computed tomography (CT) scan, the focused appendix computed tomography (FACT) scan, is the diagnostic test of choice. Barium enema with nonfilling of the appendix is also considered diagnostic of appendicitis along with the classical symptoms listed previously.

Treatment

Appendicitis is treated by surgically removing the appendix *(appendectomy)*. This procedure may be performed laparoscopically or require an open laparotomy. Before surgery, the patient is allowed nothing by mouth (NPO), and an ice bag may be placed on the abdomen to slow down the inflammation and thus avoid rupture of the swollen and inflamed appendix. **Under no circumstances should laxatives be given when appendicitis is suspected** (Safety Alert 29–1).

The patient is usually allowed out of bed within several hours of surgery if there are no complications. The patient undergoing an uncomplicated laparoscopic appendectomy may be discharged the same day after an adequate anesthesia recovery period. The convalescent period is most often uneventful, and the patient may return to his former activities within 1 to 2 weeks. The patient who had an open laparotomy needs 2 to 4 weeks for recovery.

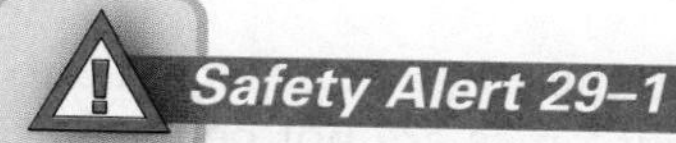

Safety Alert 29–1

Appendicitis

Never use heat to relieve abdominal pain if appendicitis is a possible cause of the pain. Heat might bring enough blood and fluid to the appendix to cause it to rupture and cause peritonitis. An ice pack can be applied to the abdomen to decrease the inflammation and pain.

NURSING MANAGEMENT

Assessment (Data Collection)

Specific assessment areas are nausea, pain level, vital signs, and assessment of the abdomen for rigidity that might indicate a ruptured appendix. A diet history for the previous 24 to 48 hours is obtained to help determine if food poisoning is a cause of the symptoms. Date and character of the last bowel movement and usual bowel pattern are obtained.

Nursing Diagnosis and Planning

Common nursing diagnoses are listed in Table 27–2. Preoperatively, Pain is the primary nursing diagnosis. Postoperatively, pain control is a top nursing priority along with prevention of infection at the surgical site.

Implementation

The patient is not medicated for pain until the cause of the abdominal pain is diagnosed. This is difficult for both the patient and the nurse, but analgesia can mask important signs and symptoms. Medication may be given for nausea and vomiting.

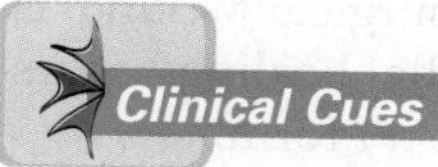

Clinical Cues

Applying a cold pack to the area of tenderness when appendicitis is suspected decreases pain and may help prevent rupture by decreasing inflammation. In the hospital, seek a physician's order for a cold pack.

An IV infusion is started for fluid administration and the patient is kept NPO for probable surgery. The abdomen is monitored for signs of rigidity indicating rupture of the appendix. Once appendicitis is diagnosed, the patient is prepared for surgery. Watch fluid and electrolyte status of the older patient. An electrolyte problem may manifest as confusion.

Evaluation

Data are gathered to determine whether expected outcomes are being met. If outcomes are not being met, the plan must be changed.

PERITONITIS

Etiology

Peritonitis is an inflammation of the peritoneum. It usually occurs when one of the organs it encloses ruptures or is perforated so that the organ's contents (including bacteria) are spilled into the abdominal cavity. **Examples of common causes of peritonitis are ruptured appendix, perforated duodenal or gastric ulcer, ruptured ectopic (tubal) pregnancy, diverticulitis with perforation, and traumatic rupture of the colon, spleen, or liver.**

Pathophysiology

As the peritoneum becomes inflamed, there is local redness and swelling of the membrane and production of serous fluid that becomes more and more purulent as the bacteria multiply. Normal peristaltic action of the intestines slows or ceases altogether, and the symptoms of intestinal obstruction occur.

Signs and Symptoms

The patient experiences nausea, vomiting, and severe abdominal pain and distention. Fever, chills, tachycardia, and pallor occur, and other symptoms of shock may emerge. **Unless the condition is treated promptly and successfully, peritonitis can be fatal.**

Diagnosis and Treatment

Diagnosis is by history, physical examination, and results of a complete blood count (CBC). A CT scan of the abdomen may be performed to rule out structural problems or tumor. Broad-spectrum antibiotics are given IV in massive doses to combat infection, IV fluids and electrolytes are administered to restore a normal balance, and gastric or intestinal suction is initiated to relieve distention. Surgical procedures needed to repair a ruptured organ are done as soon as the patient's condition will permit. The surgical wound is generally left open after surgery so that healing occurs from the inside out and abscesses don't form.

Nursing Management

Nursing care is primarily concerned with frequent assessment of the patient and prompt and accurate reporting of unexpected changes in his condition. The patient is usually placed in the semi-Fowler's position to facilitate breathing, prevent respiratory complications, and aid in localizing the purulent material in the lower abdomen or pelvis. Vital signs are taken and recorded at least every 1 to 2 hours during the critical stage. If vomiting occurs, the characteristics and amount of vomitus are noted. The emesis of fecal material indicates complete intestinal obstruction.

A common complication of peritonitis is paralytic ileus. Auscultate at least once a shift for the return of bowel sounds. If the patient passes flatus or feces rectally, this should be recorded on the chart, as it indicates return of peristalsis.

Because of the high fever and toxicity that accompany peritonitis, the patient may be delirious or disoriented and must be protected from self-injury. This includes putting side rails up and having someone at the bedside at all times. This is particularly important for the elderly patient who is prone to develop confusion and delirium in this situation. The patient should be turned *very gently* and moved in the bed with care because of extreme tenderness in the abdominal region. A high fever and the presence of the gastric tube demand frequent mouth care to protect the lips, prevent halitosis, and cleanse the mouth.

MALABSORPTION

Etiology and Pathophysiology

Many disorders interfere with the normal absorption of nutrients, water, and vitamins from the intestine (Cultural Cues 29–1). Adult celiac disease (sprue), in which the patient cannot properly metabolize gluten (a protein found in all wheat products, barley, and rye), is one cause.

Lactose intolerance is another cause because it results in diarrhea. Pancreatic disease with interference in secretion of pancreatic digestive enzymes also causes malabsorption. Some patients who have undergone chemotherapy for treatment of cancer experience alteration of the intestinal mucosa that causes malabsorption. **Whatever the cause, malabsorption creates a nutritional deficiency.**

Pathophysiologically, there is irritation of the intestinal mucosa and consequent diarrhea. Both problems limit the ability of the intestine to absorb nutrients.

Signs, Symptoms, and Diagnosis

A key sign of malabsorption is passage of stool that is bulky, frothy, and foul smelling and usually floats in the toilet. Other signs and symptoms include weight loss, weakness, and various signs of vitamin deficiency depending on the type of malabsorption the patient is experiencing. Diagnosis is by history, upper

Cultural Cues 29–1

Lactose Intolerance

Lactose intolerance is most common in Native Americans, but is seen in African Americans, Asians, and South Americans. It can affect people at any age and can affect other ethnic groups as well. It is caused by lack of the enzyme lactase, which is needed to digest lactose. Assess patients in these groups for bloating, flatulence, cramps, and loose stools or diarrhea after consuming milk or milk products.

and lower GI series, and endoscopy with biopsy. Gluten intolerance is diagnosed by blood tests for gluten antibodies.

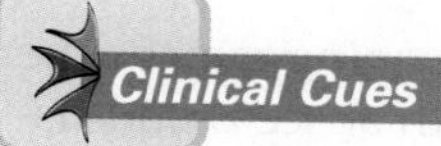

If your patient is to undergo testing for gluten intolerance, it is necessary to be eating wheat and gluten products for 2 weeks prior to testing or the tests will not be accurate.

Treatment and Nursing Management

Treatment is directed at the underlying cause. Pancreatic insufficiency can be treated by administering pancreatic enzymes with meals. Celiac disease is treated by completely omitting gluten from the diet.

Nursing management consists of supporting the patient through the diagnostic process and reinforcing teaching about diet and medications. The patient is encouraged to take supplements of vitamins and minerals for the remainder of the life span.

ANORECTAL DISORDERS

HEMORRHOIDS

Hemorrhoids are varicosities of the veins of the rectum. They may be *internal* (inside the sphincter muscles of the anus) or *external* (outside the sphincter muscles) (Figure 29–5).

Etiology and Pathophysiology

Constipation, prolonged standing or sitting, and pregnancy are predisposing causes of hemorrhoids. The habit of sitting on the toilet and straining at the stool for long periods is one of the primary factors responsible for many cases of hemorrhoids. Enlargement of the prostate, uterine fibroids, and rectal tumors are other contributing factors. Chronic liver disease with portal hypertension is another cause. Venous congestion from interference with venous return from the hemorrhoidal vessels leads to the development of hemorrhoids.

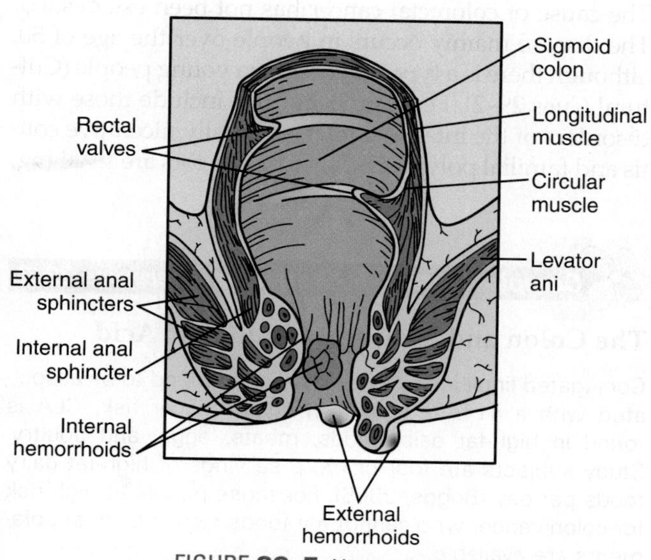

FIGURE 29–5 Hemorrhoids.

Signs, Symptoms, and Diagnosis

Local pain and itching are the most common symptoms of hemorrhoids. Bleeding from the rectum at the time of defecation may also occur. Hemorrhoidal blood is usually bright to dark red. External hemorrhoids are less likely to bleed, but they are more evident to the person examining the patient, because they appear as tumor-like projections around the rectum. Diagnosis is by physical examination.

Treatment

The symptoms of hemorrhoids may be relieved by correcting constipation, local applications of heat or cold, and sitz baths. The use of ointments that contain a local anesthetic helps relieve the itching and pain. Hydrocortisone ointment and suppositories help decrease the swelling. The patient also should be instructed to wash the anal region with warm water and soap after each bowel movement to prevent infection at the breaks in the mucosa.

Hemorrhoids can be treated by **scleropathy** (injection of a solution that causes the vessel to dry up and disintegrate). **Cryotherapy** (freezing) and **photocoagulation** (burning) are other options. **Hemorrhoidectomy** using a laser or standard surgical procedure may be performed. Another treatment method is rubber band ligation, in which a rubber band is slipped around the hemorrhoidal vessel, cutting off the blood supply. This causes the hemorrhoid to shrivel and disintegrate. All of these methods are most often done as outpatient treatments. Hemorrhoidectomy may occasionally be done as an inpatient procedure.

Nursing Management

Teaching regarding the use of hydrocortisone suppositories or cream, sitz baths to decrease swelling, and rectal hygiene are nursing measures used preoperatively. The patient is taught ways to avoid constipation and to promote regular bowel evacuation.

After surgery, thorough discharge teaching is done, and written instructions are sent home with the patient. A prescription for analgesics will also be sent home, as these patients experience quite a bit of pain. Cold or warm compresses and warm sitz baths using a rubber or air-filled ring to support the buttocks also help relieve pain. The ring may be used while the patient is lying down to remove pressure from the rectal area. Sitz baths are usually ordered twice a day. Mild, wet dressings that are commercially prepared (Tucks) also may be used on the surgical site. These dressings have a glycerin base and contain a mild astringent that reduces swelling and relieves pain.

Most patients dread the first bowel movement after a hemorrhoidectomy. There is no doubt that it will cause some pain, and the usual procedure is to administer a stool softener to make defecation less traumatic. The patient and family should be warned that the patient may become faint, and someone should stay close by.

A high-fiber diet is started right away, as it is best if formed stool is passed regularly. A sitz bath after each bowel movement will offer relief and also cleanses the affected area, keeping it free from irritation. The patient should continue to make a practice of sitting in a tub of warm water after bowel movements until healing is complete.

PILONIDAL SINUS (PILONIDAL CYST)

Etiology and Pathophysiology

The word **pilonidal** means "having a nest of hair." A pilonidal sinus is a lesion located in the cleft of the buttocks at the sacrococcygeal region. It is sometimes called a *pilonidal cyst*, but it is believed to be a subcutaneous canal (sinus) with one or more openings into the skin (rather than a true cyst or fluid-filled sac). The condition occurs when the stiff hairs in the sacrococcygeal region irritate and eventually penetrate the soft skin in the cleft of the buttocks, causing irritation. Factors that can lead to development of such a sinus include local injury, improper cleaning of the area, and obesity. People who have more than the usual amount of body hair are particularly susceptible.

Signs, Symptoms, and Diagnosis

A pilonidal sinus may cause no trouble until it becomes infected, and then the patient experiences pain in the area, with swelling and a purulent drainage. Diagnosis is by history and examination.

Treatment and Nursing Management

When symptoms are severe or persistent, the area must be incised surgically and the connecting canals opened and drained. Hairs and necrotic tissue must be removed so the area can heal. This is usually done as an outpatient surgical procedure. A drain is left in the cavity so that healing will occur from the inside to the outside.

Postoperative care includes changing of dressings and measures to avoid contamination of the wound. A stool softener and an oil retention enema usually are given before the first bowel movement to avoid strain on the sutures. Antibiotics may be given to control infection.

ANORECTAL ABSCESS AND FISTULA

Etiology and Pathophysiology

An abscess may form where there has been irritation with breaks in the skin or mucosa. Localized infection with a collection of pus forms an anorectal abscess. Tears in the mucosa of the rectum from hard, constipated stools may predispose to abscess and fistula formation. A fistula is a chronic granulomatous tract that travels in a line from the anal canal to the skin outside the anus or from an anorectal abscess to the anal canal or the area around the anus.

Signs, Symptoms, and Diagnosis

A discharge of pus from the fistula opening may be the first sign of an abscess or fistula. Both abscess and fistula are painful, and sitting or coughing aggravates the pain. If a fistula is accompanied by diarrhea, Crohn's disease is suspected because 50% of Crohn's patients develop a rectal fistula. Diagnosis is by history and physical examination.

Treatment and Nursing Management

Antibiotics may be administered to decrease the infection. Medication for pain is prescribed. Incision and drainage of an abscess may be necessary. A fistula usually requires surgical excision and repair. Nursing management involves teaching measures to prevent further incidence of constipation and infection, and rectal hygiene measures. Sitz baths are used to decrease inflammation. Education about pain medication and antibiotic regimens is provided.

CANCER OF THE COLON

Cancer of the large intestine, also called colorectal cancer, is the third most common malignancy in both men and women in the United States. The American Cancer Society says that 112,340 colon and 41,420 rectal cancer cases are expected to occur in 2007 (American Cancer Society, 2007a). Colorectal cancer is one of the most curable of all cancers if it is found in the early stages, and mortality rates have fallen over the last 30 years as detection has become easier (Complementary & Alternative Therapies 29–2).

Etiology

The cause of colorectal cancer has not been established. The disease mainly occurs in people over the age of 50, although there is a type that occurs in young people (Cultural Cues 29–2). People most at risk include those with disorders of the intestinal tract, especially ulcerative colitis and familial polyposis. Other risk factors are smoking,

Complementary & Alternative Therapies 29–2

The Colon and Conjugated Linoleic Acid

Conjugated linoleic acid (CLA) has been found to be associated with a 41% reduction in colon cancer risk. CLA is found in high-fat dairy foods, meats, eggs, and poultry. Study subjects ate four or more servings of high-fat dairy foods per day (Boggs, 2005). For those people at high risk for colon cancer who cannot eat foods high in CLA, supplements are available.

alcohol consumption, physical inactivity, obesity, and a diet high in saturated fat and/or red meat, as well as inadequate intake of fruits and vegetables (American Cancer Society, 2007b). Nursing intervention is directed at public education (Health Promotion Points 29–1).

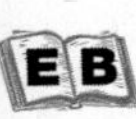

Pathophysiology

The tumor may be polypoid, protruding into the bowel lumen, or it may be annular and extend around the bowel, causing stricture. Most large bowel tumors are adenocarcinomas and are thought to arise from adenomatous polyps that visibly protrude from the mucosal surface of the bowel. The tumor may spread into adjacent structures or via the lymphatics or the bloodstream.

Signs and Symptoms

In the early stages, symptoms are typically mild and vague and depend on the location of the tumor and the function of the affected area. Weight loss may be the first sign. Later signs of colorectal cancer are the result of obstruction of the bowel and extension of the growth to adjacent structures. **Any change in bowel habits, either diarrhea or constipation, could be a sign of colon cancer** (American Cancer Society, 2007b).

Other symptoms include red blood in the stool, black tarry stools, change in stool shape (ribbon-like stool), abdominal distention without weight gain, sensation of incomplete evacuation after a bowel movement, and anemia resulting from intestinal bleeding. Abdominal pain and a sensation of pressure in the lower abdomen or rectum frequently are present. Digital examination may reveal a mass in the anus. Tumors of the rectum or lower sigmoid colon are seen by proctosigmoidoscopy.

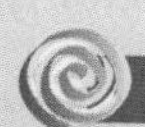

Cultural Cues 29–2

Colorectal Cancer Incidence

Colorectal cancer incidence is highest in African American men and women, with 15% more cases than in white men and women (Mayo Clinic, 2005). Worse yet, mortality rates in African Americans are approximately 40% higher than in the white population. It is not certain whether this is because white people often have better access to health care or for other reasons. Always assess an African American over 40 years of age for risk factors and signs and symptoms of colorectal cancer. Encourage annual screening after age 50.

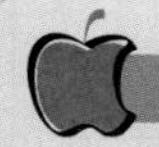

Health Promotion Points 29–1

Colon Cancer Preventive Measures

Preventive measures include a diet that is high in fiber and low in red meat and animal fat. Nutrients that offer protection against colon cancer are fiber, calcium carbonate, selenium, and vitamin C. Recent studies have indicated that NSAIDs such as aspirin or sulindac may reduce the risk of colorectal cancer.

Screening should begin at age 50 with a fecal occult blood test or fecal immunochemical test every year. A flexible sigmoidoscope examination or a double-contrast barium enema should be done every 5 years. For those who have a high risk of colon cancer (familial history, inflammatory bowel disease, or intestinal polyps), a colonoscopy should be performed at least every 10 years.

Key: *NSAIDs,* nonsteroidal anti-inflammatory drugs.

Diagnosis

Diagnostic tests include a stool guaiac test, colonoscopy examination and barium x-ray, and CT scan to determine pelvic organ involvement. If colonoscopy discovers adenomatous polyps early, they are removed, thus preventing colon cancer. Transrectal ultrasound may be utilized to determine the extent of a small rectal lesion. Carcinoembryonic antigen is elevated in 70% of patients with colorectal cancer, but since it is nonspecific to this type of cancer, it is mainly used to monitor the effectiveness of treatment.

Treatment

Treatment of colorectal cancer usually involves surgical removal of the affected portion of the intestine. **Anastomosis** (attachment of one to the other) of the remaining portions is done if the lesion is small and localized **(hemicolectomy).** Larger tumors are treated by excising the affected portion of the colon. Occasionally a surgically created opening on the abdomen **(colostomy)** is needed to provide for elimination of fecal matter. A permanent colostomy is rarely needed for cancer of the colon. After healing takes place, the colon is reconnected.

Most tumors are resected with an open approach, but laparoscopic surgery is an option for a small, localized tumor. Further treatment depends on the stage of the cancer—whether the tumor is through the bowl mucosa, through the bowel wall, or affecting lymph nodes or has metastasized to other organs.

Colectomy or Hemicolectomy. **Colectomy** simply is the removal of the diseased portion of the colon. The remaining ends of the colon are reattached (anastomosed). Hemicolectomy is removal of one half of the colon.

Abdominoperineal Resection. Abdominal resection is performed for cancer in the rectum or low sigmoid colon. It is a very extensive surgical procedure in which part of the colon and the entire rectum, anus, and regional lymph nodes are removed. Both an abdominal and a perineal incision are necessary for this procedure. Because of the nature of the surgery, a permanent colostomy is necessary. Because of the high lithotomy position used during surgery, these patients are at increased risk for thrombophlebitis postoperatively. Colostomy surgery and care are located toward the end of this chapter.

Adjunctive Treatment. Preoperative, intraoperative, or postoperative radiation and chemotherapy may be given for cancer of the rectum. Use of radiation or chemotherapy for colon cancer depends on the stage of the tumor and the presence of metastases. When metastasis is present, the patient is usually treated with 5-fluorouracil (5-FU) with or without leucovorin (folinic acid). Oxaliplatin (Eloxatin) is a new drug used with 5-FU and leucovorin for treatment-resistant tumors. Intra-arterial chemotherapy may be directed into the liver if metastasis has occurred. Two other drugs may be used as well. Bevacizumab (Avastin) is an antiangiogenesis medication that reduces blood flow to the growing tumor cells, depriving them of nutrients needed for replication. Cetuximab (Erbitux) is a monoclonal antibody that binds to protein to slow cell growth. Both are used with other chemotherapy drugs. Irinotecan (Camptosar) is available to treat recurrent colon cancer. Capecitabine (Xeloda) is given orally when the tumor has not penetrated the colon wall.

NURSING MANAGEMENT

Assessment (Data Collection)

A specific abdominal assessment is performed and a history is gathered. Questions are asked regarding bowel pattern and changes, diet pattern, and amounts of red meat and charred or grilled food usually eaten. Determine the amount of alcohol consumption and the degree of cigarette smoking. Assess for a family history of colon cancer. Diagnostic test results such as the CBC, liver enzymes, and amylase are checked for signs of anemia and possible metastatic involvement of the liver or pancreas.

Nursing Diagnosis and Planning

Common nursing diagnoses are located in Table 27–2, but diagnoses specific to cancer are also relevant. The diagnosis Fear related to prognosis of cancer is pertinent.

See Chapter 8 on care of the patient with cancer for further nursing diagnoses and expected outcomes. Individual expected outcomes are written for the specifically chosen nursing diagnoses.

Implementation

The patient is likely to be very anxious once a diagnosis of colon cancer has been made. A calm, supportive, caring attitude while giving care can be helpful. Before surgery, focus on the preoperative care and what the patient needs to be taught. Cover what to expect and provide information about postoperative care. Nursing Care Plan 29–1 describes postoperative care of the patient who has had abdominal surgery with a colectomy.

NURSING CARE PLAN 29–1

Care of the Patient Undergoing Colectomy for Colon Cancer

SCENARIO Mrs. Simpson, age 58, just returned from surgery and has a dressing over the colectomy site. She has a family history of polyposis of the colon. She had a colectomy because of a malignant lesion in the upper portion of the sigmoid colon. She was NPO even before surgery for a variety of tests. She is experiencing pain and receiving morphine by PCA pump. An NG tube was inserted and attached to suction. She is very frightened, because her father died with colon cancer. She dreads chemotherapy. Mrs. Simpson is a loan officer with a national bank, is very busy, and had put off having a physical and sigmoidoscopy until this month, when she noticed some blood in a loose stool. She had experienced some bouts of loose stools but thought these were a result of the stress she was experiencing on her job.

PROBLEM/NURSING DIAGNOSIS *Abdominal pain*/Pain related to abdominal surgery.

Supporting assessment data *Subjective:* "I'm still really hurting." *Objective:* Colectomy, abdominal incision with wound drain. Pain at 5 on 1-to-10 scale.

Goals/Expected Outcomes	Nursing Interventions	Selected Rationale	Evaluation
Pain will be controlled with analgesia during hospitalization	Assess for pain q 3–4 hr using pain scale and document location and characteristics.	Pain scale use provides more objective measure of pain.	Pain at 2–3 with use of PCA.
Pain will be controlled by oral medication at discharge	Monitor use of PCA pump.	PCA allows patient better control over pain.	Using PCA appropriately.
Patient will use relaxation techniques to decrease pain before discharge	Teach relaxation techniques to decrease anxiety.	Relaxation helps decrease pain.	Taught deep breathing relaxation exercise.
	Provide comfort measures.	Comfort measures such as a tidy room and bed and quiet environment help decrease pain.	Comfort measures provided. Continue plan.

Key: *BP,* blood pressure; *CBC,* complete blood count; *I&O,* intake and output; *IV,* intravenous; *NG,* nasogastric; *NPO,* nothing by mouth; *P,* pulse; *PCA,* patient-controlled analgesia; *PRN,* as needed; *R,* respirations; *WBC,* white blood cell.

NURSING CARE PLAN 29-1

Care of the Patient Undergoing Colectomy for Colon Cancer—cont'd

PROBLEM/NURSING DIAGNOSIS *Ordered NPO*/Imbalanced nutrition: less than body requirements related to NPO status and nasogastric tube.

Supporting assessment data *Objective:* NPO for 3–5 days; NG tube in place; IV infusing.

Goals/Expected Outcomes	Nursing Interventions	Selected Rationale	Evaluation
Patient will not develop fluid or electrolyte imbalance as evidenced by good skin turgor, moist mucous membranes, and electrolyte studies within normal range	Maintain patency of NG tube with irrigations of 30 mL normal saline every 2 hr as ordered.	NG tube with suction drains secretions from stomach, decreasing nausea and distention.	NG tube irrigated with normal saline × 5; patent.
	Keep tube above level of stomach; loop with tape and pin to gown; maintain on low continuous suction.	Tube functions best if kept above level of stomach.	Tube coiled and pinned to gown above stomach level.
	Assess amount and character of stomach secretions q shift and document.	Character of stomach secretions will reveal bleeding should it occur.	250 mL light-brown fluid drainage this shift.
	Assess for signs of dehydration.	Further dehydration can then be prevented.	Mucous membranes moist; skin turgor adequate.
	Maintain IV fluid flow.	Provides fluid, preventing dehydration.	IV flowing at 125 mL/hr.
Patient will not develop complications of IV therapy during hospitalization	Maintain I&O record.	I&O record helps evaluate fluid status.	Intake 1000 mL IV; output 895 mL this shift.
	Monitor electrolyte lab values.	Lab values indicate electrolyte imbalances should they occur.	Lab values to be drawn in A.M. No signs of electrolyte imbalance. Continue plan.

PROBLEM/NURSING DIAGNOSIS *Fresh surgical sites and risk for ileus*/Risk for infection related to colectomy and abdominal incision.

Supporting assessment data *Objective:* Colectomy and abdominal incision with drain.

Goals/Expected Outcomes	Nursing Interventions	Selected Rationale	Evaluation
Patient will not experience wound infection as evidenced by temperature and WBC count within normal range at discharge, wound clean and dry without redness, pain, or purulent drainage	Assess IV site q shift for redness, leaking, pain, and patency; document.	Assessing for signs of infection identifies infection early.	IV site clean, without redness, dry, and patent.
	Track temperature and WBC count.	Changes may indicate beginning infection.	Temp 98.8° F (37.1° C); WBC count 9400.
	Check for adequate urine output before hanging IV solution containing potassium.	Giving IV potassium before regular kidney function has returned can cause kidney failure.	Urine output 85 mL/hr.
	Assess IV site before administering each antibiotic IV piggyback medication.	Extravasation of some antibiotics can cause severe tissue irritation and phlebitis.	IV site patent without redness when antibiotic started.
	Maintain IV flow at ordered rate; check q 30 min.	Too fast an IV flow rate may cause fluid overload.	IV infusing at 125 mL/hr as ordered.
	Reinforce dressings PRN; change q 24 hr or PRN when ordered. Use strict aseptic technique for dressing changes. Clean skin around incision with ordered solution.	Maintaining sterile intact dressing decreases chance of infection.	Incision clean and dry without redness. Sterile dressing in place; reinforced once.
	Maintain patency of drain.	Drain must be patent to perform.	Drain in place; not visible.
	Monitor temperature and WBC counts.	Rising temperature and WBC counts indicate possible infection.	Temperature 97.8° F (36.6° C); CBC to be drawn in A.M. Continue plan.

Continued

NURSING CARE PLAN 29–1

Care of the Patient Undergoing Colectomy for Colon Cancer—cont'd

Goals/Expected Outcomes	Nursing Interventions	Selected Rationale	Evaluation
Patient will not experience ileus	Auscultate for bowel sounds q shift; assess for abdominal distention.	Bowel sounds indicate return of peristalsis.	Bowel sounds not present.

PROBLEM/NURSING DIAGNOSIS *Potential for bleeding from surgery*/Risk for ineffective tissue perfusion related to possible bleeding at surgical site.

Supporting assessment data *Objective:* Fresh colectomy incision.

Goals/Expected Outcomes	Nursing Interventions	Selected Rationale	Evaluation
Patient will maintain adequate tissue perfusion as evidenced by stable vital signs and adequate urine output	Assess vital signs per postop routine: q ½ hr for 2 hr, q 1 hr for 2 hr; q 2 hr for 4 hr; then q 4 hr until stable.	Vital signs can indicate hemorrhage.	P 86, R 18, BP 136/84. Stable.
	Notify physician of tachycardia with increased respirations that is not relieved by pain medication, or blood pressure 15–20 points below preoperative baseline level.	Tachycardia with increased respirations and falling blood pressure indicates hemorrhage.	
	Monitor hourly urine output; report if <30 mL for 2 consecutive hours.		Urine output 75 mL over 2 hr.
	Assess dressings for bleeding; check underneath patient.		Dressings dry; no drainage under patient.
	Assess abdomen for increasing girth or rigidity.		Abdomen not rigid; girth not increasing. Continue plan.

PROBLEM/NURSING DIAGNOSIS *Potential for lung problems*/Risk of ineffective breathing pattern related to anesthesia, analgesia, and postoperative pain.

Supporting assessment data *Subjective:* "I don't want to cough." *Objective:* Underwent general anesthesia; receiving morphine via PCA. Shallow breaths.

Goals/Expected Outcomes	Nursing Interventions	Selected Rationale	Evaluation
Patient will not develop atelectasis as evidenced by normal breath sounds in all lobes of lungs	Assist patient to turn, cough effectively, and deep breathe at least every 2 hr.	Coughing and turning assists with lung expansion.	Coughing and turning q 2 hr. Decreased breath sounds in bases of lungs.
	Monitor for proper use of incentive spirometer.	Incentive spirometer helps prevent atelectasis.	Using incentive spirometer correctly q 2 hr.
	Auscultate lungs q shift.	Auscultation tells whether all areas of the lungs are aerating.	Decreased breath sounds in bases bilaterally; no adventitious sounds.
Patient will not develop respiratory infection from retained secretions during hospitalization	Monitor temperature and assess sputum characteristics.	Temperature and sputum characteristics are indicators of whether infection is present.	Temperature 99° F (37.2° C). Continue plan.

NURSING CARE PLAN 29–1

Care of the Patient Undergoing Colectomy for Colon Cancer—cont'd

PROBLEM/NURSING DIAGNOSIS *Afraid she may have cancer*/Anxiety related to fear of cancer, its treatment, and possible death.

Supporting assessment data *Subjective:* Father died of colon cancer; expresses fear of cancer and death; dreads chemotherapy.

Goals/Expected Outcomes	Nursing Interventions	Selected Rationale	Evaluation
Patient will openly discuss fears and concerns with nurse, family, or physician	Establish trusting relationship with patient by active listening and attentive caring.	A trusting relationship helps patient express feelings.	Not wanting to talk yet; spent silent time with patient.
	Encourage "labeling" fears; talk through each one.	Voicing fears and anxieties decrease their impact.	Is withdrawn and quiet; doesn't wish to discuss situation until pathology report is back. Sat quietly with patient for 15 min. Continue plan.
Patient will verbalize positive outlook on chances for survival by discharge	Provide patient with positive statistics regarding colon cancer treated in early stages.	A positive outlook increases chances of survival if cancer is present as patient tends to fight harder.	
	Encourage patient to view cancer as a challenge rather than a defeat.	Outlook affects motivation for self-help.	
	Explain that she has a lot of control over her body and immune system and assist her with relaxation and imagery exercises.	Relaxation and imagery decrease stress and help the immune system.	
	Help patient to express positive things about herself.	Feeling positive about the self empowers the patient.	

? CRITICAL THINKING QUESTIONS

1. Why is it significant that she has familial polyposis?
2. What should other family members be told, and how would you explain the situation to them?

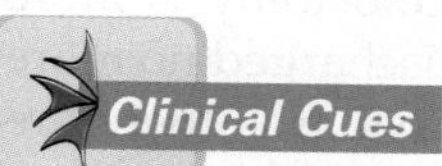

Encourage the patient to think positively about the prognosis since if the tumor is removed before it has penetrated the bowel wall, a complete cure is very likely. A lot of energy can be wasted worrying about something before one knows it is truly a problem.

Evaluation

Data are gathered regarding the nursing actions performed to see if they have been effective in helping the patient to meet the stated expected outcomes. If interventions are not working, the plan is changed.

OSTOMY SURGERY AND CARE

COLOSTOMY

In this procedure, an abdominal incision is made, and the colon is brought to the outside to drain fecal material. A colostomy may be required after a colectomy. The colostomy may be permanent or temporary. If it is a temporary colostomy, the patient must return to surgery later for anastomosis of the open ends.

Types of Ostomies

There are three basic types of colostomy surgery for intestinal disorders, and the stomas thus created are called (1) *loop colostomy;* (2) *double-barreled colostomy;* and (3) *single-barreled* or *end colostomy.*

? Think Critically About . . . What do you think might be concerns of the person who is to have a colostomy?

Loop Colostomy. As the name implies, a loop of the colon is brought through an abdominal incision and onto the surface of the body. Some kind of rod or bridge is placed under the loop to prevent it from slipping back into the abdominal cavity (Figure 29–6). The loop is formed and secured in place while the patient is in the operating room. About 2 days later, the surgeon will open the colostomy in surgery or at the patient's bedside. This may be done with an electric cauterizing instrument, a scalpel, or surgical scissors and does not require anesthesia because the bowel has no sensory nerve endings.

Once the surgeon has made the opening in the wall of the intestine, fecal material passes through the opening (stoma) in the loop of the intestine. An appliance for collection of fecal material should be on hand before the intestine is opened so that it can be attached immediately after the stoma has been created. The pouch that collects feces fits over the stoma made by the slit in the loop of intestine. After about 5 to 7 days, the surgeon may remove the bridge if the stoma has adhered to the abdominal wall.

Double-Barreled Colostomy. In a double-barreled colostomy, there are two separate stomas (Figure 29–7). The loop of intestine is completely severed, creating a *proximal stoma* and a *distal stoma.* The proximal stoma is the one closer to the small intestine, and so fecal material passes through it to the outside. The distal stoma leads to the rectum and should discharge only small amounts of mucus. The distance between the stomas varies; if they are too close together, it is difficult to get a good seal for the collection device around each one. Eventually the colon ends will be reattached.

Single-Barreled or End Colostomy. There is only one stoma in a single-barreled colostomy. It is located on the lower left quadrant of the abdomen and is the proximal end of the sigmoid colon. The end is brought to the abdominal surface, *effaced* (cuffed over itself), and sutured to the skin, making what is called a surgically mature stoma. If the colostomy is temporary, the remaining portion of bowel and rectum are left intact. If the colostomy is permanent, an abdominal perineal resection is done to remove the freed bowel, anus, and rectum.

Colostomy Locations

An ascending colostomy is one in which either one end or a loop of a portion of the ascending colon is brought to the surface of the abdomen to form a stoma. The stool from an ascending colostomy is thus watery and unformed.

An ascending colostomy usually is temporary and is done to allow the bowel distal to the ostomy to rest and heal. This is sometimes necessary for the patient with IBD, to reconstruct an intestinal birth defect, or for the patient who has experienced an intestinal tear from trauma. After the rest and healing period, the surgeon will replace and reattach the intestine ends, and fecal material can be defecated normally.

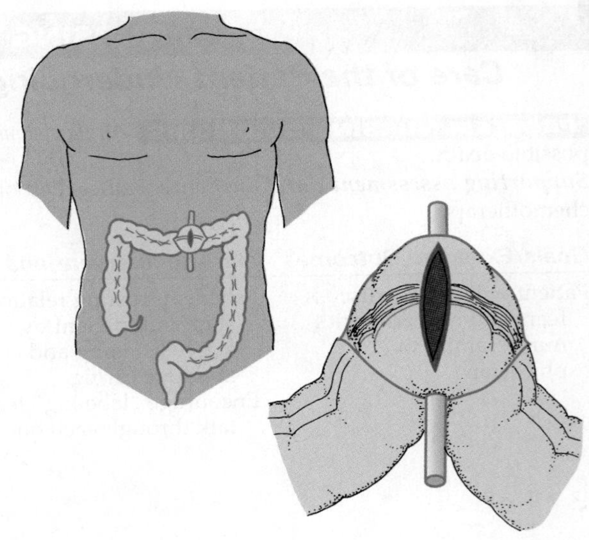

A segment ot transverse colon that is brought out through the abdominal wall and supported by a bridge. A slit in the bowel allows feces to drain from proximal colon. Support is removed 5 to 7 days after surgery or when the bowel adheres to the abdominal wall.

FIGURE 29–6 A loop transverse colostomy: first stage.

A transverse colostomy is situated toward the middle of the abdomen, which is where the transverse colon is located. This kind of colostomy usually is temporary. The stool from a transverse colostomy is semiliquid and is discharged unpredictably.

A sigmoid (descending) colostomy is located on the surface of the lower quadrant of the abdomen (see Figure 29–7). It is the most common type of permanent colostomy and usually is done to treat cancer of the rectum. The stool from a sigmoid colostomy is more solid and well formed and may be discharged no more often than once a day or every 2 days. It is therefore much easier to establish a pattern of evacuation to control the flow of fecal material through a sigmoid colostomy.

ILEOSTOMY

An **ileostomy** is performed to drain fecal material from the ileum. It is indicated when disease, congenital defects, or trauma require bypassing the entire colon. The most common indications for ileostomy are chronic IBD, such as ulcerative colitis and Crohn's disease (regional ileitis), malignancy, and the presence of many polyps in the colon *(multiple polyposes).* The last disease is hereditary, and the polyps have a high potential for malignancy.

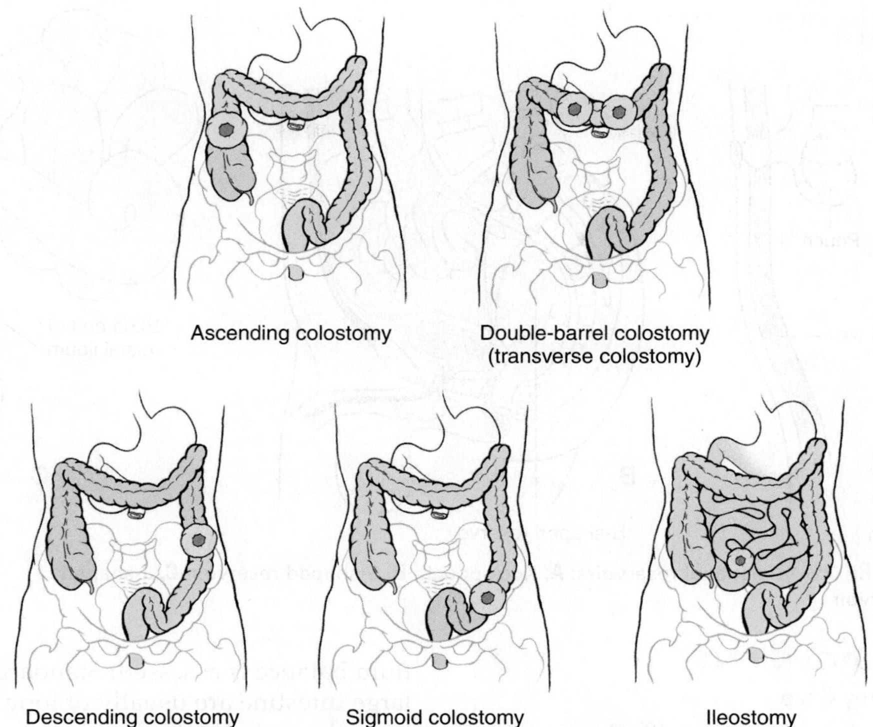

FIGURE 29–7 Types of ostomies and intestinal diversions.

The site for the stoma of an ileostomy must be carefully selected so that it is not near any bony prominences, folds of skin, or scars and is in a place where the patient can see it and care for it (see Figure 29–7). The stool from an ileostomy is liquid, and even though digestion is completed by the time the fecal material reaches the stoma, it still contains digestive enzymes that are highly irritating to the skin.

Surgeons may use other techniques to create an ileostomy. The pouch ileostomy or continent ileostomy frees the ileostomy patient from the need to wear a collection device. A small segment of the ileum is looped back on itself to form a pouch (Kock pouch), and a nipple effect is created (Figure 29–8). Pressure from the accumulating feces closes the nipple valve, preventing constant drainage through the stoma. The patient empties the pouch every 3 to 4 hours during the day by inserting a catheter into the stoma.

Not every patient can be treated by this surgical technique. It has some disadvantages and must be performed by a surgeon skilled in the procedure. Among those who are not good candidates for a continent ileostomy are patients with chronic inflammatory disease as it tends to recur. Another contraindication has to do with the patient's potential for self-care. Because a catheter must be inserted for periodic drainage of the Kock pouch, the patient must be mature enough and sufficiently able to comprehend instructions in self-care and be able to carry them out. The third contraindication is related to previous surgery. Patients who have had a conventional ileostomy cannot have a continent ileostomy done if they have less than 29 mm of terminal ileum remaining. This much is needed to construct the nipple valve.

The procedure of choice for ulcerative colitis is the creation of a pouch from the terminal ileum that is sutured directly to the anus. The anal sphincter is left intact and functional. It is a two-stage surgical procedure in which a loop ileostomy is performed and then closed 3 or 4 months later when healing is complete. The reservoir may be J-shaped or S-shaped (see Figure 29–8). Most patients then have three to eight bowel movements a day. Slight fecal incontinence may be a problem, particularly at night. This procedure is performed only on those patients under age 55 who do not have any anal sphincter deterioration. The mucosa is stripped from the small segment of the rectum that is retained in order to prevent recurrent ulcerative colitis. "Pouchitis" occurs in about 29% of patients and tends to be recurrent. A course of metronidazole (Flagyl) may adequately treat pouchitis. Otherwise antibiotics and/or steroids are employed.

Although not every patient needing an ileostomy can have a continent ileostomy, it is a safe and effective procedure for many. It eliminates the need for an external appliance, is a more natural way to handle waste, greatly reduces fear of embarrassment from leakage of gas and feces, and minimizes periostomal skin problems.

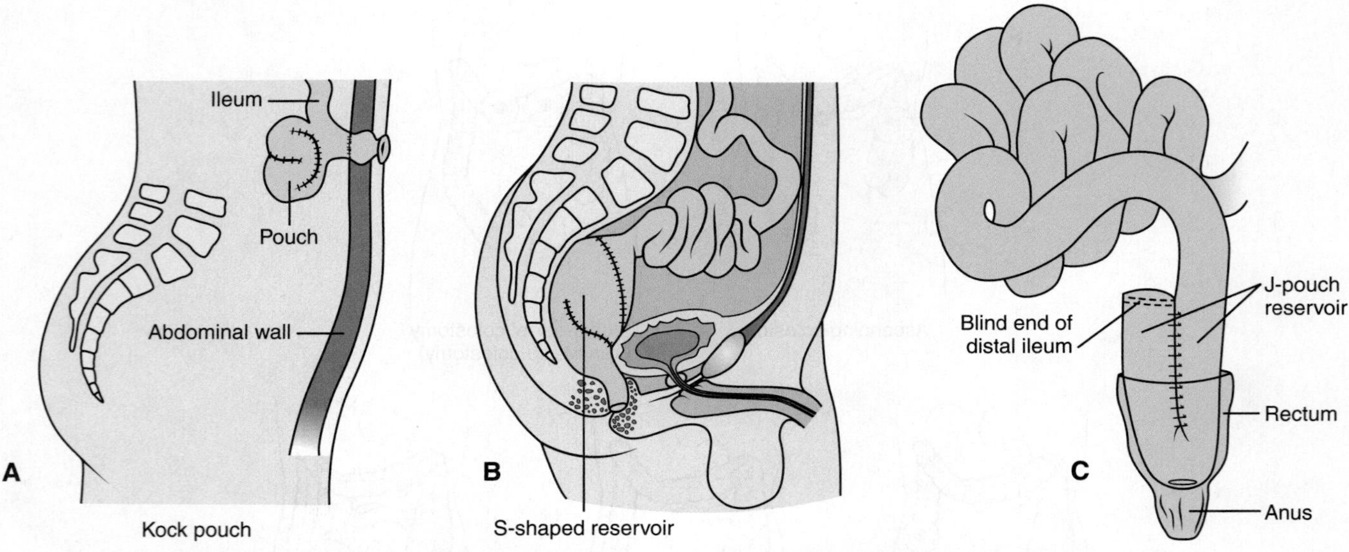

FIGURE **29–8** Ileoanal reservoirs: **A,** Kock pouch. **B,** S-shaped reservoir. **C,** J-shaped reservoir.

NURSING MANAGEMENT

Preoperative Nursing Care

Before surgery of the large intestine, efforts are made to remove as much fecal material from the colon as possible. To accomplish this, the patient is usually placed on a low-residue diet as early as 7 to 10 days before surgery. The last 24 to 72 hours before surgery, the diet is changed to liquids only. Vitamins and minerals may be given to supplement these restricted diets. Antibiotics may be given as prophylaxis against infection of the operative site.

In addition to the dietary preparation, laxatives and enemas are administered to cleanse the lower bowel further. The contents of the stomach are removed by inserting a nasogastric (NG) tube and connecting it to a suction apparatus the morning of surgery. If it is necessary to remove the contents of the small intestine, a specially designed tube that passes through the stomach and into the duodenum is inserted. This tube is called a Miller-Abbott tube (see Figure 29–3). It is attached to the suction apparatus and given the same care as a gastric tube. The tube is usually left in place after surgery to remove accumulations of mucus and gas that may cause distention and strain on the sutures.

POSTOPERATIVE NURSING MANAGEMENT

Assessment (Data Collection)

The immediate postoperative care for the intestinal surgery patient is the same as for other patients having major abdominal surgery. Frequent assessment of vital signs, surgical site, and IV site is carried out. Intestinal drainage is assessed as to amount and character. The patient is assessed for nausea in the early postoperative period. Vomiting places a strain on suture lines. Intake and output are tracked and fluid balance is assessed. Standard operations on the large intestine are usually of long duration. The prolonged period of anesthesia and exposure of the body, with loss of essential fluids, leaves the patient susceptible to shock. Urine output is assessed frequently as decreased output may be a sign of shock.

Psychosocial assessment postoperatively focuses on the patient's perception of his altered body image; the meaning of the altered body part; his usual and current coping skills, emotional state, support systems, and presurgery lifestyle; and his perception of physical prognosis and its impact on his life.

Nursing Diagnosis and Planning

Nursing diagnoses concerning the surgical procedure are much the same as for abdominal surgery (see Nursing Care Plan 29–1; see also Table 27–2). Nursing Care Plan 29–2 presents nursing diagnoses and expected outcomes for the patient with an ostomy.

Implementation

The gastric or intestinal tube is connected to suction as soon as the patient is returned to his room. The patient is NPO for the first 48 hours after surgery. Peristalsis usually becomes active after this period of time, and the NG tube can be removed. The patient will then be able to take liquids by mouth.

The passing of gas, liquids, or solids through the rectum is an indication of active peristalsis. Observe patients carefully for evidence of the return of peristalsis and chart it in the nurse's notes.

The IV site, fluids, and electrolyte levels are monitored very carefully, as the patient is especially prone to fluid and electrolyte imbalances. Pain assessment is ongoing, and the effectiveness of analgesia should be assessed after administering pain medication.

? *Think Critically About . . .* How does the effluent from a transverse colostomy, a sigmoid colostomy, and an ileostomy differ?

Care of the Stoma

The stoma is inspected for a normal pink or red color, which indicates adequate blood supply. It should look like healthy mucous membrane such as that inside the mouth. Later, the stoma will shrink in size and may be less highly colored. There may be slight bleeding around the stoma and its stem, but any more bleeding than this should be reported. Most collection devices are transparent, so that checking for color and bleeding does not require removal of the appliance. The skin around the stoma is assessed for irritation or signs of breakdown.

A noticeable lightening or blanching of the stoma may indicate inadequate blood flow through the tissues of the stoma itself. A deepening of color to a pur-

NURSING CARE PLAN 29–2

Care of the Patient with an Ostomy

SCENARIO A 22-year-old woman has a long history of ulcerative colitis that has not responded to conservative therapy. A permanent ileostomy was performed 3 days ago. She is concerned about learning to care for the ostomy and is upset, fearful, and anxious about the implications and realities it will have for her lifestyle.

PROBLEM/NURSING DIAGNOSIS *Loss of fluid and electrolytes from ileostomy*/Risk for deficient fluid volume related to new ileostomy.

Supporting assessment data *Subjective:* "I'm really thirsty." *Objective:* Ileostomy draining copious amounts of fluid.

Goals/Expected Outcomes	Nursing Interventions	Selected Rationale	Evaluation
Patient's fluid and electrolyte balance will be maintained as evidenced by sodium and potassium levels within normal range and normal skin turgor, stable weight, and balanced intake and output during hospitalization	Monitor for signs of fluid volume deficit; weight daily.	Bypassing the bowel prevents absorption of fluid and electrolytes. Weight loss may indicate fluid loss and dehydration.	Skin turgor without tenting. Weight down 2 lb from baseline before surgery.
	Monitor electrolyte values. Observe for signs of hypokalemia and hyponatremia.	Laboratory values indicate electrolyte status.	
	Accurately record intake and output and assess pattern.	Intake and output are indicators of fluid balance.	Intake 2800, output 2300; balanced.
	Instruct patient to avoid foods that may cause diarrhea: whole milk, raw fruits, iced or hot fluids.	Foods that irritate the small intestine may induce diarrhea.	Not taking solid foods as yet.
	Administer antidiarrheal agents as ordered.	Antidiarrheal agents decrease or stop diarrhea.	No diarrhea. Continue plan.

PROBLEM/NURSING DIAGNOSIS *Potential skin damage*/Risk for impaired skin integrity related to irritation of ileostomy drainage.

Supporting assessment data *Subjective:* "I don't know that I can care for this ileostomy." *Objective:* Ileostomy drainage containing enzymes and bile salts.

Goals/Expected Outcomes	Nursing Interventions	Selected Rationale	Evaluation
No evidence of skin irritation or breakdown at time of discharge	Inspect skin with each appliance change, document status.	Determines condition of skin.	Skin clean and intact without irritation.
Skin integrity will be maintained at all times	Wash skin with mild soap and water; pat dry thoroughly with a soft towel before applying the appliance.	Prevents excoriation of skin.	Skin washed and dried before appliance applied.
	Maintain an intact appliance.	Prevents effluent reaching the skin. Prevents skin breakdown.	Appliance adherence intact.
	Treat beginning skin irritation immediately.	Prevents infection and skin damage.	No skin irritation.

Continued

NURSING CARE PLAN 29-2

Care of the Patient with an Ostomy—cont'd

PROBLEM/NURSING DIAGNOSIS *Nervous about ostomy care and effect on life*/Anxiety related to self-care of ostomy and impact on lifestyle.

Supporting assessment data *Subjective:* "I'm afraid it will smell." "I'm not sure I can handle this." "How will I work?" "Can I still exercise?"

Goals/Expected Outcomes	Nursing Interventions	Selected Rationale	Evaluation
Patient will have decreased anxiety by discharge as evidence by expressed confidence in ability to handle problems of odor, appliance change, application of skin barrier, and work schedule	Establish trusting relationship, allow her to verbalize concerns and fears freely. Answer questions honestly.	Trust makes it easier to share concerns.	Answering her questions. Seems a bit less anxious.
	Assist her to identify potential problems and ways to solve them.	Anticipating problems and solutions decreases anxiety.	Is thinking about activities where she may have problems.
Within 6 mo patient will have adjusted lifestyle and be able to participate in usual activities without problems	Encourage learning of self-care; give praise for efforts and accomplishments.	Praise for self-care increases confidence.	Is participating in self-care activities of grooming. Is beginning to handle equipment and is watching appliance change.
	Enlist aid of enterostomal therapist for suggestions of how to handle ileostomy during exercise class and at work.	Enterostomal therapist knows how to instruct the patient in these areas.	Enterostomal therapist is visiting patient daily. Continue plan.

PROBLEM/NURSING DIAGNOSIS *Unfamiliar with ostomy care*/Deficient knowledge related to care of ileostomy and self-care.

Supporting assessment data *Subjective:* States she has never seen an ostomy stoma. Doesn't know anything about ostomy care; unaware of diet restrictions and precautions.

Goals/Expected Outcomes	Nursing Interventions	Selected Rationale	Evaluation
Patient will demonstrate ability to empty appliance, clean skin, apply skin barrier, and reattach a clean appliance within 3 wk	Encourage patient to look at stoma, utilize consistent teaching plan for care of stoma, appliance, and skin.	Acceptance of stoma is essential to self-care practices.	Is beginning to look at stoma.
	Demonstrate care of ileostomy step-by-step; leave written instructions with patient.	Teaching imparts needed knowledge.	Care demonstrated; written instructions left with patient.
	Have patient begin by doing one part of care and increasing the tasks each day.	Knowledge is integrated better when it is built slowly.	Is slowly learning to care for ostomy and apply appliance to ostomy.
Patient will verbalize ways to prevent odor, protect skin, and prevent problems of fluid and electrolyte imbalance	Instruct her in dietary precautions, signs and symptoms of fluid and electrolyte imbalance and what to do should they occur.	Knowledge is necessary to prevent problems and complications.	Instruction in diet precautions given; gave written instructions for what to watch for in electrolyte imbalance and what to do.
	Show various ways to prevent odor; instruct in foods to avoid because they cause offensive odor; have enterostomal therapist work with patient.	Being odor free enhances self-confidence.	Enterostomal therapist working with patient on these issues. Continue plan.

NURSING CARE PLAN 29-2

Care of the Patient with an Ostomy—cont'd

PROBLEM/NURSING DIAGNOSIS *Feels unattractive*/Disturbed body image related to altered method of elimination.

Supporting assessment data *Subjective:* States she feels that she will not be attractive to any man now that she has an ostomy.

Goals/Expected Outcomes	Nursing Interventions	Selected Rationale	Evaluation
Will begin acceptance of ileostomy before discharge as evidenced by looking at stoma, applying own appliance, and cleaning equipment	Assist her to list reasons the ileostomy was necessary; list the positive benefits of having the ileostomy versus the way things were before the surgery.	Will be able to see that life-giving benefits outweigh difficulties of having an ostomy.	Is making the list.
Within 6 months will be comfortable with new body image	Encourage discussion of male-female relationships for ostomates with ostomy group visitor and enterostomal therapist.	Knowing that other ostomates have a normal sexual life, partners, spouses, and friends will reassure her.	Will see fellow ostomate tomorrow.
	Assist her to look at positive strengths of the person she still is.	The ostomy is only one small part of her as a person.	Is making a list of her strengths. Continue plan.

? CRITICAL THINKING QUESTIONS

1. How can an ileostomy make a patient's life easier?
2. What foods would you counsel her to avoid?

plish hue may indicate obstruction of blood flow to the stoma.

Observe the stoma for signs of edema. In the early postoperative period, the stoma will be slightly edematous and larger than after complete healing has taken place. Stoma edema can be caused by a collection device that has an opening too narrow to accommodate the stoma. The opening of the collection device should be at least ⅛ inch larger than the circumference of the stoma.

Fecal output from the colostomy stoma does not occur for 2 to 4 days, as the patient has been NPO for surgery. If there is a perineal wound, the appearance, amount, and character of drainage are assessed and charted. Careful inspection for signs of infection is done. Such a wound may be left open to heal by secondary intention, in which case it may be 3 months before it is completely healed. Initially there will be a drain in the wound. Antibiotic therapy is usually given for a few days postoperatively to prevent infection.

A surgical dressing is never placed over an ileal stoma. If there is a significant decrease in ileal output accompanied by stomach cramping, the ileum may be obstructed. Such symptoms should be reported to the surgeon immediately. If the condition is not relieved, perforation or rupture of the intestine eventually may occur.

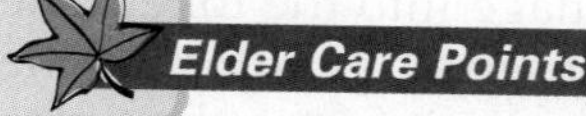

Elder Care Points

Elderly patients may require assistance with ostomy care because of poor vision or severe arthritis in the hands. In this case, a family member or significant other must be taught the techniques of care. The elderly patient needs easy-to-follow, large-print instructions for care. For the elderly patient, the focus of care is on improving the quality of life and ways to remain independent.

Measurement of Intake and Output

Accurate recording of intake and output is especially important in the care of an ostomy patient. Total output of fecal material is calculated every 8 hours. If the stool is liquid, the accuracy of measurement is very important. When the patient's condition is stable, ostomy output is regular, and the patient's nutrition and hydration status are normal, intake and output recording is discontinued.

The ileostomy patient must always be watched for signs of dehydration and fluid imbalance. This is especially important during the immediate postoperative period but remains a concern as long as the patient has the ileostomy. To prevent dehydration, fluid intake should be sufficient to compensate for the loss of fluid through the feces.

Evacuation and Irrigation

Once the patient is eating again, ileostomy drainage is usually emptied every 2 or 3 hours. The pouch should be emptied when it is half full. The patient sits on the toilet, unclamps the drainage device, and allows the effluent to drain into the bowl. The clamp is then closed, and the outside of the bag is cleansed of any debris. Ileostomies are not usually irrigated unless there is blockage by large particles of undigested food, and then only by a physician or enterostomal therapist.

A continent ileostomy with Kock pouch has a drainage tube inserted and attached to suction in the immediate postoperative period to prevent distention and allow the pouch to heal. In about 2 weeks, the patient is taught to insert a catheter into the pouch to drain the contents. As the pouch matures and its capacity increases, the time between drainings will lengthen. The pouch may be irrigated occasionally to remove fecal residue.

A sigmoid colostomy will usually drain formed stool on a relatively regular schedule. Irrigation of the colostomy gives the patient some control over when elimination takes place. The procedure is done daily or every other day at about the same time and takes close to an hour. A catheter with a cone tip is attached to a bag, which is filled with 500 to 1000 mL of warm (not hot) tap water. The bag is positioned 18 to 20 inches above the height of the stoma. The colostomy appliance is removed and an irrigating sleeve is attached to direct the drainage into the toilet. The cone tip is lubricated and inserted gently into the ostomy stoma, and the water is infused slowly to prevent cramping and distention. The cone tip is removed, and the drainage flows through the sleeve into the toilet. When drainage is complete, the sleeve is removed, skin care is performed, and a clean appliance is secured in place (Assignment Considerations 29–1). If the patient is fortunate enough to have a regular evacuation pattern, irrigation is not necessary.

The major reason for irrigating a colostomy is to establish a pattern of predictable bowel movements at the convenience of the colostomate. If the patient prefers not to irrigate, suppositories can be used to stimulate evacuation. The patient does need to wear a drainable pouch if he does not irrigate, as evacuation can be unpredictable.

Periostomal Skin Care

The area of skin around the stoma must be kept clean and protected from fecal material seeping around the opening of the collection device and pooling on the skin. Drainage from an ileostomy contains enzymes and bile salts that are very damaging to the skin. In the immediate postoperative period, the pouch should not be changed any more than is necessary to avoid trauma to the skin.

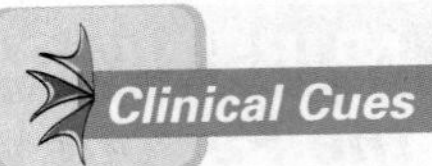

Gently placing a cotton tamponade into the stoma opening after removing the appliance will prevent ileostomy contents from getting on the skin and causing irritation.

The two major principles to follow to protect the skin are cleanliness and the provision of a protective barrier to prevent contact between the skin and the discharge from the stoma. If there is a proper seal to prevent seepage of either feces or urine around the stoma, irritation and breakdown of the skin occur much less frequently.

Appliances are generally changed twice a week in order to maintain an effective seal. When the appliance is changed, it should be removed carefully and the skin washed gently with soap and water so that it is not damaged by vigorous rubbing and scrubbing. The area should be rinsed thoroughly and dried by patting, not rubbing, the skin. In humid weather, a hair dryer on the low setting may be used to dry the skin. Possible causes of skin problems are allergic reactions, yeast infections, or irritation from changing the faceplate too frequently. A protective skin barrier paste, which serves to prevent contact between the skin and the waste being discharged through the stoma, is applied after cleansing. This may or may not be used for a sigmoid colostomy stoma.

Protective barriers are available in a number of forms and types. The enterostomal therapist or surgeon will indicate which type of barrier is most effective for the individual patient. Should the skin become highly irritated in spite of efforts to protect it, the physician will prescribe topical medications. Fungal infection of the skin sometimes occurs.

Gauze packing of a perineal wound is changed regularly. There initially will be a large amount of serous drainage from the wound.

Changing the Collection Device

There are essentially two kinds of pouches or appliances: the temporary, or disposable, pouch and the permanent, or reusable, pouch. Both types are either

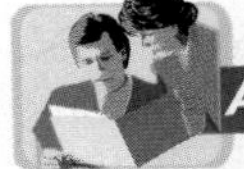

Assignment Considerations 29–1

Ostomy Care

The care of a new postoperative ostomy should not be assigned to unlicensed assistive personnel (UAPs) as assessments of the stoma, incision, and skin are essential. When ostomy care for a mature ostomy is assigned to a certified nursing assistant (CNA) or UAP, remind the person to note the color of the stoma and to report if the stoma appearance is not rosy pink. Ask that you be informed immediately if there is excoriation of the skin. Seek a report on the appearance of the stoma, the condition of the skin, and the type and amount of effluent.

drainable or closed-ended. Each is attached to a faceplate that is secured to the skin around the stoma with a special adhesive. Drainable pouches are used when regulation of the flow of waste cannot be established and the contents must be emptied frequently throughout the day (Figure 29–9). Closed-end pouches are used only for security once bowel movements have been regulated. The new appliance is trimmed to size using a template drawn from the dimensions of the stoma plus ⅛ inch. The appliance should not be constricting to the stoma, but must be tight enough so that skin isn't exposed to effluent (Skill 29–1).

Psychosocial Concerns

Your attitude toward the patient, the stoma, and care has a major impact on the attitude the patient develops about body image changes and self-care. Disposing of body waste is not a pleasant nursing task, but response to the sight and smells can be controlled. A matter-of-fact, efficient approach to caring for the stoma, effluent, and drainage device is best.

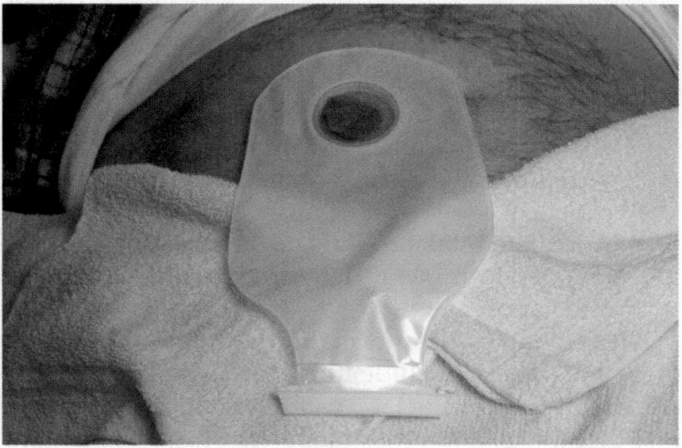

FIGURE **29–9** Ostomy collection appliance in place and sealed around the stoma.

The ostomy patient will go through the stages of grief and loss (see Chapter 8). The nurse provides active listening, emotional support, and understanding. It is essential that a trusting nurse-patient relationship be established to assist the patient with his psychosocial concerns. Only then will the patient respond to encouragement to share feelings openly.

Social interaction with others is encouraged, and contact with available support groups should be initiated. **As soon as postoperative pain is well controlled, it is best if the ostomate can talk with another who has fully adjusted to his ostomy and is living a full and active life.** A series of visits is best to provide time to formulate and answer questions. Such visits do require an order by the physician.

The ostomate should be treated warmly and acceptingly by the nurse. The patient should be guided to express his specific concerns about physical, sexual, and social problems he might encounter as a result of his ostomy. Most patients have concerns about odor, leakage, and noise from the passing of flatus. The nurse encourages joint exploration of necessary changes in lifestyle and suggests realistic alternatives.

The nurse should indicate to the patient that he might have some concerns about sexual function, thereby cueing him that it is acceptable to talk about this area of his life. Concerns should be addressed matter-of-factly, and his sexual partner should be included in discussions. The enterostomal therapist is a

Skill 29–1 Steps for Changing an Ostomy Appliance

- ✓ Gather supplies and don clean gloves.
- ✓ Remove the old appliance by pushing the skin away from the appliance and peeling the appliance downward. Place it in an appropriate trash container.
- ✓ Wash the skin around the stoma with warm water and dry it thoroughly using a soft towel. If there is paste left on the skin, let it dry and then peel it off.
- ✓ Assess the stoma and surrounding skin.
- ✓ Make a template for the appliance using the cutouts on the measuring guide that is 'included with the appliance, or use a see-through measuring grid.
- ✓ Allow 1⁄16" to ⅛" (2–3 mm) around the stoma.
- ✓ Mark the size on an index card, then cut the opening from the card. Mark it "top," "right," and "left" on the face-up side.
- ✓ Place the opening over the stoma to check accuracy. Retrim the opening as needed.
- ✓ Prepare the new skin barrier wafer by using the template and tracing the opening onto the paper backing of the wafer. Indicate "top" on the tracing.
- ✓ Cut the opening just outside the traced line.
- ✓ Remove the paper backing to expose the adhesive.
- ✓ Apply a ring of stoma adhesive paste, if using this, around the opening.
- ✓ Apply a clamp to the bottom of the new pouch if using a drainable appliance.
- ✓ Apply a coating of skin sealant to the skin for the area to be covered by the tape portion of the wafer.
- ✓ Apply the skin barrier wafer to the skin; peel back the paper covering of the tape collar around the ring and press it onto the skin.
- ✓ Attach the appliance to the flange on the wafer and gently press until it snaps into position.

wonderful resource for specific information and suggestions in this area as well.

When the patient continues with dysfunctional grieving too long, becomes clinically depressed, or cannot accept his altered body image, the nurse should seek referral for professional counseling for him. See Nursing Care Plan 29–2 for an example of an individualized care plan for an ostomy patient.

Patient Education

After teaching the patient about the physiology of his ostomy and the steps involved in taking care of the stoma and skin, the nurse teaches the patient how to control odor.

Good basic hygiene is essential. Another measure used to control odor is to eliminate from the diet certain foods known to cause problems with odor or gas. Such foods include eggs, fish, garlic, raw onions, cucumbers, radishes, sauerkraut, corn, broccoli, cabbage, cauliflower, asparagus, dairy products, beans and other legumes, soy, some spices, and chewing gum. Eating too quickly and not chewing food well can cause gas. Carbonated and alcoholic beverages also contribute to the problem.

Gas entering the pouch from the stoma will accumulate there until the pouch is opened and the gas released. This can be done by opening the lower end of the pouch and gently pressing against its sides to remove the gas. If not released, the gas may cause enough pressure to make the device separate from the stoma. Newer pouches have a charcoal-filtered valve that allows gas to escape. Reusable pouches are washed with soap and water and rinsed with cool vinegar solution.

The patient with a colostomy will slowly resume a regular diet. All ostomy patients are taught to prevent problems with diarrhea, constipation, and blockage. Dietary guidelines are more important for the ileostomy patient. Blockage of the ileostomy is fairly common (Patient Teaching 29–1). There will be odor when the drainage pouch is changed or emptied, just as there is with normal bowel movements.

Other pointers that ostomates are taught include the following:

- Ileostomy patients should not take time-release capsules and enteric-coated tablets, as there is not enough time for adequate absorption before the medication is expelled through the stoma.
- Suppositories may be inserted into a colostomy stoma. If it is a double-barreled colostomy, which stoma the suppository is placed into depends on the action of the drug. Glycerin suppositories to stimulate evacuation are inserted in the proximal stoma; a drug that is to be absorbed from the intestine, as for relief of vomiting, should be inserted into the distal stoma, where it will not be expelled.
- Adequate intake of fluids is important for all ostomates to prevent dehydration and electrolyte imbalance.

Many sources of information are available to the ostomate. These include the local branches of the American Cancer Society, ostomate clubs, enterostomal therapists, and other members of the health care

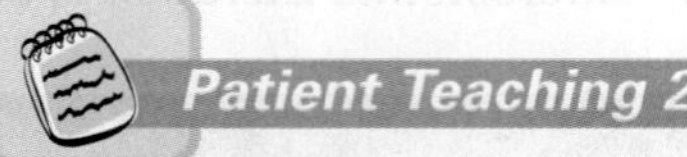

Patient Teaching 29–1

Measures to Prevent Intestinal Blockage for the Ileostomy Patient

Teach the patient the following.

- Eat six small meals a day.
- During the healing period, eat a soft diet.
- Chew food very thoroughly.
- Add other foods to your diet gradually.
- Drink more than 8 cups of fluid per day.
- Avoid the following foods:
  - Dried fruits
  - Corn, including popcorn
  - Nuts
  - Sunflower and other seeds
  - Sausages and foods with casings
  - Apple peel
  - Oranges
  - Pineapple
  - Raw cabbage
  - Celery
  - Chinese vegetables
  - Coconut
  - Mushrooms

Should you experience a blockage in the intestine or of the ostomy:

- Begin a liquid diet.
- Cut the opening in your pouch a little larger than normal because the stoma may swell.
- Take a warm bath to relax the abdominal muscles.
- Massage the abdomen and area around the stomas as this might increase the pressure behind the blockage and help it to "pop out." Most food blockages occur just below the stoma.
- Try different body positions, such as a knee-chest position, as it might move the blockage forward.
- Take oral enzymes to encourage digestion.

If you are still blocked or have no stomal output for several hours:

- Call your physician or enterostomal nurse and report the problems.
- If you cannot reach your physician or the enterostomal nurse, go to the emergency room. Take all of your pouch changing supplies with you.
- DO NOT TRY TO LAVAGE THE ILEOSTOMY.
- DO NOT TAKE A LAXATIVE.

team who have expertise in managing a stoma. Enterostomal therapists are wound care specialists, often with a master's degree, but with certification in wound and ostomy care. Information about local ostomate clubs and groups can be obtained from the United Ostomy Association, Inc., P.O. Box 66, Fairview, TN 37602-0066, telephone (800) 826-0826. A directory of enterostomal therapists to contact for local consultation can be obtained from the Wound Ostomy and Continence Nurses Society at (888) 224-9626.

Evaluation

Evaluation data are gathered regarding the actions performed to see if the expected outcomes are being met. When outcomes are not being met, the plan is revised, choosing new actions directed toward meeting the expected outcomes.

COMMUNITY CARE

Nurses in the community are in a position to do considerable teaching to promote healthy function of the GI system. Promoting a healthy diet with appropriate quantities of fiber and fluid, counseling regarding exercise programs, and teaching about the warning signs of colon cancer are all appropriate nursing interventions to be used whenever possible. Nurses can provide a good example to the public by maintaining weight within normal limits and following a healthy diet and exercise program themselves.

Nurses who work in long-term care facilities and in the home setting must use constant assessment to spot problems of the GI system. Monitoring nutritional and bowel status is standard practice for every patient. It is important to assess on a continuing basis bowel changes that might indicate colon cancer. Remembering that patients who are under care for other disorders still need to have regular cancer screenings, and speaking to the patient and physician about this can help detect early colon cancer.

Questioning patients about digestive problems, watching for undue fatigue that could be caused by anemia from intestinal bleeding, and monitoring for signs of peptic ulcer are other ways community nurses can promote health in the GI system.

Key Points

- A hernia can become incarcerated, trapping intestine and cutting off its blood supply and causing intestinal obstruction.
- An altered bowel pattern, abdominal pain with bloating, and diarrhea or constipation are typical in the patient with IBS. There is no detectable organic disease.
- Diverticulitis produces diarrhea or constipation, left lower abdominal pain, fever, and rectal bleeding.
- Treatment of diverticulitis includes parenteral antibiotics, NPO or a liquid diet, IV hydration, and surgical hemicolectomy.
- A high-fiber diet and lots of fluid are prescribed for the patient with diverticular disease.
- Mechanical bowel obstruction is mainly caused by adhesions, volvulus, intussusception, or strangulated hernia.
- Nonmechanical bowel obstruction may be a result of paralytic ileus following surgery, hypokalemia, infection, uremia, or heavy-metal poisoning.
- Inflammatory bowel disease includes ulcerative colitis and Crohn's disease. A genetic factor is implicated in IBD, and there is increased familial incidence.
- The inflammation of the mucosal lining of the intestinal tract causes ulceration, edema, bleeding, and fluid and electrolyte loss from diarrhea.
- Antidiarrheal drugs, sulfasalazine therapy, drugs to relieve abdominal cramping, and corticosteroids are all used in the treatment of IBD.
- Surgery for ulcerative colitis usually involves a proctocolectomy with ileostomy, a Kock pouch creation, or an ileoanal reservoir.
- Appendicitis (inflammation of the appendix) classically causes right lower quadrant pain accompanied by muscle guarding. Nausea and vomiting, a slight temperature elevation, and an increase in the WBC count may also occur.
- Peritonitis often occurs from a ruptured appendix. It is an inflammation of the peritoneum, and can occur from other causes.
- The inflamed peritoneum produces serous fluid that becomes more and more purulent as the bacteria multiply. Normal peristaltic action slows or ceases.
- Malabsorption in adults is usually from sprue or lactose intolerance, but IBD can also cause malabsorption when transit through the intestines is too rapid. Radiation or chemotherapy can cause malabsorption also.
- A key sign of malabsorption is stool that is bulky, frothy, and foul smelling and floats in the toilet.
- Hemorrhoids are caused by straining at stool for long periods while sitting on the toilet, prolonged standing, prolonged sitting, or pregnancy.
- A pilonidal sinus occurs at the cleft of the buttocks and can be quite painful if infected.
- Anorectal abscess or fistula is painful, and the pain is aggravated by sitting or coughing.
- Cancer of the colon or rectum is the third most common malignancy in the United States.
- Ulcerative colitis, familial polyposis, smoking, alcohol consumption, obesity, physical inactivity, and a diet high in saturated fat or red meat are risk factors for colon cancer.
- Treatment depends on tumor stage and may include surgery, chemotherapy, and radiation.
- Abdominoperineal resection is done for rectal cancer and may include a colostomy.
- A transverse colostomy is usually temporary.
- An ileostomy drains fecal material from the ileum and is usually performed for IBD problems.

- Fluid and electrolyte monitoring is important after an ostomy is performed, but is crucial for the patient with an ileostomy.
- The stoma should be a normal pink or red color, which indicates adequate blood supply.
- Proper skin care is vital to the ostomate. Use of protective powders and skin paste for application of the appliance is a normal part of ostomy care.
- The appliance must be cut to fit the stoma properly, and the opening should be ⅛" larger than the stoma.
- The ostomy patient will go through a grief process, and it is important for the nurse to provide active listening, emotional support, and understanding.

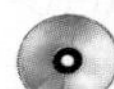

Go to your **Companion CD-ROM** for an Audio Glossary, animations, video clips, and bonus review questions.

evolve Be sure to visit the companion Evolve site at http://evolve.elsevier.com/deWit for interactive NCLEX-PN Exam Style Review Questions, WebLinks, and additional online resources.

NCLEX-PN EXAM STYLE REVIEW QUESTIONS

Choose the best answer(s) for the following questions.

1. The nurse encourages a patient with irritable bowel syndrome to keep a food diary. When asked regarding the importance of the keeping the diary, an appropriate nursing response would be:

1. "The diary will monitor caloric intake."
2. "The diary will help identify foods that cause bloating."
3. "The diary will determine food preferences."
4. "The diary will reinforce the need for better food choices."

2. A 68-year-old patient complains of left lower abdominal pain that is accompanied by diarrhea, fever, and rectal bleeding. The nurse anticipates which of the following treatment measures?

1. Administration of a bulk-forming stool softener
2. Increasing fluid intake
3. Encouraging solid foods
4. Increasing physical activity

3. ______________________ is the telescoping of one part of the bowel into another.

4. The recommended diet for patients with inflammatory bowel disease includes a combination of which of the following? *(Select all that apply.)*

1. Low fat
2. High fiber
3. High protein
4. Low calorie
5. Lactose avoidance

5. During a home visit, the nurse provides verbal instructions to a patient with a possible blockage of the ostomy. An appropriate instruction given by a nurse would be:

1. massage the stoma.
2. try different body positions.
3. take a cold bath.
4. begin a high-fiber diet.

6. Which of the following statements are true regarding Crohn's disease? *(Select all that apply.)*

1. It affects the full thickness of the small intestine.
2. It manifests as bloody diarrhea with abdominal cramping.
3. There is a cobblestone appearance in x-rays.
4. Pseudopolyps are found on the affected segments.
5. There is a greater risk for colon cancer.

7. In caring for an ostomate, which of the following statements is true regarding medication administration?

1. Time-release capsules are not given to patients with colostomy because of increased transit time.
2. Enteric-coated tablets are adequately absorbed by patients with ileostomy.
3. Glycerin suppositories are readily evacuated in the colostomy stoma.
4. An antiemetic suppository can be effectively absorbed when inserted in the distal colostomy stoma.

8. The patient with a new colostomy demonstrates early signs of acceptance in the change of body image when he:

1. allows the nurse to empty the colostomy bag.
2. refuses to look at the ostomy site.
3. gradually participates in ostomy care.
4. continues to sit on the bedpan to have a bowel movement.

9. While changing the colostomy bag, the nurse assesses the stoma and finds noticeable blanching. This most likely indicates:

1. adequate blood flow.
2. obstruction to blood flow.
3. inadequate perfusion.
4. infection.

10. The nurse admits a 23-year-old patient with possible appendicitis. The nurse anticipates which of the following signs and symptoms? *(Select all that apply.)*

1. Increased red cell count
2. Abdominal tenderness
3. Anorexia and vomiting
4. Mild fever
5. Boardlike rigidity

CRITICAL THINKING ACTIVITIES

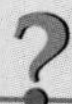

Read each clinical scenario and discuss the questions with your classmates.

Scenario A

Mrs. Blein, age 29, has had frequent bouts of diarrhea associated with physical and emotional stress since her early teens. She is admitted to the hospital with a diagnosis of possible ulcerative colitis. Her admitting physician, a gastroenterologist, feels certain that she has ulcerative colitis and that she will benefit from an ileostomy, as previous efforts on the part of several other physicians have brought no lasting relief from Mrs. Blein's symptoms. She is admitted to the hospital to establish a definitive diagnosis. Mrs. Blein is 40 pounds underweight and is suffering from severe diarrhea and fluid deficit.

1. What questions would be relevant when taking Mrs. Blein's nursing history?
2. What should be included on Mrs. Blein's nursing care plan regarding observations, measurements, and nursing interventions?
3. Discuss some benefits of an ileostomy over the alternative of continued bouts of severe diarrhea.

Scenario B

Mr. Huang, age 52, was found to have occult blood in his stool when he underwent a physical examination for a new insurance policy. Fiberoptic flexible sigmoidoscopy revealed a small lesion in the sigmoid colon; the biopsy result was positive for malignancy. He is scheduled for a hemicolectomy.

1. What are the probable postoperative nursing diagnoses that should be on Mr. Huang's care plan?
2. What are the psychosocial concerns that need to be addressed for this patient? What would be appropriate nursing interventions?
3. What further treatment will be necessary for Mr. Huang?

CHAPTER 30

Care of Patients with Disorders of the Gallbladder, Liver, and Pancreas

evolve http://evolve.elsevier.com/deWit

Objectives

Upon completion of this chapter, you should be able to:

Theory

1. Explain the plan of care for the patient with cholelithiasis.
2. Describe treatment for the patient with cholecystitis.
3. List the ways in which the various types of hepatitis can be transmitted.
4. Identify signs and symptoms of the various types of hepatitis.
5. Devise appropriate nursing interventions for the patient with cirrhosis and ascites.
6. Indicate potential causes of liver failure.
7. Differentiate the signs and symptoms of acute and chronic liver failure.
8. Describe the postoperative care of the patient who has undergone a liver transplantation.
9. Devise a nursing care plan for the patient with cancer of the liver.
10. Prepare a plan for adequate pain control for the patient with pancreatitis.
11. Compare the treatment options for cancer of the pancreas.

Clinical Practice

1. Perform preoperative teaching for a patient who is to undergo laparoscopic cholecystectomy.
2. Write a nursing care plan, including psychosocial concerns, for the patient who has hepatitis and is jaundiced.
3. Design a discharge teaching plan for the patient who has been in the hospital with a flare-up of chronic pancreatitis.

Key Terms

Be sure to check out the bonus material on the Companion CD-ROM, including selected audio pronunciations.

ascites (ă-SĪ-tēz, p. 751)
asterixis (ăs-tĕr-ĬK-sĭs, p. 757)
biliary colic (BĬL-ē-ăr-ē kō-LĬC, p. 741)
caput medusa (KĂP-ĕt mĕ-DŪ-să, p. 752)
cholecystectomy (kō-lĕ-sĭs-TĔK-tō-mē, p. 742)
cholecystitis (kō-lĕ-sĭs-TĪ-tĭs, p. 740)
choledococholithiasis (kō-lĕd-ō-kō-lĭ-THĪ-ă-sĭs, p. 740)
cholelithiasis (kō-lĕ-lĭ-THĪ-ă-sĭs, p. 740)
cirrhosis (sĭr-RŌ-sĭs, p. 751)
encephalopathy (ĕn-sĕf-ă-LŎP-ă-thē, p. 748)
esophageal varices (ĕ-sŏf-ă-JĒ-ăl VĂR-ĭ-sēz, p. 754)
fetor hepaticus (hĕ-PĂ-tĭ-kŭs, p. 757)
hematemesis (hē-mă-TĔM-ĕ-sĭs, p. 756)
hepatitis (hĕ-pă-TĪ-tĭs, p. 744)
icterus (ĬK-tĕr-ŭs, p. 752)
jaundice (JAWN-dĭs, p. 741)
palmar erythema (ĕr-ĭ-THĒ-mă, p. 752)
paracentesis (păr-ă-sĕn-TĒ-sĭs, p. 753)
prodromal stage (prō-DRŌ-măl, p. 749)
pruritus (proo-RĪ-tŭs, p. 752)
pseudocyst (soo-dō-sĭst, p. 759)
spider angioma (SPĪ-dĕr ăn-jē-Ō-mă, p. 752)
varices (VĂR-ĭ-sēz, p. 754)

DISORDERS OF THE GALLBLADDER

CHOLELITHIASIS AND CHOLECYSTITIS

Etiology

Cholelithiasis is the presence of gallstones within the gallbladder itself or in the biliary tract. The stones may vary in size, from very small "gravel" to stones as large as a golf ball. It is usually the smaller ones that cause the most trouble. Tiny stones pass into the bile ducts, where they become lodged and obstruct bile flow (Figure 30–1). When stones lodge in the common bile duct, the patient has **choledocholithiasis**. Cholelithiasis is more likely to occur in people with a sedentary lifestyle, a familial tendency, diabetes mellitus, and obesity (Cultural Cues 30–1). Cholesterol-lowering drugs increase the amount of cholesterol secreted in bile. This can increase the risk of gallstones.

Other people at risk for developing gallstones are those who have hemolytic disease, have had extensive resection of the bowel to treat Crohn's disease, or experience a rapid weight loss. Multiple pregnancies and use of oral contraceptives or hormone replacement therapy increase the chance for gallstone formation.

Cholecystitis is an inflammation of the gallbladder and is associated with gallstones in 90% to 95% of oc-

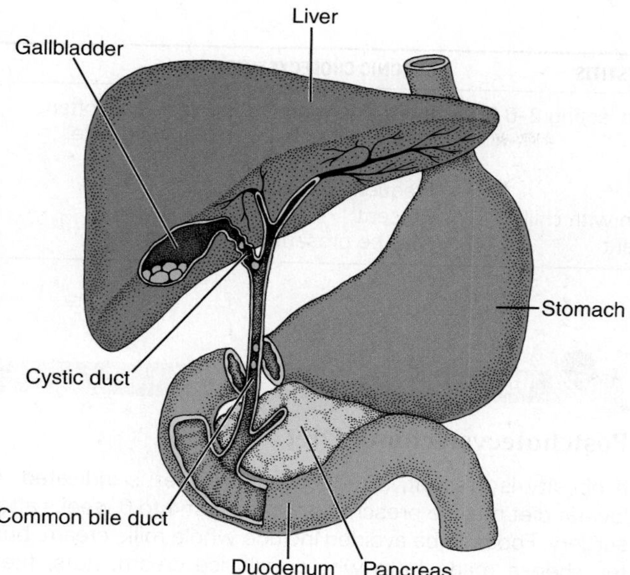

FIGURE 30–1 Gallstones within the gallbladder and obstructing the common bile and cystic ducts.

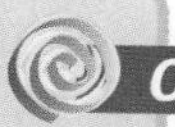

Cultural Cues 30–1

Ethnic Predisposition to Gallstones

Native Americans are genetically more prone to develop gallbladder stones than any other group. Hispanic Americans have the next highest propensity to develop gallstones. Teaching dietary changes to decrease the amount of cholesterol and total fat in the diet may be an effective means of decreasing the incidence of gallstones in these populations.

currences (Health Promotion Points 30–1). Other causes include obstructive tumors of the biliary tract and severely stressful situations such as cardiac surgery, severe burns, or multiple trauma. Trauma can compromise blood supply to the gallbladder.

Pathophysiology

Cholelithiasis (gallstones) develops when the balance between cholesterol, bile salts, and calcium in the bile is altered to the point that these substances precipitate. When cholesterol precipitates, the nucleus of a stone can be formed. The stone grows as layers of cholesterol, calcium, or pigment accumulate over the nucleus. Stasis of bile leads to changes in chemical composition and contributes to stone formation. Immobility, pregnancy, and obstructive lesions decrease bile flow. The formation of stones within the gallbladder can cause irritation and areas of inflammation in the gallbladder wall (cholecystitis). Infection can occur from organisms such as *Escherichia coli* or enterococci. The organisms enter the gallbladder through the sphincter of Oddi from adjacent structures.

Obstruction of bile flow by stones in the cystic or common bile duct causes strong muscle contractions that attempt to move the stones along. This causes severe spasms of pain.

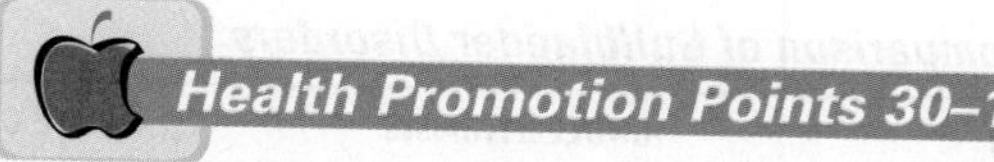

Health Promotion Points 30–1

Gallstones

Patients who have experienced signs and symptoms of gallstones or cholecystitis should be encouraged to have the gallbladder removed. Repeated inflammation and irritation from stones predispose to further bouts of cholecystitis with a negative impact on health, and may be a factor in the development of cancer of the gallbladder.

Signs and Symptoms

Symptoms of gallstones vary from none at all to severe and unbearable pain (**biliary colic**). Symptoms depend on the degree of obstruction to bile flow and extent of inflammation of the gallbladder. If a duct is obstructed by a stone, severe pain may be triggered by a fatty meal. Nausea and vomiting, fever, and leukocytosis occur with cholecystitis. Pain may be referred to the right clavicle, scapula, or shoulder. As bile backs up into the liver and blood, **jaundice** (yellow tint to skin and sclera) occurs. If obstruction is unrelieved, this condition can cause inflammation, which can progress to liver damage.

The symptom most often present in chronic cholecystitis is biliary colic. The pain sometimes is referred to the back at the level of the shoulder blades. Attacks can occur as frequently as daily or may not appear but once every year or so. Vomiting may accompany acute flare-ups, and the person may experience chills and fever. If the inflammation is not corrected or if there is an infection, the gallbladder can become filled with pus and will eventually rupture. Rupture spills gallbladder contents into the abdominal cavity and causes peritonitis.

Chronic cholecystitis causes milder symptoms between acute attacks. Symptoms are indigestion after eating fatty foods, flatulence, nausea after eating, and some discomfort in the right upper quadrant.

? *Think Critically About . . .* What questions would you ask when assessing a patient who might have cholecystitis?

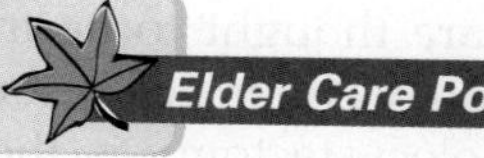

Elder Care Points

Symptoms of gallstones may be atypical in the elderly. Cholelithiasis should be considered a possibility in any elderly patient presenting with abdominal pain when another cause cannot be found. The presenting symptom of cholecystitis in this age-group may be low-grade fever rather than pain.

Table 30–1 Comparison of Gallbladder Disorders

SIGN/SYMPTOM	CHOLELITHIASIS	ACUTE CHOLECYSTITIS	CHRONIC CHOLECYSTITIS
Pain/biliary colic	Sudden onset, acute	Waves of pain lasting 2–6 hr	Intermittent during the year; pain often referred to back at shoulder blade
Nausea, vomiting	Often present	Frequent	During acute attack
Indigestion and flatulence	—	—	Frequent complaint
Low-grade fever	Present	Present, often with chills	Present
Jaundice	If duct is obstructed	May be present	May be present during attack

Diagnosis

Gallstones usually can be diagnosed with ultrasonography or computed tomography (CT) of the gallbladder and biliary tract. If the patient is jaundiced, endoscopic retrograde cholangiopancreatography (ERCP) may be done to detect common duct stones. Cholescintigraphy (hepatoiminodiacetic acid [HIDA] scan) diagnoses abnormal contraction of the gallbladder or obstruction. Liver function tests are helpful to diagnose gallbladder and biliary tract disease. Alanine aminotransferase (ALT) and aspartate aminotransferase (AST) will be slightly elevated. If there is common duct obstruction, gamma-glutamyl transpeptidase is elevated. In biliary obstruction, both direct bilirubin and alkaline phosphatase levels are elevated. The absence of bile in the intestine results in clay-colored stools that float as a result of undigested fat content.

The diagnosis of cholecystitis is aided by blood indicators of infection (elevated white blood cell count and sedimentation rate). Table 30–1 compares signs and symptoms of gallbladder disorders.

Treatment

If the patient does not respond to treatment with a low-fat diet and loss of excessive body weight, or if bile obstruction occurs, correction of the obstructed biliary tract is indicated. Sometimes small stones may be removed during ERCP, in which the common duct can be visualized.

Antibiotics are usually only given if peritonitis is present. Fluids are administered and electrolytes are rebalanced. If surgery is contraindicated, the symptoms might be controlled to some degree by a low-fat diet and restriction of alcohol intake. Meals should be spaced so that no large amounts of food are put into the intestinal tract at any one time. This avoids overstimulation of gallbladder activity (Nutritional Therapies 30–1).

The surgical procedure of choice is **cholecystectomy** (gallbladder removal). If stones are thought to be in the common bile duct, it is explored either before or during surgery. Laparoscopic cholecystectomy is the most common surgical procedure used. Four small incisions are made in the abdomen. Abdominal muscles are not cut, and the patient experiences less pain and a quicker recovery than with an "open" cholecystectomy. A laparoscope with an attached camera and a dissecting laser are used along with grasping forceps.

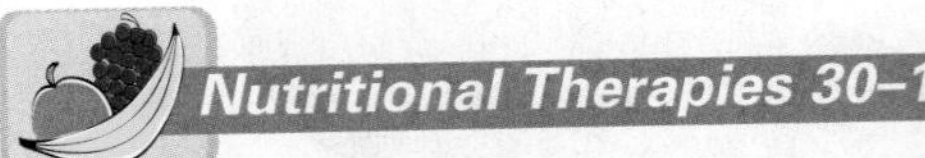

Postcholecystectomy Diet

If obesity is present, a reduced-calorie diet is indicated. A low-fat diet may be prescribed for the first 4 to 6 weeks after surgery. Foods to be avoided include whole milk, cream, butter, cheese made from whole milk, ice cream, nuts, fried foods, rich pastries, and gravies. Smaller, more frequent meals are helpful. Keeping a record of foods eaten and symptom occurrence will indicate other foods that may be a problem for a particular patient.

CO_2 is instilled into the abdominal cavity to aid visualization. The gallbladder is removed through the incision at the umbilicus. The patient will have dressings over the four small incisions on the abdomen. There is essentially no difference in complications or outcomes for either open cholecystectomy or the laparoscopic procedure. Recovery time is shorter for the laparoscopic procedure (Johansson et al., 2005). 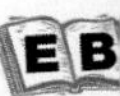

It is especially important to monitor this patient closely for internal bleeding. You and the family should watch for signs of increasing abdominal rigidity and pain and for changes in vital signs. Sometimes the retained CO_2 used during a laparoscopic procedure causes "free air" pain. Early and frequent ambulation helps the gas dissipate. The patient is discharged after recovering from the anesthesia, or 1 day postoperatively, depending on her age and condition, and must have careful discharge teaching about signs of complications (Patient Teaching 30–1).

With an open abdominal cholecystectomy, a 2- to 4-day stay in the hospital is usual and there is about a 6-week recovery period. Residual stones can lodge in the common duct after cholecystectomy. ERCP is usually used to remove residual stones.

Oral dissolution therapy is available and works best on small cholesterol stones. The drugs ursodiol (Actigall) and chenodiol (Chenix) work best. From 6 months to 2 years of oral treatment is required to dissolve the stones.

An experimental procedure called contact dissolution therapy involves injecting a drug, methyl terbutyl ether, into the gallbladder to dissolve stones in 1 to

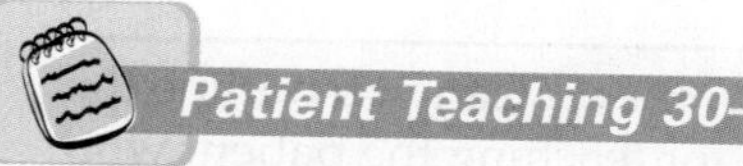

Patient Teaching 30–1

Postoperative Laparoscopic Cholecystectomy

Patient instructions:

- Remove the bandages from the puncture sites the day after surgery and shower.
- Report the following signs and symptoms should they occur:
  - Redness
  - Swelling
  - Bile-colored drainage or pus from any surgical site
  - Severe abdominal pain
  - Nausea, vomiting, chills, or fever
  - Light-colored stool, dark urine, or yellow tint to the eyes or skin as these signs may indicate obstruction to the flow of bile
- Normal activities may be resumed gradually.
- Return to work is probable at 1 week postsurgery.
- Stick to a low-fat diet for several weeks, slowly introducing fattier foods to determine if they cause unpleasant symptoms.

3 days. It is done very carefully as the drug is a flammable anesthetic that can be toxic. It is being tested on patients with noncalcified cholesterol stones (National Digestive Diseases Information Clearinghouse, 2005).

Lithotripsy, or "shock wave" therapy, is occasionally used. The procedure involves using sound waves directed through the body to break up the stones. The procedure takes 1 to 1½ hours, and the debris is then carried by the bile into the intestine. There must be no more than three cholesterol gallstones, each smaller than 1½ inches, and the patient must not be obese.

Nursing Management

Preoperative Care. Preoperatively the patient may have a nasogastric tube to relieve nausea and vomiting. Meperidine or another analgesic may be ordered to decrease pain, and antiemetics are given for nausea (Safety Alert 30–1).

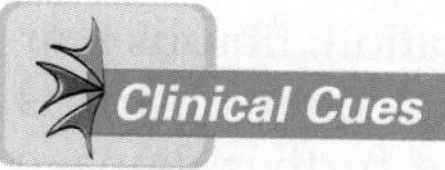

Clinical Cues

Morphine is usually not used because it is thought that it causes biliary spasm and constricts the sphincter of Oddi. An antispasmodic such as dicyclomine (Bentyl) may be used to relax smooth muscles and decrease spasm.

Intravenous (IV) fluids are begun to prevent dehydration if the patient is experiencing symptoms. Coagulation times are monitored if jaundice is present, and vitamin K, if needed, is administered prior to surgery to improve clotting ability of the blood. The patient scheduled for surgery has needs similar to those of any patient having abdominal surgery. Teaching depends to some degree on whether or not the surgery

Safety Alert 30–1

Meperidine Toxicity

A metabolite of meperidine (Demerol) is toxic, and the elderly have difficulty metabolizing and eliminating it. The buildup of the toxin in the blood can cause seizures and other mental status changes such as acute confusion. Ask for an alternate analgesic for these patients.

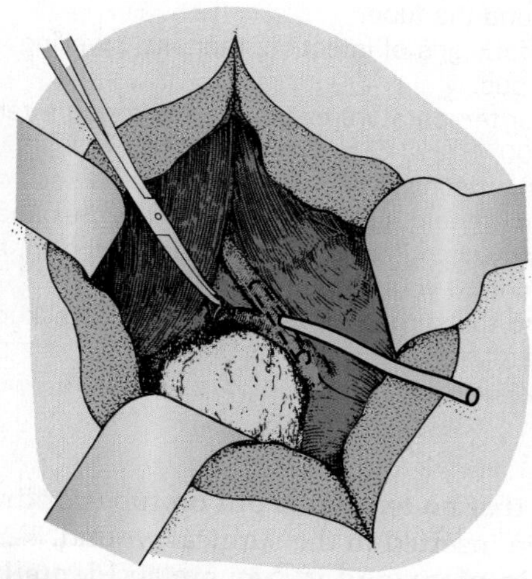

FIGURE 30–2 T-tube inserted into the common bile duct and sutured in place.

is a standard procedure or a laparoscopic procedure (see Chapters 4 and 5).

Postoperative Care. The patient is placed in the semi-Fowler's position after she recovers from anesthesia. Aside from being more comfortable and having less strain on the sutures, the patient will also be able to take deep breaths and cough more easily in this position.

A patient who has had "open" gallbladder surgery needs proper care of the drains or tubes that may be in place when she returns from the operating room. In many cases, the surgery has been performed to relieve an obstruction to the flow of bile through the bile ducts or to drain purulent material to the outside. The drainage is absorbed by the dressings over the surgical wound. These must be changed often and should be checked quite frequently for signs of fresh bleeding. The drain is left in as long as necessary and is then removed by the surgeon.

When an obstruction of the common bile duct has occurred because of stones or tumors, the surgeon may insert a small T-shaped tube (T-tube) directly into the common bile duct during an "open" cholecystectomy (Figure 30–2). This tube must be kept open at all times and is connected to a bedside drainage bag. The length of time the T-tube is left in place depends on the condition of the patient. Only a small amount of bile will be going to the duodenum. Precautions must be

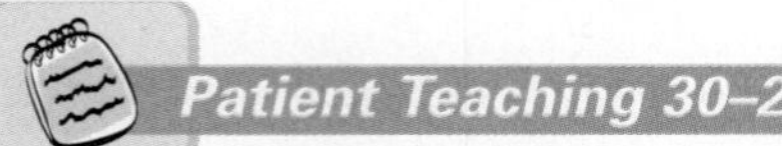

Patient Teaching 30–2

Caring for a T-Tube

Teach the patient to:

- Wear loose-fitting, older clothes.
- Coil the drainage tubing and secure it to the abdomen with tape.
- Take showers rather than baths.
- Avoid heavy lifting and strenuous activity.
- Carefully change the dressing every day, cleansing the skin around the tube.
- Inspect for signs of infection: redness, swelling, warmth, pain, or pus.
- Take your temperature every day and report a temperature >100° F (37° C) to your surgeon.
- Empty the drainage bag at the same time each day.
- Note the amount, color, and odor of the drainage.
- Report any change in drainage, abdominal pain, nausea, or vomiting to your surgeon.
- Return to the surgeon for your follow-up checkup.

taken so that no tension is put on tubes or drains that have been inserted in the surgical wound. **T-tubes are sutured in place, and if they are accidentally pulled out, the patient must be returned to the operating room and the incision reopened to replace the tube.**

With a drain and T-tube, dressings must be changed with careful handling of the tube or drain. Montgomery straps are best for holding the dressings in place. The sight of so much greenish yellow discharge (bile) on the dressings may upset the patient unless she is told that this is to be expected (Patient Teaching 30–2). The drainage bag is emptied when the dressing is changed. The patient often goes home with the T-tube in place.

Because the surgeon will be concerned with whether bile is beginning to flow through the duct and into the duodenum as it normally should, the nurse must carefully observe the color of the patient's stools. A return of the characteristic brown color to the stools is an indication that bile is entering the small intestine. If the bile duct is still obstructed, the patient will show signs of jaundice and stool will be light in color.

The "open" cholecystectomy patient is reluctant to deep-breathe and cough because of considerable pain in the operative area. She should be assisted with these exercises, and her lung sounds should be auscultated every shift to discover quickly any signs of extra secretions or atelectasis. Using a patient-controlled analgesia (PCA) pump as ordered will help the patient cooperate with turning, coughing, and ambulating and thus prevent complications.

No specific diet is recommended for the patient who has had surgery of the gallbladder, although it is wise to avoid excessive amounts of fatty foods.

? *Think Critically About . . .* Can you outline the points to be covered for teaching the patient who is about to undergo a cholecystectomy?

Complications

Constant irritation of the gallbladder may lead to cancer of the gallbladder. Inflammation and infection may produce purulent material and a fistula may form. Necrosis, gangrene, and rupture of the gallbladder causing peritonitis may occur. Choledocholithiasis may cause severe inflammation of the common duct and obstruct the pancreatic duct, inducing pancreatitis.

DISORDERS OF THE LIVER

Liver disorders occur when the liver becomes inflamed, is injured by trauma or toxins, or is invaded by tumor. Disruption of the normal functions of the liver occurs depending on how much of the liver tissue is affected. Chronic inflammation causes fibrosis of the liver cells, which then cannot function normally.

HEPATITIS

Etiology and Pathophysiology

There are five types of viral **hepatitis** (Table 30–2) that cause physical problems. A sixth hepatitis virus, hepatitis G, does not seem to cause the symptoms of hepatitis. Hepatitis is transmitted either by contaminated food and water, via infected feces, or by infected blood and body fluids. Liver cells are damaged either by direct action of the virus on hepatocytes, or by cell-mediated immune responses to the virus. Hepatitis viruses cause extensive inflammation of the liver tissue. Liver cell damage results in necrosis of hepatic cells. The Kupffer cells proliferate and enlarge. Bile flow may be interrupted because of the inflammation. Liver cells can regenerate and resume their normal appearance. The cells can function as long as there are no complications. With severe inflammation, fibrous scar tissue may form in the liver. Scar tissue often obstructs normal blood and bile flow, causing further damage from ischemia.

Hepatitis B, C, and D viruses may cause chronic inflammation and necrosis of the tissue. A carrier state of hepatitis B, C, or D may occur. In this state, asymptomatic individuals carry the virus in the liver cells. The infection can be transmitted via their blood or body fluids to others, even though the person does not have active disease.

Hepatitis A and hepatitis E viruses are transmitted primarily by the oral-fecal route. They are responsible for the epidemic forms of viral hepatitis. Hepatitis A virus is often transmitted by food handlers to customers or by mollusk shellfish from contaminated waters.

Table 30–2 **Comparison of Hepatitis-Causing Viruses**

	HEPATITIS A VIRUS (HAV)	HEPATITIS B VIRUS (HBV)	HEPATITIS C VIRUS (HCV)	HEPATITIS D VIRUS (HDV)	HEPATITIS E VIRUS (HEV)
Transmission mode	Fecal-to-oral route; poor sanitation and contaminated water and shellfish; often from infected food	Sexual contact, blood and body fluid contact; perinatal from mother to infant.	Contact with blood and body fluids, sexual contact with carrier, contact with contaminated surgical, tattooing, and piercing equipment.	Blood and body fluid contact; accompanies hepatitis B; close personal contact.	Fecal-to-oral route; contaminated water or food
Incubation period	15–60 days (average 30 days)	6 wk–6 mo (average 12–14 wk)	6–7 wk	Same as hepatitis B, which precedes it. Chronic carriers of hepatitis B are at risk throughout their carrier state.	14–60 days (average 40 days)
Infective period	Most infectious during 2 wk before onset of symptoms; not likely to be infectious after first week following onset of jaundice	Begins before symptoms appear and persists for 4–6 mo after acute illness; persists for lifetime of chronic carriers.	Begins 1–2 wk before symptoms appear; continues throughout life for chronic carriers.	Blood is potentially infectious in active hepatitis B infection; may still be present in blood of chronic hepatitis B carriers even though undetectable.	
Signs and symptoms	Acute onset *First phase (preicteric):* Malaise, fever, loss of appetite, nausea, fatigue, joint aching, skin rash, and upper abdominal discomfort May develop jaundice; malaise and fatigue	Slow onset. May be without symptoms.	Slow onset. May be without symptoms until liver damage has occurred.	Slow onset. May be without symptoms.	Abdominal pain, anorexia, dark urine, fever, hepatomegaly, jaundice, malaise, nausea and vomiting.

Hepatitis E virus infection is primarily seen in less developed countries. It is transmitted through fecal contamination of water.

Hepatitis B and C viruses are transmitted by parenteral routes and sexually as they are present in semen, vaginal secretions, and saliva of carriers. Sexual partners of patients who are carriers of hepatitis B or C virus are at high risk for contracting the virus. Hepatitis D virus coexists with hepatitis B or C virus, and is transmitted in the same ways (Health Promotion Points 30–2).

Hepatitis C virus has been the main cause of post-transfusion hepatitis, largely because before 1992 there were no known diagnostic markers for this virus. Donor blood could not be screened for this type of hepatitis. Now an enzyme-linked immunosorbent assay (ELISA) test has reduced the number of transfusion-related cases. **Intravenous drug use is a major cause of hepatitis C infection, and the virus can also be transmitted by cocaine snorting straws.** Hepatitis B and C viruses can be transmitted from mother to infant. Both can occur in hemodialysis patients. **Hepatitis B and C are the most serious forms of hepatitis, often progressing to chronic hepatitis, cirrhosis, liver cancer, and death.**

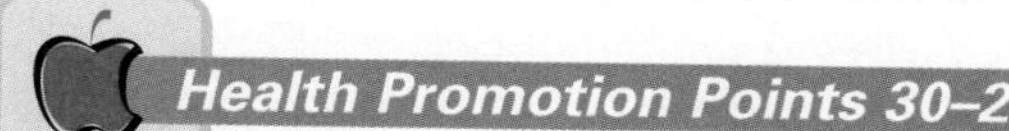

***Healthy People 2010* Hepatitis B**

It is important that all health care personnel who come into contact with patients or patient surgical and diagnostic equipment be immunized against hepatitis B as they are considered at high risk for contracting hepatitis B from blood and body fluids. Standard Precautions must be observed at all times. These practices will help meet the *Healthy People 2010* goal of reducing hepatitis B and National Patient Safety Goal #7—*Reduce the risk of health care–associated infections.*

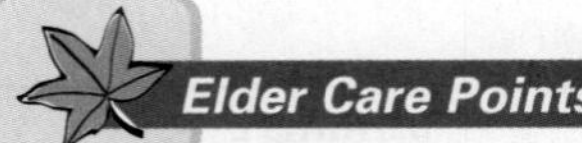

Elder Care Points

Elderly patients who have had several major surgeries and blood transfusions before 1992 are at higher risk for developing hepatitis B and C. Blood was not screened for the viruses before transfusion before that date. These patients may be carriers of these viruses.

Signs and Symptoms

The clinical signs and symptoms of hepatitis A tend to have an acute onset, whereas in hepatitis B, hepatitis C, and hepatitis D the onset is slower and more insidious. There are three phases of hepatitis with jaundice. The first, the *preicteric* phase, precedes jaundice and lasts 1 to 21 days. When symptoms do occur, they may be vague and nonspecific manifestations (see Table 30–2.) There may be a decreased sense of smell. The liver becomes tender and enlarged. The patient might think she has a mild case of influenza because the symptoms are so similar.

The *icteric* phase, characterized by jaundice, lasts 2 to 4 weeks. Urine becomes dark and stools may become light if bile flow is obstructed. Pruritus may occur from the bile pigment deposited in the skin.

The *posticteric* phase begins when jaundice is disappearing. Convalescence may take 2 to 4 months. Major complaints are malaise and fatigue. Liver enlargement may continue, but if the spleen was enlarged, it returns to normal in this phase.

Hepatitis D sometimes causes massive death of liver cells, causing liver failure and death of the patient. Hepatitis B and D become chronic in 2% to 10% of infected patients. The patient is then a constant carrier of the virus. There are no currently known signs and symptoms of hepatitis G. **Viral hepatitis without jaundice *(anicteric hepatitis)* is two to three times more common than viral hepatitis with jaundice.**

Diagnosis

Hepatitis is diagnosed by history, physical examination, and elevations in liver function tests (LFTs) (Table 30–3). Laboratory tests for the presence of serologic markers such as hepatitis A surface antigen (HAsAg) or hepatitis B surface antigen (HBsAg) may be performed. Chronic hepatitis is determined by liver biopsy. (See Table 27–1 for the liver biopsy procedure and patient care.)

Treatment

There is no specific treatment for acute viral hepatitis. Hepatitis A is treated by rest and avoidance of substances that can cause liver damage. These measures help the liver to regenerate. Consumption of alcohol must be halted. A well-balanced diet helps liver cells to heal. Four to six small meals a day may be tolerated better than three larger ones. Sucking on hard candy is recommended and adds to caloric intake. Nausea may be treated with dimenhydrinate (Dramamine) or trimethobenzamide (Tigan). Phenothiazines are not used because of their hepatotoxic effects. People who have been exposed to the patient should be notified so they can receive prophylaxis.

Table 30–3 *Laboratory Test Findings in Acute Viral Hepatitis*

TEST	ABNORMAL FINDINGS
Aspartate aminotransferase (AST)	Elevated in pre-icteric phase up to 20 times normal; decreases as jaundice subsides
Alanine aminotransferase (ALT)	Elevated in pre-icteric phase; ALT/AST ratio is >1; decreases as jaundice subsides
Gamma-glutamyl transpeptidase (GGT)	Elevated
Bilirubin	Elevated unconjugated (direct) bilirubin
Alkaline phosphatase	Some elevation
Serum albumin	Normal or decreased
Serum bilirubin (total)	Elevated to about 8–15 mg/dL (137–257 μmol/L)
Prothrombin time	Prolonged

For hepatitis B, drug therapy is used to decrease the viral load, thereby decreasing the disease progression (Table 30–4). Chronic hepatitis C virus treatment is also aimed at reducing the viral load. Treatment is directed at supportive care to enhance the patient's natural defenses and promote regeneration and healing of the liver. Hydration, sufficient rest, and adequate nutrition are the goals. Medication for nausea may be prescribed to encourage adequate nutrition. Vaccines are available to provide active immunity against hepatitis A and B for persons at high risk for infection. The vaccines produce immunity in about 95% of vaccinated individuals and protect for at least 15 years (McMahon et al., 2005). 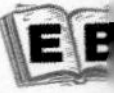

Passive immunity to type A hepatitis can be conferred by the administration of immune globulin (IG). IG is also recommended for those who have been exposed to persons infected with hepatitis B virus and have not been immunized against this virus. There is no protective vaccine for hepatitis C virus.

Hepatitis is an occupational hazard for all people who have direct contact with patients. All health care personnel should be immunized with the hepatitis B vaccine. The vaccine effectiveness lasts at least 15 years.

NURSING MANAGEMENT

Assessment (Data Collection)

Data collection for a patient with hepatitis should include a nursing history of previous contacts at home and at work and whether the contacts have

Table 30–4 ***Selected Medications Commonly Prescribed for Disorders of the Gallbladder, Liver, and Pancreas***

CLASSIFICATION	ACTION	NURSING IMPLICATIONS	PATIENT TEACHING
DIURETIC			
Potassium-sparing diuretics Spironolactone (Aldactone) Amiloride (Midamor) Triamterene (Dyrenium)	Block action of aldosterone in the distal nephron, preventing sodium uptake in exchange for potassium secretion Potassium is "spared" (not secreted) and sodium is excreted These drugs cause little diuresis	It is not necessary to supplement potassium for patients taking this type of diuretic alone. Monitor potassium levels.	Avoid foods high in potassium content: bananas, oranges, salt substitutes, dried apricots, and dates.
Loop diuretic Furosemide (Lasix)	Block reabsorption of sodium and chloride in the loop of Henle, promoting water secretion Promotes powerful diuresis	Give early in the morning. Monitor potassium levels and supplement potassium as needed. Monitor for hypokalemia, I&O. Weigh patient daily. Assess for hearing loss. Monitor for postural hypotension.	Warn that the drug will cause the need to empty the bladder frequently. Caution regarding dizziness when changing positions.
LAXATIVE: AMMONIA DETOXICANT			
Lactulose (Cephulac)	Prevents absorption of ammonia in the colon; increases water in the stool	Assess stool amount and color. Monitor serum ammonia level, electrolytes, and I&O. Assess perineal skin frequently for excoriation from diarrhea.	Advise that this drug is intended to cause bowel evacuation and diarrhea is likely.
ANTIBIOTIC			
Neomycin (Mycifradin)	Decreases protein synthesis in bacterial cells, causing bacterial death This prevents the breakdown of protein in the GI tract and helps prevent formation of ammonia	Monitor renal function and hearing. Observe for dehydration.	Explain the purpose of this drug.
VASOCONSTRICTOR			
Vasopressin (Pitressin)	Causes vasoconstriction	Monitor BP and I&O as may cause water retention.	Explain the purpose of the drug in stopping bleeding of esophageal varices.
VITAMINS			
Thiamine (vitamin B_1)	Corrects vitamin B_1 deficiency that occurs from excessive alcohol use	Assess thiamine levels.	Explain purpose of the drug.
Vitamin K (AquaMEPHYTON)	Needed for hepatic formation of coagulation factors II, VII, IX, and X	Monitor prothrombin time and INR.	Explain injection may cause discomfort.
ANTIRETROVIRALS			
Lamivudine (Epivir)	Inhibits replication of HBV	Monitor blood count, viral load, liver functions, amylase, lipase, and triglycerides. Watch for signs of lactic acidosis.	GI complaints and insomnia resolve after 3–4 wk. Drug is not a cure, but will help control symptoms. Notify physician of swollen lymph nodes, fever, malaise and sore throat. May still pass virus on to others; maintain precautions.
Ribavirin (Rebetol)	Inhibits viral protein synthesis	Ribavirin is used together with interferon alfa-2b to treat chronic HCV.	Drug may cause fainting or dizziness.
Adefovir dipivoxil (Hepsera)	Prevents DNA replication	Monitor respiratory status; assess for skin rash.	Report any difficulty breathing or itching, swelling, or redness of the eyes.

Key: *BP,* blood pressure, *GI,* gastrointestinal; *HBV,* hepatitis B virus; *HCV,* hepatitis C virus; *I&O,* intake and output; *INR,* international normalized ratio.

Continued

Table 30–4 **Selected Medications Commonly Prescribed for Disorders of the Gallbladder, Liver, and Pancreas—cont'd**

CLASSIFICATION	ACTION	NURSING IMPLICATIONS	PATIENT TEACHING
ANTIRETROVIRALS—cont'd			
Entecavir (Baraclude)	Prevents viral replication	Monitor renal function.	May cause weakness.
Telbivudine (Tyzeka)	Prevents viral replication	Monitor renal function and electrolytes.	May cause lactic acidosis and myopathy.
IMMUNOMODULATOR			
Peginterferon alfa-2b (PEG-Intron)	Inhibits viral replication and increases phagocytic action of macrophages, augmenting specific cytotoxicity of lymphocytes	Perform baseline assessments. Monitor for signs of depression; offer emotional support. Monitor for abdominal pain and bloody diarrhea. Monitor viral load.	Maintain hydration and avoid alcohol. May experience flulike symptoms.
ANTINEOPLASTIC			
Gemcitabine (Gemzar)	Produces cell death in cells undergoing DNA synthesis	Perform baseline assessments. Monitor blood count. Evaluate lab results before each dose.	Avoid crowds and exposure to infection. Promptly report fever, sore throat, signs of local infection, easy bruising, or rash.

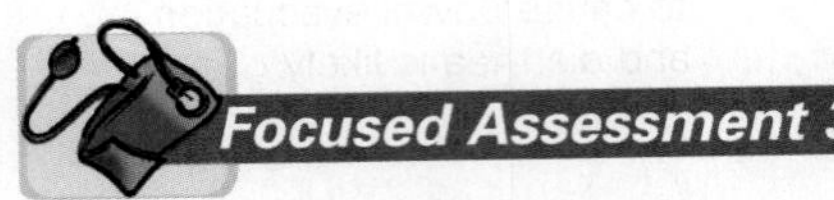
Focused Assessment 30–1

Data Collection for the Patient with a Liver Disorder

Gather the following data:

HEALTH HISTORY

- Have you ever had a parasitic infection?
- Do you have a history of cancer?
- How much alcohol do you drink?
- Do you have a history of hepatitis?
- Have you been exposed to hepatitis?
- What drugs do you take?
- Have you been exposed to pesticides or industrial chemicals? Which ones?
- Has your appetite decreased? Have you had nausea or vomiting?
- Are you more fatigued than usual?
- Have you noticed any fever?
- Have you noticed dark-colored urine?
- Have you had any light or clay-colored stools?
- Have you had excessive gas?
- Have you been bruising easily?
- Has your skin been itchy or made you feel uncomfortable?
- Has your abdomen increased in girth lately?
- Do you have abdominal pain? Where? Can you describe it?
- Have you gained weight recently?

PHYSICAL ASSESSMENT

- Inspect the skin for signs of jaundice, scratch marks, and general condition.
- Inspect sclera and mucous membranes of mouth for signs of jaundice.
- Gently palpate the abdomen for masses and for liver enlargement.
- Auscultate bowel sounds.
- Measure abdominal girth for a baseline.
- Inspect extremities for signs of edema.
- Check liver function test values and urinalysis for bilirubin presence.

been notified and immunized. Viral hepatitis must, by law, be reported to the state department of public health. This necessitates filling out paperwork for patients being treated at home. **Because the liver detoxifies many chemicals and metabolizes certain drugs, the nurse must have a complete list of medications the patient has recently taken or is currently receiving. It may be necessary to discontinue some drugs that are particularly toxic to the liver** (see Box 27–1). During assessment, the nurse will look for data that indicate a greater need for rest (Focused Assessment 30–1).

Assessment of hospitalized patients also should include data that would be helpful in identifying problems related to silent gastrointestinal (GI) bleeding, respiratory distress, and neurologic dysfunction, especially mental confusion and coma associated with hepatic **encephalopathy**. Encephalopathy is any abnormal condition of the brain. Hepatic encephalopathy occurs from circulating toxins due to liver failure.

Nursing Diagnosis and Planning

Nursing diagnoses specific to hepatitis infection might include:

- Imbalanced nutrition: less than body requirements related to anorexia, nausea, and vomiting
- Fatigue related to disease process and malaise
- Disturbed body image related to jaundice

Elder Care Points

The elderly patient is at higher risk for drug-induced hepatitis if she has chronic conditions that require the administration of various drugs that can cause liver damage over a long period of time. If an elderly person has signs of liver inflammation, the liver will not be functioning optimally and drug dosages will need to be lowered. Otherwise drugs can build to toxic levels since the liver cannot metabolize them normally.

- Pain related to inflamed liver and pruritus
- Deficient knowledge related to disease process and self-care needed
- Deficient diversional activity

Expected outcomes might be:

- Patient will maintain body weight within normal limits during illness.
- Patient will verbalize lessened fatigue after rest periods each day.
- Patient will accept changed body image by allowing visitors during convalescence.
- Patient will verbalize a decrease in pain after institution of nursing measures to decrease discomforts.
- Patient will verbalize knowledge of disease process and self-care within 2 days.
- Patient will engage in appropriate diversional activities during convalescence.

Implementation and Evaluation

Nursing interventions include monitoring the patient's progress by reviewing reports of serum liver enzyme levels and serum bilirubin values. Preventing the spread of infection is a major concern in the nursing care of patients with viral hepatitis. The patient and her family probably will need instruction in special precautions to prevent the spread of the infectious agent. This may include proper handling of body secretions, proper handwashing, and limiting contact with others.

Sedatives can have a profound effect on patients with hepatitis. They must be given with caution because a diseased liver cannot detoxify them very well. Alcohol is particularly damaging to the liver and is best avoided for 4 months following recovery from hepatitis.

The convalescence of the hepatitis patient is slow and long. Psychological support from the nurse during this period can help prevent depression. A nutritious diet is prescribed, and supplements may be helpful (Complementary & Alternative Therapies 30–1). A variety of diversional activities that are not physically taxing should be planned. Perhaps this is the time for the patient to take up a new hobby or learn a new skill. Computer access is very helpful. Handheld computer games, puzzle books, and DVDs are possible ways to keep the patient occupied. Scheduling friends to come in and play cards or board games is another possibility.

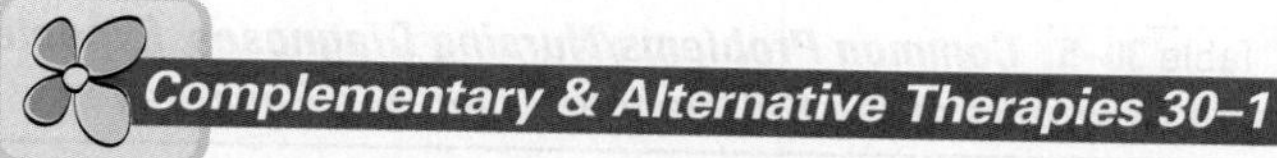

Promoting Good Liver Function

Several supplements are known to be beneficial to promoting good liver function. *N*-acetylcysteine (NAC), glutathione (GSH), choline, methionine, carnitine, and antioxidants are helpful. NAC promotes detoxification pathways; choline helps prevent deposition of fat in the liver. Carnitine allows fats to be used as energy and alleviates deposition of fat in the liver and elsewhere in the body. Consultation with the physician should always be done before taking supplements for liver disorders.

Nursing interventions for selected nursing diagnoses and problems relevant to the patient with hepatitis are found in Table 30–5. Nursing assessment and interventions for problems associated with severe liver damage are discussed in the following section on cirrhosis.

Data are gathered regarding the success of the nursing interventions and to determine progress toward meeting the expected outcomes. If the nursing interventions are not helping the patient achieve the expected outcomes, the plan is changed.

Prevention

Transmission Precautions. Both feces and blood of patients with hepatitis A contain virus during the **prodromal stage** (infected but without symptoms) and early symptomatic stage. When hepatitis is suspected, the strict use of Standard Precautions is essential, and the patient and family must use precautions at home to prevent the spread of the virus (Home Care Considerations 30–1). Close contacts of patients with hepatitis A should be given immune serum globulin as soon as possible.

Hepatitis B and D viruses are rarely transmitted by the fecal-oral route, but it is best to be very careful when disposing of a patient's stool. Standard Precautions guidelines must be carefully followed for handling, sterilizing, and disposing of equipment contaminated with blood (Safety Alert 30–2). **These viruses are transmitted by sexual contact, and homosexual men in particular are at risk.**

When a patient with viral hepatitis has been admitted to the hospital, the infection control officer must be notified as soon as possible. Notification must not be more than 48 hours after admission. Infection with type A hepatitis in a person who handles food on the job must be reported promptly. The Centers for Disease Control and Prevention have published guidelines for the care of patients hospitalized with hepatitis. These same guidelines can be modified for home care to prevent the spread of the infection.

Table 30–5 Common Problems/Nursing Diagnoses, Expected Outcomes, and Nursing Interventions for Patients with Disorders of the Gallbladder, Liver, and Pancreas

PROBLEM/NURSING DIAGNOSIS	EXPECTED OUTCOMES	NURSING INTERVENTIONS
Dehydration/Deficient fluid volume related to nausea and vomiting	Patient will cease vomiting within 24 hr. Patient will establish fluid balance within 48 hr as evidenced by moist mucous membranes and good skin turgor.	Administer antiemetics as ordered. Monitor IV infusion site and fluid rate. Encourage clear oral fluids as tolerated. Monitor electrolyte levels for imbalances. Provide mouth care q 2 hr while awake.
Malnutrition/Imbalanced nutrition: less than body requirements related to nausea, vomiting, and improper diet	Patient will ingest a 1200-calorie diet per day within 7 days after subsidence of acute vomiting. Patient will maintain present weight.	Initiate IV fluids as ordered if dehydration occurs. Keep door of room closed to keep odors out. Offer mouth care before meal time. Provide 6 small meals a day plus small, high-calorie snacks between meals. Weigh q 3 days and record. Keep hard candy at bedside for snacking.
Discomfort/Pain related to jaundice and bile pigments in skin causing itching	Patient will verbalize that itching is decreased.	Assist to bathe with tepid water three times a day. Apply lotion q 2 hr. Provide diversional activities. Teach relaxation techniques.
Lack of knowledge/Deficient knowledge related to ways in which HBV is transmitted, impact of hepatitis on the body, self-care measures, and measures to prevent transmission to others	Patient will verbalize ways HBV is transmitted, impact on body, self-care measures, and measures to prevent transmission to others before discharge.	Teach ways in which HBV is transmitted: parenteral routes, sexual contact, contact with blood and body fluids. Give explanation in understandable terms of what HBV does to the body. Reinforce teaching regarding self-care measures: hygiene, diet, rest, follow-up. Teach importance of not sharing personal articles (especially razor, toothbrush, etc.) with others. Instruct to inform health care workers of the presence of the virus until tests for it are negative. Inform that sexual partner(s) will need injection of special immune globulin for protection and then immunization.
Distress over skin color/Body image disturbance related to yellow skin color from jaundice	Patient will demonstrate acceptance of present body image by allowing visitors within 3 days.	Assure that jaundice is not permanent. Allow to ventilate feelings about the illness and present appearance. Encourage verbalization of positive aspects about self. Increase fluid intake to help flush bilirubin from blood during recovery.
Pain/Acute pain related to gallstone blockage of bile duct or pancreatic inflammation	Patient's pain level will decrease per pain scale within 1 hr of instituting nursing measures. Patient will state that pain is controlled within 8 hr.	Medicate with analgesic as ordered. Instruct in use of PCA pump if ordered. Encourage relaxation techniques to decrease discomfort. Assess q 2 hr for adequate pain relief. Administer adjunctive medications as ordered.
Respiratory distress/Risk for ineffective breathing pattern related to irritation or pressure to diaphragm from ascites or pancreatic abscess or pseudocyst	Patient will maintain adequate oxygen levels as evidenced by oxygen saturation within normal limits.	Observe for signs of respiratory distress. Auscultate lungs for crackles or abnormal lung sounds. Monitor oxygen saturation with pulse oximeter. Administer supplemental oxygen as ordered. Encourage use of incentive spirometer as ordered. Place in semi-Fowler's position as tolerated to promote better lung expansion.
Safety/Risk for injury related to hemorrhage or circulatory collapse	Patient will not experience injury while hospitalized.	Monitor laboratory values for liver enzymes, ammonia, albumin, sodium, potassium, calcium, and magnesium daily. Observe for neuromuscular irritability. Monitor vital signs closely. Observe stool for signs of bleeding. Keep urine output > 30 mL/hr. Report frank bleeding promptly.
Lack of knowledge/Deficient knowledge related to pancreatitis and its treatment and prevention of recurrence	Patient will verbalize understanding of disease process within 2 wk. Patient will verbalize understanding of treatment regimen within 1 wk. Patient will verbalize ways to prevent recurrence of pancreatitis before discharge.	Instruct in causes and progression of disease process. Explain all aspects of treatment and reason for each medication. Teach ways to prevent recurrence of pancreatitis.

Key: *HBV,* hepatitis B virus; *IV,* intravenous; *PCA,* patient-controlled analgesia.

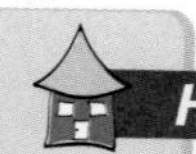
Home Care Considerations 30–1

Preventing the Spread of Hepatitis Virus

Teach the patient with hepatitis A to:

- Notify close contacts so that they can obtain immune globulin protection and then hepatitis A vaccine.
- Practice extremely good hygiene, washing with warm water and soap (liquid soap is best).
- Wash hands after using the toilet and before eating and after changing diapers.
- Not prepare food during the infectious period.
- Use separate bath and hand towels from other members of the family.
- Not share toothbrushes.
- Using gloves, disinfect the bathroom fixtures with a 10:1 bleach solution.
- Refrain from sexual contact until the physician states that the infectious period is over.

Teach the patient with hepatitis B or C to:

- Avoid sexual contact until there is no chance of transmission of the virus.
- Advise close contacts to obtain hepatitis B vaccine as indicated.
- Not share razors or toothbrushes because of the chance of blood transmission.

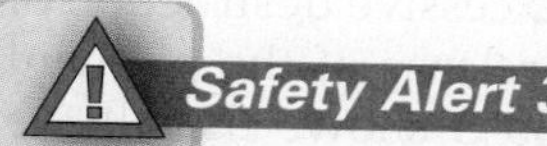
Safety Alert 30–2

Preventing Hepatitis B and C

Hepatitis C virus (HCV) is transmitted by blood and saliva. Standard Precautions and careful handling of all body fluids are recommended. The first line of defense is scrupulous handwashing, wearing rubber gloves when handling plasma-containing body fluids from a patient, and extreme care when handling used needles, syringes, and IV tubing. One does not have to be stuck with a contaminated needle or have an open wound to contract hepatitis B virus (HBV) or HCV. The mucous membranes of the eyes, nose, and mouth also can serve as portals of entry.

Avoidance of the various drugs, toxic agents, and other viruses is prudent. HBV and HCV carriers are counseled to adhere to strict hygienic principles. They should not share personal items, such as razors, likely to be contaminated with their blood. Dentists, physicians, nurses, and other health care workers must be informed of their carrier status.

Complications

In a small percentage of cases, the patient with hepatitis can develop massive necrosis of liver cells *(fulminant hepatitis)*. Death occurs in about 75% of these cases. Symptoms of fulminant hepatitis include mental confusion, disorientation, and drowsiness. These symptoms indicate hepatic encephalopathy. Ascites and edema, which usually are present, indicate liver failure.

CIRRHOSIS OF THE LIVER

Etiology

Hepatitis C virus accounts for more than 60% of the cases of cirrhosis in the United States, and excessive alcohol ingestion is the next leading cause (Durston, 2004b). *Postnecrotic cirrhosis* is caused by viral hepatitis, toxic substances, parasites, or infection. There are three other types of cirrhosis. *Laënnec's cirrhosis,* or *portal cirrhosis,* results from alcoholism. The first change caused by excessive alcohol ingestion is the deposition of fat in the liver cells. This is reversible if alcohol consumption is halted. Otherwise widespread scar formation occurs. *Biliary cirrhosis* is from chronic biliary obstruction and infection. *Cardiac cirrhosis* results from long-standing, severe right-sided heart failure in patients with cor pulmonale. Cirrhosis is the 14th most frequent cause of death in the United States and the fourth most common cause of death in people between 35 and 54 years of age (Centers for Disease Control and Prevention, 2006).

Pathophysiology

Cirrhosis is a progressive, chronic disease of the liver. The destruction of normal hepatic structures and their replacement with necrotic tissue occur. Fibrous bands of connective tissue develop in the organ. The bands eventually constrict and partition it into irregular nodules. If this process is halted before too much liver tissue is damaged, the liver tissue will regenerate. Later cirrhosis is considered irreversible. The outcome of cirrhosis of the liver is failure of its cells to perform their functions and the development of portal hypertension.

When liver cells begin to degenerate, the blood vessels within the liver also fail to function normally. This causes an obstruction to the flow of blood through the portal circulatory system, causing portal systemic hypertension. There is altered vessel permeability and fluid leakage into the abdomen, resulting in **ascites.** Ascites is an abnormal accumulation of serous fluid within the peritoneal cavity. As pressure increases in the hepatic veins, there is a shift of protein-rich plasma filtrate into the lymphatic ducts. If the pressure is high enough in the ducts, the excess fluid will ooze from the surface of the liver into the peritoneal cavity. Since the fluid has a high colloidal pressure because of its high protein content, it is not readily reabsorbed. Fluid accumulates in the cavity, causing increased abdominal girth and weight gain. Secondarily, the damaged liver's inability to synthesize albumin and the osmotic pressure within the blood vessels falls, allowing fluid to be pulled out into the tissues. The third mechanism contributing to ascites and edema is excess circulating aldosterone. The damaged liver cells cannot properly metabolize this hormone. The excess aldosterone causes sodium and water retention (Concept Map 30–1).

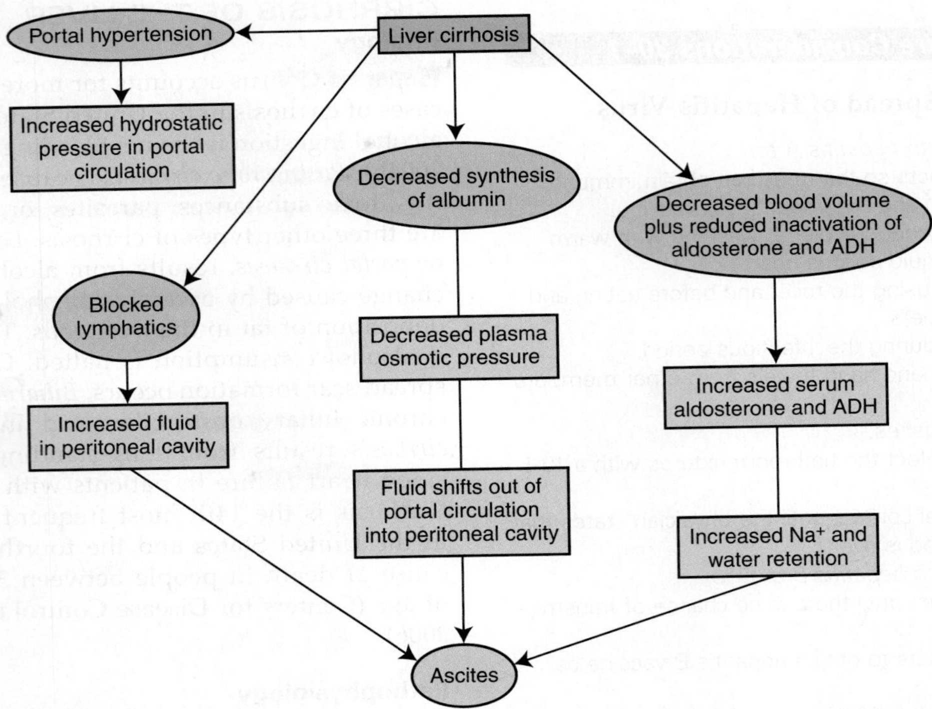

CONCEPT MAP **30–1** Relationship of systemic portal hypertension and ascites in liver cirrhosis.

Signs and Symptoms

Cirrhosis usually progresses without symptoms until severe liver damage is present. Subjective symptoms of liver cirrhosis include fatigue, weakness, headache, anorexia, indigestion, abdominal pain, nausea, and vomiting. Objective symptoms include excessive gas, skin rashes, itching, and fever. Leg and foot edema and **palmar erythema** (redness of the palms that blanches with pressure) occur. Sometimes bluish varicose veins, called **caput medusa**, radiating from the umbilicus (indicating portal hypertension) are seen. Bleeding and bruising also are associated with liver disease. Deficiencies in vitamin K, thrombin, or prothrombin interfere with clot formation. The liver often is enlarged and "knobby" and is palpable below the level of the right rib cage. Abdominal distention is present. The spleen also enlarges. Peripheral edema and ascites develop. Skin lesions, jaundice, **pruritus**, bleeding disorders, endocrine disorders, and peripheral neuropathy occur in late disease. **Spider angiomas** may appear on the face, neck, upper trunk, and arms. The angiomas may blanch with pressure.

Urine may become dark and foamy, and stools turn clay-colored, which indicates bile isn't reaching the intestine. Jaundice occurs either because the liver cannot metabolize bilirubin or because bile flow is obstructed. It indicates excessively high levels of bile pigment *(bilirubin)* in the blood. The pigment is deposited in the skin, mucous membranes, and body fluids, causing a change in color ranging from pale yellow to golden orange. The first signs of jaundice are usually seen in the sclera of the eye **(icterus)**, which takes on a yellow tint. Jaundice is not always a sign of liver damage. In *hemolytic jaundice,* there may be an increased level of bilirubin as a result of excessive destruction of red blood cells, with resultant release of the pigment into the bloodstream. Figure 30–3 shows the all the signs and symptoms of cirrhosis. **Elevations in liver enzymes usually do not occur until 65% of liver function is gone.** The patient may not seek medical attention until she develops ascites.

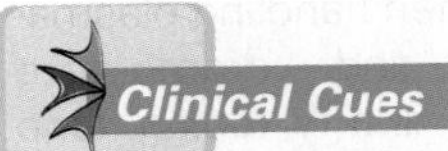

In people with dark skin, jaundice is best detected by checking the buccal mucosa, hard palate, palms, soles of the feet, sclera, and conjunctiva.

The patient who is severely jaundiced experiences a drastic change in body image. She knows her skin color attracts attention and that she looks sick. The nurse needs to provide time for sharing of feelings and affirmation of her self-worth.

Think Critically About . . . Can you list the ways in which you would collect data when checking a patient for signs of jaundice?

Diagnosis

A definitive diagnosis of cirrhosis of the liver is made by liver biopsy. Laboratory testing may show a low albumin level and elevated prothrombin time as

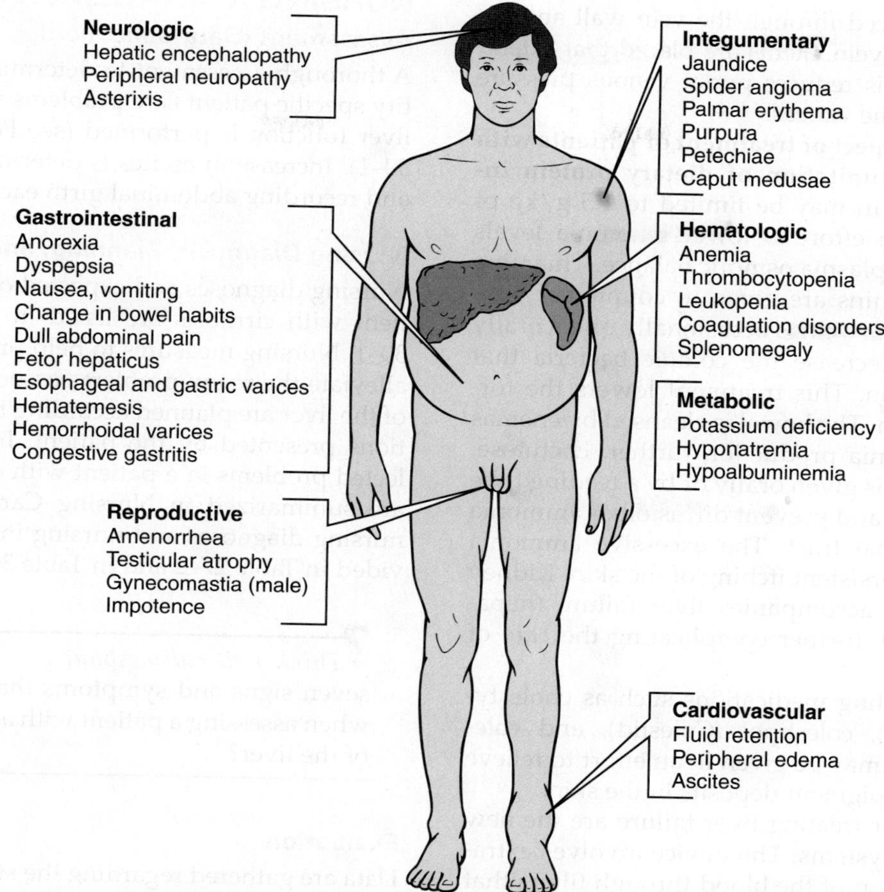

FIGURE **30–3** The many signs and symptoms of cirrhosis.

well as elevated AST, ALT, and lactate dehydrogenase values. CT and liver scan can help determine the size of the liver and presence of any masses, and outline the hepatic blood flow and any obstruction to it. Magnetic resonance cholangiopancreatography, similar to ERCP but without the use of contrast media, may be performed.

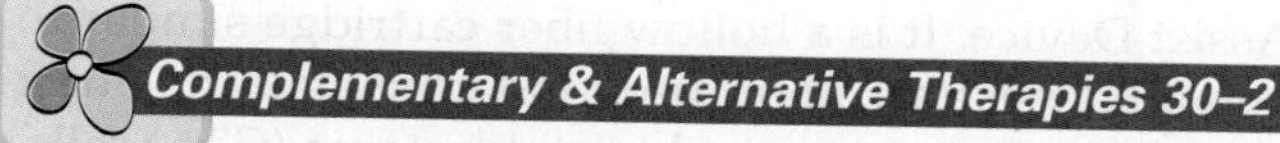

Caution with Liver Inflammation

Patients with liver inflammation or cirrhosis should avoid taking large doses of vitamins and minerals. Vitamin A, iron, and copper can worsen the liver damage.

Treatment

Treatment is aimed at stopping the liver damage and restoring the liver's functions.

The intake of alcohol and administration of drugs toxic to the liver must be restricted completely. Sedatives and opiates are either avoided or given with great caution. Rest may be prescribed to aid healing. The degree of rest and activity is dictated by the patient's stage of illness. Nutritional deficiencies are treated with supplements and diet.

When the liver cells fail to function as they should, the patient is at great risk for infection. The patient should be protected from exposure to infectious agents, and antibiotics should be given quickly when infection occurs (Complementary & Alternative Therapies 30–2).

The management of symptoms usually focuses on the effects of pathologic changes that occur as a result of degeneration of liver cells. **Medical treatment of ascites includes restriction of fluid and sodium intake and administration of diuretics.** Management of ascites was at one time entirely limited to abdominal **paracentesis** to remove accumulated fluid. This is, however, only a temporary measure that poses problems of rapid fluid shift, loss of protein, and the potential for introducing infectious organisms into the peritoneum. In years past, a procedure involving the shunting of ascitic fluid into the venous system was used. The procedure is called a peritoneal-venous shunt (LeVeen or Denver shunt). Currently, a transjugular intrahepatic portosystemic shunt (TIPS) may be used to decrease pressure between portal and hepatic veins in the liver. This is a nonsurgical procedure that creates a shunt between the systemic and portal venous systems. A catheter is inserted into the jugular vein and threaded through the superior and inferior vene cave to the hepatic vein. The catheter is then placed through the vein wall and directed to the portal vein. Stents are placed that extend into both veins. This reduces portal venous pressure and decompresses the varices.

An important aspect of treatment of patients with this condition is limitation of dietary protein intake. Dietary protein may be limited to 1.5 g/kg of body weight in an effort to lower ammonia levels while maintaining plasma osmotic balance. Thiamine and multiple vitamins are given to counteract vitamin deficiency. Neomycin is occasionally given orally or by enema to decrease the colonic bacteria that break down protein. This treatment lowers the formation of ammonia. The bowel is cleansed by enemas to decrease ammonia production further. Lactulose, an exchange resin, is given orally or by a feeding tube to induce diarrhea and prevent diffusion of ammonia out of the intestinal tract. The excessive ammonia levels can cause persistent itching of the skin. Kidney failure sometimes accompanies liver failure (hepatorenal syndrome), further complicating the care of the patient.

Cholesterol-binding medications such as cholestyramine (Questran), colestipol (Colestid), and colesevelam (Welchol) may be given in an effort to relieve pruritus from bile pigment deposits in the skin.

New options for treating liver failure are the new external support systems. The device involves extracorporeal circulation of the blood through filters that remove waste products the liver no longer can remove. Several systems currently are in clinical trials. One system is the Hepatix Extracorporeal Liver-Assist Device. It is a hollow fiber cartridge similar to hemodialysis cartridges used in kidney failure, but it contains cultured human hepatoblastoma (C3A) cells. These cells secrete liver-specific proteins and clotting factors. Liver "dialysis" may provide an alternative to liver transplantation for the chronic liver failure patient (Jones, 2003).

NURSING MANAGEMENT

Assessment (Data Collection)

A thorough assessment to determine status and identify specific patient care problems related to abnormal liver function is performed (see Focused Assessment 30–1). Increase in ascites is determined by measuring and recording abdominal girth each day.

Nursing Diagnosis, Planning, and Implementation

Nursing diagnoses and expected outcomes for the patient with cirrhosis are listed in Nursing Care Plan 30–1. Nursing measures to help prevent, minimize, or alleviate the many problems associated with cirrhosis of the liver are planned according to the specific conditions presented by the patient. Interventions for selected problems in a patient with cirrhosis of the liver are summarized in Nursing Care Plan 30–1. Other nursing diagnoses and nursing interventions are provided in Table 27–2 and in Table 30–5.

? *Think Critically About . . .* Can you identify seven signs and symptoms that you might find when assessing a patient with advanced cirrhosis of the liver?

Evaluation

Data are gathered regarding the success of the nursing interventions. If the interventions are not helping the patient meet the expected outcomes, new interventions are chosen for the plan.

Complications

Esophageal Varices. Gastrointestinal bleeding from esophageal varices (dilated, distorted blood veins) is a major complication of cirrhosis. Esophageal varices are engorged veins (similar to varicose veins) that line the esophagus. They are the result of portal congestion

NURSING CARE PLAN 30–1

Care of the Patient with Cirrhosis of the Liver

SCENARIO A 62-year-old man with a 25-year history of alcoholism is admitted with progressive alcoholic cirrhosis. His complaints include extreme fatigue, a swollen abdomen, edema of the feet and ankles, jaundice, itching, nausea and indigestion, drowsiness, and slight confusion. Esophageal varices are present.

PROBLEM/NURSING DIAGNOSIS *Potential for bleeding from esophageal varices*/Risk for ineffective tissue perfusion related to possible hemorrhage from esophageal varices and decreased clotting factors.

Supporting assessment data *Subjective:* "I can't seem to think well." *Objective:* Elevated liver function test results, known cirrhosis, spider angiomas, palmar erythema, ascites, and prolonged PT.

Goals/Expected Outcomes	Nursing Interventions	Selected Rationale	Evaluation
Patient will not experience injury while hospitalized	Call bell within reach, bed at lowest level. Monitor mental status q 4 hr.	Prevents injury from accidental fall from bed. Determines worsening of disorientation.	Bed down, call bell within reach. Mental status unchanged.

NURSING CARE PLAN 30–1

Care of the Patient with Cirrhosis of the Liver—cont'd

Goals/Expected Outcomes	Nursing Interventions	Selected Rationale	Evaluation
Patient will not experience death from hemorrhage while hospitalized.	Monitor for signs of esophageal bleeding	Alerts to bleeding.	No signs of bleeding.
	Feed only soft foods.	Prevents mechanical irritation of esophagus.	Eating soft diet.
	Give vitamin K as ordered.	Vitamin K is needed for synthesis of clotting factors.	Vitamin K administered.
	Monitor stool and vomitus for blood.		
	Monitor vital signs q 2–4 hr as ordered.	Vital sign changes, restlessness, and confusion may indicate bleeding.	Vital signs stable; is anxious, but no increased restlessness or confusion.
	Observe for increasing restlessness and confusion that might indicate hypoxia from bleeding.		
	Monitor PT and INR.	Indicate bleeding propensity.	Laboratory test results not back as yet. Continue plan.

PROBLEM/NURSING DIAGNOSIS *Confusion and drowsiness*/Disturbed thought processes related to increased ammonia level caused by liver failure.

Supporting assessment data *Subjective:* Confused as to month. *Objective:* Elevated serum ammonia and drowsiness.

Goals/Expected Outcomes	Nursing Interventions	Selected Rationale	Evaluation
Serum ammonia levels will not increase further during hospitalization	Low-protein diet as ordered.	Protein digestion produces ammonia.	Low-protein diet ordered; doesn't like it.
Serum ammonia levels will return to normal within 2 mo	Neomycin enemas as ordered.	Neomycin kills intestinal bacteria that help digest protein and produce ammonia.	Administered neomycin enema.
	Administer lactulose as ordered.	Lactulose decreases absorption of ammonia.	Lactulose administered; diarrhea occurring.
	Provide protective lubricant for anal region.	Lubricant prevents excoriation of anal area from diarrhea.	A & D ointment applied to anal area after bowel movements.
	Monitor serum ammonia levels.	Assists in determining likelihood of coma.	Lab work to be drawn in A.M. Continue plan.

PROBLEM/NURSING DIAGNOSIS *Cannot perform ADLs*/Self-care deficit related to fatigue, drowsiness, and ascites.

Supporting assessment data *Subjective:* "I'm so sleepy and weak." *Objective:* Cannot perform ADLs; very drowsy, ascites present.

Goals/Expected Outcomes	Nursing Interventions	Selected Rationale	Evaluation
Patient will be able to assist with ADLs within 2 wk.	Bathe with tepid water and apply emollients to decrease itching q shift.	Keeps patient clean and dry, decreases itching.	Baths and emollients have decreased itching slightly.
Patient will be able to perform ADLs independently within 1 mo.	Offer mouth care q 2 hr.	Mouth care improves appetite.	Mouth care given q 2 hr.
	Assist with meal trays.	Assists patient to eat.	Set up meal tray.
	Assist with toileting.	Prevents falls and aids with elimination.	Assisted with toileting. Continue plan.

Key: *ADLs*, activities of daily living; *I&O*, intake and output; *INR*, international normalized ratio; *PT*, prothrombin time.

Continued

NURSING CARE PLAN 30–1

Care of the Patient with Cirrhosis of the Liver—cont'd

PROBLEM/NURSING DIAGNOSIS *Fluid retention*/Fluid volume excess related to ascites and peripheral edema from portal hypertension.

Supporting assessment data Objective: Ascites, edema of feet and ankles, 6-lb weight gain in 2 days.

Goals/Expected Outcomes	Nursing Interventions	Selected Rationale	Evaluation
Patient will have no further increase in ascites this week	Measure abdominal girth q shift.	Determines whether ascites is increasing or decreasing.	Abdominal girth down ⅛ in.
Patient will return to normal fluid balance within 2 wk	Administer diuretics as ordered and monitor I&O.	Diuretics remove excess fluid from the body. I&O tracks fluid removal.	Diuretic administered. Intake 400 mL; output 670 mL.
	Weigh daily and record.	Daily weight indicates whether diuretic therapy is effective.	Weight down 1.5 lb.
	Turn at least q 1–2 hr. Provide good skin care.	Turning and skin care prevent pressure sores.	Turned q 2 hr; skin care provided; no reddened or excoriated areas over pressure points. Continue plan.

PROBLEM/NURSING DIAGNOSIS *Fear*/Fear related to possibility of death from liver failure.

Supporting assessment data *Subjective:* States he is afraid he is going to die.

Goals/Expected Outcomes	Nursing Interventions	Selected Rationale	Evaluation
Patient will verbalize that fear has decreased before discharge	Establish trusting relationship by attentive, caring attitude.	Displays empathy.	Listened attentively for 15 min.
	Encourage verbalization of fears; actively listen.	Verbalization helps decrease fear.	Speaking about what he has to live for.
	Encourage contact with minister, hospital chaplain, or spiritual advisor.	Spiritual advisor can provide comfort.	Minister contacted; will visit.
	Advise as to progress in decrease of ascites and ammonia.	Knowing condition is improving lessens fear of dying.	Advised ascites is decreasing.

? CRITICAL THINKING QUESTIONS

1. Can you describe the correct way to measure abdominal girth?
2. Why is good skin care even more important when a patient has edema and ascites?
3. How high would a PT or INR level have to climb before you would report it to the physician immediately?

and hypertension. In advanced cirrhosis, blood that normally flows from the intestines to the portal vein and on through the liver is shunted to other veins, including the veins of the upper stomach and lower esophagus. The added load of blood causes congestion of these veins. The congestion can lead to massive bleeding when the vein walls rupture from increased pressure or esophageal irritation. Another factor in hemorrhage is that the liver is no longer able to make vitamin K, which is an essential component in the production of clotting factors in the blood. Lack of clotting factors can lead to hemorrhage (Complementary & Alternative Therapies 30–3).

Varices may rupture and produce **hematemesis** (vomiting of bright red blood) from increased blood pressure, coughing, vomiting, or mechanical irritation from poorly chewed food. There may be bleeding from rectal varices or hemorrhoids. Esophageal varices can be deadly because of massive, rapid hemorrhage. Thirty percent to 60% of cirrhosis patients with bleeding esophageal varices die within 6 weeks of the first bleed.

Treatment options are to put pressure via balloon tamponade with a Blakemore-Sengstaken tube, administration of parenteral vasopressors such as vasopressin (Pitressin) to lower portal pressure, injection scleropathy or ligation of the bleeding vessels, emboli-

Complementary & Alternative Therapies 30-3

Milk Thistle for Cirrhosis

Milk thistle is used to treat hepatotoxicity caused by cirrhosis and hepatitis C. Liver function studies should be monitored if the patient chooses to use this herb. Silymarin, the active ingredient, acts as an antioxidant, decreasing free radicals and increasing hepatocyte synthesis (National Cancer Institute, 2005). It exerts other hepatoprotective effects. It can be used for mushroom poisoning as well.

zation of the left gastric vein, or emergency portacaval shunt surgery (Figure 30–4). Other vasoconstrictors such as terlipressin (Glypressin), somatostatin (Zecnil), and octreotide (Sandostatin) are used to reduce portal blood flow. Nitroglycerin is given to reduce vascular resistance in the liver without interfering with peripheral circulation. A beta blocker may be given to lower blood pressure. The patient is given vitamin K by injection to help rectify clotting factor deficiencies. The treatment of hemorrhage of the upper GI tract resulting from esophageal varices is discussed in Chapter 29 in the section on GI Bleeding under "Peptic Ulcer."

Encephalopathy. Portal systemic encephalopathy is another dangerous complication of cirrhosis. Encephalopathy in this instance is attributed to the buildup of ammonia and gamma-aminobutyric acid. Encephalopathy is directly related to liver failure. It produces symptoms such as delirium, convulsions, and coma. **Asterixis** (flapping tremors) may occur before coma ensues. When the patient holds out the arms and hands, there is rapid flexing and extension movements of the hands. There may be rhythmic movements of the legs with dorsiflexion of the foot and rhythmic movements in the face with strong eyelid closure. **Fetor hepaticus** (breath with a distinct sweet, almost fecal odor) occurs as liver failure progresses.

LIVER TRANSPLANTATION

Liver transplantation is considered for patients with progressive and advanced liver disease that does not respond to treatment (Legal & Ethical Considerations 30–1). It is most commonly done for nonalcoholic cirrhosis, chronic active hepatitis, sclerosing cholangitis, metabolic disorders, and biliary atresia in children. Some recovered alcoholics with cirrhosis are candidates.

Seventy percent to 80% of liver transplantation patients survive at least 3 years with good quality of life. Many transplant recipients develop cirrhosis by the fifth year. Organ transplantation, tissue matching, and measures to prevent organ rejection are discussed in Chapter 11. If the patient has encephalopathy preoperatively, an epidural sensor is placed to monitor intracranial pressure (ICP). Every attempt is made to keep ICP within normal as increased ICP levels are correlated with decreased survival rates after transplantation.

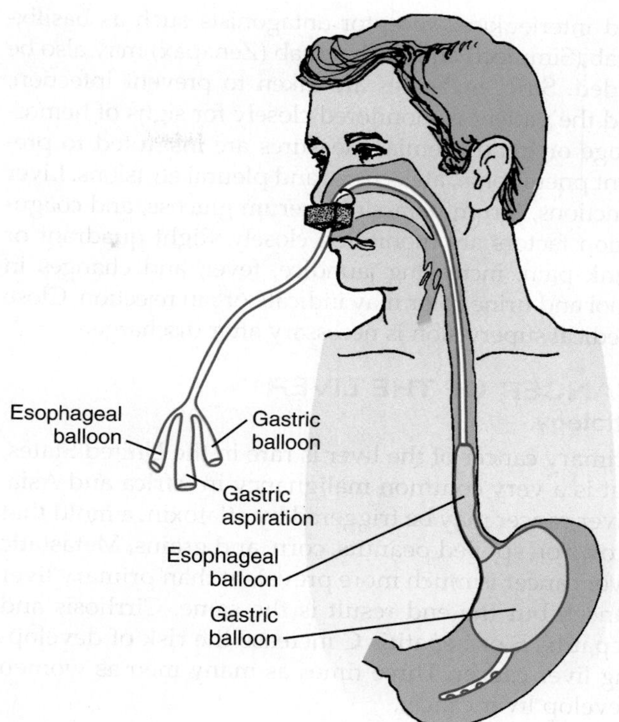

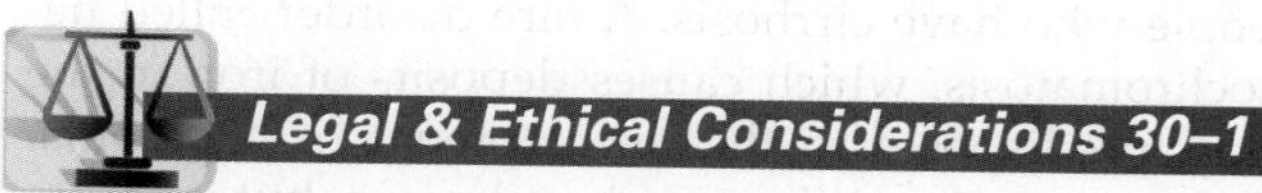
If the bleeding site is in the esophagus, as from esophageal varices, the esophageal balloon is inflated. If the bleeding site is in the stomach, the gastric balloon is inflated. Inflation of the balloon creates pressure against bleeding vessels.

FIGURE **30–4** Blakemore-Sengstaken tube.

Legal & Ethical Considerations 30–1

Liver Transplantation

Far more people with liver failure are in need of a liver transplant than there are available cadaver organs. There is a great deal of controversy about how available organs that fit a patient's genotype should be allotted. Should a person closest to the geographic location of the suitable cadaver liver receive it? Should the person who has been on the transplant list the longest be the recipient? Should the person who is closest to death be given the liver? Should the person whose liver was destroyed by alcohol or from recreational drug use be in line before the person with a metabolic or viral disease that caused end-stage cirrhosis? Should the recipient's age be a factor in the decision? These are the questions that enter into the liver transplantation decision.

Nursing Management

After surgery there will be a T-tube and Jackson-Pratt drains in place. The patient is placed on cyclosporine for life to prevent rejection of the new liver. Other immunosuppressants such as azathioprine (Imuran), corticosteroids, tacrolimus (Prograf), monoclonal antibody OKT3, and interleukin-2 receptor antagonists such as basiliximab (Simulect) and daclizumab (Zenapax) may also be added. Strict measures are taken to prevent infection, and the patient is monitored closely for signs of hemorrhage or hypovolemia. Measures are instituted to prevent pneumonia, atelectasis, and pleural effusions. Liver functions, serum potassium, serum glucose, and coagulation factors are monitored closely. Right quadrant or flank pain, increasing jaundice, fever, and changes in stool and urine color may indicate organ rejection. Close medical supervision is necessary after discharge.

CANCER OF THE LIVER

Etiology

Primary cancer of the liver is rare in the United States, but is a very common malignancy in Africa and Asia. Liver cancer may be triggered by aflatoxin, a mold that grows on spoiled peanuts, corn, and grains. Metastatic liver cancer is much more prevalent than primary liver cancer, but the end result is the same. Cirrhosis and hepatitis B or hepatitis C increase the risk of developing liver cancer. Three times as many men as women develop liver cancer.

Pathophysiology

There are two types of primary liver cancer: (1) hepatoma, which arises from the hepatocytes, and (2) cholangiocarcinoma or bile duct cancer. Benign tumors also occur in the liver. Hepatoma usually develops in people who have cirrhosis. A rare disorder called hemochromatosis, which causes deposits of iron in the body, predisposes to the development of hepatoma. Cholangiocarcinoma's cause is unknown, but it occurs more frequently in people with inflammation of the bowel, such as ulcerative colitis. The liver fluke, a parasite, is a cause of liver cancer in Africa and Asia.

Pathophysiologically, there is irritation and inflammation with disruption of the structure of normal liver cells. The cancer spreads throughout the organ and invades the portal vein and lymphatics. It can spread to the heart and lungs and may metastasize to the brain, kidneys, and spleen.

Signs, Symptoms, and Diagnosis

Symptoms may be right upper quadrant pain, fatigue, anorexia, weight loss, weakness, or fever plus signs of poor liver function. Pain may radiate to the back. Because symptoms often are vague, diagnosis occurs late and death may occur within 6 to 18 months.

Diagnostic tests are used to determine the presence of tumor and the stage of the cancer and to find areas of metastasis. Fine-needle biopsy or brush biopsy during ERCP gives a definitive diagnosis.

Treatment and Nursing Management

If no distant spread is found and there is no lymph node involvement, surgical resection may be attempted. If the tumor is primary and has not metastasized, liver transplantation is an option. Treatment is combined radiation and chemotherapy that is infused intravenously or directly into the hepatic circulation. Commonly used agents are 5-fluorouracil (5-FU), doxorubicin, and methotrexate. Chemoembolization, wherein an oily substance called lipiodol is added to the drugs given intra-arterially, makes the chemotherapy more effective. The treatment may induce toxic hepatitis, which subsides after the end of therapy. Care of the cancer patient is presented in Chapter 8. Additional care is directed at the problems of liver failure, such as ascites and encephalopathy.

Tumor ablation is used for tumors less than 5 cm in diameter. Ethanol or acetic acid is injected through the skin into the tumor. The liquid destroys the cancer cells. The procedure is carried out in the radiology department with the use of ultrasound.

Laser or radiofrequency ablation that causes heat to destroy cancer cells is performed with a local anesthetic. This procedure is used for cholangiocarcinoma. Cryotherapy that freezes the tumor area may be carried out during surgery. A probe deposits liquid nitrogen to the tumor site and destroys cancer cells.

Radioimmunotherapy is experimental and uses a radioactive isotope that attaches to a radiolabeled antibody against a protein found in liver tumors. It is given intravenously, concentrates in the liver, and irradiates the tumor internally. The side effects of thrombocytopenia and neutropenia occur 4 to 6 weeks after treatment.

Nursing care is directed at assessing for signs and symptoms of liver failure and blockage in the common bile duct. Surgical care is provided as for other abdominal surgery patients (see Chapter 5). Specific care of the cancer patient undergoing chemotherapy and radiation is located in Chapter 8.

DISORDERS OF THE PANCREAS

ACUTE PANCREATITIS

Pancreatitis is an inflammation of the pancreas. It may be acute or chronic in nature. Pancreatitis frequently accompanies obstruction of the pancreatic duct from gallstones, or from the backflow of bile into the pancreatic duct.

Etiology

Most cases of pancreatitis are related to alcoholism, although there are cases due to biliary disease. Viral infections, trauma, ERCP, penetrating ulcers, drug toxicities, metabolic disorders, scorpion stings, and a variety of other factors can cause pancreatitis. Men tend to develop pancreatitis related to alcohol. In women, it is associated more frequently with gallstones.

Pathophysiology

In some types of pancreatitis, the severe inflammation and damage are caused by escape of pancreatic digestive enzymes. The enzymes act directly on the tissue, causing hemorrhage, autodigestion, and necrosis. It is unclear how the autodigestion is activated. Reflux of bile and duodenal contents into the pancreatic duct is a possible mechanism. A gallstone stuck in the ampulla of Vater can cause edema of the sphincter of Oddi, which might permit reflux of duodenal contents. Alcohol can cause spasm of the sphincter of Oddi, blocking secretion through the pancreatic ducts. This may lead to activation of the pancreatic enzymes within the pancreas.

Pancreatic abscess or pseudocyst may develop. An abscess may form from the purulent liquefaction of the necrotic pancreatic tissue. A **pseudocyst** is a saclike structure that forms on or around the pancreas. It may contain several liters of enzymatic pancreatic exudates. If a pseudocyst ruptures, it may cause hemorrhage. Shock may occur, as well as other life-threatening complications (Concept Map 30–2).

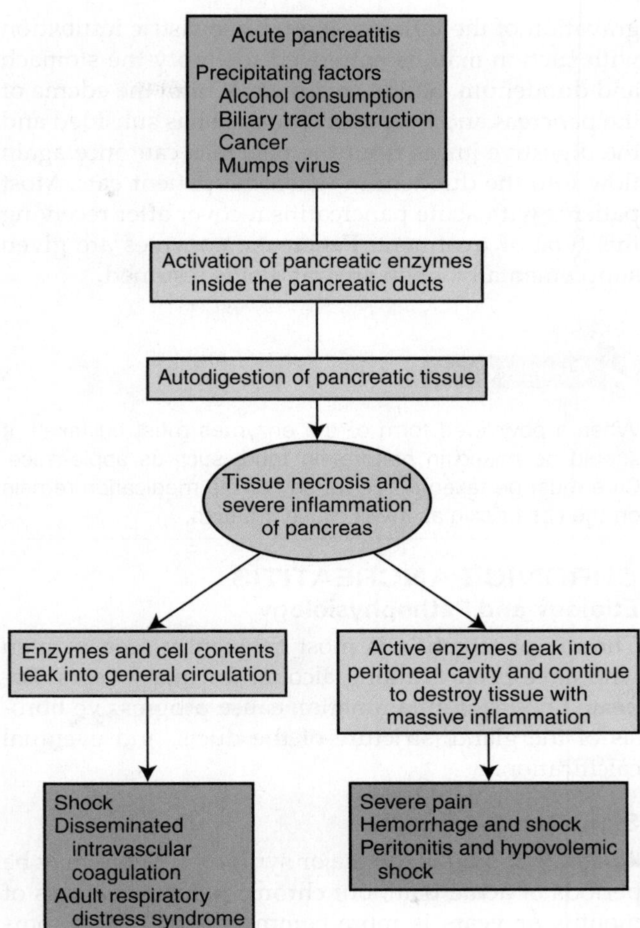

CONCEPT MAP **30–2** Pathophysiology of acute pancreatitis.

Signs and Symptoms

Pancreatitis causes abdominal pain that is usually acute, but this can vary among individuals. The pain is steady and is localized to the epigastrium or left upper quadrant. As it progresses, it spreads and radiates to the back and flank. Sitting and leaning forward may ease the pain. The severity of the pain may slowly decrease after 24 hours. **Eating makes the pain worse.** Nausea, vomiting, sweating, jaundice, and weakness often accompany pain. There may be signs and symptoms of respiratory distress, shock, tachycardia, leukocytosis, and fever.

Examination of the abdomen will reveal tenderness and guarding. If peritonitis is present, there will be distention and rigidity. Bowel sounds may be reduced or absent. A pseudocyst can be palpated as an epigastric mass in about 50% of cases. If retroperitoneal bleeding is present, there may be bruising in the flanks or a bluish discoloration around the umbilicus. Serum amylase may be two times normal and will remain elevated for 72 hours. Serum lipase remains elevated for several days. If biliary obstruction is involved, mild jaundice may be present. Laboratory values will indicate hypoglycemia, hypocalcemia, and hypokalemia.

Think Critically About . . . What assessment data might tell you that your patient's pain is from cholelithiasis rather than pancreatitis?

Diagnosis

Diagnosis is based on the presenting symptoms plus risk factors and results of tests performed to rule out other disorders. An abdominal sonogram, CT scan, and serum and urine amylase studies are usually ordered (Table 30–6).

Table 30–6 ***Laboratory Test Findings in Acute Pancreatitis***

TEST	FINDING
Serum amylase	Increased; >200 Units/L
Serum lipase	Elevated
Urinary amylase	Elevated

Treatment and Nursing Management

Treatment is supportive and consists of pain control and reduction of pancreatic secretions by placing the patient NPO. Prevention of shock, restoration of fluid and electrolyte balance, and treatment of secondary infection are other goals. Complications such as diabetes mellitus must be addressed. If abscess or pseudocyst is present, it will be surgically drained. Intravenous meperidine or morphine via PCA pump may be needed to control pain. Histamine (H_2)-receptor antagonists or a proton pump inhibitor may be given to decrease the hydrochloric acid secretion that stimulates pancreatic activity. Administration of antispasmodics such as dicyclomine (Bentyl) or propantheline bromide (Pro-Banthine) is helpful. The patient is allowed nothing by mouth during the acute phase so as to prevent stimulation of the pancreas and further aggravation of the inflammation. Nasogastric intubation with suction may be employed to empty the stomach and duodenum. Fluids are given IV until the edema of the pancreas and the pancreatic duct has subsided and the digestive juices from the pancreas can once again flow into the duodenum when the patient eats. Most patients with acute pancreatitis recover after receiving this type of treatment. Pancreatic enzymes are given supplementally when an oral diet is resumed.

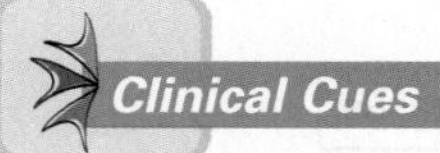

When a powdered form of the enzymes must be taken, it should be mixed in nonprotein food, such as applesauce. Care must be taken not to let any of the medication remain on the lips or skin as it will cause irritation.

CHRONIC PANCREATITIS

Etiology and Pathophysiology

Chronic pancreatitis is most frequently seen in men who have been drinking alcohol for many years. Repeated bouts of inflammation cause progressive fibrosis of the gland, stricture of the ducts, and eventual calcification.

Signs and Symptoms

Abdominal pain is the major symptom. There may be periods of acute pain, but chronic pain at intervals of months or years is more common. Other symptoms are related to pancreatic insufficiency as less and less pancreatic tissue is functional. Malabsorption with weight loss and steatorrhea, constipation, mild jaundice with dark urine, and diabetes mellitus develop.

Diagnosis

Determination of bicarbonate concentration and output in the duodenum after stimulation with secretin is the definitive test for chronic pancreatitis. Other helpful diagnostic tests are fecal fat determination, fasting blood glucose, arteriography, and radiographic examinations of the pancreas. Pancreatic cancer or another liver disorder can produce the same results on these tests. The differential diagnosis is difficult. Serum amylase and lipase may be elevated slightly or not at all. There may be increases in serum bilirubin and alkaline phosphatase. Leukocytosis and an elevated sedimentation rate are present.

Treatment

Treatment during an attack of chronic pancreatitis is the same as for acute pancreatitis. Long-term pain control presents problems. The patient is switched to nonnarcotic pain medications to try to prevent addiction, but these often are not sufficient for pain control. Pancreatic enzymes are prescribed to be taken with meals, which should be low in fat. No alcohol is to be consumed.

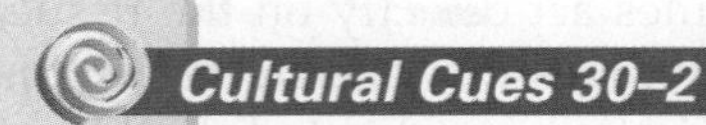

Pancreatic Cancer Deaths

More African American men die from pancreatic cancer than do men from any other ethnic group. Alcohol use and abuse is a major factor. Working with community and church leaders to discourage the immoderate use of alcohol might decrease the problem and save lives.

Chronic pancreatitis greatly interferes with the patient's usual lifestyle and often is accompanied by depression requiring psychiatric intervention.

Nursing Management

Vital signs are taken frequently, urinary output is monitored closely, and the patient is monitored for signs of shock. Observe for signs of restlessness, use of accessory muscles for breathing, irritability, confusion, or dyspnea, which indicate respiratory distress. Monitor respiratory status closely and administer oxygen as ordered. Pain evaluation and control are primary nursing responsibilities. Monitor laboratory values and note changes. Provide care regarding total parenteral nutrition (TPN) if the patient is receiving it. Glucose determinations will need to be done regularly, and administration of insulin may be necessary. Nasogastric tube care must be provided until nausea subsides. Slowly the patient will resume a bland, soft diet, and the abdomen must be assessed for tolerance of the diet. Monitor administration of fluids and for electrolyte imbalances. Reinforce teaching about the disease process. Rest is essential even if the patient does not feel ill.

A major nursing action is to be supportive of efforts to abstain from alcohol. Table 30–5 presents the problems/nursing diagnoses and specific interventions appropriate for patients with pancreatitis.

CANCER OF THE PANCREAS

Etiology

The cause of pancreatic cancer is unknown. There will be about 37,170 new cases of cancer of the pancreas in the United States in 2007. It is more common in men than in women and occurs more often in African Americans than in white Americans (Cultural Cues 30–2). Pancreatic cancer is most prevalent in the over-70 age group.

Diets high in red meats and fats may increase the risk. Cancer of the pancreas is very often fatal within 1 year. It is usually in a very advanced state when discovered, as the patient is asymptomatic in the early stages.

Pathophysiology

Cigarette smoking is the major risk factor and link identified for pancreatic cancer (Health Promotion Points 30–3). Adenocarcinoma arising from the epithe-

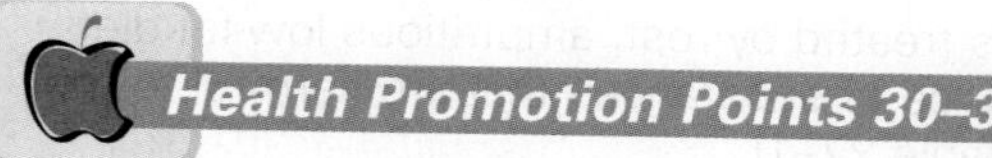

Health Promotion Points 30–3

Quitting Smoking

When a patient who smokes is encountered, it is a nursing responsibility to tactfully discuss the dangers of smoking, providing statistics on various disorders that occur so much more frequently in smokers than nonsmokers. Provide referral to community resources for quitting smoking and written materials with options on how to quit.

lial cells in the ducts is the most common form of pancreatic neoplasm. Tumor in the head of the pancreas obstructs biliary and pancreatic flow. Cancer in the body and tail of the pancreas usually remains asymptomatic until it is well advanced and invades the liver, stomach, lymph nodes, or posterior abdominal wall and nerves. Metastasis occurs early. The biliary obstruction usually causes liver failure, which in turn most often causes death.

Signs and Symptoms

Epigastric pain and weight loss are the main symptoms. Anorexia and vomiting may occur, and the patient may develop a dislike for red meat. When the disease is advanced, jaundice appears along with dark urine and clay-colored stools. There is glucose intolerance. Thrombophlebitis may cause leg or calf pain. There is a high incidence of clot formation with pancreatic cancer (Safety Alert 30–3).

Diagnosis

Diagnosis is made by ultrasonography, imaging techniques, and fine-needle biopsy. Elevated carcinoembryonic antigen levels occur 80% to 90% of the time when pancreatic cancer is present. However, serum beta-human chorionic gonadotropin and carbohydrate antigen (CA) 72-4 are the strongest indicators of pancreatic cancer. The tumor markers CA 19-9 and CA 242 are used to monitor for potential spread or recurrence.

Treatment

High doses of opioid analgesics are usually required to keep the patient comfortable. Drug dependency should not be a concern. Treating or preventing malnutrition is a major goal. Enteral feedings may need to be given via a catheter into the jejunum *(jejunostomy).* TPN may be needed to provide adequate nutrition (see Chapter 3 and Chapter 28).

Surgical treatment is appropriate for resectable tumor in about 15% to 20% of patients but has not been highly successful in curing the disease. It provides a 5-year survival rate of less than 5%. Surgery is used mainly to relieve symptoms of obstructive jaundice, severe pain, or other complications. A Whipple procedure, or radical pancreaticoduodenectomy, may be done for cancer of the head of the pancreas. The head

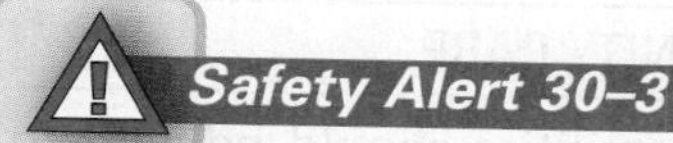

Safety Alert 30–3

Watch for Deep Vein Thrombosis

Because of the increased risk of clot formation in patients with pancreatic cancer, it is important to assess for signs and symptoms of deep vein thrombosis: pain, heat, or swelling in the calves. One leg may be swollen while the other is not. Measure the calf and ankle and compare to the other leg. Check for signs of pulmonary embolus as well: restlessness, apprehension, chest pain, and shortness of breath. Should these signs and symptoms occur, report them to the physician immediately.

of the pancreas, the gallbladder, the duodenum, part of the jejunum, and all or part of the stomach are removed. The spleen may also be removed. The remaining structures are anastomosed to the jejunum. Another option is total pancreatectomy. Because of the vast array of potential complications, the patient will usually go to the surgical critical care unit after surgery. Nursing care is the same as for any abdominal surgery, but careful observation for the many complications that can occur is essential. The patient will need enteral feedings, perhaps for life. A stent may be placed in the pancreatic duct to promote exit of pancreatic secretions and enzymes.

Cyberknife treatment, an image-guided radiosurgery, that helps target pancreatic tumor without disrupting other tissue is an option. There are several Cyberknife centers in the United States.

Gemcitabine (Gemzar) is the standard of care for treatment of nonresectable or metastatic tumors (Oettle et al., 2007). It has been considerably more effective than 5-FU used alone. A combination of drugs has proven most effective, and other commonly used drugs include mitomycin (Mutamycin), docetaxel (Taxotere), and cisplatin (Platinol).

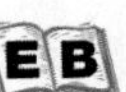

Intensive external beam radiation therapy may offer pain relief, alleviate duct obstruction, and improve food absorption. Radioactive iodine (^{125}I) seeds may be implanted in combination with systemic or intra-arterial administration of floxuridine (FUDR).

Nursing Management

Nursing care is geared toward managing the severe pain these patients experience, and managing the side effects of treatment. Postoperatively, observe for hyperglycemia, hemorrhage, bowel obstruction or paralytic ileus, wound infection, and intra-abdominal abscess. Monitor the nasogastric tube for clear, colorless, bile-tinged drainage or frank blood with an increase in output as this may indicate leakage at an anastomosis site. Provide care for the postoperative patient with abdominal surgery (see Chapter 5). Chapter 8 contains information on care of the cancer patient undergoing chemotherapy or radiation.

COMMUNITY CARE

Nurses in extended care facilities should be alert to signs of jaundice in patients. Dark-colored urine is frequently an early sign of a problem. Cancer and gallstones are both more prevalent in the elderly, and when abdominal pain occurs these disorders must be considered.

Nurses in the community should promote immunization against hepatitis B virus in all persons at risk. Teenagers and adults should be counseled about the possibility of transmission of hepatitis B virus by sexual contact and advised of measures for protection. The hepatitis A vaccine should be recommended for those traveling in areas where this disorder is prevalent and for those at risk of liver problems. Education about ways to prevent contracting hepatitis C for teens and adults is important. All health care workers should be tested for the presence of hepatitis C virus. Home care nurses must be particularly alert to the possibility of liver or pancreatic problems due to medications the patient is taking. Encouraging regular laboratory work as recommended when the patient is taking a drug known to be potentially damaging to the liver is a nursing function.

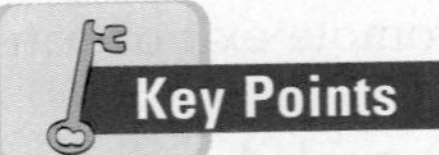

Key Points

- Typical symptoms of cholelithiasis are indigestion, flatulence, nausea after eating fatty foods, and right upper quadrant discomfort.
- Other causes of cholecystitis can be long periods of immobilization, rapid-weight-loss diets or starvation, major trauma, burns, and cardiac surgery.
- Signs and symptoms of acute cholecystitis include acute pain, fever, anorexia, nausea and vomiting, dehydration, and mild jaundice.
- Chronic inflammation causes fibrosis of the liver cells, which results in cirrhosis.
- Signs and symptoms of liver disorders are fatigue, weakness, anorexia, abdominal pain, nausea and vomiting, skin rashes, itching, fever, dark urine, light-colored stools, peripheral edema, bruising, and jaundice. Jaundice occurs when bile flow is disrupted and bilirubin levels rise in the blood.
- There are five main types of hepatitis: A, B, C, D, and E. Newly discovered hepatitis G virus does not seem to cause the disorder (see Table 30–2).
- Hepatitis B, C, D, and E viruses can be transmitted by blood contact with mucous membranes. Health care workers are at risk and must always adhere to Standard Precautions.
- Signs and symptoms of hepatitis are malaise, fever, anorexia, nausea, joint aching, skin rash, and right upper abdomen discomfort. Urine becomes dark and stool becomes light if there is obstruction of bile ducts. Jaundice and pruritus occur.
- Hepatitis is treated by rest, a nutritious low-fat diet, and avoidance of substances that are harmful to the liver (see Table 27–1).
- Cirrhosis is progressive and chronic, with destruction of normal hepatic structures and replacement with fibrotic tissue.
- When normal functions of the liver are lost, ammonia may build up in the blood, causing hepatic encephalopathy.
- Definitive diagnosis of cirrhosis of the liver is made by liver biopsy. Liver function tests, prothrombin time, and albumin levels contribute to the diagnosis.
- Bleeding esophageal varices are treated with scleropathy, banding, or surgical shunting procedures.
- Chemotherapy, radiation, and ablation therapies are used for treatment of liver cancer.
- Inflammation and damage are caused by escape of pancreatic digestive enzymes, which act directly on the tissue, causing hemorrhage, autodigestion, and necrosis.
- Signs and symptoms of pancreatitis are acute, steady pain in the epigastrium or left upper quadrant. Eating makes the pain worse. Serum lipase and amylase are elevated.
- Treatment consists of pain control, reduction of pancreatic secretions, restoration of fluid and electrolyte balance, and treatment for complications such as shock or diabetes.
- Chronic pancreatitis is related to long-term alcoholism. Abdominal pain is the main symptom.
- Long-term pain control is a difficult problem.
- Signs and symptoms of pancreatic cancer are weight loss, anorexia, vomiting, and signs of pancreatic dysfunction.
- Treatment is aimed at preventing malnutrition and controlling pain.
- Chemotherapy and radiation are employed and may improve food absorption, relieve pain, and alleviate duct obstruction.
- Pain control is a major goal.
- Gallbladder, liver, and pancreas disorders should be considered in the elderly who develop abdominal pain or have dark-colored urine.
- Nurses should promote hepatitis B immunization of all persons.
- Sex education should include the ways in which hepatitis B and C viruses are transmitted and how to avoid these viruses.
- Nurses should encourage regular laboratory testing for patients continuously taking drugs known to be harmful to the liver.

Go to your **Companion CD-ROM** for an Audio Glossary, animations, video clips, and bonus review questions.

evolve Be sure to visit the companion Evolve site at http://evolve.elsevier.com/deWit for interactive NCLEX-PN Exam Style Review Questions, WebLinks, and additional online resources.

NCLEX-PN EXAM STYLE REVIEW QUESTIONS

Choose the best answer(s) for the following questions.

1. Prior to being discharged to home, the patient with gallbladder disease is given instructions regarding the care of the drain and the T-tube. Which of the following patient statements indicates a need for further teaching?
   1. "I must empty the bag the same time each day."
   2. "Loose-fitting clothes must be worn."
   3. "I would have yellowish skin discoloration the rest of my life."
   4. "Passing brown stools indicates return to normal function."

2. ______________________ are bluish varicose veins that radiate from the umbilicus and indicate the presence of portal hypertension.

3. The nurse is caring for a 57-year-old patient with ascites due to liver insufficiency. The nurse anticipates which of the following therapeutic regimens to reduce portal hypertension?
   1. Vascular shunting of the portal venous systems
   2. Repeated abdominal paracentesis
   3. Diet restrictions and nutrient supplementation
   4. Fluid replacement therapy

4. The patient with high levels of serum ammonia asks, "Why do I have to continue taking lactulose?" The nurse accurately responds:
   1. "It destroys ammonia-producing bacteria in the intestines."
   2. "It reduces intestinal absorption of ammonia."
   3. "It restores acid-base balance."
   4. "It is used in preparation for a diagnostic test."

5. The nurse is caring for a patient who underwent a recent liver transplantation. Prior to administering the cyclosporine, the nurse reinforces the teaching for immunosuppressant therapy. Which of the following patient statements indicates a need for further instructions?
   1. "I need to report any kind of pain associated with fever and changes in stool color."
   2. "I would be able to attend a concert upon discharge."
   3. "Strict handwashing is critical in changing dressings."
   4. "These medications would be taken for life."

6. Nursing care of the patient during the acute phase of pancreatitis is geared toward reduction of pain. The following nursing interventions help alleviate pain *except:*
   1. reinforcing instructions to use the pain pump
   2. maintaining intravenous fluids
   3. providing a bland diet
   4. administering proton pump inhibitor medications

7. The nurse is caring for a patient who had undergone radical pancreaticoduodenectomy. The nurse monitors for which of the following postoperative complications? *(Select all that apply.)*
   1. Hypoglycemia
   2. Hemorrhage
   3. Bowel obstruction
   4. Intra-abdominal abscess
   5. Hyperkalemia

8. Which of the following statements by a patient indicates a need for further instructions regarding preventing the spread of hepatitis A?
   1. "Bleach solutions must be used to clean the bathroom."
   2. "Immunization with the hepatitis A vaccine affords protection from the disease."
   3. "I can share bath and hand towels with the rest of the family."
   4. "Extremely good handwashing prevents transmission of the virus."

9. The patient with hepatic failure asks, "Why am I getting neomycin?" An accurate response by the nurse would be:
   1. "The medication stimulates liver metabolism of nitrogenous compounds."
   2. "The medication decreases the colonic bacteria that break down protein."
   3. "The medication increases transit time through the intestines."
   4. "The medication helps eliminate nitrogenous compounds."

10. On initial assessment, the nurse observes rhythmic movements of the patient's arms and hands. These movements are associated with dorsiflexion of the feet. These movements, associated with hepatic encephalopathy, are referred to as:
    1. tics.
    2. asterixis.
    3. tremors.
    4. seizures.

CRITICAL THINKING ACTIVITIES 

Read each clinical scenario and discuss the questions with your classmates.

Scenario A

Mr. Moser is admitted to the hospital with a diagnosis of cirrhosis of the liver. He is 59 years of age and has been hospitalized several times for his condition. He suffers from shortness of breath as a result of a swollen and enlarged abdomen, is anemic because of minimal but constant esophageal bleeding, and appears jaundiced. He has severe abrasions on his arms, legs, and abdomen from repeated scratching to relieve his pruritus.

Mr. Moser is very depressed and will not converse with you when you enter his room with his breakfast tray the first morning you are assigned to his care. He refuses to eat and indicates his attitude by pushing the tray away and turning on his side, face to the wall.

1. What nursing measures might help relieve some of Mr. Moser's problems?
2. Why do you think he is mentally depressed?
3. How would you go about helping him emotionally?
4. What special observations must you make while caring for Mr. Moser?
5. How would you explain a paracentesis to Mr. Moser if one were ordered for him?

Scenario B

Mrs. Lincoln, age 46, is admitted to the hospital for a laparoscopic cholecystectomy. She is extremely obese and enjoys eating rich, fatty foods, even though she knows this will add to her obesity and precipitate attacks of cholecystitis. You are assigned to care for Mrs. Lincoln when she returns from surgery.

1. How will you position this patient?
2. What would you need to assess to determine whether complications are occurring?
3. What would you need to teach the patient and family before discharge?
4. What problems might occur after discharge? What should be the diet for Mrs. Lincoln?
5. How soon will Mrs. Lincoln probably be able to resume most of her usual activities?

CHAPTER 31

The Musculoskeletal System

evolve http://evolve.elsevier.com/deWit

Objectives

Upon completing this chapter you should be able to:

Theory

1. Recall the normal anatomy of the musculoskeletal system.
2. Describe how the musculoskeletal system provides the function of motion.
3. Explain how the musculoskeletal system provides protection for the body.
4. Describe the steps included in a nursing assessment of the musculoskeletal system.
5. Teach a patient about the following diagnostic tests: bone scan, arthroscopy, electromyography.

Clinical Practice

1. Gather positioning aids and place them correctly for the patient who has sustained trauma to the left knee.
2. Institute measures to reduce the chance of contracture for patients with musculoskeletal injuries.
3. Assist patients with musculoskeletal injuries with active or passive range of motion.
4. Provide care for a patient who has undergone an arthroscopy.
5. Teach a patient to properly use crutches.

Key Terms

Be sure to check out the bonus material on the Companion CD-ROM, including selected audio pronunciations.

ankylosis (ăng-kĭ-LŌ-sĭs, p. 777)
contracture (kŏn-TRĂK-chŭr, p. 774)
crepitation (KRĔP-ĭ-tā-shŭn, p. 767)
goniometry (gō-nē-ŎM-ĕ-trē, p. 769)
haversian system (p. 766)
isometric exercises (ī-sō-MĔT-rĭk, p. 778)
ossification (ŏs-ĭ-fĭ-KĀ-shŭn, p. 765)

The special branch of medical science concerned with the preservation and restoration of the functions of the skeletal system is called *orthopedics*. The principles of orthopedic nursing are applicable to the nursing care of all patients and most especially to those with limited mobility. The three main functions of the musculoskeletal system are motion, support, and protection. **Preservation of motion is probably the most important consideration to prevent orthopedic disabilities resulting from immobility.**

The bony tissues of the infant differ greatly from those of the adult because not all bone cells follow the same pattern of development from the embryonic stage to full maturity. There are two distinct groups of bone cells. The cells in the first group are designed so that they are immediately transformed into mature cells. The normal infant will have this type of firm bone cells in his skull and shoulder bones. In the second group, the bone cells form cartilage first and then are gradually replaced by mature bone cells as the person grows older. **Ossification**, or replacement of cartilage by more solid bony tissue, is not completed throughout the body until age 20 to 25.

Because the bony structures of infants and young children are softer and more pliable than those of adults, there is less danger of breaking bones during the time of life when they are learning to walk and run and are therefore more likely to have frequent falls. If a fracture does occur, it will heal more rapidly in a very young person because growth is still taking place within the bone.

Trauma and disease cause dysfunction of the musculoskeletal system. Exercise and correct diet help preserve function. To understand thoroughly the problems that can occur in the musculoskeletal system, it is necessary to recall the structures of the system and their functions.

CAUSES OF MUSCULOSKELETAL DISORDERS

Disease, trauma, malnutrition, and aging all contribute to musculoskeletal problems. Trauma may cause bruising, strain, sprain, or fracture. Poor nutrition may deprive the body of sufficient calcium and phosphorus to build strong bones. Inadequate protein intake can cause muscle wasting. Malignant tumors place a large nutritional demand on the body, and nutritional imbalances may occur that cause muscle wasting. Tumor may invade bone as either a primary or metastatic cancer.

The decrease in estrogen production after menopause in women is thought to be a contributing factor to the occurrence of osteoporosis. The use of hormone

OVERVIEW OF ANATOMY AND PHYSIOLOGY OF THE MUSCULOSKELETAL SYSTEM

What are the structures of the musculoskeletal system?

- The musculoskeletal system consists of the bones, joints, cartilage, ligaments, tendons, and muscles.
- A total of 206 bones make up the human skeleton (Figure 31–1).
- Bone is either compact or spongy. Spongy bone contains red bone marrow (Figure 31–2).
- Bones are classified as long, short, flat, or irregular.
- Each bone has markings on its surface that make it unique (Table 31–1).
- A canal system **(haversian system)** runs through the bone and contains the blood and lymph vessels.
- A joint is the articulation point between two or more bones of the skeleton. There are immovable, slightly movable, and freely movable joints.
- Ligaments join the bones of a joint together.
- Tendons are connective tissue that provide joint movement.
- Cartilage is a type of connective tissue in which fibers and cells are embedded in a semisolid gel material. Cartilage acts as a cushion. The meniscus in the knee joint is a type of cartilage.
- A bursa is a fluid-filled sac that provides cushioning at friction points in a freely movable joint.
- Skeletal muscle is made up of hundreds of muscle fibers bundled together surrounded by a connective tissue sheath.

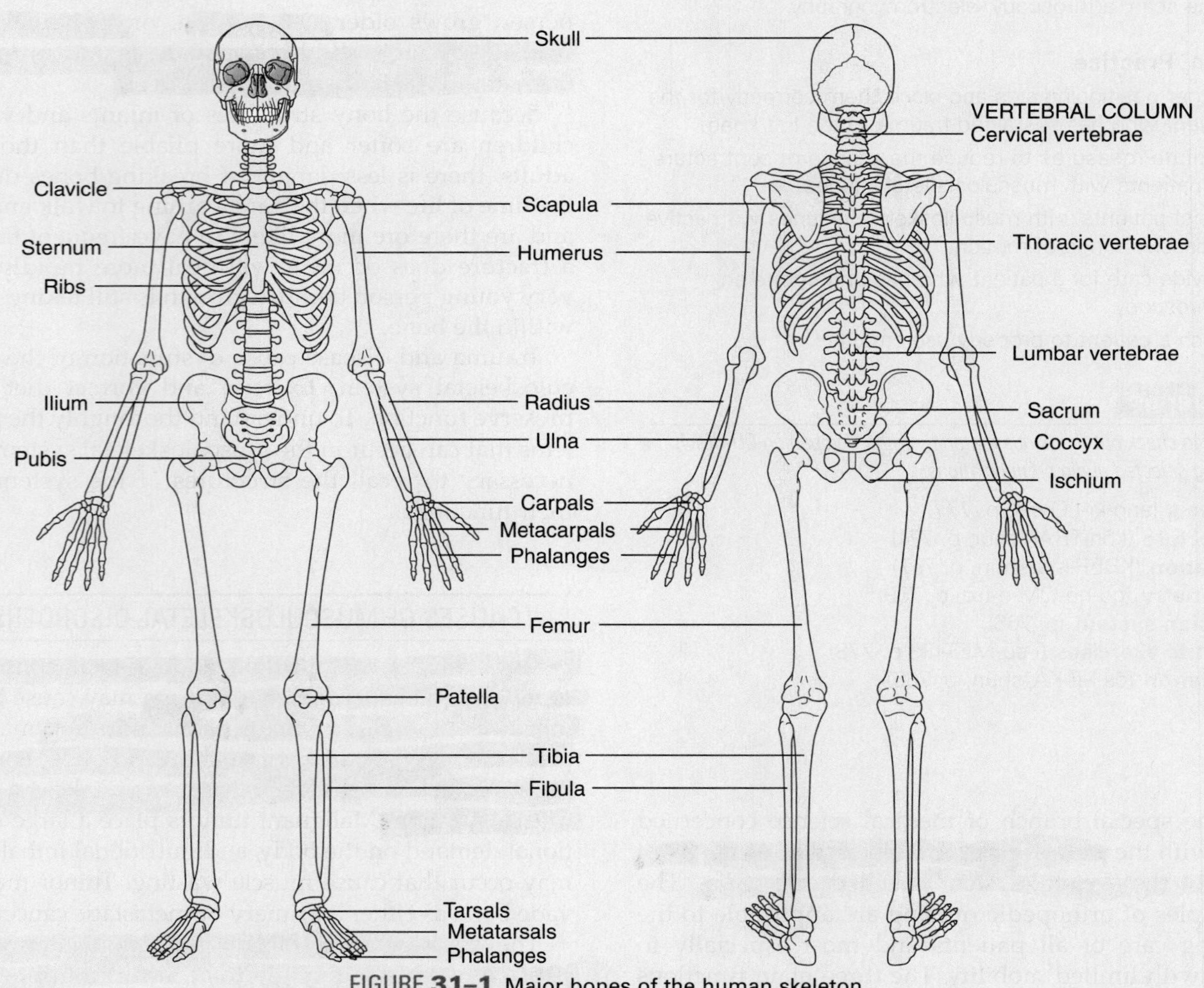

FIGURE **31–1** Major bones of the human skeleton.

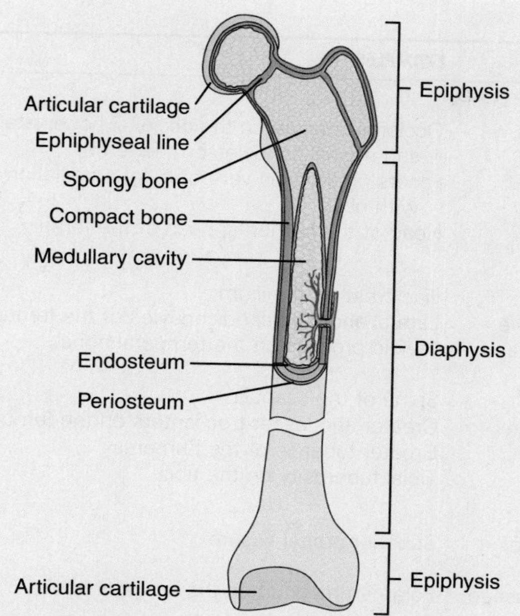

FIGURE 31–2 General features of long bones.

- Fascia is a connective tissue that surrounds and separates the muscles.
- The muscle coverings contain blood vessels and nerves.
- Muscle has properties that allow it to be electrically excited, cause it to contract, extend, or stretch, and provide elasticity.
- Skeletal muscles are attached to bones by tendons.

What are the functions of the bones?

- Bones provide shape to the body.
- The skeleton provides a rigid framework that supports the internal organs and the skin.
- The skeleton protects the internal organs of the body.
- The skeleton provides attachments for tendons and ligaments and contributes to movement of the body.
- The red bone marrow in the spongy bones forms red blood cells, white blood cells, and platelets.
- The bones store and release minerals such as calcium and phosphorus.
- The blood and lymph vessels in the canals transport nutrients to the bone cells and remove wastes.
- Bone is maintained by remodeling: existing bone is resorbed into the body and new bone is built by osteoblasts to replace it.

What are the functions of the muscles?

- Contraction of skeletal muscles is produced by synchronized contraction of many muscle fibers.
- Skeletal muscles contract, thereby providing movement and joint stability, maintaining posture, and producing body heat.
- By shortening and stretching, opposing muscle groups provide movement of the joints.

What changes occur in the musculoskeletal system with aging?

- Bone density decreases because of the resorption of minerals.
- The loss of bone mass, or *osteoporosis,* occurs with aging and is more severe in women.
- The bones of elderly people are brittle and less compact; thus, they break easily.
- When a fracture occurs, elderly bones do not heal readily because the physiologic exchange of minerals has decreased with advancing age, making the process of repair much slower.
- Thinning of the intervertebral cartilage and collapse of the vertebra result in kyphosis (dowager's hump). This is partially responsible for the decrease in height in the elderly.
- Joint cartilage thins and erodes from years of use and results in stiffness and **crepitation** (a sound like that of hair rubbed between the fingers) of the joints.
- Joint motion may decrease, limiting mobility; swelling may occur.
- Ligaments become calcified and lose their elasticity.
- Muscles decrease in mass and do not have the strength or endurance of the muscles in the younger person. Muscle cells decrease in number and the muscles atrophy.
- Tendons shrink and become sclerotic, slowing muscle movement.
- Muscle cramping, especially at night, increases because of impaired circulation and accumulation of metabolic wastes.

Table 31–1 Terms Related to Bone Markings

TERM	DESCRIPTION	EXAMPLES
PROJECTIONS FOR ARTICULATION		
Condyle (KON-dial)	Smooth, rounded articular surface	Occipital condyle on the occipital bone; lateral and medial condyles on the femur
Facet (FASS-et)	Smooth, nearly flat articular surface	Facets on thoracic vertebrae for articulation with ribs
Head (HED)	Enlarged, often rounded, end of bone	Head of the humerus; head of the femur
PROJECTIONS FOR MUSCLE ATTACHMENT		
Crest (KREST)	Narrow ridge of bone	Iliac crest on the ilium
Epicondyle (ep-ih-KON-dial)	Bony bulge adjacent to or above a condyle	Lateral and medial epicondyles of the femur
Process (PRAH-sess)	Any projection on a bone; often pointed and sharp	Styloid process on the temporal bone
Spine (SPYN)	Sharp, slender projection	Spine of the scapula
Trochanter (tro-KAN-turr)	Large, blunt, irregularly shaped projection	Greater and lesser trochanters on the femur
Tubercle (TOO-burr-kul)	Small, rounded, knoblike projection	Greater tubercle of the humerus
Tuberosity (too-burr-AHS-ih-tee)	Similar to a tubercle but usually larger	Tibial tuberosity on the tibia
DEPRESSIONS, OPENINGS, AND CAVITIES		
Fissure (FISH-ur)	Narrow cleft or slit; usually for passage of blood vessels and nerves	Superior orbital fissure
Foramen (foh-RAY-men)	Opening through a bone; usually for passage of blood vessels and nerves	Foramen magnum in the occipital bone
Fossa (FAW-sah)	A smooth, shallow depression	Mandibular fossa on the temporal bone; olecranon fossa on the humerus
Fovea (FOH-vee-ah)	A small pit or depression	Fovea capitis femoris on the head of the femur
Meatus (mee-ATE-us)	A tubelike passageway; tunnel	External auditory meatus in the temporal bone
Sinus (SYE-nus)	A cavity or hollow space in a bone	Frontal sinus in the frontal bone

From Applegate, E.J. (2006). *The Anatomy and Physiology Learning System* (3rd ed.). Philadelphia: Saunders.

replacement therapy (HRT) after menopause will decrease the incidence of osteoporosis in women, but there is controversy about the side effects of the drugs. Research found that HRT therapy increased the incidence of breast cancer (Cancer Research UK, 2003).

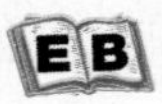

PREVENTION OF MUSCULOSKELETAL DISORDERS

Diagnosing and treating cancer in other parts of the body early can prevent the occurrence of metastases to the bone. Refraining from using steroids on a long-term basis can help prevent osteoporosis and fractures. Steroid use is a concern because of the many athletes who are using them. Individuals who must take steroids for chronic diseases such as asthma should be monitored for osteoporosis (Sebba, 2006).

EB

Weight training and exercise throughout life can decrease the incidence of osteoporosis and increase muscle strength, mass, agility, balance, and coordination, thereby preventing falls and consequent fractures. Weight-bearing exercise is needed to maintain bone mass.

Learning to lift and move objects correctly by using large muscle groups can help prevent muscle strain and sprains. Using seat belts when riding in an automobile can reduce the incidence of trauma to bone and muscle during accidents. Wearing bicycle, motorcycle, and other sports helmets will reduce the incidence of skull fractures. Consuming recommended amounts of calcium throughout the life span, obtaining sufficient vitamin D through sunshine, and maintaining adequate protein intake all help build healthy bone and muscle (Nutritional Therapies 31–1).

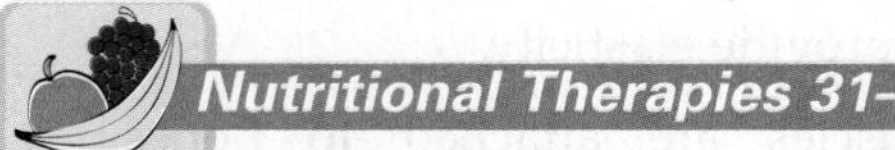

Nutrition for Bone Growth and Density

Adequate amounts of calcium and phosphorus are essential for bone growth and density. Although green vegetables are a source of calcium, that calcium is not readily absorbed. Dairy products such as cheese, yogurt, and milk are better choices. Canned sardines or salmon also provide good amounts of calcium. Magnesium and vitamin K are required for healthy bones as well. These are provided by a healthy diet containing meat and green vegetables. Spinach is a good source of vitamin K. The patient taking an anticoagulant should not alter the intake of vitamin K because it will affect coagulation times.

Calcium supplementation is not recommended for the healing of fractures. It has proven not to be readily absorbed and tends to cause kidney stones.

? *Think Critically About* . . . What could you do now to promote healthy bones during your elderly years?

DIAGNOSTIC TESTS AND PROCEDURES AND NURSING IMPLICATIONS

Specific diagnostic tests of the musculoskeletal system are listed in Table 31–2. Blood counts, blood cultures, and various tests for problems of the immune system may also be performed to detect rheumatoid arthritis or other connective tissue diseases. Other tests include an erythrocyte sedimentation rate (ESR), serum protein electrophoresis, and tests to determine the levels of serum complement and immunoglobulins (see Chapter 10).

Range of motion (ROM) testing involves both active and passive maneuvers. In active testing, the part being measured must be moved by the patient himself. In passive testing, the evaluator moves the body part while the patient is relaxed.

The measurement of ROM in a joint is called goniometry (Figure 31–3). One system of measurement that is commonly used is based on a full circle of 360 degrees. Each joint is evaluated in terms of the number of degrees it can be moved from the 0-degree position.

Muscle strength can be measured on the basis of the ability of a muscle to move the part to which it is at-

Table 31–2 ***Diagnostic Tests for Musculoskeletal Disorders***

TEST	PURPOSE	DESCRIPTION	NURSING IMPLICATIONS
X-rays of the bones or joints	Detects fracture, avulsion, joint damage	No preparation necessary. Part to be x-rayed is positioned by technician and x-rays are taken.	Explain the purpose, procedure, and possible sensations.
Tomography and xerography	Produces radiographic planes or slices; highlights contrast between structures	Specialized equipment is used; xerography uses a higher amount of radiation than normal x-rays.	Explain that the tomography procedure takes longer, as the machine takes a series of views.
Computed tomography (CT)	Detects musculoskeletal problems, especially of the spine and skull	A special machine is used and the patient is placed on a hard table. The procedure takes 30–60 min. Contrast material may or may not be used. Some patients experience claustrophobia from being encased by the machine. A computer enhances the radiographic findings.	Explain that lying perfectly still is required. The part under study is enclosed in the machine. There is a clicking sound as the machine rotates to take the next view.
Bone scan	Detects tumor, metastatic growths, bone injury, or degenerative bone disease; can detect problems earlier than x-rays	An IV injection or oral dose of a radioisotope is given, and after an interval time for the substance to be taken up by the bone, the area is scanned by scintillation camera.	Explain the purpose and procedure. Check for allergies and pregnancy. Patient will be asked to lie quietly for 30–60 min during the scanning. All metal should be removed from the area to be scanned. Explain that the dose of radiation he will receive is lower than usual with radiographs. Assure patient that he will not be "radioactive." The isotope is eliminated from the body in 6–24 hr.
Dual energy x-ray absorptiometry (DEXA)	Measures bone density of spine, hip, femur, or forearm Used to monitor changes in bone density and to diagnose metabolic bone disease	Uses minimal radiation exposure. Patient will lie supine on the imaging table with the legs supported. The scintillator camera is passed over the patient and projected onto a computer screen.	Height and weight will be measured. Instruct patient to remove all metallic objects. Test takes about 30 min.

Key: *CPK-MM,* creatinine phosphokinase isoenzyme; *IM,* intramuscular.

Continued

Table 31–2 *Diagnostic Tests for Musculoskeletal Disorders—cont'd*

TEST	PURPOSE	DESCRIPTION	NURSING IMPLICATIONS
Arthrography (arthrogram)	Provides radiographic pictures of a joint showing the outline of the joint cavity and soft tissue structures not visible on routine x-ray	A contrast agent, air, or both are aseptically injected into the joint after the area is anesthetized. Fluid may first be aspirated from the joint space. The joint is manipulated to disperse the contrast agent. X-rays are taken with the joint held in various positions.	Informed consent is often required. Explain that a needle will be inserted into the joint space after the area is anesthetized. There will be feelings of pressure and some discomfort. Administer an analgesic postprocedure if needed. Observe for swelling. Apply ice as ordered. Advise patient that crackling sounds may be heard or felt in the joint after the test and usually disappear in a day or two. Instruct patient to report any increasing pain or swelling to the physician.
Gallium/thallium scans	Detects bone problems, especially tumor invasion	The radioisotope gallium citrate (GA-70) or thallium-201 is administered before the scan. A bone scan is then performed.	The addition of the radioisotope helps locate areas of rapid bone growth activity that might indicate tumor. Explain that the radioisotope is administered 1–2 days before scanning. The procedure takes 30–60 min, during which lying still is required; sedation may be given.
Magnetic resonance imaging (MRI)	Diagnoses musculoskeletal disorders	Often preferred over bone scan. Magnetic fields and radiowaves are used to visualize tissue densities by the density of hydrogen ions. Computer enhancement depicts normal and abnormal tissue.	Instruct patient that there must be no metal on the body and no metal implants because of the strong magnetic fields used. The patient will need to lie still for 15–60 min. Older machines totally encase the patient; newer ones are more open.
Arthroscopy	Inspects the interior aspect of a joint, usually a knee, with a fiberoptic endoscope to diagnose problems of the patella, meniscus, and synovium; also used to evaluate the progress of arthritis or effectiveness of treatment	After injection of local anesthesia, an incision is made and the arthroscope is introduced into the interior of the joint; instruments for tissue biopsy or surgical procedure may be passed through the arthroscope.	Explain the purpose and procedure. A preprocedure sedative may be administered. When the patient has recovered from any sedation, he is allowed to walk but should not overuse or strain the joint for a few days. The area is observed for bleeding or swelling; ice packs may be used in the immediate postprocedure period, especially if biopsy or surgery was performed. Assessment for swelling, circulation, and sensation is done periodically to detect any complications.

Table 31–2 *Diagnostic Tests for Musculoskeletal Disorders—cont'd*

TEST	PURPOSE	DESCRIPTION	NURSING IMPLICATIONS
Arthrocentesis	Performed to extract synovial fluid for analysis or to reduce swelling	A needle is inserted into the joint space and synovial fluid is aspirated. Synovial fluid analysis may detect cells indicating infection, inflammation, rheumatoid arthritis, or lupus erythematosus. Corticosteroid may be injected after aspiration of fluid. If a large amount of fluid is aspirated, the joint is immobilized with an elastic bandage. Ice packs are applied to relieve pain and reduce swelling.	Explain the procedure. Have ice packs ready to apply afterward. Wrap with elastic bandage if ordered and show patient how to do this. It should be worn for 2–3 days. Instruct patient not to overuse the joint until pain and swelling have subsided. Administer ordered analgesics if needed after corticosteroid injection, as this can be painful.
Biopsy	Bone biopsy done to detect tumor cells Muscle biopsy done to obtain tissue for cellular analysis, which is helpful in differential diagnosis of several muscle disorders	Under local anesthesia, a piece of bone or muscle is excised and sent for pathologic analysis.	Offer emotional support during the procedures. Afterward, medicate for discomfort as needed, apply ice packs to decrease swelling, observe for bleeding; perform circulation and sensation checks distal to the area biopsied.
Culture of synovial fluid	Determines organism responsible for infection	Explain purpose and procedure. See that specimen of fluid is transported to laboratory immediately.	Synovial fluid is aspirated and sent for culture and sensitivity to determine appropriate antibiotic for therapy. Results take 48–72 hr to determine.
Electromyelography (EMG)	Detects abnormal nerve transmission to the muscle and abnormal muscle function; determines rehabilitation progress	Needle electrodes are inserted in affected muscles, and, as the muscles are stimulated, the electrical impulses generated by the muscle contractions are amplified and displayed on an oscilloscope; tracings also are made on graph paper.	Obtain a signed consent form. Caffeine-containing drinks and smoking are restricted 3 hr before the test. Muscle relaxants, anticholinergics, and cholinergic drugs should be withheld before the test; check with the physician. Explain to patient that there may be slight discomfort when the electrodes are inserted. Explain that he will be asked to relax and contract his muscles. The test usually takes about an hour. If serum enzyme tests are ordered, draw the blood before the EMG.
Calcium	Measures calcium in the blood	Used to assess calcium availability and metabolism. Calcium is needed for bone formation.	No fasting is required. Test requires 7 mL of venous blood in a red-top tube. Check for interfering factors before the sample is drawn.
Phosphate (phosphorus)	Measures phosphate in the blood	Helps assess phosphorus level in the body. Phosphorus is needed for bone formation.	Should be a fasting specimen. Requires 5–10 mL of venous blood in a red-top tube. Take to lab immediately.

Continued

Table 31–2 **Diagnostic Tests for Musculoskeletal Disorders—cont'd**

TEST	PURPOSE	DESCRIPTION	NURSING IMPLICATIONS
Alkaline phosphatase (ALP)	Detects bone disorders Isoenzymes are isolated to distinguish bone from liver, or biliary tract disorders	Helpful in determining if primary or metastatic cancer is present.	Fasting may be required for isoenzyme tests. Requires 7–10 mL of blood in a red-top tube.
Aldolase	Determines extent of muscular trauma and detects polymyositis	Enzyme test using blood.	A fasting state provides more accurate results. Requires 7–10 mL of venous blood in a red-top tube.
Creatine phosphokinase (CPK, creatine kinase, CK)	CPK-MM isoenzymes are used to test for skeletal muscle damage from trauma or disease, such as myositis	Enzyme test using blood.	IM injections will interfere with the test result. Record time and date of venipuncture on the lab slip.
Uric acid	Detects abnormally high levels of uric acid in the blood, which is a sign of gout	Collect 5–10 mL of blood in a clot (red-top) tube. *Normal range:* Female: 2.8–6.8 mg/dL Male: 3.5–7.8 mg/dL	No food or fluid restrictions.
Rheumatoid factor	Detects antibodies, indicating possible rheumatoid arthritis, lupus, or scleroderma	Collect 5–10 mL of blood in a clot (red-top) tube. *Normal range:* Adult: <1:120 titer >1:160 indicates rheumatoid arthritis	No food or fluid restrictions.
Antinuclear antibodies (ANA)	Assesses tissue antigen antibodies; useful for diagnosis of rheumatoid arthritis, lupus erythematosus, and other connective tissue disorders	Collect 2–5 mL of blood in a clot (red-top) tube. Check drugs patient is receiving for interference with this test. *Normal finding:* negative.	No food or drink restrictions.

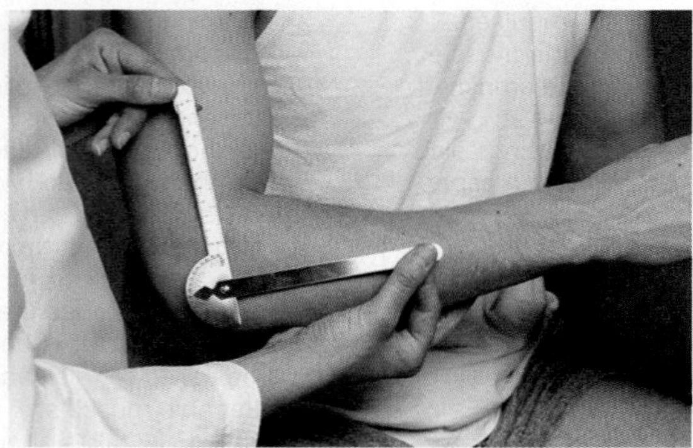

FIGURE **31–3** Measurement of joint motion with a goniometer.

tached, working against the force of gravity. A grading system is used, ranging from grade 5 (normal strength) to grade 0 (complete paralysis).

Other techniques used to evaluate musculoskeletal function include inspection, palpation, and tests for stability of a joint under stress.

Think Critically About . . . What would you tell a patient who wants to know what it is like to have a magnetic resonance imaging (MRI) scan of a knee?

NURSING MANAGEMENT

Assessment (Data Collection)

History Taking

When reviewing the patient's past history the nurse should keep in mind the significance of disorders that primarily affect other systems but secondarily affect the bones and muscles. For example, sickle cell disease and hemophilia can cause bleeding into the joints and muscles, and psoriasis is sometimes the first sign of psoriatic arthritis. Psoriatic arthritis affects a small percentage of people who have the skin disorder, psoriasis. Nutritional deficiencies can affect the mineral composition of bone and muscle, making them more susceptible to trauma and loss of function.

Family history also can be significant, as there are some bone and muscle disorders that are either inherited or have a familial tendency. For example, muscular dystrophy is inherited, and about 30% of those who have psoriatic arthritis have a family history of psoriasis (Focused Assessment 31–1).

Physical Assessment

Observe the patient for signs of joint pain, such as limping, poor posture, awkward gait, difficulty in arising or walking, and wincing upon movement. Much can be learned about the musculoskeletal system by just watching the patient, noting problems of move-

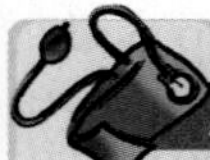

Focused Assessment 31–1

Data Collection for the Musculoskeletal System

- Have you ever suffered an injury to a bone?
- Have you ever experienced a severe muscle strain or muscle problem?
- Do you have any joints that are stiff, swollen, or painful?
- Have you experienced any sensory changes? When were they first noticed, and what did they feel like?
- When is the pain the worst? What seems to bring it on? What relieves it?
- Do you have any restriction of movement in any joint?
- Do you have trouble sleeping because of muscle or joint pain?
- Have you noticed any changes of sensation in your hands, feet, or elsewhere?
- Do you find that your fatigue level has increased?
- Do you have any problems with bathing, dressing, grooming, toileting, eating, ambulation, or going on social outings?
- Do you have any joint deformity? Bunion? Hammer toe? Deformed knuckle?
- Do you have any pain in your wrists, elbows, knees, hips, or feet?
- Is there a history of osteoporosis or arthritis in your family?
- Do you have diabetes, sickle cell disease, psoriasis, systemic lupus erythematosus, or any other chronic metabolic disease?
- Are you taking any steroid medications regularly?
- How is your calcium intake? What do you eat or drink that contains calcium? How much of it do you eat or drink?
- Are you out in the sunshine very much? Do you take a vitamin D supplement?
- What type of exercise do you do? How often do you exercise and for how long?
- Can you tell me what you see as your current problem?
- Do you have difficulty opening containers?
- Can you easily arise from a seated position?

SOCIAL HISTORY

- Is there any difficulty obtaining the medications prescribed for you?
- How do you get to the clinic/office for your appointments?
- Tell me about your work; is it very stressful? Fatiguing?
- Is the environment you are in most of the day a comfortable temperature for you?
- Do you think you will have any difficulty in following your physician's recommendations for exercise, diet, rest, or medication?

ment and changes in facial expression as the routines of bathing and grooming occur. If the patient is admitted with a fracture, obtain a history of the precipitating event so that an assessment can be made of other areas that may have been injured. Sometimes it is necessary to consult family members or someone who lives with the patient about the patient's true ability to perform the activities of daily living. **A self-care deficit is one of the primary problems for patients who suffer a problem of immobility.** Focused Assessment 31–2 provides a guide to physical assessment of the musculoskeletal system.

? ***Think Critically About . . .*** How would you gather data about an elderly patient's ability to perform self-care activities at home before he is discharged? Can you trust his statement of "I can shop, cook, clean, and do everything I need to do by myself?" If not, why not?

Nursing Diagnosis

Nursing diagnoses are chosen based on data collected. Diagnoses most commonly used for patients with musculoskeletal problems are:

- Impaired physical mobility
- Activity intolerance
- Pain
- Disturbed body image
- Self-care deficit in bathing, grooming, toileting, feeding
- Risk for disuse syndrome
- Impaired home maintenance

Several other secondary nursing diagnoses may be appropriate for patients who are highly immobile.

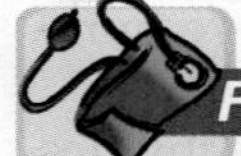

Focused Assessment 31–2

Physical Assessment of the Musculoskeletal System

Note the following points during physical assessment of the patient with a problem of the musculoskeletal system:

- **Posture:** Is there evidence of **kyphosis,** such as a rounded upper back, which is called a *dowager's hump?* Are the knuckles swollen or deformed, indicating arthritis?
- **Gait**
- **Mobility:** Is any supportive device being used, such as a cane, brace, splint, or elastic bandage?
- **Range of motion** of the neck, shoulders
- **Spine:** Tenderness of the vertebrae upon palpation
- **Appearance of joints** of elbows, hands, knees, ankles, and feet; presence of redness, warmth, deformity, or loss of motion
- **Skeletal muscle appearance** in arms and legs; degree of atrophy
- **Ability to perform activities** of daily living
- Determine whether the patient seems to be strong or weak.

Constipation, impaired tissue integrity, social isolation, and other problems caused by immobility may occur (see Chapter 9).

Planning

Caring for immobile patients requires careful planning of time. Making beds for the bed-confined orthopedic patient is best done by two people. Bathing and grooming are more time consuming when the patient has a limb immobilized or is in some sort of traction. The nurse may be a social contact for the patient as well as a caregiver, and more time is spent in interaction to meet psychosocial needs. **Planning for toileting needs at regular intervals is important for the well-being of the patient who is unable to get out of bed himself.** Neglecting such needs may cause incontinence and the time-consuming task of changing the bed and cleaning up the patient, besides being demoralizing for the patient. Incontinence puts the patient at greater risk of tissue breakdown from the moisture and irritation of urine or feces. Repositioning the patient at 2-hour intervals needs to be included in the daily work plan to prevent pressure ulcers.

Specific individual expected outcomes are written for each nursing diagnosis. Outcomes are written in collaboration with the patient and other members of the health care team. **The physical therapist and occupational therapist are very important in this process.** Possible expected outcomes for the above nursing diagnoses might be:

- Patient will have sufficient mobility for activities of daily living (ADLs) within 3 months.
- Patient will tolerate 20 minutes of activity within 2 weeks.
- Patient's pain will be controlled with analgesia before discharge.
- Patient will verbalize acceptance of change in body image within 2 months.
- Patient will resume self-care for bathing, grooming, toileting, and feeding within 6 weeks.
- Patient will not experience disuse syndrome.
- Patient will be able to care for own home with assistance within 2 months.

Implementation

Nursing interventions are chosen based on the expected outcomes desired. Specific nursing interventions are found in Table 31–3, and with the specific disorders discussed in Chapter 32.

Lifting and Turning the Patient

When working with the orthopedic patient, all movements must be *gentle* and *firm.* When moving or turning the patient, the nurse **should have sufficient help from adequately trained personnel.** Each person involved, including the patient, should understand exactly what is going to be done and the steps to be taken to accomplish the move. If the patient can help without damaging the diseased joint or limb, he should be encouraged to do so. If he is not able to help, the nurse explains the procedure to him and asks him to cooperate by relaxing completely during the procedure. Many times the patient is afraid that moving and turning will cause pain. Explanation as to the reason for moving and turning must be given so that confidence and cooperation are gained.

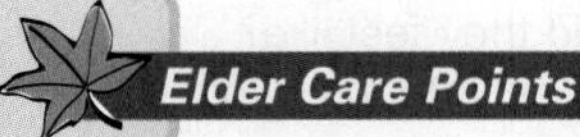

Elder Care Points

Older patients and those with poor circulation instinctively round their shoulders and tuck their limbs close to their bodies when they are chilly. Because of decreased subcutaneous fat and thin skin, the elderly often feel cooler than younger people in the same room. Feeling cold can increase feelings of pain and discomfort. Supply sufficient blankets, heat, socks, sweaters, and the like to keep the elderly person warm.

Orthopedic Bed Making

When traction is being applied to a patient's lower limb, or when he is in a large body cast or external fixation device, it is not always convenient to arrange the bed linens in the conventional manner. (See the section on traction later in this chapter for information on safe handling.) One important point to remember in changing the linen is to avoid pulling sheets from under the patient and causing friction against the skin.

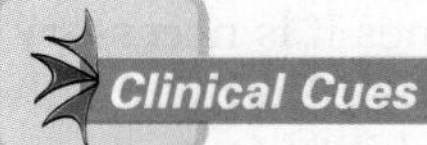

Clinical Cues

Two draw sheets may be used for the foundation of the bed in lieu of one large bottom sheet when a patient is in lower limb traction with a frame resting on the mattress. When two draw sheets are used, only the draw sheet under the patient's body needs be changed often, and the frame will not be disturbed at all. When changing the bottom sheet for the patient in traction, begin on the side opposite the limb in traction. For example, if traction is on the left leg, work from right to left and from the foot of the bed toward the head. Top covers may be folded so that the limb in traction is not covered. If extra warmth is needed for the affected limb, it can be covered with a pillowcase or towel.

Interventions to Prevent Disability

The formation of contractures (shortening of skeletal muscle tissue causing deformity), loss of muscle tone, and fixation of joints can be prevented in most cases by aggressive and consistent nursing intervention. The major components of the intervention are gradual mobilization, an exercise program, proper positioning, and instruction of the patient and family. It is the responsibility of the nursing staff to initiate the neces-

Table 31–3 ***Common Nursing Diagnoses, Expected Outcomes, and Interventions for Patients with Musculoskeletal System Disorders***

NURSING DIAGNOSIS	GOALS/EXPECTED OUTCOMES	NURSING INTERVENTIONS
Impaired physical mobility related to immobilization, loss of limb, stiffness, pain, weakness, or inability to bear weight	ROM of unaffected joints will be maintained. No signs of joint contractures at discharge.	Active ROM at least tid for all unaffected joints while on bed rest. Passive ROM on affected joints as ordered. Ensure that joints are in correct alignment when at rest and after turning. Maintain traction and body in proper alignment. Assess immobilizer for correct fit and positioning every shift; assess for signs of complications due to pressure or pins. Supervise exercise to prepare muscles for ambulation. Instruct in use of ambulatory devices as appropriate; supervise practice; assess for proper "fit" of device. Encourage use of prosthesis for ambulation; assist with practice. Assess for signs of complications in stump and assess that prosthesis is attached correctly. Maintain abduction pillow between legs if one is ordered.
Activity intolerance related to stiffness, pain, impaired mobility, fatigue	Patient will space activities and rest to conserve energy. Patient will use assistive devices to conserve energy.	Determine factors that increase fatigue. Space activities with rest periods throughout the day. Assist to set goals for slow, steady increase in exercise and activity during periods of remission of arthritis symptoms. Use heat or cold treatments to decrease stiffness and discomfort. Perform exercises after heat treatments to decrease discomfort; apply in safe manner. Apply cold as needed after exercise for discomfort. Administer medications to decrease inflammation and pain, allowing greater level of activity. Advise of assistive devices that might make ADLs easier and conserve energy. Assist in obtaining needed devices. Supervise practice with assistive device.
Pain related to injury, surgery, or joint disorder	Pain will be controlled as evidenced by patient verbalization. Pain will be decreased with medication.	Instruct in relaxation, distraction, and imagery techniques to decrease pain. Instruct in use of various heat and cold treatments to decrease pain. Administer analgesic, inflammatory, and steroid medications, as ordered, to decrease pain. Instruct in use and side effects of each drug. Advise of alternative methods of pain control, such as transcutaneous electrical nerve stimulation (TENS). Monitor patient-controlled analgesia (PCA) use for effectiveness of pain control. Assess for factors contributing to pain level such as increased pressure, infection, positioning, or swelling. Assess pain in systematic, objective manner and track course of pain and effectiveness of pain control (see Chapter 7).
Risk for injury related to hemorrhage, fat embolus, thrombophlebitis, or dislocation of prosthesis	Patient will not experience injury. No evidence of thrombophlebitis; no dislocation of hip joint.	Observe dressing for bleeding; monitor drainage in drainage device q hr for 8 hr, then q 2 hr for 24 hr. Monitor vital signs q 4 hr. Assess for signs of thrombophlebitis and possible emboli; apply antiembolic stockings, as ordered; assess q 2 hr for correct position and function of such devices. Use wedge pillow between legs for hip surgery patient as ordered; turn q 2 hr to back or unaffected side or per physician instructions. Perform neurovascular checks every hr for 8 hr, then q 2 hr.

Key: *ADLs,* activities of daily living; *ROM,* range of motion; *tid,* three times a day.

Continued

Table 31–3 Common Nursing Diagnoses, Expected Outcomes, and Interventions for Patients with Musculoskeletal System Disorders—cont'd

NURSING DIAGNOSIS	GOALS/EXPECTED OUTCOMES	NURSING INTERVENTIONS
Risk for infection related to trauma or surgical incision	No signs of infection, as evidenced by normal white blood cell (WBC) count and normal temperature; wounds clean and dry.	Follow Standard Precautions and strict contact precautions when performing patient care, and use strict aseptic technique for wound or pin care. Assess for signs of infection q shift; assess wound for redness, swelling, and tenderness. Administer prophylactic antibiotics, as ordered. Assess temperature trends and trend of WBC values for signs of infection. Assess patient for subjective signs of malaise. Sniff around cast for signs of foul odor indicating infection.
Risk for ineffective tissue perfusion related to swelling and pressure	No evidence of seriously decreased circulation distal to site of trauma. No evidence of nerve compression from swelling.	Perform neurovascular assessment q hr for 8 hr, then q 2 hr for 48 hr. Question patient regarding sensation distal to site of trauma or surgery. Apply cold to area of injury or surgery, as ordered, to reduce swelling; elevate extremity to slightly above heart level. Immediately report signs of compartment syndrome to physician and obtain order for measures to relieve pressure.
Self-care deficit in bathing, grooming, toileting, feeding related to immobilization	Patient will receive assistance for all ADLs, as needed.	Assess degree of inability to perform various self-care activities. Formulate plan to assist patient with ADLs. Answer calls for assistance with toileting promptly; do not leave on bedpan longer than necessary. Open food containers and cut food as needed for self-feeding with one hand. Do not serve extremely hot liquids to patients who have difficulty with coordination or with holding drinking containers or to immobilized patients. Provide assistive devices and help patient to be as self-sufficient as possible without incurring undue fatigue when performing ADLs. Caution patients about change in body's center of gravity when a limb is casted or amputated.
Disturbed body image related to change in appearance and/or loss of mobility or function	Patient will begin adaptation to change in appearance or loss as evidenced by verbalization of feelings of self-worth; maintenance of relationships with significant others; active interest in personal appearance; willingness to resume usual roles and participate in social activities; making plans to adapt lifestyle to meet restrictions imposed by loss.	Assess degree of body image disturbance, noting verbal or nonverbal clues to negative response to changes. Assist to verbalize feelings about effect of loss on usual roles and lifestyle. Be present and supportive during initial dressing changes on stump after amputation. Assist patient to identify strengths and abilities and positive coping mechanisms. Clarify misconceptions about limitations on mobility and activity. Promote activities that require patient to confront the body changes that have occurred, such as bathing, ADLs, or dressing changes. Demonstrate acceptance of patient and encourage significant others to do the same with touch and affection. Encourage as much independence as possible; allow to do things for self. Assist patient to explore viable options for changes in lifestyle and career. Refer for vocational retraining if needed. Encourage maximum participation in planning of care and self-care to provide a sense of control over life. Encourage participation in social activities and in a support group. Refer for psychological counseling if adaptation does not occur within 6 mo and patient is depressed or in denial.

Key: *ADLs,* activities of daily living; *CPM,* continuous passive motions; *ROM,* range of motion.

Table 31–3 ***Common Nursing Diagnoses, Expected Outcomes, and Interventions for Patients with Problems of the Musculoskeletal System—cont'd***

NURSING DIAGNOSIS	GOALS/EXPECTED OUTCOMES	NURSING INTERVENTIONS
Impaired home maintenance related to immobility or self-care deficits	Patient will obtain needed assistance with home maintenance.	Assess degree of self-sufficiency and ability to perform ADLs before discharge. Contact social worker for coordination of home care if needed. Obtain bathing and homemaker assistance as needed. Assess continued need for in-home services weekly. Instruct in-home adaptations that could aid in efforts at self-care, such as grab bars in bathroom, alterations in counter spaces for food preparation, transportation options for grocery shopping and appointments, or assistive devices for self-feeding and grooming. Assess degree of assistance significant other can provide for patient in home environment. Determine safety of home environment for patient.
Risk for disuse syndrome related to immobility or trauma	Patient will not suffer permanent joint deformity or muscle atrophy.	Position joints as ordered; keep rest of body in correct alignment. Begin exercise of affected joint as soon as physician orders. Encourage active exercise of unaffected joints tid. Perform passive ROM as ordered tid. Assist with use of CPM machine, as ordered. Medicate regularly for pain while CPM machine is in use. Use heat and cold treatments before and after exercising stiff or deformed joints. Assess joints for contractures and muscles for atrophy q 24 hr. Encourage participation in ADLs to exercise joints.

sary measures to prevent complications and to carry them out consistently. Within a matter of a few days, the structures of immobilized muscles and joints begin to undergo changes. If no effort is made to prevent these changes, the patient will become permanently disabled. The pathologic changes most commonly associated with lack of motion include:

- Contractures
- Loss of muscle tone
- **Ankylosis** (permanent fixation of a joint)

Preventing Contractures. Joint motion is the result of a shortening and stretching of opposing muscles. For example, when the flexor muscles of the leg contract and shorten, the opposing extensor muscles relax and tighten. When skeletal muscles are not regularly stretched and contracted to their normal limits, they attempt to adapt themselves to this limited use by becoming shorter and less elastic. This "adaptive shortening" is called **contracture**. Contracture formation begins within 3 to 7 days after immobilization of a body part, and the process usually is complete in 6 to 8 weeks. This means that there is no time to lose in planning and implementing nursing measures to prevent permanent and crippling disability. The most frequent contractures occurring in patients immobilized for long periods are "footdrop," knee and hip flexion contractures, "wrist drop," and contractures of the fingers and arms (Figure 31–4).

Loss of Muscle Tone. Muscle tone is defined as the readiness of the muscle to go to work—to contract and relax as needed. If a muscle is not regularly stimulated to action or if it is stretched beyond its normal limits for an extended time, it will lose its ability to contract and relax. For example, in footdrop, the calf muscles are shortened while the opposing flexor muscles are stretched. The result is loss of muscle tone and inability to produce motion. Performing ROM exercises helps prevent this.

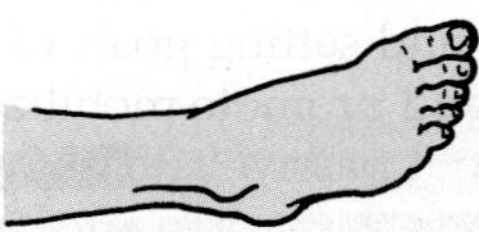

A. Footdrop, resulting from improper support of the feet while patient is confined to bed.

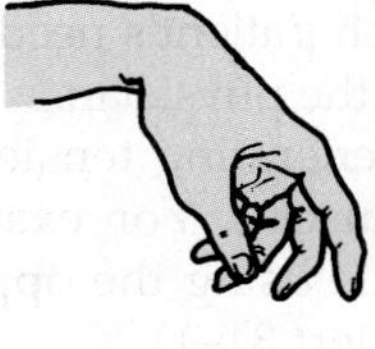

B. Wrist drop, resulting from improper support of the hand.

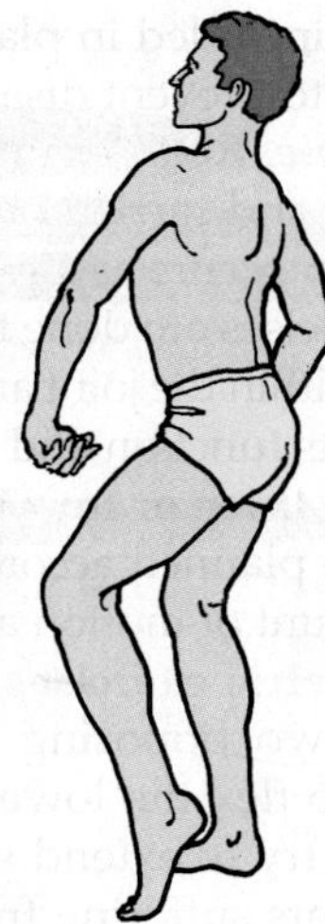

C. Flexion contracture of knee and hip force this patient to walk on tiptoe on the affected side. If both legs are involved, walking is impossible.

FIGURE **31–4** Joint contractures.

Preventing Ankylosis. Ankylosis is the result of injury or disease in which the tissues of the joint are replaced by a bony overgrowth that completely obliterates the joint. Proper positioning and movement of the joint passively can help prevent this. Sometimes it is extremely difficult to prevent this process (as, for example, in some types of arthritis). In these cases, the physician may brace the joint in the position that will be most useful to the patient, even though there is no motion in the joint.

Gradual Mobilization. The first step in nursing intervention to accomplish goals of progressive mobilization is assessment of the patient's ability to move his limbs, turn himself in bed, transfer himself from bed to chair and back again, and stand and walk. These measurable signs of independent movement can represent various stages to which it is hoped the patient will gradually progress.

Setting goals for progressive mobilization must take into account the pathologic condition causing immobility, any contraindications to movement of a body part, and the ability of the patient to understand and take part in carrying out the rehabilitation activities. In some cases, passive exercises and positioning may be necessary until the patient is able to carry out exercises and positioning on his own. If the patient is to be cared for by family members once back at home, it is essential that they be included in planning and setting goals of intervention to prevent disability and promote mobilization.

Exercise. ROM exercises, both passive and active, are planned and carried out as soon as feasible after immobilization occurs as a result of disease, injury, or surgery. The exercises are done to maintain functional connective tissue within the joint and thereby ensure that every joint retains its function and mobility. **ROM exercises should be done three or four times a day.** Other kinds of exercises are planned according to each patient's needs and the amount of motion allowed by the physician.

Isometric exercises involve generating tension between two opposing sets of muscles. For example, trying to flex the lower arm while using the opposite hand to try to extend it (Safety Alert 31–1).

Patients suffering from intense joint pain as a result of rheumatoid arthritis will need proper timing of exercises to follow administration of analgesic and anti-inflammatory drugs. If possible, the schedule for drug administration should be adjusted so that the patient receives his first dose of medication in the morning 30 to 60 minutes *before* he begins his exercises.

Sometimes after joint surgery, especially after a total knee replacement, the surgeon will order attachment of an apparatus to the affected limb that provides continuous passive motion (CPM) of the joint within set limits. The apparatus is driven by a motor and requires no effort on the part of the patient or nurse to move the limb (Figure 31–5). It usually is left on all day and is discontinued at night while the patient sleeps. When this type of apparatus is used, the nursing care plan should include specific instructions regarding its proper application and setting and regular assessment of adequacy of pain medication.

Exercises to recondition muscles for ambulation after injury or immobilization include quadriceps setting and gluteal setting (Patient Teaching 31–1).

Positioning. Even though nurses turn a patient, change his body position, and get him up in a chair to prevent pressure ulcers, circulatory stasis, and respiratory and urinary complications, nurses may not realize that changing body position does not necessarily guarantee freedom from orthopedic deformities. It also is necessary to change joint positions.

Assessing a patient's need for proper positioning should include watching for early signs of muscle tightness and resistance to joint motion. This can be done during routine ROM exercises and could signal the need for positioning a body part so that the joint is extended and muscles are stretched to their normal capacity. (Review ROM exercises in your Fundamentals of Nursing text.)

Patients with flaccid paralysis are not necessarily positioned in the same way as those with spastic paralysis. For example, a footboard is appropriate for proper positioning of the feet to prevent footdrop in a patient with flaccid paralysis. In contrast, putting the soles of the feet of a patient with spastic paralysis in contact with a footboard could trigger muscle contraction and aggravate the spasticity. Using a bed cradle to relieve pressure of the bedclothes can help prevent footdrop in these patients.

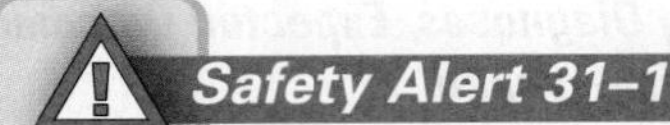

Caution with Isometric Exercises

Isometric exercise may be contraindicated in patients with hypertension, increased intracranial pressure, or congestive heart failure, as there is a significant increase in blood pressure and heart rate during the exercise.

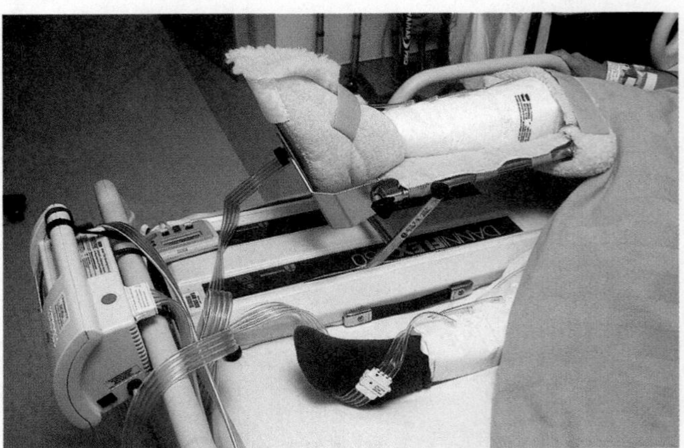

FIGURE **31–5** Continuous passive motion machine encourages joint mobility.

Patient Teaching 31–1

Quadriceps and Gluteal Muscle Exercises

For quadriceps setting:

- Instruct the patient to straighten the leg out while lying down and tense the leg muscles, straightening the knee, while raising the heel slightly. The contraction is held for a count of 5 and released for a count of 5. The exercise is done on each leg 10 to 15 times hourly while the patient is awake. Commercial breaks on television are a good reminder to do this.

For gluteal setting:

- Instruct the patient to contract the buttocks and pinch them together for a count of 4, then relax for a count of 5. Repeat 10 to 15 times hourly.

Special Beds. A type of bed that often is used for patients in cervical traction is the Roto-Rest bed (see Figure 22–12). This bed very slowly turns the patient about 300 times a day. It provides passive exercise and stimulates peristalsis without risk of injury to the patient. The bed has many other advantages, including several hatches that provide the nurse access to all of the common pressure points on the patient. There is a hatch for bowel and bladder care so that a bedpan can be placed without moving the patient. The back side of the patient can be bathed through the various hatches also. Once the nurse is familiar with the bed, it greatly simplifies care of the immobilized patient.

The FluidAir bed also is used for various types of immobilized patients. It is an air-fluidized bed and is very helpful in preventing pressure sores (Figure 31–6).

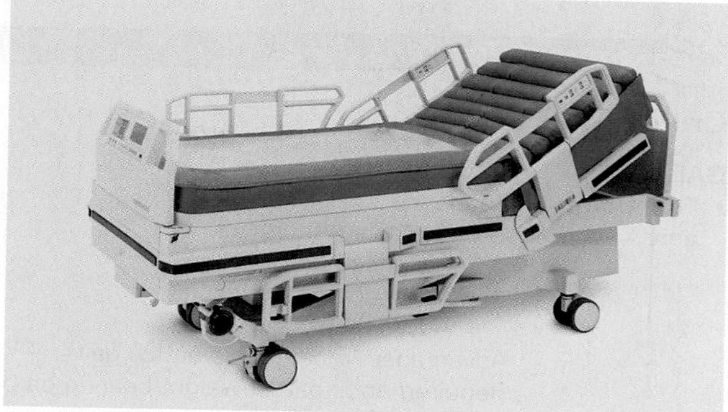

FIGURE **31–6** FluidAir bed.

Use of Slings and Splints. A sling used to support the wrist or elbow should support both joints of the arm. The sling should be positioned so that the fastening at the neck area does not rub the neck or press on a neck vessel. When a splint is applied to an extremity, it should support the joint that is to be immobilized, fit properly without impeding circulation or slipping out of place, and not cause increased pain (Figure 31–7). If in doubt about how a particular splint is to be applied, seek help from another nurse or the physical therapist.

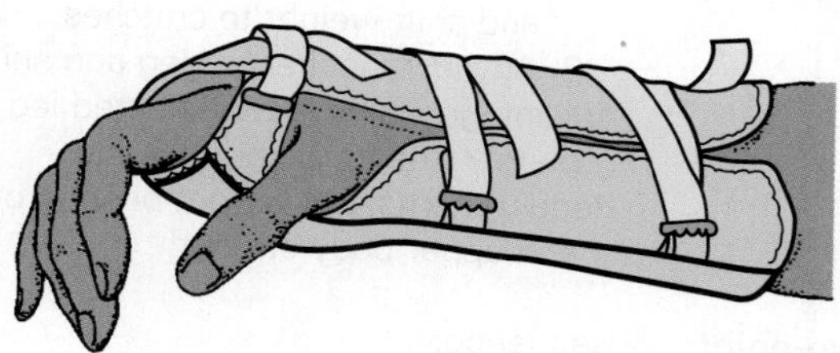

FIGURE **31–7** Wrist splint.

Teaching Ambulation with Assistive Devices

For the convalescent patient or for one who may always need support while walking, crutches can mean the difference between freedom to move about and confinement to one location. Before attempting to walk with crutches, the patient should be instructed in their use and manipulation so that he can handle them safely and effectively (Patient Teaching 31–2).

The type of crutch to be used will depend on the extent of disability or paralysis and the patient's ability to bear weight and maintain balance. If the crutches are too short or too long, they can create problems of lifting and moving about for the patient. When walking, the patient should straighten the elbow and the wrist during weight bearing. The muscles of the arms, shoulders, back, and chest are all used in the manipulation of crutches. Because this is true, many physical therapists start the patient on special exercises to strengthen these muscles several weeks before the patient begins to use the crutches (Safety Alert 31–2).

Although the physical therapist supervises the preparation and instruction of the patient before he starts to use crutches and then evaluates his ability to use them correctly, you will sometimes be responsible for assisting a patient with crutch walking while he is in the hospital. Patient Teaching 31–3 presents steps for special maneuvers on crutches.

When teaching a patient to ambulate with a cane, be certain that the cane has an intact rubber tip. The cane is the right length if the hand grip is at hip level and the elbow is bent at a 30-degree angle when weight is placed on the cane. **It should be used on the good side unless the physician orders otherwise.** The tip of the cane should be placed 6 to 10 inches (15 to 25 cm) to the side and 6 inches (15 cm) in front of the near foot when walking. The patient should look straight ahead, rather than down, when ambulating. **The cane is advanced at the same time as the affected leg.** The good leg is advanced first when going upstairs and the unaffected leg leads going downstairs.

Walker height is correct when the person's elbow is bent at a 15- to 30-degree angle while standing upright and grasping the handgrips. The walker is lifted or rolled on its wheels slightly in front of the patient while leaning the body slightly forward. A step or two is taken into the walker, and then it is lifted and placed in front of the person again.

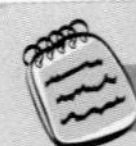

Patient Teaching 31–2

Crutch Gaits

GAIT	DESCRIPTION	PATTERN
• **Four-point gait**	Sequence: 1. Advance left crutch. 2. Advance right foot. 3. Advance right crutch. 4. Advance left foot. Advantages: most stable crutch gait. Requirements: partial weight bearing on both legs.	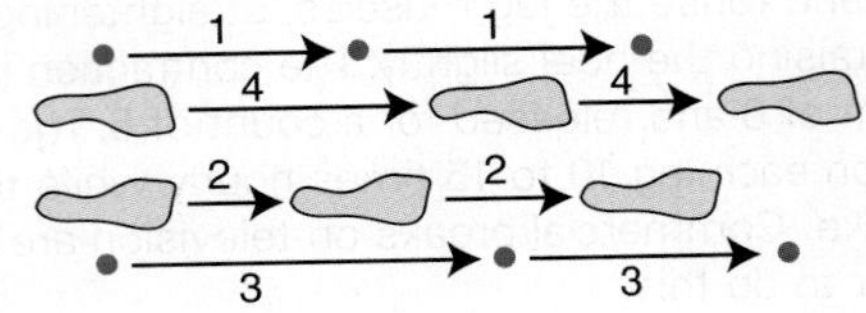
• **Three-point gait**	Sequence: 1. Advance both crutches forward with the affected leg and shift weight to crutches. 2. Advance unaffected leg and shift weight onto it. Advantages: allows the affected leg to be partially or completely free of weight bearing. Requirements: full weight bearing on one leg, balance, and upper body strength.	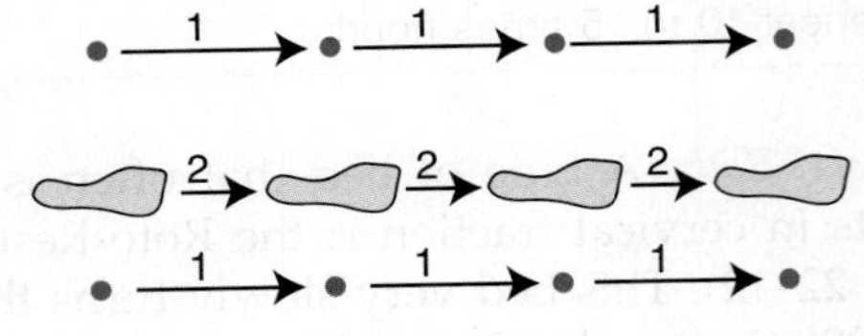
• **Two-point gait**	Sequence: 1. Advance left crutch and right foot. 2. Advance right crutch and left foot. Advantages: faster version of the four-point gait, more normal walking pattern (arms and legs moving in opposition). Requirements: partial weight bearing on both legs, balance.	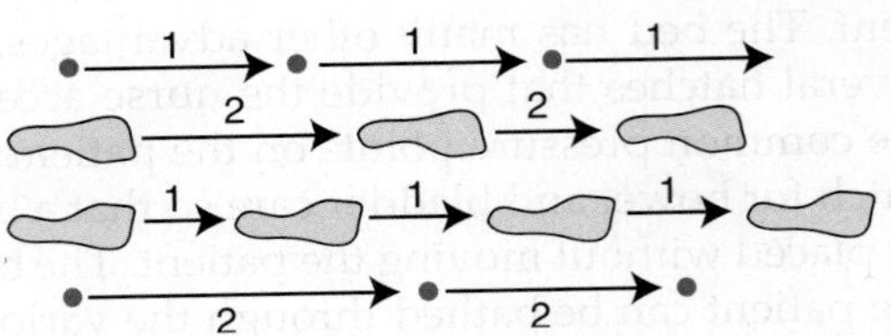

Safety Alert 31–2

Crutch Safety

Crutches should be about 16 inches (40 cm) shorter than the patient's height. When in the standing position with axillary crutches, the axillary bar should be two finger breadths below the axilla. The elbow should be flexed at a 30-degree angle when the palms of the hands rest on the hand grip. It is important that the patient not rest his body at the axilla on the top of the crutch; body weight should be borne by the arms on the hand rests of the crutches. If crutches are too long, pressure on the axilla will occur and can cause nerve damage.

To measure for crutches with the person standing and shoes on the feet, position the crutches with tips at a point 4 to 6 inches (10 to 15 cm) to the side and 4 to 6 inches in front of the patient's feet.

Psychosocial Care

Unfortunately, many orthopedic conditions require prolonged periods of confinement to bed or, at best, immobilization of a part of the body and restricted physical activities. This leads to frustration and a feeling of hopelessness and despair on the part of the patient. When the patient is young and unaccustomed to depending on others for personal care, a reaction of anger and bitterness toward his plight may occur. If the patient is a wage earner or an active member of the family upon whom others are dependent, there is the additional burden of financial and social problems. Chapter 9 discusses psychosocial care of the immobile patient.

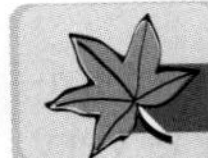

Elder Care Points

Many elderly patients are hospitalized with injuries they sustain from inability to maneuver crutches, cane, or walker. It is essential that elderly patients be taught proper methods of using assistive devices and that they receive supervised practice before they are discharged.

Evaluation

Data are gathered through reassessment to determine whether expected outcomes are being met. Determining the effectiveness of interventions to treat pain is based mainly on subjective information given by the patient, but the nurse should also be alert to nuances of body language. Observation of the patient's ability to accomplish ADLs gives clues to improvement in mobility and activity tolerance.

Diagnostic test data from x-rays and laboratory reports are used to determine the effectiveness of treatments. For example, x-rays show whether fractures are healing, whereas laboratory reports help to determine how well rheumatoid arthritis is controlled.

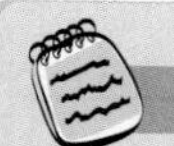

Patient Teaching 31–3

Special Maneuvers on Crutches

MANEUVER	DESCRIPTION
• Walking upstairs	1. Stand at the foot of the stairs with weight on the good leg and crutches. 2. Put weight on the crutch handles and then lift the unaffected leg up onto the first step of the stairs (angels go up). 3. Put weight on the good leg and lift the other leg and crutches up to that step. 4. Repeat for each step.
• Walking downstairs	1. Stand at the top of the stairs with weight on the good leg and crutches. 2. Shift weight completely onto the good leg and put the crutches down on the next step. 3. Put weight on the crutch handles and transfer the injured leg down on the step with the crutches (devils go down). 4. Bring the good leg down to that step. 5. Repeat for each stair step.
• Sitting down	1. Crutch-walk to the chair. 2. Turn around slowly so that the back is to the chair and the backs of the legs touch the seat of the chair. 3. Transfer both crutches to the side with the injured leg and grasp both handgrips with that one hand. 4. As weight is supported on the crutches and the good leg, reach back with the free hand and grasp the arm of the chair. 5. Lower slowly onto the chair seat, using the support of both the crutches and chair. 6. Sit back in the chair and elevate the leg. 7. Keep the knee slightly flexed when elevated, because too much extension can decrease the circulation. 8. To get up, bring both crutches along the side of the injured leg and grasp the handgrip firmly. Make sure the crutch tips are firmly on the floor. Place the other hand on the arm of the chair and push up. 9. After becoming upright, transfer one crutch to the other hand for walking.

Whenever expected outcomes are not being met, the plan of care must be revised. Collaboration among all health professionals working with the patient is vital to the creation of a realistic, workable, plan of care.

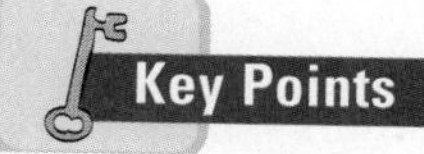

Key Points

- The main functions of the musculoskeletal system are motion, support, and protection.
- Trauma and disease cause dysfunction of the musculoskeletal system.
- Exercise and weight training throughout life can decrease musculoskeletal problems late in life.
- Using safety equipment for sports, exercise, when driving, and at work is very important to preventing trauma to the musculoskeletal system.
- Many diagnostic tests for problems of the musculoskeletal system are available (see Table 31–2).
- A thorough history and physical are necessary to determine if a musculoskeletal problem is present (see Focused Assessments 31–1 and 31–2).
- Back, knee, and shoulder pain is a frequent problem.
- Self-care deficit is one of the primary problems for patients who suffer a problem of immobility.
- Impaired physical mobility is another frequently encountered problem.
- The physical and occupational therapists are part of the collaborative team that plans care.
- Interventions to prevent disability are extremely important.
- Contractures can permanently impair the patients' ability to perform ADLs.
- ROM exercises should be done three or four times a day.
- Positioning must be performed correctly, with attention to promoting function and preserving movement.
- The nurse assists with supervising and teaching ambulation with assistive devices.
- Preventing falls is a major focus of nursing care.
- Psychosocial care of the patient with a musculoskeletal disorder should not be overlooked.
- If evaluation of the care plan does not show adequate progress toward expected outcomes, the interventions must be changed and the plan revised.

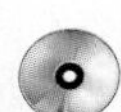

Go to your **Companion CD-ROM** for an Audio Glossary, animations, video clips, and bonus review questions.

evolve Be sure to visit the companion Evolve site at http://evolve.elsevier.com/deWit for interactive NCLEX-PN Exam Style Review Questions, WebLinks, and additional online resources.

NCLEX-PN EXAM STYLE REVIEW QUESTIONS

Choose the best answer(s) for the following questions.

1. In explaining the slowed bone healing process in the older adult, an accurate statement by a nurse would be:
   1. "Bones are more brittle and less compact."
   2. "Older women have more severe cases of osteoporosis."
   3. "There is a decreased exchange of minerals in and out of the bones."
   4. "Mineral resorption of the bones ceases in old age."
2. Permanent fixation of a joint is referred to as ______________________.
3. The nurse evaluates the patient's ability to use the cane. Which of the following indicates proper use of the cane?
   1. The cane is advanced at the same time as the good leg.
   2. The handgrip is at the hip level.
   3. The cane is used on the affected side.
   4. The patient looks down while ambulating.
4. The nurse encourages a patient to consider eating foods that are rich in calcium. The following foods are considered good sources of calcium, except:
   1. milk.
   2. green vegetables.
   3. yogurt.
   4. cheese.
5. A 50-year-old male patient complains of joint pains, difficulty rising, and limping. He has poor posture and uncoordinated gait. An appropriate nursing diagnosis would be:
   1. self-care deficit.
   2. impaired physical mobility.
   3. ineffective coping.
   4. fatigue.
6. The patient reports a sound like that of a hair rubbed between the fingers while moving her joints. A likely cause of the sound would be:
   1. rupture of ligaments and tendons.
   2. rubbing of eroded cartilage.
   3. contact between fracture surfaces.
   4. presence of inflammation.
7. The nurse is taking care of an elderly patient with severe degenerative arthritis. To accomplish progressive mobilization, an initial nursing intervention would be to:
   1. assist with transfers from bed to chair
   2. encourage increased ambulation
   3. determine ROM of all extremities
   4. reposition frequently
8. You recruit the assistance of adequately trained personnel to turn an immobile patient. In order to prevent injury to the patient and the nursing staff, which of the following measures should be taken before repositioning the patient?
   1. Encourage movement of all joints
   2. Explain the details of the move
   3. Discourage patient participation
   4. Medicate patient for anxiety
9. To manage joint discomfort associated with movement among patients with severe rheumatoid arthritis, the nurse must:
   1. encourage deep breathing exercises.
   2. administer pain medications immediately after exercise.
   3. schedule pain medication administration prior to ambulation.
   4. provide a continuous infusion of pain medications.
10. The nurse assesses the condition of a splint applied to the right arm. Which of the following clinical findings warrant immediate attention?
    1. Warm skin
    2. Presence of skin breakdown
    3. Itching
    4. Palpable distal pulses

CRITICAL THINKING ACTIVITIES 

Read each clinical scenario and discuss the questions with your classmates.

Scenario A

Miss Simpson has had trouble with her left knee for several years. She is scheduled for an arthroscopy and asks you about the procedure.

1. How would you describe the procedure to her?
2. What is the aftercare for this procedure?
3. How long is she likely to be immobile after the procedure?

Scenario B

Ms. Jackson has been experiencing muscle weakness in her right leg for a few weeks. Her health care provider has scheduled her for an electromyogram (EMG). She asks you about this procedure.

1. Is an informed consent needed for an EMG?
2. How would you describe the test to Ms. Jackson?
3. What care is needed after the procedure?

Scenario C

Ms. White, age 67, sustained a fracture of the right humerus when she fell this morning. A cast has been applied.

1. What would you tell her she needs to do at home in order to keep her joints mobile?
2. What should she do to protect the muscle mass?
3. What nutritional teaching would you provide?

CHAPTER

32 Care of Patients with Musculoskeletal and Connective Tissue Disorders

evolve http://evolve.elsevier.com/deWit

Objectives

Upon completion of this chapter, you should be able to:

Theory

1. State the factors to be assessed for the patient who has a connective tissue injury.
2. Compare the assessment findings of a connective tissue injury with those of a fracture.
3. State the care that is needed for the patient who has an external fixator in place.
4. Identify the "do's and don'ts" of cast care.
5. Describe nursing assessment and intervention for the patient in traction.
6. Identify the special problems of patients with arthritis and specific nursing interventions that can be helpful.
7. Compare the preoperative and postoperative care of a patient with a total knee replacement with that of a patient with a total hip replacement.
8. Explain the process by which osteoporosis occurs, ways to slow the process, and how the disorder is treated.
9. Differentiate care of the patient with a metastatic bone tumor from care of the patient with rheumatoid arthritis.
10. Identify important postoperative observations and nursing interventions in the care of the patient who has undergone an amputation.
11. List ways in which the elderly can increase musculoskeletal strength and protect bones.

Clinical Practice

1. Teach the patient going home with a cast about proper care of the cast and extremity.
2. Provide appropriate care for a patient in traction.
3. Teach an elderly patient with a mobility problem about ways to prevent a fall at home.
4. Set up and apply a continuous passive motion (CPM) machine for a patient who has had a total knee replacement.
5. Apply sequential compression devices on a patient for whom they are ordered.

Key Terms

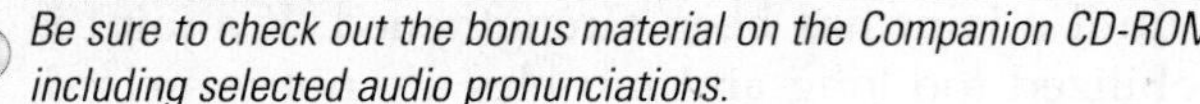
Be sure to check out the bonus material on the Companion CD-ROM, including selected audio pronunciations.

arthroplasty (ĂR-thrō-plăs-tē, p. 799)
fracture (FRĂK-shŭr, p. 784)
kyphoplasty (kī-FŌ-PLĂS-tē, p. 808)
nonunion (p. 788)
osteogenesis (ŏs-tē-ō-JĔN-ĕ-sĭs, p. 788)
osteopenia (ŏs-tē-ō-PĒ-nē-ă, p. 807)
orthoses (ŏr-thō-sēz, p. 799)
pannus (păn-nŭs, p. 797)
subluxation (sŭb-lŭk-SĀ-shŭn, p. 784)
vertebroplasty (VĔR-tĕ-brō-plăs-tē, p. 808)

CONNECTIVE TISSUE DISORDERS

Sprains, strains, and dislocations are the kinds of injuries likely to occur when ligaments, muscles, and joints are subjected to undue stress, twisting, or a physical blow. A summary of strain, sprain, and dislocation is presented.

SPRAIN

Etiology and Pathophysiology

A sprain is a partial or complete tearing of the ligaments that hold various bones together to form a joint. Sprains occur from trauma of one sort or another. A joint may be forced past its normal range of motion, or there may be twisting, as often happens during an ankle sprain. The ankle and the knee are the most common joints experiencing a sprain; the wrist comes next.

Signs, Symptoms, and Diagnosis

Grade I (mild): Tenderness at site; minimal swelling and loss of function; no abnormal motion.

Grade II (moderate): More severe pain, especially with weight bearing; swelling and bleeding into joint; some loss of function.

Grade III (severe, complete tearing of fibers): Pain may be less severe, but swelling, loss of function, and bleeding into joint are more marked.

Diagnosis is by physical examination and x-ray to rule out a fracture.

Treatment and Nursing Management

RICE is the acronym used for treatment of sprains: **rest, ice, compression,** and **elevation.** Apply ice immediately after injury and for 24 to 72 hours. Apply the ice bag for 10 to 20 minutes every 1 to 2 hours during the day. Wrap with an elastic bandage snugly, being careful not to cut off circulation, and elevate the injured part. These measures can help minimize swelling and pain and stabilize the joint in proper alignment. The goal of treatment is to protect the ligament until it heals by scarring. Ligaments do not "grow" back together. An air cast, braces, or supports are used only until a joint has been strengthened. If a joint is immobilized too long and muscles are not exercised, muscle atrophy, which begins in a matter of days, can cause permanent disability. In some cases, surgical repair may be necessary. Grade III sprains often require a cast. Patients with Grade II or Grade III sprains need to rest the joint; crutches are needed for a lower extremity sprain. Nonsteroidal anti-inflammatory drugs (NSAIDs) should be prescribed on an around-the-clock basis for the first couple days.

STRAIN

The most common muscle strain occurs in the back muscles. Back problems are discussed in Chapter 22, because they often have a neurologic component. Muscle strains do occur in other skeletal muscles and are treated the same as a joint strain—with rest and applications of heat and cold, using cold initially and heat after 48 hours. Anti-inflammatory medications are used for discomfort and, when spasm is present, a muscle relaxant may be prescribed. Time is the greatest healer. The patient is cautioned against reinjury and is taught proper ways to lift and move.

Etiology and Pathophysiology

A strain is a pulling or tearing of either a muscle, a tendon, or both. A strain occurs by trauma, overuse, or overextension of a joint. The most common sites are the hamstrings, quadriceps, and calf muscles.

Signs, Symptoms, and Diagnosis

A history of overexertion or the presence of soft-tissue swelling and pain may indicate a strain has occurred. Bleeding (ecchymosis, hemorrhagic spot) will be present if muscle is torn.

Treatment and Nursing Management

Ice and compression should be immediately applied and the part should be rested. Surgical repair may be necessary. The patient is taught to use ice for 20 minutes out of the hour only. When compression is used, the distal parts of the extremity must be checked for sensation and adequate circulation.

DISLOCATION

Etiology and Pathophysiology

A dislocation is the stretching and tearing of ligaments around a joint with complete displacement of a bone. Subluxation is a partial dislocation. This occurs from trauma. The most common sites are the shoulder, knee, and temporomandibular joint.

Signs, Symptoms, and Diagnosis

Examination revealing a history of an outside force pushing from a certain direction, severe pain aggravated by motion of the joint, muscle spasm, or abnormal appearance of a joint indicates a diagnosis of dislocation. An x-ray will reveal displacement of bone.

Treatment and Nursing Management

Reduction of displacement under anesthesia, or manual reduction is necessary. Sometimes spontaneous reduction can be achieved. Stabilization of the joint after reduction, and rehabilitation to minimize muscular atrophy and strengthen the joint are ordered.

Nursing management is aimed mainly at encouraging rest of the affected part and pain control. Heat or cold applications may be ordered.

> ***Think Critically About . . .*** How would you assess for a circulation problem or nerve injury after an ankle sprain or strain?

BURSITIS

Etiology and Pathophysiology

Bursitis occurs from injury or overuse. It often appears when a person has engaged in an uncommon activity. An example would be shoulder bursitis after digging up the garden plot in the spring. Bursitis may occur in any heavily used joint, but it most commonly occurs in the elbow, shoulder, or knee. Bursitis is an inflammation of the bursae, the saclike structures that line freely movable joints.

Signs, Symptoms, and Diagnosis

Symptoms are mild to moderate aching pain, localized to the joint, and exacerbated by activity of the joint. Swelling may be present. Diagnosis is by history of injury and physical examination. There is localized tenderness.

Treatment

Treatment is to rest the joint by altering aggravating activity, anti-inflammatory agents, ice, massage, and a compression wrap if there is soft-tissue swelling. If these measures, plus time, do not relieve the symptoms, an injection of cortisone into the bursa is administered.

Nursing Management

Assessment after a connective tissue injury focuses on determining that there is adequate blood flow to the affected part and distal to it; determining if swelling is present; assessing the degree of pain; and assessing movement of the affected part and areas distal to it to determine if a fracture is present. Nursing care consists of assisting with immobilization as needed and teaching the patient about elevation, rest, ice application, and activity restrictions.

ROTATOR CUFF TEAR

Rotator cuff injury usually results from repetitive activity, such as throwing or overhead motion. The rotator cuff is composed of four muscles. If the cuff is torn, the patient cannot perform abduction and external rotation of that shoulder. There is considerable pain. Treatment consists of rest, sling support for the shoulder, and NSAIDs for the discomfort. Some physicians treat with injections of steroids or an anti-inflammatory drug. When the acute episode is over, gentle, progressive exercise is prescribed. Heat is recommended before exercising the joint. If the tear will not heal, surgical repair is indicated.

ANTERIOR CRUCIATE LIGAMENT INJURY

Most anterior cruciate ligament (ACL) injuries of the knee occur from athletic activities, but falls and motor vehicle accidents also may cause such injury. Hyperextension, internal rotation, extremes of external rotation, and deceleration are involved in the mechanism of injury. The ligament may be torn from the femur or tibia. Often a loud "pop" can be heard at the time of injury. There is considerable swelling in the hours following the injury and the knee feels unstable and can "give way." Full extension of the leg is difficult. Diagnosis is by physical examination, x-ray, or magnetic resonance imaging (MRI) scan. Arthroscopy is performed, at which time repair may be done.

After injury, the knee is immobilized and measures instituted to reduce swelling and pain. After repair, CPM may be ordered to promote full mobility. A long leg brace with fixed knee flexion may be used as well. Isometric exercises are prescribed in the recovery period, including quadriceps setting, bent-knee leg exercises, and foot exercises. (see Patient Teaching 31–1).

MENISCAL INJURY

The meniscus is the shock absorber of the knee and lies on top of the tibia between the tibia and the femur. A meniscus tear may accompany an ACL injury. This type of injury often results from fixed-foot rotation in weight bearing with the knee flexed. After the injury, mild swelling occurs and there is joint pain. Popping, slipping, catching, or buckling of the knee can occur. Diagnosis is by physical examination to elicit a "click" and localized pain with particular movements of the joint. MRI is the most specific diagnostic test for a meniscal injury. Surgery for repair is done arthroscopically. Postoperatively, pain management is a priority. An exercise program is prescribed for muscle strengthening during recovery.

ACHILLES TENDON RUPTURE

The Achilles tendon attaches to the calcaneus (heel bone). When overstretched, it can rupture. Sports injuries or a fall from considerable height are the usual mechanisms of injury. Arthritis, diabetes, and taking some antibiotics can predispose to Achilles tendon rupture. Injury most often occurs with bursts of jumping, pivoting, and running such as occur in tennis, basketball, handball, and badminton. Symptoms are sudden pain at the back of the ankle or calf. There may be a loud "pop" or "snap" sound. A depression can be felt or seen 2 inches above the calcaneus. Pain, swelling, and stiffness follow and then bruising and weakness. There will be an inability to point the toes or stand on tiptoe. Diagnosis is by examination and squeezing the calf muscles while the patient is lying prone. The toes should point downward; if they do not, there is most likely an Achilles tendon injury.

Treatment may be by splinting, casting, or a combination with surgery. Recovery takes 6 to 8 weeks and is followed by a period of physical therapy.

CARPAL TUNNEL SYNDROME

Etiology, Pathophysiology, Signs, and Symptoms

Carpal tunnel syndrome is a nerve problem that occurs when the median nerve is compressed as it passes through the carpal tunnel in the wrist. It produces pain, numbness, and tingling of the hand, particularly at night. Repetitive movements of the hands and wrists, particularly with constant flexion of the wrist are contributing causes. Such movement occurs in certain types of factory work and in computer keyboarding. Sometimes there is no known cause.

Diagnosis, Treatment, and Nursing Management

Diagnosis is by physical examination, a compression test, and possibly electromyography to rule out other causes of symptoms. Treatment by rest, splinting, changing the angle of the wrist during repetitive movements, or steroid injection may solve the problem. Taking vitamin B_6 has been helpful in alleviating symptoms for some people. If the symptoms are of long duration, there is muscle atrophy, or if sensory loss in the fingers and hands is progressive, surgery is indicated. Surgical decompression of the medial nerve by transection of the carpal ligament is performed, usually as an outpatient procedure.

Postoperatively, blood flow must be assessed hourly by checking color, warmth of the fingertips, and capillary refill. After anesthesia has worn off, sensation of the fingers is assessed. The wrist is immobilized in a splint and the arm is elevated on pillows to reduce edema. The patient is warned to avoid heavy gripping and pinching for up to 6 weeks. Home care instructions are sent home with the patient.

BUNION (HALLUX VALGUS)

A bunion is the most common foot problem. A bunion is a painful swelling of the bursa that occurs when the great toe deviates laterally at the metatarsophalangeal joint. It may be hereditary, or it may occur from ill-fitting shoes. Bunions are more common in females than in males.

Wearing open-toed shoes of soft leather or athletic shoes that are wider in the toe area helps reduce pain. Metatarsal pads can relieve some of the pressure. Corticosteroid injections are given in the joint if active bursitis is present. Analgesics are used for discomfort. Bone realignment of the big toe with removal of bony overgrowth is performed when walking becomes too painful.

FRACTURES

Etiology and Pathophysiology

A fracture is a break or interruption in the continuity of a bone. Fractures occur mostly from trauma but can occur due to a pathologic process in which bone has degenerated, such as in osteoporosis or another metabolic problem. The amount of injury to the neighboring tissues varies according to the type of fracture, but there is always some degree of tissue destruction, interference with the blood supply, and disturbance of muscle activity at the site of injury.

Signs, Symptoms, and Diagnosis

A fracture may cause minimal to severe pain depending on the type of fracture, the bone(s) involved, and the amount of displacement. Swelling usually occurs and there may be bleeding into the tissues. Other symptoms of a fracture include pain, tenderness, deformity of the bone, ecchymoses, crepitation with any movement, and loss of function. Box 32–1 presents the most common types of fractures. Figure 32–1 illustrates the characteristics of a variety of fractures. Diagnosis is by physical examination and x-ray.

Box 32–1 *Types of Fractures*

- *Complete fracture* is when a bone breaks into two parts that are completely separated.
- An *incomplete fracture* is when a bone breaks into two parts that are not completely separated.
- A *comminuted fracture* is one in which the bone is broken and shattered into more than two fragments.
- A *closed (simple) fracture* is one in which there is no break in the skin.
- An *open (compound) fracture* is one in which there is a break in the skin through which the fragments of broken bone protrude.
- A *greenstick fracture,* common in children, is one in which the bone is partially bent and partially broken.

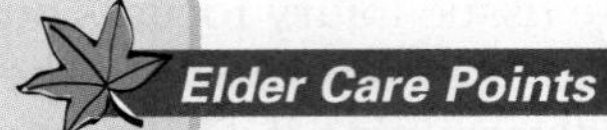

The elderly person is more at risk of sustaining a fracture because of decreased reaction time, failing vision, lessened agility, alterations in balance, and decreased muscle tone, all of which predispose to falls.

Treatment

The emergency treatment and nursing care of fractures consist of preventing shock and hemorrhage and the immediate immobilization of the part to avoid unnecessary damage to the soft tissue adjacent to the fracture. The words *splint it as it lies* mean exactly that. An inexperienced person should never attempt to straighten or set a broken bone. The injured part should be immobilized in the position in which it is found at the time of injury and should be supported firmly so that it will not be jarred when the victim is being moved. If available,

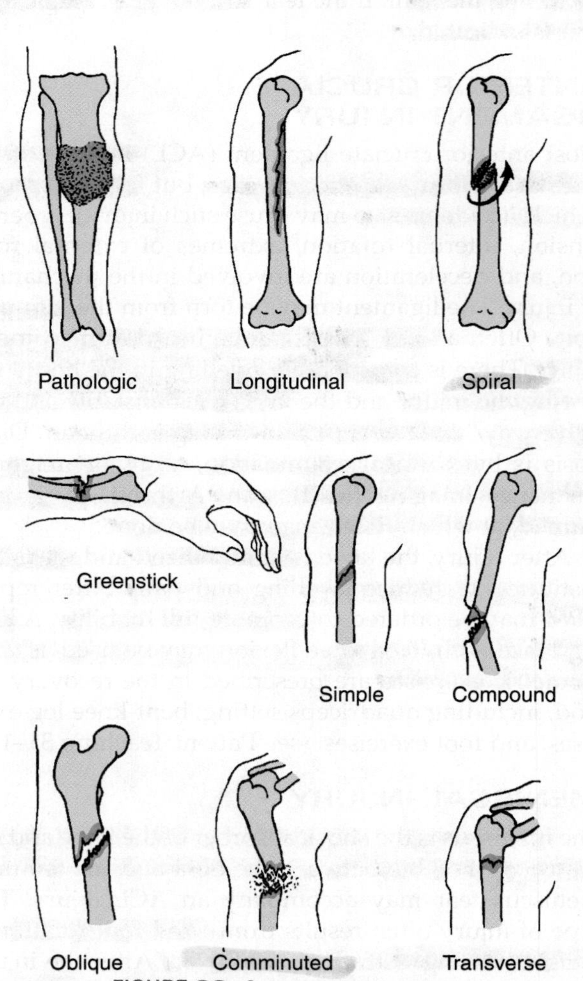

FIGURE 32–1 Types of fractures.

ice in a plastic bag can be applied to the fracture area to help minimize swelling.

In the emergency room or clinic, the patient will be examined by a health care provider, and an x-ray will be ordered if fracture is suspected. After an x-ray film of the injured part has been made and the type of fracture and extent of damage have been established, the health care provider will decide which method to use in reducing the fracture and providing immobilization. Surgery may be necessary to realign the bones and to reduce the fracture.

The primary aim in the treatment of fractures is to establish a sturdy union between the broken ends so that the bone can be restored to its former state of continuity. The healing and repair of a fracture begin immediately after the bone is broken and go through five stages:

1. Blood oozes from the torn blood vessels in the area of the fracture, clots, and begins to form a hematoma between the two broken ends of bone (1 to 3 days).
2. Other tissue cells enter the clot, and granulation tissue is formed. This tissue is interlaced with capillaries, and it gradually becomes firm and forms a bridge between the two ends of broken bone (3 days to 2 weeks).
3. Young bone cells enter the area and form a tissue called "callus." At this stage, the ends of the broken bone are beginning to "knit" together (2 to 6 weeks).
4. The immature bone cells are gradually replaced by mature bone cells (ossification), and the tissue takes on the characteristics of typical bone structure (3 weeks to 6 months).
5. Bone is resorbed and deposited, depending on the lines of stress. The medullary canal is reconstructed. This is consolidation and remodeling (6 weeks to 1 year).

To facilitate the process of repair and ensure proper healing of the bone without deformity or loss of function, the surgeon must bring the two broken ends together in proper alignment and then immobilize the affected part until healing is complete. The procedure for bringing the two fragments of bone into proper alignment is called *reduction of the fracture.*

Research is ongoing to test a way of repairing displaced fractured bones by using a liquid bonelike paste that can be injected directly into the fracture. The substance hardens in 10 minutes and within 12 hours is as strong as the natural bone—or stronger. The body seems to treat it as real bone and over time transforms it into natural bone.

Reduction, Surgery, and Stabilization. Four methods of reducing a fracture are:

- Closed reduction
- Open reduction
- Internal fixation
- External fixation

In *closed reduction,* the bone is manipulated into alignment; no surgical incision is made. A general anesthetic may be given before the fracture is reduced. An *open reduction* is done after a surgical incision is made through the skin and down to the bone at the site of the fracture. In cases of open (compound) fractures and comminuted fractures, an open reduction is necessary so that the area can be adequately cleansed and bone fragments removed.

Internal Fixation. When a fracture cannot be properly reduced by either open or closed reduction and it is impossible to guarantee adequate union of the bone fragments, the physician must perform *internal fixation* of the bone. This means that pins, nails, screws, or metal plates must be used to stabilize the position of the two broken ends. Internal fixation is particularly necessary to treat fractures in elderly patients whose bones are brittle and may not heal properly (Figure 32–2).

One of the most common internal fixation procedures is performed on a fractured hip: open reduction and internal fixation (ORIF). An incision is made, the fracture is realigned, and the bone is secured with pins, screws, nails, or plates. A drain will be in place for at least 2 days. If a prosthesis is implanted, there will be more blood loss and the patient will be receiving autotransfusion of salvaged blood after surgery. Administration of IV antibiotics to reduce the risk of infection is standard. Care includes maintaining good alignment of the affected leg, preventing complications of immobility, and keeping the patient comfortable with pain-control measures.

External Fixation. *External fixation* of fractures involves the use of a device composed of a sturdy exter-

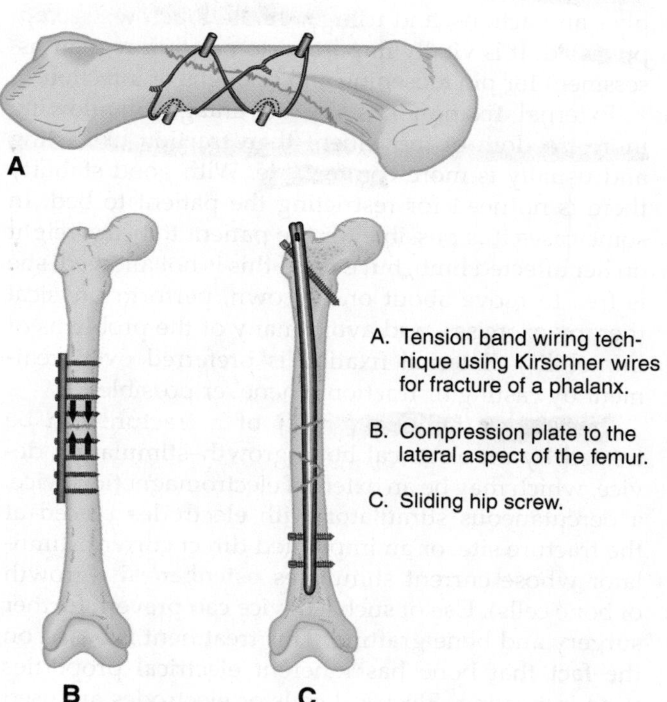

FIGURE 32–2 Examples of internal fixation.

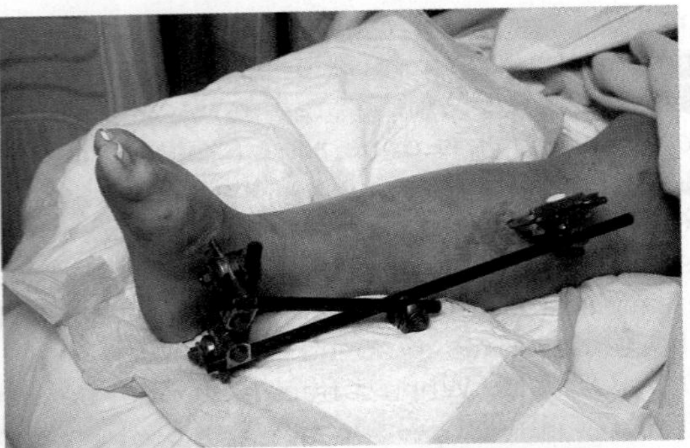

FIGURE 32–3 External fixation.

nal frame to which are attached pins that have been placed into the bone fragments. Figure 32–3 shows a fixator that is applied by inserting heavy pins on either side of the fracture and then reducing the fracture by tightening nuts attached to the connecting rods.

External fixation is indicated when:

- There are massive open fractures with extensive soft-tissue damage
- There are infected fractures that do not heal properly
- There is multiple trauma with one or more fractures and other injuries, such as burns, chest injury, or head injury.

External fixators are commonly used for fractures of an extremity or of the pelvis. The fixator frame is large and bulky and may cause the patient a body image disturbance. If there is tissue damage and dressings are used around the pins, consideration for patient comfort during dressing changes is necessary. Medication 30 minutes ahead of time, being well organized with supplies and actions, and using a gentle touch will be appreciated. It is vitally important to perform regular assessment for pin loosening and for signs of infection.

External fixation has the advantage of allowing more freedom of movement than traction or casting and usually is more comfortable. With good stability there is no need for restricting the patient to bed. In some cases it is possible for the patient to bear weight on her affected limb, but even if this is not allowed, she is free to move about on her own, perform physical therapy exercises, and avoid many of the problems of immobility. External fixation is preferred over treatment by casting or traction whenever possible.

Nonunion (failure to heal) of a fracture can be treated by an electrical bone growth–stimulating device, which may be an external electromagnetic device, a percutaneous stimulator with electrodes placed at the fracture site, or an implanted direct current stimulator whose current stimulates **osteogenesis** (growth of bone cells). Use of such a device can prevent further surgery and bone grafting. This treatment is based on the fact that bone has inherent electrical properties used in healing. Electrical coils or electrodes are used to induce weak electrical current in the bone.

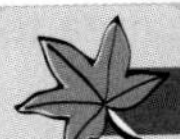

Elder Care Points

An estimated 14% to 36% of patients with hip fracture die within a year of the fracture. Most elderly people are aware of the statistic and fear for the future when a hip is fractured. Hip fracture repair should not be delayed more than 2 days because there is a 17% greater chance of dying within 30 days when that happens (Agency for Healthcare Quality and Research, 2005).

In elderly patients who have suffered a fracture of the head of the femur, the surgeon may choose to take out the broken head fragments. He replaces the fragments with a prosthesis designed with a ball to replace the head of the femur. It is shaped so that it can be fitted into or onto the shaft of the femur in such a way that the patient can bear weight on it. Although a prosthesis is not as good as a normal hip joint, many patients who have such a prosthesis are able to walk again and use the limb effectively. Total hip replacement (THR) for osteoarthritis is discussed later in this chapter.

Casts. Casts are used to hold bone fragments in place after reduction. A cast is rigid and immobilizes the body part that is mending while allowing movement of other body parts. Casts are made from a variety of materials. Fiberglass and polyester-cotton knit casts are used more frequently than the traditional plaster of Paris casts. The newer materials are lighter weight, dry quickly, and can bear weight within 30 minutes of application. They also are less bulky, do not crumble as easily, and are less likely to be damaged by wetting. In spite of all their advantages, synthetic casts do have limited use. They cost three to seven times more than plaster casts. They are less easily molded to a body part and are not suitable for immobilizing the fragments of severely displaced bones or for stabilizing serious fractures. Their rough exterior surfaces can damage the skin and tend to snag clothing and other soft materials. They are used mostly for upper-extremity fractures.

The cast brace or cast shoe permits early ambulation and weight bearing in patients who have a fracture in the shaft of the femur. It is applied 2 to 6 weeks after the fracture has been reduced, during which time skeletal traction has been used to hold the fragments in alignment during healing.

Some physicians still use plaster of Paris casts for lower extremities because these can bear more weight and will stay intact longer with weight bearing than the lighter-weight casts.

There are four main groups of casts: arm casts, leg casts, cast braces, and body or spica casts. Leg and arm casts may cover all or part of the limb (Figure 32–4). These are called *long-leg* or *short-leg* casts, depending on how much leg they cover. A *cast shoe* is a canvas sandal with a thick sole for weight bearing that fits over the bottom of the leg cast. A *spica* cast covers the

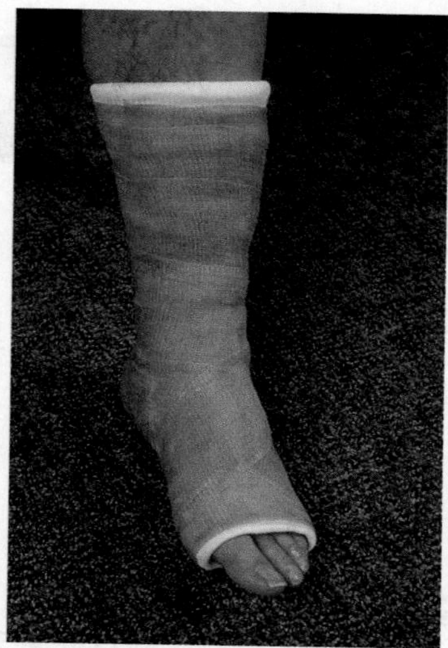

FIGURE 32–4 Synthetic limb cast.

trunk of the body and one or two extremities. There are long-leg and short-leg spicas that cover one or both legs and shoulder spicas that include the trunk and one arm.

Each type of cast presents unique problems of mobility and self-care activities. When an arm cast is applied, a sling is often used to support the arm and provide extremity elevation. Before a cast is applied, the patient's skin is thoroughly cleansed with soap and water, and any breaks in the skin are reported to the physician if he is not aware of them. Shaving is not done unless surgery is to be performed before applying the cast. In this case, a special orthopedic surgical cleanser, prepared according to hospital procedure, is used.

As soon as the cast brace is dry, the patient is allowed to get out of bed. Gradual progression from standing to partial weight bearing, full weight bearing, and walking is supervised by a physical therapist.

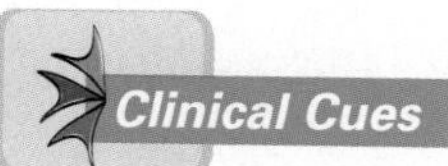

Clinical Cues

Tell the patient who is about to have a cast applied that she will feel warmth as the cast sets and dries. This is particularly true of a plaster of Paris cast. Never cover a fresh plaster of Paris cast with a blanket because that will impede the air circulation needed for it to dry.

Traction. Traction is the application of a mechanical *pull* to a part of the body for the purpose of extending and holding that part in a certain position during immobilization. Through a system of ropes and pulleys, weights are attached to a fixed point below the area of injury or disease. The apparatus is rigged so that the weights on one end and the weight of the patient's body on the other will pull the affected part in opposite directions, thus straightening and holding that part in the desired position. There are several ways to accomplish this.

The two general types of traction are *skeletal* and *skin.* In skeletal traction, the surgeon inserts pins, wires, or tongs directly through the bone at a point distal to the fracture so that the force of pull from the weights is exerted directly on the bone. Skeletal traction uses 10 or more pounds of weight. The body acts as the countertraction.

With skin traction, a bandage, such as moleskin or ACE-adherent, is applied to the limb below the site of fracture and the pull is exerted on the limb in this manner. No more than 7 to 10 lb of weight are used for skin traction.

Traction may be continuous, as in the alignment and resultant immobility of fractured bones, or it may be intermittent, as in traction on the spinal column to relieve the symptoms of a slipped disk or muscle spasms.

The system of ropes, pulleys, and weights used to provide the various kinds of traction can be very confusing at first, but the principles on which traction is based are actually very simple. Some types of traction are named for the orthopedic surgeons who first designed them. Figure 32–5 illustrates some of the different types of traction.

- *Bryant's traction* for small children with fracture of the femur uses the weight of the child's lower body to pull the bone fragments of the fractured leg into alignment. To accomplish this, the child's buttocks should just clear the mattress and the legs should be at a 90-degree angle to the trunk.
- *Buck's extension* is a simple skin traction that is used to treat muscle spasms from fractures of the hip or femur preoperatively and for dislocation of the hip.
- *Russell's traction* uses a knee sling to provide support of the affected leg. It is commonly used to treat fractures of the end of the tibia in the leg.
- *Cervical traction* can be provided through the use of tongs inserted into the skull, the use of a halo device (see Chapter 22), or a head halter.
- *Sidearm traction* is indicated when stabilization is needed to treat fractures and dislocations of the arm and shoulder.
- *Pelvic traction* with a pelvic belt or sling is indicated for pelvic fractures and other pelvic injuries.
- *Balanced suspension* with the *Thomas splint* and *Pearson attachment* is used to treat fractures of the femur and pelvis. The Thomas splint supports the thigh and knee and provides countertraction. The Pearson attachment supports the lower leg.

Care of patients with injury to the spinal column and spinal cord is covered in Chapter 22. The chapter also includes care of the patient with cervical tongs, halo traction, laminectomy, and spinal fusion.

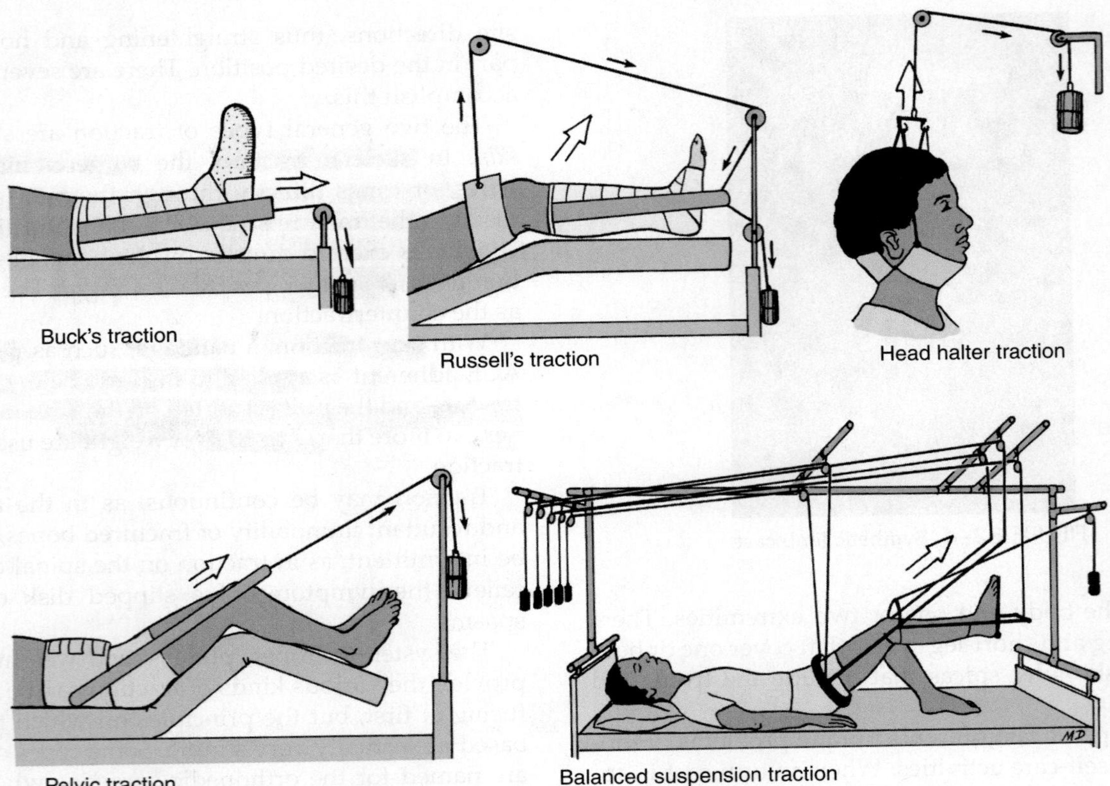

FIGURE 32–5 Examples of common types of traction.

If the skin was broken when the fracture occurred, tetanus immunization is given. Prophylactic antibiotics are usually administered when a compound fracture has occurred.

NURSING MANAGEMENT

Assessment (Data Collection)

Assessment of a suspected fracture includes noting pain, swelling, and discoloration, as well as a deformity in the contour of the bone. If there is a possibility of a fracture of an extremity, the affected limb is checked for pulse to determine whether circulation has been impaired. Nerve damage in a fractured leg is assessed by having the patient flex and extend the foot and by touching a toe and asking her which toe has been touched while obscuring her view. To determine whether the nerve pathways have been damaged by a fracture in the arm, the patient is asked to wave her hand, to identify fingers that have been touched by the examiner, and to grip the examiner's hand. Paralysis and total loss of sensation in the extremities may indicate damage to the spinal cord.

Pain is not always present when a fracture has occurred. Numbness and tingling also can accompany a fracture. **If there is some question as to whether a bone has been broken, it is best to treat the injury as if it is a fracture.** Proper first aid will be helpful and will prevent further trauma and pain regardless of the degree of injury to a bone.

Any body part encased in a cast is in danger of pressure against nerves and blood vessels and resultant nerve damage or serious obstruction to blood flow. Assessment for neurovascular status and infection is performed at least once each shift (Focused Assessment 32–1). When a fracture is fresh, this assessment should be performed every 2 to 4 hours. The cast should be inspected for problems, such as flattened areas, soft spots, cracking, and crumbling. Traction devices must be assessed to see that they are in correct position and that the weights are hanging free. The patient's body position should be assessed for proper alignment.

? ***Think Critically About . . .*** If your neurovascular assessment notes some decreased sensation and tingling in the fingers of the patient with a lower arm cast, what would you do?

Failure to notice the early signs of pressure on nerves or blood vessels and to initiate preventive measures can cause an avoidable paralysis and, possibly, gangrene. A thorough assessment of a patient in a cast should include the following:

- *Listen to the patient's complaints.* She may report numbness, a tingling sensation, increased pain with motion of her fingers or toes, or sharp lo-

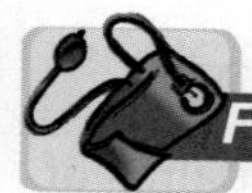

Focused Assessment 32–1

Physical Assessment of Neurovascular Status

This assessment format should be followed at least once each shift for any patient who has suffered a musculoskeletal injury.

- **Skin color** — Inspect the area around the injury and distal to the injury for increasing signs of discoloration that might indicate internal bleeding; area may be pale if arterial flow is impeded.
- **Skin temperature** — Feel the area distal to the injury with the back of the hand; if the skin is increasingly hot to the touch, report this to the physician.
- **Pulses** — Palpate pulse sites distal to the injury; compare bilaterally. Report significant differences from one side to the other to the physician.
- **Movement** — Ask the patient to move actively the affected area or the area distal to the injury. Note the amount of discomfort. If active movement is not possible, passively move the area distal to the injury. This checks for swelling and potential nerve damage.
- **Sensation** — Ask whether numbness or tingling is present (paresthesia). Touch the area distal to the injury gently with the end of a paper clip in a manner so that the patient cannot see where you are touching. Ask what this feels like and where it is felt. Loss of sensation may indicate nerve damage.
- **Pain** — Ask the patient to evaluate the pain by location, nature, and intensity. Note whether pain is increasing, evaluate whether pain-control measures are effective.
- **Capillary refill** — Press down on a nail bed distal to the injury with the side of the clip of a pen until blanching occurs; let up, and count the time it takes for color to return. Usual color should return in 3 to 5 seconds.

calized pain; any of these symptoms could be caused by pressure from a tight cast. Do not attempt to judge whether her complaints are justified. **If elevating the limb does not relieve the patient's complaints within 30 minutes, notify the physician.**

- Check frequently to see whether the cast is properly supported or if there is undue pressure on any part of the body. A sharp, localized, burning pain could mean the beginning of a pressure sore. This should be reported so that the surgeon or orthopedic technician can cut a "window" in the cast to relieve pressure.
- Lean down and smell at the edges of the cast to detect any foul odor that might indicate the presence of infection.

Every immobilized patient should be consciously assessed for the various problems of immobility. **The most commonly found problems include skin breakdown, urinary tract infection or stones, and constipation.**

Elder Care Points

When the elderly person has to be immobilized because of trauma and fractures, the complications of immobility are much more likely to occur than in a younger person. Aggressive preventive nursing care and careful assessment for signs of complications are very important. Respiratory problems can be prevented by scheduled, supervised deep breathing and coughing or the use of an incentive spirometer.

Attention to pain control is important, especially when the patient is adjusting to traction or a new cast. It is essential to try to keep the patient's mind occupied, as boredom can greatly increase discomfort.

Nursing Diagnosis and Planning

Nursing diagnoses for patients with fractures usually include:

- Pain related to disruption of bone and tissue
- Impaired mobility related to disruption of bone
- Self-care deficit related to inability to use an extremity.

Expected outcomes will be written for the specific nursing diagnoses chosen.

If the broken bone has pierced the skin and bleeding is severe, apply direct pressure over the wound or compress the appropriate pressure point. Cover the open area with a clean dressing. Try to avoid introducing infectious agents into the wound, and remember the need for the prevention and treatment of shock.

Implementation

A patient with a fracture sometimes is immobilized for an extended period, which interferes with her usual roles. She may be very worried about usual responsibilities and about employment and finances. Allowing ventilation of concerns and fears and then assisting with solving problems can often bring some peace of mind.

Because the pin sites are left open to the air during convalescence, special daily care is necessary to prevent infection. Pins must be kept clean and dry. As soon as it is feasible, the patient is taught to care for the pin sites and to report any signs of infection. Physician preferences for pin care vary, so follow the physician's orders for cleansing or check the agency's policy. Some believe that cleansing around the pins disrupts the natural barrier provided by the skin. When cleaning is ordered, the usual agent is half-strength hydrogen peroxide. Standard Precautions must be followed when providing pin care.

Think Critically About . . . If you are in the park and you observe a child fall from a tree and obviously suffer a broken forearm, what steps would you take to assist?

In emergencies, a thorough explanation of what is going to be done about a fracture is not always possible. In all other cases, however, it is best if you prepare the patient for the type of cast that will be applied, the precautions that must be taken while the cast is drying, and any special devices that may be put on her bed to help her turn and move about in the bed. An example is the trapeze bar attached to an overhead frame, which allows the patient to lift herself and turn without strain on the affected part.

Fiberglass and polyester-cotton knit casts dry very quickly; however, the newly applied plaster cast usually is not dry for about 48 hours. While the plaster is damp, its shape can be changed by careless handling or improper support. It follows, therefore, that extreme care must be used in moving the patient or the cast during this time. **During the first 24 to 48 hours after any cast has been applied to an extremity, the extremity should be elevated to minimize swelling.**

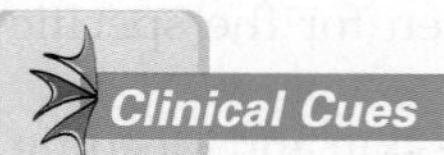

Ice bags can be used to help control swelling. Because the weight of an ice bag could make an indentation in a wet plaster cast, the ice bags should be only about half full, and they should be laid against the cast and propped in position, rather than set on top of it.

When the patient is transferred from the stretcher to the bed, there must be enough help available so that she is not "tumbled" into bed. Pillows for support should be placed on the bed *before* moving the patient onto them. Pillows are used to support the curves of large casts so that there will be no cracking or flattening of the cast by the weight of the body.

The patient in a body cast or spica is more comfortable if pillows are not put under her head and shoulders because they push the chest and abdomen against the front of the cast, causing an uncomfortable crushing sensation and dyspnea.

Bars between the legs of a cast are never to be used as handles for lifting and turning the patient. Even after the cast is dry, these braces may be dislocated or pulled out of the cast.

An effort should be made to use only the palms of the hands or the flat surface of the extended fingers when moving a wet plaster cast because fingertips can sink into the damp plaster and make impressions through the thickness of the cast, thus pressing mounds of plaster against the tissue under the cast. These can harden and, in time, lead to pressure sores. A plaster cast generates heat as it dries and assessments must be made frequently of the amount of heat generated and the sensation under the cast that the patient feels; burns can occur. A dry plaster cast is white, has a shiny surface, and will resound when tapped. A wet plaster cast is grayish and dull in appearance and will give a dull thud when tapped.

Adequate nutrition and fluids are needed to promote healing and prevent the problems of immobility (Nutritional Therapies 32–1). Stopping smoking aids healing (Health Promotion Points 32–1).

Daily Care

After the cast is thoroughly dry and the initial swelling under the cast has subsided, give attention to the cleanliness of the patient and the cast. The problems

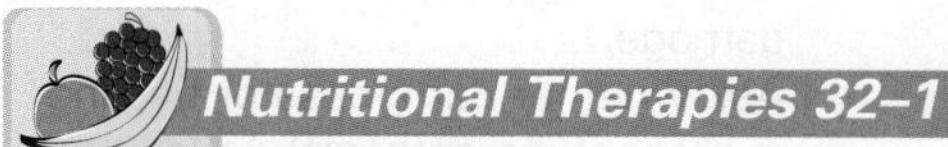

Nutrition for Immobile Musculoskeletal Patients

Protein is essential to healing and the diet should be calculated to provide 1 g/kg of body weight. Vitamins D, B, and C and calcium are included in well-balanced meals to ensure optimal soft tissue and bone healing; 500 mg of vitamin C will also help acidify the urine and prevent calcium precipitation that could form kidney stones. Fluid intake of 2000 to 3000 mL/day helps prevent bladder infection, kidney stones, and constipation. A high-fiber diet with lots of vegetables and fruits promotes good bowel function and decreases the chance of constipation. The patient in a hip spica cast or body jacket should receive six small meals a day to avoid abdominal distention and cramping.

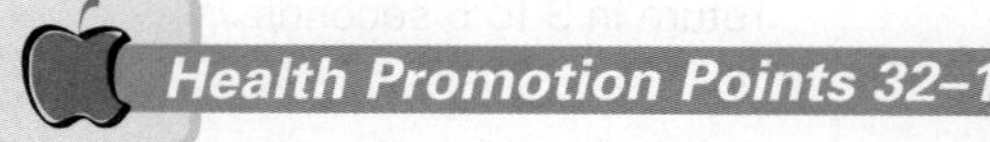

Smoking and Musculoskeletal Health

Smoking has a significant impact on the bones and joints in that it:

- Increases the risk of developing osteoporosis
- Increases the risk of a hip fracture as you age
- Increases your risk of developing exercise-related injuries
- Has a detrimental effect on fracture and wound healing
- Has a detrimental effect on athletic performance
- Is associated with low back pain and rheumatoid arthritis. (American Association of Orthopedic Surgeons, 2000.)

involved will vary according to the type of cast and the area it covers. All parts of the body not included in the cast should be bathed daily, using care not to wet a plaster cast. Patients may have permission to shower with a synthetic cast; a plastic covering is secured over the cast and taped to the skin and the patient is asked not to place the casted area directly under the stream of water.

The skin around the edges of the cast should receive special attention, including massage with lotion and close observation for signs of pressure or breaks in the skin. The edges of plaster casts tend to crumble, with bits of plaster dropping down inside the cast and causing the patient discomfort and skin irritation. This can be avoided by covering the rims of the cast with stockinette or applying tape in a "petal" fashion.

When a bedpan is used by the patient in a spica, there is the possibility of a backward flow of urine under the cast unless the head of the bed is slightly elevated. Because the patient cannot bend at the hips to sit up on the pan, the head of the bed should be elevated on shock blocks or some other device and the lumbar area of the cast supported to prevent cracking.

Itching is a common complaint. Patients must be instructed not to use sharp objects such as pencils or rulers to scratch under the cast. These can tear the skin, leaving an open break for the entrance of bacteria. An experienced orthopedic nurse has found that forceful injection of air, using a 50-mL bulb syringe or one with a plunger and directing the air under the cast, can relieve intense itching. A hair dryer on the cool setting that blows air into the cast also may relieve itching (Family Doctor, 2005).

When a cast is removed, the underlying skin is usually dry and scaly. Cleansing of these areas should be done in consultation with the physician, because the type of care to be given will depend on whether another cast is to be applied. In any case, overenthusiastic scrubbing of the area must be avoided to prevent damage to the deeper layers of skin. Nursing interventions for selected problems of a patient in a cast are summarized in Table 31–5.

Many patients with fractures and other orthopedic conditions requiring a continuous pull on a part of the body must lie on their backs, with only a limited amount of turning permitted. The patient must be kept clean and comfortable and free of pressure sores.

If the physician does not permit turning the patient far enough to allow for adequate back care, the patient may use a trapeze bar to lift herself so that back care can be given and the bottom sheet changed or tightened. She should be instructed to lift herself straight up so that the amount of pull exerted on the limb in traction will not be altered. This same maneuver can be used when the patient is placed on a bedpan. A small "fracture" bedpan should be used and the lower back supported by a small pillow or folded blanket.

Frequent observations of both the patient and the traction apparatus are necessary to protect the patient and ensure that the traction is effective. Box 32–2 presents points of care.

> ? *Think Critically About . . .* Your patient is in balanced leg traction. Can you list the points you should check before leaving the room to ensure that the traction is working properly and her safety is protected?

Evaluation

Data are gathered related to the success of the nursing interventions. If the interventions are not helping the patient meet the expected outcomes, the plan must be altered.

Complications

The healing of a fracture can be impeded by improper alignment and inadequate immobilization of the bone. Poor alignment almost inevitably leads to some perma-

Box 32–2 Points of Care for the Patient in Traction

- Keep the patient in the center of the bed in a supine position.
- Keep the body part in traction in a straight line with the trunk. Misalignment causes pain.
- *Be sure the weights are hanging free.* If the weights are resting on or against any support, such as the foot of the bed or the floor, the purpose of the traction is defeated. Be careful not to bump against the weights when walking around the foot of the bed. This can be painful to the patient and may cause damage to the healing bone. It is not necessary to lift the weights when pulling the patient up in bed. The amount of pull on the limb will remain the same as long as the weights are hanging free. Also check that the ropes run over the midline of the pulley without interference. Keep knots away from the pulleys, and arrange bedding so that it does not interfere with the ropes and pulleys.
- *Check the position of the patient, making sure her body weight is counteracting the pull of the weights.* Should the patient slip down in bed so that her feet are resting against the footboard, there will be a loss of force exerted on the limb.
- Observe all bony prominences for signs of impaired circulation and pressure or tissue necrosis.
- To prevent pressure sores, be sure slings and ropes are not pressing against or cutting into an area of the extremity.
- When a patient has skeletal traction, observe the sites of entry of pins, tongs, etc. for signs of infection.
- Devise a systematic routine for observing the patient and the apparatus at specified times during the day so that no aspect of the assessment will be overlooked.

nent deformity. Inadequate immobilization of the bone allows continued twisting, shearing, and abnormal stresses that prohibit a strong, bony union. Notify the physician if the patient states that she can feel the bone fragments grating against each other (crepitation).

Infection. Infection of the tissue at the fracture site is probably the most serious impediment to healing. It is of special concern in open comminuted fractures. Systemic infections, inadequate levels of serum calcium and phosphorus, vitamin deficiency, and generalized atherosclerosis—which deprives the healing site of adequate blood supply—also can complicate a fracture by delaying healing. It is important to monitor the patient's temperature and white blood cell (WBC) count for elevations and to monitor the appearance of the area carefully for redness, swelling, heat, or purulent drainage.

Osteomyelitis. Osteomyelitis is a bacterial infection of the bone. The causative organism is most often *Staphylococcus aureus,* which enters the bloodstream from a distant focus of infection, such as a boil or furuncle, or from an open wound, as in an open (compound) fracture. It occurs most often in older adults and is usually found in the tibia or fibula, vertebrae, or at the site of a prosthesis; however, it can also occur in other patients, at any age, when organisms are carried to the bone by the bloodstream.

Osteomyelitis has a sudden onset with severe pain and marked tenderness at the site, high fever with chills, swelling of adjacent soft parts, headache, and malaise.

Diagnosis of osteomyelitis is made on the basis of:

- Laboratory findings indicating an acute infection, for example, high sedimentation rate and WBC count
- X-rays, which may show bone destruction 7 to 10 days after onset of the disease
- History of injury to the part, open fracture, boils, furuncles, or other infections
- Biopsy, in which the bone sample exhibits signs of necrosis.

The earlier the condition is diagnosed and treatment is begun, the better the prognosis for the patient with osteomyelitis, as it can be difficult to eradicate. Specific treatment includes elimination of the infection through the use of antibiotics for 4 to 6 weeks and immobilization of the affected limb for complete rest. Surgical incision for drainage of the abscess and removal of dead bone and debris from the site of infection is necessary. Sometimes amputation is the only cure. The care of a patient with an infection is presented in Chapter 6.

Fat Embolism. Fat embolism is among the most serious complications of a fracture of a bone that has an abundance of marrow fat (e.g., the long bones, pelvis, and ribs). A high percentage of patients with multiple fractures resulting from severe trauma die of this complication. It occurs at any age but is most commonly

Safety Alert 32–1

Danger of Fat Embolism

Watch for signs of fat embolism: a change in mental status followed by respiratory distress, tachypnea, rapid pulse, fever, and petechiae (a measles-like rash over the chest, neck, upper arms, or abdomen). Signs must be reported immediately, as there is about an 80% mortality rate from this complication.

seen in young men ages 20 to 40 and in older persons between ages 70 and 80. Not all fat emboli are fatal. To be life threatening, the fat globules released when a bone is fractured must be large enough or sufficient in number to occlude a blood vessel either partially or completely. The fat embolism arises from injury of the fat-bearing bone marrow and rupture of small venules in the area, thus permitting the entrance of fat globules into the circulation. **Embolism, if it occurs, happens within 48 hours of fracture.**

Crackles and wheezes will be heard when auscultating the lungs if emboli are present (Safety Alert 32–1). Apprehension and a dropping oxygen saturation level will occur. Stay with the patient; put her in a high Fowler's position, if possible, to ease the dyspnea; remain calm; begin oxygen administration at 2 to 3 L/minute if it is available; and summon the physician immediately. Hydration with IV fluids is usually ordered along with correction of acidosis. Intubation and mechanical ventilation may be needed if oxygen levels cannot be maintained with supplemental oxygen alone.

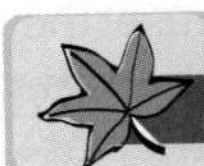

Elder Care Points

The elderly patient with a fractured hip is at high risk for fat embolism. Be especially vigilant in assessing for signs and symptoms of this complication.

Venous Thrombosis. The veins of the pelvis and lower extremities are very vulnerable to thrombus formation after fracture, especially hip fracture. Immobility, traction, and casts may contribute to venous stasis. Compression stockings, sequential compression devices, or both are used to help prevent the problems. Range-of-motion (ROM) exercises on the unaffected lower extremities is important. Prophylactic anticoagulant drugs such as aspirin, warfarin, or low-molecular-weight heparin may be ordered. Fondaparinux (Arixtra), a new class of antithrombotic drug inhibiting factor Xa, a blood clotting component, may be administered along with warfarin sodium.

Compartment Syndrome. Compartment syndrome occurs in one or more muscle compartments of the extremities. It is caused by external or internal pressure and seriously restricts circulation to the area. External pressure can occur from dressings or casts that are too tight. Internal pressure occurs from excessive IV fluid infusion, inflammation, and edema (a shifting of fluid from the vascular spaces to the intercellular spaces). The increased fluid puts pressure on the tissues, nerves, and blood vessels, thereby decreasing blood flow. Considerable pain results.

Signs and symptoms of compartment syndrome include edema, pallor, tingling, paresthesia, numbness, weak pulse, cyanosis, paresis, and severe pain. The pressure can cause permanent tissue and nerve damage if unrelieved. The physician should be notified immediately if this complication is suspected as permanent loss of function will result if the problem is not relieved.

If a cast is in place, the front will need to be split through all layers of the material. Dressings will be cut or replaced. Surgical **fasciotomy** (linear incisions in the fascia down the extremity) may be necessary to relieve the pressure on the nerves and blood vessels if other measures do not relieve the problem.

Evaluation data are gathered daily and, when expected outcomes are met, the relevant nursing diagnosis is closed on the care plan.

? *Think Critically About* . . . Your patient has an arm cast in place and is complaining of severe itching inside the cast. What could you do to help relieve the problem?

INFLAMMATORY DISORDERS OF THE MUSCULOSKELETAL SYSTEM

LYME DISEASE

Lyme arthritis occurs from a systemic infection caused by the spirochete *Borrelia burgdorferi.* The spirochete is transmitted by the bite of a deer tick. Most cases of this disease are in the New England and mid-Atlantic states, the upper Midwest, and Northern California and Oregon. The disease begins with flulike symptoms and a "bull's-eye" rash with pain and stiffness in the joints and muscles. Doxycycline, cefuroxime, or amoxicillin taken for 10 to 21 days can prevent the disease's progression. If untreated, 2 to 12 weeks later, stage II begins with carditis and nervous system disorders such as meningitis, peripheral neuritis, or a facial paralysis similar to Bell's palsy. IV antibiotics are the treatment at this point.

If undiagnosed and untreated, later chronic complications may occur. The patient may experience fatigue, cognition problems, and arthralgias. In some instances the only sign of Lyme disease is arthritis. Lyme arthritis can cause permanent damage to the nervous system and to the joints.

OSTEOARTHRITIS

Etiology and Pathophysiology

The word *arthritis,* translated literally, means inflammation of a joint. There are more than 100 different types of arthritis, ranging from hereditary disorders such as psoriatic arthritis to the more common types for which the exact cause is known. Osteoarthritis is a noninflammatory degenerative joint disease that can affect any weight-bearing joint. It usually occurs after age 40 and symptoms most commonly present between the ages of 50 to 60. Scientists identified a faulty gene that causes one form of osteoarthritis. Causes of other types are unknown. In people with osteoarthritis, there seems to be lessened production of the collagen material that strengthens the cartilage that covers and protects joints in the body. With time and use, the joint becomes thickened and withstands weight bearing poorly, with consequent damage to the cartilage. The synovial cells then release enzymes that cause further cartilage degeneration.

Arthritis causes considerable disability, and there are eight national objectives aimed at decreasing its effects (Health Promotion Points 32–2).

Signs, Symptoms, and Diagnosis

Osteoarthritis occurs asymmetrically and typically affects only one or two joints. Aching pain with joint movement and stiffness with limitation of mobility are the chief symptoms. On assessment, joint deformity and the presence of nodules may be found.

Treatment

Treatment consists of pain management, exercise, weight reduction if the patient is overweight, and maintenance of joint function. Salicylates, acetaminophen, or NSAIDs may be used. Acetaminophen in doses of 1000 mg, up to 4000 mg/day, is the standard for the patient with mild to moderate joint pain (Safety Alert 32–2).

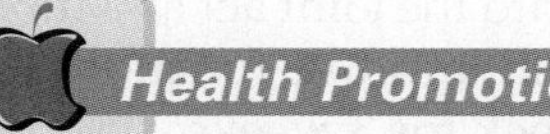

Health Promotion Points 32–2

***Healthy People 2010* Arthritis**

The following objectives are aimed at reducing the disability caused by arthritis:

2–1 Reduce the mean level of joint pain
2–2 Reduce activity limitations
2–3 Reduce personal care limitations
2–4 Increase health care provider counseling for weight and physical activity
2–5 Reduce the effect on employment
2–6 Eliminate racial disparities in total knee replacements
2–7 Increase the proportion of those seeing a health care provider for joint symptoms
2–8 Increase the proportion of those receiving arthritis education

Safety Alert 32–2

Acetaminophen Usage

All other medications and over-the-counter drugs should be checked for acetaminophen so that overdose does not occur. Taking more of this drug than recommended (no more than 4000 mg/day) can cause irreversible liver damage. The drug should not be taken when drinking alcohol. For the elderly person, the lowest effective dose should be used. Drugs are not metabolized as quickly and toxicities can easily develop in this population. Encourage an adequate intake of water, at least 2000 mL, each day to promote excretion of the drug via the kidneys.

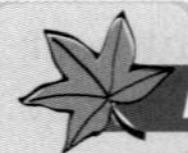

Elder Care Points

NSAIDs are not recommended for use in all elderly people because of their side effects and their interactions with other drugs an elderly patient may be taking. NSAIDs decrease the effectiveness of ACE inhibitors used for hypertension and heart failure and increase the effects of anticoagulants.

Corticosteroid injection into the joint is performed if oral medication does not control the problem. Exercises for joint mobility are encouraged. Surgery or joint replacement may be done to relieve severe pain and improve mobility. The hip and knee are the most common sites for joint replacement.

Complementary and alternative therapies have proven very helpful for many people. Acupuncture, yoga, and massage are helping to control and relieve the pain of osteoarthritis. Capsaicin cream, or ointment made from cayenne red pepper, blocks pain locally when applied topically to the inflamed joint. It can be used four times a day. It is available over-the-counter or by prescription (Complementary & Alternative Therapies 32–1).

Injections of hyaluronic acid (HA) (Orthovisc, Synvisc, Supartz, and Hyalgan) into the joint act as a lubricant and can decrease pain and improve function. The injections are given once a week for 3 weeks.

A new treatment for knee cartilage injury is the injection of autologous chondrocytes. Healthy articular cartilage cells are removed from the patient and sent to a special laboratory where they are grown for 3 to 4 weeks and then reimplanted. Patients use crutches for 6 to 8 weeks after the surgery. The procedure is successful in about 85% of all cases. It works best in patients younger than age 50 with injury to a small focal area of cartilage (Bathon, 2005).

Gentle exercise is very important in maintaining joint mobility. Walking, knitting, and swimming all help improve mobility and decrease pain. The patient should avoid placing stress on affected joints. Using assistive devices to open containers and perform other household functions is recommended.

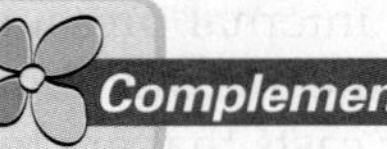

Complementary & Alternative Therapies 32–1

Glucosamine and Chondroitin

Glucosamine and chondroitin have been shown in an NIH research study to decrease the pain of osteoarthritis and to contribute to the synthesis of new cartilage. This substance may slow or halt the progression of osteoarthritis. Research is ongoing; 1500 mg of glucosamine sulfate in 500-mg doses three times per day appears to be the effective dosage for most people (Blakeley & Ribeiro, 2004).

Acupuncture can reduce pain and improve function in patients with knee and hip osteoarthritis. A randomized, controlled study showed that patients who received 23 acupuncture treatments over a period of 6 months showed improvement of 40% in pain and function scores after 14 weeks. The difference remained significant at 6 months (Berman, et al., 2004).

Ginger and turmeric, herbs that are used as spices, have anti-inflammatory, antioxidant, and antitumor properties. They are available for relief of arthritis pain in a supplement called *Zyflamend,* which can be purchased at health food stores (Weil, 2003).

Elder Care Points

Neuromuscular electrical stimulation (NMES), which can be administered at home, uses small doses of electrical current to produce involuntary muscle contractions and can decrease knee pain in elderly patients with arthritis (Gaines, Metter, & Talbot, 2004).

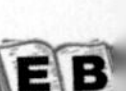

Nursing Management

Nursing interventions for osteoarthritis include teaching the patient to balance exercise and rest. Instruction for moist heat application and encouragement to maintain weight within normal limits is provided. Weight reduction decreases joint stress. Imagery, relaxation, and diversion are helpful to reduce pain. Quadriceps strengthening exercises may relieve pain and disability of the knee (see Patient Teaching 31–1).

Think Critically About . . . Where would you suggest a patient look for assistive devices available for those with arthritis?

RHEUMATOID ARTHRITIS

Etiology and Pathophysiology

Rheumatoid arthritis is an inflammatory disease of the joints. It most frequently begins between the ages of 30 and 60. There is a familial tendency. The cause is not

Table 32–1 Comparison of Rheumatoid Arthritis and Osteoarthritis

CHARACTERISTIC	RHEUMATOID ARTHRITIS	OSTEOARTHRITIS
Definition	A systemic disease, but pathologic changes and disability result from chronic inflammation of the joints	A progressive degenerative joint disease
Pathology	Chronic inflammation of synovial membranes and formation of chronic granulation tissue (pannus) in the joint; pannus capable of eroding cartilage in joints and spreading to bone, ligaments, and tendons.	Microscopic changes in the cartilage in the joint; eventually there is loss of cartilage, bony enlargement, and malalignment of joints
Etiology	Unknown; evidence that the pathologic changes are immunologic	Unknown; may be caused by "wear and tear" of aging
Rheumatoid factors (autoantibodies)	Usually present	Usually absent
Age at onset	30 to 40 years	50 to 60 years; rarely before 40
Weight	Normal or underweight	Usually overweight
General state of health	Usually anemic, "chronically ill," with low-grade fever and slight leukocytosis	Well nourished
Appearance of joints	Early: soft-tissue swelling Late: ankylosis, extreme deformity	Early: slight joint enlargement Late: enlargement more pronounced, slight limitation of motion
	Joint involvement usually symmetric and generalized	Joints usually involved are weight bearing: spine, hips, knees
Muscles	Pronounced muscular atrophy, particularly in later stages	Usually not affected
Other	Morning stiffness; pain on motion; swelling and tenderness of joints; subcutaneous nodules; typical rheumatoid changes seen on radiograph	Stiffness, relieved by moderate motion; joint malalignment; symptoms increase in cold, wet weather

known, but it is thought to be the result of an autoimmune disorder, perhaps influenced by an infectious agent.

An abnormal immune response causes an inflammatory reaction of the synovial membrane. Vasodilation, increased permeability, and the formation of exudate causes red, swollen joints. The small joints, such as those in the fingers, are often affected, but the wrists, elbows, and knees may be affected also. Rheumatoid factor (RF) which is an antibody against immunoglobulin G, appears in the blood and synovial fluid in most patients. There are remissions and exacerbations of the disease. As the disease progresses, **pannus** is formed. Pannus is granulation tissue derived from the synovium that spreads over the articular cartilage. Pannus releases enzymes and inflammatory mediators that destroy cartilage. The cartilage becomes eroded and the pannus cuts off nutrition to the cartilage. Over time, the pannus between the bone ends becomes fibrotic, causing ankylosis. Joint fixation and deformity become apparent. Along with these changes, exacerbations cause more damage and there is atrophy of muscles around the joint. Tendons and ligaments stretch and the joint becomes unstable. Muscle spasm draws the bones out of normal alignment. Contractures and deformity occur. Mobility becomes impaired if the knees or ankles are affected. Subcutaneous nodules may form and nodules may occur in the pleura, heart valves, or eyes.

Signs, Symptoms, and Diagnosis

The signs and symptoms of rheumatoid arthritis are joint pain, warmth, edema, limitation of motion, and multiple joint stiffness in the morning lasting more than 1 hour. The joints of the hands, wrists, and feet are the most commonly affected, and involvement is usually symmetrical. Subcutaneous nodules may appear over bony prominences. Systemic symptoms of low-grade fever, anorexia with weight loss, malaise, and an iron deficiency anemia resistant to iron therapy also may be present. Considerable joint deformity and consequent dysfunction can occur.

Pain or immobility of joints interferes with self-care activities. The elderly patient may not be able to maintain locomotion or perform activities of daily living (ADLs) necessary to lead an independent lifestyle. Maintaining mobility and controlling pain with the least amount of side effects are the goals for the elderly patient. Table 32–1 presents a comparison of osteoarthritis and rheumatoid arthritis.

Diagnosis is by history, examination, and blood tests for RF, plus tests to rule out other types of immune disorders. X-rays confirm the cartilage destruction and bone deformities.

Treatment

Treatment is aimed at relieving pain, minimizing joint destruction, promoting joint function, and preserving ability to perform self-care. Rest and exercise, medica-

Table 32–2 ***Medications Used to Treat Rheumatoid Arthritis***

CLASSIFICATION	ACTION/EFFECTS	EXAMPLES	NURSING IMPLICATIONS
Nonsteroidal antiinflammatory drugs (NSAIDs)	Reduce inflammation and pain	Aspirin, ibuprofen (Advil, Motrin), naproxen sodium (Aleve), COX-2 inhibitors (Celebrex)	May take 2 wk to obtain results; give with food or a full glass of water, but some are best taken 30 min before a meal or 2 hr afterward. May cause GI irritation. Teach patient to report heartburn, dyspepsia, nausea, vomiting, diarrhea, or abdominal pain. Monitor hematologic, renal, liver, auditory, and ophthalmic functions. Teach to avoid alcohol because of increased risk of GI irritation. Dosage in elderly may need to be reduced by half. Monitor weight gain and peripheral edema.
Corticosteroids	Reduce inflammation, decrease pain by suppressing the immune system	Prednisone, methylprednisolone (Medrol)	Usually rapid action. Instruct to take daily dose between 6 and 8 A.M. when natural steroids are released. Instruct not to stop taking this drug abruptly. Taper dosage downward as soon as symptoms improve. Monitor elderly closely for fluid retention, elevated blood pressure, and peripheral edema. Handle patients gently to prevent bruising; avoid using tape on skin. May cause osteoporosis, Cushing syndrome, mood changes, weight gain, cataracts, onset of diabetes, muscle weakness, and increased risk of infection.
Disease-modifying antirheumatic drugs (DMARDs)	Reduce inflammation and pain, suppress the immune system, and prevent joint and cartilage destruction	Hydroxychloroquine (Plaquenil), sulfasalazine (Azulfidine), gold salts (Ridaura), D-penicillamine (Cuprimine, Depen), methotrexate (Rheumatrex), azathioprine (Imuran), leflunomide (Arava), others	Plaquenil takes 6 mo to be effective; others take 1–6 mo. May cause rash, diarrhea, and retinal problems. Instruct that frequent eye exams are necessary. Most of the drugs can cause GI symptoms and blood dyscrasias; monitor blood counts. Gold salts can cause liver toxicity; monitor liver functions. Methotrexate can cause pulmonary, renal, and liver toxicity. Imuran and leflunomide may cause birth defects or fetal death. Alcohol use increases chance of hepatic toxicity. Monitor blood and urine weekly. Check specific drug nursing implications.
Biologic response modifiers (BMRs)	Reduce inflammation by blocking the inflammatory response	Etanercept (Enbrel), infliximab (Remicade), anakinra (Kineret), abatacept (Orencia)	1–2 wk for onset of action. Increased risk of serious infection and blood dyscrasias; monitor blood counts, temperature, and for malaise closely. May cause demyelinating disorders. Given IV or by subcutaneous injection; may cause injection site reaction. Do not immunize with live virus vaccines. Discontinue drug if sepsis or serious infection develops.

tion, immobilization with splints and use of other supportive devices during periods of severe inflammation, and hot and cold treatments are standard. Medications include salicylates, NSAIDs, corticosteroids, antimalarial drugs, methotrexate, gold compounds, sulfasalazine, D-penicillamine, and disease-modifying antirheumatic drugs (DMARDs) (Table 32–2). Surgical joint repair or replacement can be done to reduce pain and improve mobility. No drug will cure the disease, however, and medication is but one part of the overall regimen of treatment. Usually NSAIDs are the first kind of agent used for arthritis. Of these, aspirin is the drug of choice if the patient can tolerate it. The amount of aspirin prescribed is large and ranges from 15 to 25 tablets per day. The greatest disadvantage of the NSAID drugs is that they can cause serious gastrointestinal (GI) irritation, ulceration, and bleeding. Some of the NSAIDs are combined with other agents or are specially coated to minimize adverse GI side effects. These agents include aspirin compounded with antacids (Ascriptin), enteric-coated aspirin (Ecotrin), and choline salicylate (Trilisate). Although these agents are associated with a lower incidence of GI bleeding and heartburn, they are more expensive than plain aspirin.

In severe cases of rheumatoid arthritis that do not respond to other forms of drug therapy, more potent drugs may be prescribed. Although these DMARDs provide periods of remission, they also have some serious side effects in most patients.

Systemic corticosteroids have a profound antiinflammatory effect on arthritis. They were once

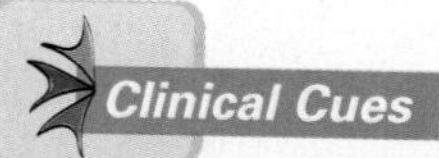

Monitor patients taking NSAIDs for GI intolerance. Assess liver, kidney, and central nervous system function frequently. Watch for signs of blood dyscrasias and check for tinnitus and hearing loss regularly. The side effects of NSAIDs can be serious and sometimes permanent. If early signs of toxicity appear, they should be reported promptly to the physician.

thought to be "miracle drugs" to treat arthritis; however, their anti-inflammatory action tends to diminish over time, thus requiring higher doses to obtain the same results. In addition, long-term steroid therapy exposes the patient to some rather severe side effects. These include diabetes mellitus, osteoporosis, hypertension, acne, cataracts, and weight gain. Because of these and other problems associated with steroid therapy, long-term oral steroid preparations are reserved for patients who cannot find relief from other drugs (Complementary & Alternative Therapies 32–2).

The injection of steroids directly into a joint (intra-articular administration) has been used successfully in treating painful flareups, shortening the period of inflammation, and relieving pain and other symptoms. When intra-articular steroid therapy is used, it is recommended that not more than three or four doses be injected into any joint within 1 year's time.

As with many other patients with chronic and incurable diseases, those with arthritis are particularly vulnerable to unproven claims for a cure and to outright quackery. Because rheumatoid arthritis sometimes goes into spontaneous remission, many patients who undergo an unorthodox treatment at the same time their disease is in remission give credit for their improvement to the treatment.

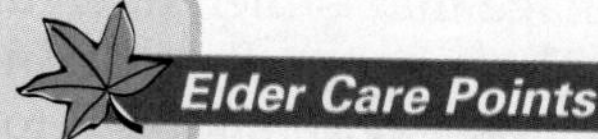

Elderly patients experience side effects of drugs more often and more quickly than younger people. These patients must be taught to watch for side effects and to report them to the physician or nurse promptly and to refrain from taking another dose until the effects have been reported. Dizziness may be experienced when taking analgesics for arthritis pain, particularly if the medication contains codeine. This predisposes the elderly patient to falls. The elderly should be cautioned to arise slowly, hold on to furniture until stable on their feet, and to wait until dizziness has cleared to ambulate. An assistive device for ambulation is of benefit to help prevent falls.

Surgical Intervention and Orthopedic Devices. In the past, surgical intervention for arthritis was reserved for patients who already had suffered severe joint deformity and loss of motion. The trend now is toward the use of surgery in the early stages of the disease to

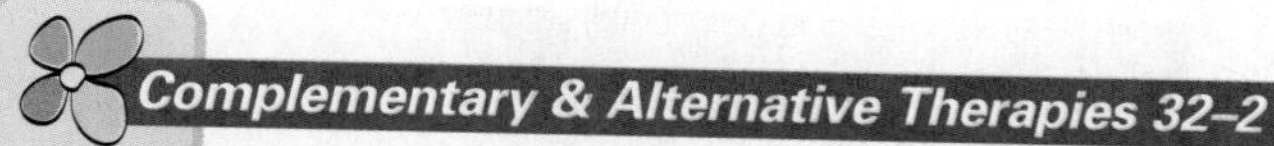

Gammalinolenic Acid for Rheumatoid Arthritis

Studies are underway on gammalinolenic acid, a fatty acid found in the seeds of evening primrose and borage plants. The substance was found to give relief to a group of rheumatoid arthritis sufferers and may one day be an accepted treatment (Gaby, 2002). Some patients find that they have fewer symptoms if they eat fish such as salmon or mackerel that are high in omega-3 fatty acids at least twice a week. Other patients experience decreased pain and swelling if they take an omega-3 fatty acid capsule once or twice a day. These substances do not seem to help all patients, however.

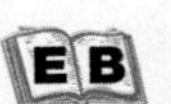

prevent, or at least modify, deformities and mechanical abnormalities.

One such surgical procedure is *synovectomy,* which is the excision of the synovial membrane of a joint. The goal of synovectomy is to interrupt the destructive inflammatory process that eventually leads to ankylosis and invasion of surrounding cartilage and bone tissues.

Researchers at Massachusetts Institute of Technology are performing a procedure called *neutron capture synovectomy,* which uses an accelerator that bombards the affected joints with subatomic particles. The technique is 10 times cheaper than standard surgery and requires little, if any, hospitalization. Although experimental, this procedure may one day be a treatment of choice.

Surgical repair of a hip joint **(arthroplasty)** is performed when there is extensive damage and ambulation is not possible. The purpose of joint repair is to restore, improve, or maintain joint function. In cases in which it is not possible to repair the damaged hip joint, total hip replacement may be done. A similar operation can be done on the knee joint.

Casts or braces and splints **(orthoses)** sometimes are used to immobilize an affected part so that it can rest during an active phase of the disease. Devices that immobilize the affected joint should allow for motion of adjacent muscles, thereby improving muscle strength and permitting more independence on the part of the patient. Braces also work to prevent deformities by maintaining optimal functional position of the joints.

Systemic lupus erythematosus is covered in Chapter 11 with the immune disorders.

Joint Replacement. An arthroplasty (joint replacement) may be done for a knee, shoulder, elbow, finger, ankle, or hip. The hip and knee are the most frequently replaced joints. Noncemented press-fit prostheses are often used now for young, heavier, and very active patients. The cement used for bone prostheses only has a life span of about 10 years; it may cause damage to the bone marrow from the heat generated during its initial "curing." A press-fit prosthesis is custom-sized

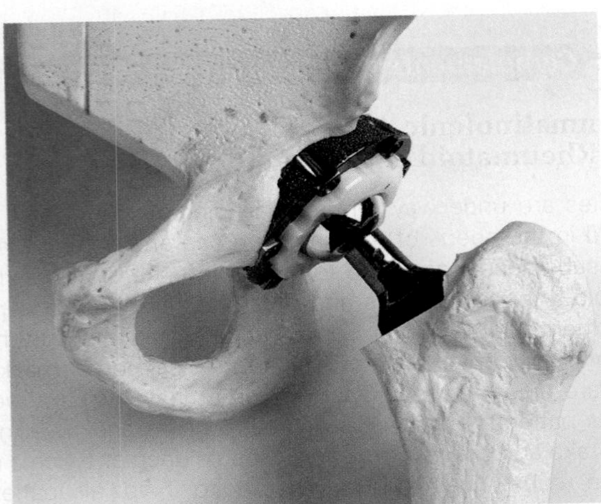

FIGURE 32–6 Hip replacement prosthesis.

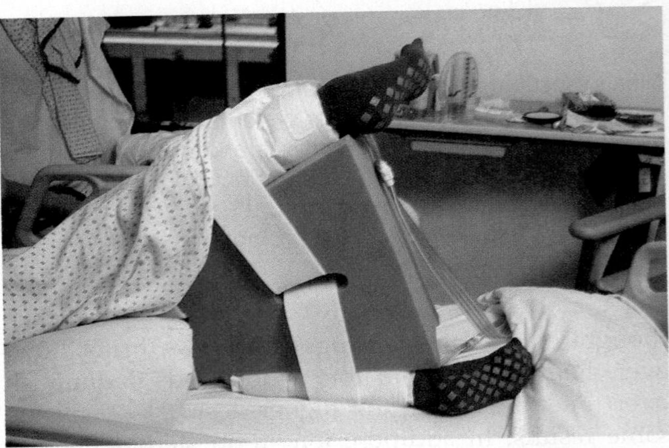

FIGURE 32–7 Abduction wedge in place to prevent dislocation of hip prosthesis.

by computer-aided design (CAD) for each patient. It doesn't require the use of cement. The outer coating is porous metal that allows new bone to "grow into" the device over a period of a few months.

Total Hip Replacement. A hip joint may be replaced with either a low-friction polyurethane socket for the acetabulum with a metallic replacement for the head of the femur or with synthetic materials combined with a porous bone implant (Figure 32–6). Partial weight bearing is permitted very soon after surgery. The porous bone implant requires 6 weeks of healing before weight bearing. Cemented prostheses patients refrain from full weight bearing for 4 to 6 weeks. Full weight bearing is avoided for 3 to 6 months. Crutches or a walker are used for ambulation, depending on the ability of the patient.

There are several kinds of prostheses to replace the hip, and the surgeon chooses the appropriate one according to an individual patient's needs. Hip replacement for osteoarthritis can be performed with minimally invasive surgery for some patients. The hospital stay is lessened for these patients.

The primary purpose of total hip replacement (THR) is to relieve chronic pain. The greatest dangers to successful replacement are infection, dislocation, and failure to function. Rehabilitation of the patient is a team effort involving the patient herself, the surgeon, nurse, and physical therapist.

Preoperative Care. Preoperatively, the patient is given specific instructions about the kind of surgery to be performed, the prosthesis to be used, the procedures to be followed after surgery, and what is expected of her to help achieve the goals of rehabilitation. She is given instructions in postoperative exercises and in the use of ambulation equipment, such as a walker, crutches, or canes. She may wish to donate a couple pints of blood several weeks before surgery in case a blood transfusion becomes necessary after surgery.

A surgical bacteriostatic scrub solution is usually prescribed for use during the daily shower for several days before hip replacement to lessen the chance of infection. The patient is told she will be placed in an orthopedic bed with an overhead trapeze bar attached after surgery and often is transported to and from the operating room on the bed if she is hospitalized before surgery. The triangular abductor pillow is shown to the patient, and its use between her legs for turning postoperatively is explained. Other care is much the same as for other types of major surgery (see Chapter 5).

Safety Alert 32–3

Precautions with Hip Abductor Wedge

Circulation should be checked after each application of the wedge to be certain that the straps are not too tight. Skin should be assessed every shift on the surface of the legs with particular attention to areas over bony prominences.

Postoperative Care. A blood salvage unit may be in place to collect blood drainage that is then filtered and returned to the patient. There is usually a drain at the surgical site with a suction device attached to it. IV fluids will be administered. A Foley catheter will usually be in place. It is imperative that all concerned with the patient's care after surgery understand what is necessary to ensure successful hip replacement and rehabilitation and to prevent dislocation of the prosthesis. Immediately after surgery, nursing intervention includes all the measures required to avoid respiratory and circulatory complications. However, extreme care must be exercised in positioning and repositioning the patient. To prevent dislocation, an abduction wedge is secured between the legs (usually in the operating room) and left in place when the patient is in bed until the surgeon requests its removal (Figure 32–7). The wedge is positioned with the narrower end between the thighs, and the straps should not go over an incision, bony prominence, or drain (Safety Alert 32–3).

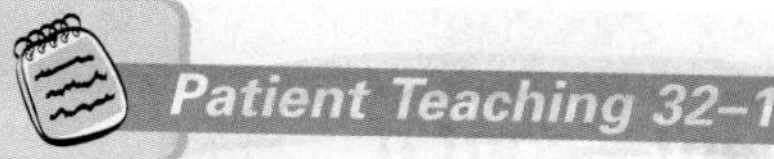
Patient Teaching 32–1

Total Hip Replacement

Before he is discharged, the patient who has undergone hip surgery should be given instructions so he can care for himself at home. These include:

- It is all right to lie on your operated side.
- For 3 months you should not cross your legs. You should put a pillow between your legs when you roll over on your abdomen or lie on your side in bed.
- It is all right to bend your hip, but not beyond a right (90-degree) angle *(demonstrate);* avoid sitting in low chairs
- Continue your daily exercise program at home in the same way you did the exercises at the hospital.

A common complication of joint replacement has been deep vein thrombosis (DVT). Low-molecular-weight heparin, enoxaparin (Lovenox), is administered to prevent this problem. It works more quickly than sodium heparin and causes less incidence of hemorrhage because it does not prevent platelets from aggregating at bleeding injury sites. Daily coagulation studies are not needed with this drug as its anticoagulant action is very predictable and stable. It is usually given in a 30-mg dose by subcutaneous injection into the abdomen twice a day.

In most cases the patient is allowed to stand at the bedside on the first postoperative day, supported by a walker and two persons. Weight bearing on the operated joint is sometimes allowed, but there should be a specific written order from the physician saying it is all right to do so. The patient will need instruction in transferring herself from bed to chair, wheelchair, and toilet. Whenever she sits, the chair seat should be raised so that the hips are not flexed beyond a 90-degree angle. Patient Teaching 32–1 shows the points to cover in discharge teaching. In addition to these instructions, the patient may be referred for outpatient or in-home physical therapy. Nursing interventions for selected problems of a patient with THR are summarized in Nursing Care Plan 32–1.

Knee Replacement. Chronic, uncontrollable pain is the main indication for knee arthroplasty. Either part or all of the knee joint may be replaced. For the best postoperative result, emphasis is placed on exercise. A continuous passive motion (CPM) machine may be used soon after surgery (Figure 31–5). To tolerate the exercise, the patient must be kept well medicated for pain. Within 2 to 5 days, quadriceps-strengthening exercises and straight-leg raising are started. Quadriceps exercise is accomplished by lying supine, straightening the legs, and pushing the back of the knees into the bed. Exercises are taught by the physical therapist, and the nurse often assists the patient in performing them. The patient then progresses to ambulation with a walker or crutches. Other pre- and postoperative care is similar to that of the patient undergoing any major surgery. After early release from the hospital, the patient continues physical therapy in the outpatient setting.

NURSING CARE PLAN 32–1

Care of the Patient After a Total Hip Replacement

SCENARIO Miko Yoshima, an 85-year-old woman, has just undergone a total hip replacement for a hip joint damaged by osteoarthritis. She normally lives alone, but has relatives within a 30-min driving distance. She had been actively gardening and taking care of herself until pain severely limited her mobility over the last few months.

(Care plan is specific to problems of hip replacement. All usual care for a postoperative patient should also be included: wound care, respiratory care, monitoring for complications, etc. See Nursing Care Plan 5–1.)

PROBLEM/NURSING DIAGNOSIS *Restricted from weight bearing*/Impaired physical mobility related to pain and activity restrictions post hip replacement.

Supporting assessment data *Subjective:* "I'm quite uncomfortable." *Objective:* Orders for non–weight bearing and up in chair tid. Abduction wedge in place when in bed.

Goals/Expected Outcomes	Nursing Interventions	Selected Rationale	Evaluation
Patient will regain sufficient mobility to care for self at home within 3 mo	Teach use of walker.	Proper use of walker will help prevent falls and injury.	PT will instruct in use of walker tomorrow.
	Encourage ROM and exercises to improve muscle strength and joint flexibility.	ROM helps prevent joint problems in unaffected joints.	Assisted to perform ROM on shoulders, upper extremities, and other leg.
		Exercises decrease muscle atrophy and help strengthen muscles for ambulation.	Encouraged ankle rotations and foot exercises on affected leg with supervision.

Key: *PT,* physical therapist; ***ROM,*** range of motion; *tid,* three times a day (Lat. *ter in die*).

Continued

NURSING CARE PLAN 32–1

Care of the Patient After a Total Hip Replacement—cont'd

PROBLEM/NURSING DIAGNOSIS *Incisional pain and joint stiffness*/Acute pain related to surgical incision and rehabilitation therapy.

Supporting assessment data *Subjective:* "My pain is at a 6 on a scale of 1 to 10." *Objective:* Face appears pinched and patient is not moving in bed at all.

Goals/Expected Outcomes	Nursing Interventions	Selected Rationale	Evaluation
Patient will experience pain control with patient-controlled analgesia (PCA) pump within 1 hr	Reinforce instructions on PCA use.	Knowledge of how to use pump provides medication for pain control.	Reinforced instructions; encouraging PCA use as needed.
Patient will have adequate pain control on oral analgesia before discharge	Assess for pain when vital signs are taken.	Constant monitoring for pain can indicate need for more medication to keep pain from escalating.	Pain level between 2 and 6/10.
	Administer medication bolus per orders PRN.	Administering a bolus of pain medication can stop pain from increasing.	Bolus administered for pain level of 6/10.
	Monitor for excessive sedation, respiratory depression, decreased level of consciousness (LOC), and confusion.	Excessive sedation, respiratory depression, decreased LOC, and confusion can indicate medication toxicity and danger for the patient.	No signs of problems of toxicity or central nervous system (CNS) depression.
	Provide comfort measures: keep linens smooth and clean, reposition q 2 hr and PRN, keep environment quiet and orderly.	Comfort measures and warmth help decrease pain perception.	Provided comfort measures. Replaced warm blankets q 2 hr, as needed.
	Keep warm with added warmed blankets. Put on socks if feet are cold.		Socks applied.

PROBLEM/NURSING DIAGNOSIS *Abduction wedge in place*/Risk for peripheral neurovascular dysfunction related to possible decreased blood flow due to compression from abduction wedge.

Supporting assessment data *Objective:* Abduction wedge firmly in place while in bed.

Goals/Expected Outcomes	Nursing Interventions	Selected Rationale	Evaluation
Patient will not experience peripheral neurovascular dysfunction before discharge	Monitor temperature, movement and sensation in affected extremity q 2 hr.	Pressure from abductor wedge can interrupt arterial blood supply and compress the peroneal nerve.	No signs of nerve compression or lack of blood flow in affected extremity.
	Check the pedal pulse in the web space between the great and second toes and have the patient dorsiflex the foot.	Compression of the nerve may cause footdrop.	
	Report any loss of sensation immediately.	Surgeon must know in order to decide what to do.	No loss of sensation reported.
	Ask patient to call if odd sensations are experienced in the affected extremity.	Quickly catching signs of beginning nerve compression may prevent damage.	Patient asked to call if sensation changes.
	Encourage performance of prescribed exercises.	Prescribed exercises improve blood flow to the muscles and nerves.	Dorsiflexed foot and rotated ankles q 2 hr.

Key: *PRN*, as needed.

NURSING CARE PLAN 32–1

Care of the Patient After a Total Hip Replacement—cont'd

PROBLEM/NURSING DIAGNOSIS *Not familiar with needed self-care*/Deficient knowledge related to precautions necessary after total hip surgery to prevent dislocation of operative hip.

Supporting assessment data *Subjective:* "No one I know has had this surgery."

Goals/Expected Outcomes	Nursing Interventions	Selected Rationale	Evaluation
Patient will verbalize movement restrictions to prevent hip dislocation within 24 hr	Explain positional restrictions: no flexion of the hip past 90 degrees, no internal rotation, no adduction of the affected leg.	Flexion, internal rotation, or adduction of the leg may cause hip dislocation. Knowledge is necessary to comply with instructions.	Explained position restrictions.
	Advise not to cross the legs or to bend over from the hips to tie shoes or pick up something off the floor.	These maneuvers cause internal rotation and more than 90 degrees of flexion.	Advised about additional restrictions after discharge.
	Instruct to only use a raised toilet seat for toileting.	Normal-height toilet seat may cause too much flexion.	States has raised toilet seat at home. Knows to use handicapped toilet stalls when out in public.
	Advise to report pain in hip, buttock, or thigh or continued limp.	Pain or continued limp may indicate dislocation.	Verbalizes understanding of symptoms to report.

PROBLEM/NURSING DIAGNOSIS *Potential for clot formation*/Risk for ineffective peripheral tissue perfusion.

Supporting assessment data *Objective:* Decreased mobility and total hip replacement.

Goals/Expected Outcomes	Nursing Interventions	Selected Rationale	Evaluation
Patient will not experience deep vein thrombosis before discharge	Encourage foot and calf exercises q 2 hr.	Encourages circulation and helps prevent clot formation.	Performing exercises q 2 hr while awake.
	Assist and encourage in prescribed physical therapy.		Working with PT.
	Administer low-molecular-weight heparin injections as ordered.	Decreases ability of blood to clot.	Heparin injections administered into abdomen as ordered.
	Assess for signs of thrombus formation, checking calf for warmth, swelling, and pain on foot dorsiflexion.	Finding a thrombus early aids in preventing further extension of clot and preventing embolus.	No redness, swelling, warmth, or pain in affected leg's calf.
	Monitor prothrombin time.	Prothrombin time indicates potential for blood clotting and thrombus formation.	Prothrombin time within desired limits.

? CRITICAL THINKING QUESTIONS

1. Besides venous thrombosis, what other complications might occur in this patient?
2. If the patient is anxious about discharge, what could you specifically do to help dispel her anxiety?

NURSING MANAGEMENT

Assessment (Data Collection)

The manifestations of arthritis are many and varied, particularly when the diagnosis is rheumatoid arthritis. Pain, limited motion, and the chronic and incurable nature of the illness have some impact on almost every aspect of the patient's life. To set realistic goals and plan for their accomplishment, the nurse will need to know about the patient's social history, her personal and family health history, current general health status, ability to do the things she wants to do, and her experience of pain and how she has been dealing with

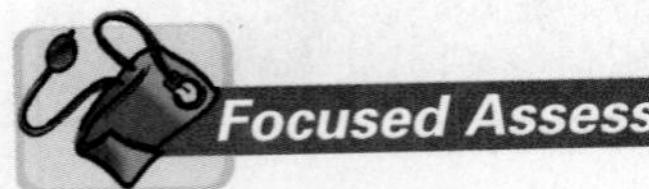

Focused Assessment 32–2

Data Collection for the Patient with Rheumatoid Arthritis

During history taking ask about:

- Family history of rheumatoid arthritis or immune disorders
- Smoking history
- Fatigue level
- Degree of malaise
- Presence of fever
- Degree of stiffness and duration after arising
- Diagnosis with accompanying disorders, such as interstitial lung disease, pericarditis, eye problems, and vasculitis
- Pain pattern and pain medication use
- Methods of coping with fatigue, malaise, and pain
- Exercise pattern
- Ability to perform ADLs; ability to work
- Ability for home maintenance
- Adaptive equipment in use
- Usual roles
- Social involvement

When gathering physical data, observe for:

- Joint deformity
- Symmetrical involvement from one side of the body to the other
- Swelling of joints
- Pain with joint movement
- Degree of limitation of joint movement

it. After a general health survey, use the guide in Focused Assessment 32–2 to gather data.

Nursing Diagnosis and Planning

Nursing diagnoses depend on the degree of disability the disease is causing. Common nursing diagnoses might include:

- Chronic pain related to inflamed joints
- Impaired physical mobility related to pain, stiffness, and joint deformity
- Risk for ineffective therapeutic regimen management related to complex medication schedule
- Disturbed body image related to joint deformities

Expected outcomes for the above nursing diagnoses might be:

- Patient's pain will be controlled with medications, heat, and exercise within 2 weeks.
- Patient's mobility will improve with the use of assistive devices and physical therapy within 3 weeks.
- Patient will maintain the medication regimen after appropriate teaching.
- Patient will demonstrate less disturbance of body image by partaking in more social activities within 1 month.

Planning care for the patient with rheumatoid arthritis should consider the length of time it takes the person to perform self-care, ambulate, and perform other functions. Allow sufficient time and do not rush the patient, as that will cause considerable frustration. Remember that any procedure that must be done may take longer as the patient may not be able to move and turn as easily as a person without rheumatoid arthritis.

Implementation and Evaluation

Nursing interventions are aimed at providing a balance of rest and exercise, freedom from pain, minimizing emotional stress, preventing or correcting deformities, and maintaining or restoring function so that the patient can enjoy as much independence and mobility as possible.

Rest and Exercise

The amount of rest needed will depend on the extent of inflammation. The more inflamed a joint is, the more rest is needed; this includes rest of the whole body, as well as of the inflamed joint. Fatigue is a common problem and usually requires that the patient change her lifestyle somewhat so that she has rest periods during the day before she becomes too fatigued or exhausted. During periods of acute exacerbation of symptoms, the patient may need continuous bed rest.

When the patient is lying down, she should maintain good body position and avoid pillows and other devices that support joints in a position of flexion. A firm mattress is recommended, with only one pillow under the head and neck.

The purpose of rest is to allow the body's natural defenses and healing powers to overcome the inflammatory process. It is necessary, however, even in the acute phase, to balance rest with exercise. The patient should sit to do tasks whenever possible. Activities should be paced and interspersed with rest. The exercise program is prescribed on the basis of assessment of each patient's status, the severity of inflammation, the particular joints affected, and the patient's tolerance for activity. Because anemia and other blood disorders can accompany arthritis, the fatigue experienced by a patient may be somewhat alleviated by correcting any underlying blood disorder.

In any exercise program, it is necessary to enlist the patient's cooperation or compliance, as the exercises must be continued at home. Teach the patient how to perform specific exercises so that they do not increase her pain. Each exercise should be done 3 to 10 times for each joint, with the lower number used

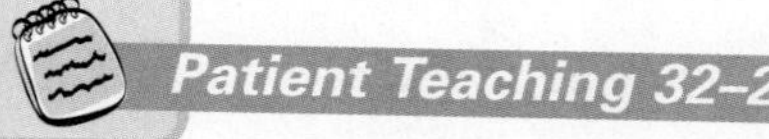

Instructions for Joint Protection

- Always stop an exercise at the point of real pain. Some discomfort can be expected, but it should be minimal. If your joints are still hurting 1 or 2 hours after exercise, you have done too much.
- Always use your biggest muscles and strongest joints. For example, push doors open with your arm instead of your hand; carry a shoulder bag instead of a hand purse.
- Try to do only those jobs that will allow you to stop and rest if you need to when pain develops. Learn to conserve your energy to do the things you really want to do.
- Exercise in a way that does not put strain on the joints. Exercising in water decreases joint strain.
- Slow down and move slowly and smoothly. Avoid rapid, jerky movements. Use the palms of the hands rather than the fingers to push up from a bed or chair when arising.
- Turn doorknobs counterclockwise to prevent extensive twisting of the elbow.
- Do not lift weights. Pick up heavier items with two hands.
- Let swollen, red, hot, and painful joints rest as much as possible. Do not use them any more than absolutely necessary.
- Change your body position frequently, alternating standing, sitting, and lying down.
- Set your own limits and compete with yourself, not with anyone else.
- Use assistive/adaptive devices, such as Velcro closures and built-up utensil handles to protect joints of the hands. Use a long-handled hair brush.

on days when pain or fatigue is increased. When joints are inflamed, exercises should not be done; rest is needed. In many instances, doing the exercises in the right way can actually diminish discomfort. If pain persists for hours after exercises have been done, the patient's status should be reassessed and the exercise program revised. When a patient is performing routine physical activities at home, carrying out general exercise, or following a prescribed exercise program at home, precautions to avoid joint injury should be followed (Patient Teaching 32–2).

Applications of Heat and Cold

There is no hard-and-fast rule to follow in deciding whether heat or cold is best for treating arthritic joints. Either one may be suitable, depending on the patient's preference and the effectiveness of each. The purpose of either hot or cold applications is to minimize pain, increase the joint's ROM, and improve exercise performance. In general, heat is better for subacute or chronic joint inflammation and cold is more effective in the acute phase when joints are hot, red, and obviously inflamed.

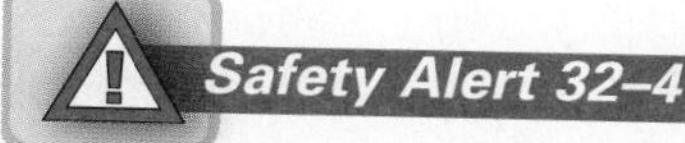

Caution with Heat Application

Patients who have decreased sensation in a body part must be very careful when applying heat or they may experience burns. Teach the family and patient to test the degree of heat being applied and to check the area after 5 minutes to make certain that burning is not occurring. A cloth should always be placed between the heat device and the skin.

Various forms of heat therapy can be used, including moist or dry heat and superficial or deep heat. For dry heat, a therapeutic infrared lamp is convenient and inexpensive for home use. For treatment of the hands, paraffin baths are effective. Wet heat can be applied by hot tub baths with the water temperature not exceeding 102° F (39° C) or by means of a towel dipped in hot water, wrung out, and applied to the joint. Whirlpool baths promote relaxation and motion with minimal pain, especially when prolonged treatment is indicated. However, immersing the whole body in warm water can cause physiologic changes in respiration and pulse rate and may be contraindicated in debilitated or elderly patients.

Think Critically About . . . If a patient asks about using a heating pad on the joint, what instructions would you give?

Whatever method of heat or cold application is used at home, the patient will need specific instructions on how to avoid injury to the skin and other hazards (Safety Alert 32–4). Information for teaching patients precautions for applications of heat and cold is summarized in Patient Teaching 32–3.

Diet

No special diet will cure or relieve arthritis, in spite of many fraudulent claims to the contrary. However, some patients find that eliminating foods from the "nightshade" family, such as tomatoes, decreases their joint pain. The patient should eat an average, well-balanced diet with no excess or limitations in amount or types of foods. Obesity can put additional stress on the weight-bearing joints and aggravate the arthritic condition. This should be explained to the patient who has a tendency to be overweight so she can be properly motivated and encouraged to lose weight and continue to keep her weight within normal limits.

Psychosocial Care

As deformities occur, sensitivity about appearance often occurs and self-esteem may drop. Encourage verbalization of feelings. Express acceptance of the pa-

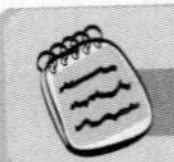

Patient Teaching 32–3

Application of Heat and Cold

For the safe application of heat or cold, follow these guidelines.

APPLICATIONS OF HEAT

- Recommended for chronic or subacute inflammation. Heat should be used for 20 to 30 minutes at a time; repeat the application every 1 to 2 hours while awake.
- Shower massager. Use shower massager for massage pulsation. Regulate water by turning on cold and adding hot water to desired temperature *before* entering the shower. Use a shower stool if balance is poor or fatigue is likely.
- Hot water bottle. Use a pad between the bottle and the skin to prevent burning.
- Heating pads. Use the type that provides moist heat; it will penetrate best. Do not go to sleep on the heating pad. Use the low settings. Heating pads often cause burns when turned up too high or used for too long.
- Reusable heat pack. Molds well to body part as it is pliable. Follow directions explicitly, and test temperature by feel of pack on skin before applying to area in need. Use a light pad or thin dishtowel between pack and skin. Heat in microwave oven. Reheat as needed. Does not retain heat long.
- Heat-producing ointments and gels. Gels containing menthol, camphor, or papain (extract from red peppers) may be applied to the sore muscle or joint as long as it does not produce skin irritation. Covering the area after application with plastic wrap helps hold the heat in longer. Wash hands thoroughly after application as these substances can cause eye irritation.

APPLICATIONS OF COLD

- Recommended for acute phase of inflammation or acute pain. Do not apply to one area for more than 10 to 20 minutes at a time; apply no more than once an hour.
- Discontinue when numbness occurs.
- Not recommended for patients with impaired circulation.
- Dry skin well after treatment.
- Ice water bath. Useful for hand or foot. Extremity can be exercised during treatment.
- Ice pack. Can be made by partially filling double plastic bag with ice. Zip-type closures work best. May use thin pad or dishtowel between pack and skin.
- Commercial cold pack can be refrozen in the freezer. Disposable chemical packs that are activated when needed also are available.
- Commercial cold packs mold to body part better than ice bag. Does not stay cold very long. Often takes two of these to finish 10- to 20-minute treatment. Return to freezer after use.
- Ice massage. Freeze ice in paper cup; peel back part of cup to use so that cup provides hand grip. Wear rubber glove or use pad to protect hand from ice. Rub ice over body part until skin feels numb, but no longer than 10 to 15 minutes at a time.

tient's appearance. Suggest clothing options that may minimize visible changes. A support group sometimes helps to reframe the disease's effects on the body. Encourage the patient to gain as much control over the disease as possible with appropriate coping mechanisms, pacing, exercise, and medication.

Resources for Patient and Family Education

It is very easy for the arthritis patient and her family to be overwhelmed with information about the illness and treatment. The Arthritis Foundation provides some excellent printed material written with the layperson in mind. Another source of information is the Arthritis Information Clearinghouse, at the National Institute of Medicine.

For the evaluation phase, gather data as to whether the care plan interventions are helping the patient meet expected outcomes. If the outcomes are not being met, choose different interventions.

GOUT

Etiology and Pathophysiology

Gout is arthritis of a joint caused by high serum levels of uric acid. Uric acid crystals precipitate from the body fluids and settle in joints and connective tissue. Gout affects men more than women and generally occurs during middle age. It is more common among populations that consume a high-protein diet. Two factors seem to be implicated: (1) a genetic increase in purine metabolism leading to overproduction or retention of uric acid; and (2) consumption of a high-purine diet. Excessive alcohol consumption causes an increased production of keto acids that inhibit uric acid excretion, causing hyperuricemia. Deposits of urate crystals occur in joints and subcutaneous tissues. The big toe is the most common site, but many other joints can be affected. Diuretic therapy sometimes causes a secondary gout because the loss of fluid increases the serum uric acid level in the body. Certain drug therapies interfere with uric acid excretion and can cause a secondary gout.

Signs and Symptoms

Typical signs and symptoms are elevated serum uric acid and tight, reddened skin over an inflamed, edematous joint, accompanied by elevated temperature and extreme pain in the joint.

Diagnosis and Treatment

History and physical examination are usually sufficient to diagnose gout, but a blood sample to check serum uric acid level is usually ordered to confirm the diagnosis.

Treatment during acute attacks consists of administration of NSAIDs for 2 to 5 days for the pain. Colchicine given orally may bring dramatic pain relief within 24 to 48 hours. Allopurinol (Zyloprim) or probenecid (Benemid) may be prescribed to prevent further attacks. Dietary management includes weight control and restriction of high-purine foods, such as anchovies, sardines, sweetbreads, liver, red meat, kidney and meat extracts. Alcohol should be restricted. Patients placed on allopurinol need periodic liver function testing as this drug can cause liver failure. A fluid intake of 2000 to 3000 mL per day is needed to protect the kidneys from urate crystal deposit and to prevent kidney stones. If the patient is overweight, an effort to get weight back within normal range should be made.

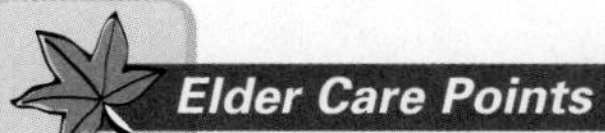

Elder Care Points

Elderly patients with decreased creatinine clearance should not take allopurinol. When the patient has both hypertension and gout, losartan (Cozaar) may be a good choice for therapy. Losartan promotes urate diuresis.

Nursing Management

Nursing care consists of teaching the patient about the disease, the medications and how to take them, the dietary adjustments that are recommended, and the need for increased fluid intake. The main nursing diagnosis will be Pain related to inflammation of joints. Other appropriate nursing diagnoses are listed in Table 31–3.

OSTEOPOROSIS

Etiology and Pathophysiology

Osteoporosis is a metabolic bone disorder that causes a decrease in bone mass and makes the person more susceptible to fractures. Fractures often are "atraumatic," meaning that they occur without being precipitated by trauma. Starting at age 35, most women lose bone mass at a rate of 1% a year; after menopause loss accelerates to 2% a year. In the United States, 10 million people have osteoporosis and another 14 to 18 million have **osteopenia** (low bone mass). It is predicted that by 2020, nearly half of all Americans will be at risk of fracture from osteoporosis or osteopenia. Causative factors for osteoporosis include long-term calcium deficiency, vitamin D deficiency, and estrogen deficiency in patients predisposed to the problem, particularly after menopause. Contributing factors are thought to be cigarette smoking, alcoholism, sedentary lifestyle, body weight below 128 lb, endocrine disorders, prolonged bed rest, and liver disease. These factors have an effect on either estrogen production or calcium metabolism. Eating disorders and inflammatory bowel disease lead to the disease because they interfere with nutrition and absorption. There is a hereditary tendency for osteoporosis. The risk of osteoporosis increases considerably in women after menopause because estrogen production is reduced.

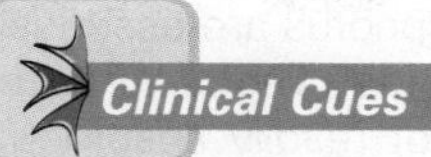

Clinical Cues

Medications such as corticosteroids, anticonvulsants, heparin, some chemotherapeutic agents, and excessive use of antacids containing aluminum may cause osteoporosis. Suggest that patients who have been on these medications be screened for osteoporosis regularly.

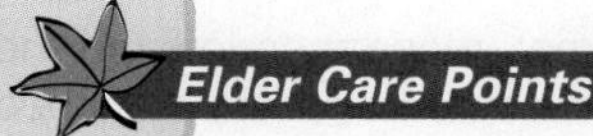

Elder Care Points

Many elderly patients are taking steroids to treat chronic diseases such as arthritis. This makes the older person more susceptible to fractures. Kyphosis from compression fractures of the spinal column resulting from osteoporosis can restrict lung expansion and cause decreased respiratory reserve.

Signs and Symptoms

Osteoporosis is a silent disease and there are no early signs or symptoms. Once the patient has developed osteoporosis, height loss, kyphosis, and back pain may occur. Compression fractures of the spine may cause debilitating pain. Often osteoporosis is diagnosed after the patient sustains a fracture from little or no known trauma.

Diagnosis

On x-rays the bone of the patient with osteoporosis appears porous. The test to determine bone density is performed by dual energy x-ray absorptiometry (DXA or DEXA) and is used to assess loss of bone density in postmenopausal women. Testing should begin at age 50.

Treatment

Treatment is aimed at stopping loss of bone density, increasing bone formation, and preventing fractures. Postmenopausal estrogen replacement therapy and adequate dietary or supplemental calcium and vitamin D in combination with weight-bearing exercise are the mainstays of treatment. Adequate calcium in the diet with 1000 mg is recommended for premenopausal women and 1500 mg after menopause (Nutritional Therapies 32–2). Calcium supplements, if required, should be taken in divided doses during the day; 400 units of vitamin D per day is recommended. Some drugstore chains have generic brands of calcium that state on the package that they are guaranteed to dissolve properly so that the mineral can be absorbed. Exposure to sufficient sunlight or vitamin D supplementation is necessary for the proper absorption and

Nutritional Therapies 32–2

Nutrition for Bone Growth and Density

Adequate amounts of calcium and phosphorus are essential for bone growth and density. Although green vegetables are a source of calcium, that calcium is not readily absorbed. Dairy products such as cheese, yogurt, and milk are better choices. Canned sardines or salmon also provide good amounts of calcium. Magnesium and vitamin K are required for healthy bones as well. These are provided by a healthy diet containing meat and green vegetables. Spinach is a good source of vitamin K. The patient taking an anticoagulant should not alter her intake of vitamin K as it will affect coagulation times.

Calcium supplementation is not recommended for the healing of fractures. It has proven not to be readily absorbed and tends to cause kidney stones.

---

metabolism of the calcium. Vitamin K is important to bone health as well, and most people obtain this through eating greens. Daily weight-bearing exercise can decrease the chance of developing osteoporosis. Walking down stairs seems to be especially helpful, but walking for 30 minutes three times a week is sufficient.

Salicylates and NSAIDs are prescribed to control back pain. A back brace may be ordered for the patient who has suffered vertebral compression fractures. The bisphosphonates, which are cousins to a bone resorption–inhibiting substance found naturally in the body, and hormone therapy, are prescribed in addition to calcium and vitamin D supplements for those with osteoporosis (Box 32–3). Fosamax must be taken first thing in the morning with a 6- to 8-oz glass of natural water at least 30 minutes before breakfast as absorption is reduced by food, coffee, or orange juice. The patient must remain in an upright position to prevent esophageal irritation. One form of Fosamax can be taken just once a week (Safety Alert 32–5). New research suggests that those patients who have been taking the medication for 5 years and have increased their bone density scores should take a "vacation" from using the drug. Bone softening has occurred in some patients who take Fosamax (Odvina, et al., 2005). Boniva, the newest of the bisphosphonates, is taken just once a month. Miacalcin or Fortical nasal spray, which contains calcitonin, slows the rate of bone loss. It is an alternative treatment for postmenopausal osteoporosis in women who cannot take estrogens. The spray is used with adequate calcium and vitamin D supplementation.

A new study of zoledronic acid (Zometa) once a year may be an effective treatment for osteoporosis. The drug is in clinical trials at the present time.

Treatment of Vertebral Fracture. Vertebral compression fractures commonly occur in patients with osteoporosis. These are often treated with pain medication, activity limitation, physical therapy, and bracing. Two new minimally invasive spine procedures that are viable treatments for those who do not respond to the conservative therapies have emerged. **Vertebroplasty** involves the percutaneous injection of polymethylmethacrylate (PMMA), a cement, directly into an osteoporotic spinal area under fluoroscopy. This stabilizes the bone and helps reduce or eliminate pain. **Kyphoplasty** consists of the percutaneous insertion of an inflatable device into the fractured vertebral body under fluoroscopy. The device is inflated, elevating the end plates and restoring the vertebral body toward its original height. Thick PMMA is then injected under low pressure into the cavity. The device is deflated and removed. This provides pain relief and reduces kyphosis (Wilke, et al., 2006).

Box 32–3 ***Drugs Used for the Treatment of Osteoporosis***

HORMONES
- Estrogen (women)
- Raloxifene (Evista) (selective estrogen receptor modulator)
- Testosterone (men)
- Calcitonin (Miacalcin) (synthetic hormone)
- Teriparatide (Forteo) (synthetic hormone)

BISPHOSPHONATES
- Alendronate (Fosamax)
- Risedronate (Actonel)
- Ibandronate (Boniva)

General Nursing Implications for Bisphosphonates
- Monitor bone density test results.
- Must take regularly: weekly or monthly.
- Observe for hypercalcemia: paresthesias, twitching, colic, or laryngospasm.
- Take with 8 oz of plain water in A.M. 30 to 60 minutes before eating, drinking, or taking any other medication that day (timing depends on the particular drug).
- Swallow the tablet whole. Do not suck or chew on it.
- Store medication in a cool location out of sunlight.
- Remain upright for 30 to 60 minutes after dose to prevent esophageal irritation (timing depends on the drug). Do not eat or drink anything during this 30 minutes to an hour.
- If dose is missed, skip the dose; do not take it later in the day. For the weekly dose medication, take it the next morning after your scheduled dose. Skip the dose if it has been 2 days since it was supposed to be taken and just resume the original schedule. If taking Boniva, take it the next morning after you remember you forgot to take it. Do not take two tablets in any 1 week; wait at least 7 days to take the next dose and then resume your original schedule.
- Take calcium and vitamin D supplements as recommended by the health care provider.
- Perform weight-bearing exercise to increase bone density.
- Advise health care provider if pregnant or planning a pregnancy.

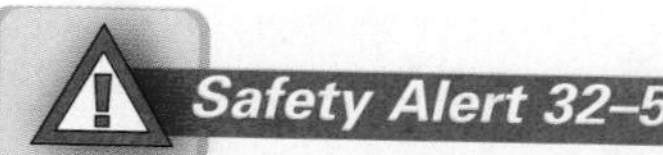

Caution with Bisphosphonate Drugs

Recently there have been some instances of jawbone death in patients who have been taking bisphosphonate drugs. Any patient taking one of this class of drugs should check with the physician regarding the possibility of this problem occurring.

The possibility of esophageal irritation or erosion is considerable if the patient does not remain in an upright position for 1 hour after taking a bisphosphonate drug. Patients need to be periodically reminded to adhere to the instructions for these medications. Adverse side effects are varied and any new onset of unusual signs or symptoms should be reported to the physician.

NURSING MANAGEMENT

Assessment (Data Collection)

Assessment for risk factors for osteoporosis should be performed with every general health assessment. Data are gathered about family history of osteoporosis, use of steroid medication, diet, and exercise pattern throughout life. Questions should be asked about history of smoking and alcohol intake.

Nursing Diagnosis and Planning

The main nursing diagnosis is "Risk for injury related to possible fracture from thinning of the bone." The expected outcome would be "Patient will not experience a fracture during her lifetime."

Implementation and Evaluation

Nursing care is focused on promoting screening for osteoporosis, teaching about the benefits of a healthy lifestyle, the need for sufficient calcium intake, and weight-bearing exercise. Educating about the harmful effects of smoking and excessive alcohol intake is also important. For the patient with osteoporosis, teaching about the medications prescribed for the disorder and their side effects, and measures to halt or reverse the disease process is the focus of care. The patient is cautioned to follow the instructions regarding staying in an upright position for 1 hour after taking bisphosphonate-type drugs. This helps prevent esophageal irritation and erosion. Osteoporosis information is readily available at the National Institutes of Health Senior Health website at www.nihseniorhealth.gov.

Evaluation is based on data collected regarding the results of the nursing actions. If expected outcomes are not being met, the plan is altered.

PAGET'S DISEASE

Paget's disease is a problem of abnormal bone resorption followed by replacement of normal marrow with fibrous connective tissue. The abnormal bone is weak and prone to fractures. The cause of Paget's disease is unknown, although it does occur in clusters in some families. Often the disease is found at the time a fracture occurs as x-rays reveal the abnormality of the bone. Diagnosis is by x-ray and laboratory testing. A 24-hour urine collection for hydroxyproline, which indicates osteoclastic activity, may be performed. Serum alkaline phosphatase is elevated if the disease is active. The disease is more common in men.

The main problem is pain, and that is the focus of treatment. Miacalcin or a bisphosphonate may be given to slow bone resorption. Orthopedic care is given for fractures and necessary joint replacements.

A firm mattress, wearing a corset or light brace to relieve back pain, and proper body mechanics are essential. The patient should avoid lifting things or twisting the body.

BONE TUMORS

Etiology and Pathophysiology

Bone is subject to both benign and malignant tumors. Tumors arise from several different types of tissue, including cartilage (chondromas), bone (osteomas), and fibrous tissue (fibromas). Benign tumors often are found on x-ray or at the time of fracture.

Malignant bone tumors are either primary or secondary to metastatic disease. Primary malignant bone tumors are most often seen in people 10 to 25 years of age. The most common type is osteosarcoma or osteogenic sarcoma. It grows rapidly and metastasizes. More than half the cases affect the knee area. However, the distal femur, humerus, and proximal tibia are other frequent sites of occurrence. Osteosarcoma may occur in men older than age 60 as a complication of Paget's disease. Other types of primary malignant tumors include Ewing's sarcoma, chondrosarcoma, and fibrosarcoma.

Signs, Symptoms, and Diagnosis

Signs and symptoms of malignant bone tumor include pain, warmth, and swelling. Metastatic bone tumors greatly outnumber primary bone malignancies. Malignancies of the prostate, kidney, thyroid, breast, and lung commonly metastasize to bone. Sites of metastases are usually the vertebrae, pelvis, ribs, and femur. Diagnosis of bone tumor is by physical x-ray, bone scan, and biopsy.

Treatment and Nursing Management

Treatment for malignant bone tumors includes surgery, radiation, and chemotherapy. Osteosarcoma has a 60% to 80% cure rate when surgery and chemotherapy are combined for treatment. Chemotherapeutic agents used include methotrexate, doxorubicin (Adriamycin), cyclophosphamide (Cytoxan), bleomycin (Blenoxane), cisplatin (Platinol), dactinomycin (Cosmegen), and ifosfamide (Ifex).

Nursing management must include psychosocial care, as the anxiety and fear that accompanies the diagnosis of a bone tumor is considerable for most patients. Nursing interventions will depend on the treatment provided. Care of the surgical patient is presented in Chapters 4 and 5. Chapter 8 covers care of the cancer patient. If a bone tumor is in an extremity, amputation may be part of the treatment.

AMPUTATION

About 80% of all limb amputations involve lower extremities. The most common reasons for amputation of a lower limb are related to peripheral vascular disease, often associated with diabetes mellitus, and resultant gangrene. Other conditions necessitating lower-limb amputation include severe trauma, malignancy, and congenital defects. Military injuries from shrapnel and land mines often result in amputation.

About 70% of upper-extremity amputations are brought on by crushing blows, thermal and electric burns, and severe lacerations. Vasospastic disease, malignancy, and infection also can necessitate amputation of an upper extremity.

The last 20 years have brought about major improvements in microvascular surgery, making reattachment or reimplantation of amputated parts possible. Teach the public what to do if an accidental amputation occurs (Patient Teaching 32–4).

Preoperative Care

Unless the amputation of a limb is an emergency procedure, the patient is prepared physically and psychologically for the removal of all or part of the extremity. If at all possible, she should participate in the decision to amputate a limb. She should understand the need for the amputation and have the opportunity to discuss realistic goals of rehabilitation with several members of the health care team.

Although the loss of a limb can be very difficult for the patient and her family to accept, they can find some consolation in knowing that the procedure is absolutely necessary and that every effort will be made to take full advantage of the patient's remaining resources. The patient may experience stages of denial, anger, and so on, similar to those of the dying process as discussed in Chapter 8. In a sense, the patient must recognize the death of the former "self," work through the grief process, and move toward acceptance of a new body image.

A member of the rehabilitation team should discuss with the patient what can be expected postoperatively with regard to pain, immobility, and readjustment to self-care.

"Phantom sensations" in the limb that has been removed are not unusual. There is no scientific explanation for these sensations, but they are nonetheless real to the amputee who experiences them.

If the patient is informed preoperatively that the sensations are not unusual, are not considered a psychiatric problem, and will be dealt with as the reality that they most certainly are, she will be less apprehensive about asking for help should the problem arise.

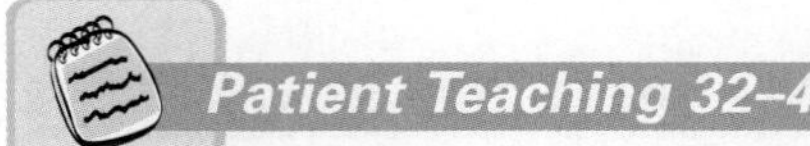

Care After an Accidental Amputation

To care for a severed body part so that reattachment may be possible:

- Rinse the detached part only enough to remove visible debris.
- Wrap the part in a clean, damp cloth.
- Place the part in a sealed plastic bag or in a dry watertight container.
- Immerse the bag or container in a mixture of water and ice (3 parts water to 1 part ice). Do not let the part get wet or freeze.
- Alternatively, place the container in an insulated cooler filled with ice.
- If no ice is available, keep the part cool; do not expose it to heat.
- Tag the bag or container with the person's name and the name of the body part and take it to the hospital with the person.

Physical preparation of the patient includes muscle-strengthening exercises in the hope that the patient can be active following amputation. These exercises are the first stages of the rehabilitation process, designed to help the patient achieve independence as rapidly as possible.

Postoperative Care

When the patient returns from the surgical suite, the two most immediate problems are hemorrhage and edema. To combat these problems, the stump is sometimes elevated for 24 to 48 hours. A lower extremity is not elevated for more than 24 hours because of the danger of hip contractures, which would prohibit rehabilitation efforts to achieve ambulation. The stump is checked at frequent intervals to determine whether bleeding is excessive. Fresh bleeding on the dressing should be reported immediately. When a cast is over the incision, other measures are relied upon to detect bleeding (i.e., pulse rate, blood pressure [BP], increasing pain, and pallor). A surgical tourniquet should be kept at the bedside in case of hemorrhage.

Postoperative wound care is essentially the same as that discussed in Chapter 5. Prophylactic antibiotics are given for 3 or 4 days. Wound drainage usually is handled with a Hemovac or similar wound drainage system. The incision should be dry, intact, and only slightly reddened along the suture line. The initial pressure dressing is removed by the surgeon 48 to 72 hours postoperatively.

Phantom limb sensations, mentioned earlier, may or may not be painful but are very disconcerting if the patient has not been previously warned that they may

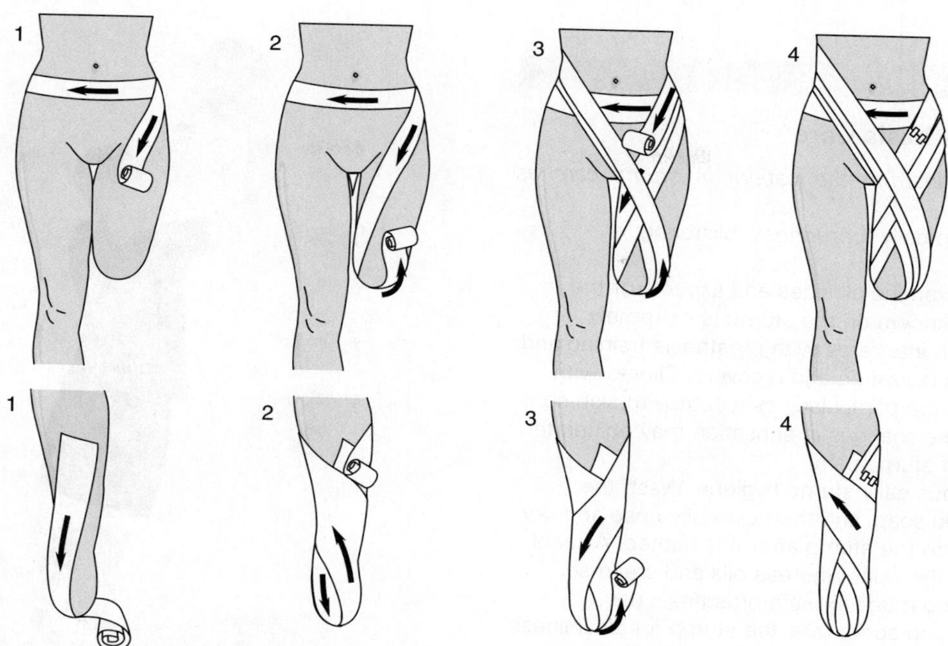

FIGURE **32–8** A common method for wrapping an amputation stump. *Top,* Wrapping for above-knee amputation (AKA). *Bottom,* Wrapping for below-knee amputation (BKA).

occur. IV infusion of Miacalcin during the week after amputation has been known to reduce phantom pain in many patients. If the pain is severe or persists, various methods are used to control it. The most effective method seems to be use of a transcutaneous electrical nerve stimulator (TENS). A new device called a stump stocking, which is a silicone liner interwoven with an electromagnetic shield works by blocking external electromagnetic impulses from outside sources. Those external impulses are thought to irritate nerve endings and trigger phantom pain (Kern et al., 2006).

Three alternative modes for managing the stump after amputation are (1) soft dressing with delayed prosthetic fitting; (2) rigid plaster dressing and early prosthetic fitting; and (3) rigid plaster dressing and immediate prosthetic fitting. Each method has its particular advantages and disadvantages. If a soft dressing is used, it is important that the stump be wrapped properly to control edema and ensure proper shrinkage of the stump for later fitting of a prosthesis. A pressure bandage wrapped in a figure-8 pattern is used most often (Figure 32–8). The bandage is anchored to the most proximal joint. It should be rewrapped three times a day, or whenever it is loose. A Jobst air splint may be used instead of the pressure bandage.

When the bandage is off, assess the skin for inflammation or breakdown. The skin should be pink in a light-skinned person without discoloration. In the dark skinned person, the skin should not be lighter or darker than other skin pigmentation. The skin should be warm but not hot.

Many complications can be avoided if the patient is able to get up and about early in the postoperative period. However, weight bearing before the stump is adequately healed can cause weakening of the suture line and rupturing of the operative wound. The patient with a lower extremity amputation should lie prone for 20 to 30 minutes every 3 to 4 hours to prevent hip contracture until she is up and about regularly. The residual limb should be extended. Patients with amputations below the knee are better able to begin early walking and weight bearing than those whose limb has been amputated above the knee. The amputation of a limb displaces the body's center of gravity and interferes with the sense of balance. Adaptation to this change in the center of gravity occurs slowly, and the patient needs to be warned to move cautiously. When the prosthesis is off during the night, the patient may need assistance in turning until she adjusts to her new center of gravity.

Proper positioning is required to prevent *abduction* contractures. Range-of-motion exercises are carried out with the amputee as with any patient who must be protected from the disabilities of immobility.

When a lower limb has been removed, the patient must learn how to balance on one leg, how to stoop and bend over without losing balance, and how to use her back muscles to maintain good posture while wearing an artificial limb. Teaching for self-care begins as soon as possible. Points for instruction in care of the stump and the prosthesis are presented in Patient Teaching 32–5.

Rehabilitation

With the help of CAD, prostheses can be manufactured that are a much better fit than ever before. Computerization has also provided a means of controlled

Patient Teaching 32–5

Stump and Prosthesis Care

The nurse should instruct the patient in stump care as follows:

- Inspect the stump daily for redness, blistering, or abrasions.
- Use a mirror to examine all sides and aspects of the stump. Skin breakdown on the stump is extremely serious because it interferes with prosthesis training and may prolong hospitalization and recovery. Clients with diabetes mellitus are particularly susceptible to skin complications, because changes in sensation may obliterate the awareness of stump pain.
- Perform meticulous daily stump hygiene. Wash the stump with a mild soap, and then carefully rinse and dry it. Apply nothing to the stump after it is bathed. Alcohol dries and cracks the skin, whereas oils and creams soften the skin too much for safe prosthesis use.
- Wear woolen stump socks over the stump for cleanliness and comfort. To maintain the size and shape of woolen socks, wash them gently in cool water with mild soap and dry flat on a towel.
- Replace, do not mend, torn socks; mending creates wrinkles that irritate the skin.
- Put on the prosthesis immediately when arising and keep it on all day (once the wound has healed completely) to reduce stump swelling.
- Continue prescribed exercises to prevent weakness.
- Lay prone with hip extension for 30 minutes three or four times a day.
- For lower extremity, replace shoes before wear becomes extreme as gait may be altered.

The nurse should instruct the client in prosthesis care as follows:

- Remove sweat and dirt from the prosthesis socket daily by wiping the inside of the socket with a damp, soapy cloth. To remove the soap, use a clean damp cloth. Dry the prosthesis socket thoroughly.
- Never attempt to adjust or mechanically alter the prosthesis. If problems develop, consult the prosthetist.
- Schedule a yearly appointment with the prosthetist.

Adapted from Lewis, S.M., Heitkemper, M.M., Dirksen, S.R., et al. (2007). *Medical-Surgical Nursing: Assessment and Management of Clinical Problems* (7th ed.). St. Louis: Mosby.

movement of various parts of a prosthesis, allowing greater mobility and ease of performing ADLs.

Usually both a physical therapist and occupational therapist work with the patient who has suffered an amputation to help regain mobility, confidence, and the ability to handle ADLs. Assist with practice at bathing, shaving, dressing, and so on. Your attitude and encouragement can make a positive difference in the adjustment the patient makes to the situation.

Elderly and chronically ill amputees can benefit from a positive, yet realistic, approach to their problems. The focus of attention should be on what the patient can do for herself and on what strengths she has in her favor. By helping the patient find short-range goals that can be accomplished without great difficulty and that indicate progress toward independence, you can be of real assistance to the amputee. For example, you can guide her toward devising ways in which personal needs such as bathing and grooming can be met. Later, encouragement to sit up, exercise the other limbs, and assist with changing of the dressing can be given. Finally, the goal can be set for wearing a prosthesis successfully and walking without assistance. A prosthesis is shown in Figure 32–9. Rehabilitation issues are covered more fully in Chapter 9.

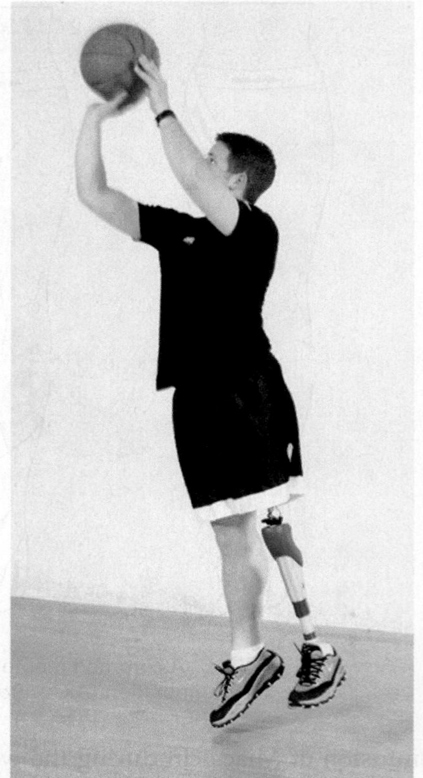

FIGURE **32–9** C-leg prosthesis in action.

COMMUNITY CARE

Rehabilitation programs for amputees, arthritis patients, and others with musculoskeletal disorders exist in most large cities and are being introduced into more communities through agencies such as the YMCA. The Arthritis Foundation has been very instrumental in working with the Ys to bring programs for exercise to local neighborhoods.

Outpatient rehabilitation programs through clinics work with patients who are regaining mobility and ability to perform ADLs with a prosthesis. Rehabilitation is moving to a program "without walls," indicating a shift from an inpatient institute to rehabilitation in the home and community.

Home care nurses are particularly instrumental in preventing musculoskeletal injury in home care patients. The premises of the elderly patient are surveyed and recommendations are made to make it safer for the patient. Flat, nonglare surfaces for walking, well-lit walkways, absence of loose rugs, installation of grab bars in showers and bathrooms, and use of communication systems to summon help are some of the measures instituted to protect the elderly patient.

When a home care patient is on crutches, the nurse should assess the patient's ability to go up and down stairs and to sit down and arise from the sitting position safely. Patient Teaching 31–3 presents the steps for performing these maneuvers correctly. Home care nurses must assess the capability and safety of elderly patients who are newly using assistive devices for ambulation and determine whether alterations in pathways in the home need to be made. Scatter rugs should be removed, and furniture may need to be moved to provide a wide enough path for the patient to move from one area to another.

Long-term care facility nurses survey patient units and group spaces daily to check for obstacles to ambulation and potential safety hazards. Slowly our communities are becoming easier to navigate for the elderly, and public places are becoming more accessible for the handicapped and safer for the frail elderly.

Perhaps with the trend in America toward considerable exercise during the middle and later years, the next generation will have fewer musculoskeletal system problems. Also, with the emphasis placed on calcium intake throughout life, the incidence of osteoporosis and fracture in the older age-group should decrease.

Key Points

- Sprains are usually treated with rest, ice, compression, and elevation (RICE).
- Bursitis occurs from injury or overuse.
- Carpal tunnel syndrome causes numbness, tingling, and pain in the hand.
- A bunion may be hereditary or from wearing ill-fitting shoes.
- Fractures occur from trauma or metabolic disease.
- A fracture should be immediately immobilized.
- Assessment of a suspected fracture includes noting pain, swelling, discoloration, and deformity in the contour of the bone.
- Fractures are treated by reduction, internal or external fixation, and immobilization by casting, traction, or splints. Surgery may be necessary for treatment.
- Frequent neurovascular assessment is necessary when a fracture has occurred or musculoskeletal surgery has been performed (see Focused Assessment 32–1).
- The most common problems in the immobilized patient are skin breakdown, urinary tract infection or stones, and constipation.
- Attention to pain control is essential.
- Complications of fractures include infection, osteomyelitis, fat embolism, venous thrombosis, and compartment syndrome.
- Signs and symptoms of compartment syndrome include edema, pallor, tingling, paresthesia, numbness, weak pulse, cyanosis, paresis, and severe pain.
- Compartment syndrome presents an emergency situation if function of the limb is to be preserved.
- Osteoarthritis occurs asymmetrically and typically affects only one or two joints.
- Treatment consists of pain management, weight control, exercise, and maintenance of joint function.
- Rheumatoid arthritis is an inflammatory disease of the joints.
- Symptoms of rheumatoid arthritis are joint pain, warmth, edema, limitation of motion, and joint stiffness. There may be systemic symptoms.
- Treatment is aimed at relieving pain, minimizing joint destruction, promoting joint function, and preserving the ability to perform self-care functions.
- Many pharmacologic agents are used to treat rheumatoid arthritis (see Table 32–2).
- Rest, exercise, and applications of heat and cold are other mainstays of arthritis treatment.
- Patient continuously taking NSAIDs must be assessed for GI bleeding, liver and kidney toxicity, tinnitus, and blood dyscrasias.
- Postoperative care after joint replacement is very important to prevent infection, prevent dislocation, and promote mobilization. Pain control is a primary consideration.
- DVT is a common complication of hip and knee joint replacement.
- Gout is caused by high serum levels of uric acid.
- Signs and symptoms of gout are tight, reddened skin over an inflamed, edematous joint accompanied by elevated temperature and extreme pain in the joint. There is an elevated serum uric acid level.
- Osteoporosis causes susceptibility to fractures.
- Calcium deficiency and estrogen depletion predispose to the development of osteoporosis.
- Treatment of osteoporosis is with calcium, vitamin D supplements, bisphosphonates, and other hormonal medications (see Box 32-3).
- Paget's disease causes weakened bone prone to fractures.
- The most common primary bone tumor is osteogenic sarcoma.
- Eighty percent of amputations involve lower extremities.
- Amputation requires great psychological adjustment on the part of the patient.
- Phantom limb pain may persist after amputation.
- Hemorrhage and infection are complications of amputation.

- Proper stump care is essential to the success of rehabilitation.
- Rehabilitation is a team effort involving many health professionals as well as the patient and family.
- The nurse can be instrumental in the community by teaching safety factors that will help prevent musculoskeletal injuries.

Go to your **Companion CD-ROM** for an Audio Glossary, animations, video clips, and bonus review questions.

evolve Be sure to visit the companion Evolve site at http://evolve.elsevier.com/deWit for interactive NCLEX-PN Exam Style Review Questions, WebLinks, and additional online resources.

NCLEX-PN EXAM STYLE REVIEW QUESTIONS

Choose the best answer(s) for the following questions.

1. A 24-year-old patient limps into the emergency department after twisting her ankle during a soccer game. On examination, there is local swelling and difficulty maintaining balance. Immediate therapeutic measures include the following except:

1. application of elastic bandage.
2. warm compress.
3. elevation of the ankle.
4. ankle rest and limited weight bearing.

2. After sustaining a rotator cuff tear, the patient's arm is placed in a sling. The patient is instructed to rest and to take ketorolac (Toradol) for pain. Which of the following patient statements indicates a need for further teaching?

1. "I will have less stomach upset if I take the pills with food."
2. "I will not be able to play tennis for a while."
3. "I need to be flat in bed for the next weeks."
4. "The sling must be worn most of the time."

3. The nurse is assuming immediate postoperative care of a 23-year-old patient who had carpal tunnel repair. On receiving the patient, the priority nursing assessment would be:

1. blood pressure.
2. color, warmth, and capillary refill.
3. condition of the dressing.
4. range of motion.

4. A nurse responds to a roadside emergency and finds a middle-aged male with pain and tenderness over the left leg. The nurse notes a closed bone deformity with inability to move the leg. While waiting for the paramedics, the most important nursing action would be:

1. immobilization of the leg.
2. realigning the bones.
3. applying warm packs.
4. elevating the extremity.

5. En route to an emergency surgery for open reduction and internal fixation of a fractured femur, the patient signs the surgical consent. During the final surgical team check for the right surgical site, the patient asks, "What does open reduction internal fixation of the femur mean?" An appropriate action by a nurse would be to:

1. ignore the patient's question and proceed as planned.
2. have the surgeon discuss the procedure with the patient.
3. administer pain medications.
4. postpone the surgical procedure.

6. A 76-year-old patient is admitted for a recent fall in which she sustained a hip fracture. While awaiting surgery, the physician would most likely order which type of traction?

1. Bryant's traction
2. Russell's traction
3. Balanced suspension
4. Buck's extension traction

7. A patient with a plaster cast of the right arm complains of itching underneath the cast. To alleviate the symptom, the nurse could:

1. encourage deep breaths.
2. insert a ruler into the cast.
3. forcefully inject 50-mL of air underneath the cast.
4. administer pain medications.

8. The nurse hears crackles and wheezes in an elderly patient who was admitted for multiple bone fractures. The patient appears apprehensive with an oxygen saturation of 84% on 3 L/min nasal cannula. The nurse stays with the patient and:

1. puts the patient in Trendelenburg position.
2. begins chest compressions.
3. prepares for probable intubation.
4. administers intravenous fluids.

9. When caring for a patient who had total hip replacement, the nurse explains the importance of using the abductor pillow to keep the hip in abduction. Which of the following patient statements indicates clear understanding of the use of the abductor pillow?

1. "I will be able to cross my legs at certain times of the day."
2. "I need to keep the pillow between my legs when turning to the nonaffected side."
3. "I can move my affected hip to position the bedpan."
4. "I must keep the abductor pillow in place when sitting."

10. Dietary management of gout includes which of the following? *(Select all that apply.)*

1. Weight reduction
2. Salt restriction
3. High-caloric intake
4. Avoiding high-purine foods
5. High-carbohydrate diet

CRITICAL THINKING ACTIVITIES  *Read each clinical scenario and discuss the questions with your classmates.*

Scenario A

Mrs. Wilson, age 38, weighs 210 lb and has been admitted to the hospital with a diagnosis of fracture of the right tibia. You have been told that when the patient returns from surgery, she will have an external fixation device in place.

1. How would you perform a neurovascular assessment?
2. How can you support the affected extremity?
3. What can you do to decrease swelling?
4. List the observations you must make while the fixator is on Mrs. Wilson's leg.
5. What complications might occur?

Scenario B

Mr. Moss, age 33, has been injured in a fall from a building on which he was working. When you are assigned to the care of this patient, you are told that the tibia and fibula of the left leg are fractured. These fractures were reduced with the patient under anesthesia, after which pins were inserted for skeletal traction. The accident occurred 3 days ago, and now you are assigned to give morning care to this patient.

1. What nursing problems will skeletal traction present?
2. What subjective and objective symptoms would you look for when assessing Mr. Moss' condition?

Scenario C

Mrs. Cox, age 50, is a moderately obese woman who comes to the orthopedic clinic for treatment of arthritis of the knees and ankles. She has great difficulty walking and would use a wheelchair if she could afford one. Her daughter states that she is becoming more and more inactive and, though her mother says she does not want to become an invalid, that she refuses to move about and do things for herself. Mrs. Cox lives alone and prefers not to live with her daughter because the grandchildren make her nervous. In fact, she prefers to be left alone because she feels that she cannot be of use to anyone. Her daughter feels that her mother could find many useful things to do in her neighborhood if she would only try.

1. How does obesity interact with arthritis in causing immobility?
2. What medications might decrease Mrs. Cox's pain?
3. What sort of exercise would be best for this patient?
4. How could you make Mrs. Cox feel more useful and motivate her to move about and get out of the house more?

Scenario D

Mr. Oliver is a 78-year-old who is discharged home after a THR. You are assigned as his home care nurse to do wound care, assess for complications, and monitor rehabilitation.

1. What teaching for self-care would you reinforce for Mr. Oliver on your first visit?
2. How would you determine whether the home environment is safe for Mr. Oliver?
3. Mr. Oliver is very depressed because he feels he will no longer be able to get out to go fishing and visit with his buddies. How would you approach the psychosocial aspects of his care?

CHAPTER

33 The Urinary System

evolve http://evolve.elsevier.com/deWit

Objectives

Upon completing this chapter the student should be able to:

Theory

1. Review the anatomy and physiology of the urinary system.
2. Identify causes of urologic problems and disorders.
3. Discuss ways in which the nurse can help patients to prevent or cope with urologic disorders.
4. Discuss the psychosocial impact of urinary incontinence.

Clinical Practice

1. Identify nursing responsibilities in the pre- and postprocedure care of patients undergoing urologic diagnostic studies.
2. Describe initial and ongoing nursing assessment of a patient's urologic status.
3. List five nursing responsibilities related to the care of a patient with an indwelling catheter.
4. Identify nursing diagnoses and interventions appropriate for a patient with urinary incontinence.

Key Terms

Be sure to check out the bonus material on the Companion CD-ROM, including selected audio pronunciations.

anuria (ă-NŪ-rē-ă, p. 825)
blood urea nitrogen (BUN) (blŭd ū-RĒ-ă NĪ-trō-jĕn, p. 820)
creatinine (krē-ĂT-ĭ-nēn, p. 818)
dysuria (dĭs-Ū-rē-ă, p. 827)
hematuria (hē-măt-Ū-rē-ă, p. 826)
micturition (mĭk-tū-RĬSH-ŭn, p. 818)
nephrotoxic (nĕf-rō-TŎK-sĭk, p. 821)
nocturia (nŏct-U-rē-ă, p. 818, 826)
oliguria (ŏl-ĭ-GŪ-rē-ă, p. 825)
polyuria (pŏl-ē-Ū-rē-ă, p. 825)
residual urine (rĕ-ZĬ-dū-ăl Ū-rĭn, p. 818)
urinary frequency (Ū-rĭ-năr-ē p. 826)
urinary hesitancy (p. 826)
urinary incontinence (Ū-rĭ-nă r-ē ĭn-KŎN-tĭ-nĕns, p. 818)
urinary retention (Ū-rĭ-nă r-ē rē-TĔN-shŭn, p. 826)
voiding (VŎYD-ĭng, p. 818)

The kidneys and urinary tract are responsible for maintaining the proper balance of fluids, minerals, and organic substances necessary for life. Therefore disorders of the kidneys and urinary tract have an effect on other body systems. Problems in the heart, lungs, or circulatory system can arise from kidney failure. Likewise, generalized diseases, such as atherosclerosis, other circulatory impairments, infections, or disturbances in the metabolic processes may seriously impair the proper functioning of the kidneys. Let's begin with a review of the structure and function of the urinary system to help you understand how disorders of the urologic system occur and how they affect the body.

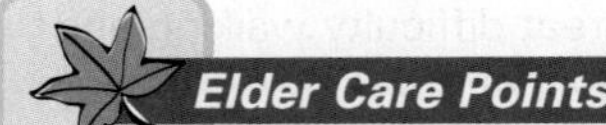

The aged kidney has less ability to concentrate the urine. This predisposes the patient to dehydration when fluid intake is restricted for diagnostic tests. The contrast agents used for x-ray tests, in conjunction with dehydration, can cause acute renal failure in the elderly patient. The nurse should carefully rehydrate the elderly patient by encouraging several ounces of oral fluid (preferable to IV if possible) every 1 to 2 hours and monitoring vital signs, urinary output, lung sounds, and respiratory effort to prevent fluid overload.

CAUSES OF UROLOGIC DISORDERS

Hypertension is a major cause of end-stage kidney disease; conversely renal disorders can also cause secondary hypertension. Because so much of the kidney's function is directly related to the capillaries and arterioles, any disorder that systemically affects the blood vessels can affect the kidneys. Atherosclerosis and diabetes mellitus both affect the capillaries and arterioles. When these vessels become sclerosed (hardened), blood flow through the kidney is decreased; kidney function diminishes and eventually this leads to chronic renal failure. Reduced blood circulation related to decreased volume (i.e., hypovolemic shock) or decreased cardiac output (i.e., cardiogenic shock) puts

OVERVIEW OF ANATOMY AND PHYSIOLOGY OF THE UROLOGIC SYSTEM

What are the structures of the urologic system and how do they interrelate?

- The kidneys, ureters, urinary bladder, and urethra are the structures of the urinary system (Figure 33–1).
- The kidneys are bean-shaped organs positioned on either side of the vertebral column at the level of the first lumbar vertebra. The left kidney is slightly higher than the right.
- The kidney consists of the cortex, the outer layer, the medulla, and the renal pelvis; the cortex contains blood vessels and nephrons; the medulla contains the collecting tubules; and the renal pelvis gathers the urine and directs it to the bladder (Figure 33–2).
- The nephron is the functional unit of the kidney; there are about 1 million nephrons in each kidney.
- The nephron consists of the glomerulus, which is a network of capillaries encased in a thin-walled sac called *Bowman's capsule*, and the tubular system.
- The tubular system of the nephron consists of the proximal convoluted tubule, the loop of Henle, the distal convoluted tubule, and the collecting duct (Figure 33–3).
- Urine is carried by peristaltic action from the kidney to the bladder by the ureters.
- The bladder, a hollow muscular organ, serves as a reservoir for urine; the inner lining of the bladder is a mucous membrane.
- The urine passes from the bladder down the urethra, which is approximately 3 to 5 cm long in women and 20 cm in men.

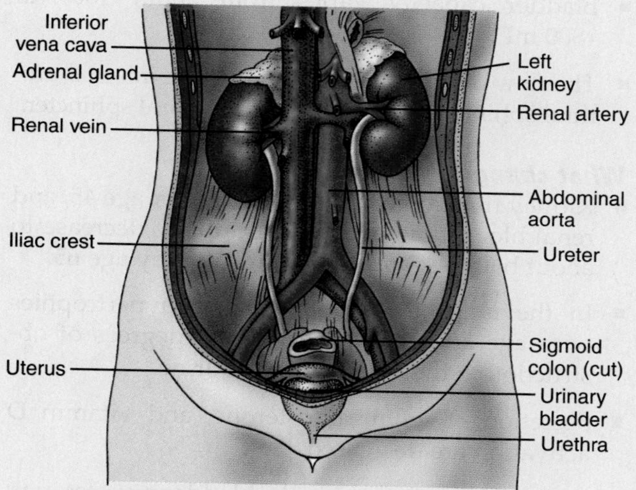

FIGURE **33–1** Structures of the urinary system.

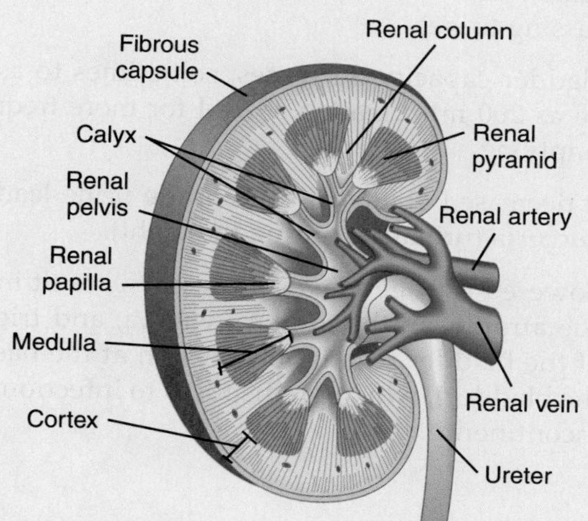

FIGURE **33–2** Structures of the kidney.

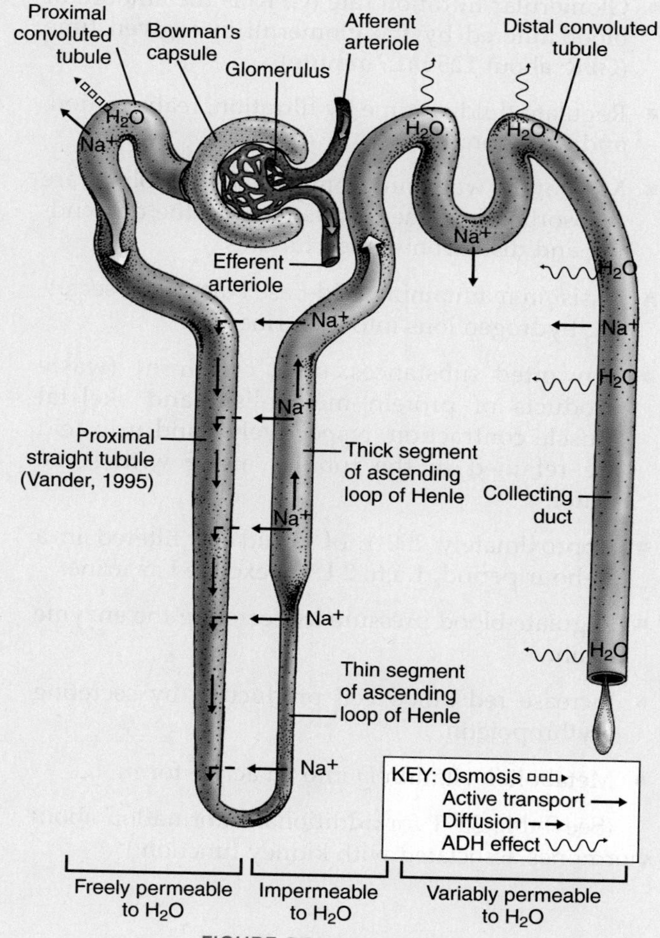

FIGURE **33–3** The nephron.

Continued

OVERVIEW OF ANATOMY AND PHYSIOLOGY OF THE UROLOGIC SYSTEM—cont'd

- The internal, involuntary, urethral sphincter is controlled by the detrusor muscle that is in the wall of the bladder.
- The external urethral sphincter voluntarily controls release of urine to the outside.
- Blood is brought to the kidney by the renal arteries, which branch off of the aorta. Blood is returned by veins to the inferior vena cava.

What are the functions of the kidneys?

- Regulate serum electrolytes by filtration and reabsorption.
- Eliminate metabolic wastes by filtration; filters about one fourth of the body's blood at any one time.
- Each nephron filters blood plasma from the bloodstream through the semipermeable glomerular membrane.
- Glomerular filtration rate (GFR) is the amount of blood filtered by the glomeruli in a given time (GFR: about 125 mL/minute).
- Regulate fluid volume by filtration, reabsorption, and excretion.
- Most of the water and some of the electrolytes are reabsorbed into the bloodstream in the descending and distal convoluted tubules.
- Assist in maintaining acid-base balance by secreting hydrogen ions into the urine.
- Unwanted substances: urea, **creatinine** (waste products of protein metabolism and skeletal muscle contraction, respectively), and uric acid are retained in the tubules along with some water.
- Approximately 200 L of liquid are filtered in a 24-hour period; 1.5 to 2 L are excreted as urine.
- Regulate blood pressure by secreting the enzyme renin.
- Increase red blood cell production by secreting erythropoietin.
- Metabolize vitamin D into an active form.

(See Table 33–1 for additional information about hormones associated with kidney function.)

What are the functions of the ureters, bladder, and urethra?

- Each ureter is a small tube about 25 cm long that carries urine collected in the renal pelvis to the bladder.
- The bladder holds the urine.
- Urine passes from the bladder through the urethra during urination **(voiding)**.
- The initial urge to void occurs when the bladder contains 150 to 200 mL of urine.
- A feeling of bladder fullness occurs and is a signal to **void** (empty the bladder).
- The **micturition** (voiding) reflex is then initiated and transmitted to the bladder.
- Bladder capacity varies from about 1000 to 1800 mL.
- The flow of urine is controlled by the internal urethral sphincter and the external urethral sphincter.

What changes occur with aging?

- Kidney function begins to lessen after age 45, and renal blood flow and GFR gradually decrease to about half the rate of a young adult by age 65.
- In the male, the prostate gland hypertrophies with age and can cause varying degrees of obstruction to the normal flow of urine.
- Secretion of renin, aldosterone, and vitamin D activation are decreased.
- Degenerative changes in the bladder muscles may lead to **residual urine** (incomplete emptying of urine), and **urinary incontinence** (involuntary passing urine).
- Bladder capacity decreases, sometimes to as little as 200 mL, creating a need for more frequent emptying.
- A decreased ability to concentrate urine leads to **nocturia** (urination during the night).
- Lowered estrogen levels in women result in tissue atrophy in the urethra, vagina, and trigone of the bladder (triangular portion at the base of the bladder), which predisposes to infection and incontinence.

Table 33–1 Hormones and Metabolic Actions Associated with Kidney Function

	ACTION
HORMONES THAT CIRCULATE IN THE BLOOD TO INFLUENCE URINE VOLUME AND CONCENTRATION	
Aldosterone	Increases the reabsorption of sodium
Antidiuretic hormone (ADH)	Increases permeability in the tubules and reabsorption of water
Atrial natriuretic hormone	Increases the secretion of sodium
HORMONES PRODUCED BY THE KIDNEY	
Erythropoietin	Stimulates the bone marrow to increase red blood cell (RBC) production; increased production of erythropoietin is triggered by a demand for oxygen or when RBC level falls below normal.
Calcitriol (active vitamin D)	Increases absorption of calcium and phosphorus
Renin	Assists in the regulation of blood pressure
HORMONES THAT AFFECT KIDNEY FUNCTION	
Parathyroid hormone	Works in conjunction with calcitriol to increase absorption of calcium and phosphorus
Cortisol	Promotes sodium and water retention

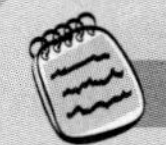

Patient Teaching 33–1

Kidney Health and Healthy Blood Vessels

If your patients have hypertension or diabetes mellitus, design a teaching session that will help them recognize that the atherosclerotic changes that occur in the blood vessels also cause decreased blood flow to the kidneys and eventually reduce kidney function. In accordance with the *Healthy People 2010* goals, emphasize that compliance with the treatment regimen is a proactive step toward preventing kidney problems that will occur later in life.

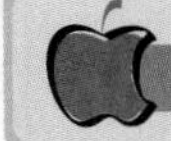

Health Promotion Points 33–1

Bladder Health

Promote bladder and urinary tract health by encouraging patients (and their children) to empty the bladder sooner rather than waiting or delaying. This prevents prolonged exposure of waste toxins on the bladder wall, which could cause cancer of the bladder. Delayed voiding also causes the bladder wall to stretch beyond normal capacity and places undue strain on the sphincters. Both can contribute to urinary incontinence later in life.

the patient at risk for acute renal failure (ARF) (Patient Teaching 33–1).

When an immune reaction occurs in the body, the glomeruli that filter the blood are exposed to antibodies and antigen–antibody complexes contained in that blood. These antibodies and antigen–antibody complexes can cause an autoimmune inflammatory reaction known as *glomerulonephritis* that damages the semipermeable glomerular membrane and interferes with normal kidney function.

Obstruction can occur because of tumors, stones, or anatomic features. Tumors may form in the bladder, ureters, or kidney and interfere with normal function by altering cell structure or impeding urine flow. Tumors most often occur in the bladder. It is hypothesized that the bladder wall has prolonged exposure to urine, which contains excreted carcinogenic chemicals that cause bladder tumors. Once urine is formed, the urinary system must be patent for urine to be excreted. Stones in the kidney or ureters may obstruct the flow of urine. In older male patients, an enlarged prostate may inhibit flow of urine from the bladder through the urethra (Health Promotion Points 33–1).

The urinary tract is very vulnerable to bacterial infection. In the high volume of blood that is filtered by the kidney, there are some bacteria. These bacteria can colonize the kidney, causing an infection. Also, bacteria can easily enter the urinary tract through the urethra, and then the infection may spread up into the kidneys.

Tubular necrosis can be caused by lack of oxygen or bacterial or chemical destruction of cells, which affects the functional ability of the nephron and decreases kidney function. Many drugs can be toxic to the kidney, and heavy metals such as mercury can cause considerable damage.

PREVENTION OF UROLOGIC PROBLEMS

One of the best ways to prevent disorders of the urologic system is to drink plenty of water. A minimum fluid intake of 2000 to 2500 mL/day is recommended to initiate good flow through the system. Emptying the bladder regularly prevents urinary stasis and eliminates toxic substances that would have prolonged contact with the bladder wall (Patient Teaching 33–2).

Controlling blood pressure within normal limits and keeping serum glucose levels normal help slow the atherosclerotic process that affects the blood ves-

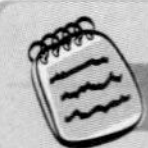

Patient Teaching 33–2

Hygiene

Instruct your patients that practicing good hygiene, showering regularly, and keeping the area around the urinary meatus clean help to prevent UTIs. Instruct female patients to wipe from front to back to prevent fecal contamination of the urethral area, and to promptly empty the bladder after sexual intercourse to help flush any bacteria that entered the urethra. Advise that seeking prompt treatment of bladder infections helps prevent the pathogens from traveling up the ureters to the kidneys.

Box 33–1 *Examples of Substances that are Potentially Nephrotoxic*

- Antiinfectives
  - Aminoglycosides (gentamicin, streptomycin)
  - Sulfonamides (trimethoprim-sulfamethoxazole)
  - Antifungals (amphotericin B)
  - Antitubercular (rifampin)
  - Cephalosporins (cefaclor)
  - Tetracyclines (doxycycline)
  - Miscellaneous (e.g., vancomycin)
- ACE inhibitors (captopril)
- Antineoplastic agents (cisplatin)
- Immunosuppressants (cyclosporine)
- NSAIDs (salicylates, ibuprofen, indomethacin)
- Other drugs (acetaminophen, furosemide, phenazopyridine HCl)
- Contrast media dye (Gastrografin)
- Anesthetics (halothane)
- Heavy metals (lithium, gold salts, lead)
- Industrial (carbon tetrachloride for cleaning)
- Environmental (pesticides, snake venom)

sels. Healthy blood vessels and a good blood supply promote good kidney function.

Carefully monitoring for adverse drug effects and avoiding the use of chemicals known to be harmful to the kidney help preserve optimal kidney function. Box 33–1 gives examples of substances that are toxic to the kidney. When drugs that can be harmful to the kidney, such as sulfa compounds, are prescribed, increasing the fluid intake to 3000 to 3500 mL/day reduces the risk of kidney dysfunction (Patient Teaching 33–3). (Increasing fluid intake must be carefully considered when the patient has other conditions, such as congestive heart failure or cirrhosis of the liver.)

? *Think Critically About* . . . What changes could you make in your dietary habits or lifestyle that might help to prevent urologic problems?

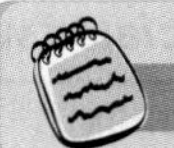

Patient Teaching 33–3

Over-the-Counter Drugs

Teach your patients to avoid routine use of over-the-counter drugs, such as acetaminophen, to decrease possibility of hepatic or renal dysfunction through unnecessary exposure to chemicals. This is in accordance with 2007 National Patient Safety Goals—to actively involve patients in their own care to ensure safety.

DIAGNOSTIC TESTS AND PROCEDURES

Patients experiencing problems with the urinary system undergo urine tests, such as a urinalysis, and culture and sensitivity, and general diagnostic tests, such as a complete blood count (CBC), blood urea nitrogen (BUN), serum creatinine, and creatinine clearance. Urea is produced when protein breaks down; it then combines with ammonia and is carried by the bloodstream to kidneys for excretion. Creatinine is a byproduct of skeletal muscle contraction. BUN and serum creatinine are interpreted together and lab values should be obtained before the use of radiologic contrast dyes. Creatinine clearance (CC) is a good measure of GFR. Cystatin C is a relatively new test used to evaluate GFR. Cystatin C is a low-molecular proteinase inhibitor that is produced at a constant rate and filtered out by the glomerulus. With impaired kidney function cystatin C levels will rise. Normal value is 0.70 to 0.85 mg/mL (depending on age). This diagnostic test shows promise of being a better indicator of GFR than creatinine clearance; however, its usefulness is currently somewhat controversial.

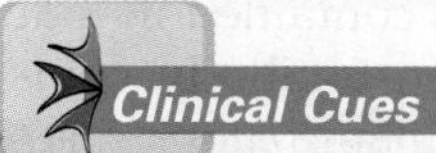

Clinical Cues

Blood urea nitrogen (BUN) level and serum creatinine are the two most common tests used to screen for kidney problems. The normal adult range for BUN is 10 to 20 mg/dL. Serum creatinine: 0.6 to 1.2 mg/dL for adult males and 0.5 to 1.1 mg/dL for adult females. An increase in BUN or serum creatinine can be a signal of decreased kidney function.

Radiologic procedures range from a single view of the kidneys, ureters, and bladder (KUB) to interventional radiology, such as balloon angioplasty. A KUB is used to locate stones and detect structural abnormalities. Angioplasty is used to open blocked vessels and increase blood flow to the organs. Urodynamic tests, such as cystometrography, are used to measure flow volume and muscle function. Biopsies of the kidney or bladder are done in combination with radiologic exams to locate lesions (Figure 33–4, Patient Teaching 33–4).

General nursing responsibilities for diagnostic testing include explaining procedures, assisting with speci-

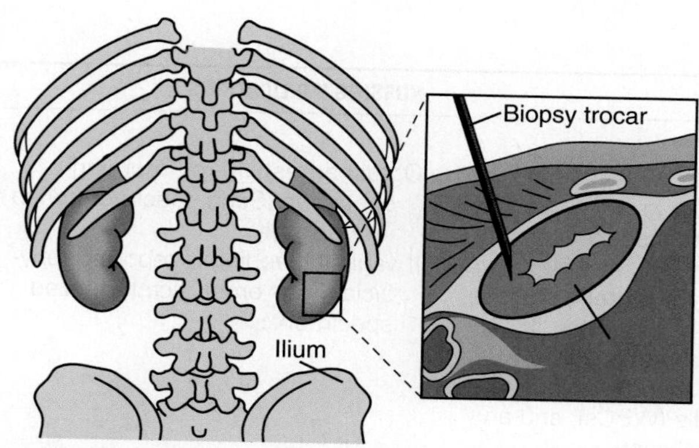

FIGURE **33–4** Renal biopsy. A needle is inserted through the skin to obtain a tissue sample.

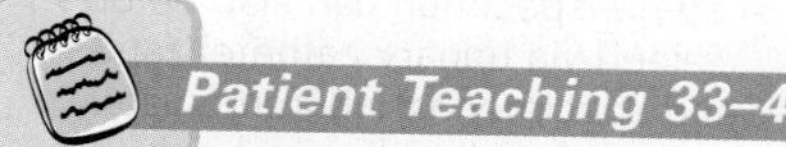

Patient Teaching 33–4

Renal Biopsy

Teaching points for patients having a renal biopsy:

- Explain purpose: To diagnosis the cause of kidney disease, to detect cancer, or to evaluate kidney transplant rejection.
- Explain procedure: Needle inserted through skin into the kidney to obtain a small sample under fluoroscopy. Local anesthetic given. Total procedure time is 10 minutes.
- Explain preparation: NPO for 6 to 8 hours preprocedure and blood tests will be done before procedure (e.g., hemoglobin and hematocrit, prothrombin time, partial thromboplastin time).
- Explain postprocedure care: Must lie on back for 6 to 24 hours (time varies according to facility protocols and physician orders), avoid activities that increase abdominal pressure (e.g., sneezing, laughing), expect that urine will have blood for first 24 hours. Drink 3000 mL fluid to flush urinary system (unless otherwise contraindicated.)
- Give home care instructions: Avoid strenuous activity (heavy lifting or contact sports) for 2 weeks. Report bleeding (e.g., bright red or with clots) immediately. Report fever, malaise, or dysuria.

From Pagana, K.D., & Pagana, T.J. (2007). *Mosby's Diagnostic and Laboratory Test Reference* (8th ed.). St. Louis: Mosby, pp. 807-810.

men collection, reinforcing any dietary and fluid restrictions, and assisting with special preparations, such as bowel evacuation. Table 33–2 lists common diagnostic tests and procedures along with nursing implications.

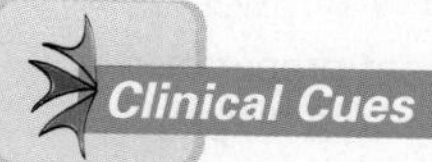

Clinical Cues

A 24-hour urine collection is usually started in the morning. Have the patient void and discard the urine, note the time on the lab slip, and then put each successive voiding into the collection container. At the time when the test is to end, have the patient void, and add this last urine to the collection bottle. Check with the lab as to whether the container must be kept on ice during the collection period. Place a sign on the patient's door and over the toilet stating "24-hour urine test in progress" so that everyone will save the urine properly.

NURSING MANAGEMENT

Assessment (Data Collection)

History and Present Illness

At the time of admission the nurse will try to obtain background data related to urinary problems. A personal history of illness or injury to any system and a family history of diabetes, cardiovascular disease, or kidney stones could be relevant to an assessment of kidney function. Previous disorders of the urinary tract, such as frequent urinary tract infections (UTIs) or problems that required surgery are particularly relevant.

Collect information about sexual health, sexually transmitted diseases, and other genital and reproductive disorders, as these may be a source of infection or blockage. Many substances can be toxic to the kidney (**nephrotoxic**); collect patient history that includes use of prescription or over-the-counter drugs or illicit substances and any occupational exposure to hazardous materials. The complete drug history should be communicated to all health care professionals and conveyed if transferred to another facility; on discharge, the patient should receive a copy of the information in accordance with 2007 National Patient Safety Goals.

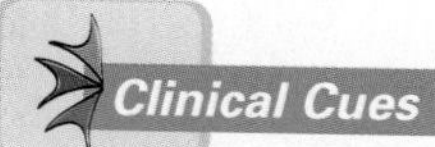

Clinical Cues

When taking a drug history, specifically ask about prescription, over-the-counter, and illicit drugs. If the patient appears hesitant to disclose illicit drug use, use a matter-of-fact approach and explain that the information is important because of potential drug-drug interactions and adverse effects on organs, such as the kidneys, heart, or liver.

Collect information about changes in urinary output, including amount and character of urine, pain or discomfort in either the bladder or the kidney region, and abnormal patterns of voiding. Focused Assessment 33–1 presents a guide to assess the urinary system.

Physical Assessment

Perform a general physical assessment, including a complete set of vital signs and a baseline weight. Observe for signs of generalized or facial edema. Gently palpate the abdomen and the bladder for distention or tenderness. Visually inspect the external genitalia particularly if there are complaints of pain, discharge, bleeding, prolapse, or if there is an indwelling or recently removed catheter.

Ongoing Assessment

Nursing responsibilities in the daily assessment of urinary function include (1) measuring intake and output; (2) evaluating abnormal flow of urine; (3) not-

Text continued on p. 825

Table 33–2 ***Diagnostic Tests for Urologic Disorders***

TEST	PURPOSE	DESCRIPTION	NURSING IMPLICATIONS
URINE			
Urinalysis	Detects bacteria, blood, casts, and other abnormalities of the urine	Normal urine is clear, straw to dark amber in color, has a pH of 4.5–6.0, a specific gravity of 1.010–1.030, and is negative for protein, glucose, ketones, and bilirubin. It should have only a rare RBC, no more than 0–4 white blood cells (WBCs), and an occasional cast.	Obtain a fresh 10-mL morning specimen. Send specimen to lab immediately. If vaginal bleeding is reported, physician may order a catheterized specimen.
Urine culture and sensitivity (C&S)	Used to verify UTI and to determine the specific infectious organism and the sensitivity to specific antibiotics	Normally, urine is sterile in the bladder. Several drops of urine are placed in a culture medium. After incubation (several days), the colonies are counted. If more than 100,000 organisms per milliliter are counted, there is a UTI. Sensitivity test: bacteria are exposed to various anti-infectives to see which is most effective in killing the organism.	Instruct patient to perform the *clean-catch* method for specimen collection. A sterile specimen can also be obtained via urinary catheterization. Send specimen to lab immediately to prevent change in pH, which can affect bacterial growth.
Urine osmolality	Determines whether the kidneys can concentrate urine; reflects hydration status	Increases in osmolality: i.e., dehydration, azotemia, chronic renal disease. Decreases in osmolality: i.e., low-salt diet, excessive water intake, diabetes insipidus. Normal findings for fasting specimen: >850 mOsm/kg.	Give a high-protein diet for 3 days before the urine collection. Restrict foods and fluids for 8–12 hr before obtaining fasting specimen. To collect a fasting urine specimen, have the patient empty bladder at 6 A.M., discard, then collect specimen at 8 A.M. Label as a *fasting specimen* and send to lab.
Uric acid	Uric acid tests are done to check for renal failure, gout, kidney stones	Uric acid is an end product of protein metabolism. Level is elevated in renal failure. Normal findings 250–750 mg/24 hr (normal diet).	Take a diet history; specifically ask about purine-rich foods (e.g., liver, beef kidneys, or sardines). Patient needs to fast the night before specimen collection. Instruct on a 24-hr urine collection. (Serum uric acid may be ordered.)
Creatinine clearance	Determines how well kidneys can excrete creatinine	Elevated serum creatinine with decreased urine creatinine indicates decreased kidney function. Normal creatinine clearance is 15–25 mg/kg body weight in 24 hr.	Collect a 24-hr urine specimen. A 5-mL venous blood sample is collected sometime during the 24-hr collection period. Instruct patient to avoid rigorous exercise (according to laboratory protocol: avoid cooked meat, tea, coffee, or drugs) during the collection period.
BLOOD			
Blood urea nitrogen (BUN)	BUN is the most common test used to evaluate kidney function and hydration status	High BUN levels can indicate poor kidney function, dehydration, or increased breakdown of body protein (i.e., severe burns or excessive exercise). Lower BUN levels are found in severe liver damage, excessive hydration, and protein deficiency. Normal BUN levels average 7–20 mg/dL, (depending on sex and age).	No fasting or patient preparation is required. Take a drug history, as many drugs can alter results. (Record drugs on lab slip as appropriate.) Requires 5 mL of venous blood. When drawing specimen, make sure it is not hemolyzed.

Key: *CBC,* complete blood count; *NPO,* nothing by mouth; *PO,* by mouth; *RBC,* red blood cell; *UTI,* urinary tract infection.

Table 33–2 ***Diagnostic Tests for Urologic Disorders—cont'd***

TEST	PURPOSE	DESCRIPTION	NURSING IMPLICATIONS
BLOOD—cont'd			
Serum creatinine	Evaluates kidney dysfunction when there are a large number of nonfunctional nephrons	Creatinine is a waste product of skeletal muscle activity. It is produced in fairly constant amounts and is excreted through the kidneys. Normal serum creatinine is 0.8–1.2 mg/dL (depending on gender).	Meats, tea, or coffee may be restricted 6 hr before the test. Cephalosporins may be stopped before the test. Record baseline height and weight. Instruct patient to avoid strenuous exercise during the test. Requires 5–10 mL venous blood and may include a 24-hr urine collection.
RADIOLOGY STUDIES			
Kidneys, ureters, bladder (KUB)	Visualizes the urinary structures or radiopaque stones	Single x-ray view of the lower abdomen done without contrast medium.	Patient needs an x-ray gown that has no radiopaque fasteners. Rule out pregnancy before examination.
Intravenous pyelogram (IVP)	Visualizes the kidneys, ureters, and bladder. Detects obstructions related to stones or tumors	An iodine-based dye is given via IV injection, then x-rays are taken at timed intervals, showing the flow of the dye through the renal system.	Check for allergy to iodine-based dye, verify BUN and creatinine results; inform physician. Bowel prep and NPO may be required. Patient may feel a hot flush or nausea when dye is injected. Postprocedure, encourage PO fluids for rehydration.
Retrograde pyelogram	Visualizes the kidneys, ureters, and bladder	Done during cystoscopy: catheters are threaded into the ureters to inject the dye backward into the kidneys.	Check for allergy to iodine-based dye, verify BUN and creatinine results; inform physician. Bowel prep and NPO may be required.
Cystogram	Visualizes the contour of the bladder	X-ray films are taken before and after sodium iodide is instilled into the bladder through a urethral catheter.	Check for allergies to iodine-based dyes. Give a clear liquid breakfast on the day of test. A Foley catheter is usually inserted before the procedure. Patient's bladder may feel very full during the examination, but bladder is drained after the x-rays are taken. Postprocedure, encourage PO fluids for flushing.
Magnetic resonance imaging (MRI)	Imaging of soft tissues to detect trauma or tumors	Noninvasive imaging uses a powerful magnetic field to scan radiowave frequencies and form 3D images. Can be done without contrast	Considered relatively safe. Metal objects are forbidden during the procedure. Pacemakers and implants are contraindicated.
Computed tomographic (CT) scan	Determines presence of a cyst, tumor, or renal calculi	A combination of x-ray and computer techniques yields cross-sectional information and indicates the density of tissues.	Contrast medium may or may not be given; check for allergy to iodine. Patient may need to be NPO before exam. Procedure lasts about 30 min; patient must remain quiet and cooperative.
Renal ultrasonography	Shows size, shape, and location of kidneys, ureters, bladder; and obstructions to flow	A handheld transducer is passed over the skin and high-frequency sound waves create visual images of the structures.	Patient may be asked to drink fluid to fill bladder before sonogram; other laboratories may require NPO for 8–12 hr before the procedure. Test takes approximately 30 min.

Continued

Table 33–2 *Diagnostic Tests for Urologic Disorders—cont'd*

TEST	PURPOSE	DESCRIPTION	NURSING IMPLICATIONS
RADIOLOGY STUDIES—cont'd			
Renal angiography	Assesses renal arterial system function and identifies areas of obstruction to blood flow	Under local anesthesia, a catheter is threaded through the femoral artery and up the aorta to the renal artery, and a contrast agent is injected. Fluoroscopy is conducted during the injection to observe for filling of blood vessels. Angiography is performed to detect complications in a transplanted kidney, to evaluate a mass, or to check the extent of kidney trauma.	Requires a signed permission form. Check for allergy to iodine-based dye. A bowel prep or NPO for 6–8 hr may be ordered. Postprocedure care includes direct pressure applied to the puncture site for 20 min, followed by a pressure dressing and additional mechanical pressure. Patient remains flat in bed for 4–12+ hr. Vital signs, popliteal and pedal pulses are checked every 15 min for the first hour and q 2–4 hr, as ordered, for signs of bleeding or shock.
Radionuclide renal scan	Detects perfusion and function; can detect abnormal areas of kidney tissue (e.g., tumors or cysts)	A radioisotope is injected into the blood and a scintillation scanner is passed over the area of the kidney. This yields a pattern of isotope uptake. Procedure may take from 1–4 hr to complete.	Explain that low-dose radiation is used and is quickly eliminated from the body. Inform patient that the procedure is not painful, but he must lie very still. There are no dietary restrictions, but the patient should drink 2–3 glasses of water before the test.
ENDOSCOPY			
Cystoscopy	Examines the interior of the bladder	Under short-acting or local anesthesia, a cystoscope is passed up the urethra into the bladder. The scope can be guided into a ureter to extract a stone or to biopsy lesions in the bladder.	Requires a signed permission form. Patient is usually NPO for several hours before the procedure. Give preoperative medication, as ordered. Postprocedure: burning, frequency, and pink-tinged urine may occur. Frank bleeding should be reported. Warm sitz baths and mild analgesics are given for voiding discomfort.
URODYNAMICS			
Cystometrography (CMG)	Measures bladder capacity, pressures, and sensations	A urinary catheter is inserted and attached to a cystometer. Fluid is instilled and the patient reports when the need to void is first noted, then mild urgency, and finally when bladder feels very full. Readings of bladder capacity and pressure are recorded and plotted.	Sterile technique must be used for catheter insertion and bladder fluid instillation. The patient is monitored for signs of postprocedure infection.
Urethral pressure study	Determines urethral pressure needed to maintain urinary continence	A catheter with pressure-sensing capabilities is inserted into the bladder. As the catheter is withdrawn, the varying pressures of the smooth muscle of the urethra are recorded.	Sterile technique must be used for catheter insertion. The patient is monitored for signs of postprocedure infection.
Electromyography of the perineal muscles	Evaluates the quality of the voluntary muscles used in voiding	Electrodes are placed either in the rectum or the urethra to measure contraction and relaxation of the muscles involved in voiding.	Inform the patient that there is mild discomfort during electrode placement and nerve conduction testing. Analgesics may be given before or after the procedure to relieve discomfort.

Key: *CBC*, complete blood count; *NPO*, nothing by mouth; *PRN*, as needed.

Table 33–2 Diagnostic Tests for Urologic Disorders—cont'd

TEST	PURPOSE	DESCRIPTION	NURSING IMPLICATIONS
MISCELLANEOUS			
Bladder scan	Noninvasive method to measure postvoid residual volume or urinary retention	Portable handheld scanner uses ultrasound to create an image and calculate bladder volume. Can be done at the bedside.	Clean the probe. Palpate for the symphysis pubis and apply gel about 1 inch above. Ensure that the probe makes good contact with the gel-covered skin. Point the probe toward the coccyx. Press the scan button for the bladder volume readout.
Renal biopsy	To obtain tissue specimen to determine cause of renal disease, to check for malignancy, or to evaluate extent of transplant rejection	The patient is placed in the prone position, with a pillow under the abdomen at kidney level. A local anesthetic is given. IVP or ultrasound is used to identify the position for biopsy needle insertion into the lower lobe of the kidney below the 12th rib. The patient must hold breath while the needle is inserted and withdrawn. A tissue sample is extracted and sent to the lab.	Requires a signed permission form. Urinalysis, CBC, and coagulation studies should be completed. Patient may be NPO for 6–8 hr before the procedure. Postprocedure, a pressure dressing is applied, and the patient remains prone for 30–60 min and on bed rest for 6–24 hr (time varies according to protocol). Vital signs are taken q 5–15 min for 1 hr and PRN until stable. Report signs of hemorrhage, back pain, shoulder ache, dysuria, or infection. Give 3000 mL of fluid unless contraindicated.

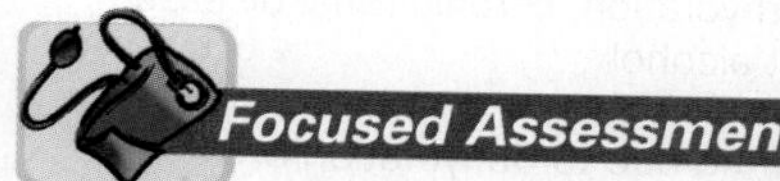

Focused Assessment 33–1

Data Collection for the Urinary System

The following questions are asked when assessing the patient with a urologic problem:

- Do you or your family have a history of hypertension, cardiovascular disease, diabetes, kidney stones, frequent urinary tract infections, or other kidney problems?
- Have you ever had genital herpes or another sexually transmitted disease?
- Do you have any pain when urinating? Any abdominal or flank pain?
- Do you have any difficulty in starting the stream of urine?
- Do you feel as though you empty your bladder completely when you urinate?
- Have you noticed any change in the appearance or smell of your urine?
- Have you needed to empty your bladder more frequently than usual?
- Have you been experiencing any urgency, accompanied by dribbling or leaking urine?
- How many times do you need to get up at night to empty your bladder? (Once a night is average.)
- Have you had any episodes of urinary incontinence?
- Have you ever noticed blood in your urine (other than when menstruating—for women)?
- Do you have any problem with sexual dysfunction?
- Are you experiencing excessive fatigue?
- Have you noticed any itching of the skin?
- How much fluid do you drink in a day?

Physical examination should include the following:

- Inspect the abdomen for any visible abnormalities.
- Palpate all four quadrants for areas of tenderness.
- Palpate above the pubic bone for evidence of bladder distention.
- Inspect genitals as appropriate (e.g., reports of bleeding, discharge, presence of or recent discontinuation of indwelling catheter).
- Examine the urine for color, clarity, volume, and smell.

ing the character of urine (i.e., color, odor, clarity); (4) noticing changes in the pattern of voiding; and (5) assessing pain and discomfort.

The following terms are commonly used to describe various changes in urine output and flow:

- **Anuria:** Absence of urine. This rarely occurs but may be associated with acute renal failure.
- **Oliguria:** Diminished or abnormally decreased flow of urine; may be due to dehydration, renal failure, or obstruction.
- **Polyuria:** Abnormally high and dilute urine output; the result of excessive solutes and increased excretion of water. Possible causes include hypercalcemia, diabetes insipidus, un-

controlled diabetes mellitus, and increased fluid intake.

- **Nocturia**: Urination that occurs during the night; may be related to the decreased ability of the aging kidney to concentrate urine.
- **Urinary frequency**: Voiding more often than every 2 hours. This can be due to inflammation, decreased bladder capacity, psychological disorders, or increased fluid intake.
- **Urinary hesitancy**: A delay in starting the stream of urine; may be related to partial obstruction.
- **Urinary retention**: Retaining or holding urine in the bladder; various causes including neurologic, psychological, medication, obstruction, or postsurgical.
- **Residual urine:** That which is left in the bladder after voiding; related to poor muscle tone or partial obstruction.

Characteristics of Urine. The color of urine can give helpful information about the status of the patient and the functioning of the kidney. Table 33–3 lists color variations in urine and the significance of abnormal coloration.

Another characteristic that should be noted is *odor.* Normal urine develops an ammonia-like odor after it has stood for a length of time, but this odor should not be present in freshly voided urine. A foul smell may indicate infection. Acetone in the urine, which occurs during metabolic acidosis, causes it to have a sweet, fruity odor.

Hematuria means blood in the urine. Microscopic hematuria occurs when blood in the urine is not visible to the naked eye. Gross hematuria is a sign of bleeding from some point in the urinary tract. Red blood in the urine is not easily missed, but if the blood has been in the bladder or kidney for a long time, it will deteriorate and cause the urine to be a smoky gray or dark brown. When assessing a patient with hematuria, the nurse should try to find out at what point the blood is noticed. If the blood is noticed as soon as voiding starts, it is likely that the blood is from somewhere in the urethra. If it is noticed at the end of urination, the site probably

Table 33–3 *Common Causes of Variations in Color of Urine*

COLOR	MEDICATION	OTHER CAUSES
Colorless or pale yellow	Diuretics	Dilute urine due to diabetes insipidus, diabetes mellitus, overhydration, chronic renal disease, nervousness, alcohol
Bright yellow	Riboflavin (multiple vitamins)	None
Dark amber to orange	Phenazopyridine HCl (Pyridium) Nitrofurantoin (Macrodantin) Sulfasalazine (Azulfidine) Thiamine (multiple vitamins)	Concentrated urine due to dehydration or increased metabolic state (e.g., fever) Urobilinogen (a by-product of bilirubin normally excreted through stool and urine) Bilirubin (a component of bile that is normally metabolized and excreted through stool and urine) Foods: excessive carrots
Pink to red	Phenothiazines (e.g., Compazine) Docusate calcium (Surfak) Phenolphthalein (Doxidan) (in alkaline urine) Phenytoin (Dilantin) Rifampin Cascara (in alkaline urine) Senna (Senokot)	Fresh red blood cells Menstrual contamination Myoglobin (a by-product of excessive exercise or skeletal tissue damage) Porphyrin (porphyria is a hereditary metabolic disorder) Foods: beets, blackberries, rhubarb, red food dyes
Brown	Cascara (in acid urine) Metronidazole (Flagyl) (if left standing) Phenothiazines (e.g., Compazine)	Extremely concentrated urine due to dehydration or increased metabolic state Red blood cells (old blood) Bilirubin Urobilinogen Myoglobin Porphyrin
Blue or green	Triamterene (Dyrenium) Amitriptyline (Elavil) Methylene blue	Bilirubin Biliverdin (a blue-green pigment that occurs in bile) Pseudomonas infection
Dark brown to black	Nitrofurantoin (Macrodantin) Iron preparations (if left standing) Levodopa (if left standing) Methocarbamol (if left standing) Quinine Senna (X-Prep, Senokot) Methyldopa (Aldomet)	Melanotic tumors Addison's disease Porphyrin Red blood cells (old blood)

is near the neck of the bladder. Bleeding throughout voiding indicates that the blood is coming from a site above the neck of the bladder, because the blood has been well mixed with the urine in the bladder.

Pneumaturia mean gas in the urine. This can occur if there is a fistula (abnormal passage) between the bladder and the bowel or vagina.

Changes in Voiding Pattern. Ask about or observe urinary frequency during the day and night. Other alterations include the size and force of the urinary stream, feeling of fullness even after voiding, and change in the amount urinated each time. Increased frequency can be a manifestation of some abnormality in the urinary drainage system, particularly in the bladder and urethra. The frequency with which a person feels the urge to urinate can be related to psychological as well as physiologic factors. Excitement, anxiety, and fear can produce increased frequency of urination. Caffeine and other diuretics found in foods and drinks and an increased intake of fluid can increase the number of times a person must urinate. Pathologic conditions that can cause increased frequency include inflammation of the bladder (cystitis) or urethra (urethritis).

Urgency is also symptomatic of inflammation. *Urgency* refers to an almost uncontrollable desire to void. Incontinence sometimes occurs because the patient is not able to get to a toilet quickly enough after the urge to urinate starts.

Pain and Discomfort. In general, the locations in which the patient with a urinary problem is most likely to experience discomfort are either the bladder area or the region over the kidney.

Bladder pain can be due to the stretching of an overfull bladder. Assessment of the size and location of the bladder is indicated when a patient reports pain in the bladder region. Normally the bladder cannot be felt. If a smooth, rounded mass is felt on palpation in the area above the pubic bone, the bladder is distended. Bladder pain also can be caused by spasms of the bladder musculature as it attempts to empty itself of clots, bits of tissue, and other cellular debris. This can occur postoperatively or when there is moderate to severe inflammation and bleeding in the urinary tract. Relief sometimes can be obtained by irrigating the bladder and tubing to remove the clots and debris.

Flank (side and back area of the body below the ribs and above the hips) pain can also be due to obstruction and distention; in this case the affected organs are the ureters and kidney pelvis. Spasmodic peristaltic contractions along the ureter can be caused by stones, clots, a tumor, inflammatory swelling, or any other condition that prevents the flow of urine from the kidney to the bladder. When evaluating flank pain, note the location and assess for radiation of pain from the kidney or ureter to the genitalia and thigh.

Another kind of discomfort may be painful urination, or dysuria. Dysuria usually is caused by inflammation in either the bladder or the urethra. It often is described as burning and can range from mild to severe. The nurse should also ask the patient when the pain occurs and if it is felt immediately before, during, or after voiding.

Nursing Diagnosis

Nursing diagnoses frequently associated with urologic problems and disturbances in urinary flow include the following:

- Impaired urinary elimination related to inflammation
- Urinary retention related to removal of indwelling catheter
- Excess fluid volume related to inability of kidneys to produce urine
- Pain related to ureteral spasm, bladder spasm, or inflammation
- Activity intolerance related to fatigue
- Insomnia related to nocturia
- Deficient knowledge related to prevention of UTI
- Fear related to cause of hematuria or possibility of malignancy
- Disturbed body image related to urinary diversion

Planning

Expected outcomes for the above nursing diagnoses might be:

- Patient will void spontaneously, with decreased symptoms (e.g., urgency, dysuria, hematuria) within 48 hours after starting antibiotics.
- Patient will spontaneously void and empty bladder within 6 hours (maximum 8) after catheter removal.
- Patient will have no signs of fluid volume overload (e.g., weight gain, edema, or crackles in lungs) within 2 days.
- Patient will report bladder pain level $<3/10$ during this shift.
- Patient will have adequate energy to independently perform activities of daily living (ADLs) before discharge.
- Patient will demonstrate decreased nocturia and will rest and sleep at least 6 consecutive hours each night within 1 week.
- Patient will identify four or five ways to prevent recurrent UTIs before leaving the clinic today.
- Patient will verbalize concerns or fears about signs and symptoms (e.g., hematuria) during this shift.
- Patient will demonstrate acceptance of stoma as evidenced by looking at stoma and handling ostomy equipment within 1 week.

Planning care of the patient with a disorder of the urologic system involves considering the effect of the disorder on the other body systems. **Fatigue and irritability are common when kidney function is im-**

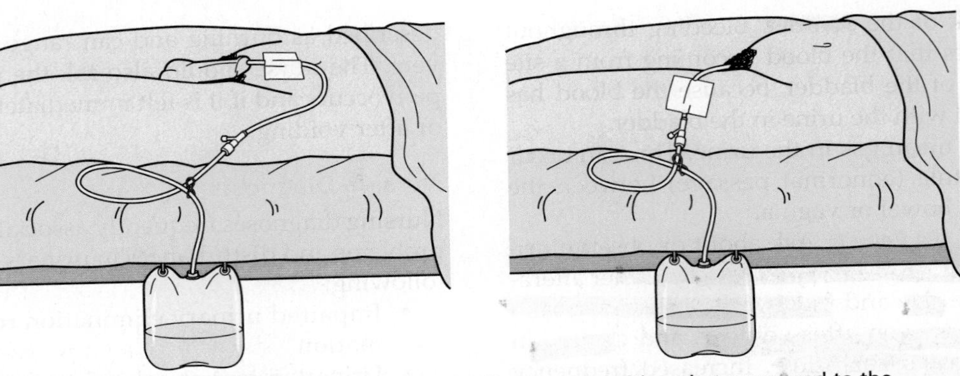

FIGURE 33–5 Catheter tubing attached to a collection bag with catheter secured to the abdomen for the male and the thigh for the female.

paired because of the buildup of waste products in the body and their effect on body cells. In addition, the nurse should educate the patient and the family to maximize participation in treatment goals and prevent complications. General nursing goals for addressing urologic disorders include:

- Absence of infection
- Absence of pain
- Restoration of normal urinary output
- Return to normal fluid balance
- Assimilation of knowledge for appropriate self-care
- Promoting resolution of body image disturbance
- Prevention of complications

Implementation

Caring for patients with urologic problems includes monitoring intake and output, body weight, and signs of edema. Monitoring the drug combinations for potential nephrotoxicity and for possible urinary retention is also very important.

The nurse must use strict aseptic technique when catheterizing patients, emptying drainage bags, handling drainage tubes and stents, and when performing peritoneal dialysis or hemodialysis. If the patient has an indwelling catheter, the meatus and catheter should be gently cleansed with soap and water and rinsed thoroughly, just as the area would be cleansed if the patient were bathing normally. All indwelling catheter drainage bags should have a backflow valve; however the drainage bag should be kept lower than the level of the insertion site to discourage backflow. **The catheter should be fastened to the upper leg with tape or a catheter strap.** Long-term catheter use in the male requires that the tube be secured to the abdomen (Figure 33-5).

Connecting tubing should be positioned so that there is no pulling on the catheter when the patient turns, moves in bed, or arises to ambulate. This prevents pulling on the balloon that holds the catheter in place, which would cause tissue irritation and predispose to infection. When the drainage bag is emptied, care should be taken not to contaminate the drainage port, and it should be cleansed before it is closed and replaced. Each patient should have a personal container into which the urine is drained for disposal. Such equipment should not be shared among patients. When irrigation of a urinary catheter is needed, evidenced-based practice dictates that it should be done using a closed-system technique whenever possible (Emr & Ryan, 2004). Opening a urine drainage system invites the entrance of bacteria. Table 34–3 lists common urinary catheters and tubes used for urologic disorders. Bedpans should be thoroughly cleansed and rinsed after use and should *not* be stored on the floor. Box 33–2 reviews principles of catheter care (Legal & Ethical Considerations 33–1).

EB

Measuring Intake and Output

The quantity of fluids entering the body, by whatever route, has a direct bearing on fluid balance. The importance of maintaining a normal fluid balance is covered in Chapter 3. Patients with urologic disorders are very likely to suffer fluid imbalances, and therefore their intake and output should be measured and the totals recorded every 8 hours during hospitalization or acute illness. In critically ill patients, the urinary output is often measured hourly. **For total output, measure all urine excreted, drainage from all tubes, any emesis, and watery stools.** An estimate of the amount of fluid lost through perspiration should also be considered if perspiration is excessive (e.g., sweating with fever). Any fluid used to irrigate catheters and tubing must be measured and the amount should be added to the total intake and subsequent output.

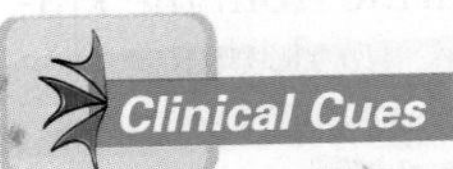

A large part of nursing intervention is to assess for decreasing urinary function. **Urine output should be at least 30 mL/hour.**

Box 33–2 Principles of Urinary Catheter and Tube Care

Apply the following principles when caring for a patient with a urinary catheter or drainage tube:

- Use aseptic technique and gentle handling when caring for any urinary drainage tube.
- Insert urethral catheters using sterile technique.
- Never open a urinary drainage system unless there is no alternative (e.g., the drainage bag must be changed for some reason).
- Empty the drainage bag by opening the drainage port at the bottom of the bag; use aseptic technique and do not allow the drainage tube to touch the collection container. After reclamping the tube, wipe away residual urine from the tube with an antiseptic swab before securing it.
- Use patient's individual collection container for draining the urine storage bag.
- Observe all tubes and level of drainage in the collection bag each time the patient is seen.
- Keep the drainage bag below the level of the catheter or insertion site. If the bag must be raised above entry level, clamp off the tube briefly while repositioning the patient and bag to prevent backflow of urine unless bag has a one-way valve.
- Perform perineal care at least twice daily, cleaning the urinary meatus and catheter with soap and water; rinse well (see agency's policy).
- Keep an intake and output record to help monitor kidney function.
- Encourage fluids to 3000 mL/day unless contraindicated.
- When irrigating, use the correct amount of sterile solution (according to agency policy, or the amount of solution that may be determined by physician's order for nephrostomy tubes, ureteral tubes, or catheters).
- Use a steady, gentle stream to irrigate. Avoid exerting pressure that may traumatize or cause discomfort.
- Do not pull back forcefully on an irrigating syringe attached to a urinary catheter or tube as this creates negative pressure that may damage delicate tissues.
- When discontinuing an indwelling catheter, never cut the catheter. Use a syringe to deflate the balloon.

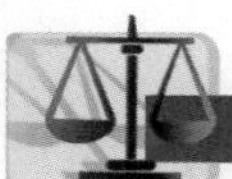

Legal & Ethical Considerations 33–1

Urinary Catheters

Urinary catheters are the most common cause of hospital-acquired (nosocomial) infection. Therefore, urinary catheters and tubes must be handled with strict aseptic technique. Alternatives to catheterization should always be considered to prevent infection, and the care should be carefully documented. In accordance with the 2007 National Patient Safety Goals, when a patient dies of a nosocomial infection, the death is investigated to determine how the patient acquired the infection and why the patient died of the infection.

Evaluation

Evaluation requires reassessment to determine whether nursing actions are achieving the desired expected outcomes. The nurse compares intake and output data over a period of days to determine clinical improvement or the presence of problems. Laboratory data, such as BUN, creatinine, potassium, and urinalysis results, provide further information to evaluate the effectiveness of treatment. A decrease in subjective symptoms, such as flank pain or dysuria, also indicates resolution of the problem.

COMMON UROLOGIC PROBLEMS

URINARY INCONTINENCE

Etiology

Incontinence affects over 17 million residents in the United States, particularly the elderly. Approximately 19% of elders who live in their own homes or with their families deal with this problem. Among institutionalized persons, 56% are incontinent; likewise, those who are incontinent appear to be more likely to be institutionalized. (Lekan-Rutledge, 2002) In the United States, more than $26 billion a year are spent on incontinence. Women experience the problem twice as frequently as men. Women who have had several children may have anatomic changes that make incontinence more likely. Men may experience the problem because of an enlarged prostate, a spinal cord injury, a neurologic disorder (e.g., dementia), or a functional disorder (e.g., difficulty manipulating clothing fasteners).

When incontinence is occurring, the first step is to identify factors that may be contributing to the patient's incontinence. Immobility, UTI, atrophic urethritis or vaginitis associated with menopause, stool impaction, prostate surgery, delirium or confusion, endocrine problems, and various types of medication, such as alpha-adrenergic agents, beta-adrenergic agonists, and calcium channel blockers may contribute to the problem of incontinence. Obesity also is a factor, as it causes increased pressure on the bladder.

Pathophysiology

Urine flow out of the bladder is controlled by two circular muscles called *sphincters.* The internal sphincter lies close to the lowermost part of the bladder, and the external sphincter surrounds the urethra. Many factors can cause loss of sphincter control.

Unconsciousness, UTI, paralysis, interference with nerve transmission to and from the brain, and loss of muscle tone of the bladder and sphincters are some of the conditions that frequently cause patients to become incontinent.

Signs and Symptoms

There are several types of incontinence: urge, stress, mixed, overflow, functional, or incontinence due to neurologic dysfunction. *Urge incontinence* is the involuntary loss of urine when there is a strong urge to urinate (urinary urgency). *Stress incontinence* occurs with urethral sphincter failure and an increase in intra-abdominal pressure caused by such things as sneezing, laughing, coughing, or aerobic exercise. *Mixed incontinence* is a combination of different types, such as stress and urge incontinence. *Overflow incontinence* occurs when there is poor contractility of the detrusor muscle or obstruction of the urethra, as in prostate hypertrophy in the male or genital prolapse or abnormality in the female. *Functional incontinence* is caused by cognitive inability to recognize the urge to urinate or self-care deficit caused by extreme depression. Inability to reach the bathroom due to restraints, side rails, or an out-of-reach walker can also result in *functional incontinence. Neurologic incontinence* is caused by disorders of the neurologic system (e.g., multiple sclerosis or spinal cord injury).

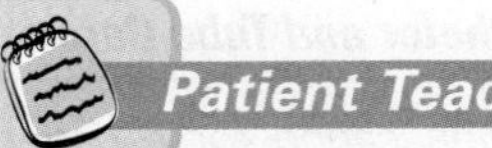
Patient Teaching 33–5

Kegel Exercises

- To locate the correct muscle, stop the flow of urine while urinating on the toilet by tightening the anus as if preventing a bowel movement.
- Practice for several days each time you urinate. Then begin the exercise program.
- While lying down, slowly count 1-2-3 while tightening the pelvic muscles.
- Release slowly to count 1-2-3. Do this 15 times.
- While sitting, repeat the above sequence 15 times; tightening while counting 1-2-3, and then slowly releasing to the count 1-2-3.
- Stand and repeat the sequence 15 times; tighten to the count 1-2-3, and slowly release to the count 1-2-3.
- Do the exercises once a day. If you can do them twice each day, improvement in continence will occur more quickly.
- Improvement may be noted in 6 to 8 weeks, but may take as long as 3 months.

Diagnosis

Diagnosis is based on a careful history, and the patient must be able to report symptoms accurately. The patient may be asked to keep a bladder diary. Routine urinalysis is also performed.

When conservative measures do not improve continence, the physician may choose to evaluate the condition with a series of diagnostic tests, including measuring post void residual, stress testing, urodynamic studies, cystogram, or cystoscopy

Treatment

Evidence-based practice indicates that stress incontinence that occurs with exercise, laughing, or coughing may be corrected by exercises to strengthen the pelvic 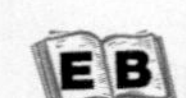 floor muscles (Dougherty et al., 2002). (Patient Teaching 33–5 describes these exercises.) Vaginal weight training with a set of five small, cone-shaped weights that are used along with pelvic muscle exercise is another option. The lightest cone, which has a string attached, is inserted into the vagina and held in place by muscle tightening for 15 minutes twice a day. When there is no problem holding this cone in place, the next heaviest cone is used. This continues until the heaviest cone can be held in place for the 15-minute period. Maintaining normal weight and using topical estrogen therapy after menopause also decreases the incidence of this disorder.

Various medications, such as phenylpropanolamine, pseudoephedrine, propantheline (Pro-Banthine), oxybutynin (Ditropan), tolterodine (Detrol), dicyclomine hydrochloride (Bentyl), imipramine (Tofranil), doxepin (Sinequan), and other tricyclic antidepressants, have been found to be helpful. Recently approved drugs for overactive bladder (OAB) include darifenacin (Enablex), oxybutynin, transdermal patch (Oxytrol), solifenacin (Vesicare), and trospium (Sanctura). Other medications that show promise, but are not yet approved by the Food and Drug Administration, include botulinum toxin A (Botox), tramadol (Ultram), baclofen (Lioresal), duloxetine (Cymbalta) and gabapentin (Neurontin). Table 33–4 provides additional information about selected medications for urinary incontinence.

Further treatment options include biofeedback therapy, and electrical stimulation therapy. A clamp-type device across the penile urethra can be used for men or occlusive devices can be inserted into the vagina or urethra for women; patients or caregivers must be able to apply and remove these devices to prevent tissue damage. Periurethral bulking is a procedure done under local anesthesia in which collagen is injected into the urethra to increase resistance (Complementary & Alternative Therapies 33–1).

Surgeries to Correct Incontinence. A variety of procedures may be performed to correct the anatomical position of the bladder, such as bladder neck suspension. These surgeries are most often performed to correct urinary incontinence in women. The *retropubic suspension* (Marshall-Marchetti-Krantz) procedure is performed to correct a cystocele (prolapse of the bladder into the vagina) and urinary incontinence. A low abdominal incision is made and the urethral position is elevated in relation to the bladder. Urethral and suprapubic catheters are in place for several days postoperatively. In the *needle bladder neck suspension* (Pereyra or Stamey) procedure, a vaginal approach is combined with a small suprapubic skin incision to elevate the urethral position in relation to the bladder. Direct visualization of the operative area is not

Table 33–4 ***Selected Medications for Urinary Incontinence and Retention***

CLASSIFICATION	ACTION	NURSING IMPLICATIONS	PATIENT TEACHING
Urinary antispasmodics, antimuscarinics Oxybutynin (Ditropan), solifenacin (Vesicare), tolterodine (Detrol), trospium (Sanctura)	Used to relieve spasms of the bladder; treats overactive bladder and incontinence	Give mouth care, as needed. Monitor I&O. Auscultate bowel sounds. Side effects include dry mouth, increased heart rate, dizziness, abdominal distention, and constipation.	Take fiber foods and fluids to prevent constipation. Do not drive if dizzy or drowsy. Use ice chips or hard candy for dry mouth. May need eyedrops to moisten dry eyes.
Bladder stimulant Bethanechol (Urecholine)	Used to treat urinary retention	Monitor for orthostatic hypotension and bradycardia. Give 1–2 hr after meals or with food for GI complaints. May cause diarrhea, cramping, or increased salivation	Immediately report severe dizziness or difficulty breathing. Rise slowly from a lying to standing position.
Medication for benign prostatic hypertrophy Tamsulosin (Flomax)	Relieves symptoms of urinary retention associated with obstruction from an enlarged prostate	May cause orthostatic hypotension. Side effects include back pain, chest pain, cough, diarrhea, nausea, dizziness, headache, weakness.	May take 6 mo for symptom relief. Do not crush, chew, or open the capsule. Immediately report a prolonged erection.

Complementary & Alternative Therapies 33–1

Biofeedback Therapy

Biofeedback therapy can be used to help your patient control bladder function by using the pelvic floor muscles. A pressure sensor is placed in the vagina. The patient is instructed to practice contracting the muscles and an electronic display demonstrates the success of the effort. The 30-minute sessions can be conducted in any office, clinic, or home setting.

possible with this procedure, and it tends to result in more complications than the retropubic suspension. However, the success rate for preventing incontinence is higher. An *artificial sphincter implant* is used more frequently to correct incontinence in males than for females. A mechanical device is placed around the urethra to open and close it.

Recently, Albo et al. (2007) in a large clinical study, the Stress Incontinence Surgical Treatment Efficacy Trial (SISTEr), demonstrated that the sling procedure was a successful option for women with stress incontinence; 86% of women were generally satisfied with the outcomes. In the sling procedure a portion of the woman's own tissue is used to reconstruct additional support for the urethra. Following the sling procedure, the nurse should monitor for urinary tract infection and difficulty voiding.

When these measures do not solve the problem, incontinence is managed by intermittent catheterization, indwelling urethral catheterization, suprapubic catheter, external collection system (such as condom catheters), protective pads and garments, or pelvic organ support devices.

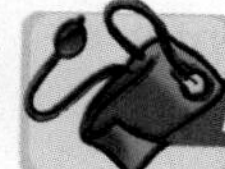

Focused Assessment 33–2

Assessment for Urinary Incontinence

Questions for initial identification and assessment of urinary incontinence.

- Can you tell me about the problems you are having with your bladder?
- Or . . . Can you tell me about the trouble you are having holding your urine (water)?
- When did the urine leakage problem start?
- How often do you accidentally leak urine?
- Are you accidentally soiling your clothing or bed linens?
- When do the accidental leaks occur? Is it happening during the day and at night? What activities or situations are associated with leakage? For example, does laughing, coughing, sneezing, or exercising cause leakage? How often do you wear a pad or other protective device?
- Are you having difficulty getting to the bathroom in time?
- Are there things about your house that are preventing you from getting to the bathroom in time? For example, do you have to climb stairs or walk a long distance?
- Do you have (or need) assistive devices (e.g., handrails) in the bathroom?

Nursing Management

Use a gentle and matter-of-fact approach when taking an incontinence history (Focused Assessment 33–2). Evidenced-based practice supports the use of protocols or guidelines for screening for urinary incontinence (Sampselle et al., 2000). The patient may be embarrassed by the symptoms, but it is likely that he will welcome the help and suggestions. Observe the clothing for stains and odors and perform a general physical assessment that includes palpation of the bladder.

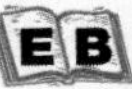

Box 33–3 *Assisting Patients to Establish a Toileting Schedule*

- Assess pattern of incontinence or instruct to keep voiding diary.
- Assist (or remind) patient to go to the toilet at set times (just before the time when incontinence usually occurs).
- Space fluid intake with the majority of fluids taken during the day.
- Discourage intake of bladder stimulants, such as alcohol and caffeine.
- Ambulate the patient for at least 10 minutes an hour or two before bedtime: the activity helps to mobilize fluid.
- At night apply a condom catheter for males and moisture-proof pants or incontinence pads for women; it is not practical to continue a voiding schedule (every 3 to 4 hours) at night.
- Give positive reinforcement for any small successes.

Inspect the genitalia if there is reason to suspect a prolapse or if there is a catheter present or recently removed.

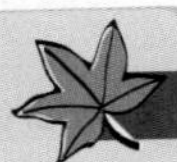

Elder Care Points

Assess elderly patients for gross motor strength, fine motor dexterity, and ability to ambulate and independently balance. The elderly patient may be having trouble walking to the bathroom or sitting on or rising from the toilet seat. In addition, complex clothing fasteners may be contributing to the patient's functional incontinence.

When incontinence is not remedied by correcting an underlying cause, the nurse attempts to help the patient by setting up a voiding and fluid schedule. Assess when the patient is experiencing incontinence. Evidence-based practice suggests that a voiding diary is a useful tool for patients who can self-report (Sampselle, 2003). For those who are unable to self-report, track the times of occurrence by closely observing when linens, pads, and clothing are wet and require changing. (Box 33–3 provides guidelines for establishing a toileting schedule.) Toileting assistance can be offered at set times just before incontinence usually occurs. Getting the patient on a voiding schedule takes a great deal of patience and persistence on the part of the nurse and the patient. Accidents will happen during the retraining period, and patients need to be assured that this is expected (Assignment Considerations 33–1). (See Chapter 22 for care of patients with incontinence related to spinal cord injury.)

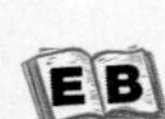

Patients may experience transient incontinence or urinary retention after removal of an indwelling catheter that has been in place for several days. Usually the catheter is clamped for intervals and then opened to drainage before it is removed to help rebuild bladder muscle tone. After this has been done for 12 to 24 hours, the catheter is removed. The patient should then be instructed to void every hour to prevent incontinence. **Any bleeding, dribbling, or incontinence of urine or inability to void within 4 to 6 hours (maximum of 8) after removal of the catheter should be reported to the physician.** It takes time to retrain the bladder to hold greater capacity. Gradually the interval between voidings is lengthened to 2, 3, or 4 hours. Techniques for insertion of urethral catheters are found in fundamentals of nursing textbooks. See Table 33–5 for Common Nursing Diagnosis, Expected Outcomes, and Interventions for Patients with Incontinence (Health Promotion Points 33–2 and Patient Teaching 33–6).

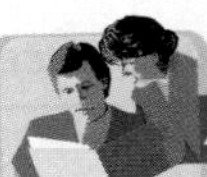

Assignment Considerations 33–1

Bladder Training

In planning and implementing a bladder training program for your confused patient, there are several ways the NA can provide valuable help. Ask the NA to record and report wet bed linens and the number of times that clothes or incontinence pads need to be changed. Once the schedule is established, direct the NA to help the patient follow the schedule by assisting him to the toilet at the designated times.

URINARY RETENTION

Urinary retention is the retaining or holding urine in the bladder. It can be acute after a surgical procedure, removal of an indwelling catheter, or with certain medications (e.g., atropine); it may be a chronic condition related to anxiety, neurologic disorders, or obstruction of urine flow through the urethra, as in enlargement of the prostate gland. A straight catheter is used for a single "in-and-out" catheterization in which the inability to empty the bladder is temporary. Also, patients who have permanent paralysis may use intermittent catheterization to empty the bladder.

Urinary retention will not cause the bladder to rupture, but urine will begin to dribble out of the urethra. Retention of urine stretches the bladder walls, causing extreme discomfort. Assess the degree of bladder distention using gentle palpation before and after intervention. Assist the patient by providing privacy and adequate time for voiding efforts. A caffeinated drink, followed by a warm bath may help. Instruct to double void; void, sit on the toilet for several minutes and void again. Schedule a trip to the toilet every 3 to 4 hours. Obtain an order for catheterization if other measures do not relieve the problem. A medication for urinary retention is bethanechol (Urecholine). Examples of medications that relieve the symptoms pro-

Table 33–5 ***Common Nursing Diagnosis, Expected Outcomes, and Interventions for Patients with Incontinence***

NURSING DIAGNOSIS	EXPECTED OUTCOMES	INTERVENTIONS
Functional urinary incontinence related to decreased muscular strength and fine motor coordination	Patient will be able to physically get to the toilet (or commode chair) and accomplish toileting (i.e., undo clothing and sit on toilet) with assistance during this shift.	Assess abilities to stand, walk, and sit. Instruct patient to call for help when needing to go to the toilet. Offer assistance q 2–4 hr. Obtain bedside commode as needed. Suggest clothing with elastic waistband or Velcro fasteners to eliminate zippers and buttons. Encourage independence, as appropriate (consider strength and motor ability).
Stress urinary incontinence related to weak pelvic muscles	Patient will increase control over incontinence within 8–12 wk.	Instruct patient to keep a voiding diary, or observe for incontinence if unable to self-report. Teach Kegel exercises. Teach to avoid bladder irritants such as coffee, nicotine. Refer to nutritionist for weight loss diet if overweight. Discuss use of incontinence pads or undergarments. Supply information about vaginal cone therapy.
Urge urinary incontinence related to bladder spasms	Patient will experience urge to void and be able to get to the toilet in time to prevent loss of urine.	Assess pattern of incontinence. Help patient establish a voiding schedule (e.g., q 3–4 hr). Give antispasmodic medications (e.g., tolterodine) as ordered. Teach patient about side effects of medication (e.g., possible urinary retention).
Self-care deficit, toileting, related to impaired cognition	Patient will participate in a routine toileting schedule during hospitalization.	Assess cognitive deficits related to toileting (e.g., unable to remember to go to toilet; senses urge to go, but cannot find the toilet). Observe for odors, stains, or wetness on clothing and linens. Assist (or remind) patient to go to the toilet q 2–3 hr. Provide visual cues to prompt toileting (e.g., commode chair at bedside, large arrows pointing toward bathroom, picture of toilet on the bathroom door). Give positive feedback for efforts.
Risk for impaired skin integrity related to moisture and irritation of urine on skin	Patient's skin will remain dry and intact without breakdown during hospitalization.	Assess for patterns of urinary incontinence (e.g., if patient cannot self-report, check q 2-3 hr). Give fluids primarily during the day and space fluids (e.g., q 2–3 hr) for predictability of voiding. Provide (or assist) with skin care (e.g., clean with mild soap and warm water; use skin barrier creams). Consult with enterostomal therapist (ET nurse) as needed (i.e., skin breakdown is progressive). Turn q 2 hr if patient is bedridden or immobile. Ensure adequate nutrition for healing and skin integrity (e.g., high-quality proteins).
Sleep deprivation related to nocturia	Patient will rest and sleep at least 6 consecutive hr each night during hospitalization.	Assess for medication (e.g., calcium channel blockers) side effects that may be contributing to incontinence. Teach patients to avoid taking fluids in late evening hours. Assist (or instruct patient) to ambulate for at least 10 min 1–2 hr before bedtime, then instruct to void before going to bed. Use incontinence pads or undergarments for women and condom catheters for men during the night.

Continued

Table 33–5 Common Nursing Diagnosis, Expected Outcomes and Interventions for Patients with Incontinence—cont'd

NURSING DIAGNOSIS	EXPECTED OUTCOMES	INTERVENTIONS
Deficient knowledge related to management of incontinence	Patient will verbalize four or five methods to manage incontinence before leaving the clinic today.	Teach patient about medication side effects (e.g., if on estrogen patient should report vaginal bleeding or signs of deep vein thrombosis, calf pain, or swelling). Teach Kegel exercises; reinforce that results may take up to 3 mo. Teach bladder training; remind that accidents are expected during training period.
Social isolation related to embarrassment	Patient will maintain usual social contact with friends and family.	Encourage verbalization of feelings (e.g., shame or embarrassment). Assist patient to identify times, settings, and activities when incontinence may occur (e.g., during exercise). Help patient make a plan to deal with incontinence during social occasions (e.g., use of incontinence briefs, mapping out toilet locations, planning fluid intake around social occasions). Refer to support groups.

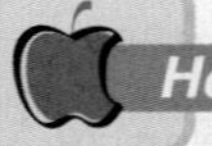

Health Promotion Points 33–2

Drinks and Substances to Avoid

Advise patients that avoiding caffeine, alcohol, carbonated beverages, and aspartame may help bladder control. These substances may stimulate or irritate the bladder.

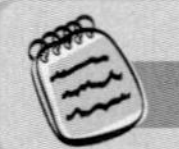

Patient Teaching 33–6

Kegel Exercises for Young Women and Men

Pelvic floor muscle exercises or Kegel exercises are generally taught to women who have stress or urge incontinence; however, younger women who are asymptomatic should also be advised that practicing these exercises will help to prevent incontinence that may occur later in life. Evidence-based practice indicates that male patients who have post-prostatectomy urinary incontinence should be taught to perform Kegel exercises (Palmer, et al. 2003).

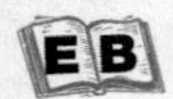

duced by benign prostatic hypertrophy (enlarged prostate gland) include, tamsulosin (Flomax), doxazosin (Cardura), and finasteride (Proscar). See Table 33–4 for information about selected medications for urinary retention.

Poor bladder tone or partial obstruction of the urethra can result in dribbling of urine or passing only the overflow, leaving the bladder partially full. During bladder retraining, **residual urine can be measured by having the patient void as much urine as possible and then immediately inserting a catheter or performing a bladder scan** (see Table 33–2 for information about bladder scan). **One hundred milliliters is considered a normal amount of residual urine.** Any amount over this can become stagnant and concentrated over time, predisposing the patient to bladder infection and the formation of stones.

? *Think Critically About . . .* The physician ordered removal of an indwelling catheter. Three hours later the patient complains of bladder fullness with inability to void. What should you do?

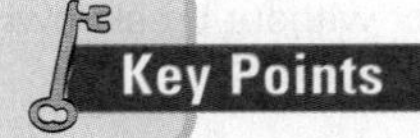

Key Points

- The urologic system is responsible for maintaining proper balance of the fluids, minerals, and organic substances necessary for life.
- The nephron is the functional unit of the kidney. It consists of the glomerulus, which is a network of capillaries encased in a thin-walled sac called *Bowman's capsule,* and the tubular system.
- Kidney function, GFR, bladder capacity, ability to concentrate urine and secrete renin, and aldosterone decrease with aging.
- Urinary incontinence and nocturia are common problems for older people.
- Infection, immunologic disorders, metabolic disorders such as diabetes mellitus, and reduced blood flow secondary to shock or atherosclerosis can result in kidney damage.
- Tubular necrosis affects the functional ability of the kidney. It can result from lack of oxygen or bacterial or chemical destruction of the nephron.
- Stones, an enlarged prostate, or tumors may obstruct the flow of urine.
- To promote healthy kidneys, advise patients to drink plenty of water, empty the bladder at regular inter-

vals, obtain prompt treatment for bladder infection, practice good hygiene, take blood pressure medication, and maintain normal serum glucose levels.

- BUN and serum creatinine are the most common screening tests for kidney function.
- Monitor intake and output, weight, and signs of edema; monitor drugs for nephrotoxic effects.
- Incontinence can be related to a variety of factors: Immobility, infection, physiologic changes related to aging, confusion, endocrine problems, and various types of medication (e.g., antihistamines).
- There are various types of incontinence: Stress, urge, overflow, mixed, functional, or neurologically induced.
- Nursing measures for incontinence include: Assist in determining and correcting underlying cause, establish a voiding and fluid schedule, coach Kegel exercises, give medications for incontinence as ordered, and advise to decrease bladder irritants (e.g., caffeine).
- Urinary retention may be related to surgery, medication, anxiety, neurologic disorders, or obstruction.
- Nursing measures include to assess for bladder distention, provide privacy, instruct to double void, and obtain an order for catheterization as needed.

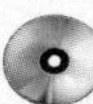

Go to your **Companion CD-ROM** for an Audio Glossary, animations, video clips, and bonus review questions.

evolve Be sure to visit the companion Evolve site at http://evolve.elsevier.com/deWit for interactive NCLEX-PN Exam Style Review Questions, WebLinks, and additional online resources.

NCLEX-PN EXAM STYLE REVIEW QUESTIONS

Choose the best answer(s) for the following questions.

1. The nurse is trying to console an elderly patient who was embarrassed for wetting the bed. "I knew that I needed to go but I cannot get out of bed by myself." The patient is most likely experiencing:

1. stress incontinence.
2. overflow incontinence.
3. functional incontinence.
4. urge incontinence.

2. The nurse is planning care for a 70-year-old Vietnamese female patient who needs assistance with toileting. Which of the following nursing diagnoses would be the priority?

1. Disturbed body image
2. Stress urinary incontinence
3. Risk for impaired skin integrity
4. Toileting self-care deficit

3. Aldosterone regulates which of the following?

1. Reabsorption of sodium
2. Secretion of renin
3. Excretion of calcium
4. Production of vitamin D

4. When starting a 24-hour urine collection, the nurse:

1. includes the first void of the 24-hour period.
2. considers the time of initial void as the start time of the test.
3. discards the last void of the 24-hour period.
4. encourages fluid intake.

5. Which of the following actions by a nursing assistant indicates inadequate knowledge regarding indwelling catheter care?

1. Keeping the drainage bag below the level of the insertion site
2. Using aseptic technique to empty the drainage bag
3. Placing the drainage bag on the bed when repositioning the patient
4. Performing the perineal care at least twice daily

6. Preoperative care of a patient about to have a renal biopsy includes the following: *(Select all that apply.)*

1. Administer bowel preparation.
2. Report abnormal coagulation studies.
3. Enforce nothing by mouth (NPO) for 6 to 8 hours before the procedure.
4. Check for allergy to iodine.
5. Insert indwelling urinary catheter.

7. In determining the specific type of urinary incontinence, an appropriate assessment question would be:

1. "Do you have any difficulty in starting the stream of urine?"
2. "Do you feel pain when you urinate?"
3. "Have you needed to empty the bladder more frequently than usual?"
4. "Have you been experiencing any urgency, accompanied by dribbling or leaking urine?"

8. To assist a patient develop a toileting schedule, the nurse must first:

1. encourage use of condom catheters or incontinence pads.
2. assess pattern of incontinence.
3. schedule bathroom privileges.
4. provide positive reinforcement for small successes.

9. Which of the following nursing interventions are appropriate for a patient with stress incontinence? *(Select all that apply.)*

1. Instruct patient to keep a voiding diary.
2. Teach patient Kegel exercises.
3. Offer patient assistance every 2 to 4 hours.
4. Obtain bedside commode as needed.
5. Teach patient to avoid bladder irritants, such as coffee and nicotine.

10. creatinine is a by-product of skeletal muscle contraction.

CRITICAL THINKING ACTIVITIES

Read each clinical scenario and discuss the questions with your classmates.

Scenario A

Mr. Jones, 65 years old, has a history of difficulty passing urine. The physician orders placement of a retention catheter. You attempt to insert a 14-Fr Foley catheter but you meet resistance and the catheter will not pass. The patient reports an uncomfortable sensation in his genital area during the attempt.

1. What is your initial action?
2. Based on your knowledge of pathophysiology, what would you suspect is preventing the passage of the catheter?
3. Once the catheter has been successfully inserted, explain why is it important to keep the drainage bag below the level of the bladder.
4. How you would perform daily catheter care for Mr. Jones?
5. Discuss four or five general principles that you will use while caring for Mr. Jones' catheter.
6. Which of the following tasks would be appropriate to delegate to a nursing assistant (NA)? State your rationale.
   a. Gathering the equipment for the catheterization procedure
   b. Inserting the Foley catheter
   c. Emptying the drainage bag at the end of the shift
   d. Checking the urinary meatus for complaints of bleeding

Scenario B

Mrs. Diaz is a 35-year-old patient who has had a nephrostomy for treatment of hydronephrosis resulting from a renal stone in the pelvis of the kidney. She returns from the surgical unit with a nephrostomy tube, a urethral catheter, and a rubber Penrose drain in place.

1. How would you explain the purpose of the nephrostomy tube?
2. What is the specific care for these drains and tubes?

Scenario C

You are working in a long-term care facility and caring for Ms. Lilley, an 85-year-old with Alzheimer's disease. She has developed urinary incontinence.

1. What factors might be contributing to your patient's incontinence?
2. Explain how to develop a toileting and fluid intake schedule for Ms. Lilley.

CHAPTER

34 Care of Patients with Disorders of the Urinary System

evolve http://evolve.elsevier.com/deWit

Objectives

Upon completing this chapter the student should be able to:

Theory

1. Describe signs and symptoms of selected urologic inflammatory disorders (e.g., cystitis, urethritis, and pyelonephritis) and nursing interventions for these patients.
2. Discuss nursing management for patients with acute or chronic glomerulonephritis.
3. Describe nursing assessments and interventions for patients with acute renal failure.
4. Describe the needs of patients on long-term hemodialysis.
5. Discuss the benefits and special problems associated with kidney transplantation.

Clinical Practice

1. Describe the postoperative nursing care of patients having surgery of the kidney.
2. List specific nursing responsibilities in the care of patients with kidney stones.
3. Describe the postoperative nursing care of patients having surgery for urinary diversion.
4. Describe interventions to increase patient compliance in the treatment of chronic kidney failure.
5. Devise a nursing care plan for the home-care patient with renal failure.

Key Terms

Be sure to check out the bonus material on the Companion CD-ROM, including selected audio pronunciations.

acute renal failure (ă-KŪT, pp. 847, 851)
azotemia (ă-zō-TĒ-mē-ă, p. 854)
chronic renal failure (KRŎN-ĭk, p. 854)
cystitis (sĭs-TĪ-tĭs, p. 837)
end-stage renal disease (p. 851)
glomerulonephritis (glō-mĕr-ū-lō-nĕ-FRĪ-tĭs, p. 841)
hemodialysis (hē-mō-dī-ĂL-ĭ-sĭs, p. 853)
hydronephrosis (hī-drō-nĕ-FRŌ-sĭs, p. 843)
lithotripsy (LĬTH-ō-trĭp-sē, p. 846)
nephrectomy (nĕF-rĔK-tō-mē, p. 843)
nephrostomy (nĕ-FRŎS-tō-mē, p. 843)
nephrotic syndrome (nĕf-RŌ-tĭk, p. 842)
peritoneal dialysis (pĕ-rĭ-tō-NĒ-ăl dī-ĂL-ĭ-sĭs, p. 853)
pyelonephritis (pī-ă-lō-nĕ-FRĪ-tĭs, p. 840)
renal stenosis (stĕ-NŌ-sĭs, p. 844)
urethritis (ū-rĕ-THRĪ-tĭs, p. 837)
uremia or **uremic syndrome** (ū-RĒ-mē-ă, p. 855)
urinary diversion (ūr-ĭ-NĂ-rē dĭ-VĔR-shŭn, p. 848)

Impairment of renal function affects most of the body's major systems because of the role the kidneys play in maintaining fluid balance, regulating the electrochemical composition of body fluids, providing protection against acid-base imbalance, and eliminating waste products. The kidneys also take part in red blood cell formation and regulation of calcium levels and, in conjunction with the endocrine system, control of blood pressure.

Many types of problems can affect the urologic system. Family history of cardiovascular disease, diabetes, or kidney stone formation is pertinent to assessment of a patient's renal status. These diseases can adversely affect the kidney; they occur more often in family members owing to genetic predisposition. Circulatory disorders, metabolic disorders such as diabetes mellitus, immunologic disorders, obstruction, bacterial infections, or toxic substances can all cause kidney dysfunction.

INFLAMMATORY DISORDERS OF THE URINARY TRACT

CYSTITIS

Etiology and Pathophysiology

Cystitis is an inflammation of the urinary bladder. It is one of the most common urinary tract infections (UTIs), especially in women; the urethra is shorter in women and the urinary meatus is in proximity to the vaginal and anal areas. The *Escherichia coli* bacterium normally resides in the intestinal tract as a nonpathogenic microorganism and it accounts for about 80% of all UTIs in females.

Cystitis and **urethritis** (inflammation of the urethra) are often seen in women after they have become sexually active. "Honeymoon cystitis" is a term you may hear; in this case, bacteria have entered the urethra due to friction during intercourse. In older women, the incidence of cystitis and urethritis increases with age as the decreased muscle tone in the urinary tract prevents complete emptying of the bladder. Urine that sits in the bladder (urinary stasis) provides a good medium for bacterial growth. The estrogen depletion that occurs with aging results in structural atrophy and urinary dysfunction.

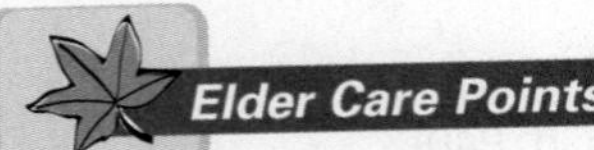

Elder Care Points

Elderly females sometimes have a urethra that becomes displaced, opening into the vaginal outlet. This occurs from relaxed musculature and atrophy of surrounding structures. These women are more prone to develop urinary tract infections.

In addition, many elderly people purposely restrict fluid intake to decrease the incidence of incontinence. Others restrict fluids to help control heart failure, renal failure, or other disorders that cause fluid retention. Restricting fluid intake decreases urine flow and makes the person more susceptible to urinary tract infection.

Signs, Symptoms, and Diagnosis

The most common symptoms of cystitis are painful urination, frequent and urgent urination, and low back pain. The urinary meatus may appear swollen and inflamed. Cystitis has a tendency to recur, producing less-acute symptoms, such as fatigue, anorexia, and a constant feeling of pressure in the bladder region between flare-ups. The urine may appear cloudy or even bloody and have a foul smell. Urinalysis and urine cultures are used to establish a definite diagnosis and to identify the specific causative organism.

Treatment

Treatment of cystitis and urethritis (see description of urethritis on p. 840) is similar. First, specimens are collected to identify the causative organism: urinalysis, urine culture and sensitivity, smear and Gram stain, or

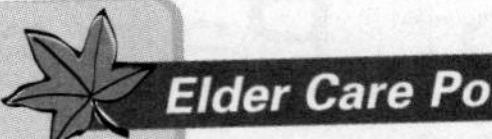

Elder Care Points

Confusion may be one of the first signs of cystitis or UTI in the elderly. If a patient who is normally alert becomes confused, assess the urine for cloudiness, foul odor, or hematuria (blood in the urine), and check for signs of infection (fever, increased white blood cell [WBC] count).

culture of the discharge. Specific antibiotics, such as trimethoprim-sulfamethoxazole (Bactrim) are used to combat infection and are combined with urinary analgesics such as phenazopyridine (Pyridium) to relieve discomfort. Postmenopausal women may benefit from topical estrogen. Table 34–1 lists the most commonly used drugs and their implications for nursing care. The patient is encouraged to drink large amounts of fluids (8 to 12 large 8-oz glasses unless contraindicated) during treatment and to continue the habit once the acute symptoms subside. Evidenced-based practice indicates cranberry-based products also have been used to prevent or treat urinary tract infections (Robbins & Bondi, 2003) (Complementary & Alternative Therapies 34–1). EB

Nursing Management

The nursing care for patients with cystitis or urethritis (see description of urethritis below) is similar. Some measures that can be taken to reduce the possibility of bacterial growth and resultant infection are presented in Patient Teaching 34–1. Measures to relieve the discomfort include sitz baths and hot water bottles on the

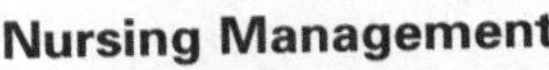

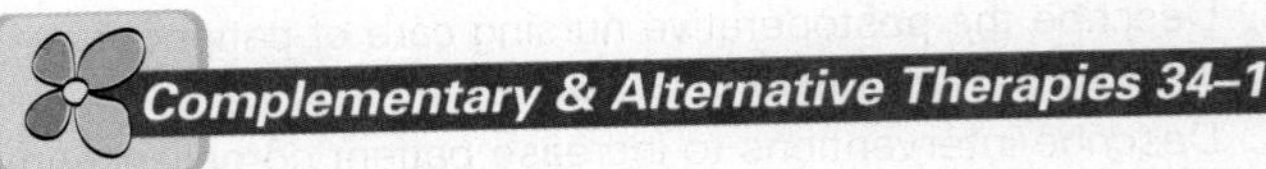

Complementary & Alternative Therapies 34–1

Vitamin C

Vitamin C can help acidify the urine and decrease the frequency of cystitis. Drinking cranberry juice has also proved to be beneficial, as it alters urine pH. German chamomile is used topically for its anti-inflammatory and antibiotic properties to soothe the inflamed genital area.

Table 34–1 *Drugs Used for Urinary Tract Infections*

CLASSIFICATION	ACTION	NURSING IMPLICATIONS	PATIENT TEACHING
MISCELLANEOUS URINARY ANTIBIOTICS			
Nitrofurantoin (Macrodantin, Furadantin)	Wide range of antibacterial action against gram-negative and gram-positive organisms; especially *Escherichia coli*	Monitor I&O. Liquid form can stain teeth; rinse mouth after administration.	Tints urine brown. Take with food and increase fluids. Can cause drowsiness; therefore, avoid driving. Report numbness or tingling
Fosfomycin tromethamine (Monurol)	Effective against most gram-negative and gram-positive organisms	Single-dose treatment. Not for use in children <12 yr old.	Can cause headaches and diarrhea.

Key: *BUN*, blood urea nitrogens; *I&O*, input and output; *WBCs*, white blood cells.

Table 34–1 Drugs Used for Urinary Tract Infections—cont'd

CLASSIFICATION	ACTION	NURSING IMPLICATIONS	PATIENT TEACHING
SULFONAMIDES			
Trimethoprim-sulfamethoxazole (Bactrim, Septra) Sulfisoxazole (Gantrisin) Sulfamethoxazole (Gantanol)	Active against gram-negative and gram-positive organisms	Assess for allergies to sulfonamides. Record I&O. Fluid intake is a minimum of 3000 mL daily. Monitor labs and symptoms related to anemia, blood dyscrasias, and renal dysfunction. (e.g., hemoglobin, hematocrit, WBCs, BUN). Sulfonamides can potentiate oral anticoagulants, methotrexate, and sulfonylureas (e.g., Glucotrol).	Drink at least 12 large glasses of water each day to prevent crystallization of urine. Immediately report to prescriber rash, abdominal pain, blood in urine, confusion, difficulty breathing or fever. Repeat urinalysis after course of medication.
FLUOROQUINOLONES			
Ciprofloxacin (Cipro) Levofloxacin (Levaquin) Newer agents Moxifloxacin (Avelox) Trovafloxacin (Trovan)	Bactericidal Considered second-line drugs; are used as alternatives to other antibiotics	Can be taken with or without food, If antacids are ordered, wait 2 hr after giving Cipro. Monitor WBC for decreased leukocytes. Can potentiate warfarin and increase theophylline levels. Use cautiously in those patients with history of seizure disorder or alcoholism.	Take all of medication. Drink at least 8 full glasses of water/day to prevent crystalluria.
CEPHALOSPORINS			
1st generation Cefazolin (Ancef) *3rd generation* Ceftazidime (Fortaz) Cefixime (Suprax) *4th generation* Cefepime (Maxipime)	Bactericidal; used to treat infections that do not respond to other, less-expensive drugs	Use cautiously in those with allergy to penicillin. *Candida* (yeast) vaginitis is a common side effect. May interfere with vitamin K metabolism; therefore, may reduce prothrombin levels. Monitor I&O, BUN, serum creatinine.	Can cause dizziness or light-headedness. Immediately report to prescriber rash, restlessness, gastrointestinal symptoms, confusion, or irregular heartbeat. Avoid alcohol.
AMINOGLYCOSIDES			
Tobramycin Gentamicin	Effective against resistant infections; use cautiously, as they are nephrotoxic, ototoxic and can cause agranulocytosis and thrombocytopenia	Monitor BUN, electrolyte, and creatinine levels. Elderly persons are especially vulnerable to problems with hearing, balance, and kidney dysfunction caused by aminoglycosides.	Use sunscreen and avoid direct exposure to sunlight. Report nausea, vomiting, tremors, or tinnitus. Take extra fluid unless contraindicated.
PENICILLINS			
Extended spectrum Carbenicillin (Geocillin) Ticarcillin/clavulanic acid (Timentin) Piperacillin tazobactam (Zosyn)	Bacteriostatic and bactericidal	Carbenicillin PO only. Ticarcillin/clavulanic acid IV only. Watch for signs of hypersensitivity (e.g., rash, itching, difficulty breathing). Do not give to patients with known allergy to penicillin. May decrease effectiveness of oral contraceptives and warfarin.	Take all of medication. Take with water 1 to 2 hr after meals to increase absorption. Immediately report to prescriber abdominal pain, decreased urine, watery or bloody diarrhea.
URINARY ANALGESICS			
Phenazopyridine (Pyridium)	Has analgesic effect on urinary mucosa	Is nephrotoxic, hepatotoxic, and can cause gastrointestinal disturbance and anemia.	Colors urine orange and can stain fabric. Discontinue if sclera becomes yellow. Maximum 2 days use.

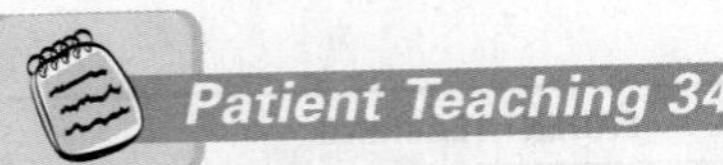

Preventing Urinary Tract Infections

The patient should be taught the following to prevent recurrence of urinary tract infections:

- Always wipe the anal area from front to back after a bowel movement.
- Avoid wearing nylon pantyhose, tight slacks, or any clothing that increases perineal moisture.
- Do not wash underclothing in strong detergents or bleaches; rinse clothing repeatedly until water is clear.
- Change wet bathing suits or wet clothing as soon as possible.
- Wear white cotton underwear.
- Showering may be preferable over bathing for women.
- Do not use bubble bath, perfumed soap, feminine hygiene sprays, or over-the-counter vaginal douche products.
- Prolonged bicycling, motorcycling, horseback riding, or traveling involving prolonged sitting can contribute to urethritis and cystitis.
- Drink at least 8 full glasses of water each day.
- Do not ignore vaginal discharge or other signs of vaginal infection. *Candida* and *Trichomonas* infections should be treated promptly to prevent their spread to the bladder.
- Empty the bladder (urinate) promptly after sexual intercourse and then drink two glasses of water to help flush out microorganisms that may have entered the urethra and bladder during intercourse.

back or directly over the bladder region. Increasing fluid intake, unless otherwise contraindicated, can help flush the bladder.

? *Think Critically About . . .* Mentally review the procedure to obtain a clean-catch urine specimen. What is the rationale of having the patient use the clean-catch method, rather than just simply voiding into a collection container?

URETHRITIS

Etiology and Pathophysiology

Urethritis is an inflammation of the urethra and can be caused by many different organisms. It is a common symptom of gonorrhea and should be investigated as soon as it is first noticed. Inflammatory involvement of the urethra from the herpesvirus is found in males and females. Nonspecific urethritis (NSU) is a sexually transmitted inflammation of the urethra caused by a variety of organisms other than gonococci; although sexually transmitted, it is not a reportable disease in the United States. NSU usually responds to treatment with antibiotics.

? *Think Critically About . . .* A young male patient is diagnosed with NSU. As you are handing him his prescription, he wants to know what he should tell his wife. What would you say to him?

In women, trauma during childbirth and the proximity of the urethra to external genitalia and the anus predispose the urethra to infection and inflammation. Chemical irritation secondary to use of spermicidal jellies, bath powders, feminine hygiene sprays, and bubble bath may also cause urethritis.

Signs, Symptoms, and Diagnosis

The chief symptoms of urethritis are burning, itching, frequency in voiding, and painful urination. There is a discharge that becomes increasingly more purulent if gonorrhea is present. The urinary meatus is swollen and inflamed.

Diagnosis is based on the presence of symptoms and a patient history that includes possible exposure to sexually transmitted diseases (STDs). Culture and sensitivity of urine are obtained to identify causative organisms, and culture specimens are used to rule out STDs.

Treatment and Nursing Management

The treatment and nursing management for urethritis are similar to cystitis and are described earlier in this chapter (see Cystitis). In addition, the nurse should be especially aware of the possibility of a gonorrheal infection until a definite diagnosis has been established and should carry out the necessary teaching to prevent spread of the infection to the eyes.

PYELONEPHRITIS

Etiology and Pathophysiology

Acute pyelonephritis is an infection of the kidneys. It is thought to occur when bacteria (such as *Escherichia coli*) from a bladder infection travel up the ureters to infect the kidneys. A frequent cause of pyelonephritis is an obstruction causing stasis of urine and stones that cause irritation of the tissue. Both situations provide an environment in which bacteria can grow.

When bacteria enter the renal pelvis, inflammation and infection occur. After the infection is treated, the inflammation subsides; however, scar tissue is left in the place of healthy tissue. With chronic infection and inflammation, more scar tissue develops and eventually kidney function becomes impaired.

Signs and Symptoms

In the acute state of pyelonephritis, the symptoms include fever, chills, headache, malaise, nausea and vomiting, and pain in the flank (lateral abdomen)

radiating to the thigh and genitalia. The chronic phase is often subtle, with gradual scarring of the kidney tissues. This results in loss of weight, low-grade fever, and weakness. Eventually the urine becomes loaded with bacteria and pus.

Diagnosis

Diagnosis is based on manifestation of symptoms, physical assessment, and urine culture and sensitivity. Special diagnostic tests, such as an x-ray of the kidneys, ureters, and bladder or an intravenous pyelogram, may be done to determine the location of the obstruction if one is suspected.

Treatment

Prompt treatment of cystitis and prevention of recurrence can help prevent acute pyelonephritis. Correction of obstruction, removal of stones, and prevention of stone formation are essential to correct chronic pyelonephritis. Bed rest, analgesics, and antipyretics are prescribed.

Specific drugs to destroy the bacteria are usually chosen according to the sensitivity of the causative organism, so that the most effective antibiotic is given, for example gentamicin, ciprofloxacin (Cipro), or trimethoprim-sulfamethoxazole (Bactrim) (see Table 34–1).

Prompt treatment of the active infection is recommended to prevent destruction and scarring of the kidney cells. With chronic pyelonephritis, the patient may live for years without significant symptoms before renal damage leads to hypertension or kidney failure.

Nursing Management

You should encourage fluid intake, record intake and output, monitor the urine for changes and keep the patient comfortable. Intravenous fluids may be given to flush the kidneys, especially if the patient is nauseated and vomiting.

? *Think Critically About . . .* What characteristics of a fresh urine specimen might indicate an infection? Why should UTIs be treated promptly?

ACUTE GLOMERULONEPHRITIS

Etiology and Pathophysiology

Glomerulonephritis is primarily seen in children and young adults and affects males more than females. It most commonly occurs about 2 to 3 weeks after a group A beta-hemolytic streptococcal infection, such as "strep throat" or impetigo; however, it can occur in response to bacterial, viral, or parasitic infections elsewhere in the body. It is an immunologic problem caused by an antigen-antibody reaction. Antigen-antibody complexes are deposited in the glomerular basement membrane. This causes cell damage and altered permeability. Renal tissue becomes scarred and function is impaired.

Signs, Symptoms, and Diagnosis

The patient with acute glomerulonephritis usually becomes suddenly ill with fever, chills, flank pain, widespread edema, puffiness about the eyes, visual disturbances, and marked hypertension.

Diagnosis is based on physical findings. Presence of marked hypertension is a late manifestation. Diagnostic tests include urinalysis, creatinine, blood urea nitrogen (BUN), and complete blood count (CBC). The urine may be smoky and will contain red blood cells and protein, and have an increased specific gravity. Serum creatinine and BUN levels rise above normal. If the condition is severe, hematocrit and hemoglobin will indicate anemia.

Treatment

A sodium-restricted diet is indicated if edema is present, and fluids may be limited if there is **oliguria** (diminished urine secretion in relation to intake) or anuria. A low-protein, high-carbohydrate diet also may be ordered.

? *Think Critically About . . .* Your patient has been told to make dietary modifications for kidney problems. He tells you that his typical daily lunch is fast-food hamburger and French fries. What suggestions could you make for this patient?

Plasmapheresis is a therapy used in autoimmune disorders, such as acute glomerulonephritis or myasthenia gravis. It removes the autoantibodies causing the disease. This procedure can be done at the bedside by a trained technician with specialized equipment. The patient's blood is accessed through a shunt or a central intravenous catheter and the blood components are separated from the plasma by filtration or centrifuge. Then the cellular components are returned to the patient and the plasma is replaced with a fluid such as normal saline or albumin.

If treatment is not successful, the disease will rapidly progress to kidney failure and death.

Nursing Management

Obtain a history of past illnesses, particularly infections, or autoimmune disorders such as lupus. Perform a general physical assessment, including vital signs, a baseline weight, and observe for fluid retention or edema. Edema that is obvious from external signs may very well be present in the internal organs.

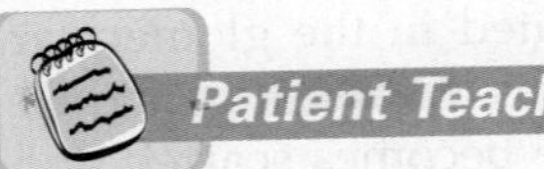

Patient Teaching 34–2

Sodium

Help your patient to recognize that a low-sodium diet involves more than avoiding the salt shaker. Demonstrate how to read food labels to identify hidden sources of sodium in items such as catsup, canned soup, and salad dressing.

For this reason, mental status must be checked frequently for indications of cerebral edema with increased intracranial pressure. Cardiac failure or pulmonary edema may develop; therefore, observe for extreme restlessness, increased respiratory difficulty, or cyanosis and be alert for sudden changes or worsening trends in blood pressure, pulse, and respiratory rate.

Decreasing the work of the kidney is a primary goal in treating acute glomerulonephritis. **Absolute bed rest usually is ordered until the clinical signs of hematuria, proteinuria, and hypertension are gone.** If the patient responds quickly to treatment and wishes to be more active, you must emphasize the need for continued rest. Low-protein diets may be ordered if the BUN is elevated to reduce nitrogenous waste by-products. Low-sodium or fluid-restricted diets may be ordered to reduce the edema (Patient Teaching 34–2).

Antihypertensives and diuretics also are ordered to control edema and hypertension. Plasmapheresis and corticosteroids may be used to reduce the antigen response and the inflammatory process. If the patient has plasmapheresis therapy, you should monitor for bleeding at the puncture site and check the shunt for a bruit (soft swishing sound) every 2 to 4 hours. Also monitor for potential complications, such as hypovolemia or electrolyte imbalance. The prognosis for acute glomerulonephritis varies, depending on the extent of permanent damage done to the kidneys or other vital organs.

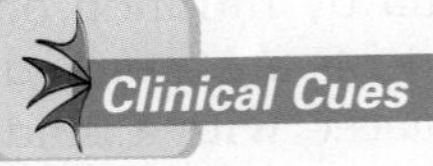

Clinical Cues

To assess for a bruit, gently auscultate the shunt with your stethoscope. You should hear an intermittent soft swishing sound that will correlate with the rhythm of your patient's pulse.

CHRONIC GLOMERULONEPHRITIS

Etiology and Pathophysiology

Chronic glomerulonephritis may develop rapidly or progress slowly over 20 to 30+ years. The exact cause is unknown; however, in chronic glomerulonephritis, the kidney atrophies; there is a decreased number of functional nephrons, and eventual kidney failure. The prognosis for this disease is ultimately poor; the speed with which it progresses to renal failure varies with the individual.

Signs and Symptoms

Generalized edema, headache associated with hypertension, fatigue, dyspnea, weight loss, loss of strength, increasing irritability, and nocturia are symptoms of glomerulonephritis. Proteinuria, hematuria, and kidney failure occur as the kidney function becomes impaired. Some patients who develop chronic glomerulonephritis may have acute exacerbations.

Diagnosis

Diagnostic testing may be prompted by findings on a routine examination; for example, retinal hemorrhage discovered during an eye examination. Testing includes urinalysis, creatinine, BUN, CBC, and electrolytes. Abnormal laboratory values include proteinuria, urinary casts (protein plugs secreted by damaged tubules), elevated creatinine and BUN levels, anemia, hyperkalemia, hypermagnesemia, increased phosphorus, and decreased serum calcium and albumin.

Treatment and Nursing Management

The treatment for chronic glomerulonephritis in the latent stage is primarily symptomatic, with emphasis on avoiding fatigue and infections, particularly of the upper respiratory tract. When renal failure develops, dialysis (filtration of the blood) and possibly a kidney transplant are the only alternative modes of therapy.

Care of the patient with chronic renal disease is discussed later in this chapter.

NEPHROTIC SYNDROME

Etiology and Pathophysiology

Nephrotic syndrome sometimes occurs after the glomeruli have been damaged by glomerulonephritis or some other disease. This damage results in increased membrane permeability and excretion of protein and decreased serum albumin (hypoalbuminemia). Hypoalbuminemia causes fluid to shift out into the body tissues and the result is severe edema. The outcome is variable. Some patients recover without further incidence, and others experience repeated episodes and eventual kidney failure.

Signs, Symptoms, and Diagnosis

Nephrotic syndrome is characterized by extensive proteinuria, hyperlipidemia (elevated blood lipids), hypoalbuminemia (low blood albumin), and severe edema. Facial edema, especially periorbital edema, may be present in the morning, whereas lower extremity edema is more evident at the end of the day. Ascites (accumulation of serous fluid in the abdomen cavity) may also occur due to fluid retention. The patient may be irritable, tired, or lethargic. Diagnostic tests include urinalysis and serum tests for protein and lipids. A renal biopsy may be used to verify the diagnosis or to evaluate the extent of kidney damage.

Treatment and Nursing Management

Treatment consists of an adequate-protein, low-fat, low-sodium diet, diuretics, supplemental multiple vitamins and minerals, and antibiotics if infection is present. Some patients are treated with cortisone and cyclophosphamide (Cytoxan).

Nursing care includes monitoring intake and output, recording daily weight, encouraging rest, providing skin care, and encouraging compliance with dietary and medication regimen.

OBSTRUCTIONS OF THE URINARY TRACT

HYDRONEPHROSIS

Etiology and Pathophysiology

Whenever the normal flow of urine is obstructed (e.g., kidney stone or enlarged prostate), there is a potential backward flow of fluid into the renal pelvis. If this condition is not relieved by removing the obstruction, the renal pelvis and ureters will become dilated and continue to fill with fluid. This condition is known as **hydronephrosis**. Soon, the kidney cells will atrophy until all normal function ceases and the kidney becomes a thin-walled cyst. It can eventually result in complete destruction of the kidneys. Hydronephrosis may be unilateral or bilateral (one or both kidneys). If it occurs on one side, the other kidney may enlarge and efficiently carry on the work of two kidneys. This is called *compensatory hypertrophy.*

Signs, Symptoms, and Diagnosis

Severe pain is present only if hydronephrosis develops rapidly. Otherwise, there are no outstanding symptoms, and the patient may develop signs of kidney failure only after serious damage has occurred. A definitive diagnosis is obtained by extensive urologic examination and detailed x-ray studies of the kidney and ureters, which usually reveal the site and cause of obstruction and distention of the renal pelvis.

Treatment

The primary goal of treatment for hydronephrosis is to remove the obstruction so the kidney may drain properly. The ideal remedy is to drain the kidney in the early stages with a **nephrostomy** tube or ureteral stent. Nephrostomy is a surgical incision into a kidney to drain the kidney artificially. This procedure may be performed to correct obstructions from large stones, or strictures of the ureters. It is also used to drain purulent material from an infected kidney. If the damage is irreparable, surgery is necessary to remove the kidney (**nephrectomy**).

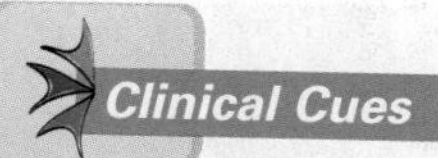

DO NOT confuse urinary drainage systems with gastrointestinal feeding or drainage systems! They can look very similar. When working with tubes and drains trace all tubes down to the patient's body surface *prior to* irrigation or instillation of fluids, feedings, or medications. Verify the purpose and type of tube or drain with the charge nurse if you are unsure.

Nursing Management

Postoperative Nursing Care. In both nephrectomy and nephrostomy, the surgical incision may be lumbar, transabdominal, or thoracic. When the patient returns from surgery, you must carefully check for the location of the surgical wound and the presence of any drains or tubes that may have been inserted during the operation. Nursing interventions focus on promoting unimpeded urine flow by properly caring for catheters and tubes.

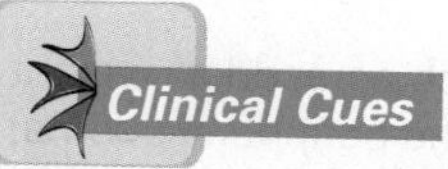

Never clamp or irrigate a nephrostomy tube without a specific order.

Hemorrhage is a danger after surgery of the kidney, because the kidneys have a very rich supply of blood directly from the aorta and vena cava. The vital signs are carefully checked and any indication of shock or hemorrhage is immediately reported. It is expected that the drainage on these dressings will be blood-tinged at first, but if bright red blood appears or if there is a sudden change in the amount of drainage, the surgeon should be notified. Dressings over the surgical wound may be reinforced. **Extreme care must be taken when changing dressings to ensure that the drains or tubes are not dislodged or pulled from the surgical incision.** If the tube dislodges, you must contact the surgeon immediately.

Positioning of the patient depends on the wishes of the surgeon, who may prefer to have the patient lie only on the affected side. Turning may be difficult at first because movement is usually painful and the patient may be reluctant. You should explain the need for frequent turning and deep-breathing so that complications may be prevented.

Adequate drainage from the opposite kidney after surgery is of great importance. Urinary output must be very carefully measured and recorded. Fluids are usually restricted immediately after surgery and then gradually increased as the remaining kidney compensates. If a nephrostomy has been done, fluids are restricted until the affected kidney can recover sufficiently to resume function.

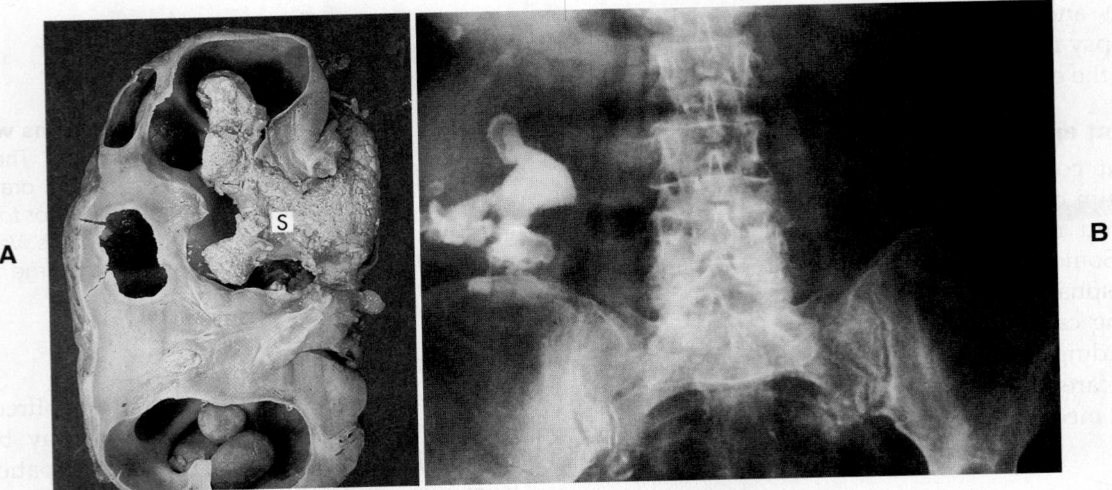

FIGURE 34–1 **A,** A renal staghorn calculus. The renal pelvis is filled and resembles the horn of a stag ("s" on the figure marks the calculus). **B,** Staghorn calculus as seen on an IVP.

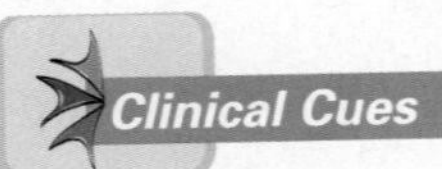

Observe for signs of fluid overload, such as sudden weight gain, crackles in lungs on auscultation, and peripheral edema; watch for and accurately record subtle changes in urinary patterns and output. Monitor labs including: electrolytes, BUN, and serum creatinine.

RENAL STENOSIS

The renal artery can become blocked or narrowed (**renal stenosis**) because of atherosclerosis or scarring. This blockage can result in hypertension or **chronic renal failure (gradual loss of kidney function).** The patient may be asymptomatic, but blood pressure should be monitored. Magnetic resonance imaging (MRI) or computed tomography (CT) scan or ultrasound may show a decreased kidney size. Anticipate that the patient will be prescribed antihypertensives to control elevated blood pressure. Balloon angioplasty or stent placement can be done to improve blood flow to the kidney.

RENAL STONES

A renal or kidney stone (lithiasis) is a crystalline mass that forms in the urinary system and, depending on the size and location, may obstruct the flow of urine. Stones can be as small as a grain of sand or large enough to fill the renal pelvis. This enlarged stone formation is called a *renal staghorn calculus* (Figure 34–1). Renal stones also vary in composition and in the environment in which they form. Some stones form more readily in acidic urine, whereas others occur in alkaline urine. There are four major types of renal stones, one of which is hereditary. Table 34–2 shows the cause and dietary interventions for each type. Identifying the type and cause of particular kinds of stones can be very effective in preventing further formation and deciding the appropriate method of treatment for each patient. However, in about half the cases, the precise cause of stone formation cannot be identified.

Etiology and Pathophysiology

Certain conditions predispose a person to having renal calculi. Among the most common causative factors are (1) supersaturation of the urine with crystalloids that do not readily dissolve (e.g., calcium, uric acid, and cystine); (2) urinary infections, which can produce bacteria and other debris that form a core for stone formation; (3) inadequate fluid intake, which results in concentrated urine and inadequate flushing of the urinary tract; (4) sluggish flow of urine, as may occur with bed rest or immobility; and (5) certain substances in the urine (e.g., urate, a salt of uric acid), which encourage the formation of crystals of calcium oxalate or calcium phosphate. In the past, patients with calcium oxalate stones were encouraged to decrease dietary calcium; however, evidence-based practice now indicates that these patients should actually be encouraged to increase fluids and dietary calcium, but decrease protein and sodium intake (Borghi et al., 2002). 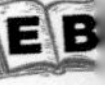

A small percentage of patients with calcium stones have a tumor of the parathyroid. This gland produces a hormone that raises the level of serum calcium, and thus calcium in the urine. Treatment of the parathyroid condition removes the cause of the stones. Risk factors for kidney stone formation include:

- Male gender
- A family history of renal stones
- History of intestinal bypass surgery for obesity. (These patients have an increased absorption of oxalate from foods.)

Table 34–2 ***Risk Factors and Treatments for Renal Stones***

STONE TYPE	RISK FACTORS	INTERVENTIONS
Calcium oxalate (most common type)	An increased intake of protein, sodium; inadequate fluid intake, prolonged immobility	Increase fluid intake. Medications to bind oxalate (cholestyramine) or calcium (e.g., cellulose phosphate). Diuretics (e.g., hydrochlorothiazide) to encourage flushing. Avoid oxalate sources such as spinach, chard, parsley, peanuts, chocolate, and strawberries.
Calcium phosphate	An increased intake of protein, sodium; inadequate fluid intake, primary hyperparathyroidism	Limit intake of foods high in protein and sodium. Treat underlying hyperparathyroidism.
Uric acid	Excess dietary purine (e.g., organ meats, gravies, red wines, and sardines) Gout (primary or secondary)	Decrease intake of purine sources. Alkalinize urine with potassium citrate or lemonade. Administer allopurinol for gout (decreases production of uric acid).
Struvite (more common in women)	Urinary tract infections	Administer antibiotics for infection and acetohydroxamic acid (inhibits the chemical action of bacteria that contributes to struvite stone formation), as ordered.
Cystine	Hereditary cystine crystal formation	Encourage oral fluids, up to 3 L/day. Medications to prevent crystallization (e.g., tiopronin). Alkalinize urine with potassium citrate or lemonade.

- Immobility for any reason, which contributes to urinary stasis and calcium loss from bones
- History of recurrent urinary tract infections

Prevention

An essential factor in preventing stone formation is an adequate flow of fluid through the kidney to prevent the formation of kidney stones. A continuous flow of dilute urine flushes the tract and removes substances that could form stones. **Ideally, the adult must put out at least 3500 mL of urine every 24 hours to prevent stone formation; likewise, preventing urinary infections and maintaining adequate drainage through tubes and catheters is also necessary.** In those cases in which the urine pH is crucial to stone formation, changing the urine pH can prevent or reduce the incidence of renal calculi. Ascorbic acid or dietary modifications (e.g., cranberry juice or prunes) can be used to acidify urine.

Signs and Symptoms

Some renal stones do not cause noticeable symptoms and can be passed without the person being aware of them. Others may lodge in the renal pelvis and cause symptoms only after the destruction of kidney cells. The kidney stones that cause severe pain are those that are small enough to move along the ureter with the urine. As the stone rolls along, sharp little spikes scrape the ureteral lining, causing excruciating pain and bleeding. **Pain is typically felt in the flank over the affected kidney and ureter, and radiates downward toward the genitalia and inner thigh. Nausea and vomiting often occur because of the severity of the pain.** Moving stones can get trapped along the ureter, causing obstruction of flow and swelling of the ureter.

> ***Think Critically About . . .*** A coworker tells you that your patient is seeking narcotics and is "faking" kidney stone pain and intentionally introducing blood into his urine sample. How would you respond to this?

Diagnosis

Diagnostic tests include urinalysis and a kidney, ureters, bladder (KUB) study to locate stones that are radiopaque (materials such as metal will appear as a white area on the x-ray) and an intravenous pyelogram (IVP) will show a gap (nonradiopaque stone) in the stream of dye being excreted in the urine. Further studies of the blood and urine might be done to determine the levels of substances, such as calcium, uric acid, and cystine that can contribute to stone formation. Treatment and prevention of recurrent renal stones must be based on identification.

Treatment

At first, the physician may try to flush the stone out by increasing the patient's IV or oral fluid intake and managing pain by prescribing opioid analgesics or nonsteroidal anti-inflammatory drugs (NSAIDs) and antispasmodics, such as propantheline bromide (Pro-Banthine) or oxybutynin chloride (Ditropan). If there is pus in the urine, an antibiotic is prescribed to deal with infection.

Some stones can be flushed by irrigation through a ureteral catheter or percutaneous nephrostomy tube or crushed by ultrasound. Usually, a stent will be placed in the ureter to allow the stone fragments to pass more freely. Extracorporeal shockwave lithotripsy (ESWL) has largely replaced surgery for renal stones. For this treatment the patient is placed in a water bath; newer machines use a water-filled mat. Shockwaves are generated, pass through the water, bounce off a reflector, and break the stone. Sedation is used to help the patient remain calm and still during the 30- to 45-minute procedure. After the procedure, the patient may experience cramping pain and is given pain medications (e.g., hydrocodone-acetaminophen [Vicodin]) if this occurs. A fluid intake of 3000 to 4000 mL is necessary to help wash the stone fragments from the kidney. The fragments travel in the urine down the ureter and into the bladder for excretion. Early ambulation helps mobilize the fluid and the stone fragments so that they can be eliminated in the urine. Newer refinements of this treatment are occurring frequently, with the goal being to break up stones effectively while minimizing the cost and discomfort for the patient.

? *Think Critically About . . .* Based on your knowledge of anatomy and physiology, what is the difference between a *urethral* catheter and a *ureteral* catheter? (Note the spelling difference!) Why is it important to know the difference between these two catheter sites?

Adjunctive therapy for ESWL includes corticosteroids and calcium channel blockers and alpha antagonists (e.g., tamsulosin), which increase the rate of stone passage. Percussion, diuresis, and inversion (PDI) therapy is used after ESWL. In this procedure, diuresis is promoted and the patient is placed in a prone, reverse Trendelenburg position and massaged or percussed to encourage stone movement.

When the stone is not passed spontaneously, cystoscopy or surgical intervention is necessary. Nephrolithotomy (incision into the kidney to remove a stone) or pyelonephrolithotomy (surgical removal of a stone from the renal pelvis) can be performed for large stones that will not pass. These procedures may be done percutaneously or with an open procedure. A special forceps is introduced through the nephroscope to retrieve the stone. A nephrostomy tube is inserted as the scope is removed and this remains in place for 1 to 5 days. A fluid intake of 3000 to 4000 mL/day is required to flush any residual stone fragments out of the kidney. The patient is monitored for infection, hemorrhage, and leakage of fluid into the retroperitoneal cavity. When a stone cannot be retrieved by percutaneous procedure, an open procedure is used. If a stone is lodged in a ureter and will not descend after fluid increases, a ureterolithotomy (surgical removal of a stone from a ureter) is performed

If the stone is 5 mm or greater, the patient could also receive a ureteral stent (usually a soft flexible silicone tube), which is inserted through a cystoscope or nephrostomy tube, or during surgery. The purpose of a ureteral stent is to maintain the patency of the ureter to allow stones to pass through. Stents are not visible on the outside of the body. They are usually removed 4 to 6 weeks in an outpatient setting. Nursing interventions include monitoring for infection, bleeding, urine output, and pain. Once stones have been removed, chemical analyses of the urine, blood, and the stone itself are necessary to plan effective preventive measures. Table 34–3 provides additional information about common catheters and tubes used for urologic disorders.

Table 34–3 *Common Catheters and Tubes Used for Urologic Disorders*

TUBE/CATHETER	PURPOSE
Urethral catheter	Drains urine from the bladder
Foley catheter	Indwelling catheter for continuous urine drainage from the bladder
Suprapubic catheter	Continuous drainage of urine from the bladder; inserted in suprapubic area of abdomen through abdominal and bladder wall
Ureteral catheter	Drains urine directly from the ureter or kidney
Ureteral stent	Tube placed in ureter to hold it open during healing; not visible on the outside of the body
Nephrostomy tube	Placed into the pelvis of the kidney to provide drainage of urine directly from the kidney

Nursing Management

During initial assessment of a patient with kidney stones, you will need to gather information about changes in urinary output, characteristics of the urine, risk factors and history, and other assessment data presented earlier in this chapter.

Attempts are made to have the patient pass the stone spontaneously, and all urine is strained to recover the stone or fragments for analysis. This is accomplished by having the patient void into a urinal or collection device and then pouring the collected urine through a fine mesh filter. Fluids are encouraged during this time to facilitate removal of the stone without surgery.

TRAUMA TO THE UROLOGIC SYSTEM

TRAUMA TO KIDNEYS AND URETERS

Etiology and Pathophysiology

Accidental injury to the kidneys, ureters, bladder, or urethra occurs frequently and should always be considered a possibility whenever there has been trauma to the abdominal cavity, lower back, or thoracic cage. Injury to the kidneys is usually caused by blunt trauma that is sustained during a motor vehicle, sports, or occupational accident. Damage can occur as a result of a direct blow, laceration from an adjacent rib or vertebrae fracture, or from sudden deceleration, which shears and tears the body tissue. Ureteral injuries are mostly associated with penetrating trauma; the right side is three times more likely than the left side to be involved. Trauma to the urinary system can range from minor contusion to severe hemorrhage that leads to hypovolemic shock.

Signs, Symptoms, and Diagnosis

Signs and symptoms characteristic of trauma to the kidneys include massive hemorrhage, hematuria, abdominal or flank pain, and possibly an enlarged mass in the kidney area. Diagnostic tests include serial urinalyses, hemoglobin and hematocrit tests, and measurements of electrolytes. Rising BUN and serum creatinine levels indicate diminishing renal function. Radiologic studies (KUB, IVP, or CT scan) can demonstrate the extent of damage to the urinary system. MRI or angiography is used in high-risk cases or if CT scan is indeterminate. Hourly measurements of urinary output and observation of the characteristics of the urine can help determine the type and extent of injury.

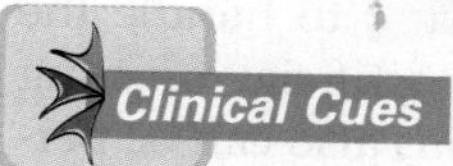

When your patient sustains significant trauma to skeletal muscle tissue, she may develop rhabdomyolysis. Damaged muscles release myoglobin into the bloodstream, and these large muscle proteins can cause **acute renal failure** (sudden loss of kidney function); however, the condition is reversible. Be alert for brown or tea-colored urine after trauma, strenuous exercise, or extensive burns, and report your findings to the physician.

Treatment

Bleeding in the kidney is often self-limiting. Lacerations and contusions without interruption of urinary function usually can be treated conservatively by bed rest. For this reason, the urologist may advocate a period of watchful waiting to see whether the kidney can be saved. If the kidney is severely damaged, the patient may undergo a nephrectomy (surgical removal of the kidney). Although this is always a serious operation, a person may live with only one kidney. The remaining kidney enlarges and is usually able to carry on the work formerly done by two kidneys.

Nursing Management

Preoperative Nursing Care. Patients with kidney trauma are likely to have damage to the colon, spleen, or pancreas. A comprehensive plan for dealing with problems associated with multiple trauma is usually necessary. Preoperatively, the patient is monitored closely for signs of hypovolemic shock, cardiovascular changes, urinary output, and size of the flank mass. Grey Turner sign is bruising over the flank or lower back and suggests retroperitoneal bleeding. For most trauma patients, a urethral catheter is inserted into the bladder. An indwelling catheter allows for close observation of urinary output. For example, critically ill patients may need hourly urine output measurements, and a drainage bag with a urometer should replace the standard drainage bag.

Postoperative Nursing Care. Postoperative nursing care for nephrectomy or nephrostomy was described earlier in the chapter (see Postoperative Nursing Care under Hydronephrosis). Refer to Nursing Care Plan 34–1 on the CD-ROM for nursing care of a patient with renal lithiasis.

TRAUMA TO THE BLADDER

Etiology and Pathophysiology

Any violent blow or crushing injury to the lower abdomen may result in rupture or perforation of the bladder wall, with resulting leakage of the urine into the pelvic tissues or peritoneal cavity. This results in severe inflammation (peritonitis). Bladder trauma is more likely if the bladder is full at the time of an accident than if it is empty.

Signs and Symptoms

Early symptoms of bladder injury are painful hematuria or inability to void, marked tenderness and spasm in the suprapubic area, or the development of a large mass in that area.

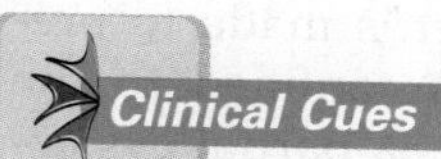

Bleeding at the urethral meatus, inability to void, or a distended bladder may indicate a urethral tear, which should be suspected in cases of pelvic or perineal trauma. Especially if bleeding is noted, notify the physician prior to inserting a catheter, because catheter insertion can extend a urethral tear.

Diagnosis and Treatment

Diagnosis is based on presence of gross hematuria, suprapubic pain, and difficulty voiding. Retrograde or CT cystography is obtained if bladder injuries are suspected. If the bladder has ruptured or is perforated, treatment consists of a suprapubic cystostomy to drain blood and urine.

Nursing Management

Care of the patient demands meticulous attention to drains and dressings to avoid infection and maintain good drainage. Cold applications to the surgical site both before and after surgery may be ordered. You should observe the patient carefully for postoperative shock and massive hemorrhage. Any mass formation in the suprapubic area before or after surgery or any change in vital signs should be reported immediately.

CANCERS OF THE UROLOGIC SYSTEM

CANCER OF THE BLADDER

Etiology and Pathophysiology

Approximately 260,000 new cases of bladder cancer are diagnosed worldwide every year. This cancer occurs more often in men (ages 60 to 80) than in women. **Smokers have double the risk of developing this cancer.** People living in urban areas or with occupational exposure (i.e., painters, hairdressers, or textile workers) to nitrates, dyes, rubber, or leather processing are at higher risk. Tumors of the bladder usually start in the superficial transitional cell layer and are considered to be papillomas (benign tumors on the epithelial tissue). Bladder tumors are removed, even though they are papillomas, because there is a high risk for invasion into the deeper tissues and metastasis.

Signs, Symptoms, and Diagnosis

The main symptom of a bladder tumor is hematuria. Frequency, urgency, or dysuria also may be present. Diagnosis is confirmed by IVP and by examining the bladder wall with a cystoscope and biopsy of the tumor (Complementary & Alternative Therapies 34–2).

Treatment

Treatment for bladder cancer is surgery, either alone or in combination with chemotherapy or radiation. The type of surgical treatment depends on the clinical stage of the tumor. Every effort is made to preserve the bladder if the tumor is confined to the mucosa or submucosa. In this case, a partial cystectomy or transurethral resection of the bladder tumor (TURB, TURBT) is performed and followed by intravesical chemotherapy (i.e., cisplatin [Platinol], doxorubicin [Adriamycin]) or bacille Calmette-Guérin (BCG) instillations (Intravesical, TheraCys). BCG was originally used as a vaccine against tuberculosis. It has been found to help patients with bladder carcinoma in situ (site of origin) by reducing tumor recurrence and by eliminating residual malignant cells after surgery. The solution is instilled into the bladder via a urinary catheter. The catheter is clamped for 2 hours and the patient's position is changed every 15 to 30 minutes. Treatments are continued weekly for 6 weeks with possible maintenance doses.

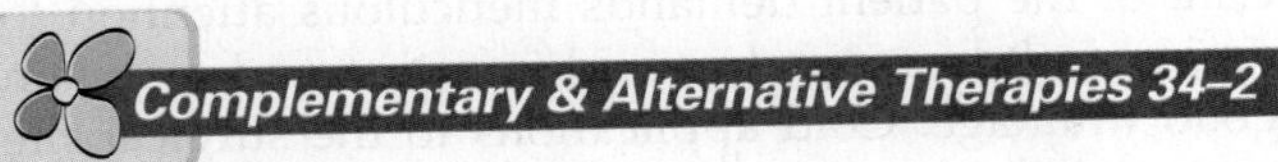

Healthy Bladder

Smoking cessation and including vegetables such as cabbage or broccoli in the diet contribute to a healthy bladder and a decreased risk of bladder cancer.

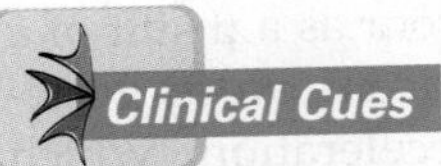

In addition to using universal precautions, when disposing of the urine after a BCG treatment, the toilet should be disinfected with bleach for 6 hours after disposing the waste.

Advise your patient that use of BCG intravesical therapy may cause future PPD (purified protein derivative) skin tests for tuberculosis to show positive.

Photodynamic therapy can be used for superficial tumors. In this therapy, a solution of light-sensitive molecules is injected IV. These molecules adhere to cancer cells longer than to normal cells. A cystoscope with a red laser light can then be used to activate the photosensitizers that destroy tumor cells.

Surgeries for Urinary Diversion. Bladder surgery may be minor, such as removing polyps from the bladder interior using a cystoscope, or major, such as cystectomy (removal of the bladder) for bladder cancer. Following cystectomy, there is always the danger of hemorrhage and infection. There also are problems involved in devising a satisfactory arrangement for urine collection. When the bladder is surgically removed, the surgeon performs a **urinary diversion** to handle the excretion of urine and creates an artificial opening (stoma) to the skin surface. Diversions also can be performed for neurogenic bladder, congenital anomalies, strictures, or trauma. There are several ways in which urinary diversion can be accomplished (Figure 34–2), including ileal conduit or ileal loop, cutaneous ureterostomy, vesicostomy, ureterosigmoidostomy or sigmoid conduit, and ileal reservoir (i.e., Kock, Indiana, Mainz, or Florida pouch). The difference in these various procedures is the segment of bowel that is used.

Cutaneous Ureterostomy and Vesicotomy. Ureterostomy is a surgical incision into the ureter that diverts the flow of urine. In a cutaneous ureterostomy, the surgeon detaches one or both ureters from the bladder and brings them to the surface of the body, usually in the region of the flank. The patient may have one or two stomas. If the patient has a cutaneous ureterostomy with two stomas (one from each ureter), the flow of urine, from each stoma, must be measured. Any tubing leading from the ureterostomy should be kept open so that urine can flow freely. The tube is checked frequently for signs of obstruction by mucus or blood clots.

A vesicotomy is an incision into the bladder just above the pubic area. After incising the bladder, the surgeon moves it forward and sutures the cut edges to the skin, forming a stoma.

Ileal Conduit. An ileal conduit is also called *urinary ileostomy* and *ileal loop* or *Bricker's procedure.* A portion of the ileum is used as a tube or conduit through which urine flows to the outside. It is important to realize that the section of ileum is separated from the intestinal tract. Urine does *not* flow through it to the intestines, as when the ureters are sutured to the sigmoid. The two open ends of the intestines where the section of ileum was removed are rejoined by anastomosis (operative union of structures). The surgeon cuts out a portion of the ileum, leaving nerve and blood supply intact so that it remains a viable tissue. The "borrowed" section of ileum is sutured together at one end to form a pouch, and the other end is brought outside to form a stoma. The ureters are attached to the ileal conduit so that urine can flow through the conduit to the outside.

Ureterosigmoidostomy or Sigmoid Conduit. A sigmoid or colonic conduit is similar to an ileal conduit, the difference being that a portion of the sigmoid colon is used to form the conduit. The ureters are implanted in the conduit.

Ileal Reservoir (Kock Pouch). This procedure creates a continent ileal reservoir. The ureters are implanted into a segment of ileum that has been isolated. Special nipple valves connect the pouch to the exterior of the skin. The pouch can then be catheterized via the nipple valve by the patient, providing continence with no exterior collection device. The distal nipple valve is

Ureterostomies divert urine directly to the skin surface through a ureteral skin opening (stoma). After ureterostomy, the client must wear a pouch.

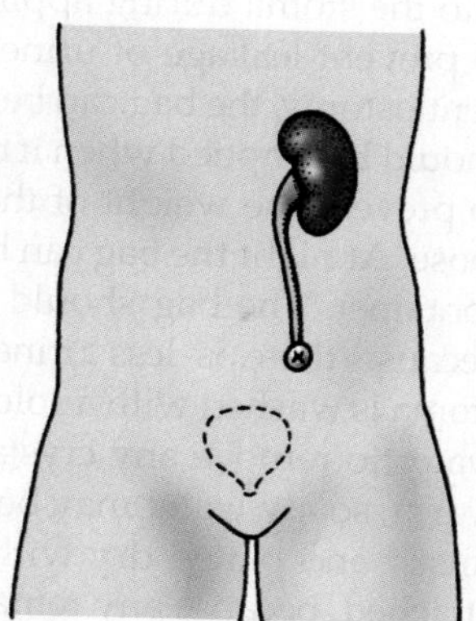

Cutaneous ureterostomy

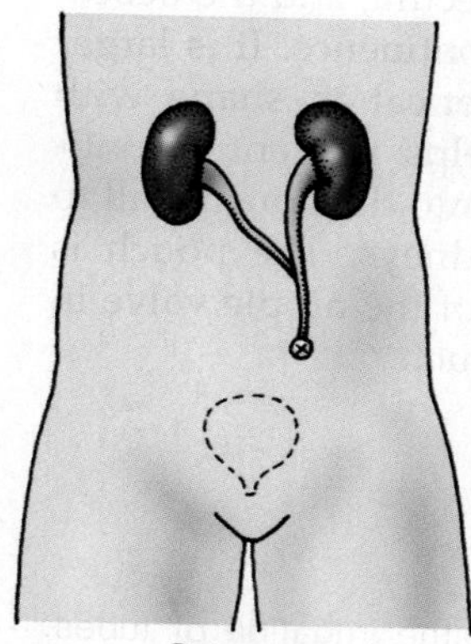

Cutaneous ureteroureterostomy

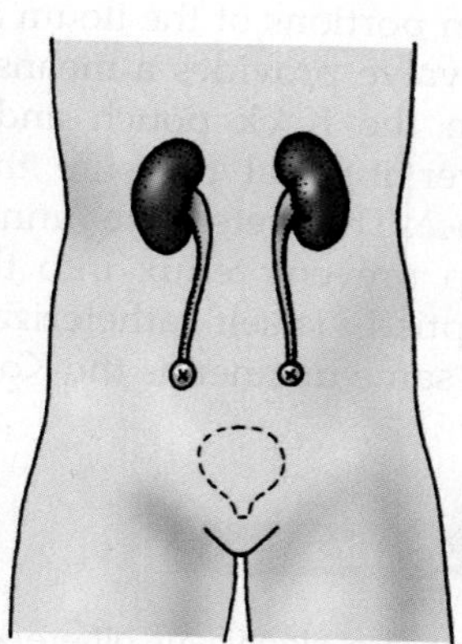

Bilateral cutaneous ureterostomy

Conduits collect urine in a portion of the intestine, which is then opened onto the skin surface as a stoma. After the creation of a conduit, the client must wear a pouch.

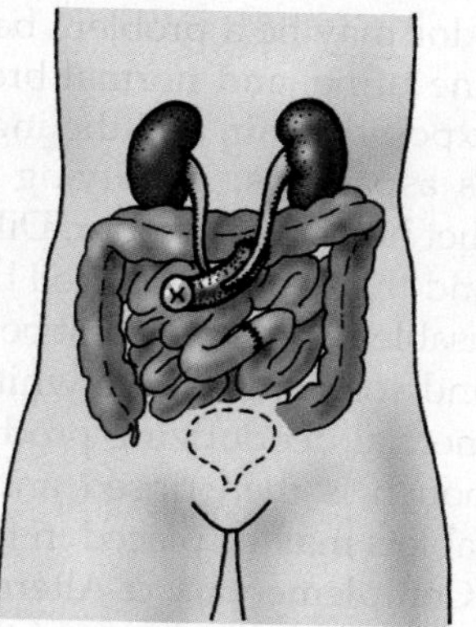

Ileal (Bricker's) conduit

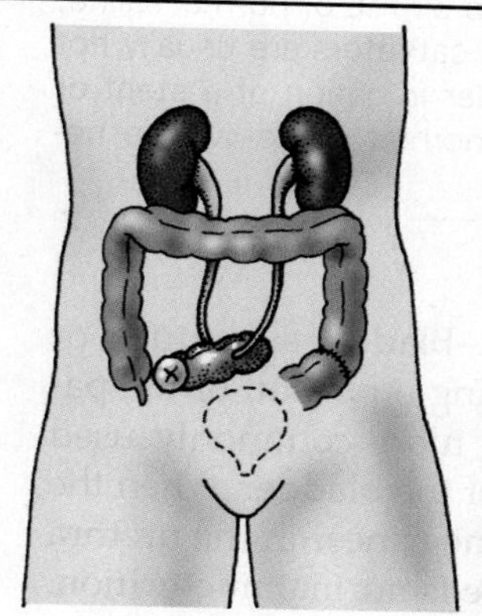

Colon conduit

Ileal reservoirs divert urine into a surgically created pouch, or pocket, that functions as a bladder. The stoma is continent, and the client removes urine by regular self-catheterization.

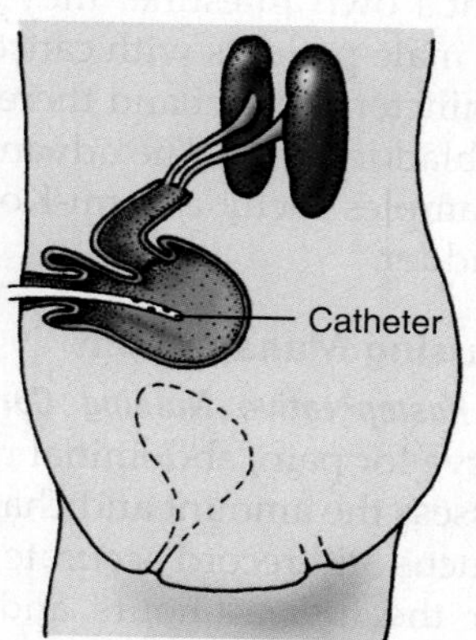

Continent internal ileal reservoir (Kock pouch)

Sigmoidostomies divert urine to the large intestine, so no stoma is required. The client excretes urine with bowel movements, and bowel incontinence may result.

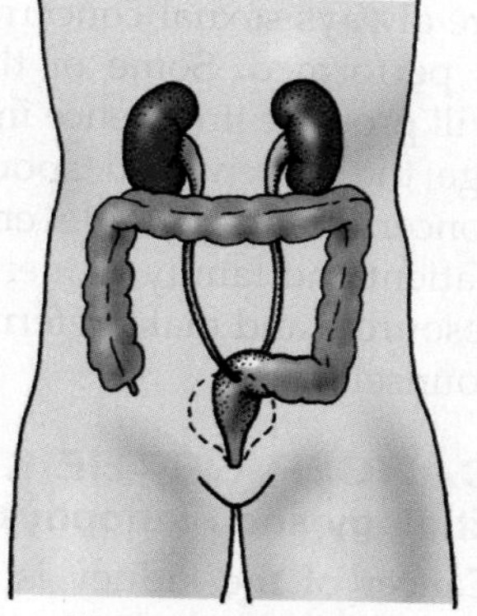

Ureterosigmoidostomy

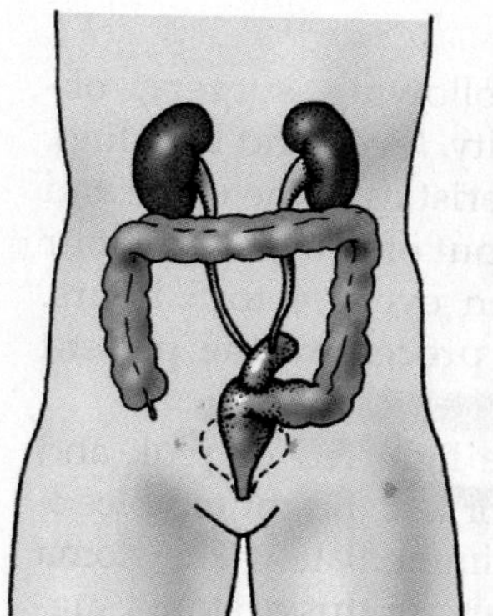

Ureteroiliosigmoidostomy

FIGURE 34–2 Surgeries for urinary diversion.

brought flush to the skin on the right side of the abdomen, forming a stoma. The patient is continent of urine, but needs to catheterize the pouch several times a day to empty the urine. An adhesive bandage or gauze pad over the stoma will absorb the secreted mucus. Daily irrigation of the pouch is performed to remove the threads of mucus in the urine that are secreted by the mucous membrane of the ileal or colonic segment of the conduit. Whitish crystals or encrustations in or near the stoma indicate alkaline urine; this should be reported so that treatment can be prescribed to prevent stone formation.

Indiana Pouch. This type of pouch is constructed from portions of the ileum and cecum, and the ileocecal valve provides a means of continence. It is larger than the Kock pouch and spherical in shape with lower internal pressure that helps prevent incontinence. The ureters are tunneled into the pouch wall to help prevent reflux into the kidneys. The pouch is emptied via self-catheterization of the nipple valve in the same manner as the Kock pouch.

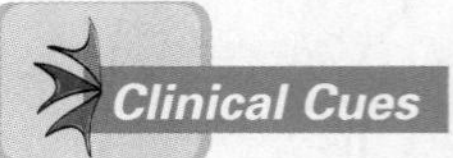

There are significant differences in the irrigation of tubes, drains, and stomas for the urinary system, so make sure to **clarify orders!** For example, the Indiana pouch should be irrigated four times a day with 30 to 60 mL of normal saline, whereas ureteral stents or ureteral catheters are usually not irrigated. If the physician does order irrigation of a stent or ureteral catheter, the amount of normal saline will be between 3 and 10 mL.

Orthotic Bladder Substitutes. Bladder substitutes or neobladders can be created using a portion of the patient's own intestine; they are more commonly used for male patients with cancer of the bladder, when the sphincter is intact and there is no cancer in the urethra or bladder neck. The advantage is normal micturition. Examples include hemi-Kock, Studer, or ileal W-neobladder.

Nursing Management

Postoperative Nursing Care. Following surgery, observe for pain, abdominal rigidity, fever, and bleeding. Assess the amount and characteristics of the urine and mucus and record accurate output of urine every hour for the first 24 hours and then every 4 to 8 hours. **Regardless of which surgical procedure the patient has had the urine should never stop flowing.**

The urine should initially be light red or pink and progress to clear within 3 days or less. Bright red bleeding or clots should be reported immediately. The stoma should be pink or red. A pale, dark, or dusky stoma suggests decreased blood flow, which should be reported immediately. Skin irritation and breakdown can be a

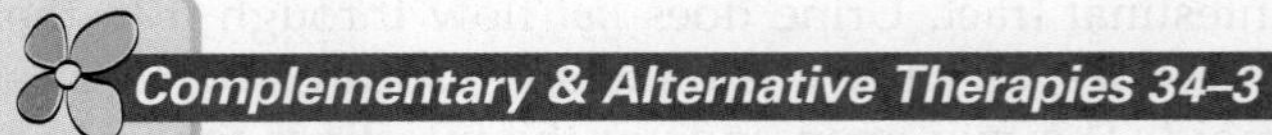

Reduce Odor

Encourage your patient to eat whole grains, nuts, plums, and prunes, and to drink cranberry juice. These foods will acidify the urine and help to decrease odors.

problem, and every effort is made to keep urine from touching the skin when the patient has an external stoma. A well-fitted and properly adhering collection appliance is essential. A thin gauze roll or tampon is placed into the stoma during appliance changing and cleaning, to prevent leakage of urine onto the skin. For a permanent ostomy, the bag can be used for 3 to 7 days. The bag should be emptied when it becomes one third to half full, to prevent the weight of the urine from pulling the bag loose. At night the bag can be connected to a larger urine container. The bag should be changed in the morning because there is less urine flow. The area around the stoma is washed with a solution of 1:1 vinegar and warm water to remove any crystals. If no crystals are present, warm, soapy water may be used. The area is thoroughly rinsed and patted dry with a towel before a new bag is attached, because any remaining moisture may interfere with the seal of the new appliance. A bath or shower may be taken with the bag on or off.

Most appliances contain an odor barrier; however, odor may be a problem because of poor hygiene, alkaline urine, and normal breakdown of urine when it is exposed to air, and the ingestion of certain foods, such as asparagus. Acidifying the urine by modifying the diet helps reduce odor. Dilute urine is also less odorous and this is accomplished by increasing fluid intake. Reusable appliances must be washed with soap and water and soaked in dilute white vinegar solution or a commercial deodorizing product for 20 to 30 minutes. The pouch is then rinsed and allowed to dry. Deodorant tablets may be placed in the appliance to decrease odor (Complementary & Alternative Therapies 34–3).

Psychological care of the patient facing malignancy and an operation that will radically change his body image should be a primary nursing concern, and there are always sexual concerns when a urinary diversion is performed. Some of the more radical procedures will produce impotence in the male. You must encourage the patient and spouse to talk about fears and concerns and provide emotional support. Help the patient and family to identify appropriate community resources and make referrals as needed for specialized counseling.

CANCER OF THE KIDNEY

Etiology and Pathophysiology

Cancer of the kidney is relatively uncommon; however, these tumors are extremely difficult to treat in the later stages. Neoplasms of the kidney occur in men (ages 50 to 70) twice as often as in women. Risk factors include smoking and exposure to lead or phosphate. Wilms' tumor is a kidney tumor that occurs primarily in children ages 2 to 3 years. Although the prognosis does depend on stage and cell type, most children with this tumor will survive.

The tumors usually begin growing in the renal cortex. They can become very large, but they are well defined and press into the renal structures rather than invade the tissue. The blood vessels also can become constricted by the tumor growth.

Signs, Symptoms, and Diagnosis

The principal symptoms of malignant tumors of the kidney are hematuria, palpable abdominal or flank mass, and flank pain, although pain and a mass may not be present in the early stages. Other symptoms that may occur are fever, fatigue, weight loss, decreased appetite, and hypertension. Tests such as renal angiogram, arteriogram, CT, MRI, and ultrasound are performed to determine whether the symptoms are being caused by a cyst (nonmalignant) or a tumor.

Treatment and Nursing Management

The only treatment that has met with any degree of success is surgical removal of the affected kidney (nephrectomy) before metastasis has occurred. Unfortunately, this is difficult to achieve, because the patient usually does not have severe symptoms until metastases have occurred. Chemotherapy with a variety of drug regimens is used for metastatic cancer. Immunotherapy is sometimes attempted for recurrent tumors. (See Chapter 8 for discussion of chemotherapy.)

In January 2006, the Food and Drug Administration (FDA) announced approval of a new drug, sunitinib (Sutent) for the treatment of advanced kidney cancer. This drug acts to deprive the tumor cells of blood and nutrients. Sorafenib tosylate (Nexavar) is another drug recently FDA approved for advanced renal cell carcinoma. Several other new types of drugs are in clinical trials.

Nursing care of the patient is the same as that for patients after nephrectomy. (Also see Chapter 8 for care of patients with cancer.)

RENAL FAILURE

Renal failure is the inability of the kidneys to maintain normal function. Renal failure is classified as acute or chronic. The final stage of chronic and irreversible renal failure is called end-stage renal disease (ESRD).

ACUTE RENAL FAILURE

Etiology

Acute renal failure (ARF) occurs suddenly as a result of physical injury, infection, inflammation, or damage from toxic chemicals. Nephrotoxic agents are those that are poisonous to kidney cells and include many drugs, iodine substances used as x-ray contrast media, heavy metals, snake venom, or exposure to industrial chemicals. These toxins may inflict damage on the renal tubules, causing acute tubular necrosis (ATN) and loss of function. They can also indirectly harm the tubules by causing severe constriction of blood vessels that serve the kidney, producing renal ischemia. ATN is responsible for 90% of acute renal failure. Other causes of renal ischemia include circulatory collapse, severe dehydration, and prolonged hypotension in certain compromised surgical or trauma patients.

Pathophysiology

The pathophysiology of ARF is not well understood. One theory is that cellular or protein debris in the tubules blocks the flow of urine and filtration stops. Another theory is that decreased blood flow results in oxygen deprivation, which causes cellular death and tubular necrosis.

There are three types of acute renal failure, depending on the cause. *Prerenal ARF* is caused by decreased blood flow, such as in hypovolemic shock, or decreased cardiac output, as in cardiogenic shock. *Intrarenal ARF* occurs from glomerular damage, ATN caused by ischemia or toxins, or vascular disease that affects the vessels in the kidney. *Postrenal ARF* is caused by obstruction in the ureters, bladder, or urethra, for example, an enlarged prostate, which causes eventual backup of urine into the kidney that leads to tissue damage. ARF is potentially reversible, especially if identified early. Often the patient regains kidney function. Concept Map 34–1 shows the manifestations of renal failure.

> ? *Think Critically About* . . . During your clinical experience, which of your patients may have been at risk for ARF? What factors placed these patients at risk?

The course of acute tubular necrosis is divided into three phases: oliguric/nonoliguric, diuretic, and recovery phases. In the oliguric/nonoliguric phase, the patient puts out either a great deal or very little urine. Oliguria is a urine output of 100 to 400 mL in 24 hours. This phase usually occurs immediately or within 1 week after an ischemic event and lasts for an average of 10 to 14 days; however, it can go on for weeks to months. and prolonged oliguria worsens the prognosis. BUN and creatinine levels rise. When this occurs, there may be volume overload, which can precipitate heart failure, multiple electrolyte imbalances, metabolic acidosis, catabolism (destructive breakdown of body tissue), and end-stage renal failure (ESRF). At this point, dialysis is needed.

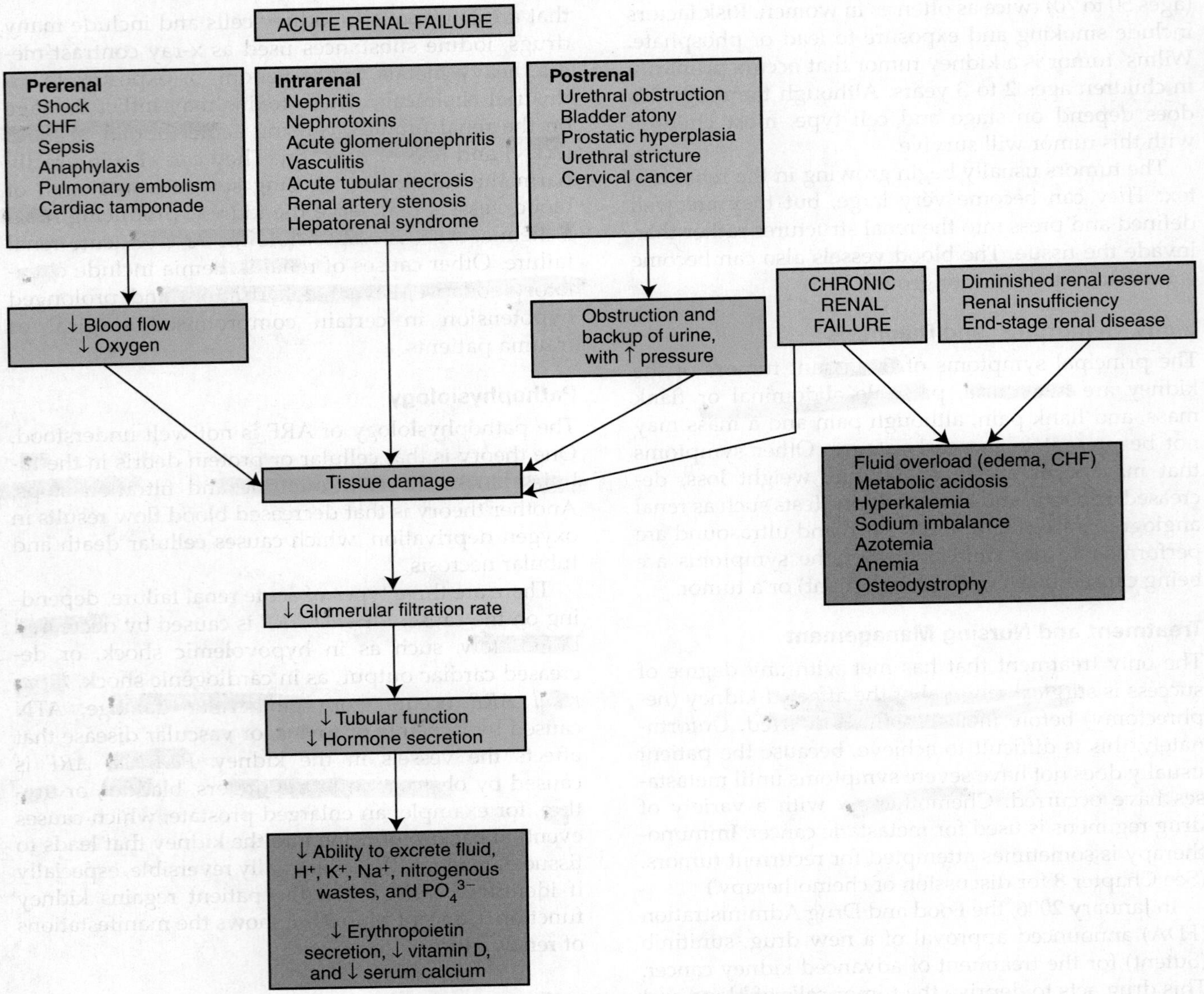

ACUTE RENAL FAILURE

Prerenal
Shock
CHF
Sepsis
Anaphylaxis
Pulmonary embolism
Cardiac tamponade

Intrarenal
Nephritis
Nephrotoxins
Acute glomerulonephritis
Vasculitis
Acute tubular necrosis
Renal artery stenosis
Hepatorenal syndrome

Postrenal
Urethral obstruction
Bladder atony
Prostatic hyperplasia
Urethral stricture
Cervical cancer

↓ Blood flow
↓ Oxygen

Obstruction and backup of urine, with ↑ pressure

CHRONIC RENAL FAILURE

Diminished renal reserve
Renal insufficiency
End-stage renal disease

Tissue damage

Fluid overload (edema, CHF)
Metabolic acidosis
Hyperkalemia
Sodium imbalance
Azotemia
Anemia
Osteodystrophy

↓ Glomerular filtration rate

↓ Tubular function
↓ Hormone secretion

↓ Ability to excrete fluid, H^+, K^+, Na^+, nitrogenous wastes, and PO_4^{3-}

↓ Erythropoietin secretion, ↓ vitamin D, and ↓ serum calcium

CONCEPT MAP **34–1** Pathophysiology of renal failure.

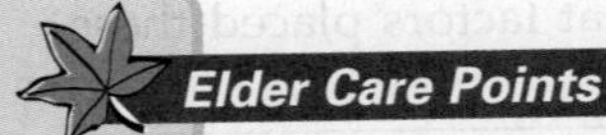

Elder Care Points

Because of the overall decreased kidney function related to aging, your elderly patient may be experiencing oliguria at urine volumes as high as 600 to 700 mL/day.

Nonoliguric ATN is often due to nephrotoxic agents. Urine output is greater, but the kidneys cannot eliminate waste products efficiently, and BUN and creatinine levels rise and electrolyte imbalances occur. Dialysis is needed less often or for shorter periods, and the prognosis is better than for oliguric failure.

The diuretic phase only occurs if dialysis has not been started early and extracellular fluid volume has built up. In this phase, the kidney is unable to concentrate urine, and output can be between 1000 and 2000 mL/day. With this increased output, there is a danger of dehydration, hyponatremia, and hypokalemia. Approximately, 25% of deaths related to ARF occur during this phase.

The recovery phase begins as the kidney function begins to normalize. The concentration of urine, urine output, and electrolyte balance begin to recover. There are 1 to 2 weeks of rapid improvement and then a period of slower recovery lasting between 3 and 12 months. About one third of ARF patients are left with residual renal insufficiency, and about 5% must continue dialysis.

Signs and Symptoms

Renal failure will have impact on the entire body, and the signs and symptoms will vary according to the phase and response to treatment. Carefully observe for any of the following:

- Changes in urine output and urine results (e.g., specific gravity, proteinuria)

- Electrolyte imbalances (e.g., hyponatremia, hyperkalemia, hypocalcemia)
- Fluid imbalance (e.g., hypotension, hypertension, edema, pulmonary edema)
- Acid-base imbalance (e.g., metabolic acidosis)
- Gastrointestinal effects (e.g., nausea, vomiting, anorexia, constipation)
- Mental status changes (e.g., lethargy, memory impairment)
- Anemia and platelet dysfunction (e.g., fatigue, bleeding signs, and bruising)
- Impaired wound healing and susceptibility to infection

Diagnosis

Diagnostic testing includes urinalysis, creatinine, BUN, CBC, electrolytes and arterial blood gases. In addition, radiologic studies, such as ultrasound, IVP, CT, or MRI can be performed if an obstruction is suspected. A renal biopsy may be obtained to assist in determining etiology or to evaluate the extent of kidney damage.

Treatment

Treatment of ARF is geared toward correcting the underlying cause and preventing or controlling complications. The goal of treatment is to restore and maintain a tolerable internal environment until the kidneys are able to recover and resume their normal functions. Symptomatic treatment includes correction of fluid and electrolyte balances, management of anemia and hypertension, and cleansing the blood and tissues of waste products with **hemodialysis** (filtration of blood across a semipermeable membrane) or **peritoneal dialysis** (filtration of blood, across the peritoneal membrane). Volume overload is treated with diuretics and sometimes low-dose dopamine to promote better kidney perfusion. Dialysis is also used to reduce volume overload if it cannot be reduced with the drugs. Electrolyte imbalances (hyperkalemia, hypocalcemia, hyperphosphatemia, and mild hypermagnesemia) are monitored and treated. Metabolic acidosis, if severe, is treated with IV sodium bicarbonate. Dialysis with buffer in the dialysate may be used.

Other problems include malnutrition, anemia, and potential for infection. The catabolic state is treated with nutritional management through total parenteral nutrition (TPN). This is necessary to provide adequate nutrients. Potassium, phosphate, and magnesium are omitted from the solution while the patient is oliguric. Anemia occurs because the kidney cannot produce normal amounts of erythropoietin. The life span of RBCs is shortened because of both the toxic wastes circulating in the blood and the hemodilution from fluid overload. To treat this anemia, the physician may order epoetin alpha (Epogen), a synthetic substance that stimulates red blood cell production. Infection frequently occurs with ARF and is the leading cause of death in these patients. You must be vigilant in monitoring for signs of infection that could be associated with IV access sites, drains and tubes, and lowered immunity state.

Continuous Renal Replacement Therapies (Continuous Hemofiltration). *Continuous renal replacement therapies* (CRRTs) can be used for intensive care unit (ICU) patients with ARF and multisystem organ involvement or those that are hemodynamically unstable. A double-lumen catheter is inserted into the subclavian, jugular, or femoral vein. The blood passes through a special hollow-fiber filter and returns to the vein. This method filters out wastes much more slowly than hemodialysis but does not cause such rapid fluid and electrolyte shifts. Continuous venovenous hemofiltration (CVVH) and continuous venovenous hemodiafiltration (CVVHDF) are newer methods and controlled by a pump. Continuous arteriovenous hemofiltration (CAVH) and continuous arteriovenous hemodialysis (CAVHD) are older methods that use the patient's own blood pressure to pump the blood; therefore, clotting during the procedure is a possible problem.

NURSING MANAGEMENT

Assessment (Data Collection)

When taking a patient's history, include questions that relate to fluid imbalance (e.g., changes in voiding patterns, weight gain, vomiting, or edema). Collect information about potential risk factors (e.g., patient or family history of renal disease or hypertension, recent surgery, trauma, or anesthesia, exposure to nephrotoxic substances, and medications, including over-the-counter). The patient should also be encouraged to describe specific symptoms (e.g., fatigue, lethargy, weakness, or pain).

All patients need a complete head-to-toe assessment at the beginning of every shift. This includes taking complete vital signs. Acutely ill patients require frequent reassessment, and patients at risk for ARF need extra vigilance for signs of fluid retention (e.g., skin turgor, edema, lungs sounds, weight, and strict intake and output) and for imbalances in electrolytes (e.g., change of mental status or cardiac dysrhythmias).

Nursing Diagnosis and Planning

Nursing diagnoses frequently associated with ARF, but not restricted to:

- Excess fluid volume related to decreased kidney function
- Imbalanced nutrition: less than body requirements, related to nausea and loss of appetite
- Activity intolerance related to metabolic changes
- Risk for infection related to indwelling urinary catheter
- Ineffective individual coping related to sudden change in health status and hospitalization

Examples of expected outcomes include:

- Patient will have no signs of fluid overload (e.g., weight gain, edema, crackles in lungs, decreased urinary output) for the next 2 hours.
- Patient will report nausea and receive sufficient calories (based on dietitian's calculation) to prevent catabolism (destructive breakdown of body tissue) during this shift.
- Patient will maintain bed rest and participate in ADLs as much as possible (e.g., brushes own teeth) during this shift.
- Patient will not have any signs or symptoms of infection (e.g., fever, cloudy urine) during hospitalization.
- Patient will verbalize two ways to cope with hospitalization during this shift.

Implementation

You must carefully monitor for signs of fluid imbalance. This includes physical assessment of edema, daily weights, and lung sounds. Strict input and out (I&O) is essential. In the acute phase, hourly measurements of urine output are necessary and sudden changes in output or an amount of less than 30 mL/hr must be reported immediately.

Equipment, such as IV control pumps, should be used for accurate and safe delivery of IV fluids. In intensive care settings, arterial monitoring or central venous lines provide additional information about fluid status. Electrolytes should be monitored and may manifest as changes in mental status or cardiac dysrhythmias. The patient may be too ill to eat and require TPN or enteral feedings. Even if the patient is unable to eat, efforts should be made to reduce noxious stimuli that exacerbate nausea, and antiemetics can be administered. Provide assistance with ADLs as needed during the acute phase and progressively provide opportunities for the patient to participate as fatigue resolves. To prevent infection, you should be vigilant for signs and symptoms of infection. Wash your hands frequently and encourage others to do so as well. Most institutions require use of surgical aseptic technique for procedures, such as Foley catheter insertion, or central line dressing changes. You can help the patient and the family cope with the stress of this serious condition by allowing them to express concerns and fears, and by providing accurate information and appropriate referrals.

Evaluation

Evaluation of outcomes for acutely ill patients must occur frequently, because the plan of care may need frequent revision. For example, **if the hourly urine output drops below 30 mL/hr, the physician must be immediately notified.** The patient should be assessed for signs of worsening, such as shortness of breath and lung crackles associated with pulmonary edema, or decreased cardiac output associated with heart failure. The patient may have to be transferred from a general medical-surgical unit to the ICU if the condition becomes unstable.

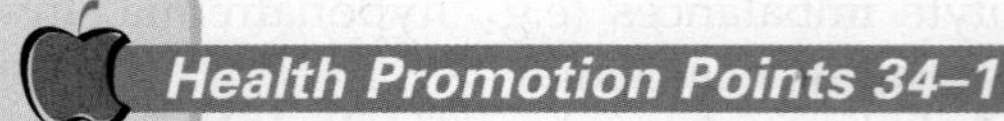

Health Promotion Points 34–1

Diabetes Mellitus

Diabetic nephropathy (kidney disease and dysfunction secondary to diabetes mellitus) is the most common cause of death in patients with diabetes mellitus. In keeping with the *Healthy People 2010* goal, "to reduce kidney failure due to diabetes," help your patients to understand the interrelationship between diabetes and kidney health. For example, you could say, "Mr. Smith, when your blood sugar goes up, protein starts to leak into your urine. This causes an increased pressure in the kidney vessels, which eventually leads to kidney damage."

CHRONIC RENAL FAILURE

Etiology

Chronic renal failure (CRF) is a progressive loss of kidney function that develops over the course of many months or years. CRF is caused by destruction of the nephrons. All the causes of ARF may also cause CRF. Hypertension, diabetes mellitus, sickle cell disease, glomerulonephritis, nephrotic syndrome, lupus erythematosus, heart failure, and cirrhosis of the liver may also contribute to CRF (Health Promotion Points 34–1).

The most common causes of CRF are glomerulonephritis and nephrosclerosis. **The primary causes of nephrosclerosis are hypertension and atherosclerotic disease of the small arteries in the kidneys.** As the blood supply decreases, the kidney cells degenerate and lose their ability to function, resulting in ESRD. Nephrosclerosis is classified as benign or malignant, depending on the severity of the disease and the speed with which hypertensive and atherosclerotic changes occur. The symptoms of nephrosclerosis are similar to those of chronic glomerulonephritis and renal failure. Treatment is the control of hypertension.

Pathophysiology

In the early stages of the disease, renal function can be adequate, but the waste products will begin to accumulate in the plasma. The patient does not experience symptoms until about 65% of the kidney tissue is damaged. As the disease progresses, nitrogenous waste products, such as urea nitrogen and creatinine, build up to higher levels in the blood. In the final or end stage of renal failure, 90% or more of kidney function is lost. **Azotemia** is the accumulation of nitrogenous products, which is signaled by an increase in BUN and serum creatinine. The patient may experience nausea and vomiting and changes in mental awareness and levels of consciousness. **The kidney is not able to excrete potassium; therefore, be alert for high levels of**

serum potassium (5 to 7 mEq/L), which can adversely affect the heart, causing dysrhythmia and arrest.

There are three stages of CRF. In stage 1 there is diminished renal reserve but no accumulation of metabolic wastes. The healthier kidney works harder. Urine concentration is decreased and polyuria and nocturia occur. Stage 2 is renal insufficiency and is signaled by a rise in circulating metabolic wastes; therefore, BUN and serum creatinine levels begin to rise. The glomerular filtration rate falls and oliguria and edema occur. Stage 3 is ESRD. Circulating metabolic wastes accumulate in the blood, homeostasis cannot be maintained, electrolyte and fluid imbalances are serious, and dialysis or kidney transplant is necessary to maintain life.

Signs and Symptoms

The symptoms of CRF do not appear early in the disease. A high normal elevation of BUN is an early warning sign, and the patient is likely to be asymptomatic. One of the earliest signs of renal impairment is the inability of the kidneys to concentrate urine. This produces polyuria and very dilute urine and the patient may report nocturia. Renal insufficiency, which occurs before renal failure, can produce occasional headaches and fatigue, but these symptoms usually either go unnoticed or unreported by the patient. At this point, the kidney function is about 20% to 40% of normal. When symptoms do become apparent, kidney function can be as little as 5% to 10% of normal. As renal insufficiency progresses, the kidneys may not be able to produce much urine at all. This causes oliguria and eventually anuria.

Uremia or **uremic syndrome** includes the clinical signs and symptoms that affect the entire body during ESRD. Uremia signs generally appear when BUN concentration passes 100 mg/dL. The presence of uremic signs is the absolute indicator for initiating dialysis and the goal is to maintain BUN below 100 mg/dL and to keep creatinine below 8 mg/dL.

The skin becomes dry, scaly, and a pallid yellowish gray. Pruritus (severe itching) occurs. Uremic frost (a late sign) appears as evaporated sweat leaves urea crystals on the eyebrows, face, axilla, and groin. Calcium is not absorbed from the intestinal tract, and this leads to the loss of calcium from the body and a corresponding drop in serum calcium. If the hypocalcemia is not corrected, the patient will eventually suffer from muscle cramps, twitching, and possibly seizures. As kidney cells cease to function, they are progressively less able to secrete phosphorus in the urine. An elevated serum phosphate level (hyperphosphatemia) serves to exaggerate the problem of inadequate calcium absorption; phosphate binds with calcium, decreasing its absorption from the intestinal tract. The patient is hypertensive from fluid overload and body weight increases. Pulmonary edema and heart failure may occur. Metabolic changes occur, including triglyceride elevation and carbohydrate intolerance. Dietary protein is restricted in an attempt to decrease the waste products that the kidney can no longer handle; therefore, serum protein decreases. Anemia is present due to decreased production of erythropoietin. Anorexia, nausea, and vomiting occur because of gastrointestinal mucosa irritation from waste products circulating in the blood. Constipation often occurs from drug therapy and fluid restriction. Complaints about restless leg syndrome are frequent, and the leg discomfort may interfere with sleep. When circulating wastes are increased, the nervous system cells become irritated and the patient can become irritable and short-tempered. Figure 34–3 shows the manifestations of uremia.

Diagnosis

Creatinine is a stable by-product of skeletal muscle activity, which is excreted completely by the kidneys; therefore creatinine clearance (CC) is a good measure of GFR. CC depends on the amount of blood passing through the kidney; narrowing of the renal arterioles, shock, or dehydration decreases the volume that is available to the kidney for filtration. CC is also affected by the functional abilities of the glomeruli. Urine is collected for a 24-hour period. Urinalysis with culture and sensitivity, hematocrit, and hemoglobin provide additional information. A renal ultrasound, a renal scan, CT scan, and a renal biopsy are additional diagnostic tests.

Treatment and Nursing Management

The management of CRF is very complex because of the impact kidney failure has on homeostasis and major body systems. Medical treatment and nursing intervention include measures to correct fluid and electrolyte imbalance and acid-base imbalance whenever possible. A restricted protein diet often is necessary, and it has been found that decreasing protein in the diet of patients with beginning renal insufficiency may help slow down the disease process. A variety of drugs, such as antacids, antihypertensives, antilipemics, epoetin alpha (Epogen) therapy, and vitamin and mineral supplements, are used to counteract the fluid and electrolyte imbalances, treat metabolic acidosis, and control the complications (Table 34–4). Diuretics are used while there is some remaining kidney function (renal insufficiency) but are not useful during ESRD. Inotropic agents, such as digitalis or dobutamine, are used in severe cases of heart failure. Antiseizure medications, such as phenytoin (Dilantin) or diazepam (Valium) also may be needed because uremic toxins can irritate the nervous system. Dialysis and kidney transplant are two major alternatives that offer hope to the patient with ESRD.

Renal Dialysis. Hemodialysis and peritoneal dialysis are two procedures commonly used to remove waste products normally excreted by the kidneys. Both procedures rely on diffusion to remove elements normally excreted in the urine. The principle of diffusion states that solute molecules that are in constant motion tend

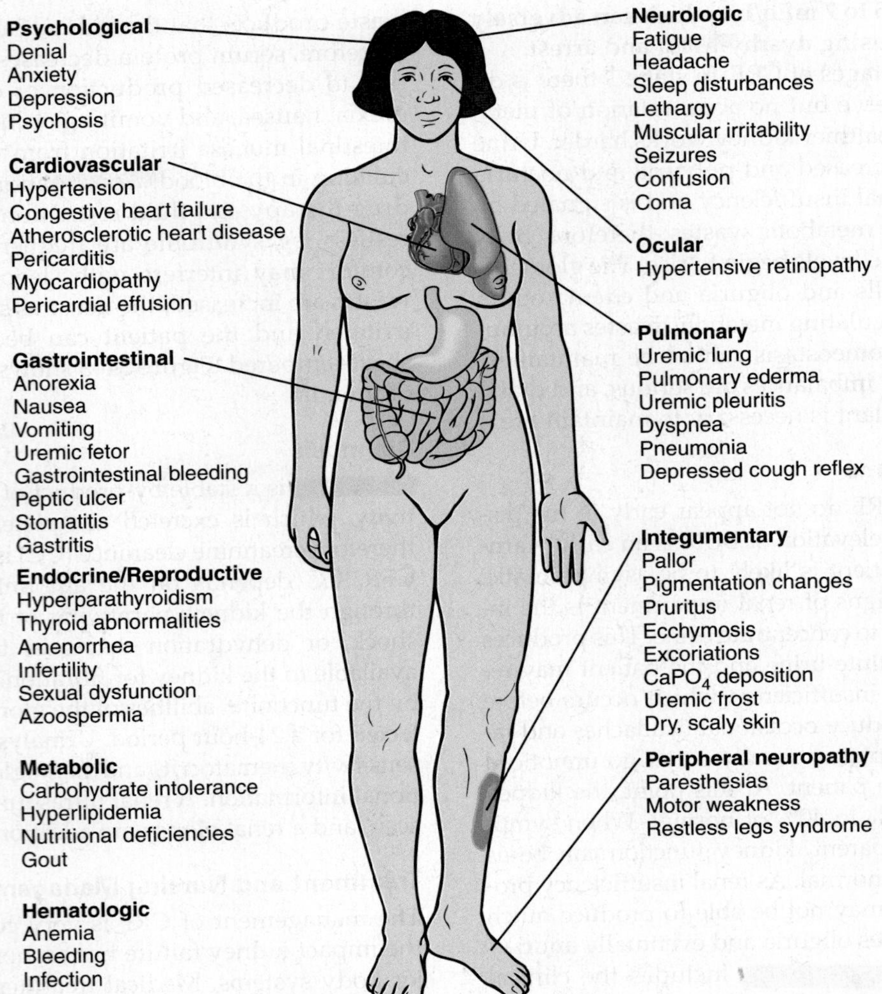

FIGURE 34–3 Systemic effects of uremia.

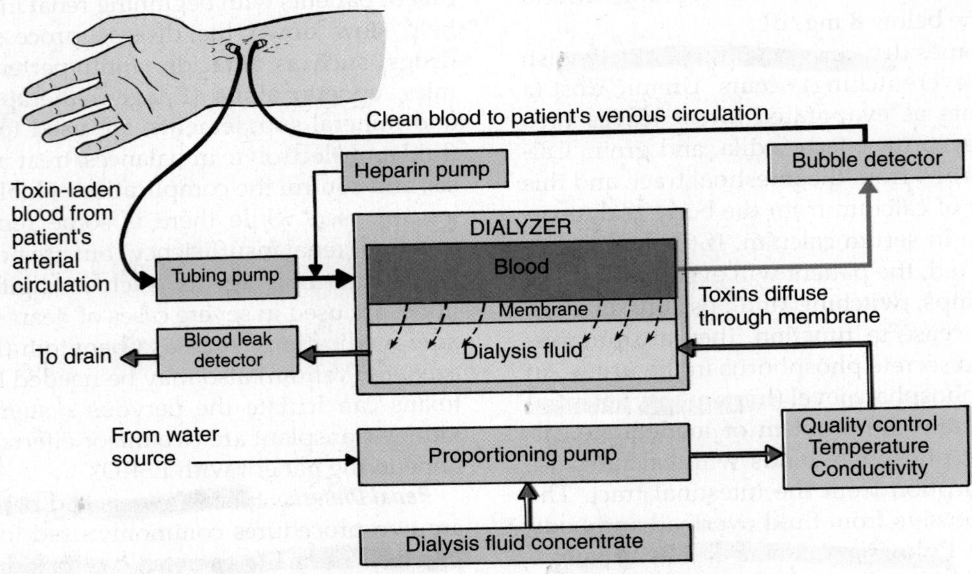

FIGURE 34–4 Schematic of hemodialysis system.

Table 34–4 **Examples of Medications for Patients with Chronic Renal Disease**

CLASSIFICATION	ACTION	NURSING IMPLICATIONS	PATIENT TEACHING
DIURETICS			
Furosemide (Lasix)	Promotes urine flow; rids body of excess fluid; used in early stages of chronic renal failure	Potentially nephrotoxic and ototoxic. Strict I&O. Monitor labs for blood dyscrasias. Side effects: Vomiting, headache, constipation, and dizziness.	Report fever, sore throat, bleeding, bruising, difficulty swallowing, rash, or change in hearing.
ANTIHYPERTENSIVES			
ACE inhibitors Enalapril (Vasotec)	Reduces angiotensin II and aldosterone, which decreases peripheral resistance and sodium reabsorption	Monitor for hypotension, blood dyscrasias, signs of infection, or bruising. African Americans have a higher incidence of angioedema (facial swelling, hoarseness), which can be fatal.	Immediately report cough, difficulty breathing, rash, tremors, blood in stool, or bleeding after brushing teeth. Report persistent dizziness or numbness and tingling.
VITAMINS			
Calcitriol (Rocaltrol)	Active form of vitamin D	Monitor serum calcium normal level 4.5 to 5.5 mEq/L. Monitor for hypocalcemia.	Report signs of hypocalcemia (e.g., twitching of mouth, numbness of fingers, laryngeal spasm, carpopedal spasm).
Folic acid and vitamin B_{12}	For red blood cell formation	Give with food to promote absorption. Side effects not expected.	Store in dry, light-protected container
MINERALS			
Iron (ferrous sulfate)	Used to treat anemia	Give with water or juice to promote absorption. Do not give with milk products.	Take with food if gastric distress occurs. Sit upright for 30 min after taking. Stool may turn black; this is a harmless side effect.
CALCIUM SUPPLEMENTS			
Calcium carbonate Calcium acetate (also binds phosphate)	Prevents problems of calcium loss Give with meals to bind phosphate	Monitor serum calcium. Monitor ECG changes for potential dysrhythmias.	Constipation is a common side effect. Nausea, vomiting, drowsiness, or headache may occur.
HEMATOPOETIC GROWTH FACTORS			
Epoetin alpha (Epogen) Darbepoetin (Aranesp)	Treatment of anemia; promotes red blood cell formation	Can cause hypertension; monitor blood pressure. May need increased doses of heparin. Subcutaneous route is preferred.	Report nausea, vomiting, edema, fatigue, or chest pain.
RESINS			
Sodium polystyrene (Kayexalate)	Treatment of hyperkalemia	Can be given mixed with food or in an enema. Monitor electrolytes. Side effects: Nausea, vomiting, constipation, and anorexia.	Report any muscle weakness, irregular heartbeat, or stomach pain.

Key: *ECG,* electrocardiogram; *I&O,* input and output.

to pass through a semipermeable membrane from the side of higher concentration to the side of lower concentration.

Hemodialysis. Hemodialysis removes nitrogenous waste products from the blood. Blood moves from the arterial circulation through a dialysate bath and back to the venous circulation. A dialysis membrane separates the blood from the dialyzing solution. The molecules of waste pass through this membrane out of the blood and into the dialyzing solution until the two solutions are equal in concentration (Figure 34–4).

A temporary access for hemodialysis can be achieved by inserting a jugular or femoral vein dialysis catheter. The jugular site has a low incidence of thrombosis; it can be used for 1 to 3 weeks and is preferred over the femoral site. These temporary access sites should be used only by trained dialysis staff for medication administration and blood draws.

Two kinds of internal access are used for ongoing hemodialysis. An arteriovenous fistula (AVF) is formed by joining an artery and a vein together (Figure 34–5, *A*). The vein is made into a large superficial vein with an arterial supply that is easily accessible by venipuncture. Most often the radial or brachial artery is joined to the cephalic vein in the arm. A period of 6 to 8 weeks after surgery is needed for the vessel walls to become thickened and usable for the repeated insertion of the hemodialysis needles. Although the AVF has fewer complications and better patency, it requires relatively healthy blood vessels; therefore, patients with diabetes, prolonged IV drug use, or peripheral vascular disease may need an alternative access site. One of the *Healthy People 2010* goals is to increase the proportion of new hemodialysis patients that use AVF as the primary mode of vascular access.

The arteriovenous (AV) access is accomplished by connecting an artery and a vein with a graft of a piece of synthetic material. The hemodialysis needles are then placed directly into the graft (Figure 34–5, *B*).

Medications frequently prescribed for the dialysis patient include multivitamins, antacids, iron and calcium supplements, antihypertensives (especially ACE inhibitors) and phosphate binders, and possibly anticonvulsants. Epoetin alpha (Epogen), a synthetic substance that stimulates red blood cell production, is given to combat the suppression of natural erythropoietin that occurs in renal failure. Darbepoetin (Aranesp) is a newer and longer acting form of erythropoietin therapy that is available. See Table 34–4 for medication information.

Complications. The problems that a patient on hemodialysis may experience include fluid overload, electrolyte imbalance, alterations in blood components leading to anemia, and platelet abnormalities that produce bleeding tendencies. Patients can experience dialysis disequilibrium syndrome. This may occur because of rapid decrease in volume and is more likely after the first several treatments. Observe the patient for changes in mental status, headache, vomiting, or seizures. Be alert for cardiac dysrhythmias, signs of air emboli, or hemorrhage. Other major problems are systemic infections or localized infections at the access site.

Hepatitis C and acquired immunodeficiency syndrome (AIDS) are dangers because of blood access and risk of contamination. Patients who had multiple blood transfusions during the early to mid-1980s may have been exposed to the human immunodeficiency virus (HIV). (Hepatitis B is also possible but less of a problem due to vaccination, antibody testing, and strict body fluid precautions. Patients and dialysis staff should receive hepatitis B vaccine.)

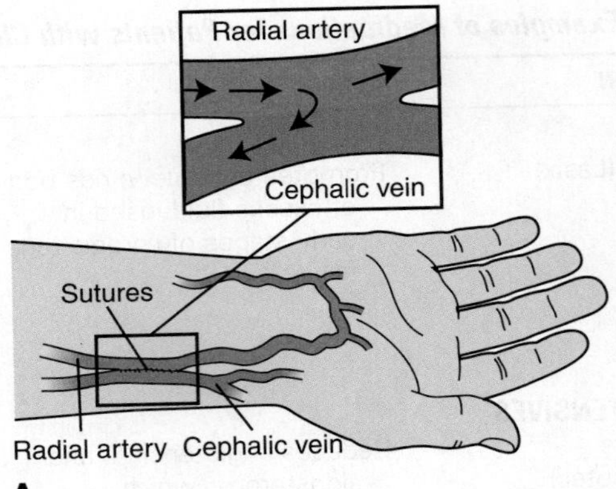

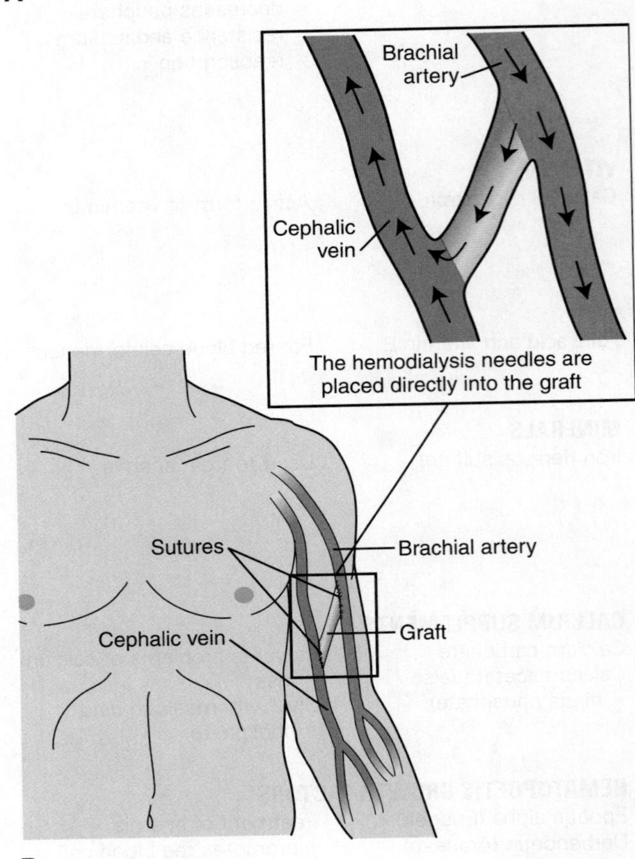

FIGURE 34–5 **A,** Arteriovenous fistula. **B,** Vascular graft access for long-term hemodialysis.

Nursing Management. When caring for the hospitalized patient who has an arteriovenous graft or an AV fistula, it is important to check the site and protect it from injury. The site should be observed at least four times a day for signs indicating clotting or infection, and the peripheral circulation distal to the graft should also be checked (capillary refill and color of nail beds). Palpate for a thrill (vibration in the vessel), by gently laying your fingers on the enlarged vessel. You should be able to feel a buzz or vibration. A bruit (soft swishing

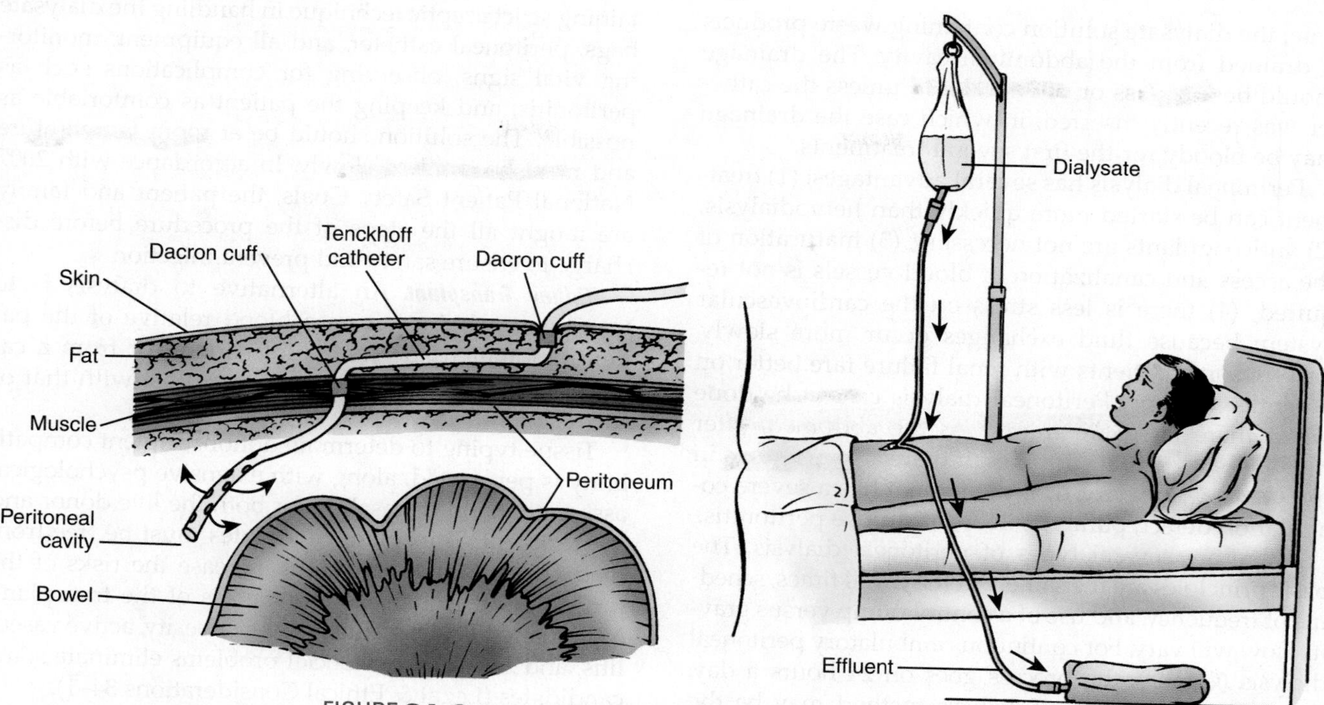

FIGURE 34–6 Peritoneal dialysis through an abdominal catheter.

sound) should be clearly heard upon auscultation. When a graft has been inserted, the extremity is elevated postoperatively and kept at a level above the heart for 24 to 72 hours. Thereafter, the patient should sleep with that extremity free (i.e., not on the side with the arm tucked underneath the body). Care is taken never to compress the extremity containing the vascular access.

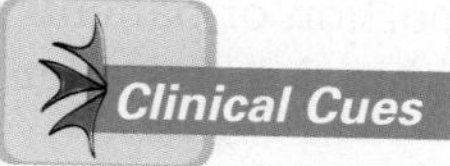

The arm or leg in which the arteriovenous shunt has been created should never be used for checking blood pressure or performing venipuncture (peripheral IVs or blood draws). Post a sign above the bed to alert other members of the health care team.

Antihypertensive drugs are not given the morning of dialysis, as they can cause severe hypotension during the treatment. Nitroglycerin (NTG) patches, digitalis, and anticoagulants also are held. You should also consult with the dialysis nurse to coordinate the timing of medications. Before the patient goes to dialysis, do a physical assessment, check for bruit and thrill at the access site, and obtain a complete set of vital signs and a weight. These measurements will be compared with post-treatment results.

The patient undergoing hemodialysis will have considerable fluid volume shifts that affect homeostasis. You will need to plan to assess this patient more frequently in the hours after dialysis treatment is completed. Postdialysis nursing care includes monitoring the access site for bleeding for 1 hour after the treatment. Assess the patient for signs of confusion or disorientation, hypotension, nausea or vomiting, headache, dizziness, or muscle cramps. Monitor and compare vital signs to pretreatment values and continue assessment of the access site for patency and signs of infection. **Invasive procedures are postponed for 4 to 6 hours after dialysis because the clotting time is extended from the heparin used during dialysis, and prolonged bleeding could occur.**

The scheduling of hemodialysis sessions varies from patient to patient, but treatments usually are done two or three times a week. Stable patients can be treated on an outpatient basis at a dialysis center.

Peritoneal Dialysis. Peritoneal dialysis is an alternative procedure that can be used instead of hemodialysis to remove waste products or toxins that have accumulated as a result of ARF or CRF. Peritoneal dialysis operates on the same principles as hemodialysis, the difference being that the semipermeable membrane is in the peritoneum and the solution is introduced into and withdrawn from the peritoneal cavity. During the procedure, dialyzing fluid, equal in osmolarity and similar in composition to normal body fluid, is introduced into the peritoneal cavity via a Tenckhoff catheter by gravity or pump (Figure 34–6). Medications such as heparin, insulin, potassium, or antibiotics may be added to the solution. The solution is left in the peritoneal cavity for a specified time (dwell time) until the concentrations of the solutions on either side of the peritoneal membrane are equalized.

After the fluid is infused, the patient can move about during the dwell time. At the end of the dwell time, the dialysate solution containing waste products is drained from the abdominal cavity. The drainage should be colorless or straw-colored unless the catheter was recently inserted, in which case the drainage may be bloody for the first several treatments.

Peritoneal dialysis has several advantages: (1) treatment can be started more quickly than hemodialysis, (2) anticoagulants are not necessary, (3) maturation of the access and canalization of blood vessels is not required, (4) there is less stress on the cardiovascular system because fluid exchanges occur more slowly, and (5) some patients with renal failure fare better on a gentler therapy. Peritoneal dialysis cannot be done when there is severe trauma to the abdomen, after multiple abdominal surgeries, if there are adhesions in the abdominal cavity, or if the patient has a severe coagulation defect, paralytic ileus, or diffuse peritonitis.

There are several types of peritoneal dialysis. The basic principles are the same, but the dwell times, schedule of frequency, and use of a control pump versus gravity flow will vary. For continuous ambulatory peritoneal dialysis (CAPD), the process goes on 24 hours a day, 7 days a week. This self-dialysis method may be the easiest for the patient and it requires no machinery. The bag of dialyzing solution is suspended above the level of the abdomen and the tubing is attached to the permanently implanted peritoneal dialysis catheter. The clamp on the tubing is opened and the dialysate solution is allowed to run into the abdomen by gravity flow. After the dwell time (4 to 8 hours), the fluid is drained. Nocturnal intermittent dialysis is accomplished either with or without use of a control pump and is performed three to five times per week for 10 to 12 hours at night. This allows the patient to be free between treatment times. Continuous cycling peritoneal dialysis combines CAPD with nocturnal intermittent dialysis for home use. An automated cycling machine allows the patient to do three exchanges at night while sleeping, then during the day there is one exchange, but the dwell time lasts all day long. Automated peritoneal dialysis is regulated by machinery and can be used in acute care settings, clinics, and at home during the night.

Complications. Potential complications of peritoneal dialysis include peritonitis, leakage, obstruction or other problems with the catheter, respiratory problems, and fluid overload or hypertriglyceridemia (disturbance of lipid metabolism).

? *Think Critically About . . .* What signs and symptoms might indicate that your peritoneal dialysis patient has peritonitis?

Nursing Management. Specific nursing care for the patient undergoing peritoneal dialysis includes obtaining the patient's weight before and after the treatment; maintaining careful intake and output records; maintaining strict aseptic technique in handling the dialysate bags, peritoneal catheter, and all equipment; monitoring vital signs; observing for complications such as peritonitis; and keeping the patient as comfortable as possible. The solution should be at room temperature and must be instilled slowly. In accordance with 2007 National Patient Safety Goals, the patient and family are taught all the steps of the procedure before discharge to ensure safety and prevent infection.

Kidney Transplant. An alternative to dialysis is to transplant a kidney from a blood relative of the patient, another tissue-compatible donor, or from a cadaver whose kidney tissue is compatible with that of the recipient.

Tissue typing to determine donor-recipient compatibility is performed, along with extensive psychological assessment and counseling for both the live donor and the recipient. Transplant candidates must be free from medical problems that might increase the risks of the procedure or jeopardize the success of the transplant. Malignancy, IV drug abuse, severe obesity, active vasculitis, and severe psychosocial problems eliminate some candidates (Legal & Ethical Considerations 34–1).

A significant factor in transplant therapy is the shortage of organs. In the United States, 96,929 persons are currently on the waiting list, which changes hourly (data accessed August 16, 2007 at www.unos.org). Stable patients who are waiting for a transplant must live close to a transplant center and be ready immediately when an organ becomes available. Hypertension is brought under the best possible control, any infection is treated, and the patient is dialyzed immediately before transplantation. One of the *Healthy People 2010* goals is to increase the proportion of patients that receive a kidney transplant within 3 years after being put on the waiting list.

There are three types of immunosuppressive drugs to prevent organ rejection: (1) cytokine inhibitors (e.g., cyclosporine [Sandimmune], tacrolimus [Prograf]); (2) antiproliferative agents (e.g., azathioprine [Imuran]); and (3) antibodies (e.g., muromonab-CD3 [Orthoclone OKT3]). Long-term problems for transplant patients are increased susceptibility to infection and a higher risk of malignancy.

Legal & Ethical Considerations 34–1

Organ Donation

Generally speaking, state law mandates that **families must be approached** about organ donation following the death of a loved one. Hospital policy may dictate that the primary nurse should initially approach the family, or there may be a specifically trained staff person that fills this role.The designated organ procurement organization is contacted after the initial approach, if the family is agreeable, so that a representative can come and give the family more details.

Renal transplant patients are transferred to critical care or specialty units after surgery, where they are closely monitored for signs of rejection: fever, increased blood pressure, and pain over the iliac fossa where the new kidney was placed (Figure 34–7). Ongoing assessment includes watching for the signs of renal failure, particularly oliguria, anuria, and rising BUN levels and serum creatinine. Protection from sources of infection is a top priority. Once the new kidney is functioning properly, the primary physician may lift any previous dietary restrictions.

Renal failure and dialysis are very expensive for the patient and family. However, lack of funds does not exclude anyone from needed care. Since July 1973, an amendment to the Social Security Act allows Medicare to pay for most of the cost of treating ESRD, including dialysis and renal transplant. Medical expenses continue after transplant, as the drugs needed to prevent rejection are very expensive.

NURSING MANAGEMENT

Assessment (Data Collection)

The assessment findings will vary because of the slow but progressive development of kidney failure and the interrelationship that kidney disease has on other body systems. Take a past medical history that includes medication, previous illness and surgeries, family history of illness, and a report of current complaints and concerns as previously discussed in Chapter 33.

Perform a general head-to toe assessment including complete vital signs and a baseline weight. Observe for changes and symptoms that include:

- Neurologic changes (e.g., lethargy, irritability)
- Cardiovascular abnormalities (e.g., dysrhythmias or hypertension)
- Respiratory abnormalities (e.g., shortness of breath or fluid in lungs)
- Gastrointestinal distress (e.g., nausea, vomiting, constipation)
- Musculoskeletal discomfort (e.g., muscle cramps, twitching, or restless leg syndrome)
- Skin changes (e.g., itching, uremic frost)

Monitor BUN, serum creatinine, electrolytes, and urinalysis. As the disease progresses, assess for impaired urine concentration, output, and anemia.

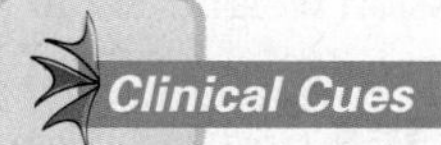

Although it is common to weigh patients in the morning with the same scale and the same amount of clothing, use your clinical judgment to initiate weights more frequently than once per day if needed. Watch for signs of fluid overload (e.g., facial or peripheral edema, shortness of breath, or crackles in lungs). One kilogram or 2.2 lb of weight gain is equal to more than 1 L of fluid.

In addition you should assess patients for sexual difficulties or concerns. Patients may experience medication side effects, such as impotence. Weight gain, peripheral edema, or presence of a shunt may alter body image or feelings of attractiveness. Fatigue caused by anemia or hormonal imbalance can result in decreased libido (sexual desire). Partners may fear that the patient is too ill to participate in sex or that the hemodialysis shunt will be damaged.

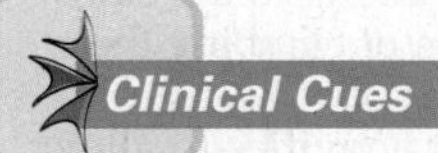

Help your patient to verbalize concerns about sexual problems by using a matter-of-fact approach (e.g., "Mr. Smith, have you or your partner noticed any changes in your sexual relations since you started your new medication?"). It is possible that you may not be able to directly solve the problem, but giving the patient the opportunity to talk about it is helpful. In addition, once you have assessed the problem, you can refer the patient to the appropriate resource if the problem is beyond your expertise (i.e., the physician may be able to change medication or the family may need psychological counseling).

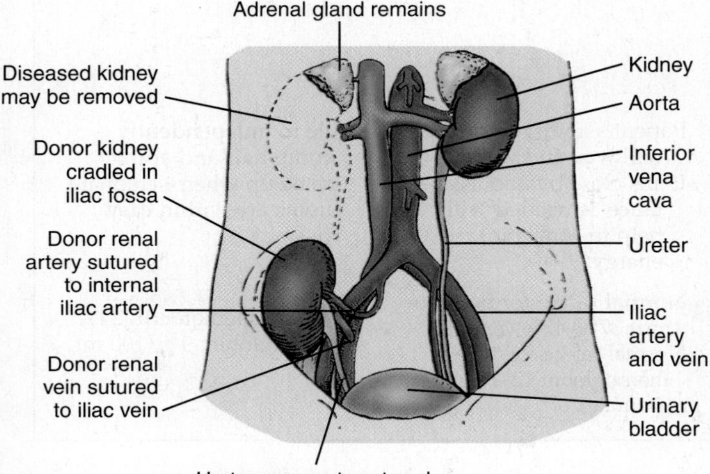

FIGURE 34–7 Placement of transplanted kidney.

Nursing Diagnosis

Many of the applicable nursing diagnoses have already been covered earlier in this text. For example, anemia, bleeding tendency, and susceptibility to infection are discussed in Chapter 16; nausea, vomiting, anorexia, gastrointestinal bleeding, and other gastrointestinal problems are covered in Chapter 28. Congestive heart failure is covered in Chapter 19. Nursing diagnoses commonly used for patients with renal insufficiency and failure are listed in Nursing Care Plan 34–1.

Text continued on p. 866

NURSING CARE PLAN 34–1

Care of the Patient with Chronic Renal Failure

SCENARIO Mrs. Stevens, age 54, has had hypertension since she was in her early 20s. She now has developed symptoms of chronic renal failure. She reports headaches, fatigue, and nausea. I have to "sleep with three pillows and I am just exhausted." She feels that "her doctor is keeping something from her" and she is withdrawn and sullen. Tearfully, she reports, "The renal diet is so complex and my husband and son cannot manage the cooking and shopping." She was referred to a nephrologist, who, after a series of diagnostic tests, recommended hemodialysis and kidney transplant when an organ is available. Admitting laboratory results include hematocrit 25%; hemoglobin 9 g/100 mL, BUN 48 mg/dL, creatinine 3 mg/dL, admission weight: 137 lb ("normal weight around 130 lb"), 3+ pitting edema, bilateral feet and ankles.

PROBLEM/NURSING DIAGNOSIS *Tired and exhausted*/Activity intolerance related to anemia.

Supporting assessment data *Subjective:* "I am just exhausted." *Objective:* Hematocrit 25%; hemoglobin 9 g/100 mL, appears tired.

Goals/Expected Outcomes	Nursing Interventions	Selected Rationale	Evaluation
Patient will identify her activity limits for this shift	Monitor for signs of weakness, or increasing fatigue.	These signs and symptoms can signal a potential decreased RBC and impaired oxygen carrying capacity.	Able to independently perform basic hygienic needs this morning.
	Check vital signs for changes when activities appear stressful or overtaxing.	Marked increase in pulse or respiratory rate during routine ADL suggests activity intolerance.	Reported feelings of fatigue and mild dyspnea after walking to the nurses' station. Vital signs at that time were BP 145/90, P 120, R 32/min. Repeat vitals after 30 min of rest: BP 140/80, P 85, R 20/min.
	Have patient use rating scale (scale 1/10) for different types of activities, such as walking to the bathroom or climbing the stairs.	The exertional scale (1/10) allows the patient (and the nurse) to rate and monitor performance and alter activities accordingly.	Ambulating in the hall was "too much" and reported an exertion level of 6/10.
	Adjust activities to allow for periods of rest.	Adequate rest facilitates recovery; activities can be increased or decreased according to the patient's level of tolerance.	Patient was assisted back to her room. Rested for 3 hr.
	Help visitors and patient to discuss what time of day and type of activities will fit the patient's current energy level (e.g., son could visit on Saturday morning and read a book with the patient).	Visitors need specific instructions to prevent overstimulating (or avoiding) the patient.	Patient's family agrees to come in midmorning hours and limit stay to 1 hr.
By discharge, patient will be able to perform ADLs independently without distress	Assist with ADLs PRN and keep personal articles within reach	Patient's ability to do ADLs will wax and wane. Items close by and assistance as needed will help to conserve energy.	Able to independently comb hair and apply makeup when personal items are within easy reach
Patient will demonstrate increased hematocrit value: 30% and increased hemoglobin 11 g/100 mL within 1 wk	Monitor for decreased hematocrit and hemoglobin values.	Normal range for hematocrit 37%–47% (female). Normal range for hemoglobin 12–16 g/dL (female).	7:00 A.M. Hematocrit: 24%; hemoglobin: 9 g/100 mL

NURSING CARE PLAN 34–1

Care of the Patient with Chronic Renal Failure—cont'd

Goals/Expected Outcomes	Nursing Interventions	Selected Rationale	Evaluation
	Give epoetin and monitor for drug side effects (e.g., increased BP, dyspnea, chest pain, seizures, headaches, or calf pain). Give iron, multivitamins, and folic acid as ordered. Instruct about foods with high iron (e.g., lean meat and vegetables) and folic acid (e.g., whole wheat bread) content.	Nutritional supplements and epoetin are given to help the body with RBC production.	Epoetin given subcutaneously, as ordered. No adverse effects noted.
	Monitor infusions of packed red blood cells, as ordered.	Transfusions may be needed if anemia is severe.	No transfusion ordered at this time. Outcomes partially met. Continue plan.

PROBLEM/NURSING DIAGNOSIS *Believes that information is being withheld and feels that family cannot manage shopping and cooking*/Powerlessness related to perceived lack of information and stress of chronic illness.

Supporting assessment data *Subjective:* "Doctor is keeping something from me." *Objective:* Appears withdrawn, sullen, and tearful.

Goals/Expected Outcomes	Nursing Interventions	Selected Rationale	Evaluation
Patient will express feelings associated with chronic illness during this shift	Encourage expression of feelings (e.g., frustration, anger).	Expression of feelings and beliefs allows the patient and the nurse to clarify how the situation impacts behavior and decision making. Taking the time to listen also builds trust and rapport.	Patient stated that she was discouraged and depressed about her illness. Expresses anger toward her physician, because she thinks, "he is not telling the whole story."
	Encourage expression of beliefs about illness and outcomes.	Patient may experience strong feelings and may or may not be able to identify the source. You may not be able to correct all situations, but just talking about the frustration will help some patients.	She "hates the idea of dialysis" and feels like it is "controlling her life."
	Observe for factors contributing to feelings (e.g., lack of information, loss of social roles) and correct if possible. Assist patient to identify factors that can and cannot be controlled	Identifying factors that cannot be controlled allows the patient to realistically work on achievable goals.	Patient identified that knowing more about dialysis would be helpful.
Patient will participate in planning care and daily goals within 2–3 days	Provide opportunities for patient to participate in activities that will increase sense of accomplishment (e.g., phoning for an appointment with social services).	A sense of accomplishment empowers the patient to act positively in own behalf.	Assisted patient in making a list of questions for her physician (e.g., What are the steps for starting hemodialysis? How long can I live on dialysis?).
	Assist patient to identify small, achievable goals and to make realistic plans.	Small goals are more readily accomplished and a feeling of success provides motivation to attempt larger goals.	Patient requested some written information about kidney transplantation and asked to speak to the transplant coordinator.

Continued

NURSING CARE PLAN 34–1

Care of the Patient with Chronic Renal Failure—cont'd

Goals/Expected Outcomes	Nursing Interventions	Selected Rationale	Evaluation
Patient will state hopes and plans for the future before discharge	Emphasize that quality of life can be good for patients on dialysis (e.g., extends time to spend with friends and family).	Emphasizing positive outcomes can create a sense of hope and optimism.	She says that she is not optimistic about getting a donated kidney, but would still like to have the knowledge and the hope that it could happen for her.
	Give positive reinforcement for statements of hope and future planning.	Positive reinforcement encourages repetition of a desirable behavior.	At the end of the shift, patient stated that making the list of questions and talking about her frustrations had helped. Outcomes partially met. Continue with plan.

PROBLEM/NURSING DIAGNOSIS *Renal diet is very complex*/ Deficient knowledge related to diet and nutrition.
Supporting assessment data "The renal diet is so complex and my husband and son cannot manage the cooking and shopping." *Objective:* Appears overwhelmed at the amount of information and seems unsure how to use it effectively.

Goals/Expected Outcomes	Nursing Interventions	Selected Rationale	Evaluation
Patient will state willingness to learn about prescribed diet during this shift	Assess readiness to learn, preferred learning styles, and barriers to learning.	Possible barriers for the patient include being upset, tired, uncomfortable, or anxious about her condition. Learning new information will be difficult under these conditions.	The patient identifies need for herself and the entire family to learn about her dietary restrictions. Patient also shows interest in attending a group class that will be conducted next month.
	Perform teaching in short sessions.	Complex information is best delivered in manageable pieces.	Limited teaching session to 10 min due to fatigue.
	Use language and terms that patient is able to understand	Medical jargon and technical terms will not help the patient understand the basic dietary information.	Verbalized understanding of terminology related to health teaching (e.g., restricted protein).
With help, the patient will create a sample diet that is within renal diet parameters within 2–3 days	Obtain a dietary consult and reinforce information provided by the nutritional expert.	A renal nutritionist must be consulted to create an individual diet plan based on lab values, nutritional requirements, and patient's eating preferences.	Nutritionist came to see the patient and discussed overall nutritional goals and plan. Arrangements have been made with the nutritionist to meet with the family next week.
Patient will apply knowledge about diet and nutrition to reduce nitrogenous waste by-products and solute overload by next outpatient dialysis appointment	Ensure that the patient has verbal and written instructions.	Written material can be reviewed at a later date; can also be shared with family members.	Written information was provided about diet and renal disease.
	Encourage expression of concerns (e.g., cost, preparation, availability of seasonal foods).	Food frequently has a sociocultural base.	Patient is concerned that family will need guidance in shopping
	Invite the family (especially the person most likely to cook and shop) to attend the teaching sessions.	Costs, food preferences, and family participation should be considered to increase the likelihood of success.	Family will attend teaching session next week

NURSING CARE PLAN 34–1

Care of the Patient with Chronic Renal Failure—cont'd

Goals/Expected Outcomes	Nursing Interventions	Selected Rationale	Evaluation
	Help her review specific information about high-quality proteins (e.g., meat, eggs) and hidden sodium sources (e.g., canned food).	Reviewing information increases retention of new information.	The patient was able to identify high-quality protein foods but continues to be confused about how sodium, phosphorus, and calcium are affecting her kidney function. Follow-up teaching sessions will be arranged this week to address the topic. Outcomes partially met. Continue with plan.

PROBLEM/NURSING DIAGNOSIS *Weight gain of 7 lb with pitting edema*/Excess fluid volume related to retention of sodium and water from inadequate kidney function.

Supporting assessment data *Subjective:* "Sleeps with three pillows." *Objective:* Admission weight: 137 lb (normal weight around 130 lb), 3+ pitting edema, bilateral feet and ankles.

Goals/Expected Outcomes	Nursing Interventions	Selected Rationale	Evaluation
Patient will have restricted fluid intake (500–700 mL plus output from previous 24 hr) during this shift	Strict I&O.	Discrepancies in I&O suggest fluid retention and overload.	Fluid intake 1000 mL, output 600 mL.
	Fluid restrictions, as ordered (intake 500–700 mL plus output from previous 24 hr). Assist to establish acceptable schedule for restricted fluids.	Kidneys may produce a small but inadequate output of urine. Limiting fluid prevents overload, whereas spacing fluid throughout the day helps to relieve subjective feelings of thirst.	Patient is aware of and compliant with fluid restrictions.
	Assist with good oral care and discourage mouth breathing; rinse mouth frequently, space fluids throughout the day.	Patient's subjective feeling of moist oral mucous membranes will increase compliance with fluid restrictions.	Subjective relief obtained from frequent, but small quantities of ice chips and periodic mouthwash.
	Instruct patient and visitors about fluid restriction.	Visitors may unintentionally offer fluid as a comfort measure if they are uninformed about therapeutic goals.	Patient actively reminds all visitors and staff "not to tempt me."
	Post a sign over the bed to alert visitors and health care team members about fluid restrictions.	Many persons can pass through a patient's room and all should be aware of precautions to prevent inadvertently offering restricted foods and fluids.	Sign placed above bed for fluid restrictions.
Patient will demonstrate signs of decreased fluid load (e.g., lungs will be clear to auscultation, foot and ankle edema decreased) within 24–48 hr	Check for signs of fluid overload: edema, crackles in lungs, orthopnea, and changes in mental status.	Peripheral fluid is observed in extremities and face. Edema within body organs (e.g., lungs or brain) manifests as functional impairment.	Fine crackles noted in base of posterior lung fields bilaterally. Reports some mild shortness of breath, especially with exertion or if lying flat in bed. Subjectively feels breathing is okay "when sitting in a chair." Resting pulse oximetry 94%. 3+ pitting edema noted bilaterally in feet.

Continued

NURSING CARE PLAN 34–1

Care of the Patient with Chronic Renal Failure—cont'd

Goals/Expected Outcomes	Nursing Interventions	Selected Rationale	Evaluation
Patient's weight will return to previous level within 10 days	Weigh daily (or more frequently if needed) and monitor trends.	An increase in weight is one of the key indicators of fluid imbalance. One kilogram, or 2.2 lb of weight gain, is equal to excess of 1 L of fluid.	Patient's A.M. weight: 137.5 lb.
Patient will demonstrate minimal peripheral edema within 7-10 days	Administer diuretic (e.g., hydrochlorothiazide), as ordered.	Diuretics can be given in CRF to reduce hypertension and edema; usually discontinued after dialysis is initiated.	Given: hydrochlorothiazide 100 mg. No adverse side effects noted.
	Restrict sodium to 2 g/day, as ordered.	Decreasing solute load decreases fluid retention.	Compliant with 2-g sodium diet. Outcomes partially met. Continue with plan.

? CRITICAL THINKING QUESTIONS

1. What diagnostic tests do you think the nephrologist would have ordered for Mrs. Stevens?
2. Why might Mrs. Stevens' renal disease not have been diagnosed earlier?
3. If Mrs. Stevens does not agree to hemodialysis, what other alternatives are available to her?
4. What concerns do you anticipate that Mr. Stevens and their son would have?

Nursing diagnoses frequently associated with chronic renal disease and dialysis include, but are not restricted to:

- Excess fluid volume related to decreased kidney function
- Imbalanced nutrition: less than body requirements, related to dietary restrictions and loss of appetite
- Fatigue related to anemia
- Risk for infection related to invasive procedures (e.g., dialysis shunt)
- Deficient knowledge related to complexity of therapeutic regimen (e.g., peritoneal dialysis at home)
- Disturbed thought processes related to accumulation of toxins
- Sexual dysfunction related to stress and medication side effects

Examples of expected outcomes include:

- Patient will have no signs of fluid volume overload (e.g., weight gain, edema, crackles in lungs) within 2 days.
- Patient will eat at least 50% of all meals during this shift.
- Patient will have adequate energy to independently perform ADLs before discharge.
- Patient will not have any signs or symptoms of infection (e.g., fever, redness, or swelling at shunt site) during hospitalization.
- Patient will list steps for peritoneal dialysis and demonstrate independent performance of procedure before discharge.
- Patient will demonstrate ability to make safe judgments (e.g., calls for help as needed) and orientation to person, place, and time before discharge.
- Patient will verbalize concerns or fears about sexual dysfunction.

Planning

In planning care for the patient with chronic renal disease, consider the stress of prolonged intensive treatment, the frustrations of dealing with an incurable illness, rigid dietary restrictions, fatigue, malaise, occasional limited mobility, and possibly sexual difficulties, all of which take their toll on the patient as well as significant others. Consider the family's needs as well as the patient's when planning nursing intervention.

General nursing goals for care of patients with chronic renal disease include:

- Positive adaptation to therapeutic regimen (i.e., dietary and fluid modifications, dialysis)
- Maintaining fluid and electrolyte balance
- Prevention of complications
- Ensuring knowledge for appropriate self-care
- Assisting with resolution of body image disturbance
- Prevention of caregiver role strain and family dysfunction related to chronic illness

THERE ARE TWO DIFFERENT TYPES OF PROTEIN		THE HEMODIALYSIS AND THE PERITONEAL MEMBRANE ARE NOT SELECTIVE, WHICH MEANS THAT VITAL AMINO ACIDS AND VITAMINS AS WELL AS UNWANTED WASTES ARE REMOVED	
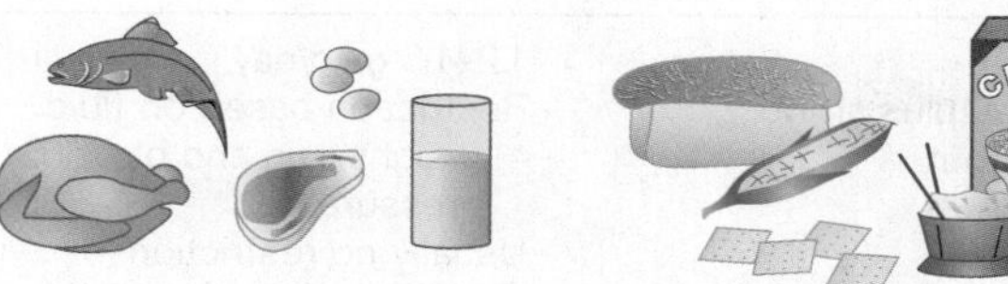	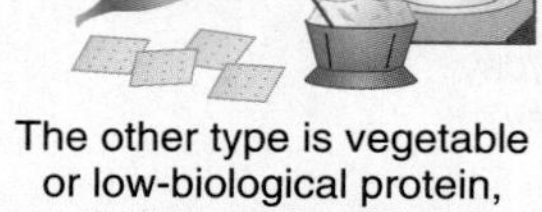	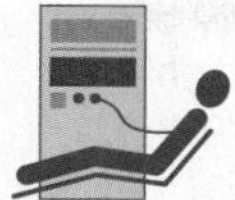	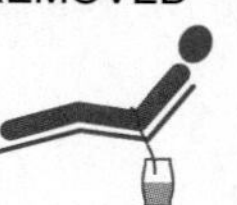
One is called animal or high-biological protein, which contains ALL essential amino acids	The other type is vegetable or low-biological protein, which contains SOME amino acids	If you are on HEMODIALYSIS, you should aim for **1.2 g of protein per kg of body weight;** e.g., if you weigh 65 kg (143 lb), your protein intake should be about 78 g/day	If you are on PERITONEAL DIALYSIS, you should aim for **1.3 g of protein per kg of body weight;** e.g., if you weigh 70 kg (154 lb), your protein intake should be about 91 g/day

EXAMPLES OF PROTEIN SOURCES					
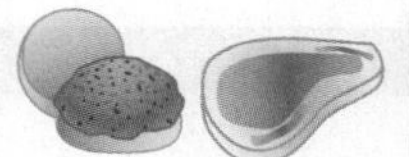	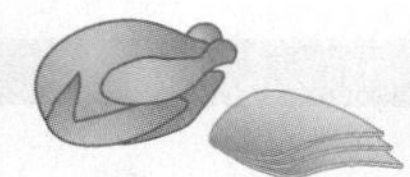	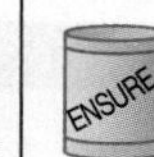 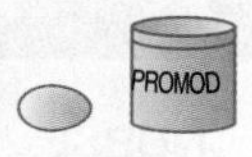	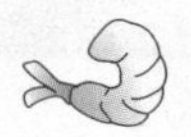 	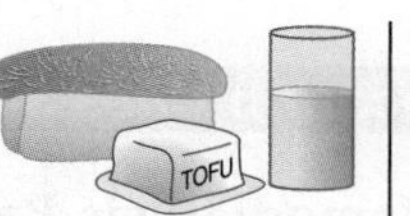	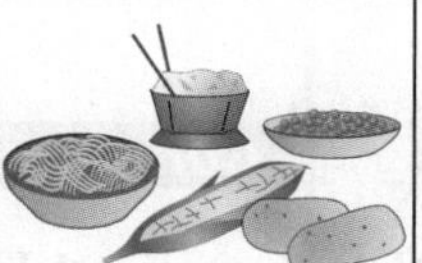
3.5 oz of extra-lean ground beef has 24 g of protein, whereas ribeye has 28 g of protein	Half of a chicken breast (3.5 oz) has 29 g of protein, turkey white meat (3.5 oz) has 30 g of protein	One can of Ensure has 13 g of protein, whereas 1 scoop of Promod has 5 g, and one egg has 6 g of protein	15 large cooked shrimp have 17 g of protein; a 3 oz can of white tuna in water has 22 g of protein	One cup of milk has 8 g of protein, whereas ½ cup of regular tofu has 10 g, and one slice of white bread has 2 g of protein	One cup of cooked corn, peas, potato, pasta, or rice has about 4 g of protein

FIGURE **34–8** Patient education: Tips on protein intake. (Modified from Darlene Michl, Sidney, British Columbia) (Source: Black, J.M., & Hawks, J.H. [2004]. *Medical-Surgical Nursing: Clinical Management for Positive Outcomes* (7th ed.). Philadelphia: Saunders. p. 965)

Think Critically About . . . What kinds of behaviors would suggest caregiver role strain for the spouse of a patient who has CRF?

Implementation

Because fluid and electrolyte balance are major concerns in the management of renal failure, you must be especially aware of hydration status. **Daily weight, measurement of I&O, determining the pattern of urination, and restricting fluid as ordered per physician (guidelines: intake 500 to 700 mL plus output from previous 24 hours) are essential to the well-being of the patient with renal damage.** In addition to these basic procedures, there should be ongoing monitoring of electrolytes, BUN, and creatinine. Hyperkalemia is present, and there is a sodium imbalance. Hypocalcemia and hyperphosphatemia occur. Specific electrolyte imbalances, their symptoms, and nursing interventions for imbalances are discussed in Chapter 3.

Think Critically About . . . How would you know whether the patient is suffering from hyperkalemia or hypocalcemia?

Maintaining adequate nutrition for the patient with CRF is a real challenge. Because of the buildup of nitrogenous wastes from protein metabolism, restriction of protein intake is necessary; only high-quality protein foods (e.g., meat and eggs) are encouraged. Figure 34–8 provides additional patient education information about protein intake. Potassium is also restricted. Sodium intake often is restricted, especially if the patient is hypertensive. Previously, aluminum carbonate (Basaljel) was used as a phosphate binder; however, concern over elevated aluminum levels has prompted the use of calcium carbonate, which acts as a phosphate binder and a calcium supplement.

The complexity of diet restrictions and modifications makes understanding and compliance very difficult for the patient and the family (Table 34–5). A major role of the nurse is to assess the patient's health status and learning needs throughout the illness and to help provide information to manage symptoms and prevent further damage whenever possible. The expertise of other professionals, especially nutritionists, is needed to help accomplish the goals of (1) minimizing uremic toxicity; (2) maintaining acceptable electrolyte levels; (3) controlling hypertension; (4) providing sufficient calories; and (5) maintaining good nutritional status. Communication Cues 34–1 provides an example of therapeutic communication with a patient who is having difficulty with dietary restrictions.

Table 34–5 ***Dietary Restrictions for the Patient with Renal Failure***

DIETARY COMPONENT	WITH CHRONIC UREMIA	WITH HEMODIALYSIS	WITH PERITONEAL DIALYSIS
Protein	0.55–0.60 g/kg/day	1–1.3 g/kg/day	1.2–1.5 g/kg/day
Fluid	Depends on urinary output, but may be as high as 1500–3000 mL/day	500–700 mL/day plus amount of urinary output	Restriction based on fluid weight gain and blood pressure
Potassium	60–70 mEq/day	70 mEq/day	Usually no restriction
Sodium	1–3 g/day	2–4 g/day	Restriction based on fluid weight gain and blood pressure
Phosphorus	700 mg/day	700 mg/day	800 mg/day

Source: Ignatavicius, D.D., & Workman, M.L. (2005). *Medical-Surgical Nursing: Critical Thinking for Collaborative Care* (5th ed.). St. Louis: Saunders, p. 1747.

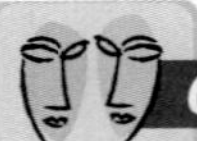

Communication Cues 34–1

Noncompliant Hemodialysis Patient

Mr. John T. is a 48-year-old male who has end-stage renal disease and is on hemodialysis twice a week. He has not been compliant with his diet and fluid restrictions and has been increased to three dialysis treatments a week. He gained 5 lb over the weekend.

NURSE: "John, I see that you have gained 5 lb since Friday. Could you tell me a little about your weekend?"

JOHN: "Yeah, but what's the difference? I just got tired of never having any fun or doing normal things with my friends. I went fishing with some buddies and we drank a lot of beer. It was hot. We barbecued our fish and some sausage and had a real feast!"

NURSE: "How are you feeling today?"

JOHN: "I feel rotten. I don't have any energy, and my thinking is slow. My legs are really swollen, and I'm having trouble breathing."

NURSE: "Do you think that might have something to do with the beer drinking and food?"

JOHN: "I suppose it does, but can't a guy have a little fun?"

NURSE: "John, you make your own decisions, but I am concerned. We have talked and you know that fluid and waste overload puts your whole body out of balance and causes damage in other organs. It's especially hard on the heart."

JOHN: "Yeah, I know you've told me. It's just so hard. You don't understand what it is like."

NURSE: "You are right, I don't have kidney disease, and I don't have the strict diet and fluid restrictions. I think it would be very difficult for me, too. I do know that I would want to take care of myself for my family and friends."

JOHN: "Well, you know that my wife left me, and I don't see much of the kids, but I sure do enjoy my granddaughter. She is the cutest little thing. I really enjoy my times with the guys at the Lodge, too."

NURSE: "Do you have any friends who are in a similar situation who you can talk to?"

JOHN: "No, none of my friends have kidney disease."

NURSE: "There is a young man who comes here for dialysis treatments who is always talking about fishing. Maybe the two of you would hit it off and could give each other some encouragement and support."

JOHN: "I don't know; I don't make new friends very easily."

NURSE: "I see on the schedule that he will be here on Wednesday. How about if we schedule your treatment for the same time? Perhaps you could get acquainted."

JOHN: "O.K. That seems fine."

NURSE: "Next week we can talk again to see how you are doing with your diet, fluid restrictions, and medication schedule."

JOHN: "Thanks, I will try to do better this week."

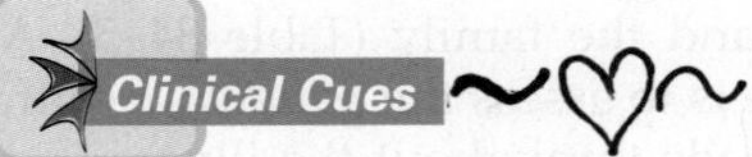

Clinical Cues

If your patient is somewhat resistant to listening to the nutritionist, support the diet teaching by showing enthusiasm and providing openings for the nutritionist to give the information. For example, the nurse says, "I'd be interested in hearing about the list of quality protein foods. This sample menu looks pretty good. Do you have more examples we could look at?"

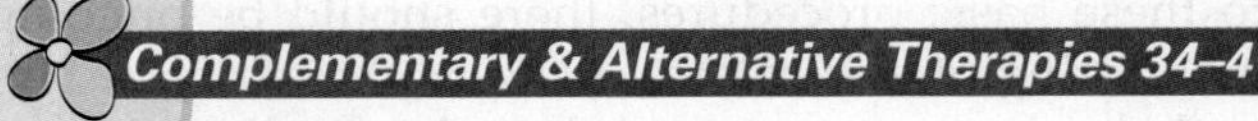

Complementary & Alternative Therapies 34–4

Acupressure and Massage

In experimental studies, acupressure and massage have helped to relieve fatigue and depression for end-stage renal patients.

Encourage communication between patient and spouse to express feelings about changes in sexual activity, role reversal, and family responsibilities. Kidney-failure patients often have self-care deficits that affect self-esteem and create an increased caregiver burden. Encourage the family to achieve a balance between supporting the patient and allowing as much independence as possible (Complementary & Alternative Therapies 34–4).

Evaluation

Evaluation of patients with chronic illness requires careful reassessment and attention to detail. The desired outcomes may occur more slowly and less dramatically compared with acute conditions; however, subtle changes in trends should be noted and considered in determining effectiveness of treatment. You use daily physical assessments, weights, I&O data, and laboratory data to monitor trends over a period of days to determine clinical improvement or the presence of problems. Daily fluctuations in subjective symptoms, such as fatigue or discomfort, along with ambivalent feelings toward the therapeutic regimen, are expected; however, if symptoms are prolonged or ongoing, the care plan should be revised.

Think Critically About . . . Your CRF patient is withdrawn and sullen at times, and is sharp and demanding at other times. How will you respond to this? How will you help the family deal with this behavior?

COMMUNITY CARE

A major function of nursing in the community is to assist hypertensive and diabetic patients to achieve good control of their disease. Adequate control of blood pressure and blood sugar helps prevent damage to the kidneys. One of the *Healthy People 2010* goals is to reduce the rate of new cases of ESRD. All nurses can promote healthy kidney function in the community by encouraging the intake of more water and prompt recognition and treatment of urinary tract infections. In addition, nurses can participate in community education to increase awareness of organ donation programs.

Nurses in outpatient clinics assist with urologic procedures, such as cystoscopy and removal or destruction of renal stones. They teach and monitor the patient with bladder or kidney cancer. Clinic nurses also do a great deal of teaching to help with problems of incontinence.

Home care nurses are constantly on the alert for signs of ARF or CRF among their patients. Many illnesses and the variety of drugs that patients receive may cause kidney damage. Many home care patients have indwelling catheters that must be periodically replaced with new ones. Home health nurses also identify problems of incontinence and have the advantage of being able to see the environmental and social factors that must be addressed.

Nurses in long-term care facilities deal with a variety of urinary problems. Bladder training for incontinence is a prime consideration. Monitoring for drug toxicities in this population is imperative, as drugs are not excreted quickly and polypharmacy can have additive effects. Keeping residents dry and odor free is very important for physical and psychological reasons. Monitoring for urinary retention or obstruction to the flow of urine is another priority in the elderly population.

Nurses who work in dialysis centers are often the primary nurses for patients in renal failure. These nurses must constantly assess patients for complications, watch for medication-related problems, and continue to reinforce diet and lifestyle modifications. Considerable psychosocial support and counseling may be necessary, as dialysis patients often experience depression, hopelessness, sexual problems, role changes, and relationship problems.

Key Points

- Teach prevention of infectious disorders, such as cystitis and urethritis (e.g., good hygiene, drinking plenty of water, and seeking prompt treatment for genital discharge or dysuria).
- Pyelonephritis: Infection of the kidney caused by bacterial invasion.
- Acute glomerulonephritis is characterized by fever, chills, flank pain, widespread edema, visual disturbances, and significant hypertension; nursing implications include encouraging bed rest, low-protein and low-sodium diet, and administering antihypertensives, corticosteroids, and diuretics as ordered.
- Symptoms of chronic glomerulonephritis include edema, dyspnea, and headache associated with hypertension.
- Hydronephrosis: Flow of urine from the kidney is obstructed; kidney dilates and fills with fluid.
- Renal stenosis: Renal artery can become blocked or narrowed because of atherosclerosis.
- Renal stones are associated with frequent urinary infections, inadequate fluid intake and concentrated urine, urinary stasis, and urate in the urine.
- Symptoms of trauma to the kidneys, ureters, and bladder may include gross hematuria, pain, or an enlarged mass in renal or bladder area.
- Risk factors for cancer of the bladder: Male gender, smoking, and exposure to industrial toxins.
- Symptoms of cancer of the kidney: Hematuria and enlargement of affected kidney are major signs.
- ARF: *Prerenal ARF* is caused by decreased blood flow (e.g., hypovolemic shock); *intrarenal ARF* occurs from damage in the kidney (e.g., glomerular damage); *postrenal ARF* is caused by obstruction (e.g., enlarged prostate), which causes backup of urine into the kidney.
- ATN can be caused by decreased oxygenation or blood flow, or nephrotoxic substances.
- Three phases of ARF: Oliguric/nonoliguric, diuretic, and recovery.
- Nephrosclerosis (hardening of renal arterioles), glomerulonephritis, diabetic nephropathy, are the most common causes of CRF.
- Treatment of CRF: Diet management, fluid and electrolyte management, hemodialysis, or peritoneal dialysis and kidney transplant.

- Hemodialysis: Use of diffusion to remove waste products normally excreted by the kidneys. Complications include fluid overload, electrolyte imbalance, anemia, platelet abnormalities, and infection.
- Peritoneal dialysis uses a dialyzing solution instilled through a catheter into the peritoneal cavity that is left in the cavity for the dwell time, and then removed.
- Nursing implications for peritoneal dialysis: Weigh patient and take vital signs before and after treatment, measure I&O, use strict aseptic technique, and monitor for infection.
- Kidney transplant is another treatment for kidney failure. Signs of organ rejection include elevated blood pressure, fever, pain over transplant area, fatigue, oliguria, increased BUN and serum creatinine.

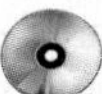
Go to your **Companion CD-ROM** for an Audio Glossary, animations, video clips, and bonus review questions.

evolve Be sure to visit the companion Evolve site at http://evolve.elsevier.com/deWit for interactive NCLEX-PN Exam Style Review Questions, WebLinks, and additional online resources.

NCLEX-PN EXAM STYLE REVIEW QUESTIONS

Choose the best answer(s) for the following questions.

1. ________________ is the accumulation of nitrogenous products with accompanying signs and symptoms.

2. Which statement would not be included in the discharge instructions for a patient who was treated for urinary tract infections (UTIs)?
  1. "Always wipe from back to front after a bowel movement."
  2. "Avoid wearing tight slacks."
  3. "Do not wash underclothing with strong detergents."
  4. "Showers are preferred over tub baths."

3. A patient with a history of throat infection becomes suddenly ill with fever, chills, flank pain, widespread edema, puffiness about the eyes, visual disturbances, and marked hypertension. The nurse would anticipate which of the following diagnostic tests?
  1. Urinalysis
  2. Creatinine kinase
  3. Serum amylase
  4. Prothrombin time

4. A 45-year-old male is admitted with renal staghorn calculus. The nurse observes that the patient is stoic and withdrawn, occasionally grimacing, and refuses any type of pain medication. The nursing diagnosis for this patient is Acute pain. An appropriate goal for this patient would be to:
  1. verbalize level of pain.
  2. have a tolerable level of pain.
  3. identify the source of pain.
  4. develop coping strategies.

5. Which of the following patients would have the highest risk for bladder cancer?
  1. A 45-year-old male smoker who is a house painter in a city
  2. An 80-year-old female nonsmoker, retired teacher in a small town
  3. A 75-year-old male smoker, retired textile worker in a city
  4. A 35-year-old female nonsmoker, hairdresser in a small town

6. A patient with nephrotic syndrome is admitted with severe generalized edema and cloudy urine. A priority nursing diagnosis would be:
  1. Impaired urinary elimination.
  2. Fluid volume excess.
  3. Disturbed body image.
  4. Altered tissue perfusion.

7. The nurse is preparing to administer bacille Calmette-Guérin (BCG) intravesically to a patient with bladder cancer. Which of the following actions would the nurse take first?
  1. Clamp the urethral catheter for 2 hours.
  2. Change position every 15 to 30 minutes.
  3. Aseptically insert a urinary catheter.
  4. Drain urinary bladder.

8. Nursing care of the patient undergoing peritoneal dialysis includes which of the following? *(Select all that apply.)*
  1. Maintain aseptic technique when accessing a peritoneal catheter.
  2. Instill warmed dialysates slowly.
  3. Weigh the patient before and after dialysis.
  4. Monitor vital signs.
  5. Check color and volume of effluent.

9. The nurse is sending the patient to the dialysis clinic. Predialysis nursing intervention includes which of the following? *(Select all that apply.)*
  1. Withholding anticoagulants
  2. Administering antihypertensive
  3. Assessing dialysis access site
  4. Checking vital signs
  5. Monitoring laboratory values

10. While caring for a patient with uremic syndrome, the nurse would anticipate which of the following clinical findings?
  1. Hypercalcemia
  2. Hypophosphatemia
  3. Polycythemia
  4. Hypoalbuminemia

CRITICAL THINKING ACTIVITIES 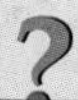 *Read each clinical scenario and discuss the questions with your classmates.*

Scenario A

Mr. Jakes, 25-years-old, comes to the clinic complaining of sudden onset of fever and chills, flank pain, and "feeling full all over and peeing dark smoke-colored urine." He tells you he had strep throat 2 weeks ago, but is otherwise healthy.

1. Based on Mr. Jakes' history and complaints, what physical assessments should you perform?
2. Why is the history of strep throat 2 weeks ago significant?
3. The physician informs Mr. Jakes that he has glomerulonephritis and prescribes complete bed rest. How long must bed rest continue?

Scenario B

Ms. Temple is a 22-year-old college student. She comes to the clinic with the complaint of a color change to her urine and urinary frequency. She begins to cry and asks if she has cancer.

1. How will you respond to Ms. Temple's anxiety about potential cancer?
2. Identify five or six other questions that you should ask Ms. Temple.
3. What are the possible causes of various color changes in the urine?

Scenario C

Mr. Mell is a 43-year-old interstate truck driver. He complains of severe right lower back pain with nausea and vomiting and pink-tinged urine. He relates a history of stones and reports, "It always feels like this until the kidney stone passes." The physician orders IV normal saline, morphine, routine labs to include BUN, creatinine, and an IVP.

1. What are three or four risk factors for kidney stones that might apply to Mr. Mell?
2. His BUN result is 17 mg/dL. What does this result indicate? What is your responsibility in reporting this data?
3. What is the care for Mr. Mell following a lithotripsy?

The Endocrine System

evolve http://evolve.elsevier.com/deWit

Objectives

Upon completing the chapter you should be able to:

Theory

1. Identify the location of each endocrine gland.
2. Illustrate the principal actions and target tissues for hormones of the hypothalamus and pituitary, thyroid, parathyroid, adrenal, and pancreas glands.
3. Verbalize three specific age-related changes in the endocrine system.
4. Describe common diagnostic tests for the endocrine system.

Clinical Practice

1. Teach patients about the diagnostic tests that might be performed for symptoms of endocrine disorders.
2. Perform a focused assessment on a patient who possibly has an endocrine disorder.
3. Identify nursing diagnoses and appropriate interventions for problems common to patients with endocrine disorders.

Key Terms

Be sure to check out the bonus material on the Companion CD-ROM, including selected audio pronunciations.

adenohypophysis (ă-DĔN-ō-hī-pō-FĂ-sĭs, p. 873)
adrenocorticotropic hormone (ă-DRĔN-ō-KŎR-tĭ-ko-TRŌ-pĭk, p. 873)
endocrine (ĔN-dō-krĭn, p. 872)
exocrine (Ĕk-sō-krĭn, p. 875)
fructosamine assay (p. 881)
glucocorticoids (gloo-kō-KŎR-tĭ-koydz, p. 875)
glucose tolerance test (p. 881)
glycosylated hemoglobin (glī-KO-sĭ-lat-ĕd HĒ-mō-glō-bĭn, p. 881)
hemoglobin A_{1c} (HĒ-mō-glō-bĭn, p. 881)
hormones (HŎR-mōnz, p. 872)
hypersecretion (hī-pĕr-SĒ-KRĒ-shŭn, p. 877)
hyposecretion (hī-pō-SĒ-KRĒ-shŭn, p. 877)
insulin (ĬN-sū-lĭn, p. 873)
mineralocorticoids (mĭn-ĕr-ăl-ō-KŎR-tĭ-koydz, p. 875)
negative feedback (p. 872)
parathormone (păr-ă-THŎR-mōn, p. 874)
pressor (p. 874)
target cells (p. 872)
target tissues (p. 872)
thyrocalcitonin (thī-rō-KAL-sĭ-TŌ-nĭn, p. 874)
thyroid panel (THĪ-royd, p. 881)
thyroxine (THĪ-rŏk-sĭn, p. 874)
triiodothyronine (trī-ī-o-dō-THĪ-rō-nĕn, p. 874)

The **endocrine** system is a complex but very interesting system important in regulating metabolism, growth and development, and sexual function and reproductive processes. The endocrine system is made up of groups of cells whose primary function is to synthesize and release **hormones** directly into the bloodstream and body fluids. These hormones are transported by the blood to various parts of the body, where they act on cells to control their physiologic functions. The cells and tissues that are affected by a specific hormone are called its **target cells** or **target tissues**.

Some of the endocrine hormones, such as the thyroid hormones, affect practically every cell in the body. Others, such as the sex hormones, exert their special effects on only one kind of organ. Moreover, hormones from one endocrine gland can affect another endocrine gland. The pituitary, for example, secretes several different kinds of hormones that affect other endocrine glands. For this reason, the pituitary gland is often referred to as the "master gland" of the body.

The endocrine system and the nervous system are the two major control systems of the body, and their regulatory functions are interrelated. However, the endocrine system typically controls body processes that occur slowly, such as cell growth, whereas the nervous system controls body processes that occur more rapidly, such as breathing and body movement.

The secretion of a particular hormone normally depends on the need for it. If an endocrine gland receives a message that its particular hormone is in short supply, it will synthesize and release more. If, on the other hand, the hormonal need of a target tissue is being satisfied, production or secretion of the hormone will be inhibited, a concept known as **negative feedback**.

Some glands, such as the adrenal medulla and posterior pituitary, receive their information about hormone levels in the body directly and respond only to stimulation of nerve endings in the glands themselves. However, the posterior pituitary gland indirectly receives notice to either release or inhibit hormones. Stimulation comes by way of the hypothalamus and the anterior lobe of the pituitary (the **adenohypophysis**). The hypothalamus contains special nerve endings that produce releasing and inhibiting hormones that are absorbed into capillaries of a portal system that transports them to the adenohypophysis. Thus the hypothalamus controls the secretion of hormones from the pituitary, which in turn controls the release or inhibition of hormones from other glands. Many of the hormones of the anterior pituitary are "tropic" hormones; that is, they tend to cause a change in the endocrine gland that is the target of the specific pituitary hormone. An example is **adrenocorticotropic hormone**, or ACTH, which acts on the adrenal cortex. (If you break down this term, you can easily see that the components of adrenal + cortex + tropic tell you exactly where or what type of hormone this is and where it comes from.) The major endocrine glands can be found in Figure 35–1; various tropic hormones and target tissues are shown in Table 35–1 on p. 878.

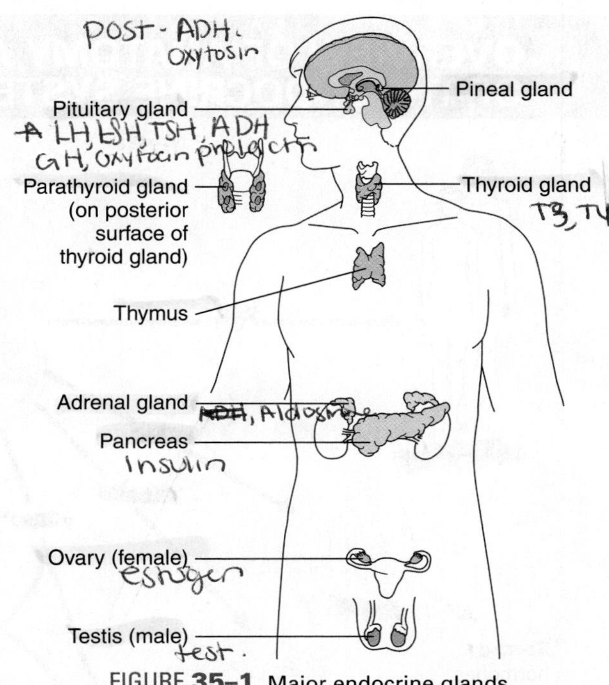

FIGURE **35–1** Major endocrine glands.

OVERVIEW OF ANATOMY AND PHYSIOLOGY OF THE ENDOCRINE SYSTEM

What are the organs and structures of the endocrine system?

- The pituitary gland connects to the hypothalamus via the hypophyseal stalk. It consists of two parts: the anterior pituitary and the posterior pituitary.
- The thyroid gland has two lobes and lies below the larynx over the thyroid cartilage in front of and on either side of the trachea.
- The parathyroid glands are four to six small glands that are located on the posterior surface of the thyroid gland.
- The adrenal glands are located on the anterior upper surface of each kidney; each is composed of the cortex and medulla.
- The pancreas sits in the upper left aspect of the abdominal cavity. Beta cells, which secrete the hormone **insulin**, are found in the islets of Langerhans.
- The ovaries are located in the pelvic cavity of the female.
- The testes hang suspended in the scrotum of the male.
- The pineal gland is in the midbrain in the cranial vault.
- The thymus gland lies at the base of the neck in the front of the thoracic cavity.

What are the functions of the endocrine system?

The endocrine system works in the body by:

- Altering chemical reactions and controlling the rates at which chemical activities take place within the cells.
- Changing the permeability of the cell membrane and selecting the substances that can be transported across the membrane.
- Activating a particular mechanism in the cell, such as the system that controls cellular growth and reproduction. The hormones produced by the endocrine system, the target organs on which they act, and the principal actions of each hormone are presented in Table 35–1.

What are the effects of the pituitary hormones?

- The effects of these hormones when secreted are illustrated in Figure 35–2.
- Any type of dysfunction of the pituitary gland will affect one or more of these hormones, as well as the target organ for that hormone.

OVERVIEW OF ANATOMY AND PHYSIOLOGY OF THE ENDOCRINE SYSTEM—cont'd

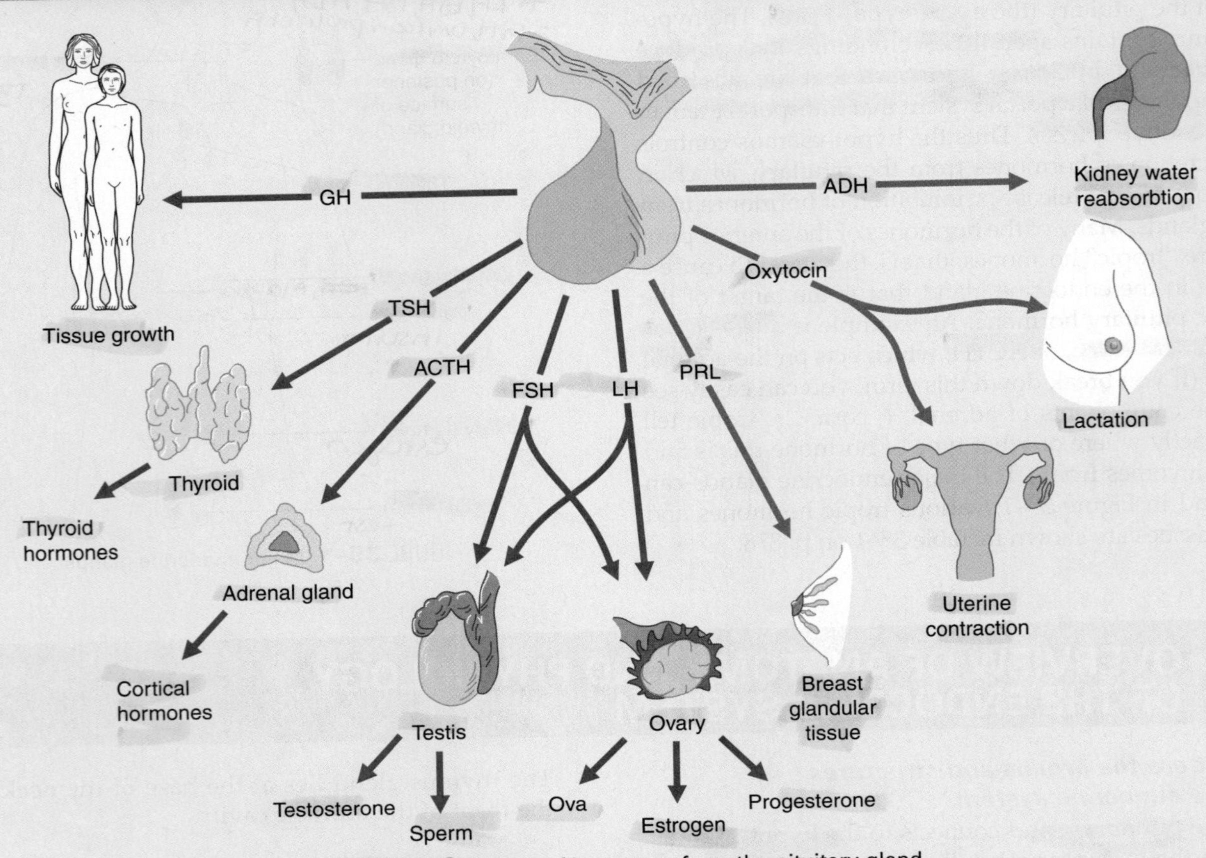

FIGURE 35–2 Effects of hormones from the pituitary gland.

What are the effects of the thyroid hormones?

- The thyroid gland secretes the hormones **thyroxine** (T_4), **triiodothyronine** (T_3), and **thyrocalcitonin.**
- T_3 is the more potent form of thyroid hormone. When T_3 is needed, it is converted from the more abundant supply of T_4.
- Intake of protein and iodine is needed to synthesize both thyroid hormones.
- Thyroid hormones activate the cellular production of heat; stimulate protein and lipid synthesis, mobilization, and degradation (breakdown); and stimulate the manufacture of coenzymes from vitamins.
- Thyroid hormones regulate many aspects of carbohydrate metabolism and affect tissue response to epinephrine and norepinephrine.

What are the functions of the parathyroid glands?

- **Parathormone,** or parathyroid hormone, is produced and secreted by the parathyroid glands.
- A low calcium level will stimulate release of parathormone, which increases the plasma level of calcium. A high calcium level will inhibit the release of parathormone.
- Parathormone acts on the renal tubules to increase the excretion of phosphorus in the urine and the reabsorption of calcium. It also acts on bone, causing the release of calcium from the bone into the bloodstream (Safety Alert 35–1 on p. 877).

What are the functions of the hormones secreted by the adrenal glands?

- The adrenal medulla (middle portion) secretes two hormones, epinephrine and norepinephrine, in response to stimulation from the sympathetic nervous system.
- Epinephrine prepares the body to meet stress or emergency situations and prevents hypoglycemia (Figure 35–3). Norepinephrine functions as a **pressor** (causing blood vessel constriction) hormone to maintain blood pressure.

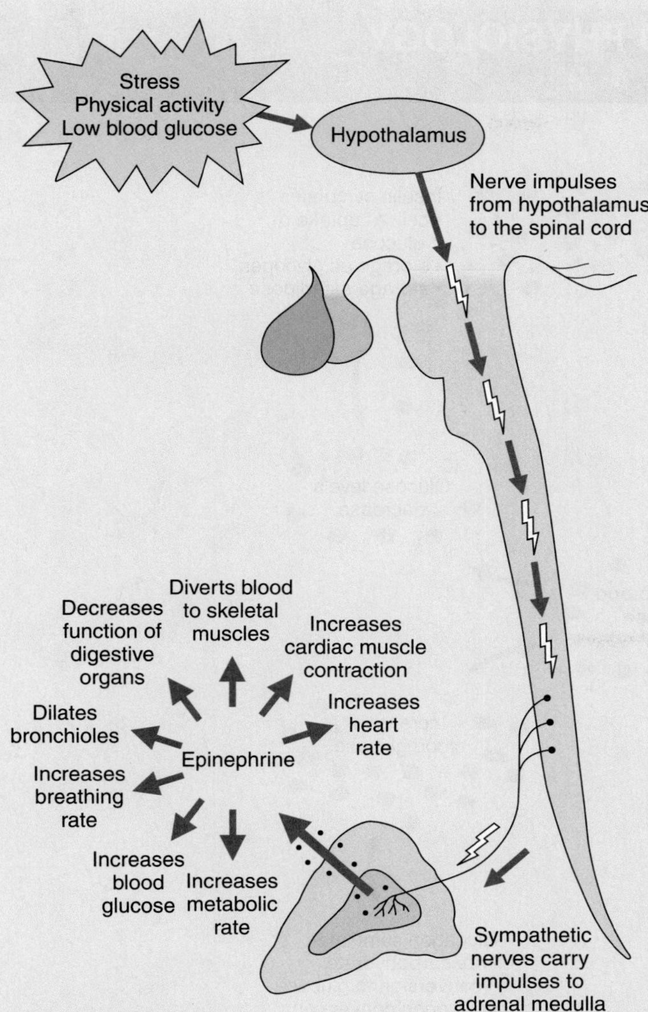

FIGURE 35–3 Epinephrine: its effects and control of its secretion.

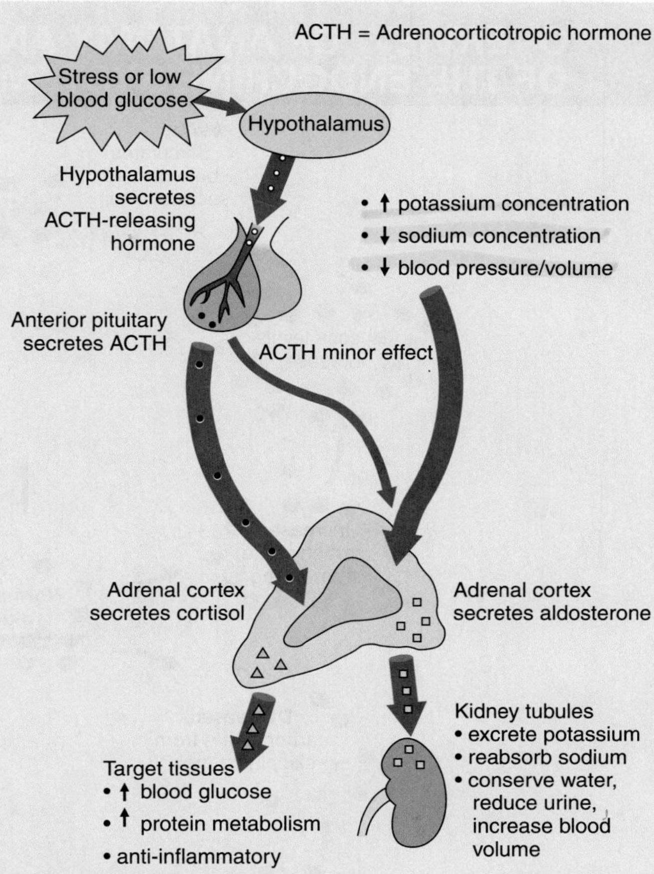

FIGURE 35–4 Regulation of aldosterone and cortisol secretion.

- The hormones secreted by the adrenal cortex are called *adrenal corticosteroids*. The word *steroid* is sometimes used to designate an adrenal corticosteroid or a synthetic compound with similar properties.
- The two major types of hormones secreted by the adrenal cortex are the **mineralocorticoids** and the **glucocorticoids** (Figure 35–4).
- Small amounts of androgenic hormones also are secreted, which have effects similar to those of the male and female sex hormones.
- The mineralocorticoids affect the electrolytes, particularly sodium, potassium, and chloride. The chief mineralocorticoid is aldosterone, which promotes conservation of water by acting on the kidney to retain sodium in exchange for potassium, which is excreted in the urine (Safety Alert 35–2 on p. 877).
- The glucocorticoids are essential to the metabolic systems for proper utilization of carbohydrates, proteins, and fats.
- The primary **glucocorticoid** is cortisol, or hydrocortisone. Cortisol acts to increase glucose levels in the blood. Cortisol also helps counteract the inflammatory response.
- Both aldosterone and cortisol are controlled by ACTH-releasing hormone from the hypothalamus and ACTH secreted by the anterior pituitary (see Figure 35–4).

What is the hormonal function of the pancreas?

- The pancreas is both an endocrine (secretes internally) and **exocrine** (secretes outwardly through a duct) gland. Its endocrine function is to produce the hormones insulin and glucagon.
- The beta cells are responsible for producing and secreting insulin. Insulin is needed for the cells of the body to be able to utilize glucose as fuel (Figures 35–5 and 35–6).

Continued

OVERVIEW OF ANATOMY AND PHYSIOLOGY OF THE ENDOCRINE SYSTEM—cont'd

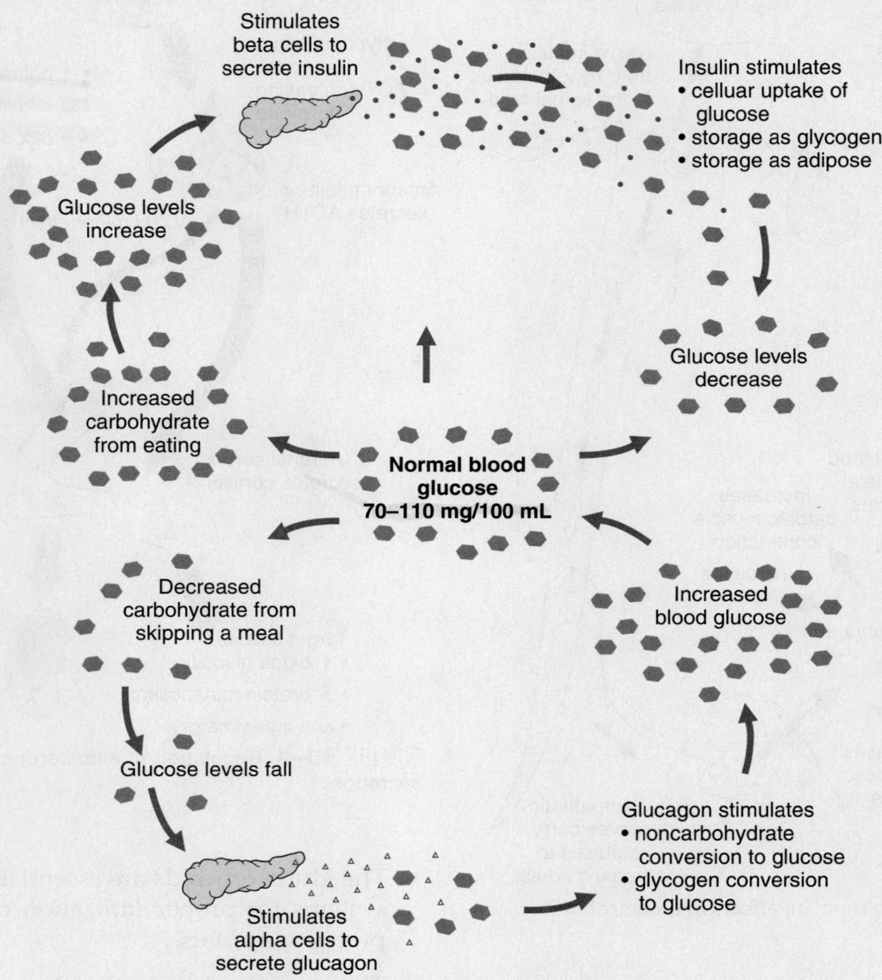

FIGURE **35–5** Effects of insulin and glucagon.

What are the effects of aging on the endocrine system?

- The pituitary gland becomes smaller.
- The thyroid becomes more lumpy or nodular; metabolism gradually declines, beginning around age 20.
- Hormones that usually decrease with age include aldosterone, renin, calcitonin, and growth hormone; also specific hormones decrease in the older female (estrogen and prolactin) and the older male (testosterone).
- Hormones that may increase with age include follicle-stimulating hormone (FSH), luteinizing hormone (LH), norepinephrine, and antidiuretic hormone (ADH).
- Hormones that remain unchanged or are only slightly decreased include thyroid hormones (T_3 and T_4), cortisol, insulin, epinephrine, parathyroid hormone, and 25-hydroxyvitamin D.
- Blood glucose levels rise with age, with fasting levels climbing about 1 mg/dL for each decade and postprandial levels increasing 6 to 13 mg/dL.
- Although insulin levels remain unchanged, decreased glucose tolerance may occur due to changes in the cell receptor sites, which can place the older adult at risk for hyperglycemia and the onset of type 2 diabetes.
- The older adult experiences hypoglycemia more quickly than a younger person and may progress to dangerously low levels of blood glucose before signs and symptoms are obvious.
- Although thyroid hormone levels may decrease with aging, the body makes up for it by decreasing the rate it is broken down; therefore, resting

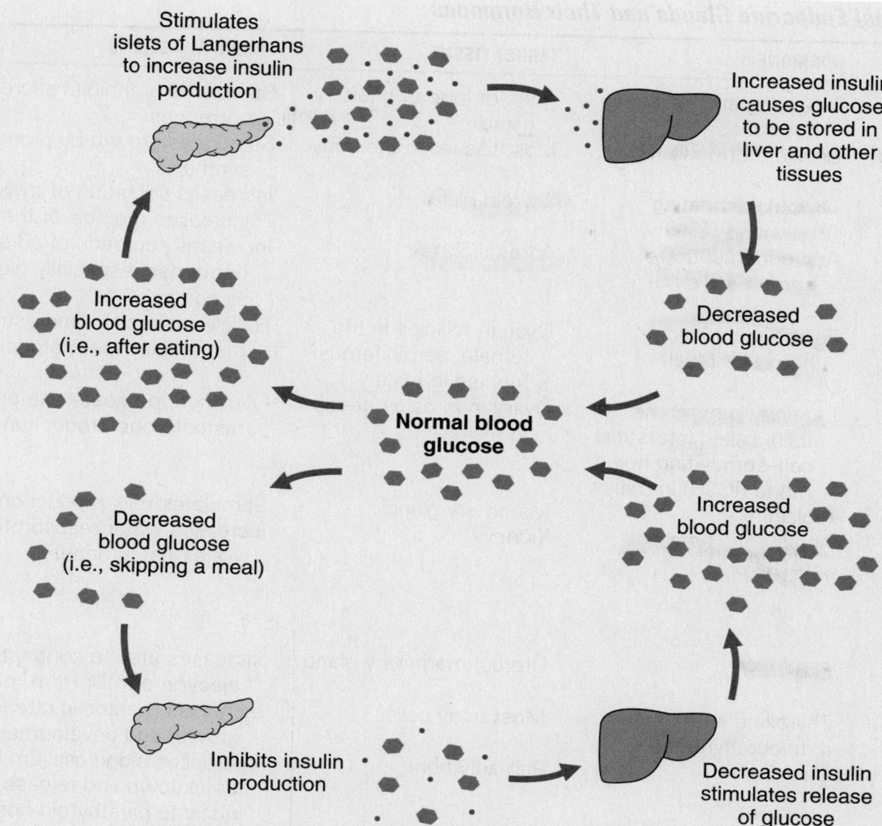

FIGURE **35–6** Interaction of blood glucose and insulin.

levels are usually normal. Thyroid disorders are, however, twice as common in the older adult. Hypothyroidism is the most common thyroid disorder, especially in older women.

- The amount of hormones secreted changes, decreasing the individual's ability to adapt to stress and respond to environmental changes as readily as someone younger.
- Because of decreasing liver and kidney function in the elderly, hormone replacement therapy must be done very cautiously to prevent overdosage.

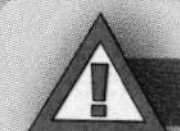
Safety Alert 35–1

Parathyroid Deficiency

A deficiency of parathyroid hormone produces muscle cramps, twitching of the muscles, and, in some cases, severe convulsions.

Safety Alert 35–2

Lifesaving Hormones

Without the mineralocorticoids, a person would die within 3 to 7 days, because these hormones directly control fluid balance, blood volume, cardiac output, exchange of nutrients, and wastes in each cell, and, in effect, all chemical processes and glandular functions within the body. Little wonder that they are said to be "lifesaving hormones."

The interrelationships between endocrine glands, the hormones they synthesize and release, and the systems affected are complex. Many steps occur between the time the need for a hormone is sensed and the time the hormone is actually released.

CAUSES AND PREVENTION OF ENDOCRINE PROBLEMS

Endocrine disorders are caused by an imbalance in the production of hormone or by an alteration in the body's ability to use the hormones produced. Dysfunction can occur at any point in the production-secretion-feedback regulation cycle.

Primary endocrine dysfunction means that an endocrine gland is either oversecreting or undersecreting hormone(s)—situations referred to as **hypersecretion** and **hyposecretion**, respectively. Tumor or hyperpla-

Table 35–1 ***The Principal Endocrine Glands and Their Hormones***

GLAND	HORMONE	TARGET TISSUE	PRINCIPAL ACTIONS
Hypothalamus	Releasing and inhibiting hormones	Anterior lobe of pituitary gland	Stimulates or inhibits secretion of specific hormones
Anterior lobe of pituitary	Growth hormone (GH)	Most tissues in the body	Stimulates growth by promoting protein synthesis
	Thyroid-stimulating hormone (TSH)	Thyroid gland	Increases secretion of thyroid hormone; increases the size of the thyroid gland
	Adrenocorticotropic hormone (ACTH)	Adrenal cortex	Increases secretion of adrenocortical hormones, especially glucocorticoids, such as cortisol
	Follicle-stimulating hormone (FSH)	Ovarian follicles in the female; seminiferous tubules in male	Follicle maturation and estrogen secretion in the female; spermatogenesis in the male
	Luteinizing hormone (LH); called interstitial cell–stimulating hormone (ICSH) in males	Ovary in females, testis in males	Ovulation; progesterone production in female; testosterone production in male
	Prolactin	Mammary gland	Stimulates milk production
Posterior lobe of pituitary (storage only: ADH and oxytocin are synthesized in the hypothalamus)	Antidiuretic hormone (ADH)	Kidney	Increases water reabsorption (decreases water lost in urine)
	Oxytocin	Uterus; mammary gland	Increases uterine contractions; stimulates ejection of milk from mammary gland
Thyroid gland	Thyroxine and triiodothyronine	Most body cells	Increases metabolic rate; essential for normal growth and development
	Calcitonin	Primarily bone	Decreases blood calcium by inhibiting bone breakdown and release of calcium; antagonistic to parathyroid hormone
Parathyroid gland	Parathyroid hormone (PTH) or parathormone	Bone, kidney, digestive tract	Increases blood calcium by stimulating bone breakdown and release of calcium; increases calcium absorption in the digestive tract; decreases calcium lost in urine
Adrenal cortex	Mineralocorticoids (aldosterone)	Kidney	Increases sodium reabsorption and potassium excretion in kidney tubules; increases water retention
	Glucocorticoids (cortisol)	Most body tissues	Increases blood glucose levels; inhibits inflammation and immune response
	Androgens and estrogens	Most body tissues	Secreted in small amounts; effect is generally masked by the hormones from the ovaries and testes
Adrenal medulla	Epinephrine, norepinephrine	Heart, blood vessels, liver, adipose	Helps cope with stress; increases heart rate and blood pressure; increases blood flow to skeletal muscle; increases blood glucose
Pancreas (islets of Langerhans)	Glucagon	Liver	Increases breakdown of glycogen to increase blood glucose levels
	Insulin	General, but especially liver, skeletal muscle, adipose	Decreases blood glucose levels by facilitating uptake and utilization of glucose by cells; stimulates glucose storage as glycogen and production of adipose tissue
Testes	Testosterone	Most body cells	Maturation and maintenance of male reproductive organs and secondary sex characteristics
Ovaries	Estrogens	Most body cells	Maturation and maintenance of female reproductive organs and secondary sex characteristics; menstrual cycle
	Progesterone	Uterus and breast	Prepares uterus for pregnancy; stimulates development of mammary gland; menstrual cycle
Pineal gland	Melatonin	Hypothalamus	Inhibits gonadotropin-releasing hormone, which consequently inhibits reproductive functions; regulates daily rhythms, such as sleep and wakefulness
Thymus	Thymosin	Tissues involved in immune response	Immune system development and function

From Applegate, E.J. (2006). *The Anatomy and Physiology Learning System* (3rd ed.). Philadelphia: Saunders, pp. 209–210.

sia of the gland may lead to hypersecretion. Hyposecretion is usually the result of a tumor or an inflammatory process that destroys glandular tissue or interferes with function. Infection, mechanical damage, or an autoimmune response may cause such an inflammatory response in a gland.

Secondary endocrine dysfunction occurs from factors outside the gland itself. Medications, trauma, hormone therapy, and other factors may cause secondary dysfunction. Such dysfunction may be temporary or permanent; function often returns to normal if the cause is corrected (for example, the medication is discontinued).

Preventing most endocrine disorders is not possible by lifestyle changes; however, there are some dietary considerations regarding the thyroid gland (Health Promotion Points 35–1).

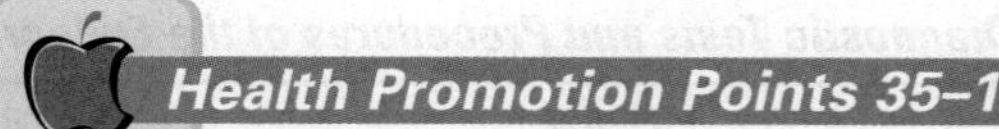

Preventing Goiter

Goiter, an overgrowth of the thyroid, may be prevented by sufficient intake of iodine. Iodine is available in foods grown near the ocean and seafood. Iodized salt is the major source for most people.

DIAGNOSTIC TESTS AND PROCEDURES

Tests of the endocrine system are performed on blood samples, urine samples, or by scans, ultrasounds, x-rays, or magnetic resonance imaging (MRI). Table 35–2 presents the various tests and procedures with their nursing implications.

Table 35–2 ***Diagnostic Tests and Procedures of the Endocrine System***

TEST	PURPOSE	DESCRIPTION	NURSING IMPLICATIONS
BLOOD TESTS			
Pituitary hormone levels: LH, FSH, GH, ACTH, TSH, prolactin	Detect oversecretion or deficiency of pituitary hormones	Sample of venous blood is drawn; requires at least 1 mL for immunoassay test; check lab procedure manual.	Monitor venipuncture site for bleeding; apply bandage or dressing.
Serum T_4 (total thyroxine) *Normal value:* 4.5–11.5 mcg/dL	Assess thyroxine in blood to evaluate thyroid function	Requires a venous blood sample of at least 1 mL.	Aspirin, iodine-containing medications, contrast media, and other drugs may affect result; check with lab.
Serum T_3 (total triiodothyronine) *Normal value:* 70–190 ng/dL	Used with T_4 to evaluate thyroid function	Requires a venous blood sample of at least 1 mL.	Same as for serum T_4.
TSH (thyroid-stimulating hormone) *Normal value:* 1–10 μU/mL	To differentiate between pituitary dysfunction and primary thyroid dysfunction; assist with diagnosis of hypothyroidism	Requires a venous blood sample of at least 1 mL.	Same as for serum T_4.
Antithyroid antibody titer *Normal value:* <1:100	Detect the presence of thyroid antibodies and distinguish between autoimmune disorders and toxic thyroid adenoma	Requires a venous blood sample.	Radioactive iodine will interfere if given within 24 hr of withdrawal of blood sample.
Calcitonin *Normal value:* <100 pg/mL	Used for differential diagnosis of cancer of the thyroid	Requires a venous blood sample.	If base level is within normal, pentagastrin may be administered by injection. Blood samples are then drawn 1½ and 5 min after injection.
Cortisol *Normal value:* 8 A.M., 6–23 mcg/dL; 4 P.M., 3–15 mcg/dL; 10 P.M., <50% of 8 A.M. value	Assess cortisol production by adrenal glands	Requires sample of venous blood.	Explain that a specimen may be collected two or three times in 24 hr to evaluate circadian effects on cortisol secretion. Keep stress to a minimum. Note time collected on laboratory slip.
Adrenocorticotropic hormone (ACTH) *Normal value:* A.M., 20–100 pg/mL; P.M., 10–40 pg/mL	Assess ACTH production from pituitary gland	Requires venous blood sample. Place specimen in ice water immediately after drawing.	Prepare ice bath before venipuncture. Note collection time on lab slip. Single specimen is best collected in morning.

Continued

Table 35–2 ***Diagnostic Tests and Procedures of the Endocrine System—cont'd***

TEST	PURPOSE	DESCRIPTION	NURSING IMPLICATIONS
BLOOD TESTS—cont'd			
ACTH stimulation test *Normal value:* after ACTH; serum cortisol >20 mcg/dL	Assess adrenal response to ACTH Used to detect adrenal cortical insufficiency (Addison's disease)	Baseline venous sample taken for cortisol determination. ACTH is administered IV or IM. Blood sample is withdrawn at 30 and 60 min for further cortisol determinations.	Note time ACTH is administered; note time each specimen is drawn. Instruct patient to avoid strenuous activity on the day before the test. Check with laboratory regarding food restrictions.
Dexamethasone suppression test *Normal value:* after dexamethasone, serum cortisol <5 mcg/dL	Help diagnose Cushing syndrome Assess response to dexamethasone	Morning baseline serum cortisol levels are measured. Oral dexamethasone is administered at bedtime. Blood sample is collected the next morning to measure cortisol levels.	Explain the procedure to the patient. Check orders for drugs to be withheld. Both cortisol levels must be drawn at the same time each day. Note time specimens were drawn and patient medications on lab slips. Instruct patient to avoid strenuous activity the day before the test.
THYROID SCANS			
Radioactive iodine uptake (RAIU) *Normal values:* <6% uptake in 2 hr; 2%–25% in 6 hr; 15%–45% in 24 hr. 24-hr urine: 40%–80% radioactive iodine excreted in 24 hr.	Assess function of thyroid gland Measures the rate of iodine uptake by the thyroid	Trace dose of radioactive iodine (RAI) is given orally. A gamma counter or scintillation counter is placed over the gland to measure the amount of RAI absorbed. Concurrent 24-hr urine specimen may be collected to assess iodine secretion.	Test must not be done during pregnancy or lactation. Explain that the amount of radioactive iodine used is small and will not make the patient "radioactive." Explain the procedure and the time it will take. Instruct how to collect 24-hr urine specimen if required.
Thyroid scan	Determine size, shape, and activity of the thyroid gland Detects hyperactive "hot" spots and hypoactive "cold" spots	After administering radioactive iodine, a scintillation camera moves back and forth across the gland to obtain an image of iodine concentration and distribution in the thyroid gland. A computer may provide a 3D image. Often done in conjunction with RAIU.	Same implications as for radioactive iodine uptake (RAIU). Patient must lie perfectly still during the scanning. Scan takes about 20 min. Rescanning is performed at intervals of 6 and 24 hr after RAI is administered.
URINE TESTS			
17-Hydroxycorticosteroids (17-OHCS) *Normal values:* females, 2–8 mg/24 hr; males, 3–9 mg/24 hr	Determine levels of glucocorticoid metabolites	Collect a 24-hr urine specimen in a container with preservative. Medications may interfere; consult with physician and laboratory about medications patient is taking.	Instruct patient in collection procedure. Note start and end time of collection on laboratory slip. Note medications patient is taking on laboratory slip.
17-Ketosteroids (17–KS) *Normal values:* females, 6-15 mg/24 hr; males, 8–22 mg/24 hr; older than age 65, 4–8 mg/24 hr	Determine amount of androgen metabolites in the urine	Collect 24-hr urine specimen. Check with laboratory regarding need to keep specimen chilled.	Same as for 17-hydroxycorticosteroids test.
Aldosterone 3–20 mcg/24 hr	Determine urinary aldosterone levels to assist in diagnosis of aldosteronism	Requires 24-hr urine specimen with preservative; specimen must be kept chilled.	Instruct in dietary and medication restrictions. Record diet and medications on laboratory slip.

Table 35–2 **Diagnostic Tests and Procedures of the Endocrine System—cont'd**

TEST	PURPOSE	DESCRIPTION	NURSING IMPLICATIONS
URINE TESTS—cont'd			
Fluid deprivation test	Detect DI	While patient is NPO, hourly urine output, specific gravity, osmolality are measured along with body weight and vital signs. Vasopressin is given Subcut; hourly measurements are continued for several hours.	Explain the procedure to the patient. Provide urine collection containers. Remind patient to void hourly.
Hypertonic saline test	Stimulates release of ADH to evaluate ADH secretion and detect diabetes insipidus (DI)	The patient is loaded with water. An infusion of hypertonic saline is administered. Urine output and urine specific gravity are measured hourly.	Tell patient to produce a urine specimen in the marked container q hr.

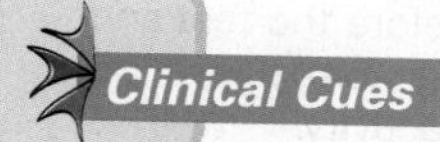

Clinical Cues

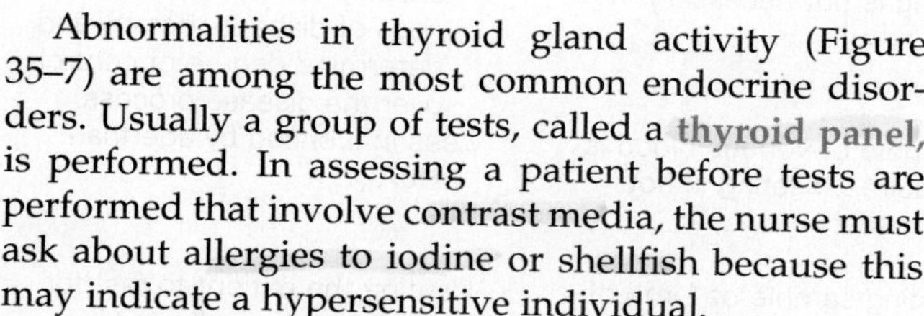

The nurse should be aware of factors that can distort test results:

- Thyroid test results are altered by iodine-based contrast media for radiologic studies.
- Betadine used for skin preparation may also affect thyroid studies.
- Oral contraceptives, aspirin, and other drugs may render thyroid hormone assays useless, because they either increase or decrease the levels of thyroid hormones (Qatanani, et. al, 2005, Samuels et. al, 2003; Toldy et al, 2004).

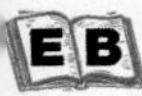

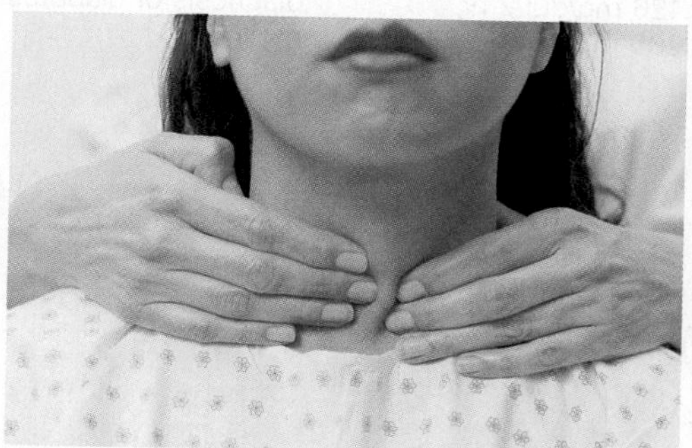

FIGURE **35–7** Posterior palpation of the thyroid gland.

Abnormalities in thyroid gland activity (Figure 35–7) are among the most common endocrine disorders. Usually a group of tests, called a **thyroid panel,** is performed. In assessing a patient before tests are performed that involve contrast media, the nurse must ask about allergies to iodine or shellfish because this may indicate a hypersensitive individual.

Laboratory testing for serum calcium and phosphate levels is usually performed to assess parathyroid function. Adrenal gland function is evaluated by laboratory testing, including electrolyte panels, glucose levels, and hormone levels; a 12-lead electrocardiogram (ECG) may be performed if cardiac dysrhythmias are suspected.

Diagnostic tests for detecting diabetes can be found in Table 35–3. Guidelines for the diagnosis of diabetes mellitus were revised in 2004. Diagnosis of diabetes mellitus can be made using any two of the following tests on different days:

- Symptoms of diabetes mellitus (Chapter 37) plus a random glucose level greater than or equal to 200 mg/dL
- A fasting glucose level of greater than or equal to 126 mg/dL or
- A **glucose tolerance test** revealing a postprandial glucose greater than or equal to 200, 2 hours after 75 g of glucose is administered

In a glucose tolerance test, the patient is given a set amount of glucose to evaluate insulin secretion and ability to metabolize glucose.

? *Think Critically About . . .* What instructions would you give to a patient who needs to collect a 24-hour urine specimen for hormonal studies?

The **glycosylated hemoglobin** test, commonly called **hemoglobin A_{1c},** measures blood glucose over a period of many weeks (Table 35–4). Glucose in the bloodstream attaches itself to the hemoglobin A molecule and remains there for the life span of the red blood cell. Physicians use test results to prescribe adjustments to a patient's treatment program in managing diabetes. **Fructosamine assay** is another test to monitor control of glucose over time. This test monitors blood glucose over a shorter time frame because it measures sugar attached to the protein albumin, which has a shorter life than hemoglobin.

NURSING MANAGEMENT

Assessment (Data Collection)

A full physical assessment and history are needed to evaluate the patient who is possibly experiencing an endocrine disorder. History taking collects data about how the patient perceives function of the various body systems affected by the endocrine glands (see Focused Assessment 35–1 on p. 863). Data elicited by history and assessment are evaluated, and the nurse then selects appropriate nursing diagnoses for the patient.

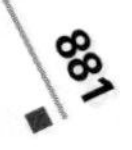

...tic Tests for Detecting and Monitoring Diabetes Mellitus

	PURPOSE	DESCRIPTION	NURSING IMPLICATIONS
... glucose *...l value:* 70–115 mg/dL; elderly: rises 1 mg/dL per decade of age	Determine level of circulating glucose; detect hyperglycemia or hypoglycemia	Requires a fasting venous blood sample.	Explain importance of fasting state to the patient.
2-hr postprandial blood glucose *Normal value:* <126 mg/dL; elderly: rises 5–10 mg/dL with age	Determine need for glucose tolerance test; determine need for change in diabetes therapy	Venous blood sample drawn 2 hr after a meal.	Explain the importance of presenting self for blood sampling exactly 2 hr after finishing a meal.
Glucose tolerance test *Normal values:* Fasting <126 mg/dL; 2 hr, <200 mg/dL	Detect abnormal glucose metabolism; assist in diagnosis of diabetes mellitus	A venous blood sample is drawn after a 10–12 hr fast; patient is given a glucose "load," usually a prepared liquid drink of 300 mL, that contains a specified amount of glucose. Venous blood samples are drawn at 30-min intervals for 2 hr. Phenytoin (Dilantin), birth control pills, diuretics, and glucocorticoids will adversely affect results; consult physician regarding taking these medications.	Instruct patient to eat a balanced diet with at least 150 g of carbohydrate for 3 days before the test and maintain a normal level of physical activity. Instruct patient to fast for 10–12 hr before beginning the test. Explain that during the test the patient cannot eat, drink, or smoke, and must stay at rest for 2 hr. During the test, instruct patient to report feelings of weakness, dizziness, nervousness, and confusion.
Glycosylated hemoglobin (HbA_{1c}) *Normal value:* 3.9%–5.2% (of total hemoglobin)	Determine degree of diabetic control of blood sugar over the preceding 6–8 wk	A sample of venous blood is required. Fasting is not necessary.	Explain to the patient the need for this test to be done periodically to monitor effectiveness of diabetic therapy and determine degree of control over the disease process.
Fructosamine assay *Normal values:* 1.5–2.7 mmol/L	Determine degree of diabetic control of blood sugar over preceding 2–3 wk	A sample of venous blood is required. Fasting is not necessary.	Less influenced by age than HbA_{1c}.
C-peptide *Normal values:* 0.78–1.89 ng/mL	Evaluate endogenous secretion of insulin when the presence of insulin antibodies interferes with direct assay of insulin	A fasting sample of 1 mL of venous blood is used.	Caution the patient to fast for 8–12 hr before the test. Water is permitted.
URINE TESTS			
Ketone bodies	Determine presence of ketones in the urine, which indicates a state of ketoacidosis	A fresh urine sample is tested with a dipstick or with Acetest tablet. Follow instructions on bottle of test material.	Instruct diabetic patient that ketone testing should be done whenever illness has interfered with normal eating and activity for more than 24 hr and whenever signs of hyperglycemia are present.

Table 35–4 ***Degrees of Control of Blood Glucose Based on Glycosylated Hemoglobin (HbA_{1c}) Levels***

GLYCOSYLATED HEMOGLOBIN LEVEL	RATING
4.9%–6.7%	Excellent
7.6%–8.5%	Good
9.4%–10.0%	Fair
12.1%–13.0%	Poor

Nursing Diagnosis

Although the responsibility for formulating the nursing diagnosis lies with the registered nurse, the LPN/LVN has an important responsibility in knowing which nursing diagnoses are appropriate for which patients. Table 35–5 presents the most common nursing diagnoses, expected outcomes, and nursing interventions for patients with endocrine problems. This table is only an overview, as further

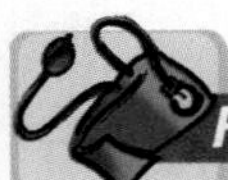

Focused Assessment 35–1

Data Collection for the Endocrine System

The nurse asks the following questions when assessing a patient with a potential endocrine problem:

- Have you gained or lost weight over the past 6 months?
- Has your appetite increased or decreased?
- Have you noticed any changes in thinking? Any difficulty concentrating? Any difficulty with memory?
- Have you become more anxious or nervous? Do you cry a lot?
- Has your personality changed?
- Has your energy level changed?
- Have you experienced muscle cramping or numbness or tingling in your hands and legs?
- Have you been experiencing diarrhea or constipation?
- Have you had more gas or abdominal bloating?
- Have you noticed any facial or ankle swelling?
- Has your voice become huskier?
- Have you been thirstier than usual? Do you find you urinate more now?
- Have you noticed any heart palpitations? Do you know if your pulse rate has changed?
- Have your sleep patterns changed? Do you need more sleep? Are you finding it difficult to sleep?
- Have your menstrual periods altered? (for women)
- Is there any history in your family of thyroid, pituitary, adrenal disease, or diabetes?
- Have you ever had radiation treatments to the head or neck?
- Have you noticed a difference in the way you react to the environmental temperature? Are you cold or hot when others are comfortable?
- Have you noticed any changes in the texture or thickness of your hair or eyebrows? What about your fingernails? Are they brittle?
- Has your skin become dry and rough?

Table 35–5 *Nursing Diagnoses, Goals/Expected Outcomes, and Nursing Interventions Commonly Used for Patients with Endocrine Problems*

NURSING DIAGNOSIS*	GOALS/EXPECTED OUTCOMES	NURSING INTERVENTIONS
Deficient fluid volume related to increased urine output (DI, HyperT, AD)	Patient will display balance between intake and output	Monitor for dehydration and signs of decreased cardiac output. Measure and record intake and output q 2 hr; maintain ordered IV fluid rate; encourage oral fluid intake.
Constipation related to loss of fluid from intestine, slowed intestinal peristalsis (DI, HypoT, AD)*	Patient will display normal bowel pattern within 2 wk	Provide high-bulk diet; encourage fluid intake; administer stool softener or laxatives, as ordered. Encourage exercise to promote better bowel function.
Disturbed body image related to changes in physical appearance (PT, HyperT)	Patient will verbalize acceptance of alteration in body appearance within 2 mo	Allow time for verbalizing feelings. Assist to identify strengths and positive aspects of self and life. Focus on strengths and positive aspects. Give sincere compliments.
Sexual dysfunction related to decreased libido, amenorrhea, or impotence (PT, HyperT)	Patient will acknowledge need for patience until therapy improves the symptoms	Help patient understand how therapy might help the problem. Assist patient to recognize and maintain personal worth as an individual. Assist to maintain roles within family or living unit. Help significant others understand patient's illness.
Deficient knowledge related to illness and treatment (all endocrine disorders)	Patient will verbalize beginning understanding of concepts taught at end of 2 wk	Teach patient and significant others about the disease and each aspect of treatment. Provide written instructions regarding medications, their side effects, and what should be reported to the physician. Provide instructions for "sick" days. Alert to signs and symptoms of too much or too little medication. Emphasize the importance of follow-up care. Stress the need for Medic-Alert tag or bracelet and wallet card.
Imbalanced nutrition: less than body requirements related to anorexia, constipation, increased metabolic rate (PT, HyperT)	Patient will regain and maintain weight within normal limits within 6 mo	Weigh twice a week. Alter diet as needed to increase fiber and carbohydrate content. Provide small, frequent meals of preferred foods. Provide patient teaching about nutritional requirements.

*Endocrine disorders to which these nursing diagnoses apply are in parentheses.

Key: *AD,* Addison's disease; *DI,* diabetes insipidus; *HyperT,* hyperthyroidism; *HypoT,* hypothyroidism; *PT,* pituitary tumors and hypopituitary syndrome.

Continued

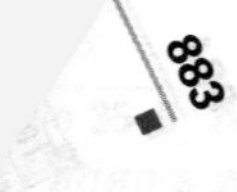

Diagnoses, Goals/Expected Outcomes, and Nursing Interventions Commonly Used ...ncrine Problems—cont'd

	GOALS/EXPECTED OUTCOMES	NURSING INTERVENTIONS
... weakness, ...ence, lethargy (PT, DI, ...ypoT, CS)	Patient will verbalize decrease in weakness and fatigue within 1 mo; patient will demonstrate improved energy within 3 mo	Provide periods of rest. Assist with activities of daily living (ADLs) as needed. Set slower pace for activities. Give patient time to respond to verbal communications. Encourage physical activity to highest level of tolerance. Monitor electrolyte and fluid status; provide electrolyte replacement as needed.
Risk for injury related to potential increased intracranial pressure (PT), inability to think clearly (HyperT, HypoT), mental and physical sluggishness (HypoT)	Patient will not experience damage from increased intracranial pressure Patient will exercise caution in making decisions, operating dangerous machinery, and moving about quickly until symptoms resolve	Conduct regular checks of neurologic status. Monitor for signs of increased intracranial pressure. Continue hormone replacement therapy as needed to decrease symptoms from tumor or hypofunction.
Readiness for enhanced sleep related to insomnia, hypermetabolic state (HyperT, CS)	Patient will use relaxation methods to induce sleep	Assist with rest periods during the day if fatigue is severe. Assure that therapy can resolve the problem. Instruct in relaxation methods to help induce sleep. Provide noise-free, sleep-inducing environment.
Ineffective coping related to emotional lability (HyperT, AD, CS)	Patient will devise plan to cope with mood swings until they resolve	Encourage verbalization of feelings and concerns. Assure patient that as disease is controlled, moods will be more stable. Help patient identify strengths and focus on them. Teach relaxation techniques to handle stressful times. Explain physiologic causes of changes in mood.
Decreased cardiac output related to fluid depletion (DI, AD), hypometabolic state (HypoT), hypermetabolic state (HyperT)	Patient will be free of signs of heart failure	Explain to patient how disease process is affecting heart function. Monitor for signs of dysrhythmia and heart failure. Assure that treatment of underlying disease should alleviate heart symptoms.
Risk for infection related to surgical incision (PT, HyperT), anti-inflammatory effect of excess cortisol (CS)	Patient will not develop infection as evidenced by normal temperature, white blood cell (WBC) count within normal range, and absence of visible signs of wound infection	Maintain strict asepsis for invasive procedures and dressing changes. Monitor temperature, WBC, and subtle signs of infection, as steroids can suppress usual signs. Advise to stay away from individuals who have colds or other infections.
Imbalanced nutrition: more than body requirements, related to altered glucose metabolism (CS), hypometabolic state (HypoT)	Patient will regain and maintain weight within normal limits within 3 mo of beginning therapy	Teach signs and symptoms of hyperglycemia and how to administer ordered insulin; teach regarding correct diet for condition. Assist in designing diet according to food preferences. Teach to balance diet and exercise.

*Endocrine disorders to which these nursing diagnoses apply are in parentheses.
Key: *AD,* Addison's disease; *CS,* Cushing's syndrome; *DI,* diabetes insipidus; *HyperT,* hyperthyroidism; *HypoT,* hypothyroidism; *PT,* pituitary tumors and hypopituitary syndrome.

nursing diagnoses may be found in the nursing care plans in the following two chapters. In all instances, the LPN/LVN plays a critical role in development of the plan of care.

Planning

Planning care for a patient with an endocrine problem will depend on what type of problem the patient has. One thing is certain: stress has an effect on the problem. Therefore, measures to help the patient decrease stress should be planned. Supplemental hormones, such as corticosteroids, are given in the early morning when such hormones will not interfere with the body's normal release and use of them. General nursing goals for the patient with an endocrine disorder are:

- Prevention of injury
- Maintenance of fluid and electrolyte balance
- Maintenance of hormone balance
- Reduction of stress
- Use of effective coping mechanisms
- Knowledge of self-care
- Tolerance to physical activity
- Promotion of normal bowel function
- Improvement of mental-emotional status
- Integration of body image

Expected outcomes are written for each individual patient depending on the nursing diagnoses chosen.

Implementation

Interventions vary depending on the type of endocrine problem present and are discussed with disorders in the following sections. Common specific nursing interventions are listed in Table 35–5.

Evaluation

Evaluation is accomplished by determining whether symptoms are resolving and by laboratory testing to see whether treatment is effective. Many of the symptoms of endocrine disorders are subjective, and the nurse must collect reliable data from the patient about symptoms, such as levels of fatigue, feeling cold or hot, and paresthesias. Each patient is questioned about the presenting symptoms and their improvement during the evaluation of care and treatment.

COMMUNITY CARE

Many patients with endocrine disorders are cared for in outpatient settings. Home care nurses often find that the patient with heart disease, neurologic problems, diabetes, or respiratory problems also has a thyroid problem. Careful assessment by the clinic nurse may uncover a developing endocrine problem.

Internet resources that may be useful for patients experiencing endocrine disorders or undergoing endocrine testing include:

- The Hormone Foundation (the educational affiliate of the endocrine society): www.hormone.org
- www.endocrineweb.com, a site maintained by physicians specializing in endocrine disorders, intended for patient information

Key Points

- The endocrine system is made up of glands and hormones that regulate metabolism, growth and development, and sexual and reproductive processes.
- The primary regulatory activities of the endocrine system are concerned with altering chemical reactions, changing the permeability of the cell membrane, and activating a particular cell mechanism. The secretion of a particular hormone normally depends on the physiologic need for it.
- Any type of dysfunction of the pituitary gland will affect one or more of its numerous hormones, as well as the target organ for that hormone.
- Age-related changes of the endocrine system include decreased size of the pituitary gland, decreased metabolic rate, decreases in some hormone levels, increases in others, and only slight changes in still others.
- Endocrine disorders are caused by an imbalance in the production of hormone or by an alteration in the body's ability to use the hormones produced. Primary endocrine dysfunction consists of either hypersecretion or hyposecretion; secondary endocrine dysfunction occurs from factors outside the gland.
- Tests of the endocrine system include examination of blood or urine, or by scans, ultrasounds, x-rays, or MRI. A thyroid panel may be ordered to evaluate thyroid function. Patients with primary hypothyroidism will have low levels of T_3 and T_4 and high levels of thyroid-stimulating hormone (TSH).
- A full physical assessment and history are needed to evaluate the patient who might be experiencing an endocrine disorder; the LPN/LVN is responsible for knowing appropriate nursing diagnoses.
- General goals for the patient with an endocrine disorder include prevention of injury, maintenance of fluid and electrolyte balance, maintenance of hormone balance, reduction of stress, and use of of effective coping mechanisms.
- Evaluation is accomplished by determining whether symptoms are resolving and by laboratory testing to see whether treatment is effective.

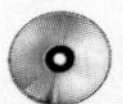
Go to your **Companion CD-ROM** for an Audio Glossary, animations, video clips, and bonus review questions.

evolve Be sure to visit the companion Evolve site at http://evolve.elsevier.com/deWit for interactive NCLEX-PN Exam Style Review Questions, WebLinks, and additional online resources.

NCLEX-PN EXAM STYLE REVIEW QUESTIONS

Choose the best answer(s) for the following questions.

1. The laboratory test that measures the amount of glucose attached to the hemoglobin during the life span of a red blood cell is known as:
   1. fructosamine assay.
   2. glucose tolerance test.
   3. glycosylated hemoglobin test.
   4. random blood sugar.

2. A 30-year-old female patient is admitted for urinary tract infection. A urine dipstick reveals presence of ketones, glucose, and nitrates. The nurse asks which of the following questions to further assess for possible diabetes mellitus?
   1. "Have you experienced muscle cramping or numbness or tingling in your hands and legs?"
   2. "Have you had more gas or abdominal bloating?"
   3. "Have you been thirstier than usual? Do you find you urinate more now?"
   4. "Have you noticed a difference in the way you react to the environmental temperature? Are you cold or hot when others are comfortable?"

3. The nurse prepares a patient for a glucose tolerance test. Which of the following instructions must be included? *(Select all that apply.)*
   1. "Eat a balanced diet."
   2. "Maintain a normal level of activity."
   3. "Fast for 24 hours before the test."
   4. "No eating, drinking, or smoking during the test."
   5. "Report dizziness, nervousness, weakness, and confusion."

4. The nurse is taking care of a patient with hyperparathyroidism. Which of the following laboratory results would confirm the diagnosis?
   1. Elevated serum calcium
   2. Increased bone density
   3. Elevated serum phosphate
   4. Increased serum potassium

5. A patient develops a hypersecreting tumor in the adrenal medulla. The most likely sign or symptom would be:
   1. hypertension.
   2. lethargy.
   3. exophthalmos.
   4. galactorrhea.

6. A patient is on corticosteroid therapy for an acute exacerbation of a respiratory disease. The initial assessment confirms a nursing diagnosis of Excess fluid volume. The underlying etiology for this nursing diagnosis would be:
   1. suppression of normal corticosteroid secretion.
   2. artificial increase in corticosteroids.
   3. increased adrenocorticotropic hormone.
   4. mineralocorticoid insufficiency.

7. The nurse formulates a care plan for a postmenopausal female who is admitted for hip fracture. Nursing assessments support the nursing diagnosis of Risk for injury. The most likely etiology for the diagnosis would be:
   1. inadequate estrogen secretion.
   2. growth hormone deficiency.
   3. progesterone deficiency.
   4. parathormone deficiency.

8. Physiologic increases in circulating antidiuretic hormone in advanced age may predispose the older adult to:
   1. dehydration.
   2. fluid overload.
   3. hypernatremia.
   4. anemia.

9. A patient is admitted with hyperthyroidism. The initial assessments suggest the nursing diagnosis of Imbalanced nutrition: less than body requirements. An appropriate expected outcome would be:
   1. patient will identify causes of weight loss.
   2. patient will maintain weight.
   3. patient will have a balanced intake and output.
   4. patient will tolerate activities of daily living.

10. A newly diagnosed diabetic patient is found to have a blood sugar of 200 mg/dL. Glycosylated hemoglobin is 12.5%. These initial findings indicate deficient knowledge. Appropriate nursing interventions would include which of the following? *(Select all that apply.)*
    1. Monitor weight and caloric intake.
    2. Teach effects of rest and relaxation.
    3. Provide small, frequent meals.
    4. Provide instructions for "sick" days.
    5. Emphasize the importance of follow-up care.

CRITICAL THINKING ACTIVITIES

Read the clinical scenario and discuss the questions with your classmates.

Scenario

Mrs. Kovash, a 64-year-old widow, comes to the endocrine clinic to be evaluated at the request of her nurse practitioner. She complains that in the past year she has "slowed down" considerably. She states, "I guess I'm just getting old." The nurse practitioner suspects that it may not be simply aging, since Mrs. Kovash has always lived a healthy and active lifestyle.

1. What type of examinations would you expect the health care provider to perform?
2. What would you teach Mrs. Kovash regarding what to expect from the laboratory blood tests?
3. What questions would you ask the patient before tests for evaluation of thyroid function?

CHAPTER

36 Care of Patients with Pituitary, Thyroid, Parathyroid, and Adrenal Disorders

evolve http://evolve.elsevier.com/deWit

Objectives

Upon completing the chapter you should be able to:

Theory

1. Give examples of four major problems associated with hyposecretion of pituitary hormones and identify three nursing interventions appropriate for each problem.
2. Outline three nursing interventions appropriate for each problem of hypopituitarism.
3. Critique appropriate nursing assessments and interventions for the patient who might experience complications of a thyroidectomy.
4. Compare and contrast the symptoms of hypoparathyroidism with hyperparathyroidism.
5. Illustrate six signs and symptoms of adrenocortical insufficiency (Addison's disease).
6. Describe four major causes of Cushing syndrome.

Clinical Practice

1. From an appropriate list of nursing diagnoses, provide nursing care for a patient with a pituitary disorder.
2. Select appropriate nursing interventions for a patient with adrenal insufficiency.
3. Implement patient teaching for the patient with hypoparathyroidism.
4. Plan postoperative assessment and nursing care for a patient who has had a hypophysectomy.
5. Initiate nursing care for a patient who has had a thyroidectomy.
6. Identify nursing diagnoses and appropriate interventions for a patient with diabetes insipidus.
7. Assist with development of a teaching plan for the patient taking a corticosteroid.

Key Terms

Be sure to check out the bonus material on the Companion CD-ROM, including selected audio pronunciations.

ablation therapy (ăb-LĀ-shŭn THĔR-ă-pē, p. 894)
acromegaly (ăk-rō-MĔG-ă-lē, p. 888)
agranulocytosis (ă-grăn-ū-LŌ-sī-TŌ-sĭs, p. 894)
anosmia (ăn-ŎS-mē-ă, p. 889)
apathetic thyrotoxicosis (ă-pă-THĔ-tĭk thī-rō-tŏk-sĭ-KŌ-sĭs, p. 893)
benign pituitary adenoma (Bē-NĪN pĭ-TŌŌ-ĭ-tĕr-ē ă-dē-NŌ-mă, p. 887)
catecholamines (kăt-ĕ-KŌL-ă-mĕnz, p. 901)
cretinism (KRĒ-tĭn-ĭzm, p. 898)
diuresis (dī-ūr-RĒ-sĭs, p. 890)
exophthalmos (ĕk-sŏf-THĂL-mŏs, p. 893)
gigantism (jī-GĂN-tĭzm, p. 888)
glucose intolerance (p. 887)
hyponatremia (hī-pō-nā-TRĒ-mē-ă, p. 891)
hypophysectomy (hī-pō-fī-SĔK-tŏ-mē, p. 888)
lability (p. 905)
nocturia (nŏk-TŪ-rē-ă, p. 890)
optic chiasm (ŎP-tĭk KĪ-ăzm, p. 888)
Sheehan syndrome (SHĒ-hăn SĬN-drōm, p. 889)
tetany (TĔT-ă-nē, p. 897)
thyroid crisis (THĪ-royd krī-sĭs, p. 894)
thyroid storm (THĪ-royd, p. 897)

DISORDERS OF THE PITUITARY GLAND

In view of the varied functions of the pituitary gland, it is difficult to classify the many syndromes that can occur as a result of a pituitary disorder. Among the more common disorders of the pituitary are

- Pituitary tumors
- Hypofunction of the pituitary gland
- Diabetes insipidus (DI)
- Syndrome of inappropriate antidiuretic hormone (SIADH) secretion

PITUITARY TUMORS

Tumors of the pituitary gland, which account for about 10% of all intracranial tumors, can produce local and systemic symptoms. Local symptoms are more likely to occur when the tumor is large and creates pressure within the brain. Smaller tumors, as well as the larger ones, can cause various endocrine dysfunctions, depending on whether they stimulate or inhibit the secretion of particular hormones.

Etiology and Pathophysiology

A tumor of the pituitary is usually a **benign pituitary adenoma.** This tumor secretes growth hormone (GH), leading to continued growth of bones and soft tissues. It also antagonizes (acts against) the effect of the hormone insulin, resulting in an increase in blood glucose and **glucose intolerance** (see Chapter 37). There is increased

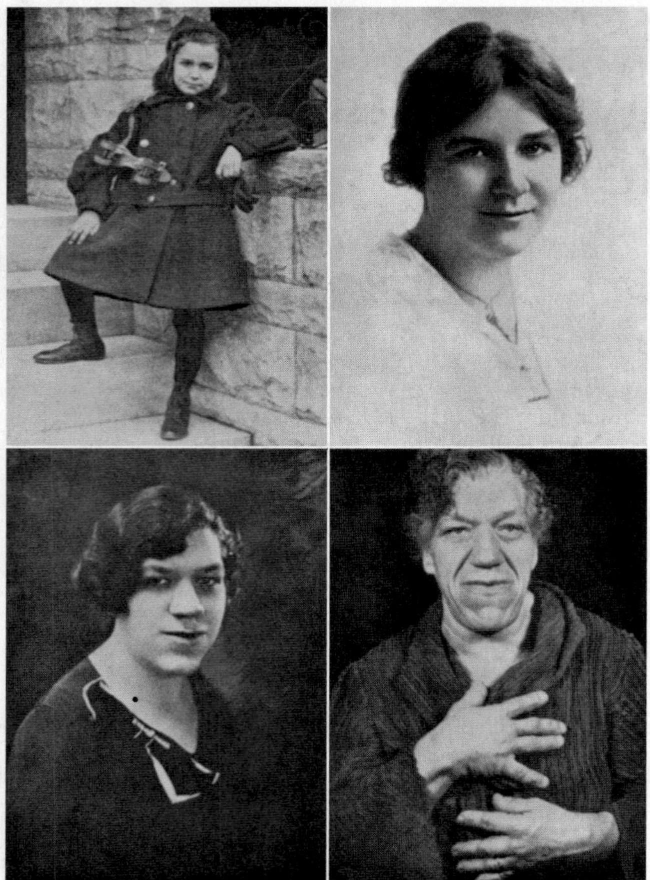

FIGURE 36–1 The progression of acromegaly.

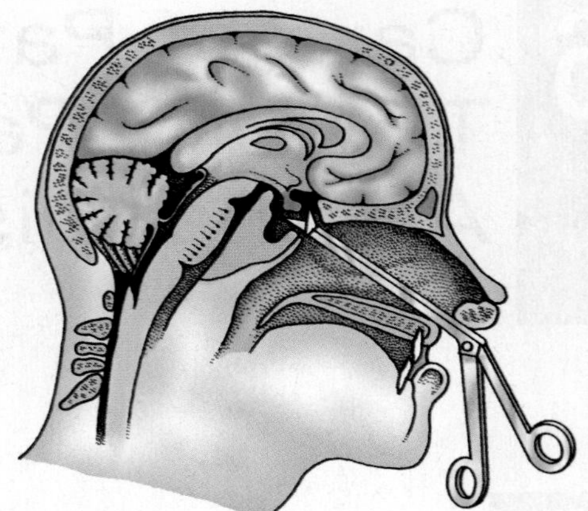

FIGURE 36–2 Transsphenoidal surgical approach for hypophysectomy.

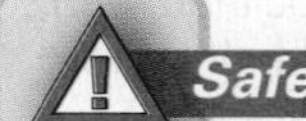

Safety Alert 36–1

Coughing

Coughing after a transsphenoidal **hypophysectomy** may lead to a cerebrospinal fluid leak.

pressure within the optic chiasm (the part of the brain where the optic nerve fibers cross), which, if not relieved, will destroy the optic nerve and produce blindness.

Signs and Symptoms

Local symptoms include headache from the pressure of the tumor, and visual disturbances from pressure within the optic chiasm. Systemic symptoms may be vague and progress very slowly. Personality changes, weakness, fatigue, and vague abdominal pain can be present for years before the condition is diagnosed correctly.

The excessive secretion of growth hormone results in **gigantism** in children, leading to excessively tall stature, as the bone growth plates have not yet closed. In adults the result is **acromegaly**. The adult's facial features change with the lips thickening, the nose enlarging, and the forehead developing a bulge (Figure 36–1). The hands and feet become enlarged; the first sign may be that the patient's shoes no longer fit. Muscle weakness may occur and osteoporosis and joint pain are common.

Diagnosis

Diagnosis of a pituitary tumor begins with a complete history and physical examination. Magnetic resonance imaging (MRI) and high-resolution computed tomography (CT) with contrast media may be used to identify, localize, and determine the extent of the tumor. A thorough ophthalmologic examination will be performed to evaluate pressure on the optic chiasm or optic nerves.

Treatment

In some cases the physician may choose to treat the pituitary tumor conservatively with hormone therapy designed to reduce levels of growth hormone. If the tumor continues to grow or presents serious hormonal imbalances, it may be treated surgically or by irradiation. Some specialists prefer to remove the tumor surgically and then apply radiation to the site to be sure that all tumor cells have been destroyed. **Hypophysectomy**, or removal of the pituitary gland, is the surgical procedure, most often done microsurgically. The usual approach is transsphenoidal via the nose (Figure 36–2).

Nursing Management

After the surgery, the patient is kept in a semi-Fowler's position. The nurse must closely monitor vital signs and the patient's neurologic status. It is important to note and communicate promptly any change in vision, mental status, level of consciousness, or strength. The nurse must also monitor for any complications, such as diabetes insipidus (DI is discussed later in this chapter). A nasal drip pad is in place and is changed as needed. Because nasal packing will be in place for 2 to 3 days, the patient must breathe through the mouth. After surgery it is important that the patient not brush teeth, cough, sneeze, blow the nose, or bend forward, as these may interfere with the healing process. The nurse will assist the patient with mouth rinses and encourage hourly deep breathing exercises to prevent pulmonary problems (Safety Alert 36–1).

HYPOFUNCTION OF THE PITUITARY GLAND

Hypofunction of the pituitary gland is a rare disorder characterized by a decrease in the level of one or more of the pituitary hormones.

Etiology and Pathophysiology

The most common cause of pituitary hypofunction is a tumor. Other causes include autoimmune disorders, infections, or destruction of the pituitary. A rare but serious postpartum complication, **Sheehan syndrome,** involves infarction of the gland secondary to postpartum hemorrhage.

The most common hormone deficiency involves a decrease in the amount of GH and gonadotropins. The result of this decrease is metabolic problems and sexual dysfunction. Decrease in GH will lead to short stature in children; in adults it leads to an increase in bone breakdown, resulting in increased bone fragility and risk for osteoporosis. The decrease in gonadotropins may lead to testicular failure in a man and, ultimately, sterility. In females, ovarian failure, amenorrhea, and infertility result.

Signs and Symptoms

Signs and symptoms depend on the cause of pituitary failure and hormones involved. If the disorder is related to a tumor, the patient may experience headaches, visual changes, **anosmia** (loss of the sense of smell), or seizures. Other signs and symptoms depend on the hormones diminished in supply, and are outlined in Table 36–1.

Diagnosis

Diagnosis of hypofunction of the pituitary gland is made by history, physical examination, and diagnostic studies. Laboratory blood tests are performed to measure levels of pituitary hormones. MRI and CT are used to determine the presence or absence of a pituitary tumor.

Treatment and Nursing Management

The mainstay of treatment for hypofunction of the pituitary gland is lifelong replacement of the hormone(s) affected. Somatropin, via subcutaneous injection, is used to replace GH. The patient experiences a feeling of increased energy and well-being, although there are side effects, such as edema, joint pain, and headache. Gonadal hormone therapy is usually offered, including testosterone for men and estrogen/progesterone for women, although associated risks may outweigh the benefits for some patients. If the disorder is caused by a tumor, surgery or radiation for tumor removal is usually performed, followed by hormone therapy.

Nursing management involves recognizing the signs and symptoms of hypofunction of the pituitary and patient teaching (Patient Teaching 36–1).

Table 36–1 ***Decreased Hormones in Pituitary Hypofunction and Associated Clinical Manifestations***

HORMONE DIMINISHED	ASSOCIATED CLINICAL MANIFESTATIONS
GH	Decreased muscle mass, reduced strength, pathologic fractures
FSH, LH	Women: menstrual irregularities, diminished libido, decreased breast size Men: testicular atrophy, diminished spermatogenesis, loss of libido, impotence, decreased facial hair, decreased muscle mass
ACTH, cortisol	Weakness, fatigue, headache, dry/pale skin, diminished axillary and pubic hair, postural hypotension, fasting hypoglycemia, decreased tolerance for stress, susceptibility to infection
Thyroid hormone	Similar to hypothyroidism, although milder: cold intolerance, constipation, fatigue, lethargy, weight gain

Adapted from Lewis, S.M., Heitkemper, M.M., Dirksen, S.R., et al. (2007). *Medical-Surgical Nursing: Assessment and Management of Clinical Problems* (7th ed.). St. Louis: Mosby.

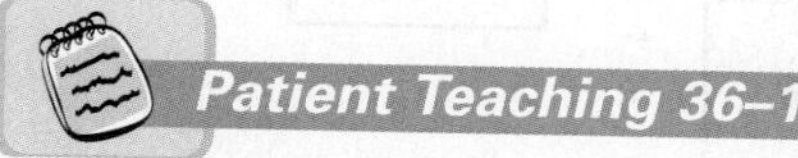

Hormone Replacement Therapy

The requirement for lifelong medication therapy (hormone replacement) must be emphasized to the patient. The patient must be educated regarding:

- Hormone administration (method and frequency)
- Side effects
- Follow-up therapy

DIABETES INSIPIDUS

Etiology and Pathophysiology

Diabetes insipidus or DI, as it is commonly referred to, is characterized by the production of copious amounts (usually more than 2.5 L/day) of dilute urine. DI occurs as a result of decreased production of the antidiuretic hormone (ADH), which regulates reabsorption of water in the kidney tubules. When ADH is not present in a sufficient amount, the water remains in the tubules and is excreted as urine. The following are three primary mechanisms of DI:

- Central DI, associated with brain tumors, head injury, neurosurgery, or central nervous system (CNS) infections
- Nephrogenic DI, caused by drug therapy (lithium) or kidney disease
- Dispogenic DI, caused by excessive water intake (sometimes associated with schizophrenia)

The pathophysiology of DI can be found in Concept Map 36–1.

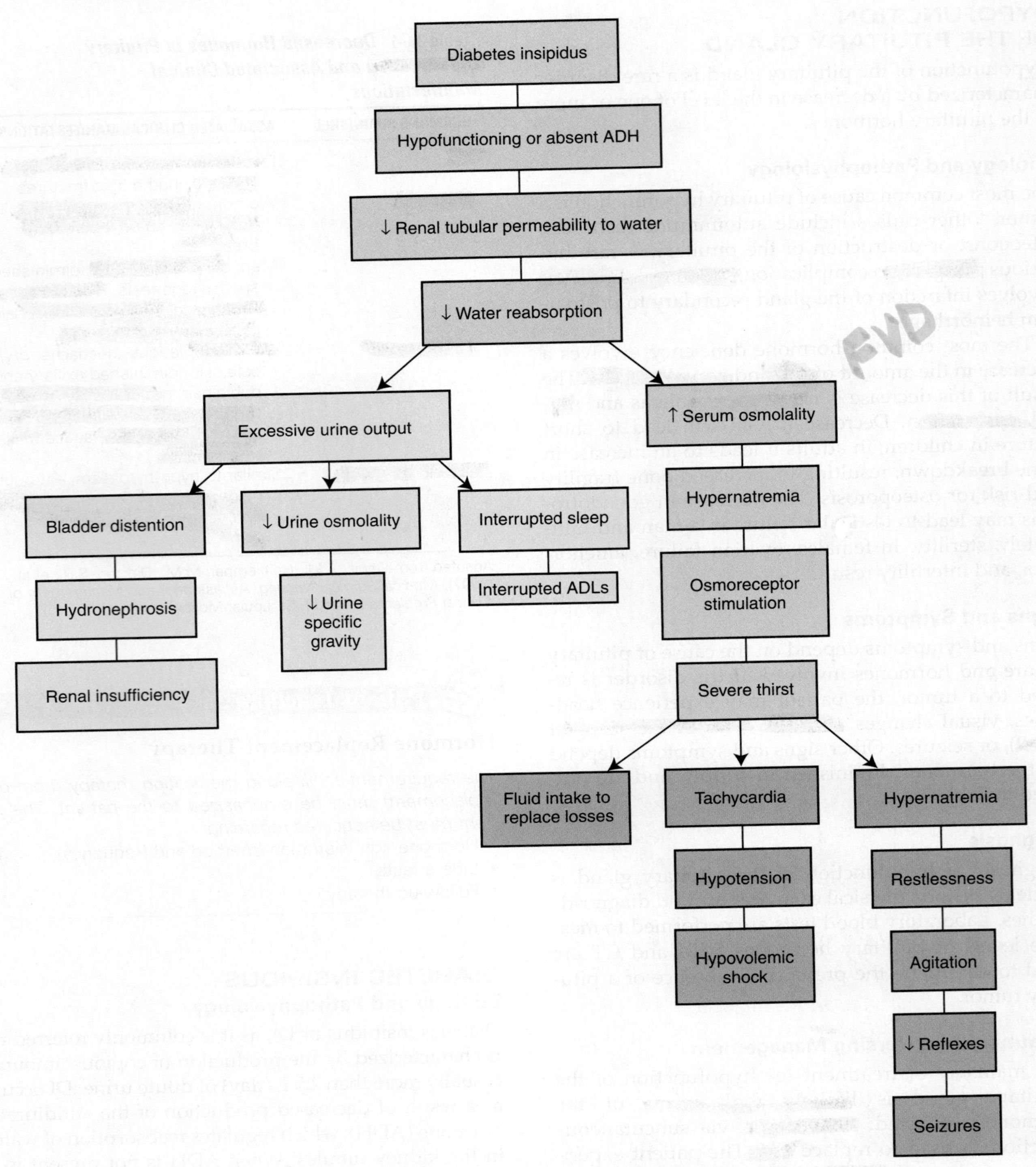

CONCEPT MAP **36–1** Pathophysiology of diabetes insipidus.

Signs and Symptoms

The patient experiences profound **diuresis** (production of a large amount of urine), often as much as 15 to 20 L in every 24-hour period. Other signs and symptoms include thirst, weakness, and fatigue, often from **nocturia** (urination at night). The patient will exhibit signs of deficient fluid volume, such as tachycardia, hypotension, weight loss, constipation, and poor skin turgor. If untreated, the patient will demonstrate signs of shock and CNS manifestations progressing from irritability to eventual coma, resulting from hypernatremia and severe dehydration.

Diagnosis

A complete history is obtained, and a physical examination and laboratory tests are performed, including urine and plasma osmolality, and urine specific grav-

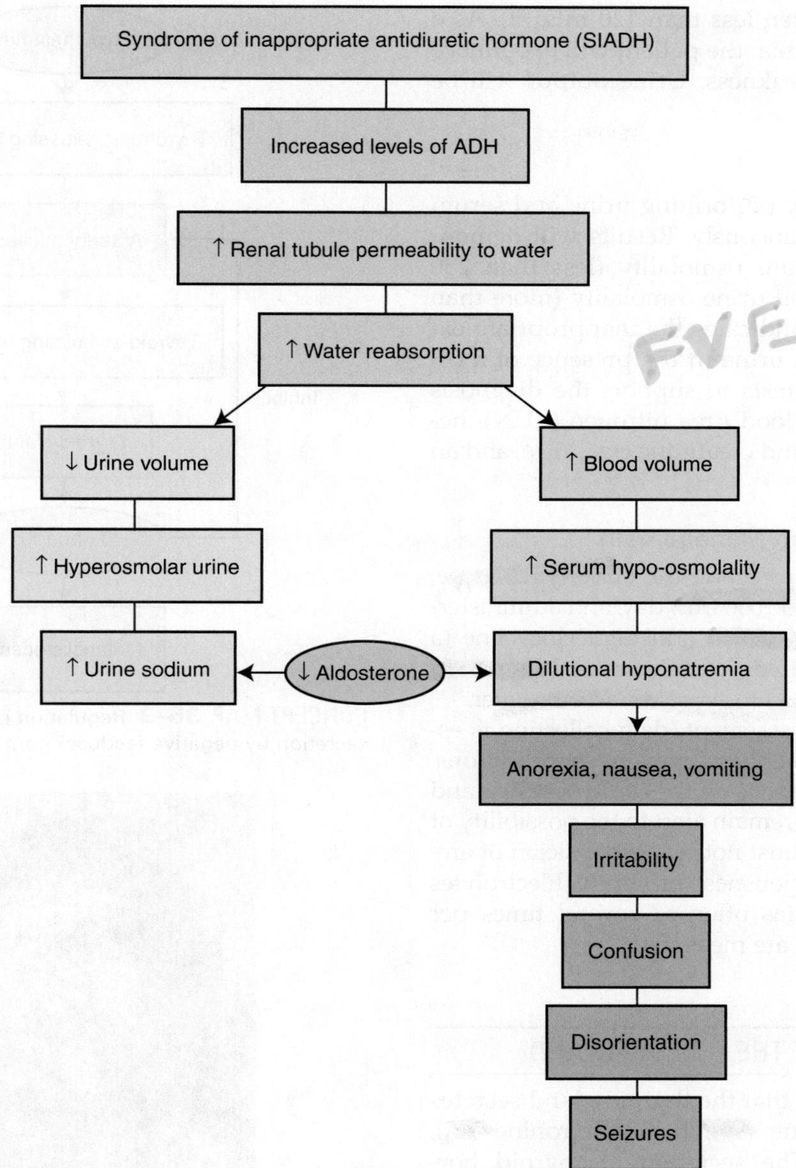

CONCEPT MAP **36–2** Pathophysiology of SIADH.

ity. A water deprivation test is done to confirm a suspected case of central DI.

Treatment and Nursing Management

Replacement of fluid and electrolytes, along with hormone therapy, represents the basis of treatment of DI. In central DI, the hormone of choice to replace insufficient ADH is desmopressin acetate (DDAVP), available orally, intravenously, or nasally. Other hormone medication choices exist, such as vasopressin (Pitressin) via nasal inhalation or by injection. For fluid replacement, hypertonic saline is used, titrated to match the patient's urinary output.

Nursing management focuses on early detection, maintenance of fluid and electrolyte balance, and patient education. Baseline vital signs and weight are important to accurately document and monitor throughout therapy. Strict (hourly) intake and output are essential to correct fluid losses and to titrate hypertonic saline infusion.

SYNDROME OF INAPPROPRIATE ANTIDIURETIC HORMONE

Etiology and Pathophysiology

SIADH is the opposite of DI. Excessive amounts of ADH are produced, resulting in fluid retention. Numerous factors can cause SIADH, including malignancies and tumors pressing on the pituitary. Concept Map 36–2 details the pathophysiology of SIADH.

Signs and Symptoms

Signs and symptoms include confusion, seizure, and loss of consciousness accompanied by weight gain and edema. Hyponatremia from fluid excess is present, with serum sodium often less than 120 mEq/L. As a result of the hyponatremia, the patient will experience muscle cramps and weakness. Urine output will be diminished.

Diagnosis

SIADH is diagnosed by performing urine and serum osmolality tests simultaneously. Results will demonstrate a decreased serum osmolality (less than 280 mOsm/kg) and elevated urine osmolality (more than 100 mmol/kg), which indicates the inappropriate excretion of concentrated urine in the presence of a dilute serum. Other lab tests to support the diagnosis include a decrease in blood urea nitrogen (BUN), hemoglobin, hematocrit, and creatinine clearance, and an elevated urine sodium.

Treatment and Nursing Management

Treatment is aimed at correcting the underlying cause, restricting fluids to 500 to 1000 mL/day, and administering sodium chloride, diuretics, and demeclocycline (a tetracycline) to increase free water clearance. Hypertonic enemas may be prescribed to draw out excess water.

Thorough nursing assessment/data collection is essential to monitor treatment and prevent complications. The nurse must closely focus on the cardiovascular and neurologic systems and remain alert to the possibility of fluid shifts. The nurse must notify the physician of any change in level of consciousness promptly. Electrolytes are monitored closely (as often as several times per day), and daily weights are measured.

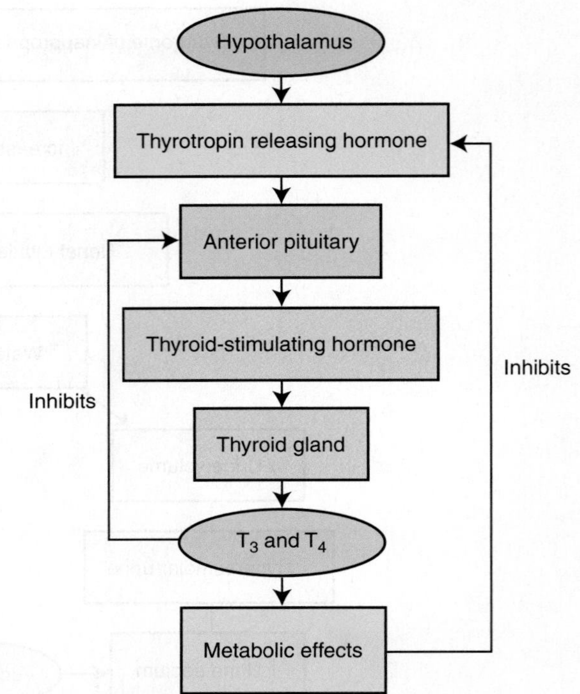

CONCEPT MAP **36–3** Regulation of thyroid hormone secretion by negative feedback control.

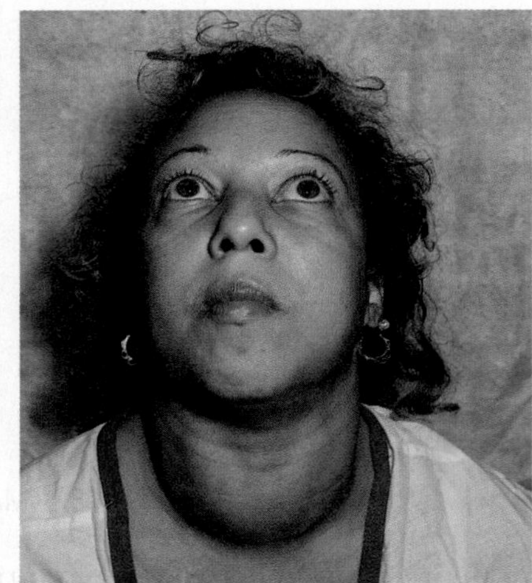

FIGURE **36–3** Goiter.

DISORDERS OF THE THYROID GLAND

Recall from Chapter 35 that the thyroid gland secretes the hormones thyroxine (T_4), triiodothyronine (T_3), and thyrocalcitonin. The secretion of thyroid hormones is regulated by the hypothalamic-pituitary-thyroid control system (Concept Map 36–3). In other words, all three organs are involved in the closed-loop negative feedback system. Internal conditions, such as low thyroid and norepinephrine (NE) serum levels, can activate the hypothalamus, as can external conditions, such as cold. In response to feedback received by the hypothalamus, thyrotropin-releasing hormone (TRH) is secreted. TRH acts on the pituitary gland, bringing about its release of thyroid-stimulating hormone (TSH). The TSH then acts on the thyroid cells, causing them to release thyroid hormones. When sufficient heat has been produced by increased metabolic activities (if cold was the stimulus), or when there are sufficient levels of thyroid hormone in the body fluids (if a deficit was the stimulus), feedback to the hypothalamus causes it to stop releasing TRH.

Abnormalities in thyroid gland activity and resultant changes in the levels of thyroid hormones are among the most common disorders affecting the endocrine system.

GOITER

Etiology and Pathophysiology

The person with a goiter has a greatly enlarged thyroid gland (Figure 36–3). The serum levels of the thyroid hormones may or may not be within normal limits. One type of goiter is caused by a deficiency of iodine in the diet. It can be prevented by providing iodine intake, such as using iodized salt. Although the administration of iodine will not cure goiter, it will stop the continued enlargement of the gland. Another type of goiter occurs as a result of unknown etiology.

Signs, Symptoms, and Diagnosis

Because there may be no systemic symptoms or changes in the metabolic rate of a person with simple goiter, the first sign that is usually noticed is an enlargement in the front of the neck. Later, if the gland continues to grow bigger, it presses against the esophagus and causes some difficulty in swallowing. The goiter also can press against the trachea and interfere with normal breathing.

The diagnosis of goiter is established by history and physical examination. Goiter can be associated with increased, normal, or decreased hormone production.

Treatment

If goiter resulting from iodine deficiency is treated early, the growth of the gland can be arrested, and in some cases the enlargement will eventually disappear. Medications prescribed include preparations containing elemental iodine (the iodide ion).

A very large goiter that continues to grow and produce local symptoms of pressure or presents the possibility of developing into a malignant growth or a toxic goiter is surgically removed in a procedure similar to the one sometimes done for hyperthyroidism, discussed next.

Nursing Management

Iodine preparations should be given well diluted and administered through a straw, as they can stain the teeth. Adverse effects of iodine preparations can include gastrointestinal upset, metallic taste, skin rashes, allergic reactions, and epigastric pain.

HYPERTHYROIDISM

Etiology and Pathophysiology

Patients at greatest risk for hyperthyroidism are adult women between the ages of 30 and 50. *Primary* hyperthyroidism is the result of an abnormality of function involving the thyroid gland itself and causes excessive circulation of thyroid T_4 and T_3 hormones. However, it is possible that only the T_3 level will be above normal if the patient has Graves' disease, toxic adenoma of the thyroid, or toxic nodular goiter. These conditions are discussed later in this chapter.

High serum levels of T_4 can be caused by either overactivity of the thyroid gland or excessive doses of T_4 given in replacement therapy. Primary hyperthyroidism is more common in women 30 to 50 years of age. *Secondary* hyperthyroidism usually is the result of an abnormality in another gland, such as the pituitary gland, that could produce too much TSH and therefore overstimulate the thyroid gland.

Primary hyperthyroidism also is known as Graves' disease or toxic goiter. Medications containing iodine, such as amiodarone, an antidysrhythmic heart medication, can predispose to hyperthyroidism. In addition, it has been discovered recently that women who smoke have nearly twice the risk of developing the disorder when compared with nonsmokers.

Signs and Symptoms

The earliest symptoms of hyperthyroidism may be weight loss, in spite of a good appetite, and nervousness. Symptoms can vary from mild to severe and may include weakness, insomnia, tremulousness, agitation, tachycardia, palpitations, exertional dyspnea, ankle edema, difficulty concentrating, diarrhea, increased thirst and urination, decreased libido, scanty menstruation, and infertility. The condition sometimes is not diagnosed in its early stages because of the vagueness of the symptoms. In some cases hyperthyroidism is misdiagnosed as a cardiovascular disease, as symptoms are similar.

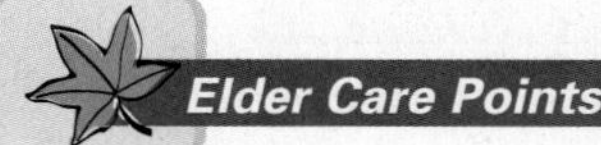

Elder Care Points

The elderly person with hyperthyroidism may exhibit milder signs and symptoms when compared with the typical adult, or he may exhibit an *atypical presentation*, such as shortness of breath, palpitations, or chest pain. In the older adult, **"apathetic thyrotoxicosis,"** or simply fatigue and slowing down, can be the only presentation.

If hyperthyroidism is not diagnosed correctly and continues untreated for any length of time, the patient can develop true organic heart disease and may experience myocardial infarction.

The symptoms manifested by a hyperthyroid patient are the result of an accelerated metabolic rate and a speeding up of all physiologic processes. Emotional upheaval occurs as a result of the action of thyroid hormones on the nervous system. The patient often reports episodes of emotional extremes with uncontrollable crying and depression followed by intense physical activity and euphoria. The patient with hyperthyroidism also exhibits an enlarged thyroid gland (toxic goiter) and abnormal protrusion of the eyeballs, or **exophthalmos** (Figure 36–4).

Diagnosis

Medical diagnosis is based on clinical manifestations of hyperthyroidism and the results of laboratory tests for thyroid hormone levels. One indicator of hyperthyroidism is assessment of the heart rate while the patient is sleeping. A rate that is consistently above 80 could signify a toxic state resulting from excessive levels of thyroid hormone.

Treatment and Nursing Management

Hyperthyroidism may be treated medically by administering radioactive iodine and antithyroid drugs, mild sedatives, and beta-adrenergic blocking agents to control tremor, temperature elevation, restlessness, and

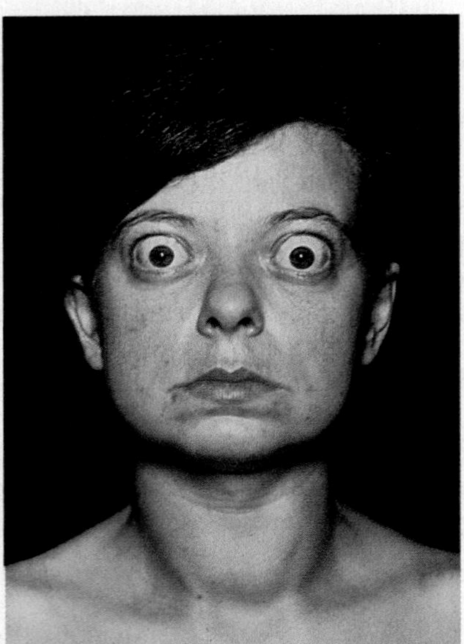

FIGURE **36–4** Graves' disease: exophthalmos.

tachycardia. Radioactive iodine (^{131}I), also known as ablation therapy, is the definitive treatment for hyperthyroidism. It is contraindicated in pregnant and nursing women, as it can disable the infant's thyroid gland. The main disadvantage of ablation therapy is the possibility of hypothyroidism caused by "overeffective" treatment. The hypothyroidism can occur immediately after treatment or long after it is completed; thus, the patient must have ongoing follow-up.

Dosage depends on the size of the gland and the thyroid's sensitivity to radiation. Patients receiving small doses can be given the drug orally for several doses on an outpatient basis. Larger doses require isolation of the patient for 8 days, which is the half-life (the time required for half the nuclei to undergo radioactive decay) of ^{131}I.

Because the iodine circulates in the blood and is excreted by the kidneys, precautions must be taken when handling needles, syringes, and other equipment likely to be contaminated with blood, and bedpans, urinals, and specimen bottles likely to be contaminated by urine.

All patients receiving radioactive iodine must be observed for signs of thyroid crisis resulting from radiation-induced thyroiditis (discussed later). If hyperthyroidism is not controlled within several months of therapy with radioactive iodine alone, the patient will require adjunctive therapy in the form of potassium iodide and antithyroid drugs.

Antithyroid drugs are prescribed as the initial treatment of hyperthyroidism in children, young adults, and pregnant women. Iodine preparations such as propylthiouracil (PTU) and potassium iodide (SSKI) have only a temporary effect. Methimazole (Tapazole) is the main drug used. The patient must take the antithyroid drug at the prescribed time and strictly according to schedule. There are dangerous side effects, such as agranulocytosis and hepatotoxicity (liver injury), which can develop rather quickly; for this reason, extreme care must be taken when these medications are given to pregnant or nursing women.

Iodine preparations also may be given for a period of 10 to 14 days before surgery of the thyroid to reduce the vascularity of the gland, minimizing the danger of releasing large amounts of thyroid hormone into the bloodstream during surgery and to decrease the risk of hemorrhage.

THYROIDECTOMY

Patients who do not respond well to antithyroid drug therapy, are unable to take radioactive iodine, or have greatly enlarged thyroid glands are candidates for a subtotal thyroidectomy. Patients with thyroid malignancy undergo a total thyroidectomy. In the subtotal procedure, two thirds of the glandular mass is removed. The remaining portion of the gland is left intact so production and release of thyroid hormones can continue. For most patients, however, surgery is a treatment of last resort, as the potential complications of hemorrhage, hypoparathyroidism, and vocal cord paralysis can be emotionally devastating.

Because many of the signs and symptoms of hyperthyroidism mimic those of cardiac disease, the nurse caring for the older adult must be alert to the possibility that such signs may be indicative of an endocrine, rather than a cardiac, disorder. Because of the effect hyperthyroidism has on physical and mental health status, caring for these patients presents a very real challenge to the nurse. Physical and mental rest is extremely important, because physical stress and emotional upset can stimulate the thyroid gland to become even more active. Adequate rest is essential to conserve strength, but it is difficult for a person with hyperthyroidism to relax and get sufficient rest.

The diet of the patient should be sufficiently high in calories to meet metabolic needs. This will vary from person to person, but continued loss of weight is an indication that more high-calorie foods are needed. It may be necessary to refer the patient to a dietitian who can work out a satisfactory diet that helps maintain normal body weight.

Patients who are being treated medically for hyperthyroidism must understand that they have an illness that requires ongoing medication and frequent monitoring to assess the effectiveness of treatment. Sometimes it is difficult for the patient's family to accept and deal with the emotional outbursts and mood changes that are present when the disease is not under control. Once hormone levels return to the normal range, the mental and physical symptoms should subside.

Many patients will be rendered hypothyroidic because of surgery or radiation therapy that alters thyroid function. It is then necessary to manage their illness with long-term thyroid replacement therapy. Nursing interventions for selected problems of patients with hyperthyroidism are summarized in Nursing Care Plan 36–1.

Preoperative Nursing Care

The responsibility of the nurse for preparation of the patient who is to have a thyroidectomy is essentially the same as for other types of major surgery. If the patient appears nervous, tense, and apprehensive, this should be reported to the surgeon. These symptoms may indicate improper control of the thyroid gland and may predispose the patient to the postoperative complication of "thyroid crisis" (see the following section).

Postoperative Nursing Care

The patient is placed in the Fowler's position (sitting upright to at least 90 degrees) to facilitate breathing and reduce swelling of the operative area. The head may be supported with sandbags on either side to relieve tension on the sutures.

Close observation of the patient is of critical importance. The vital signs are checked continuously in the immediate postoperative period, progressing to hourly once the patient is considered to be stable. The patient is watched closely for signs of bleeding and swelling at the operative area. Any rise in temperature, pulse, or respiration rate should be reported immediately, as it

NURSING CARE PLAN 36–1

Care of the Patient with Hyperthyroidism

SCENARIO Mrs. Jackson, age 35, has been having symptoms of hyperthyroidism. She complains of feeling "hot and soaked with perspiration all the time." She is 25 lb underweight, even though she reports a "ravenous" appetite. Her vital signs are P 110, bounding; RR 30 and somewhat irregular; BP 170/90. Her serum calcium level was found to be 11.5 mg/dL when she had a physical examination at her physician's office. She has been admitted for control of hypercalcemia and for more diagnostic tests. Mrs. Jackson is very apprehensive, agitated, and irritable.

PROBLEM/NURSING DIAGNOSIS *Apprehensive, agitated and irritable*/Anxiety related to excess circulating thyroid hormone as evidenced by nervousness and agitation.

Supporting assessment data *Subjective:* "I don't understand what is happening to me. I feel so nervous all of the time." *Objective:* Wringing her hands, eyes darting around the room, fidgeting in bed.

Goals/Expected Outcomes	Nursing Interventions	Selected Rationale	Evaluation
Patient will verbalize reduction of anxiety and agitation within 3 days of receiving prescribed medication	Keep environmental stimuli at a minimum.	Excessive stimuli can worsen anxiety and agitation.	Patient exhibits decrease in agitated behavior.
	No visitors other than family as requested by patient. Approach in a calm and unhurried manner.	Calm approach can lessen patient anxiety.	Patient states that she feels "less anxious."
	Provide 30-min rest periods before lunch, in afternoon, and after supper.	Rest can promote sense of calmness.	
	Change sweat-soaked linens and gown as needed.	Physical discomfort can increase anxiety.	
	Keep room as cool as possible.	Patients with hyperthyroidism experience "hot flashes."	
	Administer antianxiety medications as ordered.		Goal met.

PROBLEM/NURSING DIAGNOSIS *Does not understand what is happening*/Deficient knowledge related to lack of information about disease and treatment.

Supporting assessment data *Subjective:* Patient states that she does not know anything about hyperthyroidism or its treatment.

Goals/Expected Outcomes	Nursing Interventions	Selected Rationale	Evaluation
Patient will verbalize basic understanding of disease and treatment before discharge	Explain disease process; teach about diagnostic tests and what to expect for each one.	Effective patient teaching is the cornerstone of improving patient knowledge.	Patient verbalized basic understanding of hyperthyroidism.
	Encourage questions and supply answers.		Patient verbalized correct rationale for treatment plan, but requested more information.
	Explain options for treatment.		Continue plan.

Continued

NURSING CARE PLAN 36–1

Care of the Patient with Hyperthyroidism—cont'd

PROBLEM/NURSING DIAGNOSIS *Considerable weight loss*/Imbalanced nutrition: less than body requirements related to increased metabolic rate.

Supporting assessment data *Objective:* Has lost 25 lb over past 6 months, although appetite has increased considerably.

Goals/Expected Outcomes	Nursing Interventions	Selected Rationale	Evaluation
Patient will gain 2 lb/wk when thyroid production is under control	Weigh weekly; encourage high-calorie between-meal snacks.	Weekly weight is more reflective of true weight trends (daily weight tends to reflect water gains/losses).	Patient demonstrated 4-lb weight gain in 10 days but remains less than ideal body weight. Continue plan.
	Increase caloric intake to 3000 calories per day. Try to accommodate food preferences.	High-calorie snacks can be helpful in "sneaking in" extra calories.	

PROBLEM/NURSING DIAGNOSIS *Potential for heart damage*/Risk for injury related to excess circulating thyroid hormone and excess serum calcium.

Supporting assessment data *Objective:* Thyroid levels: T_3, 230 mg/dL; T_4, 16 mcg/dL; calcium, 16 mg/dL.

Goals/Expected Outcomes	Nursing Interventions	Selected Rationale	Evaluation
Patient will develop no permanent cardiac problems	Check vital signs q 4 hr.	Increases in pulse and blood pressure may indicate thyrotoxicosis	Patient's vital signs are within 10% of patient's baseline. Patient denies dyspnea.
	Assess cardiac function each shift and watch for symptoms of thyrotoxicosis, such as increased pulse, dyspnea, edema, and rising blood pressure; report such signs at once.	Hyperdynamic vital signs can be taxing on the heart and must be monitored closely.	
Patient will have controlled thyroid production within 2 wk	Medicate with calcium channel blocker as ordered; observe for side effects.	Beta adrenergic–blocking agents decrease sympathetic tone and decrease stimulation of the heart.	No peripheral edema present.
Patient will have normal serum calcium by discharge	Give medication to decrease calcium levels (diuretic) and monitor electrolyte levels.		Patient's thyroid and calcium levels are within normal levels. Continue plan.

PROBLEM/NURSING DIAGNOSIS *Very moody*/Ineffective coping related to labile moods.

Supporting assessment data *Subjective:* States she has been "very moody"; family says that she keeps changing her mind about things.

Goals/Expected Outcomes	Nursing Interventions	Selected Rationale	Evaluation
Patient will return to former emotional stability when thyroid production returns to normal	Assure her that mood swings are manifestations of her thyroid disorder. Stress importance of complying with treatment regimen after discharge and keeping appointments with physician.	Knowledge that emotional lability is disease related can lower anxiety. Treatment of hyperthyroidism is lifelong.	The frequency of patient's emotional instability has decreased to approximately once per week. Patient verbalized the importance of long-term follow-up.

NURSING CARE PLAN 36–1

Care of the Patient with Hyperthyroidism—cont'd

Goals/Expected Outcomes	Nursing Interventions	Selected Rationale	Evaluation
	Give positive reinforcement for correct behavior; encourage verbalization of feelings.	Positive reinforcement can encourage long-term compliance.	Patient responds to positive reinforcement. Continue plan.
	Establish trusting relationship; be accepting of behavior; spend uninterrupted time with her each shift; display acceptance of her and her behavior.	A trusted nurse-patient relationship can foster long-term compliance.	

? CRITICAL THINKING QUESTIONS

1. Taking into account Mrs. Jackson's nervousness and agitation, how would you proceed to implement a teaching session about her hyperthyroidism?
2. What specific nutritional suggestions might you offer Mrs. Jackson to help her gain weight?

may indicate a high level of thyroxine in the bloodstream. External swelling may cause constriction of the bandage around the neck.

Difficulty in swallowing or breathing also should be reported immediately, as it may indicate internal edema and pressure on the esophagus and trachea.

In many hospitals, a tracheostomy set is kept at the bedside of the postoperative thyroidectomy patient in case severe respiratory complications develop. Other symptoms to be reported are persistent hoarseness or loss of the voice, as they may indicate damage to the vocal cords. Tetany and thyroid crisis are other possible complications. These are rare, but when they do occur, the nurse must be alert for the beginning signs and report her observations immediately.

Tetany actually is a sign and results from injury to, or accidental removal of, the parathyroid glands. Recall from Chapter 35 that parathyroid hormone is important in regulating body calcium and phosphorus levels. A deficiency of parathyroid hormone produces muscle cramps, twitching of the muscles, and, in some cases, severe convulsions. These symptoms represent a medical emergency and must be reported to the physician at once. Treatment consists of IV administration of calcium gluconate during the emergency stage and subsequent maintenance doses of parathyroid hormone to maintain calcium and phosphorus balance in the body.

Thyroid storm (TS), also known as thyroid crisis or thyrotoxicosis, is another complication following a thyroidectomy. In a patient with hyperthyroidism, TS also can be triggered by other factors unrelated to surgery (Box 36–1); TS can also be caused by a patient with *hypo*thyroidism who consumes an overdose of levothyroxine.

Box 36–1 Causes of Thyroid Storm

TS usually occurs in a patient with hyperthyroidism (diagnosed or undiagnosed) and is triggered by an event such as:

- Administration of drugs or dyes containing iodine
- Childbirth (immediately postpartum)
- Congestive heart failure
- Diabetic ketoacidosis
- Inadequate hormone replacement
- Infection
- Pulmonary embolism
- Severe emotional distress
- Stroke
- Trauma or surgery

In the postoperative setting, the condition is caused by a sudden increase in the output of thyroxine caused by manipulation of the thyroid as it is being removed. Another cause of TS may be improper reduction of thyroid secretions before surgery.

The symptoms of TS are produced by a sudden and extreme elevation of all body processes. The temperature may rise to 106° F (41.1° C) or more, the pulse increases to as much as 200 beats per minute, respirations become rapid, and the patient exhibits marked apprehension and restlessness. Unless the condition is relieved, the patient quickly passes from delirium to coma to death from heart failure (Assignment Considerations 36–1).

Treatment of thyroid crisis must begin immediately after the first symptoms are noticed, rather than waiting for laboratory confirmation. Measures are taken to reduce the temperature, cardiac drugs are given to

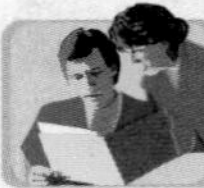

Assignment Considerations 36–1

Changes in Vital Signs

Remind the UAP to report any sudden changes in vital signs or behavior in the patient with thyroid disorders.

Think Critically About . . . What specific assessments would you perform on the patient assigned to you who returned from having a thyroidectomy 4 hours ago?

slow the heart rate, and sedatives, such as a barbiturate, are given to reduce restlessness and anxiety.

HYPOTHYROIDISM

Etiology and Pathophysiology

Hypothyroidism can be caused by inflammation of the thyroid gland (thyroiditis) or by treatment of hyperthyroidism that results in destroying too many thyroid cells and a resultant deficit of thyroid hormone. Genetic defects can cause congenital hypothyroidism (**cretinism**). Cretinism is caused by a severe lack of thyroid hormone during fetal life and infancy and is characterized by growth failure. Underactivity of the thyroid gland can also be caused by a pituitary or hypothalamus dysfunction that causes inadequate stimulation of the thyroid, inducing secondary hypothyroidism.

Signs and Symptoms

The child with hypothyroidism will have delayed physical and mental growth and will become very sluggish within a few weeks after birth. Adults who have myxedema (very low thyroid production) have a decrease in appetite but an increase in weight because of a slow metabolic rate. Other signs are bagginess under the eyes and swelling of the face. In both children and adults there is a tendency to be lethargic and to sleep for abnormally long periods during the day and night. The speech may be slurred, and the individual will appear sluggish in both mental and physical activities. Other signs and symptoms of hypothyroidism are cold intolerance; constipation and abdominal distention; flatulence; impaired memory; depression; husky voice; thinning eyebrows; hair loss; brittle nails; easy bruising; fatigue; muscle cramps; numbness and tingling; dry, scaly skin; and nonpitting edema. Gastrointestinal symptoms are the result of decreased peristaltic activity and can lead to paralytic ileus if untreated.

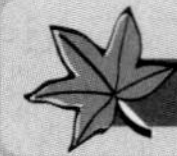

Elder Care Points

Elderly patients who exhibit lethargy, slow thought processes, and lack of enthusiasm could be demonstrating signs of hypothyroidism rather than a brain disorder such as dementia. Hypothyroidism is particularly common in older women.

Safety Alert 36–2

Thyroid Medications

Thyroid medications should not be changed by the patient to the cheapest generic brand, as even slight variations in the level of hormone can be dangerous. Prescription should be labeled "NO substitutions."

Diagnosis and Treatment

Medical diagnosis is based on clinical signs and symptoms and laboratory testing of serum levels of thyroid hormones and TSH.

Hypothyroidism can be treated effectively with replacement of thyroid hormones. The dosage is gradually increased until a proper level has been reached, and then a delicate balance must be maintained so that the patient does not suffer from either hypothyroidism or hyperthyroidism.

Nursing Management

The results of treatment of hypothyroidism are very striking, and most patients show a remarkable abatement of their symptoms. The nurse may not see many cases of hypothyroidism in the hospital because treatment usually does not require hospitalization. If the patient is admitted for some other condition or illness and is also being treated for hypothyroidism, some special considerations must be made. These patients have very rough and dry skin, and they will need massage with lotions and creams to prevent cracking and peeling of the skin. Provisions for extra warmth must also be made for those patients who have an increased sensitivity to cold as a result of their hypothyroidism. It is important that the patient receive thyroid medication every day (Safety Alert 36–2).

The nurse must also bear in mind the psychological aspects of hypothyroidism. She must avoid rushing these patients or giving them the impression of being annoyed by their sluggishness. Forgetfulness, inability to express oneself verbally, and physical inertia are mannerisms that are a direct result of the thyroid deficiency, and the nurse must recognize them as unavoidable as long as the condition is uncontrolled (Patient Teaching 36–2).

MYXEDEMA COMA

Although rare, myxedema coma is life threatening. It can be precipitated by abrupt withdrawal of thyroid therapy, acute illness, anesthesia, use of sedatives or narcotics, surgery, or hypothermia in the hypothyroid patient. Signs and symptoms are loss of consciousness along with hypotension, hypothermia, respiratory fail-

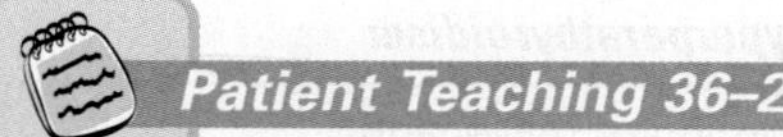

Patient Teaching 36–2

Managing Hypothyroidism

The patient with hypothyroidism requires thorough patient teaching, emphasizing the following points:

- Take levothyroxine on an empty stomach, as many medications and foods interfere with absorption.
- Take levothyroxine at the same time each day.
- Levothyroxine is lifelong therapy; it should never be stopped by anyone except the practitioner who prescribed it.
- Contact your health care provider if you experience unusual bleeding, bruising, chest pain, palpitations, sweating, nervousness, or shortness of breath.
- Signs and symptoms of myxedema coma and hyperthyroidism.

ure, hyponatremia, and hypoglycemia. Treatment is administration of levothyroxine sodium IV, fluid replacement, maintenance of an airway and respiration, IV glucose administration, corticosteroids, and provision of warmth.

THYROIDITIS

Etiology and Pathophysiology

Thyroiditis is an inflammation of the thyroid gland. There are three types: acute, such as infection-related; subacute, for example, related to upper respiratory viral infection; or chronic, the most common type. Chronic thyroiditis, also known as Hashimoto's thyroiditis, usually affects women between the ages of 30 and 50. It is an autoimmune disorder, whereby the body produces antibodies against the thyroid, which in turn destroy the gland. The reasons behind who gets Hashimoto's thyroiditis are not fully understood; however, there seems to be a genetic predisposition, and it is more prevalent in people with another autoimmune disease, such as rheumatoid arthritis.

Signs, Symptoms, and Diagnosis

The patient with Hashimoto's thyroiditis will experience a painless enlargement of the thyroid gland. The patient also will experience dysphagia caused by the inflammation.

Hashimoto's thyroiditis is based on laboratory tests, including serum thyroid hormone levels, TSH levels, and radioactive iodine uptake. Needle biopsy of the gland may be performed.

Treatment and Nursing Management

The patient with Hashimoto's thyroiditis is given thyroid hormone to prevent hypothyroidism and suppress TSH secretion. Thyroid function in this disorder is usually normal or low, rather than increased (as in acute thyroiditis). Left untreated, eventually hypothyroidism will develop. The goal of therapy is to decrease the size of the thyroid and prevent hypothyroidism. Surgery to remove part of the gland may be considered. Nursing management focuses on patient teaching and providing for comfort.

THYROID CANCER

Etiology and Pathophysiology

The incidence of thyroid cancer has become more common in recent years. The most common form of thyroid cancer is papillary carcinoma, which occurs most often in younger women. This cancer is characterized by a slowly growing tumor that can be present for years before it is diagnosed. The cause of thyroid cancer is unknown.

Signs and Symptoms

The first sign of thyroid cancer may be a nodule found on a routine physical examination. Not all nodules, however, indicate cancer: only 5% to 10% are found to be cancerous. Other signs and symptoms of thyroid cancer, such as fatigue, depression, and weight changes, can be easily missed or attributed to other causes.

Diagnosis

The diagnosis of thyroid cancer is made by examination and diagnostic tests. The practitioner may prescribe an ultrasound examination to assess thyroid size and to locate any nodules. Iodine uptake studies may be used to check for nodules also. The definitive test is called *fine needle aspiration,* in which a specimen of tissue is taken and analyzed.

Treatment and Nursing Management

The treatment for thyroid cancer is thyroidectomy. In some cases, radioactive iodine therapy (see ablation therapy, earlier in this chapter) may be used in lieu of surgery to disable the gland. Nursing management for these procedures has been discussed in a previous section of this chapter.

DISORDERS OF THE PARATHYROID GLANDS

HYPOPARATHYROIDISM

Etiology and Pathophysiology

Hypoparathyroidism is most often caused by atrophy or traumatic injury to the parathyroid glands. This can occur as a result of accidental removal or destruction of parathyroid tissue during a thyroidectomy, irradiation of the thyroids, or from idiopathic (having no known cause) atrophy of the glands. A deficiency of parathormone will result in a drop in serum calcium levels and an increase in phosphorus levels.

Signs and Symptoms

Signs and symptoms of hypocalcemia include mild tingling, numbness, muscle cramps, and mental changes, such as irritability. Tetany is a serious sign resulting from a lowered serum calcium level. In tetany, muscular twitching and spasms occur because of extreme irritability of neuromuscular tissue. If calcium levels continue to fall, the patient will suffer from convulsions, cardiac dysrhythmias, and spasms of the larynx.

Diagnosis

Medical diagnosis is established by clinical signs and laboratory data. An electroencephalogram (EEG) may demonstrate abnormalities which return to normal when the calcium level is corrected. A CT scan may reveal brain calcifications if the hypocalcemia is chronic. Changes in bone integrity may be seen on radiograph. Other labs tests that confirm the diagnosis include serum calcium, phosphate, magnesium, vitamin D, and urine cyclic adenosine monophosphate (cAMP).

Treatment and Nursing Management

Acute hypoparathyroidism is treated by measures to raise serum calcium levels to normal range. Oral or parenteral administration of calcium salts is used in the acute phase. In chronic hypoparathyroidism, treatment is aimed at restoring and maintaining normal calcium levels in the blood. This can be accomplished by parathormone replacement therapy, administration of vitamin D in massive doses to enhance absorption of calcium from the small intestine, and oral administration of calcium salts. Nursing care revolves around electrolyte replacement and patient teaching. The nurse should teach the patient to eat foods high in calcium but low in phosphorus. Milk, yogurt, and processed cheeses are high in phosphorus and therefore are not advised. The nurse must remind the patient that therapy for hypoparathyroidism is lifelong, and advise the patient to wear a Medic-Alert bracelet. Bracelets and emblems can be obtained from www.medicalert.org.

HYPERPARATHYROIDISM (VON RECKLINGHAUSEN'S DISEASE)

Etiology and Pathophysiology

Hyperparathyroidism is another common disorder of the endocrine system. The disorder occurs most often in postmenopausal women. Excessive synthesis and secretion of parathormone can occur, most often as a result of benign enlargement of the parathyroid glands (adenoma) or hyperplasia of two or more glands. Hypercalcemia (calcium level above 10.5 mg/dL) occurs with hyperactivity of the parathyroid glands.

Other causes of hyperparathyroidism are outlined in Box 36–2.

Signs and Symptoms

Signs and symptoms of hyperparathyroidism may be mild or severe and include dehydration, confusion, lethargy, anorexia, nausea, vomiting, weight loss, constipation, thirst, frequent urination, and hypertension. If hypercalcemia exists, there may be skeletal changes, including thinning of the bone and bone cysts. A fracture often causes the patient to seek medical attention.

Box 36–2 *Causes of Hyperparathyroidism*

- Parathyroid tumor (benign or malignant)
- Congenital enlargement
- Neck trauma or irradiation
- Vitamin D deficiency
- Chronic renal failure with hypocalcemia
- Lung, kidney, or GI tract cancers

Adapted from: Ignatavicius, D.D., & Workman, M.L. (2005). *Medical Surgical Nursing: Critical Thinking for Collaborative Care* (5th ed.). Philadelphia: Saunders.

Table 36–2 *Hyperparathyroidism versus Hypoparathyroidism*

	HYPERPARATHYROIDISM	HYPOPARATHYROIDISM
Serum calcium levels	+	−
Serum phosphate levels	−	+
Bone resorption	+	−
Calcium and phosphate in urine	+	−
Neuromuscular irritability	−	+ (may progress to tetany)

Key: +, increased; −, decreased.

Diagnosis

In recent years a greater number of cases of hyperparathyroidism have been diagnosed because of improved radiologic and laboratory screening procedures. Many cases are now being diagnosed in the earliest stages of the disease before the clinical manifestations of hypercalcemia become apparent. Laboratory testing for serum calcium and phosphate levels helps confirm the diagnosis.

The signs of hypercalcemia are manifested in virtually every major system in the body. Hyperparathyroidism and hypoparathyroidism are compared in Table 36–2.

Treatment

The treatment of hyperparathyroidism will depend on the severity of the symptoms produced by hypercalcemia and hypophosphatemia. Methods of therapy include the infusion of isotonic sodium chloride and administration of diuretic agents to promote excretion of excess calcium in the urine; phosphate therapy to correct the deficit; administration of mithramycin to bind calcium and enhance secretion from the body; and administration of calcitonin to decrease the rate of skeletal calcium release.

Surgical removal of a major portion of the parathyroids (subtotal parathyroidectomy) is recommended for patients who have severe systemic disorders associated with excessively high levels of parathormone. The remaining parathyroid tissue will continue to function and prevent the problem of hypoparathyroidism.

Nursing Management

Nursing management for patients receiving diuretic therapy includes accurate measuring of intake and output (every 2 to 4 hours), daily weight, monitoring of serum electrolytes, ongoing assessment of the patient for electrolyte imbalance, and appropriate nursing intervention. The patient may be placed on continuous cardiac monitoring, depending on the degree of the electrolyte imbalances.

DISORDERS OF THE ADRENAL GLANDS

PHEOCHROMOCYTOMA

Etiology and Pathophysiology

Pheochromocytoma is a rare tumor of the adrenal medulla that secretes **catecholamines** (epinephrine and norepinephrine). It often causes severe hypertension. Although the tumor usually is not cancerous, if left untreated it can lead to death.

Signs, Symptoms, and Diagnosis

Signs and symptoms of pheochromocytoma are signs of excess catecholamine release. The patient will experience signs including tachycardia, severe hypertension (as high as 250/150 mm Hg) that can be intermittent or persistent, and diaphoresis. Symptoms include anxiety, severe headache, and palpitations.

Pheochromocytoma is diagnosed by measurement of serum catecholamines and 24-hour urine measurement of catecholamine metabolites; CT and MRI may be used to locate the tumor.

Treatment and Nursing Management

Treatment is surgical removal of the tumor (adrenalectomy), which can often be performed laparoscopically. Before surgery, the patient may be in hypertensive crisis and require close monitoring of vital signs and administration of antihypertensive medications, such as prazosin (Minipress). Other nursing measures include helping the patient maintain comfort and provide emotional support. Also, the nurse will need to monitor the patient for signs of orthostatic hypotension related to medication therapy.

ADRENOCORTICAL INSUFFICIENCY (ADDISON'S DISEASE)

Etiology and Pathophysiology

Addison's disease is characterized by decreased function of the adrenal cortex resulting in a deficit of all three hormones secreted by the adrenal cortex. The major problems presented by this disorder are, however, related to insufficiencies of the mineralocorticoids and the glucocorticoids. The insufficiency of the androgenic hormones can be compensated for by the ovaries and testes.

Insufficient production of the adrenocortical hormones can result from a disorder affecting the adrenal cortex itself (primary insufficiency) or from a disorder affecting the pituitary gland that stimulates adrenal secretion (secondary insufficiency). Disorders causing a primary insufficiency include idiopathic atrophy, inflammation, infection, and nonsecreting tumors of the adrenal cortex. Secondary insufficiency is the direct result of failure of the pituitary gland to secrete adrenocorticotropic hormone (ACTH). This can occur because the pituitary is underfunctioning, the gland was surgically removed (hypophysectomy), because of certain pituitary tumors, or abrupt withdrawal of steroid therapy.

? *Think Critically About* . . . What signs and symptoms might you see in a patient who is developing Addison's disease after stopping steroid therapy?

Signs and Symptoms

In the early stages of Addison's disease, the clinical manifestations may be so vague as to be annoying to the patient but not serious enough to consult a physician. Hence it is easily missed altogether or misdiagnosed. Later, as the hormone insufficiency becomes more pronounced, the patient will begin to exhibit more severe symptoms associated with fluid and electrolyte imbalance and hypoglycemia. Considering the functions of the mineralocorticoids, a major problem is depletion of sodium (hyponatremia), which in turn causes depletion of extracellular fluid and potassium retention (hyperkalemia). The patient experiences generalized malaise and muscle weakness, muscle pain, orthostatic hypotension, and vulnerability to cardiac dysrhythmias.

Insufficiency of the glucocorticoids affects blood glucose levels and causes symptoms of hypoglycemia. There is also decreased secretion of gastrointestinal enzymes, which results in anorexia, nausea and vomiting, flatulence, and diarrhea. These symptoms, as well as anxiety, depression, and loss of mental acuity, are thought to be related to absence of the peaks of cortisol output that normally occur every 24 hours.

Diagnosis

Diagnosis of Addison's disease is made by examining blood and urine electrolytes. An ACTH stimulation test can determine if the problem lies in the adrenal gland or in the pituitary. CT and MRI scans may be used to locate tumor, calcification, or gland enlargement. Abnormal serum electrolyte levels (hyponatremia and hyperkalemia), decreased glucose tolerance, elevated white blood cell count (leukocytosis), and abnormally low levels of free cortisol are among the criteria used to diagnose Addison's disease.

Treatment

Replacement therapy to provide the missing hormones is the major component of treatment. Replacement therapy usually brings about a rapid recovery, but the patient must continue taking the hormones for the rest of her life.

Nursing Management

Nursing management of the patient with Addison's disease is concerned with:

- Intensive care and support during addisonian crisis when the patient is in a critical condition and in danger of death from fluid volume depletion, hypotension and shock, and impairment of cardiac function.
- Prevention of problems related to fatigue and orthostatic hypotension.
- Alleviation of gastrointestinal problems.
- Instruction of the patient in self-care.

Two important nursing measures are to provide both regular feedings throughout the day and adequate rest. The patient may feel well in the morning but may become progressively weaker and fatigued as the day goes on. If fasting is necessary for diagnostic studies or surgery, the patient with Addison's disease probably will need IV glucose to avoid developing profound hypoglycemia. Maintenance doses of glucocorticoids are especially important whenever fasting is required.

Gastrointestinal problems bring on the possibility of imbalanced nutrition, less than body requirements, related to anorexia, nausea and vomiting, and diarrhea. Specific fluid and electrolyte imbalances have already been discussed and are covered in more depth in Chapter 3. Stress, even relatively mild physical or emotional stress, can quickly bring on an addisonian crisis. The patient should be cautioned to avoid undue stress whenever possible and to learn effective coping mechanisms to deal with the emotional stresses everyone faces. Patient Teaching 36–3 presents guidelines for instruction of the patient with Addison's disease and Nursing Care Plan 36–2 outlines the nursing care.

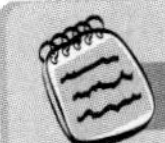

Patient Teaching 36–3

Managing Addison's Disease

The nurse should teach the patient about the signs and symptoms of inadequate or excessive steroid levels, the importance of reporting either promptly, and the following points:

- The nature of the illness and what can be done to control it.
- The purpose of each medication and the side effects to be reported.
- The importance of taking the medication every day and of never stopping corticosteroids suddenly; they need to be tapered off slowly.
- Methods of adjusting medication dosage to combat the effects of stress.
- Signs and symptoms to report to the physician immediately (worsening weakness, hypotension, confusion, infection).
- Diet adjustments to provide food throughout the day and a bedtime snack.
- The importance of following the prescribed diet to avoid gastrointestinal problems.
- Planned rest periods during the day and sufficient sleep at night, as well as avoidance of physical stress.
- The need for a Medic-Alert tag or bracelet stating Addison's disease and that the patient is on steroid therapy.

Think Critically About . . . What specific interventions would you use to help a patient with Addison's disease learn to decrease or cope with stress?

NURSING CARE PLAN 36–2

Care of the Patient with Adrenocortical Insufficiency (Addison's Disease)

SCENARIO Mr. Cox, age 49, is admitted with a tentative diagnosis of adrenocortical insufficiency (Addison's disease). He has recently experienced weight loss, weakness, poor coordination, vomiting, changes in skin coloration, and loss of body hair. During initial assessment, Mr. Cox is found to be very irritable and easily upset by the questions. His vital signs are BP 90/50, P 70 and slightly irregular, RR 16 and deep. He reports that he feels pretty good when he awakens in the morning but quickly becomes tired and his muscles begin to ache. He is concerned about his weight loss and change in appearance and also has noticed that he has been unable to "think straight." Admission laboratory data: blood glucose, 50 mg/dL; sodium, 90 mEq/L; and potassium, 5.6 mEq/L.

PROBLEM/NURSING DIAGNOSIS *Tires quickly*/Activity intolerance related to weakness and electrolyteimbalance.

Supporting assessment data *Subjective:* States that "with the least little exertion," he tires and has muscle aching.

Goals/Expected Outcomes	Nursing Interventions	Selected Rationale	Evaluation
Patient will have normal serum sodium within 24 hr	Administer glucocorticoids and mineralocorticoids as prescribed; observe for side effects	Glucocorticoids and mineralocorticoids are necessary to replace those missing due to a deficient adrenal cortex.	Patient's serum sodium level returned to normal limits within 18 hr.

NURSING CARE PLAN 36–2

Care of the Patient with Adrenocortical Insufficiency (Addison's Disease)—cont'd

Goals/Expected Outcomes	Nursing Interventions	Selected Rationale	Evaluation
	Weigh daily; measure and compare intake and output.	Daily weight is an excellent way to assess daily fluid gains/losses.	Patient gained 2 lb of weight in 3 days.
	Monitor electrolyte levels. Force fluids until steroid therapy takes effect.		
	Encourage him to maintain a nutritious diet.	Intake of nutritious foods is important to maintain adequate glucose and sodium levels.	Continue plan.

PROBLEM/NURSING DIAGNOSIS *Has adrenocortical insufficiency*/Risk for injury related to possible severe drop in blood glucose.

Supporting assessment data *Objective:* Blood glucose on admission, 50 mg/dL.

Goals/Expected Outcomes	Nursing Interventions	Selected Rationale	Evaluation
Patient will maintain blood glucose within normal limits	Observe for signs of hypoglycemia and report promptly.	Hypoglycemia can be a warning sign of impending addisonian crisis; blood glucose levels must be maintained.	Patient's blood glucose level is 110 mg/dL.
Patient will not develop crisis	Check to see that meals are served on time; provide snacks as needed.		Patient exhibits no signs/symptoms of hypoglycemia.
	Teach signs of hypoglycemia and instruct him in what to do when this occurs.	Patient teaching is a critical part of long-term care for this disorder.	Patient able to verbalize three signs and symptoms of hypoglycemia. Continue plan.

PROBLEM/NURSING DIAGNOSIS *Difficulty thinking and remembering*/Ineffective coping related to excess cortisol and mood swings.

Supporting assessment data *Subjective:* States he is unable to "think straight." *Objective:* Very irritable and impatient; tentative diagnosis of Addison's disease; serum cortisol results pending.

Goals/Expected Outcomes	Nursing Interventions	Selected Rationale	Evaluation
Patient will not develop an infection during hospitalization	Protect him from exposure to infection.	Helping the patient avoid infection will protect him.	
	Monitor vital signs, white blood cell (WBC) count, and lung fields each shift.		Patient's vital signs and WBC count are within normal limits. Lung fields clear to auscultation.
	Observe for signs of infection.	Finding infection quickly can help prevent a severe problem.	Patient has no signs of infection.
Patient will develop effective coping mechanisms; patient will use relaxation techniques before discharge	Teach relaxation techniques and supervise practice; work with patient on other ways to decrease stress in daily life.	Effective coping skills are an important determination of how successfully a patient will manage a long-term illness.	Patient verbalized techniques that help him feel relaxed. Patient beginning to practice relaxation exercise.
	Teach him how to handle anticipated stress by adjusting dosage of medications.	Decreasing stressors can assist one's coping abilities.	Patient verbalizing medication adjustments needed when stressed. Patient verbalized three methods to decrease stress.
	Encourage verbalization of concerns and fears; answer questions.	Verbalization of fears and concerns helps improve one's ability to cope.	Continue plan.
	Discuss alterations in body image and changes that can be expected with therapy.		

Continued

NURSING CARE PLAN 36–2

Care of the Patient with Adrenocortical Insufficiency (Addison's Disease)—cont'd

PROBLEM/NURSING DIAGNOSIS *Unfamiliar with Addison's disease*/Deficient knowledge related to illness, medications, and necessary changes in lifestyle.

Supporting assessment data *Subjective:* States that he knows nothing about Addison's disease, its diagnosis, or treatment. Unfamiliar with corticosteroid therapy.

Goals/Expected Outcomes	*Nursing Interventions*	*Selected Rationale*	*Evaluation*
Patient will describe, in simple terms, problems of Addison's disease	Help to identify stressors in his life and assist in determining ways to avoid them.	Decreasing stress is an important first step in managing Addison's disease.	Patient able to state basic action of each medication.
Patient will verbalize understanding of medications and dosage schedule before discharge	Answer questions and discuss expected effect of continued therapy on his ability to resume preillness activities.	Once hormone levels are normalized, the patient with Addison's can expect to resume normal activities, as long as rest periods are integrated into the schedule.	Patient verbalized medication dosing schedule.
Patient will verbalize plans for obtaining adequate rest before discharge	Help him develop a schedule that allows for periods of rest, work, social interaction, and recreation. Stress importance of balancing rest and activity.		Patient described his intention to integrate rest with desired activities.
	Provide written instructions that give warning signs and symptoms of insufficient corticosteroid medication and those of excess medication (Cushing syndrome). Instruct him to report either set of symptoms to the physician promptly so medication can be adjusted. Discuss how to adjust medication for periods of extra stress (minor illness, such as a cold, an emotional upset, or unusual physiologic or psychological stress). Instruct him to wear a form of Medic-Alert identification with data concerning steroid therapy.	Patient teaching is critical for long-term management of Addison's disease.	Patient verbalized three signs and symptoms of insufficient or excessive hormone.

? CRITICAL THINKING QUESTIONS

1. In implementing the patient teaching plan for Mr. Cox, when would you perform your patient teaching, and why?
2. Mr. Cox has put together a proposed activity schedule for after he is discharged from the hospital. He lives in a rural community and must go to the post office to get his mail each day. He asks if you would mind looking at the schedule and giving him feedback on it. The schedule reads:

   8 A.M. breakfast
   9 A.M. walk dog
   10 A.M. gardening
   11 A.M. walk to post office/get mail
   12 P.M. lunch
   1 P.M. nap
   2 P.M. watch television
   3 P.M. daughter over for visit

   What if any suggestions would you give Mr. Cox, and why?

ADDISONIAN CRISIS

Physical stress from the flu or other infection can tip the scales for the patient with Addison's disease and send her into crisis. The stress of surgery also places the patient at risk for crisis. The nurse must be especially watchful and closely monitor vital signs in these situations. Addisonian crisis requires immediate fluid replacement therapy, or the patient will go into irreversible shock. Intravenous hydrocortisone is given along with sodium, fluids, and dextrose until blood pressure becomes stable. The hydrocortisone is then tapered off slowly.

EXCESS ADRENOCORTICAL HORMONE (CUSHING SYNDROME)

Etiology and Pathophysiology

Cushing syndrome is a rare disorder. The symptoms typical of Cushing syndrome are manifestations of excess levels of the hormones from the adrenal cortex. The condition can be caused by:

- Excessive secretion of ACTH by the pituitary, which may result from faulty release of corticotropin-releasing factor (CRF) from the hypothalamus.
- A secreting tumor of the adrenal cortex.
- Ectopic production of ACTH by tumors outside the pituitary, such as lung cancer.
- Iatrogenic Cushing syndrome from prolonged use of steroid therapy.

Signs and Symptoms

Signs and symptoms presented by the patient are caused by excessive levels of this hormone (Figure 36–5). They include painful fatty swellings in the intrascapular space (buffalo hump) and facial area (moon face), an enlarged abdomen with thin extremities, bruising following even minor traumas, impotence, amenorrhea, hypertension, and weakness due to abnormal protein catabolism with loss of muscle mass.

Unusual growth of body hair (hirsutism) can occur in women, and streaked purple markings in the abdominal area can occur due to collections of body fat. Patients with Cushing syndrome who have a familial predisposition to diabetes mellitus frequently develop type 1 diabetes from the anti-insulin, diabetogenic properties of cortisol.

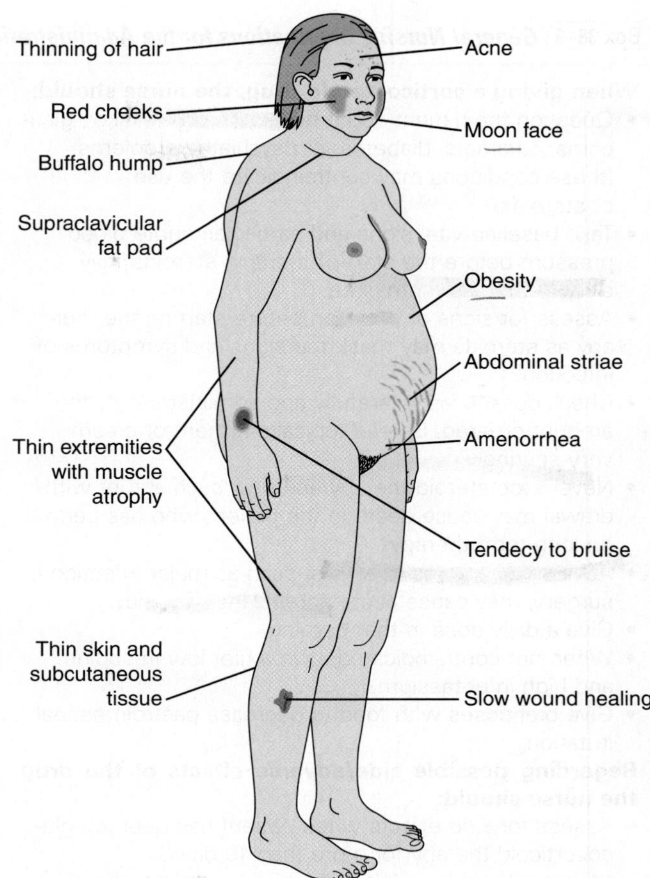

FIGURE 36–5 Common characteristics of Cushing syndrome.

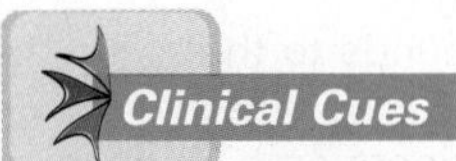

Secondary Cushing syndrome produced by long-term cortisone therapy is often reversible if the medication is tapered off and stopped. However, most people taking cortisone are taking it for other health disorders and cannot manage without it. No one should take steroids for a condition other than the specific health disorder for which they are prescribed.

Diagnosis

The diagnosis of Cushing syndrome is established by laboratory findings indicating consistently high levels of free plasma cortisol rather than the usual 24-hour fluctuations. A 24-hour urine test should be performed. If cortisol is elevated, a dexamethasone suppression test should be ordered, whereby the patient is given a steroid at night and blood and urine cortisol levels are measured in the morning.

Treatment

Pituitary Cushing syndrome can be treated by microsurgery on the pituitary gland. In some instances, the disorder can be prevented by using steroids cautiously and restricting their administration to the patient who does not respond to other forms of therapy.

If Cushing syndrome is arising from an adrenal tumor, adrenalectomy is indicated. In this instance replacement of glucocorticoids is necessary (Box 36–3).

Nursing Management

The nursing care of the patient with Cushing syndrome is primarily concerned with helping the patient cope with the many systemic problems presented by the disorder. The nurse must assist the patient with psychosocial concerns presented by emotional **lability** and depression when they occur. The patient needs assurance that the symptoms will improve with proper treatment.

Box 36–3 ***General Nursing Implications for the Administration of Corticosteroids***

When giving a corticosteroid drug, the nurse should:
- Question the patient about history of peptic ulcer, glaucoma, cataracts, diabetes, or psychiatric problems (these conditions may contraindicate the use of steroids).
- Take baseline vital signs and particularly note blood pressure before the start of therapy; steroids may elevate the blood pressure.
- Assess for signs of infection before starting the therapy as steroids may mask the signs and symptoms of infection.
- Check dosage very carefully and administer only the amount ordered. Spread topical ointment or cream very sparingly.
- Never stop steroid therapy abruptly; such abrupt withdrawal may cause death in the patient who has been on long-term therapy.
- Advise that increased stress, such as major infection or surgery, may cause acute adrenal insufficiency.
- Give a daily dose in the morning.
- When not contraindicated, give a diet low in sodium and high in potassium.
- Give oral doses with food to decrease gastrointestinal irritation.

Regarding possible side/adverse effects of the drug, the nurse should:
- Assess for side effects when patient has been on glucocorticoid therapy for more than 10 days.
- Monitor the older adult for signs of osteoporosis. Give vitamin D and recommend weight-bearing exercise to prevent osteoporosis.
- Assess for changes in muscle strength.
- Instruct to report slow healing of wounds to the physician.
- Watch for signs of depression in patients on high-dose steroid therapy.
- Monitor for signs of hypokalemia, such as nausea, muscle weakness, abdominal distention, and irregular heart rate.
- Monitor blood sugar of diabetic patients closely as glucocorticoids may cause hyperglycemia.
- Check blood pressure regularly during therapy to monitor for hypertension.
- Advise patients on long-term steroid therapy should have regular checkups for glaucoma and cataracts.
- Observe stool for signs of gastrointestinal bleeding.
- Monitor weight, as steroids may cause increased appetite and weight gain.

The nurse should teach the patient taking a corticosteroid drug to:
- Take oral doses in the morning with food.
- Not discontinue the drug abruptly but taper down the dosage before stopping it, and only with the approval of the practitioner who prescribed it.
- Watch dietary intake as patient may be hungrier and this could cause weight gain.
- Watch for signs of hypokalemia, such as muscle weakness, fatigue, anorexia, and irregular heartbeat.
- Take the drug only as prescribed.
- Eat foods such as fresh and dried fruits, juices, potatoes, meats, and nuts that are high in potassium.
- Report signs of Cushing syndrome, such as moon-shaped face, puffy eyelids, edema in the feet, increased bruising, dizziness, bleeding, and menstrual irregularity.
- Carry a Medic-Alert card and wear a bracelet stating patient is on steroid therapy when on long-term steroids.
- Avoid people with infections and stay away from crowds, especially during cold and flu season.
- Advise all other physicians and dentists seen that patient is on steroid therapy.
- Be aware that more insulin may be needed if patient is diabetic.
- Be aware that antibody response from immunization while taking steroids may be reduced; do not take a live-virus vaccine.
- Use aspirin and other NSAIDs cautiously as they will increase the risk of gastrointestinal bleeding when taken during steroid therapy.
- Be aware that steroids decrease the effect of barbiturates, phenytoin, and rifampin and that the doses of these drugs may need to be increased.
- Have clotting time monitored closely when taking an anticoagulant at the same time as the steroid.
- Be aware that taking steroids along with potassium-wasting diuretics may cause hypokalemia; increase potassium intake in diet.

COMMUNITY CARE

Nurses in long-term care facilities must be on the alert for signs of thyroid dysfunction, especially among their elderly female patients. The nurse often is the one who picks up on subtle changes in the patient that have occurred over many months.

Nurses can be instrumental in preventing secondary Cushing syndrome by cautioning patients to seek means of treatment other than long-term steroid therapy for arthritis or allergies. The nurse must teach patients receiving a new prescription for steroids that the medication must be tapered, never stopped abruptly.

Internet resources that may be useful for patients experiencing disorders discussed in this chapter include:

- Pituitary Disorders Education and Support (Web site sponsor: Massachusetts General Neuroendocrine Center): www.pituitarydisorder.net
- The American Thyroid Association: www.thyroid.org
- Cushing's Support and Research Foundation: www.csrf.net
- Cushing's help and support: www.cushings-help.com
- National Adrenal Disease Foundation: www.nadf.us

- A pituitary tumor secretes growth hormone and antagonizes the effect of insulin. Treatment consists of hormone therapy or surgery.
- Hypofunction of an endocrine gland typically mandates lifelong hormone therapy.
- Hypofunction of the pituitary gland is characterized by a decrease in pituitary hormones and metabolic and sexual dysfunction.
- DI can occur as a result of decreased production of ADH, and can lead to hypernatremia, dehydration, and coma. Replacement of fluid, electrolytes, and hormones is required.
- In SIADH, excessive amounts of ADH are produced, resulting in fluid retention. Treatment is aimed at correcting the underlying cause, restricting fluids, and administering medications. The nurse must closely focus on the cardiovascular and neurologic systems, electrolytes, and weight.
- The signs and symptoms of hyperthyroidism are the result of an accelerated metabolic rate, although the older adult may have milder or opposite symptoms. Ablation therapy is the definitive treatment, but it is contraindicated for some. Thyroidectomy is usually a treatment of last resort.
- The child with hypothyroidism will have delayed growth; adults will have a decrease in appetite and increase in weight. Myxedema coma can be precipitated by abrupt withdrawal of thyroid therapy, acute illness, or other stressors.
- The most common type of thyroiditis is Hashimoto's. Treatment includes thyroid hormones or surgery. Nursing care focuses on patient teaching and comfort.
- Thyroid cancer occurs most often in younger women. Treatment includes ablation therapy, thyroidectomy, or both.
- Hypoparathyroidism can occur from removal or destruction of parathyroid tissue. It is treated by administration of calcium, hormone replacement, and vitamin D.
- Hyperparathyroidism is characterized by excessive synthesis and secretion of parathormone. Therapies include sodium chloride and diuretics, phosphate, mithramycin, and calcitonin; subtotal parathyroidectomy may be done. Nursing care includes monitoring input and output (I&O), weight, and electrolytes.
- Pheochromocytoma is a potentially fatal adrenal medulla tumor; treatment is surgical removal of the tumor.
- In Addison's disease, there is decreased function of the adrenal cortex and a deficit of all hormones. The patient exhibits severe symptoms of fluid and electrolyte imbalance and hypoglycemia.
- Cushing syndrome involves excess levels of adrenal cortex hormones; it may be treated surgically. Nursing care is concerned with support and education.

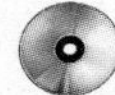

Go to your **Companion CD-ROM** for an Audio Glossary, animations, video clips, and bonus review questions.

evolve Be sure to visit the companion Evolve site at http://evolve.elsevier.com/deWit for interactive NCLEX-PN Exam Style Review Questions, WebLinks, and additional online resources.

NCLEX-PN EXAM STYLE REVIEW QUESTIONS

Choose the best answer(s) for the following questions.

1. A 50-year-old male patient output 15 L of urine within a 24-hour period. He has poor skin turgor with low blood pressure and increased heart rate. The nurse would plan to administer which of the following medications?

1. Furosemide (Lasix)
2. Desmopressin acetate (DDAVP)
3. Regular insulin
4. Spironolactone (Aldactone)

2. A 45-year-old male patient presents with muscle cramps and weakness. He is weak and confused. Serum sodium is 115 mEq/L. A critical nursing intervention would be:

1. give hypertonic enema.
2. encourage fluid intake.
3. infuse hypotonic intravenous fluids.
4. administer vasopressin.

3. A 35-year-old female patient reports episodes of emotional extremes with uncontrollable crying and depression followed by intense physical activity and euphoria. She complains of drying of the eyes and difficulty swallowing. Her symptoms confirm a nursing diagnosis of Ineffective coping. An etiology for this diagnosis would be:

1. parathyroid hormone deficiency.
2. excessive thyroid hormone secretion.
3. deficient estrogen production.
4. growth hormone deficiency.

4. A patient received large doses of radioactive iodine (^{131}I) for hyperthyroidism. Appropriate nursing interventions include which of the following? *(Select all that apply.)*

1. Monitor vital signs.
2. Restrict fluids.
3. Encourage eating high-calorie foods.
4. Properly handle contaminated materials.
5. Encourage physical activity.

5. The nurse caring for a post-thyroidectomy patient would monitor for which of the following? *(Select all that apply.)*
   1. Bleeding and swelling
   2. Hypothermia
   3. Fluid overload
   4. Difficulty swallowing
   5. Difficulty breathing
6. A post-thyroidectomy patient complains of severe muscle cramping followed by muscle twitching and convulsions. An appropriate nursing action would be to:
   1. prepare for intubation.
   2. consider calcium gluconate.
   3. force fluids.
   4. administer antibiotics.
7. The patient experiences generalized malaise and muscle weakness, muscle pain, orthostatic hypotension, and vulnerability to cardiac dysrhythmias. The nurse suspects Addison's disease and would anticipate which of the following clinical findings?
   1. Hyponatremia and hyperkalemia
   2. Hypernatremia and hyperkalemia
   3. Hyponatremia and hypokalemia
   4. Hypernatremia and hypokalemia
8. A 25-year-old female complains of amenorrhea with weakness, easy bruising, and painful fatty swelling on the back. Initial assessment would confirm which of the following nursing diagnoses?
   1. Ineffective coping
   2. Disturbed body image
   3. Social isolation
   4. Anxiety
9. The nurse provides patient instructions regarding taking iodine preparations. It is important for the nurse to include which of the following? *(Select all that apply.)*
   1. "Dilute the preparations well."
   2. "Use a straw to prevent staining of the teeth."
   3. "Watch for easy bruising."
   4. "Report severe epigastric pain."
   5. "Anticipate metallic taste."
10. A 43-year-old male develops excessive weakness and loss of coordination after a sudden withdrawal of steroid therapy. Initial assessment confirms the nursing diagnosis of Activity intolerance related to decreased corticosteroid levels. A realistic goal for this patient would be to:
    1. verbalize personal concerns.
    2. optimize level of activity and function.
    3. develop new coping strategies.
    4. gain weight.

CRITICAL THINKING ACTIVITIES  *Read each clinical scenario and discuss the questions with your classmates.*

Scenario A

Mrs. Timms has a tentative diagnosis of hyperthyroidism. She is 45 years old, 5 feet 7 inches tall, and weighs 102 lb.

1. What subjective and objective signs and symptoms would you expect Mrs. Timms to present during nursing assessment?
2. How would you go about preparing Mrs. Timms for diagnostic laboratory tests for thyroid function?
3. If Mrs. Timms' physician decided to treat her condition with large doses of radioactive iodine, what special nursing care will she require?
4. What other forms of therapy are used to treat hyperthyroidism?

Scenario B

Mr. Lau, age 37, is receiving adrenocorticoid hormones as replacement therapy for Addison's disease.

1. What kinds of problems does insufficiency of the adrenal cortex hormones bring about?
2. What should be included in your instructions to Mr. Lau to help him manage his illness?

Scenario C

Mrs. Josten, age 48, is hospitalized for a cholecystectomy. She has Cushing syndrome as well as gallbladder disease. She is 35 lb overweight and depressed.

1. What kinds of problems is Mrs. Josten likely to have as a result of her Cushing syndrome?
2. What would be your concerns in the immediate postoperative period?
3. What would you want to include in your discharge teaching plan?

CHAPTER

37 Care of Patients with Diabetes and Hypoglycemia

evolve http://evolve.elsevier.com/deWit

Objectives

Upon completing the chapter you should be able to:

Theory

1. Compare and contrast the two major types of diabetes mellitus.
2. Illustrate each of the four kinds of factors that influence the development of diabetes mellitus.
3. Describe the acute and long-term complications and results of poorly controlled diabetes mellitus.
4. Identify sources of support and information for people with diabetes and their families.

Clinical Practice

1. Teach a newly diagnosed person with diabetes about the disease, treatment, and self-care.
2. Perform a focused nursing assessment/gather data for the management of type 1 and type 2 diabetes mellitus.
3. Identify signs and symptoms of an insulin reaction (hypoglycemia) and implement appropriate nursing interventions.
4. Interpret laboratory tests used in the diagnosis and management of diabetes mellitus.
5. Assess for/gather data related to signs and symptoms that might indicate that the patient with diabetes is in early ketoacidosis.
6. Identify signs and symptoms of hypoglycemia and its treatment in people without diabetes.

Key Terms

Be sure to check out the bonus material on the Companion CD-ROM, including selected audio pronunciations.

basement membrane (p. 930)
black box warning (p. 919)
counterregulatory hormones (p. 930)
dawn phenomenon (p. 930)
endogenous (ĕn-DŎJ-ĕn-ŭs, p. 909)
exogenous (ĕks-ŎJ-ĕn-ŭs, p. 909)
gastroparesis (găs-trō-pă-RĒ-sĭs, p. 931)
glycemic (glī-SĒ-mĭk, p. 912)
glycosuria (glī-cōs-Ū-rĭ-ă, p. 911)
hyperglycemia (hī-pĕr-glī-SĒ-mē-ă, p. 911)
incretin mimetics (p. 919)
incretins (p. 919)
ketoacidosis (kē-tō-ă-sī-DŌ-sĭs, p. 909)
metabolic syndrome (p. 930)
neuroglycopenia (nū-rō-GLĪ-kō-PĒ-nē-ă, p. 932)
polydipsia (pŏl-ē-DĬP-sē-ă, p. 911)
polyphagia (pŏl-ē-FĀ-jă, p. 911)
polyuria (pŏl-ē-Ū-rē-ă, p. 911)

DIABETES MELLITUS

Diabetes mellitus is a complex group of disorders that have in common a disturbance in metabolism and use of glucose that is secondary to a malfunction of the beta cells of the pancreas. Because insulin is involved in the metabolism of carbohydrates, proteins, and fats, diabetes mellitus is not limited to a disturbance of glucose homeostasis. However, the one disorder that all people with diabetes share is intolerance to glucose.

TYPES OF DIABETES MELLITUS

It is estimated that nearly 21 million cases of diabetes mellitus exist in the United States, or approximately 7% of the population, and 6 million of these people do not even know they have diabetes! Table 37–1 summarizes the major characteristics of various forms of diabetes mellitus. This section reviews primarily type 1 and type 2.

Type 1 diabetes, formerly known as insulin-dependent diabetes mellitus, or IDDM, accounts for about 5% to 10% of all cases. Type 1 diabetes occurs when the body's immune system destroys beta cells, the cells in the pancreas responsible for making insulin. There is no known way to prevent type 1 diabetes. Persons who have this type of diabetes require injections of **exogenous** (from outside the body) insulin to maintain life because they produce little or no **endogenous** (inside the body) insulin on their own. In general, persons with type 1 diabetes are more prone to a serious complication, **ketosis,** associated with an excess production of ketone bodies, leading to **ketoacidosis** (metabolic acidosis). Moreover, type 1 diabetes is more likely to appear early in life. In fact, this type of diabetes was formerly called *juvenile diabetes* and *ketosis-prone diabetes* because of its typical early onset and potential for ketoacidosis.

Table 37–1 Clinical Categories of Diabetes Mellitus and their Characteristics

TYPE (FORMER NAMES)	CHARACTERISTICS
Type 1 (insulin dependent; IDDM; juvenile diabetes; juvenile-onset)	Little or no endogenous insulin produced. New patients can be any age but usually are young. Patient must receive exogenous insulin and follow prescribed diet and exercise program. Renal, cardiovascular, retinal, and neurologic complications likely if disease is not kept under tight control.
Type 2 (non–insulin-dependent; NIDDM; adult-onset diabetes; maturity-onset diabetes)	Rarely develop ketosis; may develop hyperglycemic, hyperosmolar nonketotic syndrome (HHNS). Patients vary in need for exogenous insulin. New patients usually over 30 and most are obese. Disorder often responds to diet and exercise.
Prediabetes (impaired glucose tolerance and impaired fasting glucose)	Glucose levels between those of normal people and those with diabetes. Are at high risk for atherosclerotic disease and cardiovascular problems. Progression to diabetes is not inevitable. Weight loss and increased physical activity can delay or prevent diabetes and return blood glucose levels to normal.
Gestational diabetes	Occurs only during pregnancy. After pregnancy, women with gestational diabetes have 20%–50% chance of developing diabetes within 5–10 years.
Statistical risk of diabetes	Those who have had impaired glucose tolerance in the past but have normal glucose tolerance now; prediabetes; latent diabetes; subclinical diabetes. Those who are predisposed to diabetes because of family history, age, race, or obesity.

Type 2 diabetes, formerly called non–insulin-dependent diabetes mellitus (NIDDM), comprises 90% to 95% of all known cases of diabetes. It is believed to begin with insulin resistance, a situation in which the cell does not properly use insulin. As the need for insulin rises, the pancreas gradually loses the ability to produce it. Type 2 diabetes has a tendency to develop later in life than type 1, and these patients rarely develop diabetic ketoacidosis. Table 37–2 compares the signs and symptoms of type 1 and type 2 diabetes.

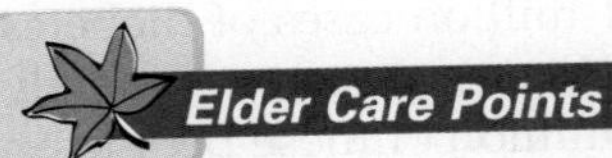

Elder Care Points

Many older patients have difficulty adjusting to the new diet, medication, and required exercise. Income is generally lower, and some patients have difficulty obtaining necessary foods or medicine because of financial constraints.

Although rare, type 2 diabetes is being diagnosed more frequently in children and adolescents, particularly in American Indians, African Americans, and Hispanic/Latino Americans. Factors associated with development of type 2 diabetes can be found in Box 37–1.

Gestational diabetes may occur as a result of the stress of pregnancy. It may be treated with diet, oral hypoglycemia agents, or insulin. After delivery, the condition must be reevaluated; approximately 5% to 10% of women with gestational diabetes go on to be diagnosed with type 2 diabetes after delivery. The baby also carries an increased risk of type 2 diabetes later in life.

Etiology and Pathophysiology

At least four sets of factors influence the development of diabetes mellitus: genetic, metabolic, microbiological, and immunologic.

Table 37–2 Comparison of Symptoms of Type 1 and Type 2 Diabetes

TYPE 1	TYPE 2
Very thirsty (polydipsia) Frequent urination (polyuria) Extremely hungry (polyphagia) Rapid loss of weight Irritability Weakness and fatigue Nausea and vomiting	May experience polydipsia, polyuria, and polyphagia More commonly experience excessive weight gain Family history of diabetes mellitus Poor healing of scratches, abrasions, and wounds Blurred vision Itching Drowsiness Increased fatigue Tingling or numbness in the feet

Box 37–1 Factors Associated with Development of Type 2 Diabetes

- Older age
- Obesity
- Family history of type 2 diabetes
- History of gestational diabetes
- Impaired glucose metabolism
- Physical inactivity
- Race/ethnicity: African Americans, Hispanic/Latino Americans, American Indians, some Asian Americans, Native Hawaiian/Pacific Islanders

Source: United States Department of Health and Human Services, Centers for Disease Control and Prevention. (2005). *National Diabetes Fact Sheet: General Information and National Estimates on Diabetes in the United States*. Atlanta, GA: USDHHS.

Genetic factors are included in the etiology of diabetes because diabetes tends to run in families, even though research has not yet pinpointed the responsible genes. It is known that the risk of having some form of diabetes increases in proportion to the number of relatives who are affected, the genetic closeness of the relatives, and the severity of their disease.

Metabolic factors involved in the etiology of diabetes are many and complex. Emotional or physical stress can unmask an inherited predisposition to the disease, probably as a result of glucogenesis induced by increased production of hormones from the adrenal cortex, especially the glucocorticoids. Perhaps even more significant than metabolic factors in the occurrence of diabetes is the association of type 2 diabetes and obesity. About 80% of type 2 diabetes patients are obese (greater than 20% above their ideal body weight), and there is a higher incidence of type 2 diabetes in persons who lead a sedentary life and eat a high-calorie diet. With weight reduction and increased physical activity, blood glucose can be restored to normal levels and maintained there—hence the importance of diet and exercise in the management of type 2 diabetes. In this type of diabetes there also seems to be a relationship to aging and a reduction in the function of the pancreatic beta cells and how they synthesize insulin.

Microbiologic factors have to do with the suspicion that some forms of type 1 diabetes are related to viral destruction of the beta cells. The mumps or coxsackie virus is thought to be the trigger. Evidence that supports viruses as causative factors include the following:

- Both IDDM and viral infections tend to have sudden onsets.
- Seasonal fluctuations in the onset of type 1 diabetes—late autumn and early spring—correspond with the times of the year when "flu" and other viral illnesses are most common.
- Viral infections can and often do attack the pancreas; many viral infections are characterized by inflammation of the pancreatic beta cells.

There are known cases in which children developed type 1 diabetes after having had a recent viral infection.

Immunologic factors are considered because research studies have presented strong evidence that some types of type 1 diabetes are an autoimmune reaction associated with the HLA-DR3 gene. At the time type 1 diabetes is diagnosed, about three fourths of the cases studied have islet cell antibodies circulating in the blood. Such antibodies are not found in normal individuals. People with diabetes who continue to produce insulin will eventually stop producing normal amounts of the hormone if islet cell antibodies remain in the blood.

? *Think Critically About . . .* What is one way in which you or your family members might decrease the risk of type 2 diabetes in later life?

Signs, Symptoms, and Diagnosis

The American Diabetes Association (ADA) recommends screening all adults, especially if overweight, for type 2 diabetes starting at age 45, to be repeated every 3 years, using fasting blood glucose as the preferred screening method. The ADA recommends screening begin at an earlier age, and at more frequent intervals, if the person has one or more risk factors associated with type 2 diabetes (American Diabetes Association, 2005).

In addition to laboratory tests (see Chapter 35), the physician depends on clinical signs and symptoms of diabetes mellitus to establish a diagnosis. The classic symptoms of the disorder, regardless of type, are related to an elevated blood glucose level, or **hyperglycemia**. This increases the concentration of the intravascular fluid, raising its osmotic pressure and pulling water from the cells and interstitial fluid into the blood. This causes cellular dehydration and the loss of glucose (**glycosuria**), electrolytes, and water in the urine. Cellular dehydration causes thirst and a resultant increased intake of water (**polydipsia**) and diuresis with increased urination (**polyuria**). Hunger (**polyphagia**) is the result of the body's effort to increase its supply of energy foods, even though the intake of more carbohydrates does not meet the energy needs of the cells.

Classic signs and symptoms of diabetes mellitus are polydipsia, polyuria, and polyphagia.

Fatigue and muscular weakness occur because the glucose needed for energy simply is not metabolized properly. Weight loss in patients with type 1 diabetes occurs for two reasons: (1) the loss of body fluid; and (2) in the absence of sufficient insulin, the body begins to metabolize its own proteins and stored fat. The oxidation of fats is incomplete and fatty acids are converted into ketone bodies: beta-hydroxybutyric acid, acetoacetic acid, and acetone. When the kidney is unable to handle accumulated ketones in the blood, the patient has what is called *ketosis*. The overwhelming presence of the strong organic acids in the blood lowers the pH and leads to a severe and potentially fatal acidosis. The metabolism of body protein when insulin is not available causes an elevated blood urea nitrogen (BUN) level. This is because the nitrogen component of protein is discarded when the body metabolizes its own protein to obtain the glucose it needs.

People with diabetes are prone to infection, delayed healing, and vascular diseases. Poor control of diabetes makes the person prone to develop an infection. The propensity for infection is thought to be partly a result of decreased normal function of leukocytes and abnormal phagocyte function. Another contributing factor to infection and delayed healing probably is decreased blood supply to the tissues because of atherosclerotic changes in the blood vessels. An impaired blood supply means a deficit in the protective cells brought by the blood to a site of injury.

It is believed that the neurologic, vascular, and metabolic complications of diabetes predispose the person to infections by allowing organisms to enter tissues that are normally better defended and less accessible. For example, a neurogenic bladder predisposes the patient to stagnant urine and accumulations of bacteria, and a leg ulcer resulting from peripheral vascular disease is without the protection of the skin as a barrier to organisms. Chronic neurologic and vascular complications of diabetes are discussed later in this chapter. Weight gain is common in persons with type 2 diabetes because of high caloric intake and the availability of endogenous insulin to use fully the food that is eaten.

? *Think Critically About . . .* If a relative complains of thirst, fatigue, and frequent urination, what questions would you ask? What would you suggest this person do?

Management of Diabetes

There is no cure for diabetes mellitus; the goal is to maintain blood glucose and lipid levels within normal limits and to control these factors as tightly as possible to prevent complications. Studies have demonstrated that there are benefits of tight **glycemic** (glucose in the blood) control for people with both type 1 and type 2 diabetes. Recall the role of hemoglobin A_{1c} from Chapter 35. For every percentage drop in hemoglobin A_{1c} level, the microvascular complications (eye, kidney, and nerve diseases) of diabetes decrease by 40%. Patients attempting tight control follow an intensive therapy plan of blood glucose testing at least four times daily and insulin injections three or more times a day, or they use an insulin pump.

There are some risks associated with perfect control of blood glucose levels, and "tight control" is not indicated for every patient. The most serious of these is hypoglycemia or insulin reaction. Weight gain is another problem with tight control, which can present other problems: extra pounds can make a patient with diabetes type 2 more insulin resistant.

Elder Care Points

The elderly experience hypoglycemia more quickly than younger people, and they are more prone to hypoglycemic episodes. The older adult may progress to dangerously low levels of blood glucose before signs and symptoms are obvious. Severe hypoglycemia in the older adult can precipitate myocardial infarction, angina, stroke, or seizures. For this reason, "tight" control may not be the best thing for the older adult.

In general, "good" or "tight" control is thought to be achieved when fasting blood glucose stays within normal limits, glycosylated hemoglobin tests show that blood glucose has stayed within normal limits from one testing period to the next, the patient's weight is normal, blood lipids remain within normal limits, and the patient has a sense of health and well-being.

The protocol for control of diabetes mellitus is highly individualized and depends on the type of diabetes a person has, his age, general state of health, ability to follow the prescribed regimen, and acceptance of responsibility for managing his illness, and a host of other factors. Both type 1 and type 2 diabetes patients must follow their prescribed diets and carry out some form of regular exercise. These are the cornerstones of management, regardless of the specific problem with glucose intolerance.

Insulin therapy can be prescribed for patients with either type 2 or type 1 diabetes. In most cases, people with type 2 diabetes can control their blood glucose by reducing caloric intake and increasing physical exercise. In addition, oral hypoglycemic agents (OHAs) or antidiabetic agents may be prescribed for patients with type 2 diabetes to manage their blood glucose levels. If control is difficult to maintain, then insulin may be added to the treatment plan.

Diet. **Diet is the cornerstone of diabetic treatment.** Weight loss is a goal for most patients with type 2 diabetes. The diet of each person with diabetes is calculated individually. There is no such thing as a "typical" person with diabetes, and because diabetes is an unstable and changing process, each patient's needs will change from time to time. It can be frustrating to the person with diabetes, because this person can eat the "perfect" breakfast 3 days in a row, which results in a "perfect" postprandial (after-meal) fingerstick value, only to eat the very same breakfast the next day and be surprised at a high blood glucose measurement! The strategies that are effective in managing diabetes can be altered by many factors (stress, illness, and many others), and the strategies that are effective for one person with diabetes may not be effective for someone else.

In general, the diet is geared toward providing adequate nutrition with sufficient calories to maintain normal body weight and to adjust the intake of food so that blood glucose is kept within safe limits. Since 1994, less emphasis has been placed on caloric intake and restriction of carbohydrates and more attention paid to the regulation of body weight and control of cholesterol and blood glucose levels in each patient (American Diabetes Association, 2005). "Sweets" (foods with high sugar content) have been added to one of the carbohydrate lists, as new evidence has revealed that eating sugar as part of the meal plan need not interfere with blood glucose control. There is also a "very lean meat" list now, and the fat group has been divided into monounsaturated, polyunsaturated, and saturated fat. Fat-modified foods, such as fat-free cookies and fat-reduced waffles, have been added. The combination food lists now contain such things as fast-food burritos, chicken nuggets, and a variety of sandwiches. These changes make the lists easier to use, and most people with diabetes now find it less difficult to stick with their designed diet.

The diet for a person with diabetes is usually designed by a certified diabetes educator (CDE) who is usually a registered dietitian (RD) or RN in collaboration with the patient. It is based on the patient's type of diabetes, height-to-weight ratio, usual dietary intake, food preferences, exercise level, and daily schedule. Meal plans are generally made up of 55% to 60% carbohydrate, 12% to 20% protein, and 30% fat. Concentrated sweets are limited, and so might be fruit juices (depending on individual tolerance), and meals should include an adequate amount of fiber. This is accomplished by taking in mostly complex carbohydrates from the carbohydrate group. Fats should be mainly polyunsaturated or monounsaturated.

Weight loss is seldom a goal for the older type 2 diabetic unless weight is more than 1½ times normal for height and frame. Older adults are more susceptible to nutritional deficiencies from teeth problems, illness, and decreased appetite. Diet is frequently managed by reducing concentrated sugars and adhering to a meal schedule. The ADA and the American Dietetic Association have worked together to devise a simplified method of calculating a diabetic diet and planning meals for a person with diabetes. The booklet containing this information is titled "Exchange Lists for Meal Planning." The principal foods are divided into three clusters. Each cluster contains foods that are similar in kind and have equal nutritional value in regard to carbohydrates, protein, and fat. For example, more than 30 fruits from which the diabetic can choose are listed, each providing 10 g of carbohydrate, a negligible amount of protein and fat, and 40 calories per serving. Other lists contain similar information for a great variety of foods. The booklet also includes instructions for substitutions among the food groups, a table for the conversion of weights and measures, and information about *trans* fats, alcohol, and type 2 diabetes in children. With this simple method of choosing a menu from the Exchange Lists, a person with diabetes or a member of her family can calculate caloric and nutritional value with ease. Copies of the 48-page booklet in English or Spanish may be purchased on the American Dietetic Association website at www.eatright.org.

It is important that the person with diabetes not develop a defeatist or negative attitude toward his diet. Emphasis should be placed on the positive aspects of the diet—on the foods she is allowed rather than those that are forbidden. Cultural preferences must be considered when helping the patient devise meal plans. A patient should not be made to feel guilty about having difficulty staying on the diet or the times when he "cheats" and eats foods that are not allowed. We all have moments when we are likely to yield to the temptation to do what we know is not in our best interest.

One of the most effective means of helping a person with diabetes follow the prescribed diet is by teaching about food values and how they affect diabetes. This can help the patient's understanding of how nutrients affect health and well-being. The physician, dietitian, and nurse can help the patient and family learn which foods are recommended and which should be avoided. Fortunately, many well-written and clearly illustrated booklets and pamphlets are available and are very helpful to the person with diabetes and his family. Organizations such as the ADA (1701 North Beauregard Street, Alexandria, VA 22311, 800-342-2383) and the Joslin Diabetes Center (One Joslin Place, Boston, MA 02215, 617-732-2400), affiliated with Harvard Medical School, will send instructive material on request. This material covers diets and warns the diabetic patient against misleading or fraudulent information about quick "cures" or special diets that are supposed to cure diabetes.

Think Critically About . . . How would you obtain accurate data about what your patient with diabetes is eating each day?

Exercise. Physical exercise is an important part of managing diabetes. Muscular activity improves glucose utilization for energy and improves circulation. In addition to lowering blood glucose levels by "burning up" the glucose, exercise makes the insulin receptors on cells more sensitive to the hormone and thus improves utilization of the available glucose. Because diabetic control also considers blood lipid levels, exercise contributes to that control by reducing triglyceride levels and increasing high-density lipoprotein (HDL) levels.

The exercise program should be designed for the individual patient. The plan should consider the age and overall physical condition of the patient, ability to carry out the exercises regularly, and how well controlled the diabetes is. For some patients a brisk walk of 1 or 2 miles daily is as much exercise as they can tolerate. Others may be able to perform more strenuous exercises, but they must be cautioned against extremes, especially if they are taking insulin. Exercise can rapidly lower blood glucose levels and cause serious hypoglycemia.

All exercise programs should begin with milder forms of exercise and gradually increase until the patient's level of tolerance or the desired therapeutic effect is reached. A program should not be started until the blood glucose is under control. The exercise program should be planned so that the exercises are performed at the same time every day, preferably after a meal when the blood glucose is highest. Blood glucose should be checked before beginning to exercise. The patient is encouraged to wear a Medic-Alert bracelet and to exercise with a friend who knows the signs and symptoms of hypoglycemia and how to treat it (Patient Teaching 37–1).

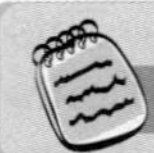

Patient Teaching 37–1

Home Treatment for Hypoglycemia

When signs of hypoglycemia are present and the patient is able to swallow, give one of the following:

- ½ cup of juice (apple or orange)
- ½ cup of 2% or skim milk
- ½ cup of regular soda (not sugar free)
- 6 or 7 hard candies, such as Life-Savers (not sugar free)
- 1 small box of raisins (2 tablespoons)
- Three glucose tablets
- 1 tablespoon of honey
- 1 tablespoon of sugar
- 5 small cubes of sugar
- 1 small tube of cake icing (2 oz)
- 1 small tube of glucose gel

If the patient is unable to swallow (groggy or unconscious):

- Turn the patient onto the side.
- Administer 1 mg of glucagon by injection after mixing the solution in the bottle until it is clear.
- Feed the patient as soon as she is awake and able to swallow.
- Give a fast-acting source of sugar (see above list) and a longer-acting source, such as crackers and cheese or a meat sandwich.
- If the patient does not awaken within 15 minutes, give another dose of glucagon and inform a physician of the situation immediately.
- If a physician cannot be contacted, call 911 or the local emergency service.

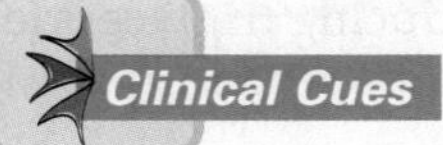

Clinical Cues

Every person with diabetes should have emergency supplies for treatment for hypoglycemia available when exercising.

Physical limitations may discourage older adults with diabetes from exercising. The older patient with diabetes is at risk of developing hypoglycemia up to 24 hours after exercising if the exercise is too strenuous. Walking, swimming, or stationary bicycle riding is considered to be among the safest activities for this group. Exercise should begin slowly and build up to 30 to 45 minutes three or four times a week. The gradual increase helps prevent hypoglycemia, stress fractures, and cardiovascular complications.

Increasing Food Intake during Exercise. During moderate exercise, such as brisk walking, bowling, or vacuuming, 5 g of simple carbohydrate should be consumed at the end of 30 minutes and at 30-minute intervals during the continued activity. (A food example with 5 g of simple carbohydrate is 1 tsp honey.) Jogging, swimming, or scrubbing floors should be preceded by consumption of 15 to 20 g of complex carbohydrate plus protein 15 to 30 minutes before beginning the exercise, and then, if the activity continues for more than 30 minutes, 10 g of simple carbohydrate should be taken every 30 minutes. Vigorous exercise, such as fast jogging, skiing, or playing tennis, requires intake of 30 to 40 g of complex carbohydrate plus protein 15 to 30 minutes ahead of time and then 10 to 20 g of simple carbohydrate intake every 30 minutes after the first half-hour.

Performing exercise when insulin or an oral antidiabetic agent is at its peak of action can bring on an acute hypoglycemic reaction. Another precaution for insulin-dependent patients is to avoid injecting insulin into an area that will soon receive extra exercise (e.g., the leg). The abdomen is a good site for insulin injection as absorption is steady, rapid, and not affected by exercise. Eating a piece of fruit before even light exercise, if done between meals, also can help prevent hypoglycemia in people with type 1 diabetes.

Once a patient begins to follow a regular exercise program, the insulin dosage and diet may need to be revised. In general, the patient may need to take less insulin and to increase caloric intake with regular exercise. Keeping a daily record of exercise, along with weight, insulin dosage, and blood glucose levels can help motivate the patient to continue exercise.

Administration of Insulin. Insulin is a potent drug that must be treated with respect by the patient and any others involved in its administration. Exogenous insulins are a liquid hormonal preparation originally obtained from the pancreas of animals. Since the advent of genetic engineering techniques, human insulin (sometimes called *humulin*) is the only available form because it is less likely to cause allergies and other problems. Human insulin is produced in the laboratory by splicing genetic material into the deoxyribonucleic acid (DNA) of a bacterium, which reproduces the insulin.

The variety of rapid-acting, short-acting, intermediate-acting, and long-acting insulins provide alternatives from which to find the one best suited for the individual patient (Table 37–3). To achieve a level of insulin throughout the day that is as near as possible to that of endogenous insulin, some patients may take both a regular and a longer-lasting insulin once or twice a day. Combination insulins, such as Humulin 70/30, combine short- and intermediate-acting insulins. These are often prescribed so that patients do not have to mix insulins. Figure 37–1 shows various regimens in split doses of insulin or split mixed doses that may give better glycemic control to patients.

Neutral protamine Hagedorn (NPH) insulin is cloudy and milky in appearance and must be thoroughly mixed before it is administered so that the patient will receive the prescribed dose. This is done by gently rolling the bottle between the palms of the hands. The bottle is not shaken, because this produces very fine air bubbles that are almost impossible to see but can alter the dosage given and may contribute to breakdown of the insulin.

The type of insulin prescribed for a patient should not be confused with its strength. Insulin labeled "U100" means that there are 100 units of insulin per milliliter of solution; that is, each milliliter contains 100 units. The

Table 37–3 Common Types of Insulins and Their Onset, Peak, and Duration of Action

PREPARATION	BRAND NAME	ONSET (HR)	PEAK (HR)	DURATION (HR)
RAPID ACTING				
Insulin inhalation powder	Exubera	0.15–0.3	0.45	6–8
Insulin aspart injection	NovoLog	0.25	1-3	3–5
Insulin lispro injection	Humalog	0.25	0.5–1.5	3–4
Insulin glulisine injection	Apidra	0.3	0.5–1.5	5
SHORT ACTING				
Regular human insulin injection	Humulin R	0.5	2–4	6–8
	Novolin R	0.5	2.5–5	8
Buffered regular human insulin injection	Velosulin BR	0.5	1–3	8
INTERMEDIATE ACTING				
Human insulin isophane suspension	NPH	1.5	4–12	24
LONG ACTING				
Insulin detemir injection	Levemir	2–4	None	20–24
Insulin glargine injection	Lantus	2–4	None	24
COMBINATION INSULIN				
70% Insulin aspart protamine suspension/30% insulin aspart injection	NovoLog Mix 70/30	0.25	1–4	24
75% Insulin lispro protamine suspension/25% insulin lispro injection	Humalog Mix 75/25	0.25	1–4	24
70% Human insulin isophane suspension (NPH)/30% human insulin injection (regular)	Humulin 70/30	0.5	2–12	24
	Novolin 70/30	0.5	2–12	24
50% Human insulin isophane suspension (NPH)/50% human insulin injection (regular)	Humulin 50/50	0.5	3–5	24

From Ignatavicius, D.D., & Workman, M.L. (2005). *Medical-Surgical Nursing: Critical Thinking for Collaborative Care* (5th ed.). Philadelphia: Saunders; Holmberg, M. (2006). An overview of insulin breakthroughs. *Pharmacy Times*, October, 2006.

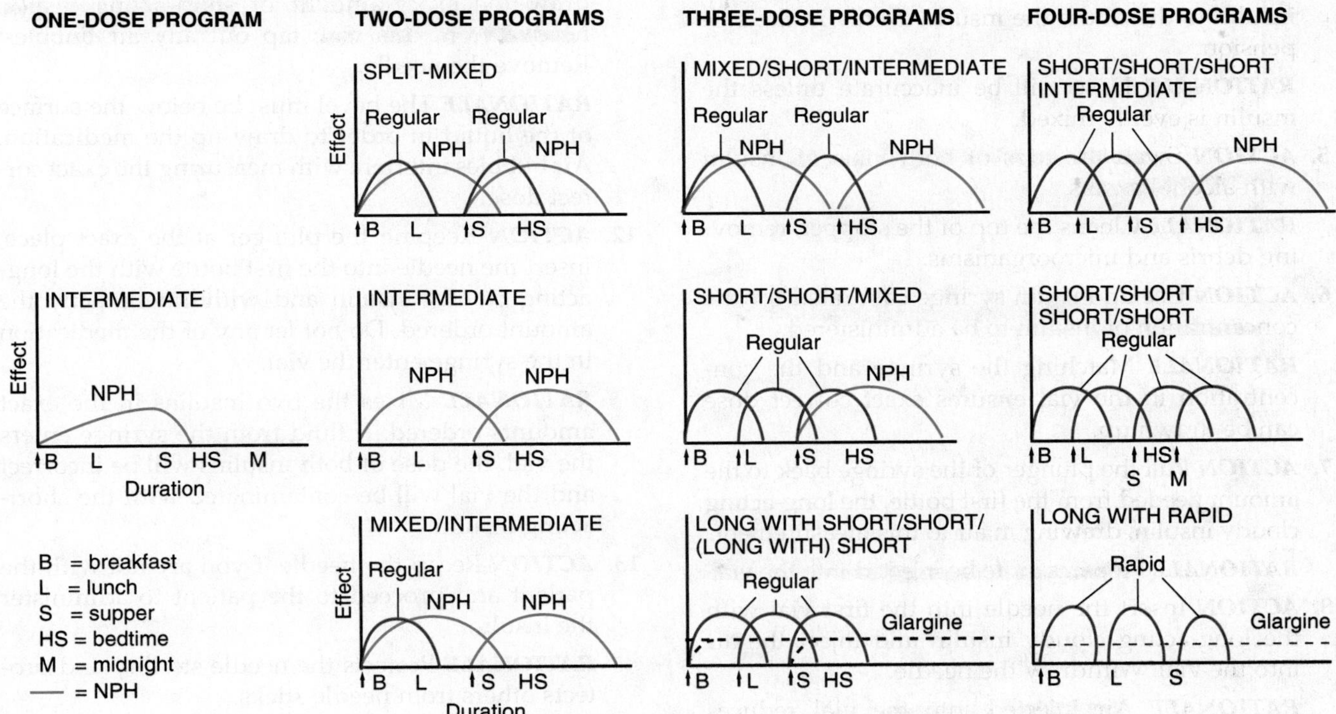

FIGURE **37–1** Insulin regimens. One injection a day of short-acting or intermediate-acting insulin may be enough to control blood glucose levels. However, split doses (two, three, or four injections of the daily dose) or split mixed doses (a mixture of short-acting and longer-acting insulins) may give better control.

syringe used for measuring and administering U100 insulin is calibrated to accommodate insulin of this strength. A "lo-dose" syringe will accommodate up to 50 U of insulin. If the dose is higher than this amount, the larger 100-U syringe is needed. If regular insulin and a longer acting insulin are to be mixed in one syringe, the regular insulin is drawn up first to prevent any contamination of the regular bottle of insulin with the longer acting variety. Skill 37–1 shows how to mix two types of insulin in one syringe.

Skill 37–1 Combining Insulins

Often short-acting insulin is ordered to be mixed with longer-acting insulin. These steps are used to mix the two insulins. The insulin syringe is used to draw up the insulins.

1. ***ACTION*** Check expiration dates on both bottles of insulin.

   RATIONALE Outdated insulin is not reliable and should not be used.
2. ***ACTION*** Check for change in color, clumping, or granular appearance of insulin and discard if such has occurred.

   RATIONALE Insulin has been contaminated or exposed to heat and is no longer good.
3. ***ACTION*** To mix insulin suspension, swirl the vial gently or rotate between palms or roll between palm and thigh.

   RATIONALE Mixes the insulin evenly without causing air bubbles, which would interfere with obtaining an accurate dose.
4. ***ACTION*** Roll the vial of the long-acting cloudy insulin to distribute the insulin evenly in the suspension.

   RATIONALE Dose will be inaccurate unless the insulin is evenly mixed.
5. ***ACTION*** Swab the tops of both vials of insulin with alcohol swabs.

   RATIONALE Cleans the top of the stopper, removing debris and microorganisms.
6. ***ACTION*** Use an insulin syringe calibrated for the concentration of insulin to be administered.

   RATIONALE Matching the syringe and the concentration in the vial ensures exact correct dose can be drawn up.
7. ***ACTION*** Pull the plunger of the syringe back to the amount needed from the first bottle, the long-acting cloudy insulin, drawing in air to this measurement.

   RATIONALE Prepares air to be injected into the vial.
8. ***ACTION*** Insert the needle into the first vial with the long-acting cloudy insulin and inject the air into the vial. Withdraw the needle.

   RATIONALE Air injected into the vial reduces the vacuum and makes it easier to withdraw the medication.
9. ***ACTION*** Pull the plunger of the syringe back to the amount of insulin needed from the second vial, the short-acting clear insulin, drawing in air to this measurement.

   RATIONALE Prepares air to be injected into the vial.
10. ***ACTION*** Insert the needle into the second vial with the short-acting clear insulin and inject the air into the vial with the needle above the surface of the medication.

    RATIONALE Air injected into the vial prevents a vacuum, which will pull regular insulin into the long-acting insulin vial; makes it easier to withdraw the medication.
11. ***ACTION*** Invert the vial and, keeping the bevel of the needle beneath the surface of the insulin, withdraw the exact amount of short-acting insulin needed from this vial; tap out any air bubbles. Remove the needle.

    RATIONALE The bevel must be below the surface of the liquid in order to draw up the medication. Air bubbles interfere with measuring the exact correct dose.
12. ***ACTION*** Keeping the plunger at the exact place, insert the needle into the first bottle with the long-acting cloudy insulin and withdraw exactly the amount ordered. Do not let any of the medication in the syringe enter the vial.

    RATIONALE Mixes the two insulins in the exact amounts ordered. If fluid from the syringe enters the vial, the dose of both insulins will be incorrect and the vial will be contaminated with the short-acting insulin.
13. ***ACTION*** Recap the needle if you are not with the patient and proceed to the patient to administer the insulin.

    RATIONALE Protects the needle sterility and protects others from needle sticks.

From deWit, S.C. (2005). *Fundamental Concepts and Skills for Nursing* (2nd ed.). Philadelphia: Elsevier Saunders.

Safety Alert 37–1

Insulin Pen Injectors

Left-handed patients must be careful when dialing the dose of insulin into a pen injector. If performed incorrectly, the numbers of the dosage will be transposed (e.g. 52 units instead of 25 units.)

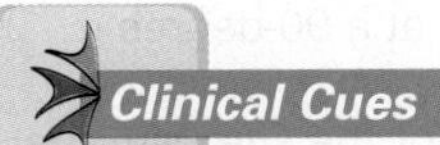
Clinical Cues

The mnemonic (memory device) "clear to cloudy" is an easy way to remember which insulin to draw up first. The clear (regular) insulin is drawn up first, followed by the cloudy (longer acting) insulin. The way to remember that clear comes first is that alphabetically, the word *clear* comes before the word *cloudy*.

Historically, the only available route for administration of insulin was injection. Insulin cannot be taken orally or given via a feeding tube, because it is destroyed by gastric juices. Researchers have tried numerous alternatives to injections of insulin, even attempting to deliver the hormone via suppository! Jet injectors, where insulin is injected via a high pressure stream instead of a needle, are available for patients who are unable to self-inject with a needle. Insulin pens, filled with insulin, are another alternative to the traditional syringe-and-needle apparatus. The patient selects the correct dose on a dial, and the insulin is delivered by a small needle at the end of the pen (Safety Alert 37–1).

The search for alternatives to injecting insulin finally came to a positive result when the Food and Drug Administration (FDA) approved a new inhaled form of insulin for people older than age 18 with type 1 or type 2 diabetes. This new insulin, brand-named Exubera, is a short-acting insulin that can be taken before meals. Side effects include shortness of breath, cough, dry mouth, and sore throat. Inhaled insulin is contraindicated for people who smoke, as more of the inhaled insulin enters their bloodstream, placing them at risk for hypoglycemia. The patient on inhaled insulin will still need to receive injections for longer-acting insulins, and therefore will most likely not be completely needle-free at this time. Injectable insulin will continue to be the most common delivery method, however, so it is critical that nurses be educated in all aspects of injectable insulin therapy. It would be wonderful for all people with diabetes if, someday, insulin injections were a thing of the past!

Insulin injections are rotated within one body area to enhance absorption. Patients are given charts showing the places on the arms, legs, buttocks, and abdomen where insulin can be injected (Figure 37–2). They are then encouraged to keep a daily record of injection sites to help remember which sites have been used and to avoid the problem of altered or erratic absorption.

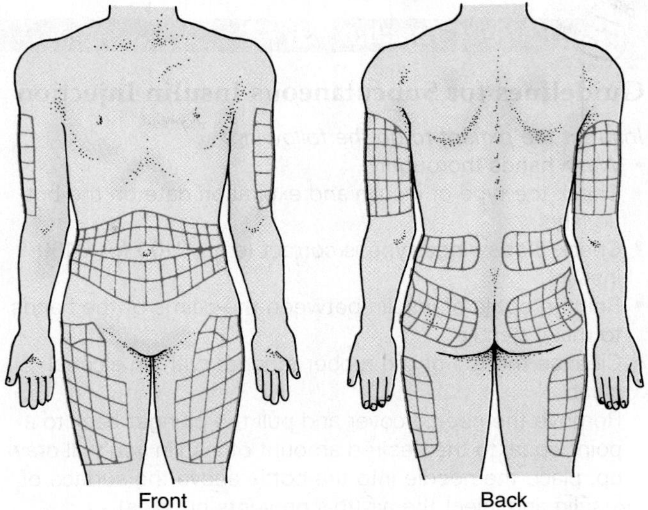

FIGURE 37–2 Rotation sites for injection of insulin.

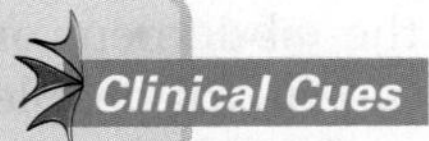
Clinical Cues

Pain at the injection site may be caused by injecting insulin that has been refrigerated. Once open, a vial of insulin in use may be stored at room temperature for up to 1 month. If insulin is refrigerated, it should be warmed by gently rotating the filled syringe between the hands.

Patient Teaching 37–2 presents guidelines for teaching a patient how to give insulin subcutaneously.

Insulin requirements change as metabolic needs are altered by diet, exercise, age, and even changes in seasons. In the summer, for example, many people are outdoors and exercising more than during the winter months. Also, as a person grows older, the level of physical activity may decrease. Insulin requirements also are altered when the patient has an infection or illness or is under added stress.

If a patient is self-monitoring blood glucose at home and the physician has recommended adjustments of insulin dosage based on daily blood glucose levels, the patient will need to be taught how to calculate the amount of insulin needed to achieve the desired blood glucose level.

? *Think Critically About . . .* How would a patient know that his insulin requirement has changed?

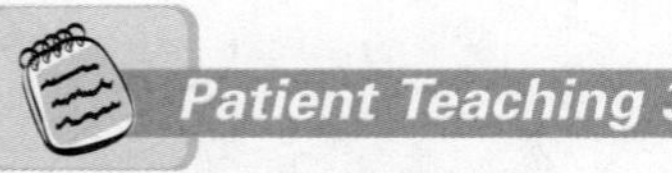

Patient Teaching 37–2

Guidelines for Subcutaneous Insulin Injection

Instruct the patient to do the following:

- Wash hands thoroughly.
- Check the type of insulin and expiration date on the bottle label.
- Check that syringe type is correct (e.g., U100 for U100 insulin).
- Roll the bottle of insulin between the palms of the hands to mix it gently.
- Cleanse the top of the rubber stopper with an alcohol swab.
- Remove the needle cover and pull the plunger back to a point equal to the desired amount of insulin you will draw up; place the needle into the bottle above the surface of insulin and inject the air (this prevents bubbles).
- Turn the bottle and syringe upside down, holding them with one hand; with the bevel of the needle well into the insulin, slowly draw up the correct amount of insulin.
- Remove air bubbles in the syringe by tapping on the barrel of the syringe, reinjecting into the bottle, and then redrawing up the correct dosage of insulin without bubbles.
- Remove the needle from the bottle; select a site for injection that has not been used in the past month.
- Clean the site with an alcohol swab; pinch up the area of skin and insert the needle all the way at a 90-degree angle; inject the insulin.
- Pull the needle straight out quickly. Blot the site with the alcohol swab; do not rub the site.
- Do not recap the needle; dispose of the syringe and needle in a puncture-proof container.

Insulin Pump. An alternative to insulin therapy by daily injections is the insulin pump. These pumps can deliver a continuous infusion of insulin through an automated system composed of a battery-driven electronic "brain," an electric motor and drive mechanisms, and a syringe (Figure 37–3). The syringe is attached to plastic tubing and a subcutaneous needle, which is inserted into the abdomen or thigh. Insulin pumps are especially useful for people with "brittle" diabetes (those whose blood glucose levels swing widely each day). Pumps are helpful in managing diabetes because they allow for improved blood glucose control; people using pumps tend to have fewer episodes and less severe hypoglycemia when compared with multiple daily injections.

The pump partially imitates the action of the beta cells by delivering insulin continuously. Current models do not yet have a mechanism by which the pump can sense the body's ever-changing needs for insulin *and* take corrective action, as happens in a normal physiologic closed-loop feedback system. However, the FDA just approved the first insulin pump with real-time continuous blood glucose monitoring, which allows the patient to take immediate corrective action based on blood glucose—a major step toward the closed-loop feedback system

(Walsh, 2006). Insulin pumps are continually being refined with a trend toward miniaturization and increased functionality. Today's pumps internally record and manage data, such as blood glucose values, insulin delivered, and carbohydrate consumption.

At present, insulin pumps are recommended only for a select few patients who are able to discipline themselves to monitor their blood glucose frequently during the day, can understand the principles of continuous insulin infusion, are compliant with their diet

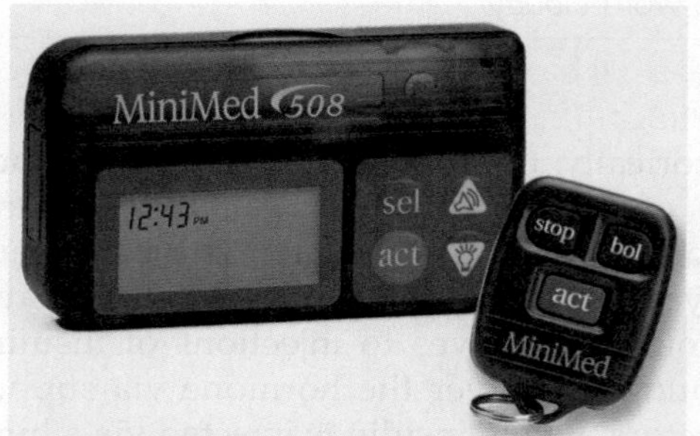

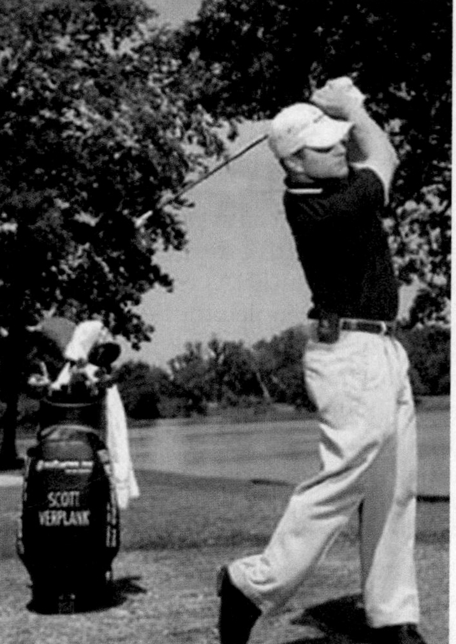

FIGURE 37–3 **A,** Medtronic MiniMed insulin pump. **B,** Professional golfer Scott Verplank wearing his MiniMed pump at Ryder Cup 2002.

Table 37–4 *Injectable Hypoglycemic Agents*

CATEGORY	EXAMPLES GENERIC NAME (BRAND NAME)	METHOD OF DELIVERY	HOW THEY CONTROL BLOOD GLUCOSE	OTHER CONSIDERATIONS
Incretin mimetics	Exenatide (Byetta)	Subcutaneous	Mimic the action of incretins Stimulate insulin secretion, suppress glucagon release, delay gastric emptying	Administer before breakfast or dinner (not lunch) to avoid severe hypoglycemia. Give 1 hr after oral hypoglycemic agents.
Synthetic hormone	Pramlintide (Symlin)	Subcutaneous	Synthetic form of the hormone amylin Slow gastric emptying, suppresses glucagon release, suppress glucose production by the liver, decrease appetite	Careful monitoring for hypoglycemia is essential. Given prior to meals and snacks >250 calories or 30 g carbohydrate; black box warning: potential to cause severe hypoglycemia; patients started on this medication should have their rapid-acting insulin dosage cut in half.

From Gates, B., Onufer, C., & Setter, S. (2007). Your complete type 2 medications reference guide. *Diabetes Health.* Retrieved July, 19, 2007, from www.DiabetesHealth.com; Bass, A., Will, T., Todd, M., et al. (2007). The latest tools for patients with diabetes. *RN, 70*(6): 39-43.

and self-care, and have no physiologic or pathologic contraindications.

A programmable implantable medication device that delivers insulin directly into the peritoneal cavity is under clinical investigation in Europe. The insulin is delivered in small bursts, much as the pancreas secretes insulin. Once surgically inserted, the device only needs to be replaced every 8 to 13 years, depending on the amount of insulin used. The device has a reservoir that is refilled with fresh insulin every 3 to 4 months; a needle is inserted through the skin to deliver the hormone. A small, easy-to-use programmer that uses radiofrequency telemetry communicates with the pump. The patient will still have to do regular blood glucose monitoring (Medtronic MiniMed, 2007).

Other Injectable Agents. Historically insulin was the only injectable medication for the management of diabetes; however, new injectable agents have been introduced. One new category of medications is called **incretin mimetics** because they mimic the action of **incretins**. Incretins are hormones released from the intestine and lower postprandial blood glucose levels in a number of ways (Table 37–4). Other injectable medications to treat diabetes are synthetic hormones, such as pramlintide. Although these medications are administered subcutaneously, none of these new medications should ever be mixed in the same syringe with insulin, and the patient must be monitored carefully for hypoglycemia (Safety Alert 37–2).

Oral Hypoglycemic Agents. Oral hypoglycemic agents (OHAs) are sometimes prescribed for patients with type 2 diabetes to help control their blood glucose. These medications are not a form of oral insulin; pharmacologically, they are from completely different classes of medications. There are now six categories of OHAs that act in different ways to help achieve blood glucose control (Safety Alert 37–3). Information about these medications can be found in Table 37–5.

Elder Care Points

The older adult metabolizes and excretes drugs more slowly than the younger patient; drugs stay active in the body longer. Some first-generation oral hypoglycemic agents (Diabinese) have a long half-life and remain active even longer in the older patient. These drugs may cause prolonged hypoglycemia in these patients and are not the best choice for older adults.

Safety Alert 37–2

Pramlintide

The medication pramlintide (Symlin) carries with it an FDA **black box warning** (a type of warning sometimes carried on prescription medications indicating the potential for serious adverse effects). This medication has the potential to cause severe hypoglycemia within 3 hours of administration. It is critically important that the nurse observe the patient closely for any signs or symptoms of hypoglycemia.

Safety Alert 37–3

Sulfa Drugs Allergy

Because the sulfonylureas are from the same family of drugs as the sulfonamide antibiotics, they must be given with caution to persons known to have an allergy to sulfa drugs.

Table 37–5 ***Oral Hypoglycemic Agents***

CATEGORY	EXAMPLES GENERIC NAME (BRAND NAME)	MAIN SITE OF ACTION	HOW THEY CONTROL BLOOD GLUCOSE	OTHER CONSIDERATIONS
Biguanides	Metformin (Glucophage) Also available in combination with other OHAs: with sulfonylurea agents (Glucovance and Metaglip), thiazolidinediones (Avandamet), and DPP-4 inhibitors (Janumet)	Liver	Keep liver from releasing excessive amounts of glucose; increases tissue cell sensitivity to insulin	Do not cause hypoglycemia or hyperinsulinemia. Do not lead to weight gain. Decrease blood lipids. Can lead to vitamin B_{12} deficiency. Janumet is contraindicated in renal failure, liver disease, and acidosis.
Alpha-glucosidase inhibitors	Acarbose (Precose) Miglitol (Glyset)	Intestine	Reduce demand for insulin by slowing absorption of complex carbohydrates, resulting in less of a blood glucose "spike"	Contraindicated in people with inflammatory bowel disease or other intestinal diseases.
Thiazolidinediones	Pioglitazone (Actos) Rosiglitazone (Avandia)	Muscle cells	Make muscle cells more sensitive to insulin; decrease liver production of glucose	Contraindicated in people with congestive heart failure. One drug from this category, Rezulin, was pulled from the market in 2000 after reports of liver damage. Avandia may increase risk of MI in some patients.*
Sulfonylureas	Acetohexamide† (generic only) Chlorpropamide† (Diabinese) Glimepiride§ (Amaryl) Glipizide‡ (Glucotrol) Glyburide‡ (DiaBeta, Micronase, Glynase PresTab) Tolazamide† (generic only) Tolbutamide† (generic only)	Pancreas	Stimulate pancreas to secrete more insulin	*First generation:* Side effects rare (5%) and include gastrointestinal and hematologic disorders, jaundice, skin rash, photosensitivity, and alcohol intolerance (vomiting, confusion, respiratory difficulty, headache) *Second generation:* Side effects GI distress and skin reactions. *Third generation:* Less likely to cause hypoglycemia, safer for those with kidney disease.
Meglitinides	Nateglinide (Starlix) Repaglinide (Prandin)	Pancreas	Stimulate insulin secretion, but shorter acting than sulfonylureas	Must be taken immediately before eating. Lower risk of hypoglycemia than sulfonylureas.
DPP-4 Inhibitors	Sitagliptin (Januvia) Vildagliptin (Galvus) is in final phase of FDA approval process	Endocrine system	Enhance a natural body system called the incretin system, which helps regulate glucose by affecting alpha and beta cells in the pancreas	Medication may cause delayed gastric empyting (can affect absorption of other medications). Reduced dosage may be required in patient with renal impairment, as medication is excreted via the kidneys.

From Gates, B., Onufer, C., & Setter, S. (2007). Your complete type 2 medications reference guide. *Diabetes Health.* Retrieved from www.DiabetesHealth.com; Krumholz, H.M. (2007). Rosiglitazone associated with increased risk for MI.
*June 13, 2007: FDA placed black box warning on both Actos and Avandia for cardiac risk. Retrieved from www.medscape.com
†First generation.
‡Second generation.
§Third generation.

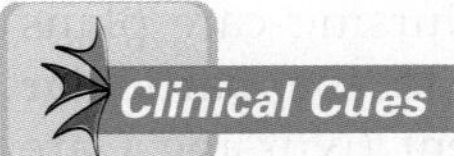

Many medications can either enhance or inhibit the effect of OHAs. Always check the other drugs a patient with diabetes is taking for drug interactions.

Patients receiving OHAs should know that these medications do not eliminate the need for following their diet and exercise program. Some may be under the notion that if they go off their diet and indulge themselves, they can just take more pills to compensate. Others who have been on a diet and exercise program for a time and then have an OHA prescribed for them think it is acceptable to stop planning their meals and exercising regularly. All OHAs are capable of producing gastric irritation, nausea, vomiting, and diarrhea. Liver damage with jaundice, bone marrow depression, and allergic skin reactions may result in some patients.

Preoperative and Postoperative Insulin Management. The emotional and physical stress of surgery can increase the blood glucose level and alter the amounts of medication needed for glycemic control. Patients with type 2 diabetes may be taken off OHAs up to 48 hours before surgery and are started on insulin by injection to achieve adequate control of their diabetes during this stressful period. The patient should be reassured that this does not indicate his diabetes is worse, and that the insulin injections are only a temporary measure. A patient with type 2 diabetes will have sliding-scale insulin orders along with his usual insulin order. Blood sugar determinations are done more frequently.

For all diabetic patients, intravenous fluids are begun as soon as the patient is ordered "nothing by mouth" (NPO) and are continued until the patient is eating again after surgery. During surgery, an insulin infusion may be used of regular or short-acting insulin, usually mixed in 5% dextrose or 0.9% NaCl solution, depending on hospital policy. Blood glucose is monitored closely during surgery and every 2 to 4 hours postoperatively; urine is checked for ketones when glucose levels are high.

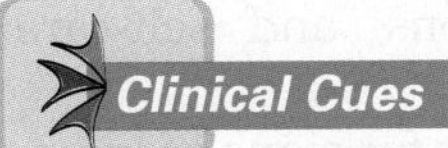

Be especially alert for signs of hypoglycemia in patients who are receiving an insulin infusion. Blood glucose is monitored hourly. The insulin infusion is adjusted according to a sliding scale: the rate of infusion is increased or decreased based on the blood glucose value.

Islet Cell Transplantation. A relatively new procedure for treatment of type 1 diabetes is transplantation of insulin-producing islet cells. This procedure was developed by several transplant centers and refined by the University of Alberta (Canada), using a protocol called the Edmonton Protocol. Once a donor pancreas is procured, a laboratory technician extracts only the islet cells and purifies them. The cells are then injected into the patient's portal vein, migrate to the liver and begin to produce insulin, functioning just as they did in the pancreas. Before implementation of the Edmonton Protocol, only about 8% of islet cell transplantations were successful; with the new protocol, nearly 60% of recipients remained insulin-free for approximately 15 months (Ryan et al., 2005). Although it is still experimental, someday this treatment may eliminate the need for insulin injections.

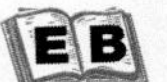

NURSING MANAGEMENT

Assessment (Data Collection)

The nurse should always assess each patient, regardless of her complaint, for signs and symptoms of diabetes mellitus. Focused Assessment 37–1 presents guidelines

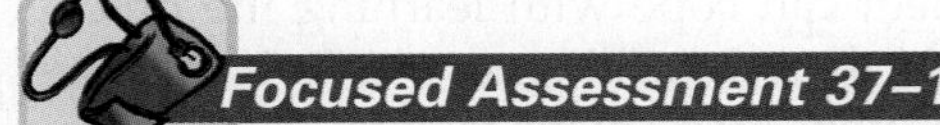

Data Collection for Diabetes

The following questions should be asked to establish a database that indicates the patient may have diabetes, has poorly controlled diabetes, or has no signs of diabetes:

- Has anyone in your family ever been told he or she has diabetes? What about your parents and grandparents?
- Have you had any recent weight loss or weight gain?
- Have you become increasingly hungry over the past few months?
- Has your thirst increased? Are you drinking more fluids than you used to?
- Do you have to urinate (go to the toilet) more than you used to?
- Have you noticed that you are more tired than you were 6 months ago?
- Do you have any trouble with scratches and wounds healing?
- Do small scratches or abrasions become easily infected?
- Have you noticed any numbness or tingling or "funny" sensations in your hands, legs, or feet?
- Is constipation becoming a problem?
- Are you having any sexual difficulties? Any impotence (men)? Any frequent vaginal infections (women)?

If the patient is known to have diabetes, ask these questions also:

- Do you feel that you can easily and correctly perform your blood glucose determinations? (Check the patient's performance using her own machine.)
- How do you calibrate your blood glucose monitor?
- Are you having any trouble sticking to your dietary plan?
- How are you planning your meals?
- Are you taking your insulin/oral medication regularly?
- Are you having any problems in relation to the medication?
- Are you keeping records of your blood glucose readings and your insulin injections? (Check the records kept.)
- Are you seeing your primary physician at regular intervals?
- Are you having your eyes examined regularly?
- Are you visiting the dentist regularly?

for history taking. The nurse should physically assess the skin for signs of poor wound healing or areas of infection. The feet should be inspected for signs of tight-fitting shoes and beginning sores. The nurse should weigh the patient and determine whether his weight is within normal limits.

For the patient newly diagnosed with diabetes, the nurse must assess whether the patient is a good candidate for using a blood glucose-monitoring machine, a glucometer. The patient must have adequate peripheral circulation to easily obtain a drop of blood for the test. Manual dexterity is needed to perform the fingerstick, to obtain a large enough drop of blood, to place the drop on the right spot, and to correctly read the meter. Patients with arthritis or visual impairment may have difficulty with these steps. The patient must be able to time the test, remember the correct sequence of the steps, and remember to do it at the designated times. Determining whether the patient can cope with learning the procedure and whether there is willingness to fit it into the daily routine are other assessment factors. Periodic assessment of glucose monitoring techniques, medication administration, and compliance with treatment regimen are essential. There is a new device available that offers continuous blood glucose monitoring. This device consists of a sensor that is surgically inserted under the skin, a radiofrequency transmitter, and a monitor. Blood glucose readings are taken every 5 minutes; the device displays the readings when a button is pushed. It also alarms if a result is too high or too low, alerting the patient to view the blood glucose value and to take corrective action (Medtronic MiniMed, 2007).

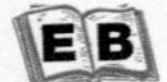

Nursing Diagnosis

The following nursing diagnoses are common for patients with diabetes mellitus:

- Imbalanced nutrition: less than (or more than) body requirements, related to alterations in insulin availability or utilization.
- Deficient knowledge related to newly diagnosed disease process, possible complications, and self-care needs.
- Risk for infection related to elevated blood glucose level.
- Ineffective coping related to denial of need for effective self-care.
- Disturbed sensory perception related to effect of elevated blood glucose on nervous system.
- Sexual dysfunction related to effect of elevated blood glucose on nervous system.
- Risk for injury related to severe decrease in tissue perfusion in feet.
- Situational low self-esteem related to diagnosis of chronic disease requiring insulin injections for survival.

There are many other nursing diagnoses related to the various complications that the patient with diabetes may develop over the years. Nursing care plans must be carefully individualized to the particular problems and needs of each patient (Nursing Care Plan 37–1).

Planning

The nurse must plan time carefully when caring for patients with diabetes. Remembering to check calibration of the glucometer before beginning testing is essential. The nurse should know the times of dietary tray delivery to plan glucose testing and insulin injections at the appropriate times throughout the day. Fingersticks for blood glucose testing should be performed 30 minutes before breakfast. If an hour has elapsed without insulin being given after the reading was obtained, the test must be repeated before insulin administration.

When a patient is NPO for tests, the nurse must plan to monitor for signs of hypoglycemia and to obtain the patient's food tray immediately when the patient is back. The insulin dose should be adjusted according to physician order during the NPO period, not withheld. Assessment for **hyperglycemia** must be planned for various times during the shift when the patient is undergoing the added stress of illness or surgery.

Making certain that the patient's insulin, appropriate syringes, or oral medication are on the unit ahead of scheduled medication time prevents delays. Every insulin dose should be verified by another nurse as it is drawn up. Asking another nurse to be present at an appointed time saves having to hunt for a nurse at the time of injection preparation. Sliding scale doses of regular insulin should be mixed in the same syringe as the standard daily dose for the patient (unless the standard daily dose is an insulin that cannot be mixed with others, such as Lantus insulin). Being certain the patient is in the room before drawing up the insulin also saves time.

Some expected outcomes for the patient with diabetes mellitus include:

- Patient will attain a body weight within normal limits within 6 months.
- Patient will demonstrate knowledge of disease process, possible complications, and self-care methods.
- Patient will constantly monitor for signs of infection.
- Patient will develop coping methods to perform self-care.
- Patient will effectively comply with treatment regimen within 2 months.
- Patient will attain blood glucose level within recommended limits within 3 months to prevent complications of diabetes.

Both long-term and short-term goals are considered when writing expected outcomes.

NURSING CARE PLAN 37–1

Care of the Patient with Diabetes Mellitus

SCENARIO Mr. Blackburn, age 49, is 5′7″ and weighs 350 lb. He was admitted to the hospital for surgical repair of a hernia. During the preoperative evaluation, his blood glucose value came back from the lab at 420 mg/dL. On further examination by the physician, Mr. Blackburn demonstrated symptoms of extreme thirst, hunger, and excessive urination. Surgery was rescheduled; further work-up confirmed the suspected diagnosis of type 2 diabetes mellitus. Mr. Blackburn was extremely upset, both at learning the diagnosis and for not being able to have his surgery. His response to the diagnosis was to ask the surgeon if he could be prescribed "some pills" and "get on with it."

PROBLEM/NURSING DIAGNOSIS *Extremely overweight*/Imbalanced nutrition: more than body requirements related to alteration in glucose utilization by cells.

Supporting assessment data *Objective:* Blood glucose 420 mg/dL; above ideal body weight.

Goals/Expected Outcomes	*Nursing Interventions*	*Selected Rationale*	*Evaluation*
Patient will develop meal plan that will assist in maintaining ideal body weight and blood sugar within normal limits	Perform dietary assessment.	Assessment is the first step before a meal plan can be devised.	
	Instruct in diabetic meal planning.		Patient states that he "doesn't get it" when asked about the Exchange Lists for Meal Planning.
	Assist with construction of an acceptable meal plan for attaining desired weight and to normalize serum glucose levels.	Any meal plan devised must take into account Mr. Blackburn's lifestyle and food preferences.	Patient able to correctly identify appropriate portion sizes of sample menu.
Glycosylated hemoglobin and fructosamine assay levels will show compliance with dietary plan within 6 mo			Glycosylated hemoglobin 5.6%. Fructosamine assay level 3.0 mmol/L. Continue plan.

PROBLEM/NURSING DIAGNOSIS *Has no knowledge about diabetes*/Deficient knowledge related to disease process, possible complications, and self-care.

Supporting assessment data *Subjective:* Patient asks physician if he could be prescribed "some pills" and "get on with it."

Goals/Expected Outcomes	*Nursing Interventions*	*Selected Rationale*	*Evaluation*
Patient will verbalize basic knowledge about disease process within 1 mo	Instruct patient about the disease process of diabetes.	Patient education about disease process is the first step toward taking control of his disease.	Patient verbalized basic knowledge of disease process.
Patient will verbalize ways to prevent the complications of diabetes within 3 mo	Instruct regarding the potential complications of diabetes and how to decrease the risk of complications.	Knowledge of ways to decrease risk of complications can help patient take preventive measures.	Patient states, "I need to lose weight." Patient acknowledges complications of diabetes but states he needs more information.
Patient will demonstrate proper foot care within 1 mo	Instruct in proper foot care techniques.	Instruction in diabetes care should include a variety of teaching methodologies based on the content and the educational preparation of the patient.	Patient demonstrates proper foot care.
Patient will demonstrate knowledge of correct meal planning within 3 mo	Instruct in meal planning. Instruct in insulin or oral medication administration. Seek feedback regarding material taught by verbalization and demonstration of skills.		Patient requests assistance with meal planning. Continue plan.

Continued

NURSING CARE PLAN 37–1

Care of the Patient with Diabetes Mellitus—cont'd

PROBLEM/NURSING DIAGNOSIS *Postoperative infection possible*/Risk for infection related to elevated blood glucose level.

Supporting assessment data *Objective:* Blood glucose 420 mg/dL.

Goals/Expected Outcomes	Nursing Interventions	Selected Rationale	Evaluation
Patient will demonstrate blood glucose levels within acceptable limits within 1 mo	Instruct in glucose monitoring technique appropriate to patient.	Proper instruction, including return demonstration, is important in ascertaining correct fingerstick values.	Blood glucose 230 mg/dL.
	Ask to chart blood glucose findings after testing.	Keeping a daily record is important in monitoring day-to-day fluctuations in blood glucose.	
Patient will demonstrate an absence of infection as evidenced by no signs of skin infection, absence of fever, and feeling of well-being	Instruct in signs of infection to report. Explain why people with diabetes are more prone to infection than the general public.	It is important to detect any potential infection early, as people with diabetes tend to heal more slowly.	T 98.8°F (37.1° C); P 110; R 24; BP 148/86; WBC 4500. Patient states he feels "grumpy." Continue plan.

PROBLEM/NURSING DIAGNOSIS *Surprised by and unprepared for diagnosis*/Ineffective coping related to denial of need for effective self-care.

Supporting assessment data *Subjective:* Patient asks physician if he could be prescribed "some pills" and "get on with it."

Goals/Expected Outcomes	Nursing Interventions	Selected Rationale	Evaluation
Patient will express desire to prevent the complications of diabetes	Assess usual coping methods for dealing with stress. Reinforce positive coping techniques.	Past methods of successful coping may be useful for this new situation.	Patient states, "I want to see my children grow up."
Patient will express commitment to the self-care techniques that when regularly practiced can help decrease the risk of complications	Refer to diabetes support group, diabetes educator, or both.	Social support, such as from a diabetes support group, can make a patient feel less isolated.	Patient expresses commitment to learn self-care techniques.
	Monitor progress toward learning and using regular self-care techniques to prevent complications.	Progress should be monitored so that adjustments in the plan can be made if needed.	
	When glycosylated hemoglobin or fructosamine assay levels indicate only poor control of disease, explore problems patient may be having with diet, exercise, medication, or glucose testing. Reinforce teaching for self-care as needed.	Control of blood glucose is multifaceted; abnormalities must be explored to determine the cause.	Goal met/reevaluate as needed.
	Offer praise and encouragement for all efforts at self-care and control of disease.	Positive reinforcement helps one make difficult lifestyle changes.	

NURSING CARE PLAN 37–1

Care of the Patient with Diabetes Mellitus—cont'd

PROBLEM/NURSING DIAGNOSIS *Feels loss of control*/Situational low self-esteem related to diagnosis of chronic disease requiring lifestyle changes or insulin injections for survival.

Supporting assessment data *Objective:* Patient with newly diagnosed diabetes.

Goals/Expected Outcomes	*Nursing Interventions*	*Selected Rationale*	*Evaluation*
Patient will verbalize own strengths within 1 mo	Encourage verbalization of feelings related to diagnosis of diabetes and need for lifestyle changes.	Verbalization of feelings is an important first step toward identifying one's own strengths.	Patient states, "I am a hard worker. I own my own business—I can certainly learn to manage this too."
	Allow expression of frustrations.	Frustration is a normal human response to a real or perceived threat.	
Patient will express that control over the disease and life is possible	Encourage exploration of strengths and positive measures of self-worth (i.e., roles, accomplishments).		Goal met/re-evaluate as needed.
	Explain how control over disease and life is possible. Provide the knowledge and tools to achieve control.	Remembering past achievements can help patients realize their strength.	
	Praise efforts at learning and practice of self-care techniques.	Positive reinforcement is a powerful tool for helping a patient accomplish acceptance of a situation.	

? CRITICAL THINKING QUESTIONS

1. The RN has planned the first teaching session for Mr. Blackburn, which you are to help implement. The topics planned for today include food exchange lists, short-term complications of diabetes, long-term complications of diabetes, foot care, and actions/side-effects/interactions of oral hypoglycemia agents. When she asks for your collaboration on the plan, what would you recommend?
2. Mr. Blackburn has visitors coming to see him. You greet them in the hallway, and notice they are carrying bags from Krispy Kreme and Baskin Robbins. How would you respond to this situation?

Implementation

Intervention is geared toward assisting the patient with self-care, performing blood glucose determinations, and administering medication when the patient is ill and cannot self-administer, observing for signs and symptoms of complications, assessing learning needs, and carrying out a teaching plan as indicated. Be sure to encourage others involved in your patient's care to be alert for signs and symptoms (Assignment Considerations 37–1).

Monitor the trend of blood glucose, glycosylated hemoglobin, and fructosamine assay readings over time, rather than focus only on the current reading. Assess how well the patient is eating and taking fluids. Intake and output recordings are appropriate if the patient is ill or having surgery. Any type of stress can alter the control of the patient's diabetes. Electrolytes also should be monitored, with particular attention to potassium levels, which can shift suddenly when insulin is insufficient.

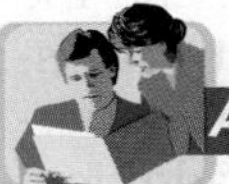

Assignment Considerations 37–1

Observations

Remind the UAP to report any breaks in the skin observed while giving physical care to the patient with diabetes. Report excessive urination or changes in vital signs such as increasingly rapid respirations.

Every patient on insulin should be monitored for hypoglycemia after insulin injections. You must know how many hours after injection of each type of insulin this might occur and should then assess the patient at that time (see Table 37–3). Patients are taught to report signs of hypoglycemia promptly to avoid a crisis.

Monitoring for signs of ketoacidosis also is essential. Some of the earliest symptoms may be polyuria,

Table 37–6 Comparison of Hypoglycemia and Ketoacidosis

	HYPOGLYCEMIA	KETOACIDOSIS
Etiology	Overdosage of insulin Skipped or delayed meal Unplanned strenuous exercise	Failure to take insulin Illness or infection Overeating or too many carbohydrates Severe stress (surgery, trauma, emotional upset)
Symptoms	Headache Weakness Hunger (polyphagia) Pallor Irritability Lack of muscle coordination Apprehension Shakiness Diaphoresis with cool, clammy skin Blurred vision Rapid heart beat Confusion Coma (late)	Increased thirst (polydipsia) Increased urination (polyuria) Acetone breath odor ("fruity") Dry mucous membranes and sunken eyeballs (dehydration) Nausea and vomiting Deep respirations (Kussmaul's respiration) Abdominal pain and rigidity Paresthesias, weakness, paralysis Hypotension Minimal urine output (oliguria) or none (anuria) (late sign) Stupor or coma (late sign)
Treatment	If patient can swallow, give 3 glucose tablets or equivalent glucose gel, 6 oz of orange juice, 6 oz regular cola, 6 oz of 2% or skim milk, or 6 to 8 Life-Savers. If patient cannot swallow, administer glucagon by injection. If at the hospital: give $D_{50}W$ solution.	Insulin and correction of electrolyte imbalances Severe cases are hospitalized for stabilization
Prevention	Eat meals 4–5 hr apart, plus prescribed snacks. Take correct dose of insulin. Test blood glucose level regularly and more frequently during illness. Eat extra food when exercising more than usual.	Take correct dose of insulin. Consult physician when ill. Follow diet; do not overeat and do not overload with carbohydrates.

fatigue, anorexia, abdominal pain, and a "fruity" smell to the breath. Look for beginning signs of dehydration with decreased tissue turgor, sunken eyeballs, and dry mucous membranes (Table 37–6). Report such findings to the physician promptly.

Patient Education

Successful management of diabetes requires that the patient be so well informed about the illness and the protocol for controlling it that responsibility is assumed for changing former dietary habits, administering medication, and monitoring progress. In addition, adjustments in lifestyle, recreational choices, and self-image will probably need to be made. The patient must be taught the correct steps for blood glucose monitoring (Figure 37–4) and how to use dipsticks to monitor urine correctly.

Noncompliance can be devastating to the patient's welfare and can mean the difference between leading a nearly normal life or becoming an invalid; eventually, it may mean the difference between life and death for the person with diabetes. Many hospitals and clinics have developed standardized teaching programs for diabetes education because the task of diabetic teaching is very challenging and complex (Figure 37–5).

Major topics covered in a standardized program usually include the following:

- Pathophysiology of diabetes mellitus, including functions of the pancreas and contributing or precipitating factors in the development of diabetes.

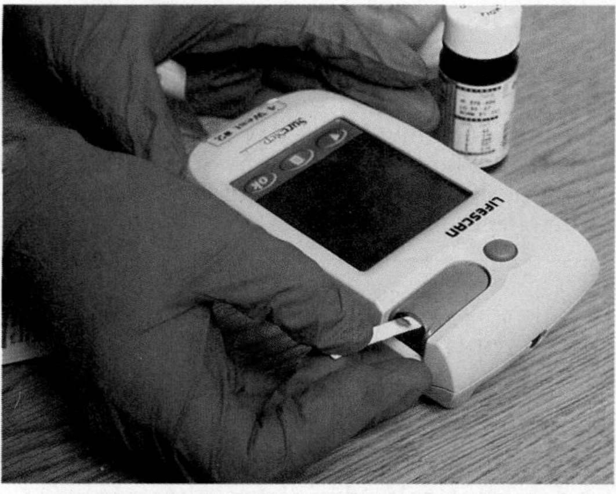

FIGURE **37–4** Blood glucose monitoring.

- How to manage a diet program using the Exchange System.
- Blood glucose monitoring at home with either a visually read test or a glucose monitoring meter.
- Foot care (Patient Teaching 37–3).
- Urine testing when blood glucose level is over 240 mg/dL to check for acetone.
- Identification tag, identification card, and medical information (Figure 37–6).
- Information on what to do on "sick" days, especially when nauseated or vomiting and unable to maintain diet (Patient Teaching 37–4).
- Community resources and help groups available to patient with diabetes and family.

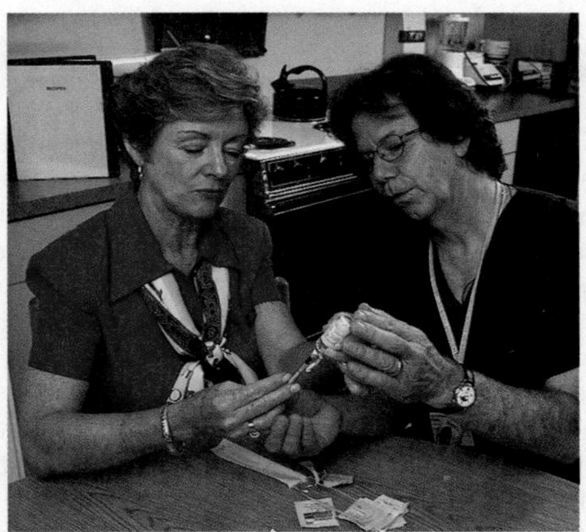

FIGURE **37–5** Nurse teaching patient with diabetes.

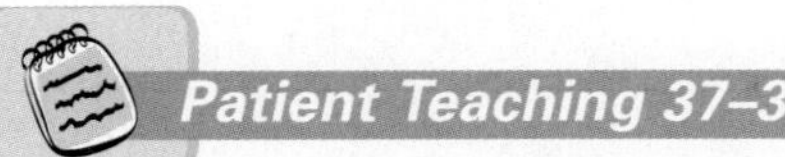

Foot Care

Every diabetic should be taught the following points for proper care of the feet.

- Inspect each foot daily for cuts, cracks, blisters, abrasions, or discoloration of the toes; report any abnormality to your health care provider. Use a mirror if unable to bend to see the bottom of the foot. Be certain to check between the toes.
- Wash the feet in warm (not hot) water, using mild soap; do not soak the feet as this can cause cracking of the skin.
- Thoroughly dry the feet after washing, paying special attention to drying between the toes. Rub in a non-scented, nonmedicated cream if the skin is dry; do not put the cream between the toes.
- Cut the nails straight across; have corns, calluses, and ingrown nails managed by a podiatrist. Smooth the nails with an emery board after cutting to prevent cuts on the legs from rough nails while sleeping.
- Wear a clean pair of cotton socks each day.
- Wear properly fitted shoes with a firm sole that do not pinch or bind the foot; never walk barefoot.
- Break in new shoes gradually.
- Never wear open sandals or sandals with straps between the toes.
- Use socks and blankets to warm the feet; do not use a heating pad or hot water bottle near them.
- Test the temperature of bath water with wrist or forearm before stepping into the tub or shower.
- Elevate the feet whenever possible to improve circulation.

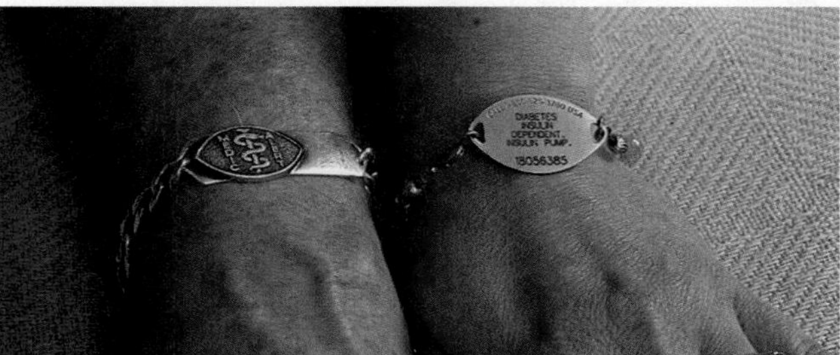

FIGURE **37–6** Medic-Alert bracelet.

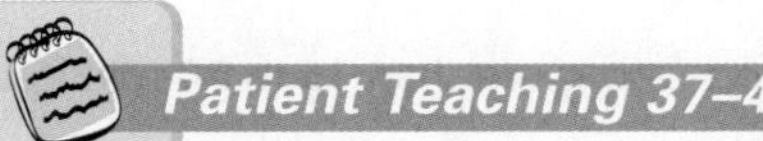

What to Do on Sick Days

The following instructions should be followed whenever you have a bad cold, flu, or minor gastrointestinal upset.

MEDICATION

- Take your insulin as prescribed. Adjust the dosage as directed, depending on your blood glucose readings.
- If taking an oral hypoglycemic, take your usual dose. Do not increase the dose unless ordered to do so by your physician. If you are vomiting and unable to take medication by mouth, the physician may place you *temporarily* on insulin.

DIET

- Eat your normal diet on schedule.
- If you have nausea and vomiting, replace carbohydrate solid foods in your normal diet with liquids that contain sugar (fruit juice, regular soft drinks, or Jell-O).
- Take at least 1 cup of water or calorie-free, caffeine-free liquid each hour. If you are nauseated, take small sips to help avoid vomiting.

MONITORING

- Test blood glucose at least every 4 hours and record result. If severely ill, check blood glucose every 2 hours.
- Test your urine for ketones if your blood sugar level is over 240 mg/dL.

NOTIFYING THE PHYSICIAN

- Call the physician right away if you are vomiting or have abdominal pain or a temperature above 100.2° F (38.8° C).
- Notify the physician if your blood glucose is above 200 mg/dL or your urine test shows ketones in the urine.
- Report to the physician if your blood glucose level that was above 200 mg/dL does not come down with an additional dose of insulin.
- If you cannot reach your physician, go to your hospital emergency room.

FURTHER TREATMENT

- Rest as much as possible.
- Treat vomiting, diarrhea, and fever with fluids and appropriate medication as recommended by your physician.

- Devices that make insulin administration easier (especially for the elderly, visually impaired, or patient with arthritis).
- Older adults have special learning needs. The nurse must be certain that the patient can hear adequately, that vision is enhanced as much as possible by aids and by lighting. Noise and distractions in the environment should be eliminated as much as possible so that the patient can concentrate more fully. Patient Teaching 37–5 presents suggestions for assisting the elderly patient to learn about diabetes and self-care.

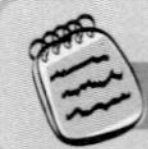

Patient Teaching 37–5

Working with the Older Adult Who Has Diabetes

The following guidelines are helpful when teaching elderly patients:

- Set a time for the teaching session that is agreeable to the patient.
- Arrange a quiet, nondistracting environment for the session.
- Be certain that the patient is comfortable before beginning.
- Keep the sessions short—no more than 15 to 20 minutes at a time.
- Limit information to a few major concepts per session.
- Go slowly and seek feedback that the patient has understood each point when finished presenting it.
- Allow time for the patient to jot down important points.
- Repeat key concepts frequently; if the patient does not understand, try rephrasing the concept.
- Use bold-type printed materials with a white or yellow background.
- Leave printed materials that are illustrated with simple drawings and that are not crowded with text.
- Printed materials should be written at a 5th- to 10th-grade reading level depending on the patient.
- If the patient becomes frustrated or distracted, stop the session and reschedule it.
- Summarize what has been taught and what has been learned at the end of the session.

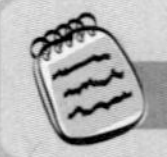

Patient Teaching 37–6

What to Do When Traveling

Instruct the patient who will be traveling to do the following:

- Carry extra medication or insulin in case a bottle gets lost or broken. Keep one set of pills or insulin with 48 hours of syringes in your purse, briefcase, or carry-on luggage, along with your blood glucose–monitoring device.
- Wear a Medic-Alert bracelet or tag, and carry a medical information card in your purse or wallet.
- Carry an emergency supply of fast-acting sugar at all times in case of a hypoglycemic episode. Also carry longer-acting foods, such as peanut butter and crackers.
- Plan ahead at least 2 days for replenishing supplies for blood glucose monitoring, insulin, and syringes in case the correct items are hard to find in a foreign city. (It is best to take supplies with you for the entire time you will be gone.)
- If you become severely ill, seek medical attention immediately before you get into a dangerous condition.
- Stick to prescribed meal plans as well as possible, substituting available foods according to food group classification.
- Obtain sufficient rest and avoid stressful situations as much as possible to prevent stress-induced hyperglycemia.
- If you are a "brittle" diabetic, it is best to travel with someone who is familiar with your condition and treatment. It is best to advise the airline or ship personnel that you have diabetes when you embark.
- Obtain your usual amount of exercise or adjust food and medication intake accordingly.
- Drink a glass of water every 2 hours to prevent dehydration.
- Check your blood glucose level frequently.
- Obtain a letter from your physician stating that you have diabetes as well as extra prescriptions for your medications.
- Protect your insulin from temperature extremes.
- Eat something at least every 4 hours.
- Call airlines and ship companies ahead of departure to request diabetic meals.
- Research food substitutions for the type of food in the places you will be traveling before departure so that you will be able easily to accommodate your personal meal plan.
- Remember time zones: going westward lengthens your day; take more insulin. Going eastward shortens your day; take less insulin.

The health care team helping the patient with diabetes should include a diabetic specialist, nurse educator, dietitian, podiatrist, periodontist, and, of course, the patient and significant others. Because of frequent updates and changes in diabetes management, all persons responsible for the care of diabetic patients should read and continue to study and learn about the current protocols. Patient Teaching 37–6 provides traveling tips for people with diabetes.

Evaluation

Evaluation is done by determining whether the expected outcomes have been met. For a patient with diabetes, this usually means assessing whether learning has taken place and whether there is compliance with the treatment regimen. Monitoring glycosylated hemoglobin and fructosamine assay levels provides data about the degree of control of blood glucose. Questioning the patient about exercise and diet provides information about those areas. Observing demonstrations of learned skills for insulin injection, proper foot care, dietary planning, and glucose monitoring tells how well these tasks have been integrated.

If the expected outcomes are not being met, then the nursing care plan must be revised. Collaboration with the physician and dietitian may be necessary to design a plan that is effective.

Complications

In general, people with diabetes are susceptible to two types of complications: short-term, or acute, problems and long-term problems.

Short-Term Problems. Acute complications arise when the blood glucose suddenly becomes either too high (hyperglycemia) or too low (hypoglycemia) (see Patient Teaching 37–1 and Table 37–6). When a patient is admitted to the hospital with hyperglycemia, decisions about the proper modes of therapy are based on whether the patient has type 1 or type 2 diabetes and the objective and subjective symptoms presented. Type 1 diabetes is more likely to be complicated by ketoacidosis, whereas type 2 diabetic patients may suffer hyperglycemic hyperosmolar nonketotic syndrome (HHNS) (HHNC, HNKC, and HHNK are also common abbreviations).

Diabetic Ketoacidosis. Diabetic ketoacidosis (DKA) is a serious condition caused by incomplete metabolism of fats due to the absence or an insufficient supply of insulin. When insulin is not present in adequate amounts to meet metabolic needs, the body breaks down protein and fat for energy. This produces an abundance of the by-products of fat metabolism, which are potent organic acids called *ketones.* In an attempt to rid itself of excess ketones, the body excretes some of them via the lungs. This produces a characteristic fruity odor to the breath. Acetone, a ketone body, is excreted in the urine, causing acetonuria or ketonuria. As the kidney excretes excess glucose and ketones, it also eliminates large quantities of water and electrolytes. These pathologic changes are responsible for metabolic acidosis, dehydration, and electrolyte imbalances.

Signs and symptoms of DKA can be life-threatening and are listed in Table 37–6. Treatment consists of fluids, insulin, and correction of electrolyte imbalances. Electrolytes, especially potassium, and serum glucose are monitored closely. **The goals of treatment are to restore the normal pH of the blood and other body fluids, correct the fluid and electrolyte imbalance, lower the blood glucose level gradually, and provide life-support measures as necessary if the patient is comatose.** Infection is the most frequent cause of DKA; however, other causes include poor compliance with the prescribed treatment regimen of diet and insulin therapy and insulin pump failure. After the patient is stabilized, the underlying cause must be determined and treatment or corrective measures implemented.

Hyperglycemic Hyperosmolar Nonketotic Syndrome. Hyperglycemic hyperosmolar nonketotic syndrome (HHNS) occurs in people with type 2 diabetes who experience high blood glucose levels because of illness or added stress, such as infection. Glucose levels between 600 and 1000 mg/dL are not unusual; in some cases the blood glucose can reach well over 1000 mg/dL. The extremely high level of glucose in the blood causes severe dehydration and circulating fluid volume depletion. Blood osmolality is considerably elevated (greater than 350 mOsm/kg). HHNS is different from DKA because a small amount of circulating insulin remains available, resulting in the absence of ketosis and acidosis. Because ketosis and acidosis are absent, the gastrointestinal symptoms do not occur and the patient does not seek early medical care in the course of illness. The patient's mental state may progress from confusion to complete coma. Also in contrast to DKA, the patient may suffer generalized or focal seizures.

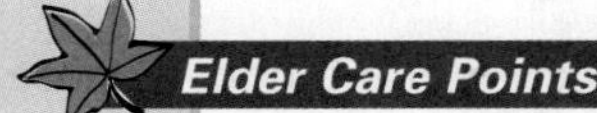

Elder Care Points

Older adults are at greater risk for HHNS syndrome, as they become dehydrated more quickly than younger patients. HHNS may be the first indicator that the patient has diabetes. It most frequently occurs after a febrile illness or gastrointestinal flu in which the patient has stopped eating properly and possibly discontinued oral hypoglycemic agents.

Things that may precipitate HHNS in a person with type 2 diabetes are (1) medications, such as steroids, thiazides, phenytoin, and beta blockers; (2) acute illnesses, such as infection, myocardial infarction, and trauma; (3) chronic illnesses, such as cerebrovascular accident, and psychiatric illnesses, such as dementia; and (4) treatments, such as total parenteral nutrition and peritoneal dialysis.

Treatment of HHNS focuses on fluid replacement and correction of electrolyte imbalances. Because fluid replacement will initially be rapid, the nurse must closely monitor cardiovascular status and auscultate lung sounds frequently. Small amounts of insulin may be used until the patient is stabilized. Blood glucose and intake and output must be monitored closely. The underlying illness that triggered the HHNS must be identified and treated. HHNS can be fatal, and mortality is directly correlated with higher elevations of blood glucose and the resultant severity of dehydration.

Rebound Hyperglycemia. Another condition sometimes encountered in patients with type 1 diabetes is rebound hyperglycemia, also known as the *Somogyi effect.* This rebound follows a period of hypoglycemia. When hypoglycemia occurs, the body secretes glucagon, epinephrine, growth hormone, and cortisol to counteract the effects of low blood sugar. This increase in circulating hormones with falling insulin levels and the rise in glucose production from the liver raises blood glucose excessively. Insulin resistance also may occur for 12 to 48 hours because of the action of the released hormones (Cooperman, 2006). Often the Somogyi effect occurs when unrecognized hypoglycemia occurs during sleep. By morning, when the patient checks the blood glucose, the released hormones have caused elevated serum glucose. The patient thus increases the insulin dose, worsening the problem. The patient may report nightmares and night sweats along with morning elevated serum glucose and ketones in the urine.

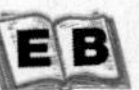

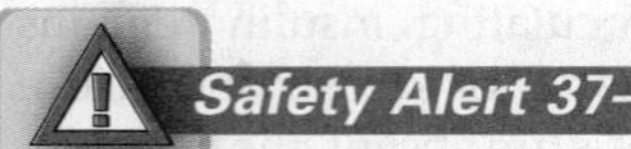

Safety Alert 37–4

Glucose

When treating a person on alpha-carboxylate inhibitors for hypoglycemia, *pure glucose* must be given, as other carbohydrates are broken down slowly, due to the nature of the medication.

Safety Alert 37–5

Hyperglycemia or Hypoglycemia

When there is doubt as to whether the patient is suffering from hyperglycemia or hypoglycemia, treatment is begun for hypoglycemia until a blood glucose determination is obtained to prevent brain damage from extremely low cerebral glucose levels.

When this phenomenon occurs, the blood glucose should be measured between 2 A.M. and 4 A.M. and again at 7 A.M. If the blood glucose is low (i.e., 50 to 60 mg/dL) and then is more than 189 to 200 mg/dL at 7 A.M., the Somogyi effect is occurring. Usual treatment is to lower the insulin dosage or move the time of the intermediate-acting insulin to bedtime. Changing or increasing the bedtime snack also helps.

The **dawn phenomenon**, a distinctly different situation, also is characterized by elevated blood glucose in the morning, but it is not related to hypoglycemia. The dawn phenomenon is caused by release of growth hormone, glucagons, and epinephrine during the night, as part of the body's natural circadian rhythm. These hormones are all **"counterregulatory hormones,"** which act to raise the body's blood sugar. The dawn phenomenon is the reason why most people with diabetes do not tolerate carbohydrates well in the morning (Diabetic-Talk.org, 2004).

Whenever a diabetic person is subjected to additional stress, as in an unrelated medical illness or when surgery is necessary, the patient's metabolic needs change, and thus the delicate balance between hyperglycemia and hypoglycemia is threatened.

Hypoglycemia. The word *hypoglycemia* means low blood glucose. Hypoglycemia is a rather common complication of type 1 diabetes mellitus. Most often it is a response to either too large a dose of insulin or too much exercise in relation to the amount of food eaten. Signs and symptoms of hypoglycemia include tremulousness, hunger, headache, pallor, sweating, palpitations, blurred vision, and weakness; symptoms may progress to confusion and loss of consciousness. Individual reactions vary considerably. Some patients are alert with a glucose level of 40 mg/dL, and others are comatose.

Treatment depends on the degree of hypoglycemia and level of consciousness. If the patient is alert enough to tolerate oral intake safely, glucose levels of 40 to 60 mg/dL respond to ingestion of food such as milk, crackers, or 4 oz of orange juice. Glucose levels of 20 to 40 mg/dL respond best to concentrated sugars, such as honey, table sugar, or juice. In the hospital, if the person is experiencing seizures or is not alert enough to tolerate oral intake safely or has a very low blood sugar, a solution of 50% glucose is given IV. When an IV access cannot be established, 1 mg of glucagon is administered intramuscularly (Safety Alert 37–4). The injection is repeated in 15 minutes if symptoms are not resolved.

People with diabetes must be taught to monitor themselves for beginning signs of hypoglycemia and always to carry a source of concentrated sugar to be taken if the symptoms occur. Glucose tablets or Life-Savers are easily portable sources of glucose (Safety Alert 37–5). Hypoglycemia is discussed in detail later in this chapter.

Long-Term Problems. The long-term consequences of diabetes mellitus are chiefly the result of damage to the large and small blood vessels. Elevated blood glucose levels over a period of years seriously damage blood vessels and the organs they serve. Diabetes remains the sixth leading cause of death in the United States for all age groups (CDC, 2004). In addition, cardiovascular disease and other causes of death often can be attributed to diabetes.

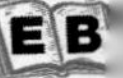

Patients who have had diabetes for more than 10 years are likely to develop one or more of the complications of the disease. The less closely the blood glucose has been controlled, the more likely the development of cardiovascular, eye, and renal complications. **Improperly treated or untreated diabetes is the leading cause of new blindness, renal failure leading to dialysis, and nontraumatic lower limb amputations.** Although not every person with diabetes will suffer from long-term complications, many will be hospitalized for one reason or another in some later stage of the disease.

Cardiovascular Disease. Thickening of the vessels, chiefly the **basement membrane** (thin layer of connective tissue under the epithelium), occurs when blood glucose is elevated over a long period. The vessels of the retina, renal glomeruli, peripheral nerves, muscles, and skin are affected. Larger vessels also are affected, which predisposes the patient to atherosclerosis and vascular occlusion. Two out of three people with diabetes die prematurely from heart attack or stroke.

Insulin Resistance Syndrome. Insulin resistance syndrome, also known as **metabolic syndrome**, is the term used to describe a syndrome whereby a patient has insulin resistance, hypertension, and increased very low–density lipoprotein (VLDL) and decreased high-density lipoproteins (HDL) cholesterol concentrations. Insulin resistance appears to combine with the abnormalities in VLDL and HDL levels in contributing to the increased risk of cardiovascular disease in patients with diabetes mellitus.

Nephropathy. Diabetic nephropathy (disease of the kidney) occurs directly from changes in the renal blood circulation. Factors that influence whether a person with diabetes will develop kidney disease include genetics, blood glucose level, and blood pressure.

After years of having to filter too much blood with elevated blood glucose, the filtering mechanism of the kidney begins to fail, allowing large particles to exit through the urine that normally would have been filtered out, such as protein. In the early phase, microalbuminuria, there are small amounts of protein in the urine. If nothing is done to prevent further damage, this progresses to a later phase, macroalbuminuria, with large amounts of protein in the urine. Finally, the patient enters end-stage renal disease, and requires either a kidney transplant or hemodialysis to perform the filtering for the kidneys.

Nephropathy can be prevented by keeping tight control of blood glucose. Research has demonstrated that tight blood glucose control reduces the risk of people developing microalbuminuria, may prevent people with microalbuminuria from progressing to macroalbuminuria, and can even reverse microalbuminuria.

Peripheral Vascular Disease. Gangrene, which often leads to amputation, is far more common in people with diabetes: more than 60% of nontraumatic amputations occur among people with diabetes. Vascular changes frequently cause very poor circulation in the feet and lower extremities. Healing of wounds in these areas is difficult because of the poor blood supply and because increased levels of glucose in the blood provide a good medium for bacterial growth, making it harder to eradicate infection. Learning and practicing excellent foot care are essential to prevent amputation. Half of all amputations can be prevented with aggressive screening to identify people at high risk and provide early intervention (Bonham, 2007).

EB

Retinopathy. Visual impairment and blindness are common sequelae of diabetes mellitus. The three most common visual problems are diabetic retinopathy, cataracts, and glaucoma. Retinal damage, which can cause visual impairment and blindness, occurs in most people with diabetes within 10 years of diagnosis. Changes in the retinal vessels lead to hemorrhages and to retinal detachment. Recent surgical techniques using photocoagulation of destructive lesions of the retina with laser beams now offer hope for preserving sight by preventing progress of diabetic retinopathy. Tight glucose control, frequent eye examinations, and treatment can help preserve vision.

Neuropathy. Approximately 60% to 70% of people with diabetes have mild to severe neuropathy. Pathologic changes in the nervous system cause deterioration, with symptoms such as paresthesia, numbness, and loss of function. Diabetic neuropathies primarily affect the peripheral nerves, causing sexual impotence in the male, constipation, neurogenic bladder, and pain or anesthesia (lack of feeling) in the lower extremities. It is for this reason that foot care and daily inspection of the feet are so important. Because the patient often cannot feel cuts, blisters, or abrasions on the foot, there is great danger that a neglected sore might become infected. Although it may be mild at the beginning, there eventually may be almost total anesthesia of the affected part, bringing with it the potential for serious injury to the patient without awareness. In contrast, some patients experience debilitating pain and hyperesthesia; some lose deep-tendon reflexes. Other problems related to diabetic neuropathies are the result of autonomic nervous system involvement. These include orthostatic hypotension, delayed gastric emptying or **gastroparesis,** diarrhea or constipation, and asymptomatic retention of urine in the bladder. Prevention of the potentially devastating long-term consequences of diabetes is a major goal of management.

HYPOGLYCEMIA

Etiology and Pathophysiology

A low blood glucose state can exist whenever the homeostatic mechanisms designed to maintain blood glucose within a rather narrow range fail to function as they should. The organs involved in meeting the challenge of carbohydrate ingestion include the intestines, liver, and pancreas (specifically, the beta cells that produce insulin). Thus any condition affecting these organs and their systems can lead to hypoglycemia. Examples other than diabetes mellitus include gastrectomy and surgical bypass procedures. These types of surgery provide more rapid access of glucose to the absorptive sites in the small bowel. Tumors of the pancreas (insulinomas), liver disease, and disorders of the adrenal cortex and pituitary gland can also produce abnormally low blood glucose levels. People who abuse alcohol and other substances are also prone to hypoglycemia.

Functional hypoglycemia, for which there is no known cause, may be a very early indicator of diabetes mellitus. In fact, studies have shown that almost one third of the people who have functional hypoglycemia may eventually develop diabetes if the hypoglycemia is not effectively controlled.

Reactive and Spontaneous Hypoglycemia. The pathophysiology of hypoglycemia and its attendant symptoms are different after eating from what they are in a fasting state. These differences are the basis for classifying the disorder into *hypoglycemia in the fed state* (also called *reactive hypoglycemia*) and *hypoglycemia in the fasting state* (also called *spontaneous hypoglycemia*).

Signs and Symptoms

Signs and symptoms of hypoglycemia include rapid heartbeat, tremulousness, weakness, anxiety, nervousness, and hunger. In reactive hypoglycemia, they occur rather suddenly, within 4 hours after a meal is eaten. Some physiologic symptoms may be mistaken for indications of a psychiatric illness. These symptoms include irritability, personality change, temper tantrums, and other psychoneurotic manifestations.

Diagnosis and Treatment

Diagnosis of hypoglycemia is done with measurement of blood sugar values. The patient's insulin levels and C-peptide levels also can be measured. The diagnosis of reactive hypoglycemia may be made using a glucose tolerance test. To diagnose spontaneous hypoglycemia, a medically supervised fast may be used. CT scan, ultrasound, and other diagnostics may be used if an insulinoma (insulin-secreting tumor) is suspected.

Hypoglycemia is treated by modifying eating patterns. Smaller and more frequent meals that are relatively free of simple sugars are recommended. The diet should be high in proteins and low in carbohydrates, and carbohydrates should be complex ones, such as those found in fruits, vegetables, and whole grains. Refined sugar and white flour are omitted. Cases in which gastric surgery and intestinal bypass are believed to be the cause of hypoglycemia may be treated with drugs that reduce intestinal motility.

Complications

Untreated fasting hypoglycemia can lead to severe **neuroglycopenia** (shortage of glucose in the brain) and possibly death. Untreated reactive hypoglycemia may cause the patient a great deal of discomfort, but usually results in no long-term complications.

Nursing Management

Nurses are in an excellent position to observe and help identify patients who might be hypoglycemic. In addition to information about the patient's physical and mental symptoms, assessment should include a rather detailed history of eating habits. Does the patient eat regularly? How often during each day? What kinds of foods constitute a typical meal? Does he crave sweets? Have there been episodes of weakness, sweating, visual disturbances, and confusion or inability to concentrate? If these symptoms have occurred, when are they most noticeable (i.e., in a fed or fasting state)?

Nursing interventions for patients with hypoglycemia include explaining the nature of the disorder and the need for diagnostic testing to confirm or rule out reactive hypoglycemia, objective and nonjudgmental observation and reporting of symptoms, and reinforcement of dietary instruction and restrictions.

COMMUNITY CARE

There is a great need for home care and monitoring of the elderly population with diabetes. If nurses could follow the progress of these patients over the years with good assessments and implement ongoing patient education programs, the incidence of complications could certainly be decreased. The public health initiative *Healthy People 2010* set forth health objectives for the nation to achieve over the first decade of the new century. One major objective of *Healthy People 2010* is to "increase the proportion of persons with diabetes who receive formal diabetes education." Nurses are in a critical position to ensure implementation of this crucial goal.

Long-term care nurses must be alert to the signs of diabetes. When a resident does not properly recover from a viral illness, in-depth assessment for signs of diabetes is wise.

Home care and clinic nurses must be persistent in assessing compliance with diabetic regimens and instrumental in teaching the public about the signs and symptoms of diabetes and the measures for self-care to prevent complications. Far too many patients with diabetes do not understand the ramifications of poor control of their disease. At present, diabetes is costing the United States more than $1 billion a year in health care expenditures. This is one area in which nurses could be instrumental in cutting health care costs.

SOURCES OF INFORMATION

With the explosion of information on the Internet, numerous materials are available to the person with diabetes, including websites, e-newsletters, support groups, and locations where print magazine subscriptions can be ordered. As with all information on the Internet, patients should realize there are legitimate and respectable sites, but there are also sites closer to "fringe" medicine and pseudoscience. The best advice is to stick to organizations that have reputable physicians associated with them.

In the print magazine category, *Diabetes Forecast* is written and edited by health care specialists and aimed at providing information for people with diabetes so that they can manage their illness more effectively. There is a charge for this publication; information can be found on the ADA website.

Internet resources that may be useful for patients with diabetes include:

- American Dietetic Association: Nutritional information, including materials available for a nominal fee ($2.50): Exchange Lists for Meal Planning (English and Spanish), Exchange Lists for Weight Management, and other materials. www.eatright.org/cps/rde/xchg/ada/hs.xsl/shop_378_ENU_HTML.htm.
- American Diabetes Association: The nation's leading nonprofit health organization providing diabetes information, research, and advocacy (in English and Spanish) www.diabetes.org.

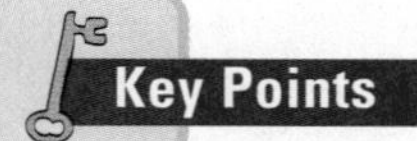

Key Points

- Diabetes mellitus involves a disturbance in glucose metabolism. Type 1 usually appears at a young age, and the patient requires insulin for life. Type 2 diabetes usually develops later in life, but is now being diagnosed more frequently in younger people. Gestational diabetes may occur in pregnancy.
- The goal in diabetes is to maintain blood glucose and lipid levels within normal limits to prevent complications.
- The cornerstone of therapy for people with diabetes is diet and exercise. Insulin must be taken by people with type 1 diabetes; OHAs may be prescribed for people with type 2.
- The diet is geared toward providing optimal nutrition and calories to maintain normal body weight and to adjust food intake to keep blood glucose within safe limits.
- The emotional and physical stress of surgery can increase the blood glucose level and alter the amounts of medication needed.
- Islet cell transplantation may someday eliminate the need for insulin injections.
- Every patient on insulin should be monitored for hypoglycemia after insulin injections. Monitoring for signs of ketoacidosis is essential.
- Older adults have special learning needs. The nurse must be certain that the patient can hear adequately, that vision is enhanced, and noise and distractions are eliminated.
- Short-term complications of diabetes include hyperglycemia and hypoglycemia.
- DKA is a serious condition caused by incomplete metabolism of fats due to the absence of insulin marked by metabolic acidosis, dehydration, and electrolyte imbalances.
- HHNS occurs in people with type 2 diabetes because of illness or stress. Glucose levels are often between 600 and 1000 mg/dL, leading to severe dehydration.
- Whenever a diabetic person is subjected to additional stress, her metabolic needs change; thus the delicate balance between hyperglycemia and hypoglycemia is threatened.
- Hypoglycemia is often a response to either too much insulin or too little exercise. If there is doubt whether the patient is suffering from hyperglycemia or hypoglycemia, treatment is begun for hypoglycemia until a blood glucose level is obtained.
- The long-term consequences of diabetes mellitus result from damage to large and small blood vessels; cardiovascular disease, nephropathy, peripheral vascular disease, retinopathy, and neuropathy can all be reduced by strict blood glucose control.
- Prevention of long-term consequences of diabetes is a major goal of management.
- Hypoglycemia can be related to diabetes mellitus, diseases of the intestines, liver, or pancreas, or alcohol or substance abuse.
- Nurses in all settings must be alert to the signs of diabetes, assess compliance with diabetic regimens, and teach the public about the signs and symptoms of diabetes.

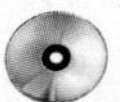

Go to your **Companion CD-ROM** for an Audio Glossary, animations, video clips, and bonus review questions.

evolve Be sure to visit the companion Evolve site at http://evolve.elsevier.com/deWit for interactive NCLEX-PN Exam Style Review Questions, WebLinks, and additional online resources.

NCLEX-PN EXAM STYLE REVIEW QUESTIONS

Choose the best answer(s) for the following questions.

1. "Tight blood glucose control" in older adults is not strongly recommended because:
   1. older adults are more prone to hyperglycemia.
   2. severe low-glucose states can precipitate other health problems.
   3. older adults can adjust quickly to changes in blood glucose.
   4. oral hypoglycemic agents have been proven to work better.

2. The nurse demonstrates understanding of medical management of diabetes mellitus when he states:
   1. "Diet and exercise are the mainstays in controlling blood glucose levels."
   2. "Oral hypoglycemic agents may be prescribed for patients with type 1 diabetes mellitus."
   3. "Insulin therapy is reserved for type 1 diabetes mellitus."
   4. "Tight blood glucose control is indicated for all patients with diabetes mellitus."

3. A patient newly diagnosed with diabetes is given diet instructions. The nurse would be more effective in motivating the patient to comply with dietary recommendations by which of the following strategies? *(Select all that apply.)*
   1. Emphasizing good food choices
   2. Applying diet prescriptions to patient-preferred foods
   3. Instilling fear and guilt when "cheating" occurs
   4. Focusing on the benefits of diet compliance
   5. Involving meal preparers in diet teaching

4. Before discussing a possible exercise regimen with a 50-year-old female who was recently diagnosed with type 2 diabetes mellitus, the nurse should initially:
   1. encourage brisk walking.
   2. recommend weight training.
   3. ensure adequate glucose control.
   4. develop an exercise schedule.

5. Which of the following patient statements regarding exercise regimen and control of blood glucose indicates a need for further teaching?
   1. "I need to exercise with a friend who knows the signs of low blood sugar."
   2. "An emergency source of glucose must be with me at all times."
   3. "Exercise must be scheduled before meals."
   4. "I could gradually increase the intensity of my exercise."

6. A patient who works as a personal trainer is diagnosed with insulin-dependent diabetes. Regarding self-administration of regular insulin, it is important for the nurse to advise the patient to:
   1. skip the oral hypoglycemic agent dose before exercise.
   2. eat a piece of fruit before a moderate exercise.
   3. exercise during the insulin peak of action.
   4. use the abdomen as an insulin injection site.

7. While the nurse is obtaining a morning blood glucose level, the diabetic patient reports having nightmares and night sweating. Her blood glucose is 200 mg/dL. The nurse notifies the physician and the morning insulin dosage is lowered. The physician most likely identified the clinical phenomenon as:
   1. dawn phenomenon.
   2. hyperglycemic hyperosmolar nonketotic syndrome.
   3. Somogyi effect.
   4. diabetic ketoacidosis.

8. ______________ is characterized by elevated blood glucose in the morning caused by the natural circadian release of growth hormone, glucagon, and epinephrine.

9. A patient presents with confusion, tremulousness, hunger, pallor, sweating, palpitations, blurred vision, and weakness. The blood glucose level is 40 mg/dL. Appropriate initial management of these symptoms would be to:
   1. recheck blood sugar.
   2. if able, give honey, sugar, or juice.
   3. give insulin.
   4. administer intravenous fluids.

10. A patient who is started on pioglitazone (Actos) asks, "How does this medication work?" The nurse accurately responds:
    1. "It slows the absorption of complex carbohydrates."
    2. "It inhibits the release of excess insulin from the liver."
    3. "It stimulates the pancreas to secrete more insulin."
    4. "It makes muscle cells more sensitive to insulin."

CRITICAL THINKING ACTIVITIES

Read each clinical scenario and discuss the questions with your classmates.

Scenario A

Mrs. Lopez is 42 years old and has had type 2 diabetes mellitus for the past 10 years. She is admitted to the hospital for treatment of an infection of the great toe on her left foot, which is the result of improper care of an ingrown toenail. She is 45 lb overweight and admits to frequent binges of eating foods not on her diet. She does not exercise regularly because she says the housework she does gives her enough exercise. When asked about the OHA and diet that have been prescribed for her, she tells you that she only takes her medicine and follows her diet "most of the time."

1. Describe the essential components of a teaching plan for Mrs. Lopez to help her manage her illness better. Why is foot care an important part of this plan?
2. What could you suggest to Mrs. Lopez to help her lose weight?
3. What do you think might motivate Mrs. Lopez to accept more responsibility for managing her illness?
4. What laboratory testing would be recommended to track Mrs. Lopez's compliance with her treatment regimen?

Scenario B

Mr. Tobin is a 22-year-old construction worker who has recently experienced fatigue, excessive thirst and urination, and weight loss. A routine urinalysis revealed glycosuria and a trace of acetone. His physician has arranged for Mr. Tobin to have an oral glucose tolerance test to determine if he has diabetes mellitus.

1. If Mr. Tobin is found to have type 1 diabetes mellitus, what kind of information will he need to manage his illness?
2. How would you explain the importance of good or tight control of his blood glucose levels to Mr. Tobin?
3. What criteria could be used to determine whether his diabetes is under control?

Scenario C

Mr. Smith, a 76-year-old male, has recently been diagnosed with type 2 diabetes mellitus. It has been difficult to control his blood sugar and his physician has added insulin to his treatment regimen. Mr. Smith was issued a glucometer by the hospital but says that the test strips are too expensive for him to buy very often. Mr. Smith lives alone, cooks for himself, and likes a glass of wine with dinner. Other than an occasional fishing trip, he does not exercise regularly.

1. How would you approach a teaching program for this patient?
2. What resources could you suggest that might assist him to purchase the test strips for the glucometer?
3. How can a glass of wine be incorporated into an acceptable meal plan for a patient with diabetes?
4. What sort of exercise program could you recommend to this patient?

CHAPTER 38

Care of Women with Reproductive Disorders

evolve http://evolve.elsevier.com/deWit

Objectives

Upon completion of this chapter, you should be able to:

Theory

1. Identify the female reproductive organs and their role in the overall health of the individual.
2. Describe normal physiology and age-related changes in the female reproductive system.
3. Discuss common menstrual disorders and their nursing interventions.
4. Discuss methods of contraception.
5. Review causes and treatment of infertility.
6. Describe changes associated with menopause, treatment options, and nursing interventions.
7. Explain the screening procedures recommended for maintaining reproductive health.
8. Compare and contrast benign and malignant disorders of the female reproductive system.

Clinical Practice

1. Explain techniques of breast self-examination and vulva self-examination to a patient.
2. Utilize the nursing process in the care of a woman with a reproductive disorder.
3. Describe the causes of and interventions for common disorders of the female reproductive tract.

Key Terms

Be sure to check out the bonus material on the Companion CD-ROM, including selected audio pronunciations.

amenorrhea (ă-mĕn-ō-RĒ-ă, p. 958)
anovulation (ăn-ŎV-ū-LĀ-shŭn, p. 959)
climacteric (klī-MĂK-tĕr-ĭk, p. 937)
cystocele (SĬS-tō-sēl, p. 957)
dowager's hump (p. 947)
dysmenorrhea (dĭs-mĕn-ō-RĒ-ă, p. 939)
dyspareunia (dĭs-pă-ROO-nē-ă, p. 947)
effleurage (ĕf-loo-RĂ-ZH, p. 939)
endometriosis (ĕn-dō-mē-trē-Ō-sĭs, p. 960)
enterocele (ĕn-TĔR-ō-sēl, p. 957)
fibroids (FĪ-broydz, p. 959)
hirsutism (HĔR-sōōt-ĭszm, p. 958)
hysterectomy (hĭs-tĕr-ĔK-tō-mē, p. 958)
lymphedema (lĭm-fĕ-DĒ-mă, p. 967)
menarche (mĕ-NĂR-kē, p. 937)
menopause (MĔN-ō-păwz, p. 937)
menorrhagia (mĕn-ō-RĀ-jă, p. 959)
menses (mĕn-sēz, p. 937)
menstruation (mĕn-strū-Ā-shŭn, p. 937)
metrorrhagia (mĕ-trō-RĀ-jă, p. 958)
mittleschmerz (MĬT-ĕl-shmărts, p. 939)
myomectomy (mī-ō-MĔK-tō-mē, p. 959)
oligomenorrhea (ŏl-ĭ-gō-mĕn-ŏ-RĒ-ă, p. 958)
polycystic ovarian syndrome (pō-lē-SĬS-tĭk, p. 958)
prolapse (PRŌ-lăps, p. 937)
pruritus (proo-RĪ-tŭs, p. 947)
rectocele (RĔK-tō-sēl, p. 957)
sentinel node biopsy (SĔN-tī-nĕl nōd BĪ-ŏp-sē, p. 964)
stress incontinence (STRĔS ĭn-KŎN-tĭ-nĕns, p. 958)

The female reproductive system depends on hormones produced by the endocrine system for correct development and reproductive function. A variety of hormones released in a specific order at specific times triggers the formation of internal and external sexual organs in the developing fetus. Puberty and sexual maturation are also dependent on accurate release of hormones at the appropriate time in the cycle. As the childbearing years draw to a close, hormone production slows until the reproductive cycle ceases altogether.

Reproductive health can be disrupted by a variety of disorders, such as infertility, spontaneous abortion, premature labor, infection, and the growth of abnormal tissue, including cancerous and noncancerous tumors. Nursing care of patients with diseases of the female reproductive system is further complicated by the emotional effects of such disorders. The reproductive organs represent the biologic aspect of sexual identity, and women may feel their personal identity is threatened by disorders of this system.

WOMEN'S HEALTH

Women's health care can be defined as the promotion of the physical, psychological, and spiritual well-being in women. The growth of the women's movement in

OVERVIEW OF ANATOMY AND PHYSIOLOGY OF THE FEMALE REPRODUCTIVE SYSTEM

What are the primary external structures of the female reproductive system?

The *vulva,* or *pudendum,* is the name given to the external female genitalia. It is made up of the following structures:

- The *mons pubis* is a rounded mound of fatty tissue that protects the symphysis pubis. It is covered with pubic hair.
- The *labia majora* are two elongated, raised folds of pigmented skin that enclose the vulvar cleft. The pubic hair extends along these folds.
- The *labia minora* are soft folds of skin within the labia majora. They are soft, shiny, and made up of fat tissue and glands, and have no hair follicles.
- The *clitoris* is located at the top of the vulvar cleft, above the urethral opening. It is made up primarily of erectile tissue and is highly sensitive to touch. It is a primary source of pleasurable sensation during sexual activity.
- The *urethral meatus,* or external opening of the urethra of the urinary bladder, is located below the clitoris within the folds of the labia minora.
- The *vaginal vestibule* is situated below the urethral meatus within the labia minora and is the entrance to the vagina.
- The *perineum* is the flat muscular surface lying between the vagina and the anus.

What are the primary internal structures of the female reproductive system?

- The *vagina* is a muscular tube lined with membranous tissue with transverse ridges called rugae. It connects the external and internal female sexual organs (Figure 38–1).
- The *uterus* (womb) is a hollow pear-shaped organ with a thick muscular wall. It lies at the upper end of the vagina. It is capable of expanding to many times its normal size to accommodate a growing fetus. The lower opening of the uterus is the *cervix,* which dilates during labor to allow for delivery of the infant.
- There are two *fallopian tubes* that branch outward from the right and left side at the top of the uterus. They form the pathway for the *ovum* (egg) from the ovary to the uterus.
- There are two *ovaries,* one located near the end of each fallopian tube. These almond-shaped glands excrete estrogen and progesterone into the bloodstream. At birth, the ovaries contain all the eggs (*oocytes*—primitive ova or eggs) the woman will ever produce, approximately 400,000 in each ovary, most of which will never mature for possible fertilization.
- The *bony pelvis,* located at the base of the body between the hips, supports the pelvic organs, including the growing uterus during pregnancy.

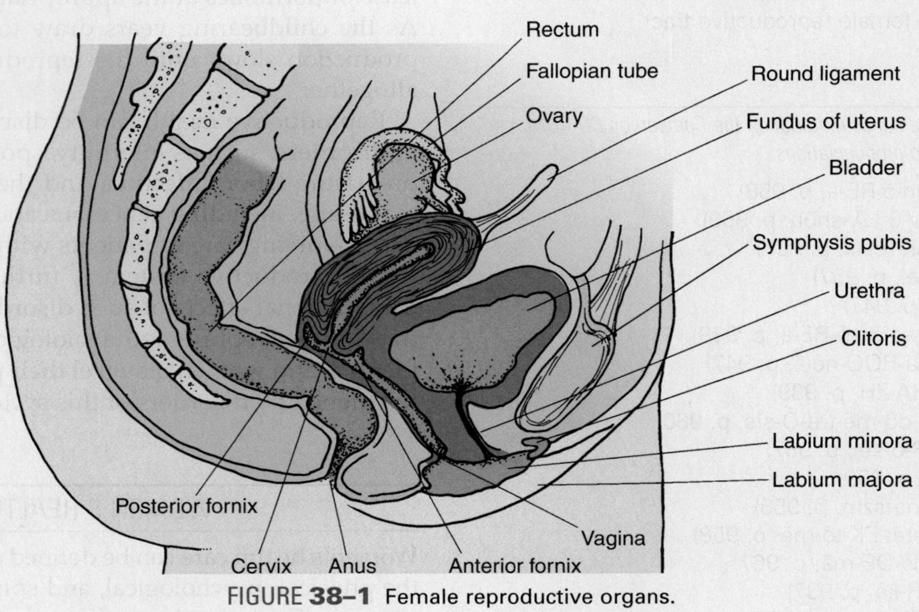

FIGURE 38–1 Female reproductive organs.

It is assisted by the *pelvic floor,* a collection of strong muscles and supportive tissues that brace the pelvis and provide both support and protection for the pelvic organs.

What are the accessory organs of the female reproductive system?

- The breasts or *mammary glands,* located on the upper chest, are the accessory organs. They are composed of fibrous, adipose, and glandular tissue, and are responsible for *lactation* (milk production), which provides nourishment for the infant.

What are the phases of the female reproductive cycle during the childbearing years?

- The *ovarian cycle* has two phases:
  - *Follicular phase*—This is the first 14 days of a 28-day cycle. *FSH* (follicle-stimulating hormone) and *LH* (luteinizing hormone) stimulate the maturing of immature ova in preparation for fertilization. Estrogen peaks when the ovum is released *(ovulation)* about 14 days before the *next* menstrual period. The ovum lives up to 24 hours after fertilization.
  - *Luteal phase*—The 15th to 28th days of the cycle. LH and progesterone are the primary hormones in this phase. The blood supply to the uterus increases in preparation for possible implantation of a fertilized ovum. If fertilization and implantation do not occur, the lining of the uterus will degrade and be shed during menstruation, and the cycle begins again.
- The *menstrual cycle* has four phases that are described in Table 38–1.

When does sexual development occur in the fetus?

- During the first weeks of pregnancy, the male and female sexual organs are undifferentiated. After the 7th week, rapid changes occur, and by the 12th week the external genitalia are formed and fully differentiated as male or female. The internal structures also are forming during this period.

What changes take place as girls mature into women and become capable of reproduction?

- The period of sexual maturation is called *puberty.* It usually occurs between ages 9 and 17 years for girls, with the average onset being 12 years of age. It involves a period of accelerated growth, then the hips begin to widen and the breasts begin to develop. Axillary and pubic hair appears. Puberty is completed by the onset of the menstrual cycle or **menses.** The beginning of menstruation is called **menarche. Menstruation** (shedding of the uterine lining) will continue at intervals of approximately 4 weeks throughout the childbearing years except when pregnancy occurs.

What changes take place as a woman enters menopause?

- Toward the end of the childbearing years, women enter the phase known as the **climacteric.** The menses become irregular in both pattern and flow and eventually cease altogether. **Menopause** has occurred when the menses have completely ceased for at least 12 months.

What changes occur with aging?

- After menopause, some atrophy of the female organs, loss of elasticity, dryness of the vaginal membranes, and reduction of bone mass occur because of the decrease in estrogen levels. Loss of natural tissue elasticity may allow internal organs to sag, or **prolapse,** into the vagina.

America was the beginning of the recognition that there are health needs unique to women, and legislation gradually emerged that included women as subjects in research studies. Research trials concerning the safe dosages and efficacy of drugs had previously been conducted on male subjects and generalized to apply to women. However, currently it is recognized that there are differences between men and women in many areas and now even the growth norms for children are published with separate charts for girls and boys.

In the late 19th century, women physicians were rarely seen, and by 1900, only 6% of all physicians were women. The women's health movement of the 1960s expanded women's rights to control their bodies and motivated women to learn more about their bodies and understand wellness. Childbirth education classes flourished and alternative birthing centers emerged. The 1972 Civil Rights Act prohibited discrimination based on sex in educational institutions, and it is estimated that by 2010 more than 30% of medical doctors will be women.

Table 38–1 *Stages of the Menstrual Cycle*

FIRST TO FIFTH DAY	SIXTH TO FOURTEENTH DAY	FIFTEENTH TO TWENTY-EIGHTH DAY
Stage I: Menstrual stage (dismantling stage) 1. Endometrium sloughs away as menstrual flow begins. 2. Progesterone and estrogen are no longer secreted. 3. New follicle starts to mature.	**Stage II:** Growth and repair (estrogen or proliferative stage) 1. Follicle grows and egg matures. 2. Endometrium returns to normal state and then begins to thicken in response to estrogen. **Stage III:** Ovulation occurs 14 days before menses, regardless of length of menstrual cycle. It takes place when follicle ruptures and releases egg. If pregnancy does not occur, the corpus luteum deteriorates, estrogen and progesterone decline, and the thickened tissue on the endometrium of the uterus is sloughed off and is discharged via the vagina as a menstrual "period."	**Stage IV:** Secretory stage (postovulatory or progesterone stage) 1. Corpus luteum secretes progesterone. 2. Endometrium continues to thicken in response to estrogen and progesterone. Prepares to receive fertilized ovum.

In 1990, the Women's Health Equity Act (WHEA) was passed, containing laws that increased women's access to health services. The Office of Research on Women's Health (ORWH) was formed as part of the National Institutes of Health.

In the 21st century, women are increasingly economically independent and empowered to make health care decisions. Health care education of the adolescent includes information concerning puberty, menstruation, and sexuality. A teen needs information concerning safe sex, contraceptives, and choices concerning high-risk behaviors. Adult women require information concerning Papanicolaou (Pap) smears, breast self-examination, nutrition, exercise, and lifestyle management. Perinatal education is important. Older women require information regarding menopause, long-term illness, and disabilities that affect health care needs. Today many older women live alone with below-poverty-level income and are without caregivers or easy access to health care. The nurse must have an understanding of these needs and of the normal physiologic changes of each age-group in order to devise a plan of care to maintain health or treat illness.

It is of utmost importance that women of all ages be knowledgeable about the function of their bodies, health care needs, and signs and symptoms of wellness as well as illness. This chapter focuses on the health of the reproductive system and reviews common gynecologic problems with suggested nursing interventions.

Young women often first enter the health care system for a Pap smear or for contraceptive advice. Support, reassurance, and understanding of cultural and personal needs are the primary responsibilities of the nurse during this first contact. A complete history, physical examination, age-appropriate screening tests with clear interpretations, referrals, and education concerning nutrition, lifestyle, and health care to meet individual needs are essential responsibilities of the nurse and the health care team.

NORMAL MENSTRUATION

During the first year following menarche, the menstrual cycle may be somewhat irregular, but by the second year a regular cycle of approximately 28 days is normally established.

Attitudes and ideas regarding menstruation are formed early. They are based on the thoughts and beliefs expressed by other women and on personal experience. Incorrect perceptions about this normal process may increase physical discomfort or cause the young woman unnecessary embarrassment or fear. Although there has been significant improvement in communication with preadolescent young women about the changes they will experience, many still need further education whenever the opportunity arises. It is important that the nurse understands her own attitudes about sexuality and the reproductive process before attempting to provide information for women on these sensitive issues. A healthy view of menarche as a natural physiologic process marking reproductive maturity should be encouraged.

Normal Menstrual Bleeding

Menstrual bleeding occurs about 14 days after ovulation and lasts between 2 and 8 days. Menstrual blood consists of endometrial tissue, blood, mucus, and vaginal and cervical cells. The amount of actual blood loss is only 40 to 80 mL. Blood flow may be heavy at first, but gradually reduces to spotting. The color may change from bright red to brown and the blood may have a musty odor. Once a menstrual pattern is established, a change from this pattern is reason to consult a health care provider. The length of the cycle can be influenced by stress, drugs, nutrition, and illness. Women should be encouraged to keep a calendar of their individual menstrual cycle to determine regularity and recognize deviations. Mild cramping may occur, and some mood swings may be associated with the hormonal changes. **Mittelschmerz** is a sharp pain in the right or left lower quadrant, sometimes felt at the midcycle around the time of ovulation, and may last a few hours. Some women are sensitive to this phenomenon and others never experience it.

Normal Vaginal Discharge

The vagina is a warm, moist, dark vault in which microorganisms can flourish. Normal vaginal secretions contain cervical mucus, endometrial fluid, exudate from Bartholin's gland and Skene's ducts, and products of normal flora. The main line of defense against infection is lactic acid, which causes an acidic pH. Any change in this pH can result in infection. An increase in secretions normally occurs during pregnancy and at the midpoint of the menstrual cycle when ovulation occurs, and a decrease in secretions normally occurs after menopause.

Normal vaginal discharge has an off-white color and is without odor. If the vaginal discharge develops an odor, changes in color or consistency, or causes irritation or burning of the vaginal mucosa, a health care provider should be consulted.

THE NORMAL BREAST

Breasts are made of adipose tissue, milk-producing glands called lobules, ducts, and fibrous tissue that rests on the chest muscle. They may not be completely symmetrical (one may be slightly larger than the other) and may feel a bit lumpy and tender, especially during the middle of the menstrual cycle. Age, pregnancy, medication, and diet can affect the way the breasts feel. As the woman ages, the denseness and adipose tissue content decreases, while birth control pills, hormone replacement therapy, and pregnancy may cause the breasts to increase in size.

MENSTRUAL DYSFUNCTIONS

Premenstrual Syndrome

Premenstrual syndrome (PMS), also known as *ovarian cycle syndrome,* is the presence of physical, psychological, or behavioral symptoms that regularly recur within the luteal phase of the menstrual cycle and significantly disappear during the remainder of the cycle. These signs and symptoms, which occur between ovulation and menstruation, include weight gain, bloating, irritability, changes in eating patterns, fatigue, mood swings, and a fear of losing control.

Premenstrual Dysphoric Disorder

Premenstrual dysphoric disorder is a more severe form of PMS and is described officially in the *Diagnostic and Statistical Manual of Mental Disorders,* fourth edition (DSM-IV), a classification of disorders that is published by the American Psychological Association. It is thought to be a decreased ability to cope with normal stressors rather than the appearance of new stressors. Functional changes such as depression and impaired concentration may interfere with the normal lifestyle or work responsibilities.

Strategies for self-care may include stress management exercises, some lifestyle changes, and maintaining a healthy diet. Consumption of refined sugar, salt, red meat, alcohol, and caffeinated beverages should be limited. Dietary supplements in the form of calcium, magnesium, and vitamin B_6 may be helpful. Exercise may increase beta-endorphin levels, which results in relief of depression and mood elevation. Peer support groups can also be helpful. Psychological counseling and prescribed medications such as diuretics or nonsteroidal anti-inflammatory medications such as ibuprofen, may provide relief. Fluoxetine (Sarafem, Prozac), a selective serotonin reuptake inhibitor, has been approved by the Food and Drug Administration (FDA) for the management of menstrual disorders. EB

Dysmenorrhea

Dysmenorrhea is painful menstruation and a very common gynecologic complaint. There are two classifications of dysmenorrhea.

Primary Dysmenorrhea. Primary dysmenorrhea usually occurs 6 to 12 months after the menarche (when the process of ovulation becomes established and regular menstruation occurs). It is thought to be due to the release of high levels of prostaglandins in the first 2 days of menstruation, causing uterine contractions and vasoconstriction that result in abdominal cramps. Backache, weakness, decrease in appetite, and central nervous system symptoms such as dizziness, headache, and poor concentration may also occur but rarely last longer than 48 hours, which coincides with the decrease in prostaglandin levels.

The most important management of the young adolescent or adult with dysmenorrhea is to promote an attitude of positive sexuality and self-worth. Correction of myths and misinformation is essential, and management is related to the woman's individual responses.

A heating pad promotes vasodilation and often relieves cramps. Back massage and soft rhythmic massage of the abdomen **(effleurage)** can also relieve discomfort. Exercises such as the *pelvic rock* relieve discomfort by releasing endorphins, suppressing prostaglandins, and shunting the blood flow away from the pelvic organs, which results in less pelvic congestion. The pelvic rock is accomplished while in the hands-and-knees position, alternating arching the back and constricting abdominal and gluteal muscles while exhaling and then hollowing the back and relaxing the muscles while inhaling. Several complementary and alternative medicine (CAM) therapies can also be helpful, such as aromatherapy and meditation. A

Table 38–2 Medications Used to Relieve Dysmenorrhea

MEDICATION	SIDE EFFECTS	NURSING IMPLICATIONS
Fenoprofen (Nalfon)	Diarrhea, abdominal distention, nausea and vomiting, dyspepsia, constipation	Contraindicated in hemophilia, bleeding ulcers, bleeding disorders. Avoid alcohol.
Ibuprofen	Nausea, dyspepsia, itching, rash	Contraindicated in hemophilia, bleeding ulcers, bleeding disorders. Do not take with aspirin. Take with meals. Avoid alcohol.
Indomethacin	Nausea, dyspepsia	Contraindicated in hemophilia, bleeding ulcers, bleeding disorders. Side effects more likely.
Mefenamic acid (potent prostaglandin synthesis inhibitor)	Diarrhea, nausea, abdominal distention	Contraindicated in hemophilia, bleeding ulcers, bleeding disorders. Incidence of GI side effects increased.
Naproxen sodium	Nausea, abdominal distress, dyspepsia, rash, itching	Contraindicated in hemophilia, bleeding ulcers, bleeding disorders. Do not take with aspirin. Take with meals. Avoid alcohol.

Key: *GI*, gastrointestinal.

balanced low-fat diet with foods that are natural diuretics, such as cranberry juice, asparagus, and watermelon, may decrease edema-related symptoms. Medications such as nonsteroidal anti-inflammatories are prostaglandin inhibitors and may relieve many discomforts. Health care providers may prescribe an oral contraceptive (OC), which provides relief from menstrual discomforts along with advantages of contraceptive protection. A new OC, Seasonale, provides longer periods of pain-free amenorrhea by allowing only four menstrual periods per year, and its use is becoming popular. Many herbal preparations and over-the-counter CAM medications are available for self-treatment. The nurse should be aware of side effects and interactions of CAM therapies with prescribed drugs.

? *Think Critically About* . . . Why should the nurse ask the patient about over-the-counter medications and herbal remedies she is taking and document their use?

Secondary Dysmenorrhea. Secondary dysmenorrhea occurs usually after 25 years of age and is caused by pelvic pathology such as endometriosis, pelvic inflammatory disease, uterine polyps, or fibroids. Pain associated with secondary dysmenorrhea is characterized by a dull lower abdominal pain that radiates to the back or thighs. The pain may occur before the menstrual period and last throughout the days of menstrual flow.

Management involves treating the cause of the pelvic pathology. Temporary relief may be obtained with the same therapies used for primary dysmenorrhea (Table 38–2).

CONTRACEPTION

Many women start sexual relationships before they are ready to have children. Others have children and do not wish to have more. For these women, information concerning techniques of contraception is essential to prevent unwanted, unintended pregnancies. Many sexually active women of childbearing age are concerned about regulating, planning, or preventing pregnancy. With the assistance of a health care provider, they can select the birth control method best suited to their physical health, sexual activity, desire to have children at a future date, cultural and religious beliefs about family regulation, and lifestyle.

Contraceptive Options

Women should make an informed decision concerning methods of reliable birth control, and nurses are responsible for providing comprehensive education concerning the advantages, limitations, and side effects of the various contraceptive drugs and devices. Some methods of birth control provide protection against sexually transmitted infections (STIs), but some do not. Newer contraceptive regimens reduce the hormone-free interval, thereby decreasing the occurrence of menstrual periods. The best contraceptive methods for adolescents and young adults are abstinence, the use of planned contraception, the correct use of condoms to prevent STIs, and lifestyle counseling. Figure 38–2 illustrates the correct application of a condom and a diaphragm. Table 38–3 reviews the various methods of contraception.

Oral Contraceptives

OCs are the most popular method of reversible hormonal contraception in use. They are effective if used properly, and offer some noncontraceptive benefits

HOW TO USE A MALE CONDOM

1. Apply condom before any contact with vagina because sperm are present in secretions *before* ejaculation.
2. Squeeze air from the tip of condom, and hold it while unrolling condom over erect penis. Leave a half-inch space at tip.
3. Use water-soluble lubricants, if needed.
4. To remove condom, hold it at the base of penis to prevent spillage as you withdraw from the vagina.
5. Dispose and use a new one each time. Be sure to check expiration date on condoms.

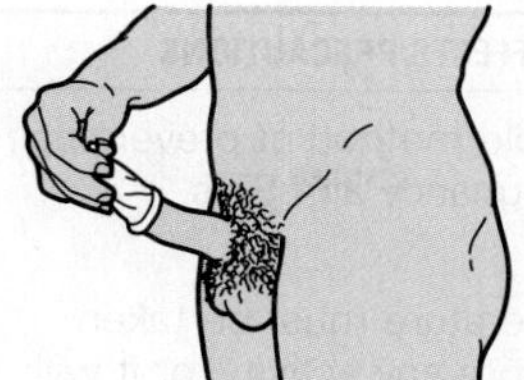

Squeeze air from tip of condom

A

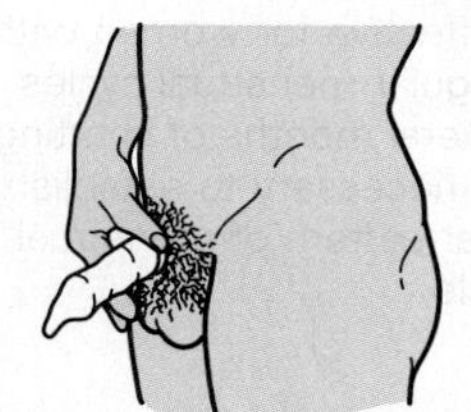

Hold condom at base of the penis to prevent spillage

HOW TO USE A DIAPHRAGM

1. The diaphragm can be inserted up to 4 hours before intercourse. Apply spermicide on the rim and inside the center of diaphragm.
2. Compress diaphragm using thumb and finger of one hand, and use other hand to spread the labia.
3. While squatting (or placing one foot on a chair), insert into vagina with spermicide toward cervix. Direct diaphragm inward and downward behind and below cervix.
4. Tuck the front rim of diaphragm into the pubic bone, and feel cervix through the center of diaphragm.
5. Leave in place at least 6 hours after intercourse.
6. To remove, assume squatting position and bear down. Hook a finger over top rim, and pull diaphragm down and out.
7. Wash diaphragm with mild soap and dry after each use. Dust with cornstarch, if needed, and inspect occasionally for small holes.

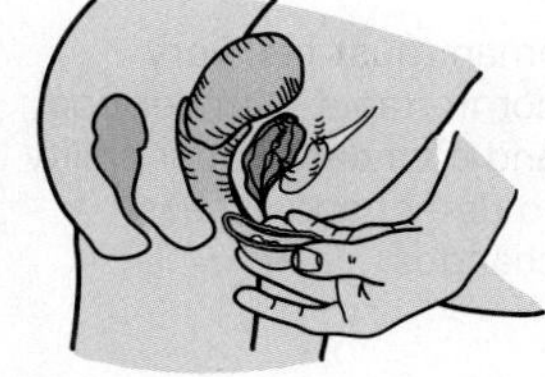

Begin to insert diaphragm into vagina with spermicide toward cervix

B

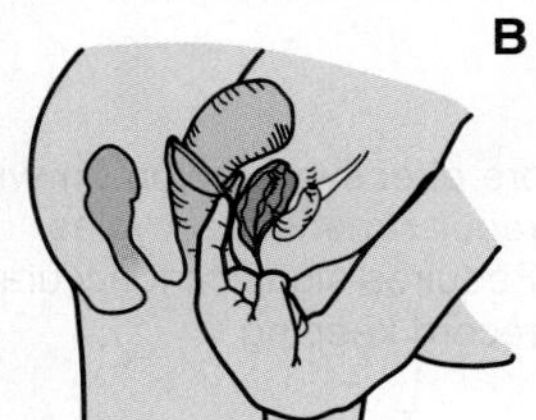

Tuck diaphragm behind the pubic bone

FIGURE **38–2** Proper application of **(A)** a condom, and **(B)** a diaphragm.

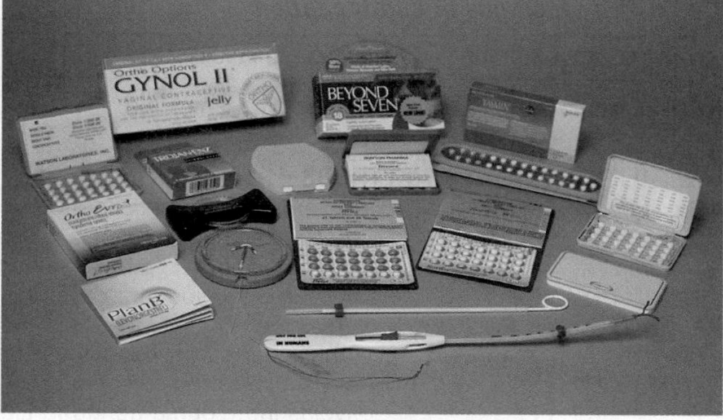

FIGURE **38–3** Contraceptives.

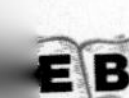

such as relief from breast tenderness, bloating, and PMS symptoms, but do have contraindications and cautions for users (Yonkers et al., 2005) (Figure 38-3). The nurse should counsel the woman concerning options and collect data that can determine which contraceptive choice is best for her. The health care provider assists the woman in making the final choice. Traditional OC regimens are based on a 28-day cycle with a 7-day hormone-free interval that allows for menstruation and gonadotropin levels to rise and ovarian follicular growth to occur (Baerwald et al., 2004). When the OC cycle is not resumed *on schedule*, the risk of unplanned pregnancy occurs. Newer OCs reduce the hormone-free interval, thereby reducing menstrual discomforts as well as decreasing the risk of contraceptive failure (Kaunitz, 2005). Seasonale, an oral contraceptive that provides delayed menstruation in which a woman has only four menstrual periods a year, is becoming popular (Davis, 2006). A new regimen (Lybrel) involves low-dose combined hormones for 365 days per year without a hormone-free interval, which allows a woman to postpone menstruation indefinately, was approved by the FDA in 2007.

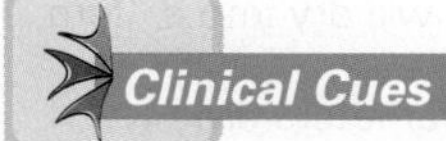

It is important to tell patients that birth control pills and most other birth control methods are not 100% effective in preventing conception. Abstinence is the only 100% effective method to prevent pregnancy.

Emergency Contraception

Known as the "morning-after pill," emergency contraception is indicated after unprotected intercourse. It is not meant to be used on a regular basis, but was developed to decrease the number of unwanted pregnancies and elective abortions. Emergency contraception prevents pregnancy by preventing ovulation or fertilization or by slowing transport of the sperm and egg or altering the uterine lining to prevent implantation (Schorn, 2006). One tablet of 1.5 mg of levonorgestrel only taken within 72 hours of unprotected sex, or two tablets of 1.5 mg levonorgestrel taken 12 hours apart, are preferable to an estrogen-progestin regimen (American College of Obstetricians and Gynecologists [ACOG], 2005). 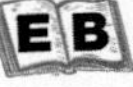 In some states, a prescription is required for emergency contraceptives, and in other states, they have over-the-counter availability (Legal & Ethical Considerations 38–1 on p. 946). The woman is advised to take an antiemetic prior to each dose to minimize nausea and vomiting. Since emergency con-

Table 38–3 ***Methods of Contraception***

CONTRACEPTIVE METHOD	HOW METHOD WORKS	SIDE EFFECTS/PRECAUTIONS	DEGREE OF EFFECTIVENESS
Abstinence	Sexual contact avoided.	Reliable method of preventing pregnancy and STIs.	100%
FERTILITY AWARENESS METHODS			
Basal body temperature (BBT)	BBT is measured and charted daily on awakening. Coitus is avoided on the day of temperature rise and for 3 subsequent days.	Temperature must be taken before any activity, or it will rise above its basal level. The special thermometer should be kept at bedside.	80%–90% for all fertility awareness methods if done correctly
Calendar or rhythm method	Woman charts her monthly menstrual cycle on a calendar and avoids intercourse during fertile period.	Not effective for woman with irregular menstrual cycles. Several months of charting are necessary to establish clear pattern of menstrual cycle.	Fertility awareness methods that monitor multiple parameters (e.g., symptothermal method) may be more effective, but most important aspect of success is faithful adherence to the method; also, the woman must feel comfortable enough with her body to make the necessary observations each month
Ovulation or Billings method	Cervical mucus changes are assessed. During ovulation, mucus is clear with high stretchability ("egg white" consistency). Degree of stretch is tested by pinching a small amount of cervical mucus between the thumb and forefinger and stretching it between them (called *spinnbarkeit*). During ovulation, mucus smeared on a glass slide will dry into a "fern" pattern.	Woman must feel very comfortable with her body and confident in her ability to detect and assess changes.	
Symptothermal method	Variety of parameters are recorded, including cervical mucus changes, BBT pattern, mittelschmerz (brief sharp abdominal pain that may occur with ovulation), increased libido (sexual drive).	More effective for women with regular menstrual cycles. Requires significant accurate record keeping.	
Chemical predictor test	A test kit that contains a chemically treated strip that will turn color when estrogen or luteal hormone levels are present in urine.	Increase in hormone levels occurs 12–24 hr before ovulation.	
MECHANICAL OR BARRIER CONTRACEPTION			
Intrauterine device (IUD)	A small, sterile, flexible plastic device that is inserted by a physician into the uterus. Can be a copper device or a device containing the hormone levonorgestrel (Mirena). Can provide 5 yr of protection.	May increase menstrual flow or cause cramping or low back pain. Increased incidence of PID in women with multiple sex partners, women whose partners have multiple partners, and women with previous incidence of PID. Patient must check placement by feeling for string once each month.	Up to 99% effective; must be removed by health care provider

Table 38–3 ***Methods of Contraception—cont'd***

CONTRACEPTIVE METHOD	HOW METHOD WORKS	SIDE EFFECTS/PRECAUTIONS	DEGREE OF EFFECTIVENESS
MECHANICAL OR BARRIER CONTRACEPTION—cont'd			
Male condom	A sheath commonly made of latex that is placed over the erect penis prior to intercourse. Oil-based lubricants such as petroleum jelly can cause latex to break down and reduce effectiveness. Some condoms, made of polyurethane, are compatible with oil-based lubricants.	Inexpensive, readily available, easy to use correctly. *Precautions:* (1) leave space at tip for semen to collect rather than being forced upward out of the condom; (2) store in a cool place and not for excessively long to avoid breakage due to aging of the latex or heat damage; (3) handle carefully to avoid spilling semen and possibly introducing it into the vagina. Effectiveness enhanced with use of spermicide. Provides protection against STIs.	88%–98% if used properly; use of spermicide increases effectiveness to 98%–99%
Female condom	Sheath with retaining ring that is placed in the vagina prior to intercourse. Open end with large entrance ring extends outside the vagina. Can be inserted up to 8 hr before intercourse.	The penis must remain inside the sheath, not between the sheath and the vaginal wall. Acceptance of the method has been slow as it is more expensive and more difficult and time-consuming to place properly than the male condom. Effectiveness enhanced with use of spermicide. Provides protection against STIs.	79%–90%; most failures occur when the penis is withdrawn too far and reenters the vagina beside rather than within the condom
Diaphragm	A latex or rubber dome-shaped cup that fits snugly over the cervix. Spermicide is applied to the cervical side of the diaphragm and it is inserted into the vagina so the fitted ring holds it securely in place at the top of the vagina to wall off the cervix. The spermicide enhances effectiveness should there be a leak around the edge or tear in the diaphragm.	A diaphragm must be fitted professionally and should be refitted annually or with a gain or loss of 7–10 lb, and particularly after pregnancy.	82%–94%
Cervical cap	Cervical cap fits over the cervix. Filled with spermicidal jelly and applied over the cervix.	Can be in place up to 48 hr before sexual intercourse. Similar to diaphragm.	82%–94%
SPERMICIDAL METHODS			
Gels, foams, creams	Work by killing sperm within the vagina. Must be applied before intercourse.	Available without prescription. More effective used as an adjunct to condoms, diaphragms, and caps.	Foam alone, 79%–90%; creams and gels alone, 79%

Key: *FDA,* Food and Drug Administration; *GI,* gastrointestinal; *PID,* pelvic inflammatory disease; *STIs,* sexually transmitted infections.

Continued

Table 38-3 Methods of Contraception—cont'd

CONTRACEPTIVE METHOD	HOW METHOD WORKS	SIDE EFFECTS/PRECAUTIONS	DEGREE OF EFFECTIVENESS
HORMONAL METHODS			
Oral contraceptives (OCs)	"The pill" contains a combination of synthetic estrogen and progestin, hormones that prevent ovulation and thicken cervical mucus, making it difficult for sperm to travel upward (also true for injectable and timed-release hormonal methods). Traditionally based on a 28-day cycle with 7 hormone-free days that result in monthly menstruation. *Seasonale* is an OC that reduces menstrual periods to 4 times a year. *Lybrel* is an OC that is taken 365 days a year and suspends menstruation indefinitely (FDA approved in 2007).	Prescription required. Must be taken faithfully to be effective. *Precautions:* Not recommended for women older than 35 who smoke or women with a history of heart or liver disease, breast or uterine cancer, blood clots or venous inflammation, or unexplained vaginal bleeding. At least three regular ovulatory cycles should be evidenced before adolescents start OC use. May cause nausea.	97%–99.9%
"Minipill"	Contains a small dose of progesterone and no estrogen. Causes endometrium to be hostile to implantation.		97%–99.9%
Low-dose regimens	*Mircette* uses low-dose estrogen for 5 of the 7 traditionally "hormone-free" days, resulting in shorter, lighter menses. *Loestrin 24 Fe* provides 24 days of combined hormones with a 4-day hormone-free interval. *Yasmin* is similar to Loestrin, but has been shown to relieve symptoms of premenstrual dysphoric syndrome. Both approved in 2006.		97%–99.9%
Injectable contraceptives (Depo-Provera)	Synthetic timed-release progesterone is injected q 12 wk, preventing ovulation.	Injections given in clinic or office. Must be repeated q 12 wk to remain effective. *Precautions:* See oral contraceptives.	99.7%
Sustained-release implants (Funk et al., 2005; London et al., 2007)	Implanon, a thin, flexible rod containing synthetic hormone, is placed under the skin of the forearm in a minor surgical procedure (replaces Norplant). Effective for 3 yr (FDA approval in 2006).	Small incision required to place and to remove. Less popular now that injection is available. *Precautions:* See oral contraceptives.	98.4%–99.4%
Emergency contraception	Taken orally the day following unprotected intercourse, it induces menses and prevents implantation in the uterus.	Not to be used as a routine form of contraception. Women receiving the "morning-after" pill should also get assistance in choosing an effective, ongoing method of contraception.	97%–99.9%
Vaginal ring	The Nuvaring (etonogestrel and ethinyl estradiol) is a flexible silicone ring inserted into vagina for 3 wk and removed for 1 wk to allow for menstruation.	Leukorrhea and vaginal infection are possible side effects. Other side effects similar to OCs but fewer GI problems since it does not pass through GI tract.	97%–99.9%

Table 38–3 **Methods of Contraception—cont'd**

CONTRACEPTIVE METHOD	HOW METHOD WORKS	SIDE EFFECTS/PRECAUTIONS	DEGREE OF EFFECTIVENESS
HORMONAL METHODS—cont'd			
Skin patch	A transdermal skin patch containing norelgestromin and ethinyl estradiol applied to dry skin of back, buttocks, upper arm, or torso. Replaced each week for 3 wk. Not applied 4th wk to allow for menstruation.	The FDA is investigating research that evidences a higher level of estrogen than expected is absorbed, giving rise to increased risk for complications (symptoms similar to OCs). This method is currently used with caution until research is completed.	97%–99.9%
Delayed menstruation	*Seasonale* is an OC that delays menstruation so that the woman experiences 4 menstrual periods a year. *Seasonique* is an OC that provides 84 days of combined hormones followed by a week of low-dose estrogen rather than a hormone-free interval. The 4 menstrual periods a year are lighter and with less discomfort.	A popular choice. Requires follow-up research concerning long-term effects.	97%–99.9%
PERMANENT CONTRACEPTION			
Tubal ligation (female)	Fallopian tubes are cut or tied to prevent sperm from reaching ovum.	Sterilization procedures are considered permanent as reversal may not be effective.	100%
Vasectomy (male)	The vas deferens (sperm ducts) are cut and tied to prevent sperm from entering ejaculatory fluid.	Use another form of birth control until two sperm analyses are negative.	100%

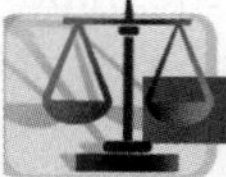

Legal & Ethical Considerations 38–1

The "Morning-After" Pill

Although the "morning-after" contraceptive pill can be sold over the counter in most states, there has been considerable unwillingness by certain pharmacists to provide it. They claim it is against their religious principles. It may not be ethical for pharmacists to withhold the medication from a woman because of their own personal beliefs.

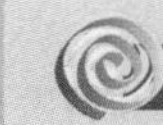

Cultural Cues 38–1

Fertility

Symbols and rites that celebrate fertility are practiced by many cultures. In the United States, throwing rice at the bride and groom is a wish for family growth. Distributing candy or cigars in celebration of a birth is also common in the United States. In some countries, rubbing the swollen abdomen of a statue of a fertility goddess is a popular practice for women seeking to conceive.

traception is not effective if the woman is already pregnant, failure to menstruate by 21 days after initiation of therapy requires evaluation for pregnancy.

A copper intrauterine device (IUD) can be inserted up to 7 days after unprotected sexual intercourse to prevent implantation of the zygote in women who prefer long-term contraception. A woman who seeks emergency contraception should be educated concerning methods of birth control and prevention of STIs.

INFERTILITY

Many women dream of having children but find difficulty in conceiving (Cultural Cues 38–1). For these women, preconception guidance and perhaps infertility treatments may be helpful. Preconception guidance involves gathering data concerning the woman and her partner in order to provide information necessary to make an informed, individualized decision concerning conception or fertility assistance. Screening for genetic disorders may be required.

Primary infertility is the inability of the couple to conceive a child after at least 1 year of active, unprotected sexual relations without using contraceptives.

Secondary infertility is the inability to conceive after having once conceived, or to maintain a pregnancy long enough to deliver a viable infant. Approximately 10% to 20% of U.S. couples have infertility, and today

Communication Cues 38–1

Emotional Impact of Infertility

The emotional impact of infertility is intense. Some couples become almost desperate to conceive. The nurse should be alert to evidence that psychological intervention may be needed to assist the couple to deal with the stress of their situation. Indications that a referral may be needed may include, but are not limited to, inability to focus on anything other than the desire to have a child, and tension in the relationship of the couple, including blaming each other.

more couples are seeking medical intervention. Infertility services also assist women without a male partner who wish to have a child.

The ability to conceive depends primarily on both partners having normal reproductive physiology, physiologically and psychologically sensitive interaction, and proper timing of intercourse. Factors in the male that contribute to infertility include problems with the sperm, abnormal ejaculation, abnormal erections, and abnormal seminal fluid. Chapter 39 presents a discussion of problems in the male reproductive system. Factors contributing to infertility in a woman include:

- Problems with ovulation
- An abnormality in the pathway between the cervix and fallopian tube
- An abnormality in the endometrium of the uterus, or malformation of the uterus
- Tumors in the reproductive tract
- Vaginal or cervical environment that is inhospitable to sperm motility or viability

Repeated pregnancy loss can be caused by an abnormality in fetal chromosomes that result in spontaneous abortion, abnormalities of the cervix or uterus, disorders of the endocrine or immune system, infections, or environmental factors, such as toxic agents. Preconception counseling helps the couple evaluate problems or risks related to conception (Communication Cues 38–1).

There are many causes of infertility; some involve a problem in the woman, and some in the partner. Diagnostic tests include a detailed health history and laboratory tests such as serum prolactin levels and other endocrine evaluations, semen analysis, sperm antibody agglutination studies, and chromosome studies. Tests for tubal patency and other possible abnormalities in both the male and female reproductive tract may also be needed.

Nursing Management

Interventions the nurse can discuss with the patient regarding infertility may include nonmedical actions such as:

- Using water-soluble lubricants during intercourse because these do not have spermicidal properties.

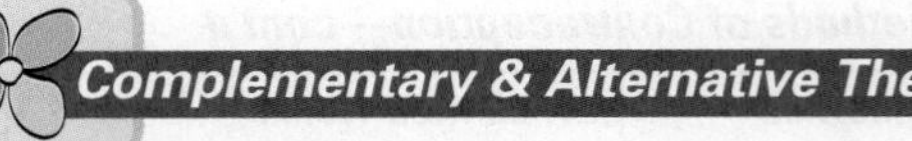

Complementary & Alternative Therapies 38–1

Herbal Products and Fertility

Since there is widespread use of complementary and alternative medicines (CAMs) such as herbs and oils, women should be instructed that use of herbs and oils such as licorice root, wormwood, fennel, ephedra, goldenseal, flaxseed, pennyroyal, cascara, sage, and periwinkle should be avoided while trying to conceive and carry a pregnancy (Breslin and Lucas, 2003).

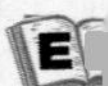

Herbal products that may be used to promote fertility include nettle leaves, dong quai, and red clover flowers. Vitamin E, calcium, and magnesium supplements have also been used. There is currently no scientific evidence that these herbal products are effective.

- Recommend that the male partner avoid environments that cause high scrotal temperatures, such as saunas, since this can reduce sperm production as well as the life span of the sperm.
- Using condoms when the woman has an elevated antisperm antibody level. After several months, condoms can be removed during the woman's fertile period.
- Referring the couple for stress management, nutrition counseling, and lifestyle analysis.

Interventions for infertility can also involve medical therapy such as the use of drugs that stimulate ovulation (Complementary & Alternative Therapies 38–1). Drugs to treat thyroid or adrenal problems in the male may enhance spermatogenesis.

Assisted Reproduction

Assisted reproductive therapies (ARTs) are available, but are associated with many ethical and legal issues such as the risk for having a multifetus pregnancy, freezing embryos for later use, and the use of a surrogate mother. Micromanipulation allows the removal of a single cell from an embryo for genetic analysis. Defective genes can be replaced. Success rates of ART vary, and the procedure is usually expensive and rarely covered by health insurance. Donor eggs or donor sperm can be used, making future legal challenges for custody a possibility. Box 38–1 lists some types of ART procedures.

MENOPAUSE

Menopause is defined by the World Health Organization as the cessation of menses for 12 consecutive months due to a decrease in estrogen production. The *perimenopausal period* or *climacteric* is the time around the actual cessation of the menstrual cycle.

Signs and symptoms of the climacteric and menopause include hot flashes (a sensation of warmth), hot flushes (a visible redness and moistness of the skin), and night sweats due to vasomotor instability resulting from low estrogen levels. These symptoms

Box 38–1 *Some Assisted Reproductive Therapies (ART) Procedures*

- **In vitro fertilization (IVF-ET):** Woman's eggs are collected from the ovary, fertilized in the laboratory, and transferred into the uterus at the embryo stage of development.
- **Zygote intrafallopian transfer (ZIFT):** After in vitro fertilization, the ovum is placed into the fallopian tube at the zygote stage of development.
- **Therapeutic donor insemination (TDI):** A donor's sperm inseminates the female.
- **Intracytoplasmic sperm injection:** Injection of one live sperm directly into the mature egg.
- **Surrogate mother:** The surrogate mother can be inseminated with the partner's sperm or an egg, fertilized by the partner's sperm in vitro. The egg is transferred to the uterus of the surrogate mother; she becomes a gestational carrier.

usually decrease as the woman's body adjusts to the lower level of estrogen. Changes in the menstrual flow and menstrual irregularity require the woman to "be prepared" for an unexpected menstrual period. The aging process as well as the decrease in estrogen levels can cause thinning of the vaginal walls *(atrophy)* as well as dryness and itching of the vagina **(pruritus)**. These changes may result in painful sexual relations **(dyspareunia)** and can also lead to increased susceptibility to infections because the vaginal pH increases.

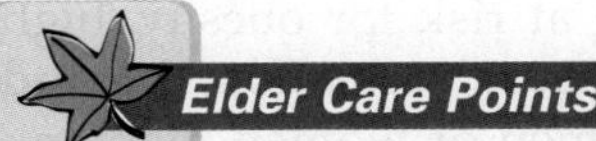

Elder Care Points

The significant reduction in estrogen after menopause (about 80% less than during the reproductive years) causes a decrease in natural vaginal lubrication. Women may be prescribed vaginal creams containing estrogen to restore moisture and elasticity to vaginal tissues. They should be cautioned not to use the estrogen cream as a lubricant for sexual intercourse as their partner may absorb the estrogen. Nonmedicated lubricants should be used for this purpose if necessary.

The psychological response to menopause has resulted in referring to that period as "the change in life" that can bring some women's personal coping skills into play and require family support in maintaining a sense of purpose in life. Other women feel a sense of freedom from the need for contraception or medication for cramping.

Our Western culture values youth and beauty, and the onset of the menopause may be seen by some women as a loss of attractiveness and the first step to old age. In other cultural groups, the wisdom gained from life's experiences is valued. Nurses must understand the perceptions of the woman and the family before designing and implementing a teaching plan.

Box 38–2 *Lifestyle Activities that Increase Risk of Osteoporosis*

- **Excess caffeine intake:** Increases calcium excretion
- **Smoking:** Decreases estrogen production
- **Excess alcohol intake:** Interferes with calcium absorption and depresses new bone growth
- **Excess cola or soft drink intake:** Results in imbalanced calcium and phosphorus or demineralizes bone

Health Risks of Menopause

The major health problems that occur at or after menopause include the development of osteoporosis and coronary heart disease.

Osteoporosis. Osteoporosis is a decrease in bone mass that increases the risk for bone fractures. The decrease in estrogen that occurs during menopause slows bone growth, and therefore bone deteriorates and thins before new bone growth occurs. Estrogen also enables vitamin D to assist in calcium absorption in the intestine, and a decrease in estrogen is associated with a decrease in calcium, which is essential to healthy bone tissue. Box 38–2 provides a list of some lifestyle activities that may increase the risk of developing osteoporosis.

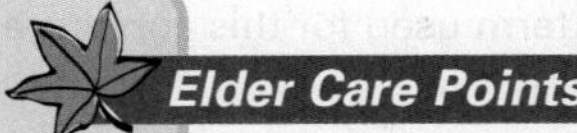

Elder Care Points

A large number of older women are now on long-term estrogen replacement therapy to prevent osteoporosis. The increased risk for endometrial cancer, as well as the possible relationship to breast cancer, makes it particularly important that these women have annual pelvic examinations and perform breast self-examination regularly.

The first signs of osteoporosis are loss of height, back pain, and the development of a **"dowager's hump"** in which vertebrae fail to support the upper body in an upright position (Figure 38–4). The ACOG Women's Health Care Physicians recommend bone density screening for menopausal women (ACOG, 2004). Refer to Chapter 32 for full coverage of osteoporosis.

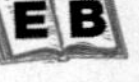

Coronary Heart Disease. Postmenopausal women are at increased risk for coronary heart disease due to changes in lipid metabolism and a rise in total cholesterol. Diet and exercise can have a positive effect in minimizing the effects of these risks. See Chapters 19 and 20 for details concerning cardiovascular diseases.

Treatment Options During Menopause

Hormone Therapy. In the past, hormone (estrogen) replacement therapy (HRT) was the cornerstone of interventions that reduced the discomforts of menopause (hot flashes and vaginal atrophy) and protected women from developing coronary heart disease and osteoporosis. Recent research has offered evidence

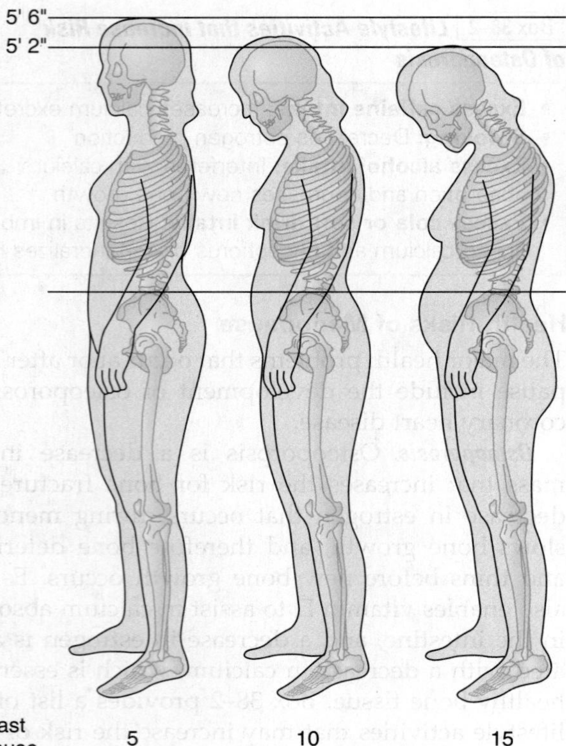

FIGURE 38–4 Osteoporosis. With progression of osteoporosis, the vertebral column collapses, causing loss of height and back pain. *Dowager's hump* is the term used for this curvature of the back.

that HRT can increase the risk of developing blood clots, stroke, and heart attack and even breast cancer. The ACOG recommends careful selection of patients for HRT and detailed education concerning risks of therapy (Hacker et al., 2004).

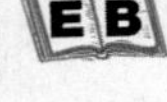

Alternative Therapies. Some CAM therapies have been helpful in relieving specific discomforts of menopause. Homeopathy, acupuncture, and certain herbs may offer relief, but each may have contraindications as well. Herbal therapy has not been fully researched or regulated, and some side effects or interactions with food or drugs are possible (Health Promotion Points 38–1). Phytoestrogens, soy products, and vitamins B, C, and E have also been helpful in relieving menopausal discomforts (Nutritional Therapies 38–1). Medications such as Fosamax can be prescribed for women with osteoporosis, but side effects should be explained carefully. After taking Fosamax, the woman must be able to sit upright for at least 30 minutes. Diet, exercise, and support groups are very effective in helping to manage menopause. When hot flashes significantly affect a woman's quality of life, nonhormonal medication may be recommended. Studies have shown that medications such as venlafaxine (Effexor) and clonidine (Catapress), soy isoflavones, and CAM therapies such as black cohosh *(Cimicifuga racemosa)* show promise for relief of hot flash symptoms (Carroll, 2006).

EB

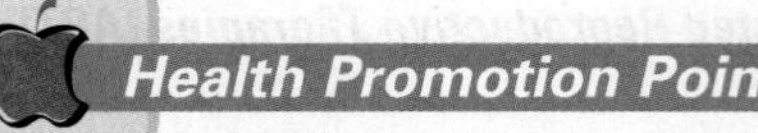

Health Promotion Points 38–1

Using CAM Therapies for Menopause

Women should be encouraged to consult with a health care provider before using complementary and alternative medicine (CAM) therapies such as soy isoflavones, black cohosh, or other herbs. For some women these substances may be contraindicated. Certain herbs may interact with other medications the patient is taking.

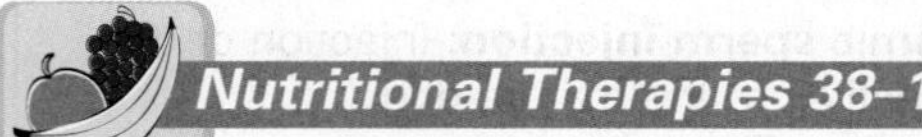

Nutritional Therapies 38–1

Managing Menopause

When phytoestrogens are recommended by the health care provider, teaching about these substances should be provided. Phytoestrogens are found in foods such as wild yams, cherries, dandelion greens, alfalfa sprouts, and black beans. Food sources of soy include tofu, soy milk, and roasted soy nuts.

HEALTH SCREENING AND ASSESSMENTS

Health screening is a form of preventive care. *Primary prevention* is designed to decrease the probability of becoming ill, such as maintaining a health or nutrition history and providing immunizations. *Secondary prevention* is designed to focus on detection of specific at-risk diseases so that early treatment may be given (such as annual mammograms). *Tertiary prevention* minimizes the impact of an already diagnosed condition.

All adult women may be at risk for obesity, high cholesterol, high blood pressure, osteoporosis, and dental disease. Pregnant women or women planning pregnancy may be at risk for a folic acid deficiency that could result in a neural tube defect in the developing fetus; therefore, prenatal vitamins, including folic acid supplements, may be prescribed.

Health screening begins with the woman's visit to her health care provider. It is your responsibility to introduce yourself, ask pertinent questions, and document all information gathered. This phase is called *"collection of data."* The data collected identify the patient and summarize her personal health history, the community in which she lives, and her available support system. Some information concerning the woman's culture, lifestyle, and usual coping mechanisms will enable the design of an individualized plan of care. All data collection should include information regarding use of nonprescription as well as prescription medications and CAM therapy.

Breast Self-Examination

Breast self-examination (BSE) should be done monthly, about 1 week after menstruation begins, or on a specific date each month after menopause. The nurse plays a major role in teaching and encouraging women to perform BSE to detect breast lumps and thickened areas. Figure 38–5 illustrates the steps in the procedure. In ad-

1. POSITIONS

Visual Inspection: Standing in each position, look for changes in contour and shape of the breasts, color and texture of the skin and nipple and evidence of discharge from the nipples.

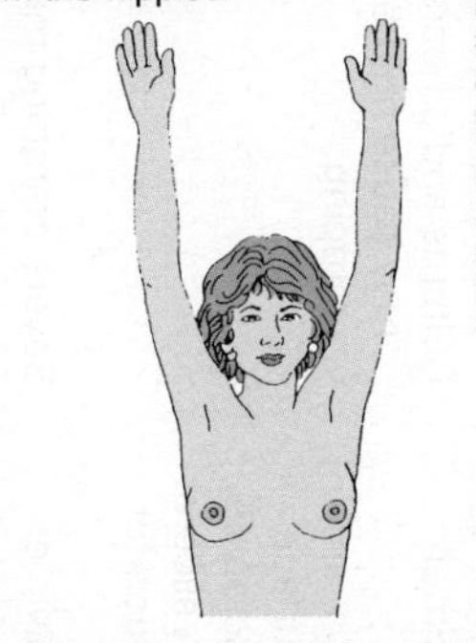

Arms raised above head

Hands on hips

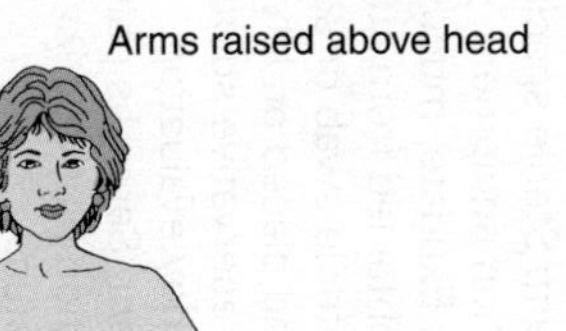

Bending forward

Arms relaxed at side

Palpation: Flat and Side-Lying:

Use your left hand to palpate the right breast, while holding your right arm at a right angle to the rib cage, with the elbow bent. Repeat the procedure on the other side. The side-lying position allows a woman, especially one with large breasts, to most effectively examine the outer half of the breast. A woman with small breasts may need only the flat position.

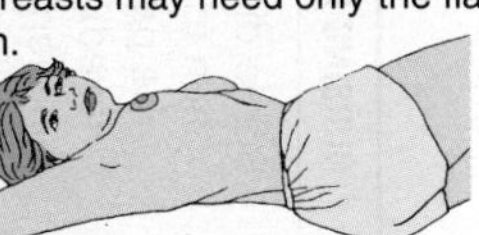

Side-lying Position: Lie on the opposite side of the breast to be examined. Rotate the shoulder (on the same side as the breast to be examined) back to the flat surface.

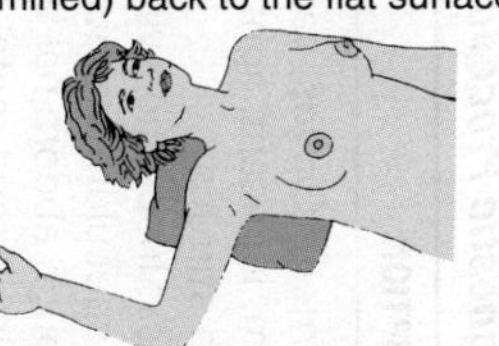

Flat Position: Lie flat on your back with a pillow or folded towel under the shoulder of the breast to be examined.

2. PERIMETER

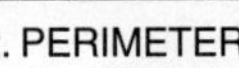

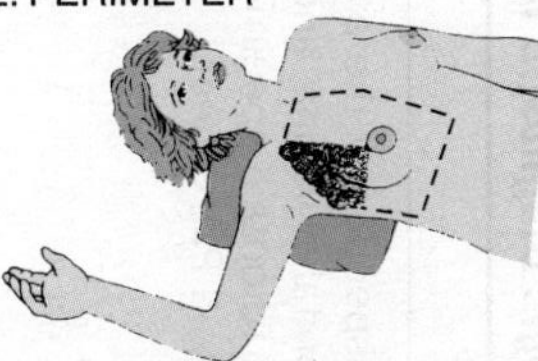

The examination area is bounded by a line that extends down from the middle of the armpit to just beneath the breast, continues across the underside of the breast to the middle of the breast bone, then moves up to and along the collarbone and back to the middle of the armpit. Most breast cancers occur in the upper outer area of the breast (shaded area).

3. PALPATION WITH PADS OF FINGERS

Use the pads of three or four fingers to examine every inch of your breast tissue. Move your fingers in circles about the size of a dime.

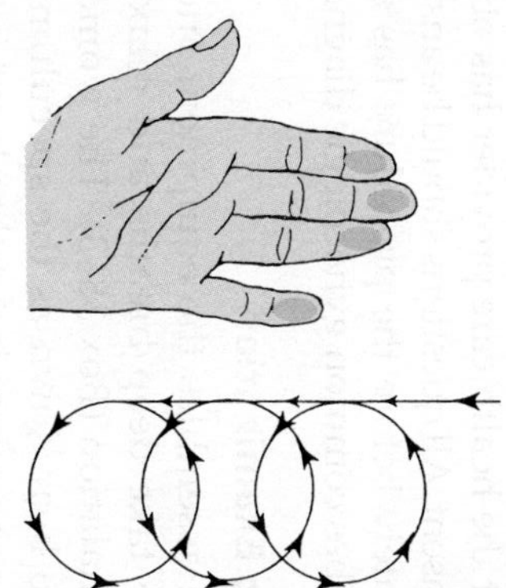

Do not lift your fingers from your breast between palpations. You can use powder or lotion to help your fingers glide from one spot to the next.

4. PRESSURE

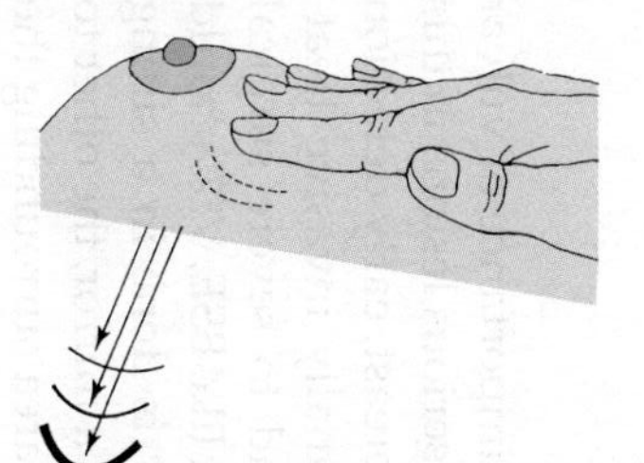

Use varying levels of pressure for each palpation, from light to deep, to examine the full thickness of your breast tissue. Using pressure will not injure the breast.

5. PATTERN OF SEARCH

Vertical Strip:

Using the following search pattern to examine all of your breast tissue, palpate carefully beneath the nipple. Any incision should also be carefully examined from end to end. Women who have had any breast surgery should examine the entire area and the incision.

Start in the armpit, proceed downward to the lower boundary. Move a finger's width toward the middle and continue palpating upward until you reach the collar bone. Repeat this until you have covered all the breast tissue. Make at least six strips before the nipple and four strips after the nipple. You may need between 10 and 16 strips.

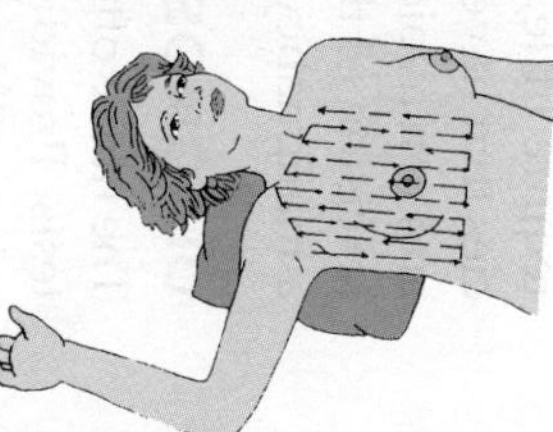

Nipple Discharge:

Squeeze your nipples to check for discharge. Many women have a normal discharge.

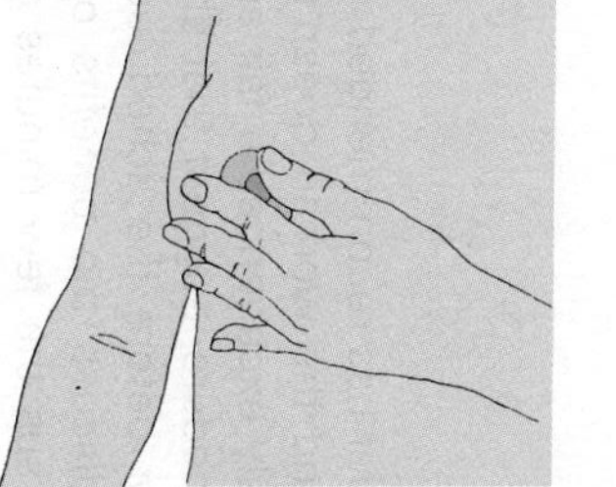

Axillary Examination:

Examine the breast tissue that extends into your armpit while your arm is relaxed at your side.

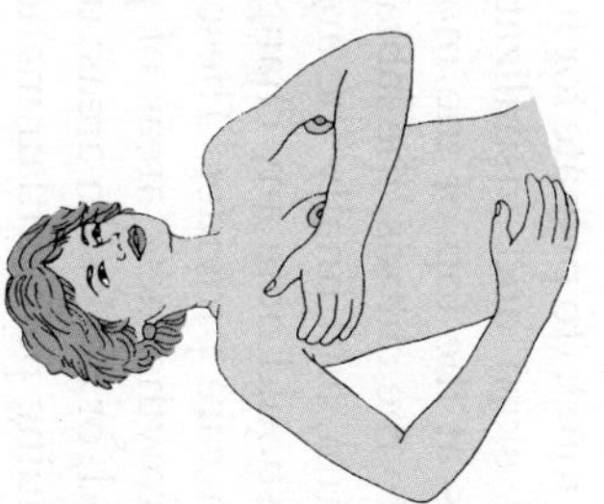

6. PRACTICE WITH FEEDBACK

It is important that you perform breast self-examination (BSE) while your instructor watches to be sure you are doing it correctly. Practice your skills until you feel comfortable and confident.

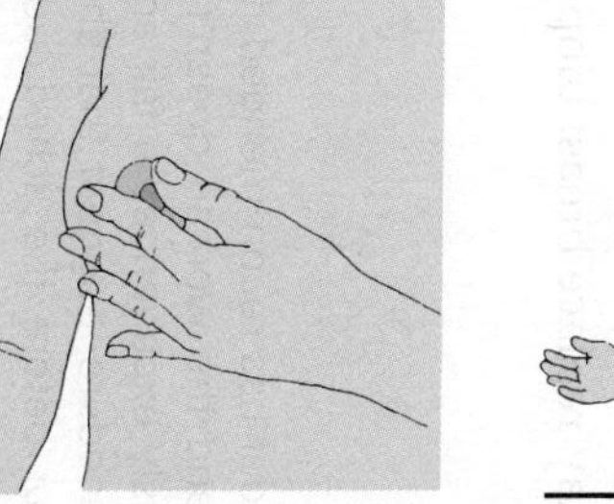

FIGURE **38–5** Recommended breast self-examination procedure.

dition, the American Cancer Society has videotapes available that demonstrate BSE.

New tests for breast cancer currently being researched include the cone-beam breast computed tomography scan that may replace current mammography. The scanner merges 300 x-rays taken in 10 seconds into 3D images. The breast is not compressed for the test. Ultrasound elastography has been supersensitive in identifying 100% of malignant tumors during trials, and the technique may replace breast biopsy.

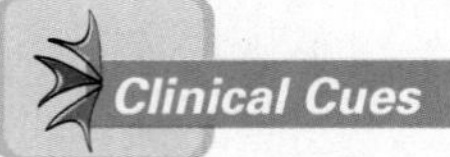

If the health care provider has recommended that a woman have a mammogram and the woman doesn't want to because she has previously experienced a fair amount of discomfort during the procedure, suggest that she take some acetaminophen an hour before the scheduled test unless contraindicated. Also discuss the benefits of discovering breast cancer early versus the few minutes of breast discomfort from the compression of the machine.

Vulvar Self-Examination

Many women are unaware of the importance of vulvar self-examination (VSE). Although serious lesions in this area are less common than in the breast, early detection allows for rapid and often minimally invasive treatment. Delay in detection can lead to severe surgical disfigurement and even death. Just like BSE, VSE should be performed monthly. It usually is done in a sitting position. One hand is used to hold a mirror, the other to separate the labia and expose the area surrounding the vagina. Using both touch (to palpate for lumps or thickening beneath the skin) and visualization, the self-examination begins at the top of the mons pubis and works downward to the clitoris, the labia majora, labia minora, the perineum, and finally the area around the anus. The woman should note any changes and report them to her health care provider. These include new moles, warts, or growths; new areas of pigmentation, especially white, red, or dark skin areas; ulcers or sores; and areas of continuing pain, inflammation, or itching. Most of these findings will not be malignancies and will require little, if any, treatment. Treatment of malignancies that have been detected early often is relatively easy and can avoid deformative surgeries such as *vulvectomy* (excision of the vulva) and prevent *metastasis* (spread of a malignancy to other areas of the body).

DIAGNOSTIC TESTS

The nurse often is asked to assist with various diagnostic tests. Providing the woman with a clear explanation of what will be done and what she can do to minimize discomfort is essential. A consent may be required with certain procedures, and the nurse is responsible for ensuring that the health care provider has obtained an informed consent. All questions should be answered clearly and accurately before the procedure has started. Table 38–4 describes common gynecologic diagnostic tests.

The Pelvic Examination

The nurse assembles the equipment and directs the woman to take deep breaths and relax all muscles during exhalation (Box 38–3). The woman can be instructed to bear down as the speculum is being inserted. The speculum is gently placed into the vagina

Table 38–4 *Common Gynecologic Diagnostic Tests and Diagnostic Procedures*

TEST	PURPOSE	DESCRIPTION	NURSING IMPLICATIONS
Pelvic examination	Visual inspection of the external genitalia, vagina, and cervix to obtain specimens such as a Pap smear.	*Equipment:* Gloves, vaginal speculum, lubricant, light, table with stirrups. *Process:* Inspection via the vaginal speculum; manual palpation through abdominal wall, vaginally, and rectally of internal organs.	Some discomfort during examination (decreased or eliminated if the patient remains fully relaxed). Nurse to ensure that patient is appropriately draped and correctly positioned in the stirrups. Examination time is usually 5–10 min.
Pap smear, thin prep	To obtain samples of cells and fluids for pathology/cytology studies.	*Equipment:* Sterile specimen collection equipment. *Process:* Exudate, mucus, and cells obtained from surface with sterile swab or scraping tool and placed on lab slide or into preservative solution for pathology evaluation.	Cultures and smears of the cervix may cause mild bleeding and cramping.
Endometrial biopsy	Postmenopausal bleeding, menstrual difficulties, infertility work-up.	*Equipment:* Same as pelvic examination plus suction biopsy apparatus. *Process:* A suction biopsy of the endometrium is performed via the cervical opening.	Severe cramping may occur during procedure. Patient is usually premedicated. Normally some vaginal bleeding follows; flow should not be heavy.

Key: *MRI,* magnetic resonance imaging; *Pap,* Papanicolaou; *PET,* positron-emission tomography.

Table 38–4 **Common Gynecologic Diagnostic Tests and Diagnostic Procedures—cont'd**

TEST	PURPOSE	DESCRIPTION	NURSING IMPLICATIONS
Colposcopy	Endoscopic examination of the vagina and cervix to evaluate abnormal cells and lesions, particularly after a positive Pap smear.	*Equipment:* Same as pelvic examination plus colposcope. *Process:* Area is visualized through the scope, with photos and possible biopsies of lesions requiring further study.	Patient is positioned as for pelvic examination. Procedure takes a few minutes. Biopsy may cause a small amount of bleeding and minor cramping. No tampons should be used until healing has occurred.
Hysteroscopy	Endoscopic examination of the interior of the uterus; may also involve procedures such as biopsy or removal of fibroids, adhesions, and septums. Endometrial laser ablation (destruction of areas within uterine lining) may also be performed.	*Process:* Hysteroscope is inserted vaginally, usually under local anesthesia. May also be done in combination with laparoscopy.	Occasional injury to cervix or uterine wall. If endometrial ablation is done, the woman will have difficulty becoming pregnant as the lining destruction is permanent.
Dilation and evacuation (D&E)	Detect cause of excessive bleeding; removal of hypertrophied uterine lining, retained placenta, or tissue remaining from incomplete abortion.	*Equipment:* Done in operating room. *Process:* The cervix is dilated and the interior of the uterus is cleansed by scraping, suction, or both.	Mild cramping and bleeding for up to 1 wk. Next period may be either early or late. Complications include uterine perforation, excessive bleeding, infection. Instruct patient to report heavy bleeding, clotting, sharp/severe abdominal pain, abnormal or foul discharge.
Mammography	To screen the breasts for abnormal growths, particularly cancer.	*Equipment:* Done in the radiology department with special x-ray equipment. *Process:* A full-field digital mammography machine records images on a computer screen and can computer-enhance questionable images for increased accuracy.	Breast discomfort from compression of the tissue during the test; occasional mild bruising. Instruct patient to wear no deodorant or lotion on the upper body and to wear clothing that allows top to be easily removed.
Ultrasound (sonogram)	*Pregnancy:* To determine gestation; screen for birth defects or placental abnormalities. *Gynecology:* Determine presence, location, and size of abdominal mass; determine whether a mass is *cystic* (fluid filled) or solid; locate intrauterine device; monitor ovulation in infertility.	*Equipment:* Ultrasound machine. *Process:* Sound wave transducer emits inaudible sound waves that record interior structures on the ultrasound screen. A videotape is made so results can be restudied and evaluated. A "picture" of the fetus may be provided to the parents.	Some tests require a full bladder, which may be uncomfortable during the test. The nurse should assist the woman to immediately empty her bladder after the examination. There are no known complications of ultrasound examination. Skin should be clean, dry, and free of lotions or powder. During pregnancy, up to two ultrasound examinations may be required. The use of independent 3- or 4-dimensional ultrasound procedures for purposes of providing mementos to parents is not recommended, as the long-term effects of the extra energy used in these examinations on the fetus has not been researched.
Pelvic/vaginal ultrasound	To detect thickness of uterine lining, size of uterus, presence of fibroids; size of ovaries, and presence of cysts or tumor.	*Process:* Ultrasound transducer is passed over pelvic area or the transducer is inserted into the vagina and guided over areas of the surface.	Advise that there will be minor discomfort if vaginal transducer is used.

Continued

Table 38–4 Common Gynecologic Diagnostic Tests and Diagnostic Procedures—cont'd

TEST	PURPOSE	DESCRIPTION	NURSING IMPLICATIONS
Breast ultrasound	Differentiates benign tumor from malignant tumor. Useful in women with dense breast tissue and fibrocystic disease.	*Process:* A noninvasive painless procedure.	An ultrasound will not detect microcalcifications that a mammogram can detect.
PET scan	Used to stage breast cancer and detect skeletal lesions.	*Process:* Performed in radiotherapy unit.	
Breast MRI	Used for women with dense breast tissue.	*Process:* Images are taken with a magnetic resonance image machine.	Premedication to lessen anxiety for women with claustrophobia may be advised. Patient must not wear metal during test.
Breast biopsy	A diagnostic test for breast cancer. Usually performed when a suspicious breast lump is detected.	*Process:* A needle aspiration can be done on an outpatient basis under local anesthesia. An incisional biopsy can be done in a same-day surgery setting under local or general anesthesia. All removed tissue or fluid is sent to lab for analysis.	Check incision for bleeding. Encourage verbalization of fears. Schedule follow-up appointment for results of lab studies.

Box 38–3 Preparing the Woman for a Pelvic Examination

- The unit should provide privacy and good lighting.
- Assemble clean gloves and supplies.
- Orient the patient to the equipment and the purpose of the examination.
- Encourage the woman to void because a full bladder will make the examination more uncomfortable.
- Position and drape the patient appropriately.
  a. Lithotomy
  b. Side-lying
  c. Knee-chest
- Stay with the woman, encouraging her with information to promote comfort.

by the health care provider. The blades are then opened to view the cervix. Specimens may be collected for laboratory examination. A Papanicolaou (Pap) smear may be obtained to determine the presence of abnormal cells *(see Skill 38–1 Assisting with a Pelvic Examination and Pap Test [Smear] on Companion CD-ROM).* After the examination, the nurse can assist the woman to a sitting, then a standing position. Disposable tissues may be provided to wipe lubricant from the perineum. The patient usually dresses and returns to speak with the health care provider. Teaching may include the purpose of the tests performed, the need for routine checkups and Pap smears from the age the woman becomes sexually active, or from ages 20 to 40, and every 1 to 3 years thereafter.

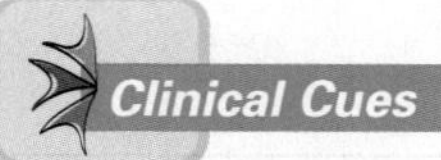

Clinical Cues

Talking to the patient and holding her hand, if possible, during the examination aids with distraction and enhances relaxation.

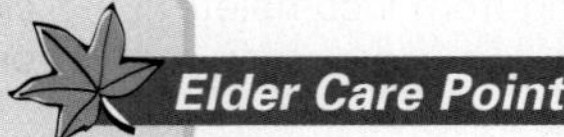

Elder Care Points

Women of advanced years may feel that they no longer need regular mammograms and Pap smears, particularly if they are not sexually active. They need to be aware that the incidence of breast and endometrial cancers increases with age and that annual screening becomes more, not less, important.

NURSING MANAGEMENT

Assessment (Data Collection)

The nurse is responsible for collecting essential data regarding the patient's reproductive history and gynecologic concerns (Focused Assessment 38–1). This can be difficult for both the patient and the nurse, as it involves discussing intimate aspects of the patient's body and personal life. The nurse should also record information on the cultural beliefs and attitudes regarding sexuality and sexual identity, reproduction, and body image as they all affect the assessment process (Cultural Cues 38–2). The nurse needs to ask questions in a tactful, yet matter-of-fact manner, as well as appreciate that the patient has the right to choose not to answer. A symptom diary can be very helpful. Note patterns of coping and available support persons.

Nursing Diagnosis

Nursing diagnoses commonly associated with gynecologic disorders include:

- Activity intolerance related to anemia from excessive blood loss, weakness, or disabling discomfort
- Excess fluid volume related to premenstrual fluid retention

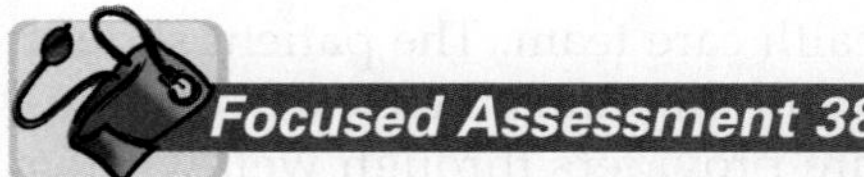

Focused Assessment 38–1

Data Collection for Gynecologic History

Sample questions when collecting data from a patient with a gynecologic problem include:

- How old were you when you began menstruating?
- Are your periods regular? How often do they occur? How long do they last?
- How heavy is your flow? Do you ever pass clots or pieces of tissue? Do you have pain before or during your period?
- Do you have cramps, headaches, or abdominal or back pain at other times of the month?
- Do you have mood swings, depression, or periods of tearfulness associated with your menstrual cycle?
- Are you having any vaginal discharge or itching?
- Do you have bleeding or spotting between your periods?
- Do you have any problems urinating, including burning, pain, or incontinence?
- How many times have you been pregnant?
- Have you had any miscarriages?
- Have you ever had a pelvic infection?
- Do you perform breast and vulvar self-examination?
- When was your last Pap smear?
- When was your last mammogram?
- Are you taking any medications routinely?
- Are you currently using any method of birth control, and if so, which method?
- Do you feel comfortable with your method or have a desire to change methods?
- Do you have any specific concerns or questions that we have not talked about?

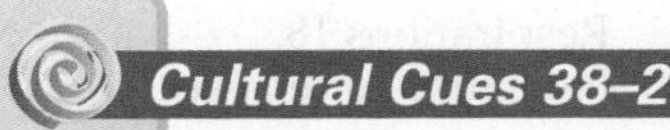

Cultural Cues 38–2

Culture and Women's Health

Cultural considerations can be particularly significant in the area of women's health care. Cultural views regarding sexuality, reproduction, and the role of women in society will have a direct bearing on the type of care sought and the amount and type of information the woman is willing and able to provide. The nurse must not pass judgment based on her own cultural bias, but must be culturally sensitive and supportive to the needs of women from diverse cultural backgrounds.

- Impaired skin integrity related to pruritus, genital lesions, and vaginal discharge
- Pain related to menstrual cycle, decreased vaginal lubrication, or vaginal irritation
- Sexual dysfunction related to dyspareunia (painful intercourse) or emotional issues
- Ineffective coping related to negative attitude about human sexuality or menstruation
- Disturbed body image related to surgery, fear of mutilating surgery, and loss of femininity
- Deficient knowledge about practices of personal feminine hygiene, normal anatomy, and physiology of the female reproductive organs, or safe methods of contraception
- Situational low self-esteem related to sterility, menopause, and surgery on a reproductive organ

Expected goals or outcomes include:

- Patient uses energy conservation techniques while maintaining activity levels within capabilities.
- Patient maintains adequate fluid volume with appropriate management techniques.
- Skin remains intact with healing of existing wounds.
- Patient verbalizes an acceptable level of pain relief and ability to engage in normal activities.
- Patient expresses satisfaction with physical intimacy patterns and experience.
- Patient develops improved method of communication, problem-solving techniques, and positive attitude to enable effective coping with signs and symptoms.
- Patient evidences enhanced body image and self-esteem with ability to accept altered body part or function.
- Patient demonstrates motivation to learn and verbalizes understanding of female hygiene and safe sex practices.
- Patient recognizes and accepts positive aspects of self.

Planning

Planning the care of a patient with a gynecologic problem depends on the specific disorder. However, prevention of infection, effective patient education, and emotional support are appropriate goals for the plan of care for all patients with a gynecologic problem. The needs of a patient facing gynecologic surgery would include pain management, education regarding the procedure and follow-up care, infection prevention, and supportive care specific to the procedure. A woman who will lose the ability to bear children because of an early hysterectomy may have very different supportive needs from those of the postmenopausal woman undergoing the same procedure. Surgery for breast cancer brings fears of a major change in body image and the possibility of death if the disease is not controlled. These issues need to be addressed in the plan of care. The plan for the patient with an infection would include an appropriate medication schedule, monitoring for effectiveness of treatment (e.g., fever, swelling, pain resolving), and monitoring for signs of an allergic response to the prescribed antimicrobial agent.

In the clinic setting, women may be attending for annual visits, reproductive or contraceptive counseling, treatment of infections or STIs, pre- and postnatal care, and a variety of other reasons. If the facility uses standardized care plans as a reference, they must be adapted to express the needs of the individual patient. Such plans are frequently used in hospitals, clinics, and other health care facilities.

The plan of care must address education, pain management needs, emotional and physical care, family impact, cultural influences, and financial constraints. Specific goals of care for any patient are based on nursing observation and assessment, prescriptions for medication and therapies, the patient's personal desires and goals, and input from other members of the health care team. The patient should agree to the goals, and they must be clearly communicated to other care providers through well-written care plans and documentation, as well as team conferences when appropriate. Nursing Care Plan 38–1 presents one example of a nursing care plan for a woman having a hysterectomy.

NURSING CARE PLAN 38–1

Care of the Patient After Hysterectomy

SCENARIO Marilyn Blair, age 52, has just returned to the unit after abdominal hysterectomy for multiple fibroids, metrorrhagia, and greatly increased uterine size that caused abdominal pain. She has an IV infusion of 1000 mL normal saline in the left forearm, an indwelling urinary catheter, an abdominal dressing, and patient-controlled analgesia (PCA) pump containing morphine. Her vital signs are BP, 138/82; P, 86; R, 16; Temp, 98.2° F (36.8° C).

PROBLEM/NURSING DIAGNOSIS *Pain and discomfort related to surgical incision*/Pain related to abdominal surgery.

Supporting assessment data *Subjective:* Pain at 7/10 on pain scale: "It hurts to turn." *Objective:* Abdominal hysterectomy incision.

Goals/Expected Outcomes	Nursing Interventions	Selected Rationale	Evaluation
Pain will be controlled by prescribed analgesia, avoiding episodes of acute pain	Instruct her in use of PCA pump. Give booster medication as ordered if needed.	When patient feels in control, anxiety is reduced and less pain medication may be required.	Analgesia via PCA pump provides good relief.
	Assess location, type, and quality of pain q 3–4 hr using a pain scale.	Assessing location and quality of pain may alert nurse to developing complications.	Pain at 3–5 on pain scale.
	Assist with repositioning and support with pillows to attain comfort. Provide quiet, darkened atmosphere for rest and sleep.	Changing position prevents stasis of circulation; comfortable, supported position promotes relaxation.	Assisted to reposition q 2 hr. Sleeping long intervals on side with pillow behind back and between knees for comfort.
	Monitor for side effects of analgesics, especially respiratory rate. Administer antiemetic as ordered at first signs of nausea to prevent vomiting and further pain.	Morphine can depress respiratory rate.	Respirations 18. No nausea or emesis.
	Check Foley catheter and tubing for patency frequently to prevent bladder distention.	Bladder distention can increase pain and cause infection due to stasis of urine in bladder.	Bladder not distended, Foley draining clear urine. Continue plan.

PROBLEM/NURSING DIAGNOSIS *Potential for hemorrhage*/Potential for deficient fluid volume related to potential hemorrhage.

Supporting assessment data *Objective*: Abdominal hysterectomy.

Goals/Expected Outcomes	Nursing Interventions	Selected Rationale	Evaluation
Vital signs (VS) will remain stable; no signs of shock or hemorrhage	Monitor VS frequently per postoperative protocol routine.	A rapid pulse and falling blood pressure can indicate development of shock.	VS are at baseline: BP 118/68; P 84; R 16.
	Check abdominal dressing and beneath patient for signs of bleeding with each set of VS; assess for bleeding from vaginal area.	Gravity can cause fluids to drain to a point beneath the patient.	Abdominal dressing clean and dry; no visible vaginal drainage.

Key: *BP*, blood pressure; *IV*, intravenous; *NPO*, nothing by mouth; *P*, pulse; *R*, respirations; *WBC*, white blood cell; *WNL*, within normal limits.

NURSING CARE PLAN 38–1

Care of the Patient After Hysterectomy—cont'd

Goals/Expected Outcomes	Nursing Interventions	Selected Rationale	Evaluation
	Assess for signs of intra-abdominal bleeding; such as increasing abdominal girth, decreasing bowel sounds, and increasing abdominal pain and rigidity.	Intra-abdominal bleeding is a complication of abdominal hysterectomy.	Abdomen soft; bowel sounds have returned; no evidence of intra-abdominal bleeding. Continue plan.

PROBLEM/NURSING DIAGNOSIS *Surgicial incision causing pain on inspiration*/Risk for ineffective breathing pattern related to pain.

Supporting assessment data *Subjective:* "It hurts to take a deep breath." *Objective:* Abdominal hysterectomy.

Goals/Expected Outcomes	Nursing Interventions	Selected Rationale	Evaluation
Patient will have no signs of atelectasis or pneumonia as evidenced by clear breath sounds in all lung fields and afebrile status	Assist patient to use an incentive spirometer, sit up to deep-breathe and cough q 2 hr while awake; give small pillow and instruct her on how to splint incision before coughing.	Cough and deep-breathing exercises can prevent development of atelectasis. Pain can prevent patient from taking deep breaths.	Able to deep breathe and cough at 8 and 10 A.M. and 12 and 2 P.M. Sitting on side of bed q 2 hr while awake.
	Enlist aid of family or significant others in reminding patient to deep-breathe.	Others can provide encouragement and support.	Family helping and reminding patient to do breathing exercises.
	Report adventitious, diminished, or absent breath sounds or crackles.	Abnormal breath sounds can be sign of developing complications.	Lung sounds clear bilaterally; all VS are WNL; Temp, 98.0° F (36.7° C). Continue plan.

PROBLEM/NURSING DIAGNOSIS *Skin disrupted by surgical incision*/Risk for infection related to surgery.

Supporting assessment data *Objective:* Abdominal surgical incision.

Goals/Expected Outcomes	Nursing Interventions	Selected Rationale	Evaluation
Patient will be without signs and symptoms of infection at discharge	Administer prophylactic antibiotics as ordered.	Antibiotics kill pathogens.	Tolerating prescribed medications.
	Monitor incision for signs of redness, swelling, purulent drainage, or hardness.	Redness, swelling, drainage, and pain at an incision site may be signs of infection.	No incisional redness, swelling, hardness, or purulent drainage.
	Keep dressing clean and dry.	A wound dressing must be kept clean and dry to prevent contamination that can cause infection.	Dressing clean and dry.
	Use careful aseptic technique when changing dressings.		
	Monitor WBC count and temperature.		WBC count WNL; afebrile.
	Assess vaginal drainage for signs of odor or change in character.	Odor or purulent appearance of vaginal drainage may indicate infection.	Vaginal drainage is minimal and without odor.
	Assess abdomen for signs of infection, increasing pain, localized tenderness, swelling, increased *erythema* (redness) around wound edges, decreased bowel sounds.	Tenderness, swelling, increased erythema, and decreased bowel sounds are signs of intra-abdominal infection.	Abdomen soft, active bowel sounds; no signs or symptoms of infection. Continue plan.

Continued

NURSING CARE PLAN 38–1

Care of the Patient After Hysterectomy—cont'd

PROBLEM/NURSING DIAGNOSIS *Potential for blood clots from inactivity*/Risk for injury related to possibility of thrombophlebitis from bed rest and abdominopelvic surgery.

Supporting assessment data *Objective:* Abdominal hysterectomy and decreased activity level.

Goals/Expected Outcomes	Nursing Interventions	Selected Rationale	Evaluation
Patient will not exhibit signs of thrombophlebitis at time of discharge	Encourage ambulation as soon as it is ordered; explain benefits of walking.	Range-of-motion exercise and early ambulation can prevent the development of thrombus formation.	Leg and ankle exercises q 2 hr while awake, and is tolerating ambulation.
	Assist with leg and ankle exercises q 2 hr.	Leg exercises increase circulation and prevent blood pooling.	
	Monitor SCDs q shift.	SCDs prevent pooling.	SCDs functioning properly.
	Encourage added fluid intake as soon as diet order allows.	Extra liquids keeps blood more fluid and less likley to clot.	Presently NPO with IV fluids.
	Inspect lower legs q shift; check for positive Homans' sign.	A positive Homans' sign may indicate development of thrombophlebitis.	Homans' sign negative. Continue plan.

PROBLEM/NURSING DIAGNOSIS *Worried that she has lost her feminity*/Disturbed body image related to removal of uterus.

Supporting assessment data *Subjective*: "I wonder how this will affect my husband's view of me." *Objective:* Abdominal hysterectomy.

Goals/Expected Outcomes	Nursing Interventions	Selected Rationale	Evaluation
Patient will express her concerns over loss of uterus before discharge	Provide openings for conversation regarding patient's concerns over loss of her uterus and its meaning to her.	Enabling patient to verbalize and express concerns will make it possible to establish a patient-centered plan of care and teaching.	Patient is able to begin discussion about her concerns; will continue tomorrow. Continue plan.
Patient will accept new body image within 3 mo as evidenced by lack of depression and reinvestment in usual activities	Explore her feelings regarding sexuality after hysterectomy.		
	Encourage expression of positive aspects of having the hysterectomy and how she as a person is unchanged.		

? CRITICAL THINKING QUESTIONS

1. Following an abdominal hysterectomy, this 52-year-old woman appears depressed and states she is worried her marital relations will "never be the same." What is the best response of the nurse?
2. Aside from an abdominal hysterectomy, what other options for the treatment of uterine fibroids are available?

Implementation

The patient's needs must always be addressed when implementing various aspects of the plan of care. Table 38–5 contains detailed information on various types of surgical procedures that are used for different gynecologic problems. Education must be done in a manner appropriate to the patient's knowledge base and her ability to learn new information. Patient teaching should form an important aspect of each nursing contact.

Evaluation

Any nursing intervention requires evaluation of its effectiveness. This can be accomplished by asking the following questions: How effective were pain control measures? How is the patient tolerating the change in diet or new therapy? Have there been any adverse reactions to medications or treatments? A decision to continue the plan of care or revise the plan of care is the outcome of evaluation.

Table 38–5 ***Gynecologic Surgical Procedures***

SURGICAL PROCEDURE	REASONS FOR PERFORMING	DESCRIPTION	NURSING CARE AND TEACHING POINTS
Dilation and evacuation (D&E)	Excessive vaginal bleeding; incomplete abortion; removal of placental fragments; therapeutic abortion.	Scraping away the inner lining of the uterus (endometrium) via the cervix.	Observe for excessive bleeding postoperatively.
Conization, or conical excision	Removal of abnormal or early cancerous tissue; biopsy.	Removal of cone of tissue with scalpel or electrical cutting wire.	Office procedure. May cause some bleeding.
Fistulectomy	Presence of rectovaginal fistula (channel between rectum and vagina) or urethrovaginal fistula (channel between bladder and vagina).	Surgical excision of the fistula and repair of the tissue to prevent passage of urine or feces into the vagina.	Observe for excessive bleeding or for vaginal fecal drainage postoperatively.
Hysterectomy	Prolapse of pelvic organs; pain associated with pelvic congestion; endometriosis; excessive/debilitating uterine bleeding; fibroids; noninvasive uterine or cervical cancer.	Removal of entire uterus, vaginally or abdominally.	Observe for excessive bleeding; paralytic ileus can occur. Ends childbearing if premenopausal, which may have profound emotional impact.
Panhysterectomy	Cancer; pain associated with pelvic inflammatory disease; recurrent ovarian cysts.	Removal of entire uterus, fallopian tubes, and ovaries.	See hysterectomy. Removal of ovaries induces menopause in premenopausal women.
Radical hysterectomy	Invasive cancer.	Removal of uterus, tubes, ovaries, upper third of vagina, and lymph nodes.	See hysterectomy and panhysterectomy. Vaginal alteration may affect ability to have sexual intercourse. Possible lymphedema due to removal of nodes.
Anterior and posterior colporrhaphy	Presence of prolapse of bladder and rectum into the vagina; may accompany a uterine prolapse.	Repair of the anterior and posterior wall of the vagina.	Observe for excessive bleeding.
Salpingectomy	Tubal pregnancy; tumor; traumatic injury.	Removal of a fallopian tube.	Will not cause infertility if other tube/ovary is intact.
Oophorectomy	Tumor; cystic disease; endometriosis; traumatic injury; severe hormonal disorder.	Removal of an ovary.	See salpingectomy. Only a portion of one ovary is necessary to provide normal hormonal balance prior to menopause.
Vulvectomy/endoscopic laparoscopy	Malignancy.	Radical vulvectomy: surgical excision of the labia, clitoris, perineal structures, femoral and inguinal lymphatic tissues.	Major disfigurement; extreme supportive measures, including professional counseling, often required.

DISORDERS OF THE FEMALE REPRODUCTIVE TRACT

PELVIC RELAXATION SYNDROME (CYSTOCELE, RECTOCELE, ENTEROCELE, AND UTERINE PROLAPSE)

When the muscles, ligaments, and fascia that support the pelvic floor weaken, the pelvic organs may descend toward the vaginal orifice. It can affect the bladder (cystocele), rectum (rectocele), bowel (enterocele), or uterus (uterine prolapse).

Etiology and Pathophysiology

Because the lack of estrogen results in weakening of tissue structures, pelvic relaxation syndrome may occur as women age. The bladder protrudes through the vaginal wall, forming a cystocele, or into the rectum, forming a rectocele. Our increasing life span results in these problems occurring more commonly. Heavy lifting, constipation, and obesity contribute to the weakening of the pelvic floor muscles and tissues. Pelvic surgery and the strain of vaginal childbirth may also contribute to the development of pelvic relaxation syndrome.

Signs and Symptoms

Symptoms relate to the specific organs involved. In a cystocele, urinary frequency or incontinence is most common. A rectocele may result in constipation, soiling, or painful defecation. A uterine prolapse may result in dyspareunia. The uterus may protrude from the vaginal orifice. The woman often complains of general symptoms that include a sense of fullness in the pelvis and backache. **Stress incontinence** (loss of small amount of urine during coughing, sneezing, or lifting objects may occur.

Diagnosis

Diagnosis is confirmed by history and physical examination. Obtain an obstetric history concerning the number of vaginal deliveries and the size of the infants, which may have contributed to the problem. A history of stress incontinence or constipation may indicate how the problem may interfere with activities of daily living. A computed tomography scan may be required if other pelvic pathology is suspected. The patient and the health care provider determine if a nonsurgical or surgical approach to management is most appropriate.

Treatment and Nursing Management

Nonsurgical Management. *Nonsurgical* management includes teaching the woman how to perform Kegel exercises in order to strengthen the pubococcygeal muscles that support the pelvic floor (refer to Patient Teaching 33–5).

Lifestyle changes include increasing fluid intake and a high-fiber diet to avoid constipation, avoiding heavy lifting, and maintaining an optimum weight. Hormone therapy may be prescribed (Complementary & Alternative Therapies 38–2). A *pessary* (a hard rubber or plastic ring) can be fitted into the vagina by the health care provider to provide support to the pelvic structures.

Surgical Management. The procedure to repair a cystocele or rectocele is called an anteroposterior repair *(colporrhaphy)*. A **hysterectomy** (removal of the uterus) may be indicated.

The management of stress incontinence includes minimally invasive surgery performed under local anesthesia, called a TVT sling procedure, wherein a transvaginal mesh sling is inserted to support the urethra. This procedure is contraindicated in women who plan to become pregnant or have a urinary tract infection or a blood-clotting problem (Stenchever, 2004). Postoperatively, the nurse must monitor bowel and bladder patency. Residual urine may be measured via catheterization after voiding. Routine postoperative pain management is provided. Refer to Chapter 34 for treatments for urinary incontinence.

POLYCYSTIC OVARIAN SYNDROME

Polycystic ovarian syndrome is a congenital condition in which many cysts develop on one or both ovaries and produce excess estrogen. High levels of testosterone and luteinizing hormone (LH), and low levels of follicle-stimulating hormone (FSH) occur. Signs and symptoms include irregular menstruation, infertility, hyperinsulinemia, and glucose tolerance problems. Excessive hair on the body **(hirsutism)** is common.

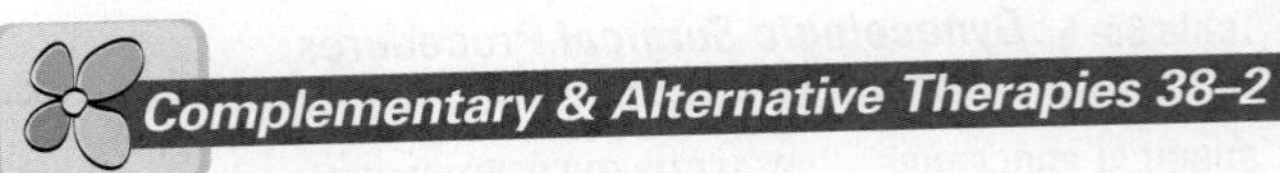

Biofeedback and TENS

Biofeedback and transcutaneous electrical nerve stimulation (TENS) may be offered by a licensed provider to help strengthen the pelvic floor muscles.

Treatment involves use of OCs to inhibit LH and testosterone production. Surgical removal of the cysts may be indicated. If pregnancy is desired, ovulation-stimulating medications are prescribed. The nurse should advise the patient concerning the importance of follow-up care to monitor the progress of this condition.

DYSFUNCTIONAL UTERINE BLEEDING

Dysfunctional uterine bleeding is uterine bleeding that occurs at times other than the normal menstrual cycle or abnormal bleeding during menstruation. Uterine bleeding may be considered abnormal if the interval between menstruations is less than 21 days or more than 45 days, the duration of menstrual flow is more than 7 days, or the amount of blood loss exceeds 80 mL.

Oligomenorrhea (decreased menstruation) usually refers to menstrual periods that occur at an interval of 45 days or longer. The cause often involves a problem with the hypothalamus, the pituitary gland, or ovarian function. Hormone therapy is the treatment of choice, and the woman should be educated concerning advantages and disadvantages of hormone therapy. The use of OCs can decrease menstrual flow. Structural abnormalities can cause obstructions or destruction of the endometrium, resulting in oligomenorrhea. The woman should be taught to keep close records of her menstrual cycle and associated symptoms.

Amenorrhea means absent menstruation. *Primary amenorrhea* refers to women who have not had a normal onset of menstrual periods (they never started to menstruate). *Secondary amenorrhea* applies to women who began normal menses that later ceased. Some causes can include anatomical defects such as *imperforate* (closed) hymen, an endocrine dysfunction affecting female hormones, chronic disease, extreme weight loss or obesity, emotional disturbances, drug side effect, excessive exercise, or poor nutrition. Amenorrhea occurs with pregnancy, but that is a normal occurrence. Goals of treatment include progression of normal pubertal development; prevention of complications such as osteoporosis, endometrial hyperplasia, or heart disease; and promotion of fertility.

Metrorrhagia is bleeding between menstrual periods. Occasionally, a brief episode of "spotting" occurs 14 days before the expected menstrual period (corresponding to the time of ovulation). This is known as "mittle staining" and is considered normal. Women who take OCs or have an IUD may have bleeding between menstrual periods, which is termed "breakthrough bleeding." The problem is usually resolved by adjustment of the medication or dosage. Causes of abnormal metrorrhagia include leiomyomas, uterine polyps, trauma, foreign body, malignancy, infection, or an interrupted pregnancy. The treatment depends on the cause. Nursing responsibilities include providing reassurance, support, and education.

Menorrhagia is excessive menstrual bleeding or duration of the menstrual period. There are many causes, including hormone imbalances, malignancies, fibroids, infections, and the use of some drugs. Treatment depends on the cause. The hemoglobin and hematocrit should always be assessed to determine the seriousness of the blood loss. Nursing interventions include education concerning follow-up care, an iron-rich diet, and information concerning treatment options available.

ABNORMAL UTERINE BLEEDING

Abnormal uterine bleeding is defined as uterine bleeding not related to the menstrual period. It is often caused by anovulation and a failure of hormonal changes during the menstrual cycle. It most often occurs at the beginning (menarche) or end (menopause) of the reproductive years. Bleeding due to continuous estrogen production can also occur due to thyroid dysfunction, polycystic ovarian disease, infection, trauma, or neoplasm. Use of some herbal products that promote estrogen activity can also cause dysfunctional or abnormal uterine bleeding.

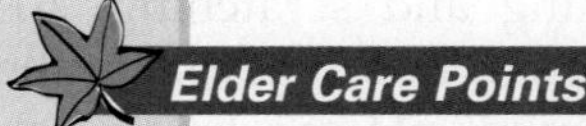

Elder Care Points

Vaginal bleeding in elderly women is a possible warning sign of cervical or uterine cancer. An immediate pelvic examination to determine and treat the cause of such bleeding is advised. The incidence of these cancers increases with age.

Monitoring the hemoglobin and hematocrit is essential, and hospitalization may be required if the hemoglobin falls below 8 g/100 mL. Severe bleeding may be treated with intravenous conjugated estrogens (Premarin) until bleeding stops or slows significantly. A dilation and evacuation (formerly known as a dilation and curettage) and endometrial biopsy may be required. The woman may be given oral contraceptives for 3 to 6 months, after which the bleeding pattern will be reassessed.

Persistent **anovulation** (failure to ovulate) with continuous estrogen stimulation of the endometrium can cause abnormal tissue changes in the uterus. Nursing interventions include educating the patient concerning the use of unsupervised CAM therapies and proper use of OCs, providing support during treatments, and ensuring that the patient is aware of treatment options.

LEIOMYOMA

Commonly known as uterine **fibroids,** leiomyomas are benign tumors of the uterine muscle. Their growth is influenced by ovarian hormones, and they are common in women taking birth control pills. They spontaneously shrink during and after menopause. Common symptoms include backache, a sense of lower abdominal pressure, constipation, urinary frequency or incontinence, and abnormal uterine bleeding. A pelvic examination and ultrasound may help confirm the diagnosis.

Medical management depends on the size and location of the fibroids, the symptoms experienced, the desire for future pregnancies, and how near the woman is to natural menopause. In mild cases, monitoring and supportive care to relieve symptoms are indicated. Nonsteroidal anti-inflammatory drugs or OCs may be prescribed. In severe cases, leuprolide (Lupron) or nafarelin (Synarel), which are gonadotropin-releasing hormone (GnRH) agonists that shrink the fibroids, and other hormones may be prescribed to suppress estrogen. These drugs may cause menopausal symptoms and bone demineralization, and their use is limited to a 6-month period to reduce the fibroids and prepare for surgery.

Uterine artery embolization involves the injection of special pellets into selected blood vessels that supply the fibroid, resulting in shrinkage of the fibroid. It is performed under conscious sedation by an interventional radiologist (an MD who is a radiologist and specializes in invasive procedures not requiring general anesthesia). Cramping, nausea, fever, and malaise (postembolic syndrome) may occur postoperatively as the fibroid degenerates. Postoperative pain may require an overnight hospitalization and treatment with fentanyl or dilaudid by patient-controlled analgesia. Maintenance of hydration and ambulation to prevent complications are encouraged postoperatively. After 6 weeks, magnetic resonance imaging (MRI) confirms the effectiveness of the procedure. Postoperative teaching includes avoiding the use of anticoagulant drugs, including aspirin; avoiding douches, sexual intercourse, and the use of tampons for 4 weeks postoperatively; monitoring urine output; preventing constipation; and returning for follow-up care.

Myomectomy is the removal of the tumor from the uterine wall and can be accomplished by use of an endoscope via an abdominal incision *(laparoscopy)* or vaginally *(hysteroscopy)*. It is performed in the proliferative phase of the menstrual cycle and does minimal damage to the uterine lining, allowing for positive pregnancy outcomes in the future. Fibroids can eventually return. *Hysteroscopic endometrial ablation* involves resection of submucosal fibroids followed by scraping and burning of tissue. This procedure significantly reduces future fertility. *Laser cauterization* of the fibroids can also be done laparascopically or vaginally but may scar the uterine wall and prevent future pregnancies. *Magnetic resonance–guided focused ultrasound surgery (MRgFUS)* is a safe way to significantly reduce symptoms of premenopausal uterine fibroids with a rapid return to quality of life (Stewart et al., 2006).

A hysterectomy may be performed if the woman does not wish future pregnancies. A laparoscopic supracervical hysterectomy preserves the cervix and

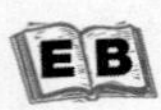

is less invasive, with fewer complications (Horbach et al., 2006). The postoperative teaching plan should include current information concerning advantages and disadvantages of hormone therapy, comfort measures for pain relief, and when to resume normal activities. The use of lubricants for vaginal intercourse and a plan for follow-up care should also be provided. Danger signs to report to the health care provider include bleeding or abnormal vaginal discharge.

ENDOMETRIOSIS

Endometriosis is a common disorder in which *endometrial tissue (the inner lining of the uterus) is found outside the uterus*, particularly on the ovaries, in the rectovaginal septum (wall separating the rectum and the vagina), and in the pelvis and abdomen. It usually undergoes the same changes as the normal endometrium during the menstrual cycle and may bleed at the time of menses, which can cause irritation, pain, and the formation of adhesions. Other symptoms may include excessive menstrual flow, bleeding between periods, painful bowel movements, and painful coitus.

Continuous hormonal contraceptive therapy and drugs such as medroxyprogesterone acetate (Depo-Provera) or norethindrone (Ortho Micronor) suppress growth of the endometrial tissue. Danazol (Cyclomen, Danocrine) and GnRH agonists such as leuprolide or nafarelin create a "pseudomenopause" by interfering with hormones that stimulate ovulation and menstruation. Menopausal symptoms such as hot flashes, decreased *libido* (sexual drive), and reduced bone density may occur. Continuous hormonal contraceptive treatment may be continued for 3 to 6 months. Surgical treatment may include a laparoscopy to remove adhesions or laser evaporation of the uterine tissue.

If the woman does not desire children in the future, a complete hysterectomy and removal of all endometrial lesions is the treatment of choice. Treatment for menopausal symptoms may be needed postoperatively.

INFLAMMATIONS OF THE LOWER GENITAL TRACT

Etiology and Pathophysiology

Inflammations or infections of the vulva, vagina, or cervix most often occur when the acid environment of the vaginal secretions changes, enabling the survival of pathogenic organisms. The acid environment of the vaginal vault is maintained by estrogen levels and the presence of *Lactobacillus*. Risk factors that alter the bacterial flora and pH environment within the vagina include aging; poor nutrition; the use of medications such as steroids, OCs, or antibiotics; and douching.

Organisms can also gain entrance to the vagina through contaminated hands, clothing, loss of skin integrity due to trauma or surgery, or sexual intercourse. Vulvar infections typically occur as a result of skin trauma caused by itching and scratching. Although *Candida albicans* is present in low levels in the vaginal area, a change in vaginal pH can lead to an overgrowth, resulting in vulvovaginitis (Table 38–6).

Table 38–6 ***Comparisons of Two Types of Common Vaginal Infections***

	BACTERIAL VAGINOSIS	YEAST INFECTION
Primary causative organism(s)	*Gardnerella* (most common).	*Candida* (formerly called *Monilia*).
Onset	May be asymptomatic.	Abrupt; preceding menstruation.
Odor	Fishy, most noticeable after intercourse.	None or mild "musty" odor.
Itching	Usually none (does not invade vaginal wall).	Severe; most prominent symptom.
Discharge	Thin, gray, may be frothy.	Thick, white, "cottage cheese" when colonization is heavy.
Sexually transmitted	Possibly; 70% of women have this organism present in vaginal flora.	Possibly. Associated with high estrogen levels; diabetes mellitus; tight underclothing that increases warmth and moisture.
Vulvar signs	Absent.	Redness; excoriation from scratching; may have edema of labia.
Vaginal signs	Vaginal pH above 4.6. Little redness; discharge adherent to vaginal wall, normal cervix.	Normal cervix, no discharge. Lesions and edema from scratching.
Treatment	Metronidazole orally, sometimes vaginally; clindamycin in second trimester if pregnant (associated with adverse pregnancy outcomes).	Miconazole, clotrimazole, or nystatin vaginally as directed. Oral treatment: fluconazole (Diflucan) 150-mg single dose. Nonprescription treatment is available.

Signs, Symptoms, and Diagnosis

A history and physical examination usually reveal the nature of the problem. Often lesions may be present, and *dysuria* (painful urination) often occurs because the acidic urine comes into contact with open lesions. An abnormal vaginal discharge may occur that often causes *pruritus* (itching discomfort). Women with cervicitis may experience bloody spotting after intercourse.

The diagnosis of the specific condition may be accomplished by culturing vaginal discharge or lesions, blood tests for specific infections, or a colposcopy or biopsy of the lesion. Drug therapy is based on the diagnosis.

Treatment and Nursing Management

You can teach the woman about the risks and prevention of genital infections as well as the treatment protocol for the specific infection. Infections of the lower genital tract are typically treated with local creams, vaginal suppositories, or systemic antimicrobials. Hand hygiene, wearing loose cotton underwear, and the use of intermittent warm, local, moist heat provide comfort and decrease irritation. Genital infections can cause the woman embarrassment, lower self-image, and negatively affect relationships. Providing psychological support is very important. Since many organisms that cause lower genital tract infections are spread by sexual intercourse, prompt treatment is essential in order to prevent the spread of infection to the upper genital tract. The importance of recognizing symptoms and seeking medical care should be stressed. A nonjudgmental attitude of the nurse will empower the woman to ask questions and seek advice. The nurse ensures that the woman fully understands directions for taking medication or applying creams, and visual aids should be used whenever possible to ensure clarity of directions. Infections of the lower genital tract that are also STIs, such as pelvic inflammatory disease, are discussed in Chapter 40.

TOXIC SHOCK SYNDROME

Toxic shock syndrome (TSS) is a rare and potentially fatal disorder caused by strains of *Staphyloccocus aureus* that produce toxins that cause shock, coagulation defects, and tissue damage if they enter the bloodstream. It is associated with the trapping of bacteria within the reproductive tract for a prolonged time. Risk factors include the prolonged use of high-absorbency tampons, cervical caps, or diaphragms.

Symptoms of TSS include:

- Sudden spiking fever
- Flulike symptoms
- Hypotension
- Generalized rash resembling a sunburn
- Peeling skin on the palms or soles

Treatment includes hospitalization and intensive care with intravenous antibiotics. The nurse plays an important role in preventing TSS by teaching the woman hand hygiene when inserting tampons, and the importance of changing tampons every 4 hours. Tampons should not be used when sleeping as they will likely remain in place longer than 4 hours.

CANCER OF THE REPRODUCTIVE TRACT

VULVAR CANCER

Vulvar intraepithelial neoplasia (VIN) refers to the growth of abnormal tissue on the vulva that may be precancerous. Cancer of the vulva is rare, and occurs most commonly in elderly women. Symptoms include red, brown, or white patches on the skin of the vulva. Treatment includes surgical removal of the pathologic tissue. Some strains of VIN are associated with the human papillomavirus (HPV). The incorporation of the HPV vaccine (Gardasil) into the standard immunization regimen for all girls will further reduce the incidence of this condition.

CANCER OF THE CERVIX

Malignant tumors of the cervix are another cancer that may occur in women. Risk factors include multiple sex partners, sexual intercourse with uncircumcised males, starting intercourse at a young age (younger than 20 years of age), multiple pregnancies, obesity, and history of HPV infection or an STI. A newly approved HPV vaccine given to girls at or before puberty may prevent the type of HPV infection that causes cervical cancer. Regular pelvic examinations and Pap smears may enable early diagnosis and provide opportunity for early and more successful intervention. Treatment may include cryosurgery, electrosurgical incision, or surgical conization of the cervix. Advanced cervical cancer may require a hysterectomy with bilateral salpingo-oophorectomy (removal of the uterus, including the fallopian tubes and ovaries) followed by radiation and chemotherapy. See Chapter 8 for discussion of care of a patient receiving radiation or chemotherapy.

CANCER OF THE UTERUS

The most common malignant tumor of the female reproductive tract is endometrial cancer. It is a slow-growing cancer that most often occurs after menopause. The treatment of choice is a hysterectomy with bilateral salpingo-oophorectomy. Treatment is often complicated by the fact that many women with cancer of the uterus may be elderly, or have chronic conditions such as diabetes. Surgery is often followed by radiation and chemotherapy. Chemotherapy agents used are doxorubicin (Adriamycin), cisplatin (Platinol), 5-fluorouracil (5-FU), carboplatin (Paraplatin), and paclitaxel (Taxol). See Chapter 8 for discussion concerning care of the patient receiving chemotherapy and radiation therapy.

CANCER OF THE OVARY

Approximately 70% of ovarian tumors are benign. Ovarian cancer is known as a "silent cancer" because signs and symptoms are often nonspecific or vague, such as fatigue or abdominal distention with no detectable precancerous changes in the ovary (Health Promotion Points 38–2). An important risk factor for the development of ovarian cancer is having a sister or mother with the disease, or inheriting the *BRCA1* or *BRCA2* gene, which is also associated with breast cancer. Exposure to asbestos, talc powder, pelvic irradiation, or mumps has also been linked to the development of ovarian cancer. Factors that may prevent ovarian cancer include one or more term pregnancies, breast-feeding, tubal sterilization, and possibly the use of OCs (Condon, 2004). Ovarian cancer is classified according to the type of tissue within the ovary that is involved. Diagnosis is often made during a routine pelvic examination. An ovarian cancer tumor marker (CA-125), assessed by a blood test, combined with pelvic ultrasound can detect ovarian cancer, but not at an early stage. Researchers at Yale Medical School have a new test under development and trials that could detect ovarian cancer in the early stages. However, at this date, the CA-125 test is not covered by most insurance companies for routine screening. Once diagnosis is established, a *panhysterectomy* (removal of the uterus, the fallopian tubes, and the ovaries) is followed by chemotherapy and radiation. Newer drugs have improved the survival rate to 50% (Cass & Karlan, 2003). Cisplatin (Platinol), and carboplatin (Paraplatin) are used for stage III and stage IV disease. Altretamine (Hexalen) is used for recurrent ovarian cancer. Paclitaxel (Taxol) and topotecan (Hycamtin) are used to treat metastatic ovarian cancer (see Health Promotion Points 38–2). See Chapter 8 concerning care of the patient with cancer.

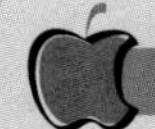

Health Promotion Points 38–2

Symptoms of Ovarian Cancer

On June 18, 2007, the American Cancer Society identified warning signs of ovarian cancer as:

- Abdominal pain
- Feeling full quickly when eating
- Feeling a frequent or urgent need to urinate

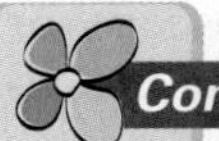

Complementary & Alternative Therapies 38–3

CAM Therapy for FBC

Relaxation techniques and herbal therapy with angelica, lady's mantle, or evening primrose oil are helpful in fibrocystic breast changes (FBC).

DISORDERS OF THE BREAST

Although the breast is not a reproductive organ, it is affected by hormonal changes related to the menstrual cycle as well as after pregnancy; therefore, it is discussed in this chapter.

BENIGN DISORDERS OF THE BREAST

Fibroadenoma

Fibroadenomas are commonly found in the teenager and young adult. Fibroadenomas are firm, rubbery, mobile nodules of fibrous and glandular tissue that may or may not be tender on palpation. They usually occur in the upper outer quadrant of the breast and do not change during the menstrual cycle. A fine needle aspiration or biopsy may be performed to determine the presence of cancerous cells.

Fibrocystic Breast Changes

Fibrocystic breast changes (FBCs) were formerly called *fibrocystic breast disorder.* This condition is common during the reproductive years. It is a palpable thickening of portions of the breast tissue associated with pain and tenderness. Multiple smooth, well-delineated cysts may form that are most painful during the premenstrual phase of the menstrual cycle. The "lumps" make BSE more difficult and are a frequent source of anxiety. Women with FBC can learn to recognize the size and shape of their normal lumps and should report any change in these findings as well as other changes to their health care provider. Treatment of fibrocystic changes is conservative and based on supportive care. Vitamin E supplements, the elimination of caffeine and alcohol, reduction of fat in the diet, and the use of nonsteroidal anti-inflammatory drugs such as ibuprofen help control discomforts found with FBC (Complementary & Alternative Therapies 38–3). Wearing a supportive bra and the use of heat are also helpful.

Intraductal Papilloma

Intraductal papilloma is the development of small elevations in the epithelium of the ducts of the breasts under the areola. The ducts erode, causing a serosanguineous discharge from the nipple. Treatment includes excision of the mass and analysis of the discharge to determine if cancer cells are present.

The nurse should clarify and reinforce the explanations of diagnostic procedures to be performed and recognize the anxiety and apprehension that the woman feels until the final diagnosis is confirmed. The woman should be encouraged to express her concerns, and supportive care should be provided.

BREAST CANCER

The United States has a high breast cancer rate, with approximately 178,480 women and 2030 men diagnosed with breast cancer in 2007 (American Cancer Society,

2007). The breast cancer rate for white women is higher than the rates for African American or Asian American women (American Cancer Society, 2003). The increased incidence of breast cancer may be due to the advanced technology that can detect cancer at an earlier stage. Although the risk of developing breast cancer increases with the woman's age, many other factors contribute to the risk (Box 38–4). Breast cancer is identified according to the structure affected and staged according to the size and degree of invasiveness (Table 38–7).

Etiology and Pathophysiology

The development of breast cancer is thought to be related to the hormones estrogen and progesterone. For example, women who start to menstruate at an early age (early menarche) and have late menopause are exposed to more estrogen spikes during monthly ovulation, whereas women who have had multiple pregnancies have fewer monthly ovulating cycles and hormonal spikes.

Recently, the genes *BRCA1* and *BRCA2* were identified as genes involved in the inherited form of breast cancer. Not all women who carry these genes will develop breast cancer, and some women who do not carry these genes will still develop breast cancer. A small percentage (5% to 10%) of newly diagnosed breast cancer is the inherited type, but 80% of the women with this gene develop breast cancer (Dell, 2005b). Genetic testing for this gene is available (Legal & Ethical Considerations 38–2).

The current breast cancer risk assessment tool developed by the National Cancer Institute (NCI) is available on the website www.cancer.gov.

The U.S. Preventive Services Task Force in 2005 did not recommend that routine genetic testing be done. BRCA testing costs about $2975 per test and is not usually covered by insurance. Significant risk factors that may warrant genetic counseling or BRCA testing include:

- In women of Ashkenazi Jewish descent:
  - A first-degree relative with breast/ovarian cancer
  - Two second-degree relatives on same side of family
- In women of non–Ashkenazi Jewish descent:
  - Two first-degree relatives with breast cancer, with one younger than age 50
  - Three first- or second-degree relatives with breast cancer
  - A first-degree relative with bilateral breast cancer
  - A history of breast cancer in a male relative (Nelson, 2004)

EB

Signs, Symptoms, and Diagnosis

Although 90% of breast lumps are detected by the woman during a BSE, most early breast cancer can be detected by mammography (x-ray examination of the breast) before it can be clinically palpated. A nipple discharge or change in the skin pattern such as "dimpled skin" on the breast may also be a sign of breast cancer. Any unilateral breast change should be immediately reported to a health care provider. Even a short delay in diagnosis can result in invasion of surrounding tissue and metastasis to other the parts of the body. Refer to Table 38–4 for details on the role of ultrasound or MRI diagnostic tests in confirming diagnosis.

Box 38–4 *Risk Factors for Breast Cancer*

- Family history of relative with breast cancer
- Early menarche, late menopause
- Late first pregnancy or no children
- Abnormal cells in previous breast biopsy
- Obesity
- Environmental exposure to hormone-modulating chemicals such as pesticides and polycyclic aromatic hydrocarbons found in meat barbequed or grilled at high temperatures.

Note that the specific cause of breast cancer has not been established. It is most likely due to genetic factors combined with environmental factors resulting in a cumulative risk level. Risk factors 1 to 4 are included on the National Cancer Institute (NCI) risk assessment tool. This can be accessed on www.cancer.org.

Prevention

A healthy lifestyle that includes exercise and a diet rich in antioxidants and phytoestrogens, such as vegetables, fruits, whole grains, and soy products, may protect against the development of many cancers. Monthly BSE (see Figure 38–5) and regular scheduled mammograms after age 40 are recommended by the ACOG. At present, the drug tamoxifen is used to prevent recurrent breast cancer but is not used as a general prophylactic measure in women with risk factors because of potential side effects such as increased bone pain, photosensitivity, headache, and increased risk for pulmonary embolism or uterine malignancies. The drug raloxifene (Evista) is FDA approved for the prevention of osteoporosis in postmenopausal women, and has now been found to play a significant role in breast cancer prevention (NCI, 2002). Aromatase inhibitors such as anastrozole or exemestane may be more effective than tamoxifen and are under current study (Speroff, 2006).

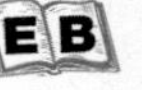

Some women who have known genetic *BRCA1* or *BRCA2* predispositions have elected to have prophylactic bilateral mastectomies. The psychological implications and effect on self-image should be carefully measured against the preventive benefits. The decision is between the woman and her health care provider.

Treatment

Treatment options are based on the type of breast cancer, stage of the disease, patient's age, physical and menopausal status, and other health factors that may

Table 38–7 *Stages of Breast Cancer*

CANCER STAGE	LOCATION	DESCRIPTION	5-YEAR SURVIVAL RATE
Stage 0	Carcinoma in situ	• Lobular carcinoma in situ (LCIS)—cancer cells in lining of a lobule. • Ductal carcinoma in situ (DCIS)—cancer cells in lining of a duct.	100%
Stage I	Early stage of invasive cancer	• Tumor is <2 cm in diameter. • Cancer cells have not spread beyond the breast.	100%
Stage II	Invasive	Any one of the following: • Tumor is <2 cm across. Cancer has spread to lymph nodes under the arm. • Tumor is between 2 and 5 cm. Cancer may have spread to lymph nodes under the arm. • Tumor is >5 cm. Cancer **has not** spread to lymph nodes under arm.	92%–81%
Stage III	Locally advanced	• Large tumor, but cancer has not spread beyond the breast and nearby lymph nodes.	
Stage IIIA		Any one of the following: • Tumor is <5 cm. Cancer has spread to underarm lymph nodes attached to each other or to other structures. • Tumor is >5 cm. Cancer has spread to underarm lymph nodes.	67%
Stage IIIB		Any one of the following: • Tumor has grown into chest wall or skin of the breast. • Cancer has spread to lymph nodes behind the breastbone. ***Inflammatory breast cancer*** is a rare type of Stage IIIB wherein breast looks red and swollen because cancer cells block the lymph vessels in the skin of the breast.	54%
Stage IIIC		Any size tumor that has: • Spread to lymph nodes behind the breastbone and under the arm. • Spread to lymph nodes under or above the collarbone.	This was defined only a few years ago, hence survival rate not yet available
Stage IV	Distant metastatic	• Distant metastatic cancer. Cancer has spread to other parts of the body.	20%

From National Cancer Institute. (2006). Survival rate information from American Cancer Society (Revised September 18, 2006). (Retrieved from www.cancer.org).

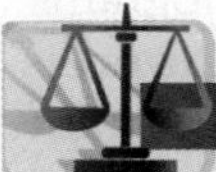

Legal & Ethical Considerations 38–2

BRCA1 and *BRCA2* Genes

If all women are tested for the presence of the *BRCA1* or *BRCA2* gene, the ethical problem is the action to take if the gene is present. Should the young woman have a prophylactic mastectomy? Should the woman be given prophylactic treatment with tamoxifen? Does the knowledge of the potential risk for cancer produce anxiety that may result in life changes that can have a negative outcome? Would there be health insurance implications?

affect the woman's ability to undergo the specific treatment. In general, the primary treatment is usually surgical removal of the tumor and varying amounts of surrounding tissue. The types of surgery include:

- *Lumpectomy* (removal of tumor only).
- Partial or *segmental mastectomy* (removal of tumor and a portion of the surrounding breast tissue and axillary lymph nodes).
- Simple or *total mastectomy* (removal of entire breast and axillary lymph nodes).
- *Modified radical mastectomy* (removal of breast, axillary lymph nodes, and lining over the chest wall muscles).
- *Radical mastectomy* (removal of breast, axillary lymph nodes, and chest wall muscles under the breast). Radical mastectomy was once very common, but high success rates with a reduction in disfigurement are now made possible by using appropriate staging of the disease when making treatment decisions.

A suggested nursing care plan for a woman undergoing a lumpectomy in a same-day surgery unit is presented in Nursing Care Plan 38–2.

If there is concern that cancer cells have invaded the lymph nodes, an axillary node dissection may be done during breast surgery, in which the lymph nodes under the affected arm are removed and sent to the laboratory. This procedure may result in swelling of the affected arm. **Sentinel node biopsy** is becoming more popular, wherein one node is removed and, if laboratory results show no evidence of cancer, the remaining nodes are left intact.

Tamoxifen (Nolvadex) blocks estrogen by binding with the estrogen receptors. This drug is usually pre-

NURSING CARE PLAN 38–2

Care of the Patient After Breast Lumpectomy

SCENARIO A 24-year-old woman is ready for discharge from the same-day surgery unit after undergoing a breast lumpectomy for a suspicious breast lesion. She expresses concern about the amount of scar tissue that will form and that her breasts may no longer be the same size after the lumpectomy.

PROBLEM/NURSING DIAGNOSIS *Worry about abnormal breast appearance*/Anxiety and Disturbed body image related to asymmetrical breasts and scar tissue as a result of undergoing a breast lumpectomy.
Supporting assessment data: *Subjective:* Concern about scar tissue and that breasts will no longer be the same size. *Objective:* Lumpectomy.

Goals/Expected Outcomes	Nursing Interventions	Selected Rationale	Evaluation
Patient will use positive coping strategies to adjust to changes in body image as evidenced by use of support system and available resources	Assess for previous problem with self-esteem.	Previous coping strategies can be revealed by discussing previous experiences.	Patient discussed previous experiences and recognizes the stages of loss she experienced.
	Assess for signs of anxiety or inability to focus.	Anxiety can be an expected result of a diagnosis that may involve a possible cancer.	Patient expressed understanding of prognosis as explained by physician.
	Encourage verbalization of feelings.	Verbalization can reduce anxiety and focus on the problem of altered body image.	Patient expressed her concerns about scar tissue and alteration in breast symmetry.
	Involve family and multidisciplinary health care team in offering support.	Providing patient with broad support base and resources assists in adjustment.	Patient expressed understanding of healing process and resources available for assistance after discharge.
	Provide accurate information concerning prognosis.	Provides an opportunity to correct misinformation.	Patient expressed understanding of need for follow-up care.
	Encourage her to help care for wound.	Looking at and touching wound indicates readiness to participate in self-care to achieve optimum wound healing.	Patient states will actively participate in wound dressing changes.

CRITICAL THINKING QUESTIONS

1. What factors influence a woman's perception of the importance of body image?
2. What other problems or issues might there be for a woman sent home the same day after a breast lumpectomy?

scribed for 5 years. Nausea and anorexia may occur, and cholesterol and triglyceride levels should be monitored. Raloxifene is a drug that had been used for osteoporosis, and is now considered to be the most effective treatment in estrogen-sensitive breast cancer.

Approximately 25% of women have a type of breast cancer tumor that manifests the human epidermal growth factor receptor-2 protein (*HER2*-positive breast cancer). Studies have shown that the monoclonal antibody trastuzumab (Herceptin) added to chemotherapy is very effective at reducing the risk of tumor recurrence (Hortobagyi, 2005). The woman should be monitored for cardiovascular side effects of this drug.

Research is ongoing concerning the customizing of treatment options for women with breast cancer. The National Institutes of Health and the NCI are researching a treatment trial called TAILORx (Trial Assigning Individual Options for Treatment). Women are assigned to treatment regimens based on genetic findings. The results of these trials may enable a change from standardized treatment to customized treatment protocols (Paik, 2006).

Radiation therapy often is done following lumpectomy or segmented mastectomy to destroy micrometastases and decrease cancer recurrence rates. Radiation therapy options include whole-breast radiotherapy using external beam radiation weekly for 7 weeks; intensity-modulated radiation therapy (IMRT), which minimizes damage to surrounding tissue; accelerated partial breast irradiation (APBI), using a balloon catheter in the local tumor site; interstitial brachytherapy, with pellets inserted around the tumor site; or external beam radiation (EBRT) after

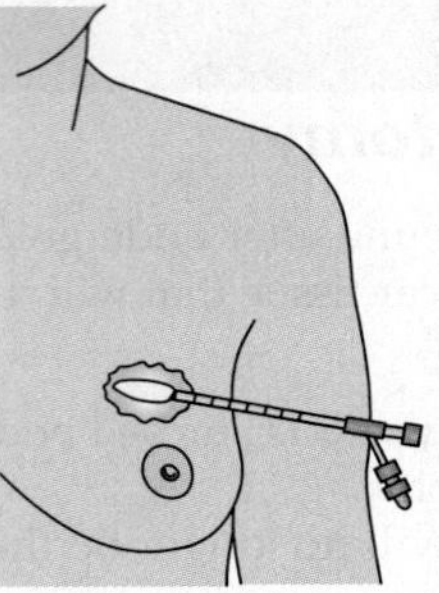

Step 1: During the lumpectomy or shortly thereafter, a deflated balloon is placed inside the cavity created by removal of the tumor.

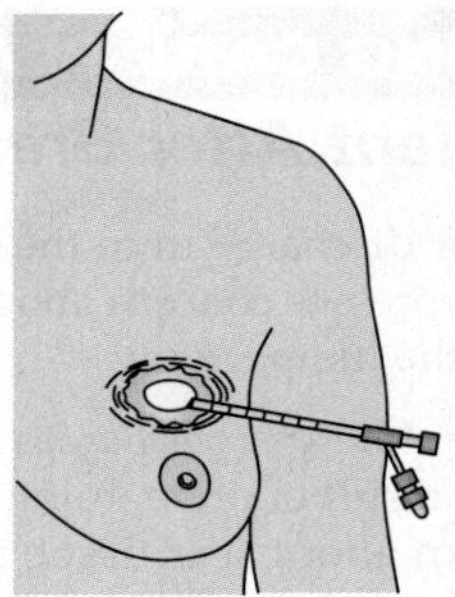

Step 2: Patient returns to clinic for 1 to 5 days of outpatient treatment, where a radioactive seed is inserted through a catheter into the balloon twice a day for 10 minutes each time. The seed targets radiation to the area where tumors are more likely to recur, while minimizing exposure to healthy tissue.

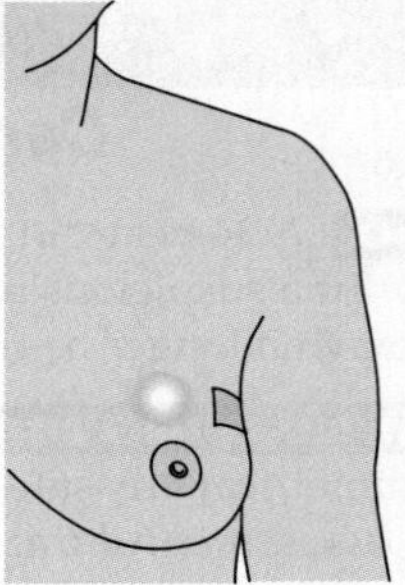

Step 3: The balloon is deflated and the catheter is removed. No source of radiation remains in the patient's body between treatments or after the final procedure.

FIGURE **38–6** Brachytherapy.

healing occurs (Figure 38–6). Chemotherapy also may be considered as part of treatment, in combination with surgery and radiation. Aromatase inhibitors such as anastrozole (Arimidex) or letrozole (Femara) or exemestane (Aromasin) reduce the risk of recurrence by inhibiting the enzyme aromatase, which results in decreased estrogen production. Aromatase inhibitors are not used in premenopausal women with functioning ovaries. An estrogen receptor agonist such as fulvestrant (Faslodex) binds with estrogen receptors and can be used when tamoxifen fails. Ovarian ablation is the surgical removal or irradiation of the ovary to stop estrogen production. The use of goserelin (Zoladex) may be an alternative to chemotherapy. See Chapter 8 concerning care of the patient receiving chemotherapy or radiation therapy.

Breast Reconstructive Surgery

Plastic surgery of the breast may be done to reduce breast size (reduction mammoplasty), enlarge breast size (augmentation mammoplasty), or reconstruct (reconstruction mammoplasty) the breast after breast cancer surgery.

Reduction Mammoplasty. Problems related to an excessively large breast include back and shoulder pain, pressure on nerves from brassiere straps, inability to buy clothing that fits, and psychological problems related to fear of ridicule or unwelcome sexual advances.

A mammogram may be necessary before surgery in women older than 40 years of age. The amount and degree of scarring should be discussed with the woman, as the scar is determined by the technique of surgery. Although data suggest that breast reduction surgery does not interfere with successful breastfeeding, it is possible milk production may be affected (Spector & Karp, 2005). Decreased nipple sensation or loss of part of the areola may also be a side effect of surgery that the woman should be aware of preoperatively. Information concerning successful breastfeeding after breast reduction surgery may be obtained from the La Leche League International.

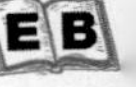

Augmentation Mammoplasty. Breast augmentation is usually initiated by the patient who wishes to improve self-image and attain a sense of increased femininity. Breast augmentation can be accomplished by insertion of a saline implant under the pectoralis muscle.

Reconstructive Mammoplasty. Reconstructive mammoplasty creates a new breast when the natural tissue has been removed during mastectomy. A nipple/areola reconstruction provides a more natural appearance. Saline implants can be used or skin and tissue may be taken from other parts of the body (autologous reconstruction), and tattooing of the nipple area provides natural-looking coloring.

Nursing Management for Breast Cancer Surgery

Preoperative Care. Most women need extensive education prior to breast surgery. Many surgeons now provide educational programs for their patients, but it is important for the nurse to determine whether, in fact, the patient did receive adequate information and if she has a good understanding of what was taught. Women often are particularly concerned about the change in their appearance following breast surgery. Talking with a Reach to Recovery volunteer or a nurse with extensive professional or personal knowledge prior to surgery can be very helpful. Teaching points will vary depending on the amount of tissue to be surgically removed and whether or not a prosthesis will be implanted either during the initial surgery or at a later date (Figure 38–7).

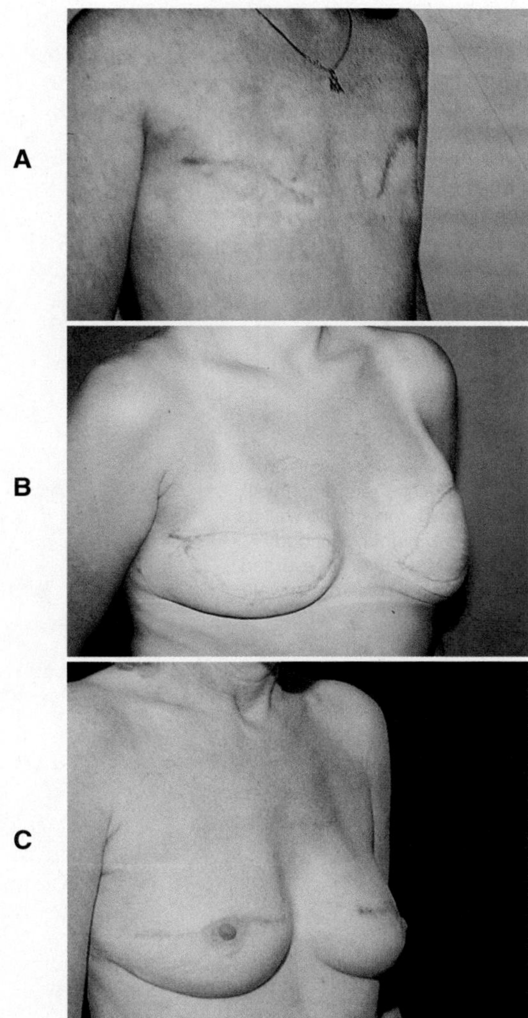

FIGURE **38–7** Reconstructive breast surgery. **A,** Appearance of the chest following bilateral mastectomy. **B,** Postoperative breast reconstruction before nipple reconstruction. **C,** Postoperative breast reconstruction after nipple and areolar reconstruction.

Postoperative Care. Postoperative care will include pain management, observation for signs of infection, and continued supportive and educational measures. Because breast tissue is very vascular, bleeding may be a problem. Surgical dressings should be observed frequently during the first 48 hours following the procedure.

Body image and disfigurement issues, as well as the focus in our society on the breast as a marker of femininity or sexual attractiveness, make treatment for breast cancer a highly emotionally charged experience. Women require ongoing supportive care, and most will benefit greatly from participating in a support group and from visits by American Cancer Society Reach to Recovery volunteers. These women have all undergone treatment for breast cancer and have been trained to do peer counseling. The local chapter of the American Cancer Society can be contacted regarding Reach to Recovery visits.

Collaborative Care. Collaborative care is essential to reduce anxiety and stress in the patient. Emotional support and accurate information are essential. The woman and her partner may differ in how much information they want to discuss. Issues concerning self-image and loss of control should be addressed.

Complications

Lymphedema. **Lymphedema** is swelling of the arm that sometimes occurs after breast cancer surgery due to the damage to and resulting congestion of the lymphatic tract. (It can also be idiopathic, or of unknown origin, or a congenital problem.) Lymphedema occurs in about 25% to 40% of women who undergo breast node biopsy or cancer surgery. Lymphedema can become a chronic condition. The use of sentinel node biopsy, with removal of additional lymph nodes only if the sentinel lymph node is positive for cancer, has reduced the occurrence of lymphedema because the less aggressive the surgery, the less damage to the lymph tissue and therefore the less chance of developing lymphedema. Nursing interventions during the postoperative nursing care of a patient with a breast node biopsy or breast cancer surgery that can reduce the risk of development of lymphedema include:

- Do not assess blood pressure in the affected arm.
- Do not give injections or do venipuncture in the affected arm.
- Provide meticulous skin care.
- Teach the patient to wear gloves in the kitchen and when gardening.
- Teach the patient to avoid heavy lifting.

The nurse should review exercises that may be helpful (Figure 38–8). Discharge teaching should focus on the need for follow-up care, exercises to improve range of motion, prevention of infection, side effects of medical therapy, and community resources available.

Lymphedema clinics are available in some states. The standard treatment is the use of a massage technique that provides lymphatic drainage, specialized pressure bandaging, and application of a compression garment. More information can be obtained from the National Lymphedema Network website at www.lymphnet.org.

The diagnosis and treatment of breast cancer in women can be a direct threat to the sense of feminity and body image. Anxiety, denial, anger, and depression are common reactions. Many women fear they will no longer be attractive to their peers. A combination of peer support and psychotherapeutic, spiritual, and educational guidance can help the woman cope with the diagnosis and treatment. Nurses play a key role in education and referral.

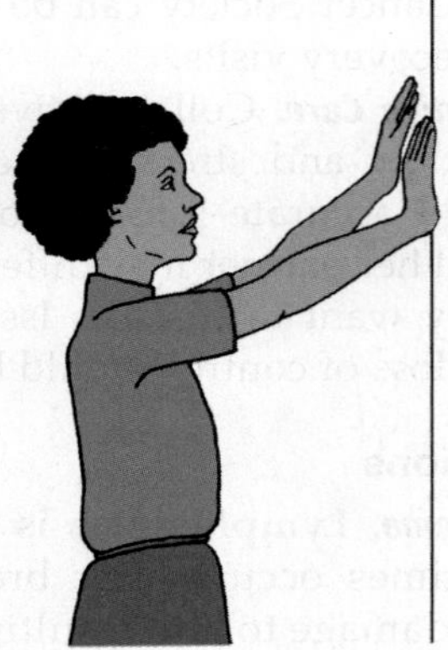

FRONT WALL CLIMBING
Patient stands facing the wall, elbows slightly bent. Palms are placed at shoulder level and fingers are flexed and unflexed as hands "walk" up the wall as high as possible. Hands are then walked back down to shoulder level. Patient moves toward wall as fingers climb higher and then away from wall as fingers move downward.

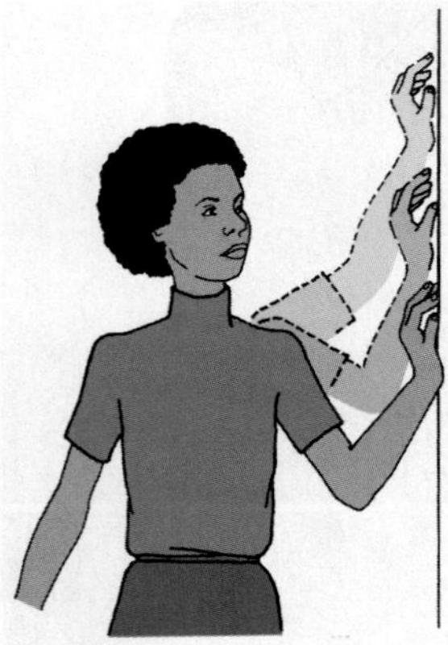

SIDE WALL CLIMBING
With operative side to wall, arm is extended until fingers touch wall. Patient moves toward the wall as fingers climb higher until body touches it. Maneuver is reversed as fingers climb back down wall.

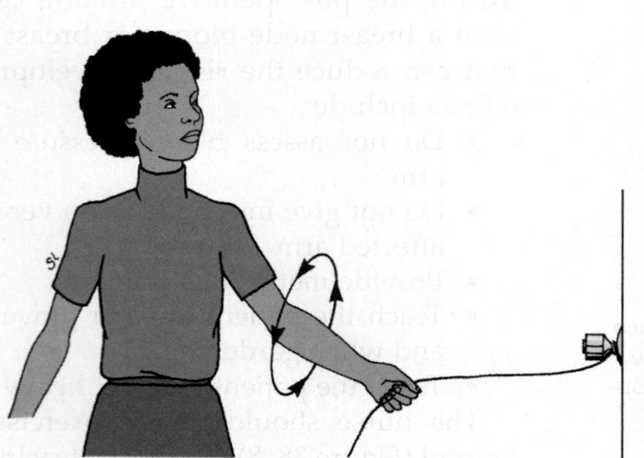

ROPE TURNING
One end of rope is tied to door knob. Patient holds other end of rope and swings it in a circular motion, being sure entire arm and not the wrist is in motion.

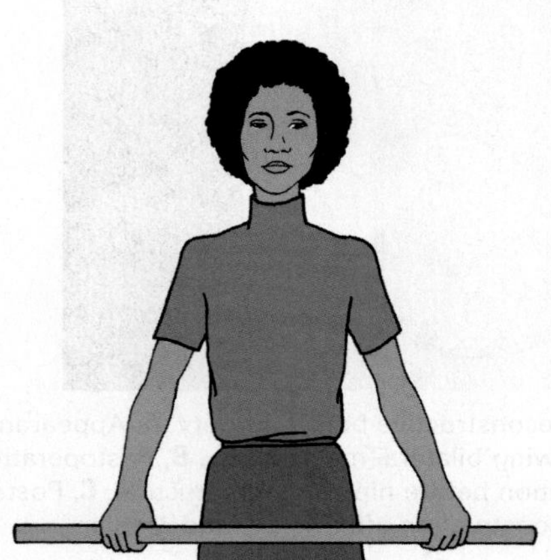

YARDSTICK OR BROOM LIFT
Holding a yardstick or broom handle with both hands, the back is placed against a wall. Arms are extended straight downward and, with elbows straight, the stick is raised by the straightened arms until knuckles touch the wall over the head.

FIGURE **38–8** Postmastectomy exercises.

HOME CARE

Home health nursing is a standard of care in the United States. Hospital stays are becoming progressively shorter, and women frequently go home very quickly after illness, surgery, or childbirth. Intravenous antibiotic therapy is being done with increasing frequency in the home setting, with many health problems being treated outside the hospital setting.

Many women recover at home following a surgical procedure. Home health nursing responsibilities would include pain management, observation of the surgical site for signs of infection (redness, swelling, pain, presence of exudate, foul odor, fever), or reopening of the surgical wound because of trauma or a poor healing response. If the procedure involves the pelvic reproductive organs, the nurse must also assess the amount and duration of bleeding, any increase in the

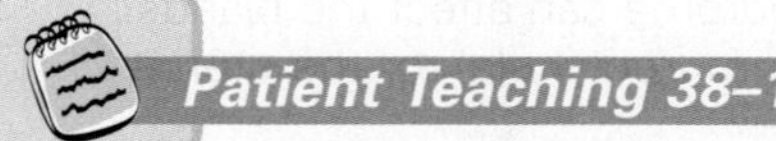

Teaching the Older Adult

Advanced age can inhibit the ability of the woman to learn at a time when information concerning comfort and health is vital. In any teaching plan, the nurse should:

- Promote readiness and motivation to learn. The woman must sense that the information applies to her and is important.
- Provide brochures; reliable sources confer credibility of information.
- Include the woman's experiences and interests; personalizing teaching makes it more meaningful.
- Ask questions to confirm understanding.
- Provide socialization and opportunity to share. Use group sessions when possible.
- Provide short teaching sessions.
- Face the patient, and talk loudly and clearly.
- Use a quiet, adequately lit environment.

volume of flow, and any change (e.g., purulence or foul odor) that indicates the presence of infection.

The majority of teaching often becomes the responsibility of the home health nurse. Even conscientious teaching by the hospital nurse frequently needs extensive follow-up because the patient's learning ability was impaired by immediate concerns such as acute pain, recovery from anesthesia, or emotional stresses associated with the diagnosis and the potential impact on daily living. The home health nurse must be prepared to give accurate, detailed information as part of home care. The nurse also should assess the patient's need for more general education regarding reproductive health, such as regular BSE and VSE, Pap smears, and need for information regarding contraception or STIs.

The home health nurse must be able to function independently and needs to communicate with the other members of the care team by phone, written documentation, and group conferences. The nurse also is often the primary source of information about appropriate support groups and informational programs that would be of assistance to the patient and her family (Patient Teaching 38–1).

COMMUNITY CARE

Community care can take many forms. In the area of general reproductive health, low-cost women's health care clinics and organizations such as Planned Parenthood offer pregnancy testing, counseling and instruction on contraception and prevention of STIs, programs concerning BSE and VSE, and screening procedures such as pelvic examinations and mammograms. Instruction and low-cost screening may also be made available by local chapters of organizations such as the American Cancer Society. These outreach programs seek to make information and services available to all women at a reasonable cost. Such programs assist in the prevention and early detection of disease, reducing the long-term effects of potentially serious illness and the cost of intrusive health care.

Community care also takes the form of educational public service announcements on radio and television and in newspapers and magazines. These give the public valuable information on sexual health and disease prevention and treatment.

School nurses can and should play a major role in reproductive education and health maintenance. Drugs, alcohol, and early sexual activity are major health care concerns for our adolescents. The school nurse is in a position to become a trusted source of accurate, nonjudgmental information for young people who are confused and lack education in the realities of reproductive health.

In recent years, a variety of programs have been developed for women at risk for serious diseases of the breast or reproductive organs. They may be sponsored by national organizations such as the American Cancer Society or by local groups or health care facilities and organizations. These programs provide both education and support groups for women undergoing treatment of serious health problems such as breast or uterine cancer, infertility, fetal loss, and other health concerns of women. The nurse can be very helpful in referring women to these community programs or by volunteering as a group facilitator or resource person.

Key Points

- Reproductive health can be disrupted by many physical disorders. Alterations in reproductive health can affect other body systems.
- Women should keep a calendar of their individual menstrual cycles to determine regularity and recognize deviations from their normal cycle.
- Premenstrual syndrome (PMS), also known as ovarian cycle syndrome, is the presence of physical, psychological, or behavioral symptoms that regularly occur in the luteal phase of the menstrual cycle.
- Premenstrual dysphoric disorder is a more severe type of PMS described officially in the DSM-IV, a classification of disorders published by the American Psychological Association.
- Personal contraceptive techniques include fertility awareness methods, basal body temperature method (BBT), calendar and rhythm methods, ovulation or Billings method, and symptothermal method.
- Mechanical contraception includes the use of the male condom, female condom, diaphragm, spermicides, cervical cap, and intrauterine device (IUD).
- Hormonal contraception methods include the use of oral contraceptives (OCs), injectable contraceptives, transcutaneous patches, intrauterine and vaginal inserts, and sustained-release implants.

- Permanent contraception includes tubal ligation (female) and vasectomy (male).
- Emergency contraception may be indicated after unprotected intercourse but is not meant for regular use.
- Menopause is described as cessation of menses for a 12-month period due to decreased estrogen production. The perimenopausal period or climacteric is the period around the actual cessation of the menstrual period. Common symptoms include irregular menstruation, hot flashes or hot flushes, fatigue, insomnia, emotional swings, depression, back pain, headache, irritability, and decreased libido.
- A decrease in estrogen can increase the risk for the development of osteoporosis and increased blood cholesterol levels.
- Osteoporosis is a decrease in bone mass that increases the risk for bone fractures.
- Breast self-examination (BSE) should be done monthly 1 week after menstruation begins or on a specific date each month after menopause.
- Risk factors for cancer of the cervix include multiple sex partners, early sexual activity, multiple pregnancies, infection with HPV, and smoking.
- Leiomyomas (fibroids) of the uterus are common among women between 25 and 40 years of age, and may cause vaginal bleeding between menstrual periods.
- Endometriosis is a condition in which endometrial tissue is found outside the uterus.
- Pelvic relaxation syndrome can affect the bladder (cystocele), the rectum (rectocele), or the uterus (uterine prolapse).
- Exercise to restore arm function is very important following mastectomy.
- School nurses can and should be a valuable resource to young women regarding issues of sexuality, reproduction, and disease.
- Disorders of the female reproductive system often affect the woman's self-image.
- Specific genes have been identified that can predict the risk of specific types of breast cancer.
- Screening measures such as mammography, BSE, VSE, and Pap smears allow early detection and treatment of cancer of the reproductive tract.
- Modern technology can assist the woman who has fertility problems.
- The nurse must understand the perceptions of the woman and family before designing a teaching plan.

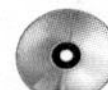

Go to your **Companion CD-ROM** for an Audio Glossary, animations, video clips, and bonus review questions.

evolve Be sure to visit the companion Evolve site at http://evolve.elsevier.com/deWit for interactive NCLEX-PN Exam Style Review Questions, WebLinks, and additional online resources.

NCLEX-PN EXAM STYLE REVIEW QUESTIONS

Choose the best answer(s) for the following questions.

1. A female patient complains of irritability, fatigue, mood swings, and fear of losing control days prior to menstruation. The initial assessment suggests a nursing diagnosis of ineffective coping related to cyclic hormonal changes. Which of the following instructions given by the nurse would likely promote patient coping?

1. "Avoid calcium-containing foods."
2. "Exercise regularly."
3. "Have occasional alcohol."
4. "Consider a sodium-rich diet."

2. Which of the following nursing interventions would help relieve symptoms of dysmenorrhea? *(Select all that apply.)*

1. Pelvic rocking exercises
2. Cold compresses
3. Effleurage
4. Low-fat diet
5. Prostaglandin inhibitors

3. A 44-year-old patient complains of irregular menses with hot flashes. She is informed that she is approaching the climacteric period. Her nurse finds the patient withdrawn and crying. An appropriate statement by the nurse would be:

1. "It is not the end of the world."
2. "You seem upset. I am here to listen."
3. "Everything will be all right."
4. "Aging is not for the faint of heart."

4. The nurse instructs a premenopausal female patient on how to perform breast self-examinations. Which of the following patient statements indicates understanding?

1. "I examine my breast about 1 week after menses."
2. "I can use my thumbs to palpate for lumps and nodules."
3. "I should pay special attention to the area between the breast and underarm."
4. "I do not have to see the physician for clinical breast examinations."

5. A postmenopausal patient complains of urinary frequency. On vaginal examination, there is a protrusion on the anterior vaginal wall. The nurse would likely suspect which of the following?

1. Cystocele
2. Rectocele
3. Uterine prolapse
4. Cyst

6. The patient reports finding multiple, smooth, well-delineated cysts in her breasts that were tender during the premenstrual phase. The nurse would most likely provide which of the following instructions? *(Select all that apply.)*
   1. "Eliminate alcohol and caffeine."
   2. "Apply a cold compress."
   3. "Reduce fat in the diet."
   4. "Take nonsteroidal anti-inflammatory agents."
   5. "Seek immediate physician consultation."

7. The nurse empowers a patient who had a right radical mastectomy by providing specific instructions regarding postoperative care of the surgical site and surgical complications. Which of the following statements by the patient would indicate a need for more teaching?
   1. "Blood pressures cannot be taken on the right arm."
   2. "I can resume intense weight training immediately after discharge."
   3. "No injections must be given in the right arm."
   4. "When gardening, I need to wear gloves."

8. A 44-year-old patient who had a right radical mastectomy expresses concerns regarding her physical appearance. Further assessment indicates a nursing diagnosis of disturbed body image. An important goal for this patient would be to:
   1. participate in activities of daily living.
   2. demonstrate acceptance of change in appearance.
   3. perform aseptic wound care.
   4. state signs and symptoms of infection.

9. The nurse is taking the gynecologic history of a postmenopausal Mexican American patient. Which of the following strategies would help develop rapport with the patient? *(Select all that apply.)*
   1. Establish direct eye contact.
   2. Involve family members.
   3. Touch the patient.
   4. Use a polite tone of voice.
   5. Respect privacy.

10. Abnormal bleeding between menstrual periods that is associated with uterine polyps, leiomyomas, trauma, and foreign body is referred to as:
    1. metrorrhagia.
    2. menorrhagia.
    3. oligomenorrhea.
    4. pseudomenopause.

CRITICAL THINKING ACTIVITIES

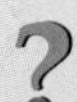

Read each clinical scenario and discuss the questions with your classmates.

Scenario

Mrs. Long is a 45-year-old college instructor, married with two teenage children. She found a lump during breast self-examination that was diagnosed as malignant. Mrs. Long does not want to have the radical mastectomy recommended by her surgeon.

1. What are some possible reasons for Mrs. Long's hesitation about having a radical mastectomy?
2. What alternative surgical procedures are available to Mrs. Long?
3. What types of resources are available to help Mrs. Long make this decision?

CHAPTER 39

Care of Men with Reproductive Disorders

evolve http://evolve.elsevier.com/deWit

Objectives

Upon completion of this chapter, you should be able to:

Theory

1. Review the effects of aging on the male reproductive system.
2. Explain the medical and nursing management of erectile dysfunction.
3. Describe factors involved in fertility, infertility, and contraception in the male patient.
4. List the most common diagnostic tests and examinations of the male reproductive system.
5. Describe the assessment of the male reproductive system.
6. Describe the pathophysiology and manifestations of common disorders of the male reproductive tract.
7. Discuss the plan of care for a patient with a disorder of the male reproductive tract.
8. Identify the psychological and emotional impact of disorders of the male reproductive tract.
9. Compare and contrast four types of surgical treatments for benign prostatic hyperplasia (BPH).
10. Review the pre- and postoperative nursing care of a patient with BPH.
11. Discuss inflammations of the male reproductive system and their treatments.
12. Illustrate the patient teaching involved for early detection of testicular and prostate tumors.
13. Describe the nursing care of a patient with prostate cancer.

Clinical Practice

1. Teach a patient about the procedure for a prostate biopsy.
2. Devise a nursing care plan for a patient with prostate cancer.
3. Devise a teaching plan for testicular examination for young adult males.
4. Provide materials describing treatment to a patient experiencing erectile dysfunction.

Key Terms

Be sure to check out the bonus material on the Companion CD-ROM, including selected audio pronunciations.

androgens (ĂN-drō-jĕnz, p. 974)
azotemia (ă-zō-TĒ-mē-ă, p. 981)
cremasteric reflex (p. 980)
cryptorchidism (krĭp-TŎR-kĭ-dĭz-ĕm, p. 987)
ejaculation (ē-jăk-ū-LĀ-shŭn, p. 973)
erection (ĕ-RĔK-shŭn, p. 973)
gonads (GŌ-nădz, p. 973)
gynecomastia (jīn-ē-kō-MĂS-tī-ă, p. 976)
impotence (ĬM-pō-tĕnz, p. 974)
infertility (ĭn-fĕr-TĬL-ĭ-tē, p. 976)
libido (lĭ-BĒ-dō, p. 974)
orchiectomy (ŏr-kē-ĔK-tō-mē, p. 987)
priapism (PRĪ-ă-pĭz-ĕm, p. 976)
prostate-specific antigen (PSA) (prŏs-tāt, p. 978)
rugae (ROO-jē, p. 973)
semen (SĒ-mĕn, p. 973)
tamponade (tăm-pon-ĀD, p. 983)
urodynamics (ū-rō-dī-NĂM-ĭks, p. 981)
vasectomy (vă-SĔK-tō-mē, p. 977)

People are more open and comfortable talking about reproductive problems or concerns than they used to be. Frequently the nurse is the first person to discover a male reproductive concern. Many diseases and disorders, as well as medications, can affect the male reproductive system. The urinary system and reproductive system are so closely linked in the male that a disorder in one system often affects the other. The nurse needs to be comfortable with his or her own sexuality and knowledgeable about the male reproductive system to be helpful to the patient.

MEN'S HEALTH

The male reproductive organs are shared with the urinary tract, and disorders in functioning of one system often affect the other. For this reason, a male who has a disorder or dysfunction of the reproductive tract is often treated by a urologist.

FERTILITY

If the anatomy and physiology of the male reproductive tract are intact, sexual function is influenced by the functioning of the hypothalamus, pituitary, and testis; the metabolism and transport of sex hormones

OVERVIEW OF ANATOMY AND PHYSIOLOGY OF THE MALE REPRODUCTIVE SYSTEM

What are the structures of the male reproductive system?

- The male **gonads** (sex glands) are the testes; they are oval shaped and are encased in the scrotum along with the epididymis, seminal vesicles, and vas deferens (Figure 39–1).
- The scrotum is covered with wrinkled skin **(rugae)** and is very sensitive to temperature, pressure, touch, and pain.
- The penis is a cylindrical, erectile organ that hangs in front of the scrotum. It contains three columns of erectile tissue that can cause it to extend and enlarge in circumference, becoming stiff. The penis is covered with skin and includes a foreskin unless circumcision has been performed. The scrotum and penis make up the external genitalia of the male.
- The prostate gland is shaped like a walnut, encircles the urethra, and is located below and to the rear of the bladder.
- The bulbourethral (Cowper's) glands are small pea-sized glands located in the urethral sphincter posterior to the urethra.

What are the functions of the organs of the male reproductive system?

- The seminiferous tubules within the testes produce sperm. Testosterone also is produced in the testes.
- The scrotum, a thin-walled, muscular sac, holds the testes, the epididymis, and the vas deferens. The scrotum, which hangs from the pubic bone, suspends the testes outside the body where they remain several degrees cooler than the body; the cooler temperature is needed for the production of viable sperm.

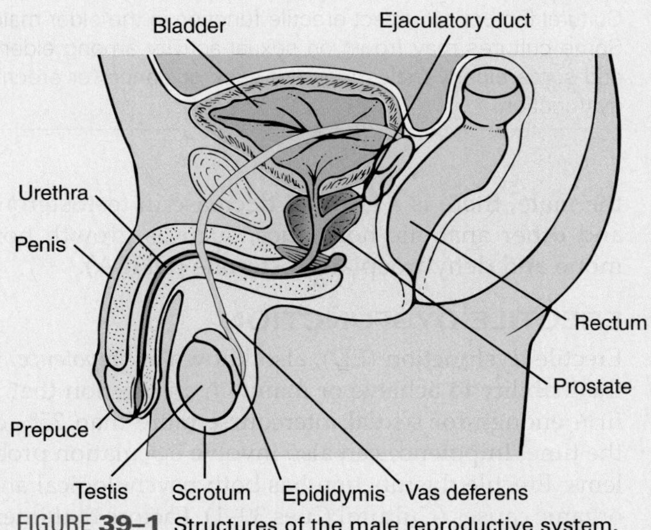

FIGURE **39–1** Structures of the male reproductive system.

- The spermatic cord attaches the testes to the body. It contains the blood vessels and nerves that supply the testes.
- The epididymis is a long tube (almost 6 m) that conducts sperm from the testes to the vas deferens. Immature sperm mature as they travel through this tube. Mature sperm are stored in the lower portion of the epididymis.
- The vas deferens is a muscular tube that connects to the epididymis. It stores sperm and then carries it to the ejaculatory duct by peristaltic movements.
- The prostatic section of the urethra receives the sperm and carries it to the penile portion of the urethra for ejaculation. Secretions from the seminal vesicles and ducts of the prostate gland are mixed with the sperm.
- The seminal vesicles produce a fluid that is thick and contains fructose to nourish the sperm and provide energy. The fluid also contains prostaglandins, which contribute to the motility of the sperm. This fluid mixes with the sperm to form seminal fluid, or **semen.** The average volume of semen ejaculated is 2.5 to 4 mL, but may vary from 1 to 10 mL.
- The prostate gland produces thin, milky, and alkaline secretions that contribute to the seminal fluid and enhance the motility of the sperm.
- The bulbourethral glands secrete an alkaline mucus-like fluid in response to sexual stimulation.
- These secretions neutralize the acid of residual urine in the urethra and provide some lubrication at the tip of the penis for intercourse.
- The penis is flaccid until sexual arousal causes the arterioles to the erectile tissue to dilate and the veins to constrict, engorging the penis with blood until it is enlarged and rigid. This is an **erection.** Erections are stimulated by anticipation, memory, visual sensations, or touch on the glans penis and skin of the genital area. If stimulation continues, **ejaculation** will occur. This is the forceful expulsion of semen from the urethra. Thoughts, emotions, some medications, or medical disorders can sometimes inhibit erection. The

Continued

OVERVIEW OF ANATOMY AND PHYSIOLOGY OF THE MALE REPRODUCTIVE SYSTEM—cont'd

penis transfers semen to the vagina of the female. It also carries urine through the urethra to be excreted.

How is sperm production controlled?

- The hypothalamus, the anterior pituitary, and the testes secrete hormones that control male reproduction.
- The hypothalamus secretes gonadotropin-releasing hormone (GnRH) in response to an unknown stimulus.
- GnRH stimulates the anterior pituitary to release luteinizing hormone (LH) and follicle-stimulating hormone (FSH). LH stimulates the testes to produce testosterone. FSH binds with cells in the seminiferous tubules, making them respond to testosterone. Testosterone and FSH stimulate the formation of sperm *(spermatogenesis).*
- The male sex hormones are called **androgens.**
- At puberty, testosterone levels rise and cause maturation of the male reproductive organs. Sperm take 70 days to mature and are constantly being produced once puberty has occurred.
- Normal sperm count is 100 million/mL. Sterility occurs when the sperm count, for one reason or other, drops to less than 20 million/mL.

What changes occur with aging?

- The scrotum becomes more pendulous and there are fewer rugae.
- Prostate enlargement may occur with risk of urethral obstruction.
- The penis becomes slightly smaller with increasing years.
- There is decreased sperm production, but fertility is intact. Ejaculate volume decreases.
- After age 60, the cycle of sexual response lengthens. Testosterone levels decrease slightly. Arousal takes longer and more direct penile stimulation is needed; the firmness of the erection may be decreased.
- Once an erection occurs, it can be sustained longer before ejaculation occurs.The time needed before another erection can occur is increased, often to between 12 and 24 hours or more.
- Transient inability to achieve an erection may occur. In the absence of disease, or side effects of medication, this will pass if the man has been consistently sexually active.
- Diabetes or hypertension, particularly if not well controlled, may cause **impotence** (inability to attain or maintain an erection).

(such as GnRH and others); and the cognitive and sensory centers in the brain. A sexual desire **(libido)** and the ability to respond to sexual stimulation with a penile erection and the ejaculation of semen containing live sperm are all necessary for fertility. Both the parasympathetic and sympathetic nervous systems influence the normal sexual response cycle.

As a man ages, there is not an abrupt cessation of gonadal hormone activity as there is in a woman. In

Elder Care Points

The decrease in testosterone with age decreases muscle strength, bone mass, libido, and erectile function and affects the psychological sense of well-being. Testosterone replacement therapy is thought to decrease visceral fat and improve bone density and muscle strength, libido, and energy, but may not improve erectile function of the penis. There is no evidence that DHEA supplements, available over the counter, benefit the older male. Studies are ongoing concerning the benefits of testosterone therapy in the aged.

Cultural Cues 39–1

Sexual Activity among Elderly Males

Cultural factors can affect erectile function in the older male. Some cultures may frown on sexual activity among elders, and some elderly males may not seek guidance for erectile dysfunction.

the male, there is a gradual decrease in testosterone and other anabolic hormones, such as growth hormone and dehydroepiandrosterone (DHEA).

ERECTILE DYSFUNCTION

Erectile dysfunction (ED), also known as *impotence,* is the inability to achieve or maintain an erection that is firm enough for sexual intercourse more than 25% of the time. Impotence can also involve ejaculation problems. Erectile dysfunction has both psychological and organic causes (Cultural Cues 39–1). Factors that interfere with the mechanisms of penile erection will cause erectile dysfunction. Any condition that impairs the

Table 39–1 ***Treatment Options for Erectile Dysfunction***

OPTION	COMMENT
Medications taken about 1 hour before intercourse	
Sildenafil (Viagra)	Side effects can include headache, dyspepsia.
Vardenafil (Levitra): rapid onset	Contraindicated in patients taking nitrates and patients with retinopathy.
Tadalafil (Cialis): longer lasting	
Apomorphine	A dopamine receptor agonist that stimulates the central nervous system, resulting in an arousal response, not yet approved by FDA.
Yohimbine	Useful if organic disease is cause of ED.
Trazodone	Has sedation as side effect.
Intraurethral prostaglandin E_1 suppository (alprostadil)	Works locally on corpora cavernosa as a vasodilator.
Intracavernosal injections of vasodilating drugs	Currently replaced by oral sildenafil therapy.
Penile implants	Can be semi-rigid rod or an inflatable prosthesis.
Negative pressure (vacuum constrictive devices)	Used to induce erection by suction. A band is placed at base of penis to maintain erection. May be cumbersome to use. Injury can occur if constriction band is left in place longer than 1 hour.
Vasoactive drugs	Can be administered by topical gel, local self-injection or insertion of medication pellet (alprostadil) into the urethra. Side effects can include pain, fibrotic nodules, and hypotension.
Papaverine gel	
Alprostadil (Caverject)	
Phentolamine (Vasomax)	
Other	
Sexual therapy	The psychosocial factors that may be causing ED are discussed with a qualified sexual therapist. Counseling should include the partner.
Complementary and alternative therapies	
Siberian ginseng	Thought to increase penile blood flow, but research-based evidence is lacking.
Ginkgo biloba	
Acupuncture	These therapies may be used in conjunction with other options. Research-based evidence of effectiveness is lacking but research is ongoing.
Aromatherapy	
Sandalwood	
Rose	
Jasmine	
Ylang ylang oil	
Imagery	
Biofeedback	
Relaxation	

Key: *ED,* erectile dysfunction; *FDA,* Food and Drug Administration.

blood supply to the penis, pathology of the nervous system or hormonal supply, or impaired psychosocial responses can interrupt the process of penile erection. Anxiety and depression can affect achieving or maintaining an erection for successful sexual performance. Organic causes can include diabetes mellitus and other endocrine disorders, disorders of the urinary tract, neurologic disorders, chronic illness (such as sickle cell anemia, hypertesion, liver disease, and cancer), medications, and drug and alcohol abuse.

A complete history and physical examination are done to rule out any physical illness that may affect sexual performance. Sleep laboratories can monitor nighttime penile erections to detect organic causes of impotence. A Doppler probe can measure adequate arterial flow in the penis, which is essential for erections, and nerve conduction tests can be performed to rule out neurologic pathology related to impotence. A review of medications taken that may have side effects that impact erectile function and a complete psychological evaluation for psychological causes of impotence are also done.

Treatment

Medical treatment depends on the cause of ED. Medical conditions are treated, medications prescribed are reviewed and adjusted, hormone therapy may be prescribed for hypothalamic-pituitary disorders, and vascular surgery may be indicated for penile blood flow obstruction. Other medical treatment options are reviewed in Table 39–1.

The primary intervention for ED is modifying reversible causes of the problem, such as treating medical conditions, sexual psychotherapy, or use of medications such as sildenafil (Viagra). Secondary interventions include use of vacuum constriction devices or self-injection of medication directly into the penis to increase blood flow and cause an erection. If these methods fail, surgical interventions include inserting a penile implant that can be rigid or flexible. One type of implant includes a pump, inflatable cylinders, and a reservoir for emptying after erection. The erection produced is usually firm enough to enable intercourse (Figure 39–2).

Postoperative care includes monitoring intake and output, and observing for deep veinthrombosis, ate-

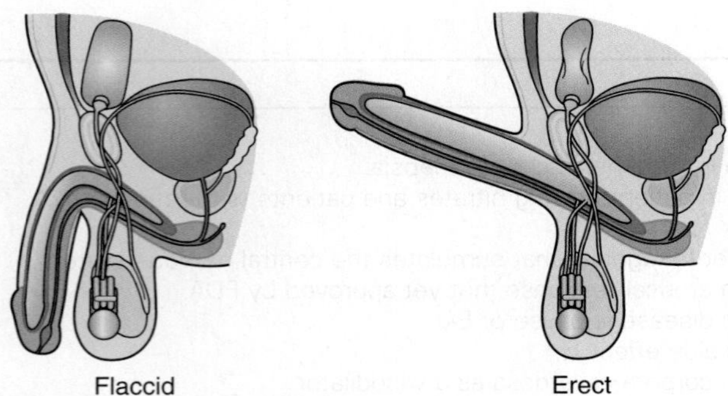

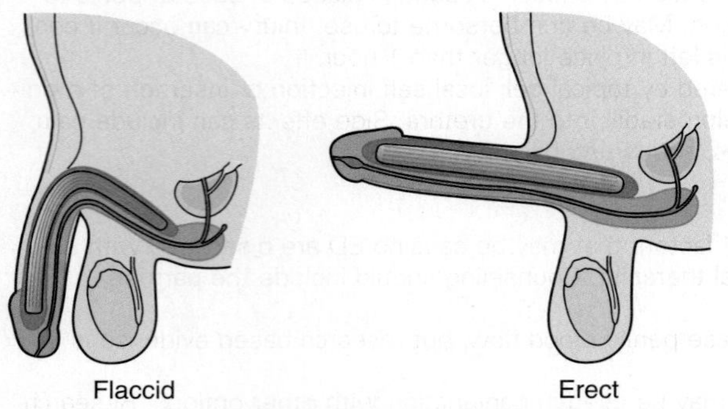

FIGURE **39–2** Penile implants.

lectasis, and other complications of anesthesia or surgery. The patient with a cardiovascular disorder or diabetes is at high risk for infection and complications from this procedure.

Complications of oral therapy include **priapism,** a persistent abnormal erection that can develop into a urologic emergency. The nurse must be aware of problems in interrelationships within the family unit. Asking open-ended questions concerning sexual function or problems can provide information that will be helpful to the plan of care. Referral to a sex therapist may be indicated to help the patient integrate his sexual belief, practices, and abilities into a healthy lifestyle. Community support groups for patients with ED and their partners may be available, such as Impotence Anonymous (I-ANON).

Elder Care Points

The elderly male who has been consistently participating in intercourse throughout the years has the best chance of maintaining this capability. When abstinence has occurred over a considerable time, ED may become a problem. With patience and treatment, this problem may be overcome. The male can reproduce as long as he can participate in intercourse.

INFERTILITY

Infertility is defined as failure of a couple to achieve a pregnancy after at least 1 year of frequent, unprotected intercourse. Approximately 25% to 30% of infertility causes may be due to male factors.

Hypothalamic-pituitary disorders and erectile dysfunction contribute to infertility, but testicular disorders are the most frequent organic cause of male infertility. Drugs, infections, systemic disease, and congenital disorders can cause testicular failure.

A semen analysis with sperm count and activity is performed. Laboratory tests performed include FSH, LH, and testosterone levels to determine if hormone therapy is indicated. A postejaculation urine specimen may be examined to diagnose retrograde ejaculation of semen into the bladder. An ultrasound of the seminal vesicles may reveal dilated vesicles and obstruction of the vas deferens near the ejaculatory duct. Surgical resection of the ejaculatory duct may be indicated. A fine-needle aspiration or biopsy of the testicles may reveal pathology that can be treated. Discussion with both partners concerning technique and timing of intercourse is indicated.

Pathology may be corrected with medications, hormone therapy, or surgery. In vitro fertilization or intracytoplasmic sperm injection (ICSI) after sperm extraction is often successful in treating male infertility.

The environment should be evaluated for toxins such as pesticides, lead, mercury, or radiation exposure, which can affect fertility. The patient should be instructed to avoid excessive heat around the scrotal area, which could decrease sperm development. Hot tubs and tight jockey shorts should be avoided. Stress reduction techniques, information concerning timing and technique of intercourse, optimum nutrition, and health practices should be reviewed with both partners. When the infertility problem is caused by the male, his self-image may be affected and therefore diplomatic, caring, and considerate family interactions are essential.

KLINEFELTER SYNDROME

Klinefelter syndrome is a genetic disorder caused by an additional X chromosome in the male. The disorder is usually diagnosed in adulthood, when the patient seeks medical care for infertility or **gynecomastia** (enlarged breasts). The patient is usually tall and slender with long legs, small testes, decreased facial and pubic hair, and a small penis. There may be mild cognitive and speech or motor delays. Persistent androgen deficiency in adulthood places the patient at risk for diabetic and cardiovascular complications. FSH and LH levels are elevated, with low plasma levels of testosterone. Genetic testing confirms the diagnosis.

A developmental assessment is done, and the patient referred to a multidisciplinary health care team for appropriate therapy. Hormonal (androgen) therapy is usually prescribed, and gynecomastasia may be treated surgically. The American Association for Klinefelter Syndrome Information and Support website is available at www.aaksis.org.

CONTRACEPTION

Contraception is a method of preventing unwanted pregnancy. The only 100% effective method of contraception is abstinence. Abstinence is encouraged for adolescents and young adults and taught in many school programs. However, the nurse must be able to provide contraceptive options for the many couples who prefer not to have additional children added to the family. Contraception is the responsibility of *both* the male and the female. Female contraception is discussed in Chapter 38, Table 38–3.

Reversible Contraception

Reversible contraception involves the use of spermicidal creams, gels, or foams applied before intercourse to kill sperm in the vagina. These are more effective if used in conjunction with a condom. A male condom is an effective reversible contraceptive technique if it is applied and used properly. The condom sheath is typically made of latex. Proper application includes timing of application and removal, and providing a space at the tip for semen to collect. Oil-based lubricants such as petroleum jelly can cause latex to deteriorate and reduce reliability. Condoms made of polyurethane are compatible with oil-based lubricants. Latex condoms provide some protection against sexually transmitted infections (STIs).

Permanent Contraception: Vasectomy

Sterilization of the male by vasectomy is a popular method of permanent contraception. The term **vasectomy** refers to a surgical procedure performed on the vas deferens for the purpose of interrupting the continuity of this duct, which conveys the sperm at the time of ejaculation. This is considered a permanent procedure, but occasionally a vasectomy can be successfully reversed by vasovasotomy at a later time if a man's life circumstances change.

The procedure is done on an outpatient basis in a clinic or physician's office with a local anesthetic. An incision is made into the scrotal sac on each side, and the vas is lifted out. A segment of the vas is cut out, the ends are bound, and the incision is closed.

Instruct the patient to use ice applications and acetaminophen or ibuprofen for scrotal pain and swelling the first 12 to 24 hours postoperatively. The patient should wear jockey shorts or a scrotal support for comfort. Sexual intercourse may be resumed in about 1 week or whenever the patient finds it comfortable. Two negative sperm counts are needed postvasectomy before the patient is infertile.

Since seminal fluid is manufactured in seminal vesicles and the prostate gland, there is no decrease in semen ejaculation following a vasectomy. However, the semen does not contain sperm. The sperm cells that are produced are reabsorbed by the body. Vasectomy has no effect on libido or sexual performance, and provides no protection from STIs. Some patients consider storing fertile sperm in a sperm bank before a vasectomy. Since reversal of a vasectomy may or may not be successful, using frozen sperm at a later date to father a child remains an option. Ethical and legal problems are under continued review.

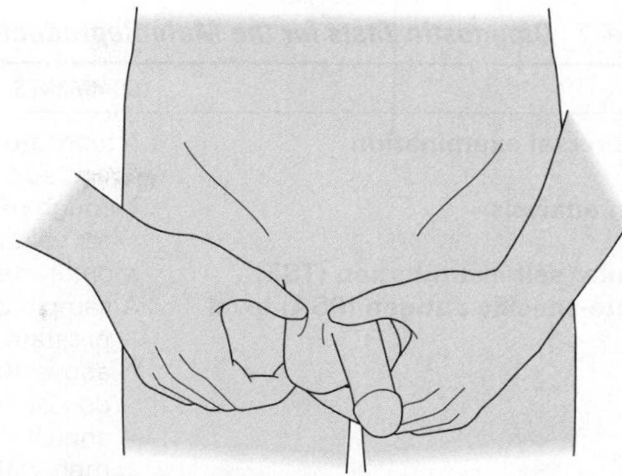

FIGURE **39–3** Testicular self-examination.

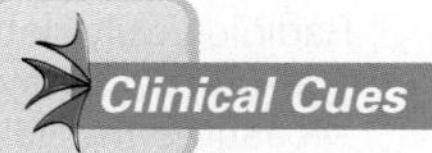

Ask the patient to use another method of birth control until sperm counts are negative, because active sperm are still present in the vas. A second sperm count should be done 1 year later to verify that the vas deferens is not intact.

HEALTH SCREENING, ASSESSMENTS, AND DIAGNOSTIC TESTS

Regular self-evaluation of the testes is encouraged, such as testicular self-examination for early detection of cancer. The nurse can encourage the patient to perform self-examination and teach proper techniques and follow-up care (Figure 39–3). (Privacy should be provided during examination and obtaining specimens.)

Think Critically About . . . Can you think of five relatives or friends for whom you could provide information on testicular self-examination? How would you approach them on this subject?

Tests for general state of health, such as complete blood cell count, urinalysis, chemistry profile, and thyroid tests, are done initially for problems concerning the male reproductive tract. Serum acid phosphatase is usually elevated in the patient with prostate cancer. Serum alkaline phosphatase is elevated if malignancy of the prostate has metastasized to the bone. A kidney-ureters-bladder x-ray, an intravenous pyelogram, and cystoscopy with uroflowmetry studies also may be done (refer to Chapter 33 for more information on these tests).

Smears of urethral discharge and serum tests are done to detect STIs. Tumor protein marker studies are performed for patients with testicular cancer for

Table 39–2 *Diagnostic Tests for the Male Reproductive System*

TEST	COMMENTS
Digital rectal examination	A lubricated, gloved finger is inserted into the rectum to evaluate the consistency and size of the prostate and detect any nodules.
Semen analysis	Through masturbation, the patient provides a specimen of semen, which is analyzed for volume and for sperm content and motility.
Testicular self-examination (TSE)	Monthly self-examination is encouraged (see Figure 39–3).
Prostate-specific antigen (PSA) level	A sample of blood is examined for the level of glycoprotein produced only by the prostate. An elevated level is found in benign prostatic hyperplasia,and levels above 10 mg/mL may be indicative of prostate cancer. However, abnormal levels do not indicate a positive diagnosis. The American Cancer Society recommends annual digital rectal exams and PSA levels for males over 50 yr of age or young men with high-risk factors.
Transrectal ultrasound	Recommended when PSA and/or digital rectal exam results are abnormal. May also be used to guide needle biopsies of the prostate.
Urography	Radiologically detects changes caused by ureter abnormalities and follows urine excretion pathway.
Uroflowmetry	Measures the volume of urine expelled from the bladder per second. Detects outflow tract obstruction. Patient voids into a urine flowmeter. Privacy is provided.
Prostate tissue analysis (biopsy)	Specimens of prostate tissue or fluids can be obtained by perineal or transrectal needle aspiration. If procedure is outpatient based, the patient is taught to report hematuria or change in urine flow after the procedure.
Cystoscopy	A lighted instrument is inserted through the urethra into the bladder. Used to detect prostate hypertrophy and bladder tumors. This is done as a sterile procedure.
Urethral smears	Used for laboratory microscopy study to identify pathogens. Prostate massage increases secretions in the urethra. A sterile swab is inserted into the urethra to obtain the specimen.
ENDOCRINE STUDIES	
Luteinizing hormone (LH) level	LH secreted by the pituitary stimulates Leydig cells in the testes to produce testosterone. High levels may indicate testicular failure.
Prolactin level	Prolactin, a hormone secreted by the pituitary, potentiates testosterone production.
Follicle-stimulating hormone (FSH) level	FSH is secreted by the anterior pituitary gland and stimulates the Sertoli cells in the seminiferous tubules to complete formation of mature sperm. Increased FSH levels indicate decreased spermatogenesis.
Testosterone level	Testosterone is secreted by the Leydig cells of the testes. High levels may indicate a testicular tumor. Low levels may occur in the aging male. Because testosterone levels are highest in the morning and lowest in the evening, it is important to obtain a morning sample.

follow-up to determine the success of treatment or recurrence of the disease. The primary tumor markers are alpha-fetoprotein (AFP) and the beta subunit of human chorionic gonadotropin (beta-hCG). A **prostate-specific antigen (PSA)** test detects levels of a glycoprotein produced by the prostate that is elevated in prostate cancer.

Diagnostic tests that relate to the male reproductive organs are summarized in Table 39–2.

NURSING MANAGEMENT

Assessment (Data Collection)

Because of the predominance of certain kinds of reproductive disorders in males in certain age groups, the age of the patient is relevant to nursing assessment. In males over the age of 50, the assessment is directed more toward detecting prostate problems, whereas younger males are carefully assessed for STIs and testicular cancer.

It may be awkward for the new nurse to obtain a sexual and reproductive history, but with experience in interviewing male patients of all ages, she will soon become more comfortable and adept at obtaining necessary data. Because questions about urinary problems are usually less sensitive than those dealing with sexual dysfunction, it is best to begin with questions of this kind and then lead into more sensitive ones.

Open-ended questions that start out with "Tell me about . . ." or "When did you first notice . . ." give the patient room to discuss only those things he is comfortable talking about. It also is helpful to relate his problem to the inconvenience it has caused in his daily life. For example, tenderness and discomfort in the scrotal area could make sitting at a desk or walking very difficult and interfere with getting assigned work done. Frequent urination can cause distracting and sometimes embarrassing interruptions in his work schedule or recreational activities.

Good communication depends on the sender and receiver of messages using mutually understood language. Many people do not know the medical names of their sex organs. If the nurse suspects that the patient does not understand what particular part of the body she is talking about, or if the nurse herself is not familiar with the term the patient is using, it is important to phrase questions differently or ask for clarifica-

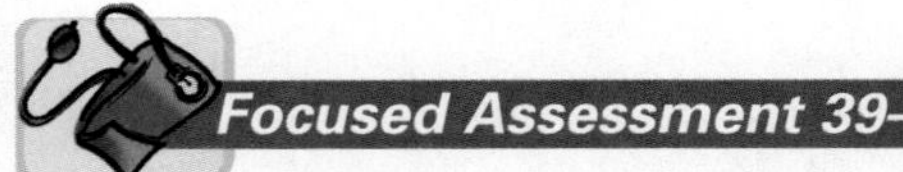

Data Collection for the Male Reproductive System

Ask the following questions:
- Have you noticed any changes in patterns of urination; any differences in the stream of urine?
- Do you ever have any discharge coming from the penis?
- Have you felt any masses or bumps in the scrotum or groin?
- Do you have any tenderness or pain in the scrotum or penis?
- Do you have any rectal or perineal pain?
- Do you perform regular testicular exams?
- Have you had past infections of the reproductive system?
- What drugs do you take regularly?
- Do you have difficulty obtaining or maintaining an erection?

tion from the patient. Focused Assessment 39–1 provides a list of questions helpful in eliciting needed information.

? *Think Critically About . . .* How would you begin your assessment interview with a 52-year-old male patient? Would you have any difficulty asking the questions necessary to obtain a good reproductive organ history and information about present problems?

Nursing Diagnosis

Nursing diagnoses commonly used for problems of the male reproductive system may include:
- Urinary retention related to urinary obstruction
- Anxiety related to inability to empty bladder completely or dribbling
- Pain related to pressure of pelvic mass or distended bladder; surgical incisions; or bladder spasms
- Sexual dysfunction related to inability to achieve erection
- Ineffective sexuality pattern related to decreased libido
- Disturbed body image related to changes in sexual function
- Potential fluid volume excess related to bladder irrigation.
- Risk for infection related to stasis of urine

Additional nursing diagnoses may be appropriate for the patient undergoing surgery or who has cancer. Refer to Chapters 4, 5, and 8 for more information.

Planning

Expected outcomes are written for individual patients based on the nursing diagnoses chosen. Interventions are planned to help the patient meet the expected outcomes. The nurse plans her interaction with the patient based on his age, educational level, degree of comfort in discussing reproductive problems, and culture.

Expected outcomes for the patient with problems of the male reproductive system are:
- Patient will have normal urinary flow without obstruction.
- Patient will have normal urinary elimination after surgery.
- Pain will be resolved after surgical recovery.
- Patient will have intact self-esteem 3 months after surgery.
- Patient will have bladder spasms controlled with medication.
- Patient will explore avenues for achieving sexual satisfaction.
- Patient will focus on positive traits and capabilities to increase a positive body image.
- Patient will not experience a fluid imbalance. Patient will not experience any infection from stasis of urine or surgery.

Implementation

Nursing actions for selected problems of the male reproductive system are found within the sections on specific disease that follow. Privacy should always be provided when assessing the genitals, performing catheter care, or doing dressing changes. There are wide variances in the degree of modesty in men. The female nurse must be especially cautious and display a matter-of-fact, respectful manner when providing care. Sensitivity to embarrassment is necessary. Rather than stating "Don't worry; I'm used to this," it might be better to state, "I understand that this may be embarrassing for you; I will try to be as quick about it as I can."

If a male patient who is experiencing sexual dysfunction or is about to undergo surgery that may affect his sexuality makes sexual comments or advances to a female nurse, she should be tactful and matter of fact in setting limits on such behavior without taking it personally. Some patients express such comments when they feel that their sexuality is threatened.

Evaluation

Evaluation is carried out by assessing the effectiveness of the nursing actions in helping the patient achieve the expected outcomes. If the actions and treatments are not achieving the desired effect, a revision in the plan of care is necessary.

DISORDERS OF THE MALE REPRODUCTIVE TRACT

HYDROCELE

There is normally a small quantity of fluid in the space between the testis and tunica vaginalis within the scrotum (Figure 39–4). A larger-than-normal amount of fluid accumulating in this space is known as *hydrocele.*

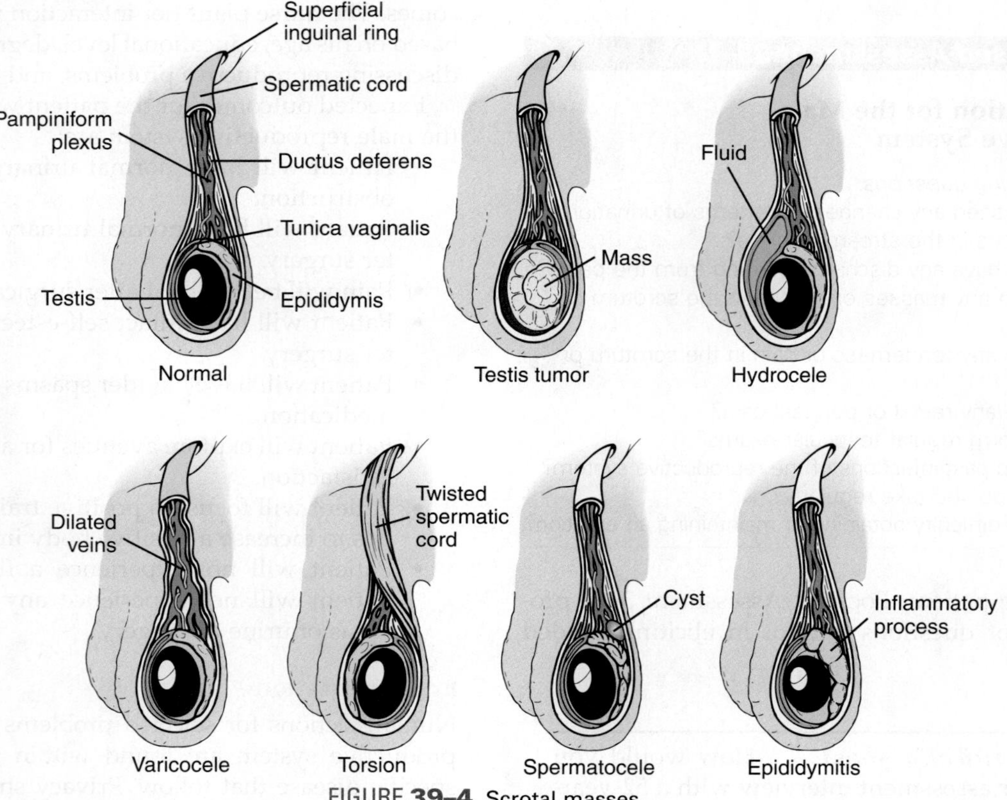

FIGURE **39–4** Scrotal masses.

The fluid accumulation may be caused by infection, such as epididymitis or orchitis, or it may occur after trauma and involves interference with lymphatic drainage of the scrotum. Many times the cause is unknown. Hydrocele causes enlargement of the scrotum and usually is painless, but the weight and added bulk can cause discomfort.

Treatment, when indicated, is aspiration or surgical incision and drainage of the sac. A pressure dressing and a drain are left in place postoperatively. The patient will need to wear an athletic support for several weeks.

VARICOCELE

Dilation and clumping of the tributary vessels of the spermatic vein cause this somewhat painful swelling (see Figure 39–4). It usually occurs on the left side of the scrotum due to retrograde flow of blood from the left renal vein. The discomfort is rarely enough to warrant surgery. If infertility has been a problem, surgical correction via injection of a sclerosing agent or ligation of the spermatic vein may improve the infertility problem.

Nursing measures to help the patient cope with fatigue, weakness, and fever are appropriate, because these problems often are associated with urogenital infections. Fluid intake should be increased to help prevent fluid deficit, reduce fever, increase urinary flow, and remove debris and bacteria.

TESTICULAR TORSION

Testicular torsion is a twisting of the testes and spermatic cord (see Figure 39–4). It is commonly caused by elevated hormone levels in young adult males but can also be the result of scrotal trauma. Signs include sudden acute scrotal pain and an absence of the **cremasteric reflex** (retraction of the testicles when the inner thigh is stroked). Nausea and vomiting may also occur. A Doppler ultrasound scan may reveal diminished blood flow and confirm the diagnosis. To avoid testicular ischemia and necrosis, emergency surgery is done to secure the testicle within the scrotum or possibly remove the testicle. The nurse provides routine postoperative wound care with emphasis on providing support and relieving anxieties concerning the patient's sexual self-image and future sexual performance.

PRIAPISM

Priapism is a prolonged penile erection resulting in a large, hard, and painful penis unrelated to sexual desire or activity. The cause can be neurologic, vascular, or the result of medications such as those designed to increase sexual performance. The most common disease that causes priapism is sickle cell disease, which causes a local accumulation of erythrocytes that result in engorgement of the corporal bodies. Circulation to the penis may be compromised, and voiding may be impaired while the penis remains erect, so prompt treatment is essential.

Treatment can be conservative, to promote dilation of vessels and relief of pressure. Warm baths or enemas and urinary catheterization may be prescribed. Aspiration of the corpora cavernosa with a large-bore needle may be necessary to prevent ischemia of the penis.

The nurse should provide supportive care to the patient, who not only may be in pain, but may be embarrassed by the loss of erectile control and fearful of the effect of this condition on future sexuality.

PEYRONIE'S DISEASE

Peyronie's disease is a condition in which a plaque of nonelastic fibrous tissue develops in the tunica portion of the dorsal corpus cavernosa of the penis. The loss of elasticity in that section of the penis results in the inability to have a uniform erection of the penis. The penis will curve upward when erection occurs. Inability to penetrate the vagina may result, and the erection may become painful as well as embarrassing.

Treatment may include conservative measures such as topical applications or oral medications such as colchicines or tamoxifen. Local radiation or injections to soften the lesion are also options. The size of the lesion and the level of erectile dysfunction may indicate a need for surgical intervention.

BENIGN PROSTATIC HYPERPLASIA

Etiology and Pathophysiology

Enlargement of the prostate, also known as benign prostatic hyperplasia (BPH), occurs because of endocrine changes associated with aging and involves an enlargement of the prostate gland. Increasing age and functioning testes are the main risk factors, although some genetic factors may be involved. Also, about one third of U.S. men, ages 40 to 79 years, have some urinary tract problems attributed to BPH (Goldman et al., 2004).

Signs and Symptoms

BPH produces no symptoms until the growth becomes large enough to press against the urethra (Figure 39–5). Then the patient begins to experience difficulty in urinating evidenced by a decrease in the caliber of the stream of urine, hesitancy, and dribbling after voiding. There may be frequency, nocturia, and urgency due to irritation of the distended bladder wall. In the later stages there may be complete obstruction of the urinary flow.

Incomplete emptying of the bladder results in urinary retention (more than 60 mL of residual urine). Gradual dilation of the ureter *(hydroureter)* and kidneys *(hydronephrosis)* can occur. Urinary tract infections can result from urinary stasis as the retained urine acts as a medium for organism growth. Nitrogen products can accumulate in the blood **(azotemia)** and cause renal failure if the urinary obstruction is not relieved. The American Urological Association has developed a tool to assess symptoms related to urinary obstruction, which aids in clarifying the severity of the problem.

Diagnosis

A digital rectal examination will reveal an enlarged prostate. The "gold standard" test for bladder outlet obstruction is increased bladder pressure relative to urinary flow. Pressure flow studies can be performed **(urodynamics).** A postvoiding catheterization to determine residual urine volume is also a helpful diagnostic aid. A transrectal ultrasound differentiates BPH from prostate cancer, and a serum creatinine level can rule out renal insufficiency.

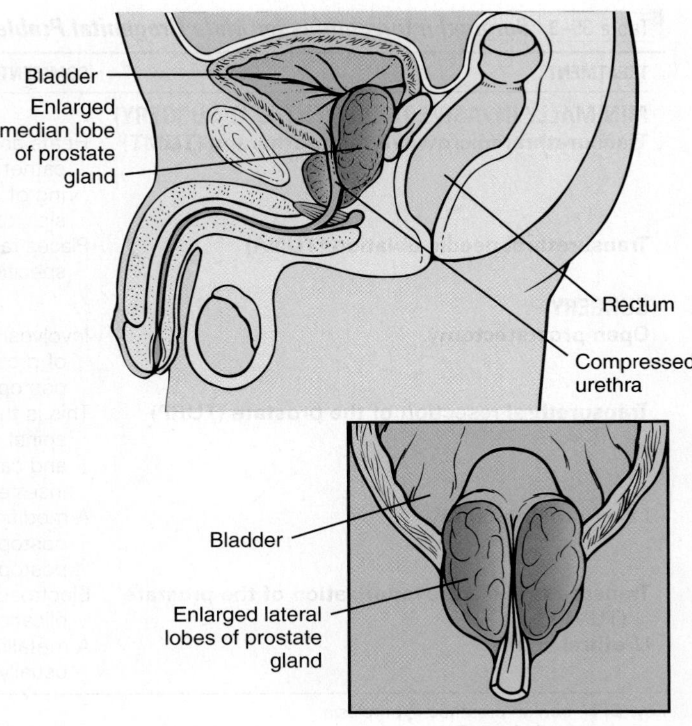

FIGURE **39–5** Benign prostatic hyperplasia.

Treatment

Treatment is based upon the severity of the symptoms and condition of the patient. In cases of mild symptoms, treatment includes careful follow-up care, dietary modifications such as decreasing caffeine and artificial sweetener consumption, limiting spicy foods and alcohol intake, avoiding decongestants and anticholinergic medications, and planning a timed voiding schedule with limited bedtime fluid intake.

Drug Therapy. Drug therapy includes:

- *α-Adrenergic blockers,* which promote relaxation of smooth muscle and reduce blood pressure. Side effects of doxazosin (Cardura), terazosin (Hytrin), tamsulosin (Flomax), and alfuzosin (Uroxatral) include dizziness and orthostatic hypotension.
- *5α-Reductase inhibitors,* such as finasteride (Proscar) and dutasteride (Avodart), can decrease prostate size up to 20% in 1 year. Side effects include decreased libido, decreased ejaculate volume, and ED. These medications lower PSA levels, and the PSA tests must be interpreted differently. Combination therapy with doxazosin and finasteride has been successful.

Herbal Therapy. Plant extracts such as saw palmetto *(Senenoa repens)* have been shown to relieve symptoms

Table 39–3 ***Surgical Interventions for Male Urogenital Problems***

TREATMENT	COMMENTS
MINIMALLY INVASIVE TREATMENT (DAY SURGERY)	
Transurethral microwave thermotherapy (TUMT)	Heats and coagulates prostate tissue via a transurethral probe. A urinary catheter may be left in place for 1 wk after treatment to facilitate passing of necrotic tissue and prevent urinary retention. Antibiotics, analgesics, and bladder antispasmodics are prescribed after the procedure.
Transurethral needle ablation (TUNA)	Places radiofrequency needles directly into the prostate to coagulate specific tissue areas. Hematuria may occur for 1 wk after this procedure.
SURGERY	
Open prostatectomy	Involves an external abdominal incision that allows complete visualization of prostate tissue. There is risk for infection and erectile dysfunction, postoperative pain, and a longer recovery period.
Transurethral resection of the prostate (TURP)	This is the "gold standard" of treatment for BPH and is performed under spinal anesthesia. A resectoscope is inserted into the urethra to excise and cauterize obstructive prostate tissue. A large three-way catheter is inserted to provide hemostasis and allow urinary drainage.
Laser prostatectomy	A modified TURP; uses a laser beam to destroy prostate tissue. Minimal postoperative bleeding occurs, but a catheter may be required for 1 wk postoperatively to prevent urinary retention due to edema.
Transurethral electrovaporization of the prostate (TUVP)	Electrosurgical vaporization and desiccation destroy prostate tissue. Complications include hematuria and retrograde ejaculation.
Urethral stent	A metallic stent is placed in the urethra to hold the urethra open. This is usually a temporary measure as displacement is common.

Key: *BPH*, benign prostatic hyperplasia.

and increase urine flow in some patients. Side effects may include an increase in blood pressure and gastrointestinal disturbances. Saw palmetto should not be taken if the patient is receiving hormone replacement therapy. Pumpkin seeds are also thought to decrease prostate size. Research concerning the role of complementary and alternative medicine therapies in the treatment of BPH is ongoing.

Surgery. The nurse should review the surgical options that were presented by the health care provider to assure that the patient has a clear understanding of treatment options (Table 39–3).

Think Critically About . . . A patient has been experiencing increasing difficulty in emptying his bladder; he has BPH. Tests indicate that he has hydronephrosis. His physician has recommended prostate surgery, but he is reluctant to have surgery. How would you interact with him to help him see the potential consequences of not having surgery? What other options are available to this patient that might prevent further organ damage?

Nursing Management

Preoperative Care. Urinary drainage is accomplished by insertion of a catheter using sterile technique. If the obstruction is severe, a urologist may insert a special rigid catheter. A high fluid intake is encouraged, and antibiotics are routinely prescribed. The nurse should interview the patient to assess the understanding of the procedure to be performed and the impact on his lifestyle, self-image, and sexual function.

Preoperative teaching includes deep-breathing exercises, range-of-motion leg exercises, the general preoperative and postoperative routine, and explanation of the care of the incision, catheters, irrigation system, and drains (see Chapter 4).

Postoperative Care. The postoperative nursing care of the patient varies according to the type of prostate surgery performed (Figure 39–6). The general principles of postoperative nursing care that apply to all patients having major surgery are necessary for the patient undergoing a prostatectomy. Potential postoperative complications are bleeding, urinary incontinence, and bladder spasms. Because hemorrhage always is a danger, vital signs are taken every 2 hours initially, then every 4 hours. The patient is monitored for pallor and rising pulse, which, along with blood pressure changes, may indicate excessive bleeding and shock. A high-fiber diet and a stool softener may be prescribed to prevent straining, which increases intra-abdominal pressure and can cause further bleeding.

Patients with suprapubic prostatectomy and transurethral resection of the prostate (TURP) will return from surgery with a three-way urethral catheter connected to continuous bladder irrigation with sterile normal saline (Figure 39–7).

Blood-tinged urine is usual for the first few days following the surgery. To decrease clot formation, the bladder irrigation flow rate is adjusted to keep the urine diluted to a reddish pink, clearing to a pink tinge within 48 hours. Some pieces of tissue and small clots will be

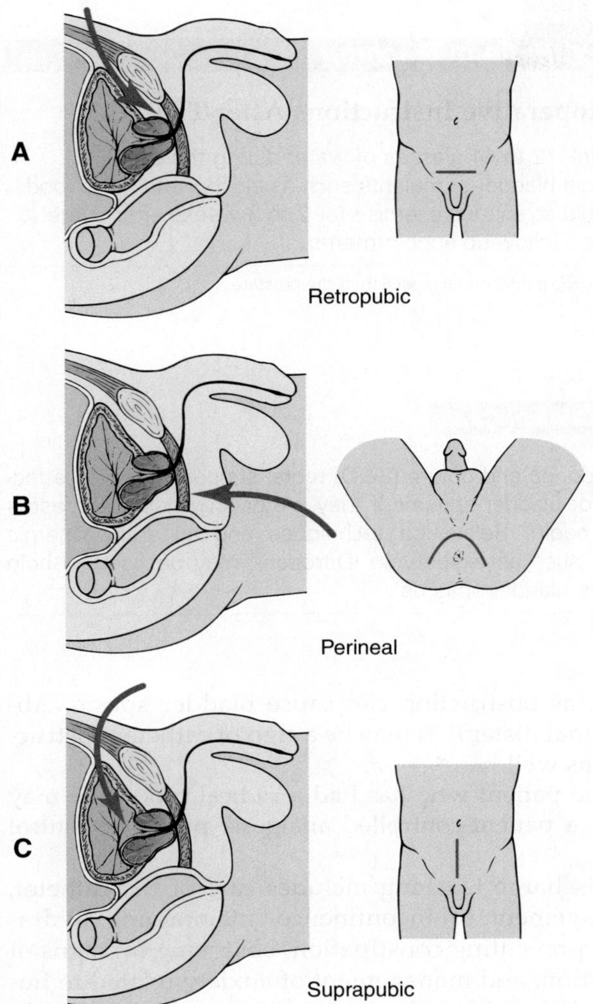

FIGURE 39–6 Three approaches to perform a prostatectomy. **A,** Retropubic approach involves a midline abdominal incision. **B,** Perineal approach involves an incision between the scrotum and anus. **C,** Suprapubic approach involves an abdominal incision.

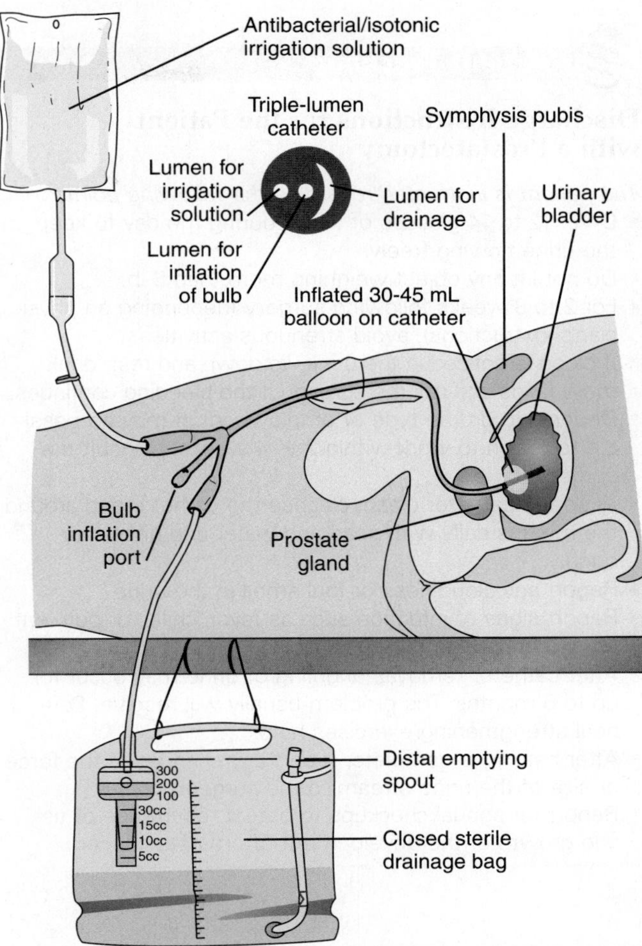

FIGURE 39–7 Continuous bladder irrigation (CBI) system.

seen in the drainage. Additional intermittent irrigation with 20 to 30 mL of normal saline may be needed to clear the catheter of obstruction (see Nursing Care Plan 39–1 on p. 985). Hemorrhage is a possible complication and occurs most frequently in the first 24 hours. Strict sterile technique must be used when irrigating the bladder, and the catheter should be connected to a closed drainage system to prevent infection.

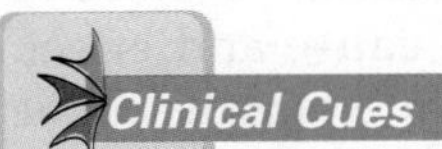

Clinical Cues

When caring for a bladder irrigation system:

- Use sterile normal saline unless otherwise ordered.
- Monitor rate of irrigation.
- Monitor and record input and output.
- Check drainage tubes for kinks and clots.
- Observe for signs of bladder spasms and medicate promptly PRN.

Persistent bleeding turning the urine darker than cherry red or bright red, or viscous drainage with many clots, should be reported immediately to the surgeon. Traction may be applied to the catheter to supply pressure **(tamponade)** to prevent excessive bleeding. The surgeon does this by pulling against the balloon and then taping the catheter to the thigh or abdomen. The nurse checks frequently to see that the catheter and tubing are not kinked and that outflow is appropriate. Irrigation is continued for 2 to 3 days. The patient may have some urinary frequency and burning after catheter use is discontinued. Some blood in the urine is not unusual for several more days.

The patient who has had a suprapubic prostatectomy will have a suprapubic catheter in addition to a urethral catheter. Each catheter is attached to a separate sterile drainage system. After the urethral catheter is removed (sometime after the third day), the suprapubic catheter is clamped, and the patient attempts to void. Residual urine is measured afterward by unclamping the suprapubic catheter. When there is no more than 75 mL of residual urine after voiding, the suprapubic catheter is removed. Drib-

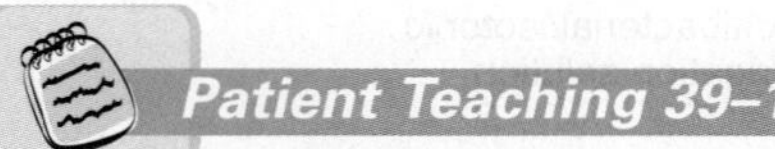

Discharge Instructions for the Patient with a Prostatectomy

The patient is instructed regarding the following points:
- Drink 12 to 14 glasses of water during the day to keep the urine flowing freely.
- Do not lift any object weighing more than 8 lb.
- For 2 to 3 weeks following surgery (depending on physician's instructions), avoid strenuous activities.
- If blood is noticed in the urine, lie down and rest; drink more fluids and call the surgeon if the bleeding continues.
- Depending on the type of employment, it may be possible to return to work within 2 to 4 weeks. Consult the surgeon.
- Keep the catheter clean; cleanse the catheter and around the meatus daily with soap and water and rinse thoroughly.
- Report any cloudiness or foul smell in the urine.
- Report signs of infection such as fever, chills, or purulent wound drainage.
- After catheter removal, dribbling of urine may occur for up to 6 months. The problem usually will resolve. Perineal strengthening exercises help.
- After healing is complete, report any changes in the force or size of the urine stream to the surgeon.
- Report for annual checkups to detect recurrence of tissue growth or the development of prostate cancer.

bling of urine often occurs after prostatectomy due to decreased sphincter tone, but usually stops within about 6 months. Patients who experience incontinence are taught perineal muscle strengthening (Kegel) exercises for this problem and are given instruction in bladder training (see Patient Teaching 33–5). Teaching begins 24 to 48 hours after surgery. Kegel exercises and coping strategies should be taught to enable early return to a normal lifestyle.

When the urethral or suprapubic catheter is removed, the patient must be carefully monitored for ability to void. Intake and output are tracked closely. Any difficulty in voiding within 6 hours after removal must be reported to the surgeon promptly as a distended bladder may cause bleeding.

The nurse monitors the incisional dressings and changes them as often as necessary to keep the patient dry and comfortable. Urine is very irritating to the skin, and any area that is exposed to urine drainage is thoroughly cleansed before a new dressing is applied.

Prophylactic antimicrobials and analgesics are administered in the early postoperative period. Bladder spasms often are a problem for the post-TURP and post–suprapubic prostatectomy patient. Before giving medication, the nurse checks to see that the tubing is not kinked and the catheter is draining well, as obstruction can cause bladder spasm. Abdominal distention may be a sign of catheter obstruction as well.

The patient who has had a radical procedure may have a patient-controlled analgesia pump to control pain.

Discharge teaching includes care of the catheter, management of incontinence, maintaining hydration, preventing constipation, observing for signs of infection, and management of anxiety related to impaired sexual function and self-image (Patient Teaching 39–1). *Retrograde ejaculation* (semen discharged intro the bladder) may cause the urine to appear cloudy. Frequent planned urination and avoidance of irritating foods such as citrus, caffeine-containing products, and alcohol should be initiated (Patient Teaching 39–2). BPH can recur, so annual digital rectal examinations should be continued (Nursing Care Plan 39-1).

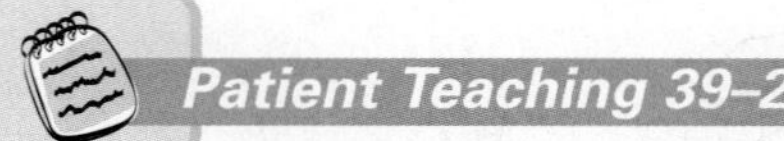

Postoperative Instructions After TURP

- Drink 12 to 14 glasses of water during the day.
- Avoid bladder stimulants such as alcohol and spicy foods.
- Avoid strenuous exercise for 2 to 3 weeks after surgery.
- Keep follow-up appointments.

Key: *TURP,* transurethral resection of the prostate.

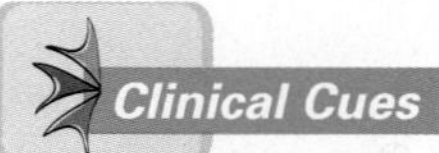

Belladonna and opium (B&O) rectal suppositories are effective for bladder spasms if they are given when the spasms first begin. Relaxation techniques and an anticholinergic drug, such as oxybutynin (Ditropan), may be used to help relieve bladder spasms.

INFLAMMATIONS AND INFECTIONS OF THE MALE REPRODUCTIVE TRACT

Many of the inflammations and infections affecting the male reproductive system are similar to those of the female reproductive system in cause and effect. For example, urethritis in the male and female can be caused by common pyrogenic and colonic bacteria and by *Neisseria gonorrhoeae.* The male also can be infected with *Trichomonas vaginalis* or *Chlamydia,* which are transmitted by sexual contact. There always is the possibility that the sexual partners will reinfect one another until both are treated simultaneously.

NURSING CARE PLAN 39–1

Care of the Patient After Prostatectomy

SCENARIO A 65-year-old man is admitted to the postoperative unit after a prostatectomy. His vital signs are stable, and a bladder irrigation system is set up at the bedside. The patient is awake and oriented, and the physician's orders include diet as tolerated.

PROBLEM/NURSING DIAGNOSIS *Prostatectomy*/Risk of deficient fluid volume secondary to postoperative hemorrhage and limited fluid intake.

Supporting assessment data *Objective:* Transurethral prostatectomy.

Goals/Expected Outcomes	Nursing Interventions	Selected Rationale	Evaluation
Patient evidences normal fluid volume and stable vital signs	Monitor vital signs.	A change in vital signs can indicate fluid deficit.	Vital signs stable.
	Monitor intake and output.	Encouraging oral fluids as tolerated and recording amount and type of output enable identification of fluid volume status.	Intake = 3500 mL; output = 3200 mL. Taking sufficient oral fluids.
Patient evidences clear to pink urinary drainage with no clots	Perform closed bladder irrigation as prescribed.	Irrigation removes accumulating clots that can obstruct urine outflow and precipitate further hemorrhage.	Irrigation outflow pink with few clots.
	Administer IV fluids as prescribed.	IV therapy can help maintain fluid balance.	IV infusion at 150 mL/hr.

PROBLEM/NURSING DIAGNOSIS *Does not know anything about wound care*/Deficient knowledge related to lack of knowledge regarding self-care after discharge.

Supporting assessment data *Subjective:* "No, I've never had to do any wound care before. What do I have to do?"

Goals/Expected Outcomes	Nursing Interventions	Selected Rationale	Evaluation
Patient will list signs of infection, explain need for increased fluid intake, demonstrate care of wounds, dressings, and catheter, and follow medication regimen	Instruct to report signs of infection: fever, chills, malaise, increased pain, purulent drainage, excessive swelling.	Finding infection early means early treatment.	Able to provide accurate feedback of all instructions.
	Instruct to avoid heavy lifting, driving, and sexual activity until permitted by urologist.	Heavy lifting or sexual activity may cause disruption of tissue and bleeding.	States he understands and will comply with restrictions.
	Instruct to report new onset of burning on urination or cloudy urine.	Burning on urination or cloudy urine may indicate bladder infection.	No burning on urination or cloudy urine.
	Explain what each medication is for and when and how to take it.	Helps with compliance with medication regimen.	States understands when and how to take the medications.
	Provide written information about signs and symptoms of urethral stricture or infection and instruct to report these.	Written instructions can be reviewed at home and help to get quick attention for problems.	Given written instructions regarding complications and what to report to surgeon.

Key: *IV,* intravenous.

Continued

NURSING CARE PLAN 39-1

Care of the Patient After Prostatectomy—cont'd

PROBLEM/NURSING DIAGNOSIS *Worried about being able to achieve an erection*/Risk for sexual dysfunction related to inability to achieve erection.

Supporting assessment data *Subjective data:* "Do you think my wife will leave me if I can no longer have an erection to meet her sexual needs?" *Objective data:* Prostatectomy 6/25.

Goals/Expected Outcomes	Nursing Interventions	Selected Rationale	Evaluation
Patient will discuss concerns before discharge	Encourage verbalization of problems and concerns.	Verbalization of concerns helps with identifying solutions.	Verbalizes concern about the possibility of not being able to obtain an erection.
	Provide information on alternative ways to achieve erection.	Gives the patient useful information in case of need.	Provided with information about the alternate ways to achieve erection.
Patient will discuss concerns with his spouse before discharge	Counsel in other ways to achieve intimacy. Include spouse or significant other in discussions.	Addressing individual needs of patient encourages learning and retention.	Agrees to include spouse in discussions regarding his sexual concerns.
	Assist to make plan to meet sexual needs.	Provides tools to cope with sexual problems.	

CRITICAL THINKING QUESTIONS

1. What are the priority nursing interventions if the nurse notices that the urinary outflow is less than the irrigation input after bladder irrigation?
2. Why is it important to attend to complaints of pain from bladder spasms as soon as possible? What is the medication generally used for this type of pain?

Nonspecific genitourinary infections in the male, including nongonococcal urethritis (NGU), may be caused by various organisms but present substantially the same clinical picture. Among the symptoms of nonspecific urethritis are mucopurulent discharge from the urethra, painful urination of varying degrees of severity, and occasionally the appearance of blood in the urine. A microscopic examination of a smear from urethral secretions may not show any specific organisms, but there may be an excessive number of white cells.

EPIDIDYMITIS

Epididymitis is an inflammation of the epididymis and may result from an infection of the prostate. The patient with epididymitis complains of groin pain plus swelling and pain in the scrotum. In men below the age of 35, the major cause of epididymitis is *Chlamydia trachomatis*, a sexually transmitted organism. Sometimes an inflammatory epididymitis occurs after vigorous exercise. Symptoms are scrotal pain, swelling, induration of the epididymis, and eventual edema of the scrotal wall. The adjacent testicle may become involved. Antibiotics, ice packs, analgesics, and elevation of the scrotum are the prescribed treatment protocol. Treatment of the partner is recommended if the source is *Chlamydia* infection.

ORCHITIS

Orchitis is inflammation of the testicle and may affect one or both testes. It may be caused by local or systemic infection (viral or bacterial) or by trauma. *Mumps orchitis* occurs in about 20% of adult males who contract mumps. Bilateral orchitis is serious and very often causes sterility. Gamma globulin usually is given to lessen the severity of mumps orchitis. The symptoms and treatment parallel those of epididymitis.

PROSTATITIS

Prostatitis is an inflammation of the prostate that occurs from an infectious agent or other causes. A newly established National Institutes of Health (NIH) classification (Goldman et al., 2004) system includes:

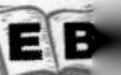

- *Type I: Acute bacterial prostatitis* with recovery of bacteria from fluid and signs of illness such as fever
- *Type II: Chronic bacterial prostatitis* with recovery of bacteria from fluid and no signs of systemic illness
- *Type III: Nonbacterial prostatitis:* recovery of leukocytes; microscopic purulence of prostate fluid is present but few or no bacteria are recovered
- *Type IV: Prostatodynia:* no bacteria or leukocytes in prostate fluid but persistent symptoms of prostate discomfort, including poor urinary flow, frequency, and dysuria

Symptoms are often mistaken for BPH, and since blood PSA levels are often elevated in prostatitis, misdiagnosis of prostate cancer can occur. Type I prostatitis is diagnosed by a positive urine culture. Prostate massage is contraindicated in order to prevent bacteremia. Symptoms include low back and perineal pain, dysuria, and urinary frequency.

Types II and III prostatitis can be diagnosed with a segmented culture of the initial stream urine, midstream urine, prostate fluid before and after massage, and postmassage urine specimen. Symptoms include recurrent urinary infections, pelvic pain, and sexual dysfunction. Type IV is diagnosed by prostate biopsy. It may be asymptomatic or considered "chronic pelvic pain syndrome" (Goldman et al., 2004).

For type I prostatitis, a culture will determine the appropriate antimicrobial therapy. Parenteral antibiotics may be necessary, but oral fluoroquinolones or trimethoprim-sulfamethoxazole treatment for 1 month may be required. Type II prostatitis is more difficult to treat because chronic infection renders the prostate fluid alkaline and resistant to some antibiotics. Penicillin, cephalosporins, aminoglycosides, and nitrofurantoins are ineffective. Fluoroquinolones or trimethoprim-sulfamethoxazole therapy for 1 to 3 months is recommended. For type III prostatitis, the bioflavinoid quercetin and rofecoxib may have clinical benefits. There is no evidence that antibiotics are helpful. Research is ongoing.

The NIH and the National Institute of Arthritis, Diabetes, Digestive and Kidney Diseases funds the Chronic Prostatitis Collaborative Research Network, which is a multidisciplinary medical team conducting randomized clinical trials and research concerning the diagnosis and treatment of prostatitis (Goldman et al., 2004).

CANCER OF THE MALE REPRODUCTIVE TRACT

CANCER OF THE PENIS

Cancer of the penis is rare, occurring mostly in males with human papillomavirus infections or males who were not circumcised (Cultural Cues 39–2). A nontender nodule may appear on the penis, and biopsy will show a squamous cell–type carcinoma. Laser resection of the lesion is the treatment of choice unless the cancer has spread. Radical resection of the penis followed by radiation and chemotherapy may be required.

TESTICULAR CANCER

Testicular cancer, although rare, occurs most commonly in men ages 15 to 40 and is the leading cause of cancer death in men 25 to 35 years of age. It is most frequently found in whites and is quite rare in African Americans.

Men most at risk for testicular cancer are those who have had an undescended or partially descended testicle. This condition, called **cryptorchidism,** occurs during fetal development. As the unborn male child matures, the testes first appear in the abdomen at about the level of the kidneys. They develop at this site until approximately the seventh month of fetal life, when they start to move downward to the upper part of the groin. From there they move into the inguinal canal and then into the scrotum. If the descent of a testis is halted in its progress, it is known as *undescended testis* or cryptorchidism. Sometimes the undescended testicle will drop into the scrotum when the boy starts walking. If it remains undescended, surgical correction is required because bathing of the testicle in the warm environment of the abdomen will cause sterility. Treatment of cryptorchidism consists of surgical correction in a procedure called *orchidopexy.*

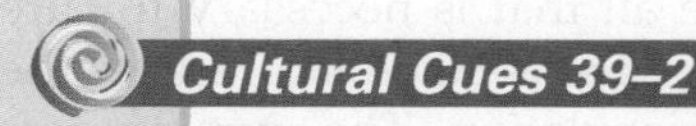

Cultural Cues 39–2

Incidence and Mortality Rate of Penile Cancer

Penile cancer is very rare in this country. Testicular cancer is more common in whites, whereas prostate cancer occurs most frequently among African American men, with a high mortality rate.

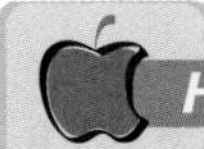

Health Promotion Points 39–1

Testicular Self-Examination

- Should be performed monthly.
- Perform after bathing when scrotal skin is relaxed.
- Roll each testicle between thumb and fingers.
- Report lumps to health care provider.

Men who were exposed to diethylstilbestrol (DES) in utero also are at higher risk for testicular cancer. All males between the ages of 15 and 40 should practice testicular self-examination regularly on a monthly basis (Health Promotion Points 39–1).

If a mass is found and thought to be malignant, diagnostic tests for tumor marker proteins such as elevated levels of AFP, beta-HCG, alkaline phosphatase, and lactate dehydrogenase are obtained to confirm diagnosis. Computed tomography (CT) scans and/or ultrasound should be performed to detect sites of metastasis, as testicular cancer spreads rapidly via lymph and blood vessels.

When testicular cancer is suspected, **orchiectomy** (unilateral removal of the testicle) is performed. There are three stages for classifying the malignancy. In *Stage I,* the tumor is confined to the affected testis. In *Stage II,* malignant cells have spread to the regional lymph nodes, usually on the same side as the affected testis. In *Stage III,* there is metastasis to other organs, such as the lungs and liver.

If the testicular tumor is limited to the scrotal sac and there is no metastasis, surgical removal of the testis (orchiectomy) may be all that is necessary to cure the patient of his disease. Care is taken to preserve the nerves associated with ejaculation. The nursing care focuses on teaching and providing psychological support. Ice bags and scrotal support provide comfort, and the importance of follow-up care is stressed. Removal of only one testis will not affect the patient's ability to produce the male hormone testosterone or render him impotent, as there remains another testis to carry on normal testicular function.

Further treatment for testicular cancer may include chemotherapy and radiation. Refer to Chapter 8 for a detailed discussion of radiation and chemotherapy in the care of cancer patients. In addition to routine preoperative and postoperative nursing care and attention to the special needs of a cancer patient, the nurse helps the patient with testicular cancer deal with problems related to his masculinity and sexual activity. He will need time to think about and discuss the effects of surgery that have been explained to him by the surgeon.

Some men view an orchiectomy as a loss of manhood. The nurse can be instrumental in assisting the patient to accept the procedure. Time for questions and discussion of concerns should be provided for the patient and his sexual partner. Sperm banking prior to surgery is an option for the young patient who may wish to produce children in the future. Continued follow-up care is essential.

PROSTATE CANCER

Carcinoma of the prostate is the second most common cause of cancer deaths in men (following lung cancer). There are approximately 218,890 new cases per year in the United States (American Cancer Society, 2007). It is usually a slow growing cancer that is dependent on the hormone androgen. When palpated, a malignant nodule feels hard and immovable. Needle biopsy and tests to determine whether metastatic spread has occurred are performed to determine the best treatment. Whenever a biopsy shows a prostate tumor to be malignant, the entire prostate and its capsule may be removed.

? *Think Critically About . . .* What sort of psychological care would the patient undergoing a prostatic biopsy need from the nurse? What might be some of the patient's concerns?

An elevated PSA screening test indicates prostate pathology but is not diagnostic for prostate cancer. A PSA level of 4 to 10 ng/mL and the percentage of free PSA are helpful in diagnosing prostate cancer. A transrectal ultrasound may be done. In cases in which the PSA levels rise above 10 ng/mL, a bone scan may be done; if the level is above 20 ng/mL, an abdominal CT may be indicated to detect metastasis. A prostascint scan using single-photon emission computed tomography (SPECT) is an imaging technique that targets PSA and detects the spread of prostate cancer.

Box 39–1 *Staging and Treatment Options for Prostate Cancer*

STAGE A

- Detected in about 10% of men with prostatic cancer. Tumor not palpable but detected by pathologic examination of biopsy specimen or surgically removed prostate tissue.
- In Stage A1 or in men over 70 who are not good candidates for surgical removal, watchful waiting is suggested. Monitor with physical examination and PSA tests every 3 to 6 months. Watchful waiting is recommended only for men with a life expectancy of less than 10 years.
- In Stage A2 or for patients younger than age 70, radical prostatectomy is recommended.

STAGE B

- Detected in about 15% to 20% of cases diagnosed. Palpable tumor is confined to the prostatic capsule and involves no more than one lobe of the prostate.
- Radical prostatectomy, radiation therapy, or implantation of a radioactive seed are the options.

STAGE C

- Detected in about 40% of cases diagnosed. Local extension of tumor beyond the prostate, but no evidence of distant metastases.
- Radical prostatectomy, radiation therapy, or both are options. Hormone therapy may also be used.

STAGE D

- Detected in 30% to 35% of new cases. The cancer is no longer localized and has spread to regional lymph nodes or beyond the pelvis to the bone or other organs.
- Prostatectomy is not an option as disease has spread beyond the prostate. Hormone therapy is the treatment of choice. Radiation or chemotherapy may be combined with the hormone therapy.

Prostate cancer has a staged classification that is based upon the size of the tumor and degree of metastasis. The regional stage of prostate cancer (local involvement) offers almost a 100% survival rate. Box 39–1 presents the stages and the recommended treatment.

Some studies have shown that a low-fat diet, soy products, and vitamin E and selenium supplements may reduce the risk of developing prostate cancer, but research is ongoing.

Since prostate cancer is relatively slow growing, conservative treatment may involve monitoring and follow-up care. Annual digital rectal exams are done, and PSA levels are monitored. When surgical therapy is indicated, a radical prostatectomy is considered the most effective treatment for long-term survival before metastasis occurs. Other treatment options are listed in Table 39–4.

A multidisciplinary approach integrates surgery, radiation, and androgen restriction. Following sur-

Table 39–4 Treatment Options for Prostate Cancer

TREATMENT	COMMENTS
Radical prostatectomy	The prostate gland, seminal vesicles, and portions of the neck of the bladder are removed. ED and incontinence are two long-term complications.
Cryosurgery	A freezing technique destroys prostate tissue. Complications include urethral damage, ED, and incontinence.
Radiation therapy	May be prescribed when the patient is not a candidate for surgery or may be offered in combination with surgery and hormone therapy.
External beam radiation	Most popular form of radiation therapy, given weekly on an outpatient basis for 2 mo. Side effects can include skin irritation, GI cramping and bleeding, ED, and bone marrow suppression. Cure rates for patients with localized cancer are comparable to radical prostatectomy.
Brachytherapy	The implantation of radioactive seeds into the prostate gland. It may be offered in combination with external beam radiation.
Hormone therapy	Designed to reduce androgens. Leuprolide (Lupron, Viadur), goserelin (Zoladex) and triptorelin (Trelstar) are common drugs used; produces a chemical castration.
Chemotherapy	Used for hormone-resistant cancer or late-stage cancer. The prostate has limited response to chemotherapy.
Bisphosphonates	Reduce bone complications in advanced stages of prostate cancer. Drugs may include zoledronic acid (Zometa), risedronate (Actonel), etidronate (Didronel), or alendronate (Fosamax).

Key: *ED*, erectile dysfunction.

gery, PSA levels are monitored, and a decrease may indicate treatment success.

Radiation therapy may be added to surgical treatment for malignancy. Chapter 8 presents a detailed discussion concerning care of the cancer patient receiving radiation and chemotherapy. The nurse should provide a sensitive, caring approach to the patient and family to help them cope with the diagnosis and make informed choices. Preoperative care involves restoration of urinary drainage, prevention of urinary tract infection, and understanding the options for treatment and their impact on sexual function. Postoperative care is reviewed in Patient Teaching 39–1 and Nursing Care Plan 39–1.

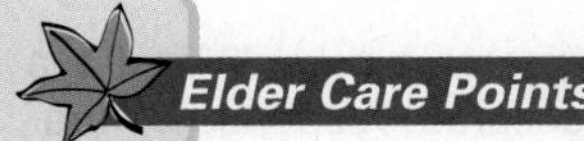

Elder Care Points

For the elderly patient undergoing chemotherapy or radiation:

- Monitor for infections.
- Promote assisted ambulation.
- Institute fall precautions.
- Encourage use of incentive spirometer.
- Minimize pain.
- Reorient to environment as needed.

COMMUNITY CARE

Nurses in the community can be instrumental in teaching and promoting the use of testicular self-examination in men between the ages of 15 and 40. Teaching the benefits of and encouraging all men over 50 to have an annual digital rectal examination and PSA test may help reduce the death rate from prostate cancer by promoting earlier detection and treatment.

Each nurse should be knowledgeable enough about BPH and prostate cancer to direct patients who are trying to make a decision about treatment options to reliable information. The Agency for Health Care Policy and Research has available a publication detailing outcomes of BPH treatments (www.ahrq.gov).

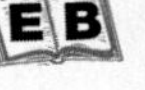

Nurses in long-term care facilities must be watchful for urinary obstruction in elderly male residents. Alert men should be questioned regularly about problems with urination; men with cognitive impairment who do not have a normal urinary stream should be placed on intake and output recording to detect any problems with urinary obstruction. Palpation just above the symphysis pubis may reveal a distended bladder.

All nurses can be instrumental in teaching perineal muscle (Kegel) exercises to decrease the incidence of incontinence. Incontinence is one of the prime causes of loss of self-esteem in the elderly and can be corrected in many cases. Correcting incontinence also greatly decreases the nursing care time that needs to be spent with the patient, thereby cutting health care costs.

Home care nurses supervise or assist with dressing changes for the patient who has radical surgery, monitor side effects and complications in patients undergoing radiation, teach self-care, and provide psychosocial support for patients with prostate cancer and sexual dysfunction. Collaboration with the physician, social worker, and community agencies can provide avenues of help for these patients.

Nurses in the community can assist patients who are suffering from erectile dysfunction by including assessment for this problem when working with male patients. Knowledge about treatment options, a matter-of-fact optimistic attitude, and a comfortable manner when speaking about this topic can provide hope and guidance. Sometimes this problem is brought to light when speaking with the spouse of the older patient. Many times a satisfying sexual life can be reinstituted for these couples, providing added fulfillment and joy in the later years.

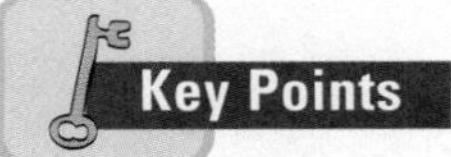

- The urinary and reproductive systems in the male are closely linked, and a disorder in one system often affects the other.
- Cancer of the testicle is linked to history of undescended testicle or to exposure in utero to DES.
- PSA levels become elevated when prostate disease is present. Normal values in males over age 15 are 0.81 to 0.89 ng/mL.
- Transrectal ultrasonography of the prostate is performed when a nodule is found or when PSA levels rise. It is performed as an outpatient procedure without anesthesia and takes about 20 minutes.
- Nursing care is planned based on patient's age, educational level, degree of comfort in discussing reproductive problems, and culture.
- Patient education concerning disorders of the reproductive tract should include information about the impact on sexual activity.
- Elderly patients suffering from urinary retention may have fluid and electrolyte imbalances that cause confusion.
- Elderly patients who have consistently participated in intercourse through the years have the best chance of maintaining this capability into old age.
- Nurses can be instrumental in teaching and promoting use of monthly testicular self-examination and monitoring for prostate cancer by digital rectal examination and PSA testing.
- Nurses in long-term care facilities must watch for signs of urinary obstruction in elderly men.

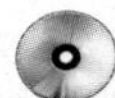
Go to your **Companion CD-ROM** for an Audio Glossary, animations, video clips, and bonus review questions.

evolve Be sure to visit the companion Evolve site at http://evolve.elsevier.com/deWit for interactive NCLEX-PN Exam Style Review Questions, WebLinks, and additional online resources.

NCLEX-PN EXAM STYLE REVIEW QUESTIONS

Choose the best answer(s) for the following questions.

1. A 22-year-old man complains of sudden acute scrotal pain. Initial examination reveals absence of the cremasteric reflex. Doppler ultrasound reveals a diminished blood flow. This condition would most likely be:
   1. varicocele.
   2. testicular torsion.
   3. hydrocele.
   4. priapism.

2. A 65-year-old man complains of difficulty urinating, described as decreased caliber of the urine stream. He also has accompanying hesitancy, dribbling, and urgency. A digital rectal examination (DRE) reveals an enlarged prostate. Appropriate nursing interventions include which of the following? *(Select all that apply.)*
   1. Teach to decrease caffeine and artificial sweeteners.
   2. Teach to limit spicy foods and alcohol intake.
   3. Apply a condom catheter.
   4. Restrict fluid intake.
   5. Plan a timed voiding schedule.

3. The physician prescribs finasteride (Proscar) to a patient with benign prostatic hyperplasia. The nurse must discuss which of the anticipated side effects of the medication?
   1. Increased libido
   2. Increased ejaculate volume
   3. Erectile dysfunction
   4. Increased PSA levels

4. The nurse admits a patient with a tentative diagnosis of benign prostatic hyperplasia. An appropriate question to determine urinary patterns would be:
   1. "Have you noticed any changes in the stream of urine?"
   2. "Do you ever have any discharge coming from the penis?"
   3. "Do you have any tenderness or pain in the scrotum or penis?"
   4. "Do you perform regular testicular examinations?"

5. A patient with cancer of the prostate asks, "What is a radical prostatectomy?" An accurate response by the nurse would be:
   1. "A freezing technique that destroys prostate tissue."
   2. "A urethral resectoscope is used to remove prostate tissue."
   3. "Surgical removal of the prostate gland, seminal vesicles, and portions of the bladder neck."
   4. "A transurethral probe heats and coagulates prostate tissue."

6. The nurse is taking care of a 40-year-old Hispanic American man who had a bilateral orchiectomy. Clinical interviews with the patient confirm mounting concerns regarding his "manhood." The nurse would effectively approach the patient's disturbance in body image effectively by:
   1. establishing eye contact.
   2. demonstrating sensitivity to nonverbal cues.
   3. asking specific questions.
   4. involving nonessential members of the family.

7. A patient who had transurethral resection of the prostate (TURP) complains of mounting bladder spasms. An appropriate initial nursing action would be to:
   1. medicate with a belladonna and opium suppository.
   2. check the urinary catheter tubing for kinks and obstruction.
   3. teach relaxation exercises.
   4. encourage use of patient-controlled analgesia.

8. The loss of elasticity in a section of the penis that results in the inability to have a uniform erection is referred as ____________________.

9. A 25-year-old African American man was hospitalized for a prolonged penile erection unrelated to sexual desire or activity. A likely cause would be:
   1. diabetes mellitus.
   2. sickle cell disease.
   3. hemophilia.
   4. urinary infections.

10. A postprostatectomy patient expresses concerns regarding his ability to have intimate relations with his wife. The nurse identifies a nursing diagnosis of Risk for sexual dysfunction. Nursing interventions would be geared toward which of the following nursing goals?
   1. Identify signs and symptoms of infection.
   2. Have him verbalize personal concerns with his partner.
   3. Demonstrate good aseptic wound care.
   4. Help him develop alternative coping strategies.

CRITICAL THINKING ACTIVITIES

Read each clinical scenario and discuss the questions with your classmates.

Scenario A

Your brother, who is 20 years old, tells you of a friend who has just learned that he has testicular cancer and is scheduled for surgery tomorrow. Your brother is concerned about the effect the surgery will have on his friend's "manhood." He also says that, if ever he has that kind of cancer, he doesn't want to know about it, and he certainly wouldn't allow surgery.

1. What information could you give your brother about testicular cancer and self-examination of the testes?
2. How could you explain that removal of a testis does not render a man less masculine?

Scenario B

Mr. Watts, age 67, has been admitted to the hospital to undergo a transurethral resection of the prostate. He is assigned to your care on his second postoperative day. Mr. Watts seems disoriented and restless, and when you begin to give him his bath, he tells you that his bladder is full and he needs to urinate. You check the catheter and find that it apparently is not draining as it should.

1. What would you tell Mr. Watts about his need to void?
2. What would you do about the catheter, which seems obstructed?
3. What observations should you make while caring for this patient?
4. What special precautions should be taken for his safety?

CHAPTER 40

Care of Patients with Sexually Transmitted Infections

evolve http://evolve.elsevier.com/deWit

Objectives

Upon completion of this chapter, you should be able to:

Theory

1. Identify the signs and symptoms of common sexually transmitted infections.
2. Discuss the danger of contracting human papillomavirus (HPV) or pelvic imflammatory disease (PID).
3. Explain the procedure for the various tests for STDs.
4. Describe the characteristics of genital herpes, its treatment, and the resources available to those who need information about it.
5. Compare the symptoms of gonorrhea in male and female patients.
6. Describe the treatment of gonorrhea and the potential consequences of failure to treat this infection.
7. List the ways in which human immunodeficiency virus (HIV) is transmitted.
8. Identify the three stages of syphilis and discuss treatment and the importance of early detection and intervention.

Clinical Practice

1. Devise a teaching plan for the patient who has experienced a first incidence of genital herpes.
2. Instruct a female patient on ways to prevent contracting or transmitting HIV.
3. Teach a female patient and a male patient ways to prevent sexually transmitted diseases.

Key Terms

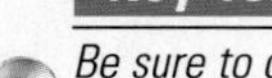
Be sure to check out the bonus material on the Companion CD-ROM, including selected audio pronunciations.

agglutination (ă-GLŪ-tĭ-NĀ-shŭn, p. 994)
bacterial vaginosis (băk-TĒ-rē-ăl vă-jĭ-NŌ-sĭs, p. 993)
chancre (SHĂNG-kĕr, p. 999)
gram negative (p. 1000)
gram positive (p. 1000)
oophoritis (oof-ō-RĪ-tĭs, p. 994)
pelvic inflammatory disease (PĔL-vĭk ĭn-FLĂ-mă-tŏ-rē dĭ-ZĒZ, p. 993, 994)
peritonitis (pĕr-ĭ-tō-NĪ-tĭs, p. 994)
salpingitis (săl-pĭn-GĪ-tĭs, p. 994)
sexually transmitted infection (p. 992)

The term **sexually transmitted infections** (STIs) refers to those particular infections spread by intimate physical contact. Modes of transmission include sexual intercourse and contact with the *genitals* (sexual organs), rectum, or mouth. STIs can also be transmitted via blood contact, and can be transmitted to the fetus via the placenta or to the newborn during the birth process.

The incidence of STIs continues to rise throughout the world. Although all sexually active people must be considered potentially at risk, and people with multiple sexual partners are at very high risk for contracting an STI, the largest population group affected by STIs is adolescents and young adults (Workowski & Berman, 2006). 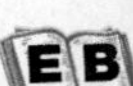 Teens are engaging in sexual practices at an earlier age and have an opportunity for multiple partners. They are often unaware of signs and symptoms of STIs and are reluctant or unable to access confidential health care. **Inflamed tissue and open lesions associated with STIs increase the risk of developing human immunodeficiency virus (HIV) infection that can result in acquired immunodeficiency syndrome (AIDS). AIDS is a progressive infection for which there is currently no cure** (see Chapter 11).

> *Think Critically About . . .* What safer sex practices can help prevent the spread of STIs

STIs have a major impact on reproduction and general health. Because they are communicable, these infections are of concern both to the patient and to general public health. **One of the goals of *Healthy People 2010* is to increase efforts to "promote responsible sexual behaviors, strengthen community capacity and increase access to quality services to prevent STI and their complications." Another *Healthy People 2010* goal is to "prevent HIV infection and its related illness and death."** The progress in reaching these national goals will be reevaluated in 2010 (U.S. Department of Health and Human Services, 2000).

Refer to Chapters 38 and 39 for details on anatomy and physiology of male and female reproductive systems.

RISK FACTORS FOR TRANSMISSION OF STIs

Although men and women are equally susceptible to STIs, **women are diagnosed with STIs at a much higher rate.** Biologically, young, sexually active women have a large proportion of columnar epithelium lining the cervix and a vaginal pH that can be altered by frequent douching or by **bacterial vaginosis,** a common condition in women. An alteration of vaginal pH can place the woman at higher risk for an STI. Male secretions and semen are in contact with female mucous membranes for a longer period of time than female secretions are in contact with male mucous membranes during and after the sexual act. Therefore, women have an increased risk for STI infection (Cultural Cues 40–1). The mucus plug in the cervix of women (that protects the upper genital tract) becomes more permeable around the menstrual period, which can result in an increased risk for infections in the upper genital tract, such as **pelvic inflammatory disease** (PID).

Contraceptive choice may influence a woman's increased risk of STIs because the use of oral contraceptives alters the cervical secretions, resulting in a more alkaline environment in the vagina and thus a more favorable setting for growth of organisms that cause STIs. The use of long-acting contraceptives may reduce the use of condoms, thus increasing the risk of exposure to STIs in both partners (Cultural Cues 40–2).

Women may not seek medical care as quickly as men for symptoms of an STI. Often a vaginal discharge is considered a normal variance and health care may not be sought until the infection spreads and symptoms of PID occur. In men, urinary tract infections associated with sexual activity may be the first sign of an STI. Men may seek earlier health care intervention because the signs and symptoms are obvious and distressing. STIs can have long-term effects in the form of sterility, complicated pregnancy, or neonatal infection.

The development of a female-controlled microbicide would help women take control of preventing STIs as well as pregnancy without the need for male compliance. Health care screening services and easy access to health care are important in preventing the spread of STIs.

PREVENTION OF HPV

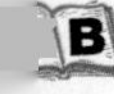

The Advisory Committee on Immunization Practices of the Centers for Disease Control and Prevention (CDC) has recommended routine human papillomavirus (HPV) vaccinations for all 11- to 26-year-old girls. Gardasil can be used for girls as young as 9 years of age. Three doses are required. (The second dose is given 2 months after the first, and the third dose is given 6 months later.) Although the vaccine is effective in preventing genital warts and precancerous lesions of the cervix, it does not protect against other HPV infections, and so recommendations for routine cervical cancer screening are still valid.

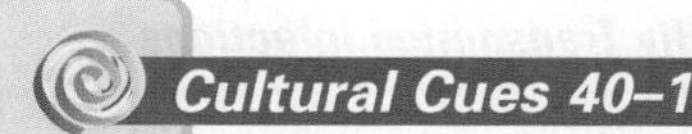

Cultural Cues 40–1

Media Effects on STIs

Custom and culture can also affect the development of STIs. STI rates increase in societies in which the media (television, magazines, movies, and Internet chat rooms) focus on sexuality and premarital sexual experiences with an increased mixing of people with varying behaviors and values, including greater sexual freedom.

Key: *STIs,* sexually transmitted infections.

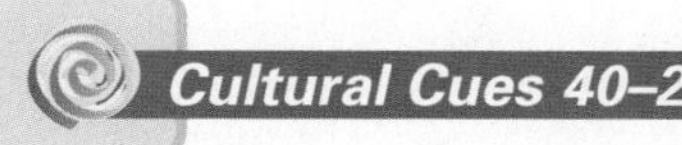

Cultural Cues 40–2

Contraception Choices

In societies or cultures in which women are passive, they may not insist on condom protection before intercourse. The condom offers protection from sexually transmitted infections, but the man often decides if it is to be used or not.

LESIONS OF STIs

In men, the lesions related to STIs may appear under the prepuce, on the head or body of the penis, or on the scrotum, perianal area, rectum, or inner thighs. In women, lesions of STIs can appear on the vulva, vagina, cervix, perianal area, or inner thighs. Lesions around the mouth can occur in cases of oral sexual practices. Lesions can also be found far from the genital area. For example, lesions of syphilis include a classic rash on the palms of the hands and soles of the feet. Lesions of *Neisseria gonorrhoeae* may spread and cause pustules on the extremities as part of an "arthritis-dermatitis" syndrome (Goldman & Ausiello, 2004). Examples of common organisms involved in STIs are listed in Box 40–1.

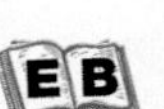

REPORTING STIs

STIs must be reported to the local public health agency in accordance with state and local statutory requirements. The CDC and local health authorities establish these regulations and provide regular updates and reporting forms to health care providers for monitored infections. Syphilis, gonorrhea, chlamydia, chancroid, lymphogranuloma venereum, hepatitis B, PID, HIV infection, and AIDS are reportable diseases in all parts of the United States according the the public health guidelines from the CDC. The requirements for report-

Box 40–1 *Causes of Sexually Transmitted Infections*

BACTERIA
- *Neisseria gonorrhoeae*
- *Chlamydia trachomatis*
- *Treponema pallidum* (syphilis)
- *Haemophilus ducreyi* (chancroid)
- *Mycoplasma hominis*

VIRUSES
- Human herpesvirus 2 (herpes simplex virus type 2)
- Hepatitis B virus
- Human immunodeficiency virus (HIV)
- Human papillomavirus (HPV)

YEASTS AND FUNGI
- *Candida albicans*
- *Candida glabrata*
- *Candida tropicalis*

PARASITES
- *Trichomonas vaginalis* (trichomoniasis)

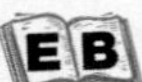

Data from www.cdc.gov/std/trichomoniasis/default.htm.

ing others STIs differ by state, and clinicians must be familiar with state and local reporting requirements. This tracking information is used to determine community resource needs and is evaluated in terms of the national goals of *Healthy People 2010.*

COMMON INFECTIONS OF THE FEMALE REPRODUCTIVE TRACT

PELVIC INFLAMMATORY DISEASE

Pelvic inflammatory disease (PID) refers to any inflammation in the pelvic cavity. If the infection is located in the fallopian tubes, it is called **salpingitis.** Infection of the ovary is called **oophoritis;** involvement of the pelvic peritoneum is called pelvic **peritonitis.** The organisms causing the infection are usually introduced from the outside, traveling through the uterus to infect pelvic organs. Therefore PID is much more common in sexually active women, particularly women with multiple sexual partners. Most of these infections are commonly caused by two sexually transmitted organisms, *Neisseria gonorrhoeae* and *Chlamydia trachomatis,* and the most common complication is infertility due to fallopian tube damage. However, PID can also be the result of an infection following pelvic surgery or childbirth and is not *always* an STI.

Symptoms of acute PID include severe abdominal and pelvic pain and fever, frequently accompanied by a foul-smelling purulent vaginal discharge, and the woman appears acutely ill. Chronic PID usually causes backache, a feeling of pelvic heaviness, and disturbances in menstruation. However, mild cases may produce no symptoms but still cause significant reproductive damage. Acute PID usually is treated with intravenous antimicrobials, symptom relief, and patient support and teaching. Refer to Chapter 38 for other common inflammations and infections of female reproductive tract.

OVERVIEW OF SEXUALLY TRANSMITTED INFECTIONS

STIs are primarily passed through some type of intimate contact, either genital to genital, mouth to genital, or genital to rectum. They occur in both heterosexual and homosexual relationships. Some infections, such as HIV or hepatitis B, also may be passed through blood contact, the sharing of contaminated needles, or, though rare, transfusion with contaminated blood. Accidental transmission may occur via needle or sharps injuries to medical personnel or by direct exposure to open wounds or body fluids.

Blood-borne infections may be transmitted to the fetus prior to birth. The newborn is at risk for contracting any STI that may reside in the vagina at the time of birth. Depending on the organism, such exposure can lead to a variety of serious problems for the infant, including pneumonia and blindness.

? ***Think Critically About . . .*** What are the four major modes of transmission for STIs?

In many states screening for some STIs, particularly syphilis, is required for a marriage license. However, it is expensive to screen for all STIs. The greatest hope for controlling STIs is public awareness, and willingness to take responsibility for prevention and for treatment should infection occur.

COMMON DIAGNOSTIC TESTS

Table 40–1 lists the more common STIs and contains information about modes of transmission, diagnosis, symptoms, treatment, and nursing responsibilities.

A variety of tests are used to detect STIs. Noninvasive diagnostic techniques have been developed that use urine samples. *Smears and cultures* may be taken directly from the site (e.g., vaginal, cervical, or urethral swabs). In some instances, organisms also can be cultured from the blood. *Biopsies* are microscopic tissue examinations performed on a sample taken from the affected area and are usually done to differentiate between benign and malignant tissues, but can also provide a differential diagnosis in diseases that have specific unusual cellular changes or organisms present.

Numerous types of blood tests can help detect STIs. They look for specific antibodies formed by the presence of certain microorganisms or for the effects of antigens (substances in the bloodstream that stimulate the production of antibodies). Such effects include the tendency for **agglutination,** the clumping together of cells in a variety of characteristic patterns.

Text continued on p. 1000

Table 40–1 Common Sexually Transmitted Infections

INFECTION	MODES OF TRANSMISSION	SYMPTOMS	MEDICAL DIAGNOSIS	MEDICAL TREATMENT	NURSING INTERVENTIONS
Chlamydia trachomatis	Direct sexual contact. May be transmitted to the newborn during vaginal delivery. Most common STI in the United States.	*Male:* Often asymptomatic. Dysuria frequency of urination, watery, mucus-like discharge. Causes about half the cases of epididymitis and nongonococcal urethritis. *Female:* Approximately 75% have no symptoms. Yellow vaginal discharge, urinary frequency, dysuria. May have unusual odor after intercourse. Can result in PID, ectopic pregnancy, and sterility. *Neonate:* Exposure can cause eye infections and pneumonia.	By cervical culture, DNA probe, enzyme immunoassay, or nucleic acid amplification. Also screened for gonorrhea as co-infection is common.	A 7-day course of antibiotics such as doxycycline (Vibramycin), ofloxacin (Floxin), or levofloxacin (Levaquin). A single dose of azithromycin (1 g PO) for patients with compliance problem. Erythromycin for pregnant women.	*Education:* Encourage patients to seek attention for any unusual vaginal or penile discharge. Partner(s) must be treated concurrently. Condom use for prevention of future infection, with abstinence until course of treatment completed. Must complete antibiotics to ensure effective treatment and prevent development of PID. Screening of all pregnant women and sexually active young women is recommended by CDC.
Human papillomavirus (HPV) Condylomata acuminata (venereal warts) caused by HPV	Spread during sexual contact. Highly contagious. Can be transmitted to newborn during vaginal delivery.	Warts are flat or raised, rough, cauliflower-like growths on the vulva, penis, perianal area, vaginal or rectal walls, or cervix. The flat variety is more likely to lead to tissue changes that contribute to cervical or penile cancer. *Neonate:* Laryngeal papillomas.	Biopsy, colposcopy, anoscopy, Pap smear.	Freezing, laser therapy, surgical removal, cryotherapy. Topical podophyllin, imiquimod, and podofilox are alternative treatments for external warts. Topical TCA or interferon is used for difficult cases. Some lesions can cause cancer.	*Education:* Teach about mode of infection and use of condoms to prevent spread. Regular Pap smears due to increased risk of cervical cancer. Vaccine has been developed and is recommended for all young women to prevent infection.

Key: *AIDS,* acquired immunodeficiency syndrome; *ARC,* AIDS-related complex; *CD4,* T helper cell; *CDC,* Centers for Disease Control and Prevention; *DNA,* deoxyribonucleic acid; *FDA,* Food and Drug Administration; *FTA-Abs,* fluorescent treponemal antibody absorption; *HBIG,* hepatitis B immune globulin; *HBsAg,* hepatitis B surface antigen; *IM,* intramuscular; *Pap,* Papanicolaou; *PID,* pelvic inflammatory disease; *PO,* oral; *RPR,* rapid plasma reagin; *STI,* sexually transmitted infection; *TCA,* trichloroacetic acid; *VDRL,* Venereal Disease Research Laboratory.

Continued

Table 40–1 ***Common Sexually Transmitted Infections—cont'd***

INFECTION	MODES OF TRANSMISSION	SYMPTOMS	MEDICAL DIAGNOSIS	MEDICAL TREATMENT	NURSING INTERVENTIONS
Genital herpes 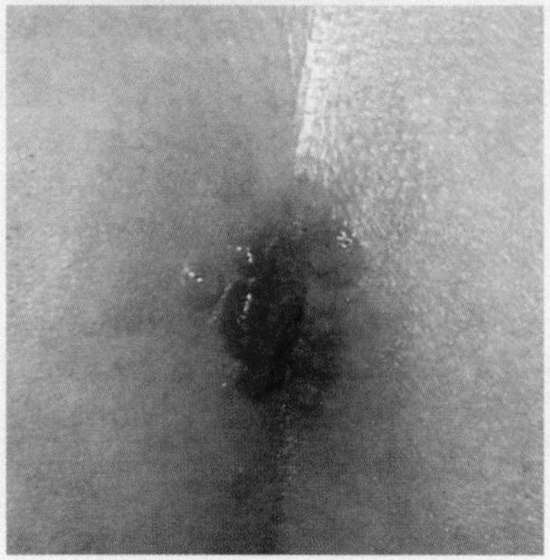	Caused by herpes simplex virus (HSV) types 1 and 2. Highly contagious, spread by direct contact; not limited to sexual contact. Self-inoculation also possible, for example, from lip ulcer (fever blister) to genitals. Invades nerve cells located near the site of infection. Lies dormant, flare-ups erratic and unpredictable. Some patients have frequent recurrence, others rarely or none. Neonate may be infected during delivery if mother has active disease (more common if initial episode occurs during pregnancy).	*Primary:* Fever, headache, malaise, myalgia, burning genital pain, dysuria (female), painful intercourse. Vesicles in genital area that ulcerate, crust over, and resolve spontaneously in about 2 wk. *Secondary:* Burning genital pain, possible numbness and tingling 24 hr before lesions appear, vesicles. *Male:* Lesions may appear on glans penis, shaft of penis, prepuce, scrotal sac, inner thighs. *Female:* Vulva, vaginal surface, buttocks, cervix. Cervical lesions may be small and superficial with diffuse inflammation, or a single, large, necrotic ulcer. Increased risk of cervical cancer. Primary infection during pregnancy associated with high risk of premature labor and spontaneous abortion. *Neonate:* Severity ranges from clinically inapparent to local infections of eyes, skin, or mucous membranes to severe disseminated infection. The latter may be neurologic and can cause severe damage or death.	Lesions usually easily identified by experienced clinician. Can be confirmed by viral cultures.	No known cure. Treatment with acyclovir, valacyclovir, or famciclovir may reduce symptoms and accelerate healing. For individuals with frequent recurrence, continuous treatment may reduce frequency. Topical acyclovir is not as effective as systemic.	Lesions must be kept clean and dry to prevent secondary infection. Increased fluids will dilute urine for greater comfort during voiding. Topical anesthetics and oral analgesics may help manage pain. Strict gloving and observation of Standard Precautions are necessary. *Education:* Use of condoms with spermicide to help prevent spread, avoidance of sex if lesions present; scrupulous hand hygiene; importance of informing health care provider if patient becomes pregnant that she has been diagnosed with genital herpes (if disease is active, infant will be delivered by cesarean section to protect it from exposure).

Gonorrhea (GC) 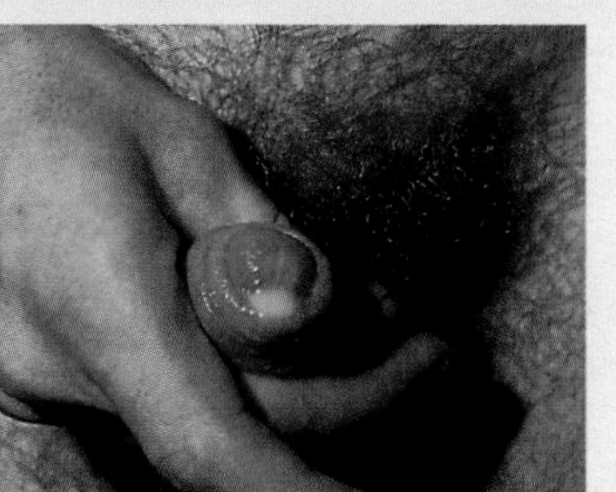	Easily transmitted by direct sexual contact. Transmitted to the newborn during vaginal delivery if mother has active disease. Autoinoculation via fingers to eye possible. Occasionally becomes blood-borne.	Incubation: 2–6 days after exposure. May be asymptomatic. *Male:* Dysuria with frequency; scant to copious purulent discharge from penis, unilateral testicular pain. If untreated, discharge increases and may continue for months; may develop urethral stricture, epididymitis. Can advance to inflammation of prostate and testes; can cause sterility. *Female:* Vaginal discharge, burning on urination. Untreated, results in PID. May involve rectum, eyes, oropharynx. *Neonate:* Due to exposure at birth to mother's vaginal secretions, is at risk for ophthalmia neonatorum, which can cause blindness, and other infections within 2–5 days after birth. *Children:* Infection in children over 1 yr of age is likely due to sexual abuse.	Confirmed by presence of the causative organism, *Neisseria gonorrhoeae,* in vaginal or urethral smear, rectal or pharyngeal culture. Nucleic amplification test using urine sample is accurate.	A single dose of ceftriaxone IM is treatment of choice.* Cefixime, tablets are awaiting FDA approval. Hospitalize if PID or severe illness occurs. Empirical treatment for chlamydia is recommended by CDC.	Observation of Standard Precautions and frequent hand hygiene if contact with any body fluids. *Education:* Teach about prevention and treatment, specifically importance of completing treatment, naming all contacts so everyone can be treated, and having follow-up cultures to ensure that treatment has been effective. Encourage safer sex practices (use of condoms, limiting sexual contacts) to prevent reinfection. Be sure patient understands how to take prescribed medication. Teach CDC recommendations for sexually active young women to be screened for GC infection. Men are not screened routinely as symptoms may be more obvious.

Continued

Table 40–1 ***Common Sexually Transmitted Infections—cont'd***

INFECTION	MODES OF TRANSMISSION	SYMPTOMS	MEDICAL DIAGNOSIS	MEDICAL TREATMENT	NURSING INTERVENTIONS
Hepatitis B	Caused by hepatitis B virus (HBV). Transmission via sexual contact, blood contact, and to the fetus via the placenta in an infected mother.	May have anorexia, malaise, nausea, vomiting, abdominal pain, dark urine, jaundice, skin rashes, arthralgias, arthritis. Acute infection may be asymptomatic, and may resolve, resulting in permanent immunity. However, infection may be persistent and result in a chronic carrier state. Long-term patients may develop chronic persistent or chronic active hepatitis, cirrhosis, hepatocellular carcinoma, hepatic failure, and death. Infants born infected are at high risk for chronic hepatitis B infection.	Serologic testing for HBV infection gives definitive diagnosis.	No specific therapy is available. HBIG is given prophylactically following known exposure. Hepatitis B vaccine (Hep B) is recommended for people at risk for exposure, including health care workers. Hep B vaccine is currently given as part of normal childhood immunizations with a 3-dose regimen beginning at birth. Postexposure interval before vaccination administration should not exceed 7 days for needle-stick and 14 days for sexual exposure.	Appropriate handling of all blood or body fluids to prevent transmission of infection. Prevention of needle-stick injuries. *Education:* Universal vaccination of newborns with single-antigen Hep B vaccine before discharge; routine screening of all women for HBsAg. Final dose of 3-dose regimen should be given between 6 and 12 mo of age for infants from Alaska, Pacific Islands, Africa, and other endemic areas.
Human immunodeficiency virus (HIV), AIDS, ARC	HIV is transmitted by intimate contact with body secretions of an infected person or exposure to infected blood or by perinatal transmission from mother to newborn.	Initially, flulike symptoms several weeks after HIV exposure. Antibodies appear in blood a few months to 1 yr later. A latent period follows with gradual reduction in CD4 cells. CD4 cell decline results in reduced immune function, resulting in opportunistic infections, such as Kaposi sarcoma, *Pneumocystis jiroveci* (formerly *Pneumocystis carinii*) pneumonia, and oral candidiasis. CD4 count below 200/mm^3 is diagnostic of AIDS.	Diagnosis of HIV infection based on reactive enzyme immunoassay (EIA) confirmed by a more specific assay (e.g., Western blot or immunofluorescent assay). AIDS and ARC may be diagnosed based on lab results and/or specific diagnostic criteria. An anal Pap test screen for HIV-infected men may prevent progression to anal cancer. FDA has approved a rapid test for HIV screening that provides results in less than 1 hr. A positive rapid HIV test requires further testing for confirmation.* EB	Currently there is no cure. Drug regimens interrupt reproduction of viruses. Zidovudine (ZVD) and protease inhibitors such as indinavir and other combination drugs are prescribed.	People who have tested HIV positive or been diagnosed with AIDS or ARC should receive specific professionally trained counseling on lifestyle practices, treatment protocols, and follow-up procedures. Provide support and information to improve general health. Safe sexual practices should be used to prevent spread. Avoid breastfeeding. Cesarean section for birth if pregnant.

Syphilis	Direct body contact; organism (*Treponema pallidum,* a spirochete) requires warm, wet environment to survive; can be destroyed with plain soap and water. Can penetrate intact mucous membrane. Placental transmission to fetus in about 50% of women with active disease during pregnancy.	Syphilis has three stages. *Primary* (after 3-wk incubation period): **Chancre** (hard, painless sore) on the mucous membrane of the mouth or genitals, often unnoticed in women. Chancre teeming with spirochetes, very contagious at this stage. Spirochetes enter bloodstream 3–7 days after infection and begin to multiply rapidly. May have bacteremia. Symptoms disappear within 3–8 wk. *Secondary* (6 wk later): Symptoms vary. May have generalized skin rash. Serology test is positive. Symptoms may disappear as the disease enters latent period. *Tertiary* (late: 1–20 yr after infection): Spirochetes have had access to all body tissues. "Gumma" lesions (a soft encapsulated tumor) appear on any organ; damage can cause a variety of symptoms. Progressive neurologic or aortic pathology. *Congenital:* Stillbirth, intrauterine growth restriction, multiple organ damage, including central nervous system.	*Screening:* VDRL and RPR tests, performed on blood or spinal fluid if neurosyphilis is suspected. May be negative in primary, but always positive in secondary and tertiary phases. *Confirmation:* FTA-Abs blood test. Tests for other STIs should also be done.	Antibiotics. Single-dose benzathine penicillin G or adequate blood levels of penicillin given over an 8- to 14-day period, or ceftriaxone 1 g IM for 14 days.	*Education:* Caution patients not to ingest alcohol for 24 hr prior to VDRL or RPR (may cause false-positive result). Remember that chancre is highly infectious (gloved contact only). Encourage naming of contacts so everyone can be treated. Encourage condom use to prevent reinfection. Explain importance of follow-up (usually 3- and 6-month VDRL) to ensure treatment has been effective. Follow-up usually at 1, 2, 3, 6, 9, and 12 months for HIV-positive individuals.
Trichomoniasis	Sexually transmitted.	Pruritus; frothy gray-green vaginal discharge; dysuria.	Laboratory observation of protozoa; ulceration on cervix or vaginal wall.	Metronidazole (Flagyl), single dose for woman and partner.	*Education:* Educate concerning safe sex practices and importance of seeking early care for symptoms.

*2007 Centers for Disease Control and Prevention Treatment Guidelines.

Staining procedures differentiate organisms by using dyes that have been found to stain some bacteria in specific ways. An example of this would be a Gram stain, in which bacteria are first stained with crystal violet, then treated with a strong iodine solution, decolorized with ethanol or ethanol acetone, and then counterstained with contrasting dye. Those retaining the initial stain are considered **gram positive;** those losing the stain but accepting the counterstain are considered **gram negative.** Current development of noninvasive testing and screening procedures using urine samples will increase public acceptance of mass screening. See Chapter 6 for further discussion on testing for infectious agents.

Identifying microorganisms is a complex procedure. When collecting or assisting in the collection of specimens, the nurse has several specific responsibilities to ensure that the samples will allow accurate studies to be performed. These include:

- Ensure that appropriate laboratory request slips have been prepared according to the health care provider's specific orders. If antimicrobials have been started, note this on the laboratory slip.
- Check the laboratory manual for any specific restrictions or preparations for the tests ordered. For example:
  - Urethral swabs should not be done within 1 hour of the last void as organisms will have been flushed away.
  - Female patients should not douche before vaginal cultures or smears.
- Some tests will give a false-positive reading if the patient is on specific medications or has other types of infection present. Check the patient's history.
- Antimicrobials may cause cultures to be negative even though the drug or the dose may not be sufficient to cure the infection. Document the medication history.
- Stool present in the rectum can prevent good rectal swabs from being obtained.
- Cultures and smears usually are obtained with a *sterile* swab and sent to the laboratory.
- Prepare the patient. (See information on preparing the patient for a pelvic examination in Chapter 38.)
- Explain what tests have been ordered and any specific home preparation. Answer all questions.
- Provide appropriate draping and privacy, and remain with the patient during the procedure.
- Provide emotional support as needed.
- Make sure that specimens are appropriately labeled and delivered to the laboratory with the corresponding laboratory slips.

NURSING MANAGEMENT

Assessment (Data Collection)

Screening for potential STIs or risk for acquiring such an infection should be part of any patient history data collection. However, it often is difficult to get accurate information (Communication Cues 40–1). Patients may not disclose symptoms such as inflammation, a rash, or a discharge if they fear it is related to sexual activity. Adolescents may fear parental disapproval, rejection, or disciplinary action if they admit to being sexually active and may hide symptoms. Fear of finding a serious disorder such as HIV also may make the patient reluctant to cooperate with data collection.

Obtaining a history on a patient seeking treatment for an STI requires tact and sensitivity. Such a history involves very intimate questions and may involve a variety of cultural and personal issues (Focused Assessment 40–1). The nurse must maintain an open and nonjudgmental attitude.

> *Think Critically About . . .* What factors make it difficult to take an accurate history or provide education for a patient with an STI?

Physical examination involves exposure of the most private parts of the anatomy. Such an examination is usually performed by both a health care provider and a nurse, particularly when there are gender differences between the medical personnel and the patient. It is the nurse's responsibility to provide appropriate draping and to give the patient privacy when he or she is undressing for the examination.

Patients may request that a family member or significant other be allowed to remain with them, and they have this right. The nurse should escort such individuals into the room and have them sit or stand by the patient in a manner that allows them to provide support. The nurse also should make sure that any required equipment, supplies, specimen containers, and laboratory slips are ready in the examination room.

Communication Cues 40–1

Gathering Information

When someone is diagnosed with a sexually transmitted infection, the public health department is responsible for collecting the names of sexual partners so that they can be reached and treated. Many people do not wish to give out this information. Professionals who deal with these issues regularly, such as public health nurses, often have special training in obtaining an appropriate history.

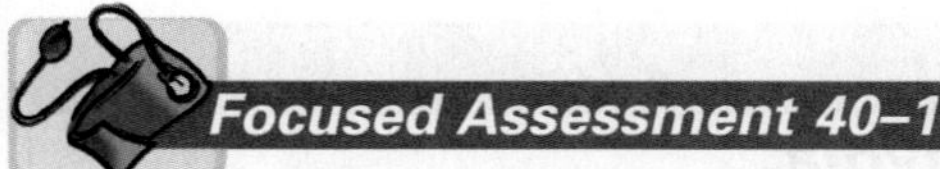

Focused Assessment 40–1

Data Collection for STIs

The following questions are asked when assessing the patient with or at risk for an STI:

- Are you currently sexually active?
- At what age did you become sexually active?
- Do you currently have more than one sexual partner?
- Have you had other partners in the past?
- (If yes to either of the last two questions) Do you understand the risks associated with having multiple sexual partners?
- (If a sexually active female) Are you having regular gynecologic examinations with Pap smears? If yes, when was your last examination?
- (If a sexually active female) Are you currently pregnant or trying to become pregnant?
- Are you checked at least annually for STIs even if you don't have symptoms?
- (If currently in a non-monogamous relationship) Are you using condoms to help prevent sexually transmitted infections?
- Have you ever had a sexually transmitted disease? If yes, ask for specific information (what, when, how treated, was follow-up done?).
- Do you have symptoms or reasons to believe you might have one now? If yes, ask for specific information (symptoms, duration, partner[s] symptomatic?).

Key: *Pap,* Papanicolaou; *STIs,* sexually transmitted infections.

Nursing Diagnosis

Nursing diagnoses for the patient who has an STI may include:

- Deficient knowledge related to modes of transmission, signs and symptoms, and treatment
- Pain related to inflammation
- Anxiety related to intimate examination and personal information required
- Fear of being HIV positive
- Noncompliance related to repeated infection with STIs and refusal to use condoms

Planning

Expected outcomes for the patient with an STI may include:

- Patient will verbalize knowledge of self-care to prevent recurrence or other STI
- Patient will be free of pain after treatment
- Patient will cope adequately with history taking and physical examination
- Patient will have decreased fear of HIV diagnosis after examination and treatment
- Patient will comply with safer sex practices
- Patient will comply with treatment requirements

In addition to managing the treatment protocol and any pain related to an STI, patient education and emotional support are primary aspects of planning for patients with or at risk for STIs.

Education in this area often is hampered by the patient's reluctance to discuss sexual issues. This may result from cultural views or more personal feelings. Patients of all ages may wish to protect themselves or their partners from possible condemnation or embarrassment through disclosure of sensitive information. The nurse must maintain a nonjudgmental attitude and give assurance that information will be kept confidential within the health care system.

When planning education, consider the patient's existing knowledge base and ability to understand information provided. Select appropriate teaching aids, such as pictures, pamphlets, and three-dimensional models, to assist in the education of the patient.

Emotional support is another important aspect of care for the patient with an STI. Allow time in the teaching plan for listening to the patient's concerns and answering questions. Be prepared with information on support groups, counseling services, and informational programs that may be of assistance. In the case of serious infections, such as HIV, support programs and professional counseling are of particular importance to the patient.

Implementation

Symptom Relief

STIs carry a variety of symptoms, some of which may cause mild discomfort or significant pain. Review Chapter 7 on pain management techniques. Table 40–1 lists details concerning common STIs and suggestions for specific nursing interventions. Nursing Care Plan 40–1 gives specific nursing interventions for a patient with chlamydia.

Prevention of Spread

The spread of STIs is a major health concern in the United States. People often become sexually active at a young age, and it is not uncommon for individuals to have had a variety of sexual partners over the years (Health Promotion Points 40–1). Strategies for prevention and control of STIs are given in Box 40–2.

Evaluation

Initially, each patient teaching contact should be evaluated for effectiveness by reviewing information discussed to determine whether learning has taken place. Over time, it is necessary to evaluate whether the patient is indeed following the recommendations. Follow-up cultures that are negative are a good indicator that treatments were followed as prescribed. During the follow-up interview, the nurse can inquire about use of safer sex practices and evaluate retention of information previously taught.

NURSING CARE PLAN 40–1

Care of the Patient with Chlamydia

SCENARIO A 21-year-old woman is admitted to the clinic and diagnosed with a chlamydia infection.

PROBLEM/NURSING DIAGNOSIS *Doesn't know what chlamydia is*/Deficient knowledge related to new diagnosis of chlamydia infection.

Supporting assessment data *Subjective:* "What is chlamydia?" *Objective:* Positive test for chlamydia.

Goals/Expected Outcomes	Nursing Interventions	Selected Rationale	Evaluation
Patient will verbalize understanding of disease prevention, transmission, and treatment protocols	Assess readiness to learn about chlamydia.	Readiness to learn is essential for successful learning to occur.	Patient asking questions about her diagnosis.
	Determine knowledge base concerning chlamydia.	Learning plan should build on existing knowledge.	Patient discussing her understanding.
	Identify barriers to learning.	Language barriers, cultural beliefs, and embarrassment can alter learning effectiveness.	Patient speaks fluent English and is willing to discuss illness.
	Teach the medication regimen.	Compliance with medication regimen is essential for successful treatment.	Patient verbalizes understanding of when and how to take medication.
	Review safer sex practices.	Safer sex practices can prevent exchange of body fluids and minimize risk of STI transmission.	Patient demonstrates understanding of safer sex practices.
	Schedule follow-up appointments.	Follow-up testing is an essential part of confirming successful treatment of chlamydia.	Patient promises to return for follow-up care.

PROBLEM/NURSING DIAGNOSIS *Vaginal discharge*/Impaired tissue integrity related to testing positive for chlamydia.

Supporting assessment data *Subjective:* "I've had a small amount of vaginal discharge." *Objective:* Chlamydia test is positive.

Goals/Expected Outcomes	Nursing Interventions	Selected Rationale	Evaluation
Patient will evidence signs of successful treatment of chlamydia as evidenced by absence of symptoms and completion of medication regimen	Assess for signs and symptoms of chlamydia such as vaginal discharge and dysuria.	Absence of symptoms may indicate successful treatment.	Patient does not evidence continued signs of the disease.
	Assess for risk factors for reactivation of disease.	Minimizing risk factors can prevent reinfection.	Patient states she is now in a monogamous relationship.
	Encourage woman to identify partners to enable treatment.	Treating sexual partners can minimize risk for reinfection and spread of infection.	Patient has contacted other partners, who have come in for examination.
	Teach safer sex practices and risk for recurrence.	Use of safer sex practices can minimize reinfection.	Patient evidences understanding of safer sex practices.

? CRITICAL THINKING QUESTION

1. What are the long-term problems associated with untreated chlamydia?

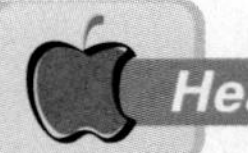

Health Promotion Points 40–1

Preventing STIs

Although the only absolute prevention is abstinence, certain behaviors significantly reduce the risk of contracting an STI. These include the use of condoms with a spermicide containing nonoxynol-9, which both acts as a barrier and has viricidal and bactericidal action; limiting sexual contacts, preferably to one partner; and avoiding sexual contact if one of the partners is known to be infected or if lesions are observed in the genital, perianal, or oral regions. If the patient or a patient's sexual partner is an IV drug user, education regarding nonsharing of needles is important.

Key: *IV*, intravenous; *STIs*, sexually transmitted infections.

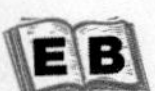

Box 40–2 *Prevention of STIs*

The prevention and control of STIs are based on the following major strategies:

- Early education of adolescents concerning abstinence programs and safer sex practices.
- Education and counseling of people at risk on ways to avoid STIs through changes in sexual behaviors.
- Identification of asymptomatically infected people and of symptomatic people unlikely to seek diagnostic and treatment services.
- Effective diagnosis and treatment of infected people.
- Evaluation, treatment, and counseling of sex partners of people who are infected with an STI.
- Preexposure vaccination of patients at risk for vaccine-preventable STIs such as hepatitis B and HPV.

Key: *HPV*, human papillomavirus; *STIs*, sexually transmitted infections.
Adapted from www.cdc.gov/std/hpv/default.htm.

COMMUNITY CARE

Most communities have clinics, often through the public health system, that provide screening and treatment for STIs. These may be low cost or no cost, and they provide a valuable service by assisting the community to control the spread of STIs.

Patient education is an important service provided by community clinics. The health department and organizations such as Planned Parenthood are just two of the community agencies that routinely provide pamphlets, posters, and classes on preventing and treating STIs. Confidential screening and education on safer sexual practices are important services provided by these clinics. Public service announcements, such as the television spots on HIV/AIDS awareness, are another source of public education. In many areas, information and education are made available through the schools and colleges and are directed both at students and families and at the general community.

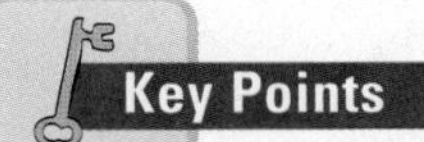

Key Points

- STIs are primarily passed through intimate contact with body fluids. Needle-sticks or blood transfusions with contaminated blood can also spread STIs. An STI can also be transmitted to the newborn during the birth process.
- STIs have a major impact on reproductive and general health.
- One goal of *Healthy People 2010* is to "prevent HIV infection and its related illness and death."
- STI infections can be caused by bacteria, viruses, or protozoa.
- Contraceptive choice influences a woman's risk for STIs.
- A properly used condom offers protection from the transmission of STIs.
- STIs can cause sterility, complicated pregnancy, or neonatal infection.
- Many STIs are reportable to the public health department.
- PID is an inflammation of the pelvic cavity often caused by STIs and can cause sterility.
- Education concerning safer sex practices can prevent STIs.
- The health department, community clinics, the media, and schools offer educational information and literature concerning prevention of STIs.

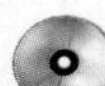

Go to your **Companion CD-ROM** for an Audio Glossary, animations, video clips, and bonus review questions.

evolve Be sure to visit the companion Evolve site at http://evolve.elsevier.com/deWit for interactive NCLEX-PN Exam Style Review Questions, WebLinks, and additional online resources.

NCLEX-PN EXAM STYLE REVIEW QUESTIONS

Choose the best answer(s) for the following questions.

1. An acutely ill 36-year-old patient complains of severe abdominal and pelvic pain and fever. A foul-smelling, purulent vaginal discharge is sent to the laboratory for culture and sensitivity. The nurse identifies the nursing diagnosis as acute pain; an appropriate intervention would be to:

1. administer antibiotics.
2. provide relief measures.
3. teach preventive measures.
4. offer support.

2. The nurse talks with the parents of a 9-year-old girl regarding the human papillomavirus (HPV) vaccinations. The information session must include which of the following statements? *(Select all that apply.)*

1. The vaccine is a one-dose immunization.
2. The vaccine prevents genital warts.
3. The vaccine prevents precancerous lesions of the cervix.
4. The vaccine protects against other full-blown HPV infections.
5. The vaccine eliminates the need for routine cervical cancer screening.

3. Changes in the vaginal pH increase the female predisposition to various forms of infections. Which of the following decrease vaginal resistance to infections?

1. Vaginal douching
2. Tampons
3. Latex condoms
4. Spermicidal agents

4. The impact of disclosing the diagnosis of sexually transmitted infections warrants specific nursing responsibilities. These nursing responsibilities include which of the following? *(Select all that apply.)*

1. Recognize a false-positive reading.
2. Provide emotional support.
3. Ensure accuracy of laboratory request slips.
4. Check specific restrictions or preparations for tests.
5. Provide expert advice.

5. The nurse is taking the clinical history of an adolescent with a tentative diagnosis of nongonoccocal urethritis. Initial assessment confirms a nursing diagnosis of fear. A likely etiology for the diagnosis would be:

1. potential death.
2. parental disapproval.
3. peer rejection.
4. loss of reproductive function.

6. A patient was prescribed a 7-day course of doxycycline (Vibramycin) for chlamydial infection. Which of the following patient statements indicates understanding of the treatment regimen?

1. "I can take the medication at bedtime."
2. "I need to take the entire prescription even if symptoms subside."
3. "I can sunbathe."
4. "I must take the medication on an empty stomach."

7. While inserting an indwelling urinary catheter, the nurse finds raised, rough, cauliflower-like growths on the vulva and vaginal walls. A likely causative agent would be:

1. herpes simplex virus.
2. human papillomavirus.
3. *Treponema pallidum.*
4. *Neisseria gonorrhoeae.*

8. Which of the following statements is true regarding the Venereal Disease Research Laboratory (VDRL) test?

1. VDRL tests are used for screening and diagnosis.
2. False-negative reactions are associated with malaria, leprosy, and viral pneumonia.
3. The VDRL values increase quantitatively after completion of therapy.
4. False-positive reactions are associated with lupus.

9. A neonate is at risk for ____________ when exposed to a birth canal infected with *Neisseria gonorrhoeae.*

10. A patient presents with itching and frothy gray-green vaginal discharge, and difficulty urinating. The physician would most likely prescribe which of the following?

1. Doxycycline (Vibramycin)
2. Metronidazole (Flagyl)
3. Ceftriaxone (Rocephin)
4. Benzathine penicillin G (Bicillin L-A)

CRITICAL THINKING ACTIVITIES

Read each clinical scenario and discuss the questions with your classmates.

Scenario A

A friend confides that she has a rash in her genital area that occurred since she began having sex with her latest boyfriend. She is afraid she may have syphilis or genital herpes and doesn't know what to do.

1. What would you say to convince her that she needs to see an experienced clinician for diagnosis and treatment?
2. Where can she go if she does not want to see her regular health care provider?

Scenario B

A patient confides in you that he has three girlfriends, all of whom are taking oral contraceptives, so he sees no reason to use condoms.

1. What could you tell him about the risks of multiple sexual partners and the importance of using condoms to prevent sexually transmitted infections?

CHAPTER 41 The Integumentary System

evolve http://evolve.elsevier.com/deWit

Objectives

Upon completing this chapter, you should be able to:

Theory

1. Review the structure and functions of the skin.
2. Discuss the changes that occur with aging that affect the skin barrier.
3. Discuss the various causes of integumentary disorders.
4. Identify important factors in the prevention of skin disease.
5. Plan specific measures to prevent pressure ulcers.
6. Interpret laboratory and diagnostic test results for skin disorders.
7. State nursing responsibilities in the diagnosis of skin disorders.
8. Describe the proper staging of a pressure ulcer.
9. Write outcome objectives for a patient with a nursing diagnosis of Impaired skin integrity.
10. Develop a teaching plan appropriate for adolescents and young adults for the prevention of skin cancer.

Clinical Practice

1. Teach three patients to perform a self-assessment of the skin.
2. Perform a focused integumentary assessment on a patient.
3. Provide ordered therapeutic measures for a patient with an integumentary disorder.

Key Terms

Be sure to check out the bonus material on the Companion CD-ROM, including selected audio pronunciations.

biopsy (BĪ-ŏp-sē, p. 1010)
erythrasma (ĕ-rĭth-RĂZ-mă, p. 1011)
exudate (ĔKS-ū-dāt, p. 1010)
keloid (KĒ-loid, p. 1012)
keratoses (kĕr-ă-TŌ-sēs, p. 1012)
macule (MĂK-ūl, p. 1014)
papule (PĂP-ūl, p. 1014)
plaque (plăk, p. 1014)
pustule (PŬS-tūl, p. 1014)
senile lentigines (SĒ-nīl lĕn-TĬJ-ĭ-nēz, p. 1007)
senile purpura (SĒ-nīl PŬR-pū-ră, p. 1013)
vesicle (VĔS-ĭ-kŭl, p. 1014)
wheal (WĒL, p. 1011, 1014)

The skin is an organ that is essential for the maintenance of life and good health. It functions very much like a built-in suit of armor. The skin is the first line of defense against invasion by pathogenic bacteria living in the environment.

Disorders that primarily affect the skin are numerous, but the skin also reflects systemic diseases. A knowledge of the patient's health history greatly improves the chances of accurately diagnosing any skin abnormality.

When an area of the skin is destroyed by disease or trauma, its protective functions are immediately impaired. This impairment makes the body susceptible to infection. If very large areas of skin are destroyed, as in an extensive burn, fluid and electrolyte balance is disturbed. Protein and body heat are lost from burned areas.

Skin diseases are very common in humans. They also are extremely exasperating because they often are difficult to diagnose and cure. Skin ailments tend to recur. The physical effects of skin diseases are not often serious. However, when the disorder renders the patient unattractive, there is a psychological impact that threatens self-image and damages self-esteem.

The word *dermatology* refers to the study of diseases of the skin. A *dermatologist* is one who specializes in the treatment of skin disorders. Many dermatologists have some standing orders or written instructions they wish followed when their patients are hospitalized. The nurse must check standing orders and agency protocols when caring for patients with skin disorders. To understand the discussion of the skin disorders better, a review of the anatomy and functions of the skin is necessary.

Disorders that affect pediatric patients, such as impetigo, eczema, and ringworm, are discussed further in pediatric nursing texts.

CAUSES OF SKIN DISORDERS

More than 3000 disorders of the skin have been officially named, and many more are not included in any official nomenclature. The majority of the recognized and named skin disorders arise from some pathology in

OVERVIEW OF ANATOMY AND PHYSIOLOGY OF THE INTEGUMENTARY SYSTEM

What is the structure of the skin, hair, and nails?

- The skin consists of two layers of tissue, the epidermis and the dermis (Figure 41–1).
- The skin is attached to underlying structures by subcutaneous tissue.
- The epidermis consists of squamous epithelium and contains no blood vessels; cells receive nutrients by diffusion from vessels in the underlying tissue.
- Cell growth occurs from the bottom of the epidermis and pushes cells above to the surface, where they eventually die and slough off or are washed off. This layer is called the stratum corneum.
- The bottom layer of the epidermis contains melanocytes that contribute color to the skin.
- The dermis, also called the corium, is thicker than the epidermis and consists of dense connective tissue.
- The dermis contains both elastic and collagenous fibers that give it strength and elasticity.
- The dermis contains blood vessels and nerves as well as the base of hair follicles, glands, and nails that are derived from the epidermis.
- A hair consists of a shaft and a root made up of dead keratinized epithelial cells.
- The hair root is below the surface of the epidermis and is enclosed in a hair follicle that is embedded in the dermis.
- Fibroblasts that produce new cells to heal the skin are contained in the dermis.
- Glands contained in the skin are *sebaceous* (sweat producing) or *ceruminous* (wax producing).
- Nails are dead stratum corneum with a very hard type of keratin.

What are the functions of the skin and its structures?

- The skin acts as a protective covering over the entire surface of the body.

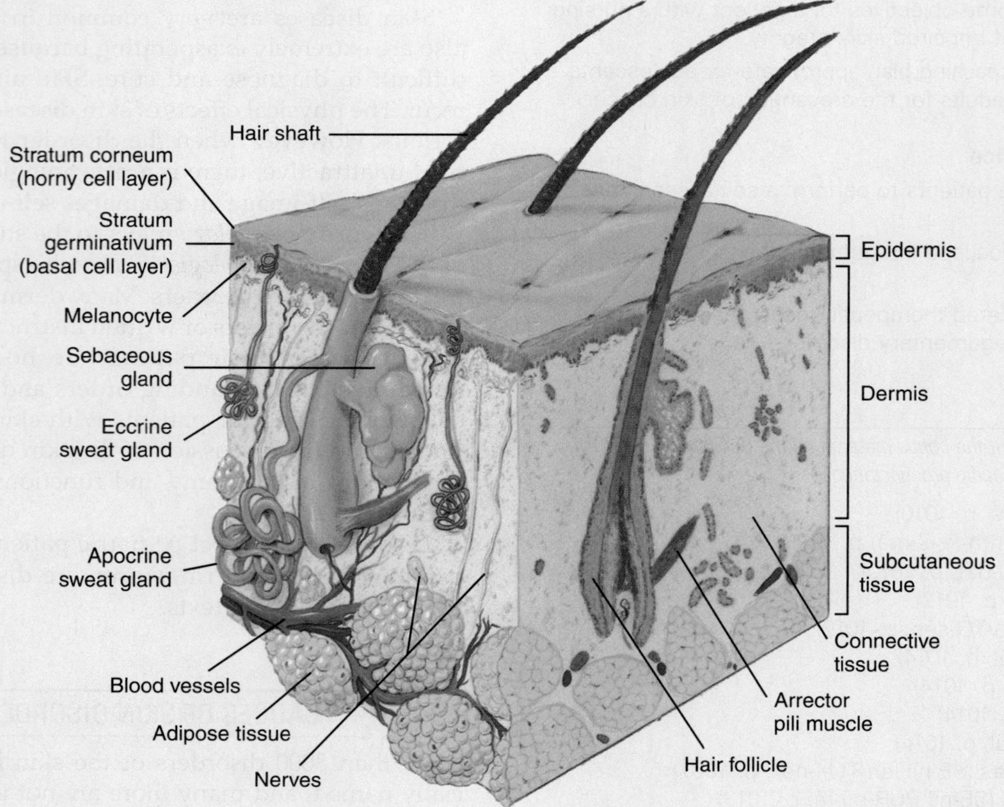

FIGURE 41–1 Structure of the skin.

- The keratin in the skin makes it waterproof, preventing water loss from the underlying tissues and too much water absorption during swimming and bathing.
- Skin provides a barrier to bacteria and other invading organisms.
- Skin protects underlying tissues from thermal, chemical, and mechanical injury.
- The skin helps regulate body temperature by dilating and constricting blood vessels and by activating or inactivating sweat glands.
- When the skin is exposed to ultraviolet light, molecules in the cells convert the rays to vitamin D.
- Melanin pigment absorbs light and acts to protect tissue from ultraviolet light.
- The nerve receptors in the dermis transmit feelings of heat, cold, pain, touch, and pressure.
- Hair follicles contained in the skin produce hair.
- Sebaceous glands secrete sebum that functions to keep hair and skin soft and pliable. Sebum also inhibits bacterial growth on the surface of the skin and, because of its oily nature, helps prevent water loss from the skin.
- Sweat glands act to excrete water and salt when the body temperature increases; sweat evaporates, producing a cooling effect.
- Sweat glands in the axillae and external genitalia secrete fatty acids and proteins as well as water and salts. They become active at puberty and are stimulated by the nervous system in response to sexual arousal, emotional stress, and pain.
- Hair color is produced by melanocytes in the skin and depends on the type of melanin produced.
- The shape of the hair shaft determines whether hair is straight or curly.
- Hair assists the body to retain heat.
- Nails cover the distal ends of the fingers and toes.
- Each nail has a free edge, a nail body, and a nail root that is covered by skin.
- The cuticle of each nail is a fold of stratum corneum.

What changes occur in the skin and its structures with aging?

- The number of elastic fibers decreases and adipose tissue diminishes in the dermis and subcutaneous layers, causing skin to wrinkle and sag.
- Loss of collagen fibers in the dermis makes the skin increasingly fragile and slower to heal.
- The skin becomes thinner and more transparent.
- Reduced sebaceous gland activity causes dry skin that may itch.
- The thinned skin and decreased sebaceous gland activity reduce temperature control and lead to an intolerance of cold and a susceptibility to heat exhaustion.
- A reduction in melanocyte activity increases risk of sunburn and skin cancer.
- The number of hair follicles decreases and the growth rate of hair declines; the hair thins.
- Decreased numbers of melanocytes at the hair follicle causes gradual loss of hair color.
- Nail growth decreases, longitudinal ridges appear, and the nails thicken; nails become more susceptible to fungal infections.
- Some areas of melanocytes increase in production, producing brown "age spots" or "liver spots," properly named **senile lentigines** (Figure 41–2).

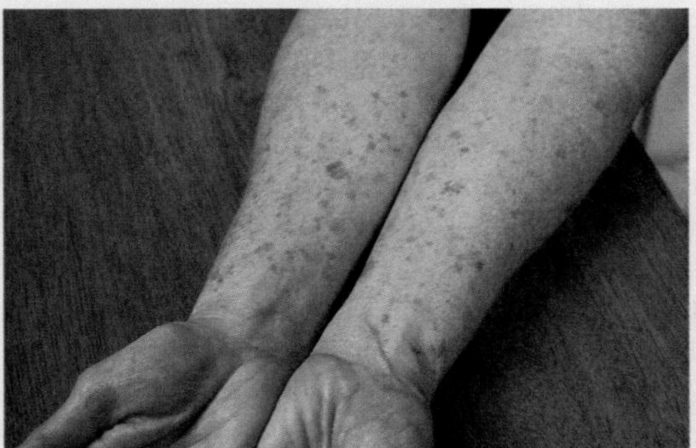

FIGURE 41–2 Senile lentigines (age spots or liver spots).

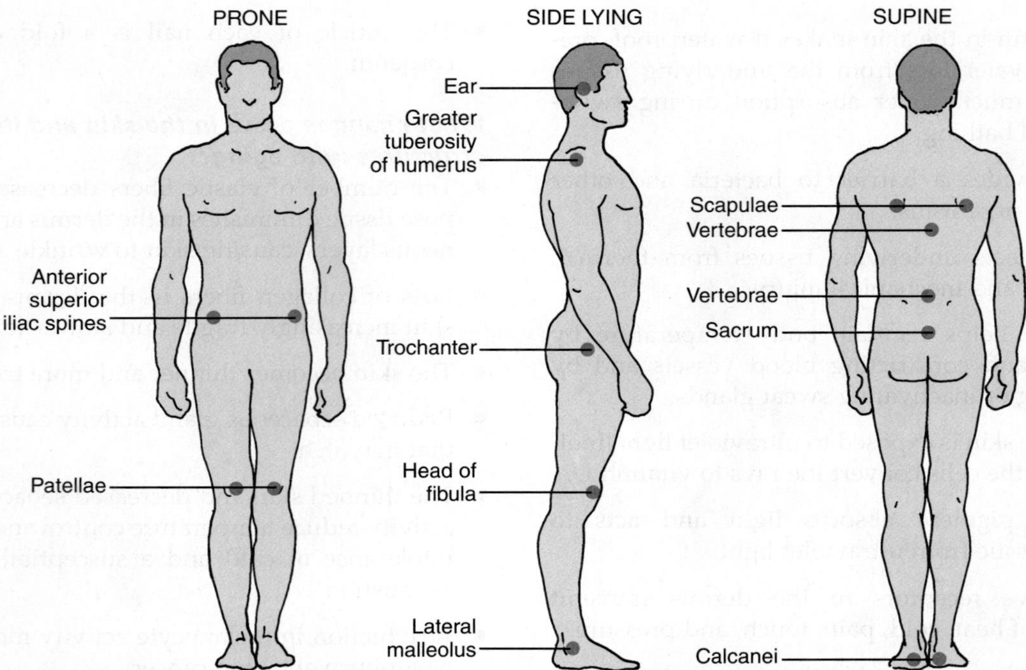

FIGURE **41–3** Bony prominences most susceptible to skin breakdown depending on position.

the skin itself. The remainder are manifestations of some systemic disease. Skin disorders may occur from immunologic and inflammatory disorders, proliferative and neoplastic disorders, metabolic and endocrine disorders, and nutritional problems. Physical, chemical, and microbiologic factors also can damage the skin.

Many patients with dermatologic disease are not hospitalized and are seen only in physicians' offices and outpatient clinics. Others do not seek medical attention but treat their skin disorder themselves with home remedies and over-the-counter drugs. In some cases self-care measures are successful, but they also have the potential for aggravating the condition or only temporarily relieving its more severe symptoms. This can lead to delay in treatment and allows the disease to progress to a chronic and sometimes untreatable state.

When a patient is on bed rest, or constantly sitting because of paralysis, pressure against the skin in various areas interferes with circulation. Because cells die very quickly without adequate blood supply, a pressure ulcer can develop. Depending on the patient's general condition, weight, and other factors, skin damage may occur within a few hours to a few days. Areas most prone to pressure ulcer formation are those over bony prominences. When the patient is placed in a position in which the bone is pressing on the skin where the skin is against the bed, the circulation to that area is compromised (Figure 41–3). Shearing action can cause damage to the skin if the patient is slid along the sheets for positioning rather than lifted. Box 41–1 presents risk factors for pressure ulcers.

Box 41–1 ***Risk Factors for Pressure Ulcer Formation***

MAJOR FACTORS
- Bed or chair confinement
- Impaired mobility
- Bowel or bladder incontinence
- Inadequate nutrition
- Decreased level of consciousness or confusion

CONTRIBUTING FACTORS
- Obesity
- Diabetes mellitus
- Dehydration
- Edema
- Excessive sweating
- Extreme age with fragile skin
- Shearing injury
- Unrelieved pressure on bony prominences

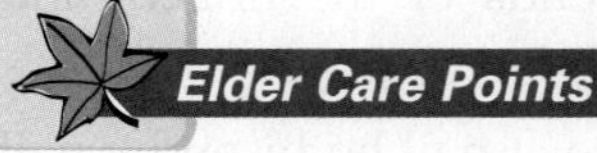

Elder Care Points

The elderly are very prone to skin tears from shearing injuries or from bumping into things. A skin tear can occur just from holding a limb improperly when moving a patient. They occur because of the fragility of the skin. This should be kept in mind any time you are assisting an elderly person to reposition, ambulate, or transfer. Padding on areas of the arms of chairs and wheelchairs is helpful in preventing skin tears.

Caring for those who have a skin disorder can be particularly challenging because of the recurrent nature of many skin disorders, the potential these disorders have for disfigurement, and the added burden they can place on the patient if the skin disease can be spread to others.

PREVENTION OF SKIN DISORDERS

CLEANLINESS

The ritual of the daily bath is almost an obsession with the average American (Assignment Considerations 41–1). Nurses are perhaps guiltier than most in their insistence on using soap and plenty of hot water for bathing patients. No one will quarrel with the value of cleanliness, but it can be overdone, and the method of cleansing the skin deserves some consideration.

First, recognize that there are various skin types. **Blondes and redheads with a fair complexion usually have very delicate skin that requires special care to prevent drying and irritation.** On the other hand, people with dark hair usually have skin that is more oily and less susceptible to excessive drying and irritation.

If the skin appears dry and scaly, frequent bathing with soap and hot water only aggravates the condition. Oils and creams are available that cleanse the skin quite effectively and help replace the natural oils at the same time. The person with oily skin will need to clean the skin frequently, use a liberal amount of soap and water, and avoid applying additional oils to the skin.

DIET

Adequate intake of vitamins and minerals is essential to the maintenance of healthy skin. Even borderline deficiencies in these nutrients will cause the skin to take on a sallow and dull appearance. Severe nutritional deficiencies lead to skin breakdown and the development of sores and ulcers. Dehydration causes loss of skin turgor and predisposes to pressure ulcers. People who are so concerned with their physical appearance that they refuse to eat properly for fear of gaining weight fail to realize that they are robbing themselves of one of the sources of real beauty—a healthy and radiant complexion.

AGE

Young people are not the only ones who should be concerned with the care of their skin. As we grow older, our skin undergoes certain changes that easily lead to irritation and breakdown if proper care is not given. The oil and sweat glands become less active, and the skin has a tendency to become dry and scaly. It also loses some of its tone, becoming less elastic and more fragile. Frequent cleansing of the skin becomes unnecessary as the skin ages, and alcohol and other drying agents must be used sparingly, if at all. As we grow older, we should establish a regular routine of massaging oil, cream, or oily lotion into the skin, if not for the sake of vanity, at least for the sake of preserving a very important organ.

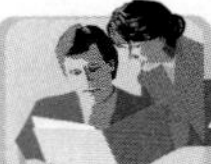

Assignment Considerations 41–1

Observation While Bathing

When assigning baths and personal care to unlicensed assistive personnel, ask the person to please advise you if there is any reddening, bruising, break in the skin, or new lesion noticed. Remind the person to handle elderly patients gently and to protect their limbs when transferring them from bed to chair and back so that skin tears do not occur. Do not rely on assistive personnel to totally assess the skin. This should be performed by the nurse.

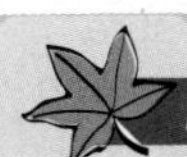

Elder Care Points

The elderly patient who has dry skin does not need a full bath every day; cleansing of the axillae and genital-rectal area between bathing days should be sufficient. Elderly patients should use a mild lotion-based soap, such as Dove, or a body wash such as Aveeno, for bathing. After showering or the bath, a lotion or cream that helps seal in moisture should be applied while the skin is still damp. Moisturizing lotion or cream should be reapplied at bedtime.

ENVIRONMENT

Several environmental factors can have a direct effect on the health of the skin. These include prolonged exposure to chemicals, excessive drying from repeated immersions in water, very cold temperatures, and prolonged exposure to sunlight. Some of these are occupational hazards. A change of jobs may be necessary to eliminate contact with a factor that is causing a skin disorder. See the discussion of contact dermatitis in allergic reactions in Chapter 11.

Overexposure to the ultraviolet rays of the sun can seriously and permanently damage the superficial and deeper layers of the skin. The damage results in severe wrinkling and furrowing, as well as loss of elasticity, and the skin assumes a tissue-paper transparency. In addition to the potential for premature aging and degenerative changes, solar damage also can result in malignant changes. Ultraviolet rays from the sun have long been known to be carcinogenic (Health Promotion Points 41–1). This is especially true for fair-skinned people who have subjected their skin to prolonged exposure to sunshine. Although sunburns are particularly harmful, it is the normal daily exposure of unprotected fair skin to sun that causes long-term damage (Complementary & Alternative Therapies 41–1).

PREVENTION OF PRESSURE ULCERS

Preventing pressure ulcers is far more desirable and less time-consuming than treating them. Efforts to preserve the integrity of the skin are the responsibility of the nursing staff, as well as the patient himself

Health Promotion Points 41–1

Sun Exposure Precautions

Health teaching to inform the public about the dangers of solar ultraviolet radiation should include the following information.

- Although fair-skinned people who freckle easily are more likely to suffer sun-damaged skin, people of all complexions and races can and do burn if exposed to sufficient sunlight.
- Although a good tan might be considered by many to be desirable, dermatologists say that there is no such thing as a "healthy tan." Tanning causes damage to the skin. If one insists on lying out in the sun, the initial exposure should be slow and gradual, and an adequate sunscreen with a skin protection factor (SPF) of at least 15 as well as UVA and UVB protection should always be used. Too much sun too soon only leads to blistering and peeling.
- Select a sunscreen preparation on the basis of skin type and ability to tan, as well as its active ingredients and the amount of time to be spent in the sun. Remember that the sunscreen can be washed off by water or perspiration or rubbed off on sand and towels and must be periodically reapplied. Apply sunscreen liberally.
- Avoid exposure to the sun during the time its rays are most hazardous; that is, between 10 A.M. and 2 P.M. standard time or 11 A.M. and 3 P.M. during daylight saving time. Local radio and television stations often give information about current weather conditions and the chances for being burned by the sun at particular times during each day.
- You can be sunburned on a cloudy or overcast day.
- Light, loosely woven clothing will not give adequate protection from the sun's rays.
- Remember that snow, water, and sand can reflect the sun's rays and increase the intensity of exposure.
- Do not try to gauge how much you are being burned while in the sun. It may be 6 to 8 hours before a painful burn becomes obvious.
- Wear sunglasses and a hat when you go out in the sun, and, when possible, wear protective clothing.
- Never use a tanning booth.

if he is able to participate in his own care. Box 41–2 presents interventions for preventing pressure ulcers based on Agency for Healthcare Policy and Research (AHCPR) clinical practice guidelines.

DIAGNOSTIC TESTS AND PROCEDURES AND NURSING RESPONSIBILITIES

SKIN BIOPSY

Removing a sample of tissue **(biopsy)** from a skin lesion usually is performed with a local anesthetic. It can be done by shaving a top layer off a lesion that rises above the skin line *(shave biopsy)*, by removing a core from the center of the lesion *(punch biopsy)*, or by excising the entire lesion *(excisional biopsy)*.

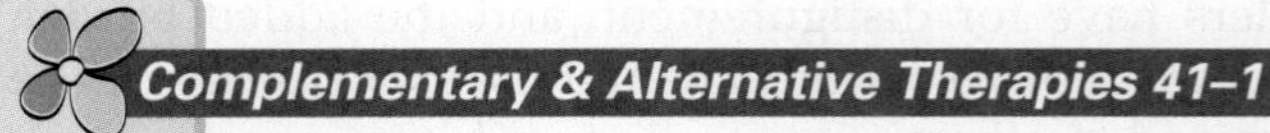

Complementary & Alternative Therapies 41–1

Ultraviolet Radiation Protection

Research is underway to test a fern plant extract packaged in a pill form to prevent sunburn. It may help protect the skin from ultraviolet (UV) radiation. The fern extract is from *Polypodium leucotornos,* and is a natural antioxidant with tumor inhibition properties. It is sold under the name Heliocare by Teva. A small study published in the December 2004 issue of the *Journal of the American Academy of Dermatology* stated that there were positive results. Such a pill would offer total body protection and wouldn't wash off (*Chicago Sun-Times,* 2006).

Safety Alert 41–1

Skin Drainage or Weeping

Whenever there is a question of a pathogenic process, weeping or drainage from skin lesions, or the suspicion of scabies, Standard Precautions should be employed when touching the patient's skin to prevent self-contamination or transmission of an organism.

Skin biopsy is used to differentiate benign from malignant lesions and to help identify the causative organism in bacterial and fungal infections. No special patient preparation is necessary beyond a simple explanation of the procedure and its purpose. If a local anesthetic is to be used, the patient is asked about any personal or family history of allergies. After the procedure, the patient is given instructions for the care of the biopsy site. Usually the bandage is changed daily. The site may or may not be treated with a topical antibiotic solution or ointment. Sutures from an excisional biopsy will need to be removed in 10 to 14 days.

CULTURE AND SENSITIVITY TESTS

When a bacterial, viral, or fungal infection of the skin is suspected, the dermatologist may wish to know the causative organism and the drug most appropriate for treating the specific infection. A sampling of **exudate** (drainage) is taken from the lesion and sent to the laboratory for culturing. Once the organism has been cultured, colonies can be tested for sensitivity to certain anti-infective agents. These tests take the guesswork out of treating infectious skin disease and very quickly determine which drug will be most effective in treating it. Care must be taken when handling the specimen and its container to avoid contaminating people who will later be handling the specimen (Safety Alert 41–1).

MICROSCOPIC TESTS

Various stains and solutions are used to prepare skin, hair, scales, or nail material for study. These tests can

Box 41–2 Guidelines for the Prevention of Pressure Ulcers

- Assess the skin of all patients at risk at least once a day, paying particular attention to the bony prominences (see Figure 41–3). Document the findings.
- Reposition patients every 2 hours; use a written schedule for systematically turning and repositioning each patient. Patients in wheelchairs should be repositioned more frequently (every 15 minutes is preferable).
- Utilize positioning devices, such as pillows, foam wedges, and padding, for bed rest patients, to keep body prominences from being in direct contact with one another; include positioning devices in the written plan of care.
- For patients on bed rest who are completely immobile, use devices that totally relieve pressure on the heels, by raising the heels off the bed. Do not use donut-type devices.
- When the side-lying position in bed is used, avoid positioning directly on the trochanter.
- For bed rest patients, maintain the head of the bed at the lowest degree permitted by medical condition. Limit the time the head of the bed is elevated.
- Use lifting devices, such as a trapeze or bed linen, to move rather than drag patients who cannot assist during transfers and position changes.
- For patients with limited mobility, utilize a pressure-reducing device on the bed, such as a foam, static air, alternating air, gel, or water mattress. Such devices should be used for any patients at risk for developing pressure ulcers.
- For wheelchair-bound patients, use a pressure-reducing device such as those made of foam, gel, air, or a combination of items. Do not use donut-type devices.
- Positioning of wheelchair-bound patients should include consideration of postural alignment, distribution of weight, balance and stability, and pressure relief by device or repositioning.
- Use a written plan for the use of positioning devices and schedules for wheelchair-bound patients.
- Skin cleansing should occur at the time of soiling and at routine intervals based on patient need and preference. Avoid hot water, and use a mild cleansing agent that minimizes irritation and dryness of the skin. Cleanse gently, minimizing the force and friction applied to the skin.
- Any person at risk for developing a pressure ulcer when sitting in a chair or wheelchair should be repositioned, shifting the points under pressure at least every hour; patients who are able should be taught to shift weight every 15 minutes.
- Keep the environmental humidity above 40% and avoid exposure to cold. Treat dry skin with moisturizers.
- Do not massage bony prominences.
- Minimize skin exposure to moisture due to incontinence, perspiration, or wound drainage. When sources of moisture cannot be controlled, underpads or briefs that absorb moisture and present a quick-drying surface to the skin should be used. Utilize an incontinence management program for incontinent patients.
- Minimize skin injury due to friction and shear forces by proper positioning and correct transferring and turning techniques. Reduce friction injuries by using lubricants, protective films, protective dressings, and protective padding. Use lift devices to reposition patients rather than sliding them on the bedding.
- Correct inadequate dietary intake of protein and calories with nutritional intervention either by oral supplementation or enteral or parenteral feedings.
- If a potential for improvement of mobility and activity status exists, institute a rehabilitation program. Maintain current activity and mobility status with a range-of-motion exercise program.

identify fungal, bacterial, and viral organisms. To check for organism infestations, scrapings are suspended in mineral oil and examined under the microscope.

SPECIAL LIGHT INSPECTION

Inspection of the skin is one of the principal means by which skin lesions are diagnosed. To facilitate the diagnosis of certain kinds of skin disorders, special lights may be used by the examiner. A *cold light* is one in which the light is transmitted through a quartz or plastic structure to dissipate the heat. Because there is no danger of burning the skin, the cold light can be applied directly to the skin to illuminate its layers for visualization of malignant changes.

A *Wood's light* is a specially designed ultraviolet light. The nickel oxide filter holds back all but a few violet rays of the visible spectrum. This special light is especially useful to diagnose fungal infections of the scalp and chronic bacterial infection of the major folds of the skin (**erythrasma**). Under a Wood's light, fungal lesions and erythrasma are fluorescent. Erythrasma usually is seen on the inner thighs, scrotum, and axilla, under the breasts, and in the area between the toes.

DIASCOPY

Diascopy uses a glass slide or lens pressed down over the area to be examined, blanching the skin and thereby reducing the erythema caused by increasing blood flow to the area. The shape of the underlying lesion is then revealed.

SKIN PATCH TESTING

When a rash is suspected to be of an allergic nature, patch testing is used to identify the responsible allergen. Test chemicals or substances are introduced to unaffected skin, usually on the forearm or back, by superficial scratches or pricks. If a localized reaction producing a **wheal** (smooth, slightly elevated area that is pale or reddened) occurs, the test is positive.

NURSING CARE FOR DIAGNOSTIC TESTS

Obtain an informed consent, if one is needed, for biopsies. Explain the procedure and any local anesthetic that will be used. Check for allergies to the anesthetic or skin prep solution. Properly label the biopsy specimen and send it to the laboratory. Apply a dressing and give both verbal and written postoperative instructions to the patient. Tell the patient approximately when the results will be back and that he will be notified. Advise if a follow-up visit is necessary. Patch tests are sometimes evaluated at a later time.

NURSING MANAGEMENT

Assessment (Data Collection)

History Taking

Diagnosing skin disorders often requires diligent detective work to identify factors that predispose a patient to or actually cause some type of skin disease. Data gathering on the potential etiologic factors mentioned is necessary. Focused Assessment 41–1 presents a guide for history taking.

Scabies, lice, and other parasites can be transmitted through close personal contact with infected persons at work, recreation, home, or schools. It is important to know if exposure has occurred. If the patient has recently been exposed to severe cold, his skin may be drier than usual and he may complain of severe itching *(winter itch).*

Many drugs can produce skin eruptions in certain individuals. Drug allergy or reaction can produce lesions and rashes that imitate those found in a long list of diseases, including measles, chickenpox, fungal infections, skin cancers, and psoriasis.

Itching and pain are the most common complaints. If the disorder is due to an allergy, the patient also may complain of shortness of breath, cough, or some gastrointestinal symptoms. The patient also may be able to relate what other factors, such as stress or excitement, could be related to the appearance of the skin lesions.

Physical Assessment

A thorough inspection of the skin under good lighting is essential. Provide privacy and have the room at a moderate temperature so that the patient does not become chilled. Dress the patient in a gown that allows access to all areas of the skin.

Seborrheic **keratoses** are common in the elderly. They appear as wartlike, greasy lesions on the trunk, arms, scalp, and sometimes the face. They are not a cause for concern.

Darkly pigmented people will have areas that are darker than other parts of the skin. This is due to hormonal influences. The darker areas are the nipples, areola, scrotum, and labia minora. This is true among both African Americans and Asians. The hair of African Americans differs in texture. It varies from being long and straight to being short, thick, and tightly curled. It is very dry and fragile and requires daily grooming with oil. If an African American child suffers from malnutrition, sometimes the hair will turn a coppery red. Asians tend to have straight, fine hair. When the skin of a darkly pigmented person is damaged, scar tissue may hypertrophy, forming a **keloid** (a thick ridge of scar tissue that stands up from the surrounding skin) (Figure 41–4).

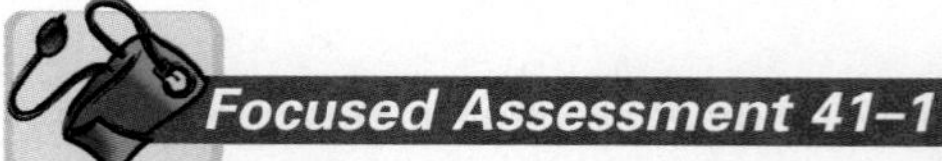

Focused Assessment 41–1

Data Collection for Skin Disorders

The following questions should be asked when seeking data on a skin disorder.

- When did the rash or lesion first appear?
- Can you think of any event or different food you ate or substance you were using just before it appeared?
- What is your usual dietary pattern? What do you eat and drink?
- Have you noticed if anything makes it worse?
- What seems to make it better?
- Have you been using any chemicals lately for household cleaning or in pursuit of your hobbies?
- Have you been out in the country or the woods lately?
- Have you been traveling? Did you visit a tropical area?
- What drugs are you taking? Do you take any over-the-counter medications?
- Have you ever had a drug reaction?
- Have you ever had radiation therapy?
- Do you have a history of any skin disorders in your family?
- Do you have any allergies?
- Are you experiencing itching? Pain?
- Have you had any gastrointestinal problems that began about the same time that the rash or lesion appeared? What about a runny or stuffed-up nose? Cough?
- How do you feel about having this problem? Has it had an impact on your social life or work?

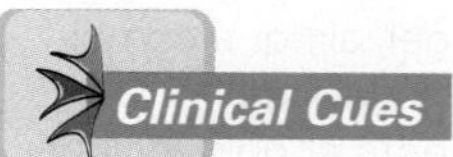

Clinical Cues

When trying to differentiate between a macule and a papule, shine a flashlight at a right angle to the lesion. A papule will cast a shadow. If there is no shadow the lesion is a macule. To determine whether there is fluid in a lesion, place the tip of a penlight against the side of the lesion. If the light illuminates it with a red glow, it's fluid filled. If there is no light illumination, the lesion is solid.

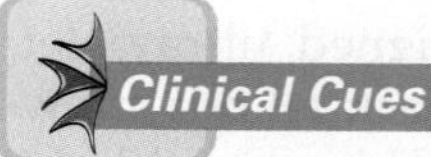

Clinical Cues

Pallor in the dark-skinned person presents as an ashen-gray tone to the skin. In the brown-skinned person, pallor gives the skin a yellow-brown color.

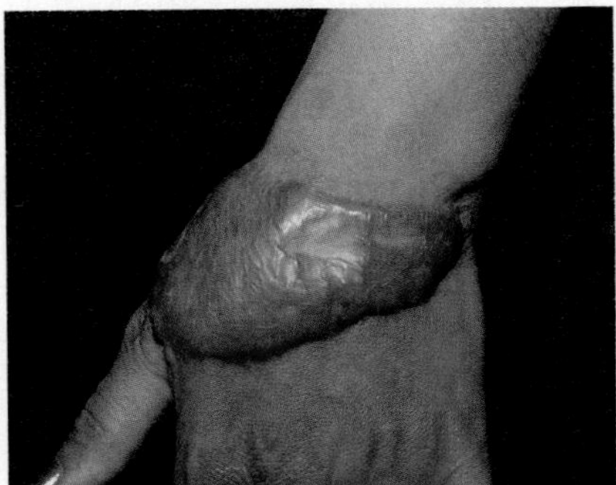

FIGURE **41–4** A keloid scar.

The skin should be lightly palpated to detect changes in texture and surface elevations. Palpation also is used to detect pain, areas of increased warmth, and tenderness. When checking the temperature of the skin, the back of the hand should be used. Skin turgor is assessed by lifting a fold of skin on the forearm, chest, or abdomen between two fingers and seeing how fast it falls back into place (Focused Assessment 41–2). Table 41–1 shows characteristics of various types of skin lesions.

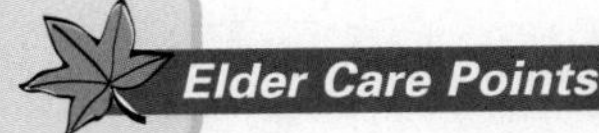

Elder Care Points

When checking skin turgor on an elderly patient, test the upper chest because the skin of the arms and hands of the elderly has often lost elasticity and is not a reliable index. Gently pinch a small amount of skin and lift up and let go. Note the time it takes for the skin to move back to its normal position. If the skin stays "tented" or takes more than 8 to 10 seconds to return to normal position, the patient is dehydrated.

Elderly patients bruise more easily as the skin becomes thinner and collagen is lost. Patches of **senile purpura,** deep red areas, may occur even from minor injuries.

Teaching Self-Examination

All people who have warts, moles, scars, or birthmarks should be taught how to do monthly evaluations of the lesions to detect malignant changes in their earliest stages. Examination can be done by the patient or by someone in the family if the patient cannot see well or has difficulty inspecting the area of the body where the lesions are located (Patient Teaching 41–1).

? *Think Critically About . . .* Can you describe how you specifically assess a patient who indicates that a rash has appeared on the legs?

Staging of Pressure Ulcers

Skin should be thoroughly assessed when the patient is admitted. Skin checks are performed every shift on immobile patients, noting the condition of skin over bony prominences. Findings must be accurately documented (Legal & Ethical Considerations 41–1). Once every 24 hours, usually during the bath, the skin is totally assessed. When a reddened area is found, it is checked for blanching by pressing gently in the center of the area to see if it turns from red to white or to a paler color on darker skin. Blanching usually indicates that the redness is temporary and will resolve when pressure on the area is relieved.

Several kinds of preprinted forms can be used to assess the risk of developing pressure ulcers. These assessment tools take into account the general condition of the skin, control of urination and defecation, mobility, men-

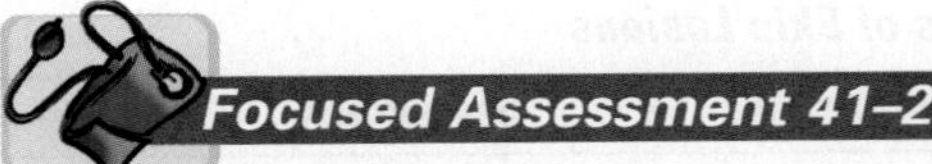

Focused Assessment 41–2

Physical Assessment of Skin

Perform physical examination of the entire skin surface. Proceed from head to toe. Compare from one side of the body to the other. Note the following data.

- Check the patient for:
  - General appearance of skin surface: texture, elasticity, thickness
  - Condition of areas between skinfolds
  - Type of lesions and distribution, size, and appearance; photograph or measure and document measurements
  - Appearance of skin adjacent to lesions; note whether reddened areas blanch when mild pressure is applied
  - Localized or generalized skin edema
  - Characteristics of secretions: color, viscosity, amount
  - Odor: description of odor; strong or faint; source—local or generalized
  - Temperature changes: location of hot spots or cold areas of the skin
- Check the back and the soles of the feet, including between the toes.
- Observe patient for scratching, rubbing, or picking at lesions.
- Observe for scratching of the scalp or pubic areas.
- Inspect the hair for texture, brittleness, thinning, and cleanliness.
- Inspect the nails for chipping, splitting, discoloration, and ragged or inflamed cuticles.

Use the metric system when measuring lesions; document all findings.

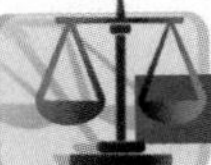

Legal & Ethical Considerations 41–1

Skin Lesion Documentation

All data gathered when assessing the skin and any lesions should be accurately documented as to location, size, appearance, and characteristics. Measure lesions using a ruler device and note the measurements in the chart. For pressure ulcers, many facilities take photos and enter those in the chart so that healing progress can be demonstrated.

Table 41–1 ***Types of Skin Lesions***

LESION	DESCRIPTION	LESION	DESCRIPTION
Macule	Circumscribed, flat area with a change in skin color; <1 cm in diameter *Examples:* Freckles, petechiae, measles, flat mole *(nevus)*	**Plaque**	Circumscribed, elevated superficial, solid lesion; >1 cm in diameter *Examples:* Psoriasis, seborrheic and actinic keratoses
Papule	Elevated, solid lesion; <1 cm in diameter *Examples:* Wart *(verruca)*, elevated moles	**Wheal**	Firm, edematous, irregularly shaped area; diameter variable *Examples:* Insect bite, urticaria
Vesicle	Circumscribed, superficial collection of serous fluid; <1 cm in diameter *Examples:* Varicella (chickenpox), herpes zoster (shingles), second-degree burn	**Pustule**	Elevated, superficial lesion filled with purulent fluid *Examples:* Acne, impetigo

From Lewis, S.M., Heitkemper, M.M., Dirksen, S.R., et. al. (2007). *Medical-Surgical Nursing: Assessment and Management of Clinical Problems* (7th ed.). St. Louis: Mosby.

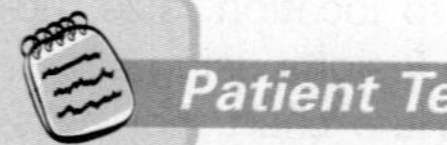

Patient Teaching 41–1

Self-Assessment of the Skin

The skin should be examined every few months. If you are unable to see your back or other areas, have a family member or close friend examine the skin of that area for you. If you have any warts, moles, or discolorations of the skin, check them each month for:

- A darkening or spreading of color or increasing unevenness of color.
- An increase in size or diameter.
- A change in shape; that is, has the lesion become elevated, or have its formerly regular edges become irregular?
- Redness or swelling of surrounding skin, or any other noticeable change around the lesion.
- Itching, tenderness, or other change in sensation.
- Crusting, scaling, oozing, ulceration, or other change in the surface of the lesion.
- When assessing for melanoma, check for the "ABCDs": A = asymmetrical; B = irregular border; C = color change; D = diameter greater than ¼ inch.

If any changes have occurred, consult your physician right away.

tal status, and nutritional status. They provide a more systematic approach to evaluating a patient's potential for pressure ulcer development. Many agencies use either the Braden scale system or the Norton system for systematic assessment of the skin (Figure 41–5).

Ascertaining the stage of ulceration can be useful to document that an ulcer was present on admission. Classifying an ulceration also can be helpful to evaluate the effectiveness of treatment and progress toward healing and repair. The AHCPR, a division of the U.S. Depart-

Patient's Name ______	Evaluator's Name ______			Date of Assessment				
SENSORY PRECEPTION Ability to respond meaningfully to pressure-related discomfort	**1. Completely limited:** Unresponsive (does not moan, flinch, or grasp) to painful stimuli, due to diminished level of consciousness or sedation. OR Limited ability to feel pain over most of body surface.	**2. Very Limited:** Responds only to painful stimuli. Cannot communicate discomfort except by moaning or restlessness. OR Has a sensory impairment that limits the ability to feel pain or discomfort over half of body.	**3. Slightly Limited:** Responds to verbal commands, but cannot always communicate discomfort or need to be turned. OR Has some sensory impairment that limits ability to feel pain or discomfort in one or two extremities.	**4. No Impairment:** Responds to verbal commands. Has no sensory deficit which would limit ability to feel or voice pain or discomfort.				
MOISTURE Degree to which skin is exposed to moisture	**1. Constantly Moist:** Skin is kept moist almost constantly by perspiration, urine, etc. Dampness is detected every time patient is moved or turned.	**2. Very Moist:** Skin is often, but now always moist. Linen must be changed at least once a shift.	**3. Occasionally Moist:** Skin is occasionally moist, requiring an extra linen change approximately once a day.	**4. Rarely Moist:** Skin is usually dry, linen only requires changing at routine intervals.				
ACTIVITY Degree of physical acitivity	**1. Bedfast:** Confined to bed	**2. Chairfast:** Ability to walk severely limited or non-existent. Cannot bear own weight and/or must be assisted into chair or wheelchair.	**3. Walks Occasionally:** Walks occasionally during day, but for very short distances, with or without assistance. Spends majority of each shift in bed or chair.	**4. Walks Frequently:** Walks outside the room at least twice a day and inside room at least once every 2 hours during waking hours.				
MOBILITY Ability to change and control body position	**1. Completely Immobile:** Does not make even slight changes in body or extremity position without assistance.	**2. Very Limited:** Makes occasional slight changes in body or extremity position but unable to make frequent or significant changes independently.	**3. Slightly Limited:** Makes frequent though slight changes in body or extremity position independently.	**4. No Limitations:** Makes major and frequent changes in position without assistance.				
NUTRITION <u>Usual</u> food intake pattern	**1. Very Poor:** Never eats a complete meal. Rarely eats more than a third of any food offered. Eats two servings or less of protein (meat or dairy products) per day. Takes fluids poorly. Does not take a liquid dietary supplement. OR Is NPO and/or maintained on clear liquids or IVs for more than 5 days.	**2. Probably Inadequate:** Rarely eats a complete meal and generally eats only about half of any food offered. Protein intake includes only three servings of meat or dairy products per day. Occasionally will take a dietary supplement. OR Receives less than optimum amount of liquid diet or tube feeding.	**3. Adequate:** Eats over half of most meals. Eats a total of four servings of protein (meat, dairy products) each day. Occasionally will refuse a meal, but will usually take a supplement if offered. OR Is on a tube feeding or TPN regimen that probably meets most of nutritional needs.	**4. Excellent:** Eats most of every meal. Never refuses a meal. Usually eats a total of four or more servings of meat and dairy products. Occasionally eats between meals. Does not require supplementation.				
FRICTION AND SHEAR	**1. Problem:** Requires moderate to maximum assistance in moving. Complete lifting without sliding against sheets is impossible. Frequently slides down in bed or chair, requiring frequent repositioning with maximum assistance. Spasticity, contractures, or agitation leads to almost constant friction.	**2. Potential Problem:** Moves feebly or requires minimum assistance. During a move, skin probably slides to some extent against sheets, chair, restraints, or other devices. Maintains relatively good position in chair or bed most of the time but occasionally slides down.	**3. No Apparent Problem:** Moves in bed and in chair independently and has sufficient muscle strength to lift up completely during move. Maintains good position in bed or chair at all times.					
				Total Score				

At risk = 15-18; Moderate risk = 13-14; High risk = 10-12; Severe Risk = 9.
Key: IV, intravenously; *NPO,* nothing by mouth; *TPN,* total parenteral nutrition.

FIGURE 41–5 Braden scale for predicting pressure sore risk.

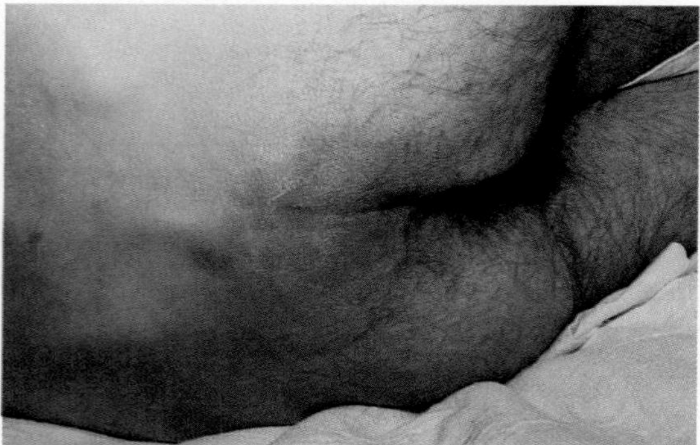

FIGURE 41–6 Stage I pressure ulcer.

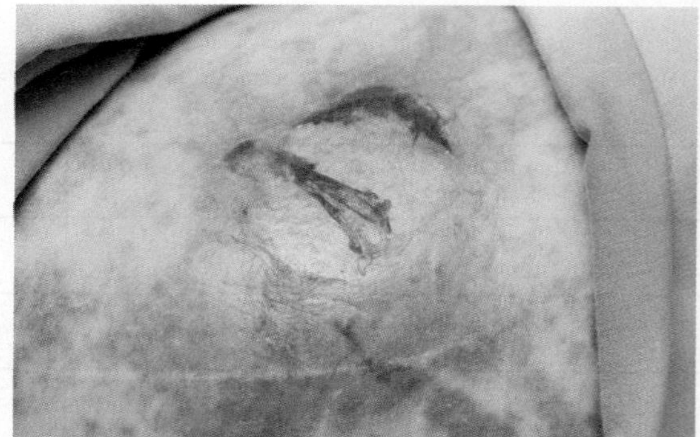

FIGURE 41–7 Stage II pressure ulcer.

ment of Health and Human Services, has issued clinical practice guidelines for the prediction and prevention of pressure ulcers and a staging system for classification:

- **Stage I:** An area of reddened, deep pink, or mottled skin. The skin may feel very warm and firm or tightly stretched across the area. The area does not blanch with finger pressure. The redness remains for over half as long as the area was subjected to pressure (Figure 41–6).
- **Stage II:** Partial-thickness skin loss involving the epidermis and/or dermis. The skin appears blistered or abraded, or has a shallow crater. The area surrounding the damaged skin is reddened and probably will feel hot or warmer than normal (Figure 41–7).
- **Stage III:** The skin is ulcerated. There is a crater-like ulcer, and the underlying subcutaneous tissue is involved in the destructive process. The ulcer may or may not be infected. Bacterial infection is almost always present at this stage, however, and accounts for continued erosion of the ulcer and the production of drainage (Figure 41–8).
- **Stage IV:** There is deep ulceration and necrosis involving deeper underlying muscle and possibly bone tissue. At this stage, the ulcer usually is extensively infected. The ulcer can be dry, black, and covered with a tough accumulation of necrotic tissue, or it can be made up of wet and oozing dead cells and purulent *exudate* (Figure 41–9).

When *eschar* (blackened, dead tissue) is present, it must be débrided to properly stage the ulcer.

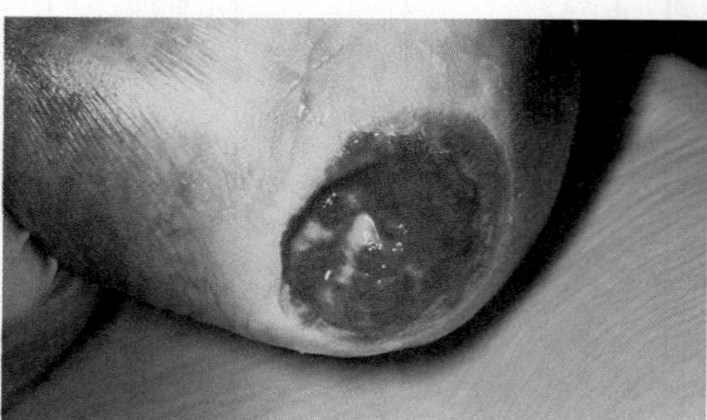

FIGURE 41–8 Stage III pressure ulcer.

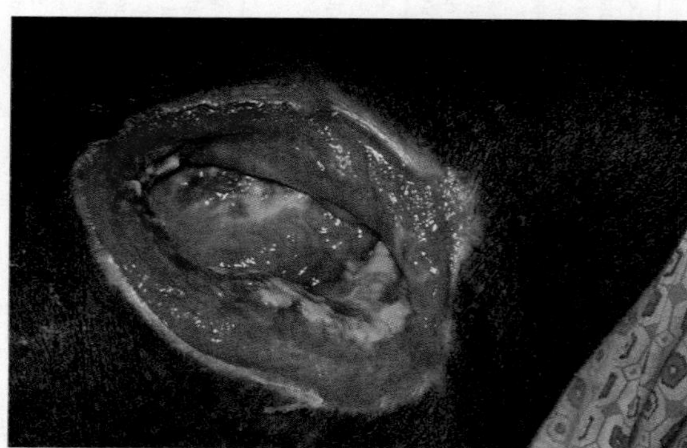

FIGURE 41–9 Stage IV pressure ulcer.

Nursing Diagnosis and Planning

Nursing diagnoses are based on the analysis of the data gathered from assessment. Diagnoses commonly associated with skin disorders are presented in Table 41–2.

Nursing goals for patients with skin disorders are to:

- Restore the skin to normal
- Decrease pain and itching
- Protect the skin from further damage
- Prevent infection
- Prevent scarring as much as possible

Nursing goals may be long or short term. Specific expected outcomes are written for the individual nursing diagnoses chosen for the patient (see Table 41–2).

Planning of the daily work schedule should include consideration of time necessary for dressing changes, soaks, special baths, and other skin treatments.

Implementation

Some general rules when caring for patients with a skin disease may be helpful as a guide until specific orders are obtained:

- Bathing with soap is usually contraindicated in all inflammatory conditions of the skin.
- Dressings covering the skin lesions that have been applied by a physician should not be re-

Table 41–2 ***Common Nursing Diagnoses, Expected Outcomes, and Nursing Interventions for Patients with Skin Disorders***

NURSING DIAGNOSIS	GOALS/EXPECTED OUTCOMES	NURSING INTERVENTIONS
Impaired skin integrity related to injury and treatment; excoriation or scaling; infectious process	Patient's skin will be intact within 2 wk (4 mo for burns). Number of lesions will decrease within 2 mo. Patient will exhibit no signs of infection within 3 mo.	Cleanse skin and apply topical medications as prescribed. Monitor for signs of adverse reaction to topical medication. Preserve integrity of grafted areas with aseptic dressing technique and splinting. Apply light treatments as prescribed. Provide medicated baths as prescribed.
Pain related to itching, soreness, or tenderness of lesions, exposure of denuded skin to air, or involvement of nerve tissue	Patient's pain will be controlled by medication and relaxation or distraction techniques.	Apply topical medication as ordered. Administer analgesia as ordered PRN. Teach relaxation techniques. Provide distraction activities.
Chronic low self-esteem related to disrupted skin surface and lesions	Patient will show increase in self-esteem by socializing with others within 3 wk.	Suggest ways to cover lesions. Help patient list positive aspects and achievements. Encourage socialization with others. Show acceptance and matter-of-fact attitude when dealing with patient's lesions.
Risk for infection related to loss of intact skin barrier	Patient will not experience skin infection before lesions are healed.	Cleanse skin carefully and gently. Use aseptic technique when attending to lesions. Apply ordered topical medication. Encourage patient to keep hands off affected skin areas. Encourage hand hygiene for patient.
Anxiety related to chronic, recurring nature of skin disorder; reaction to diagnosis of cancer; slow healing	Patient will verbalize feelings within 3 wk. Patient will explore options for treatment of cancer. Patient will acknowledge that although healing is slow, disorder is self-limited and will resolve.	Provide atmosphere of acceptance. Allow patient time to verbalize feelings. Assist to recognize positive coping techniques by looking at ways patient has coped with anxiety in the past. Provide information on treatment and prognosis for skin malignancy. Provide information on the skin disorder, treatment options, and prognosis.
Deficient knowledge related to cause and treatment of skin disorder	Patient will verbalize knowledge of factors related to appearance of skin disorder. Patient will verbalize knowledge of treatment for disorder. Patient will demonstrate self-care techniques.	Explain the etiology of the skin disorder and measures to prevent recurrence, if possible. Instruct in various methods of treatment. Teach signs of side effects of medications. Instruct in self-care techniques for medication application, dressing changes, and so on. Obtain feedback of information and skills taught.
Sleep deprivation related to itching or pain	Patient will obtain at least 7 hr of rest per day.	Administer medication to relieve itching. Keep environment cool to decrease itching sensation. Caution patient to take cool or tepid baths or showers to decrease itching. Caution not to scratch lesions as this often makes itching worse. Advise in ways to use distraction to decrease focus on itching (i.e., card or game playing, intense concentration on learning something, or reading an absorbing book). Administer hypnotic as ordered. Administer analgesics as ordered. Encourage use of meditation, relaxation, or imagery techniques to decrease pain. Provide restful, quiet, environment. Use massage as appropriate to promote relaxation and sleep. Allow usual bedtime rituals that help patient induce sleep.
Social isolation related to long treatment process; disfigurement	Patient will maintain social contact with family and friends. Patient will reintegrate into community within 3–24 mo.	Encourage family and friends to send cards, call, and visit. Encourage patient to continue dialogue with family and friends. Refer to psychologist or social worker for grief work and reintegration of new body image. Refer to support group for expression of feelings and realization patient is not alone with such problems. Encourage return to employment or job training. Encourage return to church or community activities.

moved when the patient is admitted unless there are specific orders to do so.

- Do not attempt to remove scales, crusts, or other exudates on the skin lesions until the physician has had an opportunity to examine the patient.
- Observe the skin very carefully at the time of the patient's admission, and record observations on the chart or report them to the nurse in charge.
- Avoid excessive handling or rubbing of the skin against the sheets and bedclothes when changing the bed.
- Lotions or other skin products should not be used on the skin unless the physician has approved their use.

Once the physician has determined the type of lesions present, specific treatments will be ordered to relieve the patient's symptoms and promote healing. The two most commonly used treatments are special dermatologic baths and wet compresses or dressings. In addition, lotions, salves, or ointments may be applied locally at frequent intervals.

Although the vast majority of skin diseases are *not* contagious, nurses should be careful to observe rules of cleanliness and Standard Precautions when caring for any patient with a skin eruption. **Special care is needed to avoid spreading infection from the fluid in all pustules and in the vesicles of fever blisters and cold sores.**

Giving Medicated Baths

Among the agents that may be added to the bath water are sodium bicarbonate, sodium chloride, cornstarch, oatmeal, medicated tars, oils, potassium permanganate, and special bath preparations (Safety Alert 41–2).

During the bath, the patient must be protected from chilling, because the bath usually lasts from 30 minutes to an hour, and most patients with skin diseases have a lowered resistance to cold. **When the patient is removed from the tub, the skin is dried by patting rather than by rubbing.** If medication is to be applied locally, it should be put on as soon as the bath is completed in order to keep *pruritus* (itching) at a minimum. **Medication is applied in a thin layer unless otherwise ordered.**

The medicated bath has a very soothing and relaxing effect on the patient and also helps relieve the itching and burning commonly associated with skin diseases. The nurse should encourage the patient to rest in bed and perhaps to take a short nap after each bath.

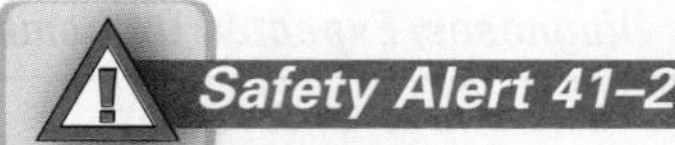

Prevent Falls

A nonslip bath mat should be used in the tub when giving medicated baths. The substance used for the bath can make the tub very slippery. Showers should have nonslip mats in them as well, especially when showering an elderly person.

Laundry Requirements

The bed linens and gowns used for patients with severe skin diseases may need special laundering to eliminate all traces of soap. If the patient is to be cared for at home, vinegar may be added to the rinse water to neutralize the soap. One tablespoon of vinegar is used for each quart of water. Only detergent without perfume or other additives should be used. Dryer sheets should not be used as they contain chemicals that often cause skin problems. Residue from dryer sheets can remain in the dryer and affect laundry that has been washed separately for the sensitive-skinned person. New clothes should be washed before wearing when skin sensitivity is a problem. Washing removes chemical fabric finish products.

Application of Wet Compresses or Dressings

Wet dressings may be applied to the skin in various ways. The two general types used are *open dressings* and *closed dressings*. Open compresses must be changed repeatedly and are never allowed to dry. They usually need to be remoistened every 20 to 30 minutes. The solution used should be at room temperature or warmer. This type of dressing is used when the dermatologist wishes to have air circulating to the skin lesions. Closed dressings are thoroughly soaked with the prescribed solution and wrapped with an airtight, waterproof material. It is recommended that you obtain specific instructions from the dermatologist before applying wet dressings to any skin lesions.

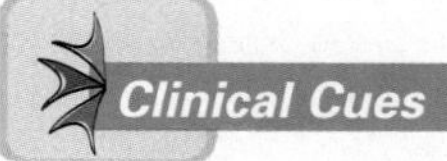

When changing wet dressings, inspect the skin adjacent to the wound for signs of maceration from the moisture. Such a problem could cause the wound to enlarge.

Application of Topical Therapy

Many skin lesions are treated by directly applying medications to the surface of the affected area. This method is called topical therapy. Lotion, cream, ointment, powder, or gel may be used. The physician prescribes the kind of medication to be used and the way in which the drug is to be applied. Patients with skin conditions do not always consult a physician and sometimes choose to treat themselves at home. **All patients should be instructed in the proper application of topical medications** (Box 41–3). Occlusive dressings must not be applied over the area after ap-

Box 41–3 Guidelines for Applying Topical Medications*

POWDERS

- Dry the area thoroughly before applying powder to prevent caking.
- Do not apply to raw and denuded areas.
- Some powders, such as cornstarch, can actually serve as culture media for the growth of bacteria.

OINTMENT

- Use only a small amount and gently massage into the skin until a thin film covers the area. An exception is when ointment is used as an occlusive dressing, as for a burn.
- Ointments tend to leave a greasy feeling to the skin. They are best for chronic lesions, because they help the skin retain moisture and natural oils.
- Avoid putting ointment on areas where the skin is creased and overlaps itself.

GELS

- A gel is a semisolid mixture that tends to liquefy when applied to the skin. It is absorbed into the skin and dries quickly, leaving a thin, nonocclusive film.
- If applied to abraded or sensitive areas, alcohol in the base can cause a burning or stinging sensation.

LOTIONS

- These are actually powders suspended in water; they will leave a residue once the liquid evaporates from the skin. This residue should be washed off before a fresh dose is applied.
- Be sure powder is uniformly dispersed in solution before applying, then use a firm stroke to distribute the medication evenly. Do not "dab" on lotions, as this can be irritating to the skin.

ALL TYPES

- Always apply topical medications sparingly and in a thin film that extends beyond the affected area about ¼ inch. Thick layers of topicals are wasteful, and some of these drugs, such as corticosteroids, are very expensive.
- Too much of some topicals (e.g., antifungal agents) can chemically irritate the skin and delay healing. Thick layers also tend to soften the skin too much.

If the skin condition appears to be getting worse after a topical agent is applied, or if the patient develops eczema, suspect an allergic contact dermatitis caused by the drug.

*Allergies must be assessed before applying a topical medication.

plication of the medication unless ordered by the health care provider. Other nursing interventions are included with the discussion of the various skin disorders in the next chapter and in Table 41–2.

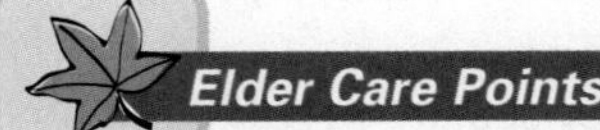

Elder Care Points

Elderly people usually have very dry skin. The skin should be moisturized twice a day with an appropriate oil, lotion, or cream. When applying moisturizer after the bath, do it immediately after patting the patient dry to seal in moisture. Be gentle when massaging moisturizer into the skin so you do not bruise the patient or cause a skin tear.

Think Critically About . . . If a patient has an order for a topical cream to be applied to an area of rash on the right upper thigh, how would you apply this cream? (Describe every step you would take in detail.)

Evaluation

Evaluation of treatment and nursing interventions for skin disorders is based on improved appearance of the skin, absence of signs of infection, relief from itching and pain, and signs of healing. Many skin disorders are slow to respond to treatment, and patience is required on the part of the patient and the nurse. Even a minor fungal skin infection may take from 7 to 14 days to clear with topical medication. A fungal infection of a nail may take up to a year to clear. A major part of evaluation is to determine that treatment is not aggravating the condition. On occasion this happens when the patient who has sensitive skin reacts badly to medication, heat, or light treatments.

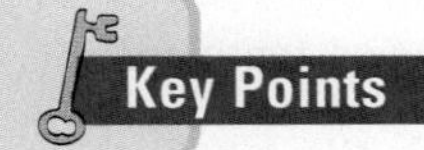

Key Points

- The skin is essential for the maintenance of life; it is the first line of defense against pathogenic organisms.
- Skin disorders are difficult to diagnose, cure, and control.
- Skin has two layers, the epidermis and the dermis.
- New cells to heal the skin are contained in the dermis.
- With age the skin becomes thinner and more fragile, less elastic, and drier.
- There are many causes of skin disorders, both primary disorders and secondary disorders related to systemic diseases.
- Pressure ulcers occur from unrelieved pressure over bony prominences.
- Factors in the prevention of skin diseases include cleanliness, appropriate diet, proper skin care, and environment.
- Damage to skin by the sun is cumulative.
- Several types of diagnostic measures are used to diagnose skin disorders: Biopsy, culture, microscopic

examination of scrapings or tissue, special light inspection, diascopy, and skin patch testing.
- A thorough health history is key in the diagnosis of skin disorders.
- A careful physical assessment of the skin provides much necessary information.
- All patients should be taught self-examination of the skin.
- Pressure ulcers are staged from I to IV.
- Topical lotions, gels, creams or ointments should be applied in a thin layer.
- Standard precautions are used when touching patients with weeping lesions or when drainage is present.
- Treatments for skin disorders include medicated baths, special laundry precautions, application of compresses or dressing, and topical therapy. Systemic therapy may be used for some fungal infections and for serious bacterial infections.

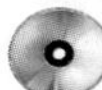
Go to your **Companion CD-ROM** for an Audio Glossary, animations, video clips, and bonus review questions.

evolve Be sure to visit the companion Evolve site at http://evolve.elsevier.com/deWit for interactive NCLEX-PN Exam Style Review Questions, WebLinks, and additional online resources.

NCLEX-PN EXAM STYLE REVIEW QUESTIONS

Choose the best answer(s) for the following questions.

1. Which of the following physiologic changes in aging predispose the older adult to skin breakdown? *(Select all that apply.)*

1. Decreased melanocytes
2. Loss of collagen
3. Increased elastic fibers
4. Decreased adipose tissues
5. Reduced sebaceous gland activity

2. ____________ are brown "age spots" or "liver spots" due to concentrated increased melanocytes production.

3. A patient with a suspicious skin lesion is prepared for a punch skin biopsy. When asked about the procedure, the nurse accurately explained:

1. "It is shaving a top layer off a lesion that rises above the skin line."
2. "It is removing a core from the center of the lesion."
3. "It is removing the entire lesion."
4. "It is aspirating a tissue sample."

4. The nurse admits a patient with a tentative diagnosis of chronic bacterial infection of the major folds of the skin. The physician confirms the diagnosis by:

1. Wood's light inspection.
2. diascopy.
3. cold light inspection.
4. skin patch testing.

5. The nurse documents that there is a skin loss involving the epidermis and dermis. The skin appears blistered with a shallow crater. The surrounding areas are red and warm to touch. What is the stage of the pressure ulcer?

1. Stage I
2. Stage II
3. Stage III
4. Stage IV

6. A nurse is observing a nursing assistant provide skin care to an older adult patient. Which of the following actions by the nursing assistant indicates a need for further training?

1. Using soap over the entire skin every second or third day
2. Alerting the nurse about a wet dressing
3. Reporting changes in a skin lesion
4. Applying prescribed lotions or other skin products

7. The nurse is developing a plan of care for a wheelchair-bound patient. To prevent development of pressure ulcers, which of the following nursing interventions must be implemented? *(Select all that apply.)*

1. Maintain postural alignment.
2. Use pressure-relieving devices.
3. Teach to shift weight every 15 minutes.
4. Use donut-type devices.
5. Reposition in the chair every hour.

8. The nurse is giving instructions to a caregiver regarding the proper application of skin ointment. The following instructions given by a nurse are appropriate except:

1. use sparingly.
2. gently massage into a thin film.
3. avoid creased areas.
4. apply a thick layer.

9. The nurse reminds teenagers regarding the importance of protecting the skin from ultraviolet rays. Appropriate sun protection information includes which of the following? *(Select all that apply.)*

1. Use a sunscreen with a skin protection factor (SPF) of at least 15.
2. Apply sunscreen thinly.
3. Wear light, loosely worn clothing.
4. Gauge exposure while in the sun.
5. Wear sunglasses and a hat.

10. The patient presents with a rash of unknown origin. Which of the following assessment questions would help determine the underlying cause of the lesion? *(Select all that apply.)*
    1. "When did the rash or lesion first appear?"
    2. "Can you think of any event or different food you ate or substance you were using just before it appeared?"
    3. "What drugs are you taking? Do you take any over-the-counter medications?"
    4. "Have you ever had radiation therapy?"
    5. "Do you have a history of any skin disorders in your family?"

CRITICAL THINKING ACTIVITIES 

Read each clinical scenario and discuss the questions with your classmates.

Scenario A

You have been asked to give a presentation to your younger sister's ninth-grade class on skin care and prevention of skin cancer.

1. What specific information would you include on the subject of general skin care?
2. What would you say about lying out in the sun?
3. What information would you give regarding the use of tanning booths?
4. What would you say about protection when out in the sun?

Scenario B

Mrs. Hess, an 83-year-old resident of a long-term care facility, has very dry skin. She asks you to look at spots on her hand that are brown and "ugly."

1. What could this lesion on Mrs. Hess' hand be?
2. What would you tell her?
3. Mrs. Hess asks you why she bruises so easily. She says she hates these reddish purple areas she gets on her arms and legs. What would you answer?
4. What nursing measures should be instituted for skin care for Mrs. Hess' dry skin?

CHAPTER

42 Care of Patients with Integumentary Disorders and Burns

evolve http://evolve.elsevier.com/deWit

Objectives

Upon completing this chapter, you should be able to:

Theory

1. Describe the etiology of dermatitis.
2. Plan psychosocial interventions for the patient who has psoriasis.
3. Compare the treatment of fungal skin or nail disorders to the treatment of bacterial skin disorders.
4. List the main nursing care points for patients with herpesvirus infections.
5. Discuss the types of acne and their treatment.
6. Compare the characteristics of the various types of skin cancer.
7. Compose a teaching plan for a family of an immobile patient to prevent pressure ulcers.
8. Prepare care plan interventions for each stage of a pressure ulcer.
9. List important assessment points for the patient who has sustained a burn.
10. Explain emergency burn care.
11. Identify the measures used for burn treatment during the acute or emergent phase.
12. Describe the process of rehabilitation for the patient with a major burn.

Clinical Practice

1. Teach a family about care for the patient and home when scabies is present.
2. Assess the skin of family members for signs of skin cancer.
3. Provide care for a Stage III or Stage IV pressure ulcer.
4. Apply Standard Precautions and sterile technique for the care of a burn.
5. Assist with the planning of care after the acute stage of a major burn, paying attention to both physical and psychosocial needs.

Key Terms

Be sure to check out the bonus material on the Companion CD-ROM, including selected audio pronunciations.

allograft (ĂL-ō-grăft, p. 1043)
autograft (AW-tō-grăft, p. 1043)
autoinoculation (ăw-tō-ĭn-Ō-kŭ-LĀ-shŭn, p. 1026)
biologic dressing (bī-ō-LŎJ-ĭk, p. 1042)
biosynthetic (bī-ō-SĬN-thĕt-ĭk, p. 1043)
carbuncles (KĂR-bŭn-kŭlz, p. 1026)
dermabrasion (dĕrm-ă-BRĀ-zhŭn, p. 1024)
dermatophytosis (DĔR-mă-tō-fī-TŌ-sĭs, p. 1028)
eschar (ĔS-kăr, p. 1033)
escharotomy (ĔS-kă-RŌ-tō-mē, p. 1038)
furuncles (fyoo-RŬN-kŭlz, p. 1026)
mycoses (mī-KŌ-sēz, p. 1028)
onychomycosis (ŏn-ĭ-kō-mī-KŌ-sĭs, p. 1028)
purulent (PŬ-roo-lĕnt, p. 1034)
serosanguineous (SĔR-ō-săng-GWĬN-ē-ŭs, p. 1034)
tinea pedis (TĬN-ē-ă pē-dĭs, p. 1029)
xenograft (ZĒ-nō-grăft, p. 1043)

Many skin diseases result from infection with bacteria, viruses, or fungi or from infestation with parasites. Diseases of this kind require special precautions to avoid spreading the infectious organism or the parasite. The Center for Infectious Diseases, a division of the Centers for Disease Control and Prevention, recommends that Contact Isolation, as well as Standard Precautions, be implemented for a number of these diseases (Box 42–1).

A variety of topical and systemic medications are used to treat infectious and parasitic skin diseases. A culture and sensitivity test or biopsy is used to determine the causative organism and appropriate drug therapy.

INFLAMMATORY INFECTIONS

DERMATITIS

Etiology, Pathophysiology, Signs, and Symptoms

Contact dermatitis is a delayed allergic response involving cell-mediated immunity. An inflammatory disorder results. On contact with the skin, the allergen is bound to a carrier protein and forms a sensitizing antigen. T cells become sensitized to the antigen. Local skin irritation is evident within a few hours or days after exposure to an antigen. Erythema and swelling, pruritus, and the appearance of vesicular lesions follow. Many chemicals, cosmetics, soaps, latex, and poison ivy or oak can cause such a reaction.

Box 42–1 Review of Contact Isolation Requirements

Specifications for Contact Isolation are as follows:

- A private room is indicated. In general, patients infected with the same type of organism may share a room.
- Gloves are worn when entering the room. Change gloves after contact with infective material, such as wound drainage or feces, and before treating a different location on the body. Wash hands before donning clean gloves.
- Remove gloves when leaving the room, and wash hands with an antimicrobial agent.
- Gowns are indicated if soiling is likely, particularly if there is drainage from an uncovered wound or the patient is incontinent.
- Articles contaminated with infective material should be discarded in a biohazard waste receptacle or bagged and labeled before being sent for decontamination and reprocessing.
- Patient care equipment should be used only for the one patient and should be left in the room until no longer needed.

Skin disorders that require Contact Isolation include:

- Diphtheria, cutaneous
- Furunculosis, group A *Streptococcus*
- Herpes simplex, disseminated, severe primary, or neonatal
- Herpes zoster (varicella-zoster)
- Varicella (chickenpox)
- Impetigo
- Infection or colonization by bacteria with multiple drug resistance (any site)
- Pediculosis
- Scabies
- Skin wound or burn infection, major (draining and not covered by dressing, or dressing does not adequately contain purulent material), including those infected with *Staphylococcus aureus*
- Vaccinia (generalized and progressive eczema vaccinatum)

A variety of topical and systemic medications are used to treat infectious and parasitic skin diseases. A culture and sensitivity test or biopsy is used to determine the causative organism and appropriate drug therapy.

Atopic dermatitis affects about 10% of the population and is more common in infancy and childhood, but does affect some adults. It results from a complex activation process that involves mast cells, T lymphocytes, Langerhans cells, monocytes, B cells that produce immunoglobulin E, and other inflammatory cells that release histamine, lymphokines, and other inflammatory mediators.

Stasis dermatitis generally occurs on the legs as a result of venous stasis and edema and is seen in conjunction with varicosities, phlebitis, and vascular trauma. Erythema and pruritus occur first, and then there is scaling, development of petechiae, and *hyperpigmentation* (excessive pigmentation). Lesions may become ulcerated, particularly around the ankles and tibia.

Seborrheic dermatitis is a common inflammation involving the scalp, eyebrows, eyelids, ear canals, nasolabial folds, axillae, chest, and back. It is most common on the scalp. The cause is unknown. Lesions appear as scaly, white or yellowish plaques with mild pruritus. Dermatitis is not contagious unless a secondary infection has occurred in the lesions.

Diagnosis and Treatment

Diagnosis of dermatitis is done by inspection and a complete history looking for possible exposure to causative substances. Atopic dermatitis does seem to have a genetic, allergic association as it is more prevalent in families.

In general, treatment is aimed at avoidance of the contact irritant or allergen, good skin lubrication, preservation of skin moisture, and control of inflammation and itching. Topical agents are often used. Corticosteroids may be used topically, or sometimes orally or by injection to intervene in a severe episode of dermatitis. (See Box 36–3 for nursing implications for corticosteroids.)

Nursing Management

Nursing care is geared toward teaching patients to avoid contact irritants and to properly care for their skin. Instructing in the proper way to apply topical agents is important. Caution any patient who is experiencing pruritus to avoid becoming hot and to bathe in tepid water. The skin should be patted rather than rubbed dry.

ACNE

Etiology, Pathophysiology, Signs, and Symptoms

Acne is a disorder of the skin characterized by papules and pustules over the face, back, and shoulders. There are many kinds of acne, but the two major types are *acne vulgaris* and *acne rosacea.* Of the two, acne vulgaris is the more common. It typically begins in early puberty, continues through the teens, and then begins to subside. Occasionally it persists, or it can recur several years later.

Acne rosacea usually begins between the ages of 30 and 50. It is characterized by erythema (redness), papules, pustules, and telangiectases. It occurs on the face over the cheeks and bridge of the nose. Comedos do not occur. Factors that cause facial flushing precipitate worsening. Tea, coffee, alcohol (especially wine), caffeine-containing foods, spicy foods, sunlight, and emotional stress cause flare-ups.

Some types of acne are related to cosmetics or to chemicals in the environment. For example, occupational acne is due to prolonged contact with oils and tars.

Acne vulgaris occurs when the ducts leading from the sebaceous glands become plugged with sebum, the oily secretion of the glands. Factors that contribute to the development of acne include hereditary disposition, increased androgen levels, and premenstrual hormonal fluctuations. Use of heavy creams, certain drugs, and exposure to increased heat also contributes to the disorder.

The onset of acne vulgaris in adolescents is related to increased release of sex hormones, which stimulate activity of the sebaceous glands, causing increased production of sebum. It is not known why in some persons the ducts from these glands become plugged, but the increased production of sebum triggers the formation of blackheads and whiteheads. These lesions are not a sign of uncleanliness. The color of blackheads is the result of particles of melanin, the skin's own pigment, combined with sebum and keratin.

Accumulations of sebum, skin particles, and dead skin cells can cause an inflammatory reaction. Bacterial infection leads to the formation of pustules. An extensive inflammation can lead to the formation of cysts, with swelling above and below the surface of the skin.

Diagnosis and Treatment

Diagnosis is by history and physical examination. Mild, noninflammatory cases of acne vulgaris respond well to efforts to remove blackheads and whiteheads by promoting dryness and peeling of the top layer of skin. The medication is applied directly on the skin. Nonprescription drugs, such as lotions, creams, and gels that contain sulfur, benzoyl peroxide, and sulfur combined with resorcinol usually are effective for noninflammatory acne.

Among the topical medications, retinoic acid (tretinoin [Retin-A]) is the best agent for papular and pustular acne problems. It should be used once or twice a day. Benzoyl peroxide is the most frequently used topical agent for acne and is available both by prescription and over the counter. A newer drug, azelaic acid (Azelex) is available and is applied topically twice a day.

Antibiotics such as tetracycline and erythromycin also are sometimes prescribed topically and orally for cystic acne to inhibit the growth of bacteria in the plugged ducts. Isotretinoin (13-*cis*-retinoic acid) given to treat cystic acne has been especially effective in controlling cases that are resistant to other forms of treatment. The drug is marketed under the trade name Accutane. Almost all patients experience some adverse reaction to this drug. It is not recommended for pregnant women as it can cause birth defects. Accutane is taken by mouth daily for 2 to 4 months and inhibits activity of the sebaceous glands. Its effects are sustained for months to years after it has been discontinued. **Accutane is used only for severe cystic acne that is resistant to all other treatment. There are serious adverse side effects, including organ damage and mental problems.** Close monitoring with laboratory testing is very important for the patient taking Accutane.

The appearance of the patient with deep scarring and pitting as a result of cystic acne can be improved by **dermabrasion.** This dermatologic procedure involves mechanically scraping away the outer layers of skin and smoothing out its surface by applying motor-driven wire brushes or diamond wheels. Chemical dermabrasion is done by applying phenol or trichloroacetic acid to remove the scars.

Acne rosacea is treated by avoiding the triggers for flare-ups and with topical antibiotics, metronidazole (MetroGel), and retinoids. Sometimes oral antibiotics are prescribed.

Nursing Management

Nursing intervention is primarily concerned with teaching the patient about the nature of her particular skin disease and giving support while she is trying to cope with its physiological and psychosocial effects. She should feel that her problems are being taken seriously, even though they are certainly not life threatening. Acne can be particularly distressing to adolescents, who are often deeply concerned about their appearance and acceptance by their peers.

There are many misconceptions about acne and its treatment. It is not a contagious disease. It is not due to uncleanliness or poor personal hygiene. Diet can contribute to the formation of lesions, but this is true of relatively few people who usually can find a relationship between the intake of certain foods and the appearance of the lesions of acne. In general, however, chocolate, colas, and the fried foods of which most adolescents are so fond need not be eliminated from the diet in an effort to prevent or cure acne. A well-balanced diet is all that is recommended in the management of acne.

The face should be washed gently and with a mild soap. Scrubbing the skin and using a harsh soap is damaging to the skin and contributes to inflammation. Special medicated soaps do not seem to be any better than a mild face soap. If the hair is oily, it should be shampooed frequently and kept off the face.

It is not a good idea to squeeze pimples and pustules. This can press the sebum and accumulated material more firmly in the clogged duct, increase the chance of inflammation, and spread an infection to other parts of the skin and body. Blackheads and whiteheads are best removed by applying a prescription medication that causes peeling of the skin. The hands should be kept off of the face.

Because the management of acne can go on for years and requires periodic evaluation by a dermatologist, patients and their families will need continued support and encouragement to follow the prescribed regimen. They will need to know the expected results of prescribed medications, any adverse reactions that might occur, and symptoms that should be reported immediately.

? *Think Critically About . . .* What skin care measures would you recommend to a young teenager who is just beginning to experience face blemishes such as blackheads or whiteheads? The kids at school are calling him "scab face."

PSORIASIS

Etiology, Pathophysiology, Signs, and Symptoms

Psoriasis is a noncontagious, chronic, and recurring skin disorder that typically appears as inflamed, edematous skin lesions covered with adherent silvery white scales (Figure 42–1). These scales are the result of an abnormally rapid rate of proliferation of skin cells. When the scales are removed, there is pinpoint bleeding. The plaques most often appear on the skin of the elbows, knees, and base of the spine. It also may affect the scalp, in which case it can be confused with seborrheic dermatitis. When the fingernails are involved, there can be pitting of the surface of the nails. The palms and soles also can be affected, making it difficult for the patient to carry out activities of daily living. In some cases the skin eruptions are accompanied by inflammation of the joints, especially those of the fingers and toes. This is called psoriatic arthritis. Psoriasis affects about 2% of the U.S. population. There is a genetic predisposition for the disease. It is likely that an immunologic event triggers the disorder as the first lesion commonly appears after an upper respiratory infection. T cells are mistakenly activated and they trigger immune responses that speed up the growth cycle of skin cells.

Researchers have recently established a link between psoriasis and cardiovascular disease. In the study, patients with psoriasis had a higher incidence of myocardial infarction than the controls with the highest incidence in those with severe psoriasis. The risk is higher in those developing psoriasis before age 40 (Gelfand, 2006).

Diagnosis and Treatment

Diagnosis is by history, physical examination, and ruling out other skin disorders. Each case of psoriasis is treated individually. The disease is unpredictable, tends to go into remission spontaneously, and sometimes will clear up temporarily with or without treatment.

Mild cases usually respond to steroid creams (triamcinolone acetonide [Kenalog]), but there is a possibility that eventually the disease will become resistant to steroids. Sunlight in moderate doses can help, because the ultraviolet (UV) rays slow down the rate at which epithelial cells are produced. Extremes of UV radiation can have the opposite effect, resulting in an aggravation of the condition. Calcipotriene (Dovonex), a vitamin D analogue cream, helps to regulate skin cell production, decreasing the incidence of psoriasis plaques.

Tar preparations also act to impede the proliferation of skin cells and have long been used to heal psoriasis

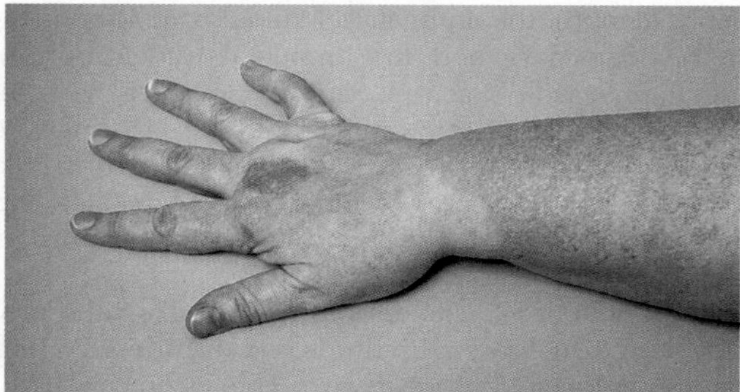

FIGURE 42–1 Psoriasis lesion on the hand.

lesions. They may be administered in the form of baths, topical applications, or shampoos. Combinations of artificial UV radiation and a coal tar product often are prescribed for severe cases. This usually requires hospitalization so that the dosage of each component of therapy can be measured precisely. A form of therapy called PUVA combines application of one of a class of drugs called psoralens, which penetrates the skin, and exposure to ultraviolet light type A (UVA).

Antimetabolites have been used to treat severe psoriasis, helping to control the disorder by their antiproliferative action. Methotrexate is the most commonly used antimetabolite for this purpose. Acitretin (Soriatane) or cyclosporine are sometimes used. New biologics such as etanercept, alefacept, efalizumab, and infliximab that block T-cell activation are showing promising results with few complications (Bowles, 2005). 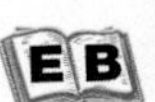

Nursing Management

Patients with psoriasis will need instruction about the nature of their disease, the purpose of the prescribed treatment, and information about ways to avoid aggravating it. **The skin should be kept as moist and pliable as possible. Humidifiers to increase moisture in the environment are sometimes helpful.** Lubricating lotions and creams should be approved by the dermatologist before they are applied.

Minor scratches and abrasions and bacterial infections can trigger the formation of lesions at a new site. **Because any irritation or break in the skin seems to stimulate the growth of psoriatic plaques in a person susceptible to psoriasis, the patient should be cautioned to avoid injury of any kind.** This includes hangnails, damaged cuticles, blisters from poorly fitting shoes, and potentially harmful agents in the environment such as radiation and chemicals.

STEVENS-JOHNSON SYNDROME

Stevens-Johnson syndrome (SJS) is an allergic reaction with skin manifestations. It is usually triggered by a medication. The signs and symptoms appear within 14 days of starting drug therapy. Offending drugs are the anticonvulsants carbamazepine (Tegretol) and phenytoin (Dilantin), the antimalarial sulfadoxine/pyrimethamine (Fansidar), and the antibiotic trimethroprim/sulfamethoxazole (Bactrim, Septra). However over-the-counter medications can cause SJS. Lesions that may be mistaken for chickenpox develop on the face, trunk, palms, extensor surfaces of joints, soles of the feet, and dorsum of the hands. The lesions have irregular borders and may have blistered, necrotic centers.

Treatment of SJS is to discontinue the drug and provide supportive care with fluids and nutrition. Wound care is similar to that for a burn. The lesions are painful, and analgesia is provided. Sedatives may be necessary. If not treated early, SJS can cause death.

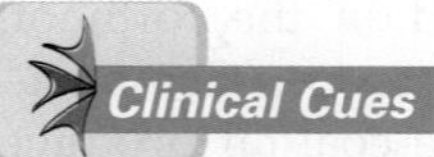

Assess the skin of every patient daily. If new skin lesions appear, seek an opinion from a physician. Check the medication profile and medication history to see what medications the patient has been receiving. Alert the physician if the patient has been taking a medication known to cause SJS.

BACTERIAL INFECTIONS

Etiology, Pathophysiology, Signs, and Symptoms

Cellulitis is an infection of the dermis and subcutaneous tissue and is generally caused by *Staphylococcus.* It may occur as an extension of a skin wound, as an ulcer, or from furuncles or carbuncles.The area will be erythematosus, swollen, and painful. It is treated with systemic antibiotics, and Burow's soaks may be used to relieve pain. Burow's solution is an astringent and topical antiseptic also called aluminum acetate solution.

Furuncles (boils) are inflammations of hair follicles. The organism responsible is usually *Staphylococcus aureus.* Any skin area with hair can be affected. Initially there is a deep, firm, red, painful nodule 1 to 5 cm in diameter. The nodule changes to a large and tender cystic nodule accompanied by cellulitis. The lesion may drain large amounts of pus and necrotic tissue.

Carbuncles are a collection of infected hair follicles and most often occur on the back of the neck, the upper back, and the lateral thighs. It begins as a firm mass and evolves into an erythematosus, painful, swollen mass. It may drain through many openings in the mass. Abscesses may develop with fever, chills, and malaise.

Diagnosis, Treatment, and Nursing Management

Diagnosis is by history and examination. Treatment of both furuncles and carbuncles is application of warm compresses to provide comfort, promote localization, and cause spontaneous drainage. Abscess formation requires incision and drainage. Recurrent episodes are treated with systemic antibiotics.

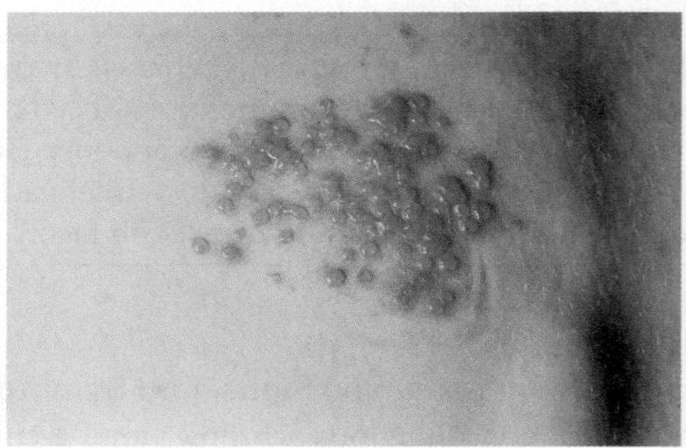

FIGURE 42–2 Herpes simplex virus lesions.

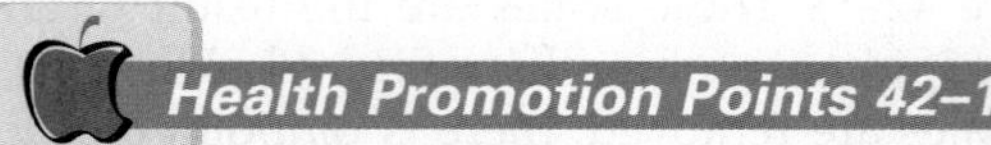

Preventing Spread of Herpesvirus

Patients with genital herpes need to be aware that the disorder can be transmitted even when no lesions are present.

When a person has a "cold sore," the virus can be transferred to others. Contact with the lesion should be avoided. Care should be taken not to share drinking glasses and eating utensils, lipstick, or other items that touch the lesion.

Nursing interventions are aimed at healing the infected areas and preventing recurrence. Rinsing very well after bathing to eliminate soap residue is recommended. The patient is taught to avoid using cosmetic products and over-the-counter topical remedies on the affected areas. A clean washcloth and towel should be used for bathing each day until the carbuncle or furuncle is healed. Linens should be washed in hot soapy water and thoroughly dried before reuse.

VIRAL INFECTIONS

The herpesviruses are an extensive family of viruses, many of which are capable of causing disease in humans.

HERPES SIMPLEX

Herpes simplex virus type 2 (HSV-2) is most often associated with genital herpes, whereas herpes simplex virus type 1 (HSV-1) lesions are primarily nongenital (Figure 42–2). **It should be understood, however, that either type can cause lesions in the genital area as well as other regions of the body.** **Autoinoculation** of the virus is possible by direct contact; for example, lips to fingers to genitals or lips to fingers to eyes (Health Promotion Points 42–1).

Etiology and Pathophysiology

When initial infection occurs, the virus is imbedded in a nerve ganglion that innervates the site of the lesion. Reactivation of the virus causes new lesions to occur at the same site. The virus travels along the nerve to the site of the original infection. Reactivation is brought about by exposure to ultraviolet light, skin irritation, fever, fatigue, or stress.

Signs and Symptoms

An infection with HSV-1 appears as lesions on the lips and nares that are commonly called cold sores or fever blisters. As with other types of herpesvirus infections, no drug will completely cure the infection.

Diagnosis, Treatment, and Nursing Management

Diagnosis is by physical examination and history. Sometimes topical and oral acyclovir (Zovirax), famciclovir (Famvir), or valacyclovir (Valtrex), available by prescription, hastens healing. The symptoms of itching and burning that accompany oral herpes infection sometimes can be minimized by applying warm compresses to the sores, followed by local application of tincture of benzoin or spirits of camphor to aid drying and facilitate healing. The disease usually is self-limiting, which means that it does not progress and will subside on its own, but it can recur. Contagion is possible up to 5 days after appearance of the lesion. Docosanol cream (Abreva), sold over the counter, is a helpful treatment for this disorder.

Patients should be cautioned to use good personal hygiene to avoid spreading the virus to the eyes and genital area and other body parts. Handwashing is a very simple, but essential, part of preventing spread of the virus.

HERPES ZOSTER

Etiology and Pathophysiology

The causative organism for this skin disorder is herpes varicella-zoster. The virus causes chickenpox (varicella), mostly in young children, and shingles (herpes zoster) in all ages. In herpes zoster, the herpesviruses replicate in the peripheral nerve ganglia, where they lie dormant until reactivated by trauma, malignancy, or local radiation (Figure 42–3). There are approximately 750,000 cases a year in the United States. The incidence in immunocompromised individuals (those with cancer or HIV/AIDS) is about 50%. A vaccine is available for children to prevent chickenpox.

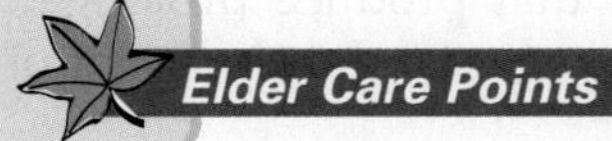

Elder Care Points

Approximately 50% of individuals who live past 80 years of age develop shingles. There is a vaccine available (Zostavax) that is about 50% effective in preventing shingles and appears effective in attenuating the disorder if it occurs (National Institutes of Health, 2005).

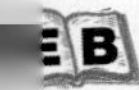

Elderly patients should be taught the early signs and symptoms of herpes zoster so that they can seek early treatment. If the disorder is full-blown when medical assistance is sought, postherpetic pain syndrome often occurs. Early treatment can prevent that

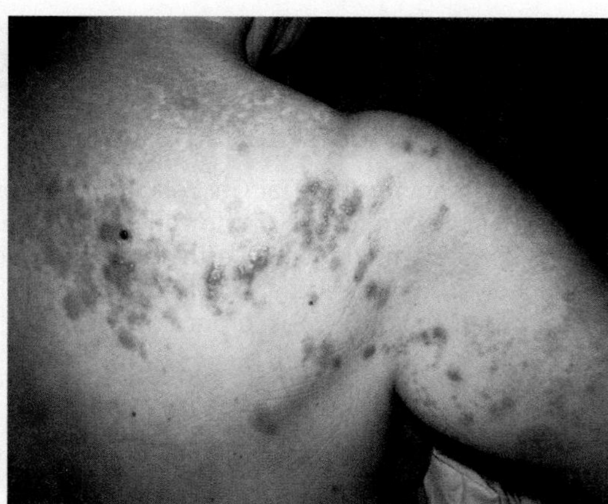

FIGURE **42–3** Herpes zoster (shingles).

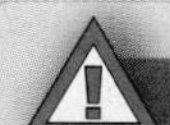

Safety Alert 42–1

Danger of Herpes Zoster Transmission

No health care worker, or visitor, should be in contact with a patient who has chickenpox or shingles if they have never had the disease. A pregnant woman should not care for a patient with chickenpox or herpes zoster either. The virus is very contagious and can harm a fetus.

Signs and Symptoms

Herpes zoster begins with vague symptoms of chills and low-grade fever and possibly some gastrointestinal disturbance. There may be only aching or discomfort along the nerve pathway with or without erythema. About 3 to 5 days after onset, small groups of vesicles appear on the skin. They usually are found on the trunk and spread halfway around the body, following the nerve pathways leading from the spinal nerve to the skin (Safety Alert 42–1).

The vesicles eventually change from small blisters to scaly lesions and are accompanied by pain and itching. The lesions usually affect only one side of the body or face. The pain of shingles often is quite severe. Pain can persist for several days or weeks after the skin lesions are completely healed. The pain of postherpetic syndrome is not easy to control.

Diagnosis and Treatment

Diagnosis is by history and physical examination. There is no cure for herpes zoster. The condition can persist for months, especially in older and debilitated patients. Herpes infections may be recurrent as immunity does not occur. **The earlier the condition is diagnosed and treatment begins, the better are chances to decrease the amount and duration of the associated pain** (Easter, 2004).

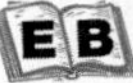

Symptomatic treatment usually involves administering an analgesic to relieve pain. Capsaicin, an over-the-counter analgesic that is applied topically five

Complementary & Alternative Therapies 42–1

Tai Chi Boosts Immunity to Shingles

Recent research showed that Tai Chi resulted in a level of immune response close to that of the varicella vaccine and that Tai Chi boosted the positive effects of the vaccine. The study involved a clinical trial of 112 adults aged 59 to 86 who took part in a 16-week program of Tai Chi (NIH, 2007).

times a day, decreases pain for some patients. A paste made from aspirins and water placed on the lesions decreases pain for others. Antibiotics may be prescribed prophylactically against secondary bacterial infection of the lesions. Most physicians prescribe oral acyclovir (Zovirax), famcyclovir (Famvir), or valacyclovir (Valtrex) to diminish the extent or duration of the lesions. Valacyclovir is used only in otherwise healthy patients. Famciclovir (Famvir), if given within the first 2 to 3 days of the outbreak, seems to shorten the duration of the chronic pain that frequently follows shingles. Systemic corticosteroids are often used to decrease pain and in an attempt to prevent postherpetic pain syndrome. Their use is controversial. Tricyclic antidepressants and gabapentin (Neurontin), an anticonvulsant drug, have been used with variable success at controlling pain.

Narcotic analgesics are avoided if possible, because they can lead to addiction when used for an extended time. If the pain persists and is intractable, the physician prescribes a corticosteroid to reduce inflammation. Vidarabine, administered intravenously (IV), is sometimes given to patients who have an immune deficiency. It is usually effective in reducing, if not completely relieving, the pain.

Even though shingles may be difficult to live with while it is running its course, the only lasting complication from the disease is postherpetic neuralgia. However, the prognosis is obviously less favorable in patients who have an underlying malignancy or who are immunocompromised. If the virus attacks the eye, however, it can cause blindness.

Nursing Management

Nursing intervention is aimed at providing emotional support and symptomatic relief from the pain and itching and at preventing a secondary bacterial infection (Complementary & Alternative Therapies 42–1). Cold compresses, calamine lotion, and diversional activities are sometimes helpful. Rest and adequate nutrition can promote healing and shorten the acute phase of shingles. Teaching imagery, deep muscle relaxation, or use of distraction activities may help decrease pain. Contact transmission precautions are utilized along with all Standard Precautions when providing care for the patient.

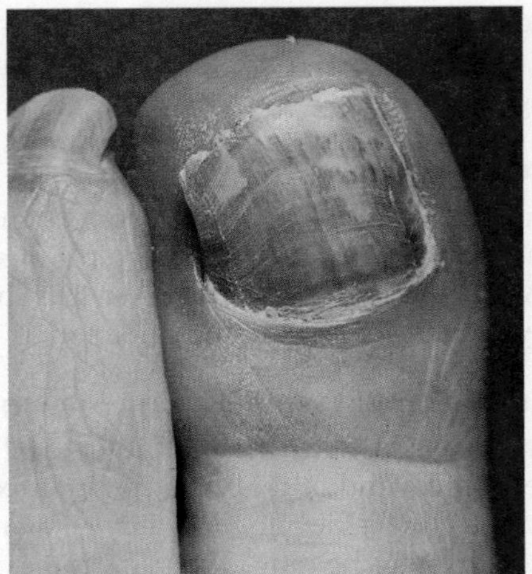

FIGURE **42–4** Onychomycosis (nail fungus).

FUNGAL INFECTIONS

Fungal infections are called **mycoses;** systemic fungal infections involving the lungs and other internal organs are called *systemic mycoses.* There are actually two groups of fungi: (1) fungi that are truly pathogenic to humans; and (2) opportunistic infections (that can cause an infection when the host has an altered immune system).

True pathogenic fungi can cause infection in an otherwise healthy person, but relatively few fungi are able to do this. Fungal infections are rarely fatal if they involve only the superficial tissues of the body. Nevertheless, mycotic skin infections can be exasperating because they are difficult to diagnose and are often resistant to treatment.

The most common types of fungal infections involving the skin are *tinea pedis* (athlete's foot or **dermatophytosis**), *tinea cruris* (jock itch), *tinea of the scalp* (commonly known as ringworm), and *tinea barbae* (barber's itch). *Moniliasis* (thrush) is a fungal infection that can attack the mucous membranes of the mouth, rectum, and vagina (*candidiasis*). (This condition is discussed more fully in Chapter 38.)

The skin fungal infections produce itching, some swelling, and a breakdown of tissue. Because fungi thrive in warm, moist places, a tropical climate or other environmental factors that produce prolonged heat and moisture can encourage the development of fungal infections.

The elderly are prone to develop fungal infections of the fingernails or toenails **(onychomycosis)** (Figure 42–4). Hands and feet should be thoroughly dried after becoming wet, with special attention to drying between the toes after the bath or shower. Nails should be cut straight across without rounding the edges. Wearing clean socks daily helps prevent fungal growth. In the toenails, the condition may become quite painful. Treatment requires oral antifungal medication daily for several months or topical agents daily for a

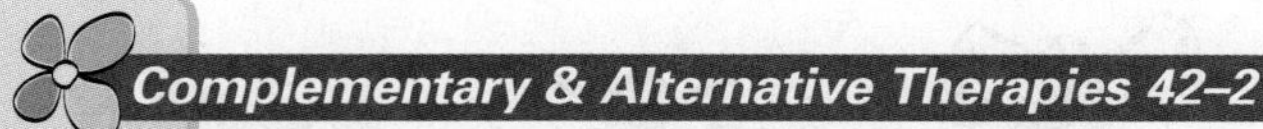

Complementary & Alternative Therapies 42–2

Treatment of Nail Fungus

Tea tree oil used topically daily on the nail and cuticle has been successfully used for treatment of yeast and fungal infection (Combest, 2007). It must be used very regularly to be effective, and may take weeks or months to cure the infection. Another inexpensive treatment that may work with consistent daily use is the topical application of Vicks VapoRub twice a day. This salve contains camphor, menthol, and eucalyptus. It seems to arrest the development of further fungal growth, allowing a fungus-free nail to grow. It takes about 6 months of treatment and is not effective for everyone.

year or more (Complementary & Alternative Therapies 42–2). There are many side effects of the oral antifungal medications. Liver function should be monitored during drug administration.

Diagnosis of fungal infections is confirmed by microscopic examination of skin scrapings that have been treated with potassium hydroxide (KOH) solution. Fungal specimens generally show the typical filaments of fungal organisms. Patients should be taught how to prevent recurrence of fungal infections (Patient Teaching 42–1).

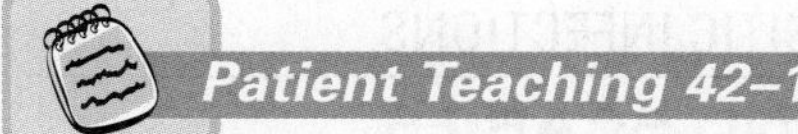

Patient Teaching 42–1

Prevention of Recurrent Fungal Infection

Instruct the patient to do the following.

- Wear shoes that provide ventilation for the feet. Wear cotton socks when rubber-soled shoes or sneakers must be worn.
- Wash and dry the feet at least daily, being careful to dry completely the skin between the toes.
- Sprinkle an antifungal powder on the feet and between the toes if there is a tendency to have athlete's foot. An antifungal spray may be used rather than powder.
- Change hose or socks daily; do not wear them more than one day without washing.
- Change underpants or shorts daily; do not wear them more than one day without washing.
- Use only clean towels, changing them at least every other day.
- Change bed linens at least once a week and wash in hot water.
- Do not use the combs, hairbrushes, or hair clips or ties of others, and do not allow them to use yours.
- Inspect pets regularly for ringworm. Have a veterinarian check the animal if an infection is suspected.

TINEA PEDIS

Tinea pedis (athlete's foot) affects the feet, particularly between the toes. The infection may spread to the entire foot and cause blistering, peeling, cracking, and itching. If it continues unchecked, it can spread to other parts of the body. The condition can be complicated by a severe bacterial infection.

Etiology, Pathophysiology, Signs, and Symptoms

Most cases of tinea pedis are contracted and spread in swimming pools, spas, showers, and other public facilities of this type (Health Promotion Points 42–2). *Trichophyton mentagrophytes* or *Trichophyton rubrum* are the usual infecting agents. These organisms may be normal flora that spread easily under conditions of excessive warmth and moisture. The skin between the toes becomes inflamed and develops cracks that become painful fissures. Itching is often present.

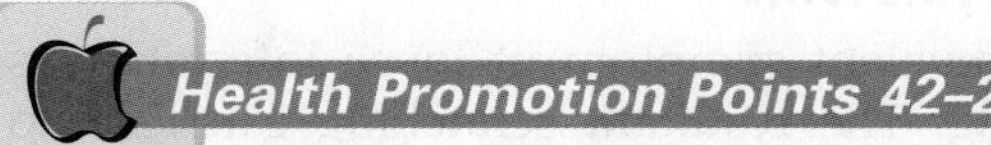

Health Promotion Points 42–2

Preventing Athlete's Foot (Tinea Pedis)

People should be taught that after using swimming pools and spas, the feet should be washed and dried thoroughly. When showering away from home, the feet should be carefully dried, including between the toes. If feet become sweaty while exercising or working, the feet should be washed and dried, or at least dried, and clean, dry socks put on.

Diagnosis and Treatment

Diagnosis is by physical examination. Treatment of tinea pedis consists of keeping the area dry, clean, and exposed to the air and sunlight as much as possible. Clean cotton socks should be worn every day, and the affected areas between the toes should be separated by gauze or cotton. Soaks of Burow's solution help. Various topical antifungals can be prescribed, including ciclopirox (Loprox), miconazole, clotrimazole (Mycelex), econazole (Spectazole), ketoconazole (Nizoral), and naftifine (Naftin). Some medicated powders, such as undecylenic acid/zinc undecylate (Desenex), work to keep the feet dry and also help control fungal growth. Other treatments are available without prescription. Systemic treatment for stubborn infection includes oral itraconazole (Sporanox) or terbinafine (Lamisil).

Nursing Management

Encourage the patient to keep the feet clean and dry and to wear clean cotton socks every day. Daily application of the topical agent must be done diligently in order to eradicate the problem. The patient should only use her own towel, and the shower or tub should be thoroughly cleaned and disinfected after bathing to prevent transmission to other family members. Personal footwear should be used in public places (e.g., at the swimming pool and in the showers at fitness centers).

PARASITIC INFECTIONS

PEDICULOSIS AND SCABIES

Etiology and Pathophysiology

The parasites that cause pediculosis and scabies are found throughout the world in all types of climates. They can infest anyone. The parasites are particularly troublesome, however, where people live under crowded conditions and are negligent in their personal hygiene. The occurrence of pediculosis and scabies in the United States has recently increased significantly because of the growth of the homeless population, and communal living. These parasites are often found among schoolchildren. The parasites are also found in nursing homes, dormitories, and sometimes hospitals.

Three basic types of lice that infest human beings are (1) the head louse, *Pediculus humanus capitis* (Figure 42–5, *A*); (2) the body louse, *Pediculus humanus corporis;* and (3) the pubic or crab louse, *Phthirus pubis* (Figure 42–5, *B*). In addition, human beings also may be infested by *Sarcoptes scabiei,* the mange mite that produces scabies (Figure 42–5, *C*). The lice are oval and 2 to 4 mm long. All types are acquired by contact with infested people or their clothing, bed linen, and bedding. Pets have also been known to carry lice and the scabies mite.

Signs and Symptoms

The most prevalent symptom of louse infestation is severe itching. The resultant scratching can lead to excoriation of the skin and secondary infection causing impetigo, furunculosis, and cellulitis. Systemic infections are not commonly associated with louse infestation, but they can and do occur in the forms of glomerulonephritis, septicemia, pneumonia, and cystic abscesses. If the lice infest the eyelids and eyelashes, the eyelids become red and swollen. Swelling may also occur in the lymph glands of the neck of a person heavily infested with head lice. The body louse can transmit typhus fever, trench fever, and some other diseases. Other types of lice are not known to be transmitters of disease.

The scabies mites burrow under the top layers of the skin and live their entire life there. They are more likely to be found in the skin between the fingers and toes, in the groin, and in other areas where there may be folds of skin. Excretions from the mites produce irritation with intense itching and blistering. Secondary infection is not uncommon with scabies, and some deaths have occurred when the scabies infestation has led to pneumonia or septicemia.

Diagnosis

Diagnosis is by body inspection and by examination of skin scraping of a lesion under the microscope. Lice eggs are deposited at the base of the hair shaft and can be seen on close inspection. Scabies causes curved or linear white or erythematosus ridges in the skin that are easily visible.

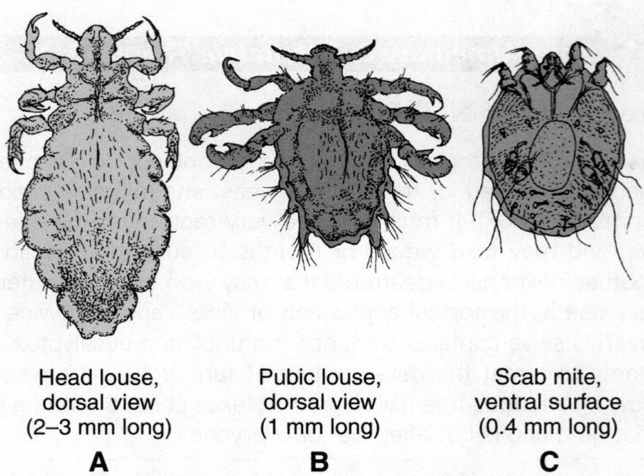

FIGURE **42–5** Types of lice that infest human beings.

Treatment

The prescription drugs most commonly used and considered most effective against lice and scabies are permethrin (Nix Elimite), pyrethrins (RID), and malathion (Ovide). These substances must be carefully used and the patient's liver functions monitored as they can be very toxic. They are available as creams, lotions, and shampoos. Lindane has been found to be especially harmful and is no longer recommended. A fine-toothed (nit) comb is then used to remove the nits (eggs) that may have remained on the hair.

Nursing Management

Contact Isolation is recommended. In addition, clothing, bedding, hats, stuffed animals, and other infested articles must be decontaminated to prevent reinfection. Laundering in hot water and machine drying using the hottest cycle is effective. Dry cleaning of nonwashable bed coverings or clothing can be effective. Mattresses, upholstered furniture, carpets, and other articles should be sprayed with a specific disinfectant. All combs and brushes should be soaked in very hot water for more than 5 minutes. For items that cannot be cleaned, such as some stuffed animals, sealing them in plastic bags with the air expelled for 14 days can be effective. You must instruct all family members about the infection and ways to prevent reinfestation.

? *Think Critically About . . .* How would you approach and instruct the parents of an 8-year-old who has scabies?

DISORDERS OF SKIN

SKIN CANCER

Skin cancer is often neglected because there is no pain associated with it and patients fear that treatment will involve extensive or disfiguring surgery.

More than 800,000 cases a year of basal cell cancers occur in the United States. These are highly curable cancers. It is expected that 59,940 persons will have been diagnosed with melanoma, the most serious type of skin cancer, in 2007, and that 8110 deaths from melanoma will occur (American Cancer Society, 2007). There has been about a 6% a year increase in melanoma since 1973. Most melanoma deaths could have been averted through early diagnosis and treatment. Information on Kaposi sarcoma and T-cell lymphoma is located in Chapter 11 in the discussion of disorders of the immune system.

Etiology and Pathophysiology

Several factors predispose an individual to developing skin cancer. Among these are internal changes in the cells that may be due to hereditary factors and external influences such as chronic exposure to ultraviolet (UV) radiation, to chemicals such as coal tar, pitch, creosote, or arsenic compounds, or to other irritants in the environment (Heistein & Ruberg, 2005). Sunburn as a child is a particular risk factor. Because children tend to inherit their skin characteristics from their parents, susceptibility to skin cancer tends to run in families. Blue-eyed blondes and redheads seem to be most susceptible, probably because they lack sufficient pigment to protect the skin cells from outside irritants. The incidence of skin cancer in African Americans is very low.

A major cause of skin cancer today is the alteration in the ozone layer of the earth's atmosphere that allows more UV radiation to reach the earth's surface. This type of radiation is inflicting much quicker damage to skin with much less sun exposure than in years past. Another problem is that the quickly proliferating skin cells of the younger generation are even more susceptible to this type of damage, and it is mostly the young who spend large amounts of time in the sun. Nurses should instruct all people about the dangers of sunning without an appropriate protective sunscreen (Health Promotion Points 42–3). Whatever the cause, the skin cells mutate into abnormally growing cells forming a malignancy.

Signs, Symptoms, Diagnosis, and Treatment

Signs and symptoms vary according to the type of lesion. Diagnosis is by examination, biopsy, and pathology study. The three main types of skin malignancy are basal cell carcinoma, squamous cell carcinoma, and melanoma. *Basal cell carcinoma* usually appears first as a small, scaly area and tends to become larger as the disease progresses (Figure 42–6). It occurs most often on the face and trunk. As the scales shed, there is a small amount of bleeding and a scab will form. When the scab is shed, the affected area becomes wider, and it is bordered by a waxy, translucent, raised area. **If such a sore has not healed within a month, it may be a basal cell carcinoma.** This spreading may continue very gradually during several months or years. Even though these malignancies do not metastasize, they can invade underlying tissues, and death can result from complications such as infection or hemorrhage from encroaching into a blood vessel. Small lesions can be removed under local anesthesia in a doctor's office. Larger lesions respond well to radiation therapy.

Squamous cell carcinoma is caused by sunlight, affects the epidermis, and can become invasive and metastasize to other areas of the body. It appears on the head and neck most frequently. The tumor begins as a small nodule that rapidly becomes ulcerated (Figure 42–7). Treatment must begin early if the condition is to be relieved before the skin cells sustain extensive damage. Surgical procedures involve total removal or destruction of the lesions and the surrounding tissues that have been invaded. Radiation therapy is advised for patients who are poor surgical risks or who are fearful of surgery.

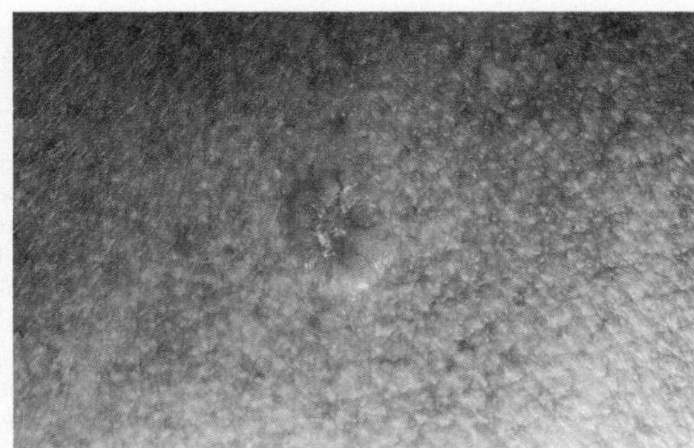

FIGURE **42–6** Basal cell carcinoma.

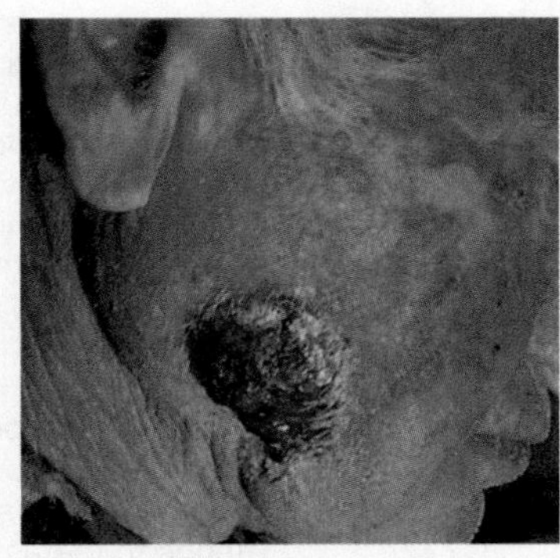

FIGURE **42–7** Squamous cell carcinoma.

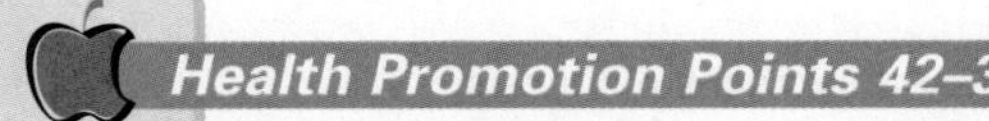

Health Promotion Points 42–3

Tanning Salon Dangers

Warn patients and the community about the dangers of using a tanning salon. Many use tanning beds that deliver dangerous UV radiation to the skin. **Dermatologists adamantly state that no one should use artificial tanning equipment.**

Key: *UV,* ultraviolet.

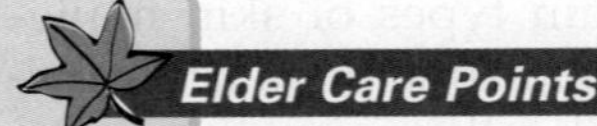

Elder Care Points

Actinic keratoses occur very frequently on the skin of the elderly. They appear on fair-skinned people as a small, scaly, red or grayish papule particularly on areas of skin that are often exposed to the sun. These lesions should be removed as they can evolve into a squamous cell carcinoma that can grow rapidly and metastasize.

Malignant melanoma is the least common form of skin cancer. It arises from pigment-producing cells and varies in its course and prognosis according to its type (Figure 42–8). Causative factors are genetic predisposition, solar radiation, and steroid hormone influence. There are several types of melanoma, but the three major kinds of malignant melanoma are superficial spreading, nodular, and lentigo maligna melanoma. In general, the superficial lesions can be cured, but the deeper lesions tend to metastasize more readily through the lymphatic and circulatory systems. Characteristics of the three main types of skin cancer are shown in Table 42–1.

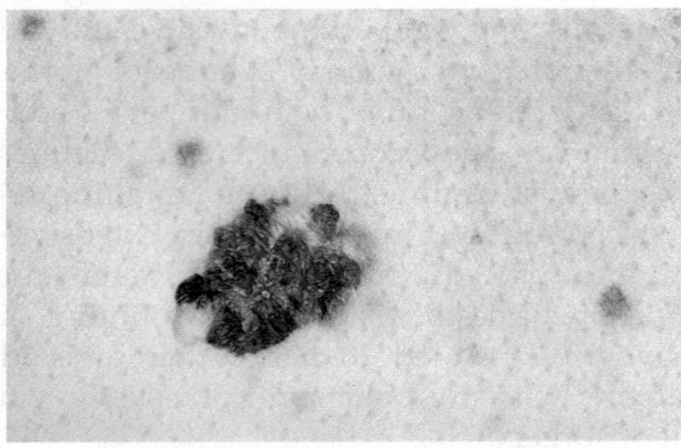

FIGURE **42–8** Melanoma.

Malignant melanoma always requires surgical removal of the tumor and excision of adjacent tissues and possibly nearby lymphatic structures. Chemotherapy may be employed to destroy tumor cells believed to have migrated beyond the tumor site. Radiation therapy usually is not indicated unless there is extensive metastasis. The radiation does not eliminate the disease, but it can relieve symptoms by reducing tumor size. Interferon alfa-2b has been found to prolong life in patients who have undergone malignant melanoma surgery and are at high risk for systemic recurrence. The medication is given for 1 year after the surgery (American Cancer Society, 2005).

A new drug combination is proving hopeful for patients with metastatic melanoma. The new treatment uses paclitaxel and carboplatin, with an agent that blocks the growth of blood vessels. This combination delayed new growth for 6 months in phase II clinical trials.

The type of removal of cancerous skin tissue will depend on the type of malignant growth present. **In all but the most extensive growths, treatment is relatively simple and completely successful if started early.** Although benign precancerous lesions do not inevitably develop into malignant lesions, the most advisable course of action is to remove them when they are first diagnosed. Removal is performed by surgery, *electrodesiccation* (tissue destruction by heat),

Table 42–1 ***Three Major Types of Skin Cancer***

TYPE	CHARACTERISTICS
Basal cell carcinoma	Slowly enlarging, firm, scaly papule. Crusted or ulcerated center that may be depressed; has pearly (semitranslucent) raised border. Dilated capillaries around lesion. Accounts for 70% of all skin cancers. Rarely spreads and is easily treated.
Squamous cell carcinoma	Appearance variable. Frequently seen as well-defined, irregularly shaped nodule or plaque. May be elevated, nodular mass, or fungated mass. Varying amounts of scale and crusting. May have ulcerated center. Predominantly on sun-exposed areas: head, neck, hands; 75% occur on the head. Spreads rapidly.
Malignant melanoma	
Superficial spreading melanoma (SSM)	Appears in a variety of colors: white, red, gray, black, blue over a brown or black background. Has irregular surface and notched border. Small tumor nodules may ulcerate and bleed. Horizontal growth can continue for years. Vertical growth worsens prognosis.
Nodular malignant melanoma (NMM)	Nodule with uniformly grayish black color, resembles a blackberry. May be flesh-colored with specks of pigment around base of nodule. Itching, oozing, and bleeding may occur. Prognosis less favorable than superficial type.
Lentigo maligna melanoma (LMM)	Relatively rare. Arises from a lesion that resembles a large flat freckle that is of variable color from tan to black. Has irregularly spaced black nodules on the surface. Often located on the back of the hand, on the face, and under fingernails. Develops very slowly; may ulcerate. Tends to metastasize; prognosis poor.

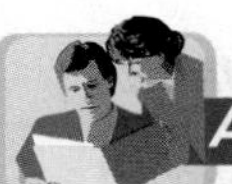

Assignment Considerations 42–1

Report Different Skin Lesions

When assigning hygiene care to unlicensed assistive personnel, ask them to report any odd-looking lesions they find on the patient's skin. Skin cancers are often discovered on further assessment of suspicious lesions.

cryosurgery (tissue destruction by freezing with liquid nitrogen), topical application of 5-fluorouracil (5-FU), interferon therapy, laser therapy, and molecular therapy. Radiation therapy is sometimes used to destroy the cancer.

Nursing Management

While performing daily care of patients, you often are in a position to notice these lesions in their early stages and should do your best to persuade the person with such a lesion to seek prompt medical attention (Assignment Considerations 42–1). Because victims of skin cancer run a high risk of eventually developing another malignancy, either at the original site or elsewhere in the body, they should visit a physician at least once a year after the skin cancer has been cured. Although most skin cancers are easily curable, they should not be considered harmless and something to forget about after treatment. See Chapter 8 for further information on care of the cancer patient.

Another nursing function is educating the patient about the type of cancer, and helping to decrease fear (see Patient Teaching 41–1). For many people, the diagnosis of "cancer"—even of an easily cured skin lesion—causes a change in body image and, possibly, in self-esteem. You can assist patients to talk about concerns and the future, point to community resources and support groups, and answer questions about treatment.

? ***Think Critically About*** . . . If you noticed a skin lesion on a person in line with you at the grocery store that looked like a skin cancer, how would you alert the person to the danger of such a lesion and the need for medical attention?

PRESSURE ULCERS

Basic measures for pressure ulcer prevention and assessment are provided in Chapter 41. Pressure relief, positioning, padding, use of pressure relief devices, adequate nutrition, and excellent skin care are the hallmarks of pressure ulcer prevention (see Boxes 41–1 and 41–2). Box 42–2 presents measures for best practice for preventing pressure ulcers. Pressure ulcer prevention has been addressed by *Healthy People 2010* (Health Promotion Points 42–4).

Box 42–2 *Best Practice for Preventing Pressure Ulcers*

POSITIONING
- Pad contact surfaces with foam, silicon gel, or air pads.
- Do not keep the head of the bed elevated above 30 degrees.
- Use a lift sheet to move the patient in the bed. Avoid dragging or sliding the patient.
- When positioning a patient on his or her side, do not position directly on the trochanter.
- Reposition an immobile patient every 2 hours while in bed and every 1 hour while sitting in a chair.
- Do not place a rubber ring or donut under the patient's sacral area.
- When moving an immobile patient from a bed to another surface, use a designated slide board well lubricated with talc.
- Place pillows or foam wedges between two bony surfaces.
- Keep the patient's skin directly off plastic surfaces.
- Keep the patient's heels off the bed surface.

NUTRITION
- Ensure a fluid intake between 2000 and 3000 mL/day.
- Help the patient maintain an adequate intake of protein and calories.

SKIN CARE
- Use moisturizers daily on dry skin, and apply when skin is damp.
- Keep moisture from prolonged contact with skin.
- Dry areas where two skin surfaces touch, such as the axilla and under the breasts.
- Place absorbent pads under areas where perspiration collects.
- Use moisture barriers on skin areas where wound drainage or incontinence occurs.
- Do not massage bony prominences.
- Humidify the room.

SKIN CLEANING
- Clean the skin as soon as possible after soiling occurs and at routine intervals.
- Use a mild, heavily fatted soap.
- Use tepid rather than hot water.
- While cleaning, use the minimal scrubbing force necessary to remove soil.
- Gently pat rather than rub the skin dry.

From Ignatavicius, D.D., and Workman, M.L. (2005). *Medical-Surgical Nursing: Critical Thinking for Collaborative Care* (5th ed.). Philadelphia: Elsevier Saunders, p. 1582.

Treatment and Nursing Interventions

When a patient has developed a pressure ulcer, its treatment depends on the stage of the ulcer (see Chapter 41). Ulcers are cleaned whenever the dressing is changed. Many hospitals and larger long-term care facilities have a wound care nurse specialist who oversees wound treatment.

Débridement. Removal of any **eschar** (dead, necrotic tissue) present has to occur for a pressure ulcer to heal. The exception is a heel ulcer with dry eschar that has no edema, erythema, drainage, or boggy tissue. Débride-

Health Promotion Points 42–4

Healthy People 2010 Pressure Ulcers

Objective 1-16 concerning pressure ulcers states: "Reduce the proportion of nursing home residents with current diagnosis of pressure ulcers." A concerted effort must be made to prevent and heal pressure ulcers on all residents.

Table 42–2 *Appropriate Dressings for Pressure Ulcers**

Appropriate dressings depend on the stage of the wound. A large variety of dressing products is available on the market. Follow agency policy, keeping in mind the following guidelines:

Stage I	Thin film dressing to protect the area from shearing forces and to retain moisture.
Stage II (noninfected)	Hydrocolloid dressing that protects against bacterial contamination and retains moisture. Can be left on for 7 days.
Stage III (draining ulcer)	Choose a dressing that will absorb exudate and maintain a moist environment.
Stage IV	Chemical enzyme formula may be used to help débride eschar. Sometimes a wet-to-dry dressing is used to help mechanically débride necrotic tissue.

**A nonocclusive dressing is always used for an infected wound.*

Table 42–3 *Color of Purulent Exudate and Probable Pathogen*

THIS COLOR EXUDATE	MAY INDICATE THE PRESENCE OF
Beige with a fishy odor	*Proteus*
Brown with a fecal odor	*Bacteroides*
Creamy yellow	*Staphylococcus*
Green-blue with a fruity odor	*Pseudomonas*

ment can be done surgically with forceps and scissors or mechanically. Mechanical débridement is accomplished by whirlpool baths, wet-to-dry saline dressings, dextranomer beads sprinkled over the wound, or other proteolytic enzymes or chemical products that break down the dead tissue and absorb the exudate. When wet-to-dry dressings are used, the patient should be medicated for pain before the dressing is pulled from the wound, pulling necrotic and some viable tissue with it. This method is falling out of favor because of the damage that occurs to new granulation tissue. Carefully read the instructions for whatever product is being used. Surgical débridement may be done in the patient's room, the physician's office, or the surgical suite depending on the depth and extent of the wound. Surgical débridement may require a skin graft to cover the area exposed. Whenever surgical débridement, forceful irrigation, or whirlpool débridement is to occur, be certain to provide sufficient analgesia for the patient as the procedure is painful (AHCPR, 1994).

Cleansing and Dressing. After sharp débridement with bleeding, clean, dry dressings are used for 8 to 24 hours, then moisture-retaining dressings are applied. Normal saline and light mechanical action with sponges or irrigation equipment is a way of cleansing that prevents disruption of granulation tissue. Other antiseptic solutions are not used as they are toxic to new granulation tissue. At least 250 mL of solution and a 30-mL syringe with a small catheter or 18-gauge needle attached is used to irrigate and to reach undermined areas and tunnels. A reddened wound bed requires gentle irrigation with a 30- to 50-mL needleless syringe to prevent damage to newly developing tissue. Select the wound dressing appropriate for the characteristics of the wound (Table 42–2).

Pressure ulcers should be measured and documented when they are discovered and at least once a week thereafter. Document the characteristics of the wound and any exudate present. Exudate is usually **purulent** (containing pus) or **serosanguineous** (containing serum and blood). Serosanguineous exudate is amber colored and blood tinged. Purulent drainage may be one of several colors (Table 42–3).

Common dressing materials include polyurethane films, hydrogel dressings, hydrocolloid wafers, alginates, biologic dressings, and gauze dressings. Use hypoallergenic tape when tape is necessary. Choose a dressing that keeps the ulcer moist and the surrounding skin dry. Prevent abscess formation by loosely filling all cavities with dressing material. Pressure must be kept off the wound for it to heal.

Other Treatment Methods. Application of electrical stimulation is the only other therapy that has sufficient supporting evidence of its effectiveness. A low-voltage current is applied to the wound area and can increase blood vessel growth and promote granulation tissue. The therapy is used 1 hour a day five to seven times a week. Electrical stimulation may be used for stage III and stage IV pressure ulcers that have proved unresponsive to conventional therapy. This type of treatment may also be used for nonhealing stage II ulcers. Electrical stimulation therapy is to be applied only by a certified wound care specialist.

In some agencies, vacuum-assisted wound closure is being used. A suction tube covered by a special sponge is sealed into place for 48 hours. Low-negative suction pressure is applied through the tube. This seems to stimulate the formation of granulation tissue. This treatment is used for chronic ulcers (Gupta, 2004).

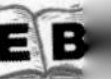

For an ulcer that will not heal with other methods, hyperbaric oxygen therapy may be prescribed if the equipment is available in the community. The patient is placed in the hyperbaric oxygen chamber for the treatments. Tissue becomes flooded with more oxygen than is normally available when breathing atmospheric-pressure air. This is an effective treatment for other difficult-to-heal wounds as well.

Patient name ______________________ Patient ID# ______________________
Ulcer location ______________________ Date ______________________

Directions
Observe and measure the pressure ulcer. Categorize the ulcer with respect to surface area, exudate, and type of wound tissue. Record a subscore for each of these ulcer characteristics. Add the subscores to obtain the total score. A comparison of total scores measured over time provides an indication of the improvement or deterioration in pressure ulcer healing.

Length × width	**0** 0 cm^2	**1** <0.3 cm^2	**2** 0.3–0.6 cm^2	**3** 0.7–1.0 cm^2	**4** 1.1–2.0 cm^2	**5** 2.1–3.0 cm^2	**Subscore**
		6 3.1–4.0 cm^2	**7** 4.1–8.0 cm^2	**8** 8.1–12.0 cm^2	**9** 12.1–24.0 cm^2	**10** >24.0 cm^2	
Exudate amount	**0** None	**1** Light	**2** Moderate	**3** Heavy			**Subscore**
Tissue type	**0** Closed	**1** Epithelial tissue	**2** Granulation tissue	**3** Slough	**4** Necrotic tissue		**Subscore**
							Total score

Length × Width: Measure the greatest length (head to toe) and the greatest width (side to side) using a centimeter ruler. Multiply these two measurements (length × width) to obtain an estimate of surface area in square centimeters (cm^2). *Caveat:* Do not guess! Always use a centimeter ruler and always use the same method each time the ulcer is measured.

Exudate Amount: Estimate the amount of exudate (drainage) present after removal of the dressing and before applying any topical agent to the ulcer. Estimate the exudate (drainage) as none, light, moderate, or heavy.

Tissue Type: This refers to the types of tissue that are present in the wound (ulcer) bed. Score as a "4" if there is any necrotic tissue present. Score as a "3" if there is any amount of slough present and necrotic tissue is absent. Score as a "2" if the wound is clean and contains granulation tissue. A superficial wound that is reepithelializing is scored as a "1." When the wound is closed, score as a "0."

4 **Necrotic tissue (eschar):** black, brown, or tan tissue that adheres firmly to the wound bed or ulcer edges and may be either firmer or softer than surrounding skin
3 **Slough:** yellow or white tissue that adheres to the ulcer bed in strings or thick clumps, or is mucinous
2 **Granulation tissue:** pink or beefy red tissue with a shiny, moist, granular appearance
1 **Epithelial tissue:** for superficial ulcers, new pink or shiny tissue (skin) that grows in from the edges or as islands on the ulcer surface
0 **Closed/resurfaced:** the wound is completely covered with epithelium (new skin)

Directions: Observe and measure the pressure ulcers at regular intervals using the PUSH Tool. Date and record PUSH subscale and total scores on the Pressure Ulcer Healing Record below.

Pressure Ulcer Healing Record																
Date																
Length × width																
Exudate amount																
Tissue type																
Total score																

Version 3.0: 9/15/98

FIGURE **42–9** The Pressure Ulcer Scale for Healing (PUSH) tool 3.0.

Documentation. All aspects of risk assessment, preventive measures instituted, objective description and measurement of pressure ulcers, treatment, and progress toward healing are documented regularly in the patient's chart. The Pressure Ulcer Scale for Healing (PUSH) tool is a good way to objectively document your findings (Figure 42–9). Photographs are often taken of the ulcer on discovery and during treatment to document progress.

SKIN TEARS

A skin tear is a traumatic wound that occurs primarily on the extremities of older adults. The wound occurs as a result of friction alone or shearing and friction forces that separate the epidermis from the dermis or separate both structures from the underlying tissue. Skin tears are a painful injury, and they are preventable. More than 1.5 million occur each year in institutionalized adults in health care facilities (Baranoski, 2005). The greatest risk 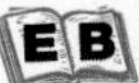

Box 42–3 Risk Factors for Skin Tears in the Elderly

Assess for the following factors.
- Dry skin with dehydration
- Areas of ecchymoses
- Presence of friction, shearing, or pressure from bed or chair
- Impaired sensory perception
- Impaired mobility
- Taking multiple medications
- Prolonged use of corticosteroids
- Presence of renal disease, congestive heart failure, or stroke impairment
- Incorrect removal of adhesive dressings
- Rough handling when being bathed, dressed, transferred, or repositioned

of skin tears occurs among the 35.9 million people over the age of 65. With age, the epidermis thins and becomes less elastic, making it susceptible to tearing with little trauma. Those individuals who require total care are at the highest risk. About half of skin tear injuries occur with no apparent cause. These are probably due to wheelchair injuries, bumping into objects, transfers, and falls. The long-term care environment, because of the age and debility of residents, has the greatest number of skin tear occurrences. Risk factors for skin tears, other than age over 65, are presented in Box 42–3.

The Payne-Martin classification system classifies skin tears as:

- Category I: A skin tear without tissue loss
- Category II: A skin tear with partial tissue loss
- Category III: A skin tear with complete tissue loss in which the epidermal flap is missing (National Guideline Clearing House, 2006).

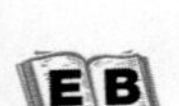

Preventive measures include a "safety conscience" when working with elderly patients or residents. Box 42–4 presents preventive measures.

Nursing Management

When a skin tear is discovered, steps for its management are:

- Gently cleanse the skin tear with saline.
- Allow the area to air-dry, or pat dry gently and carefully.
- If the skin tear flap has dried, remove it using scissors and sterile technique.
- If the skin tear flap is viable, gently roll the flap back into place using a moistened cotton-tipped applicator.
- If bleeding has stopped, apply Steri-Strips sparingly. Or, a petroleum-based protective ointment may be used over the flap. Apply an appropriate dressing. BAND-AID Liquid Bandage has proven beneficial.
- If bleeding continues, dress with alginate and a secondary dressing. Liquid Bandage is another alternative dressing.

Box 42–4 Measures to Prevent Skin Tears

- Have patients wear long sleeves and long pants to protect the extremities, or protect the fragile skin on extremities with stockinette.
- Provide adequate lighting to reduce the risk of bumping into furniture or equipment.
- Maintain the patient's nutrition and hydration; offer fluids between meals.
- Lubricate the skin with cream or lotion twice a day, paying special attention to the arms and legs.
- Use an emollient soap for bathing, and do not use soap every day on extremities if no soiling has occurred.
- Use a lift sheet to move and turn patients.
- Avoid wearing rings or bracelets that could snag the skin.
- Use transfer techniques that prevent friction or shear.
- Pad bed rails, wheelchair arms, leg supports, or other equipment where the patient might bump an extremity.
- Support dangling arms and legs with pillows or blankets.
- Use nonadherent dressings on fragile skin. Use gauze wraps or stockinettes to secure dressing. If tape must be used, use a paper or nonallergenic tape and apply it without tension.
- Mark the dressing with an arrow showing the direction it should be removed.
- Remove tape and dressing with extreme caution:
  - Use a solvent or saline to loosen the adhesive bond.
  - Slowly peel tape away from anchored skin (stabilize skin).
- If a thin hydrocolloid or solid wafer skin barrier is used as a protective barrier between the skin and the dressing, allow it to fall off naturally.

- Manage the same as a skin graft. The flap should not be disturbed for about 5 days to allow the skin flap to readhere.
- Assess and measure the size of the skin tear.
- Document assessment and treatment.

The wound must be watched for signs of infection. Extra padding for the involved extremity can protect the area further.

BURNS

Etiology and Pathophysiology

Burns are injuries to the skin caused by exposure to extreme heat, hot liquids, electrical agents, strong chemicals, or radiation. Inhaling smoke or fumes also causes injury. About 500,000 Americans seek care for burns each year. The majority of burns are relatively minor, but approximately 40,000 patients are hospitalized each year. Fire and burns kill approximately 4000 victims each year in the United States (American Burn Association, 2007).

Burns cause an acute inflammatory response (see Chapter 6). Serious burns have local and systemic effects. When a burn area is large, the inflammatory response can result in a massive shift of water, electrolytes, and protein into the tissues. This causes severe edema. Evaporation from denuded areas is four times that from intact skin. Hyperkalemia occurs when potassium is released from the damaged cells. Hyponatremia is caused by the stress response and potassium shifts. Metabolic acidosis develops. The loss of fluids from the vascular space leads to hypovolemia with low blood pressure and possible hypovolemic shock. There will be an increased hematocrit due to concentration of the blood, which is missing the components that have shifted into the tissues. The increased viscosity of the blood causes slowing of blood flow in the small vessels, which in turn causes tissue hypoxia. There is danger of kidney failure from both the hypovolemia and the cellular debris that the kidneys must clear from the body. Lung tissue injury from inhalation of heat and smoke may cause alveolar edema.

The decreased perfusion to other organs causes changes in the gastric mucosa that impairs its integrity. A type of ulcer called Curling's ulcer can occur within 24 hours.

The stress response to the trauma releases catecholamines, aldosterone, cortisol, and antidiuretic hormone. A hypermetabolic state results, and unless nutrition needs can be met, the body falls into negative nitrogen balance. A low-grade fever may develop as core temperature rises.

Signs, Symptoms, and Diagnosis

Burn severity depends on the cause, the temperature and duration of contact, the extent of burned area, and the anatomical site of the burn. Signs and symptoms vary from slight reddening of the skin to full loss of tissue down to bone with black, charred areas. Blisters may form. Diagnosis of the depth of burn is made based on a classification system.

Classification of Burns. The classification of burns is based on the amount of the body surface that has been burned and the depth of the burn. The extent of a burn is roughly calculated outside of the hospital according to the *"rule of nines"* and is expressed as a percentage of total body surface (Figure 42–10). The figures used in this method are fairly accurate for gross assessment in adults. The Lund-Browder classification or the Berkow chart can be used to compute the depth of the burn as well as the extent of the injury according to relative age, and the total burn estimate is used as the basis for treatment.

The depth of a burn is more difficult to determine, because various graduations of injury are sustained in a major burn. Some small patches may be more deeply burned than the areas adjacent to them. Burn depth originally was classified according to degrees, a first-degree burn being the most superficial and a fourth-degree burn being the deepest.

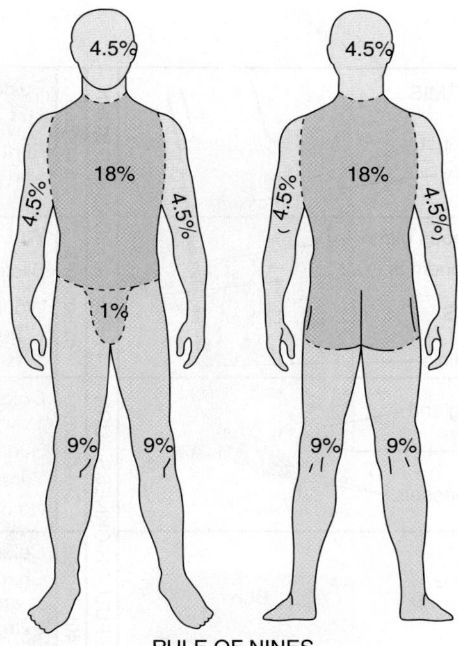

FIGURE 42–10 Chart used for burn area estimate ("rule of nines").

A more current method to evaluate the depth of burns is based on the layers of skin that have been damaged (Figure 42–11). *Partial-thickness wounds* are those in which the epidermal appendages (sweat and oil glands and hair follicles) are not destroyed and the wound will heal by itself if no further injury occurs from either infection or inappropriate treatment (see Table 5–1 for the phases of wound healing) (Figure 42–12). Grafting may or may not be necessary. *Full-thickness wounds* involve all layers of skin and the destruction of the epidermal appendages (Figure 42–13). Wounds of this type will require grafting for the wound to heal and for optimal function to be restored. Table 42–4 provides a guide for estimating the depth of a burn.

Electrical burns damage tissue deep within the body. The extent of damage is not always visible. There is an entrance site and an exit site, but the course of the injury is difficult to know. An electrical injury may result in the loss of one or more limbs.

Chemical burns result from accidents in homes or industry. The severity of the injury depends on the duration of contact and the concentration of the chemical. The amount of tissue exposed to the chemical and the action of the chemical affect severity. Alkalis cause greater injury and burn by liquefying tissue. Industrial cleaners and fertilizers are alkalis. Acids damage the tissue by coagulating cells and proteins. Chemicals for swimming pools, rust removers, and bathroom cleaners are acids. Organic compounds damage tissue by their fat solvent action.

Radiation skin injury is most often from therapeutic radiation treatment. In industries in which radioactive isotopes are used, the degree of injury depends on the amount and type of energy deposited over

EPIDERMIS
Sweat duct
Capillary
Sebaceous gland
Nerve endings
DERMIS
Hair follicle
Sweat gland
Fat
Blood vessels
Bone

		WOUND APPEARANCE	WOUND SENSATION	COURSE OF HEALING
PARTIAL-THICKNESS BURN	1st-degree	Epidermis remains intact and without blisters. Erythema; skin blanches with pressure.	Painful	Discomfort lasts 48-72 hours. Desquamation in 3-7 days
PARTIAL-THICKNESS BURN	2nd-degree	Wet, shiny, weeping surface. Blisters. Wound blanches with pressure.	Painful. Very sensitive to touch, air currents	Superficial partial-thickness burn heals in < 21 days. Deep partial-thickness burn requires > 21 days for healing. Healing rates vary with burn depth and presence/absence of infection.
FULL-THICKNESS BURN	3rd-degree	Color variable (i.e., deep red, white, black, brown). Surface dry. Thrombosed vessels visible. No blanching	Insensate (↓ pinprick sensation)	Autografting required for healing
FULL-THICKNESS BURN	4th-degree	Color variable. Charring visible in deepest areas. Extremity movement limited	Insensate	Amputation of extremities likely. Autografting required for healing

FIGURE **42–11** The tissues involved in burns of various depths.

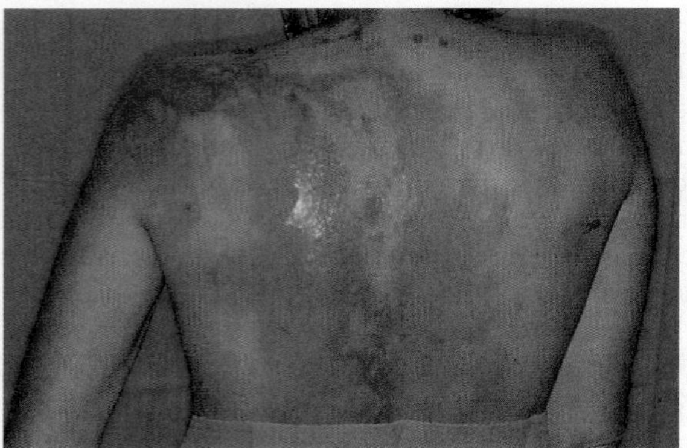
FIGURE **42–12** Partial-thickness burn injury.

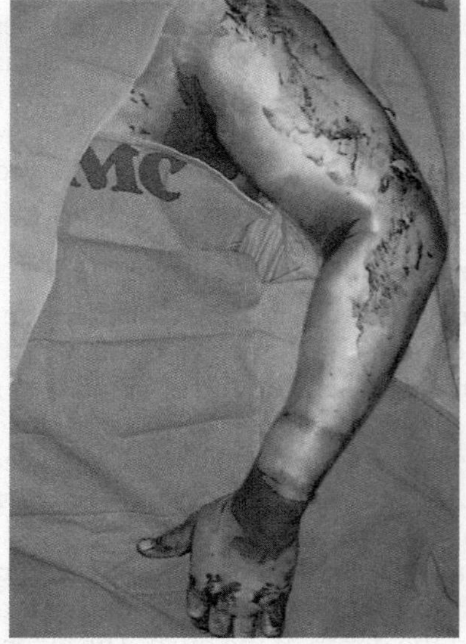
FIGURE **42–13** Full-thickness burn injury.

time. See Chapter 8 for care of skin damaged by radiation treatments.

A dry, scablike crust forms over a superficial burn. Eschar is a hard, leathery layer of dead tissue that results when there has been a full-thickness injury. It is dark brown to black. The eschar is a source of infection, and it impairs healing. Removal of eschar and skin grafting are usually done within 1 week after the burn (Figure 42–14). If there is a circumferential burn that is cutting off circulation in a limb because of the edema, an incision is made through the eschar down to the viable tissue **(escharotomy)**.

Emergency Treatment

First, all burn patients are treated as trauma patients. Establishment and maintenance of an airway is the first priority. They may have other life-threatening injuries besides their burns. All burns should be considered potentially life threatening until they are thoroughly assessed. **The recommended treatment for minor burns is submersion in cool water or applications of cool compresses as soon as possible after the injury** (Health Promotion Points 42–5). Submersion should be for at least 5 minutes. Do not use ice or ice water as that may cause further damage. The cool water helps relieve pain and edema and reduces the chances for a deeper burn. Cover the burn with a sterile dressing, clean cloth, or freshly laundered sheet. For minor burns, give ibuprofen or acetaminophen to help with the pain. Every emergency room has guidelines that indicate whether a burn victim needs to be transferred to a burn center.

Clothing that is stuck to the burn area is not removed before the patient is in the hospital. Do not

Table 42–4 *Classification of Burn Depth*

CHARACTERISTIC	SUPERFICIAL	SUPERFICIAL PARTIAL-THICKNESS	DEEP PARTIAL-THICKNESS	FULL-THICKNESS	DEEP FULL-THICKNESS
Color	Pink to red	Pink to red	Red to white	Black, brown, yellow, white, red	Black
Edema	Mild	Mild to moderate	Moderate	Severe	Absent
Pain	Yes	Yes	Yes	Yes and no	Absent
Blisters	No	Yes	Rare	No	No
Eschar	No	No	Yes, soft and dry	Yes, hard and inelastic	Yes, hard and inelastic
Healing time	3–5 days	Approximately 2 wk	2–6 wk	Weeks to months	Weeks to months
Grafts required	No	No	Can be used if healing is prolonged	Yes	Yes
Example	Sunburn, flash burns	Scalds, flames, brief contact with hot objects	Scalds; flames; prolonged contact with hot objects, tar, grease, chemicals	Scalds; flames; prolonged contact with hot objects, tar, grease chemicals, electricity	Flames, electricity, grease, tar, chemicals

From Ignatavicius, D.D., and Workman, M.L. (2006). *Medical-Surgical Nursing: Critical Thinking for Collaborative Care* (5th ed.). Philadelphia: Elsevier Saunders, p. 1620.

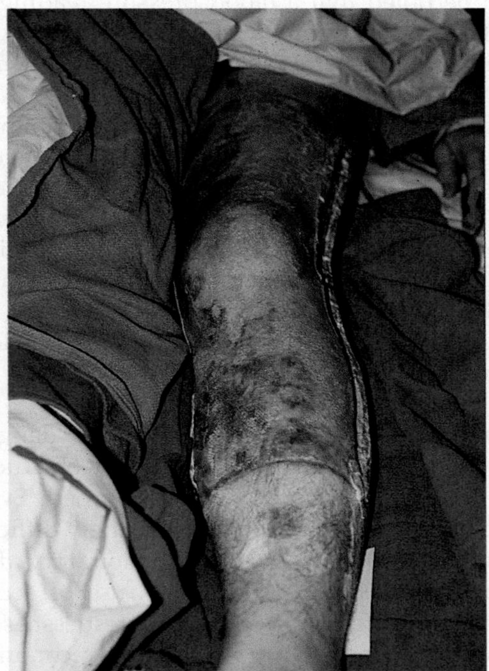
FIGURE **42–14** Escharotomy of the lower extremity.

apply salves or ointments or any greasy substance to a burned area. Because the removal of greasy substances is very painful, inappropriate treatment can cause unnecessary suffering and increase the possibility of infection. Blisters should not be disturbed initially, as they serve as a protective covering over the wound. If the burn is extensive, the patient must be transported to a hospital as soon as possible. The American Burn Association has identified criteria for minor and major burn injuries. It recommends that all major burn injury patients be treated in a burn center.

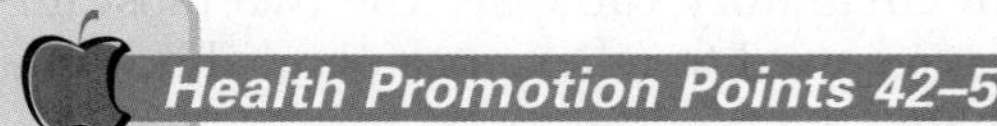

Burn First Aid Assistance

If you come upon a person who is on fire, place her supine on the ground and roll her over and over until the flame is extinguished. If a heavy tarp or rug is available, smother the flames with that. See that 911 is called as soon as possible. Cool the burned areas with cool water continuously for at least 5 minutes. Cover the burns with sterile dressings or clean cloth. Keep the person warm. Do not remove burned cloth from the wounds. Stay with the person until help arrives (Mayo Clinic, 2006).

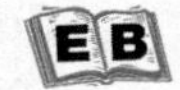

Hemorrhage does not usually occur with burns. If a burned patient shows signs of bleeding, she must be checked for some other type of injury, such as a penetrating wound, fracture, or laceration that occurred at the same time that she was burned.

The seriously burned victim is generally given nothing by mouth until arrival at a medical facility. If there will be a delay of several hours before transport is possible, and the patient is conscious and able to swallow, then fluids are given. A solution of ½ teaspoon each of salt and baking soda in 1 quart of water is ideal. The patient is encouraged to drink small amounts of the solution at 10- to 15-minute intervals unless nausea develops and vomiting seems likely. Intravenous fluid therapy and more extensive medical treatment are started as soon as possible. Rings, bracelets, and watches should be removed from injured extremities to avoid a tourniquet effect when swelling occurs.

Emergent Phase

The emergent phase averages 24 to 48 hours, but may last as long as 3 days. It begins with fluid loss and edema formation and lasts until edema fluid is mobilized and diuresis begins.

The first hour of treatment after burning can be crucial to the eventual outcome of a serious burn. Other life-threatening injuries must be treated first.

If possible, details of the nature of the accident should be obtained so that a more thorough assessment can be made. A thorough assessment is necessary. The cause of the burn and whether there is any possibility of thermal damage to the respiratory tract can help identify more closely the specific needs of the patient (Box 42–5). Once the depth and extent of the burn area have been estimated, efforts are made to establish multiple IV lines. Oxygen is administered if pulse oximetry indicates a problem with respiratory function or if inhalation injury is suspected. Assessment for carbon monoxide inhalation should be made by checking the mucous membranes for a cherry-red color.

Box 42–5 ***Signs and Symptoms Indicating Respiratory (Inhalation) Injury***

- Facial burns
- Singed nasal or facial hair
- Rapid, shallow respirations
- Coughing
- Increasing hoarseness
- Smoky-smelling breath
- Black, sooty (carbonaceous) sputum
- Decreased oxygen saturation
- Burning pain in throat or chest
- Restlessness, anxiety, confusion

Fluid Resuscitation and Prevention of Shock. **A major concern in the care of a burn victim is to prevent shock due to circulatory collapse.** The two most important measures used to relieve profound shock in a burn patient are:

- Replacement of lost fluids and electrolytes (fluid resuscitation)
- Enhancement of tissue perfusion

The loss of fluids and electrolytes results from the sudden capillary leak and shifting of the blood plasma and tissue fluids from their normal site to the area of the burn. This shift occurs in the first 24 to 48 hours postburn. The fluids are then lost by movement from the vascular space to the interstitial spaces. Fluid resuscitation needs are based on one of several burn formulas. The Parkland formula for fluid resuscitation is:

$$4 \text{ mL Ringer's lactate (RL)} \times \% \text{ burn} \times \text{weight in kg}$$

One half of the required fluid should be given within 8 hours of the time of the burn. The second half is given over the next 16 hours. After that, fluids are based on specific volume and electrolyte imbalances and response to treatment. **Fluid replacement is calculated from the time of injury, not from the time of arrival at the medical facility.** An important nursing function is to keep IV access sites patent and sutured in place, and see that the fluids are administered at the ordered rates. Urine output provides one measure of adequacy of fluid resuscitation. A Foley catheter is inserted to monitor hourly urine output and provide data to determine whether fluid resuscitation is adequate. The minimum urine flow for an adult is 30 mL/hr. For a child, minimum urine flow is 0.5 mL/kg/hr. The state of sensorium or level of consciousness is another measure. Constantly assess the patient's level of alertness and clarity of thinking. Ask questions about who she is, where she is, her age, what happened, and the like. After the first 24 hours, 5% dextrose in water (D_5W) for an adult or 5% dextrose in one half normal saline ($D_{5\frac{1}{2}}NS$) for a child is administered to maintain a serum sodium level of 135 to 145 mEq/L.

Unless fluids are replaced immediately, the cardiac output will drop and the resultant profound shock may be fatal to the patient. The patient's vital signs must be checked hourly and recorded accurately. It should be noted that a blood pressure reading taken by cuff from an extremity may not be reliable. An arterial line may be inserted for more accurate monitoring of blood pressure changes.

Fluid intake and output, and daily weights, are measured as long as the patient has open wounds. Laboratory data are checked frequently for evidence of either a deficit or surplus of specific electrolytes.

There are significant dangers to fluid resuscitation, particularly when the patient gets either too much or too little fluid volume based on her calculated needs. It is very important to monitor the signs of adequate fluid resuscitation and know when to increase or decrease the fluids based on clinical findings.

Respiratory Support. In addition to the dangers of shock, there is a potential for respiratory obstruction if upper airway passages have been burned. Swelling will occur, and it will become increasingly difficult for the patient to breathe. Signs of respiratory distress such as increased respiratory rate, use of accessory muscles, nasal flaring, retractions, restlessness, and confusion may occur. Early intubation is recommended for an extensive upper airway injury.

Lower airway injury (damage to lung parenchyma) is caused by breathing in smoke and soot from the fire. This type of injury may also require intubation and ventilation and may be life threatening.

Patients who should be watched closely for signs of developing respiratory problems include those who have:

- Burns of the face and neck
- Singed nasal hair
- Darkened membranes in the nose and mouth
- A history of having been burned in an enclosed space

Watch for increasing hoarseness, *stridor* (high-pitched musical sound on inspiration), and falling oxygen saturation (below 95%). Humidified oxygen is given if the patient is experiencing respiratory distress; intubation and mechanical ventilation may be required. Keep necessary equipment at hand and constantly assess the patient's respiratory effort. Employ the use of an incentive spirometer, coughing, turning, and ambulation to maintain good respiratory function. Respiratory therapy treatments may be ordered.

Pain Management. As soon as IV lines are established and fluid resuscitation is begun, pain control can begin. Measures to relieve pain include the administration of morphine or hydromorphone hydrochloride (Dilaudid) IV. The massive fluid shifts that occur after a burn injury make absorption from an intramuscular site unpredictable in the first 24 hours postburn. An antianxiety drug also may be given. Pain medication is given before any other burn interventions are started. Give small incremental doses of opioids IV and monitor the patient's pain level and vital signs.

Burn Treatment. Wound care is started with cleansing and débridement as necessary. Topical antimicrobial therapy is started and tetanus prophylaxis is given. A tetanus toxoid injection is the only intramuscular injection given initially.

Acute Phase

The acute phase extends from the time of fluid mobilization and diuresis to when the burned area is completely covered by skin grafts or when burns are healed. Goals during this phase include management of pain and anxiety, prevention of wound infection, promotion of nutritional intake, and rehabilitation therapy.

Prevention of Infection. Although wound infection is no longer the major cause of death in burn victims (the main cause of death is pneumonia), its prevention is important to recovery. Today patients are taken to the operating room very early postburn. Burn eschar is excised away from the wound and the area is covered with a biologic or biosynthetic skin. If wound sepsis occurs, IV antibiotics specific to bacteria in the wound are given and topical antibacterial soaks are applied to the wound. Thirty years ago most patients with burns over 50% of the body did not survive. Today, because of fluid resuscitation, burn wound excision and grafting techniques, new skin coverings, and nutritional supplementation, a patient may survive a 99% burn.

Wounds are carefully assessed at each dressing change. Signs that indicate infection include:

- Strong odor
- Color change to dark red or brown
- Redness around edges extending to nonburned skin
- Texture change
- Exudate and purulent drainage
- Sloughing of graft

Such signs should be reported as culture or biopsy is needed.

Although the physician chooses the type of medication to be applied topically or administered systemically, the nursing staff are responsible for continued assessment of the burn wounds to determine the effectiveness of the prescribed treatments.

The patient's vital signs must be checked at regular intervals and recorded accurately. The condition of the wounds also should be checked systematically to determine whether healing is taking place as it should and infection is being avoided.

A very wet wound that has a foul odor indicates infection. A greenish blue exudate from the wound is a sign of *Pseudomonas* infection. Signs of inflammation, such as redness and swelling of the tissues adjacent to the wound, may indicate *cellulitis* (acute inflammation of the subcutaneous tissues).

Healthy granulation tissue does not emit exudate. During the granulation stage of repair, the wound should look slightly pink and somewhat shiny. If there are any deviations from this description, notify the physician and culture the wound.

Infection Control. An aseptic environment is needed for burn care. Standard Precautions are used for all burn care, and protective isolation techniques are used. Those in attendance usually wear sterile caps, gowns, shoe covers, and gloves while caring for the patient. Contact Isolation measures are used for infected wounds. Gloves are worn for all contact with open wounds, and are changed when handling wounds on different areas of the patient's body and between handling soiled and sterile dressings. **Patient care items are not shared, and great attention is paid to maintaining asepsis for all patient care.** Bed linen is changed daily and whenever soiled, and a bed cradle or some other device is used to support the weight of the top covers to keep them off the burned areas.

Wound Treatment. In general, two methods may be used to treat a burn wound: the *open technique,* which leaves the wound undressed; or the *closed technique,* in which the wound is covered with a dressing.

Open Technique. When the wound is left undressed, it usually is covered with a topical ointment to prevent infection and promote healing. The wound is cleansed at least once daily and the topical agent is reapplied, usually every 8 hours. Nonsterile disposable gloves are used for washing the wound. Aside from preventing infection, the nurse also must provide additional warmth when the open method of treatment is used. Much body heat is lost through the parts of the body where the skin has been destroyed, and the patient is chilled easily. Heat lamps or radiant heat shields will usually provide the extra warmth needed and may be used in place of covers.

Wet compresses or soaks to cleanse the burned area and remove excess exudate and drainage must be used with extreme care and under sterile conditions to minimize the danger of infecting the wound.

Closed Technique. Topical medication is applied either to the wound directly or to dressings that are then placed on the wound. Dressings are composed of layers of sterile gauze saturated with one of the topical medications, biologic dressings, synthetic dressings, and artificial skin. The wound is then wrapped with a stretch gauze, such as Kling, or with elastic mesh webbing. Table 42–5 lists the most common topical medications and their nursing implications. The wound may be cleansed at the bedside, on a shower table in the burn unit treatment room, or in a whirlpool bath. Cleansing is done at least once a day.

Patients who have dressings are freer to move about and do things for themselves than those who do not have their wounds covered. An advantage of covering wounds is that when dressings are changed, dead tissue that is stuck to the bandage is débrided. The main disadvantages of the closed method are the need for frequent dressing changes and the trauma to the regenerating tissue.

Systematically assess scar tissue formation and help the patient adjust to the fact that burn scars may take as long as 12 to 24 months to mature completely.

Escharotomy. When tissue perfusion or quality of respiration is compromised because of eschar constriction, an escharotomy is performed. **An incision into the burn eschar with a scalpel or electrocautery relieves pressure caused by circumferential burns that encircle an extremity or that constrict movement of the chest.** The incisions extend into the subcutaneous tissue. If the pressure is not relieved, arterial blood flow in the extremity will be compromised, possibly causing necrosis; nerve damage from the pressure also may occur. An escharotomy on the chest improves lung expansion and oxygenation. The procedure does not cause discomfort as the nerve endings have been destroyed by the burn. No anesthesia is required.

Be alert for compartment syndrome. This occurs when there is increased pressure within a compartment (e.g., arm, leg) that causes compromise of circulation to the area. Fluid accumulation from edema is the cause in burn patients. Monitor for increasing pain, paleness and tenseness of the tissue, numbness or tingling, discoloration in the distal portion of the extremity, and decreased sensation *(paresthesia)*.

Surgical removal of eschar and applications of biologic dressings are done within the first week after the burn injury. **Biologic dressings** are materials obtained

Table 42–5 *Topical Medications Commonly Used for Burns*

MEDICATION	ACTION	NURSING IMPLICATIONS
Silver sulfadiazine (Silvadene, Flamazine)	Interferes with DNA synthesis by binding to bacterial cell membrane.	Assess for allergy to sulfonamides. Observe for rash, itching, or burning, which may indicate allergic reaction. Observe for leukopenia, which may indicate an adverse reaction. Is not well absorbed into eschar. Not effective against *Pseudomonas* infections. Observe for suprainfection of wound evidenced by "soupy" appearance.
Mafenide acetate (Sulfamylon)	Bacteriostatic agent; effective against both gram-positive and gram-negative organisms.	Assess for allergy to sulfonamides. Observe for signs of allergic reaction. May cause metabolic acidosis; monitor blood gases and electrolyte levels. Application may cause pain for 30–40 min; medicate before applying. Penetrates eschar and is effective against *Pseudomonas*. Very effective for electrical burns.
Silver nitrate	Antimicrobial action.	Dressings must be kept continually wet with 0.5% solution. Stings on application; stains fabric. Monitor electrolyte levels as may cause imbalances. Penetrates wound only 1–2 mm.
Sodium hypochlorite solution (Dakin's)	Bactericidal action; inhibits blood clotting and may dissolve clots.	Observe for signs of irritation. Keep dressings moist with the solution at all times. Helps dry wounds and assists débridement.
Povidone-iodine (Betadine)	Bactericidal for gram-positive and gram-negative organisms.	May cause metabolic acidosis and elevated serum iodine levels; monitor electrolytes, serum iodine, and blood gases closely. May cause rash and burning sensation. Stains fabric.
Collagenase (Santyl) with polymixin B (Polysporin) powder	Digests collagen in necrotic tissue; powder prevents infection.	Monitor for wound infection.
Gentamicin sulfate (Garamycin)	Interferes with protein synthesis in bacterial cell.	Monitor for ototoxicity and nephrotoxicity. Use with caution if decreased renal function is present. Monitor creatinine clearance during treatment. Used when there is resistance to other drugs.
Polymyxin B–bacitracin	Wide-spectrum antibiotic action.	May cause itching, burning and inflammation. Will not penetrate eschar. Must be applied q 2–8 hr.
Nystatin	Interferes with fungal DNA replication.	May cause itching or allergic reaction. Requires long-term use to clear fungal infection.

from cadavers or from animals. It is most desirable to graft the patient's own skin **(autograft),** but, when this is not possible, a homograft (the skin of another person **[allograft]**, obtained from a cadaver), a heterograft (**xenograft**, usually obtained from a pig), or artificial **(biosynthetic)** skin can be used as a temporary measure. The many synthetic dressings available consist of silicone, plastics, or alginate (brown seaweed combined with other substances) and remain in place for 1 to 14 days. **The patient's own skin is the only permanent graft material.** Some success has been achieved in growing skin cells harvested from the patient in cultures, but this is a slow, expensive process. The epithelial sheets grown are then used for grafting.

Débridement. Débridement involves removing the eschar and necrotic material from underlying tissues. It is usually done in the operating room. Whirlpool tubs are used 3 to 4 days after grafting procedures. Hibiclens, which is nonirritating, may be added to clean the wounds. The whirlpool action facilitates the cleansing process. Pain medication is given before the bath. Enzyme compounds, such as collagenase (Santyl), containing proteolytic agents may be applied topically to digest necrotic tissue. They are used in conjunction with a polysporin powder to prevent bacteria from entering the bloodstream from the wound. Surgical débridement and grafting may require IV anesthetic agents, sedation, nitrous oxide, or narcotic analgesia.

Grafting. When autografting is performed, there is a donor site from which a split-thickness piece of skin has been removed. That piece of skin may be used intact, or it may be cut into a mesh pattern (Figure 42–15). It takes longer for a mesh graft area to heal as the skin cells need to grow into the holes between the links of skin. The donor site may be covered by a film dressing to hasten healing and decrease pain. Often the donor site is more painful than the graft site. Once the donor site has healed completely, skin may be harvested from that site again. Hospital length of stay has been greatly reduced from years past. Today the length of stay is estimated to be 1 day to 4 days per 1% of burn.

Pressure dressings are worn as soon as grafts heal to decrease scarring that can inhibit mobility. The pressure dressing may be an elastic wrap or a custom-fitted, elasticized piece of clothing that provides uniform pressure over the burned area. These pressure dressings must be worn 23 hours a day, every day, until the scar tissue is mature. Scar maturity takes 12 to 24 months. Daily exercise and splint applications are done to prevent contracture formation. After burns are fully healed and the scar tissue has matured, plastic surgery may be performed to try to rebuild lost structures such as the nose or an ear or to enhance appearance.

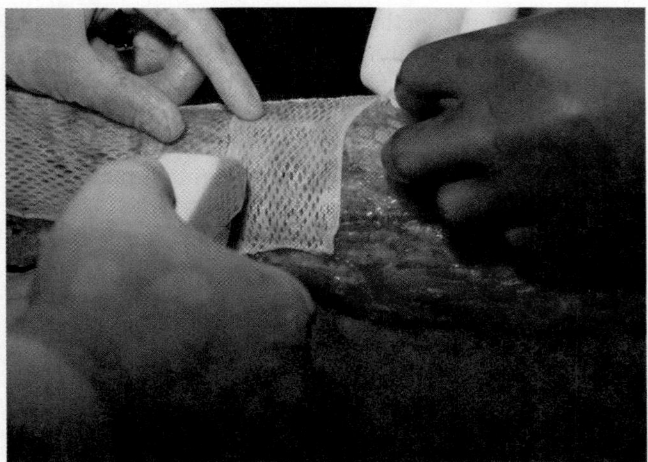

A

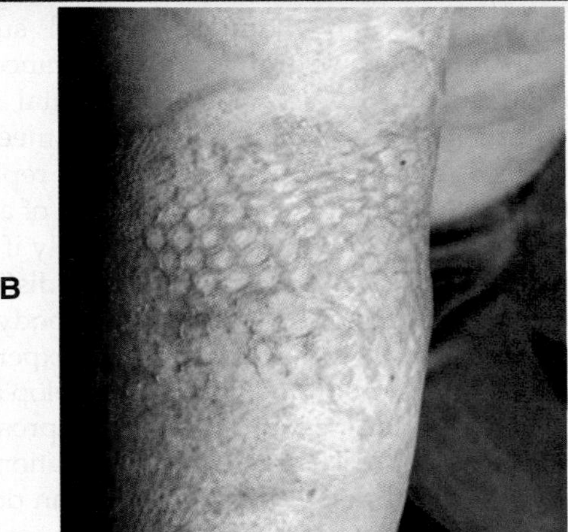

B

FIGURE 42–15 Typical appearance of meshed autografts. **A,** Appearance during application of meshed autograft. **B,** Appearance of meshed autograft after healing.

Nursing Interventions

Managing Pain. The nurse must use gentleness and care in handling the patient as he turns her or administers treatments. Not only does this reduce the amount of pain the patient must suffer, but also the less the patient is handled, the less danger there is of contaminating the wounds. Morphine or hydromorphone hydrochloride (Dilaudid) is administered via a patient-controlled analgesia pump when possible. Boluses may be necessary before treatments or surgical procedures and at bedtime. Burn treatment can be very painful. Sedatives such as lorazepam (Ativan), midazolam (Versed), and haloperidol (Haldol) may be used along with analgesia.

? *Think Critically About . . .* What would you do if when taking vital signs, you find that the pulse on the burned arm is weaker than that on the other nonburned extremity?

Managing Itch. Nonpharmacologic measures to reduce itching, such as relaxation techniques, meditation, guided imagery, and music therapy, are used along with pain medication. Therapeutic touch may prove helpful. Accupressure and acupuncture may assist with pain and itch relief.

Nutritional Support. Enteral feedings may be started as early as 4 hours after the start of fluid resuscitation for a major burn victim. The patient with large burns often develops paralytic ileus as a response to the trauma. The stomach stops working when this occurs, and a nasogastric tube must be inserted and attached to intermittent suction. Bowel sounds should return 48 to 72 hours later, and then intake may begin with increased protein, high-calorie drinks if tolerated.

A diet high in protein and calories is necessary for healing. The patient has increased metabolic needs directly proportional to the size of the burn area. Nutritional needs may be increased 50% to 150% above normal. Caloric needs may be as high as 5000 calories per day. Failure to meet the nutritional needs results in malnutrition and delayed healing. Only high-calorie liquids are given to drink. Dietary supplements include vitamins, especially vitamin C; minerals such as iron and calcium; and electrolytes. Perseverance and ingenuity in making meals and supplemental foods appealing are needed to help the patient meet her metabolic needs and to promote healing and repair.

Psychosocial Support. The emotional shock of a burn can be quite serious and long lasting, especially if there is some loss of mobility and independence, or disfigurement involving the face or other parts of the body usually visible to others. Many burn patients experience post-traumatic stress syndrome. Strive to develop an attitude of acceptance of the patient, a calm approach to dressing changes and discussions of scar formation, and an optimistic emphasis on what the patient can do and will be able to do in the future. As is true in most long-term and slowly progressing disorders, the severely burned patient can become bored and apathetic and might even lose the will to live. Diversional and occupational therapy and a coordinated effort on the part of all members of the health team are needed to help the burn patient recover and adjust to the effects of her injury.

Psychological care is very important for the burn patient. When a patient has difficulty coping with the physical and psychosocial effects of a severe burn, effective nursing intervention can help her deal with her fears, anxieties, and sense of loss. Assist the patient through the grief process. Encourage the patient to relate what is experienced and her feelings about what has happened or is happening. Questions about how the nurse and others who care for her can be most helpful and what changes in the environment might help are appropriate. It may be possible to change some elements of the environment. For example, noise, lights, or certain people—visitors or staff—may be very irritating to the patient; these factors usually can be adjusted. If the patient is unhappy about being isolated, bringing in a television, radio, computer games, and books may help. Regardless of whether every change desired by the patient can be made, at the very least assurance is given that there is someone who will listen and empathize.

The patient's self-esteem can be reinforced by emphasizing the strengths the nurse has noticed when she is coping with pain, inconvenience, or some other unpleasant situation. Involving the patient in performing self-care as much as possible and giving some sense of control over the situation are helpful. Words and actions can communicate your concern and caring.

If the burns were caused by a suicide attempt, or activity that the victim had been warned not to do, psychiatric therapy will probably be necessary to deal with feelings of guilt.

The patient's body image may have been severely disrupted. This will require considerable adjustment. Assist the patient to grieve over the loss and integrate the present body image. Referrals to a psychologist, psychiatrist, social worker, or religious leader are made to help the patient address this issue. Nursing interventions for selected problems in a burn patient are summarized in Nursing Care Plan 42–1.

Complications

When a sizable burn occurs, blood flow is shifted to the brain, heart, and liver because of the fluid shifts that occur. The gastrointestinal tract receives decreased blood and gastric motility is impaired. Monitor peristalsis and be alert to signs of paralytic ileus. Severe abdominal distention may occur. Curling's ulcer may develop, inducing gastrointestinal bleeding. Stools are monitored for signs of occult blood. A histamine (H_2)-receptor antagonist, such as cimetidine (Tagamet), ranitidine (Zantac), famotidine (Pepcid), or nizatidine (Axid), may be administered IV to prevent this complication.

Contractures always are a threat to a patient with major burns and sometimes to one with minor burns. Proper positioning and regular exercise are essential to prevent musculoskeletal deformities following a burn. Painful as the motion of physical therapy exercises may be, the muscles and skin must be exercised and stretched every day if normal motion is to be maintained. Sometimes it is necessary for the patient to continue visiting the physical therapist for several months after discharge from the hospital. Ambulation two or three times a day is begun as soon as the fluid shift has stabilized for patients who have no fractures or serious injuries to the feet or legs.

Rehabilitation

The rehabilitation phase begins with wound closure and ends when the patient reaches the highest level of function possible. This phase may last for years. When the patient is ready to accept some responsibility for self-care, preparation for release from the hospital begins. Teach how to apply topicals without contaminating the wound and how to change dressings if these are used. A family member, if available, is included in burn care education.

Maturing scars usually appear red, hard, and raised before they eventually begin to fade and soften. Pressure garments and masks help prevent thick and disfiguring scars but are uncomfortable

NURSING CARE PLAN 42–1

Care of the Patient with a Burn

SCENARIO Mr. Young, age 33, sustained partial- and full-thickness burns over both arms when a container of gasoline he was carrying ignited. He also suffered superficial partial-thickness burns on his hands and face. In the emergency room, his wounds were cleaned and a topical agent was applied; no dressings were applied. IV lines were established, and fluids were administered to avoid potential fluid and electrolyte imbalance. He received morphine for pain and on admission to the unit was fairly comfortable, conscious, and oriented. He is in the emergent phase.

PROBLEM/NURSING DIAGNOSIS *Superficial partial- and full-thickness burns on the arms, hands, and face/*Deficient fluid volume related to fluid shift and loss of fluids via open wounds.

Supporting assessment data *Objective:* Partial-thickness burns over hands and face with full-thickness burns on arms. Burn areas becoming edematous.

Goals/Expected Outcomes	Nursing Interventions	Selected Rationale	Evaluation
Patient will have adequate circulating blood volume as evidenced by blood pressure, pulse, and urine output	Monitor vital signs q 2 hr.	Falling BP and rising pulse can indicate hypovolemia.	Vital signs stable.
	Monitor urine output, report drop below 0.5 mL/kg/hr.	Urine output is another indicator of hypovolemia as kidneys will be less perfused.	Urine output at 45 mL/hr.
	Monitor lab values for electrolyte imbalances.		K^+ = 4.5 mEq/L; Na^+ = 140 mEq/L.
	Maintain IV fluids on schedule.	Adequate fluid resuscitation prevents hypovolemia.	IV fluids on schedule.
	Encourage fluid intake of 3000 mL q 24 hr when bowel sounds are present.		Bowel sounds absent. Continue plan.

PROBLEM/NURSING DIAGNOSIS *Open wounds with dead tissue/*Risk for infection related to burn damage to skin.

Supporting assessment data *Objective:* Skin on face, hands, and arms damaged by burns.

Goals/Expected Outcomes	Nursing Interventions	Selected Rationale	Evaluation
Patient will not experience infection of burn wounds as evidenced by normal vital signs and negative wound cultures	Assess for medication allergy.	Medication ordered may be contraindicated.	No allergies to medication.
	Use strict aseptic technique when working with patient.	Infection is the greatest cause of burn wound depth.	Strict aseptic technique provided to wounds.
	Apply topical silver sulfadiazine as ordered to wounds tid.	Suppresses bacterial growth and promotes healing.	Wounds cleansed, silver sulfadiazine applied, and wounds redressed.
	Monitor WBC count for signs of infection; assess and cleanse wounds tid.	Cleansing wounds helps prevent infection and promotes healing.	WBC count = 10,200. No signs of wound infection.
	Encourage adequate nutrition.	High caloric intake with sufficient vitamins and minerals is needed for healing.	Not taking food as yet. Continue plan.

PROBLEM/NURSING DIAGNOSIS *Extensive burns and painful care procedures/*Pain related to burn wounds and cleansing procedures.

Supporting assessment data *Subjective:* States is in constant pain at an 8–10 level. *Objective:* Grimacing and holding body rigid.

Goals/Expected Outcomes	Nursing Interventions	Selected Rationale	Evaluation
Patient's pain will be controlled to tolerable levels with analgesia	Administer IV analgesia as ordered, giving boluses as appropriate before procedures and at bedtime.	IV narcotic analgesia is best for burn pain control initially.	Pain at 2–4 on pain scale. Bolus given for pain of "4" before dressing change.
Patient's pain will be controlled with oral medication before discharge	Teach relaxation and imagery techniques to assist with pain control.	Relaxation and imagery techniques have proven helpful in pain control.	Began instruction on relaxation technique.
	Supply diversionary activities to diminish pain awareness.	TV, card games, visitors, computer games, and reading help divert attention from pain.	Is watching TV; not ready for greater activity yet. Continue plan.

Key: *ADLs*, activities of daily living; *IV*, intravenous; *PT*, physical therapy; *WBC*, white blood cell.

Continued

NURSING CARE PLAN 42–1

Care of the Patient with a Burn—cont'd

PROBLEM/NURSING DIAGNOSIS *Cannot use hands and arms*/Self-care deficit: hygiene, feeding, toileting, and grooming related to inability to use hands and arms.
Supporting assessment data *Objective:* Burns on hands and arms being treated and grafted. Unable to use hands and arms for self-care activities.

Goals/Expected Outcomes	Nursing Interventions	Selected Rationale	Evaluation
Patient will assist with self-care activities within 3 mo	Assist with hygiene, toileting, grooming, and feeding.	Cleanliness helps prevent infection and increases well-being.	Assistance with ADLs provided.
	Allow him to make decisions as much as possible to lessen feelings of helplessness.	Participation in care decreases feelings of dependency and increases feelings of control.	Choosing time for bath. Unable to use hands and arms at this time. Continue plan.
	Allow him to do as much as he is able to do.		

PROBLEM/NURSING DIAGNOSIS *Fears he will not be able to work at job and support family*/Situational low self-esteem related to burned hands and worries about role in family as "bread winner."
Supporting assessment data *Subjective:* "With my hands and arms burned, I won't be able to work anymore. I'm not much of a man anymore if I can't take care of my family." *Objective:* Unable to use hands and arms because of burns.

Goals/Expected Outcomes	Nursing Interventions	Selected Rationale	Evaluation
Patient will verbalize frustrations and concerns before discharge	Establish trusting relationship, actively listen to concerns and frustrations.	A trusting relationship helps him believe what you say to him.	Expressed concerns about helplessness.
	Help him establish his active role in recovery of use of hands and arms.	Collaboration helps improve his self-esteem.	States wants to recover self-sufficiency.
	Allow him to do whatever ADLs are possible for him.	Assisting with his own care helps increase self-esteem.	Unable to assist yet.
	Praise him for his efforts with PT exercises and use of splints.	Praise encourages his actions.	Passive PT only so far.
	Help him establish small, accomplishable goals on a weekly basis.	Accomplishing small goals increases self-esteem.	Is thinking about goals for next week.
	Offer emotional support and encouragement that is realistic.	Realistic encouragement supports hope.	Offering encouragement with PT.
Patient will discuss possible job retraining if needed	Refer for job retraining if needed.		Need for job retraining unknown at this time. Continue plan.

? CRITICAL THINKING QUESTIONS

1. With partial-thickness burns on his hands, do you think Mr. Young will be able to use his hands as a mechanic again?
2. Since he had burns on his face, what specific assessments should be made to see if there has been an inhalation injury?
3. Will he probably need skin grafting? If so, where? Is it likely that autografts could be used?

(Figure 42–16). The patient may resist wearing them unless she understands their intended purpose. Your encouragement and reinforcement of their need can help.

Pain and itching often continue beyond the point at which the wound appears to have healed completely. Exercises to prevent contractures can cause pain because they stretch the skin at a time when it is very tender. Splints to prevent musculoskeletal complications also can be uncomfortable for the burn patient. Analgesics will allow the patient to get sufficient rest, but they should be administered judiciously. If a patient begins to depend too much on one kind of analgesic, alternative drugs can be given.

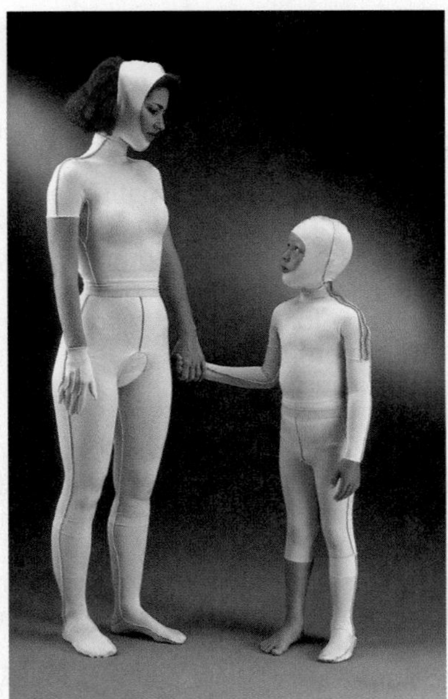

FIGURE **42–16** Pressure garments are individually fitted.

Itching can be controlled by giving regular doses of medication to prevent the problems, rather than waiting until the itching becomes intense and interferes with rest.

The patient who has experienced a major burn is transferred to a rehabilitation facility. Continued physical therapy and psychological care are essential to help the patient achieve her optimal level of function. Some patients must learn to use adaptive devices or alter the way they formerly accomplished tasks.

Participation in a support group of burn victims is sometimes helpful. In this way the patient and family realize that they are not alone in their struggles with the many problems that the injury has brought.

Assessment of the home environment and family interaction is essential before discharge home. Knowing how the patient formerly coped with stressful situations helps professional personnel involved support her. Having friends visit and making short trips out in public is helpful in dealing with the reactions of others to burn scars and disfigurement.

Reintegration into roles, community activities, and employment takes considerable time. Referral for job retraining may be required if the patient will be unable to return to a former occupation because of residual physical deficits. The nurse and health care team members can be very instrumental in helping the patient with these tasks. Rehabilitation goals and principles are covered in Chapter 9.

NURSING MANAGEMENT

Care of the burn patient is interdisciplinary and includes the services of the physician, surgeon, nurses, dietitian, respiratory therapist, physical therapist, occupational therapist, psychologist or psychiatrist, and social worker. Other health professionals are added to the team as needed. Collaborative planning meetings are scheduled at least once a week initially. Input for the plan of care is contributed by all members of the team.

Assessment (Data Collection)

A thorough assessment of all body systems is performed on admission and continues for all systems affected by the trauma. Areas where complications might occur are also assessed on a daily basis.

Nursing Diagnosis

Nursing diagnoses commonly used for burn patients include:

- Risk for deficient fluid volume related to evaporative loss, plasma loss, and shift of fluid into the tissues secondary to the burn injury
- Acute pain (and chronic pain) related to loss of tissue from burn injury and treatments
- Risk for infection related to impaired skin integrity, suppressed immune response, and normal flora on surrounding skin
- Imbalanced nutrition: less than body requirements related to increased caloric demands and inability to orally ingest sufficient calories
- Self-care deficit: bathing/hygiene, grooming, feeding, or toileting related to pain and immobility
- Anxiety related to pain, guilt associated with injury, financial concerns, appearance, treatment, and prognosis
- Disturbed body image related to disfigurement secondary to burn injury
- Ineffective coping related to alteration in roles
- Disabled family coping related to care and support of burn victim
- Deficient knowledge related to home care

Other nursing diagnoses may be added if complications occur.

Planning

Appropriate expected outcomes are written for the individual patient and may include:

- Patient will maintain fluid, acid-base and electrolyte balance.
- Patient will experience adequate pain control.
- Patient will not evidence infection.
- Patient will regain nutritional balance.
- Patient will experience as much functional restoration as possible.
- Patient will decrease anxiety.
- Patient will develop new coping mechanisms.
- Patient will integrate the altered body image.
- Family will develop ways to cope with caring for patient at home.
- Patient and family will learn to provide good care at home.

Implementation

Specific interventions are chosen for each patient problem/nursing diagnosis. Interventions will depend on the depth and extent of the burn injury. Decreasing fear and anxiety and teaching self-care are as important as the interventions for physical problems (see Nursing Care Plan 42–1).

Patient-Family Education

The patient and family are taught about daily skin and wound care before discharge. They must be familiar with dressing instructions, lubrication of grafts, and donor site care. Moisturizing with an alcohol-free skin moisturizer is necessary at least three times a day. Pressure dressings or garments must be worn for 23 hours daily. Direct sunlight should be completely avoided for 1 year after injury because of increased sensitivity to ultraviolet rays.

Medication dosages, precautions, and potential side effect information are sent home with the patient. Nutritional needs and particular diet recommendations are discussed. Adequate protein and calories are very important to full recovery. Referral is made to support groups or peers and counseling as needed for readjustment to life after the burn incident. The need for follow-up care is stressed, and appointment dates and times are established.

Evaluation

Evaluation is performed by collecting data regarding the success of the interventions in reaching the expected outcomes. If outcomes are not being met, the plan's interventions are changed.

COMMUNITY CARE

Nurses in the community can do much to educate the public about the dangers of unprotected sun exposure and the signs of skin cancer. Skin self-screening is taught at every opportunity. School nurses perform assessments for signs of lice and scabies. They teach families how to deal with these problems and how to prevent their spread.

Teaching fire safety to schoolchildren helps decrease fire injury. Home care nurses must continually assess patient homes for fire dangers and reinforce teaching to prevent home fires.

Long-term care nurses seek to promote good skin integrity in all residents, handling the elderly with special care so as not to tear the skin. Patients who are immobile are turned diligently to prevent pressure ulcers, and skin is inspected regularly. Elderly patients are encouraged to use skin emollients to moisten and protect the skin surface. Nurses vigilantly assess changes in skin lesions that may indicate a cancer.

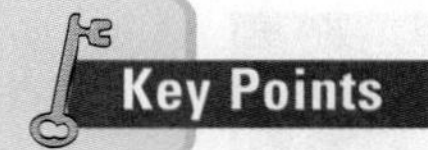

- Bacteria, viruses, fungi, or parasites can cause a skin disorder.
- There are several types of dermatitis, all of which tend to cause erythema and itching.
- When dermatitis occurs, a thorough history is necessary to locate the offending agent.
- Patient education for most skin disorders involves teaching the patient to avoid causative factors, how to apply topical medications, and to avoid becoming hot.
- Viral skin disorders are caused by herpesviruses. Care must be taken to prevent autoinoculation.
- Herpes zoster is very painful and can result in a postherpetic neuralgia.
- Anyone who has not previously had chickenpox or been immunized for it should not care for a patient with herpes zoster.
- Herpes zoster lesions follow nerve pathways and should be treated early.
- Fungi prefer warm moist places, and fungal infections may be difficult to eradicate.
- Tinea pedis is one of the most common fungal infections and occurs on the feet.
- Treatment of pediculosis and scabies requires treating both the patient and objects that may harbor the parasites.
- Acne is a troublesome disorder that often occurs at puberty.
- The accumulation of sebum and dead skin cells causes the inflammatory reaction.
- The lesions of acne should not be squeezed; drying agents that cause peeling work best to rid the skin of blackheads and whiteheads.
- Acne patients need to be taught proper skin care regarding cleansing and the use of topical medications.
- Psoriasis appears as inflamed, edematous skin lesions with adherent silvery-white scales.
- There is a genetic predisposition to psoriasis. It can be controlled, but not cured.
- Skin cancer has increased in incidence, but is highly curable if treated in the early stages.
- Exposure to ultraviolet radiation (sunlight) is a major cause of skin cancer. Alteration of the earth's ozone layer is a contributing factor.
- Everyone should wear sunscreen with UVB protection and at least an SPF of 15, when outdoors. A hat and sunglasses are recommended.
- Basal cell, squamous cell, and melanoma are the usual carcinomas arising from the epidermis.
- Actinic keratoses are a premalignant lesion common on the skin of the elderly.
- If squamous cell carcinoma is not treated early, it can become invasive and metastasize.
- Melanoma is the most aggressive of the skin cancers and needs to be treated early to prevent metastasis.
- All patients should be screened for skin cancer lesions and taught prevention measures and self-screening.
- Pressure ulcers are a potential problem for all immobile patients.

- Careful assessment of risk factors, staging, and treatment is the way to prevent and control pressure ulcers.
- Treatment of a pressure ulcer depends on the stage and location of the ulcer.
- Irrigation cleansing or hydrotherapy cleansing is needed for stage II to IV pressure ulcers.
- Only normal saline should be used to irrigate pressure ulcers as chemicals can be toxic to newly formed granulation tissue.
- Pressure ulcers should be measured and documented on discovery and then measured and documented regularly to show progress in healing.
- Skin tears are a serious problem for elderly patients, and many can be prevented.
- If discovered early, the flap of a skin tear can be approximated, promoting quicker healing.
- Burns are caused by extreme heat, hot liquids, electrical agents, strong chemicals, or radiation.
- The classification of a burn determines its treatment.
- The greatest danger from a major burn is fluid shifts causing hypovolemic shock.
- Early fluid resuscitation is essential to prevent death when a patient suffers a major burn.
- Eschar must be removed for a burn wound to heal.
- Early grafting with biologic or synthetic substances helps burn wounds heal more quickly.
- Only real skin acts as a permanent graft.
- Pain control is a major nursing action for the burn patient.
- Each burn patient is assessed for an inhalation injury.
- Burn care is divided into phases: emergency care, emergent care, acute care, and rehabilitation.
- Burn care is very complex because so many systems can be affected by the systemic effects of a large burn.
- It is a priority to monitor the burn patient for signs of respiratory problems and infection.
- Burns are cared for in an aseptic manner.
- Burn patients have both physical and psychosocial problems that must be addressed.
- Wound débridement can be very painful, but is essential to healing of the wounds and the prevention of infection.
- Contracture prevention begins at the time of admission; special splints and positioning are used to preserve anatomical alignment and prevent contracture.
- Nutritional support is another major focus of burn care as patients may need as many as 5000 calories a day in order to heal.
- When skin grafts are healed, pressure dressings or garments are used to prevent excessive scarring.
- There is a long rehabilitation period after a major burn in which readjustment to life and roles as well as further physical rehabilitation occurs.
- Nurses can do much to educate about skin disorders, burn prevention, and prevention and detection of skin cancer.

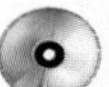
Go to your **Companion CD-ROM** for an Audio Glossary, animations, video clips, and bonus review questions.

evolve Be sure to visit the companion Evolve site at http://evolve.elsevier.com/deWit for interactive NCLEX-PN Exam Style Review Questions, WebLinks, and additional online resources.

NCLEX-PN EXAM STYLE REVIEW QUESTIONS

Choose the best answer(s) for the following questions.

1. A patient complains of itching on reddened, hyperpigmented areas over the right ankle and right tibia. The leg has non-pitting edema with varicosities. A likely diagnosis would be:

1. stasis dermatitis.
2. seborrheic dermatitis.
3. atopic dermatitis.
4. contact dermatitis.

2. In managing dermatitis, the nurse provides which of the following instructions? *(Select all that apply.)*

1. Avoid the irritant or allergen.
2. Provide adequate skin lubrication.
3. Wash skin frequently with germicidal soaps.
4. Maintain skin moisture.
5. Apply steroid-based preparations.

3. ______________________ is characterized by erythema, papules, pustules, and telangiectases over the cheeks and bridge of the nose among 30- to 50-year-olds.

4. A teenager visits a dermatologist for acne vulgaris and asks the physician, "What is the nature of my skin condition?" Which are true statements regarding acne vulgaris? *(Select all that apply.)*

1. Acne vulgaris results from accumulations of sebum in occluded sebaceous glands.
2. Acne vulgaris is caused by increased levels of androgens and fluctuating premenstrual hormones.
3. Application of heavy creams and heat exposure contribute to the development of acne.
4. Alcohol, caffeine-containing foods, spicy foods, sunlight, and emotional stress cause flare-ups.
5. These lesions are not a sign of uncleanliness.

5. A male patient presents with inflamed, edematous skin of the elbows and knees accompanied by swelling of the joints of the fingers and toes. On examination, the skin is covered with adherent silvery white scales. Which of the following questions would provide more information regarding the patient's condition?

1. "What do you do for a living?"
2. "How much do you smoke?"
3. "Have you had an upper respiratory tract infection recently?"
4. "Have you recently changed your laundry detergent?"

6. A patient has skin lesions of face, trunk, palms, extensor surfaces of joints, soles of the feet, and dorsum of the hands. On inspection, the lesions have irregular borders and blistered, necrotic centers. With a tentative diagnosis of Stevens-Johnson syndrome, appropriate medical management would include which of the following?
   1. Methotrexate
   2. Trimethroprim/sulfamethoxazole (Bactrim, Septra)
   3. Narcotic analgesics
   4. 13-*cis*-retinoic acid (Accutane)
7. The nurse responds to a hospital-wide emergency for a 50-kg burn victim who has a calculated 30% burned total body surface area. The nurse uses the Parkland formula and administers lactated Ringer's solution. What is the rate of infusion during the first 8 hours?
   1. 38 mL/hr
   2. 188 mL/hr
   3. 250 mL/hr
   4. 375 mL/hr
8. While performing the initial assessment, the patient with extensive burn injuries suddenly develops increasing hoarseness and stridor. Pulse oximetry is 86%. The initial nursing action would be to:
   1. encourage the patient to take deep breaths.
   2. provide positive ventilation with humidified oxygen.
   3. administer respiratory treatments.
   4. suction respiratory secretions.
9. A school-age female with evidence of severe itching in the scalp is checked for pediculosis. Careful assessment confirms a nursing diagnosis of Deficient knowledge related to unfamiliarity with managing the disease. Important instructions given by the nurse would include which of the following? *(Select all that apply.)*
   1. "Machine wash clothes and bedding using the coldest cycle."
   2. "Share combs and hairbrushes."
   3. "Soak all combs and brushes in very hot water for more than 5 minutes."
   4. "Seal items that cannot be washed in air-expelled plastic bags for 14 days."
   5. "Instruct all family members about the infection and ways to prevent reinfestation."
10. The nurse at a long-term care facility launches an information campaign to prevent skin tears among the residents. The nurse would include which of the following information? *(Select all that apply.)*
    1. Encourage long sleeves and long pants.
    2. Provide adequate lighting.
    3. Use germicidal soap every day on extremities.
    4. Support dangling arms and legs with pillows or blankets.
    5. Remove tape and dressing with extreme caution.

CRITICAL THINKING ACTIVITIES 

Read each clinical scenario and discuss the questions with your classmates.

Scenario A

Mrs. Nash, age 32, has been assigned as your patient on the evening shift. She has severe dermatitis, probably allergic. Her physician has ordered a topical lotion, dermatologic baths twice a day, and an antihistamine to relieve itching.

1. What kinds of data would you include in your ongoing assessment of Mrs. Nash's skin disorder?
2. What nursing care problems is Mrs. Nash likely to present?
3. What objectives and nursing measures to meet them would you include in Mrs. Nash's nursing care plan?
4. What would you teach Mrs. Nash about the application of topicals when she returns home?

Scenario B

Ms. Moore, age 22, was badly burned when her clothing caught fire while she was grilling hamburgers on her patio. She has partial-thickness and full-thickness burns over her abdomen and down the front of both upper legs.

1. What is the priority of care after assessment when Ms. Moore reaches the emergency room?
2. What nursing measure should be taken to prevent infection of her burns?
3. What nursing measures would be included in the patient's nursing care plan to ensure that she did not suffer from an undetected fluid and electrolyte imbalance?
4. How is Ms. Moore's pain treated? Why?
5. List some specific things you and the other nurses could do to help her handle her sense of loss and altered self-image as a result of the appearance of the burns and scars.

CHAPTER 43 Care of Patients in Disasters or Bioterrorism Attack

evolve http://evolve.elsevier.com/deWit

Objectives

Upon completion of this chapter, you should be able to:

Theory

1. State the difference between an emergency situation and a disaster.
2. Discuss an emergency preparedness plan for a health care facility.
3. Compare the three stages of psychological response that occur with a disaster.
4. Describe the parameters used in the triage system for victims after a disaster.
5. Identify responsibilities and duties of the nurse in the care of disaster victims.
6. Explain safety measures to be employed for a chemical emergency or an earthquake.
7. Demonstrate knowledge of measures to be taken in the event of a nuclear disaster.
8. Explain safety measures to be used in the event of a bioterrorism attack.
9. Differentiate the signs and symptoms of the various agents that could be used for a terrorist attack.
10. Interpret the measures used for debriefing of health care personnel after a disaster.

Clinical Practice

1. Participate in a disaster drill.
2. Teach a group of adults how to prepare safe water after a disaster has disrupted the water supply.
3. Identify the measures you would take for your own safety when assisting others after a disaster has occurred.

Key Terms

Be sure to check out the bonus material on the Companion CD-ROM, including selected audio pronunciations.

bioterrorism (p. 1057)
debriefing (p. 1070)
decontamination (dē-kŏn-tăm-ĭ-NĀ-shŭn, p. 1062)
disaster (p. 1051)
mass casualty (p. 1053)
triage (TRĒ-ăhzh, p. 1053)

DISASTER PREPAREDNESS AND RESPONSE

An emergency is an extraordinary event such as a multivictim incident involving an explosion or a train crash. A rapid and skilled response is necessary to manage the wounded. There may be walking wounded, critically wounded, and fatally wounded victims. This type of event usually can be handled by the community's hospital emergency rooms. A disaster may occur naturally as a result of severe weather or an earthquake. A man-made event such as terrorism or a war attack may result in disaster. Either type may overwhelm the community's existing emergency resources. A disaster causes mass casualties, psychological as well as physical trauma, and permanent changes within the community.

A disaster exists when the number of casualties exceeds the resource capabilities of the area. Natural disasters include epidemics, earthquakes, explosions, hurricanes, tornadoes, fires, floods, and transportation accidents. Man-made disasters may result from attacks with chemical, biologic, nuclear, and conventional weapons. Terrorist attacks are classified as disasters.

The governmental agencies for disaster planning are the Department of Homeland Security, the Office of Domestic Preparedness, and the U.S. Public Health Service. The American Red Cross is a voluntary organization that traditionally provides the basic essentials of shelter, food, and first aid during a natural disaster (Figure 43–1). In most communities, the local Office of Emergency Services (OES), the Red Cross, and the Salvation Army work together to formulate disaster plans. They coordinate their services with each other and with other agencies in planning for essential services, such as shelter, transportation, communication, and welfare. The Centers for Disease Control and Prevention has a website with information on all types of disasters, weather events, and mass casualty events (www.bt.cdc.gov).

Special courses in civil defense and disaster nursing are usually offered by the OES, the Red Cross, and professional organizations. These courses help nurses and volunteer workers in the community understand the function of each agency in a particular type of disaster and serve to coordinate the planning for each kind of emergency care.

Think Critically About . . . Which community agency in your area has training courses for disaster situations?

Whether the disaster is natural or war-caused, it will involve physical injuries, loss of property, and interruption of the normal activities of daily living. People often will need food, clothing, shelter, medical and nursing or hospital care, and other basic necessities of life.

All nurses should be instrumental in encouraging people in the community to prepare disaster supplies in their homes with all the recommended items (Health Promotion Points 43–1). Most people know about these recommendations, but few are truly prepared. Every family should have a contact person out of the geographic area where extended family members can call to receive information about the welfare of their relatives. Communication into and out of the disaster region is often cut off. Each member of a family living together should know whom they are to call if separated from one another.

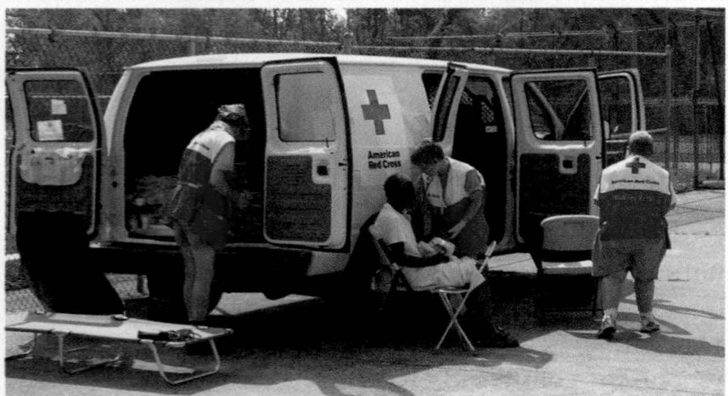

FIGURE **43–1** September 19, 2005. A Red Cross volunteer checks on a resident affected by the extreme heat in Algiers, Louisiana, after Hurricane Katrina. ©American Red Cross.

COMMUNITY PREPAREDNESS

The law enforcement agency, the city or county emergency management department, and the state public health department are responsible for coordinating efforts to assist people when a disaster happens. The American Red Cross may disperse personnel and supplies to assist with essential needs and medical care. If the state requests assistance, Homeland Security determines if the Federal Emergency Management Agency (FEMA) is to be called. If so, FEMA brings personnel and aid to the area. If a disaster is of major proportions, a Disaster Medical Assistance Team (DMAT) may be activated at the state or federal level. These units bring medical, paraprofessional, and support personnel along with medical equipment and supplies to sustain an operation for a minimum of 72 hours. The team provides

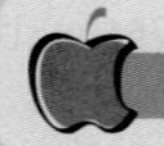

Health Promotion Points 43–1

Preparing Disaster Supplies

Community members should be encouraged to prepare for a disaster. Preparations should include a minimum of 3 days' supplies. The following should be gathered and placed in one area:

- Water in plastic containers: 1 gallon per person per day. Change the supply every 6 months.
- Nonperishable food that requires no refrigeration, preparation, or cooking and little water, including:
  - Ready-to-eat canned meats, fruits, and vegetables
  - Canned juices, milk, and ready-to-eat soups
  - Sugar, salt, pepper
  - Peanut butter, jelly, crackers, granola bars, trail mix
  - Foods for infants or elderly on special diets
  - Hard candy, instant coffee, tea bags, cookies in tins
- Disposable dishes and eating utensils or camping or military "mess kit"
- First aid kit containing an assortment of bandages, scissors, tweezers, needle, antiseptic, thermometer, and moistened towelettes
- Supply of essential prescription medications
- Nonprescription drugs: Pain reliever, antacid, vitamins, laxative, anti-inflammatory
- Battery-operated or wind-up radio
- Flashlight and extra batteries
- Hand sanitizer and soap
- Disinfectant wipes

TOOLS

- Nonelectric can opener
- Work gloves
- Disposable gloves
- Utility knife
- Pliers
- Matches in waterproof container
- Paper and pencil
- Aluminum foil
- Whistle
- Plastic sheeting and duct tape
- Shut-off wrench to turn off household gas and water
- Fire extinguisher: ABC type
- Signal flare
- Tube tent, blanket or sleeping bag
- Jacket
- Change of clothes
- Shoes

OTHER ITEMS

- Cash or traveler's checks
- Copies of insurance cards
- Copies of official identification
- Pet food, water, and medications

Some agencies advocate keeping a 3- to 6-week supply of food and water on hand. Food items should be used and replaced every 6 months to maintain freshness.

Sources: Federal Emergency Management Agency and the American Red Cross (2006). Shelter in Place in an Emergency. Retrieved from www.redcross.org/preparedness/cdc_english/Sheltering.asp.

Safety Alert 43–1

Fire!

In the event of a wildfire, if told to evacuate, leave quickly! If at home and the smoke detector goes off, do not wait to dress or gather belongings—get out of the dwelling. If fire or smoke is evident, drop to the floor and crawl to the exit. Cover mouth and nose with a moistened cloth if smoke is present. Feel any door before opening it. If it is hot, find another way out. If clothes catch on fire, drop to the ground and roll to suffocate the fire. Keep rolling until flames are out.

Safety Alert 43–2

Earthquake!

If an earthquake strikes and you are indoors, stay there. Get under a desk or table, or stand in a corner or door frame. Cover your head with your arms. If outdoors, get into an open area away from trees, buildings, walls, and power lines. If driving, pull over to the side of the road and stop away from trees, buildings, and power lines. Stay inside the vehicle. If you are in a crowded public place, do not rush for the doors. Move away from display shelves containing objects that could fall and large-pane windows. If you are in a high-rise building, stay away from windows and outside walls. Avoid using the elevators. Get under a table or desk.

After the shaking has stopped, assist those injured, applying first aid as needed. Do not use the telephone unless there is a life-threatening injury or fire. If uninjured, check for gas leaks. If you find any, turn off the utility at once. Turn off water if water pipes are broken. Turn on the portable radio for instructions and news reports.

triage (sorting out of casualties by priority of need for treatment), evacuation, primary health care, and assistance to local health care facilities that are overwhelmed. The emergency management team sets up a communications system, and the Emergency Medical Services (EMS) personnel at the scene notify the emergency departments at the hospitals of the situation. With pagers, telephone trees, and instant computer alert messages, essential personnel are notified of a disaster or **mass casualty** (many-victims incident).

Community residents are instructed about what to do in the event that an earthquake, wildfire, hurricane, tornado, or flood occurs in their area (Safety Alerts 43–1, 43–2, and 43–3). If advised to evacuate the area, residents should gather essential belongings, medications, pets, and keepsakes and leave immediately. If tornado sirens are sounded, people should take refuge in a basement or in an inner room without windows, such as a closet or a bathroom, to avoid flying debris. Getting into the bathtub and covering oneself with cushions or a mattress can also protect a person from flying debris. If outside, it is best to lie in a culvert or ditch below ground level.

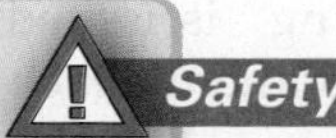

Safety Alert 43–3

Tornado, Hurricane, and Flood!

Choose ahead of time where you could go if evacuation is necessary. Evacuate when you are told to do so. Listen to a NOAA Weather Radio or local radio or television stations for evacuation instructions. Keep a road map handy because you may have to take unfamiliar routes. Take these items with you:

- Prescription medications and medical supplies, glasses, hearing aid, and the like
- Bedding and clothing, including sleeping bags and pillows
- Bottled water, battery-operated radio and extra batteries, first aid kit, and flashlight
- Maps and documents, such as driver's license, Social Security card, proof of residence, insurance policies, wills, deeds, birth and marriage certificates, and tax records, if they are at home

Key: *NOAA,* National Oceanic and Atmospheric Administration.

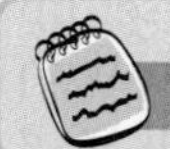

Patient Teaching 43–1

Preparing for a Hurricane

People living in a hurricane-prone area should be taught to:

- Prepare a disaster kit and keep it refreshed every 6 months.

When a hurricane "watch" is issued:

- Bring inside any outdoor furniture, trash cans, potted plants, toys, and the like that could be picked up by the wind.
- Protect the windows with hurricane shutters or ½″ outdoor plywood boards.
- Fill your car's gas tank.
- Have cash on hand.
- Check batteries and stock up on canned food, first aid supplies, drinking water, and medications.
- Do not stay in a mobile home.

When a hurricane "warning" is issued:

- If not advised to evacuate, stay inside and away from windows.
- Be aware that the calm "eye" of the storm is deceptive. The worst winds will blow from the opposite direction once the "eye" passes over.
- Be alert for flying debris. Stay in a room, bathroom, or closet with no windows.

After the hurricane passes:

- Stay away from floodwaters once the hurricane is past. Do not drive through flowing water. If caught in the car and the water is rising, get out and go to higher ground immediately.
- Do not let children play in the floodwater.
- Stay away from standing water as there may be a downed power line touching it.
- Use tap water for drinking and cooking *only* when local officials say it is safe.

Adapted from National Oceanic and Atmospheric Administration. Hurricanes: Unleashing Nature's Fury. Retrieved from www.nws.noaa.gov/om/brochures/hurr.pdf.

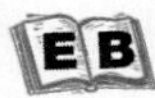

If a hurricane "watch" or a "warning" is issued, people should prepare appropriately (Patient Teaching 43–1).

HOSPITAL PREPAREDNESS

The Joint Commission requires that hospitals have an emergency preparedness plan in place. There are guidelines for systems notification and for the parameters for emergency preparedness by type of facility. Emergency room physicians undergo formal training for disaster events. Emergency room nurses are encouraged to obtain certification in emergency preparedness. The emergency plan is to be tested with drills at least twice a year (Couig, et al., 2005). Know what is in the emergency preparedness plan at the facility where you work or are assigned. A catastrophic event or a terrorist incident involving weapons of mass destruction (WMDs) requires volunteer assistance from all levels of health care providers in the area.

The emergency preparedness plan will identify who will be in charge and the chain of command for the facility. The designated communications officer will set up the communication system and will be in touch with the other agencies called in for help. There will be a hospital incident commander (physician or administrator) who assumes responsibility for launching the institutional plan. This person's role as commander is to take a global view of the entire situation, to bring in needed human and supply resources, and facilitate the flow of patients through the system. Usual hospital routine will be altered to accommodate care for high numbers of patients. Departmental roles will be changed. Patients ready for discharge may be moved to non–patient care areas to free up beds for the wounded. Physical therapy and other departments may close down usual operations and become the minor treatment area for the nonurgent patients (Halpern & Chaffee, 2005).

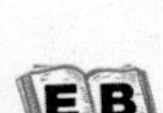

A medical command physician will focus on determining the number, acuity, and medical needs of the casualties arriving from the scene of the disaster. This person will organize the emergency health care team response to the injured or ill patients. Specialists trained for the particular type of disaster will be called in to help as the need is foreseen. Decisions will be made about who is to be evacuated to a facility with a higher level of care.

A triage officer, usually a physician, with the assistance of triage nurses, will rapidly evaluate each person presenting to the hospital and send the patient to the appropriate area for immediate or eventual treatment. The emergency department supervisor or charge nurse collaborates with the medical command physician and triage officer to organize nursing and ancillary personnel to meet patient needs. A telephone tree will be activated to call in off-duty staff. In addition to the above personnel, there will be a supply officer, communications officer, infection control officer, and public information officer. The public information officer will manage the media. Hospital staff at all levels will be called on to assist with whatever care is needed. Long-term care facilities may need to evacuate residents, or they may need to take in people from other facilities or the community.

? *Think Critically About* . . . If a disaster occurred in your community and you were not injured, where would you call, or go, to see how you could help?

FIELD HOSPITALS AND SHELTERS

In 2005, the United States experienced a major disaster with Hurricane Katrina and the subsequent hurricane, Rita, which quickly followed. Katrina, the tsunami in Indonesia, and the major earthquake in Pakistan have shown the importance of disaster services.

When the local hospitals are unusable, field hospitals are established in tents or large public facilities. Shelter areas are designated by emergency management personnel and/or the military and are set up to provide sleeping areas, food, water, and sanitation facilities (U.S. Department of Health and Human Services, 2002).

Although the medical community is more concerned with treating injuries and illness than with the issues of housing and community services, attention must be directed to safe water, and food supply as well.

PSYCHOLOGICAL RESPONSES TO DISASTER

Since the 1940s, many studies have been conducted to determine the needs and problems of people trying to cope with a major disaster. Typical responses are not unlike those of any person who is overwhelmed with sudden and profound change, death, or destruction of a former way of life.

One would expect people to panic when they are caught up in a major disaster, but this is not a common reaction, except when there is life-threatening danger that occurs in a matter of moments and without warning. More typical of psychological responses to a major disaster are the following three stages:

- Stage I is the *impact stage.* Survivors are stunned, apathetic, and disorganized. For several hours after the initial event, they may have difficulty following directions and will need strong support and firm guidance.
- Stage II is the *recoil stage.* During this stage, individuals are very compliant, want to be helpful, and may minimize or ignore their own injuries. At this stage, some people may need to be protected from themselves if they are indeed injured or physically and emotionally exhausted.
- In Stage III, called the *post-trauma stage,* some survivors become elated, grateful that they are

Table 43–1 *Disaster Triage System*

CLASSIFICATION	TRIAGE TAG	TYPICAL CONDITIONS	TREATMENT
Class I: Emergent	Red tag	Immediate threat to life, such as airway compromise or hemorrhagic shock	Immediate
Class II: Urgent	Yellow tag	Major injuries, open fractures, large wounds	Within 30 min to 2 hr
Class III: Nonurgent	Green tag	"Walking wounded": closed fractures, sprains, strains, contusions, abrasions	>2 hr
Class IV: Dead or expected to die	Black tag	Dead, or imminently dying with little chance of survival	None

still alive. Others might feel guilty when they realize they did not suffer as much as their friends and neighbors. At this stage, the attention of the survivors turns toward rebuilding, and they have a strong sense of brotherhood and community spirit (Halpern & Chaffee, 2005).

Later on, victims of a disaster probably will begin to complain about the help provided by various agencies, governmental and private. If the disaster could have been avoided or at least mitigated by an efficient emergency preparedness or similar agency, the psychological effects may be more severe and psychological recovery will take longer. Some victims may later experience post-traumatic stress disorder and need additional counseling and psychological care.

TRIAGE

After a disaster, care of victims is prioritized according to a triage system that is different from regular emergency department triage. Those victims with life-threatening conditions and a good chance of survival are cared for first (Table 43–1). These Class I or life-threatened, emergent, patients are identified with a red tag. Class II patients are treated next and have conditions that are urgent and require treatment within a 2-hour time frame. Class II patients are identified with a yellow tag. Class III patients come last and are considered nonurgent; treatment can be delayed for 4 to 6 hours. They are identified with a green tag.

When there are more victims of a disaster than medical personnel to treat them, those who are mortally wounded or are not expected to survive are generally not treated until those more likely to survive are treated. These patients are issued a black tag (Figure 43–2). This is a difficult choice for most nurses, but in a disaster, the good of the most must prevail over that of the few.

Even though triage may have been done out in the field, it is performed again at the emergency care facility. Green-tagged patients usually comprise the greatest number in most large-scale disaster situations. They need to be managed until they are able to be treated. If not managed, they can be a health hazard by walking in with infection, radioactivity, and the like. A special bracelet with a disaster number may be applied to tagged patients.

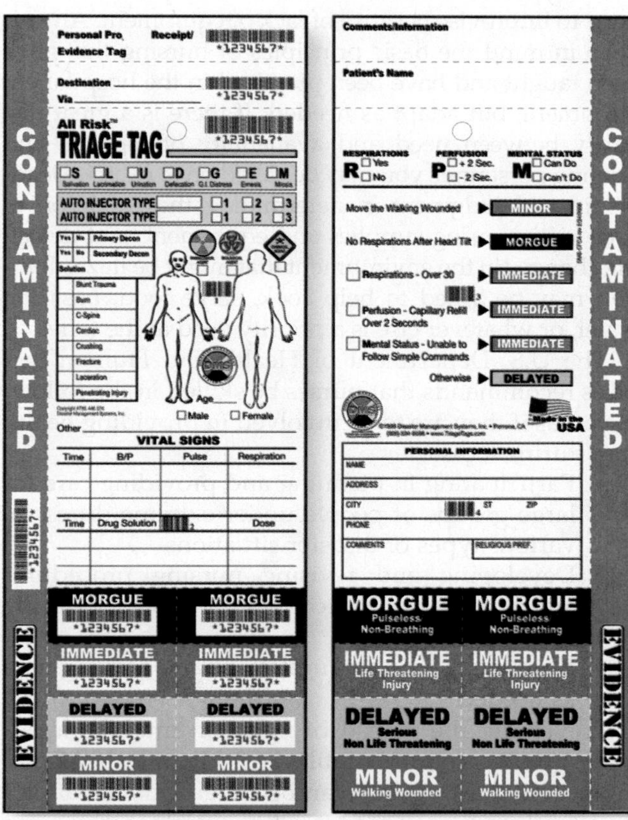

FIGURE 43–2 Example of triage tags.

NURSING RESPONSIBILITIES

A booklet published under the direction of the U.S. Department of Health and Human Services (2002) includes the following list of nursing responsibilities in case of a disaster. All nurses should:

- Be prepared for self-survival and for performing emergency nursing measures.
- Evaluate the environmental and physical risks (i.e., damaged building structure, etc.).
- Know the community disaster plans and organized community health resources.
- Know the meaning of warning signals of disaster and the action to be taken.
- Know measures for protection from radioactive fallout.
- Know measures for prevention and control of environmental health hazards.

- Be prepared to interpret health laws and regulations.
- Know and interpret community resources for citizen preparedness, such as first aid and medical self-help courses.

Nursing Roles

In the emergency room, you will perform needed procedures such as inserting catheters, nasogastric tubes, and possibly intravenous (IV) lines and drawing blood. In many types of disaster, outside the hospital you may need to improvise because of lack of equipment. Always keep in mind the basic principles of nursing that have been taught and have been practiced in the hospital environment, but adapt as needed. If there is a great disparity between need and availability of medical and nursing personnel, you may be called on to exercise leadership and judgment in determining the condition of each victim, using supplies and equipment, and detecting changes in the environment that might be hazardous. You may be asked to help cook, serve food, pass out water, or whatever else is a priority need at the time.

The U.S. Department of Health and Human Services recommends that nurses be skilled in the following areas if they are to be involved in providing health care during a disaster:

- Participating in planning and providing care for large groups of people under extreme duress in various types of disaster situations
- Developing and revising nursing procedures aimed at providing comfort and safety during and after a disaster
- Knowing your own limitations and seeking help as needed

Preventing the spread of infection must be a primary nursing concern. Table 43–2 identifies the communicable diseases that can become epidemic after a disaster. Infection control is a top priority when large groups of people are together in a shelter because the incidence of communicable disease is much greater.

The emotional and physical comfort and safety of large numbers of disaster victims must be attended to with limited supplies, equipment, utilities, and personnel. You must understand the emotional stress caused by personal fear, problems of displacement and separation of families, increasing anxiety, and continuing danger. You will need to help people of different cultural backgrounds and religious beliefs accept and adapt to temporary living conditions in crowded and often adverse situations.

Recognizing and understanding the effect of disrupted social and economic patterns, such as personal and material losses, emotional trauma, and crowded living conditions, helps you to deal with the people involved more effectively. It is helpful to encourage people to verbalize their concerns and fears and to guide them in performing certain tasks.

Providing basic instruction to people displaced by disaster about appropriate self-care within the current environment and encouraging them to further provide for their own needs, as well as those of others, are essential nursing responsibilities in any disaster situation.

Care of Special Populations

Infants, elderly, disabled, and immunocompromised groups will need more support and assistance in obtaining items that may not be with them. Diapers, formula, bottles, and powdered milk will need to be obtained for infants. The elderly may be without their prescriptions for chronic or other serious health conditions. Medications will need to be obtained for them. Eyeglasses may be lost, and many elderly cannot really see much without them. Hearing aids may be lost or batteries may die. Having new batteries on hand can greatly ease feelings of panic and anxiety. Developmental concerns should be considered along with physical and psychosocial responses to disaster.

The disabled may need a means of mobility if they are separated from their belongings. They may need assistance with bathing, eating, and general activities of daily living. Immunocompromised people need special attention and care to prevent infection when in large crowds. You can direct people to where they can obtain assistance, or obtain needed items for them. Safety for these groups is a priority.

Water and Food Safety

Disruption or contamination of the water supply is probable when a disaster occurs. Floodwater or storm water should not be used to wash dishes, brush teeth, wash and prepare food, wash hands, make ice, or make baby formula. People have to be taught how to purify water (Health Promotion Points 43–2).

If there is a power outage, and people can stay in their homes, they will need to know how to keep their food supply safe to eat (Todd, 2006) (Box 43–1).

Nursing Management

Observing, recording, and reporting information about patients to appropriate authorities must be carried out in an organized manner. General physical and mental conditions of patients and signs and symptoms that may be indicative of changes in their conditions must be accurately observed. Stresses in relationships between patients, their families, and personnel must be kept to a minimum.

Performing nursing procedures in a disaster situation demands skill and judgment to provide for the good of the greatest number of people. The nurse must administer medications and treatments as directed and improvise supplies, equipment, and techniques as

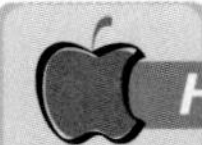

Health Promotion Points 43–2

Preparing Safe Water

When the normal water supply is disrupted, water may be purified by:

- Bringing it to a rolling boil for 3 to 5 minutes. Let the water cool before drinking.
- Adding household liquid bleach containing 5.25% sodium hypochlorite. Add 16 drops of bleach to a gallon of water and let stand for 30 minutes.
- Distilling the water. To distill, fill a large pot halfway with water. Tie a cup securely to the handle on the pot's lid so that the cup will hang right side up when the lid is upside down. Set the lid upside down on the top of the pot so that the cup hangs down into the pot below the lid (the cup should not dangle in the water). Boil the water for 20 minutes. The water that drips from the lid into the cup is distilled. This method frees water of microbes that may remain after bleach treatment.

From American Red Cross (2006). Water Treatment. Retrieved from www.redcross.org/services/disaster/0,1082,0_563,00.html.

necessary. She also must carry out precautionary measures, including maintaining a safe and sanitary environment and separating patients with communicable diseases. Instituting emergency first aid measures also is essential and usually requires using available supplies and observing aseptic technique under very chaotic conditions.

Working toward restoring community and family life after the disaster, according to available resources, involves the nurse and other members of the health care team. Individual self-help and work therapy are encouraged, as are activities of daily living, with adaptations designed to attain and maintain a clean and healthy environment. Existing community facilities and resources must be used as much as possible for continued patient care.

You can promote the effectiveness of the health service agency in disaster preparedness by knowing and interpreting the agency's disaster plan. Understand the relationship between the agency plan, the local government plan, and the community agencies plans. Trying to maintain and restore community health by controlling environmental health hazards is an important responsibility for every nurse.

? *Think Critically About . . .* Are you and your family prepared for a disaster? Do you have a disaster kit on hand? If you have children, do you have measures in place for their care by others if you are unable to reach them? Is there a contact person out-of-state for family to call and let know their status?

Box 43–1 *Keeping Food Safe to Eat*

Perishable foods should not be held above 40° F (4.4° C) for more than 2 hours. A refrigerator will ordinarily keep food chilled to below 40° F for 2 to 4 hours. It is wise to have a quick-response digital thermometer on hand.

If a power outage occurs, do the following:

- Keep the refrigerator and freezer doors closed. A freezer that is half full will keep food safe for up to 24 hours; a full freezer will keep food safe for 48 hours.
- If it appears that the outage will be for more than 2 to 4 hours, pack refrigerated milk, dairy products, mayonnaise, meats, fish, poultry, eggs, gravy, stuffing and leftovers into coolers and surround them with ice.
- When uncertain as to how long the power has been out, check the internal temperature of foods in your refrigerator with the quick-response thermometer. If the internal temperature is above 40° F, throw the food away.
- Throw away food that may have come into contact with flood or storm water.
- Throw away food that has an unusual odor, color, or texture.
- Food containers with screw-on caps, snap-on lids, crimped caps (soda pop bottles), twist-off caps, and snap-open caps, as well as home-canned foods, should be discarded if they have come into contact with floodwater because they cannot be disinfected.
- If cans have come into contact with floodwater or storm water, remove the labels and wash them with hot soapy water or dip them in a solution of 1 cup of bleach in 5 gallons of clean water. Relabel the cans with a marker.

Adapted from Food Safety in a Power Outage. (2003). Giant Foods, Inc., Landover, MD. Retrieved from www.redcross.org/services/disaster/0,1082,0_564_,00.html.
Further information is available from the Emergency Preparedness and Response website at www.bt.cdc.gov/disasters/foodwater.asp.

PREPARING FOR BIOTERRORISM AND NUCLEAR ATTACKS

Bioterrorism involves the deliberate release of microorganisms or toxins derived from living organisms that cause disease or death to humans or animals or plants on which we depend for food. The pathogens most likely to be released into a community are anthrax, plague, smallpox, botulism, viral hemorrhagic fevers, and tularemia. These are category A because they pose a threat to national security. These organisms cause a high death rate and can cause public panic. They require special preparedness by the public health system. Emergency departments stockpile antibiotics and antidotes in case of need.

Chemical agents such as the Sarin gas used in the Tokyo subway can also be used by terrorists. Other poisonous gas use is possible in terrorist attacks as well.

Table 43–2 ***Communicable Diseases with Epidemic Potential (All Except Tetanus) in Natural Disasters***

DISEASE	TRANSMISSION	AGENT	CLINICAL FEATURES	INCUBATION PERIOD	DIAGNOSIS	TREATMENT	PREVENTION/CONTROL
WATERBORNE							
Cholera	Fecal/oral, contaminated water or food	*Vibrio cholerae* serogroups O1 or O139	Profuse watery diarrhea, vomiting	2 hr–5 days	Direct microscopic observation of *V. cholerae* in stool	Intensive rehydration therapy; antimicrobials based on sensitivity testing	Hand washing, proper handling of water/food and sewage disposal
Leptospirosis	Fecal/oral, contaminated water	*Leptospira* species	Sudden-onset fever, headache, chills, vomiting, severe myalgia	2–28 days	*Leptospira*-specific IgM serologic assay	Penicillin, amoxicillin, doxycycline, erythromycin, cephalosporins	Avoid entering contaminated water; safe water source
Hepatitis	Fecal/oral, contaminated water or food	Hepatitis A and E viruses	Jaundice, abdominal pain, nausea, diarrhea, fever, fatigue, and loss of appetite	15–50 days	Serologic assay detecting anti-HAV or anti-HEV IgM antibodies	Supportive care; hospitalization and barrier nursing for severe cases; close monitoring of pregnant women	Hand washing, proper handling of water/food and sewage disposal; hepatitis A vaccine
Bacillary dysentery	Fecal/oral, contaminated water or food	*Shigella dysenteriae* type 1	Malaise, fever, vomiting, blood and mucus in stool	12–96 hr	Suspect if bloody diarrhea; confirmation requires isolation of organism from stool	Nalidixic acid, ampicillin; hospitalization of seriously ill or malnourished; rehydration	Hand washing, proper handling of water/food and sewage disposal
Typhoid fever	Fecal/oral, contaminated water or food	*Salmonella typhi*	Sustained fever, headache, constipation	1–3 days	Cuture from blood, bone marrow, bowel fluids; rapid antibody tests	Ampicillin, co-trimoxazole, ciprofloxacin	Hand washing, proper handling of water/food and sewage disposal; mass vaccination in some settings
ACUTE RESPIRATORY							
Pneumonia	Person to person by airborne respiratory droplets	*Streptococcus pneumoniae, Haemophilus influenzae,* or viral	Cough, difficulty breathing, fast breathing, chest indrawing	1–3 days	Clinical presentation; culture respiratory secretions	Co-trimoxazole, chloramphenicol, ampicillin	Isolation; proper nutrition; if cause is *Streptococcus,* polyvalent vaccine to high-risk populations
DIRECT CONTACT							
Measles	Person to person by airborne respiratory droplets	Measles virus *(Morbillivirus)*	Rash, high fever, cough, runny nose, red and watery eyes; serious postmeasles complications (5%–10% of cases)—diarrhea, pneumonia, croup	10–12 days	Generally made by clinical observation	Supportive care; proper nutrition and hydration; vitamin A; control fever; antimicrobials in complicated cases with pneumonia, dysentery; treat conjunctivitis, keratitis	Rapid mass vaccination within 72 hr of initial case report (priority to high-risk groups if limited supply); vitamin A in children 6 mo–5 yr of age to prevent complications and reduce mortality

Bacterial meningitis (meningococcal meningitis)	Person to person by airborne respiratory droplets	*Neisseria meningitides* serogroups A, C, W135	Sudden-onset fever, rash, neck stiffness; altered consciousness; bulging fontanel in patients <1yr of age	10–12 days	Examination of CSF—elevated WBC count, protein; gram-negative diplococci	Penicillin, chloramphenicol, ampicillin, ceftriaxone, cefotaxime, co-trimoxazole; supportive therapy; diazepam for seizures	Rapid mass vaccination
WOUND-RELATED							
Tetanus	Soil	*Clostridium tetani*	Difficulty swallowing, lockjaw, muscle rigidity, spasms	2–10 days	Entirely clinical	Tetanus immune globulin	Thorough wound cleansing, tetanus vaccine
VECTOR-BORNE							
Malaria	Mosquito (*Anopheles* species)	*Plasmodium falciparum, P. vivax*	Fever, chills, sweats, head and body aches, nausea and vomiting	7–30 days	Parasites on blood smear observed using a microscope; rapid diagnostic assays if available	Chloroquine, sulfadoxine-pyrimethamine	Mosquito control; insecticide-treated nets, bedding, clothing
Dengue fever	Mosquito *(Aedes aegypti)*	Dengue virus-1, -2, -3, -4 *(Flavivirus)*	Sudden-onset severe flulike illness, high fever, severe headache, pain behind the eyes, and rash	4–7 days	Serum antibody testing with ELISA or rapid dot-blot technique	Intensive supportive therapy	Mosquito control; insecticide-treated nets, bedding, clothing
Japanese encephalitis	Mosquito (*Culex* species)	Japanese encephalitis virus *(Flavivirus)*	Quick-onset, headache, high fever, neck stiffness, stupor, disorientation, tremors	5–15 days	Serologic assay for JE virus IgM-specific antibodies in CSF or blood (acute phase)	Intensive supportive therapy	Mosquito control, isolation of cases, mass vaccination
Yellow fever	Mosquito *(Aedes, Haemogogus)*	Yellow fever virus *(Flavivirus)*	Fever, backache, headache, nausea, vomiting; toxic phase—jaundice, abdominal pain, kidney failure	3–6 days	Serologic assay for yellow fever virus antibodies	Intensive supportive therapy	Mosquito control, isolation of cases, mass vaccination

Key: *CSF,* cerebrospinal fluid; *ELISA,* enzyme-linked immunosorbent assay; *HAV,* hepatitis A virus; *HEV,* hepato-encephalomyelitis virus; *IgM,* immunoglobulin M; *JE,* Japanese encephalitis; *WBC,* white blood cell.

From Waring, S.C., & Brown, B.J. (2005). The threat of communicable diseases following natural disaster: A public health response. *Disaster Management and Response, 3*(2), 44–45.

CHEMICAL DISASTER

A chemical emergency can occur from a transportation accident, an explosion at a chemical plant, or a deliberate terrorist attack. Determining that a chemical attack or accident has occurred is difficult in that most chemical agents vaporize quickly from their liquid form. Many have no odor or have a familiar odor such as that of onion, garlic, or almonds. Indications that a chemical attack has occurred might include:

- Foglike or low-lying cloud suddenly appearing in the atmosphere
- Many dead birds, domestic animals, or insects within a particular area
- Many dead, dying, or sick people in an area or downwind from a suspicious cloud or fog
- EB An atypical, unexplained odor for the location (Stopford, 2006)

There are five categories of chemical agents that might be used in a terrorist attack: pulmonary agents, cyanide agents, vesicant agents, nerve agents, and incapacitating agents (Table 43–3). Chemicals are dispersed as a gas or liquid or are aerosolized and may contaminate skin, clothing, and any object they touch. The vapor from a liquid or solid toxic chemical is harmful as well.

Those exposed to toxic chemicals should be decontaminated in the field before transport to a medical facility. This is usually done with running water and scrubbing. Otherwise decontamination should be done outside the medical facility (Patient Teaching 43–2).

Depending on the chemical agent, there may be an antidote that can be used. One set of protocols for toxic chemical exposure are listed in Table 43–4. Each hospital should have a set of protocols in place. Symptomatic supportive care is supplied with oxygen and IV fluids. Keep the public informed of what to do in the event of a chemical disaster (Safety Alert 43–4).

NUCLEAR DISASTER

A nuclear disaster may be the result of an accident at a nuclear power plant, a disruption of a nuclear power plant by terrorists, or a nuclear or "dirty bomb" (one containing radioactive substances). Nurses need to know what to do in this type of event. The amount of damage to each person depends on the type of radiation, the dose received, the length of time of exposure, and the route of the exposure. **Time, distance, and shielding are key to the quantity of radiation an individual will receive.** The shorter the time of exposure, the farther away from the radiation source, and whether or not the person was shielded by materials that are impermeable to radiation rays are extremely pertinent (see Chapter 8). Individual characteristics among those exposed will have some bearing as well. Some types of radiation produce particles and other types produce rays. Which type is involved is impor-

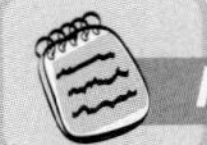

Patient Teaching 43–2

Removal and Disposal of Contaminated Clothing

If you are in an area where a chemical spill has occurred and the liquid or solid comes into contact with your clothing, you will need to both remove and bag contaminated clothing and decontaminate your skin. Chemicals will penetrate the clothing and contaminate the skin. If the exposure to a chemical was by vapor (gas), you will only need to remove your clothing and the source of the toxic vapor. Perform the following steps:

- Quickly take off clothing that has a chemical on it. Any clothing that has to be pulled over the head should be cut off instead of pulling it over the head.
- When helping others remove clothing, be careful not to touch any contaminated areas. Remove clothing as quickly as possible.
- As quickly as possible, wash any chemicals from your skin with large amounts of soap and water. If the eyes are burning, rinse with plain water for 10 to 15 minutes.
- If contact lenses are worn, remove them and place with the contaminated clothing.
- After washing yourself, carefully place all contaminated clothing and contact lenses into a plastic bag. Avoid touching contaminated areas, use tongs, a stick, or tool to place the clothing in the bag. Place the implement within the bag as well when finished using it.
- Thoroughly wash eyeglasses worn at time of chemical contamination before wearing again. Wash hands thoroughly again after cleaning glasses.
- Carefully seal the bag and place it within another plastic bag and seal that one.
- Dress in clothing that has not been contaminated (i.e., clothes that have been in the closet or dresser drawers).
- When health department or emergency personnel arrive, have them handle the bags and arrange for disposal.

Adapted from Centers for Disease Control and Prevention. (2003). Chemical Agents: Facts about Personal Cleaning and Disposal of Contaminated Clothing. Atlanta: Centers for Disease Control and Prevention. Retrived from www.bt.cdc.gov/planning/personalcleaningfacts.asp.

Safety Alert 43–4

Chemical Disaster!

When a chemical disaster has occurred in your neighborhood, you should do the following unless you are told to evacuate immediately:

- Close all windows and doors to the dwelling.
- Turn off all fans, heaters, and air conditioning systems.
- Close the fireplace damper.
- Wet some towels and jam them in the cracks under the doors. Use plastic garbage bags or plastic sheeting and duct tape to cover doors, windows and skylights, electrical outlets, exhaust fans or vents, window air conditioners, and heat registers.
- Go to an above-ground room with the fewest windows and doors.
- Take your emergency kit and a portable radio with you.
- Stay put until you are told all is safe or you are asked to evacuate.

Table 43–3 ***Chemical Agents: Symptoms and Care***

AGENT	CLINICAL PRESENTATION	DECONTAMINATION PROCEDURES	PERSONAL PROTECTIVE EQUIPMENT
Phosgene	*Ocular:* Severe pain, conjunctivitis and keratitis. *Dermal:* Pain and blanching with erythematous ring, followed by necrosis; absorption through skin can cause pulmonary edema. *Respiratory:* Immediate upper airway irritation; inhalation and systemic absorption may cause pulmonary edema, necrotizing bronchiolitis, and pulmonary thrombosis. *Gastrointestinal:* No human data available.	Decontamination immediately after skin and ocular exposure is the only way to prevent or decrease tissue damage because phosgene is absorbed within seconds. Negative-pressure room. Patients whose clothing or skin is contaminated with liquid or solid phosgene can contaminate health care providers by direct contact or through off-gassing vapor. Decontaminate before bringing into health care facility. Flush eyes with water 5–10 min. Do not cover eyes with bandages. All clothing is removed and skin washed with soap and water. If showers are available, showering with water alone is adequate. Place contaminated clothing and personal belongings in biohazard bag. Contain decontamination runoff.	Pressure-demand, self-contained breathing apparatus. Butyl rubber gloves, eye protection, and protective clothing.
Mustard (sulfur and nitrogen)	The sooner after exposure that symptoms occur, the more likely they are to progress and become severe. *Ocular:* Eyelid swelling and inflammation. *Dermal:* Erythema. *Pulmonary:* Laryngitis, shortness of breath, productive cough. *Gastrointestinal:* Do not induce vomiting.	Decontaminate before bringing into health care facility. Negative-pressure room. Contain decontamination runoff. Patients whose clothing or skin is contaminated with liquid or solid mustard can contaminate health care providers by direct contact or through off-gassing vapor. Place contaminated clothing and personal belongings in biohazard bags.	Pressure-demand, self-contained breathing apparatus. Butyl rubber gloves, eye protection, and protective clothing.
Lewisite and mustard-lewisite mixture	Damages skin, eyes, and airways by direct contact. *Dermal:* Pain and skin irritation within seconds to minutes after contact; erythema and blisters within several hours; starts as small blister in center of erythematous area that expands to include entire inflamed area. *Ocular:* Vapor causes pain and blepharospasm; edema of conjunctiva and eyelids; high doses may cause corneal damage; liquid lewisite causes severe eye damage on contact. *Respiratory:* Burning nasal pain, epistaxis, sinus pain, laryngitis, cough, and dyspnea may occur; necrosis can cause local airway obstruction. *Gastrointestinal:* Inhalation or ingestion may cause nausea and vomiting. *Cardiovascular:* High-dose exposure may cause capillary permeability and subsequent intravascular fluid loss, hypovolemia, and organ congestion. *Renal:* High levels of lewisite may cause renal failure caused by hypotension. *Hepatic:* High levels may cause hepatic necrosis and hypoperfusion.	Decontaminate before bringing into health care facility. Negative-pressure room. Contain decontamination runoff. To significantly reduce tissue damage, the eyes and skin must be decontaminated within 1–2 min after exposure. Place contaminated clothing and personal belongings in biohazard bags.	Pressure-demand, self-contained breathing apparatus. Butyl rubber gloves, eye protection, and protective clothing.

Data from Center for the Study of Bioterrorism & Emerging Infections. (2002). Bioterrorism agent fact sheets. (Retrieved December 18, 2001 from www.bioterrorism.slu.edu); and McKinney, W., Bia, F., and Stewart, C. (2000). Bioterrorism: An update for clinicians, pharmacists and emergency management planners. In Emergency Medicine Consensus Reports. Atlanta: American Health Consultants.

Continued

Table 43–3 Chemical Agents: Symptoms and Care—cont'd

AGENT	CLINICAL PRESENTATION	DECONTAMINATION PROCEDURES	PERSONAL PROTECTIVE EQUIPMENT
Nerve gases	*Respiratory:* Bronchial constriction and spasm; severe respiratory distress or apnea; miosis; rhinorrhea. *Gastrointestinal:* Do not induce emesis.	Decontaminate before bringing into health care facility. Negative-pressure room. Contain decontamination runoff. Patients whose clothing or skin is contaminated with liquid or solid nerve agents can contaminate health care providers by direct contact or through off-gassing vapor. If exposed to liquid nerve agent, irrigate eyes 5–10 min with water or saline within minutes of exposure to limit injury. If exposed to liquid nerve agent, cut and remove all clothing and wash skin immediately with soap and water. If shower is not available, wash with 0.5% bleach solution. If exposed to vapor only, remove outer clothing and wash exposed skin with soap and water or 0.5% bleach solution. Place contaminated clothing and personal belongings in biohazard bags.	Pressure-demand, self-contained breathing apparatus. Butyl rubber gloves, eye protection, and protective clothing.
Cyanide	*Cardiovascular:* Dysrhythmias caused by acidosis. *Inhalation exposure:* Refer to Table 43–4 for treatment protocols. *Dermal:* Chemical burns may occur; treat as thermal burns. *Ocular:* Irrigate for at least 15 min; corneal injuries may occur. *Ingestion:* Abrupt onset of syncope, seizures, coma, gasping respirations, and cardiovascular collapse, causing death within minutes.	Decontaminate before bringing into health care facility. Negative-pressure room. Contain decontamination runoff. Patients whose clothing or skin is contaminated with cyanide can contaminate health care providers by direct contact or through off-gassing vapor. Patients exposed only to vapor require no decontamination. Avoid dermal contact with gastric contents that may contain ingested cyanide-containing materials. Remove contaminated clothing and wash with soap and water.	Pressure-demand, self-contained breathing apparatus. Butyl rubber gloves, eye protection, and protective clothing. Cyanide penetrates most rubbers, but butyl rubber provides good skin protection for a short period.
Chlorine	Acute exposure can cause coughing, eye and nose irritation, tearing. Airway constriction, pulmonary edema and hemoptysis may occur. *Dermal:* Skin irritation, burning pain, inflammation, and blisters. Treat as thermal burns. Liquefied, compressed chlorine can cause frostbite. Treat by rewarming affected areas in a water bath of 102°–108° F (38.8°–42.2° C) for 20–30 min. Continue until flushing has returned to affected area. *Ocular:* Do not irrigate frostbitten eyes; if exposed to vapor, irrigate for at least 15 min; check for corneal damage.	Health care providers are at minimal risk of secondary contamination from patients who have been exposed to chlorine gas. Clothing or skin soaked with industrial strength bleach or similar solutions may be corrosive to personnel and may release chlorine gas. Remove contaminated clothing and wash with soap and water. Flush exposed skin and hair with plain water for 2–3 min; then wash twice with soap and water.	

tant. Particles will adhere to airborne dust particles, may be inhaled, and will settle on clothes, crops, water supplies, and other surfaces.

Decontamination of those exposed is essential before treatment to protect health care personnel and the safety of the health care facility. **Decontamination** is done with showering and scrubbing the skin. Radiation exposure to rays does not require decontamination, although it can cause serious health effects or death as it does internal damage to tissues. However,

Table 43–4 ***Treatment Protocols for Specific Chemical Agents***

PHOSGENE PROTOCOL
- Restrict fluids
- Obtain chest x-rays and blood gases
- Oxygen/PEEP

MUSTARD PROTOCOL
- Airway obstruction?
  - Tracheostomy
- Large burns?
  - Establish IV: Do not push fluids as with thermal burns
  - Drain vesicules: Unroof large blisters and irrigate with topical antibiotics
- Treat other symptoms
  - Antibiotic eye ointment
  - Morphine PRN

LEWISITE PROTOCOL
- Treat affected skin with British anti-lewisite (BAL) ointment, if available
- Treat affected eyes with BAL ointment, if available
- Treat pulmonary symptoms
  - BAL in oil, 0.5 mL/25 lb/body weight to max. of 4 mL, deep IM; repeat q 4 hr × 3
  - Morphine PRN
- Severe poisoning: Shorten interval for BAL injections to q 2 hr

CYANIDE PROTOCOL
- Administer cyanide poisoning kit for significant cyanide toxicity and persistent high anion gap metabolic acidosis
- Use clinical response to determine administration
- Give amyl nitrite until IV access obtained, then give sodium nitrite followed by sodium thiosulfate
  - Amyl nitrite:
    - Crush 1 or 2 ampules in gauze and hold close to the nose (may also place in the lip of the face mask or within the Ambu bag)
    - Inhale for 30 sec/min until IV access is obtained
  - Sodium nitrite
    - Adults: Give 300 mg (10 mL) IV as a 3% solution over 5–20 min
    - Children: Give 0.19–0.33 mL/kg
    - Dilute and infuse slowly if hypotensive
    - May repeat once at half the initial dose within 30–60 min
  - Sodium thiosulfate
    - Adults: Give 12.5 g (50 mL) IV as a 25% solution over 10–15 min
    - Children: Give 0.95–1.85 mL/kg
    - May be given half the initial dose after 30–60 min

NERVE AGENT PROTOCOL
1. Severe respiratory distress?
   - **No:** Go to step 6
   - **Yes:** Intubate and ventilate
     - Atropine
       - Adults: 6 mg IM or IV
       - Infants/children: 15 mg/kg
     - 2-PAM C1
       - Adults: 600–1000 mg IM or slow IV
       - Infants/children: 15 mg/kg
2. Major secondary symptoms?
   - **No:** Go to step 6
   - **Yes**
     - Atropine
       - Adults: 4 mg IM or IV
       - Infants/children: 15–25 mcg/kg
     - 2-PAM C1
       - Adults: 600–1000 mg IM or slow IV
       - Infants/children: 15–25 mg/kg
   - Open IV line
3. Repeat atropine as needed
4. Repeat 2-PAM C1 as needed
   - Adults: 1 g IV over 20–30 min
   - Repeat q 1 hr × 3 PRN
   - Infants/children: 15 mg/kg
5. Seizures
   - **No:** Go to step 6
   - **Yes:** Diazepam 10 mg slow IVP
6. Reevaluate q 3–5 min; if symptoms worsen, repeat from step 3

CHLORINE PROTOCOL
- Dyspnea?
  - Oxygen by mask
  - Chest x-ray
- Bronchodilators
- Consider phosgene poisoning
- Give supportive therapy and treat other problems

Key: *IM,* intramuscular(ly); *IV,* intravenous(ly); *IVP,* intravenous push; *2-PAM C1,* prilodoxime chloride; *PEEP,* positive end-expiratory pressure; *PRN,* as needed.
Adapted from Newberry, L. (Ed.). (2003). *Sheehy's Emergency Nursing: Principles and Practice* (5th ed., p. 195). St. Louis: Mosby.

if the exposure is from a terrorist attack, it would not be immediately known if the exposure to radiation was in the form of particles or rays. Therefore, everyone exposed, or suspected of being exposed, will need to be decontaminated. Personnel performing triage and decontamination must be protected from radioactive particulates and contaminated dust (Figure 43–3). Usually, specially trained units supply personnel to handle decontamination. If such a unit is not available, health care personnel may be involved in decontamination procedures. Minimal protective equipment includes protective gear for clothes and shoes, double gloves (one under clothing and taped to the skin, and one over the clothing cuffs), and a high-efficiency particulate arresting (HEPA) air-filtering respirator mask with a full facepiece. If no such mask is available, a fit-tested N-95 respirator mask such as used for tuberculosis precautions is better than no mask. Radiation detection badges are worn underneath the protective clothing. Each person will be assessed after disposing of the protective garb in specially marked biohazard containers to make certain radiation contamination has been eliminated (Shields, 2003).

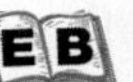

Exposure to high doses of external radiation rays that penetrate the body even for a few minutes may result in acute radiation sickness syndrome. Three subsyndromes may be seen depending on the dose of

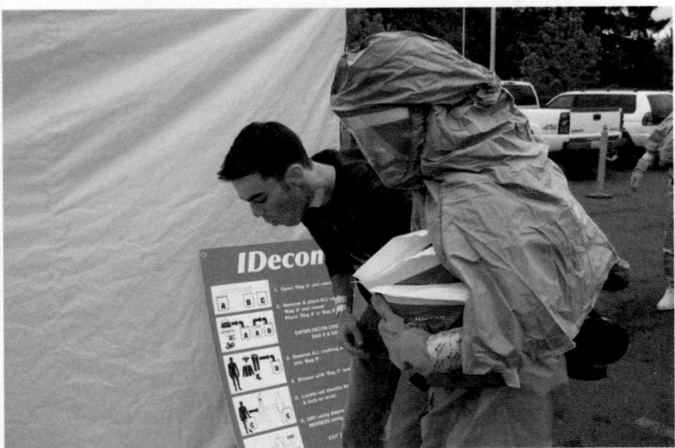

FIGURE 43–3 Assisting a victim of a radioactive event to a decontamination showering area. (This was a drill.)

radiation received: bone marrow syndrome, gastrointestinal syndrome, and cardiovascular/central nervous system syndrome. Bone marrow tissue is affected first, then with increased dosage, the gastrointestinal lining is affected. The person who receives a high enough dose of radiation to cause cardiovascular/central nervous system syndrome will experience effects on the bone marrow and gastrointestinal system as well. The effects are progressive as the dosage increases. Signs and symptoms may include nausea, vomiting, diarrhea, leukopenia, signs of bleeding or hemorrhage, lethargy, confusion, ataxia, convulsions, hair loss, and respiratory complications with fever and pneumonia (Table 43–5). Treatment of life-threatening injuries takes precedence over the radiologic damage (Fell-Carlson, 2003a).

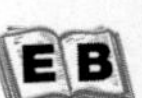

Table 43–5 ***Acute Radiation Syndrome***

			SUBCLINICAL RANGE	WHOLE BODY RADIATION FROM EXTERNAL RADIATION OR INTERNAL ABSORPTION			
				SUBLETHAL RANGE		LETHAL RANGE	
PHASE OF SYNDROME	FEATURE	0–100 RAD	100–200 RAD	200–600 RAD	600–800 RAD	600–3000 RAD	>3000 RAD
Initial or prodromal	Nausea, vomiting	None	5%–50%	50%–100%	75%–100%	90%–100%	100%
	Time of onset		3–6 hr	2–4 hr	1–2 hr	<1 hr	<1 hr
	Duration		<24 hr	<24 hr	<48 hr	<48 hr	<48 hr
	Lymphocyte count/μL			<1000 at 24 hr	<500 at 24 hr		
	CNS function	No impairment	No impairment	Routine task performance; cognitive impairment for 6–20 hr	Simple and routine task performance; cognitive impairment for >24 hr	Progressive incapacitation occurs	Progressive incapacitation occurs
"Manifest illness" (obvious illness)	Signs and symptoms	None	Moderate leukopenia	Severe leukopenia, purpura, hemorrhage Pneumonia Hair loss after 300 rad	Severe leukopenia, purpura, hemorrhage	Diarrhea, fever, electrolyte disturbance	Convulsions, ataxia, tremor, lethargy
	Time of onset		>2 wk	2 days–2 wk	2 days–2 wk	2–3 days	2–3 days
	Critical period		None	4–6 wk	4–6 wk	5–14 days	1–48 hr
	Organ system	None		Hematopoietic and respiratory (mucosal) systems	Hematopoietic and respiratory (mucosal) systems	GI tract Mucosal systems	CNS
Hospitalization	%	0%	<5%	90%	100%	100%	100%
Fatality	%	0%	0%	0%–80%	90%–100%	90%–100%	90%–100%
Time to death				3 wk–3 mo	3 wk–3 mo	1–2 wk	1–2 days

Key: *CNS,* central nervous system; *GI,* gastrointestinal.
From Employee Education System for the Office of Public Health and Environmental Hazards, Department of Veterans Affairs. (2003). (2006). *Pocket Guide for Responders to Ionizing Radiation Terrorism*. Bethesda, MD: Armed Forces Radiobiology Research Institute. Retrieved from www.afrri.usuhs.mil/www/outreach/pocketguide.htm.

Once injuries are managed and decontamination is complete, nursing care is supportive with strict infection control procedures in place. Maintaining an accurate record of the onset and duration of the clinical symptoms is essential for the physician to decide on treatment strategies. Record hair loss, inflamed mucosa, and locations of erythema hourly and, if possible, record skin symptoms with a camera. Serial blood counts will be performed. Nausea is treated with antiemetics. Blood problems may be treated with blood component transfusions.

When the radiation exposure has been in the form of particulates that have entered the body, treatment depends on the type of radiologic substance. The four types of agents used to reduce the radiation damage by reducing exposure to the radiologic substance are chelating agents, isotope-specific blocking agents, mobilizing agents, and diluting agents.

Chelating agents bind with the radioactive material and allow it to be excreted without being absorbed into the tissues. Examples of chelating agents used are edetate calcium disodium (ethylenediamine tetraacetic acid; EDTA) and diethylenetriamine pentaacetic acid (DTPA). Radioactive iodine exposure is treated with potassium iodide, an isotope-specific blocking agent, to prevent the thyroid cancer this type of radiation causes. Mobilizing agents are used when radioactive material has been ingested. Examples include emetics, gastric lavage, cathartics, and enemas, all of which reduce the time the radiologic material is in the gastrointestinal tract. Diluting agents reduce the concentration of the radioactive material. Water is the best example of a diluting agent. Special precautions need to be used when administering a mobilizing or diluting agent as the fluids produced could be radiologically contaminated.

BIOLOGIC DISASTER

Many biologic agents could be used in a terrorist attack. These agents are the most lethal and contagious. Biologic agents are divided into three groups (Centers for Disease Control and Prevention [CDC], 2001; Persell et al., 2002):

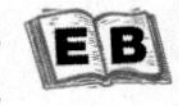

- *Category A agents:* Easily disseminated, and some may be transmitted from person to person as well. These could cause mass casualties and require a well-organized and extensive health care system response for management. Examples are anthrax, smallpox, botulism, plague, tularemia, and viral hemorrhagic fever (Table 43–6).
- *Category B agents:* Delivered through water and food sources. These produce moderate amounts of illness and low death rates. Public health department action is needed for management. Examples are Q fever, brucellosis, glanders, ricin toxin, epsilon toxin of *Clostridium perfringens,* and *Staphylococcus aureus* enterotoxin B.

Table 43–6 *Agents of Bioterrorism: Category A*

PATHOGEN AND DESCRIPTION	CLINICAL MANIFESTATIONS	TRANSMISSIBILITY	TREATMENT
ANTHRAX *(Bacillus anthracis)*			
Inhalational Bacterial spores multiply in the alveoli Toxins cause hemorrhage and destruction of lung tissue High mortality rate	Incubation period: 1–2 days to 6 wk Abrupt onset Dyspnea, diaphoresis, fever, cough, chest pain, septicemia, shock, meningitis, respiratory failure, widened mediastinum (seen on chest x-ray)	No person-to-person spread Found in nature and most commonly infects wild and domestic hoofed animals Spread through direct contact with bacteria and its spores Spores are dormant, encapsulated bacteria that become active when they enter a living host	Antibiotics prevent systemic manifestations Effective only if treated early Ciprofloxacin (Cipro) is the treatment of choice Penicillin Doxycycline Postexposure prophylaxis for 30 days (if vaccine not available) Vaccine has limited availability
Cutaneous 95% of anthrax infections Least lethal form Spores enter skin through cuts or abrasions Handling of contaminated animal skin products Toxins destroy surrounding tissue	Incubation period: up to 12 days Small papule resembles an insect bite Advances to a depressed, black ulcer Swollen lymph nodes in adjacent areas Edema		
Gastrointestinal Ingestion of contaminated, undercooked meat Intestinal lesions in ileum or cecum Acute inflammation of intestines	Nausea, vomiting, anorexia, hematemesis, diarrhea, abdominal pain, ascites, sepsis		

From Lewis, S.M., Heitkemper, M.M., Dirksen, S.R., et al. (2007). *Medical-Surgical Nursing: Assessment and Management of Clinical Problems* (7th ed.). St. Louis: Mosby.

Continued

Table 43–6 *Agents of Bioterrorism: Category A—cont'd*

PATHOGEN AND DESCRIPTION	CLINICAL MANIFESTATIONS	TRANSMISSIBILITY	TREATMENT
BOTULISM *(Clostridium botulinum)*			
Spore-forming anaerobe Found in soil Seven different toxins Lethal bacterial neurotoxin Can die within 24 hr	Incubation period: 12–72 hr Abdominal cramps, diarrhea, nausea, vomiting, cranial nerve palsies (diplopia, dysarthria, dysphonia, dysphagia), skeletal muscle paralysis, respiratory failure	Spread through air or food No person-to-person spread Improperly canned foods Contaminated wound	Induce vomiting Enemas Antitoxin Mechanical ventilation Penicillin No vaccine available Toxin can be inactivated by heating food or drink to 85° C for at least 5 min
PLAGUE *(Yersinia pestis)*			
Bacteria found in rodents and fleas Forms Bubonic (most common) Pneumonic Septicemic (most deadly)	Incubation period: 2–4 days Hemoptysis, cough, high fever, chills, myalgia, headache, respiratory failure, lymph node swelling	Direct person-to-person spread Transmitted through flea bites Ingestion of contaminated meat	Antibiotics only effective if administered immediately Drug of choice: streptomycin or gentamicin Vaccine under development Hospitalization Isolation for containment
SMALLPOX			
Variola major and minor viruses United States ended routine vaccination in 1971 Global eradication declared in 1980	Incubation period: 7–17 days Sudden onset of symptoms Fever, headache, myalgia, malaise, back pain Lesions progress from macules to papules to pustular vesicles	Highly contagious Direct person-to-person spread Transmitted in airborne droplets Transmitted by handling contaminated materials	No known cure Cidofovir (Vistide) under testing Isolation for containment Vaccine available for those exposed Vaccinia immune globulin (VIG) available
TULAREMIA *(Francisella tularensis)*			
Bacterial infectious disease of animals Mortality rate about 35% without treatment	Incubation period: 3–10 days Sudden onset Fever, swollen lymph nodes, fatigue, sore throat, weight loss, pneumonia, pleural effusion, ulcerated sore from tick bite	No person-to-person spread Aerosol or intradermal route Spread by rabbits and ticks Contaminated food, air, water	Gentamicin treatment of choice Streptomycin, doxycycline, and ciprofloxacin are alternatives Vaccine in developmental stage
HEMORRHAGIC FEVER			
Caused by several viruses, including Marburg, Lassa, Junin, and Ebola Ebola virus is life threatening	Fever, conjunctivitis, headache, malaise, prostration, hemorrhage of tissues and organs, nausea, vomiting, hypotension, organ failure	Carried by rodents and mosquitos Direct person-to-person spread by body fluids Virus can be aerosolized	No intramuscular injections No antiplatelet drugs Isolation for containment Ribavirin (Virazole) effective in some cases No known treatment available

- *Category C:* Agents that have not been weaponized as yet, but have the potential for high morbidity and mortality. These agents are plentiful and easy to produce and disseminate. Examples include *Hantavirus,* tick-borne encephalitis, yellow fever, and multidrug-resistant tuberculosis.

Symptoms from exposure to a biologic agent are not immediate. There are various incubation periods. So, unless someone knows that he has been exposed to a strange powder or substance, decontamination does not take place. Nurses particularly need basic knowledge about the category A agents because they are easily disseminated and easily spread from person to person.

Anthrax

Anthrax is caused by the gram-positive bacteria *Bacillus anthracis,* which forms spores. It is primarily a disease of sheep and cows. Animal vaccination programs have controlled naturally occurring anthrax in the United States. There are three forms of the disease: cutaneous, gastrointestinal, and inhalational. Aerosolized inhalable anthrax is most likely to be used for a terrorist attack. The greatest chance of inhaling the spores after aerosolization is during the first day after the event, before the particles hit the ground. Symptoms in those who have inhaled the spores will resemble a nonspecific influenza at first. A rapid downhill progression is then seen with respiratory failure, shock, and possibly death over a 2- to 5-day period. Features that differentiate anthrax illness from flu are shortness of breath, a nonproductive cough, chest discomfort, myalgia, and fatigue. The lack of a sore throat and rhinorrhea and the appearance of nausea and vomiting may occur with flu as well. Treatment is with ciprofloxacin (Cipro) or doxycycline (Vibramycin) for 14 days. Antibiotics are adjusted after culture and sensitivity results are known. Treatment continues for 60 days if infection is proven as the disease can continue to develop from germinating spores up to that time. Otherwise prophylaxis lasts for 10 to 14 days when cultures are completed and results obtained. Other care is supportive for respiration, fluid and electrolyte balance, and comfort. Extended precautions are not necessary as anthrax is not transmissible from person to person. Further information is available at www.bt.cdc.gov/agent/anthrax.

Botulism

Botulism is caused by the botulinum toxins produced by *Clostridium botulinum*. Seven different toxins may be produced. There are three forms of botulism that adults get: food-borne, wound, and inhalational. Foods can become contaminated with botulism spores when canned or processed under conditions favorable for toxin production (e.g., insufficient heat). Toxin production by spores contaminating tissue in a wound can occur. Inhalational botulism does not occur naturally and would most likely indicate a terrorist attack.

Double vision, drooping eyelids, and difficulty swallowing and speaking may be the early symptoms of botulism. A triad of symptoms is classic for the disorder:

- Symmetrical descending flaccid paralysis progressing to respiratory weakness
- Absence of fever
- Alertness and orientation without sensory deficits

Respiratory support may require intubation and mechanical ventilation. If a large number of persons are infected, the community health care resources would be taxed to provide adequate care for all. Treatment is with botulinum antitoxin if the toxin type is A or B. The CDC and public health departments stock these antitoxins. Early treatment is required as the antitoxin does not reverse the muscular paralysis that has already occurred. The adult antitoxin costs about $25,000. Supportive therapy may be needed for several weeks until new synapses can grow to replace those damaged by the toxins. The website www.bt.cdc.gov/agent/botulism provides a summary of botulism information (Bioterrorism Institute, 2005).

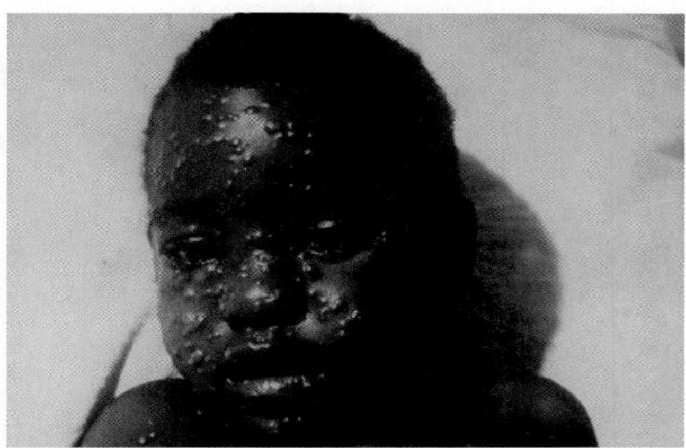

FIGURE 43–4 Face lesions on a boy with smallpox.

Plague

Plague is caused by a gram-negative bacillus, *Yersinia pestis.* It is naturally transmitted by infected fleas that bite rodents or people. Pneumonic plague is the most likely type to be spread by a terrorist attack with aerosolized plague organisms. Fortunately, plague bacilli are killed by sunlight and remain viable in aerosolized form for only about an hour after release. Clinical signs are an abrupt onset of pneumonia with bloody sputum *(hemoptysis)* that follows a rapidly progressive course. Disseminated intravascular coagulation (DIC) can develop leading to multiorgan failure. Death is likely within 24 hours of infection if treatment is not started.

Gentamicin (Garamycin) is the drug of first choice for this organism. Ciprofloxacin and doxycycline are used to treat pneumonic plague and are given for 7 to 10 days. Plague can be transmitted from person to person, and respiratory droplet precautions along with standard precautions are necessary until 48 hours after treatment has been initiated.

The bubonic form of plague starts with skin infection and progresses to the lymph nodes. It is transmitted by infected flea bites. This form of plague is not likely to be used as a biologic weapon.

Smallpox

Smallpox is caused by variola virus. It is communicable, has no known effective treatment, and has a high mortality rate. The disease was declared eradicated worldwide in 1980. There are still laboratory strains of the virus in some laboratories. Because it is so lethal and highly contagious, it is listed as a category A agent.

Smallpox has an average incubation period of 12 to 14 days. Symptoms begin with fever for 1 to 4 days and then a rash occurs. High fever may be accompanied by headache, backache, malaise, vomiting, and delirium. The rash contains firm, deep-seated vesicles or pustules all in the same stage of development on any one area of the body (Figure 43–4). The rash starts on the buccal and pharyngeal mucosa, spreads to the face, hands, and forearms, and then spreads to the rest of the body over several days. A cough may develop. Lesions progress

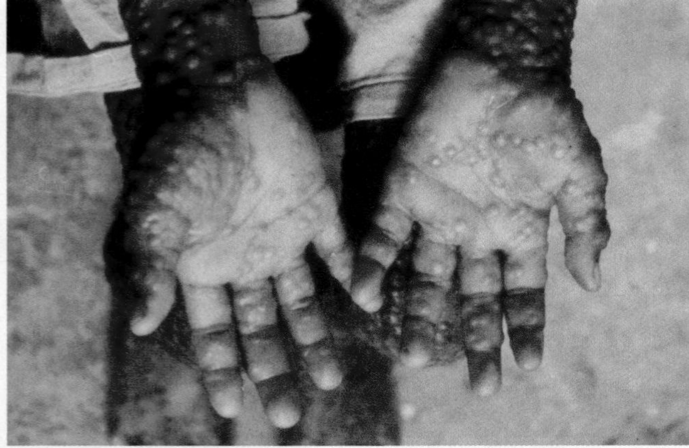

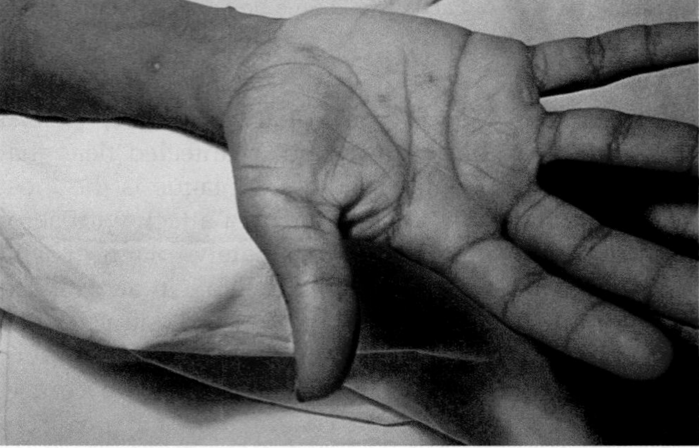

FIGURE **43–5** Comparison of smallpox and chickenpox lesions. **A**, Smallpox. **B**, Chickenpox.

from macules to papules to vesicles to pustules to scabs, with each stage lasting 1 or 2 days. It must be differentiated from chickenpox. With chickenpox, the lesions appear before illness symptoms and are usually concentrated on the trunk initially. Chickenpox lesions are usually more superficial and are "flimsy" rather than firm as in smallpox. Chickenpox lesions do not usually occur on the palms and the soles of the feet; smallpox lesions do occur in those areas (Figure 43–5). Chickenpox lesions are often in various stages within the same area of the body, whereas smallpox lesions are all in the same stage within a body area.

Smallpox is communicable from the onset of rash until all scabs have separated from the skin. Patients should be treated with strict Airborne Infection Isolation and Contact Precautions, and placed in a negative-pressure room with a HEPA-filtered exhaust system. All linens and gowns *must* be incinerated to prevent spread of the disease (Bioterrorism Institute, 2005).

Although there is no treatment for smallpox, receiving the smallpox vaccine within 4 days of exposure can reduce the severity of the disease. The vaccine is not available in large amounts, and for that reason isolation and quarantine of infected patients will be the most likely course of action. Smallpox vaccine has significant possible side effects. If health care workers are to be vaccinated, you will receive all the necessary information about the vaccine and how to take care of the vaccination site. Medical management is supportive, with antimicrobial drug treatment for secondary infection of lesion sites, fluid and electrolyte replacement, and nutritional therapy. Those vaccinated against smallpox before 1972 have no immunity now. The vaccine provides immunity for only 3 to 5 years, but those who had multiple vaccinations may have some residual immunity.

? *Think Critically About . . .* Can you explain to someone how to distinguish smallpox lesions from those of chickenpox?

Tularemia

Tularemia is caused by a gram-negative coccobacillus, *Francisella tularensis.* It is a vector-borne illness that is transmitted by an infected tick, mosquito, or deer fly bite, by direct exposure to contaminated animal tissues and fluids, or by ingestion of contaminated food or water. A variety of small mammals are natural reservoirs of the organism. It is seen throughout the United States except in Hawaii. If aerosolized, it could be inhaled, and this is the most likely form for a terrorist attack. The disease is not spread by person-to-person contact.

Tularemia occurs in three different forms: cutaneous, pneumonic, and typhoidal. The pneumonic form is the one most likely to occur in a terrorist attack. The pneumonia caused by the inhaled form is difficult to differentiate from other pneumonias. Symptoms include abrupt onset of fever, chills, headache, muscle aches, nonproductive cough, and sore throat. Laboratory testing can establish the correct diagnosis.

Treatment or prophylaxis is with streptomycin and gentamicin (Garamycin), the drugs of first choice. Doxycycline (Vibramycin), chloramphenicol (Chloromycetin), and ciprofloxacin (Cipro) may also be used. The course of treatment should extend through 10 to 14 days depending on the drug used. Tularemia is fatal if not treated with the proper antibiotics. Standard Precautions are used, but the inhalational form is not transmitted person to person and no other extended precautions are necessary. A vaccine for protection from tularemia is under review by the U.S. Food and Drug Administration.

Viral Hemorrhagic Fevers

The hemorrhagic fevers are a group of illnesses caused by four families of viruses: arenaviruses, filoviruses, flaviviruses, and bunyaviruses. The viruses, which are within the category A agents, cause Ebola, Marburg, and Lassa hemorrhagic fevers. Junin, Machupo, Guanarito, and Sabia hemorrhagic fevers occur more frequently in the Southern Hemisphere. There are no vaccines available for these diseases. These occur in different geographic parts of the world. Reservoirs for the viruses are rodents and arthropods. Human infection usually occurs by being bitten by an infected arthropod, by contact with infected animal carcasses, or by inhaling aerosolized rodent excreta. Once contracted, the virus can be transmitted from person to person by blood and body fluids. Contact and Airborne Infection Isolation Precautions are necessary. Only special biosafety laboratories can test for the viral hemorrhagic fevers. Such tests are performed at the CDC. It is thought that an aerosolized form of Ebola or Marburg virus might be used for a terrorist attack. Travelers from a region experiencing an outbreak could also carry the virus into this country (Centers for Disease Control and Prevention, 2006b).

The incubation period is from 2 to 42 days, depending on the virus, and there is a prodromal syndrome lasting less than a week. Signs and symptoms are marked fever, fatigue, dizziness, muscle aches, and loss of strength. Symptoms may progress to abdominal pain, nonbloody diarrhea, weakness, and exhaustion. Later bleeding begins, starting with bleeding under the skin and petechiae and progressing to spontaneous bleeding and DIC. Many body systems are affected. Hypotension, conjunctivitis, pharyngitis, plus skin rash may reflect increasing capillary permeability. Shock, nervous system malfunction, seizures, delirium, and coma may occur. Mortality rates can be very high with Ebola, but are not always so with the other viruses.

There is no specific treatment for these hemorrhagic fevers; treatment is supportive. The antiviral ribavirin may be useful in treating Lassa fever. Contact and Airborne Expanded Precautions are essential. Double gloves, impermeable gowns, leg and shoe coverings, face shields, eye protection, and an N-95 mask are required for patient contact. A negative-pressure room is desirable.

Prevention measures include use of insect repellant, bed nets, window screens, and proper clothing and eradication of rodents from living spaces. Mosquito abatement is performed in areas of outbreak when possible. All linens and gowns used for patient care must be incinerated.

NURSE'S ROLE IN BIOTERRORISM PREPAREDNESS AND RESPONSE

The nurse's role includes:

- Recognizing clusters of cases or unusual cases suggestive of biologic terrorism
- Promptly evaluating and assisting with medical management
- Promptly communicating with the local public health department and infection control department
- Working closely with law enforcement, emergency management, public health, and other government agencies

Recognizing a Bioterrorism Event

The most likely bioterrorism agents are presented in Table 43–6. Many of these agents do not produce symptoms right away. Certain signs or events may present a warning that a bioterrorism attack has occurred. Some of the signs include:

- Rapidly progressing flulike illness, particularly in the young and previously healthy
- Rapidly progressive respiratory illness, especially in young, previously healthy people
- Unusual or extensive rashes, especially if preceded by flulike symptoms
- Flaccid muscle paralysis
- Severe bleeding disorders
- A large group of patients with food-borne illness
- Sudden death of many animals in the community (Bioterrorism Institute, 2005)

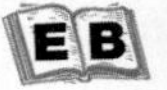

Nursing Management

When such patterns are discovered, implement the hospital and community response plan. **Strictly adhere to infection control procedures and policies.**

If your assessment has aroused suspicion of a bioterrorism event, ask these questions:

- Was there a sudden onset of severe respiratory or gastrointestinal problems?
- Has the illness progressed rapidly?
- Has the patient been healthy otherwise?
- Are others among the patient's family, friends, or colleagues ill?

If the answers indicate that an infectious agent is present, immediately take the following steps:

- Notify your supervisor and the infection control department of the situation.
- Put a surgical mask on any patient who is coughing.
- Pay strict attention to Standard Precautions and hand hygiene and encourage the patient and family to do the same.
- Don an N-95 or P-100 respirator mask (one certified by the Occupational Safety and Health Administration [OSHA]).
- If indicated, isolate the patient in a negative-pressure room; obtain specimens for laboratory testing.
- Use all recommended personal protective equipment whenever caring for the patient and pay strict attention to Standard and Expanded Precautions.

When a known terrorist airborne event has occurred and victims are triaged to the hospitals and emergency field medical units, they will need to be decontaminated before being brought into the medical facility. Outside shower areas will be set up to accomplish the decontamination. Whether the agent used in the attack is biologic or nuclear, the outside of the body must be thoroughly scrubbed. Personnel in biohazard suits handle this task (Figure 43–6). Clothing must be removed and sealed in plastic biohazard bags to prevent contamination of others. The skin should be scrubbed in every area with warm soapy water for at

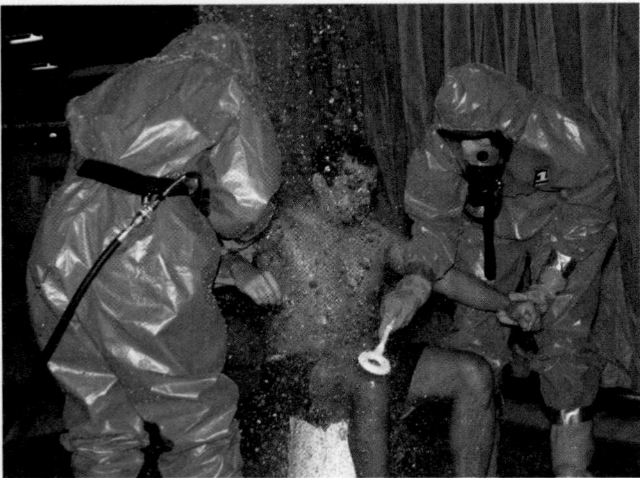

FIGURE 43–6 A volunteer undergoes decontamination during a disaster drill. Copyright © AP/WIDE WORLD PHOTOS.

least 30 seconds. The hair should be soaped and shampooed several times (Bioterrorism Institute, 2005).

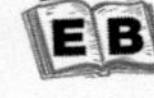

A calm demeanor will be needed as people will be very scared, anxious, and possibly hysterical. Giving firm directions with a kindly tone can help. Let people know what will happen next. Active listening and assisting with problem solving provided needed psychosocial support. Provide assistance with coordinating the locating of children and other family members if a family has been separated. Psychological support should be integrated into care. Direct people to the available support services needed to meet physical and psychological needs.

Debriefing

After disaster mobilization is no longer needed, there will be a **debriefing** for the personnel involved in handling disaster management and for the health care personnel.

Critical incident stress debriefing (CISD) teams provide sessions for small groups of personnel to help with the promotion of effective coping strategies. These people are trained in crisis management and psychological care. After the turmoil and the emotional impact of the disaster, including its aftermath, personnel may find it difficult to return to their normal routine. Their lives have been disrupted, and each person involved has gone through considerable stress in trying to meet the needs of others. Without intervention, some may develop post-traumatic stress disorder, which can have many psychological and physical effects that interfere with the person's ability to function. A member of the CISD team may meet with the nurses. A session usually lasts 1 to 3 hours. There is strict confidentiality of any information shared during the sessions. Unconditional acceptance of the thoughts and feelings expressed by individuals is one of the ground rules for the group. Participants are educated about self-care concepts and given suggested coping strategies that can be used immediately.

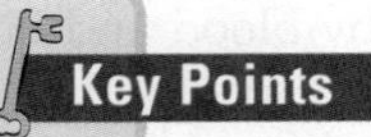

Key Points

- Most communities have a disaster plan in place; small unincorporated rural areas may not have such a plan of their own.
- It is important to know the facility's disaster plan.
- The Department of Homeland Security, Office of Disaster Preparedness, Office of Emergency Services, Federal Emergency Management Agency, local emergency preparedness department, the Red Cross, the Salvation Army, local law enforcement, the military, and fire fighters all work together when a major disaster occurs.
- Nurses should be proactive in encouraging people to stock a disaster kit at home.
- Nurses should help teach the public about what to do when a disaster occurs.
- A chain of command is set in place when a disaster occurs, and it must be followed to ensure that appropriate notification and information is provided to the Office of Emergency Services.
- Besides physical injury, people suffer psychological trauma when involved in a disaster situation.
- Triage for a disaster is based on saving those with life-threatening conditions and a likelihood of survival first.
- First aid, safety measures, and prevention and control of health hazards are priorities.
- Special populations such as the elderly, infants, disabled, and immunocompromised individuals need considerable help to stay safe and meet basic life requirements.
- Nurses should be prepared to teach people how to purify water.
- Knowledge of food safety when there has been a power outage or a flood is essential.
- Nurses should know what to do in the event of a chemical spill or explosion, bioterrorism event, or nuclear disaster.
- Nurses should know how to recognize that a biologic terrorism event has occurred and whom to notify.
- Decontamination of individuals affected by a chemical, radiologic, or bioterrorism event is performed before they are allowed into the health facility.
- Debriefing by a trained team after a disaster helps prevent long-term psychological problems among the personnel involved in caring for people affected by the event.

Go to your **Companion CD-ROM** for an Audio Glossary, animations, video clips, and bonus review questions.

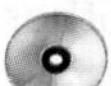

Be sure to visit the companion Evolve site at http://evolve.elsevier.com/deWit for interactive NCLEX-PN Exam Style Review Questions, WebLinks, and additional online resources.

NCLEX-PN EXAM STYLE REVIEW QUESTIONS

Choose the best answer(s) for the following questions:

1. A ______________________ exists when the number of casualties exceeds the resource capabilities of the area.

2. The nurse is attending to the needs of a family during a hurricane. The family members seem compliant and helpful and tend to minimize or ignore their own injuries. The nurse would focus on:
   1. assessing physical injury and promoting rest and relaxation.
   2. providing support and firm guidance.
   3. perpetuating the strong sense of brotherhood and community spirit.
   4. evaluating overall effectiveness of disaster management.

3. During a disaster, victims are sorted by priority of need for treatment. A nurse finds a person who is imminently dying with little chance of survival and applies a black tag. This person would:
   1. be treated immediately.
   2. have treatment within 30 minutes to 2 hours.
   3. wait for treatment for greater than 2 hours.
   4. not be treated at all.

4. Which of the following statements is true regarding green-tagged patients?
   1. They no longer need health management.
   2. They potentially pose a health hazard.
   3. They would only be reassessed in the emergency department.
   4. They are seen and treated immediately.

5. The deliberate release of microorganisms or toxins derived from living organisms that cause disease or death to humans, animals, or plants on which we depend for food is referred to as ______________________.

6. A patient is tentatively diagnosed with chickenpox. During skin assessment, the nurse would likely find which of the following to confirm the diagnosis?
   1. Skin lesions are firm.
   2. Skin lesions are found on palms and soles.
   3. Skin lesions occur in various stages.
   4. Skin lesions occur with other signs and symptoms.

7. Which of the following conditions is considered easily disseminated and may be transmitted from person to person?
   1. Tuberculosis
   2. Brucellosis
   3. Smallpox
   4. Hantavirus

8. A 34-year-old patient complains of double vision, drooping eyelids, and swallowing difficulties. He is alert and oriented with some difficulty speaking. He is afebrile. The medical management of this condition would include:
   1. gentamicin (Garamycin).
   2. botulinum antitoxin.
   3. doxycycline (Vibramycin).
   4. streptomycin.

9. To review disaster preparedness information, the nurse asks, "In the event of a hurricane watch, which of the following measures must be done?" *(Select all that apply.)*
   1. Bring inside any outdoor furniture, trash cans, potted plants, toys, and the like that could be picked up by the wind.
   2. Fill your car's gas tank.
   3. Have cash on hand.
   4. Check batteries and stock up on canned food, first aid supplies, drinking water, and medications.
   5. Stay in a mobile home.

10. While admitting a young, previously healthy patient with a rapidly progressive respiratory illness, the nurse became suspicious of a bioterrorism event. To confirm the suspicion, the nurse would ask which of the following questions?
    1. "Was there a sudden onset of severe behavioral problems?"
    2. "Has the illness progressed rapidly?"
    3. "Is the patient young or old?"
    4. "Is the patient a local resident?"

CRITICAL THINKING ACTIVITIES  *Read each clinical scenario and discuss the questions with your classmates.*

Scenario A

A hurricane has hit the town in which you live. There is widespread wind damage in much of the town, many streets are flooded, and a lot of people are injured. The power is out and the phones are dead. Your neighbor has a gash in his lower leg and is bleeding.

1. Describe how you would stop the bleeding.
2. How would you transport him to a health care facility? What precautions would you take on the journey?
3. If teenagers want to go out and wade in the floodwater and see if they can rescue stranded people or animals, what would you tell them?

Scenario B

A civic organization or church to which you belong knows that you have had training in disaster nursing. They have asked you to come and teach a group about what to do in the event of a bioterrorism attack.

1. Outline your teaching plan in detail.
2. If questions arise about a nuclear disaster, what would you say about measures they could take?

CHAPTER 44

Care of Patients with Trauma or Shock

evolve http://evolve.elsevier.com/deWit

Objectives

Upon completion of this chapter, you should be able to:

Theory

1. State the key components of assessing a trauma patient.
2. List five basic principles of first aid.
3. Discuss prevention of injuries from extremes of heat and cold.
4. Describe specific interventions in the emergency care of accidental poisoning by ingestion and inhalation.
5. Describe emergency care of victims of insect stings, tick bites, and snakebites.
6. Review the appropriate nursing actions and care needed for the patient who has experienced a respiratory or cardiac arrest.
7. Describe actions to take in a choking emergency.
8. List the four categories of shock and give an example of each.
9. Identify signs and symptoms of shock.
10. Compare the treatment of cardiogenic, hypovolemic, and neurogenic shock.

Clinical Practice

1. Observe how the triage nurse in the emergency room sets priorities for patient care.
2. Observe how the emergency team works together on a major accident victim.
3. Role play with fellow students, practicing techniques to calm a combative patient.

Key Terms

Be sure to check out the bonus material on the Companion CD-ROM, including selected audio pronunciations.

anaphylaxis (ă-nă-fă-LĂK-sĭs, p. 1083)
angioedema (ăn-jē-Ō-ĕ-DĒ-mă, p. 1093)
automated external defibrillator (AED) (ĂW-tō-mā-tĕd ĕks-tĕr-năl dē-fĭb-rĭ-LĀ-tŏr, p. 1085)
corrosive (kŭ-rō-sĭv, p. 1085)
hypovolemia (hī-pō-vō-LĒ-mē-ă, p. 1092)
inotropic (ĭn-ō-trō-pĭk, p. 1091)
multisystem organ dysfunction syndrome (MODS) (p. 1094)
perfusion (pĕr-FŪ-zhŭn, p. 1089)
ptomaines (tō-mănz, p. 1082)
shock (shŏk, p. 1089)
systemic inflammatory response syndrome (SIRS) (p. 1094)
tamponade (tăm-pon-ĀD, p. 1078)
triage (TRĒ-ăhzh, p. 1074)
vasoactive (vă-zō-ĂK-tĭv, p. 1093)

PREVENTION OF ACCIDENTS

HOME SAFETY

According to statistics compiled by the National Safety Council, accidents in the home account for one fourth of all fatal accidents. People under 5 and over 65 years of age are the principal victims of fatal mishaps occurring in the home. Because these individuals spend a large majority of their time inside the house, safety hazards must be identified and removed if accidental deaths are to be avoided.

Nurses, physicians, and others concerned with safety and welfare must take an active part in educating the public about ways to prevent home accidents. The two most dangerous rooms in the house are the kitchen and the bathroom. Box 44–1 shows some of the most common home hazards and how they can be eliminated.

? *Think Critically About . . .* Can you find three ways to increase safety in your own home?

HIGHWAY SAFETY

Motor vehicle accidents are the leading cause of accidental death in the United States. Every year, thousands of Americans are killed in motor vehicle accidents and millions are disabled by some kind of injury sustained in a traffic accident.

The two principal causes of motor vehicle accidents are human failure and mechanical failure. Human failure is by far the greater danger. Improper driving, which is responsible for almost 90% of all accidents, can be caused by the influence of alcohol and/or drugs, fatigue, excessive speed, distractions, or emotional instability. Mechanical failure often is not detected as the cause of an accident; however, there has been much interest recently in built-in safety devices and inspection for safety hazards in new automobiles. The use of seat belts and air bags, and better enforcement of laws

Box 44–1 *Home Safety*

KITCHEN

- For a gas, coal, or wood-burning stove, have vents or flues; keep windows open a crack. Never light the stove with kerosene or gasoline. Turn off all flames after cooking. Repair any gas leakage.
- Use pot holders. Keep handles of pots and pans turned away from edge of stove.
- Keep knives, sharp instruments, and poisons, such as bleach and household cleansers, out of children's reach. Keep matches out of reach of children. Place child safety locks on all cupboard doors within reach where dangerous substances are stored.
- Wipe up spills on floor.
- Keep electric appliances in good working order.
- Place broken glass in a heavy paper sack to prevent cuts through plastic bags.

STORAGE AREAS

- Always keep cellars, attics, and garages neat.
- Clean and disinfect the area where garbage is kept, and dispose of garbage frequently.
- Never place poisonous substances in drinking glasses, cold drink bottles, or other containers that have been used for food or drink.
- Always label poisonous compounds; read labels of poisons you have purchased and store the containers out of reach.

LIVING ROOM

- Be sure floors are not slippery. Use rubber mats under rugs to prevent slipping.
- Replace frayed or torn carpets.
- Cover electric sockets.
- Replace frayed electrical cords. Keep electrical cords off floor where people walk.
- Place heaters a safe distance from walls. Use screens around fireplace. Keep fireplace matches out of reach of children.
- Pad sharp edges on furniture as necessary.
- Check ashtrays for lit matches or cigarettes when going to bed or leaving the house.

FURNACE

- Have the furnace checked every year, especially for leaks in the tank of an oil-burning furnace.
- Never light the furnace with gasoline or kerosene.
- Change filters monthly.

BATHROOM

- Use a rubber mat in the tub.
- Store medicines out of children's reach. Keep all medicines capped and labeled. Throw out old medicines. Keep phone number of poison center close to telephone.
- Install child safety locks on cupboards where dangerous substances or medicines are stored.
- Be cautious in using appliances plugged into a wall plug near water.
- Keep hot water heater set at 120° F (48.8° C) or lower.

BEDROOM

- Do not smoke in bed.
- Use rubber mats under scatter rugs.

STAIRWAYS

- Cover with carpeting or rubber safety treads.
- Replace torn or frayed carpeting. Keep stairs clear of toys and cleaning equipment.
- Install handrails and proper lighting.
- Use gates at top and bottom if there are young children.

GENERAL AREAS

- Install smoke alarms throughout the house.
- Install carbon monoxide alarms.
- Make sure candles are away from drapes or other flammable materials. Never leave a lit candle unattended.

against drunk driving, have made a significant impact on decreasing vehicular deaths. There are mixed reviews on the role of speed limits and traffic accidents. Better safety devices should decrease mortality rates, but there has been no statistically significant difference on highways. It is thought that the increase in speed limits may be offsetting the benefits of the safety measures. Improvements in emergency medical services, which provide prompt and effective first aid and emergency care of accident victims, have significantly decreased vehicular deaths.

A distracted driver is an unsafe driver. Natural distractions such as passengers, environmental noise, and weather are difficult to control. Other distractions are under scrutiny and are being regulated. Many states have passed legislation requiring hands-free electronic devices such as cell phones and have placed restrictions on installation or use of other technology. Other wireless communications and entertainment devices in vehicles, such as navigation systems, televisions, DVD players, and computers, are becoming more common and are a threat to safe driving.

Vehicular deaths do not always involve automobiles. Motorcycles, motor scooters, all-terrain vehicles (ATVs), and other recreational vehicles contribute to trauma and death. Following safety precautions can greatly decrease morbidity and mortality related to recreational accidents. Utilization of vehicles in authorized locations by individuals of an appropriate age, wearing recommended/required safety gear, with the training and ability to handle the vehicle can significantly reduce accidents and fatalities.

WATER SAFETY

Weekends and vacations are an opportunity for Americans to enjoy water sports. With increased participation has come a proportionate increase in accidental deaths and injuries in or on the water. Many water accidents involve Jet Skis or wave riders. People who use these recreational items should take a safety test before unsupervised use.

Many water accidents can be prevented if the simple rules of water safety are observed. These rules include using good judgment about the choice of swimming area, ensuring proper supervision of children and adults who are not strong swimmers, diving only in areas where the water is sufficiently deep and is free of rocks or other obstacles, never swimming alone, and avoiding overexertion or swimming distances beyond one's ability. A life jacket and appropriate rescue equipment should be available for each occupant of a boat. All water skiers and Jet Ski users should wear life jackets. Above all, one should know how to handle an emergency should it arise. Panic frequently increases the danger for both the victim and the would-be rescuer.

The victim of a diving injury preferably should not be removed from the water until emergency medical personnel are in attendance. The chance of a neck and spinal cord injury is considerable. The victim is placed on a flat surface and moved as a unit, taking care to rigidly stabilize the neck.

Rescue of a drowning person requires clear thinking and deliberate action. First, the rescuer should call for help. If possible, he should try to reach the victim without going in water over his head. It is often possible to reach the victim by extending an arm, towel, rope, pole, or any long and sturdy object that is available. When the victim has grasped the object, she can be pulled slowly to safety. If a boat is available, it should be used to rescue the person who is beyond reach by other methods.

A swimming rescue is very difficult, even for the most experienced swimmer. Because the victim is frightened, she may demonstrate abnormal strength and be quite capable of drowning both herself and the rescuer. After the rescued person is brought out of the water, she must be given cardiopulmonary resuscitation (CPR) if she is not breathing and is pulseless. If she is breathing, she should be placed on her side in the recovery position (Figure 44–1) and covered with a blanket or coat. Her head should be turned to one side so that if she vomits, she will not aspirate the vomitus into her lungs.

Because near-drowning victims usually aspirate water, pulmonary edema may occur and the victim should be transported to a medical facility promptly for evaluation and treatment. Bacterial or fungal pneumonia may follow aspiration of fresh water. There is danger of delayed cardiac irregularities in all people who have been rescued from drowning, no matter how short a time they might have been struggling in the water.

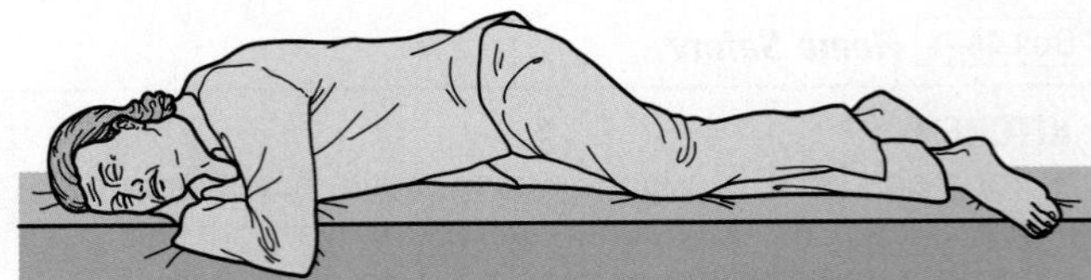

FIGURE **44–1** Recovery position.

EMERGENCY CARE

Emergency care may be provided in the emergency room, in a clinic, or out in the community. Those emergencies affecting the heart, thorax and lungs, musculoskeletal system, head and spine, eye and ear, skin (burns), and gastrointestinal (abdominal injuries) and genitourinary systems are discussed within the chapters related to the specific body system. Acute alcohol or drug intoxication is discussed in Chapter 46 on substance abuse disorders. General emergency nursing and disorders that affect the entire body are presented in this chapter.

TRIAGE: INITIAL SURVEY

In dealing with an emergency situation, it is important to have a plan in mind on how to proceed. People with injuries that are in need of immediate care can best be helped when the most urgent problems are handled first. This process of setting priorities for treatment is known as **triage.** One of the most common methods for triage of patients uses "ABCDE" as a memory trigger for the sequence of assessment (Focused Assessment 44–1). *A* is airway, *B* is breathing, and *C* is circulation. *D* can mean either the need for defibrillation or, in a trauma setting, assessment of neurologic disability. *E* is exposed, reminding health care providers to expose all areas of the body so that injuries are not missed by being hidden by clothing.

GENERAL PRINCIPLES OF FIRST AID

As a health care provider, your skill and knowledge will be depended on in situations in which immediate intervention is needed. Some general principles will allow you to provide the best care possible. Keep calm and think before acting. Concentrate on what should be done first and the manner in which to proceed step by step. Move slowly and deliberately so that you can gain time to think things through and at the same time instill confidence in those you are trying to help. The guidelines in Table 44–1 explain specific actions to take when called on to provide first aid.

Most states have adopted "Good Samaritan" laws that protect medical personnel from liability from rendering emergency medical care for victims of accidental injury. These laws guard against liability for care given as long as medically trained individuals

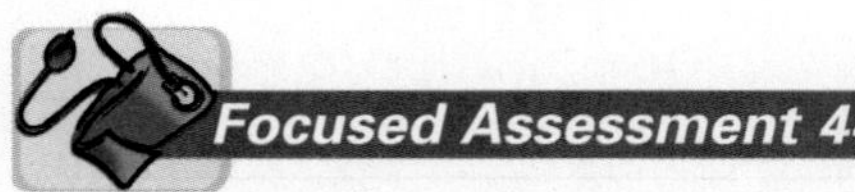

Focused Assessment 44–1

Evaluation of Accident and Emergency Patients

AREA OF ASSESSMENT	MODE OF ASSESSMENT	RATIONALE
Primary Survey	**ABCDE**	A systematic approach is needed for assessment.
A: Airway	Look and listen for signs of breathing. If breathing is present, assess for signs of respiratory distress, gasping, wheezing, *stridor* (high-pitched sound made by partial airway obstruction), choking. Check mouth for easily removable foreign body.	Adequate air exchange is necessary for the body's oxygen needs. The tongue may block the airway in an unconscious patient.
	Do *not* tilt head and hyperextend neck; if trauma patient, immobilize cervical spine.	Any patient with an unknown degree of trauma is at risk for cervical spine injury. Movement may worsen the injury.
B: Breathing	Put ear close to nose and mouth and listen for breathing. Watch chest and abdomen for rhythmic rise and fall. Note rate and quality of respirations.	Normal breathing requires no intervention. Abnormal breathing should be further evaluated and assisted as needed.
C: Circulation/hemorrhage	Feel for pulse in carotid or femoral artery; note rate and quality. Check for bleeding.	Absence of a pulse indicates cardiac arrest or obstructive shock. A rapid bounding pulse may indicate fright or hypovolemia. A rapid thready pulse may indicate further blood loss, leading to shock.
D: Disability or, if nontrauma patient, defibrillation	If nontrauma patient, place defibrillator pads and follow the AED instructions.	In the presence of primary cardiac arrest, early defibrillation significantly increases the chance for survival.
	If trauma patient: Note if alert, oriented to time, place, person. Note response to verbal stimuli. Check for Medic-Alert ID. Assess ability to move all extremities.	Additional assessment of trauma patients helps identify injuries.
E: Exposure	Remove clothing to look for injuries that may be covered, especially if the patient is not alert or cannot communicate. Look for life-threatening injuries. Keep patient warm.	The only way to verify if there are other injuries is to look. Protect patient privacy.
Secondary Survey	**HEAD TO TOE**	Initiated after life-threatening injuries are addressed.
Head, face, neck, neurologic status	Look for bleeding, bruising, abrasions. Inspect pupils, assess level of consciousness. For *obtunded* (decreased responsiveness) patients, use the Glasgow Coma Scale.	Alterations in level of consciousness can be caused by head trauma, stroke, hypoglycemia, drug overdose.
	Maintaining cervical spine precautions, assess for neck injury.	Neck injuries may be hidden by the cervical collar.
Chest	Listen to breath sounds. Look for equal chest expansion.	Tension pneumothorax can develop after a chest injury.
	Note bruising or abrasions.	External trauma may indicate internal damage.
Abdomen/genitourinary system	Auscultate for bowel sounds. Palpate for tenderness, guarding, and fullness. Look for bloody urine.	Abdominal trauma can result in ruptured spleen or bladder, or liver fracture.
Limbs	Assess adequacy of circulation in all extremities.	Dislocations or fractures can compress nerves and blood vessels.
Log roll	Using at least four people, stabilize the neck and head and gently log roll the victim to assess the back of the head, neck, back, and buttocks.	Bleeding and fractures may obscure additional injuries that are located on the back. Missed injuries can be life threatening.

Key: *AED*, automatic external defibrillator; *ID*, identification.

act in good faith and to the best of their ability. Individuals who choose to provide care are held to the standard of care consistent with their level of training. If a nursing assistant stops to provide emergency care, he will be held to a different standard than the physician who stops at the same accident scene. Both are expected to do the best they can in the circumstances. A bad outcome is not proof of improper care. Even in states in which there are no such protective laws, malpractice suits of this kind very rarely occur. For many people, the advantages derived from knowing that they have used their skills and experi-

Table 44–1 ***General Principles of First Aid***

ACTION	REASONING
• Before attending to the victim or victims of an accident, quickly survey the accident scene to determine whether there are further hazards to yourself and the victims.	Spillage of gasoline after a motor vehicle accident can cause a fire or explosion, or there may be danger to the victim, yourself, and onlookers from oncoming traffic and secondary collisions. In both highway and home accidents, live electrical wires may be in the vicinity. Whenever there is a high risk of death from hazardous conditions in the immediate environment, the victims should be moved at once, regardless of the nature of their injuries. One factor that often is overlooked is the heat of the pavement in the summertime. Victims may receive severe burns from lying on a sun-baked street or sidewalk while waiting for the ambulance. Although it may not be safe to move the victim to a shaded area, it is advisable to place clothing, newspaper, or some other protective covering between her skin and the hot pavement.
• If there are several victims of the accident, make a quick check on each one before beginning treatment.	The most serious and life-threatening injuries must be treated first; those victims who do not seem to be in immediate danger can be attended to by someone else who is capable of watching them and reporting to you any change in their condition.
• Look for a Medic-Alert bracelet or necklace.	If the victim is wearing one or has some other identification showing specific medical needs, bring this to the attention of the ambulance or hospital personnel.
• Try to determine the mechanism of injury: for example, the column of the steering wheel, a drug or poison, or electric current.	This will give clues about the type of injury sustained and the treatment required. When evaluating the victim, begin at the head and work downward to the toes. Refer to the evaluation checklist in Focused Assessment 44–1.
• Do not move the victim unless she is in immediate danger or until you have immobilized injured parts.	This is particularly true if spinal injury is suspected. Moving the victim can cause further injury if precautions are not taken.
• Do not remove an object that has penetrated a part of the body and is still in place.	A knife, piece of metal, or sliver of wood that is protruding from the chest or abdomen should be left as is until it can be removed in a control situation by trained professionals. Removal of the object can cause further damage and make bleeding worse. Bandages are applied around the object to stabilize it and control bleeding as necessary.
• Do not try to give anything by mouth to a person who is unconscious or has a decreased level of consciousness.	Aspiration of the material into her air passage may occur, causing breathing difficulty or complete airway obstruction.
• Explain to the victim in a calm and positive tone of voice what you are doing for her and why. Give honest answers, but do not alarm her unduly. You must sound as if you are in control of yourself and the situation.	Giving reassurance to the victim will decrease anxiety and promote cooperation. Forcing yourself to remain calm can increase your own ability to function in an emergency situation.

ence to help someone in need outweigh the risk of a lawsuit.

? *Think Critically About* . . . If you came upon an automobile accident in which several people were involved and stopped to render aid, how would you assess the situation for safety of yourself and the victims? How would you act to ensure as safe a scene as possible for evaluation of the victims?

CONTROL OF BLEEDING

The only emergency conditions that have priority over control of hemorrhage are cessation of breathing and a sucking wound of the chest (a wound in the chest wall allowing air to pass through with each breath, causing a bubbling or sucking sound). Severe bleeding can rapidly lead to irreversible hypovolemic shock from loss of blood, causing circulatory collapse.

Blood issuing from an artery is bright red and will gush forth in spurts at regular intervals. Blood loss from an artery is more rapid than from a vein. Blood from a severed or punctured vein leaks slowly and steadily and is dark red. To control bleeding, **apply pressure to the wound or compress the artery above the wound** (Box 44–2).

Even major bleeding can usually be stopped by applying pressure directly over the wound. When in a community setting, use non-sterile exam gloves if available. When in a health care work setting, Centers for Disease Control and Prevention and Occupational Safety and Health Administration requirements mandate use of personal protective equipment that includes barrier devices such as gloves when in contact with body fluids (Safety Alert 44–1). The palm of the hand is used, preferably after a clean cloth or sterile

Box 44–2 *Techniques to Control Bleeding*

- Position the body part that is bleeding over a firm surface and immobilize the part.
- Place a sterile dressing or a clean cloth over the wound.
- With the flat palm of the hand or several fingers, apply direct pressure to the wound continuously for 5 minutes.
- Check for stoppage of bleeding after 5 minutes; if bleeding is occurring, apply pressure continuously for another 10 minutes.
- When bleeding has stopped, gently remove hand pressure and apply a pressure dressing over the existing cloth or dressing by folding another dressing or piece of cloth several times and tying it firmly over the wound.
- Check circulation distal to the wound to be certain that the pressure dressing is not so tight that circulation below the wound is cut off.
- Reinforce the dressing as needed by applying yet another layer of dressing as blood soaks through; do not remove previously applied dressings.
- If direct pressure will not stop the bleeding, and the bleeding is considerable, apply pressure over the artery leading to the wound. (Cut off arterial flow only as a last resort.)
- Check for adequate pressure over the artery by identifying that there is a lack of pulse distal to the wound and possibly a sensation of tingling and numbness in the wound area.

dressing has been placed over the open wound. However, if no dressing is available and the victim's life is in danger from blood loss, trying to avoid contamination of the wound is not as important as controlling the hemorrhage. Once the bleeding has stopped, a compression dressing and bulky bandage are gently but snugly secured in place. Do not wrap the body part so tightly as to constrict circulation completely. The amount of blood leaking from a wound can be minimized somewhat by elevating the injured part and immobilizing it so that clots are not disturbed and the pumping action of neighboring vessels is decreased.

Once the bleeding has been controlled, the pressure dressing is left in place so as not to disturb clots and renew the bleeding. If blood soaks through the original dressing, additional dressings are applied over the soaked ones. None of the dressings should be removed until medical help is available.

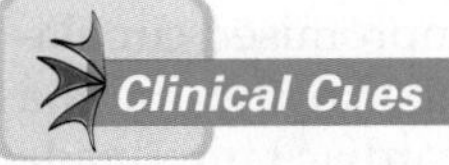

Many patients are on antiplatelet drugs such as aspirin and clopidogrel (Plavix) or anticoagulants such as warfarin (Coumadin) to treat heart and vascular conditions. If there is injury, bleeding will be significant and may be difficult to stop.

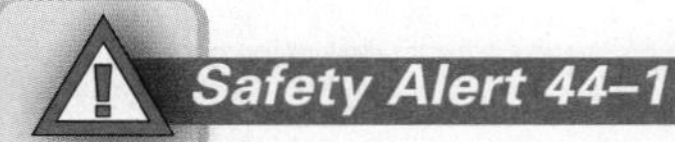

Protective Gear

Use of protective gear such as gloves will help keep the rescuer from contact with blood that might contain pathogens. In a community setting, personal protective equipment may not be present where needed. If gloves are not available, create a barrier with plastic or multiple layers of cloth. Hands and any other skin in contact with blood should be washed as soon as possible.

If bleeding is copious and cannot be stopped with a pressure bandage and immobilization, the artery leading to the wound can be compressed to decrease or perhaps stop altogether the flow of blood from the wound. Pressure points for control of arterial bleeding are shown in Chapter 15, Figure 15–3. If the pressure point has been covered properly, there should be no pulse below the point of pressure and the victim should notice tingling and numbness in the area. Pressure points in the neck and head must be used with caution, because there is danger of interrupting blood supply to the brain or of blocking the intake of air.

NECK AND SPINE INJURIES

Presence of neck or spinal injury should be suspected in any situation in which the individual has sustained multiple injuries, a fall, or blunt force impact or is unconscious. In emergency or accident situations, it is not uncommon for severe bleeding, absence of respirations, or other life-threatening conditions to distract the rescuer and cause him to overlook the possibility that the victim also might have a spinal cord injury (Safety Alert 44–2). If this happens, and the rescuer proceeds to treat the more obvious injuries and moves the victim before properly immobilizing the neck and back, permanent damage and paralysis may result.

Types of accidents in which spinal injury should be suspected are motor vehicle, diving, biking, and sledding mishaps or any situation in which the neck receives significant force. Rescuers must move a person who has been injured by diving into shallow water, because she may be in danger of drowning. Efforts to remove her from the water and to resuscitate her must be gentle and undertaken only after the neck and back have been properly supported to avoid further damage to the spinal cord. The victim of a sledding or skiing accident may not show signs of injury because of bulky clothing, but she should be moved only after careful evaluation and immobilization, as indicated.

Only trained personnel familiar with the techniques of applying and maintaining traction on the head while the collar or other device is being applied should do spinal immobilization (Figure 44–2). When

Safety Alert 44–2

Cervical Spinal Immobilization

In any traumatic injury in which there is the potential for spinal injury, victims are treated as spinal cord–injured patients until a spinal injury is ruled out. Cervical spine immobilization is implemented before the person is moved to a stretcher.

a cervical collar is not available and the victim must be moved to safety, the neck may be immobilized with any material handy, such as a coat, shirt, or towel, rolled in the shape of a collar. The purpose of the collar is to keep the neck as straight as possible, preventing it from flexing or hyperextending. Treatment for neck and spinal cord injuries is covered in Chapter 22.

ABDOMINAL TRAUMA

Abdominal injuries resulting from improperly worn seat belts, penetrating objects, blunt instruments, and sharp cutting edges are all potential sources of hemorrhage and damage to internal organs. **A bluish tinge around the umbilicus may indicate abdominal hemorrhage.** If internal hemorrhage is suspected, the victim should be observed closely for symptoms of shock and handled very gently when being moved.

Peritoneal lavage is performed to diagnose intra-abdominal bleeding. A lavage catheter is inserted into the peritoneal space and the contents of the cavity are aspirated with a large syringe. If no blood is aspirated, a liter of warmed saline solution is infused, allowed to remain in place for a time, and then drained by gravity flow from the cavity. The drainage is evaluated for the presence of blood.

External wounds with evisceration are covered with a piece of nonadhering material such as plastic wrap or aluminum foil until the patient can be treated in an emergency facility. This will keep the protruding intestinal contents moist and relatively free of contamination. After the occlusive covering is applied, a clean folded towel or sheet is placed over it to retain body heat in the protruding organs. No attempt should be made to replace the abdominal organs through the wound. The victim is transported to a medical facility as quickly as possible.

MULTIPLE TRAUMA

Trauma occurring simultaneously in several parts of the body is considered multiple trauma. The most common cause of multiple trauma is motor vehicle accidents, with most victims being male and in their teens. In the elderly, falls are the most common cause of multiple trauma.

Head injury is present in most incidences of multiple trauma. Fractures and chest and abdominal injuries

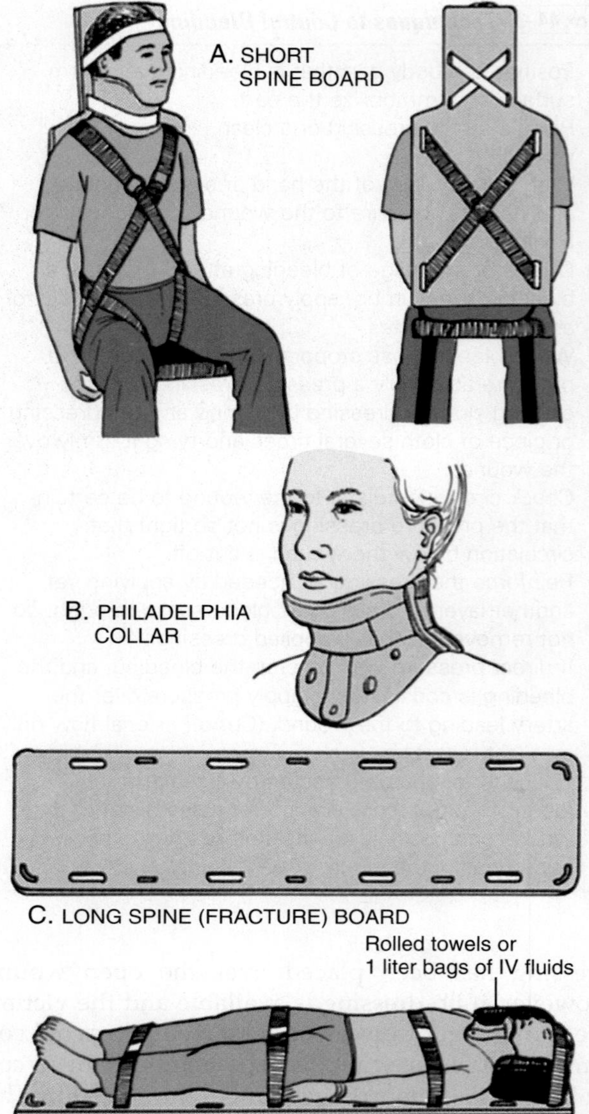

FIGURE **44–2** Spinal immobilization.

may accompany the head trauma. Focused Assessment 44–1 gives the sequence of assessment for the trauma patient. Airway management is always the first priority for any patient in distress. In head trauma, adequate ventilation and oxygenation may be compromised due to decreased level of consciousness. If head trauma is present, suspect cervical spine injury and use C-spine precautions when performing airway interventions. The secondary survey listed in Focused Assessment 44–1 helps identify additional injuries. Threats to breathing may include injuries such as pneumothorax, rib fractures, or open chest wounds. Compromised circulation usually results from hemorrhage in the trauma patient. Tension pneumothorax and cardiac **tamponade** (compression) can also compromise circulation. Inadequate circulation leads to inadequate supply of oxygen and nutrients to the tissues. Lack of perfusion to the tissues is the etiology of shock.

Think Critically About . . . What do you have available at home or in your car that could be used to hold pressure on a bleeding wound or stabilize the neck? Are you prepared to respond to an emergency?

INJURIES DUE TO EXTREME HEAT AND COLD

HEATSTROKE

Heatstroke, a rare condition also called *sunstroke,* is the result of a serious disturbance of the heat-regulating center in the brain. Heatstroke is further defined as exertional or nonexertional. Exertional heatstroke tends to occur in young, healthy individuals who engage in prolonged physical activity in a hot environment. The increased metabolic demands exhaust the body's ability to regulate temperature. Nonexertional heatstroke occurs more commonly in the very young and very old and those who cannot control their ambient temperature or water intake. Normally, the body is able to regulate body temperature even with increased activity or changes in environmental temperatures by increasing perspiration and by using other internal mechanisms. In heatstroke, these mechanisms fail to function properly and the patient's temperature rises, the skin becomes dry and hot, and there may be convulsions and collapse. Alteration in neurologic function is a finding common to both types of heatstroke. Other symptoms include visual disturbances, dizziness, nausea, and a weak, rapid, irregular pulse. Because the body temperature may go as high as 108° to 110° F (42.2° to 43.3° C), the patient may die if her condition is not treated.

Prevention

In hot weather or if active in warm weather, take the following precautions. Drink plenty of fluids that are nonalcoholic, noncaffeinated, and low in sugar content. Don't wait until thirsty to drink fluids. Drinking the wrong kind of fluids can increase the amount of fluid lost. Stay indoors with cooling systems. If air conditioning or adequate cooling is not available in the home, go to the library, mall, or other public place with air conditioning.

If staying indoors is not an option, appropriate dress is needed. In the heat, wear lightweight, light-colored, loose-fitting clothing. Limit outdoor activities to morning and evening hours, using sun protection such as wide-brimmed hats, sunglasses, and sunscreen. Try to rest often in shaded areas, limiting the amount of exertion if possible.

Treatment

A person suffering from heatstroke should be placed in the shade and cooled immediately by being sprinkled with water and fanned. The longer the body temperature remains elevated the worse the outcome, so rapid cooling measures should be implemented. There is no one cooling mechanism that has been proven to be superior to another. Whatever is available, cools quickly without inducing shivering, and can be implemented immediately should be utilized. Standard cooling measures include removal of extra clothing or coverings, application of ice packs to the groin and axillae, use of a cooling blanket, and infusion of cold fluids. Ice water enemas and gastric lavage have not been shown to be any more effective than less invasive measures. Chlorpromazine (Thorazine) is not recommended; benzodiazepines are a better choice for control of seizures and shivering.

HYPOTHERMIA

Hypothermia is a serious lowering of the total body temperature caused by prolonged exposure to cold. People most at risk for hypothermia are the elderly, very young and thin children, the mentally ill, the homeless, and others unable to alter their ambient environment.

Hypothermia is a chilling of the entire body. The extremities can withstand lower temperatures (20° to 30° F lower) than the torso, where vital organs are located. When the core (central) temperature drops even 2° or 3° F, physiologic changes that can lead to fatal cardiac dysrhythmias and respiratory failure occur.

Symptoms of hypothermia range from mild shivering and complaints of feeling cold to loss of consciousness and a deathlike appearance. Indeed, people in profound hypothermia may be presumed dead because the body's protective mechanisms have drastically slowed its metabolic processes. The body uses less than half its normal requirement for oxygen in severe hypothermia. Pulse and respiration are barely detected, reflexes are absent, and the person is unconscious.

Prevention

Prevention of hypothermia includes eating high-energy foods, exercising, wearing layers of clothing, and covering the head. From one half to two thirds of the body's heat is lost through the head. Elderly persons particularly need protection against the effects of extreme cold (Box 44–3). Hypothermia in these individuals can easily be misdiagnosed because its symptoms resemble those of so many diseases to which the elderly and weak are most susceptible. Mild hypothermia (90° to 95° F [32° to 35° C] body temperature) is usually tolerated fairly well. Moderate hypothermia (84° to 90° F [29° to 32° C] body temperature) results in a mortality rate of about 21%. Severe hypothermia (core temperature below 82° F [28° C]) has an even higher mortality rate.

Most clinical thermometers used in hospitals and clinics do not register temperatures below 94° F (34.5° C), and many times the temperature is taken orally rather than rectally. In the emergency room, rectal, bladder, or esophageal probes will be used to monitor

Box 44–3 ***Prevention of Hypothermia in the Elderly***

- Room temperature should not be lower than 65° F. An indoor thermometer should be kept in the house and checked daily during the cool seasons.
- An energy audit by the utility company can identify ways to prevent heat loss from the home. Check with the gas or electric company.
- If heating the entire house presents economic problems, suggest heating one or two rooms adequately and closing off the other rooms of the house.
- Suggest aids, such as throw or quilted snuggle bag (a quilt with snaps or zipper that becomes a bag), extra socks, and warm hats to be worn indoors.
- Recommend wearing several loose layers of clothing to retain body heat.
- Head covering should be worn even while sleeping, as two thirds of the body's heat is lost through the head.
- Advise against using fireplaces in extremely cold weather unless no other heat source is available; a substantial amount of heat is lost through the flue. If a fireplace is used, close the damper as soon as the fire is competely extinguished.
- Arrange for someone to check in daily with elderly persons who live alone.
- Suggest an early alert system be installed, allowing the individual to call for help by pressing a button. This allows the elder to contact someone when they may not be near a phone.

temperature throughout the warming process. Any other temperature measurement may not reflect true core temperature.

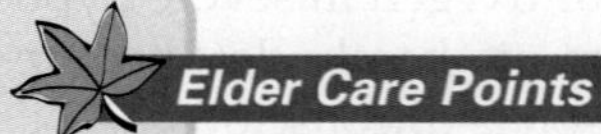

Anyone in the cold long enough without adequate protection can become hypothermic. With aging, the body's ability to withstand the cold is lessened. Older people may also be less active, which generates less body heat. The elderly are at risk for accidental hypothermia after exposure even to mild cold weather or a small drop in temperature.

Treatment

Once hypothermia is diagnosed, rewarming is begun. The method varies according to the age and physical condition of the patient. The core must be rewarmed first to prevent lactic acid in the extremities from being rapidly shunted to the heart, which can cause ventricular fibrillation. **The heart is extremely sensitive when cold, and the patient must be handled carefully to prevent dysrhythmias.** If rewarming is done in an emergency care facility, monitoring equipment must be readily at hand. Rewarming outside a health care facility should be more gradual. This must be done properly to avoid sending cold blood that has pooled in the extremities back to the heart, where it can cause deadly arrhythmias. The person is warmed by wrapping her in a blanket or submerging her in a tepid bath.

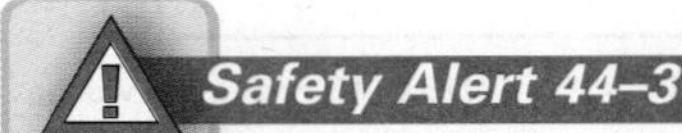

Frostbite

Do not try to hasten the warming process by using water that is hotter than recommended, as this can add to the damage.

FROSTBITE

Frostbite is a localized injury to tissue caused by freezing. Exposure of the tissues to extreme cold constricts the blood vessels, damages vessel walls and tissue cells, and leads to the formation of blood clots. Frostbite occurs most often in the fingers, toes, cheeks, and nose, where exposure usually is greatest and blood supply is most easily hampered. Frostbite is categorized by degree of injury much like burns. The appearance of a first-degree injury includes reddened skin, swelling, waxy appearance, hard white plaques, and sensory deficit. Second-degree injury also has redness and swelling and formation of blisters filled with clear or milky fluid that form within 24 hours of injury. In third-degree injury, the blisters are blood-filled and over several weeks black eschar forms. Fourth-degree injury involves full-thickness damage affecting muscles, tendons, and bone, resulting in tissue loss.

Prevention

Like hypothermia, frostbite can be prevented by wearing protective clothing and avoiding exposure to extreme cold. Sometimes this is not possible if a person is caught unaware or unprepared. Those who are intoxicated or under the influence of drugs may not realize they are suffering from frostbite. If the person also is suffering from hypothermia, she cannot think clearly and does not realize that her skin is being exposed to severe cold.

Treatment

Once the patient is removed from the cold, the affected area should be warmed by immersion for about 10 minutes in water heated to between 100° and 110° F (38° to 43° C) (Safety Alert 44–3). Handle the frostbitten part gently. *Never* rub or massage skin that has been frozen. The practice of rubbing snow or ice on the part is dangerous and completely without benefit. Rubbing or rough handling can cause further damage to the fragile tissues. Wrap the affected area in bulky clean or sterile bandages, being sure to separate skin areas, as between the fingers. Elevate the affected area. Avoid alcohol or sedatives as they tend to further depress function.

Débridement of dead tissue and skin grafting will be necessary if the deeper tissues have been destroyed.

The extent of the tissue injury may not be known for several months.

POISONING

Poisoning from gases, chemicals, drugs, and other toxic substances accounts for many deaths in the United States every year. Prevention of accidental poisoning begins with a realization that there are literally hundreds of thousands of poisonous substances in our environment. Every home has a variety of poisons sitting on the shelves of the medicine cabinet, under the kitchen sink, or in the laundry room, utility room, and garage. **Children are the most frequent victims of poisoning, and medicines account for half of all accidental poisonings of children under the age of 5.** Aspirin has consistently been the leading cause of death in accidental poisoning in children of this age. Other poisons frequently ingested by children include bleaches, soaps and detergents, insecticides, and vitamin and iron preparations. In the past decade, there has been an increase of poisoning in children who have ingested a parent's prescribed medications.

Since the government began requiring "childproof" caps on all medications and many poisonous substances ordinarily found in households, the incidence of poisoning in children has decreased somewhat, but carelessness on the part of adults continues to be a major factor in the accidental poisoning of children. Despite this progress in prevention of accidental poisoning in children, acute poisoning still is the most frequently encountered pediatric emergency in this country.

Prevention

As a member of the health team, the nurse must do all he can to educate the public in the ways in which accidental poisoning can be prevented. He should remember the simple rules given in Health Promotion Points 44–1 and use every opportunity to teach them to his friends and neighbors.

Symptoms

The symptoms of poisoning vary according to the substance ingested and the time that has elapsed since it first entered the body. Poisoning should be suspected if the victim becomes ill very suddenly and there is an open poison or drug container nearby. In children, one should be alert to the possibility of poisoning when there is a peculiar odor to the breath or when there is evidence that the child has eaten leaves or wild berries. Always remember that children are naturally very curious and that a substance need not taste good for a child to place it in her mouth and swallow.

Other symptoms of poisoning include pain or burning sensation in the mouth and throat, nausea, vomiting, disorientation, visual disturbances, loss of consciousness, or a deep, unnatural sleep.

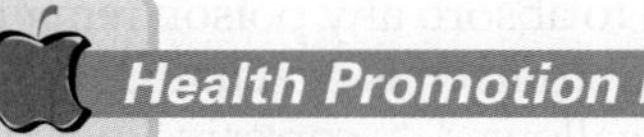

Health Promotion Points 44–1

Poison Prevention

- Destroy all medicines that are no longer being used. An overdose can be fatal, especially to a child. In some instances, drugs undergo chemical changes with age and become toxic compounds.
- Store poisons and inedible products separately from edible foods.
- Do not transfer poisonous substances from their original container to an unmarked one. NEVER place a poison in a container (such as a soft drink bottle) that is normally used for edible solids or liquids.
- Never tell a child that the medicine she is being given is candy. Tell her it is a medicine to make her feel better and that it must be taken only as the doctor has directed.
- Always read the labels of chemical products before using them.

Treatment

Call the poison control center first, at 1-800-222-1222. All cases of poisoning demand immediate action. The longer the delay before treatment, the greater the chance of the poison being absorbed in the body and permanently damaging body tissues.

Always save the container and any of its contents that may help in identifying the poison. If the container cannot be found and the type of poison is not known, try to save a sample of any vomitus for analysis and identification.

INGESTED POISONS

Generally, the first step is *dilution* of the poison, immediately followed by *removal* of the stomach contents. In the absence of a stomach pump, vomiting can be induced, but this is contraindicated for certain kinds of poisons, such as corrosive chemicals and petroleum products. A liquid such as water or milk can usually serve to dilute the poison.

Vomiting is induced by placing a spoon or an index finger down the back of the throat to stimulate the gag reflex. An emetic such as 2 tablespoons of salt in a glass of warm water or 15 to 30 mL of syrup of ipecac diluted in a glass of water can be used, but gastric lavage in the emergency room is more effective. The smaller amount is given to children, and the larger amount is for adults. Be sure that during the vomiting episode the victim is positioned so that the vomitus will not be aspirated into the lungs.

Antidotes to specific poisons often are printed on the labels of the containers. A phone call to the nearest hospital emergency room can provide specific instructions on what to do until the patient can reach the emergency room and be treated by a physician. If possible, the specific antidote should be given as soon as the stomach has been emptied of the poison. In the emergency room, activated charcoal is given to absorb any poison remaining in the stomach and the stomach is evacuated.

When a patient has swallowed a corrosive poison, such as a strong acid or alkali, vomiting is contraindicated, because there is the danger of further irritating and damaging the upper intestinal tract. In addition, the corrosive substance also may be aspirated into the respiratory tract during vomiting. Corrosive substances should be diluted with milk or water given orally. Never induce vomiting if the victim is unconscious. Never induce vomiting unless **directed to do so by the poison control center or an emergency health care professional.**

FOOD POISONING

The toxins of bacteria present in contaminated food produce this type of poisoning. The term *ptomaine poisoning,* so frequently associated with food poisoning, is actually misleading. **Ptomaines** are substances formed by the decomposition, or "spoilage," of protein foods. The digestive system is able to cope with these substances, and they do not necessarily cause illness. Decomposing food is not of itself necessarily harmful, but because foods in the process of decomposition frequently harbor pathogenic organisms and serve as excellent media for their growth, they should be avoided.

Types of Food Poisoning

Food poisoning may be bacterial or chemical. The chemical types, however, are not true food poisonings, but toxic conditions caused by poisonous mushrooms, toxic berries, or foods that have not been cleansed of insecticides or other chemicals.

Staphylococcus aureus frequently grows in creamed foods that have not been refrigerated adequately. **Custards, cream pies, mayonnaise, and processed foods commonly used for picnics often are the source of this type of food poisoning.** The illness rarely is fatal, and symptoms are usually limited to nausea, vomiting, diarrhea, and abdominal cramps. The patient should be kept quiet and given sedation and parenteral fluids as necessary.

Prevention

Cleanliness, good personal hygiene, and proper preparation and handling of foods are essential to prevent food poisoning. The recommendations found in Health Promotion Points 44–2 are from the National Institutes of Health. Following guidelines such as these will help prevent the spread of organisms commonly associated with food poisoning, as stated in the *Healthy People 2010* goals (Health Promotion Points 44–3).

Symptoms and Treatment

Food poisoning should be suspected when more than one person in a group, family, or community is affected by an acute febrile gastrointestinal disturbance. The onset is sudden, with nausea, vomiting, diarrhea, and abdominal cramps. Food is withheld, drugs are administered to control diarrhea, and sedation and parenteral fluids are given.

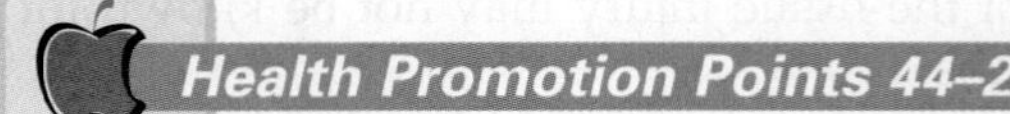

Safe Food Handling

- Carefully wash your hands and clean dishes and utensils.
- Use a thermometer when cooking. Cook beef to at least 160° F, poultry to at least 180° F, and fish to at least 140° F.
- DO NOT place cooked meat or fish back onto the same plate or container that held the raw meat, unless the container has been thoroughly washed.
- Promptly refrigerate any food you will not be eating right away. Keep the refrigerator set to around 40° F and your freezer at or below 0° F. DO NOT eat meat, poultry, or fish that has been refrigerated uncooked for longer than 1 to 2 days.
- DO NOT use outdated foods, packaged food with a broken seal, or cans that are bulging or have a dent.
- DO NOT use foods that have an unusual odor or a spoiled taste.

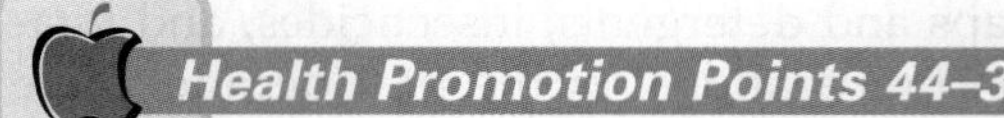

***Healthy People 2010* Food Safety**

Focus area # 10: Food Safety. To reduce food-borne illnesses.

The Food and Drug Administration and the Food Safety and Inspection Service, U.S. Department of Agriculture have implemented guidelines to reduce the numbers of people who become ill as a result of the food they eat. Standards for food handling from farm and field to home or factory are in place to prevent contamination of food with illness-causing organisms. In addition to concerns regarding microorganism contamination, the agencies have also implemented standards for labeling of foods to identify potential allergens.

These agencies are tracking instances of illness linked to food consumption to be able to immediately implement changes needed to protect the public.

INHALED POISONS

When a person has inhaled a poisonous substance, call for emergency help. Never attempt to rescue a person without notifying others first. If it is safe to do so, rescue the person from the danger of the gas, fumes, or smoke. Open windows and doors to remove the fumes. Take several deep breaths of fresh air, and then hold your breath as you go in. Hold a wet cloth over your nose and mouth. Do not light a match or use a lighter because some gases can catch fire.

After rescuing the person from danger, loosen clothing from around the neck and chest. Check and monitor the person's airway, breathing, and pulse. If necessary, begin rescue breathing and CPR. Even if the person seems perfectly fine, get medical help.

Symptoms that may indicate an individual has inhaled a poison may include excessive coughing; shortness of breath, wheezing, and a burning sensation of the nose and throat; pale or bluish color to skin; dizziness, headache, nausea, and vomiting; and chest pain or tightness. **If carbon monoxide has been inhaled, the mucous membranes will be cherry red.** If there is any suspicion of inhalation of a poison, make sure the victim receives appropriate medical care.

BITES AND STINGS

ANIMAL BITES

Family pets, especially dogs and cats, are the most common source of animal bites. When a wild animal, such as a squirrel or fox, attacks and bites a human being without provocation, one should always suspect rabies as the cause of the animal's unusual behavior. All animal and human bites should be treated as potentially dangerous because of the presence of pathogenic microorganisms in the mouth that can cause a serious infection.

Treatment

Wounds from animal bites should be rinsed immediately with soap and hot running water for 5 to 10 minutes. The affected area is then treated with antibiotic ointment, covered with a clean bandage, and immobilized. Medical attention should be given to the wound as soon as possible. Antibiotics may be given to prevent infection. If the victim has not had a tetanus shot in the past 5 years, a booster will be given.

Because the possibility of rabies must always be considered in an animal bite, the animal must be confined and observed for signs of the disease. The local animal control agency should be contacted to catch the animal if necessary. If it has been killed, animal control will take the body for examination. If a diagnosis of rabies in the animal has been confirmed or if there is no proof that the animal has been immunized against rabies, the victim is given a series of injections to build up antibodies against the virus. A series of five intramuscular injections are given over a period of 3 weeks for an individual who has never been vaccinated against rabies. Only two doses of vaccine are needed for those who have previously been vaccinated.

SNAKEBITE

Although bites from poisonous snakes are rare in the United States, they do occur and can be fatal if not treated promptly and effectively. There are four kinds of poisonous snakes in this country: copperheads, rattlesnakes, coral snakes, and cottonmouths (or water moccasins). Copperheads, rattlesnakes, and cottonmouths are all called pit vipers because they have pits or depressions behind their nostrils; coral snakes are small snakes with characteristic red, black, and yellow bands. Coral snakes do not have fangs; they inject their venom by a chewing motion.

A venomous snakebite usually can be distinguished by two fang marks (though there may be only one on a small surface, such as the toe or finger), severe pain and swelling in the area, discoloration at the site of injection of venom, nausea and vomiting, respiratory distress, and shock. Nonpoisonous snakebites usually appear as either small scratches or lacerations.

Treatment

Nonpoisonous snakebites are treated as simple wounds and require only a cleansing of the wound with soap and water and the application of a mild antiseptic. Venomous snakebites should receive medical attention as quickly as possible. The victim of a poisonous snakebite should be kept as quiet and calm as possible while being transported. Under no condition should she be given an alcoholic beverage or stimulant.

Current treatment for poisonous snakebite consists of washing the wound, lowering the extremity or area and immobilizing it, keeping the victim calm, and seeking medical attention as quickly as possible. Applying suction to the area can be helpful if initiated within several minutes of the bite. Incisions over the wound are not recommended. A tourniquet above the wound to prevent the venom from traveling through the body is not routinely recommended. It may be helpful if there is significant delay in obtaining medical care.

Once the snakebite victim reaches a hospital or clinic, the wound is débrided and irrigated to remove the venom and damaged tissues. Skin grafting may be required later. The victim is given antivenin, medications to counteract the specific pharmacologic action of the venom, and other drugs to avoid complications and provide relief.

INSECT BITES AND STINGS

Systemic reactions to the bites and stings of insects and bees account for more deaths each year in the United States than do snakebites. A systemic reaction is caused by hypersensitivity to the venom of bees, wasps, hornets, fire ants, or harvester ants. Symptoms of a systemic reaction include hives, swelling, general weakness, tightness in the chest, abdominal cramps, constriction of the throat, loss of consciousness, and possibly death from severe **anaphylaxis.** Whenever a person suffers from any of these symptoms after a sting or insect bite, treatment must be started immediately. The shorter the interval between the time of the sting or bite and the development of symptoms, the more likely the possibility that death will result. Ice packs may be applied to the area of the bite or sting while medical help is being sought.

Some spider bites are also of concern. The black widow and the brown recluse spiders are the best known that have a potentially serious bite. The symptoms of a black widow bite may not be obvious initially; the bite may feel like a pinprick with some slight redness and swelling. Within a few hours intense pain and stiffness will occur. Other symptoms include chills, fever, nausea, and severe abdominal pain. The brown recluse spider bite produces a mild stinging, redness, and pain within several hours. A fluid-filled blister forms at the site of the bite. The tissue sloughs off, leaving a deep, hard-to-heal ulcer.

Elder Care Points

Anyone over the age of 65 should seek medical attention if bitten by a brown recluse spider. The elderly are more at risk for developing complications related to the bite.

Treatment

First aid treatment for a systemic reaction is to inject aqueous epinephrine (1:1000 solution) in dosages of 0.3 to 0.4 mL for adults and 0.15 to 0.3 mL for children. An antihistamine, such as diphenhydramine (Benadryl), also is given. An ice pack may be applied to reduce swelling and relieve pain. Patients who appear to be in shock should be kept warm and should remain lying down with the legs elevated and the head flat. If symptoms persist after 20 minutes and the patient has not yet reached a medical facility, a second injection of epinephrine should be given.

The female worker honeybee injects a venom sac that may remain embedded in the victim's skin. This sac may be removed by gently scraping the site with a fingernail or knife blade, being careful not to squeeze the sac and force the venom into the tissues. **The "stinger" should be removed as quickly as possible.**

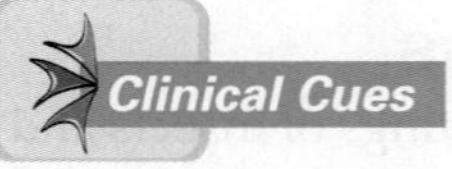

Clinical Cues

Do not use tweezers to remove an insect stinger; this may cause squeezing of the venom sac and worsen the symptoms. A convenient flat edge that can be used to scrape out the stinger is a credit card or any plastic item with a smooth edge.

An emergency kit that contains the drugs, syringe, constricting band, towelette, and tweezers needed for prompt treatment of a systemic reaction to stings and bites is available by prescription. Individuals known to be hypersensitive to insect and bee venom should keep such a kit with them at all times and be thoroughly familiar with its use *before* the need for it arises (Health Promotion Points 44–4). These people also should wear some kind of medical identification that indicates their hypersensitivity. Any person who has had a systemic reaction or even a severe local reaction with swelling beyond two joints should receive hyposensitization therapy to increase her tolerance to insect and bee stings.

Applying a paste of baking soda and water or household ammonia and a cold compress treats less serious stings of bees, wasps, yellow jackets, and hornets. Meat tenderizer also has been found effective in relieving the symptoms of minor insect sting reactions. Topical cortisone cream can also be applied to relieve inflammation and itching.

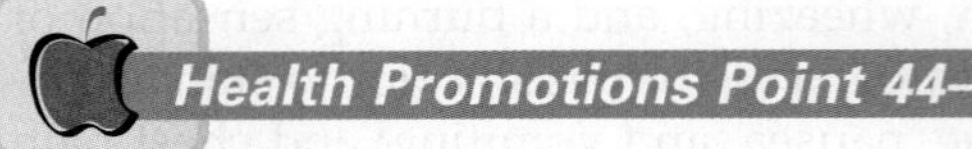

Health Promotions Point 44–4

Anaphylaxis Kit

Individuals who have known allergies to insect bites or other common environmental allergens should carry an anaphylaxis kit. Family and friends should know how to use the contents in case the individual is unable to treat herself.

Bites from venomous spiders, scorpions, and other poisonous insects are treated in the same manner as poisonous snakebites. Antivenin specific to the spider, scorpion, or other poisonous creature is available at hospital emergency rooms and clinics that serve rural areas.

Ticks, which can carry diseases such as Rocky Mountain spotted fever or Lyme disease, are removed by grasping the tick as close to the skin as possible with tweezers and pulling it straight out without twisting. Some people believe that placing a drop of turpentine, mineral oil, or petroleum jelly on its body will make the tick let go before pulling it out. After the tick is removed, wash the area with soap and water and apply a mild disinfectant. If there is some question as to whether the tick may be carrying an infectious disease, a physician should be consulted.

ELECTRIC SHOCK AND BURNS

ELECTRIC SHOCK

When an electric current passes through the body, it can cause severe damage to the entire body, including cessation of breathing, circulatory failure, and serious burns. The current travels along the path of least resistance, and may be conducted through the heart. The amount of voltage and current involved, the length of time in contact with the electricity source, and the condition of the skin all play a role in how much damage may occur as a result of an electric shock.

Emergency treatment of electric shock involves CPR if breathing has ceased or the heart has stopped, treatment of burns if present, and treatment of any other injuries. Many times with an electric shock, an explosion or fall is associated with the event that may cause additional injuries. The proper procedure for separating a victim from a live conductor of electricity is shown in Figure 44–3. **Remember that water serves as a conductor of electricity, and wet objects can transmit a fatal electric current to a person trying to rescue the victim of electric shock.** A person who is struck by lightning suffers from electric shock (Safety Alert 44–4). All electric shock victims must be observed for cardiac dysrhythmias after the injury.

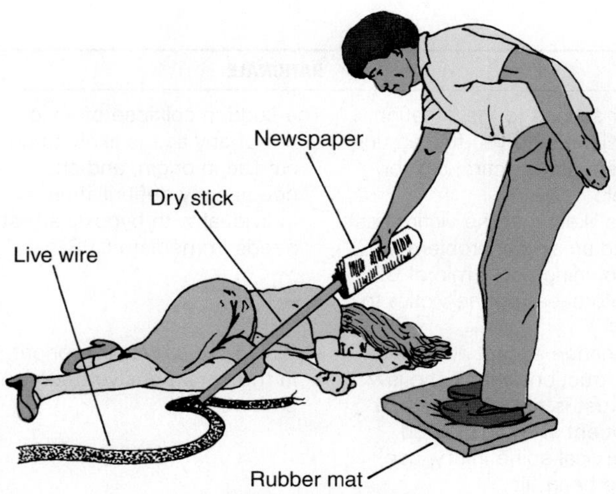

FIGURE **44–3** Separating a victim from a live electrical wire while avoiding similar shock.

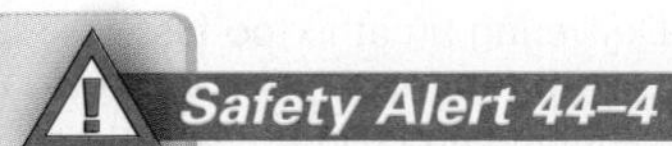

Lightning

If outdoors when lightning occurs, avoid water, high ground, open spaces, and metal objects. Do not seek shelter under canopies, small picnic or rain shelters, or trees.

CHEMICAL BURNS

Strong chemicals capable of burning the skin and mucous membranes will continue to destroy tissue unless they are diluted and removed immediately. **For this reason, one must act quickly to irrigate any area burned by chemicals with large amounts of water (with some exceptions) until all traces of the chemical have been removed.** Once this has been done, the burned area is covered with a dressing, and the patient is transported to a hospital. If possible, the following information should be made available to the treating physician: (1) offending agent, physical form, and concentration; (2) route and volume of exposure; (3) timing and extent of irrigation; and (4) coexisting injuries.

Treatment begins with ending the contact of the agent with the skin. This is usually accomplished by irrigation with copious amounts of water. However, water is not used for burns caused by dry lime or phenol. Dry lime should be brushed from the skin and clothing unless there is enough water to remove *all* traces of the powder. The nurse should use gloves to protect the hands. Small amounts of water will react chemically with the lime to produce a highly **corrosive** (destroys gradually) substance. Phenol (carbolic acid) is not water soluble. The phenol is first removed by alcohol and the burned area is then rinsed with water.

If a corrosive chemical has been ingested, the poison control center should be contacted for instructions and proper dosage of an antidote. Vomiting should **not** be induced or encouraged by overloading the stomach. No attempt should be made to neutralize an ingested chemical substance, as this can cause further damage to the esophagus and stomach.

THERMAL INJURY

If the burn is caused by heat, removal of the heat source and cooling the skin is always the first step in treatment. Use cool water to help prevent further heat injury and to provide some pain relief. See Chapter 42 for additional information on burn management.

CARDIOPULMONARY RESUSCITATION

The first priority in administering emergency medical care is to assess the airway, then check for signs of breathing. The second priority is to determine whether the heart is beating by assessing circulation. When neither breathing nor circulation is present, cardiopulmonary resuscitation, usually abbreviated CPR, is indicated.

Table 44–2 presents the most recent changes to the techniques of CPR. For the most up-to-date science, refer to a current CPR handbook. Supervised practice is recommended at least once a year to maintain previously learned skills. Most health care providers do not routinely implement CPR in their daily or weekly practice. Any skill not practiced will become more difficult to perform when needed. Most organizations providing CPR training only require recertification every 2 years. Studies show that skills are not retained for that length of time unless reviewed.

Many phenomena cause sudden cessation of breathing and circulation, from electric shock to drowning to heart attack and cardiac arrest. Prompt action is vitally important to the success of CPR. When a person stops breathing spontaneously and her heart stops beating, "clinical death" has occurred. Within 4 to 6 minutes, the cells of the brain, which are most sensitive to lack of oxygen, begin to deteriorate. If the oxygen supply is not restored immediately, the patient suffers irreversible brain damage and "biologic death" occurs. Intentional use of hypothermia within hours of cardiac arrest has been shown to improve survival and neurologic function. This practice has been slow to be implemented by the medical community and is more likely to be initiated by a critical care specialist (Abella et al., 2005).

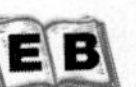

CPR is indicated when the person shows signs of cardiac arrest. **These signs include (1) absence of response to stimuli, (2) absent respirations, and (3) absence of a carotid pulse.** To make the steps in CPR easier to remember, use the "ABCs." The letter *A* reminds one of "airway," *B* of "breathing," and *C* of "circulation," and now *D* for defibrillation is part of the sequence. Resuscitation for infants and children is somewhat different; see Table 44–3 for details.

The use of the **automated external defibrillator (AED)** is covered in CPR courses for health care providers.

Table 44–2 ***Changes to Health Care Provider CPR for Adults***

MANEUVER	OLD	NEW	RATIONALE
Activate emergency response system	Call first, call fast. Adjusting response to situation was mentioned but not emphasized	Tailor actions to the situation; if alone, and you find an unresponsive victim, call for help If it is likely that the victim has had an airway problem (i.e., drowning), do 2 min of CPR before leaving the victim to call	The sudden collapse of a victim of any age is likely to be cardiac in origin, and she needs early defibrillation. An individual with hypoxic arrest needs immediate CPR.
Airway	Head tilt, chin lift; use jaw thrust if cervical injury is suspected	No change except additional instructions that if the jaw thrust is not effective in a patient with suspected cervical spine injury, use the head tilt	Opening the airway is a priority in the unresponsive trauma patient.
Check for breathing	Check for adequate breathing	Same	Changes were made to the infant and child procedures (see Table 44–3).
Breaths			
Initial	Recommendations for tidal volumes were given Breaths were to be given over 1–2 sec	Deliver each breath (using a barrier device) over 1 sec. The volume of each breath should be adequate to cause the chest to rise	Delivering breaths too fast or with too much volume is not helpful and can be harmful.
Rescue breathing without chest compressions	10–12 breaths/min (approximately 1 breath q 5–6 sec)	Same	Health care providers should be aware that lay rescuers are not taught to check for signs of circulation or a pulse; therefore, they are not taught to do rescue breathing without chest compressions.
Rescue breathing with CPR and advanced airway	Ventilation rate of 12–15 breaths/min	Ventilation rate of 8–10 breaths/min	During CPR, the blood flow to the lungs is less than normal so a slower respiratory rate is adequate.
Pulse check	≤10 sec, carotid	Same	Lay people are not taught this step.
Chest compressions			
Compression landmarks	Center of chest, between nipples	Same	Proper hand position is important to deliver adequate compressions
Compression method	2 hands: heel of one hand, other hand on top	Same	Pushing hard, pushing fast, and allowing for the chest to recoil between compressions has been found to be the most effective.
Compression depth	1½–2 inches	Same	
Compression rate	Approx 100/min	Same	
Compression/ventilation ratio	15:2	30:2 (1 or 2 rescuers)	Minimizing interruptions to compressions gives the best blood flow. Rescuers should change compressors q 2 min to prevent fatigue and decreased efficiency of compressions.
AED use	Use immediately	For an unwitnessed arrest with an out-of-hospital response, may provide 5 cycles/2 min of CPR before shock if 4–5 min have elapsed since arrest	Providing oxygenation prior to defibrillation may make the effort more successful.

Key: *AED*, automated external defibrillator; *CPR*, cardiopulmonary resuscitation.

Table 44–3 ***Differences in CPR Between Infants and Children (Health Care Provider, Single Rescuer)***

INFANTS	CHILDREN
Use "puff" breaths to make the chest gently rise.	Use sufficient breath to just make the chest rise for each of the two breaths delivered.
Check for a brachial pulse in the arm between the shoulder and the elbow for no more than 10 sec.	Check the carotid pulse for no more than 10 sec.
Locate chest compression position with fingers in center of chest just below nipple line. If possible, the preferred position is holding the infant in both hands with both thumbs in the center of the chest.	Locate chest compression position: lower half of the sternum, between nipples.
Using two fingers, compress chest 30 times at a rate of 100/min. If two-hand method is used, squeeze the chest, pressing the sternum with the thumbs. Compress approximately ⅓–½ the depth of the chest.	Use one hand and align shoulders over your hand. Deliver 30 compressions at a rate of 100/min. Compress approximately ⅓–½ the depth of the chest.
Tilt head back and cover infant's mouth and nose with barrier device; give two breaths at end of each 30 compressions.	Pinch off nose, cover mouth with barrier device, and give two breaths between sets of 30 compressions (15 compressions for two health care rescuers).
Check pulse and breathing at end of five cycles; continue CPR if no pulse or breathing is detected.	Check pulse and breathing at end of five cycles; use pediatric AED if available, or continue CPR if no pulse or breathing is detected.

Key: *AED*, automated external defibrillator; *CPR*, cardiopulmonary resuscitation.

AEDs are now located in many public buildings, health clubs, airlines, malls, and sporting venues. Health care providers are expected to have knowledge in the use of an AED. As soon as the AED is brought to the scene, turn on the device; it will audibly give instructions on what to do next. The most recent American Heart Association guidelines recommend that single shocks be delivered instead of the previously recommended sequential three shocks. Also approved in the new guidelines is the use of AEDs in children 1 to 8 years old.

When the AED indicates that it is analyzing the rhythm, all CPR, rescue breathing, and direct contact with the victim must stop. If the AED identifies a shockable rhythm, it will either automatically charge, or give instructions to charge the device. Once the AED is charged, the instructions will state "stand clear" of the victim. It is important that no one is touching the victim when the charge is delivered. Anyone in direct contact will also be electrically shocked. Continue resuscitation efforts until Emergency Medical Service (in the community) or Advanced Life Support (in a health care setting) providers arrive to take over your efforts.

The most common cause of airway obstruction in the unconscious person is the tongue. The head tilt–chin lift maneuver repositions the trachea and tongue so that the airway is open. Because this maneuver also repositions the cervical spine, the jaw thrust method of opening the airway should be used if a spinal injury in the neck area is suspected. For this, kneel at the head of the victim with your elbows on the ground on either side of the victim's head, and place your thumbs on her lower jaw near the corners of the mouth and pointing toward her feet; place your fingertips around the bone of the lower jaw, and lift (Figure 44–4).

Although transmission of the human immunodeficiency virus (HIV) is highly unlikely via saliva, many people are hesitant to give mouth-to-mouth rescue

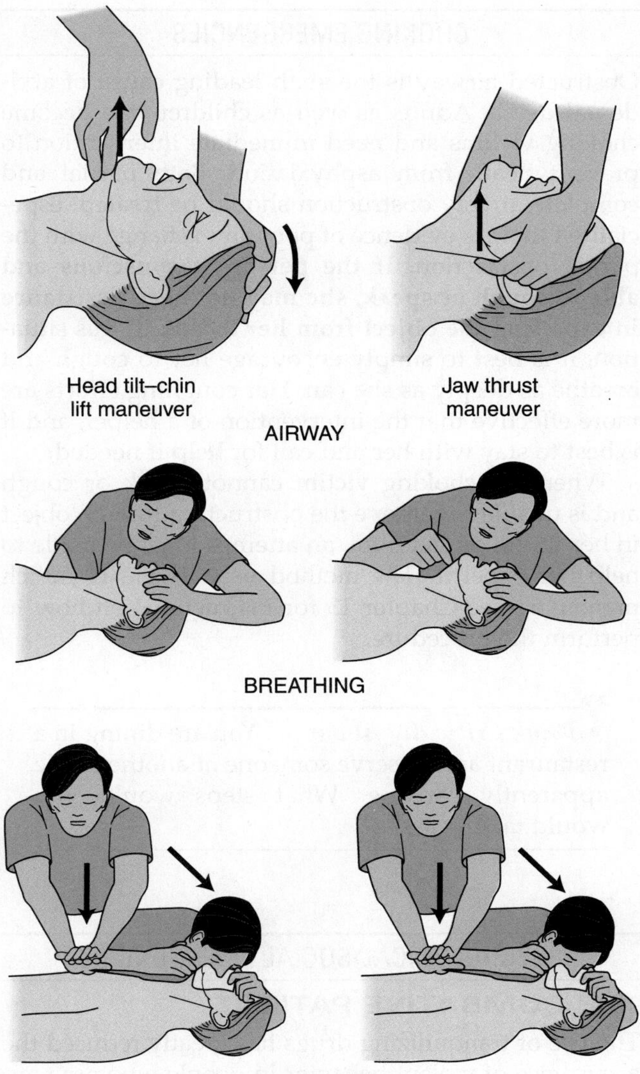

FIGURE 44–4 Cardiopulmonary resuscitation.

breathing to strangers. If no barrier device is available and bystanders are reluctant to administer mouth-to-mouth breathing, chest compressions alone are of some value. The recoil of the chest at the end of a compression will cause a small amount of air to be pulled into the lungs. A pocket mask that can be carried in a purse, pocket, or car is available and can be used to provide a barrier while giving rescue breathing. In a health care setting, where responding to emergencies is part of the job, barrier devices must be utilized. Know where the personal protective equipment is located for use in an emergency.

Two-person CPR is currently being taught only to health care providers (Figure 44–4). If a health care provider stops to render aid with another individual, he needs to understand that lay rescuers are not being taught two-person CPR methods. If a lay rescuer is participating in the rescue, take turns doing single-rescuer CPR until other help arrives.

CHOKING EMERGENCIES

Obstructed airway is the sixth leading cause of accidental death. Adults as well as children can become choking victims and need immediate intervention to prevent death from asphyxiation. Both partial and complete airway obstruction should be treated, especially if there is evidence of poor air exchange with the partial obstruction. **If the person is conscious and able to cough or speak, she may not need assistance in expelling the object from her throat.** In this situation, it is best to simply encourage her to cough and breathe as deeply as she can. Her coughing efforts are more effective that the intervention of a helper, and it is best to stay with her and call for help if needed.

When the choking victim cannot speak or cough and is unable to remove the obstructing foreign object in her throat on her own, an attempt must be made to help her expel it. The method used is the Heimlich maneuver; see Chapter 13 for instructions on how to perform the procedure.

Think Critically About . . . You are dining in a restaurant and observe someone at another table apparently choking. What steps would you would take to assist?

PSYCHOLOGICAL/SOCIAL EMERGENCIES

THE COMBATIVE PATIENT

The use of tranquilizing drugs has greatly reduced the occurrence of violent behavior in people who are temporarily unable to control their emotions because of a psychological disorder. When a person becomes greatly agitated and experiences an uncontrollable urge to act violently, she may be extremely frightened and usually welcomes help in regaining control if it is offered in the correct way. Box 44–4 shows ways to approach a combative patient. Language barriers and hearing difficulties need to be considered as possible contributors to an escalating situation. When an emergency patient seems to be out of control and combative, it might be that she perceives herself to be in danger from the emergency staff as well as from her injuries, or she may be under the influence of drugs or alcohol. However, if physical restraint becomes necessary, one should be sure that enough people are on hand to control the patient.

Box 44–4 *Strategies for Approaching a Combative Patient*

- Offer help on a one-to-one basis. Several people trying to talk to the patient or subdue her at once may only add to her fright and disorientation.
- Establish eye contact.
- Use the person's name frequently.
- Explain who you are and what you are trying to do.
- Express genuine concern about the situation.
- Use a soft voice.
- Make sure the patient can hear and understand what is being said.
- Observe for signs of drug or alcohol use.

Patients who are not diagnosed as mentally ill can also become "violent" when nurses and other health care personnel fail to respect their rights and needs or when they are feeling threatened. **Everyone has a right to privacy and to know what is happening to her.** Patients should be told what procedures are planned and why they are necessary. Approaching the patient in a nonthreatening manner, using a calm tone of voice, and remaining calm will help maintain control over the situation. It may be necessary to help the patient by exerting some outside controls. These may be verbal or physical, but physical force should be used only after it is apparent that talking with the patient is not effective. One may simply tell the patient to stop screaming, to sit down, or to put down an object that is apparently intended to be used as a weapon. If verbal control does not work, it may be necessary to restrain the overwrought patient. If restraints are used, the patient should not be left alone after being restrained, as this action will give the impression that she is being punished for wrongdoing rather than being assisted in controlling herself. The Joint Commission has standards related to the use of restraints, and many states have regulations regarding the use of restraints. All policies and procedures should be followed regarding restraining patients.

DOMESTIC VIOLENCE/ABUSE

Sometimes the emergency room patient is a victim of abuse. Signs of battering include bruises, swellings, lacerations, fractures, hematomas, blackened eyes, abdomi-

Box 44–5 *Questions to Detect Abuse*

- Have you been hit or hurt in any way in the past year?
- Who injured you? Has it occurred before?
- Are you afraid of anyone?
- Do you feel safe at home?
- Does your partner use drugs or alcohol? How does his or her behavior change after using them?

nal injuries (especially during pregnancy), burns, and open wounds. Bruises or fractures in various stages of healing and signs of old lacerations and wounds in the presence of new ones indicate a need for a thorough assessment for battering. Often the victim may explain all of the injuries as the result of logical accidents rather than disclose that battering by an intimate partner has occurred. Psychologically the person may display signs of depression, low self-esteem, anxiety, and stress. Box 44–5 presents the types of questions that might be asked to elicit more information. Asking these questions after establishing rapport with the patient may encourage honest sharing of thoughts and feelings.

Although many more women are battered by their intimate partners, men sometimes also suffer from battering. If battering is revealed, the person is referred to an appropriate shelter and the incident is reported to the appropriate agency. **Some states have laws requiring health care providers to report domestic violence.**

Child Abuse

Any time a child is brought into the emergency room with unexplained or questionably explained injuries, a thorough physical assessment is performed for signs of physical abuse. If such signs are found, the case is referred to the proper authorities. **Child abuse or suspicion of child abuse must be reported by law.**

Elder Abuse

Unfortunately, elder abuse is common. Elderly patients also should be assessed for signs of abuse. The attitude of the elderly patient toward the caregiver should be assessed to determine whether there is any element of fear. The same signs of physical abuse listed for domestic abuse should be searched for, as well as signs of malnutrition, uncleanness, or severe depression. **The law requires that signs of elder abuse be reported.**

PSYCHOLOGICAL TRAUMA

Any intense event results in an emotional response. Natural disasters or massive injury from a man-made event have both physical and emotional effects. Whether the event is a widespread occurrence affecting many people or an individual trauma, emotional distress is very real. The phrase "they are in shock" is used to explain the emotional state of the vitims following one of these events. Although emotions can trigger physical signs and symptoms, the condition is usually not life

Box 44–6 *Classifications of Shock*

- Cardiogenic
  - Coronary
  - Noncoronary
- Hypovolemic
- Distributive
  - Anaphylactic
  - Neurogenic
  - Acute adrenal insufficiency
  - Insulin or hypoglycemic
  - Septic
- Obstructive

threatening unless the individual affected has a preexisting condition that puts her at risk.

Signs and symptoms of emotional shock include headaches, nausea, and chest pain. Preexisting medical conditions may worsen due to the stress. A calm presence and seeing to immediate physical needs can reassure the victim that someone is in charge and that there is control over the situation. Severe emotional traumas may take years of therapy to process. Emotional injury is not as obvious as physical trauma, but can have lasting effects. Physiologic shock is discussed in the next section.

SHOCK

Shock is a condition that starts at the cellular level and gradually spreads to enough cells to affect enough tissues to produce clinical signs and symptoms. The hallmark of shock is lack of **perfusion** (blood supply) to tissues, depriving them of oxygen and nutrients. There are multiple ways in which perfusion to tissues can be impaired. The different types of shock are categorized as to the mechanism causing the lack of perfusion. Shock can be labeled as hypovolemic, cardiogenic, distributive, or obstructive (Box 44–6). For perfusion to be maintained, adequate blood volume must be present, the blood vessels must be intact, and the pump (the heart) must be working correctly. Any abnormality in the components of the system can result in inadequate perfusion to tissues.

Stages of Shock

There are several stages in the progression of shock. Initially, cellular changes occur and may cause no signs or symptoms detectable by usual assessment methods. Some authorities consider this the first or initial stage of shock. Other authors list the compensatory stage as the first stage. During this stage, the body is able to maintain blood pressure (BP) and tissue perfusion due to compensatory mechanisms. The next stage is the progressive stage, when BP is affected and the body is no longer able to preserve blood flow to tissues. The last stage of shock is the refractory or ir-

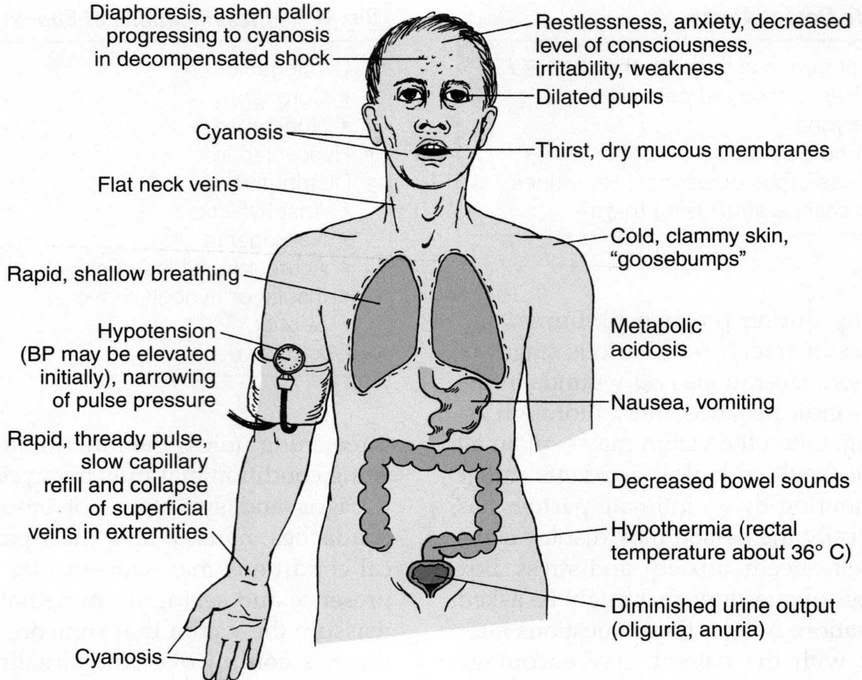

FIGURE **44–5** Clinical signs of shock.

reversible stage, when treatment is not effective. If the early stages of shock are recognized and aggressive treatment is started, the syndrome may be reversed. If shock is not treated until the progressive stage, treatment is usually not effective.

Signs and Symptoms

Recognition of impending shock is essential for early intervention. Early treatment results in better outcomes. Typical clinical symptoms of shock result from lack of oxygen to essential organs. Signs and symptoms associated with shock are those that accompany decreased cardiac output, such as confusion, restlessness, diaphoresis, rapid thready pulse, increased respiratory rate, cold clammy skin, and diminishing urinary output to less than 20 mL/hr (Figure 44–5).

CARDIOGENIC SHOCK

Cardiogenic shock occurs when the heart is incapable of pumping enough blood to meet the needs of the body (Concept Map 44–1). Cardiogenic shock is classified as coronary or noncoronary based on the reason for the dysfunction. Myocardial infarction is the primary cause of coronary cardiogenic shock due to direct damage of the heart muscle from a heart attack. Heart muscle can be rendered ineffective as a pump by noncoronary causes such as cardiomyopathy and valvular dysfunction.

Treatment

Shock is usually treated by infusion of volume. In cardiogenic shock, however, increased volume will overwhelm an already inefficient pump. Treatment for this type of shock is aimed at increasing pump efficiency without an increase in workload. Chemical and mechanical means are used to support the impaired heart muscle. Sympathomimetic agents (isoproterenol, dopamine, dobutamine), cardiac glyclosides (digoxin), calcium, and phosphodiesterase inhibitors (amrinone,

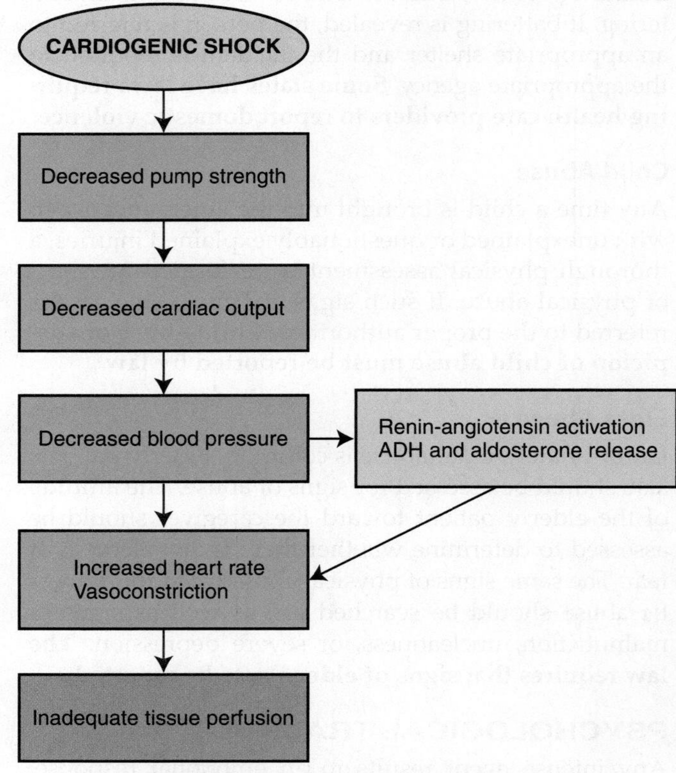

CONCEPT MAP **44–1** Cardiogenic shock.

Table 44–4 ***Clinical Manifestations of Blood Loss***

VOLUME LOST	CLINICAL MANIFESTATIONS
10%	None
20%	At rest, no signs or symptoms; slight postural hypotension when standing; tachycardia with exercise.
30%	Blood pressure and pulse normal when supine; postural hypotension and tachycardia with exercise.
40%	Below-normal blood pressure, central venous pressure, and cardiac output at rest; rapid, thready pulse and cold, clammy skin.
50%	Shock and potential death.

Adapted from Lewis, S.M., Heitkemper, M.M., Dirksen, S.R., et al. (2007). *Medical-Surgical Nursing: Assessment and Management of Clinical Problems* (7th ed.). St. Louis: Mosby.

milrinone) are all used to increase the contractility of cardiac muscle (positive inotropy). The difficulty with this is that as the heart works harder, it requires more oxygen. If it is already damaged so that inadequate circulation is occurring, pushing the heart to do more will only worsen the problem. In conjunction with the positive inotropes listed, vasodilators are judiciously used to decrease cardiac workload.

When the heart ejects blood into the systemic circulation, it has to overcome the pressure of the closed aortic valve and the resistance of the peripheral blood vessels. Think of watering the lawn with a hose that has an adjustable nozzle attached. If the nozzle is turned so that it has a larger opening, the pressure that it takes to get the water out of the hose is less than if the nozzle is turned to the smallest setting. With the smaller opening, much more pressure is exerted to expel the water. If the blood vessels that the heart is pumping blood into are dilated, the heart does not have to work as hard to expel the blood. This lessens the oxygen demand of the cardiac muscle. Vasodilator medications are used to open up blood vessels. When blood vessels dilate, the pressure in the system decreases, which drops BP. Vasodilators must be used cautiously in order to enhance cardiac performance without compromising BP. Medications are available that both increase contractility of the heart (have a positive **inotropic** effect) and also vasodilate. They are called inodilators and are used to help the heart pump better while decreasing the workload.

Mechanical means can also be utilized to support cardiac function. The intra-aortic balloon pump (IABP) is a mechanical left ventricular assist device that supports cardiac function. The balloon is inserted via the femoral artery and is positioned in the thoracic aorta above the renal arteries. The machine is timed to inflate the balloon during the resting phase of the cardiac cycle, during diastole. The balloon displaces 20 to 30 mL of blood during inflation. At the onset of systole, when the heart is trying to eject blood, the balloon deflates. On deflation, blood rushes out of the left ventricle to fill up the space vacated by the balloon. In effect, the deflation of the balloon causes a vacuum in the vessel, practically sucking the blood out of the heart. This greatly decreases the workload of the heart because it does not have to generate a lot of pressure to eject blood. The added bonus is that the coronary arteries receive their blood supply during diastole, at the time the balloon is inflated. That blood displaced by the balloon is pushed into the coronary arteries, providing better perfusion and oxygenation of the cardiac muscle.

Nursing care for the patient in cardiogenic shock includes the administration of medications that will help optimize heart function as well as manage any mechanical supports being used for the heart. A thorough baseline assessment of the cardiovascular system is needed so that changes can be identified and reported quickly. Ongoing interaction with the patient and family to keep them informed of what is happening is not only good nursing practice, it also helps the patient in decreasing her anxiety level, which can help the heart by reducing heart rate.

HYPOVOLEMIC SHOCK

The amount of blood loss that leads to hypovolemic shock varies depending on the ability of the patient's body to compensate for the lost fluid volume. A blood loss of even 500 mL in an adult who had normal circulating volume may cause hypovolemic shock. Table 44–4 shows the amount of blood loss and consequent clinical manifestations. Loss of whole blood is not the only fluid loss that can lead to a shock state. Any significant loss of volume can result in hypovolemic shock (Concept Map 44–2). Loss of plasma from a burn, severe nausea, vomiting and diarrhea, and internal oozing secondary to pancreatitis are all potential sources of hypovolemia.

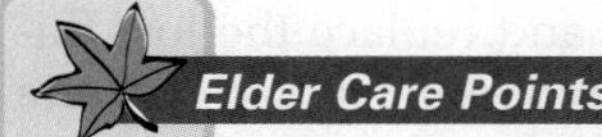

Elder Care Points

The elderly may develop shock with smaller blood loss because of decreased vascular tone and impaired cardiac function.

Treatment

Hypovolemic shock is treated by stopping the source of volume loss if possible and replacing the lost fluids. If hemorrhage is present, intravenous (IV) fluids will be rapidly infused until blood products are available for transfusion. If a large volume of blood is lost, clotting factors will also need to be replaced. Packed red cells are given to replenish cell volume. Fresh frozen plasma

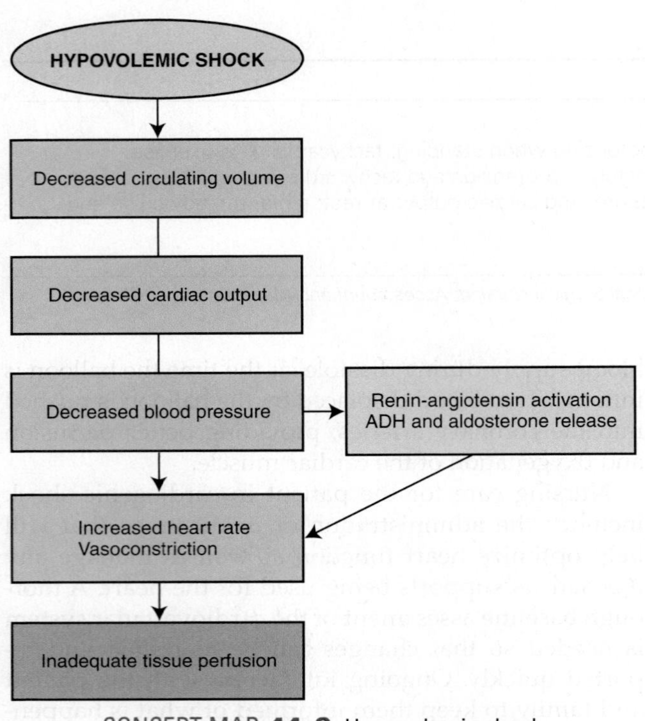

CONCEPT MAP **44–2** Hypovolemic shock.

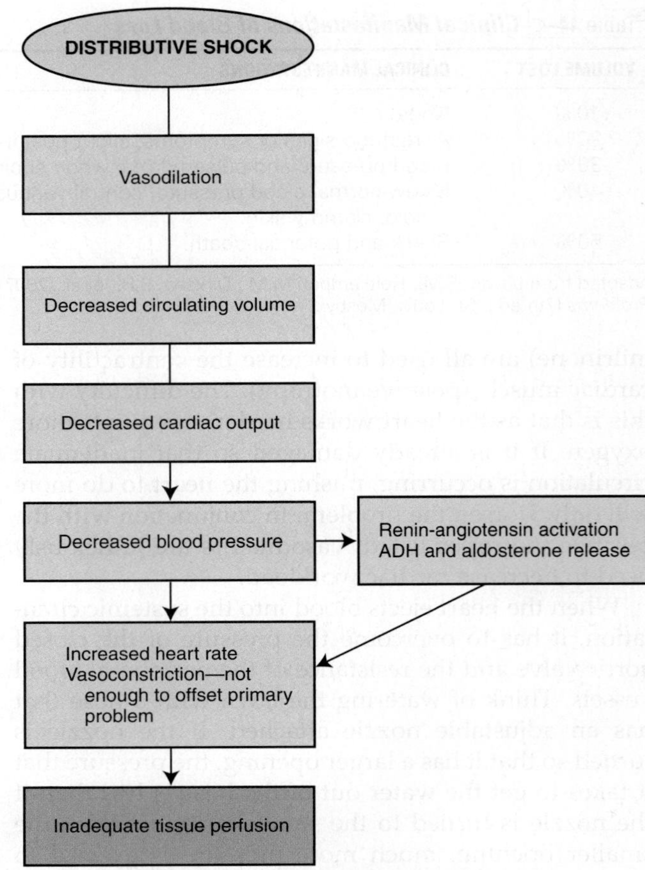

CONCEPT MAP **44–3** Distributive shock.

is given for replacement of clotting factors. Units of packed cells contain citrate as an anticoagulant. If multiple units of blood are rapidly infused, the citrate can bind with ionized calcium, decreasing the amount of circulating calcium. This can result in depressed cardiac function and in alteration in coagulation. Whole blood is made up of multiple components, so when replacement is necessary, many factors must be considered and tailored to the patient's specific need.

If fluid loss is from gastrointestinal sources, isotonic solutions will be utilized to replenish the fluid and electrolytes. Burn patients require replacement of lost plasma that is rich in protein. Both crystalloids containing salt and colloids such as albumin will be administered to rehydrate burn victims.

The primary interventions for **hypovolemia** are to stop the fluid loss if possible and replace the lost fluids. **In all situations of hypovolemic shock, volume replacement is essential.** To infuse large volumes of fluid and/or blood products, adequate IV access is extremely important. Two large-bore peripheral IV sites are needed, or placement of a central line with multiple lumens. Having vascular access in place that will allow for the infusion of necessary fluids is a life-saving intervention.

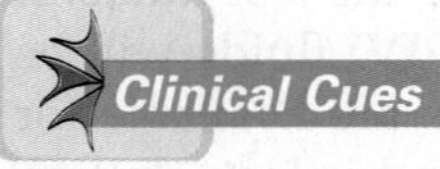

If large volumes of fluid are required for fluid resuscitation, warming of the fluids can help prevent hypothermia.

DISTRIBUTIVE (VASOGENIC) SHOCK

Distributive shock, also called vasogenic shock, involves a maldistribution of the fluid within the vascular system. As described earlier, the circulatory system consists of a pump (the heart), fluid (the blood), and the pipes for the fluid to flow through (the blood vessels). If the blood vessels change size and the volume of fluid stays the same, the pressure within the system changes. If the vessels dilate, there is more room for the same amount of fluid and the pressure decreases. All forms of distributive shock involve vasodilation of blood vessels, resulting in a "relative hypovolemia." This means that although there has not been actual volume loss, it physiologically seems that way. The way in which the alteration in distribution of the fluid happens are the various forms of distributive shock (Concept Map 44–3).

ANAPHYLACTIC SHOCK

Acute allergic reactions that are life threatening result in anaphylactic shock. For the body to produce this hypersensitive reaction, a previous exposure to the antigen must have occurred. Hypersensitivity reactions have been classified in several ways. The traditional classification system identified four different types of reactions based on the mechanisms involved and the time it takes for the reaction to happen. A newer classification system has been proposed that is more specific as to the components of the immune system that are involved and has seven categories. In either classification, anaphylaxis is an acute condition involving more than one organ system.

As mentioned earlier, shock is the syndrome resulting from inadequate tissue perfusion. In anaphylactic shock, the antigen-antibody reaction that occurs releases vasoactive substances that cause massive vasodilation as well as increased capillary permeability. This combination of factors results in hypotension. These mediators can also cause bronchoconstriction and angioedema of the laryngeal tissue, causing an acute airway emergency. Other signs and symptoms may include skin rash and flushing of the skin all over the body.

Treatment

If possible, the antigen should be removed immediately. With a bee sting, prompt removal of the stinger may help. If the anaphylaxis is due to an ingested or inhaled substance, removal may not be possible and symptoms must be treated immediately.

Treatment of anaphylactic shock includes airway management, including intubation when necessary, and administration of epinephrine intravenously or, if there is no IV access, intramuscularly. Epinephrine helps maintain BP, counteracts the effects of the released mediators, and inhibits further release of mediators from mast cells and basophils.

Administration of fluid volume is also needed. Although the actual circulating volume reduction due to leaking capillaries is not enough to cause hypotension, this loss in addition to the vasodilation is more than enough to cause a significant drop in BP. Therefore, fluid administration is important for BP support. An infusion of dopamine may be implemented to increase peripheral vascular tone, causing vasoconstriction and shunting blood back into the central circulation, improving flow to the brain, heart, lungs, and kidneys.

NEUROGENIC SHOCK

Neurogenic shock is the rarest form of shock and results from the blocking of sympathetic outflow from the vasomotor center of the brainstem, usually caused by spinal injury or anesthesia. Most blood vessels are never completely constricted or completely dilated. The in-between state is known as vascular tone. It allows for constriction or dilation as necessary. The sympathetic nervous system is in charge of maintaining this state of readiness. When spinal cord injury happens or high levels of spinal anesthesia are administered, the sympathetic impulses regulating the state of the blood vessels are blocked and passive vasodilation occurs. The volume of fluid circulating in the blood vessels is the same, but the space within the blood vessels has gotten larger. This decreases pressure within the blood vessels, resulting in a lower BP leading to hypotension and a shock state.

Treatment

Treatment includes giving volume to "fill up the tank" and giving vasoconstrictor medications to decrease the amount of vasodilation that is present. Many times the cause of this condition is not immediately fixable, so supportive care is given to maintain BP and perfusion.

ACUTE ADRENAL INSUFFICIENCY

The presence of cortisol in the body allows the blood vessels to function properly in response to epinephrine and other catecholamines by constricting. Conditions that decrease the amount of circulating cortisol interfere with the ability of the blood vessels to constrict. Patients with Addison's disease have a decrease or absence of adrenal cortical secretions, primarily cortisol. Since cortisol is released in response to adrenocorticotropic hormone (ACTH) from the pituitary gland, abnormalities in ACTH release can also cause a reduction in circulating cortisol. Another situation that can cause symptoms of acute lack of cortisol results from prescribed treatment. Steroids are given to treat many autoimmune diseases, and the body becomes dependent on this outside source of cortisol. If administration of the medication is stopped abruptly, acute cortisol insufficiency will occur.

Decreased levels of cortisol result in decreased sensitivity of the blood vessels to sympathetic stimulation. It is the sympathetic stimulation that maintains vascular tone. Lack of vascular tone causes vasodilation, producing hypotension. Cortisol helps maintain blood pressure and cardiovascular function, so the acute lack of it will decrease BP and produce typical signs and symptoms of shock.

Treatment

Treatment of acute cortisol deficiency is to give corticosteroids such as betamethasone, cortisone, hydrocortisone, or methylprednisolone intravenously. Oral and inhaled forms are available for chronic treatment. This allows the body to respond appropriately in maintaining the amount of vasoconstriction needed to have an adequate BP. The immediate treatment of the hypotension includes administration of IV fluids and BP support.

INSULIN OR HYPOGLYCEMIC SHOCK

Hypoglycemia from whatever cause will block the sympathetic outflow from the vasomotor center in the brainstem with the same result as in neurogenic shock—dilation of blood vessels resulting in a drop in BP. The brain needs a constant supply of glucose to function properly. If glucose levels drop, level of consciousness is altered and blood vessels dilate. This results in the classic clinical picture of a patient who has received too much insulin: altered level of consciousness; cold, clammy skin; hypotension that can cause dizziness; and tachycardia. Most patients experiencing hypoglycemia have diabetes, but some individuals become hypoglycemic who are not diabetic.

Treatment

Administration of glucose is the treatment for hypoglycemia. If the patient is awake, glucose in the form of ½ cup of juice or regular soda may be given. Glucose tablets or hard candy may also be used to provide a ready source of glucose. If a patient has a decreased level of consciousness, IV glucose may need to be given. Alteration in level of consciousness often results in impaired swallowing. Attempts to give glucose by mouth could result in aspiration. If an IV is not in place, intramuscular glucagon can be given by medical personnel or trained family members.

Correction of the blood glucose level will allow the normal sympathetic pathways to regain function and the blood vessels to respond appropriately. This will restore BP.

SYSTEMIC INFLAMMATORY RESPONSE SYNDROME (SIRS)

The response of the body to a break in the protective skin layer or invasion of a microorganism is to initiate the inflammatory response that has been discussed in Chapter 10. The inflammatory response is part of the cascade of events that is part of the body's immune response. Once the threat has been dealt with, feedback mechanisms shut off the supply of chemicals that were released and the immune system goes back into a state of readiness. In some situations this does not happen, and the substances that cause inflammation continue to be released. This clinical picture is known as **systemic inflammatory response syndrome (SIRS).** The signs and symptoms include tachycardia, tachypnea, hypotension, oliguria, fever, and signs of poor perfusion. All of these signs and symptoms occur without a documented source of infection.

The Society of Critical Care Medicine, the American College of Chest Physicians, the European Society of Intensive Care Medicine, the American Thoracic Society, and the Surgical Infection Society sponsored an international conference in 2001 to update previous definitions of sepsis. They made few changes to the document originally created in 1991. It is difficult for clinicians to discuss diagnosis and treatment of sepsis because it is difficult to quantify. The conference was intended to allow physicians to use the same diagnostic criteria around the world so that interventions and epidemiology could reliably be compared.

According to the findings in the 2001 conference, the diagnosis of sepsis is based on documented OR ***suspected*** infection and some of the following (partial list): fever (or hypothermia in patients who are unable to mount an immune response), elevated heart rate, tachypnea, altered mental status, significant edema, hyperglycemia, hypotension, oliguria, ileus, and decreased capillary refill. Although none of these findings is specific to the diagnosis of sepsis, the symptoms paint a clinical picture of a very sick patient who meets the criteria for sepsis.

Once sepsis is suspected, appropriate treatment should promptly be started. This includes antibiotic therapy, fluid resuscitation, BP management, and support of oxygenation, which may require intubation and mechanical ventilation. To receive adequate monitoring and treatment, patients who are septic need to be cared for in a critical care environment.

It is thought that SIRS is the first part of a continuum that leads to sepsis, then severe sepsis, and ultimately **multisystem organ dysfunction syndrome (MODS).** When the immune system initiates the inflammatory response, it also initiates the clotting cascade. The body is responding to an unknown threat and prepares to fight off foreign organisms and/or to stop bleeding, so both systems are activated. In sepsis, the heightened coagulant state of the body leads to multiple small clots forming in the microcirculation, which is known as disseminated intravascular coagulation (DIC). These small clots clog up the circulation to organs. This clotting leads to organ damage throughout the body. When two or more organ systems show signs of abnormality, the condition is called MODS.

The extensive clotting that occurs throughout the body in DIC uses up most of the clotting factors in the blood. As a result, bleeding occurs easily. Patients may ooze blood from previously dry wounds, from their gums, and around IV catheters, and bruise very easily. The clinical sign most noticeable is bleeding from any break in the skin.

If an event occurs that triggers clotting, normally the process to dissolve the clot is also activated. This allows the clot to stop the bleeding and then be reabsorbed when no longer needed, conserving the clotting factors for reuse. One of the substances involved in the breakdown of the clot is activated protein C. Scientists have been able to duplicate this chemical in the laboratory. Drotrecogin alfa (activated) (Xigris) is given to decrease clotting in the extremely small blood vessels and keep the blood flowing. Although it may seem contradictory to give a medication that will dissolve clots when the patient is bleeding, the clots that have formed in the small blood vessels are harming the patient, and keeping the clotting factors from being available in the areas they are needed. Administration of this medication is an attempt to disrupt the abnormal clotting.

The usual clinical progression starts with symptoms indicating SIRS, moving into sepsis, then severe sepsis and MODS complicated by DIC. If this sequence of events continues, mortality rates range from 28% to 80%. The wide range is due to multiple variables such as age, preexisting illnesses, and access to treatment. Early recognition and treatment of this cascade of events are the most significant factors in reducing mortality.

Safety Alert 44–5

Infection Control

Hospitalized patients with urinary catheters, intravenous lines, surgical wounds, and other situations that disrupt the protective barrier of the skin are at increased risk of infection. Most are somewhat immunocompromised due to their reason for hospitalization. A hospital-acquired infection can lead to sepsis. Following infection control principles will safeguard these patients.

One of the primary infection control principles is consistently following hand hygiene standards. This is so important that one of the 2008 National Patient Safety Goals is "Comply with current World Health Organization (WHO) Hand Hygiene Guidelines or Centers for Disease Control and Prevention (CDC) hand hygiene guidelines."

SEPTIC SHOCK

Septic shock is part of the distributive (vasogenic) category of shock and is an inflammatory condition caused by a systemic bacterial infection. The inflammatory process, in addition to causing clotting and activation of the immune system, releases chemicals that cause vasodilation and increased capillary permeability. The vasodilation, as with the other forms of distributive shock, causes BP to fall. The addition of leaking capillaries causing fluid loss increases the severity of the hypotension. The infecting organism secretes toxins from its cell wall that also react with the blood vessels and cell membranes, causing further increased capillary permeability and further loss of fluid from the vascular space, cellular injury, and greatly increased cellular metabolic rate.

Bacteria are organisms that are commonly associated with the infections leading to sepsis and septic shock. Gram-negative bacteria such as *Pseudomonas aeruginosa, Escherichia coli,* and *Klebsiella pneumoniae,* and gram-positive bacteria such as *Staphylococcus* and *Streptococcus,* are normally present in the environment, and exposure to them is common. In a hospital environment, it is essential to protect patients from *nosocomial* (hospital-acquired) infections. These infections can lead to sepsis with deadly outcomes. Meticulous care must be taken with IV sites, Foley catheters, and other devices that disrupt the body's protective mechanisms (Safety Alert 44–5).

Treatment

To provide adequate treatment of sepsis, early detection is required. Each nurse must consider which patients are at greatest risk for sepsis. Postsurgical infections and peritonitis are two problems that can lead to sepsis. Patients who have delayed seeking treatment for an infection of any kind also are at risk. An immunocompromised patient with multiple tubes and IV lines is also at risk. When a patient has been identified as being at risk for sepsis, monitor for slight changes in condition such as warm, dry, flushed skin; full, bounding pulse; normal to high BP; and elevated urine output. The temperature may be normal or slightly elevated, although some patients do experience a high temperature with sepsis. Some patients, often the elderly, experience hypothermia when septic.

When the patient is known to have sepsis, the nurse must be vigilant for signs of septic shock. **Watch the urine output. If it begins to decrease hourly, notify the physician.** Monitor breath sounds for crackles, and check for an increasing heart rate and decreasing BP. Assess for increased fatigue, feelings of anxiety, and changes in mental status. Watch for dependent edema. If shock becomes established, the skin will become cool and clammy and the peripheral pulses will be weak and thready. Urine output will drop, and BP will fall as hypovolemia becomes more pronounced. Watch for signs of bleeding that may indicate DIC. **Treatment involves controlling and eliminating the infection and supporting the patient with fluids, BP control, and oxygen and preventing complications.**

OBSTRUCTIVE SHOCK

Another way in which tissue perfusion can be impaired is when there is a mechanical obstruction to blood flow. This can be caused by such conditions as pericardial tamponade, tension pneumothorax, aortic dissection, constrictive pericarditis, or massive pulmonary embolus. In all of these conditions, a physical obstruction prevents adequate filling or emptying of the heart, or there is a problem in the blood vessels, preventing forward flow of blood. For each of these conditions, the abnormality must be corrected to restore cardiovascular function.

Treatment

All causes of obstructive shock prevent the heart from pumping blood either by squeezing the heart, which prevents filling and emptying, or by blocking the forward flow of blood through the blood vessels. The only treatment is to fix the problem, if possible.

Pericardial tamponade is treated by inserting a needle into the pericardial sac and removing the fluid that is compressing the heart. Tension pneumothorax is also treated by needle decompression. A needle or thoracostomy tube is inserted to release the air trapped in the chest that is putting pressure on the heart.

Aortic dissection must be quickly recognized and the patient taken immediately to the operating room for repair of the vessel. Aortic dissection is one of many causes of chest pain and diagnosis can be difficult.

Constrictive pericarditis does not usually have a sudden onset. It is usually a chronic problem that can have acute episodes. Medical treatment with antiinflammatory medications may help, but the only definitive treatment is surgery.

Massive pulmonary embolus is usually fatal. A less severe pulmonary embolus will be treated with heparin to prevent further clot formation. Thrombolytic therapy in pulmonary embolus is controversial. Care should be taken in administration of anticoagulant medications. Patient Safety Goal 3E 2008 is to reduce the likelihood of patient harm associated with the use of anticoagulation therapy.

Any threat to adequate blood flow must be treated quickly to prevent damage to tissues from oxygen deprivation. The brain is the most sensitive to changes in blood flow and the most easily damaged by lack of oxygen. Prompt recognition and reporting of changes in the patient's condition are essential to maintaining life and function for patients at risk for shock.

NURSING MANAGEMENT

The stages of shock progress rapidly, making it imperative that nursing management includes being aware of patients that may be at risk for developing shock and taking immediate action with the first symptoms that appear. Since shock involves the entire body, the nurse must be ready to systematically evaluate the function of multiple body systems. Maintaining adequate fluid volume and BP are key components in adequately managing shock.

Controlling blood sugar in seriously ill patients has been shown to improve outcomes. Patients undergoing a severe illness exhibit elevated glucose levels as the body tries to mobilize energy to respond to the physiologic threat. A recent study found that maintaining glucose levels between 80 and 110 mg/dL in a group of patients requiring intensive care significantly reduced the incidence of kidney injury. It also accelerated weaning from mechanical ventilation, and accelerated discharge from the intensive care unit and the hospital (Van den Berghe et al., 2006). Other studies have replicated these findings. 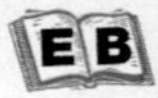

Assessment (Data Collection)

Ongoing evaluation of the patient's level of consciousness, vital signs (including temperature), skin signs, and urine output are all essential to the recognition of shock and management of the condition. Serial assessment data are compared to the previous data and the baseline assessment. Watching for changes and trends in physical and laboratory findings is extremely important. This information is used to make treatment decisions.

Many hosptials have implemented rapid response teams to help with the assessment and management of patients that are unstable. Goal 16 of the 2008 National Patient Safety Goals is to improve recognition and response to changes in a patient's condition. To do this "the organization selects a suitable method that enables health care staff members to directly request additional assistance from a specially trained individual(s) when the patient's condition appears to be worsening."

Nursing Diagnosis, Planning, and Implementation

The primary nursing diagnosis for all shock is ineffective in tissue perfusion. The reason for the alteration will vary depending on the type of shock the patient is experiencing. The planning of care for the patient in shock should include measures to monitor and maintain a patent airway, body temperature, and skin integrity (Nursing Care Plan 44–1).

NURSING CARE PLAN 44–1

Care of the Patient Exhibiting Symptoms of Shock

SCENARIO Bob Jones, a 22-year-old, was involved in a motor vehicle accident, sustaining abdominal injury and multiple fractures.

PROBLEM/NURSING DIAGNOSIS *Multiple trauma*/Decreased cardiac output related to shock syndrome.

Supporting assessment data *Objective:* BP 80/40, P 150, skin pale and clammy.

Goals/Expected Outcomes	*Nursing Interventions*	*Selected Rationale*	*Evaluation*
Patient will have adequate BP to maintain vital organ perfusion	Monitor vital signs, CVP (when used), urine output, pulse oximetry q 5 min to 1 hr as indicated by patient condition.	Prolonged hypotension will cause end-organ damage.	BP is maintained at >90 mm Hg systolic and urine output is ≥30 mL/hr.
	Maintain patent IV sites. Administer fluids as ordered.	Volume replacement is essential and requires adequate access.	IV access is adequate to administer IV fluids as ordered.
	Note quality/strength of peripheral pulses with vital signs.	Weak, thready pulses indicate decreased cardiac output.	Pulses are appropriately monitored.
	Monitor laboratory and x-ray results.	Evaluate patient's response to therapy.	Labs indicate therapy is working.

Key: *ABGs,* arterial blood gases; *ARDS,* acute respiratory distress syndrome; *BP,* blood pressure; *CVP,* central venous pressure; *IV,* intravenous; *P,* pulse; *SaO_2,* percentage of hemoglobin saturated with oxygen.

NURSING CARE PLAN 44-1

Care of the Patient Exhibiting Symptoms of Shock—cont'd

PROBLEM/NURSING DIAGNOSIS *Very low blood pressure*/Risk for impaired gas exchange related to altered blood flow.

Supporting assessment data *Objective:* BP 80/40, blood loss secondary to trauma.

Goals/Expected Outcomes	Nursing Interventions	Selected Rationale	Evaluation
ABGs and respiratory rate are within patient's normal range	Maintain patent airway. Elevate head of bed if tolerated by BP.	Enhances lung expansion.	Note any increased work of breathing.
	Administer oxygen to keep SaO_2 ≥92%.	Maximize the oxygen-carrying capacity of the available hemoglobin.	ABGs indicate adequate oxygenation and ventilation. SaO_2 is ≥92%.
	Auscultate breath sounds q 2–4 hr.	The patient is at risk for ARDS.	Lungs remain clear or changes are identified and reported promptly.
	Investigate alterations in level of consciousness.	Decreased levels of oxygen can cause alterations in sensorium.	No change in level of consciousness.

PROBLEM/NURSING DIAGNOSIS *Very anxious about injuries*/Patient/family fear and anxiety due to uncertainty of condition related to presence of a life-threatening situation.

Supporting assessment data *Subjective:* Patient states that he is scared and wants to know if he will live.

Goals/Expected Outcomes	Nursing Interventions	Selected Rationale	Evaluation
Patient/family will express concerns and fears	Maintain a calm and reassuring presence.	This will reduce anxiety and the patient's oxygen need.	Patient/family is reassured when the nurse is present.
	Explain activities, medications, treatments, and equipment simply and honestly.	The greatest need of families and patients is that of information.	The patient/family states that all of their questions were answered.
	Demonstrate concern and respect for patient and family.	Extending an attitude of concern makes it easier for patients/families to discuss concerns.	The patient/family discussed concerns with the health care team.

? CRITICAL THINKING QUESTIONS

1. What complications is this patient at risk for developing?
2. If this patient were 72 instead of 22, how would that change your care?

Regardless of the label, the treatment goals in shock are to restore circulating volume and to stop the initiating cause if possible. In most types of shock, BP responds to administration of IV fluids. The exception to this is cardiogenic shock in which the pump cannot manage the fluids that are already present and pump support is needed.

If an IV is not in place, volume can be redistributed to the central circulation by laying the patient flat and elevating the legs 10 to 12 inches or placing her in the Trendelenburg position. Traditional guidelines recommend this positioning. Current research is questioning this time-honored therapy since the practice is more tradition based than evidence based. There are findings that indicate that Trendelenburg positioning may not be helpful for shock resuscitation (Bridges & Jarquin-Valdivia, 2005). 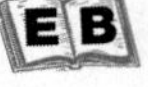

Evaluation

If interventions are effective, then there should be improvement in tissue perfusion. This can be evaluated by looking at BP, urine output, and level of consciousness. These are key indicators of adequacy of blood flow to vital organs. Since the main malfunction in shock is inadequate blood flow to the tissues, it is logical to look at tissue perfusion indicators to evaluate if treatment is having an effect. Other indicators to monitor include capillary refill, color and temperature of the skin, and the amplitude of pulses in the extremities.

With adequate fluid and medication administration, BP should be maintained above 90 mm Hg systolic. This should provide enough blood flow to the kidneys to generate 20 to 30 mL of urine output per hour. If there has been no neurologic insult, the patient should return to her previous level of consciousness.

Shock is a life-threatening condition that requires careful nursing assessment and intervention to improve outcomes for patients. Continuous assessment and reassessment give valuable information as to the effectiveness of treatment and allow for appropriate management of the patient's care.

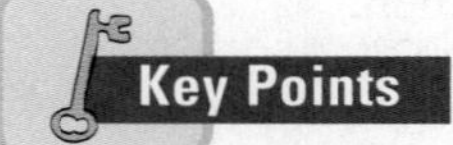

Key Points

- Nurses play a key role in educating the public about home, highway, and recreational safety.
- Cervical spine precautions should be taken with all trauma patients.
- Bleeding can be controlled with appropriately applied pressure.
- Extreme heat and extreme cold can both produce injury. Prevention is key.
- Have the phone number of the poison control center readily available.
- Insect bites can be life threatening for those that have allergies to the venom.
- Burns need prompt cooling and treatment for the best outcomes.
- Knowledge of first aid and CPR is useful on and off of the job and can save lives.
- Airway management and artificial breathing are key to successful resuscitation.
- Current American Heart Association guidelines require two breaths for every 30 chest compressions.
- The ABCs (airway, breathing, and circulation) are always priorities.
- The Heimlich maneuver is performed for clearing an obstructed airway.
- A calm, respectful approach to combative patients can help control the situation.
- Health care workers are required to report signs of abuse.
- Shock occurs when tissues do not get enough oxygen.
- Early recognition of shock is important to allow for prompt treatment.
- The clinical signs and symptoms of shock are produced when enough tissues are compromised to produce organ dysfunction.
- The major categories of shock are cardiogenic, hypovolemic, distributive, and obstructive.
- Blood pressure support in cardiogenic shock involves support for the pump (the heart) rather than adding volume.
- Blood pressure support in all other kinds of shock includes infusion of large volumes of IV fluid.

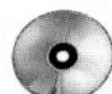

Go to your **Companion CD-ROM** for an Audio Glossary, animations, video clips, and bonus review questions.

evolve Be sure to visit the companion Evolve site at http://evolve.elsevier.com/deWit for interactive NCLEX-PN Exam Style Review Questions, WebLinks, and additional online resources.

NCLEX EXAM STYLE REVIEW QUESTIONS

Choose the best answer(s) for the following questions:

1. To control a gushing bleed, the nurse must initially:
  1. elevate the injured part.
  2. compress the artery above the wound.
  3. wrap the body part tightly.
  4. snugly secure a bulky dressing.

2. The nurse reinforces the need for prompt action in the event of any type of poisoning. The initial course of action would be to:
  1. save the container and any of the contents.
  2. save a sample of vomitus for analysis.
  3. call poison control.
  4. induce vomiting.

3. ____________________ are substances formed by the decomposition of protein foods.

4. A 70-year-old patient is hospitalized for excessive coughing, shortness of breath, wheezing, and a burning sensation of the nose and throat. Mucous membranes are cherry red. The nurse would most like suspect:
  1. ptomaine ingestion.
  2. carbon monoxide inhalation.
  3. corrosive chemicals ingestion.
  4. food poisoning.

5. A 50-year-old Korean man is admitted for acute alcohol intoxication. Anticipating combative behaviors, the nurse musters communication skills that would help in obtaining clinical information. Effective approaches to this patient would include: *(Select all that apply.)*
  1. establishing eye contact.
  2. using the person's name frequently.
  3. expressing genuine concern about the situation.
  4. using a loud, commanding voice.
  5. involving essential family members.

6. The nurse is caring for a patient with cardiogenic shock. Ongoing assessments confirm the nursing diagnosis of Decreased cardiac output. An appropriate nursing intervention would be to:
  1. force fluids.
  2. administer inotropic medications.
  3. encourage activity.
  4. give antibiotics.

7. The nurse identifies Deficient fluid volume as the priority nursing diagnosis for a patient hospitalized for severe gastrointestinal bleeding. An etiology for the nursing diagnosis would be:
   1. maldistribution of body fluids.
   2. ongoing blood loss.
   3. increased capillary permeability.
   4. decreased pump efficiency.

8. When taking care of a septic patient, the nurse must watch for which of the following signs and symptoms of impending septic shock?
   1. Increasing urine output
   2. Decreasing heart rate
   3. Increasing blood pressure
   4. Changes in mental status

9. A critically ill patient presents with fever, low blood pressure, increased heart rate, increased respirations, and oliguria. There is no documented infection. The most likely diagnosis would be:
   1. disseminated intravascular coagulation (DIC).
   2. systemic inflammatory response syndrome (SIRS).
   3. multisystem organ dysfunction syndrome (MODS).
   4. septic shock.

10. A patient bitten by a stray dog and was rushed to the emergency room. Which of the following measures must be done first?
   1. Apply antibiotic ointment on affected sites.
   2. Cover with a clean bandage and immobilize.
   3. Rinse wound with soap and hot running water for 5 to 10 minutes.
   4. Give tetanus booster shot if patient has not had one in the past 5 years.

CRITICAL THINKING ACTIVITIES

Read each clinical scenario and discuss the questions with your classmates.

Scenario A

While watching a sporting event from the stands, you notice the person sitting in front of you has slumped over. You touch her shoulder and ask if she is all right. There is no response and you see no signs of breathing.

1. What should you do next?
2. Describe the appropriate airway maneuver you would use for this person.
3. The victim has no pulse and is not breathing. What do you do now?
4. An AED is on scene. What is your role in use of this equipment?

Scenario B

You are on your way home from work and you see a car hit a teenage boy on a bicycle. You stop to help the bicyclist. He is unconscious, has a large scalp laceration that is bleeding profusely, and has an obviously fractured left leg.

1. Where do you start?
2. If you need to open his airway, what method would you use?
3. What should you do about the scalp laceration and broken leg?
4. What is your legal obligation in this setting?

Scenario C

While working as a student nurse in the hospital's emergency unit, you notice that patients who have been injured or are very ill sometimes become hostile and combative. Some try to assault members of the emergency team and others use abusive and threatening language.

1. Discuss with your classmates some reasons why patients may behave in these ways when they are injured or very ill.
2. What are some ways in which so-called violent patients who are not mentally ill can be handled so as to calm them and prevent assault on and encourage cooperation with the emergency staff?
3. What resources are available to help manage combative patients?
4. What information would be helpful to have regarding the patient's history when making treatment decisions?

Scenario D

Your 80-year-old male patient admitted yesterday for pneumonia has become confused, hypotensive, oliguric, clammy, and pale.

1. What are the possible explanations for his clinical signs and symptoms?
2. What are your priorities for his care?
3. Discuss what treatment is indicated.
4. How will you know if your treatment has been effective?

CHAPTER 45 Care of Patients with Anxiety, Mood, and Eating Disorders

evolve http://evolve.elsevier.com/deWit

Objectives

Upon completion of this chapter, you should be able to:

Theory

1. Discuss the significance of anxiety in the general adult population.
2. Differentiate between normal anxiety and anxiety disorders.
3. Describe the signs and symptoms and treatment for anxiety disorders.
4. Discuss assessment, nursing diagnoses, and nursing interventions for patients with anxiety disorders.
5. Discuss the variances of normal mood and discuss mood alterations that become debilitating.
6. Discuss assessment, nursing diagnoses, and nursing interventions for patients with bipolar disorder and major depressive disorder.
7. Discuss factors that are essential when assessing a suicidal patient.
8. Consider the impact of family, peer, and media pressure on patients with eating disorders.
9. Discuss assessment, nursing diagnoses, and nursing interventions for patients with eating disorders.

Clinical Practice

1. Watch the movie, "As Good as It Gets" and discuss behaviors that are debilitating for the main character.
2. Design a teaching plan for a patient with a mood disorder to increase medication compliance.
3. Write a care plan to include at least six interventions for the safety of a suicidal patient.

Key Terms

Be sure to check out the bonus material on the Companion CD-ROM, including selected audio pronunciations.

affect (ĂF-ĕkt, p. 1107)
anorexia nervosa (ăn-ō-RĔK-sē-ă nĕr-VŌ-să, p. 1114)
bipolar disorder (bī-PŌ-lăr dĭs-ŌR-dĕr, p. 1105)
bulimia nervosa (bū-LĒ-mē-ă nĕr-VŌ-să, p. 1114)
dual diagnosis (dū-ăl dī-ăg-NŌ-sĭs, p. 1109)
dysthymia (dĭs-THĪ-mē-ă, p. 1105)
electroconvulsive therapy (e-LĔK-trō-kŏn-VŬL-sĭv THĔR-ă-pē, p. 1110)
flight of ideas (p. 1105)
generalized anxiety disorder (jĕn-ĕr-ăL-ĪZD ăng-ZĪ-ĭ-tē dĭs-ŎR-dĕr, p. 1101)
hypersomnia (hī-pĕr-SŎM-nē-ă, p. 1108)
hypomania (hī-pō-MĂN-ēa, p. 1105)
insomnia (ĭn-SŎM-nē-ă, p. 1108)
lanugo (lă-NOO-gō, p. 1115)
major depressive disorder (MĀ-jŏr de-PRĔ–sĭv dĭs-ŎR-dĕr, p. 1109)
mania (MĀ-nē-ă, p. 1105)
obsessive-compulsive disorder (ŏb-SĔS-ĭv cŏm-PŬL-sĭv dĭs-ŎR-dĕr, p. 1102)
phobic disorder (FŌ-bĭk dĭs-ŎR-dĕr, p. 1101)
post-traumatic stress disorder (pōst-trăw-MĂT-ĭk strĕs dĭs-ŎR-dĕr, p. 1102)
psychomotor retardation (sī-kō-MŌ-tĕr rē-tăr-DĀ-shŭn, p. 1109)

ANXIETY AND ANXIETY DISORDERS

Anxiety is considered normal and healthy unless it becomes debilitating and prevents a person from functioning in everyday life. Abnormal or debilitating anxiety is intense and feels life threatening to the individual. One of four people will experience symptoms of an anxiety disorder during his or her lifetime.

Anxiety is often self-limiting and alleviated without specific medical or nursing interventions. However, intervention may be necessary to prevent potential harm toward self or aggression toward others. Nurses can be very instrumental in helping a patient recover from a panic level of anxiety. Table 45–1 describes the various levels of anxiety and Figure 45–1 depicts the relationship between stress, anxiety and related behaviors. Remaining calm and supportive provides a safety net for the patient. Anticipate that panic-level anxiety is very challenging and will often require medication. Patients with anxiety need teaching about how to prevent further attacks. They need to be taught how to relax and should attempt to determine the underlying cause of their anxiety. Anxiety can recur at a greater level of severity; therefore, early intervention is important.

? *Think Critically About . . .* Recall a time when you felt very anxious. What were your feelings and behaviors? What strategies did you use to manage your own anxiety?

Table 45–1 **Nursing Management for Levels of Anxiety**

LEVEL OF ANXIETY	ASSESSMENT	NURSING GOAL	NURSING MANAGEMENT
Mild	Increased alertness, motivation, and attentiveness.	To assist patient to tolerate some anxiety.	Help patient identify and describe feelings. Help patient develop the capacity to tolerate mild anxiety, and use it conscientiously and constructively.
Moderate	Perception narrowed, selective inattention, physical discomforts.	To reduce anxiety; long-term goal directed toward helping patient understand cause of anxiety and new ways of controlling it.	Provide outlet for tension such as walking, crying, working at simple, concrete tasks. Encourage patient to discuss feelings.
Severe	Behavior becomes automatic; connections between details are not seen; senses are drastically reduced.	To assist in channeling anxiety.	Recognize own level of anxiety. Link patient's behavior with feelings. Protect defenses and coping mechanisms. Identify and modify anxiety-provoking situations.
Panic	Overwhelmed; inability to function or communicate; possible bodily harm to self and others; loss of rational thought.	To be supportive and protective.	Provide nonstimulating, structured environment. Avoid touching. Stay with patient. Medicate patient with tranquilizers if necessary.

Adapted from Zerwekh, J., & Claborn, J. (2003). *NCLEX-PN: A Study Guide for Practical Nursing.* Dallas: Nursing Education Consultants (p.112).

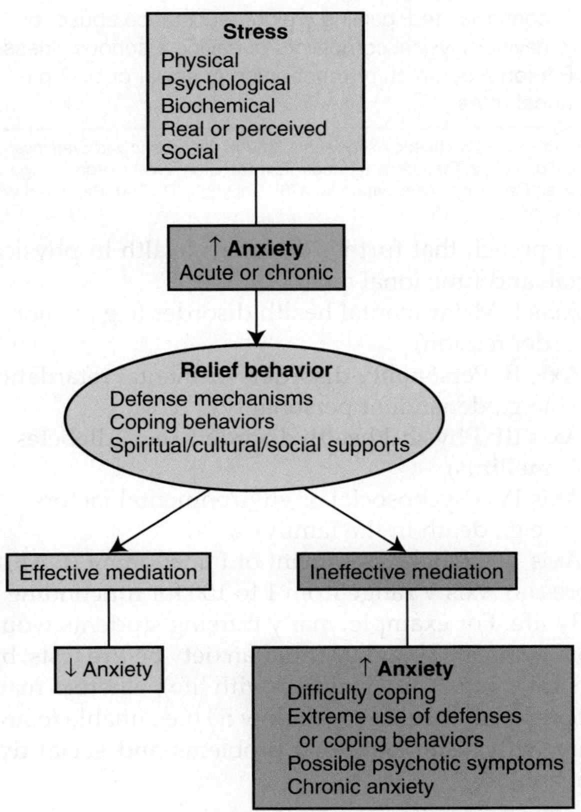

FIGURE **45–1** Stress, anxiety, and behavioral effects.

GENERALIZED ANXIETY DISORDER

A person who experiences persistent, unrealistic, or excessive worry about two or more life circumstances (e.g., worry over children, finances, employment, and health) for 6 or more months is exhibiting symptoms associated with **generalized anxiety disorder** (GAD). GAD usually develops slowly and is chronic in nature. For example, John Evans has GAD. He worries about his work performance. John worries that his children are not happy, smart, popular, or excelling and he worries constantly about their future. He worries about the bills and his elderly parents. There are no actual serious problems, and despite his wife's support and reassurance, he can't stop worrying and he experiences the signs and symptoms of excessive physiologic response such as tachycardia, restlessness, sweating, fatigue, muscular tension, and shortness of breath. His cognitive symptoms include difficulty with problem solving and poor concentration. John also demonstrates limited coping skills.

PHOBIC DISORDER

A person with a **phobic disorder** experiences excessive fear of a situation or object. This fear can lead to avoidance or extreme anxiety that interferes with normal responsibilities and routines. For example, Max Payne has a specific type of phobia known as social anxiety disorder. Max is chronically unable to hold a job; he fears scrutiny of his abilities and is afraid of being embarrassed. Work settings cause him to feel pressured, overwhelmed, and distressed and he experiences physical symptoms such as trembling, blushing, and nausea.

He avoids opportunities by creating a variety of excuses, and this further lowers his self-esteem. He acknowledges that his fears are unreasonable.

OBSESSIVE-COMPULSIVE DISORDER (OCD)

When a person has an **obsessive-compulsive disorder,** he experiences an *obsession* (recurrent or intrusive thought) that he cannot stop thinking about, and these thoughts create anxiety. A *compulsive act* (act that the person feels compelled to perform), for example, repetitive hand washing, is performed in an attempt to reduce that anxiety. Time spent in these thoughts and rituals can become overwhelming to the point of interfering with normal life. For example, Jane Forman is constantly thinking about a boyfriend who left her. She doesn't want to think about him; however, she *ruminates* (repeatedly talks or thinks about the same topic) about their relationship. She scrubs and cleans everything that he might have touched. Jane begins to miss work and stops socializing with friends because she can't stop cleaning.

POST-TRAUMATIC STRESS DISORDER (PTSD)

Individuals with **post-traumatic stress disorder** have experienced an extreme life-threatening event(s) that produces intense horror, with recurrent symptoms of anxiety and nightmares or flashbacks (Cultural Cues 45–1). Holly Harris was a rape victim 2 months ago. She frequently relives the traumatic experience, although she tries to avoid thinking or talking about what happened. She feels detached from others and disinterested in her normal activities. She fears she may not ever be able to have loving feelings toward a man, and feels bleak about the future in general. She experiences irritability and difficulty sleeping and concentrating. She is hypervigilant and startles very easily.

Diagnosis of Anxiety Disorders

To help clinicians define and diagnose behavioral disorders more consistently, the American Psychiatric Association publishes a regularly updated manual that establishes guidelines for how diagnoses are made. The *Diagnostic and Statistical Manual of Mental Disorders,* fourth edition, Text Revision (DSM-IV-TR) provides a set of diagnostic criteria (specific behaviors) and a specific time frame for each mental health disorder. For example, a patient might feel mildly anxious for 1 or 2 days before surgery, but mild anxiety for a short period before such an event would be considered normal; therefore, that patient would not meet the criteria for any of the anxiety disorders. In contrast, a person who is dysfunctional because of continuous worry and restlessness, is losing sleep, and has difficulty concentrating for at least 6 months over a job or other potential problems would meet the criteria for GAD (Box 45–1). The DSM-IV-TR also uses a multiaxial approach that further describes health in physical, social, and functional areas:

Axis I: Major mental health disorder (e.g., major depression)
Axis II: Personality disorders or mental retardation (e.g., dependent personality)
Axis III: Physical health disorders (e.g., diabetes mellitus)
Axis IV: Psychosocial or environmental factors (e.g., death in the family)
Axis V: Global Assessment of Functioning (GAF)

Scores on Axis V range from 1 to 100 for functioning in daily life. For example, many nursing students would score between 81 and 90 (mild anxiety before tests, but generally active and satisfied with life), whereas many people in jail would score below 50 (i.e., unable to hold a job with history of legal problems and social dysfunction).

Treatment of Anxiety Disorders

People with anxiety disorders can be treated with supportive therapy and *anxiolytic* (antianxiety) medications. Supportive therapy may include individual therapy and education about relaxation techniques and stress management.

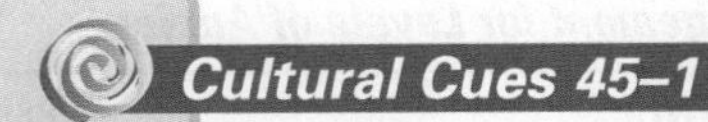

PTSD and Immigrant Patients

Patients who have emigrated from war-torn countries such as Vietnam or Afghanistan are at risk for post-traumatic stress disorder (PTSD). Language and a reluctance to seek professional help for psychiatric problems are barriers to care. In accordance with *Healthy People 2010,* health programs should include culturally appropriate and linguistically competent care.

Box 45–1 *Diagnostic Criteria for Generalized Anxiety Disorder*

1. Excessive anxiety and worry occurring very frequently for at least 6 months.
2. Difficulties controlling worry.
3. Worrying frequently results in three or more of the following symptoms for the past 6 months.
   a. Restlessness
   b. Fatigue
   c. Difficulty concentrating
   d. Irritability
   e. Muscle tension
   f. Sleep disturbance
   The focus of the anxiety and worry is not about having a panic attack, being embarrassed in public, being contaminated, gaining weight, substance abuse, or having physical complaints or having a serious illness.
4. Person has difficulty functioning in social or occupational roles.

From American Psychiatric Association. (2000). *Diagnostic and Statistical Manual of Mental Disorders,* (4th ed.). Text Revision. Washington, DC: American Psychiatric Association (p. 476).

Table 45–2 Medications Used to Treat Anxiety

CLASSIFICATION	ACTION	NURSING IMPLICATIONS	PATIENT EDUCATION
BENZODIAZEPINES			
Alprazolam (Xanax) Chlorodiazepoxide (Librium) Diazepam (Valium) Lorazepam (Ativan) Oxazepam (Serax)	Has depressant action on the CNS and inhibits stimulation of the brain. Used for anxiety disorders and insomnia.	Watch for signs of orthostatic hypotension. Watch for side effects: palpitations, dry mouth, nausea and vomiting, and occasional nightmares. Elderly patients have significantly increased risk for falls.	Do not take any other CNS depressants, including alcohol. Potentially addictive; use only as prescribed. Can cause drowsiness and lethargy. Do not stop taking these medications abruptly.
NONBENZODIAZEPINE			
Buspirone (BuSpar)	Interacts with serotonin receptors (see Chapter 48 for discussion of neurotransmitters). Used for anxiety and sleep disorders.	Always a scheduled medication, never PRN. May cause headaches, dizziness, or drowsiness, but much less so compared to the benzodiazepines.	Takes 7–10 days for symptoms to subside and several weeks for optimal results. No evidence of tolerance or physical dependence. Do not stop taking this medication abruptly.
SSRIs (see Table 45–4)			

Key: *CNS*, central nervous system; *PRN*, as needed; *SSRIs*, selective serotonin reuptake inhibitors.

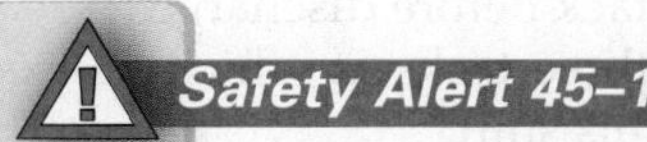

Unexpected Agitation and Rage

For 7% of patients receiving benzodiazepines, unexpected agitation and occasional rage can occur. Patients at high risk for this phenomenon include pediatric, geriatric, autistic, and HIV-positive patients. Also, those with poor impulse control, those receiving IM or IV doses, or those taking drugs such as alprazolam are at an increased risk.

Key: *HIV*, human immunodeficiency virus; *IM*, intramuscular; *IV*, intravenous.

Safety Alert 45–2

Serotonin Syndrome

SSRIs have the potential to cause serotonin syndrome. This is a potential life-threatening condition that could start 30 minutes to 48 hours after taking the medication. Symptoms include change of mental status, increase in pulse and fluctuation in blood pressure, loss of muscular coordination, and hyperthermia. Treatment includes stopping medication, adminstering IV fluids, and decreasing temperature.

Key: *IV*, intravenous; *SSRIs*, selective serotonin reuptake inhibitors.

These patients need much reassurance, and a nurse who is a good listener. Chapter 7 presents guidelines for a relaxation exercise. Evidence-based practice indicates that for certain anxiety disorders, such as OCD, patients should be referred for cognitive behavioral therapy (CBT). In this therapy patients are assisted to face their anxieties and 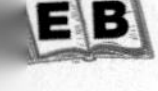 to prevent their ritualistic behavior. (Geffken, et al., 2004).

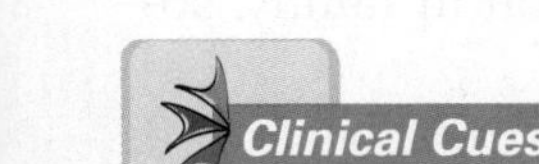

Your patient may need referral to stress management class; however, there are a few basic suggestions that you can make to help your patient cope with stress. These include talking to a friend, listening to music, taking a warm bath or shower, or doing a large muscle activity like walking or throwing ice cubes against the back fence. Evidenced-based practice suggests that music reduces anxiety, blood pressure, heart rate and tension (Burgner, 2005). 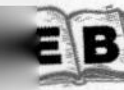

Benzodiazapines are commonly prescribed for anxiety disorders (Safety Alert 45–1). Drugs from this category are alprazolam (Xanax), chlordiazepoxide (Librium), oxazepam (Serax), lorazepam (Ativan), and diazepam (Valium). Patients taking these drugs must be advised to use them with caution because *tolerance* (increased dosage to achieve the desired effect) and physical and psychological dependency can occur.

Buspirone (BuSpar), in a class by itself, takes longer to reach therapeutic efficacy (3 to 4 weeks). The advantage of BuSpar is the decreased risk of dependency and less sedation. The selective serotonin reuptake inhibitors (SSRIs) are becoming first-line drugs for anxiety because they have fewer adverse effects (Safety Alert 45–2). Examples from this category include citalopram (Celexa) and sertraline (Zoloft). Table 45–2 presents a list of common medications used to treat anxiety.

NURSING MANAGEMENT

Assessment (Data Collection)

You should assess the patient for subjective feelings of fear, apprehension, isolation, or the need for increased space. Assess the patient's ability to concentrate and make rational judgments, and explore the source of preoccupation and worries. Physical symptoms may include trembling, feeling shaky, increased muscle tension, muscle soreness, easy fatigability, and restlessness (Cultural Cues 45–2). Patients may be hypervigilant, have difficulty sleeping, and be very irritable. In addition, an autonomic nervous system response can cause an increase in blood pressure, dyspnea, palpitations, dry mouth, dizziness, and nausea.

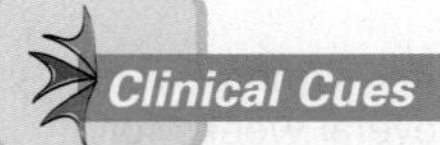

Clinical Cues

You have a PRN (as-needed) order for a short-acting anxiolytic. How will you know when to give it? Observe the patient for signs of anxiety (e.g., pacing, restlessness, and facial expressions of fear or concern). Approach your patient with a gentle and caring manner and assess for feelings of apprehension and his ability to concentrate. For example, "Mr. Smith, you seem a little restless. Let's sit for a while and you can tell me what is going on." If therapeutic communication is not successful, and the patient shows progressively escalating signs of trembling, agitation, irritability, or inability to relax and converse, it would be appropriate to offer him the medication.

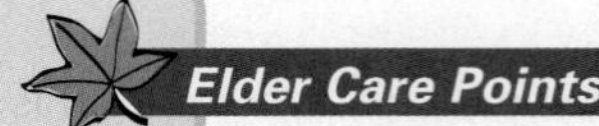

Elder Care Points

The elderly population often expresses somatic complaints rather than openly verbalizing emotional distress. You may observe the anxious elder complaining of an upset stomach, inability to sleep, fatigue, or increased need to urinate. Medications (e.g., sertraline [Zoloft], levothyroxine [Synthroid], theophylline [Slo-Phyllin]) that the elder is taking may increase feelings of anxiety. Certain medical conditions, such as problems with the thyroid gland, problems with the cardiac system, and altered blood sugar, can also mimic anxiety disorders.

Nursing Diagnosis

Nursing diagnoses for anxiety include, but are not limited to:

- Anxiety related to threat to self-concept
- Fear related to threat in the environment
- Impaired social interaction related to extreme anxiety in social situations
- Ineffective coping related to panic attack
- Ineffective role performance related to perceived inability to complete work responsibilities
- Powerlessness related to loss of control when facing specific phobic object (e.g., spider)
- Complicated grieving related to multiple loss of fellow soldiers (i.e., war trauma)

Planning

Expected outcomes are written for the specific individual nursing diagnoses chosen to resolve the patient's problems. For the nursing diagnoses above, they might include:

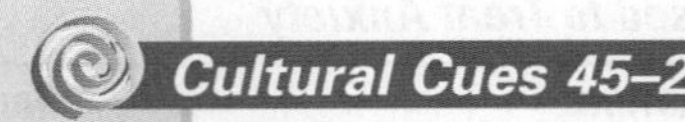

Cultural Cues 45–2

The Hispanic/Latino Patient

The Hispanic/Latino patient may believe that an emotional trauma will result in a fright sickness called *susto*. Symptoms of susto include crying, insomnia, restlessness, nightmares, diarrhea, and fever. Treatment is brushing the body with a rough object. The patient might also believe in *brujeria*, which is a magical or supernatural illness. Symptoms include paranoia, delusions, hallucinations, and being controlled by others. The patient may reject the physician in favor of a *brujo* (witch) for reversal of the spell or hex.

- Patient will demonstrate decreased symptoms of anxiety (e.g., pacing, crying) within 3 days.
- Patient will verbalize feelings of safety before discharge.
- Patient will attend group meeting today accompanied by primary nurse.
- Patient will practice three coping strategies to use during a panic attack before discharge.
- Patient will identify three tasks at which he excels at work, during this shift.
- Patient will verbalize increased feelings of control when encountering phobic object within 1 month.
- Patient will express grief and loss related to multiple losses before discharge.

Planning care for a patient with an anxiety disorder involves promoting a physically and psychologically safe environment. For example, provide a quiet, clean, and noncluttered environment and verbal reassurance ("Mr. Smith, you are safe here. The staff is here to help you.") Methods to reduce the symptoms of anxiety include therapeutic communication (e.g., active listening, being physically present, offering emotional reassurance, and giving clear and concise instructions) and pharmacologic methods (Complementary & Alternative Therapies 45–1) (Nutritional Therapies 45–1). As the acute anxiety passes, the focus of care is to help the patient recognize that certain behaviors such as avoidance are being overutilized. The patient is then assisted to develop new methods of coping and to resume participation in family, social, and occupational roles.

Implementation

When intervening with a patient who is experiencing extreme levels of anxiety, the most helpful response you can use is a calm, reassuring attitude. Stay with the patient and attend to physical needs as necessary. Attempt to make the immediate surrounding environment less stimulating. For example, dim the lights, turn off the television or radio, and limit the number of people in the area. Be sure to use clear, simple statements and repeat as necessary.

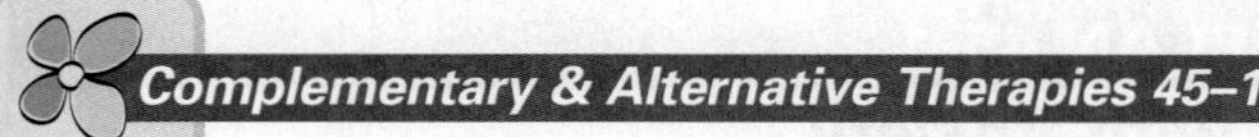

Complementary & Alternative Therapies 45–1

Essential Oils

Essential oils that have a calming and soothing effect include basil, bergamot, chamomile, jasmine, rose, and lavender. These oils can be used in an aromatic bath or as massage oil.

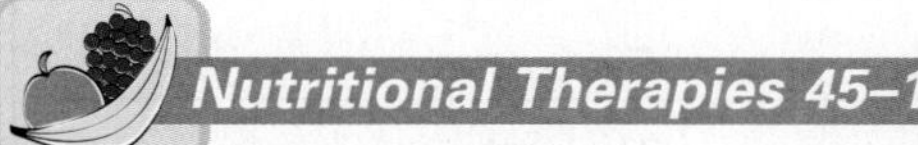

Nutritional Therapies 45–1

Promoting Relaxation

Advise your patient that stimulants such as coffee and colas should be avoided to help decrease anxiety and nervousness. Consumption of raw nuts and seeds, whole grains, and fresh fruits and vegetables helps to build the body's reserve and strength. Bananas, rice, milk, and pasta contain tryptophan, which helps to induce relaxation.

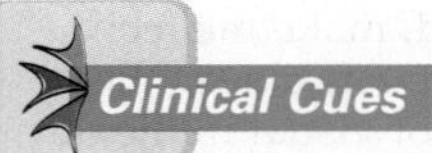

Clinical Cues

Anxiety is contagious and can spread rapidly from person to person until the entire unit is affected; likewise, the nurse is not immune to having these feelings. Fortunately, you can use therapeutic communications skills to help the patient de-escalate. Use a calm voice and a relaxed body position, and convey confidence in your own ability to maintain control of your own anxiety. This helps the patient to mimic your calm behavior and control his anxiety.

When the anxiety is under control, you can assist in helping the patient to use problem-solving strategies. The long process of determining root causes of the anxiety can take years of therapy, but you can make referrals as needed and provide support. Nursing Care Plan 45–1 describes nursing management of anxiety.

Evaluation

Ongoing evaluation of patients with anxiety is necessary. This includes the status of the patient before discharge from the hospital, clinic, or emergency room. Carefully document that outcome criteria were met and symptoms were relieved. If symptoms are not totally resolved, you should clearly document that the patient's level of anxiety is not a threat to self or others at the time of discharge. Also include the plan for follow-up care and a plan to obtain emergency care if needed. For example, the patient was discharged to home, accompanied by his wife. He reports mild anxiety continues, but feels much better due to the Ativan; he also knows to avoid stressful situations. He has a follow-up appointment in 2 weeks with Dr. Smith. If problems occur in the interim, he and his wife know to return to the emergency room.

MOOD DISORDERS

The incidence of mood disorders is very high. Unfortunately, these disorders are often inaccurately diagnosed and treated. **Dysthymia** refers to a disturbance in mood that may manifest in either depression or elation (mania). An individual experiencing clinical depression is more than just sad. Depressed or dysthymic individuals feel a sense of hopelessness and despair that cannot be alleviated by usual means. This hopelessness can lead to thoughts of suicide.

Mania, on the other hand, is an elevation in mood that includes increased grandiosity or irritability that is present for at least 1 week. A manic person may exhibit *pressured speech* (talking that is loud and rapid and difficult to interrupt) and flight of ideas (goes from topic to topic with little or no connection). There is an inability to concentrate, a decreased need for sleep or nutrients, and an increase in goal-directed activity, impulsive spending, and hypersexuality. Behavior, often described as *labile* (unstable and frequently changing) in manic patients can escalate rapidly from a mood of frivolity and joking to agitation and extreme paranoia. The agitation and irritability seen in manic patients can often lead to aggressive behavior. Manic individuals may require hospitalization for an inability to eat or sleep for days that leads to complete physical and mental exhaustion and aggressive behavior. Sometimes individuals will rapidly switch from being extremely depressed to being euphoric and manic. This condition is called bipolar disorder and occurs equally in men and women. It often is initially diagnosed in young adults, but it may be diagnosed at any time during the life span.

BIPOLAR DISORDER

Bipolar disorder is suspected when a patient experiences episodes of extreme sadness, hopelessness, and helplessness interspersed with periods of extreme elation and hyperactivity. According to the DSM-IV-TR, two types of bipolar disorder are recognized. Bipolar I disorder is characterized by episodes of major depression with at least one episode of manic or hypomanic behavior. Bipolar II disorder is characterized by one or more depressive episodes with at least one episode of hypomania. **Hypomania is an inflated or irritable mood for at least 4 days. Patients may display loud, rapid speech, and flight of ideas, decreased need for sleep, distractibility, and an increase in goal-directed activity, but hospitalization is not indicated because it does not involve psychotic behavior.**

Treatment

Lithium carbonate is the drug of choice used to stabilize manic behavior. Lithium has a narrow therapeutic range, so serum lithium levels must be determined 8 to 12

NURSING CARE PLAN 45–1

Care of the Patient with Anxiety

SCENARIO Janet Jones, age 32, was brought to the clinic by her new supervisor for an episode of "uncontrolled hysteria" following a minor error. Janet tearfully explains that she is "so incompetent that she needs to quit," but her husband will ridicule her for quitting another job. The supervisor tells you that it is Janet's second day on the job and she was doing okay, but Janet weeps and states that she has "too much anxiety to continue working."

PROBLEM/NURSING DIAGNOSIS *Uncontrollable emotional response*/Anxiety related to perceived threat to self-concept.
Supporting assessment data *Subjective:* States she has too much anxiety to work. *Objective:* Crying, appears distraught.

Goals/Expected Outcomes	Nursing Interventions	Selected Rationale	Evaluation
Patient will verbalize what triggered anxiety	Maintain a calm, nonjudgmental manner.	Anxiety is contagious; being calm helps her to mimic your composure.	The patient was calm and composed at the end of the shift.
Patient will verbalize at least three methods to reduce anxiety	Keep immediate surroundings low in stimuli.	Decreasing stimuli helps patient to refocus on internal control.	Preferred to be in her room away from the other patients.
	Stay with patient.	Promotes feeling of support and security.	"I feel less anxious when I am by myself for a while."
	Administer anxiolytics (e.g., Ativan) as ordered.	Medications alter anxiety at the biochemical level.	One dose of PRN Ativan was given with relief in 30 min.
	When anxiety is sufficiently reduced, explore possible reasons for the anxiety with the patient.	Assisting the patient to gain insight is a step toward learning to cope with anxiety.	States, "Men, especially my husband, make me feel very self-conscious." Being out of visual range of male patients makes her feel less anxious.
	Teach patient how to recognize increasing levels of anxiety (e.g., increased pulse, feeling of apprehension, narrowing of perception).	Early recognition of symptoms allows the patient to interrupt before escalation.	Identified that heart pounds when anxiety is starting. Outcome met. Continue plan.

PROBLEM/NURSING DIAGNOSIS *Unable to cope at work*/Ineffective coping related to perceived stress of new job and possible lack of spousal support.
Supporting assessment data *Subjective:* States she "needs to quit" her job. *Objective:* Continues emotional display and unable to see alternatives to quitting.

Goals/Expected Outcomes	Nursing Interventions	Selected Rationale	Evaluation
Patient will describe two new coping methods	Support patient's efforts to explore the meaning of behavior and the significance of the current crisis in her life.	Places the situation in context and makes it seem less overwhelming.	The patient says that her new job is stressfully for her. She acknowledges her pattern of quitting jobs is frustrating for her husband, but he is not supportive in helping her overcome her anxiety.
	Identify previously used coping mechanisms.	Use of a familiar and successful coping mechanism can help her to deal with the current crisis.	Past coping mechanism is to quit and thereby avoid the stress. Patient acknowledges that this coping strategy is being overused.
	Teach new ways to cope (relaxation techniques, talking to a friend).	New coping mechanisms are needed to prevent overuse of the familiar ones (i.e., crying and quitting are being overused).	Patient practiced relaxation exercise, but states, "it will not be enough to help me with my job anxieties."

NURSING CARE PLAN 45-1

Care of the Patient with Anxiety—cont'd

Goals/Expected Outcomes	*Nursing Interventions*	*Selected Rationale*	*Evaluation*
Patient will identify a supportive network to help her cope	Encourage patient to develop a supportive network. Refer to support groups.	Increased social support facilitates coping, provides secondary source when husband is unsupportive.	Mother-in-law was identified as a support person. Declines referral to support group at this time. Outcome partially met. Continue plan.

PROBLEM/NURSING DIAGNOSIS *Unable to fulfill work commitments*/Ineffective role performance related to feelings of incompetence.

Supporting assessment data *Subjective:* States, "I'm so incompetent." *Objective:* Perception of performance does not match the report of the supervisor.

Goals/Expected Outcomes	*Nursing Interventions*	*Selected Rationale*	*Evaluation*
Patient will identify at least two strengths that she brings to her job	Use active listening.	Attentive listening increases patient's self-esteem and encourages expression of feelings.	Expressed feelings of frustration and embarrassment about her work performance.
Patient will verbalize or demonstrate competency in job performance within 1 mo	Encourage patient to verbalize her feelings and help her identify what is triggering those feelings.	Insight into feelings will assist patient to make a plan to overcome her fears.	Acknowledges that she is overly sensitive to criticism and her response is disproportionate, but continues to be unsure how to change her feelings or response.
	Assist to identify strengths and weaknesses related to job performance.	Patient may not recognize her own strengths; these should be pointed out. She needs to be aware of her weaknesses, but not focus solely on those points.	Identifies personal strengths of intelligence and willingness to learn.
	Assist patient to develop small and realistic work-related goals.	Realistic goals are more achievable, and success will help to decrease feelings of incompetence.	Identifies work-related goal of being able to get dressed and go to work as the initial step. Outcomes partially met. Continue plan.

? CRITICAL THINKING QUESTIONS

1. What interventions would you use to improve the communication between Janet and her husband?
2. How would you respond to Janet's comment that she is "just too anxious to work"?

hours after the first dose, then two or three times per week for the first month and then weekly to monthly. See Table 45–3 for nursing implications for lithium. Because it may take 2 to 3 weeks for lithium to become effective, antipsychotics such as chlorpromazine (Thorazine) or haloperidol (Haldol) are given to decrease the initial level of hyperactivity. Anticonvulsant drugs such as divalproex sodium (Depakote) and carbamazepine (Tegretol) are effective in the treatment of mania and quetiapine (Seroquel), which is an atypical antipsychotic (see Table 48–2 and Table 48–3) is also used for mania. Lamotrigiene (Lamictal) is effective for the depressive episodes. All of these can be used safely in combination with lithium. In addition to stabilizing the patient with medication, it is sometimes necessary to hospitalize patients with manic symptoms, particularly if they are a danger to themselves or others, or are suffering from exhaustion caused by extreme hyperactivity.

NURSING MANAGEMENT

Assessment (Data Collection)

Assessing for mood disorders involves observing for mood and affect, and physical signs and symptoms. You assess mood by asking the patient questions about feelings and observing facial expressions and verbalizations. **Affect** is a term used to describe a person's external expression of emotion. A person with a flat or blunted affect may report feeling fine, but you notice that his facial expression and overall demeanor convey sadness. The sadness described by depressed indi-

Table 45–3 Nursing Implications for Patients on Lithium

CLASSIFICATION	ACTION	NURSING IMPLICATION	PATIENT TEACHING
Antimanic	Alters the release, synthesis, and reuptake of neurotransmitters in the brain (i.e., dopamine, norepinephrine, and serotonin) (see Chapter 48 for discussion of neurotransmitters). Does not cure bipolar disorder, but helps to decrease the manic behavior.	Takes 7–14 days to reach therapeutic level (1.0–1.5 mEq/L.) Blood levels should be drawn 8–12 hr after the first dose, then two or three times/wk for the first mo and then weekly to monthly until a maintenance level is reached. Sodium depletion or dehydration could cause toxicity; therefore, monitor fluid intake and dietary sodium. Diuretics should be avoided. Monitor renal and thyroid function periodically.	Normal salt intake. Drink 2500–3000 mL of fluids per day. Take with meals to decrease gastric distress. Avoid caffeinated drinks because of diuretic effects. Immediately report diarrhea, vomiting, tremors, or lack of coordination.

viduals is intense and creates feelings of worthlessness and hopelessness. The mood of a manic patient, on the other hand, is one of grandiosity and general well-being. In the midst of a manic episode, the patient may feel invincible and recklessly engage in extremely dangerous behavior.

Many physical signs and symptoms are classic for mood disorders. An initial question concerns sleep. A depressed patient may report sleeping all of the time **(hypersomnia)** or falling asleep easily, but then waking up after 2 to 3 hours and being unable to get back to sleep **(insomnia)**. Manic patients are unable to sleep, and it is not unusual for them to tell you they have not slept for days.

Nursing Diagnosis

Typical nursing diagnoses for mania may include, but are not limited to:

- Imbalanced nutrition: less than body requirements, related to shortened attention span while trying to eat
- Risk for other-directed or self-directed violence related to labile emotional state
- Sleep deprivation related to hyperactivity
- Impaired verbal communication related to flight of ideas and pressured speech
- Interrupted family processes related to inability to perform child care duties.
- Disturbed thought processes related to loosening of associations
- Noncompliance related to refusal to take medications during manic phase

Planning

Expected outcomes are written for the specific individual nursing diagnoses chosen to resolve the patient's problems. For the nursing diagnoses above, they might include:

- Patient will consume at least 1500 calories during a 24-hour period.

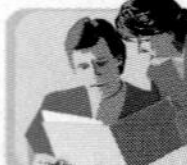

Assignment Considerations 45–1

Hygienic Care of Manic Patients

On a medical-surgical unit, the nursing assistants (NAs) are likely to be accustomed to assisting patients with hygienic needs in the morning. When caring for a manic patient, inform the NA that the patient may have a shortened attention span and a tendency to be argumentative; therefore, the NA should accomplish the hygienic care in small steps over the course of the day (e.g., washing hands and face on waking, brushing teeth after breakfast, combing hair midmorning, and talking a shower midafternoon).

- Patient will refrain from hurting self or others during this shift.
- Patient will sleep and rest at least 6 hours within a 24-hour period.
- Patient will demonstrate a decrease in pressured speech and flight of ideas before discharge.
- Patient and family will identify and use substitutes and resources for child care until the patient is able to resume family responsibilities.
- Patient will demonstrate ability to communicate using logical and related thoughts before discharge.
- Patient will identify two methods of ensuring medication compliance before discharge.

Planning care for a patient with mania involves promoting safety, adequate nutrition, and sleep. Patients in a manic state can be a source of danger to others on the unit. They can quickly escalate from good-natured humor into active aggression. Often it is necessary to assign a nurse or nursing assistant to stay with the patient until the medications have reduced agitation and hyperactivity (Assignment Considerations 45–1).

Implementation

Nursing interventions for the manic patient include keeping the patient safe, providing a high-calorie intake, administering antimanic medications, and providing for a restful sleep. Manic patients often come into the hospital malnourished. Small, frequent, high-calorie meals and finger foods are often necessary because the manic patient will not sit down long enough to eat. Close observation and documentation of mood, verbalizations, and behavior are very important. It may be necessary to place a manic patient in a quiet area away from others, to decrease environmental stimulation.

When communicating with a manic patient, it is essential that you maintain a calm demeanor. Until the medications are effective, therapeutic communication consists of setting limits. When setting limits, it is necessary that you clearly state your initial expectations of the patient's behavior. For example, you might say, "Mr. Smith, I am talking to Ms. Jones right now, so please stop interrupting us and wait for me in the dayroom. I will be with you as soon as we are finished." State the consequences for noncompliance with the request, and always follow through. For example: "Mr. Smith, I have asked you to stop interrupting us. I will ask you again. Please stop interrupting us. If you interrupt us one more time, I am not going to help you with your project today and you will have to wait until tomorrow. So, please wait for me in the dayroom." To avoid being manipulated by the patient, it is important that all staff members be consistent. Sometimes, because of the severity of the mania, the manic patient is unable to comply with simple requests. In these instances, it is necessary to distract the patient rather than attempt to use reason.

When the patient is stabilized, providing him with information about medications and the rationale for their long-term use is important to increase medication compliance. Compliance is important because it is not unusual for the patient to stop taking medications once the symptoms subside. *Refer to Nursing Care Plan 45–2 on the **Companion CD-ROM** for nursing management of a patient with bipolar disorder (manic phase).*

Evaluation

Ongoing evaluation of patients with bipolar disorder is necessary. You must determine whether the outcome criteria for the patient's physical needs (safety, nutrition, and rest) were met. In addition, are the symptoms resolving? Is the patient able to communicate effectively and resume social and occupational roles? Do the patient and the family have a plan to maintain medication and follow-up appointments?

MAJOR DEPRESSIVE DISORDER

Major depressive disorder is diagnosed when at least five symptoms characteristic of depression have been present for at least 2 weeks. **These symptoms include an overwhelming feeling of sadness, inability to feel pleasure or interest in daily activities, weight gain or loss not attributed to dieting, sleep disturbances, fatigue or loss of energy, feelings of worthlessness, difficulty in making decisions or concentrating, and suicidal thoughts. The depressed patient often presents with psychomotor retardation, in which speech, movements, and thought processes are slowed. However, it is not uncommon to see agitation and irritability in a depressed person.** These symptoms may be *subjective* (described by the patient) or *objective* (observable by others).

Before making a diagnosis of depression, the physician must be certain that there are no medical conditions present that could mimic depression, such as hypothyroidism or chronic fatigue syndrome. In addition, patients who have suffered a stroke or myocardial infarction, have cancer, or are newly diagnosed with a chronic disease such as diabetes all need to be screened for depression, because major illness can lead to depression. Moreover, many classifications of medications may induce a pharmacologic type of depression. Examples are antihypertensives, sedatives, anxiolytics, antipsychotic medications, steroids, and hormones. In addition, substance abuse, especially alcohol, often produces symptoms that mimic depressive symptoms. In other cases, drinking large amounts of alcohol will actually cause a person to feel depressed because alcohol is a central nervous system depressant. In either instance, a diagnosis of alcohol dependence needs to be considered. When a person has an emotional problem such as depression and abuses a substance such as alcohol, he has a **dual diagnosis.** See Chapter 46 for more on substance abuse.

? *Think Critically About . . .* How would you differentiate symptoms of depression and hypersomnia from the medication side effects of drowsiness or sedation?

There is increasing evidence that major depressive disorder is caused by a biochemical imbalance. However, most scientists agree that the majority of chronic illnesses result from a combination of heredity and environment. What is not understood is how these elements interact to precipitate an episode of major mental illness. While the signs and symptoms of mild depression usually subside, research findings indicate that an attack of major depression is very likely to recur with even greater severity; therefore, regardless of the cause, symptoms of depression need to be addressed and not ignored.

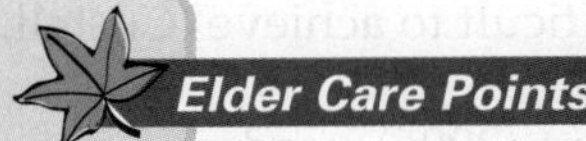

Elder Care Points

Although risk factors for depression, such as loss of friends and body changes, increase with age, symptoms of major depression are not a normal part of the aging process. Research shows that the majority of older adults are not depressed most of the time. Our senior citizens want to enjoy good mental health, but cost and access are barriers to mental health services.

Treatment

Patients who are depressed respond best to a combination of antidepressant medication and psychotherapy (Complementary & Alternative Therapies 45–2). Hospitalization may be necessary if there is a high potential for suicide. Since the 1960s, medications have made a great difference in the lives of people who are depressed. The four main categories of medications used to treat depression are the monoamine oxidase inhibitors (MAOIs), tricyclic antidepressants, SSRIs, and other chemically unique antidepressants. Tricyclics and MAOIs are very effective in treating depressive symptoms. However, they can cause some serious side effects (i.e., tricyclics can cause cardiac dysrhythmias and bone marrow depression; MAOIs can cause a hypertensive crisis when combined with tyramine-containing foods such as red wine or chocolate) that are unpleasant for the patient and cause noncompliance.

Clinical Cues

The class of drugs known as MAOIs (e.g., isocarboxazid [Marplan], phenelzine [Nardil], tranylcypromine [Parnate]) are rarely prescribed because there is a danger of hypertensive crisis when combined with some common foods or medications. Any patients taking MAOIs should be advised to avoid foods high in tyramine, such as aged cheeses, red wine, sherry or beer, pickled or smoked fish, fermented meats, and artificial sweeteners. If the medication is discontinued for any reason, dietary restrictions should continue for at least 14 days. Other medications used, such as ephedrine, stimulants, alcohol, narcotics, tricyclic antidepressants, or antihypertensives, should be reported to the physician because of potential drug-drug interactions.

SSRIs cause fewer side effects and are becoming first-line drugs, but they are very expensive and do not work for every patient. Other newer drugs, such as mirtazapine (Remeron) and venlafaxine (Effexor), show promise, but there is less research on these chemically unique drugs; therefore, SSRIs are preferred. Evidence-based practice indicates that medications should be started at the low dose and increased gradually; however, it is also important that the patient receives a sufficient dose for an appropriate length of time; if the patient experiences medication failure compliance is more difficult to achieve (Costell, 2003).

EB

Recently, Zarate and others (2006) used one dose of intravenous ketamine (Ketalar) with treatment-resistant depression and subjects showed improvement in 2 hours. It is unlikely that Ketalar will be widely used to treat depression because of the potential side effects (i.e., hallucinations, euphoria); however, this research could lead to new rapid-acting antidepressants.

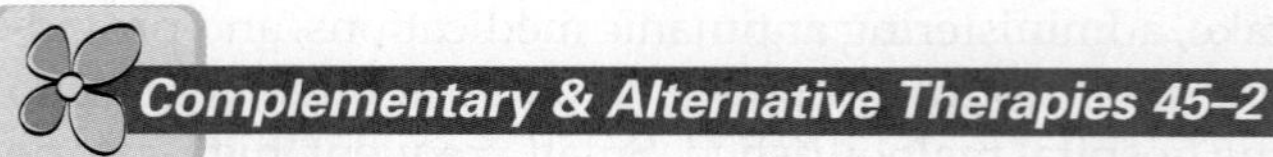

St. John's Wort

Herbal remedies such as St. John's wort have been used for mild to moderate depression and anxiety; however, patients should be advised that taking MAOIs or SSRIs with St. John's wort can cause adverse drug-herb interactions.

Key: *MAOIs*, monoamine oxidase inhibitors; *SSRIs*, selective serotonin reuptake inhibitors.

For a list of nursing implications of commonly prescribed antidepressant medications, see Table 45–4.

Electroconvulsive therapy (ECT) is the oldest form of brain stimulation therapy used for severe depression. After several regimens of medication are unsuccessful, or if the patient is severely depressed and suicidal, ECT is considered. Evidenced-based practice shows that more than 50% of patients respond well to ECT (Rother, 2003) Basically, ECT consists of electric shock delivered to the brain via electrodes applied to the temples. This shock artificially induces a grand mal seizure lasting 30 to 90 seconds. How this mechanism actually relieves depression is not understood. The patient typically receives 6 to 12 treatments spread over several weeks. ECT is frequently done on an outpatient basis in the early morning. EB

Signed consent is required in most states, and the risks associated with the procedure (i.e., increased intracranial pressure, increased blood pressure, especially for those with essential hypertension, and cardiac dysrhythmias) should be explained. Short-term memory loss, occasional headaches, and confusion are expected but will resolve in minutes to hours after the procedure, and this should also be explained to the patient and family before treatment. The patient should take nothing by mouth for 6 to 8 hours before the procedure. Basic preoperative preparation includes obtaining a signed consent, and removing dentures, jewelry, hairpins, contact lenses, and hearing aids. The patient will receive a preoperative medication such as atropine sulfate and a short-acting general anesthetic. After the procedure is completed and seizure activity has ceased, monitor vital signs and reorient the patient; anesthesia personnel may be present during the recovery period. Before discharge, the patient is given something to eat and the family is reminded about the expected short-term memory loss.

Other newer forms of brain stimulation therapy are not yet widely used, but do show promise. Repetitive transcranial magnetic stimulation (rTMS) and magnetic seizure therapy (MST) are noninvasive methods; a magnet is placed on the skull and then areas of the brain are stimulated by pulsations. Vagus nerve stimulation (VNS) and deep brain stimulation (DBS) use a surgically implanted pacemaker to stimulate nerve tissue.

Table 45–4 Nursing Implications for Antidepressant Drugs

CLASSIFICATION	ACTION	NURSING IMPLICATIONS	PATIENT EDUCATION
TRICYCLICS			
Amitriptyline (Elavil) Clomipramine (Anafranil) Imipramine (Tofranil) Maprotiline Nortriptyline (Pamelor)	Inhibit the reuptake of neurotransmitters (serotonin and norepinephrine) (see Chapter 48 for discussion of neurotransmitters.) Used to treat major depression.	Watch for side effects: dry mouth, blurred vision, tachycardia, postural hypotension, constipation, urinary retention, and esophageal reflux. Usually taken at bedtime. Monitor patient for suicidal ideation. An overdose of these medications could be fatal.	Mood elevation may take 7–28 days. Full recovery from major depression may take 6–8 wk. Avoid taking alcohol and working around machines and heavy equipment. Drowsiness, dizziness, and hypotension will subside after the first few weeks. Do not stop taking these medications abruptly.
MAO INHIBITORS			
Isocarboxazid (Marplan) Phenelzine (Nardil) Tranylcypromine (Parnate)	Inhibits the MAO enzyme, thereby preventing the breakdown of dopamine, norepinephrine, and sertonin.	Common side effects: weight gain, postural hypotension, edema, change in cardiac rate and rhythm, urinary retention, constipation, insomnia, weakness, and fatigue. Monitor blood pressure very closely during the first few weeks of treatment. Take a medication history to identify use of medications that increase the heart rate, such as ephedrine, stimulants, alcohol, narcotics, TCAs, or antihypertensives; report findings to physician or RN.	Avoid foods high in tyramine, such as aged cheeses; red wine, sherry, and beer; pickled or smoked fish; fermented meats; and artificial sweeteners, because drug-food interactions can cause a life-threatening hypertensive crisis. If the medication is discontinued for any reason, dietary restrictions should continue for at least 14 days. Go to the emergency room immediately for headaches.
SELECTIVE SEROTONIN REUPTAKE INHIBITORS			
Citalopram (Celexa) Escitalopram (Lexapro) Fluoxetine (Prozac) Paroxetine (Paxil) Sertraline (Zoloft)	Block the reuptake of serotonin. Used for depression, anxiety disorders, and bulimia.	These medications elevate mood faster than the TCAs or MAOIs. They are not as sedating and do not have the anticholinergic side effects of TCAs or MAOIs. Common side effects include nausea, nervousness, insomnia, anxiety, and sexual dysfunction.	Take with food if GI distress occurs. Take drug in the A.M. for optimal effects. Full therapeutic effects may take up to 4 wk. Decreased libido or impotence may occur; check with physician rather than stopping medications abruptly.
ATYPICAL ANTIDEPRESSANTS			
Trazodone (Desyrel)	Block the reuptake of norepinephrine, serotonin, and dopamine. Used to treat depression in patients who are not responding to other antidepressants.	Side effects are similar to the SSRIs.	Immediately contact your doctor if *priapism* (a painful, prolonged erection of the penis) occurs.
Bupropion (Wellbutrin)		Bupropion, in doses >450 mg/day, can cause seizures; assess for history of head trauma or seizure disorder.	Immediately contact your physician if seizures occur.
Nefazodone		Nefazodone can cause liver failure.	Report yellowing of the skin or sclera, anorexia, or malaise.
Mirtazapine (Remeron)		Mirtazapine can cause agranulocytosis.	Immediately report sore throat, fever, or other infection signs.
Venlafaxine (Effexor)		Venlafaxine, in doses >300 mg/day, potentiates risk of sustained hypertension; assess for history of hypertension.	Continue taking BP medications as ordered.
Duloxetine Cymbalta		Side effects are similar to the SSRIs.	Monitor for hypoglycemia

Key: *BP,* blood pressure; *GI,* gastrointestinal; *MAO,* monoamine oxidase; *MAOIs,* monoamine oxidase inhibitors; *SSRIs,* selective serotonin reuptake inhibitors; *TCAs,* tricyclic antidepressants.

NURSING MANAGEMENT

Assessment (Data Collection)

You should collect information about feelings of sadness, hopelessness, and a loss of interest in usual activities. In accordance with 2008 National Patient Safety Goals, nurses are responsible for identifying patients at risk for suicide. Assess for changes in ability to fulfill family, social, or occupational obligations. Appetite must be assessed along with recent weight loss or gain and changes in normal patterns of eating. A person who is depressed may also have many somatic complaints, such as headache, stomachache, dizziness, nausea, indigestion, constipation, and change in sexual responsiveness. The inability to concentrate and indecisiveness are also hallmarks of mood disorders.

Nursing Diagnosis

Common nursing diagnoses for patients experiencing depression include, but are not limited to:

- Fatigue related to psychomotor retardation
- Hopelessness related to inability to achieve career goals
- Spiritual distress related to questioning the meaning of life
- Complicated grieving related to divorce
- Chronic low self-esteem related to past failures
- Self-care deficit, bathing/hygiene, dressing, grooming, feeding related to lack of motivation
- Risk for self-directed or other-directed violence related to repressed anger and grief

Planning

Expected outcomes are written for the specific individual nursing diagnoses chosen to resolve the patient's problems. For the nursing diagnoses above, they might include:

- Patient will participate in at least one unit activity today and gradually increase participation as depression and fatigue resolves.
- Patient will identify two short-term goals that would contribute to achieving overall long-term career goals by the end of shift.
- Patient will verbalize renewal of faith in a higher power after two or three visits from hospital clergy.
- Patient will express feelings of loss and sadness about divorce within 1 month.
- Patient will relate at least one "success story" about self every day for 1 week.
- Patient will participate with assistance (e.g., verbal coaching) in activities of daily living (ADLs) (e.g., brush own teeth) for 1 week and gradually increase independent completion of ADLs before discharge.
- Patient will refrain from harming self or others during this shift.

Planning care for a patient with depression involves promoting safety, adequate nutrition, and rest. Initially, the patient may require assistance in performing ADLs until the severe depression subsides. Mental energy and concentration to work on complex psychological issues are not available to a person who is still in the depths of depression. However, as the energy level improves, you need to help the patient begin to set some small goals such as meeting his own hygienic needs, and gradually work toward the greater goal of reentry into the workforce. It is important to remember that an increased energy level also increases the risk for self-harm.

Implementation

The priority nursing intervention for a depressed patient is to protect the patient from acting on impulses to harm himself. Medications to treat an underlying depression often are indicated, and you must help the patient understand that sometimes pharmacologic intervention is necessary to combat depression at the biochemical level; reversing depression is not merely a matter of thinking happy thoughts. Also, comparing the need for medication to that for a condition such as diabetes or a heart problem may help the patient to feel less stigmatized. **Once the antidepressant medications begin to take effect, the risk for self-harm actually increases because the patient now has sufficient energy to complete the act.** Genuine caring and concern and close monitoring are very important.

Depressed patients can be difficult to be with because of their self-defeating thoughts and verbalizations. Set limits on the amount of time spent ruminating in negative thoughts and redirect the patient to discussions of the here and now. For example, focus on the small successes that the patient has achieved during the shift, such as combing his own hair or attending a group session.

> ***Think Critically About . . .*** What types of goals would be suitable for a 25-year-old female nursing student who is depressed? She is taking Zoloft, an SSRI, and feeling better, but continues to be overwhelmed.

Most depressed people complain of some type of sleep deprivation. You should provide an environment that is conducive to sleep and educate the patient and family about the importance of regular sleep.

Evaluation

Daily evaluation of the patient's depression includes determining whether the outcome criteria for the patient's physical needs were met. These include safety and issues related to decreased energy levels, such as helping with ADLs. Also evaluate the patient's ability to participate in social activities and to express feelings. Part of this overall assessment will include determining the effectiveness of medications. Sometimes it takes several different trials of a combination of drugs to achieve the desired effect. In addition, many of the medications take 2 to 4 weeks to become effective, and the initial side effects of drowsiness and nausea may discourage long-term compliance. *Refer to Nursing Care Plan 45–3 on the* **Companion CD-ROM** *for care of a patient with depression.*

NURSING MANAGEMENT OF THE SUICIDAL PATIENT

Assessment (Data Collection)

Risk factors for suicide include family history of suicide, history of a previous attempt, terminal illness, addiction to drugs or alcohol, diagnosis of major depressive disorder or bipolar disorder, and excessive stress. Suicide assessment includes determining the level of risk (low, moderate, or high) for accomplishing the act of suicide, the presence of a distinct plan, and means of acting on the plan. Be caring in your approach; however, do not be afraid to be direct. You cannot cause the patient to commit suicide with your questions. Moreover, the patient is likely to feel relieved that you are not afraid to hear about and are capable of dealing with this painful disclosure.

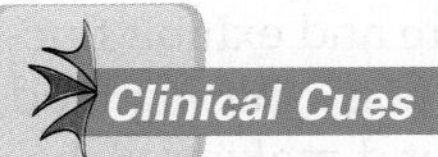

Clinical Cues

If you are working on a busy medical-surgical unit, you may wonder how you will have time to provide the support, therapeutic listening, and attentive observation that a depressed, suicidal patient may need. If you are identifying signs of suicidal thoughts or behaviors, first ensure patient safety, and then immediately report these behaviors to the physician or RN. The patient may need a psychiatric consult, transfer to a medical-psychiatric unit, or initiation of intensive suicide precautions (i.e., one-on-one observation); these measures are beyond the routine care provided on a med-surg unit.

The probability of a completed suicide attempt increases with male gender, weapon availability (guns or knives), poor support system, social isolation, and the influence of mood-altering chemicals. However, all suicide threats and gestures should be taken seriously. Focused Assessment 45–1 lists examples of questions to ask potentially suicidal patients. Patients who are actively suicidal are considered unstable, and if you gather data that support this suspicion, the facts should be immediately reported to the physician or RN.

Think Critically About . . . Women are two times more likely to attempt suicide, but men are four times more likely to complete the suicide act. Why might older white males have the highest rate for completed suicide?

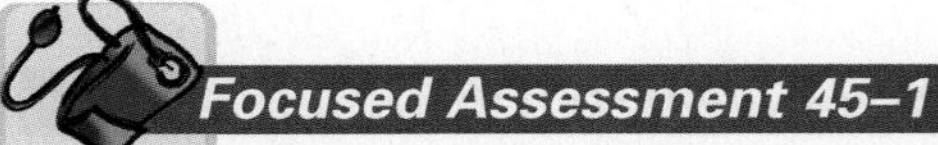

Focused Assessment 45–1

Questions to Ask a Potentially Suicidal Patient

- Are you feeling suicidal?
- Do you have a plan? How do you plan to take your life?
- Can you think of any event that may have caused you to feel this way?
- Do you have a lethal weapon in your possession?
- Who is a part of your support system?
- Do you drink or use drugs on a regular basis?
- Has anyone in your family made a previous suicide attempt?
- Are you currently taking any antidepressants?
- Have you experienced a major loss within the last year?
- What is your history with past close relationships?
- Have you given away any of your possessions recently?
- Have you been having difficulty remembering things lately?

Nursing Diagnosis

Common nursing diagnoses for patients at risk for suicide include, but are not limited to:

- Risk for self-directed violence related to impulsive behavior
- Risk for suicide related to history of previous suicide attempt
- Powerlessness related to history of dependency in relationships
- Hopelessness related to viewing the future as bleak and grim
- Spiritual distress related to loss of belief in God
- Ineffective individual coping related to overuse of avoidance
- Chronic low self-esteem related to unmet dependency needs

Planning

Expected outcomes are written for the specific individual nursing diagnoses chosen to resolve the patient's problems. For the nursing diagnoses above, they might include:

- Patient will refrain from injuring self during this shift.
- Patient will refrain from suicide attempts during this shift and will stop verbalizing suicidal ideations before discharge.
- Patient will identify three examples of dependency in his relationships and describe how this dependency affects his life during this shift.
- Patient will verbalize one or two future events that he could look forward to and enjoy (e.g., birth of a niece) during this shift.
- Patient will demonstrate renewal of his usual spiritual activities (e.g., attending church) within 2 months.
- Patient will identify at least two additional coping mechanisms during this shift.
- Patient will list at least two ways to meet his own needs during this shift.

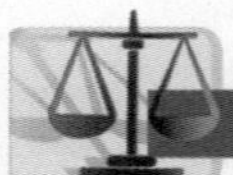

Legal & Ethical Considerations 45–1

Safe Environment for a Suicidal Patient

Although patients have the right to bring and keep personal items, you have the legal responsibility for maintaining a safe environment for a suicidal patient. Belts, shoelaces, and even undergarments such as a bra could be used in a self-strangulation attempt and should be taken away as necessary.

Planning care for a patient at risk for suicide involves ensuring a safe environment by determining the level of risk and initiating the appropriate suicide precautions (Legal & Ethical Considerations 45–1). As the risk for suicide decreases, the focus of nursing care shifts to assisting the patient to develop alternative methods to cope and problem solve.

Implementation

Protecting a suicidal patient from self-harm is a priority nursing intervention. Suicide precautions for a high level of risk consist of placing the patient in a seclusion room with one-to-one (1:1) observation, which is ordered by the physician, although it can temporarily be initiated by the nursing staff until the physician is notified. The purpose of 1:1 observation is to ensure the safety of the patient by assigning one person to be with the patient continuously. Suicidal patients may require 1:1 observation in which the observer is close enough (arm's length) to immediately intervene if the patient attempts self-harm (e.g., head banging). As the level of risk decreases, the patient is allowed to have more personal space (may be permitted into the dayroom), but visual contact must be maintained at all times. In addition, all items with a potential for self-harm must be removed, such as sharp or pointed objects, glass objects, or pills. Observe the patient for "cheeking," which is a ploy to avoid taking his medication by holding the pill in the cheek pouch rather than swallowing it. Suicidal patients have been known to hoard medication and then use it in an attempt to overdose.

When assessment indicates that the suicide intent is less lethal, maintaining close observation and contracting with the patient to refrain from taking action is sufficient. A no-suicide contract, preferably written, should be initiated and renewed as needed. Active listening and a caring attitude are necessary to build a trusting relationship with a severely depressed, suicidal patient. Even if the patient is unwilling to talk to you, you must indicate to the patient both verbally and nonverbally that you care and are available to listen. Your attention and presence convey your respect, and this helps the patient to build self-esteem and a sense of self-worth.

Evaluation

Unstable, suicidal patients need to be reassessed and evaluated frequently (i.e., every 15 to 30 minutes), and the plan of care should be adjusted accordingly to ensure safety and prevent self-harm. As the patient stabilizes and the level of risk decreases, you will evaluate patient outcomes related to gaining new coping skills, renewing hope and a sense of purpose, improving communication skills to get needs met, and preparing to resume life in a community setting. The status of the patient just before discharge should be carefully documented to reflect the absence of suicidal ideations and a follow-up plan with a specific method to access emergency care if suicidal feelings return.

EATING DISORDERS

ANOREXIA NERVOSA

Anorexia nervosa is characterized by the patient's refusal to maintain minimal body weight or eat adequate quantities of food. There is a disturbance in the perception of body shape and size and an extreme fear of becoming fat. The patient strives for perfection and control by controlling caloric intake. These patients may act immature and are socially insecure and exhibit fluctuating moods. Intricate food rituals (e.g., shifting food around the plate, collecting recipes, and making elaborate meals for others) develop, and the patient may have superstitions about food (e.g., ice cream goes straight to your hips). Excessive exercise is commonly used as another means of staying thin.

In many cultures, the emphasis on a slim body has influenced young women's body image. It occurs in about 1 of 100 to 200 females in late adolescence or early adulthood. About 10% of cases occur in males. Anorexia nervosa is a dangerous disorder; 6% to 20% of patients with this diagnosis will die from starvation or suicide. Other psychiatric conditions such as anxiety or depression can accompany anorexia nervosa.

? *Think Critically About* . . . How does your own culture influence your body image?

BULIMIA NERVOSA

Patients with bulimia nervosa induce vomiting after consuming large quantities of food. This binge eating occurs in a frenzied state and usually in secrecy; afterward, the patient experiences feelings of shame and self-criticism. Laxatives may be taken to purge the system after the binge. Ninety percent of patients with bulimia are young women. Bulimia and anorexia nervosa can occur simultaneously in some patients, and both conditions are difficult to cure.

Treatment of Eating Disorders

The goal of treatment in eating disorders is to restore nutritional health and a normal body weight. If weight is below 75% of ideal body weight and the patient is medically unstable, the first step is hospitalization to correct fluid and electrolyte imbalances and severe weight loss. After the medical condition is stabilized, behavior modification is the focus of treatment. Therapy is long term, requiring 1 to 6 years for reversal of the disorder. Both inpatient treatment and outpatient treatment are required with individual, group, and family therapy. Support groups can provide opportunities for growth and sharing of feelings and information. The long-term goal is for the patient to achieve a sense of self-worth and self-acceptance that is not exclusively based on appearance.

NURSING MANAGEMENT

Assessment (Data Collection)

Collect information about compulsive dieting, severe weight loss, or an unrealistic body image. The patient and the family may be in denial. Amenorrhea and electrolyte imbalances occur, and as the disease progresses, a host of other symptoms appear. Problems related to vitamin and nutrient deficiencies, occur including dry skin, constipation, muscle wasting, and facial puffiness. **Lanugo** (downy hair covering the body) may occur. Cardiac dysrhythmias, hypotension, and hypothermia can be life threatening.

Individuals with bulimia nervosa may maintain a normal weight. Assess for tooth marks on the knuckles from repeated attempts to induce vomiting and dental caries from exposure to stomach acid. Other signs and symptoms include fluid and electrolyte imbalances, complaints of heartburn, vomiting of blood, or constipation due to dehydration.

Nursing Diagnosis

Common nursing diagnoses for patients with eating disorders include, but are not limited to:

- Imbalanced nutrition: less than body requirements related to refusal to eat and fear of gaining weight
- Risk for deficient fluid volume related to self-induced vomiting
- Disturbed body image related to sociocultural and media influence
- Impaired social interaction related to immature behavior
- Chronic low self-esteem related to repeated negative feedback from parents
- Ineffective coping related to using maladaptive dietary practices to cope with stress
- Interrupted family processes related to supporting the emotional growth and development of the adolescent family member

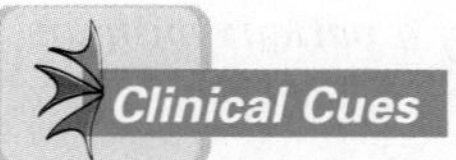

The patient with an eating disorder is attempting to gain a sense of control by controlling dietary intake; therefore, it is important to avoid power struggles over food. Use a matter-of-fact approach and help the patient to experience control in non–food-related areas. For example, "Jane, go ahead and finish your lunch and then you can show me what CDs you decided to take on your school trip."

Planning

Expected outcomes are written for the specific individual nursing diagnoses chosen to resolve the patient's problems. For the nursing diagnoses above, they might include:

- Patient will take at least _____ calories per day for 1 week and gradually increase caloric consumption to regain 85% of ideal body weight within _____ months.
- Patient will refrain from self-induced vomiting during this shift.
- Patient will discuss four or five ways in which culture and media are influencing her self-image within 3 days.
- Patient will demonstrate age-appropriate behavior when relating to peer group within 3 to 4 months.
- Patient will identify examples of negative feedback from parents and discuss how that feedback is affecting her during today's group session.
- Patient will identify three alternative coping strategies to replace maladaptive dietary practices before discharge.
- Patient and family will identify three family activities (nonfood and nonexercise related) that provide support to the adolescent (e.g., discussing a homework assignment)

Planning care for a patient with an eating disorder involves ensuring a safe environment and helping to restore weight and correct nutritional deficiencies. As the physical needs are met, the focus of nursing care shifts to assisting the patient to develop a more realistic body image, increase self-esteem, increase feelings of control, and practice new coping skills.

Implementation

The initial interventions for eating disorders are targeted toward physical health and safety. Suicide precautions are initiated if necessary, and fluid and electrolyte imbalances are corrected. Nutritional status, weight gain, and behaviors such as excessive exercise or self-induced vomiting are monitored. You uses a supportive, nonjudgmental approach to assist the patient in building self-esteem, assertiveness, a realistic body image, and age-appropriate peer relationships. Power struggles and discussions of food should be avoided. *Refer to Nursing Care Plan 45–4 on* *the **Companion CD-ROM** for care of a patient with anorexia nervosa.*

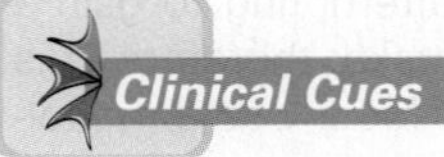

Evidence-based practice indicates that patients can learn to interrupt negative thoughts and substitute positive affirmations (Peden et al., 2005). Teach your patients to use a personal positive affirmation statement (or a thought) that can be said out loud (or thought) on a regular daily basis. For example, you may even want to use a positive affirmation to build your own confidence while you are in nursing school. Wake up every morning and say to your mirror, "I am a good student and I am going to be a great nurse!"

Evaluation

In the acute phase, patients with eating disorders need evaluation of outcome criteria that ensure safety, nutritional, and electrolyte and fluid balance needs. Changing beliefs about food or body image, building self-esteem, learning new coping skills, and restructuring eating habits may take months or even years; therefore, even small gains should be carefully documented. Evaluate the patient's readiness to resume life in a community setting with healthier eating habits and the family's ability to support the patient's efforts. In accordance with the *Healthy People 2010* goals, follow-up, support, and ongoing evaluation are needed to decrease the relapse rates for persons with eating disorders.

COMMUNITY CARE

As hospital stays are becoming shorter, many patients with anxiety, mood, or eating disorders will be hospitalized only long enough to stabilize their life-threatening symptoms. They will then be seen in outpatient clinics, in long-term care, at home, or in day hospitals. Medication compliance is a major nursing responsibility. Once a patient feels better and the crisis is over, there may be a tendency to stop taking medications. Regular visits to the clinic or physician and a social support system are essential.

- There are four levels of anxiety: mild, moderate, severe, and panic.
- Examples of anxiety disorders include generalized anxiety disorder, phobic disorder, obsessive-compulsive disorder, and post-traumatic stress disorder.
- Assess for physical symptoms of anxiety: increased blood pressure, pulse, respirations, and urinary output; dry mouth, nausea, diarrhea, trembling, muscular tension, restlessness, hypervigilance, and insomnia.
- Assess for the psychological symptoms of anxiety: feelings of impending doom, fear, guilt, anger, helplessness, irritability, and low self-esteem.
- Interventions for patients with anxiety disorders include remaining calm, decreasing environmental stimuli, teaching relaxation techniques and stress management, medicating with anxiolytics as necessary, and determining root causes of anxiety as indicated.
- Bipolar disorder is characterized by episodes of extreme sadness, hopelessness, and helplessness alternating with periods of extreme elation and hyperactivity.
- Assess for physical indicators: hypersomnia or insomnia, change in appetite, and somatic complaints such as headache, stomachache, dizziness, nausea, indigestion, and change in sexual responsiveness.
- Assess for psychological indicators: irritability, grandiosity, delusions, labile emotions, flat affect, sadness, indecisiveness, and inability to concentrate.
- Interventions for patients in the acute manic phase include ensuring the safety of the patient and others, providing a high-calorie diet and finger foods, setting limits on behavior, administering and monitoring the effectiveness of antimanic medications, and encouraging rest and sleep.
- Major depressive disorder is diagnosed when at least five symptoms characteristic of depression have been present for at least 2 weeks.
- Assess for physical indicators: weight loss or weight gain, sleep disturbances, fatigue or loss of energy, and psychomotor retardation.
- Assess for psychological indicators: feelings of sadness, worthlessness, hopelessness, or excessive guilt; inability to feel pleasure or disinterest in daily activities; difficulty in making decisions or concentrating; and recurrent thoughts of death or suicide.
- Interventions for depressed patients include active listening, assessing for suicidal ideations, attending to physical needs, administering and monitoring the effectiveness of antidepressant medications, assisting in setting goals, and educating about medications and ECT.
- Assess for suicide plan, including lethality level and means to act on the plan.
- Interventions for suicidal patients in the acute phase include developing a trusting relationship, one-on-one observation, removing dangerous objects, and initiating a no-suicide contract.
- Anorexia nervosa is the extreme fear of becoming fat, with a disturbance in perception of body size.
- Bulimia nervosa is characterized by the practice of inducing vomiting after binge eating.
- Assess for physical symptoms: amenorrhea, electrolyte imbalances, dry skin, constipation, muscle wasting, facial puffiness, lanugo, dysrhythmias, hypotension, hypothermia, and dental caries (related to self-induced vomiting).
- Assess for psychological and behavioral symptoms: denial of problem, compulsive dieting, preoccupation with food, unrealistic body image, low self-esteem, and shame (related to binge eating).
- Interventions for patients with eating disorders include monitoring nutritional intake and weight gain,

monitoring behaviors such as excessive exercise and self-induced vomiting, and assisting to build self-esteem and assertiveness.
- Medication compliance, regular visits to the clinic or physician, and a social support system are essential to prevent rehospitalization.

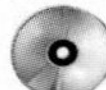
Go to your **Companion CD-ROM** for an Audio Glossary, animations, video clips, and bonus review questions.

evolve Be sure to visit the companion Evolve site at http://evolve.elsevier.com/deWit for interactive NCLEX-PN Exam Style Review Questions, WebLinks, and additional online resources.

NCLEX EXAM STYLE REVIEW QUESTIONS

Choose the best answer(s) for the following questions:

1. A patient is irritable, pacing, crying, and becoming increasingly more agitated. The physician orders a PRN medication for acute anxiety. The nurse knows that the most likely medication to be ordered is:
   1. amitriptyline (Elavil).
   2. buspirone (BuSpar).
   3. lorazepam (Ativan).
   4. quetiapine (Seroquel).

2. A 40-year-old male patient presents with restlessness, muscle tension, and fatigue. He has difficulty concentrating and is frequently worrying about his family and his elderly parents. The patient is displaying symptoms of:
   1. phobic disorder.
   2. obsessive-compulsive disorder.
   3. general anxiety disorder.
   4. post-traumatic stress disorder.

3. A patient is having recurrent, intrusive, and anxiety-producing thoughts that he cannot stop. Which of the following terms most accurately describes what the patient is experiencing?
   1. Compulsion
   2. Delusion
   3. Panic attack
   4. Obsession

4. The nurse determines the need to medicate an elderly patient for anxiety. Which of the following strategies would help the nurse make the clinical decision?
   1. Listen to verbalization of apprehension.
   2. Be sensitive to somatic complaints.
   3. Initiate therapeutic communication.
   4. Observe for escalation of agitation.

5. A patient with manic disorder must take lithium carbonate. Which of the following patient statements would indicate a need for further teaching?
   1. "I will need to decrease my salt intake."
   2. "I need to drink lots of water."
   3. "The medication must be taken with meals."
   4. "I need to report diarrhea, vomiting, tremors, or lack of coordination."

6. A patient is hospitalized for dehydration and weight loss. He is very restless and exhibits flight of ideas with easy distractibility. The nurse identifies the priority nursing diagnosis of Imbalanced nutrition: less than body requirements. Which of the following interventions is most appropriate?
   1. Give three high-calorie meals on a regular schedule.
   2. Offer finger foods, such as a meat and cheese sandwich.
   3. Provide a pleasant, odor-free environment.
   4. Encourage family meals and socialization while eating.

7. The nurse is admitting an adolescent with a tentative diagnosis of anorexia nervosa. Which of the following behaviors characterizes this disorder?
   1. Eating in secrecy
   2. Excessive exercise
   3. Suicidal ideations
   4. Difficulty making choices

8. A male patient demonstrates an overwhelming feeling of worthlessness, difficulty in making decisions or concentrating, and suicidal thoughts. The nurse determines the suicide risk by asking which of the following questions? *(Select all that apply.)*
   1. "Are you feeling suicidal?"
   2. "Do you have a plan? How do you plan to take your life?"
   3. "Why do you want to commit suicide?"
   4. "What would you accomplish by killing yourself?"
   5. "Do you drink or use drugs on a regular basis?"
   6. "Have you considered how your family would feel?"
   7. "Have you recently given away any of your belongings?"

9. A patient taking a selective serotonin reuptake inhibitor suddenly develops a rapid pulse, fluctuating blood pressure, fever, loss of muscle coordination, and mental status changes. The nurse anticipates that the physician is most likely to order which of the following?
   1. Infuse intravenous fluids and administer an antipyretic.
   2. Obtain an ECG and start oxygen per nasal cannula.
   3. Administer an antidote and encourage PO fluids.
   4. Monitor the patient closely and continue the medication.

10. A patient is taking phenelzine (Nardil), an MAOI used to treat depression. The patient should be instructed to avoid which of the following?
   1. Red meat
   2. Milk products
   3. Grapefruit
   4. Artificial sweeteners

CRITICAL THINKING ACTIVITIES

Read each clinical scenario and discuss the questions with your classmates.

Scenario A

You are working in a clinic, and the mother of an adolescent who was recently diagnosed with cancer becomes hysterical. You briefly assess her and find she is at a panic level of anxiety.

1. Explain why closed questions (questions that can be answered with a yes or no, or with very specific answers) and short simple sentences delivered in a firm, kind tone would be effective while she is at a panic level of anxiety.
2. What signs and behaviors would indicate that your interventions are successfully helping this mother to reduce her anxiety?

Scenario B

You are caring for an elderly couple in their home. The husband suffered a stroke 6 months ago. One day the wife takes you aside and tells you that she is concerned about her husband. She says that he is not sleeping well and that his appetite is poor. On further questioning, you find that he is verbalizing a desire to "end it all."

1. What questions would you ask the husband? What questions would you ask the wife?
2. What type of community supports might be available for this couple?

Scenario C

Bill Jones, a 35-year-old, comes into the emergency room after a high-speed chase with the police. He is using vulgar, profane language and is unable to sit down even for a few minutes. Bill switches rapidly from being fun loving and humorous to angry and aggressive. The psychiatrist tells you that Bill has bipolar disorder and orders a dose of intramuscular Thorazine.

1. How would the team approach Bill to give him the injection?
2. What are the major safety concerns for this patient while he is in the emergency room?
3. What other nursing interventions are necessary at this time?

Scenario D

You are assigned to care for Joyce, a 17-year-old who has been admitted for treatment of anorexia nervosa. She tells you she would like to delay breakfast to take a walk around the unit. You kindly, but firmly tell her that she cannot delay breakfast. Later you walk into her room and she is doing jumping jacks; the breakfast is untouched. She tells you she really can't eat this morning because she feels so fat.

1. How will you respond to Joyce?
2. What can you do to help her gain a more realistic body image?

CHAPTER

46 Care of Patients with Substance Abuse Disorders

evolve http://evolve.elsevier.com/deWit

Objectives

Upon completion of this chapter, you should be able to:

Theory

1. Discuss the significance of substance use disorders in the general adult population.
2. Explain the difference between abuse of and dependence on psychoactive substances.
3. Outline the physical, behavioral, and psychological indicators of substance use disorder.
4. Discuss the significance of denial and rationalization in substance use disorder.
5. Describe the effects of substance use disorders on family and friends.
6. Discuss symptoms and complications of withdrawal from alcohol.
7. Identify at least four nursing diagnoses that would be appropriate for a patient with a substance use disorder.

Clinical Practice

1. Visit a 12-step group and identify the advantages and disadvantages for patients.
2. Develop a teaching plan for a community presentation on smoking cessation.
3. Write a care plan with at least three nursing diagnoses and five nursing interventions per diagnosis for a patient who is at risk for alcohol withdrawal.
4. Outline a care plan with at least three nursing diagnoses and five nursing interventions per diagnosis for a patient who is taking central nervous system stimulants (e.g., cocaine).

Key Terms

Be sure to check out the bonus material on the Companion CD-ROM, including selected audio pronunciations.

abuse (ăb-ūz, p. 1120)
addiction (ă-DĬK-shŭn, p. 1120)
co-dependency (KŌ-dĭ-PĔN-dĕn-sē, p. 1121)
confabulation (kŏn-fă-bū-LĀ-shŭn, p. 1125)
denial (dĕ-NĪ-ăl, p. 1121)
dependency (dĭ-PĔN-dĕn-sē, p. 1120)
detoxification (dĕ-tŏk-sĭ-fĭ-KĀ-shŭn, p. 1122)
enabling (ĕn-ĀB-lĭng, p. 1121)
Korsakoff's syndrome (SĬN-drōm, p. 1124)
psychoactive substances (sī-kō-ĂK-tĭv sŭbz-tăn-sĕz, p. 1119)
rationalization (ră-shŭn-ăl-ī-ZĀ-shŭn, p. 1121)
substance abuse (sŭbz-tăn-sē ăb-ūz, p. 1119)
substance use disorder (sŭbz-tăn-sē ūz dĭs-ŌR-dĕr, p. 1119)
tolerance (TŎL-ŭr-ŭns, p. 1120)
Wernicke's encephalopathy (ĕn-sĕf-ă-LŎP-ă-thē, p. 1124)
withdrawal (p. 1120)

SUBSTANCE AND ALCOHOL ABUSE

Substance abuse (excessive use of drugs or alcohol that creates problems) has the potential for causing death and medical problems for the patient, and also causes many emotional and physical problems for family, co-workers, and friends. There are many theories about the cause of substance and alcohol abuse. In 1956, alcoholism was recognized by the American Medical Association as a medical disease rather than a moral weakness. Change in attitude takes time, and there are still many stigmas associated with alcoholism and use of other substances that have potential for abuse. Research conducted in the mid-1980s identified a genetic predisposition to alcoholism. Neurobiologic theories suggest that some people are born deficient of endorphins (the brain's own morphine-like substances) or that other people have hormonal influences that make them more susceptible to peer pressure. Social and psychological theories suggest that users are trying to avoid adult responsibilities and use substances as a dysfunctional coping method.

? *Think Critically About . . .* What personal experiences have you or your family had with substance abuse, and how might this experience affect your care of the patient and the family?

A **substance use disorder** is diagnosed when individuals have problems with alcoholism or substance abuse. This term implies that there is a recognizable set of signs and symptoms related to the ingestion of a psychoactive substance. **Psychoactive substances** are any mind-altering agents capable of changing a person's mood, behavior, cognition, level of consciousness, or perceptions. Box 46–1 lists the diagnostic criteria for substance abuse.

This chapter includes some of the more commonly abused substances: alcohol, narcotic analgesics, opiates (e.g., heroin) cocaine, amphetamines (includes methamphetamines), nicotine, cannabis (marijuana), hallucinogens (e.g., lysergic acid diethylamide [LSD]), and inhalants.

TERMINOLOGY

Several terms are used to describe substance use disorders. **Abuse of substances** implies that an individual is using a psychoactive substance in a nontherapeutic manner or is illicitly using prescription drugs. **Dependency** on substances implies that there are physical and psychological symptoms of addiction. *Psychological dependence* implies the craving or compulsion to take a substance to feel good. When **addiction** or *physical dependence* occurs, the individual needs the substance to prevent symptoms of withdrawal, not merely to sustain the feeling of euphoria that was present with early use of the drug. When **tolerance** occurs, there is a need for increased amounts of substances to achieve the desired effect.

For many categories of drugs, a certain group of symptoms will be present when the patient attempts to stop using a drug. This phenomenon is called **withdrawal,** and in some instances it can be fatal. **Withdrawal symptoms are *usually* the opposite of the symptoms caused by use of the chemical.** For example, when an individual has been abusing drugs that depress the central nervous system (CNS), such as alcohol, you should expect an elevation in pulse and blood pressure, nervousness, and heightened anxiety. People who are withdrawing from stimulants will experience drowsiness, headache, lethargy, nausea, alterations in eating and sleeping patterns, and sometimes cravings.

Box 46–1 *Diagnostic Criteria for Substance Abuse*

The patient has one or more of the following behaviors within a 12-month period:

1. Repeated substance abuse that causes a failure to meet usual obligations (e.g., frequently absent from school, unable to care for children, poor work performance).
2. Repeated substance abuse creating potential danger of physical harm (e.g., driving under the influence of substances)
3. Repeated legal problems related to substance abuse (e.g., arrests for possession)
4. Continued substance abuse despite disruption to interpersonal relationships (e.g., physically fighting with co-workers)

Adapted from American Psychiatric Association. (2007). *Diagnostic and Statistical Manual of Mental Disorders* (4th ed.). Text Revision. Washington, DC: American Psychiatric Association. Copyright © 2000. Reprinted with permission.

Dual diagnosis is a term that indicates that the patient has been diagnosed with a substance abuse problem and a mental health disorder. In accordance with the *Healthy People 2010* goals, there is a need to increase the percentage of people with dual diagnosis who receive treatment for both disorders.

? *Think Critically About* . . . Treating dual diagnosis patients can be challenging and difficult. For example, your patient has schizophrenia and admits to drinking alcohol and using "lots of drugs all of the time." What are the additional challenges to think about when this patient is discharged to a community setting?

PHYSICAL SIGNS AND SYMPTOMS

Symptoms of substance abuse vary greatly, depending on the substance and on the duration of use (Figure 46–1). Blood pressure, pulse, and respiration may be decreased or increased. The temperature may be elevated. Impaired coordination, unsteady gait, or problems with fine motor control may be observed when the individual is trying to perform simple tasks such as walking or eating. Pupils may be dilated or constricted, and the sclera may be bloodshot. Observe the skin for needle tracks, bruises, excessive perspiration, and excoriation. Grooming could vary from extreme neatness to being unkempt.

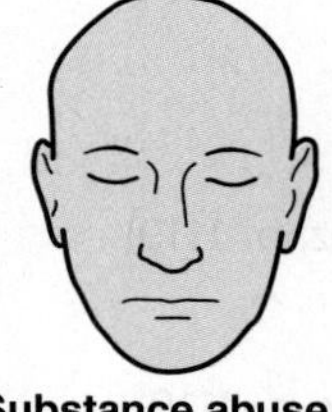

FIGURE 46–1 Signs and symptoms of substance abuse.

Table 46–1 Common Defense Mechanisms

DEFENSE MECHANISMS	CHARACTERISTICS	EXAMPLE
Denial	A simple and primitive defense mechanism. Person ignores reality and absolutely refuses to be swayed by evidence.	An alcoholic states, "I do not have a problem with alcohol. I never drink before 5 P.M."
Displacement	Discharging intense feelings for one person onto another object or person who is less threatening.	A woman has an argument with her co-worker and goes home and kicks the dog.
Identification	Modeling behavior after someone else.	A student starts dressing and talking like a popular schoolmate.
Intellectualization	Excessive reasoning and logic to counter emotional distress.	A nursing student is upset by the death of a patient, but talks at length about the equipment on the code cart.
Reaction-formation	An intense feeling that is unknowingly acted out in an opposite manner.	You treat someone whom you unconsciously dislike in an overly friendly manner.
Regression	Returning to an earlier level of behavior when severely threatened.	A 7-year-old child resumes bed-wetting and thumb sucking during the first few days of hospitalization.
Repression	Unconsciously blocking an unwanted thought or memory from open expression.	A student truly does not remember cheating on an important exam.
Splitting	Viewing people or situations as all good or all bad.	A patient praises a nurse one day and then hates and scorns her the next day.
Sublimation	Rechanneling an impulse into a more socially desirable acceptable activity.	A student has generalized angry feelings about school so she takes up kick boxing as an after-school sport.

BEHAVIORAL SIGNS AND SYMPTOMS

The individual may be disoriented or have a decreased level of consciousness. There may be little or no direct eye contact. Speech may be slurred, incoherent, or loud and boisterous. Mood or affect will vary from calm and complacent to extremely agitated and hostile. It would not be unusual to observe some paranoid ideation, particularly with illegal substance use. **Delusions, hallucinations, or illusions could be present.**

Think Critically About . . . What is your current idea about a typical substance abuser? Has this image of a substance abuser changed since you entered nursing school?

PSYCHOLOGICAL SIGNS AND SYMPTOMS

Denial and **rationalization** are common defense mechanisms used by substance abusers. A typical example of denial would be: "I drink a few on the weekend." "I just have a few drinks to relax" is a classic example of rationalization. To be effective in treating these patients, you must remember that substance abusers usually do not seek help voluntarily. Denial and rationalization become very entrenched behaviors and are difficult to eradicate. A review of defense mechanisms is presented in Table 46–1.

EFFECTS OF SUBSTANCE ABUSE ON FAMILY AND FRIENDS

Anyone living in proximity to a substance-dependent person will be affected. People who are abusing substances are unavailable for emotional intimacy because life becomes centered on the substance of choice rather than relationships or responsibilities. **Family members experience a multitude of feelings, including anger, rage, embarrassment, guilt, shame, and hopelessness. The family also uses denial and rationalization to cope.**

Two terms commonly associated with the family and friends of a substance abuser are enabling and co-dependency. **Enabling is "helping" a person so that the consequences of her unhealthy behavior are less severe; enabling "helps" the unhealthy behavior to continue.**

In maintaining their own denial about the situation, enablers cover up for their troubled loved one and attempt to maintain a status quo. Calling in sick for the abuser is one common example of enabling behavior. Enabling keeps the substance-dependent person from facing consequences and ultimately supports the continuation of denial. Enablers often have a difficult time understanding that their behavior is counterproductive to the overall health and well-being of the substance abuser and the family. Self-righteousness is a typical attitude observed in enablers and is difficult to confront.

Think Critically About . . . How might a family enable their loved one? Is enabling ever helpful?

Co-dependency is another behavior that occurs. **The co-dependent is any family member or friend who overcompensates and tries to "fix the situation" or control the substance abuser.** For example, a teenage son may repeatedly go to the bar and retrieve his drunk mother when she binges and then assume all household and child care duties until she can function. Because overcompensating does not work, co-dependents feel powerless and attempt to control even more. A vicious, self-destructive cycle is established and is difficult to break. The overcompensating also keeps the substance abuser from facing reality objectively.

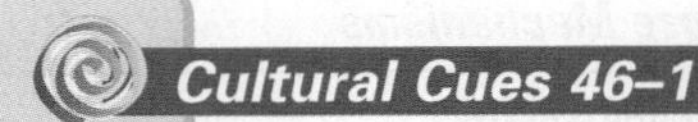

Cultural Cues 46–1

Culture and Alcohol

In cultures where drinking alcohol is interwoven into ritual and social custom, there are fewer alcohol-related problems than in cultures that hold ambivalent attitudes about alcohol consumption. How does your own cultural background influence your attitudes toward alcohol consumption?

DISORDERS ASSOCIATED WITH SUBSTANCE ABUSE

ALCOHOL ABUSE AND DEPENDENCE

Alcohol is a CNS depressant and is the most commonly abused substance. It is widely available, legally sanctioned, and relatively inexpensive, and abuse of this substance is found at all socioeconomic levels (Cultural Cues 46–1). A 12-oz bottle of beer, a 6-oz glass of wine, and a 1.5-oz single shot of whiskey contain the same amount of alcohol. It takes approximately 1 hour for the body to metabolize one standard drink.

Symptoms in the early stages of alcoholism are vastly different from symptoms in chronic, end-stage alcoholism. Results also vary depending on when the assessment was done.

For example, is the individual acutely intoxicated or in the early stages of withdrawal? Taking a thorough preoperative history is absolutely essential because it is not uncommon for a patient to return from surgery to a busy surgical unit and develop symptoms of alcohol withdrawal. An event of this type complicates postoperative recovery and can be fatal. **Early symptoms may manifest within 6 to 12 hours after the last drink; these include anxiety, irritability, and agitation.** Major withdrawal symptoms can occur 2 to 3 days after the last drink and may last 3 to 5 days. **Progressive symptoms include increased blood pressure and pulse, tremors, nausea and vomiting, diaphoresis, delirium, hallucinations, and seizures**. Medications such as chlordiazepoxide (Librium), lorazepam (Ativan), oxazepam (Serax), or diazepam (Valium) and intravenous (IV) fluids can be given to prevent severe withdrawal.

Alcoholism is a major health problem and is a factor in many other instances of death and morbidity. **Some of the medical conditions include *cirrhosis* (liver damage), cardiomyopathy, gastrointestinal bleeding, pancreatitis, hypertension, stroke, sleep disturbances, malnutrition, peripheral neuropathies, cognitive impairment, *leukopenia* (decreased white blood cells), *thrombocytopenia* (decreased platelets), and chronic infection.** Alcohol is also frequently associated with traffic accidents, murder, spousal abuse, child abuse, rape, and suicide. Concurrent abuse of other substances *(polysubstance abuse)* is frequent. Until alcoholism reaches advanced stages, it is often easy to conceal the problem from the general community.

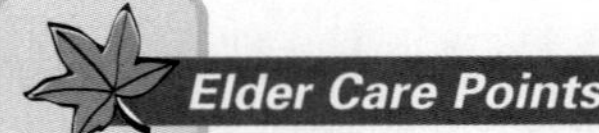

Elder Care Points

The elderly are at great risk for alcohol abuse. Drinking can be an attempt to alleviate depression, pain, or loneliness. Remember that the function of vital organs, especially the liver and kidneys, is diminished with increasing age. Therefore, the by-products of alcohol are not cleared from the body as efficiently, and many medical problems occur.

Diagnosis

To establish a diagnosis of alcohol dependence, the following criteria must be met: presence of withdrawal, significant impairment in family relationships and occupational productivity, *blackouts* (a temporary loss of recent memory that occurs while drinking), drinking in spite of serious consequences to health or occupation, and evidence of tolerance.

Making the diagnosis of alcohol dependence is not necessarily difficult. The difficulty lies in getting the patient to admit that there is a problem. Unless there is *self-diagnosis* **(*"I am an alcoholic"*)**, treatment will be for the benefit of the treatment team and the family, but will not foster long-term recovery for the patient.

? ***Think Critically About . . .*** You are caring for a patient with a history of alcohol abuse, who has been admitted for surgery. After a visitor leaves, you notice the smell of alcohol on the patient's breath. How would you handle this situation?

Treatment

At one time it was thought that allowing alcoholics to experience a painful withdrawal would frighten them so much they would never drink again. Today we know that **withdrawal can be life threatening,** especially withdrawal from alcohol and certain anxiolytics, such as benzodiazepines. Treatment consists of two phases. Initial priorities consist of detoxifying and stabilizing the patient. **Detoxification refers to the process of ridding the body of the substance without causing harmful ill effects.** Chlordiazepoxide (Librium) or diazepam (Valium) is given in titrated doses. Phenytoin (Dilantin) and magnesium sulfate (if magnesium levels are low) may be given to prevent seizures. Promethazine (Phenergan), prochlorperazine (Compazine), ibuprofen (Motrin), or dicyclomine (Bentyl) may be given for the symptoms of nausea, vomiting, pain, or cramps. Intravenous fluids are used to correct dehydration, and nutritional therapy such as multivitamins and thiamine is prescribed. Table 46–2 lists the medications used to treat substance abuse.

Once the patient is stable and able to participate in a treatment program, therapy consists of confronting the patient's denial and encouraging self-diagnosis. Disulfiram (Antabuse) is a drug that causes unpleasant reactions if the patient decides to return to drinking anytime within 2 weeks after starting Antabuse. Even small quantities of alcohol that might be inhaled from shaving lotion could trigger serious reactions such as chest pain, nausea and vomiting, hypotension, weakness, blurred vision, and confusion. Naltrexone (ReVia) can be used to block the craving for alcohol and to prevent relapse in the recovery phase; nalmefene (Revex) is

Table 46–2 *Medications Used to Treat Substance Abuse*

CLASSIFICATION	ACTION	NURSING IMPLICATIONS
MEDICATIONS USED TO TREAT ACUTE ALCOHOL WITHDRAWAL		
Benzodiazepines		
Chlordiazepoxide (Librium) Diazepam (Valium) Lorazepam (Ativan) Oxazepam (Serax)	Have depressant action on the CNS and inhibit stimulation of the brain. Used for acute withdrawal and to prevent seizures.	Dilute with normal saline and give IV dose slowly. Watch for phlebitis. Have respiratory resuscitation equipment available. Can cause drowsiness and lethargy. Watch for signs of orthostatic hypotension. May cause paradoxical excitement, especially in the elderly.
Antiseizure		
Phenytoin (Dilantin)	Suppression of neuronal activity that might cause seizures. Used for all types of seizures except absence seizures.	Give IV bolus dose slowly (50 mg/min). Use IV normal saline, not D_5W. Can cause purple glove syndrome (pain, discoloration, and tissue damage) if given into hand vein. Therapeutic level is 10–20 mcg/mL.
Magnesium sulfate	Depresses activity of the CNS.	Maximum infusion rate is 150 mg/min. Give IV infusion over 4 hr. Overdose signs include sedation, confusion, intense thirst, and muscle weakness. IV calcium gluconate is the antidote for magnesium intoxication.
Vitamins		
Thiamine	Contributes to enzyme production for carbohydrate metabolism. Used to correct thiamine deficiency found among alcoholics.	Assess for symptoms of Wernicke's encephalopathy (confusion, ataxia, memory loss). Dilute IV dose and give slowly.
MEDICATIONS USED TO DISCOURAGE RELAPSE		
Naltrexone (ReVia)	Competitively binds to opiate receptors to prevent narcotic's effects. Used for alcohol rehabilitation.	Advise patient about side effects of naltrexone: dizziness, fatigue, headache, nausea, nervousness, sleeplessness, and vomiting. Screen for history of liver problems. Caution that concurrent use of heroin can cause withdrawal symptoms or even death.
Acamprosate calcium (Campral)		Advise patient about side effects of Campral: diarrhea, fatigue, nausea, and flatulence.
Nalmefene (Revex)	Similar to naltrexone.	Must be administered IM or IV. Side effects include nausea, vomiting, tachycardia, hypertension.
MEDICATIONS USED TO TREAT HEROIN ABUSE OR DISCOURAGE RELAPSE		
Opioid Analgesic		
Methadone Buprenorphine (Suboxone, Subutex)	Produces mild euphoria; used as a heroin substitute in rehabilitation programs.	Extreme caution with use in: elderly or debilitated patients, or patients with renal or hepatic impairment, hypothyroidism, Addison's disease, head injury, urethral stricture, enlarged prostate, or respiratory conditions. Advise patient about side effects of dizziness or drowsiness. Monitor for constipation and encourage fluids and fiber. Methadone tablets should be dissolved in orange juice. Buprenorphine is taken sublingually.

Key: *CNS,* central nervous system; *D_5W,* 5% dextrose in water; *IV,* intravenous.

Continued

Table 46–2 ***Medications Used to Treat Substance Abuse—cont'd***

CLASSIFICATION	ACTION	NURSING IMPLICATIONS
MEDICATION USED TO TREAT HEROIN OVERDOSE		
Narcotic Antagonist		
Naloxone (Narcan)	Competes with opioid receptors and blocks (or reverses) the action of narcotics. Used for patients who have narcotics overdose.	Abrupt reversal of CNS depression may cause nausea, vomiting, increased pulse and blood pressure. Short half-life; watch for recurrent respiratory depression. May have to give repeated doses q 2–3 min or an IV infusion.
MEDICATIONS USED TO TREAT NICOTINE ADDICTION		
Nicotine polacrilex (Nicorette) Nicotine transdermal (Nicotrol)	Delivers lower doses of nicotine. Used in smoking or tobacco cessation programs.	Apply patch immediately after opening to avoid evaporation. Do not cut or fold patch. Instruct patient to chew gum slowly for about 30 min. Advise patient about gradual withdraw from gum after 3 mo; not recommended for use longer than 6 mo. Advise patient to suck on lozenge until dissolved; no chewing, biting, or swallowing. Do not eat or drink for 15 min after finishing lozenge. Advise patient that patch should not be used longer than 3 mo. If no benefit within 4 wk, unlikely that continued use will produce desired effects; consult health care provider.
Bupropion (Zyban)	Weakly blocks reuptake of serotonin, epinephrine, and dopamine (see Chapter 48 for discussion of neurotransmitters.) At lower doses, used in smoking cessation programs; at higher doses is used as an antidepressant.	Advise patient that Zyban may cause insomnia; do not take at bedtime. Do not chew, divide, or crush tablets. Treatment usually lasts 7–12 wk. May not notice therapeutic effect for 1 wk. Avoid alcohol while taking this drug.
Varenicline (Chantix)	Blocks nicotine from binding at the receptor sites.	Teach patient to begin taking Chantix 1 wk before stop date. Side effects include nausea or decreased appetite, headaches, insomnia, or vivid dreams.

similar to naltrexone, but lasts longer and is more potent. An oral form of Revex has been used in research studies, but it is currently only available in parenteral form. Acamprosate (Campral) has been used successfully in Europe and has been recently approved for use in the United States; patients show significantly higher rates of completing therapy programs. Group therapy helps break through denial and also gives the patient a new sense of belonging and identity. Behavioral therapy helps with self-discipline and discourages impulsive behavior. Limit setting is one of the hallmarks of behavioral therapy, and it is essential that all members of the team participate and completely agree about the limits.

? ***Think Critically About . . .*** A woman brings her 85-year-old father into the clinic and insists that he be admitted to a detox program. The man tells you, "At my age, with my health problems, my fixed income and everything else I have to worry about, having a drink or two is the least of my problems." Discuss your personal reactions and your professional responsibilities in dealing with this family.

Referral to a 12-step program, such as Alcoholics Anonymous (AA), is also integral to most treatment plans. AA has been in existence for over 50 years and has helped millions of alcoholics throughout the world; although there is no "cure," there is hope for ongoing recovery. Evidenced-based practice shows that active participation in AA results in decreased alcohol consumption (Back, 2007). Box 46–2 lists the 12 steps of AA.

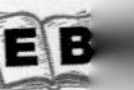

Complications

A serious effect of chronic alcohol abuse is damage to brain cells. A condition that is reversible with treatment is **Wernicke's encephalopathy.** This condition precedes **Korsakoff's syndrome (substance-induced persisting dementia)**, which is irreversible. If the individual has a history of alcohol use and displays the symptoms of confusion, ataxia, and significant memory loss, Wernicke's encephalopathy is suspected. Treatment involves giving large doses of thiamine (vitamin B_1) and abstaining from alcohol. Thiamine acts as a nerve insulator in the body and is absent in the diets of most chronic alcoholics.

The individual presenting with Korsakoff's syndrome has grossly impaired memory and gait distur-

Box 46–2 ***The Twelve Steps of Alcoholics Anonymous***

1. We admitted we were powerless over alcohol—that our lives had become unmanageable.
2. Came to believe that a Power greater than ourselves could restore us to sanity.
3. Made a decision to turn our will and our lives over to the care of God *as we understood Him.*
4. Made a searching and fearless moral inventory of ourselves.
5. Admitted to God, to ourselves and to another human being the exact nature of our wrongs.
6. Were entirely ready to have God remove all these defects of character.
7. Humbly asked Him to remove our shortcomings.
8. Made a list of all persons we had harmed and became willing to make amends to them all.
9. Made direct amends to such people wherever possible, except when to do so would injure them or others.
10. Continued to take personal inventory and when we were wrong, promptly admitted it.
11. Sought through prayer and meditation to improve our conscious contact with God, *as we understood Him,* praying only for knowledge of His will for us and the power to carry that out.
12. Having had a spiritual awakening as the result of these steps, we tried to carry this message to alcoholics, and to practice these principles in all our affairs.

From Alcoholics Anonymous. (2005). *The Big Book Online* (4th ed.). New York: AA World Services, Inc. (pp. 59–60). The Twelve Steps are reprinted with permission of Alcoholics Anonymous World Services, Inc. (AAWS) Permission to reprint the Twelve Steps does not mean that AAWS has reviewed or approved the contents of this publication, or that AAWS necessarily agrees with the views expressed herein. A.A. is a program of recovery of alcoholism *only*—use of the Twelve Steps in connection with programs and activities which are patterned after A.A., but which address other problems, or in any other non-A.A. context, does not imply otherwise.

bance. **Confabulation** (making up stories) frequently is seen as an attempt to communicate. A brain scan will show brain atrophy; currently there is no treatment to reverse this condition.

ABUSE OF OTHER CENTRAL NERVOUS SYSTEM DEPRESSANTS

Other CNS depressants subject to abuse and dependence are barbiturates and anxiolytics, including benzodiazepines. Drugs in this category may be purchased illegally, or initially they may be prescribed by a physician for insomnia or to ease anxiety. It is not uncommon to see these drugs used in conjunction with alcohol, but this practice can be fatal because of the additive effects.

Benzodiazepines (e.g., lorazepam [Ativan], oxazepam [Serax], temazepam [Restoril]) have familiar side effects: drowsiness, hypotension, relaxation, and slurred speech. The chronic user may display lack of motivation, memory loss, poor concentration, irritability, aggression, anxiety, and an increased appetite with weight gain. Flunitrazepam (Rohypnol) is classified as a benzodiazepine and may look like a packaged prescription medication because it is produced and used in Europe and Mexico for insomnia; however, it is illegal in the United States. Rohypnol gained notoriety in the 1990s as the date-rape drug. It produces *anterograde amnesia* (inability to remember events that happened while under the influence of a substance), along with muscle relaxation, drowsiness, and slowed motor performance.

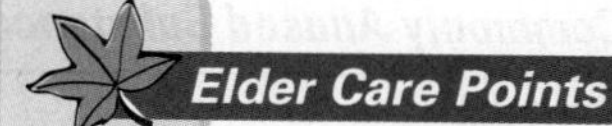

Elder Care Points

Insomnia is not atypical in the elderly population. Great care must be taken when prescribing sedatives and hypnotics for this group. Decreased liver and renal function can quickly lead to toxicity and dependence. Benzodiazepines, in particular, have a long half-life and are not excreted readily by the body. Therefore, patients with poor liver and renal function are subject to a cumulative effect and may experience toxic side effects. Patient education is very important.

Treatment

As with detoxification from alcohol, the patient may be given a drug from a similar category in titrated doses. The amount depends on the severity of the addiction. With the long half-life of benzodiazepines, the initial symptoms of withdrawal may not appear for 3 to 5 days. Table 46–3 presents the symptoms of intoxication with and withdrawal from CNS depressants. Long-term treatment consists of referral to a 12-step program (i.e., Narcotics Anonymous) and perhaps individual and/or group psychotherapy. Patients need to be taught alternative ways to induce sleep and relieve anxiety.

ABUSE OF OPIATES

Opiate analgesics can also be obtained both legally and illegally. The process of addiction may begin with a prescription drug for severe pain. If these individuals rely totally on narcotics to relieve chronic pain and have a tendency to abuse drugs, addiction may occur. On the other hand, if narcotics and a variety of measures are used to alleviate the pain, there may be some increased tolerance and physical dependence (Complementary & Alternative Therapies 46–1). However, tolerance and physical dependence can be treated by slowly decreasing dosages of the opiates.

Treatment

The greatest danger with opiates is an overdose. Treatment for an overdose usually consists of administration of a narcotic antagonist, such as naloxone (Narcan).

Withdrawal from opiates is not life threatening, but patients can experience considerable discomfort (i.e., abdominal cramps, irritability, profuse sweating, yawning, muscle aches, fever and chills, and cravings). Treatment involves helping the individual withdraw from the drug. Methadone maintenance programs are successful in helping patients who have a heroin ad-

Table 46–3 ***Characteristics of Commonly Abused Substances***

SUBSTANCE	USUAL METHODS OF ADMINISTRATION	SYMPTOMS	EFFECTS OF OVERDOSE	WITHDRAWAL SYNDROME
Alcohol	Oral	Drowsiness, ataxia, initial euphoria and aggressive or belligerent behavior, muscular incoordination. At higher alcohol levels, slurred speech, marked ataxia and muscular incoordination, marked cognitive impairment.	Amnesia, tremors, hypothermia, seizures, respiratory failure, coma, death.	Nausea, vomiting, anorexia, agitation, hallucinations, seizures, increased body temperature, increased blood pressure and heart and respiratory rate, possible death.
Opiates (narcotic analgesics)	Oral, inhalation, IV	Euphoria, drowsiness, decreased respiration, constricted pupils.	Decreased respirations, shallow breathing, clammy skin, seizures, possible death.	Watery eyes, runny nose, yawning, anorexia, irritability, tremors, panic, cramps, nausea, chills, and sweating.
CNS stimulants (cocaine, amphetamines)	Inhalation, oral, IV, smoked	Increased alertness, excitation, euphoria, increased pulse and blood pressure, insomnia, anorexia.	Agitation, hyperthermia, hallucinations, convulsions, cardiac dysrhythmias, possible death.	Apathy, long periods of sleep, irritability depression, disorientation.
CNS depressants (anxiolytics and barbiturates)	Oral	Slurred speech, disorientation, drunken behavior without odor of alcohol.	Shallow respiration, clammy skin, dilated pupils, weak, rapid pulse, coma, possible death.	Anxiety, insomnia, tremors, delirium, convulsions, possible death.
Cannabis (marijuana)	Inhaled, oral	Euphoria, relaxed inhibitions, increased appetite, disoriented behavior.	Fatigue, paranoia, psychosis.	None.
Hallucinogens (LSD, PCP)	Oral	Illusions, hallucinations, impaired perception.	Effects are increased and intensified, psychosis, flashbacks, possible death.	None.

Key: *CNS,* central nervous system; *IV,* intravenous; *LSD,* lysergic acid diethylamide; *PCP,* phencyclidine.

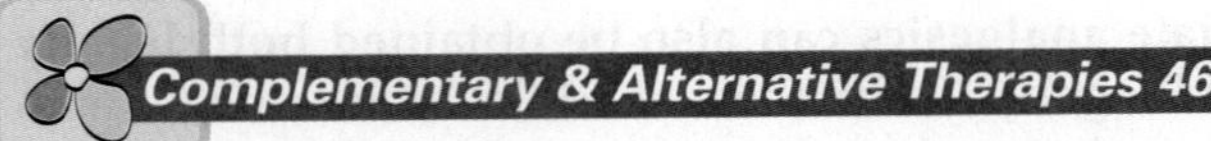

Complementary & Alternative Therapies 46–1

Pain

Assist your patients to explore adjunctive therapies to alleviate pain. These include meditation, visualization, biofeedback, hypnosis, and acupuncture. Aromatherapy with fragrant oils such as jasmine or patchouli can stimulate endorphins (natural pain killers produced by our bodies).

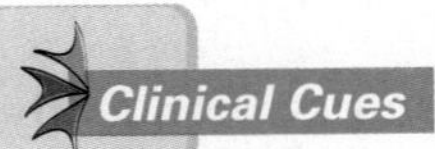

Clinical Cues

A dose of IV Narcan can produce dramatic and rapid results. Your lethargic overdosed patient may arouse very suddenly with nausea, vomiting, tachycardia, and an increased blood pressure. Don't assume that the danger is over! The half-life of Narcan is short, and the opiate action will resume and cause respiratory depression; therefore, anticipate that a continuous Narcan infusion may be ordered.

diction. Recently, buprenorphine (Suboxone or Subutex) was approved in the United States for opiate substitute therapy. See Table 46–2 for nursing implications related to medications to treat opiate overdose and recovery.

Think Critically About . . . Why is it usually necessary to have a different approach for individuals who obtain their drugs legally versus those who obtain their drugs illegally on the street?

If a street drug such as heroin is the substance of choice, rehabilitation is difficult unless the environment and social factors (e.g., breaking off relationships with friends who abuse substances) are also changed. It is not unusual for an individual addicted to heroin to require up to 2 years in some type of supervised alternative living program. Group, individual, and behavioral therapy and a referral to a 12-step program (i.e., Narcotics Anonymous) are also essential to success.

Support groups are useful to any individual who is trying to make a major life change (e.g., a housewife reentering the workforce after 30 years) or to someone who has experienced a major life-changing event (e.g., the death of a child). Substance abusers who are trying to change to a totally different lifestyle can also benefit from this extra support. The purpose of support groups is to help promote healthy relationships, learn and practice new coping skills, and reduce stress and anxiety. Support groups borrow from the principles of group therapy: universality (we have similar experiences), cohesiveness (we have a feeling of belonging), catharsis (expressing feelings make us feel better), altruism (you help me, I'll help you), information giving (this worked for me, it might help you), improved social skills (you can say this in group, now say it to your family), and intrapersonal learning. Nurses should refer and encourage patients to use this valuable resource.

Think Critically About . . . Why might some people feel very threatened by the idea of entering a support group? What are your personal feelings about disclosing information in a group?

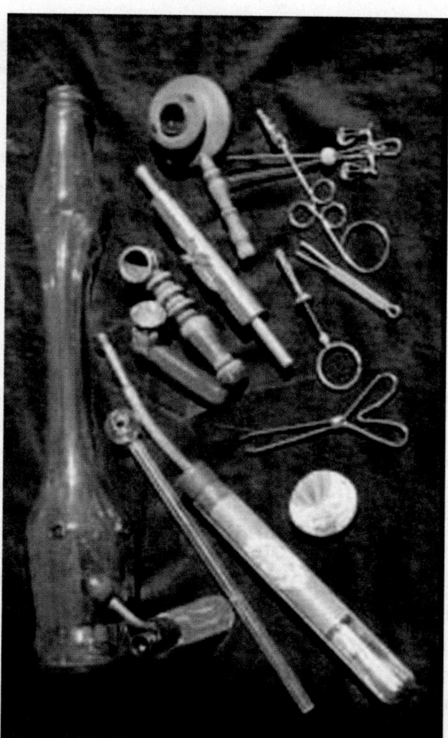

FIGURE 46–2 Drug paraphernalia.

ABUSE OF STIMULANTS

The two common categories of CNS stimulants are cocaine and amphetamines. Both categories of drugs have legitimate medical uses, but are also abused. **Amphetamines can cause an increase in pulse rate and blood pressure, general excitation, anorexia, and hyperactive reflexes and can produce life-threatening conditions such as cardiac dysrhythmias, seizures, or hyperthermia.** Misuse can range from small and infrequent amounts to ingestion of large amounts, which cause prolonged sleeplessness and anorexia. Sleep deprivation of this magnitude can lead to extreme agitation and hostility, as well as a transient psychosis, and can be fatal.

Methamphetamine, known as "speed," "meth," "crank," or "crystal," is injected or smoked. White males ages 20 to 35 have the highest abuse rate for methamphetamines. It is very addictive, and users end up taking progressively larger doses. "Meth labs" are unfortunately easy to establish in any average household, garage, trailer, or the like, where common chemicals are "cooked" creating a harmful residue on the walls and in the air that lingers well after the cooking process is finished. Chronic users may develop toxic psychosis and experience paranoia, hallucinations, and delusions. They are also at risk for *pericarditis* (inflammation of the heart lining).

Cocaine use has increased dramatically. It is highly addictive and can cause death, even in small doses. Cocaine is a short-acting substance and is more commonly used for binges. It produces euphoria, increased energy, and a sense of well-being. The stimulating effects are very fast acting and energizing. However, the effects after the "high" are equally intense, and individuals are subject to severe emotional lows. The powder is either "snorted" (intranasal administration) or dissolved and taken intravenously. "Crack," a purified form of cocaine, is smoked by placing it in a pipe or smoking it with marijuana or tobacco (Figure 46–2). This "freebasing" of cocaine reduces it to its purest form. This is the most dangerous type of administration; it produces an immediate rush and accounts for many overdoses and lethal reactions.

Treatment

Treatment for abuse of CNS stimulants is similar to treatment for alcohol abuse. Initially the treatment protocol is symptom specific and managed by medications. Anxiolytics or antipsychotics may be used for agitation or aggressive behavior, and antidepressants may be used for the depressive symptoms. Experimental studies are being conducted on the use of familiar drugs as potential treatments for cocaine addiction: methylphenidate (Ritalin), amantadine (Symmetrel), fluoxetine (Prozac), propranolol (Inderal), and ondansetron (Zofran). A combination of behavioral and group therapy and referral to a 12-step program is necessary to treat the inevitable depression. These patients must also be taught ways to cope with the psychological craving that often leads to relapse (Complementary & Alternative Therapies 46–2).

ABUSE OF NICOTINE

Nicotine is very addictive and causes increased respiration, decreased pulmonary function, and a chronic cough. It contributes to the development of

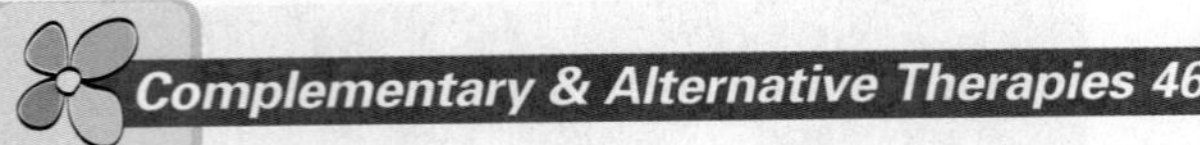

Complementary & Alternative Therapies 46–2

Acupuncture

Auricular acupuncture uses hair-thin needles placed at various sites on the outer ear to stimulate the body's self-regulating system. This technique has been used to assist substance abusers in their recovery programs.

lung cancer and other lung diseases, such as emphysema; pipe smokers and people who chew tobacco are more prone to oral cancer. Smoking has been implicated in many other health conditions, including heart disease, stroke, many cancers, hypertension, premature wrinkling of the skin, bad breath, and discoloration of the fingernails. In addition, secondary smoke is dangerous to others who are in close proximity to the smoker. **Withdrawal symptoms can begin as soon as 24 hours after the cessation of smoking and include irritability, tension, decreased heart rate, and insomnia.** Cigarettes are legal and accessible, and the craving continues long after the patient quits smoking; therefore, most smokers stay in denial about the effects of nicotine (Cultural Cues 46–2). Frequently it is not until later years that the devastating effects are apparent.

Treatment

Nicotine replacement therapy ([NRT] patches, lozenges, gum, sublingual tablets, inhalant, and nasal spray), self-help groups, hypnosis, and acupuncture are among the treatments available for nicotine addiction. In 1997, bupropion (Zyban) was approved as a stop-smoking aid in the United States. Varenicline (Chantix) is a new medication that acts to blocks nicotine from binding at the receptor sites. Cessation smoking programs support the *Healthy People 2010* goals and emphasize the positive effects of quitting, such as better overall health for the individual and the family, an increased sense of smell and taste, and saving money. Making a plan is essential and includes setting a stop date, asking friends and family for help, anticipating how to combat cravings, and removing all tobacco products and accessories from the house, car, and workplace. Evidence-based practice suggests that nurses can actively participate in helping patients succeed in smoking cessation programs. Wynd used guided imagery (exercises that included deep breathing, recalling childhood memories, and visualizing future outcomes) as part of a smoking cessation program with significant abstinence results (Wynd, 2005). 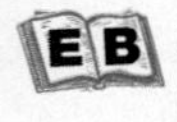 Buchanan et al. researched and demonstrated the efficacy of a multicomponent intervention for smoking cessation that included an on-site visit, follow-up phone calls, enhanced education about NRT and identification of a support partner (Buchanan et al., 2004). 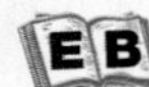

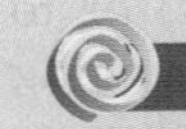

Cultural Cues 46–2

New Consumer Markets

There has been a decrease in smoking in the United States in the past 25 years. In 1966, the U.S. Surgeon General's health warnings were placed on all cigarette packages. Since then, similar warnings have been put on other tobacco products. Television and radio advertising for cigarettes was banned in 1971. Education and an increase in cigarette taxes, along with restrictions on smoking in public places, have also contributed to the decrease. Nevertheless, new potential consumer markets are being targeted around the world. For example, cigarette manufacturers have now identified China as a good alternative consumer market, and as a result, many Chinese men and teenagers have developed this high-risk habit.

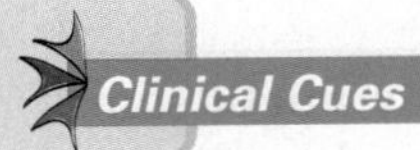

Clinical Cues

On admission to the hospital or at every clinic visit, ask your patients if they smoke and if they have thought about quitting. In accordance with the *Healthy People 2010* goals, this opens up opportunities to discuss smoking cessation programs and provide literature.

? *Think Critically About* . . . Do you have any bad habits such as smoking, drinking alcohol, or drinking too much coffee? How does your personal behavior affect what you will say to your patients about making changes for a healthier lifestyle?

ABUSE OF CANNABIS

The leaves and flowering tops of the *Cannabis sativa* (marijuana) plant are dried and loosely rolled in cigarette paper and smoked. It is commonly used as a "gateway substance" (substance that leads the way or opens the gate to more dangerous and serious substance abuse) by teenagers and as a recreational drug by adults. There is active and controversial discussion of legalizing marijuana for medical purposes. The active ingredient in marijuana is effective in controlling nausea in patients who are receiving chemotherapy, and studies also indicate that it lowers intraocular pressure in patients who have glaucoma.

Marijuana is typically smoked, but it can also be ingested. It acts quickly (15 minutes), and the effects last for up to 4 hours. **General effects are a mild euphoria, increased appetite, and increased sensitivity to sound, colors, and other environmental elements. Impaired coordination, mental concentration, and altered judgment are also present.** In large doses, the person may experience psychotic symptoms. Marijuana is thought not to be physically addictive, but it may lead to psychological dependence and a lack of motivation and ambition. There is no particular withdrawal syndrome for cannabis, so treatment must focus on issues related to the dangers of substance abuse in general.

Think Critically About . . . Substance abuse crosses all ethnic, gender, age, and socioeconomic backgrounds. You have three patients: a homeless elderly Asian American female, a well-to-do African American teenager, and a middle-aged white male who works as a carpenter. You must assess all three for marijuana (and other substances) use. First, identify your own biases and then describe your approach.

ABUSE OF HALLUCINOGENS AND INHALANTS

Two common drugs that cause hallucinations are lysergic acid diethylamide (LSD) and phencyclidine hydrochloride (PCP, or angel dust). These hallucinogens are thought to be somewhat less physiologically addictive compared to other psychoactive substances; however, there are extremely unpredictable effects. Hallucinogens cause distortion of the senses, an inability to separate fact from fantasy, impaired sense of time, and severely impaired judgment. Users never know whether they will have a good "trip" or a bad one. Uncontrolled *flashbacks* (feelings and sensations associated with use despite being drug-free) can occur. This group of drugs is very dangerous because use is known to cause panic, paranoia, and death from extremely impaired judgment.

Inhalants are psychologically and physiologically addictive. Commonly abused inhalants include glue, nail polish remover, aerosol-packaged products (e.g., deodorants), and paint thinner and other types of solvents. Symptoms of use are acute confusion, excitability, and sometimes hallucinations. Prolonged use of inhalants causes permanent damage to all body organs and a psychological dependence. Inhalants are most frequently used by teens and children because they are inexpensive and easily accessible.

Think Critically About . . . You are caring for a 14-year-old who admits to you that he has been experimenting with glue sniffing. He tells you that he has stopped and he asks you not to share this information with his parents. How will you handle this situation? Who can you consult to clarify your legal and ethical obligations?

Treatment

Medical treatment and intervention for both hallucinogens and inhalants may include provision of safety for the individual who may be experiencing a bad "trip." Emergency measures may be necessary to provide respiratory support for an individual who has impaired gas exchange as a result of inhalants.

Box 46–3 *CAGE Assessment*

A commonly used screening tool for alcohol abuse is the CAGE assessment. Two or more "yes" answers have a 90% correlation with an alcohol abuse problem.

- **C** Are you thinking about **C**utting down on your drinking?
- **A** Are you **A**nnoyed when someone criticizes you for drinking?
- **G** Do you feel **G**uilty about your drinking?
- **E** Do you have to have an **E**ye opener (i.e., to get rid of a morning hangover)?

From Ewing, J.A. (1984). Detecting alcoholism: The CAGE questionnaire. *JAMA, 252*(14), 1905–1907. Copyright © 1984. American Medical Association.

NURSING MANAGEMENT

Assessment (Data Collection)

A general physical assessment, including vital signs, is necessary. Any life-threatening physical problems must be quickly identified and treated. For example, patients can and do die from cardiac dysrhythmias associated with stimulant abuse, whereas patients who have overdosed on heroin are at risk for respiratory arrest. Obtain a substance and alcohol history that includes the type of substance used, the amount taken, and the pattern of use. A quick and simple assessment tool for alcohol abuse is the CAGE questionnaire (Box 46–3). It includes four questions, and a "yes" answer to two or more of the four questions correlates with alcohol abuse.

Also obtain information about past and current function in family, social, and occupational roles. Remember that denial is a primary defense mechanism used in these disorders. Therefore, it often is necessary to also ask the family to describe their perception of the user's problem and the extent of substance use. At the appropriate time, assess the impact of the user's behavior on the family and explore the presence of codependent or enabling behaviors. Examples of questions to ask either the individual or the family member(s) are listed in Focused Assessment 46–1.

Nursing Diagnosis

Nursing diagnoses for substance use disorders include, but are not limited to:

- Disturbed thought processes related to chronic alcohol consumption
- Ineffective denial related to physical and psychological dependence on a substance
- Interrupted family processes related to substance addiction that overrides family responsibilities
- Risk for injury related to impaired judgment
- Ineffective role performance related to impaired ability to complete assigned work duties
- Noncompliance related to abstinence from a substance

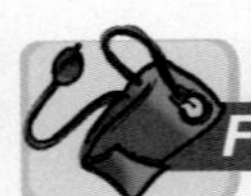

Focused Assessment 46–1

Data Collection for Substance and Alcohol Use

Ask the following questions during history taking to determine past and present substance and/or alcohol use:

- What substances (alcohol, tobacco, or illicit substances) are you currently using?
- What other types of drugs (prescription and nonprescription) do you routinely take?
- How much do you drink or how much do you use?
- How often do you drink or use substances?
- Have you ever tried to cut down or control your substance use or drinking?
- When did you last drink or use drugs of any kind?
- Have you noticed that now it takes more of the substance or drink to get the same effect you got several months ago?
- Have you noticed any withdrawal symptoms?
- Have you ever been treated for liver disease, hepatitis, heart disease, anemia, or overdose?
- Have you had any recent falls, accidents, or injuries?
- Have you ever stopped drinking or using drugs for a period of time?
- Have you ever been in treatment for substance abuse?
- Is there a family history of alcoholism or substance abuse?
- What is your marital status? If married, are you happily married?
- Have you ever been in trouble with the law?
- What is your occupation? Are you experiencing any difficulties at work?

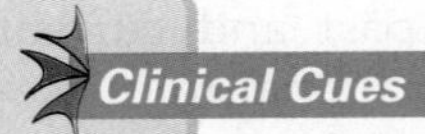

Clinical Cues

Patients will enter the health care system with medical complaints or injuries who also have unidentified substance abuse problems. When taking a routine admission history, ask about the use of substances. This information is needed to evaluate drug-drug interactions and any potential toxic effects on the body organs (i.e., heart, kidneys, liver). Use a matter-of-fact tone of voice: "Sir, what kind of prescription, over-the counter, or illicit (street) drugs do you use? Do you smoke or drink alcohol?" In accordance with 2008 National Patient Safety Goals, your findings contribute to a complete list of medications that should be communicated to the health care team within the organization, sent to other facilities if the patient is transferred, and provided to the patient when discharged.

Planning

Expected outcomes are written for the specific individual nursing diagnoses chosen to resolve the patient's problems. For the nursing diagnoses above, they might include:

- Patient will demonstrate less confusion and memory loss after receiving thiamine and abstaining from alcohol before discharge.

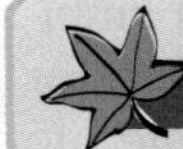

Elder Care Points

When working with elderly patients, be on the alert for substance use disorders; this group is at high risk because of loneliness, multiple losses, and limited resources. Health care providers frequently overlook substance abuse in elderly patients because behaviors may be attributed to aging, depression, or dementia. Stevenson and Masters suggested a "best predictor model" for older women who had a high risk for alcohol abuse (Stevenson & Masters, 2005). They 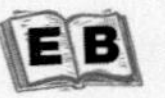 found that scores of 1 or higher on the T-ACE questionnaire (similar to CAGE), regular use of over-the counter drugs, ingestion of large amounts of coffee and using alcohol to induce sleep were associated with alcohol abuse.

- Patient will discuss how reliance on substances is affecting her quality of life during today's group therapy session.
- Patient and family will communicate needs and identify sources of support to sustain family during weekly sessions with social service counselor.
- Patient will remain safe from harm or injury during this shift.
- Patient will resume job duties within ____ months.
- Patient will participate in a 12-step program at least three times per week.

Collaborative goal setting is very important when working with an individual who is addicted to a substance. In addition to working with the patient, it is necessary that you collaborate with the family. Setting goals with the patient and excluding the family or friends often leads to failure or relapse. Planning care for a patient with a substance use disorder includes promoting safety (physical and psychological), providing a safe withdrawal from the substance, and ensuring adequate nutrition and sleep. To prevent relapse, considerable education regarding substance abuse becomes a priority goal. The education may be started in a treatment center, but needs to be continued after discharge for at least 1 year. People who abuse substances need opportunities to learn and practice new coping skills in a supportive environment.

Implementation

Nursing intervention depends on the severity of the addictive process. Initial interventions for the patient focus on physical recovery. For example, cardiac monitoring, pulse oximetry, IV access, and other emergency measures may be indicated. Potentially fatal effects of drugs and/or alcohol, such as cardiac dysrhythmias, hypotension, and respiratory depression, must receive priority attention. Another priority intervention is to ensure that the patient does not suffer ill consequences from a poorly managed detoxification. Detoxification is managed medically by giving antianxiety agents, such as chlordiazepoxide (Librium). Close monitoring of vital signs is important because signs of alcohol withdrawal include an increase in blood pressure and heart rate. Preventing the patient from experiencing a seizure, delirium tremens, or "DTs" is an essential part of the detoxification process.

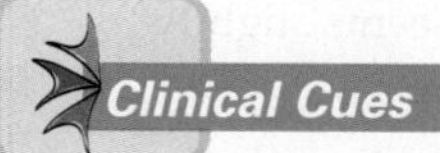

Clinical Cues

When monitoring and reporting changes in blood pressure, keep several factors in mind: patient's baseline, trends (if available), and medications (last dose and type). Also assess for accompanying subjective symptoms such as dizziness or lightheadedness (hypotension), headache, or blurred vision (hypertension).

Orienting the patient to person, place, and time is necessary, and so is providing for physical safety. A person who is intoxicated may need to be placed in a protected environment until judgment and coordination return. Seeing that the patient gets adequate sleep and a balanced diet high in proteins and multivitamins is also part of early intervention (Assignment Considerations 46–1).

Once the substance is cleared from the body, nursing intervention is directed toward helping the patient lead a drug-free life. This includes alleviating the symptoms and confronting denial. You must also observe for signs of suicide. These patients often feel they cannot live without the euphoria and consolation of the substance experience.

Patients who are in the early recovery process from substance abuse benefit greatly from therapeutic conversations with the nurse, and a caring, concerned attitude is very important. They must grieve the loss of the substance, and they also feel guilt and shame for acts that were committed while under the influence. To help the patient "work through" these feelings, you need to be an active listener, offering support and validation as necessary. Mandating a patient to stop is usually not an effective intervention; however, you should support the patient's decision to stop. Assist by reminding her that the physical symptoms of withdrawal will not last forever. The craving will last longer than the withdrawal symptoms, but is manageable if a change toward a healthy lifestyle is desirable. Help your patient to identify ways to cope with the craving. For example, help her to make a list of activities that she could use to distract her attention from the craving, such as calling a friend, taking a brisk walk, cleaning the house, or eating a nutritious snack. Help her identify settings, circumstances, or relationships that were part of her substance abuse pattern, then identify alternative settings and relationships that are now part of her new lifestyle. For example, polysubstance use might routinely occur in a bar or lounge with friends after having a few beers, but is less likely to occur in a movie theater with friends who are having popcorn.

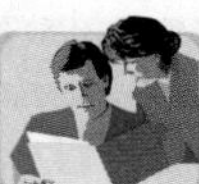

Assignment Considerations 46–1

1:1 Observation

Frequently a nursing assistant (NA) is assigned to sit with a patient who needs one-to-one (1:1) observation. Before assigning the NA to this task, clarify with the physician or RN the purpose of 1:1 observation and the stability of the patient. For example, recall that opioid withdrawal is not life threatening, but the restless patient may be temporarily placed on 1:1 observation to prevent *elopement* (leaving) to seek drugs to satisfy the intense craving. It would be appropriate to assign an NA to stay with this patient. In contrast, an agitated patient who is withdrawing from alcohol is not physically stable and her care should be managed by an RN.

If the patient is addicted to heroin, the recovery process will be lengthy because of the lifestyle changes that are necessary. Typically, with heroin addiction, there has been considerable legal involvement and maladaptive coping. Each situation must be considered individually. The patient needs to be educated about the disease process and needs to learn new coping methods. See Nursing Care Plan 46–1 for nursing diagnosis, goals, and interventions for patient with a substance use disorder.

Nursing Intervention with the Family

A trusting relationship needs to be developed with the family or they may continue to focus on the patient rather than focus on their own recovery. Families need to learn in what manner they might have been enabling their loved one, and they need time to practice new behaviors that will require the substance abuser to be responsible for herself. Family members should be encouraged to express how the crisis is affecting them. There may be need to refer families to legal or social services if the person is abusing illegal drugs or if there was an arrest for driving while intoxicated. The family feels shame and guilt and shares the stigma associated with substance abuse. Encourage them to seek support from groups such as Al-Anon or Alateen. Family members may consider substance abuse a moral weakness, rather than a disease. Educating them about the neurobiologic theories may help them to reconsider their attitudes and relieve some guilt. **To be effective in working with substance abusers, nurses must examine their own attitudes and make certain the patients and families are treated with respect.**

? *Think Critically About . . .* A patient tells you that he drinks socially, but his wife and children tell you that he drinks to the point of intoxication at least three times a week. What would you say to the family? What would you say to the patient?

NURSING CARE PLAN 46–1

Care of the Patient with a Substance Abuse Disorder

SCENARIO Jerry Sanders is a 42-year-old man brought in by his supervisor for admission to a "detox" unit. The supervisor last saw Mr. Sanders drinking about 10 hours ago. He states that Jerry is a good worker but could lose his job. Mr. Sanders jokingly replies, "My boss is a worrier. I'm just a social drinker. My wife and kids know I'm okay." The supervisor states that the wife frequently makes excuses but seems unaware of the problem. Mr. Sanders seems slightly anxious and irritable. He appears thin and malnourished.

PROBLEM/NURSING DIAGNOSIS *Showing early signs of withdrawal*/Risk for injury related to effects of drug, complications of withdrawal.

Supporting assessment data *Subjective:* None. *Objective:* Slightly anxious and irritable. Last known drink 10 hours ago.

Goals/Expected Outcomes	Nursing Interventions	Selected Rationale	Evaluation
Patient will remain free from any injury this shift Patient will withdraw from drugs or alcohol without any undue effects	Assess for early symptoms of withdrawal (e.g., agitation, irritability, anxiety) and notify physician or RN of first signs.	Early detection of withdrawal allows for prompt intervention to prevent life-threatening complications.	Is anxious and irritable.
	Administer medications (e.g., chlordiazepoxide [Librium]) as prescribed by physician.	Decreases neurologic irritability at the biochemical level.	Thirty minutes after administration of Librium, patient appears more relaxed.
	Remain with patient during times of confusion and disorientation.	Provides support and decreases agitation.	Currently alert and oriented.
	Restrain and/or place in seclusion as ordered if the patient becomes a danger to self or others.	May temporarily be unable to control aggressive or self-harm impulses. May attempt to leave.	Is verbally hostile and denies substance abuse problems, but shows no signs of physical aggression.
	Ensure safe environment (i.e., call bell within reach, bed in lowest position).	Safety is a priority, and patient judgment and coordination may be temporarily impaired.	Did not sustain any injury during the shift. Outcomes met. Continue plan.

PROBLEM/NURSING DIAGNOSIS *Not admitting to problem*/Ineffective denial related to minimization of the symptoms of addiction.

Supporting assessment data *Subjective:* States "My boss is a worrier. I'm just a social drinker." *Objective:* Supervisor's report and Mr. Sanders' perception of the problem are mismatched.

Goals/Expected Outcomes	Nursing Interventions	Selected Rationale	Evaluation
Patient will acknowledge the abuse of substances and the unhealthy impact on his life	Approach the patient in a nonjudgmental manner.	Helps to build trust and rapport	Is agreeable to talking but is unable to disclose feelings.
	Gently confront the denial as you gain the trust of the patient.	Breaking through denial is essential to recovery.	Denial continues.
Patient will openly acknowledge the need for substance abuse treatment	Help the patient see the need for treatment and abstinence.	May be unaware of or is ignoring the long-term consequences.	Denies need for treatment.
	Inform the patient about the negative aspects of addictive processes.	Helps the patient to make an informed decision.	Verbally acknowledges that substances are harmful for others, "but I don't drink that much."
	Encourage patient to list the harmful effects that he has experienced.	Increases insight and facilitates self-diagnosis.	Denies that substances are harming him.
Patient will agree to attend 90 12-step meetings in 90 days	Encourage attendance at a 12-step program to help break through the denial.	Provides support by others who have experienced the same difficulties.	Agrees to go to a 12-step program, but thinks it is unnecessary. Outcomes not met. Continue plan.

Key: *IV*, intravenous.

NURSING CARE PLAN 46-1

Care of the Patient with a Substance Abuse Disorder—cont'd

PROBLEM/NURSING DIAGNOSIS *Wife is affected, but is not openly acknowledging problem*/Dysfunctional family process: alcoholism, related to altered family roles, unexpressed feelings, family history of alcoholism.

Supporting assessment data *Subjective:* Per supervisor, wife frequently makes excuses but seems unaware of the problem. *Objective:* Wife is absent; supervisor is advocating for treatment.

Goals/Expected Outcomes	Nursing Interventions	Selected Rationale	Evaluation
Family will be able to identify and share feelings	Invite family to participate.	Family may be unaware, or need assistance to break through their denial.	Wife and children did come in to talk with physician and social worker about Mr. Sanders' condition.
	Assess for presence of denial, shame, or guilt.	Feelings of denial, shame, and guilt are expected, but may be repressed.	Family members expressed support for Mr. Sanders, but are unable to disclose personal feelings.
	Encourage expression of genuine feelings.	Opportunity for expression of feelings helps to build trust and rapport.	Trust and rapport are being established, but communication between family members continues to be ineffective.
	Teach how to recognize feelings and safe ways to express them (e.g., "I love you, but I am not going to stay here while you drink.")	New communication methods are needed to help the family break old patterns.	Currently family is not openly acknowledging how Mr. Sanders' behavior affects each member, but they agree to attend group therapy.
	Educate the family about the altered roles present in addictive families. (e.g., child taking care of the parent).	Family members may be unaware of how the illness is affecting role function.	Family is not identifying dysfunctional roles, but appear open to exploring the family situation.
	Define the term *enabling* for family members.	Identifying and defining enabling helps family to recognize this behavior.	Entire family appears to be in denial at this time; denies enabling behaviors.
	Encourage family members to state at least one time when they engaged in enabling behavior.	Increases insight into own behavior.	
	Offer family members alternative choices to enabling behavior (e.g., telling him that he must call in sick for himself).	Family needs new ways to cope with old problems.	Family open to learning more about disease process and how to cope with Mr. Sanders' behavior.
Family will role play at least one situation of potential enabling	Have family members practice and role play alternative responses to enabling behavior.	Practice in a safe environment allows family to test new skills.	Family having difficulty with role play.
Family will agree to attend at least six 12-step meetings	Encourage family members to attend a 12-step support meeting.	Provides support by sharing with others who are experiencing the same problem.	Family agrees to go to a 12-step group this weekend. Outcomes not met. Continue plan.

Continued

Evaluation

Recovery from a substance use disorder is a lengthy process. Ridding the substance from the body can take weeks, particularly if there is coexisting liver damage. Often the patient is malnourished, physically exhausted, and in poor general health. Return to an optimum healthy state may take 6 months to 1 year. Recovery of psychological or emotional health takes even longer. If the patient started abusing drugs at a very young age, emotional development was arrested. Coping mechanisms to deal with anxiety or emotional pain were never developed; the individual used the drug(s) instead.

Consequently, nurses working in the hospital may only see early physical recovery. Evaluating overall effectiveness of substance abuse treatment is measured in years rather than weeks. Admitting a pa-

NURSING CARE PLAN 46-1

Care of the Patient with a Substance Abuse Disorder—cont'd

PROBLEM/NURSING DIAGNOSIS *Drinking excessive alcohol and not eating enough to meet daily needs*/Imbalanced nutrition: less than body requirements, related to poor food intake, inadequate absorption of nutrients, poor appetite.

Supporting assessment data *Subjective:* None. *Objective:* Appears thin and malnourished.

Goals/Expected Outcomes	Nursing Interventions	Selected Rationale	Evaluation
Patient will self-select a nutritious diet	Assess ability to feed self.	May have impairment in fine motor coordination.	Is able to independently feed self; shows some fine tremors in hands.
Patient will gain 5 lb within 1 mo; signs of peripheral neuropathy (numbness and tingling) will disappear	Watch for nausea, vomiting, diarrhea. Administer antacids, antiemetics, and IV fluids as ordered.	Alcohol can cause gastritis and alterations in absorption.	Currently no nausea or vomiting.
	Document intake and output and food intake. Weigh patient.	To monitor nutritional status and progress toward goal.	Weighs 140 lb (ideal body weight 165 lb). Finishes food trays.
	Collaborate with patient to determine food preferences.	Increases likelihood of consumption.	Eats all types of food.
	Encourage small, frequent meals, high in proteins with 50% carbohydrates.	Small meals are easier to tolerate, and foods rich in nutrition will replace loss due to poor dietary practices.	States that he sometimes forgets to eat, but knows he should gain some weight ("Will try harder").
	Administer multivitamins, especially thiamine (vitamin B_1) and niacin, as ordered.	Patient is at risk for Wernicke's encephalopathy.	Agrees that supplements are a good idea and will continue to take them after discharge.
	Consult nutritionist.	Collaboration with specialist ensures best plan.	Consultation with nutritionist deferred because patient agrees to eating everything on food trays. Outcomes partially met. Continue plan.

? CRITICAL THINKING QUESTIONS

1. What are some questions that would be appropriate to ask the wife (if she is willing to come in or speak on the phone)?
2. Mr. Sanders is currently far from being ready for self-diagnosis. What are some things that might signal that he is breaking through the denial?

tient to a hospital and guiding her safely though detoxification is a very necessary, but small, beginning step in the overall process (Legal & Ethical Considerations 46–1).

COMMUNITY CARE

Nurses who work in emergency rooms and busy outpatient clinics often see individuals who present for medical problems related to substance abuse. Often these patients are treated only for their presenting medical problem. In these instances, the medical treatment team is reinforcing the patient's denial system. In accordance with the *Healthy People 2010* goals, a proactive approach would be to use these incidental contacts to screen for substance abuse and appropriately refer these patients to prevent costly long-term complications.

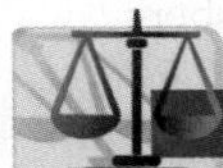

Legal & Ethical Considerations 46–1

Substance Abuse among Health Care Workers

Those in the health care field are particularly vulnerable to substance abuse because of the availability of drugs and the tendency to care for others while ignoring personal problems. Approximately 40 states have established confidential programs to assist impaired health care providers to get help for the problem rather than immediately forfeiting their professional license. Signs and symptoms to be aware of among health care workers include frequently calling in sick or always working (to have access to drugs), sloppy patient care, frequently leaving for breaks, offering to give pain medications, and patients complaining of no relief after receiving pain medications.

As is the case with the general patient population, inpatient hospital stays for individuals who are addicted are usually short. If the patient has some type of insurance, it is not unusual for the insurance company to pay only for medical detoxification. Any further treatment that is necessary would be performed on an outpatient basis.

Making a decision to become sober and/or substance free often requires lifestyle changes. Changes of this magnitude are not made overnight. Addicted individuals often need ongoing medical support as well as support from the recovery community. Encourage your patients who are attempting recovery to seek out help and make the recovery process a number-one priority. As a nurse, you can be instrumental in facilitating public awareness, and in educating patients about the responsible use, and ultimate hazards, of mood-altering substances. Nurses should also be politically attuned to and advocate for legislation that regulates product availability and marketing of substances such as tobacco and alcohol.

Key Points

- Substance use disorder is diagnosed when ingestion of psychoactive substances such as alcohol or drugs results in recognizable signs and symptoms.
- Psychoactive substances are mind-altering agents capable of changing or altering a person's mood, behavior, cognition, arousal level, level of consciousness, and perceptions.
- Abuse implies use of a psychoactive substance in a nontherapeutic manner or the illicit use of prescription drugs.
- Dependence implies the presence of physical or psychological symptoms of addiction; when the substance use is stopped, withdrawal symptoms appear.
- Withdrawal symptoms occur when there is an attempt to stop using a substance. Symptoms of withdrawal from CNS depressants include increased blood pressure and pulse, nervousness, and heightened anxiety. Symptoms of withdrawal from CNS stimulants include drowsiness, headache, lethargy, nausea, alterations in eating and sleeping patterns, and cravings.
- Medical conditions related to alcohol abuse include liver damage, cardiomyopathy, hypertension, gastrointestinal bleeding, stroke, sleep disturbances, malnutrition, peripheral neuropathies, chronic infection, cognitive impairment, Wernicke's encephalopathy, and Korsakoff syndrome.
- Assess for physical, psychological, and behavioral symptoms of abuse or withdrawal.
- Take a history from the patient and the family to determine type, amount, and pattern of use.
- General nursing interventions include observing for life-threatening conditions, safely managing detoxification, orienting the patient to reality, providing a balanced diet high in protein and multivitamins, setting limits, confronting denial, identifying enabling behaviors and teaching new coping mechanisms, and referring the patient to a 12-step program.
- Denial and rationalization are primary defense mechanisms used by the substance abuser.
- Substance abuse affects family and friends; they may experience anger, rage, guilt, embarrassment, shame, and hopelessness.
- The family also uses denial and rationalization to cope. Enabling behaviors ("helping" a person so that the consequences of her unhealthy behavior are less severe) or co-dependency (family member or friend attempts to control the behaviors of the substance abuser) further inhibit recovering.
- Elderly people may drink to alleviate depression and loneliness. Decreased liver and renal function can quickly lead to toxicity and dependence.
- Nurses can participate in screening, advocating for legislation related to alcohol and tobacco, and educating the general public about the consequences of substance abuse.

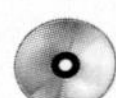
Go to your **Companion CD-ROM** for an Audio Glossary, animations, video clips, and bonus review questions.

evolve Be sure to visit the companion Evolve site at http://evolve.elsevier.com/deWit for interactive NCLEX-PN Exam Style Review Questions, WebLinks, and additional online resources.

NCLEX EXAM STYLE REVIEW QUESTIONS

Choose the best answer(s) for the following questions:

1. Which of the following medications would be useful in the treatment of nicotine withdrawal?

1. Naloxone (Narcan)
2. Buprenorphine (Subutex)
3. Bupropion (Zyban)
4. Sertraline (Zoloft)

2. When the nurse has to administer increasing doses of the same narcotic analgesic medication to alleviate pain in a patient hospitalized for chronic cancer pain, the patient is said to be developing:

1. psychological dependence.
2. withdrawal.
3. tolerance.
4. addiction.

3. When asked regarding alcohol consumption, a patient responds, "I really do not have a problem with drinking. I just have a few swigs now and then." The nurse identifies the response as a form of:

1. intellectualization.
2. sublimation.
3. displacement.
4. denial.

4. The teenage son of an alcoholic cares for his younger siblings. When asked about his father's whereabouts, the boy often responds, "He is working somewhere and will not be back for a while." The priority nursing diagnosis is:
   1. Ineffective individual coping.
   2. Dysfunctional family processes: alcoholism.
   3. Readiness for enhanced family coping.
   4. Parental role conflict.

5. The wife of a substance abuser demonstrates enabling behavior. Which of the following outcomes would be appropriate for the nursing diagnosis of Ineffective denial related to husband's substance problem?
   1. Wife will identify family behaviors related to substance abuse.
   2. Wife will accept responsibility for the husband's behaviors.
   3. Wife will verbalize ways to enhance husband's self-esteem.
   4. Wife will list reasons for husband's substance abuse.

6. A postoperative patient who is a self-confessed drinker is given chlordiazepoxide (Librium) for increased blood pressure, increased pulse, tremors, nausea and vomiting, and diaphoresis. When asked regarding the rationale for the medication, the nurse accurately responds:
   1. "It prevents clot formation."
   2. "It reduces symptoms of alcohol withdrawal."
   3. "It decreases pain associated with the surgery."
   4. "It stimulates wound healing."

7. A self-confessed alcoholic asks, "Why do I have to take disulfiram (Antabuse)?" The nurse would accurately respond:
   1. "It blocks the craving for alcohol."
   2. "The medication causes unpleasant symptoms when you drink."
   3. "The medication keeps you from having seizures."
   4. "It controls symptoms of nausea, vomiting, pain, or cramps."

8. Cocaine users experience a fast-acting euphoria, increased energy, and heightened sense of well-being, but they also experience the severe, intense emotional lows when the drug is metabolized. This compulsion to keep "feeling good" is best described as:
   1. addiction.
   2. psychological dependence.
   3. withdrawal.
   4. tolerance.

9. The nurse is teaching a community group about substance abuse among children and teens. Which statement by an audience member indicates a need for additional teaching?
   1. "Inhalants are most frequently used by children and teens."
   2. "Marijuana causes mild euphoria, increased appetite, and altered judgment."
   3. "African American teenagers have the highest rate of abuse for methamphetamines."
   4. "Withdrawal from heroin is not life threatening."

10. A patient is in the early recovery process and is attempting to lead a drug-free life. Which of the following interventions is appropriate to assist the patient?
    1. Remind the patient of the discomfort and pain that occurred during detoxification.
    2. Tell the patient that there is no need to feel guilty or ashamed.
    3. Help the patient to identify relationships that were part of the substance use pattern.
    4. Advise the patient that stopping forever is the only choice for a drug-free life.

CRITICAL THINKING ACTIVITIES  *Read each clinical scenario and discuss the questions with your classmates.*

Scenario A

Mr. Samm, a 65-year-old white man, is recently widowed and misses his wife very much. He comes to the physician's office and he is stumbling. His speech is slurred, and his breath has an alcohol-like odor. He begins to cry and states he has changed his mind. He does not want to see the physician, but is going to drive home.

1. How will you ensure his safety?
2. What type of assessment will you perform on this patient?

Scenario B

Ms. Brown, age 29, is an ambulatory postoperative patient. She admits to a past history of illicit substance abuse, but claims to be drug-free for several months. You notice that she leaves the floor and when she returns her coordination is slightly impaired and she seems inappropriately euphoric and giddy. Shortly thereafter, you observe her hiding a plastic bag; you suspect that she may be taking an illicit substance.

1. How would you handle this situation?
2. What types of documentation should you perform?

Scenario C

Mr. Martinez, a 32-year-old construction worker, was admitted for emergency orthopedic surgery yesterday evening following an on-the-job accident. He begins yelling profanity and is irritable and argumentative. He seems to be having trouble concentrating on your questions. His wife says he forgot to tell the physician that he drinks 12 beers every night.

1. What do you suspect is wrong with Mr. Martinez?
2. What other signs and symptoms would you watch for if you suspect alcohol withdrawal?
3. List the nursing interventions to care for Mr. Martinez during the initial phase of withdrawal.

CHAPTER

47 Care of Patients with Cognitive Disorders

evolve http://evolve.elsevier.com/deWit

Objectives

Upon completion of this chapter, you should be able to:

Theory

1. Discuss the incidence and significance of cognitive disorders in the aged population.
2. Differentiate between delirium (acute cognitive disorder) and dementia (chronic cognitive disorder).
3. Describe the signs and symptoms of Alzheimer's disease in relation to the early, middle, and late stages.
4. From the diagnoses listed, choose appropriate nursing interventions and expected outcomes when caring for patients with Alzheimer's disease.
5. Discuss the assessment skills that are necessary to accurately monitor a cognitive disorder.
6. Identify at least three nursing diagnoses that would be appropriate for a patient with delirium.
7. Identify nursing interventions that can be used to assist the family and friends of patients who have cognitive disorders.

Clinical Practice

1. Develop a care plan with at least six interventions for a patient who is confused and disoriented.
2. Design a teaching plan for a family member who is caring for an elderly parent with Alzheimer's disease in the family home.

Key Terms

Be sure to check out the bonus material on the Companion CD-ROM, including selected audio pronunciations.

Alzheimer's disease (ĂWLTZ-hī-mĕrz dĭ-ZĒZ, p. 1139)
cognition (kŏg-NĬ-shŭn, p. 1137)
confabulation (kŏn-fă-bŭ-LĀ-shŭn, p. 1138)
delirium (dĕ-LĬR-ē-ŭm, p. 1137)
delusion (dĕ-LŪ-shŭn, p. 1138)
dementia (dē-MĔN-shē-ă, p. 1137)
global amnesia (GLŌ-băl ăm-NĒ-zē-ă, p. 1148)
hallucination (hă-lū-sĭ-NĀ-shŭn, p. 1138)
illusion (ĭ-LŪ-shŭn, p. 1138)
sundowning (SŬN-doun-ing, p. 1146)
vascular dementia (VĂS-kū-lăr dē-MĔN-shē-ă, p. 1141)

OVERVIEW OF COGNITIVE DISORDERS

Cognition refers to mental processes of perception, memory, judgment, and reasoning. It includes the ability to perceive and process information. **A cognitive disorder is diagnosed when there is a significant change in cognition from a previous level of functioning.** Cognitive disorders greatly affect the quality of life for affected individuals, families, and friends. Although these disorders do occur across the life span, they are often linked to the neurobiologic changes that accompany aging. These disorders are increasingly common with the aging of the population since the mid-1980s. Disorders of cognition include delirium and dementia.

Delirium (acute confusion) is characterized by a change in overall cognition and level of consciousness over a short time. Dementia, on the other hand, is characterized by several cognitive deficits, memory in particular, and tends to be more chronic. Both conditions are classified according to *etiology* (cause or origin of disease). Examples of etiologies for delirium are ingestion of a toxic substance or a serious infection. An example of etiology for dementia is multiple small blood clots that cause brain tissue damage (known as **vascular dementia**). **Alzheimer's disease** (a degenerative disease of the brain) is another example of dementia, although the exact cause is unknown. A simple way to remember the difference between the two conditions is that **delirium is an acute condition that requires immediate treatment and dementia is a chronic condition.** Reversing the symptoms of delirium depends on timely diagnosis and treatment. It also is important to note that **delirium can coexist with dementia.** If delirium is recognized and promptly treated, the patient with preexisting dementia should be restored to a previous level of functioning.

DELIRIUM

Many conditions or physiologic alterations can cause delirium. **Some examples are cerebrovascular accident; drug overdose, toxicity, or withdrawal; tumors; systemic infections; fluid and electrolyte imbalances; and malnutrition. The onset of acute delirium is sudden.** The patient may be very alert or lethargic, depending on the cause of the delirium, and may appear very confused. The attention span changes and overall awareness of the environment is decreased. Orientation is impaired as well as recent and immediate memory. Speech may be incoherent, and overall thinking is disorganized and distorted. The patient will not be able to communicate his thoughts to you in a mean-

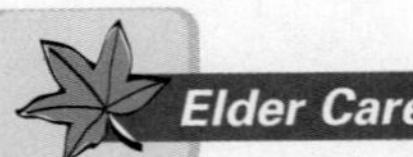

In hospitalized older adults with preexisting dementia, it is not unusual to see a patient who has been previously conscious and oriented become drowsy, disoriented, combative, and unable to recognize family and friends. The astute nurse suspects delirium or acute confusion. One of the first interventions is to note what type of medications the patient is receiving. Anticholinergic medications have potent central nervous system effects and can cause a sudden episode of confusion. Is the dose too high for age and physiologic functioning? Is there a cumulative effect? Are the medications interacting? Delirium and dementia can coexist, and the acute condition needs to be recognized and treated, not merely dismissed as part of the overall dementia.

ingful way. In delirium, a patient may experience **illusions** (misinterpretations of reality). For example, a pen appears to be a knife, or a shadow on the floor appears to be a menacing monster. If your patient appears to be talking to someone who is not there, it is likely that he is experiencing **hallucinations** (seeing or hearing things that are not there). If he insists that you are an FBI agent, this is an example of a **delusion** (belief in a false idea).

Problem-solving ability and judgment may be diminished, but not completely absent. Consequently, the patient may not make good decisions, or may become combative or hostile if the nurse or family member attempts to intervene. The general features of delirium are the same for all the causes, and nursing care is basically the same; the main difference is in diagnosis and treatment of the underlying cause. In this chapter the prototype condition of substance-induced delirium is discussed.

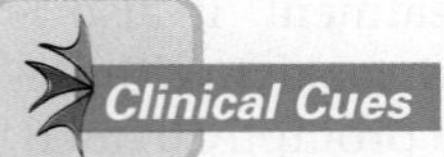

Does your patient have depression, dementia, or delirium? Recall from Chapter 45 that a patient with depression can have poor personal hygiene, can have difficulty with concentration, and may be very quiet and withdrawn or very agitated. You will have to observe for subtle differences to detect depression, dementia, or delirium. For example, your depressed patient may speak very little, but the speech is generally logical and will contain sad and negative thoughts and feelings of hopelessness. The patient with dementia may confabulate or will have difficulty finding words. The patient with delirium will be incoherent or loud.

SUBSTANCE-INDUCED DELIRIUM

Substance-induced delirium can be caused by withdrawal from a substance, intoxication with a substance, or side effects from a medication. For a review of intoxication and withdrawal delirium, see Chapter 46. Many classes of medications can produce symptoms of delirium. Some common examples are anesthetics, analgesics, sedative-hypnotics, any products with anticholinergic activity (tricyclic antidepressants, antihistamines, theophylline derivatives, and antipsychotics), and histamine (H_2)-receptor blockers (e.g., famotidine, cimetidine, and ranitidine). Commonly prescribed beta blockers and nonsteroidal anti-inflammatory drugs (NSAIDs) can also cause symptoms of delirium.

Diagnosis and treatment depend on thorough history taking. If the patient is unable to give you a history, elicit help from the family. It is not unusual for a person to be taking large amounts of over-the-counter medications and forget to mention them because the medications were not prescribed by a physician. Pay attention to drug interactions and incompatibilities and consult with the pharmacist as needed. Early recognition can assist in a faster recovery. If the medication accumulates over several days, elimination of the substance from the body takes much longer and places the patient in even greater danger.

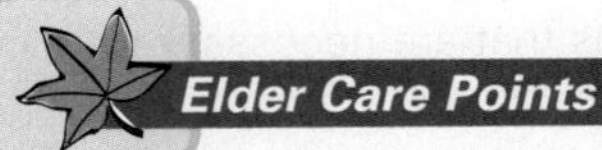

Older adults have a high risk for substance-induced delirium because of overall decreased metabolism and reduction in liver and kidney function. A general principle that providers should use in prescribing medications to elders is to give the smallest amount possible and increase the amount only as symptoms indicate. Therefore, you must carefully observe and report subtle changes in behavior, vital signs, and laboratory results.

DEMENTIA

There are several different types of dementia, and these conditions are also classified according to the underlying cause. **Examples include Alzheimer's disease, frontotemporal lobe dementia, Huntington's disease, Korsakoff's syndrome, vascular dementia, acquired immunodeficiency syndrome (AIDS) dementia complex, and Parkinson's disease.** The onset for dementia is slow, and the condition may progress over a long time (months to years). The patient is generally alert and has a normal attention span. Orientation to person, place, and time and recent memory may be impaired. In later stages of dementia, patients lose remote memory as well. You would observe that the patient has difficulty with abstracting thoughts and a poverty of thoughts. **Confabulation** (making up experiences to fill conversational gaps) and impaired judgment are common. Hallucinations, delusions, and illusions usually are not present. These patients experience fragmented sleep rather than a reversed cycle (Complementary & Alternative Therapies 47–1). Often, there is a notable change in personality. The two most common prototypes are Alzheimer's disease and vascular dementia.

Complementary & Alternative Therapies 47–1

Herbs

Herbs that have a sedative effect include chamomile, hops, and valerian. These can be used in a tea or taken in capsules. A popular method of promoting sleep is to place a few drops of lavender onto the pillowcase. If your patients are using herbs or alternative therapy, advise them to inform their physician because of potential drug-herb interactions, or for contraindications due to medical conditions.

ALZHEIMER'S DISEASE

Etiology and Pathophysiology

Alzheimer's disease **(AD) is the most common degenerative disease of the brain.** Approximately 4.5 million Americans have AD, and there is no known cause or cure. AD typically affects people over the age of 65, but can also strike younger people. The incidence increases as age advances. In AD, there is a loss of neurons in the frontal and temporal lobes. The atrophy in these areas accounts for the patient's inability to process and integrate new information and to retrieve memories. Brain biopsies of AD patients have revealed that nerve cells are tangled and twisted and there is an abnormal buildup of proteins. Production of neurotransmitters (e.g., acetylcholine, serotonin) is relatively decreased for these patients. (See Chapter 48 for a discussion of neurotransmitters.) Genetic factors and exposure to environmental elements such as metals, infection, or toxins, as well as a previous head injury, may also play a role (Health Promotion Points 47–1).

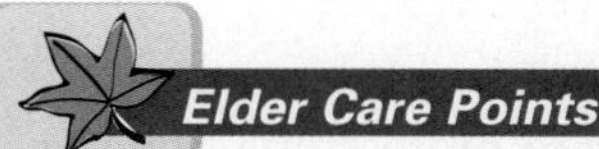

The 85-year-old-and-over age-group is currently the fastest growing age-group in the United States. It is estimated that 50% of this group have Alzheimer's disease.

Signs and Symptoms

The disease has a slow onset and variable rate of progression. Eventually, it is fatal. Behavioral patterns and symptoms associated with AD are typically divided into four stages: mild (early stage), moderate (middle stage), moderate to severe (middle to late stage), and late stage. Early signs and symptoms of beginning mental deterioration include forgetfulness, recent memory loss, difficulty learning and remembering, inability to concentrate, and a decline in personal hygiene, appearance, and inhibitions. Later the patient becomes quite confused and unable to make judgments, has difficulty communicating, suffers losses in motor function, and becomes dependent on others.

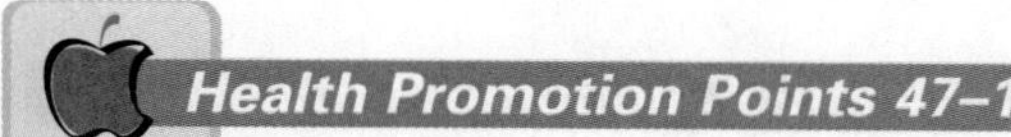

Diet and Memory

Help patients and families to understand that a diet with large amounts of meat and high-sodium foods along with a sedentary lifestyle and high blood pressure are factors associated with poor memory recall.

Box 47–1 *Behavioral Patterns in Various Stages of Alzheimer's Disease*

EARLY (MILD) STAGE
- Slow, progressive loss of intellectual ability
- Difficulty in learning new things
- Mild depression
- Personality and social interactions remain intact

MIDDLE (MODERATE) STAGE
- Increase in memory loss
- Decreased ability to perform usual ADLs
- Variable mood
- Noticeable personality change
- Social withdrawal
- Monitor for safety
- Conversation is disorganized

MIDDLE TO LATE (MODERATE TO SEVERE) STAGE
- Unable to recognize familiar objects and family
- Needs repeated instructions for simple tasks
- Needs total care—can be very burdensome for the family
- Wanders away
- Incontinent
- Outbursts of anger, hostility, paranoia

LATE STAGE
- Unable to speak or ambulate
- Profound memory loss
- Difficulty swallowing
- Weight loss
- Bedridden
- Fetal position
- End-stage consequences of poor nutritional state and bedridden status: pressure sores, respiratory failure, contractures, pneumonia

Key: *ADLs,* activities of daily living.

Common behavioral manifestations associated with stages of AD are presented in Box 47–1.

Patients have a progressive loss of common cognitive functions. For example, Mr. Allan Jennings is an 85-year-old retired attorney. You observe that Mr. Jennings has trouble remembering words *(anomia)* or verbally expressing himself *(aphasia)*, and he is unable to write down his thoughts *(agraphia)* or understand written language *(alexia)*. If he holds a common object such as a spoon, he doesn't seem to recognize it *(agnosia)*, and he can't put on his shirt, although he has the strength and motor movement to dress himself *(apraxia:*

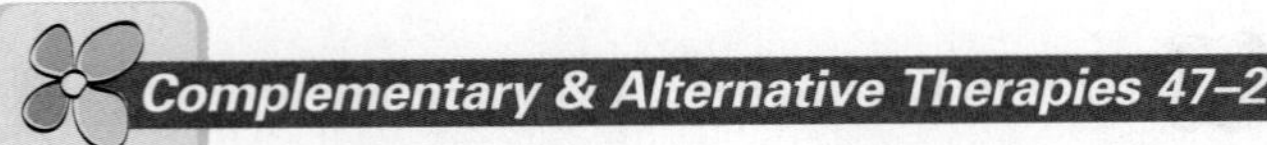

Complementary & Alternative Therapies 47–2

Animal-Assisted Therapy

Animal-assisted therapy may help patients to improve memory (e.g., calling the therapy dog's name), coordination (e.g., throwing a ball for the dog), object identification (e.g., directing the dog to get the ball), language (e.g., talking to the dog), and attention (e.g., caring for the dog).

inability to perform an activity despite motor function) (Complementary & Alternative Therapies 47–2).

? *Think Critically About . . .* It is not uncommon for patients with dementia to act in a sexually inappropriate way because of loss of social reserve. Your elderly male patient is reaching to fondle your breasts when you turn him to do hygienic care and linen changes. How will you handle this?

Diagnosis

In making the diagnosis, the physician will use a detailed medical and family history and conduct a thorough physical, neurologic, and functional assessment. Your patient may undergo magnetic resonance imaging (MRI) to rule out pathologic lesions. The diagnostic use of positron emission tomography (PET) and single-photon emission computed tomography (SPECT) are controversial, but considered. Apolipoprotein E4 genotyping is used to confirm the diagnosis of late-onset AD. Research is being conducted on new diagnostic tests for AD. These include noninvasive optical testing and the identification of biomarkers that detect AD before the manifestation of symptoms. Box 47–2 lists the diagnostic criteria for AD in the *Diagnostic and Statistical Manual of Mental Disorders,* fourth edition, Text Revision (DSM-IV-TR). It is currently proposed that the diagnostic criteria for AD be revised so that the diagnosis can be made earlier and with greater specificity (Dubois et al, 2007). The new diagnostic procedures will combine imaging studies, biomarkers and evidence of memory deficits.

Treatment

Current medications do not cure AD, but may improve intellectual functioning and slow the progression of the disease (Complementary & Alternative Therapies 47–3). These include donepezil (Aricept), galantamine (Razadyne), memantine (Namenda), and rivastigmine (Exelon), which has recently been approved as a transdermal patch. A new drug tramiprosate (Alzehemed) is in clinical trials. Table 47–1 describes medications used to treat cognitive disorders and their nursing implications.

Box 47–2 *Diagnostic Criteria for Dementia (Alzheimer's Disease)*

The following diagnostic criteria should be used to determine dementia in a patient:

A. The patient has multiple cognitive deficits, including memory impairment (difficulty learning new or recalling old information) and one (or more) of the following:
   (a) Aphasia (language disturbance)
   (b) Apraxia (impaired motor ability)
   (c) Agnosia (failure to recognize objects)
   (d) Disturbance in activities such as planning, organizing, sequencing, or abstracting
B. The cognitive deficits cause impairment in social or occupational functioning and represent a decline from a previous level of functioning
C. Neurologic signs and symptoms (e.g., gait abnormalities)
D. The deficits do not occur exclusively during the course of a delirium

Adapted from American Psychiatric Association. (2000). *Diagnostic and Statistical Manual of Mental Disorders* (4th ed.). Text Revision. Washington, DC: American Psychiatric Association (p. 157).

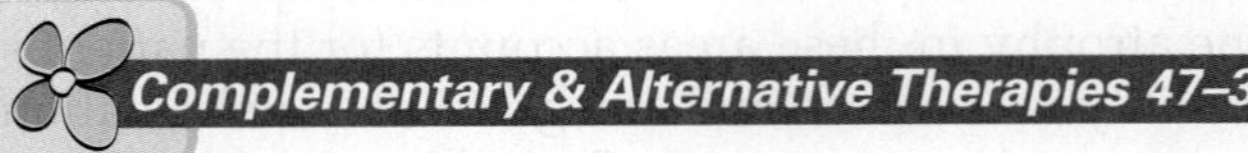

Complementary & Alternative Therapies 47–3

Ginkgo Biloba

In clinical trials, *Ginkgo biloba* has shown some modest, but inconsistent improvements in patients with AD, vascular dementia (VaD), and memory impairment. Common side effects include nausea, vomiting, diarrhea, headaches, and irritability. Advise the patient about possible drug-herb interactions if he is taking aspirin and NSAIDs.

Key: *AD,* Alzheimer's disease; *NSAIDs,* nonsteroidal anti-inflammatory drugs.

NURSING MANAGEMENT

Assessment (Data Collection)

You may be the first health care professional who encounters a patient who is in the early stages of AD. For example, the family may tell you, "We think Dad is experiencing some difficulties with daily tasks, and we also think he is attempting to hide his forgetfulness." Ask the patient and the family questions about memory, ability to perform activities of daily living (ADLs), and any subtle changes in personality. Give specific common examples (e.g., "Does he forget to turn off the stove or to lock the doors?"). Refer this type of patient to the RN or physician because he needs an in-depth assessment and an extensive physical examination. Assessment should include the necessary data to plan measures to protect the patient.

Nursing Diagnosis and Planning

Nursing diagnoses are identified to maximize safety and to minimize complications due to loss of cognitive function. For example, risk for injury, impaired social interaction, wandering, confusion, self-care deficits,

Table 47–1 Medications Used to Treat Cognitive Disorders

CLASSIFICATION	ACTION	PATIENT EDUCATION	NURSING IMPLICATIONS
Donepezil (Aricept) Galantamine (Razadyne) Memantine (Namenda) Rivastigmine (Exelon) Transdermal patch has been recently approved	Causes elevated acetylcholine levels in the brain and slows progression of Alzheimer's disease symptoms (see Chapter 48 for discussion of neurotransmitters).	Take with food to decrease GI distress. Slows progression of symptoms, but is not a cure. Take frequent drinks of cool liquids or use sugarless gum or candy for dry mouth. Increase fiber and fluids to prevent constipation. Common side effects (nausea, vomiting, headaches and dizziness, GI bleeding, urinary frequency, anorexia) should be reported to physician.	Be alert for abdominal pain, fatigue, hypotension, and agitation. Monitor CBC, liver and renal function tests. Signs of overdose include severe nausea and vomiting, bradycardia, hypotension, convulsions, or severe muscle weakness. Rivastigmine patch: first patch should be applied on the day following the last oral dose, then rotate sites, replace every 24 hours.
Tacrine (Cognex)		Immediately report jaundice, nausea and vomiting, or malaise.	Used in the past, but is rarely prescribed now due to liver toxicity. If prescribed, liver function tests should be monitored weekly for 18 wk after starting the medication.
Nefiracetam (Translon) CX516 (Ampalex)			May improve memory; currently being researched.
Tramiprosate (Alzehemed)			Interferes with amyloid (abnormal protein combination) deposition

Key: *CBC,* complete blood count; *GI,* gastrointestinal.

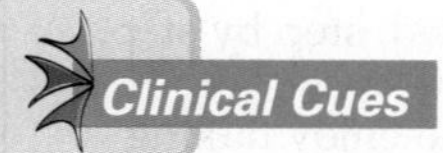

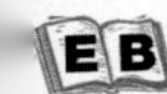

When caring for confused patients, evidenced-based practice supports the need for careful observation and documentation of patterns of behavior. This process, dementia care mapping, can be used to improve care (McEvoy, 2004). For example, you observe that your confused patient consistently tries to get out of bed on the right side, despite the fact that there is more room on the left. This suggests that the patient has an automatic habit of getting out on the right side; these data can now be used to adapt the room and increase patient safety.

and caregiver role strain are some of the diagnoses that are used for patients with AD.

Planning care for a patient with AD is based on the stage of the disease, and the family should be encouraged from the beginning to participate in developing the long-term goals. As the disease progresses, the patient will sustain losses in every area of function.

Implementation and Evaluation

Patients with AD need interventions that enhance memory. For example, put up holiday decorations that are appropriate to the season, or use photos of family and friends to help them reminisce. Although safety is a primary concern, restraints are rarely appropriate for these patients; creative interventions that are specific to the individual and family can ensure safety while preserving dignity. For example, one family placed a pleasant musical bell on the front door to prevent the confused elder from leaving the house undetected. Supporting the family will be a priority, particularly if the patient is being cared for at home. Help the family to have realistic expectations and refer them to respite care and support groups. Placing written name tags on commonly used household objects, such as the bathroom door or the patient's room door, seems to help the patient function better within the home setting. Visual cues such as the picture of the toilet on the bathroom door are helpful as the disease progresses.

AD patients may seem to require very infrequent evaluation, because the disease can progress very slowly and obvious changes in behavior or success in meeting goals may seem very gradual. However, vigilant evaluation will help you detect subtle changes in behavior that may signal delirium or progression of the disease. Also, any small successes can and should be shared with the family. Refer to Nursing Care Plan 47–1 for additional nursing management. Data are gathered regarding the success of the interventions in meeting the expected outcomes. If outcomes are not being met, the plan must be revised.

VASCULAR DEMENTIA

Vascular dementia was formerly known as multi-infarct dementia. It is the second most common type

NURSING CARE PLAN 47–1

Care of the Patient with Alzheimer's Disease

SCENARIO Mrs. Jane Best, an 85-year-old with Alzheimer's disease, lives with her daughter. The daughter works full time and occasionally leaves Mrs. Best at a senior citizen day care center where you are working. "Mom is confused and withdrawn most of the time and needs reminders to eat and coaching to go to the bathroom. I really try my best, but Mom can be difficult." The daughter appears tired, but is very patient with her mother. You observe Mrs. Best wandering alone and trying to go outside. You have to redirect her several times, and she mistakes you for her daughter.

PROBLEM/NURSING DIAGNOSIS *Intellectual and memory impairment*/Chronic confusion related to cognitive impairment.

Supporting assessment data *Subjective:* Per daughter, patient is "confused most of the time." *Objective:* Mistakes you for her daughter.

Goals/Expected Outcomes	Nursing Interventions	Selected Rationale	Evaluation
Patient will function at an optimal level for the degree of cognitive losses at this time	Identify yourself.	Patient may not recognize people previously introduced.	Patient repeatedly mistakes nurses for her daughter. Does recognize physician.
Patient will follow concrete instructions	Speak clearly and calmly and use short phrases and repeat as needed.	Facilitates communication.	Speaking slowly and clearly and repeating helps patient to understand.
	Face the patient directly when you talk.	Stimulation of two senses (visual and auditory) facilitates understanding.	Use of arrows to bathroom also appears helpful.
	Use pictures to communicate.		
	Be consistent in approach and assign the same staff and maintain daily structure and routine.	Familiar faces and repetitive patterns decrease confusion.	Patient functions best when A.M. routine is followed and primary nurse helps her.
	Break down all tasks into simple steps and encourage completion of one step at a time.	Single steps are less complex and easier to achieve.	This A.M. patient was able to brush own teeth if instructed, step by step.
	Encourage reminiscing about the past.	Remote memory is more likely to be intact than recent memory.	Appears to enjoy talking about "Maggie's cat." Outcomes met. Continue plan.

PROBLEM/NURSING DIAGNOSIS *Unable to independently perform ADLs*/Bathing/self-care/feeding deficit related to cognitive and perceptual impairment.

Supporting assessment data *Subjective:* Per daughter, "needs reminders to eat and coaching to go to the bathroom." *Objective:* Needs repetitive verbal prompting.

Goals/Expected Outcomes	Nursing Interventions	Selected Rationale	Evaluation
Patient will perform ADLs independently or with minimal assistance from caregivers	Assess the patient's ability to perform ADLs independently or with minimal assistance.	Provides baseline for daily planning (abilities may wax and wane).	Is able to physically perform most ADLs, but needs verbal coaching for each step.
	Encourage patient to maintain independence in performing ADLs.	Maximal independence should be maintained for as long as possible to increase self-esteem and stimulate mental processes.	Daughter reports that "it is really faster, just to do everything for her" but acknowledges the benefit of allowing her independence.
	Allow patient to wear own clothes.	Familiar objects decrease confusion.	Usually recognizes own clothing, but needs coaching for dressing; can manipulate Velcro fasteners.
	Use clothing with zippers and Velcro.	Ease of equipment decreases frustration.	
	Praise for any and all accomplishments.	Reinforces desired behavior.	Appears to enjoy interaction and feedback.

Key: *ADLs,* activities of daily living; *ID,* identification; *NA,* nursing assistant.

NURSING CARE PLAN 47–1

Care of the Patient with Alzheimer's Disease—cont'd

Goals/Expected Outcomes	Nursing Interventions	Selected Rationale	Evaluation
	Use simple, direct explanations when demonstrating the specific behavior you want the patient to complete.	Verbal and visual cues help to decrease confusion.	Follows instructions, but rarely asks for help.
	Maintain toileting schedule.	Bowel and bladder routine decreases incontinence.	Toileting schedule q 4 hr; patient usually continent.
	Encourage the use of finger foods.	Simplifies eating while maintaining intake.	Eats all food if encouraged. Has difficulty cutting meat with knife and fork. Outcomes met. Continue plan.

PROBLEM/NURSING DIAGNOSIS *Withdrawn*/Impaired social interaction related to anxiety and depression, apathy, and confused state.

Supporting assessment data *Subjective:* Per daughter, confused or withdrawn most of the time. *Objective:* Walking alone.

Goals/Expected Outcomes	Nursing Interventions	Selected Rationale	Evaluation
Patient will participate in group activities Patient will demonstrate socially acceptable behavior	Assess preferred patterns of social activity from earlier years.	Ideally, current socialization should mimic past patterns.	Social contact usually limited to family. Occasionally went to church.
	Provide group activities that are simple, such as singing or simple crafts.	Simple activities decrease frustration and are a vehicle to interaction.	Appears to enjoy movie night and musical groups.
	Stay with the patient during social activities as needed.	Provides support and reassurance.	Does not initiate conversation with others, but will respond if spoken to.
	Do not force a patient who is becoming agitated to participate in any social activity.	Socialization can be stressful, and forcing is counterproductive.	Readily agreed to go to all activities today.
	Gradually increase social interaction with other staff and patients.	Gradual exposure increases comfort level and familiarity.	Will sit with others, but does not initiate any interaction. Will speak to other patients if they speak to her.
	Reminisce rather than focus on events of the day.	Remote memory more likely to be intact than recent memory. Elder people frequently enjoy reminiscing as a social event. Gives clues to what can stimulate their interest.	Smiles and looks happy when making references to "Maggie's cat." Outcomes met. Continue plan.

PROBLEM/NURSING DIAGNOSIS *Daughter is the primary caregiver*/Risk for caregiver role strain, related to high emotional and physical demands, safety concerns for the relative, and caregiver isolation.

Supporting assessment data *Subjective:* "I really try my best, but Mom can be difficult." *Objective:* Daughter works full time and appears tired, but very patient with her mother.

Goals/Expected Outcomes	Nursing Interventions	Selected Rationale	Evaluation
Caregiver will verbalize ways to perform the caregiver role without becoming exhausted	Assess caregiver's ability to meet the needs of the patient.	Baseline for planning.	Daughter expresses willingness to care for her mother, but does work full time.
Caregiver will openly express feelings	Actively listen to caregiver's fears and concerns.	Allowing expression helps to build trust and rapport, also helps speaker and listener to clarify issues.	Fears for mother's safety; is concerned about wandering.

Continued

NURSING CARE PLAN 47–1

Care of the Patient with Alzheimer's Disease—cont'd

Goals/Expected Outcomes	Nursing Interventions	Selected Rationale	Evaluation
	Educate the caregiver about cognitive disorders and the patient's specific cognitive deficits.	Accurate information allows daughter to have realistic expectations.	Written information given and discussion of cognitive disorders provided for daughter.
	Help caregivers be realistic about the prognosis for their loved one.	Being realistic about prognosis helps the family to begin the process of anticipatory grieving.	Daughter appears unsure about the future, knows that her mother is going to get worse.
	Make caregiver aware of community resources such as respite care.	Community supports are available to provide care, education, support, and advice.	Referred to support group for caregivers of Alzheimer's disease patients.
	Encourage participation in support groups.	Sharing with people who are experiencing similar problems decreases feelings of alienation and allows sharing of information.	
	Support caregiver in taking steps to maintain own health.	Daughter must be healthy in order to continue supporting her mother.	Daughter discussed respite care and plans to take occasional breaks. Continue plan.

PROBLEM/NURSING DIAGNOSIS *Unfamiliar environment*/Wandering related to cognitive impairment and loss of judgment.

Supporting assessment data *Subjective:* Per daughter, "Mom is confused." *Objective:* Wandering by herself and trying to get outside despite repetitive redirection.

Goals/Expected Outcomes	Nursing Interventions	Selected Rationale	Evaluation
Patient will remain within the boundaries of the center (or the family property) unless accompanied by others	Place in a limited-access unit. Put complex locks on the doors. Allow access to fenced yard.	Securing the environment allows the patient to roam safely, but without restraints.	Patient remained safe in secure unit. Went out to grounds with NA in the A.M.
	Use identification bracelets or sew ID labels on clothes.	ID methods facilitate location and return if she does get lost.	Discussed sewing labels into clothes with daughter.
	Label all rooms and doors.	Patient may be wandering because she can't find the bathroom, bedroom, etc.	Arrows to bathroom appear especially useful.
	Remove visual cues that trigger wandering (e.g., car keys, coat).	Visual cues such as car keys can trigger a past familiar behavior (e.g., driving to work).	Asked for coat, was reassured that it was in the storage closet.
	Notify police and neighbors to be on the alert.	Police and neighbors can quickly contact caregiver.	Discussed with daughter about notifying neighbors and police. Outcomes met. Continue plan.

? CRITICAL THINKING QUESTIONS

1. How would you react if Mrs. Best's daughter complains about the care that Mrs. Best is receiving at the senior center?
2. What interventions could you initiate to protect patients like Mrs. Best from physical injury related to confusion?

Cultural Cues 47–1

Race Factors

African Americans have a 14% to 100% greater risk for AD than do whites. African Americans are also at greater risk for developing VD compared to whites. Patients with risk factors for VD, such as hypertension and diabetes, should be identified and educated to optimize healthy lifestyle practices.

Key: *AD*, Alzheimer's disease; *VaD*, vascular dementia.

of chronic cognitive disorder. *Vascular dementia* is a broad term used to describe any type of dementia caused by vessel disease. People who are predisposed to this type of dementia have a history of hypertension, hyperlipidemia, diabetes mellitus, and abuse of nicotine and alcohol (Cultural Cues 47–1).

Any type of vessel disease in the brain will cause brain damage. Lack of oxygen to the brain tissue because of *mini-strokes* (clots or hemorrhage) can cause death of brain tissue in a short time. The parts of the brain originally affected by cell death will be permanently damaged.

The onset can be gradual or abrupt, and the neurologic impairment is localized rather than global. The progression of symptoms is more rapid than in AD. Neurologic deficits are present in whatever part of the brain has been destroyed. Prompt treatment of hypertension and vascular disease is necessary to prevent long-term complications.

AIDS DEMENTIA COMPLEX

AIDS dementia complex (ADC) is caused by infection with human immunodeficiency virus (HIV). The central nervous system can be affected, and the patient may also have *peripheral neuropathy* (disturbance in the function of peripheral nerves that results in numbness or muscle weakness). ADC affects cognition, behavior, mood, and motor ability. There is great variability in the manifestation of symptoms. In the beginning, symptoms can be easily mistaken for depression: apathy, loss of interest, difficulty concentrating and slowed thinking, and irritablity. Early symptoms may also include unsteady gait and poor hand coordination for things such as writing. In the later stages, the patient can develop bowel and bladder incontinence, confinement to bed, and psychosis or mania. ADC is diagnosed by computed tomography or MRI, spinal tap, and a mental status examination. Treatment includes anti-HIV drugs, and symptoms are treated with antidepressants, antipsychotics, and anxiolytics.

NURSING MANAGEMENT

Assessment (Data Collection)

On admission, an extensive mental status examination should be conducted by the physician and the RN to obtain a baseline for the patient's thought content, intellectual functioning, mood, affect, and judgment. After the baseline is established, the Mini-Mental Status Exam (MMSE) can be used for ongoing assessment. The MMSE is a popular shortened version of the mental status examination that was developed by Folstein et al. in 1975. It can be used for patients who have cognitive disorders or thought disorders to assess orientation, memory, and ability to follow commands. It consists of 11 easily scored items and should take about 5 to 10 minutes to administer. Examples of items would include "What day is it? What city is this? What am I holding? (common objects such as a pen, or paper clip would be displayed).

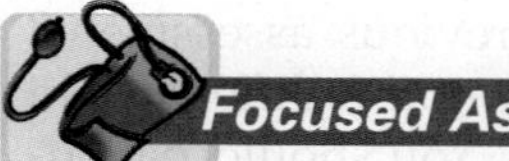

Focused Assessment 47–1

Quick Assessment Guide for Delirium and Dementia

Use the mnemonic JAMCO (Judgment, Affect, Memory, Cognition, Orientation).

JUDGMENT
- Does patient have insight into his behavior? Is the patient aware of danger or safety issues?

AFFECT
- Is affect blunt, flat, inappropriate, suddenly changed, or variable?

MEMORY
- Is memory intact? Does the patient have remote memory, but not recent or immediate? Is memory better during the day?

COGNITION
- Is the patient able to process abstract thoughts? Are thoughts fragmented or disorganized?
- Does the patient make up answers to questions *(confabulate)* to hide deficits?

ORIENTATION
- Is the patient oriented to person, place, and time?
- Does the patient recognize family and friends?

Differentiating between delirium and dementia is often difficult for the nurse because the patient is not a reliable historian. A mood disorder, such as depression, may also further complicate the picture. (For a review of the symptoms of depression, see Chapter 45.) Accurate recognition of these three conditions requires excellent assessment skills. An effective way to assess whether a patient has delirium or dementia is to note function in the following five areas: **judgment, affect, memory, cognition, and orientation (JAMCO)** (Focused Assessment 47–1). First, what is the status of the patient's *judgment?* Your patient insists on driving, despite the fact that he has had several minor accidents within the past 2 weeks. This connotes poor judgment, and you must work with the patient and the family to seek alternative transportation.

Assessing and documenting *affect* (emotional or feeling tone) are also important. Has there been a sudden change in mood from the previous assessment? The family will often say that they note a difference in mood when they visit the patient. You should pay attention to what family members tell you and elicit their opinions about the changes that they are seeing in their loved one.

Clinical Cues

Mood and affect are frequently assessed simultaneously. Mood is the current state of emotion that a person is experiencing. Affect is the demonstration of emotion, usually by facial expression and body position. Ordinarily, we expect affect and mood to match, so when we are in a "good mood" we would display a cheerful affect. Likewise, depressed people often display a flat or sad affect. In a flat affect, the face is devoid of expression and the patient may appear to have little or no energy for interaction. A sad affect is usually apparent, and the patient may cry, frown, or have a worried, preoccupied expression.

When assessing *memory,* it is important to note recent and remote memory. In some types of dementia, a patient may not be able to remember what was on the breakfast tray, but may be able to talk at great length about events in his younger years. When assessing delirium, you may find that both recent memory (a few hours before) and immediate memory (a few minutes before) are absent.

Think Critically About . . . Think of one or two ways you can assess immediate, recent, and remote memory. How would you know whether the patient's memory is accurate?

Cognition is the ability to abstract and process information. Obviously, there are links and overlaps to memory and perception when assessing cognition. The family should also be consulted whenever possible for valuable baseline information about the patient's past performance. For example, a patient's son tells you, "My mother was a former math teacher; now she cannot seem to balance her checkbook, and that was something that she could easily do in the past."

Finally, is the patient *oriented* to person, place, and time? Are there times when the patient is disoriented? It is not unusual for a patient to be completely oriented during the daytime hours and become confused and disoriented at night. This phenomenon is known as **sundowning** and needs to be documented (Complementary & Alternative Therapies 47–4).

Think Critically About . . . What implications does sundowning have for planning care and activities for the patient?

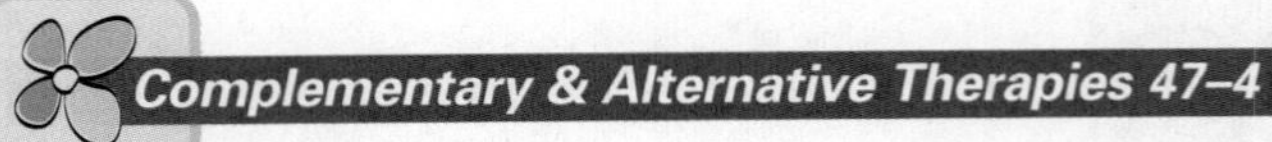

Complementary & Alternative Therapies 47–4

Agitated Patient

Music, recordings of soft ocean sounds, light touch or hand massage (avoid touching if the patient is violent or angry), or aromatherapy may help to calm an agitated patient with sundown syndrome. Having your patient sit by a light box in the early morning may also help, particularly if the patient has depression.

A mental status assessment needs to be completed at least once per shift, so that any change can be detected promptly and appropriate interventions taken. This assessment should include orientation to person, place, and time and the other elements of JAMCO. The MMSE can be used at the nurse's discretion to validate mental status changes or according to the agency's policy for long-term care patients. When abrupt changes are noted, the RN and the physician should be notified to perform more detailed assessments.

In cases of delirium or acute confusion, you must assess the patient's medication history, look for any signs of infection, and assess current fluid and electrolyte status. Also, if you have reason to suspect that the patient may have sustained a fall, assess for head trauma.

Nursing Diagnosis

Nursing diagnoses for patients with cognitive disorders include, but are not limited to:

- Acute confusion related to delirium induced by infection
- Chronic confusion related to slow progressive memory loss
- Disturbed thought processes related to biochemical changes in the brain
- Impaired social interaction related to inability to recognize friends and family
- Self-care deficits, bathing/hygiene/eating related to decreased psychomotor abilities
- Risk for injury related to faulty judgment
- Sleep deprivation related to age-related sleep pattern changes
- Disturbed sensory perception related to hallucinations
- Wandering related to disorientation to time and place
- Risk for caregiver role strain related to prolonged 24-hour responsibility of caregiving

Planning

Expected outcomes are written for the specific individual nursing diagnoses chosen to resolve the patient's problems. For the nursing diagnoses above, they might include:

Clinical Cues

When assisting elderly and confused patients to eat, slowly give one bite of an item, allow adequate time for chewing and swallowing, and then give another bite of a different food item. This varies the taste and texture and enhances the enjoyment of eating. Also remember to include some time for socialization.

- Patient will demonstrate orientation to person, place, and time within 24 to 48 hours after starting antibiotic therapy.
- Patient will recognize self and primary caregiver (e.g., daughter) during hospital stay.
- Patient will remain calm and follow simple instructions during this shift.
- Patient will interact with family and friends during weekly visits.
- Patient will perform ADLs with assistance as needed during this shift.
- Patient will be safe and free from harm during this shift.
- Patient will rest and sleep for at least 6 hours every 24-hour period.
- Patient will decrease behaviors that suggest hallucinations (e.g., listening to voices) within 1 week.
- Patient will remain on unit or within fenced grounds during this shift.
- Family will identify signs and symptoms of caregiver role strain during counseling session at the end of the week.

In accordance with 2008 National Patient Safety Goals, nurses must identify patients that have safety risks; this includes patients with cognitive disorders. Planning care for a patient with delirium involves accurately assessing the acute condition, stabilizing the patient, reducing environmental stimuli, providing reality orientation, and assisting the physician in determining the cause. Planning care for a patient with dementia frequently involves the caregivers and should be done with long-term goals in mind. Patients in the early stages of AD may be experiencing difficulties with ADLs; however, they may attempt to hide their condition. Forgetting to turn off the stove or to lock the doors is not uncommon. Regardless of the cause, the loss of cognition is devastating, and it is important to maintain the patient's dignity, provide for safety and optimal level of functioning, and promote quality of life.

Implementation

Interventions to provide safety and minimize anxiety for patients with dementia and delirium are similar. **However, when caring for a patient whose sudden change in behavior may be due to delirium, time is of the essence.** Assess the patient frequently, document your findings, and be certain the physician is notified. Because the level of consciousness may be

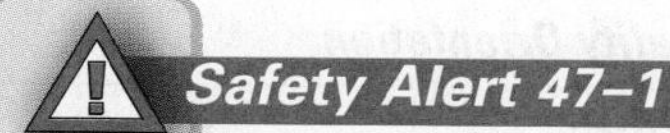
Safety Alert 47–1

Antipsychotic Drugs

Nurses should be aware that atypical antipsychotics such as olanzapine (Zyprexa) and risperidone (Risperdal) are approved for use in schizophrenia, but are not approved for use with older patients who display behavioral changes related to dementia. Clinical trials showed an increased risk of death in this population with use of these drugs.

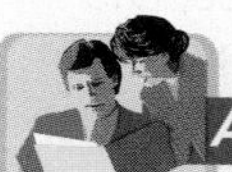
Assignment Considerations 47–1

Reality Orientation

Nursing assistants (NAs) can be instrumental in the ongoing orientation of confused patients. First, identify those patients who would benefit from reality orientation. Then give the NA specific instructions about how to orient to person, place, and time (e.g., "Hi, Mrs. Collins. I am Judy, the nursing assistant at Sunshine Care Center. It is 8 A.M. on Wednesday, June 28, 2008. It's a nice warm summer day today."). Instruct the NA in how to use visual cues to orient patients (e.g., "Mrs. Collins, this calendar will help you remember the day, month, and year.").

clouded, reduce distractions in the environment. For example, research shows that having the television on creates background noise that increases confusion. It may be necessary to medicate patients with anxiolytics if their anxiety is great, or with antipsychotics if the misinterpretation of the environment causes them to be aggressive (Safety Alert 47–1). Patients may be able to remember their own name, but may be confused about place and time. A patient who is experiencing acute confusion or delirium will benefit from repeated orientation to person, place, and time (Assignment Considerations 47–1). It is not adequate to repeat this information once or twice. It must be repeated frequently and in a calm, soothing manner.

Your calm attitude is very important in reducing the anxiety that is inevitably present for the patient. Box 47–3 lists guidelines to conduct reality orientation for confused patients.

A patient experiencing acute confusion may become combative, or may attempt to crawl out of bed or remove therapeutic equipment. In 1992, the Food and Drug Administration issued a warning stating that restraints should no longer be considered as first-line management of a patient's behavioral problems (Legal & Ethical Considerations 47–1). When using restraints, your patients may be at risk for physical problems such as immobility, strangulation, or asphyxiation, or for psychological issues such as anger, humiliation, loss of autonomy, and decreased functioning. In fact, evidenced-based practice suggests that use of side rails may actually increase the risk for injury because patients attempt to go around or climb over the perceived

Box 47–3 Guidelines for Reality Orientation

WHAT IS REALITY ORIENTATION?

- Reality orientation is a therapeutic program implemented **consistently** by all nursing staff to orient a patient to person, place, and time. This method includes the use of verbal communication techniques, as well as written signs indicating the current date, month, or room identification. Clocks with large letters are included to help the patient know the correct time.
- Special group sessions are also used to orient patients. These sessions focus on person, place, and time as well as certain holiday events. These groups improve orientation and provide opportunities for social interaction.

WHEN TO USE REALITY ORIENTATION

- The use of reality orientation is appropriate when a patient is experiencing acute confusion or delirium. A sudden episode of confusion is very frightening, and orienting the patient is a way to allay fear and anxiety.
- Patients experiencing dementia or chronic confusion often have global amnesia and do not benefit from repeated verbal reality orientation. Gentle reminders of the day or time are helpful, but need to be repeated often and without the expectation that the patient will remember something that was said 5 minutes ago.
- All aspects of reality orientation are helpful for all patients with cognitive disorders. However, in patients experiencing acute confusion, the ultimate expectation is that the patient will become completely oriented and return to a previous level of functioning. With chronic confusion, the goal is to preserve dignity and maintain optimum function.

EXAMPLES OF WAYS TO IMPLEMENT REALITY ORIENTATION AND REDUCE CONFUSION

- Under no circumstances should nurses ever chastise or become frustrated when a patient cannot remember. This has no therapeutic value.
- Verbalize to patients in a consistent and caring manner who you are, where they are, and the date and time: "Hi, Mr. Jones. I am your nurse, Betty, at the Davis Nursing Care Center. It is 8 A.M. on Wednesday, October 25, and it is time for breakfast."
- Look directly at the patient when you are speaking.
- Ask only one question at a time.
- Ask questions that can be answered with a "yes" or "no": "Would you like to eat in the dining room?"
- Eliminate environmental distractions when talking to a patient.
- Break down tasks such as dressing into simple one-step tasks.
- Ask the patient to do only one task at a time.
- Gently touch the patient to convey acceptance.
- If possible, provide caregivers who are familiar to the patient.
- Provide general orientation to the calendar year by using holiday decorations.
- Decrease the noise level in the environment by avoiding paging systems and call lights that ring or buzz.
- Label photos of people familiar to the patient with the names of the people who are in the photos.
- Limit visitors to one or two at a time.
- Place the patient's name in large block letters in his room and on clothing.
- Use symbols rather than words on signs indicating location of dining room or bathroom.
- When misperceptions are present, clarify them for the patient: "No Mr. Jones, I am not your daughter; I am your nurse, Betty. Your daughter will be here after you eat your lunch."
- When special low-stimulus units designed for patients with chronic confusion are not available, use yellow tape to mark specific boundaries for the patient.
- Give frequent reassurances.
- Keep the patient's room well lit.
- Encourage the use of hearing aids and prescription glasses.
- Have clocks, calendars, and personal items in clear view of the patient.
- Encourage reminiscing about happy times in life.

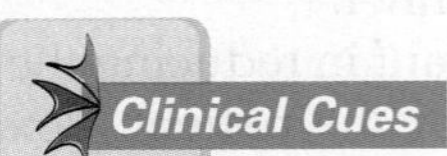

An inappropriately placed mirror can be a source of overstimulation when your patient is agitated and confused. It is startling and upsetting for the patient to glance over and see a scared and anxious person looking back at him!

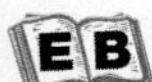

barrier (Capezuti, 2004). It is recommended that institutions have policies and procedures that address the safe and legal use of restraints. Box 47–4 presents guidelines on the use of restraints and alternatives to restraints. (Legal & Ethical Considerations 47–2).

An individual with chronic confusion in the late stages of dementia will not benefit from repetitive information. If **global amnesia** (generalized loss of memory) is present, the patient will not be able to remember family, friends, or events, regardless of how

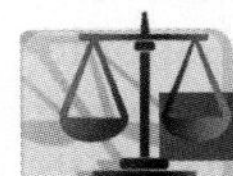

Legal & Ethical Considerations 47–1

Use of Restraints

Remember, having to restrain a patient is considered an unusual circumstance that requires clear documentation and adequate elaboration as to the events leading to the need for restraints, all alternatives tried before restraint, the type of restraint, strict accounting for time in and out of restraints, and the care given to the patient while in restraints. (Don't forget to offer and document bathroom breaks, fluid and food, and skin care!)

many times you repeat the information. Moreover, expecting the patient to remember leads to frustration for you and the patient. Use of pictures or symbols, such as arrows pointing to the bathroom, can facilitate daily tasks and clarify communication. In addition,

Box 47–4 Alternatives and Guidelines for the Use of Restraints

ALTERNATIVES TO RESTRAINTS

Acute Care Settings

- Encourage family members and friends to stay with the patient.
- Assign a nurse or nursing assistant for one-on-one observation.
- Encourage oral feedings instead of intravenous or nasogastric feedings. (Avoid inserting tubes that can be pulled out.)
- Remove catheters and drains as soon as possible.
- Decrease glaring lighting, reduce noise, and minimize stimulation.
- Keep the patient close to the nurse's station.
- Be certain the call button is within easy reach.
- Place the bed in the lowest setting, and use three side rails to keep the patient from rolling out.
- Check on the patient frequently to offer nutrition, fluids, pain relief, and toileting assistance as appropriate.

Long-Term Care Facilities

- Place the mattress on the floor to prevent the patient from falling out of bed.
- Talk to the patient, even when the patient is not responding to you or is responding in an inappropriate way.
- Incorporate relaxation techniques into the care plan, such as back massage and hydrotherapy.
- Use therapeutic communication techniques to encourage the patient to verbalize feelings.
- Encourage ambulation whenever feasible.
- Encourage participation in recreational, physical, and occupational therapy.
- Encourage participation in as many ADLs as possible.
- Initiate diversional activities, such as listening to radio, television, and music.
- Maintain a schedule for toileting.

GUIDELINES FOR THE SAFE USE OF RESTRAINTS

- Use the least restrictive type of restraint that will accomplish the objective.
- Obtain informed consent from the patient or the patient's relatives before using restraints.
- Have an institutional policy on restraints written and available for the patient and family.
- Make certain that all staff have adequate in-service training on the use of restraints.
- Use hand mitts for patients who are receiving IV therapy or have catheters or nasogastric tubes.
- If hand mitts do not work, consider wrist restraints.
- All restraints must have a doctor's order.
- Restraints must not be used to punish or control the patient.
- Apply restraints snugly, but ensure that circulation is not impeded.
- Check the area distal to the restraint every 2 hours (or according to the agency policy) for circulation and function.
- Remove the restraints and change the patient's position at least every 2 hours.
- Apply active or passive ROM to the affected joints and muscles.
- Secure restraints to the bed frames, not the side rails.
- Tie restraints with knots that can be quickly released.
- Consider restraints as a temporary solution.
- Clearly document in the patient record the reason for the restraint, the type selected, and the time frame for use.
- Document care given to the patient while in restraints.

Key: *ADLs*, activities of daily living; *IV*, intravenous; *ROM*, range of motion.

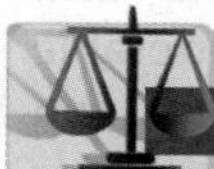

Legal & Ethical Considerations 47–2

Patient Charts

Many facilities have converted to computerized charting. Although computer entry can be quick and convenient, the format may be too restrictive to allow you to provide adequate detail. Chart defensively!

creative therapies such as video histories, use of familiar songs, and pet and aroma therapy may enrich the quality of life for these individuals (Complementary & Alternative Therapies 47–5 and 47–6).

Think Critically About . . . Is it always necessary to encourage a patient to see and acknowledge reality? What about elderly patients who have severe dementia and believe they are living in their own homes, even though they are in a nursing home?

Nurses who care for patients with dementia need to be aware of the importance of maintaining the dignity of the patient and family. In the later stages of dementia, there are numerous deficits in self-care, such as grooming and toileting. It is very important to treat both patients and families with respect. **Call the patient by name, provide for privacy, and individualize your care for this patient based on culture and history.** It is well documented in the nursing literature that when patients are seen as people or human beings, nurses are likely to be more compassionate and caring.

Elder Care Points

When working with the elderly, do not confuse clear and supportive communication with "elderspeak." Elderspeak is a style of speech that includes baby talk, exaggerated tones and slow speed, elevated pitch and volume, and simplified vocabulary. Being overly nurturing ("Come on, sweetie, let's eat now.") or overly controlling ("Sit down and finish your food!") is perceived as patronizing and demeaning without improving communication.

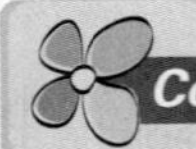

Complementary & Alternative Therapies 47–5

Smell

The limbic or "old brain" is associated with the sense of smell. Use of familiar smells reinforces remote memories. For example, the smell of pine or fir can trigger past memories of happy Christmas times spent with family and friends.

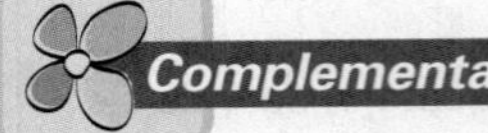

Complementary & Alternative Therapies 47–6

Massage

Massage has been used to reduce the agitation in Alzheimer's disease patients. Additional benefits include meeting the human need for nurturing touch, decreasing mild depression, reducing mental stress, improving circulation, and relieving muscle tension and stiffness.

Nursing Assessment and Interventions for the Family

The family should be assessed for knowledge deficit related to the illness and care of the family member with dementia. For example, if the patient lives at home, the family will need to realize that **a person with dementia responds much better if there are daily routines and a structured environment.** Assist them to develop a schedule that includes adequate time for hygiene care, meals, medications, and activities such as walking. Home care nurses are in an excellent position to make suggestions to help the family create a safe environment. For example, potentially hazardous areas can be evaluated and then suggestions made for gates across stairwells, or better lighting in dark hallways.

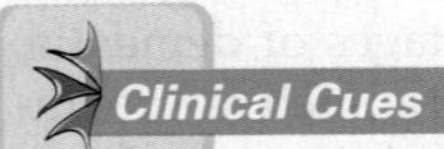

Clinical Cues

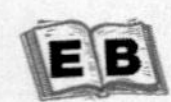

Evidence-based practice suggests that structured activities, such as "Simple Pleasures" (Buettner et al.,1996) benefits patients and families. In this classic intervention, family members or volunteers are asked to make items such as fleece-covered hot water bottles. Handling the handmade item reduces agitation in the patient with dementia. The family sees the impact of the gift and the family-patient interaction is improved.

If the patient has a tendency to wander or get lost, the family will live in a constant state of hypervigilance to ensure the safety of their loved one. Help family members to recognize potential wandering behaviors: looking for keys and preparing to go to "work," restlessness and pacing, getting lost going to the bathroom or the bedroom, or performing a task without actually accomplishing anything (e.g., moves dirty dishes from place to place without actually washing them). Nurses can make practical suggestions such as sewing identification labels into clothing, or using a bell that signals when an exit door is opened. Box 47–5 presents additional tips for families.

Families should also be assessed for signs of caregiver role strain. Observe and assist family members to recognize that when they are personally experiencing denial, irritability, anxiety, sleeplessness, and anger, these are signs that the illness of the elder is taking its toll on the caregivers. Family members often are exhausted from the daily requirements of round-the-clock care. Evidence-based practice (Talerico, 2005) suggests that families who receive intensive support and counseling are able to manage the care of the AD patient in the home for longer periods of time. Encourage caregivers to consider day care or respite care. These options give the family members a much-needed psychological and physical rest. In addition, families should be encouraged to use support groups. Refer families to local chapters of the Alzheimer's Association for assistance (www.alz.org or 1-800-272-3900).

? *Think Critically About . . .* How would you help a family member to recognize and acknowledge the need for respite care?

Families also need to be encouraged to talk openly and frankly about quality of life, and end-of life issues such as advance directives. Preferably these talks should be completed before the diagnosis of dementia, when the patient still has cognitive functioning. If not, the family caregiver becomes the spokesperson and needs to be encouraged to get a power of attorney and a living will for the patient. Families need considerable support in these matters. **Observing someone you love deteriorate neurologically is very difficult.** Refer to Nursing Care Plan 47–1 for additional nursing management information.

Evaluation

Evaluating the care for a patient with cognitive disorders is accomplished by determining whether the expected outcomes were met. Because confusion is present in all cognitive disorders, keeping the patient free of injury is of primary importance. Returning the patient to a previous level of cognitive and psychomotor functioning whenever possible is essential. Eliminating or determining the cause of acute delirium is a main priority for the health care team during the assessment process. An additional expected outcome, particularly with patients with dementia, is that the family will be able to verbalize the stages of illness and maintain realistic expectations for their loved one.

Box 47–5 Suggestions for Families Caring for a Person with Alzheimer's Disease

- Make and keep a copy of the daily schedule, and stick to the schedule as closely as possible.
- Establish bedtime rituals.
- Orient the person as necessary to maintain safety and promote maximum functioning.
- Avoid multiple caregivers.
- Simplify the environment to minimize illusions and confusion; keep decorative items to a minimum.
- Keep the environment as quiet as possible.
- Schedule rest breaks throughout the day for yourself and your loved one.
- Change your expectations; forcing thought and interaction causes frustration.
- Offer the person help when needed, and distraction as necessary.
- Always supervise the use of medications.
- Use sense of touch; there is an increased need for touch.
- Always approach the person from the front before touching.
- Use distraction if agitated. Walking, gardening, rocking in a rocking chair, sanding wood, and folding laundry are good examples of distraction.
- Use many of the safeguards for young children, such as storing all cleaning solutions, pesticides, medications, and nonedible items in locked cabinets.
- Put protective caps on all unused electrical outlets.
- Remove all sharp objects.
- Remove all throw rugs, and keep hallways and stairs free of clutter.
- Keep the house well lit.
- Allow smoking only under very close supervision.
- Attach safety grab bars in the bathroom.
- Protect windows and doors with Plexiglas.
- Rather than restrict the person from wandering, provide a safe area in which to wander. For example, gates could be installed in a fenced backyard.

COMMUNITY CARE

If patients with dementia or delirium are hospitalized, the inpatient stay will typically be for a short time. For a variety of reasons, financial and personal, many families are choosing to keep their elders at home. Nurses who make home visits will often encounter families attempting to care for a relative who is experiencing either of these conditions. Teaching must be done about the causes and stages of these illnesses. In addition, families are eager for practical knowledge that will make the living arrangement more acceptable. Box 47–5 includes some tips for caring for a patient with dementia at home.

In the later stages of dementia, nursing home placement sometimes is necessary. Many nursing homes have special units set aside for AD patients. In these units, safety precautions are a primary concern. Entrance and exit doors have special codes so that patients cannot wander off the unit. Nurses in these units spend considerable time educating families about the stages of AD and helping families with the inevitable grieving process.

In addition to observing patients with delirium in the acute hospital setting, nurses often interact with these patients in outpatient clinics, emergency rooms, or physician's offices. Excellent assessment skills are necessary to prevent any further decline. In accordance with the *Healthy People 2010* goals, nurses should be actively screening and identifying older adults who are at risk for mental health crisis, in order to make appropriate referrals for treatment or services.

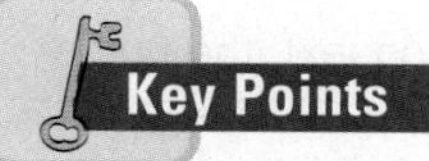

Key Points

- Cognition includes the mental processes of perception, memory, judgment, and reasoning.
- Delirium is acute confusion; signs and symptoms may include a shortened attention span, disorientation, impairment in recent and remote memory, incoherent speech, disorganized thinking, and possible presence of delusions, hallucinations, and illusions.
- Dementia is chronic confusion that has slow onset (months to years); signs and symptoms include impairments in memory, poverty of thoughts, difficulties with abstract thoughts and judgments, confabulation, and changes in personality. In later stages, global amnesia is present. Attention span and alertness are normal, and there are usually no hallucinations, delusions, or illusions.
- Assess *j*udgment, *a*ffect, *m*emory, *c*ognition, and *o*rientation (JAMCO). **Judgment** is the presence of judgment and insight. **Affect** is the demonstration of emotion, and is usually apparent in facial expression or body position. (Mood is the current state of emotion that a person is experiencing.) **Memory** is assessed for impairments in recent, remote, and immediate memory. **Cognition** is the ability to abstract and process information. **Orientation** to person, place, and time should be assessed.
- Alzheimer's disease is the most common degenerative disease of the brain and usually affects people over the age of 65.
- Vascular dementia describes any type of dementia caused by vessel disease, which causes brain damage. Onset is usually more abrupt, and neurologic impairment is localized rather than global.
- Goals of treatment for cognitive disorders include achieving an optimal level of functioning, ensuring safety, educating caregivers, and preserving the dignity of the patient and family.
- Nursing interventions depend on the stage of illness. General interventions include maintaining a calm and soothing manner, ensuring environmental safety, using appropriate reality orientation, and monitoring the effects of medications.

- Elders are sensitive to the cumulative effects of medications because of decreased metabolic and liver function.
- Elders should be prescribed the smallest amount of medication possible, and doses should be increased only when symptoms indicate the need.
- Families are frequently electing to care for their elders at home; teach the family about cognitive disorders and provide practical knowledge about living arrangements.

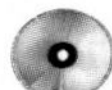
Go to your **Companion CD-ROM** for an Audio Glossary, animations, video clips, and bonus review questions.

evolve Be sure to visit the companion Evolve site at http://evolve.elsevier.com/deWit for interactive NCLEX-PN Exam Style Review Questions, WebLinks, and additional online resources.

NCLEX EXAM STYLE REVIEW QUESTIONS

Choose the best answer(s) for the following questions:

1. If a patient is prescribed tacrine (Cognex), the nurse should advise the patient that weekly follow-ups for at least 18 weeks are needed because the medication can be:

1. hepatotoxic.
2. cardiotoxic.
3. nephrotoxic.
4. ototoxic.

2. A nursing student is caring for a patient who has Alzheimer's disease. Which of the following actions indicates that the student needs more education and training?

1. Uses season-appropriate holiday decorations and a calendar with large numbers
2. Labels family photos with names of family members and discusses photos with patient
3. Encourages the patient to acknowledge that he is not living in his own home
4. Helps the patient to perform one task at a time, giving step-by-step instructions

3. A patient with a tentative diagnosis of dementia is admitted with pneumonia. While obtaining the clinical history, the nurse observes that the patient is making up experiences to fill conversation gaps. The patient is demonstrating:

1. flight of ideas.
2. delusional thinking.
3. confabulation.
4. sundown syndrome.

4. An elderly man with dementia displays a sudden change in behavior with slurred speech and combativeness. He appears to be having hallucinations. What is the priority nursing diagnosis?

1. Disturbed thought processes
2. Disturbed sensory perception
3. Risk for injury
4. Chronic confusion

5. The nurse is caring for a confused patient in an acute medical-surgical unit. Which of the following alternatives to restraints would be appropriate for the patient and the setting?

1. Put the patient's mattress on the floor.
2. Keep the patient close to the nurse's station.
3. Put four side rails up instead of tying the patient down.
4. Use hand mitts and a soft vest with Velcro fasteners.

6. A confused elderly man is hospitalized for a recent fall. He is accompanied by his wife, who cries, "I can no longer take care of him!" Initial assessment confirms a nursing diagnosis of Caregiver role strain. Which nursing interventions would be appropriate? *(Select all that apply.)*

1. Encourage verbalization of feelings.
2. Refer to respite care or day care programs.
3. Tell the wife to calm down and maintain composure.
4. Reassure the wife that everything will be okay.
5. Offer to assist with admission to a nursing home.
6. Assess for alternative family support and resources.

7. Which of the following measures would reduce the sundowning phenomenon?

1. Install grab bars in the shower stalls and tub.
2. Remove throw rugs and clear walkways.
3. Orient the patient to the time of day at sundown.
4. Have the patient sit by a bright light in the morning.

8. The caregiver of a male patient with Alzheimer's disease is given instructions regarding donepezil (Aricept). Which of the following statements by the caregiver indicates a need for further instructions?

1. "The medication must be given with food."
2. "The medication eventually cures the disease."
3. "I must increase fiber and fluid in his diet."
4. "I need to provide frequent sips of cool liquids."

9. The nurse is assessing the dietary preferences of a patient with chronic confusion. Which assessment question would be the most appropriate to use with this patient?

1. "Do you have cultural preferences with regards to food?
2. "What would you usually eat during a typical day?"
3. "Do you prefer water or milk with your meals?"
4. "What did you think about the dinner that was served last night?"

10. The nurse observes that a patient with dementia cannot put on his shirt, although he has the strength and motor movement to dress himself. Which of the following interventions would be appropriate to accomplish dressing while maximizing the patient's dignity?
    1. Verbally coach the patient using simple directions.
    2. Leave the patient alone and give extra time and privacy.
    3. Have the wife help the patient to get dressed.
    4. Give the patient a shirt with Velcro fasteners.

CRITICAL THINKING ACTIVITIES

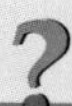

Read each clinical scenario and discuss the questions with your classmates.

Scenario A

Mrs. Oneida Lampert, 82 years old, has Alzheimer's disease. Her daughter tells you that Mrs. Lampert has "good days and bad days" but seems to be more forgetful and more withdrawn. "Do you have any suggestions for me? I know Mom is going to get worse, but I'd like to care for her at home as long as possible."

1. What are some questions you should ask the daughter?
2. What can you do to help the daughter with the practical issues of caring for Mrs. Lampert at home?

Scenario B

You are caring for Mr. Dixon, who is a 75-year-old patient residing in a nursing home for the past 6 months. Today he becomes uncharacteristically combative when the nurse's aide attempts to give him a bath. You have never observed Mr. Dixon exhibit this type of behavior before.

1. What would your initial nursing interventions be?
2. How might you explain Mr. Dixon's sudden change in behavior?

Scenario C

Jill Botello, a 40-year-old schoolteacher, accompanies her father, Sam Miller, to the physician's office where you are working. Mr. Miller, currently 65 years old, was diagnosed with vascular dementia 2 years ago. His condition is progressively deteriorating, and Ms. Botello tells you that she is fearful that this type of dementia could happen to her.

1. How would you respond to Ms. Botello?
2. What type of preventive education might be helpful for Ms. Botello?

CHAPTER

48 Care of Patients with Thought and Personality Disorders

evolve http://evolve.elsevier.com/deWit

Objectives

Upon completion of this chapter, you should be able to:

Theory

1. Discuss the incidence of thought disorders in the general population.
2. Describe the signs and symptoms of schizophrenia.
3. Discuss at least four nursing diagnoses and the major nursing interventions that would be appropriate for a patient with a thought disorder.
4. Describe two or three behaviors evident for each of the various personality disorders.
5. Discuss at least four nursing diagnoses and the major nursing interventions that would be appropriate for a patient with borderline personality disorder.
6. Discuss how the nurse can identify and modify personal feelings that can occur when caring for a patient with borderline personality disorder.

Clinical Practice

1. Watch the movie *A Beautiful Mind* and develop a teaching plan to help the wife understand the husband's bizarre and erratic behavior.
2. Develop a care plan with at least six nursing interventions for a patient who is paranoid and suspicious.
3. Develop a care plan with at least six nursing interventions for a patient who is manipulative.

Key Terms

Be sure to check out the bonus material on the Companion CD-ROM, including selected audio pronunciations.

akathisia (p. 1157)
alogia (p. 1156)
anhedonia (p. 1156)
atypical antipsychotics (ā-tĭ-pĭ-kăl ăn-tē-sī-KŎT-ĭks, p. 1158)
avolition (p. 1156)
borderline personality disorder (BŎR-dĕr-līn pĕr-sō-NĂL-ĭ-tē dĭs-ŎR-dĕr, p. 1165)
command hallucinations (KŎM-mănd hă-lū-sĭ-NĀ-shŭns, p. 1159)
conventional antipsychotics (kŏn-VĔN-shŭn-ăl ăn-tē-sī-KŎT-ĭks, p. 1156)
delusion (dĕ-LŪ-zhŭn, p. 1154)
dystonic reaction (dĭs-TŎN-ĭk rē-ĂK-shŭn, p. 1156)
hallucination (hă-lū-sĭ-NĀ-shŭn, p. 1154)
illusion (ĭ-LŪ-shŭn, p. 1155)
loose associations (p. 1161)
milieu therapy (mēl-yoo THĔR-ă-pē, p. 1167)
negative symptoms (NĔG-ă-tĭv, p. 1156)
neologisms (NĒ-ō-lō-jĭzm, p. 1161)
oculogyric crisis (p. 1156)
personality disorder (pĕr-sō-NĂL-ĭ-tē dĭs-ŎR-dĕr, p. 1165)
positive symptoms (p. 1155)
psychotherapy (sī-kō-THĔR-ă-pē, p. 1167)
psychotic features (sī-kŏ-tĭk, p. 1154)
schizophrenia (skĭt-sō-FRĒ-nē-ă, p. 1154)
splitting (p. 1166)
tardive dyskinesia (TĂR-dĭv dĭs-kĭ-NĒ-zē-ă, p. 1157)
thought disorder (p. 1154)
word salad (p. 1161)

OVERVIEW OF THOUGHT DISORDERS

The *Diagnostic and Statistical Manual of Mental Disorders,* fourth edition, text revision (DSM-IV-TR) defines **thought disorders** by the presence of psychotic symptoms. **Schizophrenia** is the most common thought disorder. **Examples of psychotic features are hallucinations (hearing, seeing, or feeling something that is not really there), delusions (false fixed ideas), and disorganized speech and/or behavior.**

The incidence of thought disorders is not as high as that of mood disorders, but they tend to be more chronic and debilitating. It is estimated that 1% of the general population is affected with schizophrenia, and in the United States this represents 2 million Americans. Other types of thought disorders are brief psychotic disorder, schizoaffective disorder, delusional disorder, shared psychotic disorder, psychotic disorder due to a medical condition, substance-induced psychotic disorder, and psychotic disorder not otherwise specified (NOS).

NEUROTRANSMITTERS

Neurotransmitters are chemical messengers that are produced and stored in the nerve terminal *(axon)* (Figure 48–1). An electrical impulse causes the release of the neurotransmitter, and it then moves into the gap *(synaptic cleft)* between the nerve endings and attaches to receptor sites on the receiving nerve cell *(dendrite)*. This causes a reaction in the dendrite, the receptor sites close, and the neurotransmitter travels back across the gap into storage *(reuptake)*.

Many of the medications used to treat mental disorders are thought to affect the activity (production,

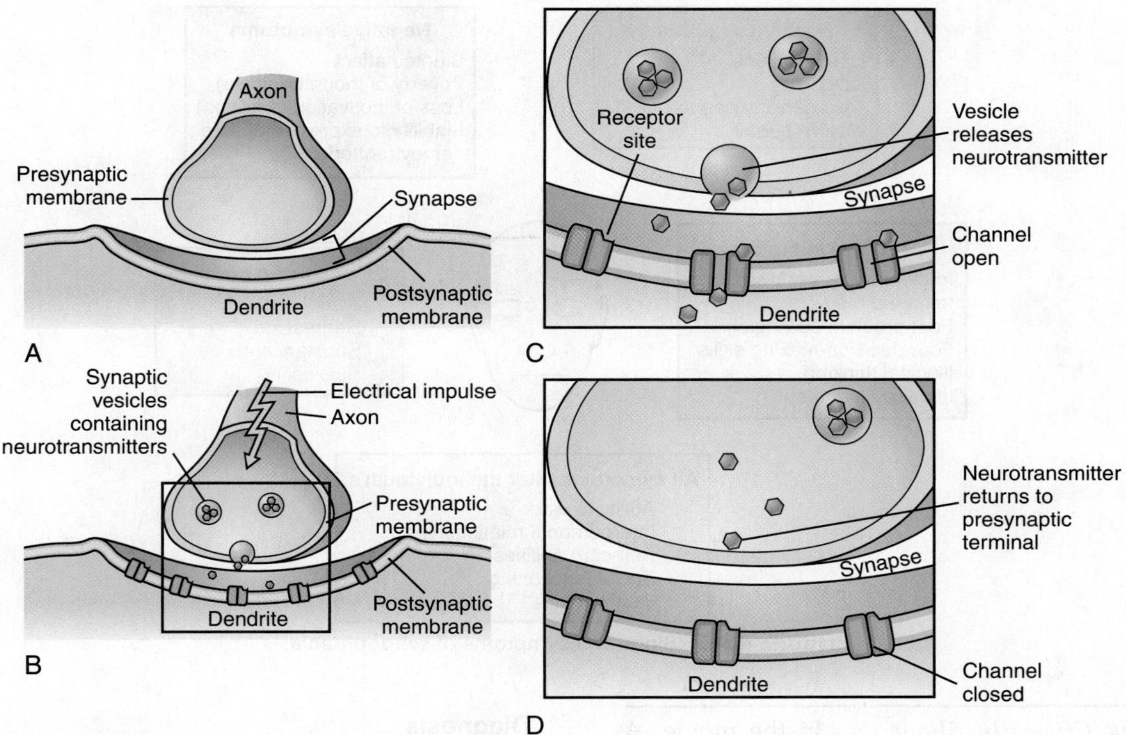

FIGURE **48–1** Neurotransmitters. **A,** Axon with stored neurotransmitters and dendrite with receptor sites. **B** and **C,** Electrical impulse causes release of neurotransmitter. **D,** Receptor sites close and neurotransmitter returns to storage.

release, destruction, or blocking [or reuptake] at the receptor site) of neurotransmitters. Serotonin is a neurotransmitter of the central nervous system. It is important in sleep, pain perception, and emotional states. Lack of serotonin can lead to depression. Norepinephrine and acetylcholine are neurotransmitters of the autonomic nervous system. Norepinephrine plays an important role in the *"fight or flight" reaction* (constriction of the blood vessels, dilation of the pupils, increased heart rate, increased awareness and vigilance). Acetylcholine causes decreased heart rate and force of contraction and plays a role in the sleep-wake cycle. Dopamine is located mostly in the brainstem. It is thought to play a role in controlling complex movements, motivation, and cognition. For patients with schizophrenia, it is thought that there is an imbalance of neurotransmission of dopamine and serotonin. Antipsychotic drugs work by blocking dopamine receptors.

SCHIZOPHRENIA

Etiology and Pathophysiology

The exact cause of schizophrenia is unknown; however, current research favors the theory that there is a neurobiologic basis with a genetic component. As with most chronic conditions, an unfavorable social environment contributes to a poor prognosis. Schizophrenia usually develops in late adolescence or the early 20s.

Signs and Symptoms

The signs and symptoms are divided into positive (present) and negative (absent) symptoms (Figure 48–2). **Positive symptoms** are **present** in schizophrenic patients, **but should not be there. These include the presence of hallucinations, delusions, and disordered thinking or loose associations between thoughts.** Voices *(auditory hallucinations)* will be telling the person what to do, and delusions develop as the disorder progresses.

Delusions can be either grandiose or persecutory. An individual who believes she is a queen is having *delusions of grandeur.* Individuals with *delusions of persecution* believe that they are being persecuted by agencies, other people, or supernatural beings. An **illusion** is a misinterpretation of something that really exists. For example, an electrical cord appears to be a snake, or a pencil is misinterpreted to be a knife blade. When *ideas of reference* occur, the individual believes that events or situations are occurring because of or specifically for her. A common idea of reference is to believe that people on the television are sending special telepathic messages. Positive symptoms are much more responsive to medication therapy compared to the negative symptoms; however, some patients will tell you that "the voices are always there, but if I take my medications the voices are less intrusive."

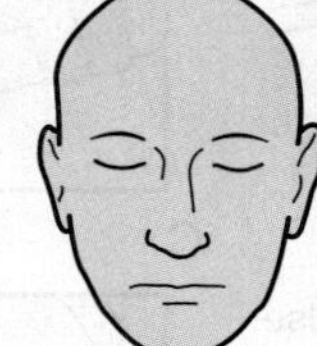

FIGURE **48–2** Signs and symptoms of schizophrenia.

? *Think Critically About . . .* In the movie, *A Beautiful Mind,* what are the early symptoms and behaviors that the main character displays? Later symptoms? Why might friends and family fail to recognize that there is a problem when schizophrenia first develops? Describe how you might feel, and how it would change your life, if someone you loved developed schizophrenia in early adulthood?

Negative symptoms are abilities or personal characteristics that are **absent** or lost to the patient. For example, think of elements of personality that make people motivated, socially outgoing, happy and active in daily life, and then take away those elements. The results are negative symptoms: **apathy, social isolation, psychomotor retardation, blunted affect, poverty of thoughts** (alogia), **lack of motivation** (avolition), **and inability to experience pleasure or joy** (anhedonia). These symptoms are notoriously more difficult to treat because the symptoms, in and of themselves, inhibit the individual from seeking help. Negative symptoms are also linked to acquisition of important social skills. For example, if your teenage patient withdraws because of feelings of persecution, she will miss the important socialization tasks that occur during adolescence, such as exploring identity and preparing to live independently away from her parents.

In addition, these patients also have cognitive impairments that manifest as difficulty with memory, judgment, problem solving, and decision making. Concurrent mental health problems such as anxiety and depression can also occur. Overall there is an impact on the individual's quality of life, and some will have great difficulty functioning in society.

Diagnosis

There are different types of schizophrenia (paranoid, catatonic, disorganized, undifferentiated, and residual), and diagnosis is based on guidelines in the DSM-IV-TR. Table 48–1 provides a description of the different types of schizophrenia.

Treatment

Antipsychotic medications (neuroleptics) treat the positive symptoms of schizophrenia (Table 48–2). The conventional antipsychotics include fluphenazine (Prolixin), haloperidol (Haldol), chlorpromazine (Thorazine), perphenazine (Trilafon), thioridazine (Mellaril), thiothixene (Navane), and trifluoperazine (Stelazine). These antipsychotics are very effective in stopping the auditory hallucinations, enabling the patient to connect thoughts in a logical manner, and eliminating the delusional system. They do cause serious and unpleasant side effects and are becoming less commonly prescribed. However, some patients respond well to these drugs and, particularly for older patients who have taken them for a long time, it is likely that a successful drug regimen will continue (Cultural Cues 48–1).

The side effects for these medications include the familiar anticholinergic effects (i.e., dry mouth, flushing, urinary retention and constipation). In addition, these drugs have **extrapyramidal side effects (EPS): dystonia, pseudo-parkinsonism,** and **akathisia** (Figure 48–3). **Dystonia or** dystonic reaction is an acute muscle contraction, especially of the tongue, face, neck, and back. Oculogyric crisis, a fixed upward gaze or muscle spasm of the eye, can occur. **Pseudo-parkinsonism or drug induced-parkinsonism** includes a shuffling gait, flat affect, slowed movements, tremors,

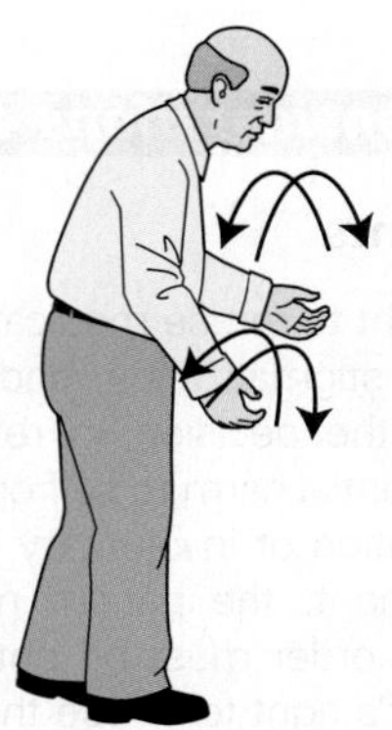

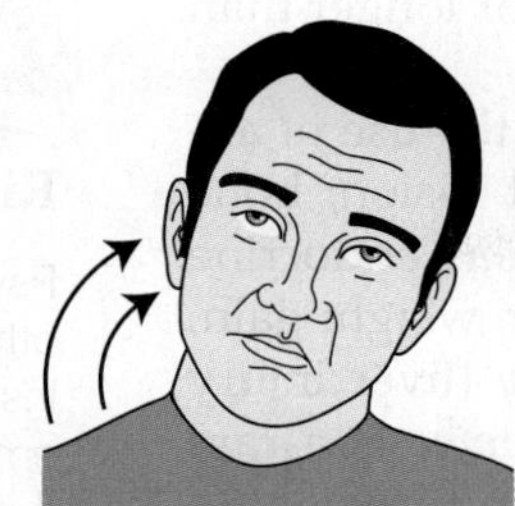

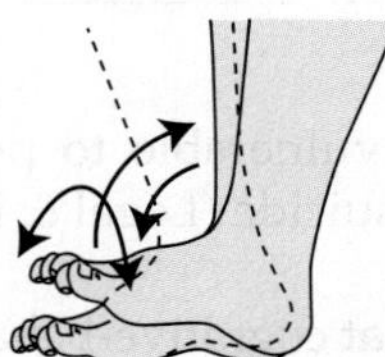

Tardive dyskinesia
• Protrusion and rolling the tongue
• Sucking and smacking movements of the lips
• Chewing motion
• Facial dyskinesia
• Involuntary movements of the body and extremities

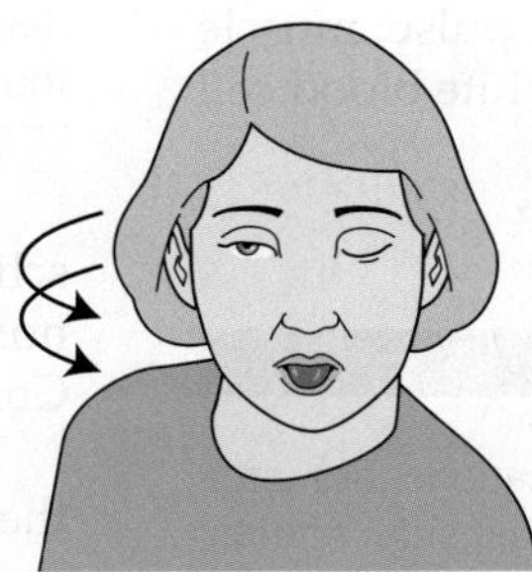

FIGURE **48–3** Characteristics of pseudo-parkinsonism, acute dystonia, akathisia, and tardive dyskinesia.

Table 48–1 ***Types of Schizophrenia***

TYPE	BEHAVIORAL MANIFESTATIONS
Paranoid	Exhibits extreme suspiciousness, delusions of grandeur, and delusions of persecution. Can be hostile and aggressive. Auditory hallucinations are common.
Catatonic	Exhibits a stuporous condition associated with rigidity, unusual posturing, and waxy flexibility. Also demonstrates echopraxia and echolalia. Exhibits unpredictable behavior because behavior is controlled by delusions and hallucinations.
Disorganized	Exhibits flat affect, silliness, and incoherence. Has gross thought disturbances, including word salad and neologisms. Delusions and hallucinations are common.
Undifferentiated	Exhibits symptoms found in more than one type, but does not meet adequate criteria for paranoid, catatonic, or disorganized types.
Residual	Exhibits negative symptoms (i.e., apathy, social isolation, psychomotor retardation, blunted affect, poverty of thoughts, and lack of motivation) of schizophrenia, with no evidence of hallucinations, delusions, or disorganized thoughts.

Table 48–2 ***Medications Used to Treat Schizophrenia***

CONVENTIONAL MEDICATIONS	NEWER (ATYPICAL) MEDICATIONS*
Chlorpromazine (Thorazine)	Clozapine (Clozaril)†
Fluphenazine (Prolixin)	Aripiprazole (Abilify)
Haloperidol (Haldol)	Olanzapine (Zyprexa)
Loxapine (Loxitane)	Quetiapine (Seroquel)
Molindone (Moban)	Risperidone (Risperdal)
Perphenazine (Trilafon)	Ziprasidone (Geodon)
Thioridazine (Mellaril)	Paliperidone (Invega)
Thiothixene (Navane)	
Trifluoperazine (Stelazine)	

*These drugs have fewer side effects than the conventional medications.
†First atypical antipsychotic, now rarely prescribed due to potential agranulocytosis. Weekly monitoring of white blood cell count is necessary.

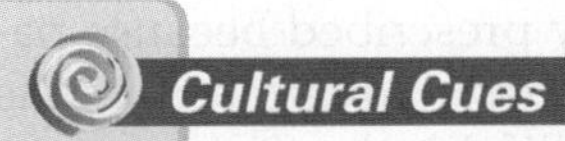

Cultural Cues 48–1

Race and Dosage

African Americans and Asian Americans may need dosage adjustments because of genetic differences in metabolism of antipsychotic medications.

and drooling. **Akathisia** manifests as motor restlessness (e.g., tapping a foot, rocking, pacing) or apprehension and irritability. Treatment for akathesia, dystonia, or pseudo-parkinsonism is to lower the dosage or change the medication, and to give benztropine (Cogentin) or diphenhydramine (Benadryl).

Tardive dyskinesia is a primary concern because **symptoms are irreversible once they have developed.** Symptoms include tongue protrusion, lip smacking, sucking, chewing, blinking, lateral jaw movements, grimacing, shoulder shrugging, pelvic thrusting, wrist and ankle flexion or rotation, foot tapping and toe movements, and rapid, purposeless and irregular movements. Movements are often described as writhing and wormlike. Monitor for signs of tardive dyskinesia, particularly in patients who have been taking a conventional antipsychotic medication for longer than 6 to 12 months.

Other adverse effects associated with the use of antipsychotic medications include blurred vision; bone marrow suppression; cardiac dysrrhythmias; endocrine changes such as elevation of blood sugar, weight gain, and breast enlargement; and *hepatoxicity* (liver injury and jaundice). *Neuroleptic malignant sydrome* is a rare reaction; however, it is life threatening, and frequently the patient will be transferred to the intensive care unit. Symptoms include high fever, increased pulse, muscle rigidity, stupor, incontinence, elevated white blood cell count, hyperkalemia, and renal failure.

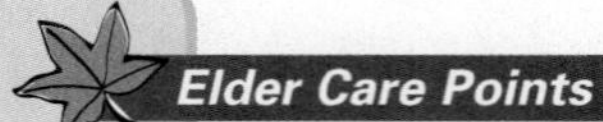

Elder Care Points

Elders who are taking antipsychotic medications are at a higher than usual risk for developing serious side effects. Baseline cardiac, renal, hepatic, and hematologic studies need to be done before initiating psychotropic drugs. The beginning dosages should be one half to one third of the normal adult dosage. Elders need to be watched very closely for difficulty swallowing, constipation and fecal impactions, weight gain, memory impairment, and orthostatic hypotension.

Examples of newer medications, sometimes referred to as **atypical antipsychotics,** include ziprasidone (Geodon), risperidone (Risperdal), quetiapine (Seroquel), and olanzapine (Zyprexa). Advantages of these newer drugs are fewer side effects, especially tardive dyskinesia, and some success with treating the negative symptoms. Olanzapine comes in a quickly dissolving oral form that is a potential alternative to an injection. This form is more expensive; however, it eliminates the risk of needlestick injury if the patient is combative, and it discourages *"cheeking"* (attempts to avoid swallowing by holding the pill in the cheek pouch). Clozapine (Clozaril), the first of the atypicals, is effective but is now less frequently prescribed because patients can develop *agranulocytosis* (decreased white blood cells). Aripiprazole (Abilify) is the first in a new class of antipsychotics, the dopamine system stablizers. The most recently approved medication for schizophrenia is paliperdone (Invega). Table 48–3 presents medication side effects and nursing implications for drugs used to treat thought disorders.

Negative symptoms are treated with a therapeutic environment, including a therapeutic relationship with the nurse, and education regarding basic living skills. **Historically, individuals with schizophrenia were shunned and stigmatized** because of unusual and bizarre behavior. Evidence-based practice indicates that with early intervention (e.g., enroll in social skills training at the earliest onset of symptoms), these individuals can cope with symptoms and maintain independent and productive lives outside of an institution (Wilson et al. 2005). If left untreated, individuals with

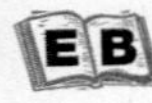

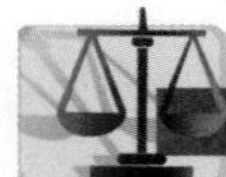

Legal & Ethical Considerations 48–1

Rights of Psychiatric Patients

Psychiatric patients do have the right to refuse medication and other therapies. Denial, paranoia, stigmatization, and lack of insight into illness contribute to the decision to refuse. In emergency situations, such as potential harm to self or others, the physician can order administration of involuntary medications. For routine ongoing treatment, the patient must be deemed incompetent and a court order must be obtained if the staff are to override the patient's right to refuse therapy.

schizophrenia are particularly vulnerable to poverty, homelessness, drug abuse, and suicide (Legal & Ethical Considerations 48–1).

There is growing evidence that cognitive-behavioral therapy (CBT) should be used in conjunction with medication in the treatment of schizophrenia. (Weiden, et al. 2006). In CBT, the therapist helps the patient to identify stressors, to make plans, and to modify behaviors. For example, the patient is assisted to recognize that hallucinations increase during the late evening hours. The plan might include listening to music and going to bed earlier. If the voices continue or get louder the patient knows to say, "Stop!"

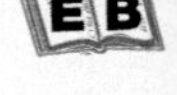

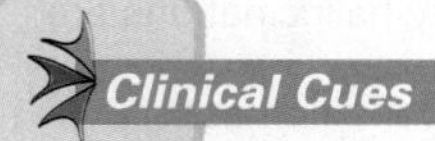

Clinical Cues

Nursing students often have difficulty applying therapeutic communication skills with schizophrenic patients because these patients have trouble answering questions, conversing coherently, or expressing feelings. Remember to offer yourself ("Ms. Elliott, if you would like to talk or play cards, I can spend some time with you today.") and attempt to understand ("Ms. Elliott, I am having a little difficulty understanding what you are saying, but I can tell you are trying to say something important."). Spending even a few seconds with a paranoid schizophrenic patient is therapeutic because your attention builds trust and rapport and allows her to practice social skills. Also remember that the purpose of therapeutic communication is to meet the patient's needs, not to have your questions answered.

NURSING MANAGEMENT

Assessment (Data Collection)

When collecting information from patients who have thought disorders, the interview must be brief. Because there is a problem with logical thought processing, it is difficult for the individual to remain focused for very long. Mental status assessment tools, such as the Mini-Mental Status Exam (MMSE) (Chapter 47), are useful in evaluating thinking processes and the ability to abstract information. Assessment of a thought disorder involves observing the person's ability to think in a logical manner and the presence of psychotic

Table 48–3 ***Nursing Implications for Antipsychotic Medications Used to Treat Thought Disorders***

COMMON SIDE EFFECTS	NURSING IMPLICATIONS
ANTICHOLINERGIC SIDE EFFECTS SEEN WITH ANTIPSYCHOTICS	
Dry mouth	Provide adequate fluids. Suggest sugarless hard candy or gum and good oral care.
Urinary retention and hesitancy	Monitor voiding and elimination patterns.
Constipation	Administer stool softener. Encourage fluids and fiber foods.
Blurred vision	Remind patient that blurred vision will cease once the body becomes accustomed to the drug.
Photophobia	Remind patient to wear sunglasses when in the sun.
Sexual dysfunction	Remind patient to alert treatment team for sexual difficulties.
COMMON EXTRAPYRAMIDAL SIDE EFFECTS SEEN WITH ANTIPSYCHOTICS	
Pseudo-parkinsonism: Masklike facies, stiff and stooped posture, shuffling gait, drooling, fine tremors, and pill-rolling movement.	May need to switch to a different antipsychotic. Administer anticholinergic medications such as trihexyphenidyl (Artane) or benztropine (Cogentin).
Akathisia: Characterized by pacing and motor restlessness.	Notify physician. Antipsychotic may need to be changed or an anticholinergic added to the drug regimen. Symptoms disappear when the drug is discontinued.
OTHER ADVERSE NEUROMUSCULAR EFFECTS	
Tardive dyskinesia: Typically manifests after 6–12 mo or more of medication therapy. It is characterized by tongue protrusion, lip smacking, sucking, chewing, blinking, lateral jaw movements, grimacing, shoulder shrugging, pelvic thrusting, wrist and ankle flexion or rotation, foot tapping and toe movements, and rapid, purposeless, and irregular movements.	Prevention by assessment; encourage checkups every 3 mo. Discontinuing the drug does not always relieve the symptoms. No specific treatment other than discontinuing the drug. Give soft foods. Have patient wear soft shoes or slippers.
Neuroleptic malignant syndrome: A rare, but potentially fatal reaction to antipsychotic medications. It is characterized by high fever, increased pulse, muscle rigidity, stupor, diaphoresis, hyperkalemia, incontinence, elevated white blood cell count, and renal failure.	Early detection increases survival rate. Stop all medications. Give supportive, symptomatic care. Decrease body temperature. Hydrate (oral and IV). Correct electrolyte imbalance. Medicate for dysrhythmias as ordered. Renal dialysis for renal failure.
CARDIOVASCULAR SIDE EFFECTS	
Orthostatic hypotension	Check blood pressure and pulse before giving medications.
Tachycardia	Inform patient to dangle feet before getting out of bed to prevent falls.
Paliperidone (Invega) can cause cardiac dysrhythmias (i.e., QT prolongation)	Inform patient that tolerance will develop in several weeks. Report to physician or RN any history of cardiac disease before starting the medication. Increase fluid intake to expand vascular volume as ordered.
MISCELLANEOUS SIDE EFFECTS	
Sleepiness and fatigue	Inform patient that tolerance to the dosage will develop in 1–2 wk. Administer medication at bedtime.
Photosensitivity	Avoid direct sunlight. Wear protective clothing and sunscreen when outside.
Weight gain	Monitor food intake.
Hives and contact dermatitis	Notify physician if there is a rash; may need to discontinue or change the drug.

Key: *IV*, intravenous.

features. Assessing the content and themes of hallucinations and delusions is important to ensure safety. For example, the patient may be receiving **command hallucinations** in which the voices are directing her to harm herself or others. Your patient may be experiencing delusions of persecution and be suspicious of staff and therefore refuse to eat. In addition, you should observe for stressors that seem to trigger or exacerbate disorganized behavior, such as an unfulfilled promise from a family member.

Patients with thought disorders may have difficulty verbalizing physical symptoms, and routine physical assessment should be performed to identify or monitor potential health problems. In addition, an initial and ongoing assessment of functionality, including activities of daily living and social skills, should be conducted. For example, the patient may have a disheveled appearance and dress in a bizarre fashion. Clothes may be worn in layers, backward, or inside out and be inappropriate to the season, or the patient

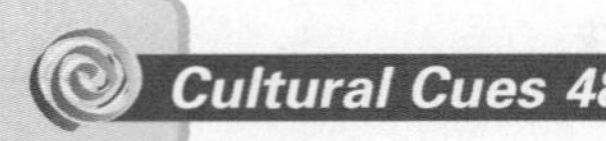

Cultural Beliefs

If your patient is a Mormon (member of the Church of Jesus Christ of Latter-Day Saints), she may wear a protective undergarment that is consider a blessed garment to be worn at all times. The patient will prefer to wear the hospital gown over the garment. If the patient declines to remove the garment for a bed bath, assist or allow the patient to partially remove portions of the garment as you perform the hygiene (part of the body should be touching the garment at all times).

may disrobe and stride about naked (Cultural Cues 48–2). One of the nursing goals would be to help the patient recognize and adopt socially appropriate attire. Table 48–4 provides definitions of terms associated with assessment of a thought disorder.

Nursing Diagnosis

Typical nursing diagnoses for thought disorders may include, but are not limited to:

- Disturbed thought processes (delusions) related to panic level of anxiety
- Disturbed sensory perception (hallucinations) related to biochemical imbalance
- Impaired verbal communication related to cognitive impairment
- Impaired social interaction related to extreme distrust
- Self-care deficit, bathing/dressing/eating related to cognitive deficits
- Noncompliance related to medications
- Risk for other-directed or self-directed violence related to command hallucinations

Planning

Expected outcomes are written for the specific individual nursing diagnoses chosen to resolve the patient's problems. For the nursing diagnoses above, they might include:

- Patient will verbally acknowledge that delusional thinking and beliefs (e.g., accuses others of being FBI agents) occur during times of intense anxiety, before discharge.
- Patient will spend decreased time attending to hallucinations (e.g., less time talking to self, less time listening for voices) before discharge.
- Patient will communicate basic needs more clearly within 1 week.
- Patient will attend the community meeting for _____ minutes today.
- Patient will wash her face and hands with supervision this morning.
- Patient will identify three methods that will help her to continue medications (after discharge) at first follow-up appointment.
- Patient will refrain from hurting self or other during this shift.

Table 48–4 Definition of Terms Used in Assessing Thought Disorders

TERM	DEFINITION
Delusions	Experiences *grandeur* (inflated sense of self-importance); *persecution* (feels that others intend harm). Patient has false, fixed beliefs that cannot be changed by logical reasoning.
Echolalia	Involves involuntary repetition of words spoken by others. Seen in catatonic schizophrenia.
Echopraxia	Involves imitating the motions of others. Seen in catatonic schizophrenia.
Flat affect	An obvious reduction in intensity of affect or absence or near absence of emotional expression.
Hallucinations	Patient experiences various sensory perceptions—auditory (hearing), visual (seeing), gustatory (tasting), olfactory (smelling), tactile (feeling or touching)—without corresponding stimuli in the environment. Auditory hallucinations are common in schizophrenia.
Ideas of reference	A type of delusion in which events, objects, or other people in the immediate environment have a particular and personalized significance. For example, the individual believes that the television newscaster is speaking directly to her.
Illusions	Patient misinterprets reality. For example, patient may perceive a curtain as a person in a long, flowing dress.
Loose association	Expression of ideas that do not have a logical association or connection.
Neologisms	Involves making up new words to express confused thoughts. Seen in schizophrenics with a serious thought disturbance.
Waxy flexibility	A state seen in catatonic schizophrenia in which the person maintains a limb in one position for a long time.
Word salad	A disorganized mix of words, phrases, and fragments that lack comprehension. Seen in severe schizophrenia.

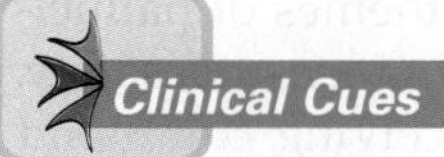

Monitor your own appearance and clothing when you are working with patients who have thought disorders. First, be a role model for clean, matching, and appropriate clothing. Second, avoid flashy and dangling jewelry because patients are easily distracted by such objects. Third, watch what you put around your neck. An agitated patient can grab a long necklace, a scarf, a tie, or a stethoscope during a takedown.

Planning care for a patient with a thought disorder involves promoting safety, monitoring medications intended to relieve agitation or psychosis, and ensuring adequate nutrition and sleep. **Care for these disorders will be long term, with intermittent treatment for acute episodes.** Patients need to be educated about the medications and coping skills necessary to function outside of a hospital setting. It is not unusual for a patient to stop taking medications because the voices returned with a warning that all medications are poison. Noncompliance with medications often leads to rehospitalization.

Think Critically About . . . Can you think of some ways that nurses could devise to help individuals with thought disorders comply with the medication regimen?

Implementation

A priority intervention in working with schizophrenic is to administer antipsychotic medications. As with any medication, nursing responsibility includes not only giving the medication, but also monitoring the effectiveness and any adverse effects (Patient Teaching 48–1). Antipsychotics have many serious side effects, some of which can be life threatening.

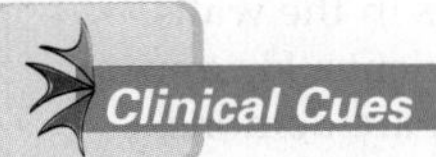

Clinical Cues

In accordance with 2007 National Patient Safety Goals, there should be at least two identifiers before giving medication or blood products or taking blood samples. When patients are not able to state their correct legal name (because of confusion or psychosis), an alternative method would be to have two health care providers verify the patient's identity.

When dealing with an actively psychotic patient, use a calm and caring approach. Do not touch the patient without warning or permission, especially if she is agitated or paranoid. During active hallucinations, state reality and help the patient return to reality. "Ms. Elliott, you seem to be listening to something. I am not hearing any voices. Come and talk to me." Evidence-base practice (Buccheri et al., 2004) suggests strategies for helping patients to manage persistent auditory hallucinations. These include monitoring what triggers the hallucinations, talking with someone, listening to music, watching TV, saying "stop," using earplugs, doing deep breathing or relaxation exercises, and doing a favorite activity.

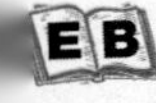

You may have great difficulty understanding the patient because of **neologisms** (making up new words), **word salad** (disorganized mix of words, phrases, and fragments), or **loose associations** (expression of ideas that do not logically connect) (Cultural Cues 48–3). Use therapeutic communication and be attentive, respond to the underlying feelings, and gently verbalize concern. "Ms. Elliott, you seem really anxious to tell me something. I am trying to understand."

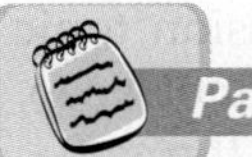

Patient Teaching 48–1

Antipsychotic Medications

Patients taking antipsychotic medications should be advised not to use ginseng or caffeine sources such as coffee. Taking these substances while on antipsychotic medications may result in decreased therapeutic effect, an undesirable enhancement of an intended effect, or untoward side effects.

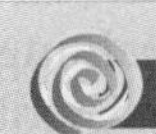

Cultural Cues 48–3

Language

During times of stress, it is natural to revert to your first language. If your patient speaks English as a second language, obtain the assistance of a translator to determine if the patient is having disturbances in communication (e.g., the patient's verbalizations might sound like word salad, but are actually a mixture of English and another language). Also, you can be charged with giving substandard care if you fail to call for a translator when the patient is unable to speak or understand English.

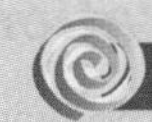

Cultural Cues 48–4

Eye Contact

Lack of direct eye contact does not necessarily signal disinterest or an unwillingness to communicate. Direct eye contact may be considered a sign of disrespect by people from different cultural backgrounds (i.e., Asian, Hispanic/Latino).

Think Critically About . . . You are caring for a patient who does not trust you. How does her distrust affect medication compliance? How will you establish trust and rapport with this patient?

General nursing interventions for the negative symptoms include establishing trust and teaching the patient and family how to manage the signs and symptoms. An attitude of acceptance is necessary to promote trust. Begin by offering yourself and being available to the patient even if she initially rejects your overtures to establish a therapeutic relationship ("I'm here if you want to spend some time talking today.") You should model conventional social behaviors such as greeting the patient by name ("Good morning, Ms. Elliott,") and making friendly eye contact (Cultural Cues 48–4). Give your patient positive feedback for making attempts to overcome negative symptoms: "You seemed very interested in the group discussion topic today." Do not make promises that you cannot keep, and if you make a promise, be sure to follow through.

Consistently invite your patient to join groups even if she rejects the initial invitations ("Ms. Elliott, we are going to play cards. Would you like to join us?"). Acknowledge and thank the patient for her efforts to interact, even if she spends only a few seconds with you ("Thank you for talking to me today.") Leave the door open for future interactions: "I understand if you don't want to talk today; maybe we can try tomorrow." Although these patients may have difficulty sustaining an interaction for even 1 or 2 minutes, your persistent effort builds the therapeutic alliance and increases the patient's self-esteem.

Administering medications and teaching the patient and family about antipsychotic medications are two additional nursing interventions. In addition, the side effects of the medications must be monitored. Nursing Care Plan 48–1 lists specific nursing diagnoses, expected outcomes, and nursing interventions for individuals with thought disorders.

Evaluation

To evaluate the effectiveness of nursing interventions, it is necessary to determine expected outcomes and then monitor the patient's progress. **Compliance with antipsychotic medications will decrease hallucinations and delusions (positive symptoms) and improve sleep.** Achieving expected outcomes for the negative symptoms of schizophrenia is a much longer process than for the positive symptoms (Complementary & Alternative Therapies 48–1). **Outcomes for the negative symptoms would include a decrease in psychomotor retardation, increase in self-care, improved affect, and an increase in motivation. In addition, the patient would exhibit a trusting attitude toward others and a decrease in social withdrawal.** Box 48–1 lists additional interventions for patients who are angry, hostile, aggressive, manipulative, or paranoid.

NURSING CARE PLAN 48–1

Care of the Patient with Schizophrenia

SCENARIO Jake Green is a 29-year-old man who was diagnosed with schizophrenia 8 years ago. He was taken to the emergency room yesterday after he destroyed his own trailer home. Jake states, "There were demons in the walls." He is disheveled and unkempt and appears paranoid and reluctant to interact with the staff or other patients. He appears to be hearing voices and tells you, "I am Jesus, saving you, saving you; hear the demons. You, all of you are demons, yourselves are demons."

PROBLEM/NURSING DIAGNOSIS *Delusions continue*/Disturbed thought processes related to delusional thinking, loosening of associations, or neurobiochemical imbalances.

Supporting assessment data *Subjective:* States "You, all of you are demons, yourselves are demons." *Objective:* Believes he is Jesus and believes others are demons.

Goals/Expected Outcomes	Nursing Interventions	Selected Rationale	Evaluation
Patient will be able to talk for 5 min without discussion of delusions	Assess the themes of delusions.	Delusional themes suggest fears and safety issues.	Has a belief that he is being persecuted by demons.
Patient will be able to distinguish between reality and nonreality before discharge	Assess for situations that trigger anxiety and stress.	Anxiety and stress are theorized to increase delusions and disorganized behavior.	Currently very anxious and actively delusional; assessment for associated triggers continues. Patient is making continuous reference to demons.
	Reflect the underlying feelings ("It's frightening if you feel someone is trying to hurt you.").	Acknowledging feelings validates the patient's experience without agreeing with the delusional content.	Appears suspicious and fearful.
	State reality as you perceive it ("I believe that the hospital is a safe place.").	Corrects misperceptions without directly arguing against patient's perspective.	Reassured that the hospital is a safe place, but he continues to be fearful.
	Avoid arguing about the patient's delusional system.	Arguing causes patient to verbally defend own beliefs and potentially strengthens the delusional system.	Occasionally, patient appears to recognize certain staff members, but overall is highly delusional.

Key: *ADLs*, activities of daily living; *NA*, nursing assistant.

NURSING CARE PLAN 48–1

Care of the Patient with Schizophrenia—cont'd

Goals/Expected Outcomes	Nursing Interventions	Selected Rationale	Evaluation
	Redirect discussions to real people and events.	Helps patient to stay in the here and now.	Continues unwavering in his beliefs in demons. Does respond when called by name (Jake); however, continues to verbalize the belief that he is Jesus.
	Administer antipsychotic medications as ordered and monitor for effectiveness and side effects.	Counteract psychosis at the biochemical level.	Agrees to take risperidone (Risperdal) if administered by certain nurses. Outcomes not met. Continue plan.

PROBLEM/NURSING DIAGNOSIS *Not attending to basic ADLs*/Self-care deficit related to cognitive impairment.
Supporting assessment data *Subjective:* None. *Objective:* Is disheveled and unkempt.

Goals/Expected Outcomes	Nursing Interventions	Selected Rationale	Evaluation
Patient will independently perform self-care within 1 wk Patient will dress appropriately and maintain appropriate hygiene before discharge	Encourage the patient to independently perform ADLs according to current level of ability.	Performing ADLs helps the patient to focus on real tasks and decreases time spent in delusional thinking.	Is not initiating ADLs, but will perform brief tasks (e.g., washing face) with coaching.
	Make available only the clothes the patient is to wear.	Limiting choices decreases confusion and indirectly suggests appropriate attire.	Is continuously changing clothes unless locked out of room.
	Intervene as necessary if patient is unable to complete daily care.	Initially the patient may not be able to complete ADLs due to impaired thought processes.	NA verbally directed patient to shower. Patient became hostile; therefore, shower deferred for today. Will try to have his brother assist him tomorrow.
	Offer positive reinforcement for any completed portion of ADLs.	Increases likelihood that desired behavior will be repeated.	Acknowledges feedback by looking up when spoken to.
	Assist the patient to make a structured plan if necessary.	Having a plan provides structure, goals, and ways to achieve goals, which helps the patient to complete tasks.	Verbally advised that shower is deferred for today, but that brother will help tomorrow. Agrees to wash hands and face today. Outcomes not met. Continue plan.

PROBLEM/NURSING DIAGNOSIS *Hearing voices of demons*/Disturbed sensory perception related to neurobiochemical imbalance and anxiety.
Supporting assessment data *Subjective:* States, "hear the demons." *Objective:* Appears to be hearing voices.

Goals/Expected Outcomes	Nursing Interventions	Selected Rationale	Evaluation
Patient will verbalize three ways to cope with hallucinations this week Patient will verbalize a decrease in hallucinations before discharge	Observe behavior that suggests that hallucination is occurring (e.g., talking to self, listening intently).	Staff can interrupt the hallucination in progress.	Observed in listening position and talking to self. Is actively hallucinating today (more than yesterday), appears upset; reason unclear.

Continued

NURSING CARE PLAN 48-1

Care of the Patient with Schizophrenia—cont'd

Goals/Expected Outcomes	*Nursing Interventions*	*Selected Rationale*	*Evaluation*
	Assess for theme of hallucinations, especially command hallucinations (e.g., voices that say, "Kill others.").	Knowing themes helps to anticipate violent or unexpected behavior.	Hearing command hallucinations ("I have the word, the word to save you.").
	Redirect when hallucinations occur. (e.g., "Talk with me.").	Interrupts hallucination in progress.	Patient does attend to voice when spoken to; although he appears fearful, he will stay for 10–15 sec if he is given adequate space (e.g., 5 ft).
	Help patient recognize the feelings that are present before the hallucination.	Anxiety, fear, and stress are theorized to exacerbate hallucinations.	Unclear why patient is so agitated today; he is unable to verbalize specific feelings.
	State reality (e.g., "I understand that you hear voices. I do not hear those voices.").	Helps patient to recognize and stay in the here and now.	Patient is actively hallucinating; only able to attend to NA's voice for a few seconds.
	Teach patient to identify and use strategies to interrupt the hallucinations (e.g., seek out nursing staff, sing, listen to music).	Allows patient to cope with hallucinations. (For some patients, hallucinations never completely resolve.)	Unable to identify or teach alternative coping methods. Appears less agitated if not approached by other patients.
	Administer antipsychotic medications and monitor effectiveness and side effects.	Counteracts psychosis at the biochemical level.	Agrees to take risperidone (Risperdal) if administered by certain nurses. Outcomes not met. Continue plan.

PROBLEM/NURSING DIAGNOSIS *Paranoid and avoiding others*/Social isolation related to mistrust, bizarre behavior, or cognitive impairment.

Supporting assessment data *Subjective:* "…all of you are demons." *Objective:* Reluctant to interact with the staff or other patients.

Goals/Expected Outcomes	*Nursing Interventions*	*Selected Rationales*	*Evaluation*
Patient will engage in social interaction with others on the psychiatric unit (meals, outings, groups) within 2 wk	Convey a warm, accepting attitude.	Builds therapeutic relationship.	Has some trust toward selected nurses.
	Spend some structured time with the patient every day.	Encourages social interaction with a set time and purpose.	Able to tolerate 10–15 sec of contact with nurses. Responds to name.
	Determine patient's interests.	Patient more likely to engage if interested in activities.	Family states that Jake is interested in baseball. Does show some interest in watching sports on television.
	Model social interaction and conversation.	Patient may be unaware of how to converse with others.	Is not initiating any conversations. Is able to attend group meeting for <1 min.
	Create opportunities for socialization (i.e., card games).	Patient may not know how to independently engage others.	
	Acknowledge and thank patient for any efforts to interact and participate in groups.	More likely to repeat behavior if encouraged and acknowledged.	Unable to participate in any group interaction today.

NURSING CARE PLAN 48–1

Care of the Patient with Schizophrenia—cont'd

Goals/Expected Outcomes	Nursing Interventions	Selected Rationales	Evaluation
	Encourage the patient to interact with others, even if only briefly.	Brief contacts allow for gradual trust and familiarity to decrease suspiciousness.	Declined going to group music class this afternoon. Appears more restless and suspicious compared to yesterday. Patient unable to verbalize source of distress, no known event or trigger identified. Will continue to observe. Outcomes not met. Continue plan.

? CRITICAL THINKING QUESTIONS

1. Why is it important for a patient like Jake to have consistent social support after he is discharged from the hospital?
2. What can nurses do to help decrease the social stigma of chronic mental illnesses such as schizophrenia?

OVERVIEW OF PERSONALITY DISORDERS

Personality disorders are enduring patterns of behavior in which there is no loss of contact with reality or impaired cognition. Symptoms of personality disorders are usually first observed in late adolescence and early adulthood. Four characteristics of personality disorders are:

1. Inflexible and maladaptive response to life events
2. Serious difficulty in areas of personal and work relationships
3. Tendency to evoke interpersonal conflict
4. Tendency to evoke a negative empathic response from others

An actual diagnosis may not be made until the person reaches the late 20s or 30s; by then the entrenched behaviors are quite evident. It is not uncommon to note failed marriages, poor work histories, and considerable difficulty with interpersonal relationships. Box 48–2 presents the DSM-IV-TR diagnostic criteria for a personality disorder.

The DSM-IV-TR describes 10 different personality disorders. Depending on the descriptive characteristics, these disorders are clustered into three separate categories. Cluster A includes behaviors that are considered **odd** or **eccentric** (schizotypal, schizoid, and paranoid). Cluster B describes behaviors that are considered **dramatic, emotional,** and **erratic** (antisocial, borderline, histrionic, and narcissistic). Individuals with Cluster C behaviors appear **anxious and fearful** (avoidant, dependent, and obsessive-compulsive). A final type of personality disorder is personality disorder NOS. Box 48–3 provides a brief description of each of these personality disorders. In this chapter we review borderline personality disorder because it is more commonly diagnosed, and caring for patients with a borderline personality presents many challenges.

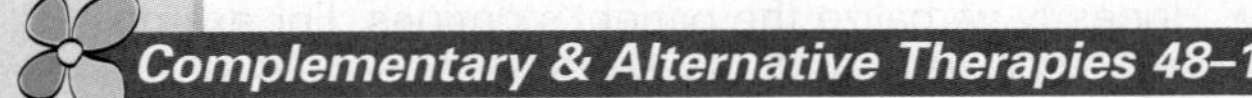

Music Therapy

Music therapy can be used with selected patients to treat positive and negative symptoms of schizophrenia. Participation in music groups increases socialization and stimulates interest. Encourage participants to express how the music makes them feel and to discuss their favorite kinds of music. Focused projects such as a performance event help patients to meet individual goals and experience success.

BORDERLINE PERSONALITY DISORDER

Borderline personality disorder is defined by the DSM-IV-TR as "a pattern of instability in interpersonal relationships, self-image and affect, and marked impulsivity" (American Psychiatric Association, 2000). Individuals with this disorder attach quickly and easily to others and fear **real or imagined abandonment.** Emotions and relationships are very intense. In response to potential abandonment from caregivers or significant others, it is not unusual to see **self-mutilating behavior** (e.g., cutting on hands and wrists, cigarette burns) or **suicidal gestures.** Evidence-based practice suggests that the therapeutic goals for patients who self-mutilate include acquiring new coping methods, better impulse and emotional control and increasing self-awareness (Starr, 2004).

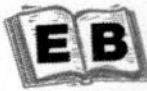

Box 48–1 ***Specific Nursing Interventions for Patients Who Are Angry, Hostile, Aggressive, Manipulative, or Paranoid***

ANGRY, HOSTILE, AND AGGRESSIVE BEHAVIOR

- Continuously assess for nonverbal cues (pacing, fidgeting, and increase in verbalizations) and intervene early.
- Maintain a calm, self-assured attitude, even if you are frightened.
- Listen and acknowledge that you care and want to help.
- Be culturally aware of how your patient is interpreting eye contact.
- Allow the patient to have adequate personal space.
- Encourage the patient to find a quiet, safe place.
- Maintain your own safety—have adequate staff visually present in the background. However, only one person should attempt verbal de-escalation.
- Stand to the side or sideways to present yourself as a smaller target. Your hands should be relaxed at your sides or with the palms turned upward.
- Be aware of the exits and position yourself so that the patient is not blocking the exit.
- Ask for permission before touching. Defer therapeutic touching if the patient is highly agitated.
- Honestly verbalize the patient's options. For example, say, "You can stay in the dayroom if you can remain calm; otherwise it will be necessary for you to go to the quiet (seclusion) room."
- Set a time frame for verbal de-escalation. If progress is made within the time limit, continue. If not, remind the patient of the initial time limit.
- Offer appropriate PRN medications as ordered. If the patient continues to escalate and the behavior becomes aggressive, physical restraints may be necessary.
- Application of physical restraints requires a team approach by trained staff.
- Inform the patient of the staff's intentions and actions. Accurately document the entire episode, including all efforts to use the less restrictive measures before resorting to physically restraints.

MANIPULATIVE BEHAVIOR

- Set clear and realistic limits on specific behaviors.
- Establish realistic and enforceable consequences.
- Make certain that all staff are informed of the limits and are in agreement.
- Specific limits need to be documented in the plan of care/nurses' notes.
- The decision to discontinue limits should be made by the entire staff and should be made only when the patient has demonstrated consistent behavior.
- Be self-aware and establish clear boundaries.

PARANOID BEHAVIOR

- Assign only one or two staff to the patient.
- Initially make brief contact with the patient, and do not make unnecessary demands.
- Increase credibility by being honest, adhering to a stated schedule and following through on commitments.
- Do not touch a patient who is paranoid.
- Do not mix medications with food.
- Supply food in commercially wrapped packages if the patient is refusing to eat.

Key: *PRN*, as needed.

? ***Think Critically About . . .*** You are assigned to escort a young female patient to the smoking area. As she is finishing her cigarette, she touches the hot ash to her wrist and sustains a burn before you can stop her. She publicly announces to the staff and the other patients that you were negligent in watching her. How would you handle this?

Splitting, a primitive defense mechanism, involves the initial idealization of a caregiver or friend, followed by a hasty devaluing of that same person. For example, the patient may say, "You are the best nurse I have ever had. No one else understands me like you do." When the nurse returns after 2 days off, the patient would say, "I can't believe you didn't call me when you were off. I felt horrible and began cutting on my wrists, and it is your fault."

The patient with borderline personality disorder also may idealize one or two team members and devalue others. It is very important that the staff decide on an approach to use with a particular patient. To implement the plan properly, all team members must be consistent with the approach. **Impulsivity** in at least two of the following areas also is characteristic of borderline personality disorder: **gambling, overeating, spending impulsively, abusing substances, engaging in unsafe sex,** or **driving recklessly.** Engaging in one or more of these impulsive behaviors is often the reason for admission to a hospital.

Box 48–2 ***General Diagnostic Criteria for a Personality Disorder***

The patient with a personality disorder demonstrates an ongoing, inflexible pattern of behavior that is *very* different from the individual's culture. Onset usually occurs in adolescence or early adulthood. The behavior occurs in a wide range of personal and social situations and causes distress in social or occupational functioning. Two (or more) of the following areas are affected:

1. Cognition (i.e., perceiving and understanding self, others, and events)
2. Affect (i.e., the range, intensity, and appropriateness of emotional response)
3. Interpersonal functioning
4. Impulse control

From American Psychiatric Association. (2007). *Diagnostic and Statistical Manual of Mental Disorders* (4th ed.). Text Revision. Washington, DC: American Psychiatric Association.

Box 48–3 Description of Personality Disorders

CLUSTER A (ODD AND ECCENTRIC)

- *Schizotypal:* Exhibits difficulty with close relationships, distortions in thinking and feeling, and odd or eccentric behavior.
- *Schizoid:* Exhibits withdrawal from social relationships and a restricted affect.
- *Paranoid:* Exhibits distrust and suspiciousness of others and feels others wish her harm or evil.

CLUSTER B (DRAMATIC, EMOTIONAL, AND ERRATIC)

- *Antisocial:* Exhibits disregard for, and violation of, the rights of others; lacks empathy.
- *Borderline:* Exhibits instability in interpersonal relationships and self-concept, labile emotions, and marked impulsivity.
- *Histrionic:* Exhibits pattern of extreme emotionality and attention-seeking behavior.
- *Narcissistic:* Exhibits grandiose behavior, intense need for admiration, and lack of empathy.

CLUSTER C (ANXIOUS AND FEARFUL)

- *Avoidant:* Exhibits social inhibition, feelings of inadequacy, and fear of rejection.
- *Dependent:* Exhibits behavior that is submissive and clinging; needy.
- *Obsessive-compulsive:* Exhibits behavior that is concerned with excessive orderliness, perfectionism, and need for control.

Treatment

Treatment for people with this disorder involves long-term psychotherapy, such as individual counseling and group or family therapy. The purpose of **psychotherapy** is to help the participants identify problem areas and work to change behavior and attitudes or modify feelings. Patients with personality disorders can also benefit from milieu therapy. **Milieu therapy** uses the structured environment of a hospital or group home setting to help patients participate as active members of the milieu community and practice social behaviors. Medications are not indicated for personality disorders, although they are sometimes prescribed when there is a concurrent mood disorder.

NURSING MANAGEMENT

Assessment (Data Collection)

You need to collect information about how the individual views herself and others. Obtain a history of former relationships and identify how the individual typically expresses feelings. It is important not to make a hasty judgment and label a person with a personality disorder. For example, adolescents may impulsively act out with substances and have identity problems, but these traits often disappear with maturity. In addition, when a patient is labeled as "borderline," nurses may view the patient as "hopeless." Box 48–4 lists examples of behaviors nurses might observe when assessing a personality disorder.

Box 48–4 Guide for Assessing Patients with Personality Disorders

Observe and assess for the following:

- Low self-esteem
- Constant seeking of praise and admiration
- Self-centeredness
- Extreme envy of others
- Anger and possible rage when others do not share the same point of view
- Acting without thinking; impulsivity
- Consistent poor judgment in making decisions
- Unreliability
- Evidence of self-destructive behavior
- Treatment of others as objects, not people
- Expression of a need to control others
- Excessive use of manipulation to get needs met

Nursing Diagnosis

Typical nursing diagnoses for personality disorders may include, but are not limited to:

- Impaired social interaction related to immature and manipulative behavior
- Chronic low self-esteem related to childhood abuse and neglect
- Ineffective coping related to controlling emotional state outbursts
- Anxiety related to perceived threats of abandonment
- Risk for self-mutilation related to feelings of guilt and rejection

Planning

Expected outcomes are written for the specific individual nursing diagnoses chosen to resolve the patient's problems. For the nursing diagnoses above, they might include:

- Patient will discuss one example of how her behavior alienates others by the end of the week.
- Patient will share two things that she likes about herself in today's group meeting.
- Patient will identify three methods to cope with intense emotions (e.g., anger at staff or significant others) within 1 week.
- Patient will identify situations that provoke feelings of abandonment (e.g., favorite nurse is on vacation) and state two methods to reduce accompanying anxiety during this shift.
- Patient will substitute a safe behavior (e.g., talking to nurse, counting to 100) for self-mutilating behavior when experiencing feelings of guilt or rejection during hospitalization.

Planning for the care of a patient with a borderline personality disorder requires involvement of the entire team to define goals and to avoid the patient's inevitable attempts at staff manipulation (Assignment Considerations 48–1). If possible, some staff debriefing time will help everyone to maintain a professional and

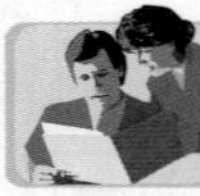

Assignment Considerations 48–1

Interpersonal Skills

When planning care for your patients, incorporate the strengths and interpersonal skills of your team members and make assignments appropriately. For example, your patient is a 23-year-old woman who needs an escort to attend a group therapy class outside of the unit. She is known for her attempts to manipulate male staff members; therefore, assign a mature female nursing assistant who is familiar with the patient's manipulative behavior.

---

optimistic focus when working with patients who have this disorder. Long-term goals are appropriate for behavioral and lifestyle changes.

Implementation

For individuals with borderline personality disorder, setting limits is a priority intervention. Individuals must be taught healthy and nonmanipulative ways to get their needs met. To work effectively with borderline personality disorder, the staff need to maintain good boundaries without being controlling, rigid, and inflexible. Patients with this disorder often ask you to "bend the rules" or grant special privileges. **The staff needs to consistently set limits with caring and empathy, offer a rationale, and decline negotiation.** If the patient views the limit setting as punitive, the behavior is certain to recur at a later time. This does not mean that the patient will always gladly accept the limit setting and be grateful for your concern. It does mean that you are assisting the patient in developing some internal sense of boundaries and subsequent changes in behavior.

It is also necessary to maintain a safe environment for patients with borderline disorder because they can be impulsive and do not have internal control. It may be necessary to initiate suicide precautions or help the patient who is self-mutilating to stop this behavior. See Chapter 45 for information on suicide precautions.

Patients with personality disorders have an ability to "get under the skin" of caregivers. If you note a particularly intense reaction to a patient (excessive sympathy, empathy, anger, or frustration), it is important to talk about these feelings with a more experienced nurse or a peer whom you trust. **Identify and express the feelings that the patient's behavior evokes in you.** Your awareness of your own feelings will help you to modify your reactions and focus on the therapeutic aspects of your relationship with the patient. See Nursing Care Plan 48–2 for nursing di-

NURSING CARE PLAN 48–2

Care of the Patient with Borderline Personality Disorder

SCENARIO Delia Gates, a 35-year-old, is recovering from surgery. She has a history of borderline personality disorder. The psychiatric clinical nurse specialist has been advising the staff on how to set boundaries with Ms. Gates and has made arrangements for the patient to attend a hospital-based support group. During her hospital stay, Ms. Gates has been flattering and excessively friendly toward you. When you try to talk to her about her upcoming discharge, she angrily accuses you of "trying to kick her out of the hospital" and calls you a "two-faced faker." Twenty minutes later you are summoned to Ms. Gates' room and you find that she has pulled out her IV line and has macerated the IV site with a staple from a magazine. She is crying, "This is all your fault."

PROBLEM/NURSING DIAGNOSIS *Cannot cope with discharge teaching*/Ineffective coping related to loss of a relationship, real and perceived stressors, or inability to get needs met in a healthy way.

Supporting assessment data *Subjective:* States "This is all your fault." *Objective:* Has emotional outburst and copes by blaming others and harming self.

Goals/Expected Outcomes	*Nursing Interventions*	*Selected Rationale*	*Evaluation*
The patient will verbalize and practice alternatives to manipulative behavior during this shift	Set firm limits as necessary (e.g., "You can go to the hospital shop for 20 minutes.").	Helps patient to recognize appropriate behavior; ideally, the patient learns to set limits for herself.	Is frustrated and angry this A.M. at the end of 20-min limit. She attempts to extend time limit by cajoling and begging ("I really need just a few more minutes.").
	Explain consequences of manipulative behavior in a calm, rational manner.	Helps patient to connect actions and consequences.	Explained to patient that 20 min was the agreed limit and last-minute attempts to change the agreement would result in loss of off-unit privileges.

Key: *IV*, intravenous.

NURSING CARE PLAN 48–2

Care of the Patient with Borderline Personality Disorder

Goals/Expected Outcomes	Nursing Interventions	Selected Rationale	Evaluation
	Use clear, direct communication (e.g., "Delia, the support group will start in 10 minutes. Please get ready now.").	Clarifies and models good communication.	Continues to have trouble with direct communication.
	Assist to redirect angry feelings into constructive activities, such as art or exercise.	Helps patient to learn alternative ways to cope with feelings.	Appears to enjoy drawing and painting; says she will consider drawing next time she is angry.
	Role play direct communication.	Provides opportunity to practice new coping skill.	States that role play is "stupid" and refuses to try, but keenly observes others when the technique is demonstrated.
	Assist to identify manipulative behaviors and discuss how these behaviors affect self and others.	Insight into how behavior affects others helps patient to recognize consequences and to alter behavior.	Acknowledges that "men are easier to manipulate than women because they want sex," but is unable to state why this type of manipulation is problematic.
	Assist to identify and define major stressors.	Identification and delimiting of stressors help patient to learn to cope and intervene early.	Identifies past problems with parents and men: "Always felt ignored and wanted more attention than they ever gave me." "I get pretty easily stressed out over guys."
	Assist in developing a realistic plan to minimize stressors.	Planning empowers patient to control behaviors and outcomes.	States that finding a "really nice guy" would be the best solution, but acknowledges that may not happen. Might be willing to try seeing a counselor after discharge if she does not meet "a nice guy." Outcomes partially met. Continue plan.

PROBLEM/NURSING DIAGNOSIS *Is hurting herself to get attention*/Risk for self-directed violence with self-mutilating behavior related to inability to directly verbalize needs and feelings.

Supporting assessment data *Subjective:* None. *Objective:* Uses staple to macerate IV site.

Goals/Expected Outcomes	Nursing Interventions	Selected Rationale	Evaluation
The patient will not demonstrate self-mutilating behaviors during this shift	Encourage the patient to identify, label, and express feelings.	Patient is having strong feelings. Verbalization is healthier than acting out.	Is able to verbalize feelings of anger and rejection.
	Assist patient to become aware of escalating levels of anxiety and the desire to self-mutilate.	Self-awareness will help patient to know when to use an alternative coping mechanism.	Reports noticing that her heart is beating faster when she is anxious, and she is beginning to associate the tachycardia with the urge to cut herself. She has reported the concurrent anxiety and the urge to the nurse.

Continued

NURSING CARE PLAN 48–2

Care of the Patient with Borderline Personality Disorder—cont'd

Goals/Expected Outcomes	*Nursing Interventions*	*Selected Rationale*	*Evaluation*
	Encourage the use of diversional activities, such as journal writing, crafts, or reporting to the nurse when the desire to self-mutilate is present.	Alternative methods will help patient to stop self-mutilating.	There were no attempts to self-mutilate during this shift. Outcomes met. Continue plan.
	If the patient self-mutilates, care for the wound in a matter-of-fact manner.	Matter-of-fact attitude does not provide the secondary gains of sympathy or solicitousness.	

PROBLEM/NURSING DIAGNOSIS *Ms. Gates shows unstable response toward nursing staff*/Impaired social interaction related to disturbance of self-concept, inability to maintain a healthy relationship.

Supporting assessment data *Subjective:* Calls nurse a "two-faced faker." *Objective:* Demonstrates splitting by being flattering and excessively friendly, then being accusing and blaming.

Goals/Expected Outcomes	*Nursing Interventions*	*Selected Rationale*	*Evaluation*
The patient will verbalize elements of healthy relationships during this shift	Teach the patient the essential components of a healthy relationship, such as trust and honesty.	Patient is unaware of how to establish or function in a relationship.	Participated in a discussion today about friendship and romantic relationships.
Patient will participate in and respect the boundaries of the nurse-patient relationship during this shift	Make patient aware that intensity of emotions (e.g., excessive flattering) is not an essential part of healthy relationships (e.g., "Ms. Gates, thank you for your kind compliments, but I am your nurse and it makes me feel a little uncomfortable when you say…").	Insight into how her behavior is affecting others will help her modify her responses.	Is initially angry and appears hurt when given feedback about excessive flattery, but later says that she understands and will try to restrain from making too many compliments.
The patient will be able to identify and set personal boundaries before discharge	Teach the patient the necessity of personal boundaries and how to maintain them (e.g., "Telling people directly what you need helps to decrease misunderstandings. For example, tell your boyfriend that you need to talk to him about the breakup.").	Patient is unaware of how boundaries are set or how to function in an adult relationship.	Agrees that talking to the boyfriend about the breakup would be a better alternative to cutting herself.
	Role model boundaries for the patient by being consistent and congruent in your interactions and enforcing limits (e.g., "Ms. Gates, I can't talk to you now, but I will meet with you after lunch.") Then follow through as promised.	Allows patient to see how to perform new behavior.	Continues to be angry about limits placed on her.
	Observe patient setting boundaries and give appropriate feedback as necessary.	Provides opportunities for patient to practice new skills; feedback allows patient to modify behavior.	Has been observed setting limits with regards to other patients (e.g., told another patient, "I'll braid your hair if you will please stop crying for at least 10 minutes."). Outcomes met. Continue plan.

NURSING CARE PLAN 48–2

Care of the Patient with Borderline Personality Disorder—cont'd

PROBLEM/NURSING DIAGNOSIS *Patient feels angry and rejected*/Chronic low self-esteem related to unmet dependency needs, perceived abandonment, or rejection.

Supporting assessment data *Subjective:* States "you are trying to kick me out of the hospital." *Objective:* Hurts self to get her needs for attention met.

Goals/Expected Outcomes	*Nursing Interventions*	*Selected Rationale*	*Evaluation*
The patient will consistently verbalize positive and realistic comments about self and others before discharge	Assist the patient in setting goals that are realistic.	Realistic goals increase success, which increases self-esteem.	Is having trouble with realistic goals. Continues to state, "I just need to find a really nice guy to solve all my problems."
	Assist in developing a plan.	Planning helps patient to meet goals.	Unable to complete plan.
	Assist to identify strengths and accomplishments for self and others.	Realistic identification of positive aspects reinforces self-esteem and helps to limit idealization of others.	Identifies that she is creative (i.e., drawing and hair styling). States her mother's greatest strength is her intelligence.
	Encourage independent action and decision making.	Independence increases self-esteem.	Was able to decide that going to the hospital shop for 20 min was better than not going at all.
	Teach the patient basic assertiveness techniques.	Learning assertiveness increases patient's ability to advocate for self.	Is having some difficulty differentiating between assertiveness and aggressiveness.
	Teach patient how to give and receive positive feedback.	Giving and receiving feedback helps patient to communicate needs and to recognize what others need from her.	Was able to give and receive feedback in group therapy session today. Outcomes met. Continue plan.

? CRITICAL THINKING QUESTIONS

1. What is the pitfall of labeling a patient as "borderline"?
2. Do you think Delia's behavior represents a risk for suicide? Why or why not?

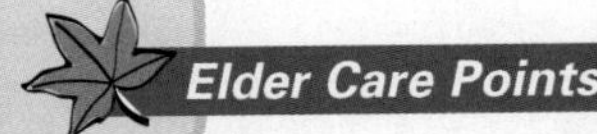

Elder Care Points

Although elderly schizophrenics are few, they can present unique challenges for nurses who work in long-term care. Because of the negative symptoms of social withdrawal, apathy, and sometimes paranoia, schizophrenic elders are not as likely to seek out nurses for help. They may ignore physical problems and often will not seek help for pain associated with physical disabilities.

agnoses, expected outcomes, and nursing interventions for an individual with a borderline personality disorder.

Evaluation

Achievement of long-term outcomes is demonstrated by new coping strategies for handling stressors, verbalizing anger without acting out, increasing independent decision making, and decreasing manipulative behaviors to get needs met. It is expected that in times of stress, the patient will revert to previously learned behaviors. When the stress has passed, you should encourage the patient to continue implementing new behaviors.

COMMUNITY CARE

At one time individuals with thought disorders were hospitalized indefinitely. With the introduction of antipsychotic medications, hospitalization is reserved for medication stabilization; then patients are released to a less restrictive type of care. Therefore, it would not be unusual for nurses to care for individuals with thought disorders in a variety of settings, such as nursing homes, clinics, or home care.

Patients with personality disorders are not hospitalized unless they present an imminent danger to themselves via self-mutilation or suicidal gestures. Again, nurses come into contact with personality disorders in a variety of settings outside the hospital. Setting limits and appropriate boundaries continues to be an effective intervention, regardless of the setting.

Patients with chronic mental illness are at high risk for social problems and may have limited encounters with health care professionals. For example, patients with schizophrenia are at a high risk for homelessness, and patients with personality disorders, particular antisocial personality disorder, are more likely to be incarcerated. In accordance with the *Healthy People 2010* goals, a greater percentage of people who are homeless and those who are in jail need mental health screening and access to treatment.

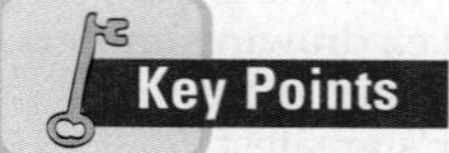

Key Points

- Thought disorders are characterized by disorganized thought and behavior and hallucinations. Mood and interpersonal relationships are altered.
- These disorders include schizophrenia, brief psychotic disorder, schizoaffective disorder, delusional disorder, schizophreniform disorder, shared psychotic disorder, psychotic disorder due to medical condition, substance-induced psychotic disorder, and psychotic disorder NOS.
- Schizophrenia is the most commonly diagnosed thought disorder and usually develops in late adolescence or the early 20s.
- The positive symptoms of schizophrenia (hallucinations, delusions, and disordered thinking) can be treated with antipsychotic medications.
- The negative symptoms of schizophrenia (apathy, social isolation, psychomotor retardation, blunted affect, poverty of thoughts, and lack of motivation) are responsive to some of the newer atypical medications but are more difficult to treat. Long-term social skills training and ongoing family and community support are essential.
- General nursing management includes establishing trust and rapport, encouraging social skills, administering medications and monitoring effects, and educating the patient and family about the illness and the therapeutic regimen.
- Personality disorders are characterized by enduring traits. The four hallmarks of personality disorders are inflexible and maladaptive response to life events, serious difficulty in personal and work relationships, a tendency to evoke interpersonal conflict, and a tendency to evoke a negative empathic response from others.
- Borderline personality disorder is the most prevalent personality disorder.
- Assess the patient's view of self and others, expression of feelings, and behaviors that are interfering with routine life and relationships.
- General nursing management of patients with personality disorders includes building trust, setting limits, teaching coping skills, preventing self-mutilation or self-harm, and encouraging insight into behavior.
- Elders who are taking antipsychotics are at a greater risk for developing extrapyramidal symptoms, tardive dyskinesia, and neuroleptic malignant syndrome. Beginning doses should be one half to one third of the normal adult dose.

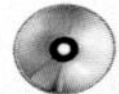

Go to your **Companion CD-ROM** for an Audio Glossary, animations, video clips, and bonus review questions.

evolve Be sure to visit the companion Evolve site at http://evolve.elsevier.com/deWit for interactive NCLEX-PN Exam Style Review Questions, WebLinks, and additional online resources.

NCLEX EXAM STYLE REVIEW QUESTIONS

Choose the best answer(s) for the following questions:

1. An elderly male patient on antipsychotic medications develops a flat affect with drooling and a shuffling gait. He has slowed movements, tremors, motor restlessness, apprehension, and irritability. An appropriate medication would be:

1. benztropine (Cogentin).
2. haloperidol (Haldol).
3. chlorpromazine (Thorazine).
4. perphenazine (Trilafon).

2. A patient states, "The people on the screen are sending me telepathic messages!" This is an example of:

1. a delusion of persecution.
2. a delusion of grandeur.
3. an idea of reference.
4. an illusion.

3. The nurse discusses the effects of a patient's antipsychotic medication. Which of the following patient statements indicates a need for further teaching?

1. "The medication helps me to think more logically."
2. "The medication makes my mouth dry. "
3. "The medication improves my memory."
4. "The medication helps to stop the voices."

4. A patient reports that he has been taking thioridazine (Mellaril) for more than 12 months. The most serious complication would be:

1. pseudo-parkinsonism.
2. tardive dyskinesia.
3. anticholinergic effects.
4. akathisia.

5. When talking with a patient who is having active hallucinations, the nurse must:
   1. assess the content and themes of hallucinations.
   2. provide immediate feedback.
   3. take the patient to a secluded area.
   4. set boundaries and explain rationale.

6. The patient is suspicious and believes that he is surrounded by terrorists. He tells the nurse, "They put anthrax in the food and there is a bomb in the bathroom." The most therapeutic response is:
   1. "Who do you think is doing all these things?"
   2. "Let's go together and check the bathroom."
   3. "Tell me why you believe these things are happening."
   4. "I believe that the hospital is a safe place."

7. A patient demonstrates negative symptoms of apathy, social isolation, and lack of motivation. To establish trust, the nurse must: *(Select all that apply.)*
   1. offer self and be available.
   2. reorient to person, place, and time.
   3. keep all promises.
   4. invite the patient to join groups.
   5. leave the door open for future interactions.
   6. encourage independence in ADLs.

8. A patient is readmitted for an acute psychotic episode. He appears to be having command hallucinations. The priority nursing diagnosis is:
   1. Disturbed sensory perception.
   2. Risk for self- or other-directed violence.
   3. Disturbed thought processes.
   4. Ineffective coping.

9. A nursing student is caring for a patient with a personality disorder. Which of the following statements indicates that the student needs additional training and education on setting boundaries?
   1. "I can spend 20 minutes talking with you and then I have to pass to medications."
   2. "I understand that you are bored, but you have to complete the task."
   3. "If you promise not to cause trouble, I'll give you the magazine."
   4. "When someone is speaking in group, it is polite to listen while they speak."

10. A student nurse realizes that a patient with borderline personality "gets under my skin." An appropriate action by the student nurse would be to:
    1. disregard the feelings.
    2. change patient assignments.
    3. talk with an experienced nurse.
    4. confront the patient.

CRITICAL THINKING ACTIVITIES  *Read each clinical scenario and discuss the questions with your classmates.*

Scenario A

You are caring for Mrs. Leiber, a 65-year-old who has a fixed delusional system with many religious overtones. You notice that she is pacing and becoming increasingly agitated. She begins to yell in a loud voice about God and salvation and not being saved.

1. How might you approach Mrs. Leiber and assist her to de-escalate?
2. What behaviors would cause you to consider physically restraining Mrs. Leiber?

Scenario B

Mr. John Hammer, a 42-year-old, was recently discharged from a psychiatric facility after an extended stay. He comes to the clinic for a renewal of his antipsychotic medications, accompanied by his elderly father, who reports that his son is noncompliant with medications and has limited social interaction.

1. What nursing interventions could increase Mr. Hammer's compliance with therapy?
2. What type of community referrals would be appropriate for this patient and his family?

Scenario C

A 32-year-old patient, Betsy Johnston, arrives at the clinic with a superficial scratch on the wrist. She begins to cry, "You are the best nurse here. You're always so kind and understanding. Would you call my boyfriend and tell him that I am here? I cut myself, because we just broke up." You know Ms. Johnston because she has been in the clinic many times with similar minor injuries. In the past, she has been manipulative and verbally abusive toward the staff.

1. What behaviors suggest that Ms. Johnston may have a personality disorder?
2. How would you respond to her request to call the boyfriend?

APPENDIX 1

Standards of Practice and Educational Competencies of Graduates of Practical/ Vocational Nursing Programs

These standards and competencies are intended to better define the range of capabilities, responsibilities, rights and relationship to other health care providers for scope and content of practical/vocational nursing education programs. The guidelines will assist:

- Educators in development, implementation, and evaluation of practical/vocational nursing curricula.
- Students in understanding expectations of their competencies upon completion of the educational program.
- Prospective employers in appropriate utilization of the practical/vocational nurse.
- Consumers in understanding the scope of practice and level of responsibility of the practical/ vocational nurse.

A. PROFESSIONAL BEHAVIORS

Professional behaviors, within the scope of nursing practice for a practical/vocational nurse, are characterized by adherence to standards of care, accountability for one's own actions and behaviors, and use of legal and ethical principles in nursing practice. Professionalism includes a commitment to nursing and a concern for others demonstrated by an attitude of caring. Professionalism also involves participation in lifelong self-development activities to enhance and maintain current knowledge and skills for continuing competency in the practice of nursing for the LP/VN, as well as individual, group, community, and societal endeavors to improve health care.

Upon completion of the practical/vocational nursing program the graduate will display the following program outcome:

Demonstrate professional behaviors of accountability and professionalism according to the legal and ethical standards for a competent licensed practical/ vocational nurse.

Competencies which demonstrate this outcome has been attained:

1. Comply with the ethical, legal, and regulatory frameworks of nursing and the scope of practice as outlined in the LP/VN nurse practice act of the specific state in which licensed.
2. Utilize educational opportunities for life-long learning and maintenance of competence.
3. Identify personal capabilities and consider career mobility options.
4. Identify own LP/VN strengths and limitations for the purpose of improving nursing performance.
5. Demonstrate accountability for nursing care provided by self and/or directed to others.
6. Function as an advocate for the health care consumer, maintaining confidentiality as required.
7. Identify the impact of economic, political, social, cultural, spiritual, and demographic forces on the role of the licensed practical/vocational nurse in the delivery of health care.
8. Serve as a positive role model within health care settings and the community.
9. Participate as a member of a practical/ vocational nursing organization.

B. COMMUNICATION

Communication is defined as the process by which information is exchanged between individuals verbally, non-verbally, and/or in writing or through information technology. Communication abilities are integral and essential to the nursing process. Those who are included in the nursing process are the licensed practical/vocational nurse and other members of the nursing and health care team, client, and significant support person(s). Effective communication demonstrates caring, compassion, and cultural awareness, and is directed toward promoting positive outcomes and establishing a trusting relationship.

Upon completion of the practical/vocational nursing program the graduate will display the following program outcome:

Effectively communicate with patients, significant support person(s), and members of the interdisciplinary health care team incorporating interpersonal and therapeutic communication skills.

Competencies which demonstrate this outcome has been attained:

1. Utilize effective communication skills when interacting with clients, significant others, and members of the interdisciplinary health team.
2. Communicate relevant, accurate, and complete information.
3. Report to appropriate health care personnel and document assessments, interventions, and progress or impediments toward achieving client outcomes.
4. Maintain organizational and client confidentiality.
5. Utilize information technology in support and communicate the planning and provision of client care.
6. Utilize appropriate channels of communication.

C. ASSESSMENT

Assessment is the collection and processing of relevant data for the purposes of appraising the client's health status. Assessment provides a holistic view of the client which includes physical, developmental, emotional, psychosocial, cultural, spiritual, and functional status. Assessment involves the collection of information from multiple sources to provide the foundation for nursing care. Initial assessment provides the baseline for future comparisons in order to individualize client care. Ongoing assessment is required to meet the client's changing needs.

Upon completion of the practical/vocational nursing program the graduate will display the following program outcome:

Collect holistic assessment data from multiple sources, communicate the data to appropriate health care providers, and evaluate client responses to interventions.

Competencies which demonstrate this outcome has been attained:

1. Assess data related to basic physical, developmental, spiritual, cultural, functional, and psychosocial needs of the client.
2. Collect data within established protocols and guidelines from various sources, including client interviews.
3. Assess data related to the client's health status, identify impediments to client progress and evaluate response to interventions.
4. Document data collection, assessment, and communicate findings to appropriate member(s) of the health care team.

D. PLANNING

Planning encompasses the collection of health status information, the use of multiple methods to access information, and the analysis and integration of knowledge and information to formulate nursing care plans and care actions. The nursing care plan provides direction for individualized care, and assures the delivery of accurate, safe care through a definitive pathway that promotes the client's and support person(s)'s progress toward positive outcomes.

Upon completion of the practical/vocational nursing program the graduate will display the following program outcome:

Collaborate with the registered nurse or other members of the health care team to organize and incorporate assessment data to plan/revise patient care and actions based on established nursing diagnoses, nursing protocols, and assessment and evaluation data.

Competencies which demonstrate this outcome has been attained:

1. Utilize knowledge of normal values to identify deviation in health status to plan care.
2. Contribute to formulation of a nursing care plan for clients with non-complex conditions and in a stable state, in consultation with the registered nurse and as appropriate in collaboration with the client or support person(s) as well as members of the interdisciplinary health care team using established nursing diagnoses and nursing protocols.
3. Prioritize nursing care needs of clients.
4. Assist in the review and revision of nursing care plans with the registered nurse to meet the changing needs of clients.
5. Modify client care as indicated by the evaluation of stated outcomes.
6. Provide information to client about aspects of the care plan within the LP/VN scope of practice.
7. Refer client as appropriate to other members of the health care team about care outside the scope of practice of the LP/VN.

E. CARING INTERVENTIONS

Caring interventions are those nursing behaviors and actions that assist clients and significant others in meeting their needs and the identified outcomes of the plan of care. These interventions are based on knowledge of the natural sciences, behavioral sciences, and past nursing experiences. Caring is the "being with" and "doing for" that assists clients to achieve the desired outcomes. Caring behaviors are nurturing, protective, compassionate, and person-centered. Caring creates and environment of hope and trust where client choices related to cultural, religious, and spiritual values, beliefs, and lifestyles are respected.

Upon completion of the practical/vocational nursing program the graduate will display the following program outcome:

Demonstrate a caring and empathic approach to the safe, therapeutic, and individualized care of each client.

Competencies which demonstrate this outcome has been attained:

1. Provide and promote the client's dignity.
2. Identify and honor the emotional, cultural, religious, and spiritual influences on the client's behalf.
3. Demonstrate caring behaviors toward the client and significant support person(s).
4. Provide competent, safe, therapeutic, and individualized nursing care in a variety of settings.
5. Provide a safe physical and psychosocial environment for the client and significant other(s).
6. Implement the prescribed care regiment within the legal, ethical, and regulatory framework of practical/vocational nursing practice.
7. Assist the client and significant support person(s) to cope with and adapt to stressful events and changes in health status.
8. Assist the client and significant other(s) to achieve optimum comfort and functioning.
9. Instruct client regarding individualized health needs in keeping with the licensed practical/vocational nurse's knowledge, competence, and scope of practice.
10. Recognize client's right to access information and refer requests to appropriate person(s).
11. Act in an advocacy role to protect client rights.

F. MANAGING

Managing care is the effective use of human, physical, financial, and technological resources to achieve the client identified outcomes while supporting organizational outcomes. The LP/VN manages care through the processes of planning, organizing, and directing.

Upon completion of the practical/vocational nursing program, the graduate will display the following program outcome:

Implement patient care, at the direction of a registered nurse, licensed physician, or dentist through performance of nursing interventions or directing aspects of care, as appropriate, to unlicensed assistive personnel (UAP).

Competencies which demonstrate this outcome has been attained:

1. Assist in the coordination and implementation of an individualized plan of care for clients and significant support person(s).
2. Direct aspects of client care to qualified UAPs commensurate with abilities and level of preparation and consistent with the state's legal and regulatory framework for the scope of practice for the LP/VN.
3. Supervise and evaluate the activities of UAPs and other personnel as appropriate within the state's legal and regulatory framework for the scope of practice for the LP/VN as well as facility policy.
4. Maintain accountability for outcomes of care directed to qualified UAPs.
5. Organize nursing activities in a meaningful and cost-effective manner when providing nursing care for individuals or groups.
6. Assist the client and significant support person(s) to access available resources and services.
7. Demonstrate competence with current technologies.
8. Function within the defined scope of practice for the LP/VN in the health care delivery system at the direction of a registered nurse, licensed physician, or dentist.

As approved and adopted by NAPNES Board of Directors May 5, 2007.

APPENDIX 2

NFLPN Nursing Practice Standards for the Licensed Practical/Vocational Nurse

"*Nursing Practice Standards*" is one of the ways that NFLPN meets the objective of its bylaws to address principles and ethics and also to meet another Article II objective, "To interpret the standards of practical (vocational) nursing."

In recent years, LPNs and LVNs have practiced in a changing environment. As LPNs and LVNs practice in expanding roles in the health care system, "*Nursing Practice Standards*" is essential reading for LPNs, LVNs, PN, and VN students and their educators, and all who practice with LPNs and LVNs.

NURSING PRACTICE STANDARDS FOR THE LICENSED PRACTICAL/VOCATIONAL NURSE

PREFACE

The Standards were developed and adopted by NFLPN to provide a basic model whereby the quality of health service and nursing service and nursing care given by LP/VNs may be measured and evaluated.

These nursing practice standards are applicable in any practice setting. The degree to which individual standards are applied will vary according to the individual needs of the patient, the type of health care agency or services, and the community resources.

The scope of licensed practical nursing has extended into specialized nursing services. Therefore specialized fields of nursing are included in this document.

THE CODE FOR LICENSED PRACTICAL/VOCATIONAL NURSES

The Code, adopted by NFLPN in 1961 and revised in 1979, provides a motivation for establishing, maintaining, and elevating professional standards. Each LP/VN, upon entering the profession, inherits the responsibility to adhere to the standards of ethical practice and conduct as set forth in this Code.

1. Know the scope of maximum utilization of the LP/VN as specified by the nurse practice act and function within this scope.
2. Safeguard the confidential information acquired from any source about the patient.
3. Provide health care to all patients regardless of race, creed, cultural background, disease, or lifestyle.
4. Uphold the highest standards in personal appearance, language, dress, and demeanor.
5. Stay informed about issues affecting the practice of nursing and delivery of health care and, when appropriate, participate in government and policy decisions.
6. Accept the responsibility for safe nursing by keeping oneself mentally and physically fit and educationally prepared to practice.
7. Accept responsibility for membership in NFLPN and participate in its efforts to maintain the established standards of nursing practice and employment policies that lead to quality patient care.

INTRODUCTORY STATEMENT

Definition

Practical/Vocational nursing means the performance for compensation of authorized acts of nursing that utilize specialized knowledge and skills and that meet the health needs of people in a variety of settings under the direction of qualified health professionals.

Scope

Licensed Practical/Vocational nurses represent the established entry into the nursing profession and include specialized fields of nursing practice.

Opportunities exist for practicing in a milieu where different professions unite their particular skills in a team effort: to preserve or improve an individual patient's functioning and to protect health and safety of patients.

Opportunities also exist for career advancement within the profession through academic education and for lateral expansion of knowledge and expertise through both academic/continuing education and certification.

STANDARDS

Education

The Licensed Practical/Vocational Nurse

1. Shall complete a formal education program in practical nursing approved by the appropriate nursing authority in a state.
2. Shall successfully pass the National Council Licensure Examination for Practical Nurses.
3. Shall participate in initial orientation within the employing institution.

Legal/Ethical Status

The Licensed Practical/Vocational Nurse

1. Shall hold a current license to practice nursing as an LP/VN in accordance with the law of the state wherein employed.
2. Shall know the scope of nursing practice authorized by the nurse practice act in the state wherein employed.
3. Shall have a personal commitment to fulfill the legal responsibilities inherent in good nursing practice.
4. Shall take responsible actions in situations wherein there is unprofessional conduct by a peer or other health care provider.
5. Shall recognize and have a commitment to meet the ethical and moral obligations of the practice of nursing.
6. Shall not accept or perform professional responsibilities that the individual knows he or she is not competent to perform.

Practice

The Licensed Practical/Vocational Nurse

1. Shall accept assigned responsibilities as an accountable member of the health care team.
2. Shall function within the limits of educational preparation and experience as related to the assigned duties.
3. Shall function with other members of the health care team in promoting and maintaining health, preventing disease and disability, caring for and rehabilitating individuals who are experiencing an altered health state, and contributing to the ultimate quality of life until death.
4. Shall know and utilize the nursing process in planning, implementing, and evaluating health services and nursing care for the individual patient or group.
    a. Planning: The planning of nursing includes:
        (1) Assessment/data collection of health status of the individual patient, the family, and community groups
        (2) Reporting information gained from assessment/data collection
        (3) The identification of health goals.
    b. Implementation: The plan for nursing care is put into practice to achieve the stated goals and includes:
        (1) Observing, recording, and reporting significant changes that require intervention or different goals
        (2) Applying nursing knowledge and skills to promote and maintain health, to prevent disease and disability and to optimize functional capabilities of an individual patient
        (3) Assisting the patient and family with activities of daily living and encouraging self-care as appropriate
        (4) Carrying out therapeutic regimens and protocols prescribed by personnel pursuant to authorized state law
    c. Evaluations: The plan for nursing care and its implementations are evaluated to measure the progress toward the stated goals and will include appropriate person and/or groups to determine:
        (1) The relevancy of current goals in relation to the progress of the individual patient
        (2) The involvement of the recipients of care in the evaluation process
        (3) The quality of the nursing action in the implementation of the plan
        (4) A re-ordering of priorities or new goal setting in the care plan
5. Shall participate in peer review and other evaluation processes.
6. Shall participate in the development of policies concerning the health and nursing needs of society and in the roles and functions of the LP/VN.

Continuing Education

The Licensed Practical/Vocational Nurse

1. Shall be responsible for maintaining the highest possible level of professional competence at all times.
2. Shall periodically reassess career goals and select continuing education activities that will help achieve these goals.
3. Shall take advantage of continuing education and certification opportunities that will lead to personal growth and professional development.
4. Shall seek and participate in continued education activities that are approved for credit by appropriate organizations, such as the NFLPN.

Specialized Nursing Practice

The Licensed Practical/Vocational Nurse

1. Shall have had at least 1 year's experience in nursing at the staff level.
2. Shall present personal qualifications that are indicative of potential abilities for practice in the chosen specialized nursing area.
3. Shall present evidence of completion of a program or course that is approved by an appropriate agency to provide the knowledge and skills necessary for effective nursing services in the specialized field.
4. Shall meet all of the standards of practice as set forth in this document.

GLOSSARY

Authorized (acts of nursing) Those nursing activities made legal through state nurse practice acts.

Lateral Expansion of Knowledge An extension of the basic core of information learned in the school of practical nursing.

Peer Review A formal evaluation of performance on the job by other LP/VNs.

Special Nursing Practice A restricted field of nursing in which a person is particularly skilled and has specific knowledge.

Therapeutic Regimens Regulated plans designed to bring about effective treatment of disease.

Career Advancement A change of career goal.

LP/VN A combined abbreviation for Licensed Practical Nurse and Licensed Vocational Nurse. The LVN is the title used in California and Texas for the nurses who are called LPNs in other states.

Milieu One's environment and surroundings.

Protocols Courses of treatment that include specific steps to be performed in a stated order.

APPENDIX 3 AHA: The Patient Care Partnership

Understanding Expectations, Rights, and Responsibilities

When you need hospital care, your physician and the nurses and other professionals at our hospital are committed to working with you and your family to meet your health care needs. Our dedicated physicians and staff serve the community in all its ethnic, religious, and economic diversity. Our goal is for your and your family to have the same care and attention we would want for our families and ourselves.

The sections explain some of the basics about how you can expect to be treated during your hospital stay. They also cover what we will need from you to care for you better. If you have questions at any time, please ask them. Unasked or unanswered questions can add to the stress of being in the hospital. Your comfort and confidence in your care are very important to us.

WHAT TO EXPECT DURING YOUR HOSPITAL STAY

HIGH-QUALITY HOSPITAL CARE

Our first priority is to provide you the care you need, when you need it, with skill, compassion, and respect. Tell your caregivers if you have concerns about your care or if you have pain. You have the right to know the identity of physicians, nurses, and others involved in your care, and you have the right to know when they are students, residents, or other trainees.

A CLEAN AND SAFE ENVIRONMENT

Our hospital works hard to keep you safe. We use special policies and procedures to avoid mistakes in your care and keep you free from abuse or neglect. If anything unexpected and significant happens during your hospital stay, you will be told what happened, and any resulting changes in your care will be discussed with you.

INVOLVEMENT IN YOUR CARE

You and your physician often make decisions about your care before you go to the hospital. Other times, especially in emergencies, those decisions are made during your hospital stay. When decision making takes place, it should include:

Discussing Your Medical Condition and Information About Medically Appropriate Treatment Choices. To make informed decisions with your physician, you need to understand:

- The benefits and risks of each treatment
- Whether your treatment is experimental or part of a research study
- What you can reasonably expect from your treatment and any long-term effects it might have on your quality of life
- What you and your family will need to do after you leave the hospital
- The financial consequences of using uncovered services or out-of-network providers

Please tell your caregivers if you need more information about treatment choices.

Discussing Your Treatment Plan. When you enter the hospital, you sign a general consent to treatment. In some cases, such as surgery or experimental treatment, you may be asked to confirm in writing that you understand what is planned and agree to it. This process protects your right to consent to or refuse a treatment. Your physician will explain the medical consequences of refusing recommended treatment. It also protects your right to decide if you want to participate in a research study.

Getting Information From You. Your caregivers need complete and correct information about your health and coverage so that they can make good decisions about your care. That includes:

- Past illnesses, surgeries, or hospital stays
- Past allergic reactions
- Any medicines or dietary supplements (such as vitamins and herbs) that you are taking
- Any network or admission requirements under your health plan

Understanding Your Health Care Goals and Values. You may have health care goals and values or spiritual beliefs that are important to your well-being. They will be taken into account as much as possible throughout your hospital stay. Make sure your physician, your family, and your care team know your wishes.

Understanding Who Should Make Decisions When You Cannot. If you have signed a health care power of attorney stating who should speak for you if you become unable to make health care decisions for yourself, or a "living will" or "advance directive" that states your wishes about end-of-life care, give copies to your physician, your family, and your care team. If you or your family need help making difficult decisions, counselors, chaplains, and others are available to help.

PROTECTION OF YOUR PRIVACY

We respect the confidentiality of your relationship with your physician and other caregivers, and the sensitive information about your health and health care that are part of that relationship. State and federal laws and hospital operating policies protect the privacy of your medical information. You will receive a Notice of Privacy Practices that describes the ways that we use, disclose, and safeguard patient information and that explains how you can obtain a copy of information from our records about your care.

PREPARING YOU AND YOUR FAMILY FOR WHEN YOU LEAVE THE HOSPITAL

Your physician works with hospital staff and professionals in your community. You and your family also play an important role in your care. The success of your treatment often depends on your efforts to follow medication, diet, and therapy plans. Your family may need to help care for you at home.

You can expect us to help you identify sources of follow-up care and to let you know if our hospital has a financial interest in any referrals. As long as you agree that we can share information about your care with them, we will coordinate our activities with your caregivers outside the hospital. You can also expect to receive information and, when possible, training about the self-care you will need when you go home.

HELP WITH YOUR BILL AND FILING INSURANCE CLAIMS

Our staff will file claims for you with health care insurers or other programs such as Medicare and Medicaid. They also will help your physician with needed documentation. Hospital bills and insurance coverage are often confusing. If you have questions about your bill, contact our business office. If you need help understanding your insurance coverage or health care plan, start with your insurance company or health benefits manager. If you do not have health care coverage, we will try to help you and your family find financial help or make other arrangements. We need your help with collecting needed information and other requirements to obtain coverage or assistance.

APPENDIX

4 Most Common Laboratory Test Values

Reference Intervals for Hematology

TEST	CONVENTIONAL UNITS	SI UNITS
Acid hemolysis (Ham test)	No hemolysis	No hemolysis
Alkaline phosphatase, leukocyte	Total score, 14–100	Total score, 14–100
Cell counts		
Erythrocytes		
Males	4.6–6.2 million/mm^3	4.6–6.2 × 10^{12}/L
Females	4.2–5.4 million/mm^3	4.2–5.4 × 10^{12}/L
Children (varies with age)	4.5–5.1 million/mm^3	4.5–5.1 × 10^{12}/L
Leukocytes, total	4500–11,000/mm^3	4.5–11.0 × 10^9/L
Leukocytes, differential counts*		
Myelocytes	0%	0/L
Band neutrophils	3–5%	150–400 × 10^6/L
Segmented neutrophils	54%–62%	3000–5800 × 10^6/L
Lymphocytes	25%–33%	1500–3000 × 10^6/L
Monocytes	3%–7%	300–500 × 10^6/L
Eosinophils	1%–3%	50–250 × 10^6/L
Basophils	0%–1%	15–50 × 10^6/L
Platelets	150,000–400,000/mm^3	150–400 × 10^9/L
Reticulocytes	25,000–75,000/mm^3 (0.5%–1.5% of erythrocytes)	25–75 × 10^9/L
Coagulation tests		
Bleeding time (template)	2.75–8.0 min	2.75–8.0 min
Coagulation time (glass tube)	5–15 min	5–15 min
D-Dimer	<0.5 mcg/mL	<0.5 mg/L
Factor VIII and other coagulation factors	50%–150% of normal	0.5–1.5 of normal
Fibrin split products (Thrombo-Welco test)	<10 mcg/mL	<10 mg/L
Fibrinogen	200–400 mg/dL	2.0–4.0 g/L
Partial thromboplastin time, activated (aPTT)	20–25 sec	20–35 sec
Prothrombin time (PT)	12.0–14.0 sec	12.0–14.0 sec
Coombs' test		
Direct	Negative	Negative
Indirect	Negative	Negative
Corpuscular values of erythrocytes		
Mean corpuscular hemoglobin (MCH)	26–34 pg/cell	26–34 pg/cell
Mean corpuscular volume (MCV)	80–96 μm^3	80–96 fL
Mean corpuscular hemoglobin concentration (MCHC)	32–36 g/dL	320–360 g/L
Haptoglobin	20–165 mg/dL	0.20–1.65 g/L
Hematocrit		
Males	40–54 mL/dL	0.40–0.54
Females	37–47 mL/dL	0.37–0.47
Newborns	49–54 mL/dL	0.49–0.54
Children (varies with age)	35–49 mL/dL	0.35–0.49
Hemoglobin		
Males	13.0–18.0 g/dL	8.1–11.2 mmol/L
Females	12.0–16.0 g/dL	7.4–9.9 mmol/L
Newborns	16.5–19.5 g/dL	10.2–12.1 mmol/L
Children (varies with age)	11.2–16.5 g/dL	7.0–10.2 mmol/L
Hemoglobin, fetal	<1.0% of total	<0.01 of total
Hemoglobin A_{1C}	3%–5% of total	0.03–0.05 of total
Hemoglobin A_2	1.5%–3.0% of total	0.015–0.03 of total

From Borer, W.Z., & McCloskey, L.J. (2007). Reference intervals for interpretation of laboratory test values. In Rakel R. *Conn's Current Therapy 2007*, Philadelphia: Saunders.

*Conventional units are percentages; SI units are absolute cell counts.

Continued

Reference Intervals for Hematology—cont'd

TEST	CONVENTIONAL UNITS	SI UNITS
Hemoglobin, plasma	0.0–5.0 mg/dL	0.0–3.2 μmol/L
Methemoglobin	30–130 mg/dL	19–80 μmol/L
Erythrocyte sedimentation rate (ESR)		
Wintrobe		
Males	0–5 mm/hr	0–5 mm/hr
Females	0–15 mm/hr	0–15 mm/hr
Westergren		
Males	0–15 mm/hr	0–15 mm/hr
Females	0–20 mm/hr	0–20 mm/hr

Reference Intervals* for Clinical Chemistry (Blood, Serum, and Plasma)

ANALYTE	CONVENTIONAL UNITS	SI UNITS
Acetoacetate plus acetone		
Qualitative	Negative	Negative
Quantitative	0.3–2.0 mg/dL	30–200 μmol/L
Acid phosphatase, serum (thymolphthalein monophosphate substrate)	0.1–0.6 U/L	0.1–0.6 U/L
ACTH (see Corticotropin)		
Alanine aminotransferase (ALT), serum (SGPT)	1–45 U/L	1–45 U/L
Albumin, serum	3.3–5.2 g/dL	33–52 g/L
Aldolase, serum	0.0–7.0 U/L	0.0–7.0 U/L
Aldosterone, plasma		
Standing	5–30 ng/dL	140–830 pmol/L
Recumbent	3–10 ng/dL	80–275 pmol/L
Alkaline, phosphatase (ALP), serum		
Adult	35–150 U/L	35–150 U/L
Adolescent	100–500 U/L	100–500 U/L
Child	100–350 U/L	100–350 U/L
Ammonia nitrogen, plasma	10–50 μmol/L	10–50 μmol/L
Amylase, serum	25–125 U/L	25–125 U/L
Anion gap, serum calculated	8–16 mEq/L	8–16 mmol/L
Ascorbic acid, blood	0.4–1.5 mg/dL	23–85 μmol/L
Aspartate aminotransferase (AST), serum (SGOT)	1–36 U/L	1–36 U/L
Base excess, arterial blood, calculated	0±2 mEq/L	0±2 mmol/L
Bicarbonate		
Venous plasma	23–29 mEq/L	23–29 mmol/L
Arterial blood	21–27 mEq/L	21–27 mmol/L
Bile acids, serum	0.3–3.0 mg/dL	0.8–7.6 mmol/L
Bilirubin, serum		
Conjugated	0.1–0.4 mg/dL	1.7–6.8 μmol/L
Total	0.3–1.1 mg/dL	5.1–19.0 μmol/L
Calcium, serum	8.4–10.6 mg/dL	2.10–2.65 mmol/L
Calcium, ionized, serum	4.25–5.25 mg/dL	1.05–1.30 mmol/L
Carbon dioxide, total, serum or plasma	24–31 mEq/L	24–31 mmol/L
Carbon dioxide tension (P_{CO_2}), blood	35–45 mm Hg	35–45 mm Hg
β-Carotene, serum	60–260 mcg/dL	1.1–8.6 μmol/L
Ceruloplasmin, serum	23–44 mg/dL	230–440 mg/L
Chloride, serum or plasma	96–106 mEq/L	96–106 mmol/L
Cholesterol, serum or EDTA plasma		
Desirable range	<200 mg/dL	<5.20 mmol/L
Low-density lipoprotein (LDL) cholesterol	60–180 mg/dL	1.55–4.65 mmol/L
High-density lipoprotein (HDL) cholesterol	30–80 mg/dL	0.80–2.05 mmol/L
Copper	70–140 mcg/dL	11–22 μmol/L
Corticotropin (ACTH), plasma, 8 A.M.	10–80 pg/mL	2–18 pmol/L
Cortisol, plasma		
8 A.M.	6–23 mcg/dL	170–630 μmol/L
4 P.M.	3–15 mcg/dL	80–410 μmol/L
10 P.M.	<50% of 8 A.M. value	<50% of 8 A.M. value
Creatine, serum		
Males	0.2–0.5 mg/dL	15–40 μmol/L
Females	0.3–0.9 mg/dL	25–70 μmol/L

*Reference values may vary, depending on the method and sample source used.

Reference Intervals for Clinical Chemistry (Blood, Serum, and Plasma)—cont'd

ANALYTE	CONVENTIONAL UNITS	SI UNITS
Creatine kinase (CK), serum		
Males	55–170 U/L	55–170 U/L
Females	30–135 U/L	30–135 U/L
Creatinine kinase MB isoenzyme, serum	<5% of total CK activity <5% of ng/mL by immunoassay	<5% of total CK activity <5% of ng/mL by immunoassay
Creatinine, serum	0.6–1.2 mg/dL	50–110 μmol/L
Estradiol-17β, adult		
Males	10–65 pg/mL	35–240 pmol/L
Females		
Follicular	30–100 pg/mL	110–370 pmol/L
Ovulatory	200–400 pg/mL	730–1470 pmol/L
Luteal	50–140 pg/mL	180–510 pmol/L
Ferritin, serum	20–200 ng/mL	20–200 mcg/L
Fibrinogen, plasma	200–400 mg/dL	2.0–4.0 g/L
Folate, serum	3–18 ng/mL	6.8–4.1 nmol/L
Erythrocytes	145–540 ng/mL	330–120 nmol/L
Follicle-stimulating hormone (FSH), plasma		
Males	4–25 mU/mL	4–25 U/L
Females, premenopausal	4–30 mU/mL	4–30 U/L
Females, postmenopausal	40–250 mU/mL	40–250 U/L
Gastrin, fasting, serum	0–100 pg/mL	0–100 mg/L
Glucose, fasting, plasma or serum	70–100 mg/dL	3.9–5.55 nmol/L
γ-Glutamyltransferase (GGT), serum	5–40 U/L	5–40 U/L
Growth hormone (hGH), plasma, adult, fasting	0–6 ng/mL	0–6 mcg/L
Haptoglobin, serum	20–165 mg/dL	0.20–1.65 g/L
β-Hydroxybutyrate	0.3–2.8 mg/dL	20–280 μmol/L
Immunoglobulins, serum (see table of Reference Intervals for Tests of Immunologic Function)		
Iron, serum	75–175 mcg/dL	13–31 μmol/L
Iron-binding capacity, serum		
Total	250–410 mcg/dL	45–73 μmol/L
Saturation	20–55%	0.20–0.55
Lactate		
Venous whole blood	5.0–20.0 mg/dL	0.6–2.2 mmol/L
Arterial whole blood	5.0–15.0 mg/dL	0.6–1.7 mmol/L
Lactate dehydrogenase (LD), serum	110–220 U/L	110–220 U/L
Lipase, serum	10–140 U/L	10–140 U/L
Lutropin (LH), serum		
Males	1–9 U/L	1–9 U/L
Females		
Follicular phase	2–10 U/L	2–10 U/L
Midcycle peak	15–65 U/L	15–65 U/L
Luteal phase	1–12 U/L	1–12 U/L
Postmenopausal	12–65 U/L	12–65 U/L
Magnesium, serum	1.3–2.1 mg/dL	0.65–1.05 mmol/L
Osmolality	275–295 mOsm/kg water	275–295 mOsm/kg water
Oxygen, blood, arterial, room air		
Partial pressure (Pa_{O_2})	80–100 mm Hg	80–100 mm Hg
Saturation (Sa_{O_2})	95%–98%	95%–98%
pH, arterial blood	7.35–7.45	7.35–7.45
Phosphate, inorganic, serum		
Adult	3.0–4.5 mg/dL	1.0–1.5 mmol/L
Child	4.0–7.0 mg/dL	1.3–2.3 mmol/L
Potassium		
Serum	3.5–5.0 mEq/L	3.5–5.0 mmol/L
Plasma	3.5–4.5 mEq/L	3.5–4.5 mmol/L
Progesterone, serum, adult		
Males	0.0–0.4 ng/mL	0.0–1.3 mmol/L
Females		
Follicular phase	0.1–1.5 ng/mL	0.3–4.8 mmol/L
Luteal phase	2.5–28.0 ng/mL	8.0–89.0 mmol/L
Prolactin, serum		
Males	1.0–15.0 ng/mL	1.0–15.0 mcg/L
Females	1.0–20.0 ng/mL	1.0–20.0 mcg/L

Continued

Reference Intervals for Clinical Chemistry (Blood, Serum, and Plasma)—cont'd

ANALYTE	CONVENTIONAL UNITS	SI UNITS
Protein, serum, electrophoresis		
Total	6.0–8.0 g/dL	60–80 g/L
Albumin	3.5–5.5 g/dL	35–55 g/L
Globulins		
α_1	0.2–0.4 g/dL	2.0–4.0 g/L
α_2	0.5–0.9 g/dL	5.0–9.0 g/L
β	0.6–1.1 g/dL	6.0–11.0 g/L
γ	0.7–1.7 g/dL	7.0–17.0 g/L
Pyruvate, blood	0.3–0.9 mg/dL	0.03–0.10 mmol/L
Rheumatoid factor	0.0–30.0 IU/mL	0.0–30.0 kIU/L
Sodium, serum or plasma	135–145 mEq/L	135–145 mmol/L
Testosterone, plasma		
Males, adult	300–1200 ng/dL	10.4–41.6 nmol/L
Females, adult	20–75 ng/dL	0.7–2.6 nmol/L
Pregnant females	40–200 ng/dL	1.4–6.9 nmol/L
Thyroglobulin	3–42 ng/mL	3–42 mcg/L
Thyrotropin (hTSH), serum	0.4–4.8 μIU/mL	0.4–4.8 mIU/L
Thyrotropin-releasing hormone (TRH)	5–60 pg/mL	5–60 ng/L
Thyroxine (FT_4), free, serum	0.9–2.1 ng/dL	12–27 pmol/L
Thyroxine (T_4), serum	4.5–12.0 mcg/mL	58–154 nmol/L
Thyroxine-binding globulin (TBG)	15.0–34.0 mcg/mL	15.0–34.0 mg/L
Transferrin	250–430 mg/dL	2.5–4.3 g/L
Triglycerides, serum, after 12-hr fast	40–150 mg/dL	0.4–1.5 g/L
Triiodothyronine (T_3), serum	70–190 ng/dL	1.1–2.9 nmol/L
Triiodothyronine uptake, resin (T_3RU)	25%–38%	0.25–0.38
Troponin I	0.05–0.50 ng/mL	0.05–0.50 ng/mL
Urate		
Males	2.5–8.0 mg/dL	150–480 μmol/L
Females	2.2–7.0 mg/dL	130–420 μmol/L
Urea, serum or plasma	24–49 mg/dL	4.0–8.2 nmol/L
Urea, nitrogen, serum or plasma	11–23 mg/dL	8.0–16.4 nmol/L
Viscosity, serum	1.4–1.8 × water	1.4–1.8 × water
Vitamin A, serum	20–80 mcg/dL	0.70–2.80 μmol/L
Vitamin B_{12}, serum	180–900 pg/mL	133–664 pmol/L

*Reference values may vary, depending on the method and sample source used.

Reference Intervals* for Therapeutic Drug Monitoring (Serum or Plasma)

ANALYTE	THERAPEUTIC RANGE	TOXIC CONCENTRATIONS	PROPRIETARY NAME(S)
Analgesics			
Acetaminophen	10–40 mcg/mL	>150 mcg/mL	Tylenol, Datril
Salicylate	100–250 mcg/mL	>300 mcg/mL	Aspirin, Bufferin
Antibiotics			
Amikacin	20–30 mcg/mL	Peak >35 mcg/mL Trough >10 mcg/mL	Amkin
Gentamicin	5–10 mcg/mL	Peak >10 mcg/mL Trough >2 mcg/mL	Garamycin
Tobramycin	5–10 mcg/mL	Peak >10 mcg/mL Trough >2 mcg/mL	Nebcin
Vancomycin	5–35 mcg/mL	Peak >40 mcg/mL Trough >10 mcg/mL	Vancocin
Anticonvulsants			
Carbamazepine	5–12 mcg/mL	>15 mcg/mL	Tegretol
Ethosuximide	40–100 mcg/mL	>250 mcg/mL	Zarontin
Phenobarbital	15–40 mcg/mL	40–100 ng/mL (varies widely)	Luminal
Phenytoin	10–20 mcg/mL	>20 mcg/mL	Dilantin
Primidone	5–12 mcg/mL	>15 mcg/mL	Mysoline
Valproic acid	50–100 mcg/mL	>100 mcg/mL	Depakene

*Values may vary depending on the method and sample collection device used. Always consult the reference values provided by the laboratory performing the analysis.

Reference Intervals for Therapeutic Drug Monitoring (Serum or Plasma)—cont'd

ANALYTE	THERAPEUTIC RANGE	TOXIC CONCENTRATIONS	PROPRIETARY NAME(S)
Antineoplastics and Immunosuppressives			
Cyclosporine	100–300 ng/mL	>400 ng/mL	Sandimmune
Methotrexate, high-dose, 48 hr	Variable	>1 μmol/L, 48 hr after dose	
Tacrolimus (FK-506), whole blood	3–20 mcg/L	>15 mcg/L	Prograf
Bronchodilators and Respiratory Stimulants			
Caffeine	3–15 ng/mL	>30 ng/mL	Elixophyllin
Theophylline (aminophylline)	10–20 mcg/mL	>30 mcg/mL	Quibron
Cardiovascular Drugs			
Amiodarone (obtain specimen more than 8 hr after last dose)	1.0–2.0 mcg/mL	>2.0 mcg/mL	Cordarone
Digoxin (obtain specimen more than 6 hr after last dose)	0.8–2.0 ng/mL	>2.4 ng/mL	Lanoxin
Disopyramide	2–5 mcg/mL	>7 mcg/mL	Norpace
Flecainide	0.2–1.0 mcg/mL	>1 mcg/mL	Tambocor
Lidocaine	1.5–5.0 mcg/mL	>6 mcg/mL	Xylocaine
Mexiletine	0.7–2.0 mcg/mL	>2 mcg/mL	Mexitil
Procainamide	4–10 mcg/mL	>12 mcg/mL	Pronestyl
Procainamide plus NAPA (*N*-acetyl procainamide)	8–30 mcg/mL	>30 mcg/mL	
Propranolol	50–100 ng/mL	Variable	Inderal
Quinidine	2–5 mcg/mL	>6 mcg/mL	Cardioquin Quinaglute
Tocainide	4–10 ng/mL	>10 ng/mL	Tonocard
Psychopharmacologic Drugs			
Amitriptyline	120–150 ng/mL	>500 ng/mL	Elavil, Triavil
Bupropion	25–100 ng/mL	Not applicable	Wellbutrin
Desipramine	150–300 ng/mL	>500 ng/mL	Norpramin
Imipramine	125–250 ng/mL	>400 ng/mL	Tofranil
Lithium (obtain specimen 12 hr after last dose)	0.6–1.5 mEq/L	>1.5 mEq/L	Lithobid
Nortriptyline	50–150 ng/mL	>500 ng/mL	Aventyl, Pamelor

Reference Intervals* for Clinical Chemistry (Urine)

ANALYTE	CONVENTIONAL UNITS	SI UNITS
Acetone and acetoacetate, qualitative	Negative	Negative
Albumin		
Qualitative	Negative	Negative
Quantitative	10–100 mg/24 hr	0.15–1.5 μmol/day
Aldosterone	3–20 mcg/24 hr	8.3–55 nmol/day
δ-Aminolevulinic acid (δ-ALA)	1.3–7.0 mg/24 hr	10–53 μmol/day
Amylase	<17 U/hr	<17 U/hr
Amylase/creatinine clearance ratio	0.01–0.04	0.01–0.04
Bilirubin, qualitative	Negative	Negative
Calcium (regular diet)	<250 mg/24 hr	<6.3 nmol/day
Catecholamines		
Epinephrine	<10 mcg/24 hr	<55 nmol/day
Norepinephrine	<100 mcg/24 hr	<590 nmol/day
Total free catecholamines	4–126 mcg/24 hr	24–745 nmol/day
Total metanephrines	0.1–1.6 mg/24 hr	0.5–8.1 μmol/day
Chloride (varies with intake)	110–250 mEq/24 hr	110–250 mmol/day
Copper	0–50 mcg/24 hr	0.0–0.80 μmol/day
Cortisol, free	10–100 mcg/24 hr	27.6–276 nmol/day

*Values may vary, depending on the method used.

Continued

Reference Intervals for Clinical Chemistry (Urine)—cont'd

ANALYTE	CONVENTIONAL UNITS	SI UNITS
Creatine		
Males	0–40 mg/24 hr	0.0–0.30 mmol/day
Females	0–80 mg/24 hr	0.0–0.60 mmol/day
Creatinine	15–25 mg/kg/24 hr	0.13–0.22 mmol/kg/day
Creatinine clearance (endogenous)		
Males	110–150 mL/min/1.73 m^2	110–150 mL/min/1.73 m^2
Females	105–132 mL/min/1.73 m^2	105–132 mL/min/1.73 m^2
Cystine or cysteine	Negative	Negative
Dehydroepiandrosterone		
Males	0.2–2.0 mg/24 hr	0.7–6.9 μmol/day
Females	0.2–1.8 mg/24 hr	0.7–6.2 μmol/day
Estrogens, total		
Males	4–25 mcg/24 hr	14–90 nmol/day
Females	5–100 mcg/24 hr	18–360 nmol/day
Glucose (as reducing substance)	<250 mg/24 hr	<250 mg/day
Hemoglobin and myoglobin, qualitative	Negative	Negative
Hemogentisic acid, qualitative	Negative	Negative
17-Hydroxycorticosteroids		
Males	3–9 mg/24 hr	8.3–25 μmol/day
Females	2–8 mg/24 hr	5.5–22 μmol/day
5-Hydroxyindoleacetic acid		
Qualitative	Negative	Negative
Quantitative	2–6 mg/24 hr	10–31 μmol/day
17-Ketogenic steroids		
Males	5–23 mg/24 hr	17–80 μmol/day
Females	3–15 mg/24 hr	10–52 μmol/day
17-Ketosteroids		
Males	8–22 mg/24 hr	28–76 μmol/day
Females	6–15 mg/24 hr	21–52 μmol/day
Magnesium	6–10 mEq/24 hr	3–5 mmol/day
Metanephrines	0.05–12 ng/mg creatinine	0.03–0.70 mmol/mmol creatinine
Osmolality	38–1400 mOsm/kg water	38–1400 mOsm/kg water
pH	4.6–8.0	4.6–8.0
Phenylpyruvic acid, qualitative	Negative	Negative
Phosphate	0.4–1.3 g/24 hr	13–42 mmol/day
Porphobilinogen		
Qualitative	Negative	Negative
Quantitative	<2 mg/24 hr	<9 μmol/day
Porphyrins		
Coproporphyrin	50–250 mcg/24 hr	77–380 nmol/day
Uroporphyrin	10–30 mcg/24 hr	12–36 nmol/day
Potassium	25–125 mEq/24 hr	25–125 mmol/day
Pregnanediol		
Males	0.0–1.9 mg/24 hr	0.0–6.0 μmol/day
Females		
Proliferative phase	0.0–2.6 mg/24 hr	0.0–8.0 μmol/day
Luteal phase	2.6–10.6 mg/24 hr	8–33 μmol/day
Postmenopausal	0.2–1.0 mg/24 hr	0.6–3.1 μmol/day
Pregnanetriol	0.0–2.5 mg/24 hr	0.0–7.4 μmol/day
Protein, total		
Qualitative	Negative	Negative
Quantitative	10–150 mg/24 hr	10–150 mg/day
Protein/creatinine ratio	<0.2	<0.2
Sodium (regular diet)	60–260 mEq/24 hr	60–260 mmol/day
Specific gravity		
Random specimen	1.003–1.030	1.003–1.030
24-hr collection	1.015–1.025	1.015–1.025
Urate (regular diet)	250–750 mg/24 hr	1.5–4.4 mmol/day
Urobilinogen	0.5–4.0 mg/24 hr	0.6–6.8 μmol/day
Vanillylmandelic acid (VMA)	1.0–8.0 mg/24 hr	5–40 μmol/day

Reference Intervals for Toxic Substances

ANALYTE	CONVENTIONAL UNITS	SI UNITS
Arsenic, urine	<130 mcg/24 hr	<1.7 μmol/day
Bromides, serum, inorganic	<100 mg/dL	<10 mmol/L
Toxic symptoms	140–1000 mg/dL	14–100 mmol/L
Carboxyhemoglobin, blood	Saturation, percent	
Urban environment	<5%	<0.05
Smokers	<12%	<0.12
Symptoms		
Headache	>15%	>0.15
Nausea and vomiting	>25%	>0.25
Potentially lethal	>50%	>0.50
Ethanol, blood	<0.05 mg/dL	<1.0 mmol/L
	<0.005%	
Intoxication	>100 mg/dL	>22 mmol/L
	>0.1%	
Marked intoxication	300–400 mg/dL	65–87 mmol/L
	0.3%–0.4%	
Alcoholic stupor	400–500 mg/dL	87–109 mmol/L
	0.4%–0.5%	
	>500 mg/dL	
Coma	>0.5%	>109 mmol/L
Lead, blood		
Adults	<20 mcg/dL	<1.0 μmol/L
Children	<10 mcg/dL	<0.5 μmol/L
Lead, urine	<80 mcg/24 hr	<0.4 μmol/day
Mercury, urine	<10 mcg/24 hr	<150 nmol/day

Reference Intervals for Tests Performed on Cerebrospinal Fluid

TEST	CONVENTIONAL UNITS	SI UNITS
Cells	<5 mm³; all mononuclear	<5 × 10^6/L, all mononuclear
Protein electrophoresis	Albumin predominant	Albumin predominant
Glucose	50–75 mg/dL (20 mg/dL less than in serum)	2.8–4.2 mmol/L (1.1 mmol/L less than in serum)
IgG		
Children <14 y	<8% of total protein	<0.08 of total protein
Adults	<14% of total protein	<0.14 of total protein
IgG index		
$\left(\frac{\text{CSF/serum IgG ratio}}{\text{CSF/serum albumin ratio}}\right)$	0.3–0.6	0.3–0.6
Oligoclonal banding on electrophoresis	Absent	Absent
Pressure, opening	70–180 mm H_2O	70–180 mm H_2O
Protein, total	15–45 mg/dL	150–450 mg/L

Reference Intervals for Tests of Gastrointestinal Function

TEST	CONVENTIONAL UNITS
Bentiromide	6-hr urinary arylamine excretion >57% excludes pancreatic insufficiency
β-Carotene, serum	60–250 ng/dL
Fecal fat estimation	
Qualitative	No fat globules seen by high-power microscope
Quantitative	<6 g/24 hr (>95% coefficient of fat absorption)
Gastric acid output	
Basal	
Males	0.0–10.5 mmol/hr
Females	0.0–5.6 mmol/hr
Maximum (after histamine or pentagastrin)	
Males	9.0–48.0 mmol/hr
Females	6.0–31.0 mmol/hr
Ratio: basal/maximum	
Males	0.0–0.31
Females	0.0–0.29
Secretin test, pancreatic fluid	
Volume	>1.8 mL/kg/hr
Bicarbonate	>80 mEq/L
D-Xylose absorption test, urine	>20% of ingested dose excreted in 5 hr

Reference Intervals for Tests of Immunologic Function

TEST	CONVENTIONAL UNITS	SI UNITS
Complement, serum		
C3	85–175 mg/dL	0.85–1.75 g/L
C4	15–45 mg/dL	150–450 mg/L
Total hemolytic (CH_{50})	150–250 U/mL	150–250 U/mL
Immunoglobulins, serum, adult		
IgG	640–1350 mg/dL	6.4–13.5 g/L
IgA	70–310 mg/dL	0.70–3.1 g/L
IgM	90–350 mg/dL	0.90–3.5 g/L
IgD	0.0–6.0 mg/dL	0.0–60 mg/L
IgE	0.0–430 ng/dL	0.0–430 mg/L
Autoantibodies, serum, adult		
Antinuclear antibody	<1:40	
Anti dsDNA antibody		0–41 IU/mL
Anti CCP	0–19 units	
Rheumatoid factor	0–30 mg/dL	

Lymphocyte Subsets, Whole Blood, Heparinized

ANTIGEN(S) EXPRESSED	CELL TYPE	PERCENTAGE (%)	ABSOLUTE CELL COUNT
CD3	Total T cells	56–77	860–1880
CD19	Total B cells	7–17	140–370
CD3 and CD4	Helper-inducer cells	32–54	550–1190
CD3 and CD8	Suppressor-cytotoxic cells	24–37	430–1060
CD3 and DR	Activated T cells	5–14	70–310
CD2	E rosette T cells	73–87	1040–2160
CD16 and CD56	Natural killer (NK) cells	8–22	130–500
Helper/suppressor ratio: 0.8–1.8			

Reference Values for Semen Analysis

TEST	CONVENTIONAL UNITS	SI UNITS
Volume	2–5 mL	2–5 mL
Liquefaction	Complete in 15 min	Complete in 15 min
pH	7.2–8.0	7.2–8.0
Leukocytes	Occasional or absent	Occasional or absent
Spermatozoa		
Count	60–150 × 10^6 mL	60–150 × 10^6 mL
Motility	>80% motile	>0.80 motile
Morphology	89–90% normal forms	>0.80–0.90 normal forms
Fructose	>150 mg/dL	>8.33 mmol/L

APPENDIX 5

Standard Precautions*

Assume that every person is potentially infected or colonized with an organism that could be transmitted in the health care setting and apply the following infection control practices during the delivery of health care. *Category 1B/1C*

A. HAND HYGIENE

1. During the delivery of health care, avoid unnecessary touching of surfaces in close proximity to the patient to prevent (1) contamination of clean hands from environmental surfaces and (2) transmission of pathogens from contaminated hands to surfaces.
2. When your hands are visibly dirty, contaminated with proteinaceous material, or visibly soiled with blood or body fluids, wash your hands with either a nonantimicrobial soap and water or an antimicrobial soap and water. *Category 1A*
3. If your hands are not visibly soiled, or after removing visible material with nonantimicrobial soap and water, decontaminate your hands. The preferred method of hand decontamination is with an alcohol-based hand rub. Alternatively, hands may be washed with an antimicrobial soap and water. Frequent use of alcohol-based hand rub immediately following handwashing with nonantimicrobial soap may increase the frequency of dermatitis. *Category 1B*

   Perform hand hygiene:
   - Before having direct contact with patients
   - After contact with blood, body fluids or excretions, mucous membranes, nonintact skin, or wound dressings
   - After contact with a patient's intact skin (e.g., when taking a pulse or blood pressure or lifting a patient)
   - If your hands will be moving from a contaminated body site to a clean body site during patient care
   - After contact with inanimate objects (including medical equipment) in the immediate vicinity of the patient
   - After removing gloves
4. Wash your hands with nonantimicrobial soap and water or with antimicrobial soap and water if contact with spores (e.g., *Clostridium difficile* or *Bacillus anthracis*) is likely to have occurred. The physical action of washing and rinsing your hands under such circumstances is recommended because alcohols, chlorhexidine, iodophors, and other antiseptic agents have poor activity against spores. *Category II*
5. Do not wear artificial fingernails or extenders if duties include direct contact with patients who are at high risk for infection and associated adverse outcomes (e.g., those in ICUs or operating rooms). *Category 1A*
   - Develop an organizational policy on the wearing of nonnatural nails by health care personnel who have direct contact with patients outside of the groups specified above.

B. PERSONAL PROTECTIVE EQUIPMENT (PPE)

Observe the following principles of use:

- Wear PPE when the nature of anticipated patient interaction indicates that contact with blood or body fluids may occur. *Category 1B/1C*
- Prevent contamination of clothing and skin during the process of removing PPE. *Category II*
- Before leaving the patient's room or cubicle, remove and discard PPE. *Category 1B/1C*

Gloves

Wear gloves when it can be reasonably anticipated that contact with blood or other potentially infectious materials, mucous membranes, nonintact skin, or potentially contaminated intact skin (e.g., of a patient incontinent of stool or urine) could occur. Wear gloves with fit and durability appropriate to the task. Wear disposable medical examination gloves for providing direct patient care. Wear disposable medical examination gloves or reusable utility gloves for cleaning the environment or medical equipment. Remove gloves after contact with a patient and/or the surrounding environment (including medical equipment) using proper technique to prevent hand contamination. Do not wear the same pair of gloves for the care of more than one patient. Do not wash gloves for the purpose of reuse since this practice has been

*Sections pertinent to adult health care nursing extracted from Siegel, J.D., Rhinehart, E., Jackson, M., et al. (2007). *Guideline for Isolation Precautions: Preventing Transmission of Infectious Agents in Healthcare Settings 2007*, Atlanta: Centers for Disease Control and Prevention.

associated with transmission of pathogens. Change gloves during patient care if your hands will move from a contaminated body site (e.g., perineal area) to a clean body site (e.g., face).

Gowns

Wear a gown that is appropriate to the task to protect skin and prevent soiling or contamination of clothing during procedures and patient care activities when contact with blood, body fluids, secretions, or excretions is anticipated. Wear a gown for direct patient contact if the patient has uncontained secretions or excretions. Remove gown and perform hand washing before leaving the patient's environment. Do not reuse gowns, even for repeated contacts with the same patient. Routine donning of gowns on entrance into a high-risk unit (e.g., ICU, NICU unit) is not indicated.

Mouth, Nose, and Eye Protection

Use PPE to protect the mucous membranes of your eyes, nose, and mouth during procedures and patient care activities that are likely to generate splashes or sprays of blood, body fluids, secretions, and excretions. Select masks, goggles, face shields, and combinations of each according to the need anticipated by the task performed. During aerosol-generating procedures (e.g., bronchoscopy, suctioning of the respiratory tract [if not using in-line suction catheters], endotracheal intubation) in patients who are not suspected of being infected with an agent for which respiratory protection is otherwise recommended (e.g., *Mycobacterium tuberculosis,* SARS, or hemorrhagic fever viruses), wear one of the following: a face shield that fully covers the front and sides of the face, a mask with attached shield, or a mask and goggles (in addition to gloves and gown).

Patient Care Equipment and Instruments/Devices

Establish policies and procedures for containing, transporting, and handling patient care equipment and instruments/devices that may be contaminated with blood or body fluids. Remove organic material from critical and semicritical instruments/devices, using recommended cleaning agents before high-level disinfection and sterilization to enable effective disinfection and sterilization processes. Wear PPE (e.g., gloves, gown), according to the level of anticipated contamination when handling patient care equipment and instruments/devices that are visibly soiled or may have been in contact with blood or body fluids.

Care of the Environment

Establish policies and procedures for routine and targeted cleaning of environmental surfaces as indicated by the level of patient contact and degree of soiling. Clean and disinfect surfaces that are likely to be contaminated with pathogens, including those that are in close proximity to the patient (e.g., bed rails, overbed tables) and frequently touched surfaces in the patient care environment (i.e., door knobs, surfaces in and surrounding toilets in patients' rooms) on a more frequent schedule compared to that for other surfaces (e.g., horizontal surfaces in waiting rooms). Use EPA-registered disinfectants that have microbiocidal (i.e., killing) activity against the pathogens most likely to contaminate the patient care environment. Use in accordance with manufacturer's instructions. Review the efficacy of in-use disinfectants when evidence of continuing transmission of an infectious agent (e.g., rotavirus, *C. difficile,* norovirus) may indicate resistance to the in-use product and change to a more effective disinfectant as indicated.

Textiles and Laundry

Handle used textiles and fabrics with minimum agitation to avoid contamination of air, surfaces, and persons. If laundry chutes are used, ensure that they are properly designed, maintained, and used in a manner to minimize dispersion of aerosols from contaminated laundry.

Safe Injection Practices

The following recommendations apply to the use of needles, cannulas that replace needles, and, where applicable, intravenous delivery systems. Use aseptic technique to avoid contamination of sterile injection equipment. Do not administer medications from a syringe to multiple patients even if the needle or cannula of the syringe is changed. Needles, cannulae, and syringes are sterile, single-use items; they should not be reused for another patient nor to access a medication or solution that might be used for a subsequent patient. Use fluid infusion and administration sets (i.e., intravenous bags, tubing, and connectors) for one patient only and dispose of appropriately after use. Consider a syringe or needle/cannula contaminated once it has been used to enter or connect to a patient's intravenous infusion bag or administration set. Use single-dose vials for parenteral medications whenever possible. Do not administer medications from single-dose vials or ampules to multiple patients or combine leftover contents for later use. If multidose vials must be used, both the needle or cannula and syringe used to access the multidose vial must be sterile. Do not keep multidose vials in the immediate patient treatment area and store in accordance with the manufacturer's recommendations; discard if sterility is compromised or questionable. Do not use bags or bottles of intravenous solution as a common source of supply for multiple patients.

Infection control practices for special lumbar puncture procedures: wear a surgical mask when placing a catheter or injecting material into the spinal canal or subdural space (i.e., during myelograms, lumbar puncture, and spinal or epidural anesthesia.

Worker Safety

Adhere to federal and state requirements for protection of health care personnel from exposure to bloodborne pathogens.

APPENDIX 6

Standard Steps for All Nursing Procedures

At the Beginning of the Procedure

Step A. *Perform the task according to protocol.*

Mentally review the steps of the task beforehand. If you are uncertain how to do a task, ask your team leader, resource nurse, instructor, or charge nurse. Plan for efficiency of time and effort while delivering safe care.

Step B. *Check the order, collect the equipment and supplies, and wash your hands.*

Verify that the procedure is to be done for the patient. Check the agency's policies and procedures manual for the accepted method of performing the procedure. Process equipment and supply charges. Take all equipment and supplies to the patient's room.

Step C. *Identify and prepare the patient.*

Greet the patient, introduce yourself, and check the patient's identification band. Use two identifiers during the identification process. Explain what you are going to do in terms the patient can understand. Elicit questions and answer clearly. Provide necessary teaching related to the procedure to be performed.

Step D. *Provide privacy and institute safety precautions; arrange the supplies and equipment.*

Close the door or curtains and drape the patient before beginning the procedure or discussing information the person might want kept confidential. Check equipment for breaks or wear and for safety. Set up the equipment and supplies in an orderly, methodical fashion. Raise the bed to an appropriate working height. Raise the side rail before turning the patient and be certain that the wheels are locked. Perform hand hygiene to prevent contaminating the patient with organisms from the chart, the nurses' station, and the supply room.

During the Procedure

Step E. *Use Standard Precautions and aseptic technique as appropriate.*

Protect yourself from blood and body fluids by wearing gloves. If there is a danger of splashing blood or body fluids, wear protective glasses or goggles and an impermeable cover gown or apron. Be very careful with sharp instruments and needles so as not to nick your skin. (See Appendix 5: Standard Precautions.)

At the End of the Procedure

Step X. *Remove gloves and other protective equipment.*

After making certain the patient is clean and dry, dispose of used supplies, remove goggles and other protective equipment, and discard or store appropriately. To remove gloves without contaminating yourself, begin by pulling one glove off without touching your skin; hold the removed glove in the palm of the remaining gloved hand and then reach to the inside of the other glove and roll it down the hand. Dispose of the gloves in the trash. Perform hand hygiene immediately.

Step Y. *Restore the unit. Collect the used equipment; dispose of, clean, or store items in the proper places.*

Make the person comfortable, tidy the bed and unit, place the call light and personal items within reach, and provide for safety by lowering the bed. Remove used equipment. Soiled linens are placed in a soiled-linen hamper. Reusable items are cleaned and returned to the storage or processing area (central supply). Discontinue use of the equipment on the computer so no further charges will be made. Remove unsightly, odorous, or potentially infectious trash from the room. Inquire if anything else is needed. Perform hand hygiene before leaving the room.

Step Z. *Record and report the procedure.*

Document assessment findings and the details of the procedure performed, or care given, in the chart. Include any problems encountered and the patient's response to the care or treatment. The recording should be accurate, specific, concise, and appropriate and should include the specific time the procedure was performed and how it was done. Report abnormalities encountered to the charge nurse or physician.

Bibliography

GENERAL RESOURCES

Ackley, B.J., & Ladwig, G.B. (2006). *Nursing Diagnosis Handbook: A Guide to Planning Care* (7th ed.). St. Louis: Mosby.

Alfaro-Lefevre, R. (2004). *Critical Thinking and Clinical Judgment* (3rd ed.). St. Louis: Elsevier.

Agency for Health Care Policy and Research. (1994). *Pressure Ulcer Treatment.* Rockville, MD: U.S. Department of Health and Human Services, Public Health Service.

American Cancer Society. (2007). *Cancer Facts and Figures 2007–2008.* Atlanta: American Cancer Society.

American Cancer Society. (2007). *Colorectal Cancer Facts & Figures.* Atlanta: American Cancer Society.

American Heart Association. (2006). *Handbook of Emergency Cardiovascular Care.* Dallas, TX: American Heart Association.

American Heart Association (Eds.). (2006). *Heart Disease and Stroke Statistics–2006 Update.* Dallas: American Heart Association.

American Pain Society. (2003). *Principles of Analgesic Use in the Treatment of Acute Pain and Cancer Pain* (5th ed.). Glenview, IL: American Pain Society.

American Psychiatric Association. (2000). *Diagnostic and Statistical Manual of Mental Disorders,* Fourth Edition, Text Revision. Washington, DC: American Psychiatric Association.

Applegate, E. (2006). *The Anatomy and Physiology Learning System* (3rd ed.). Philadelphia: Elsevier Saunders.

Arias, K.M. (2000). *Quick Reference to Outbreak Investigation and Control in Health Care Facilities.* Gaithersburg, MD: Aspen.

Bauer, B., & Hill, S. (2000). *Mental Health Nursing: An Introductory Text.* Philadelphia: Saunders.

Beers, M., & Berkow, R. (Eds.). (2005). *The Merck Manual of Diagnosis and Therapy* [Online edition]. Retrieved from www.merck.com/mrkshared/mmanual/home

Bioterrorism Institute, Ltd. (2005). *Bioterrorism Basics for Nurses CE Program.* Columbus, OH: Bioterrorism Institute.

Black, J.M., & Hawks, J.H. (2005). *Medical-Surgical Nursing: Clinical Management for Positive Outcomes* (7th ed.). Philadelphia: Elsevier Saunders.

Brooks, G.F., Butel, J.S., & Morse, S.A. (2001). *Jawetz, Melnick & Adelberg's Medical Microbiology* (22nd ed.). New York: Lange Medical Books/McGraw-Hill.

Brunicardi, F.C., Andersen, D.K., Billiar, T.R., et al. (2005). *Schwartz's Principles of Surgery* (9th ed.). New York: McGraw-Hill.

Burke, K.M., LeMone, P., & Mohn-Brown, E. (2003). *Medical-Surgical Nursing Care.* Upper Saddle River, NJ: Prentice Hall.

Carpenito-Moyet, L.J. (2005). *Nursing Diagnosis: Application to Clinical Practice* (11th ed.). Philadelphia: Lippincott Williams & Wilkins.

CDC National Center for Injury Prevention and Control (2004). *10 Leading causes of death, United States.* Retrieved from http://webapp.cdc.gov/cgi-bin/broker.exe

Centers for Disease Control and Prevention. (1992; revised 1993). Revised classification system for HIV infection and expanded surveillance case definition for AIDS among adolescents and adults. *MMRW Morbidity and Mortality Week Report,* 1992; 41(RR-17).

Centers for Disease Control and Prevention. (1998). Update: Universal precautions for prevention of transmission of human immunodeficiency virus, hepatitis B virus, and other blood-borne pathogens in health-care settings. *MMRW Morbidity and Mortality Week Report,* June 1988, 377.

Centers for Disease Control and Prevention. (2003). *HIV/AIDS surveillance report 2002.* Retrieved from www.cdc.gov/hiv/stats/hasr1302.pdf

Centers for Disease Control and Prevention. (2005). *Recommendations for isolation precautions in hospitals.* Retrieved from www.cdc.gov/ncidod/hip/ISOLAT/isopart2.htm

Christensen, B., & Kockrow, E. (2005a). *Adult Health Nursing* (5th ed.). St. Louis: Mosby.

Christensen, B., & Kockrow, E. (2005b). *Foundations of Nursing* (5th ed.). St. Louis: Mosby.

Cleri, L.B., & Haywood, R. (2002). *Oncology: Pocket Guide to Chemotherapy* (5th ed.). New York: Mosby Medical Communications.

Corbett, J.V. (2004). *Laboratory Tests and Diagnostic Procedures with Nursing Diagnosis* (6th ed.). Upper Saddle River, NJ: Prentice Hall.

Dambro, M.R. (2005). *2005 Griffith's 5-Minute Clinical Consult.* Philadelphia: Lippincott Williams & Wilkins.

DeVita, V.T., Hellman, S., & Rosenberg, S. (2001). *Cancer Principles and Practice of Oncology* (6th ed.). Philadelphia: Lippincott.

deWit, S.C. (2005). *Fundamental Concepts and Skills for Nursing* (2nd ed.). Philadelphia: Elsevier Saunders.

Dorland, I., & Newman, W.A. (2003). *Dorland's Illustrated Medical Dictionary* (30th ed.). Philadelphia: Saunders.

Ebersole, P., & Hess, P. (2004). *Toward Healthy Aging: Human Needs and Human Response* (6th ed.). St. Louis: Mosby.

Ebersole, P., Hess, P., Touhy, T., et al. (2005). *Gerontological Nursing and Healthy Aging* (2nd ed.). St. Louis: Mosby.

Ellsworth, A.J., Witt, D.M., Dugdale, D.C., et al. (2004). *Mosby's Medical Drug Reference.* St. Louis: Mosby.

Fischbach, F., & Dunning, M.B. (2006). *Common Laboratory & Diagnostic Tests* (4th ed.). Philadelphia: Lippincott Williams & Wilkins.

Fontaine, K.L. (2005). *Complementary and Alternative Therapies for Nursing Practice.* Upper Saddle River, NJ: Prentice Hall.

Fortinash, K., & Holoday-Worret, P. (2007). *Psychiatric Nursing Care Plans* (5 ed.). St. Louis: Mosby.

Frisch, N.C., & Frisch, L.E. (2006). *Psychiatric Mental Health Nursing.* Clifton Park, NY: Thomson Delmar Learning.

Giger, J.N., & Davidhizar, R.E. (2004). *Transcultural Nursing: Assessment & Interventions* (4 ed.). St Louis: Mosby.

Goldman, L., Bennet, J., & Ausiello, D. (Eds.). (2004). *Cecil Textbook of Medicine* (22nd ed.). Philadelphia: Saunders.

Gould, B.E. (2006). *Pathophysiology for the Health Professions* (3rd ed.). Philadelphia: Saunders.

Guyton, A.C., & Hall, J.E. (2005). *Textbook of Medical Physiology* (11th ed.). Philadelphia: Elsevier Saunders.

Harkreader, H., Hogan, M.A., & Thobaben, M. (2007). *Fundamentals of Nursing: Caring and Clinical Judgment* (3rd ed.). Philadelphia: Saunders.

Herlihy, B., & Maebius, N.K. (2007). *The Human Body in Health and Illness* (3rd ed.). St. Louis: Saunders.

Hill, S., & Howlett, H. (2005). *Success in Practical/Vocational Nursing: From Student to Learner* (5th ed.). Philadelphia: Elsevier Saunders.

Hodgson, B.B., & Kizior, R.J. (2008). *Saunders Nursing Drug Handbook 2008.* Philadelphia: Saunders.

Hoefler, P.A. (2004). *NCLEX-RN Exam Essentials Review* (11th ed.). Laurel, MD: Meds Publishing.

Huether, S.E., & McCance, K.L. (2008). *Understanding Pathophysiology* (4th ed.). St. Louis: Mosby.

Additional references may be found in the on-line Bibliography at http://evolve.elsevier.com/deWit. These resources are updated periodically as additional information becomes available.

Note: Some references cited in text may appear only in the General Resources and not in the list for that chapter.

Ignatavicius, D.D., & Workman, M.L. (2005). *Medical-Surgical Nursing: Critical Thinking for Collaborative Care* (5th ed.). Philadelphia: Elsevier Saunders.

Jarvis, C. (2004). *Physical Examination & Health Assessment* (4th ed.). Philadelphia: Saunders.

Joint Commission on Accreditation of Healthcare Organizations. (2003). *Universal Protocol for Preventing Wrong Site, Wrong Procedure, Wrong Person Surgery.* Chicago: The Joint Commission.

Joint National Committee on Prevention, Detection, Evaluation, and Treatment of High Blood Pressure. (2003). *The Seventh Report of the Joint National Committee on Prevention, Detection, Evaluation and Treatment of High Blood Pressure.* Available at: www.nhlbi.nih/gov/guidelines/hypertension

Kee, L.L. (2005). *Laboratory & Diagnostic Tests with Nursing Implications* (7th ed.). Upper Saddle River, NJ: Pearson Prentice Hall.

Klein, D.G., Moseley, M.J., & Sole, M.L. (2004). *Introduction to Critical Care Nursing* (4th ed.). Philadelphia: Saunders.

Kübler-Ross, E. (1969). *On Death and Dying.* New York: Macmillan.

Kumar, V., Abbas, A.K., & Fausto, N. (Eds.). (2004). *Robbins and Cotran Pathologic Basis of Disease* (7th ed.). Philadelphia: Saunders.

Lantus Prescribing Information. Retrieved from http://products.sanofi-aventis.us/lantus/lantus.html

Lehne, R.A. (2006). *Pharmacology for Nursing Care* (6th ed.). Philadelphia: Saunders.

Lewis, S.L., Heitkemper, M.M., Dirksen, S.R., et al. (2007). *Medical-Surgical Nursing: Assessment and Management of Clinical Problems* (7th ed.). St. Louis: Mosby.

Linton, A., Matteson, M., & Maebius, N. (2003). *Introduction to Medical-Surgical Nursing* (3rd ed.). Philadelphia: Saunders.

London, M., Ladewig, P., Ball, J., et al. (2007). *Maternal & Child Nursing Care* (2nd ed.). Upper Saddle River, NJ: Pearson/Prentice Hall.

Lowdermilk, D.L., & Perry, S.E. (2007). *Maternity and Women's Health Care* (8 ed.). St. Louis: Mosby.

Mahan, K., & Escott-Stump, S. (2004). *Krause's Food, Nutrition, & Diet Therapy* (11th ed.). Philadelphia: Saunders.

Malarkey, L.M., & McMorrow, M.E. (2005). *Saunders Nursing Guide to Laboratory and Diagnostic Tests.* Philadelphia: Elsevier Saunders.

Mandell, G.L., Bennett, J.E., & Dolin, R. (2005). *Mandell, Douglas, and Bennett's Principles and Practice of Infectious Disease* (6th ed.). Philadelphia: Elsevier Saunders.

Meiner, S., & Lueckenotte, A. (2005). *Gerontologic Nursing* (3rd ed.). St. Louis: Mosby.

Micozzi, M.S. (2006). *Fundamentals of Complementary and Integrative Medicine* (3rd ed.). Philadelphia: Saunders.

Monahan, F.D., Sands, J.K., Neighbors, M., et al. (2007). *Phipps Medical-Surgical Nursing: Health and Illness Perspectives* (8th ed.). St. Louis: Mosby.

Mosby's Drug Consult. (2007). (17th ed.). St. Louis: Mosby.

National Cancer Institute. (2002). *Cancer trials information.* Retrieved from www.nic.nih.gov/clinicaltrials

National Center for Biotechnology Information. (2005). Diseases of the immune system. In *Genes and Diseases.* Retrieved from www.ncbi.nlm.nih.gov/books/bv.fcgi?rid=gnd.chapter.51

National Council of State Boards of Nursing. (2005). *NCLEX-PN Examination: Test Plan for the National Council Licensure Examination for Licensed Practical/Vocational Nurses.* Chicago: National Council of State Boards of Nursing.

National Pressure Ulcer Advisory Panel. (2006b). *PUSH tool 3.0.* Retrieved from http://222.npuap.org/positn5.html

National Stroke Association. (2004). *Stroke prevention.* Retrieved from www.stroke.org/site/PageServer?pagename=PREVENT

Nevidjon, B., & Sowers, K. (2000). *A Nurse's Guide to Cancer Care.* New York: Lippincott.

Newberry, L. (Ed.). (2003). *Sheehy's Emergency Nursing: Principles & Practice* (5 ed.). St. Louis: Mosby.

Nurses' Legal Handbook. (2004). Philadelphia: Lippincott.

Office of Disease Prevention and Health Promotion. (2005). *Healthy People 2010.* Rockville, MD: U.S. Department of Health and Human Services.

O'Neill, P.A. (2002). *Caring for the Older Adult: A Health Promotion Perspective.* Philadelphia: Saunders.

O'Toole, M. (Ed.). (1997). *Miller-Keane Encyclopedia and Dictionary of Medicine, Nursing, and Allied Health* (6th ed.). Philadelphia: Saunders.

Pagana, K.D., & Pagana, T.J. (2008). *Mosby's Diagnostic and Laboratory Test Reference* (9th ed.). St. Louis: Elsevier Mosby.

Perry, A.G., & Potter, P.A. *Clinical Nursing Skills and Techniques.* (6th ed.). St. Louis: Mosby.

Phipps, W.J., Monahan, F., Sands, J., et al. (2003). *Medical-Surgical Nursing: Health and Illness Perspectives* (7th ed.) St. Louis: Mosby.

Preusser, B.A. (2005). *Winningham & Preusser's Critical Thinking in Medical-Surgical Settings: A Case Study Approach* (3rd ed.). St. Louis: Mosby.

Price, S.A., & Wilson, L.M. (2003). *Pathophysiology: Clinical Concepts of Disease Processes* (6th ed.). St. Louis: Mosby.

Psychiatric Nursing Made Incredibly Easy!, (2004). Philadelphia: Lippincott.

Purnell, L.D., & Paulanka, B.J. (2003). *Transcultural Health Care: A Culturally Competent Approach* (2nd ed.). Philadelphia: Davis.

Rinehart, W., Sloan, D., & Hurd, C. (2005). *Exam Cram: NCLEX-PN.* Indianapolis: Que Publishing.

Roth, J.J., & Hughes, W.B. (2004). *The Essential Burn Unit Handbook.* St. Louis: Quality Medical Publishing, Inc.

Rothrock, J.C. (2007). *Alexander's Care of the Patient in Surgery* (13th ed.). St. Louis: Mosby.

Scott, J., Gibbs, R., Karlan, B., et al. (Eds.). *Danforth's Obstetrics and Gynecology* (9 ed.). Philadelphia: Lippincott Williams & Wilkins.

Skidmore-Roth, L. (2006). *Mosby's Handbook of Herbs & Natural Supplements* (3rd ed.). St. Louis: Mosby.

Skidmore-Roth, L. (2009). *Mosby's Nursing Drug Reference.* St. Louis: Elsevier Mosby.

Smeltzer, S.C., Bare, B.G. Hinkle, J.L., et al. (2006). *Brunner & Suddarth's Textbook of Medical-Surgical Nursing* (11th ed.). Philadelphia: Lippincott Williams & Wilkins.

Snyder, M., & Lindquist, R. (2006). *Complementary/Alternative Therapies in Nursing* (5th ed.). New York: Springer.

Spratto, G.R., & Woods, A.L. (2004). *PDR Nurse's Drug Handbook.* Clifton Park, NY: Delmar Learning.

Stanhope, M., & Lancaster, J. (Eds.). (2004). *Community and Public Health Nursing* (6th ed.). St Louis: Mosby.

Stuart, G.W., & Laraia, M.T. (2005). *Principles and Practice of Psychiatric Nursing.* St. Louis: Elsevier Mosby.

Swearingen, P.L. (2004). *All-in-One Care Planning Resource: Medical-Surgical, Pediatric, Maternity, and Psychiatric Nursing Care Plans.* St. Louis: Mosby.

Thibodeau, G.A., & Patton, K.T. (2005). *The Human Body in Health & Disease* (4th ed.). St. Louis: Elsevier Mosby.

Ulrich, S.P., & Canale, S.W. (2005). *Nursing Care Planning Guides for Adults in Acute, Extended and Home Care Settings* (6th ed.). Philadelphia: Saunders.

U.S. Department of Health and Human Services. (2000). Healthy People 2010. *With understanding and improving health and objectives for improving health* (2nd ed.). Washington, DC: U.S. Department of Health and Human Services.

U.S. Department of Health and Human Services. (2002). *Disasters and emergencies.* Retrieved from www.hhs.gov/disasters/index.shtml

U.S. Department of Health and Human Services, Centers for Disease Control and Prevention. (2005). *National Diabetes Fact Sheet: General Information and National Estimates on Diabetes in the United States.* Atlanta, GA: USDHHS. Retrieved from www.diabetes.org/uedocuments/NationalDiabetesFactSheetRev.pdf

U.S. Department of Health and Human Services, National Center for Health Statistics. (2007). *Health, United States.* Retrieved from www.cdc.gov/nchs/hus.htm

Varcarolis, E.M. (2004). *Manual of Psychiatric Nursing Care Plans.* Philadelphia: Saunders.

Varcarolis, E.M. (2006). *Foundations of Psychiatric Mental Health Nursing: A Clinical Approach* (5 ed.). Philadelphia: Saunders.

Weber, J., & Kelley, J. (2007) *Health Assessment in Nursing* (3rd ed.). Philadelphia: Lippincott Williams & Wilkins.

Wenzel, R.P. (2003). *Prevention and Control of Nosocomial Infections* (4th ed.). Philadelphia: Lippincott Williams & Wilkins.

Wilkinson, J.M. (2005). *Prentice Hall Nursing Diagnosis Handbook with NIC Interventions and NOC Outcomes* (8th ed.). Upper Saddle River, NJ: Prentice Hall.

Zerwekh, J., & Claborn, J. (2007). *Illustrated Study Guide for the NCLEX-PN* (5th ed.). St. Louis: Mosby.

Chapter 1

Carey, B. (2005). In the hospital, a degrading shift from person to patient. *The New York Times,* August 16, 2005. Retrieved from www.nytimes.com/2005/08/16/health/16dignity.html?th=&emc=th&pagewanted=print

Centers for Medicare and Medicaid Services. (2006). *Medicare and you.* Washington, DC: U.S. Department of Health and Human Services.

Consumer Reports reader survey ranks top PPOs, HMOs based on satisfaction. (2005). *Kaiser Daily Health Policy Report,* August 12. Retrieved from www.kaisernetwork.org/daily_reports/print_report.cfm?DR_ID=31989&dr_cat=3

Fink, J. (2005). The power of low-tech nursing. *RN, 68*(6), 43–45.

Gullickson, C. (2005). Nursing in the gray zone. *Nursingmatters, 16*(9), 14.

Hansten, R., & Jackson, M. (2004). *Clinical Delegation Skills* (3rd ed.). Sudbury, Mass: Jones and Bartlett.

Hathaway, L. (2005). Safely delegating to unlicensed assistive personnel. *LPN 2005, 1*(5), 13–14.

Medicaid: A Primer. (2006). Washington, DC: The Kaiser Commission on Medicaid and the Uninsured.

National Council of State Boards of Nursing. (2005b). *Working with others: A position paper.* Chicago: National Council of State Boards of Nursing. Retrieved from www.ncsbn.org

Porter, B. (2005). 6 things I learned when Mom was ill. *RN, 68*(7), 43–45.

Seago, J.A., Spetz, J., Chapman, S., et al. (2004). *Supply, demand, and use of licensed practical nurses. National Center for Health Workforce Analysis.* Retrieved from bhpr.hrsa.gov/healthworkforce/reports/lpn/LPN1_5.htm

Spector, N. (2005). *Practical nurse scope of practice* [White Paper]. Chicago: National Council of State Boards of Nursing. Retrieved from www.ncsbn.org

Chapter 2

Alfaro-Lefevre, R. (2004). *Critical thinking indicators.* Retrieved from www.AlfaroTeachSmart.com

Del Bueno, D. (2005). A crisis in critical thinking. *Nursing Education Perspectives, 26,* 278–282.

Spector, N. (2005a). Focus group on licensed practical nurse scope of practice at National Council of State Boards of Nursing. *JONA's Healthcare Law, Ethics and Regulation, 7,* 1–13.

Spector, N. (2005b). *Practical nurse scope of practice* [White Paper]. Chicago: National Council of State Boards of Nursing. Retrieved from www.ncsbn.org

Turner, P. (2005). Critical thinking in nursing education and practice as defined in the literature. *Nursing Education Perspectives, 26,* 272–277.

Chapter 3

Anderson, R. (2005). When to use a midline catheter. *Nursing2005, 35*(4), 28.

Astle, S.M. (2005). Restoring electrolyte balance. *RN, 68*(5), 34–39.

Bixby, M. (2006). Third-spacing: Where has all the fluid gone? *Nursing Made Incredibly Easy!,* 4(5), 42–53.

Goertz, S. (2006). Gauging fluid balance with osmolality. *Nursing2006, 36*(10), 70–71.

Gorski, L.A., & Czaplewski, L.M. (2004). Peripherally inserted central catheters. *Home Healthcare Nurse, 22,* 758–771.

Gorski, L.A., & Czaplewski, L.M. (2005). Managing complications of midlines and PICCs. *Nursing2005, 35*(6), 68–69.

Hadaway, L.C. (2004). Preventing and managing peripheral extravasation. *Nursing2004, 34*(5), 66–67.

Hadaway, L.C. (2006). Keeping central line infection at bay. *Nursing2006, 36*(4), 58–63.

Hayes, D.D. (2004a). Balancing act. *Nursing Made Incredibly Easy!, 2*(1), 52–57.

Hayes, D.D. (2004b). Magnesium's balancing act. *Nursing Made Incredibly Easy!,* 2(4), 44–49.

Hayes, D.D. (2004c). Phosphorus: Here, there, everywhere. *Nursing Made Incredibly Easy!,* 2(6), 36–41.

Krueger, A. (2007). Need help finding a vein? *Nursing2007, 37*(6), 39–41.

Marders, J. (2005). Sounding the alarm for I.V. infiltration. *Nursing2005, 35*(4), 19–20.

Miller, J. (2006). K Potassium in the balance: Understanding hyperkalemia and hypokalemia. *LPN2006, 2*(5), 43–49.

Mills, L.S.E. (2005). Don't forget to drink the water. *LPN2005, 1*(4), 10–13.

Moureau, N.L. (2004). Tips for inserting an I.V. in an older patient. *Nursing2004, 34*(7), 18.

Nursing Made Incredibly Easy! Eds. (2004). Calcium in the balance. *Nursing Made Incredibly Easy!,* 2(2), 47–53.

O'Neill, P. (2007). Helping your patient to restrict potassium. *Nursing2007, 37*(4), 64hn6–64hn8.

Posthauer, M.E. (2006). Hydration: An essential nutrient. *Advances in Skin & Wound Care, 18*(1), 32.

Quillen, T.F. (2005). . . . About hypercalcemia. *Nursing2005, 35*(7), 74.

Rosenthal, K. (2004). What you should know about needleless I.V. systems. *Nursing2004, 34*(9), 76.

Rosenthal, K. (2005a). Documenting peripheral I.V. therapy. *Nursing2005, 35*(7), 28.

Rosenthal, K. (2005b). Initiating intravenous therapy. *LPN2005, 1*(3), 4–10.

Rosenthal, K. (2005c). Providing safe CVAD site care. *LPN2005, 1*(4), 5–9.

Rosenthal, K. (2006a). Navigating safely through a minefield of CVD complications. *Nursing Made Incredibly Easy!,* 4(1), 56–58.

Rosenthal, K. (2006b). When your patient develops phlebitis. *Nursing2006, 36*(2), 14.

Rosenthal, K. (2006c). The whys and wherefores of I.V. fluids. *Nursing Made Incredibly Easy!,* 4(3), 8–11.

Rosenthal, K. (2007a). Reducing the risks of infiltration and extravasation. *Nursing2007, 37*(9), 4–8.

Rosenthal, K. (2007b). Totally TPN. *Nursing Made Incredibly Easy!, 5*(5), 59–62.

Sudakin, T. (2006). Supporting nutrition with T.E.N. or T.P.N. *Nursing2006, 36*(12), 52–55.

Woodruff, D.W. (2006). Take these 6 easy steps to ABG analysis. *Nursing Made Incredibly Easy!,* 4(1), 4–7.

Chapter 4

Adamow, S.M. (2004). The OR of tomorrow. *ADVANCE for Nurses,* 2(5), 19–20.

Armstrong, M. (2004). Caring for the patient with piercings. *RN, 67*(6), 46–52.

Barzoloski-O'Connor, B. (2007). Infection control: From scrub to rub: Hand hygiene in the OR. *OR Nurse, 1*(1), 10–12.

Carter-Templeton, H. (2006). Awake to danger: Temperature rising. *Nursing Made Incredibly Easy!,* 4(4), 10–11.

Dixon, B.A., & O'Donnell, J.M. (2006). Is your patient susceptible to malignant hyperthermia? *Nursing2006, 36*(12), 26–27.

Domrose, C. (2005). Senior surgery: Outcomes improving for elderly patients. *NurseWeek, 13*(22), 10–11.

Dunn, D. (2006). Age-smart care: Preventing perioperative complications in older adults. *Nursing Made Incredibly Easy!,* 4(3), 30–39.

Evans, S. (2006a). Paging Doctor Robot! *ADVANCE for Nurses,* 3(14), 25–26.

Evans, S. (2006b). Sterile field. *ADVANCE for Nurses, 3*(22), 12–14.

Evans, S., (Ed.). (2007). Perfect harmony: Music therapy eases anxiety and pain in the perioperative setting. *ADVANCE for Nurses, 4*(2), 25–26.

Evans, T. (2000). Neuromuscular blockage: When and how. *RN, 63*(5), 56–59.

Goodman, T. (2005). Pressure damage in surgery. *ADVANCE for Nurses, 2*(11), 37–41.

Halliday, A.B. (2006). Shades of sedation: Learning about moderate sedation and analgesia. *Nursing2006, 36*(4), 37–41.

Keefe, S. (2005). Cell salvaging. *ADVANCE for Nurses, 2*(8), 17–19.

LPN2006 Eds. (2006). You're a witness: Know your role in obtaining informed consent. *LPN2006, 2*(4), 15–16.

Mace, S. (2006). Keeping count: "Radio tags" help eliminate retained foreign bodies. *NurseWeek, 19*(22), 14–15.

Nursing2007 Eds. (2007). How herbal products increase surgical risks. *Nursing2007, 37*(9), 24–25.

Odom-Forren, J. (2006). Winning the battle against surgical site infections. *LPN2006, 2*(3), 44–47.

OE Magazine Eds. (2005). Medical history made with robot surgical assistant. *OE Magazine,* June 23, 2005. Retrieved from oemagazine.com/newscast/s005/062305_newscast01.html

Perry, K., & Jagger, J. (2005). Pass with care in the OR. *Nursing2005, 35*(2), 70.

Schwartz, A.J. (2006). Learning the essentials of epidural anesthesia. *Nursing2006, 36*(1), 44–49.

Schweon, S. (2006). Stamping out surgical site infections. *RN, 69*(8), 36–40.

Smydra, K.E., & Votodian, A.M. (2007). Perioperative management of obese patients. *ADVANCE for Nurses,* 4(2), 21–24.

Tabor, W. (2007). On the cutting edge of robotic surgery. *Nursing2007, 37*(2), 48–50.

Chapter 5

Agency for Healthcare Research and Quality. (2005). Pain management is often inadequate for elderly patients hospitalized for surgery. *Agency for Healthcare Research and Quality Bulletin, 296*(4), 16–17.

Appleby, S.L., Eberhard, M.H., & Spears, M.A. (2007). A home care wound care challenge. *Home Healthcare Nurse, 25*(6), 362–368.

Barclay, L., & Lie, D. (2004). Electroacupuncture helpful for postoperative nausea and vomiting. *Medscape Medical News,* September 29, 2004. Retrieved from www.medscape.com/viewarticle/489936?src=mp

Beattie, S. (2007). Wound dehiscence. *RN,* 70(6), 34–37.

Cofer, M.J. (2005). Unwelcome companion to older patients: Postoperative delirium. *Nursing2005, 35*(1), 32hn1–32hn3.

Crum, E. & Valenti, J. (2007). Can a bloodless surgery program work in the trauma setting? *Nursing2007, 37*(3), 54–56.

D'Arcy, Y. (2006). Managing postop pain in a patient who's delirious. *Nursing2006, 36*(6), 17.

Day, M.W. (2005). Pulmonary embolism. *Nursing2005, 35*(9), 88.

Doughty, D.B. (2004). Preventing and managing surgical wound dehiscence. *Home Healthcare Nurse, 22*(6), 365–367.

Dunn, D. (2004). Preventing perioperative complications in older adults. *Nursing2004, 34*(11), 36–41.

Hess, C.T. (2005). The art of skin and wound care documentation. *Home Healthcare Nurse, 23*(8), 502–514.

Hunter, S., Thompson, P., Langermo, D., et al. (2007). Understanding wound dehiscence. *Nursing2007, 37*(9), 28–30.

Keefe, S. (2005). Postoperative ileus. *ADVANCE for Nurses,* 2(14), 26–27.

Mabrey, M.E. (2004). Using insulin to prevent hyperglycemia in surgical patients. *Nursing2004, 34*(10), 22.

Moz, T. (2004). Wound dehiscence and evisceration. *Nursing2004,* 34(5), 88

Nursing2007 Eds. (2007). Scopolamine: Putting a patch on postop nausea. *Nursing2007, 37*(1), 30.

RN Eds. (2005). Reduce surgical infection: A step-by-step guide. *RN, 68*(5), 32hf1–32hf2.

Sarvis, C. (2007). Postoperative wound care. *LPN2007, 3*(5), 34–38.

Waresak, M. (2004). Reducing postprocedure emesis. *Nursing2004, 34*(6), 28.

Wilson, J.A., & Clark, J.J. (2004). Obesity: Impediment to postsurgical wound healing. *Advances in Skin & Wound Care, 17*(8), 426–432.

Chapter 6

Batazy, A., Toivola, M., Adhikari, A., et al. (2006). Do N95 respirators provide 95% protection level against airborne viruses, and how adequate are surgical masks? *American Journal of Infection Control, 34*(2), 51–57.

Boyce, J.M., & Pittet, D. (2002). Guidelines for hand hygiene in healthcare settings: Recommendations of the Healthcare Infection Control Practices Advisory Committee and the HICPAC/SHEA/APIC/IDSA Hand Hygiene Task Force. Infection Control and Hospital *Epidemiology, 23*(12 Suppl), S3–S40.

Brunicardi, F.C., Andersen, D.K., Billiar, T.R., et al. (2005). *Schwartz's Principles of Surgery* (9th ed.). New York: McGraw-Hill.

Centers for Disease Control and Prevention. (2002). Guidelines for the prevention of intravascular catheter-related infections. *MMWR Recommended Reports, 51*(RR-10), 1–26.

Chettle, C.C. (2007). *P. Aeruginosa* proves to be a tough foe. *NurseWeek, 20*(11), 14–16.

Chettle, C.C. (2007). Are you prepared for a flu pandemic? *NurseWeek, 20*(2), 16–18.

Chettle, C.C. (2006). Life-threatening fungal infections on the rise. *NurseWeek, 19*(8), 19–20.

Coughlin, A.M. (2007). Combating community-acquired pneumonia. *Nursing2007,* 64hn1–64hn3.

D'Alessandro, M. (2007). Scrub, scrub, rub: Hand-rub dispensers will have a new home in health facility hallways. *Advance Newsmagazine for LPNs.* Retrieved from http://lpn.advanceweb.com/common/Edial/PrintFriendly.aspx?CC=84618

Davey, V.J. (2007). Questions and answers on pandemic influenza. *American Journal of Nursing, 107*(7), 50–55.

Fenstermaker, L. (2007). Community-associated MRSA. *ADVANCE for Nurses, 4*(7), 17–19.

Nursing2007 Eds. (2007). Does a high WBC count always signal infection? *Nursing2007, 37*(5), 56hn15–56hn16.

Nursing Made Incredibly Easy! Eds. (2007). Vancomycin: Champion against drug-resistant infection. *Nursing Made Incredibly Easy!, 5*(5), 23–27.

Oriola, S. (2006). *C. difficile:* A menace in hospitals and homes alike. *Nursing2006, 36*(8), 14–15.

Perry, J., & Jagger, J. (2005). Sharps safety update: "Are we there yet?" *Nursing2005,* 17.

Rutala, W.A. (Ed.). (2004). *Disinfection, Sterilization and Antisepsis: Principles, Practices, Challenges, and New Research.* Washington, DC: APIC.

Safdar, S., & Maki, D.F. (2005). Risk of catheter-related bloodstream infection with peripherally inserted central venous catheters used in hospitalized patients. *Chest, 128,* 489–495.

Smith, N. (2007). Campaign targets stealthy sepsis. *NurseWeek, 20*(6), 12–13.

Todd, B. (2007). Outbreak: *E. coli O157:H7. American Journal of Nursing, 107*(2), 29–32.

Valente, S.M. (2007). Keep *C. difficile* infection at bay. *Nursing2007,* 37(10), 56hn1–56hn2.

Vos, M.C., & Verbrugh, H.A. (2005). MRSA: We can overcome, but who will lead the battle? *Infection Control and Hospital Epidemiology, 26*(2), 117–120.

Walker, B. W. (2007). New guidelines for fighting multidrug-resistant organisms. *Nursing2007, 37*(5), 20.

Chapter 7

Agency for Healthcare Research and Quality: National Clearinghouse Guidelines (2006). *Clinical practice guideline for the management of postoperative pain.* Retrieved from www.guidelines.gov/summary/summary.aspx?doc-id+3284&nbr=0025 10&string=hea+AND=therap

American Pain Society. (2003). *Principles of Analgesic Use in the Treatment of Acute Pain and Cancer Pain* (5th ed.). Glenview, IL: American Pain Society.

Arnstein, P. (2006). Placebos: No relief for Ms. Mahoney's pain. *American Journal of Nursing, 106*(2), 54–65.

D'Arcy, Y. (2005). Pain management standards, the law, and you. *Nursing2005, 35*(4), 17.

D'Arcy, Y. (2007a). Managing pain with nonpharmacologic therapies. *LPN2007I, 3*(5), 10–13.

D'Arcy, Y. (2007b). New pain management options: Delivery systems and techniques. *Nursing2007, 37*(2), 26.

D'Arcy, Y. (2007c). Safe pain relief at the push of a button. *Nursing Made Incredibly Easy!, 5*(5), 9–12.

D'Arcy, Y. (2007d). Taking a new look at NSAIDs. *LPN2007, 3*(3), 11–13.

D'Arcy, Y. (2007e). The fentanyl patch: Convenient, effective pain control. *LPN2007, 3*(3), 4–5.

D'Arcy, Y. (2007f). Using the WHO analgesic ladder to choose pain medication. *LPN2007, 3*(2), 4–7.

French, D.D., Cameron, M. (2006). *Superficial heat and cold for low back pain.* Retrieved from www.clinicalevidence.com/ceweb/conditions/msd/1103-114.jsp#REF12

Joint Commission on Accrediation of Healthcare Orgnizations. (2004). *Pain assessment and management standards.* Retrieved from www.jcaho.org

Keller, D.L. (2006). Pain relievers. *RN, 69*(4), 22–28.

Lipson, G., Dibble, S.L., & Minarik, P.A. (Eds.). (1996). *Culture & Nursing Care: A Pocket Guide.* San Francisco: UCSF Nursing Press.

Malkowski, M.G., Mielenz, T., & Wang, J.H.C. (2007). Regulating mood to lessen pain. *Agency for Healthcare Quality and Research Bulletin, 319,* 5–6.

McCaffery, M., & Pasero, C. (1999). *Pain: Clinical Manual* (2nd ed.). St. Louis: Mosby.

McCaffery, M., & Pasero, C. (2003). Breakthrough pain: It's common in patients with chronic pain. *American Journal of Nursing, 73*(4), 83–85.

McCarberg, B., & O'Connor, A. (2007). *A new look at heat treatment for pain disorders,* part 1. Retrieved from www.ampainsoc.org/pub/bulletin/nov04/innol.htm

Manworren, R.C.B. (2006). A call to action to protect range orders. *American Journal of Nursing, 106*(7), 65–68.

O'Connor, A., & McCarberg, B. (2005). *A new look at heat treatment for pain disorders, part 2.* Retrieved from www.ampainsoc.org/but/bulletin/wino4inno1.htm

Pasero, C. (2007). IV opioid range orders for acute pain management. *American Journal of Nursing, 107*(2), 52–59.

Pasero, C., & McCaffery, M. (2004). Comfort-function goals: A way to establish accountability for pain relief. *American Journal of Nursing, 74*(9), 77–81.

Perret, D.M., Rim, J., & Christian, A. (2006). A geriatrician's guide to the use of physical modalities in the treatment of pain dysfunction. *Clinics in Geriatric Medicine, 22*(2), 331.

Vallerand, A.H., Hasenau, S.M., & Templin, T. (2004). Barrriers to pain management. *Home Healthcare Nurse, 22,* 831–840.

Wentz, J.D. (2003a). Assessing pain at the end of life. *Nursing2003, 33*(8), 22.

Wentz, J.D. (2003b). Understanding neuropathic pain. *Nursing2003, 33*(1), 22.

Wheeler, M.S. (2006). Pain assessment and management in the patient with mild to moderate cognitive impairment. *Home Healthcare Nurse, 24,* 354–359.

Chapter 8

Bingley, A.F., McDermott, E., Thomas, C., et al. (2006). Making sense of dying: A review of narratives written since 1950 by people facing death from cancer and other diseases. *Palliative Medicine, 20,* 183–195.

Bloch, A., Cassileth, B.R., Holmes, M.D., et al. (Eds.). (2004). *Eating Well, Staying Well During and After Cancer.* Atlanta: American Cancer Society.

Byock, I. (1997). *Dying Well: The Prospect for Growth at the End of Life.* New York: Riverhead Books.

Callanan, M., & Kelley, P. (1997). *Final Gifts: Understanding the Special Awareness, Needs, and Communications of the Dying.* New York: Simon & Schuster.

Cash, J.C. (2006). Changing paradigms: Intensity modulated radiation therapy. *Seminars in Oncology Nursing, 22*(4), 242–248.

Cigna, J.A. (2007). Home care physical therapy for the cancer patient. *Home Healthcare Nurse, 25*(3), 158–161.

Davison, D. (2006). Oral mucositis. *Clinical Journal of Oncology Nursing, 10,* 283–284.

Dest, V. (2006). Cancer therapies. *RN, 69*(6), 31–36.

Duggleby, W., & Raudonis, B.M. (2006). Dispelling myths about palliative care and older adults. *Seminars in Oncology Nursing, 22*(1), 58–63.

Eilberg, A. (2006). Facing life and death: spirituality in end-of-life care. *Journal of Jewish Communal Service,* Spring, 157–162.

Evans, R.C., & Rossner, A.L. (2005). Alternatives in cancer pain treatment: The application of chiropractic care. *Seminars in Oncology Nursing, 21*(3), 184–189.

Fabbro, D.E., Dalal, S., Bruera, E., et al. (2006). Symptom control in palliative care—Part II: Cachexia/anorexia and fatigue. *Journal of Palliative Medicine, 9,* 409–421.

Gift, A.G. (2007). Symptom clusters related to specific cancers. *Seminars in Oncology Nursing, 23*(2), 136–141.

Goldwein, J.W., & Somer, B. (2006). BiologicTherapies. OncoLink: Abramson Cancer Center of the University of Pennsylvania. Retrieved from www.Oncolink.com

Haylock, P.J., Mitchell, S.A., Cox, T., et al. (2007). The cancer survivor's prescription for living. *American Journal of Nursing, 107*(4), 58–70.

Hester, D. (2006) The quiet man: A dying patient reminded me of why I became a nurse. *Nursing, 36*(4), 64cc5–64cc5, 1p.

Hogle, W.P. (2006). The state of the art in radiation therapy. *Seminars in Oncology Nursing, 22*(4), 212–220.

Hynes, R. (2007). Finding the words: When a nurse understands grief. *American Journal of Nursing, 107*(5), 88.

Kemp, C. (2005). Cultural issues in palliative care. *Seminars in Oncology Nursing, 21*(1), 44–52.

Kinlaw, K. (2005). Ethical issues in palliative care. *Seminars in Oncology Nursing, 21*(1), 63–68.

Kornmehl, C.L. (2007). *The value of exercise during radiation therapy for breast and prostate cancer.* Retrieved from www.articlealley.com/article_134929_23.html

Kramer, K. (2005). You cannot die alone (interview of Dr. Elisabeth Kübler-Ross, 1990). *Omega, 50,* 83–101.

Kübler-Ross, E. (1969). *On Death and Dying.* New York: Macmillan.

Langemo, D., Anerson, J., Hanson, D., et al. (2007). Understanding palliative wound care. *Nursing2007,* 65–66.

Lu, W. (2005). Acupuncture for side effects of chemoradiation therapy in cancer patients. *Seminars in Oncology Nursing, 21*(3), 190–195.

Lynch, M.P. (2005). *Essentials of Oncology Care.* New York: Professional Publishing Group, Ltd.

Marangolo, M., Bengala, C., Conte, P.F., et al. (2006). Dose and outcome: The hurdle of neutropenia [Review]. *Oncology Reports, 16*(2), 233–248.

Maritess, C., Small, S. & Waltz-Hill, M. (2005). Alternative nutrition therapies in cancer patients. *Seminars in Oncology Nursing, 21*(3), 173–176.

Meyskens, F.L., & Tully, P. (2005). Principles of cancer prevention. *Seminars in Oncology Nursing, 21*(4), 229–235.

Milligan, L. (2006). Epidemiology & cancer. *ADVANCE for Nurses, 3*(13), 15–17.

National Cancer Institute. (2006). *Biological therapies for cancer: Questions and answers.* Retrieved from www.cancer.gov/cancertopics/biologicaltherapy

National Cancer Institute. (2006). *Eating hints for cancer patients: Before, during, and after treatment.* Retrieved from www.cancer.gov/cancertopics/eatinghints/page3#C10

Perez, C. (2007). *Aromatherapy helps heal cancer patients.* Retrieved from http://link.dhn.bottomlinesecrets.com

Peters, L., & Sellick, K. (2006). Quality of life of cancer patients receiving inpatient and home-based palliative care. *Journal of Advanced Nursing, 53*, 524–533.

Phillips, J.M. & Williams-Brown, S. (2005). Cancer prevention among racial ethnic minorities. *Seminars in Oncology Nursing, 21*(4), 278–285.

Rich, S. (2005). Providing quality end-of-life-care. *Journal of Cardiovascular Nursing, 20*, 141–145.

Rosenfield, R.L., & Stahl, D. (2006). Pain management of bone metastases in breast cancer. *Journal of Hospice & Palliative Nursing, 8*, 233–244.

Rutledge, D.N., & Kuebler, K.K. (2005). Applying evidence to palliative care. *Seminars in Oncology Nursing, 21*(1), 36–43.

Sapir, R., Cetane, R., Kaufman, B., et al. (2000). Cancer patient expectations of and communication with oncologists and oncology nurses: The experience of an integrated oncology and palliative care service. *Supportive Care in Cancer, 8*, 458–463.

Schofield, P., Carey, M., Love, A., et al. (2006). "Would you like to talk about your future treatment options?" Discussing the transition from curative cancer treatment to palliative care. *Palliative Medicine, 20*, 397–406.

Shaw, G. (2006). Pharmacogenomics for chemotoxicity. *Drug Discovery and Development, 9*(2), 10.

SIGN breast cancer guideline. (2006). *Practice Nurse, 31*(2), 10.

Smith, J.J., Tully, P., & Padberg, R.M. (2005). Chemoprevention: A primary cancer prevention strategy. *Seminars in Oncology Nursing, 21*(4), 243–251.

Springhouse Eds. (2006). *Nursing2006 Drug Handbook.* Springhouse, Pa: Springhouse.

Stagg, D. (2007). Luke's last day. *ADVANCE for Nurses, 4*(13), 55.

Steffey-Stacy, E.C. (2006). Frameless, image-guided stereotactic radiosurgery. *Seminars in Oncology Nursing, 22*(4), 221.

Taylor, E.J. (2005). Spiritual complementary therapies in cancer care. *Seminars in Oncology Nursing, 21*(3), 159–163.

Treasure, J. (2005). Herbal medicine and cancer: An introductory overview. *Seminars in Oncology Nursing, 221*(3), 177–183.

Wetherbee, S.L. (2006). New weapons to snuff out kidney cancer. *Nursing2006, 36*(12), 59–63.

Chapter 9

Algase, D., Beel-Bates, C., & Beattie, E. (2003). Wandering in long-term care. *Annals of Long-term Care, 11*(1), 33–39.

Arango-Lasprilla, J.C., & Niemeier, J. (2007). Cultural issues in the rehabilititation of TBI survivors: Recent research and new frontiers. *Journal of Head Trauma Rehabilitation, 22*(2), 73–74.

Banotai, A. (2006). Safe swallowing. *ADVANCE for Nurses, 3*(11), 24.

Baranoski, S. (2006). Pressure ulcers: A renewed awareness. *Nursing2006, 36*(8), 36–41.

Cowles, L. (2006). The first step. *ADVANCE for Nurses*, 3(12), 10–12.

De la Plata, C.M., Hewlitte, M., de Oliveira, A., et al. (2007). Ethnic differences in rehabilitation placement and outcome after TBI. *Journal of Head Trauma Rehabilitation, 22*(2), 113–121.

Fang Yu, T.R. (2005). Factors affecting outpatient rehabilitation outcomes in elders. *Journal of Nursing Scholarship, 37*, 229–236.

James, E. (2006). Steps toward recovery. *ADVANCE for Nurses*, 3(11), 25–26.

Keefe, S. (2005). No limits: Taking a total rehabilitation nursing focus to the client's doorstep. *ADVANCE for Nurses, 2*(20), 38–39.

London, F. (2006). When the patient refuses to learn self-care skills. *Home Healthcare Nurse, 24*, 17–18.

Luggen, A.S. (2003). Arthritis in older adults: Current therapy with self-management as centerpiece. *ADVANCE for Nurse Practitioners, 11*(3), 26–35.

Powers, S.E. (2006). The family caregiver program. *Home Healthcare Nurse*, 24(8), 513–516.

Rubenstein, L., & Trueblood, P. (2004). Gait and balance assessment in older persons. *Annals of Long-term Care, 12*(2), 39–46.

Theodus, P. (2003). Fall prevention in frail elderly nursing home residents. A challenge to case management: Part I. *Lippincott's Case Management, 8*(6), 246–251.

Chapter 10

Beers, M., & Berkow, R. (Eds.). (2005). *The Merck Manual of Diagnosis and Therapy* [Online edition]. Retrieved from www.merck.com/mrkshared/mmanual/home

Carlock, C. (2007). Thimerosal, vaccines, and ethical interventions. *NurseWeek, 20*(10), 38.

Dell, D., & Doll, C. (2006). Caring for a patient with lymphedema. *Nursing2006, 36*(6), 49–51.

Dulak, S.B. (2006). Stop the assault on skin in HIV. *RN, 69*(6), 25–29.

Durston, S. (2006). Caring for the immunocompromised patient. *LPN2006, 2*(4), 31–37.

Hayden, M.L. (2004). In defense of the body: How the immune system protects us from harm. *Nursing Made Incredibly Easy!*, 2(3), 30–37.

Nowlin, A. (2005). The promise of stem cells. *RN, 68*(4), 48–52.

Rosenthal, K. (2005). A jump start for the immune system. *Nursing Made Incredibly Easy!, 3*(6), 10–12.

Rosenthal, K. (2006). Administering immune globulin. *Nursing2006, 36*(3), 20–21.

U.S. Department of Health and Human Services. (2003). *Understanding the Immune System: How It Works* (NIH Publication No. 03-5423). Bethesda, Md: U.S. Department of Health and Human Services.

Chapter 11

Botwinik, J. J., & Kessenich, C. R. (2006). Systemic lupus ergythematosus: An overview. *ADVANCE Magazine for LPNs.* Retrieved from lpn.advanceweb.com/common/editorial/PrintFriendly.aspx?CC=79537

Centers for Disease Control and Prevention. (2003). *HIV/AIDS surveillance report 2002.* Retrieved from www.cdc.gov/hiv/stats/hasr1302.pdf

Centers for Disease Control and Prevention. (2006a). *CDC trials of pre-exposure prophylaxis for HIV prevention.* Retrieved from www.cdc.gov/hiv/resources/factsheets/prep.htm

Centers for Disease Control and Prevention. (2006b). *A glance at the HIV/AIDS epidemic.* Retrieved from www.cdc.gov/hiv/resources/factsheets/At-A-Glance.htm

Centers for Disease Control and Prevention. (2007). *Factsheet: HIV and its transmission.* Retrieved from www.cdc.gov/hiv/resources/factsheets

Cibulka, N.J. (2006). Mother-to-child transmission of HIV in the United States. *American Journal of Nursing, 106*(7), 56–63.

Dell, D.D., & Doll, C. (2006). Caring for a patient with lymphedema. *Nursing2006, 36*(6), 49–51.

De Santis, J. (2006). HIV/AIDS update. *ADVANCE for Nurses, 3*(7), 15–19.

Dulak, S.B. (2006). Stop the assault on skin in HIV. *RN, 69*(6), 25–27.

Durston, S. (2006). Caring for the immunocompromised patient. *LPN2006, 2*(4), 31–37.

Enrique, M., & McKinsey, D. (2004). Readiness for HIV treatment. *American Journal of Nursing, 104*(10), 81–84.

Hayden, M.L. (2004). In defense of the body. *Nursing Made Incredibly Easy!*, 2(3), 30–39.

Hayden, M.L. (2005). The itchy, runny, sneezy misery of allergic rhinitis. *Nursing Made Incredibly Easy!*, 3(2), 64.

Keefe, S. (2006). Home HIV testing. *ADVANCE for Nurses, 3*(14), 32–33.

Kirton, C. (2005). The HIV/AIDS epidemic: A case of good news, bad news. *Nursing Made Incredibly Easy!, 3*(2), 29–41.

Lymphoma Information Network. (2005). *How is Hodgkin's lymphoma and the non-Hodgkin's lymphomas different?* Retrieved from www.lymphomainfo.net/lymphoma/comparison.html

National Center for Biotechnology Information. (2005). Diseases of the immune system. In *Genes and Diseases.* Retrieved from www.ncbi.nlm.nih.gov/books/bv.fcgi?rid=gnd.chapter.51

Nowlin, A. (2005). The promise of stem cells. *RN, 68*(4), 48–52.

Nutankalva, L., McNeil, J.I., Reddy, R.B. (2004). *Gender differences in cancers in HIV-infected patients.* (Posler, H-1765). Presented at the 44th Interscience Conference on Antimicrobia Agents and Chemotherapy. Retrieved from www.thebodypro.com/confs/ic22c2004/print/hoffman4.html

Rosenthal, K. (2005). A jump start for the immune system. *Nursing Made Incredibly Easy!, 3*(6), 10–12.

U.S. Department of Health and Human Services. (2003). *Understanding the immune system how it works* (NIH Publication No. 03-5423). Washington, D.C.: U.S. Department of Health and Human Services.

Chapter 12

Ayers, D.M., & Lappin, J.S. (2004). Act fast when your patient has dyspnea. *Nursing2004, 34*(7), 36–41.

Beattie, S. (2006). Back to basics with O_2 therapy. *RN, 69*(9), 37–40.

Centers for Disease Control and Prevention. (2005). Guidelines for using the QuantiFERON-TB gold test for detecting *Mycobacterium tuberculosis* infection, United States. *MMWR 2005 54*(No. RR-15), 1–47.

Centers for Disease Control and Prevention. (2007a). Guidelines for preventing the transmission of *Mycobacterium tuberculosis* in health-care setting, *MMWR, 54*(RR17), 1-141.

Centers for Disease Control and Prevention. (2007b). *2007-08 Recommendations of the Advisory Committee on Immunization Practices (ACIP).* Retrieved from www.cdc/flu/professionals/vaccination/#ACIP10-08-2007

Farquhar, S.L., & Fantasia, L. (2005). Pulmonary anatomy and physiology and the effects of COPD. *Home Healthcare Nurse, 23,* 167–175.

Hughes, N.L. (2006). Respiratory protection, Part 2. *American Journal of Nursing, 106*(2), 88–89.

McCarron, K. (2006). Take a deep breath: Assessing atelectasis. *LPN2006, 2*(3), 20–25.

McCormick, M. (2007). Every breath you take: Making sense of breath sounds. *Nursing Made Incredibly Easy!,* 5(1), 7–9.

Nursing Made Incredibly Easy!, Eds. (2007). Take a look inside the lungs with bronchoscopy. *Nursing Made Incredibly Easy!,* 5(2), 11–12.

Nursing2007 Eds. (2007). Smoking cessation. *Nursing2007, 37*(5), 57–58.

Pruitt, W.C. (2005). Teaching your patient to use a peak flowmeter. *Nursing2005, 35*(3), 54–55.

Rushing, J. (2006). Assisting with thoracentesis. *Nursing2006,* 36(12), 18.

Rushing, J. (2007). Obtaining a throat culture. *Nursing2007,* 37(3), 20.

Smith, S.K. (2005). Is your patient getting enough oxygen? *LPN2005, 1*(2), 10–12.

Chapter 13

Aung, K., Ojha, A., & Lo, C. (2005). *Pharyngitis, viral.* Retrieved from www.emedicine.com/topic1812.htm

Centers for Disease Control and Prevention. (2007). *CDC urges hospitals and healthcare facilities to increase efforts to reduce drug-resistant infections.* Retrieved from www.cdc.gov/od/oc/media/pressrel/4061019.htm?s_cid=mediarel_r061019_x

Dixon, B., & Tasota, F.J. (2003). Inadvertent tracheal decannulation. *Nursing2003, 33*(1), 96.

Graf, P., Hallen H., & Juto, J. E. (1995). Benzalkonium chloride in a decongestant nasal spray aggravates rhinitis medicamentosa in healthy volunteers. *Clinics of Experimental Allergy,* 25(5), 395–400.

Harvard Reports on Cancer Prevention. (1996). *Volume 1: Human causes of cancer: Environmental pollution.* Retrieved from www.hsph.harvard.edu/cancer/resources_materials/reports/HCCPreport_1environmental.htm

Iqbal, N., Lo, S., Frazier, A.J., et al. (2006). *Laryngeal carcinoma.* Retrieved from www.emedicine.com/radio/topic384.htm

Mayo Foundation for Medical Education and Research (2006). *Strep throat.* Retrieved from http://health.yahoo.com/topic/infectiousdisease/overview/article/mayoclinic/7A8C6CBF-246F-423C-9D9F889E25F2EE05

Mossad, S.B., Macknin, M.L., Medendorp, S.V., et al. (1996). Zinc gluconate lozenges for treating the common cold. A randomized, double-blind, placebo-controlled study. *Annals of Internal Medicine, 125*(2), 81–88.

National Reye's Syndrome Foundation. (2005). *What is the role of aspirin.* Retrieved from www.reyessyndrome.org/aspirin.htm

Pruitt, W.C. (2004). The ins and outs of tracheostomy care. *Nursing Made Incredibly Easy!,* 2(6), 58–62.

Schiech, L. (2007). Looking at laryngeal cancer. *Nursing2007, 37*(5), 50–55.

Seckel, M.A. (2005). All about airways. *ADVANCE for Nurses,* 2(1), 23, 28.

Warltier, D. C., ed., Marret, E., Flahault, A., et.al. (2003). Effects of postoperative, nonsteroidal antiinflammatory drugs on bleeding risk after tonsillectomy meta-analysis of randomized, controlled trials. *Anesthesiology, 98*(6), 1497–1502.

Chapter 14

Abboud, R.T. (1992). The effect of postural drainage positioning on ventilation homogeneity in healthy subjects. *Physical Therapy.* Retrieved from www.thefreelibrary.com_/print/PrintArticle.aspx?id+12920110

Agnes, K., & Condon, M. (2006). Tuberculosis guidelines update. *American Journal of Nursing, 106*(6), 104.

American Lung Association. (2005). *Search LungUSA.* Retrieved from www.lungusa.org/site/apps/s/content.asp

American Lung Association. (2006a). *Occupational lung disease fact sheet.* Retrieved from www.lungusa.org/pp.asp?c=dvLUK90oE&b=34334

American Lung Association. (2006b). *Pneumonia.* Retrieved from www.lungusa.org/site/apps/s/content.asp?c=dvLUK90OE&b=34706&ct=67310

Anders, K. (2004). Chest drainage to go. *Nursing2004, 34*(5), 54–55.

Ayers, D.M.M., & Lappin, J.S. (2004). Act fast when your patient has dyspnea. *Nursing2004, 34*(7), 36–41.

Barclay, L. (2004). *Acid-suppressive therapy may increase risk of community-acquired pneumonia.* Retrieved from www.medscape.com/viewarticle/492096

Barclay, L. & Lie, D. (2004). *ACCP revises guidelines for prevention of thomboembolism.* Retrieved from www.medscape.com/viewarticle/48942

Barclay, L., & Vega, C. (2004). *Acid-suppressive therapy may increase risk of community-acquired pneumonia.* Retrieved from www.medscape.com/viewarticle/492096

Borkovec, T.D., & Costello, E. (1993). Efficacy of applied relaxation and cognitive—behavioral therapy in the treatment of generalized anxiety disorder. *Journal of Consulting and Clinical Psychology, 61*(4), 611–619.

Canaday, P., & Collins, J. (2004). *Asthma.* Retrieved from www.emedicinehealth.com/articles/asthma

Carroll, C.M. (2005). Helping your patients manage adult-onset asthma. *LPN2005, 1*(2), 28–37.

Carroll, P. (2005). Keeping up with mobile chest drains. *RN,* 68(10), 27–31.

Centers for Disease Control and Prevention. (2001). *Severe acute respiratory syndrome (SARS).* Retrieved from www.cdc.gov/ncidod/sars/faq.htm

Centers for Disease Control and Prevention. (2005a). *Avian flu facts for travelers.* Retrieved from www.cdc.gov/travel/other/avian_flu/key_facts_travelers_notice.htm

Centers for Disease Control and Prevention. (2005b). *Frequently asked questions about SARS.* Retrieved from www.cdc.gov/ncidod/sars/faq.htm

Centers for Disease Control and Prevention. (2006). *West Nile virus (WNV) infection: Information for clinicians.* Retrieved from www.cdc.gov/westnile/resources/fact_sheet_clinician.htm

Centers for Disease Control and Prevention. (2007). *Antibiotic/antimicrobial resistance.* Retrieved from www.cdc.gov/drugresistance/prevtips.htm

Chaulk, C.P., & Kazandjian, V.A. (1998). Directly observed therapy for treatment completion of pulmonary tuberculosis. *The Lancet, 355*(9212), 1345–1350.

Chulay, M. (2005). VAP prevention: The latest guidelines. *RN, 68*(3), 52–56.

Cigna, J.A., & Turner-Cigna, L.M. (2005). Rehabilitation for the home care patient with COPD. *Home Healthcare Nurse, 23*, 578–585.

Coughlin, A.M. (2005a). Let's clear the air about suctioning. *LPN2005, 1*(6), 42–45.

Coughlin, A.M. (2005b). Tips for preventing and treating influenza. *LPN2005, 1*(3), 6–10.

Coughlin, A.M. (2006). Go with the flow of chest tube therapy. *Nursing2006, 36*(3), 36–39.

Covey, M.K. (2004). Exercise and COPD. *American Journal of Nursing, 104*(5), 40–43.

D'Arcy, Y. (2005). Easing pain from blunt thoracic trauma. *Nursing2005, 35*(12), 17.

Dest, V.M. (2006). Lung cancer: The battle continues. *RN*, 69(11), 30–35.

Domrose, C. (2006). Stemming the tide: Diligence is key in treating TB. *NurseWeek, 19*(25), 8–9.

Edmondson, D. (2007). Smoke out lung cancer. *Nursing Made Incredibly Easy!, 5*(2), 42–52.

eMedicine Health. (2005). *Lung cancer overview.* Retrieved from www.emedicinehealth.com/articles/15405-a.asp

FDA. (2007). *FDA approves novel medication for smoking cessation.* Retrieved from www.fda.gov/bbs/topics/NEWS/2006?NEW01370.html

Frankes, M.A., & Evans, T. (2004). TB—your vigilance is vital. *RN, 67*(11), 30–35.

Gallo, C.M. (2005). Plant the seeds of success for smoking cessation. *Nursing2005, 35*(9), 68–70.

Gavaghan, S.R., & Jeffries, M. (2006). Your patient's receiving noninvasive positive-pressure ventilation. *Nursing2006, 36*(5), 46–48.

Gerontologic Nursing Center. (2004). Excerpt from Guyatt, G., Schunemann, H.J., Cook, D., et al. (2004). Applying the grades of recommendation for antithrombotic and thrombolytic therapy. *Chest 2004, 12*, 179S–187S.

Goldrick, B.A. (2005). Update: Tuberculosis in the United States. *American Journal of Nursing, 105*(7), 85–86.

Goodwin, R. S. (2007). *Prevention of aspiration pneumonia: A research-based protocol.* Retrieved from www.neurosy.org/disease/aspiration/pneu.shtml

Gronkiewicz, C. (2007). Women face special lung cancer risks. *NurseWeek, 20*(4), 16–18.

Gross, P.A., Hermogenes, A.W., Sacks, H.S., et al. (1995). The efficacy of influenza vaccine in elderly persons. A meta-analysis and review of the literature. *Annals of Internal Medicine, 123*(7), 518–527.

Holcomb, S.S. (2006). The stuffy head blues. *Nursing Made Incredibly Easy!, 4*(2), 64.

Holcolmb, S.S. (2007). When your patient has pneumonia. *Nursing2007, 37*(6), 43cc1–48cc3.

Hughes, N. (2006). Respiratory protection, Part I. *American Journal of Nursing, 106*(1), 96.

Jacobs, M. (2005). Ease the stress of managing ARDS. *Nursing Made Incredibly Easy!, 3*(1), 6–18.

Jacobs, M., & Meyer, T. (2006).The push is on in pulmonary hypertension. *Nursing Made Incredibly Easy!, 4*(3), 42–51.

Lawson, P. (2005). Zapping VAP with evidence-based practice. *Nursing2005, 35*(5), 66–67.

Lindgren, V.A., & Ames, N.J. (2005). Caring for patients on mechanical ventilation. *American Journal of Nursing, 105*(5), 50–60.

Liu, P.T., Stenger, S., Li, H., et al. (2006). Toll-like receptor triggering of a vitamin D-mediated human antimicrobial response. *Science*, 10(11), 1126.

Manno, M.S. (2005). Managing mechanical ventilation. *Nursing2005, 35*(12), 36–41.

McCarron, K. (2006a). Puzzled about the state of airlessness? *Nursing Made Incredibly Easy!*, 4(1), 60–63.

McCarron, K. (2006b). Take a deep breath: Assessing atelectasis. *LPN2006, 2*(3), 20–25.

McCarron, K. (2007). Solving the puzzle of bronchospasm. *Nursing Made Incredibly Easy!, 5*(1), 20–25.

McCormick, M. (2007). Every breath you take: Making sense of breath sounds. *Nursing Made Incredibly Easy!*, 5(1), 7–10.

Mesothelioma Research Foundation of America. (2005). *Mesothelioma causes.* Retrieved from www.mesorfa.org/about-meso/causes.php

Munro, S.A., Lewin, S.A., Smith, H.J., et al. (2007). *Patient adherence to tuberculosis treatment: A systematic review of qualitiative research.* Retrieved from www.medscape.com/viewarticle/560907

National Center for Health Statistics. (2006). *Chronic obstructive pulmonary disease (COPD).* Retrieved from www.cdc.gov/nchs/fastats/copd.htm

National Human Genome Research Institute. (2006). *Learning about cystic fibrosis.* Retrieved from www.genome.gov/pfv.cfm?pageID=10001213

National Institute of Allergy and Infectious Diseases (NIAID). (2005). *NIAID researchers show how promising TB drug works.* Retrieved from www.niaid.nih.gov/news/newsreleases/2005/tb_pa_824.htm

Nursing Made Incredibly Easy! Eds. (2005). Need to get something off your chest? *Nursing Made Incredibly Easy!, 2*(2), 55–57.

Nursing Made Incredibly Easy! Eds. (2006). Skin deep: Screening for TB. *Nursing Made Incredibly Easy!, 4*(2), 5–9.

Pruitt, B. (2005). Keeping respiratory syncytial virus at bay. *Nursing2005, 35*(11), 62–64.

Pruitt, B. (2006a). Best practice interventions: How you can prevent ventilator-associated pneumonia. *Nursing2006, 36*(2), 36–41.

Pruitt, B. (2006b). Weaning patients from mechanical ventilation. *Nursing2006, 16*(9), 36–41.

Pruitt, B. (2007a). Clearing the air with chest tubes. *LPN2007, 3*(5), 50–55.

Pruitt, B. (2007b). Fending off influenza. *Nursing2007*, 37(10), 44–47.

Pruitt, W.C. (2003). Basics of oxygen therapy. *Nursing2003, 33*(10), 43–45.

Pruitt, W.C. (2004). Manual ventilation by one or two rescuers. *Nursing2004, 34*(11), 43–45.

Pruitt, W.C. (2005a). Teaching your patient to use a peak flowmeter. *Nursing2005, 35*(3), 54–55.

Pruitt, W.C. (2005b). Why is this patient coughing up blood? *Nursing Made Incredibly Easy!, 2*(3), 50–53.

Puhan, M.A., Scharplatz, M., Troosters, T., et al. (2005). Respiratory rehabilitation after acute exacerbation of COPD may reduce risk for readmission and mortality—A systematic review. *Respiratory Research*, 6(54), 6–54.

Roiter, G. (2005). Sarcoidosis: Scattered symptoms make detection difficult. *NurseWeek, 18*(17), 24–25.

Rushing, J. (2006). Using bag-valve-mask ventilation. *Nursing2006, 36*(1), 72.

Science. (2006). *How you can successfully treat TB without drugs.* Retrieved fro www.mercola.com/s006/mar/18_03/18/2006

Sharma, S. (2004a). *Chronic obstructive pulmonary disease.* Retrieved from www.emedicine.com/med/topic373.htm

Sharma, S. (2004b). *Emphysema.* Retrieved from www.emedicine.com/med/topic373.htm

Sheff, B. (2005a). Avian influenza: Are you ready for a pandemic? *Nursing2005, 35*(9), 26–27.

Sheff, B. (2005b). Connecting the DOTS to treat pulmonary TB. *Nursing2005, 35*(10), 24–25.

Sheff, B. (2006). *Haemophilus influenzae* type B (Hib). *Nursing2006, 36*(1), 31.

Smith, S. (2005). Is your patient getting enough oxygen? *LPN2005, 1*(2), 10–13.

Todd, B. (2006). The QuantiFERON-TB gold test. *American Journal of Nursing, 106*(6), 33–34, 37.

Weichel, A.S. (2000). *Antimycobacterial therapy for tuberculosis.* Retrieved from www.findarticles.com/p/articles/mi_m3225/is_3_61/ai_59480939

Chapter 15

Beattie, S. (2007). Bone marrow aspiration and biopsy. *RN, 70*(2), 41–43.

Ferrell, B.R., et al. (1996). Bone tired: The experience of fatigue and impact on quality of life. *Oncology Nursing Forum, 23,* 1539–1547.

McCarron, K. (2007). Clues in the blood: Know your CBCs. *Nursing Made Incredibly Easy!,* 5(3), 13–17.

Chapter 16

Agency for Healthcare Research and Quality. (2001). *Chronic renal failure, epoetin for anemia.* Retrieved from www.ahrq.gov/clinic/to/epcrftp.htm

American Pain Association. (1999). *Guideline for the Management of Acute and Chronic Pain in Sickle-Cell Disease.* Glenville, IL: American Pain Association.

British Columbia Ministry of Health. (2006). *Investigation & Management of B_{12} and Folate Deficiency.* Victoria, BC: Guidleines & Protocols Advisory Committee.

Burrus, N. (2005). Managing the risks of thrombocytopenia. *Nursing2005, 35*(6), 32hn1–32hn5.

Conrad, M.E. (2005). *Iron deficiency anemia.* Retrieved from www.emedicine.com/med/topic1188.htm

Conrad, M.E. (2005). *Pernicious anemia.* Retrieved from www.emedicine.com/med/topic1799.htm

Dorman, K. (2005). Sickle cell crisis! Managing the pain. *RN, 68*(12), 33–36.

Evans, S. (2006). The hard cell. *ADVANCE for Nurses, 3*(19), 30–32.

Francis, J.L. (2005). Striking back at heparin-induced thrombocytopenia. *Nursing2005, 35*(9), 48–51.

Holcomb, S.S. (2005). Anemia. *Nursing2005, 35*(3), 53.

Knippen, M.A. (2006). Transfusion-related acute lung injury. *American Journal of Nursing, 106*(6), 61–62.

Kyles, D. (2007). Is your patient having a transfusion reaction? *Nursing2007, 37*(4), 64hn1–64hn3.

Levi, M., & ten Cate, H. (1999). Disseminated intravascular coagulation. *New England Journal of Medicine, 341*(8), 586–592.

Mangan, P. (2006). Teach your patient about multiple myeloma. *Nursing2006, 6*(4), 64hn1–64hn4.

Mank, A., & Van der Lelie, H. (2003). Is there still an indication for nursing patients with prolonged neutropenia in protective isolation? An evidence-based nursing and medical study of 4 years experience for nursing patients with neutropenia without isolation. *European Journal of Oncology Nursing, 7*(1), 17–23.

Montoya, V.L., Wink, D., & Sole, M.L. (2005). Anemia: What lies beneath. *Nursing Made Incredibly Easy!, 2*(1), 37–45.

Moz, T. (2006). It's in the blood: Helping your anemic patients thrive. *LPN2006, 2*(1), 42–47.

Munson, B.L. (2004). . . . About idiopathic thrombocytopenic purpura. *Nursing2004, 34*(11), 76.

Munson, B.L. (2005). . . . About polycythemia vera. *Nursing2005, 35*(5), 28.

National Heart, Lung, and Blood Institute. (2005). *Clinical alert: Drug treatment for sickle cell anemia.* Retrieved from www.nlm.nih.gov/databases/alerts/sickle_cell.html

Paper, R. (2003). Can you recognize and respond to von Willebrand disease? *Nursing2003, 33*(7), 54–56.

Pfadt, E., & Carlson, D.S. (2005). Transfusion-associated graft-versus-host disease. *Nursing2005, 35*(2), 88.

Platt, A., & Beasley, J. (2005). Puzzled about sickle-cell disease? *Nursing Made Incredibly Easy!, 3*(6), 60–64.

Robinson, P. (2005). Is surgery safe for a patient with hemophilia? *Nursing2005, 35*(5), 32hn1–32hn3.

Rogers, B. (2005). Looking at lymphoma & leukemia. *Nursing2005, 35*(7), 56–63.

Rushing, J. (2006). Assisting with bone marrow aspiration and biopsy. *Nursing2006, 36*(3), 68.

Shelton, B.K. (2003). Evidence-based care for the neutropenic patient with leukemia. *Seminars in Oncology Nursing, 19*(2), 133–141.

Taher, A., & Kazzi, Z. (2005). *Anemia, sickle cell.* Retrieved from www.emedicine.com/emerg/topic26.htm

Trent, J.T., & Kirsner, R.S. (2004). Leg ulcers in sickle cell disease. *Advances in Skin & Wound Care, 37,* 410–414.

Woodruff, D.W. (2006). Dangerous drug interactions: HIT: Now you see 'em, now you don't. *Nursing Made Incredibly Easy!, 4*(1), 53–55.

Wu, L., & Martinez, J.(2005). *Leukemias.* Retrieved from www.emedicine.com/oph/topic489.htm

Chapter 17

American Diabetes Association. (2001). *Standards of medical care for patients with diabetes mellitus.* Retrieved from www.medscape.comviewarticle/412643

Arbor Clinical Nutrition Updates (Ed.). (2006). Vitamin D and cardiovascular disease. *254,* 1–3. Retrieved from www.arbor-com.com

Brooks, L. (2007). *New guidelines for treatment of hypertension in the prevention and management of ischemic heart disease.* Retrieved from www.medscape.com/viewarticle/448277

Cushman, M. (2005). Leukocyte count in vascular risk prediction. *Archives of Internal Medicine, 165*(5), 487–488.

Dulak, S.B. (2004). Hands-on help assessing heart sounds. *RN, 67*(8), 24ac1-24ac-4.

Felker, G.M., Cuculich, P.S., & Gheorghiade, M. (2006). The Valsalva maneuver: A beside "biomarker" for heart failure. *American Journal of Medicine, 119*(2), 117–122.

Galvan, L. (2005). Assessing venous ulcers and venous insufficiency. *Nursing2005, 35*(11), 70.

Galvan, L. (2004). Using compression therapy for venous insufficiency. *Nursing2005, 25*(12), 24–25.

Gami, A.S., Witt, B.J., Howard, D.E., et al. (2007). Metabolic syndrome and risk of incident cardiovascular events and death. *American College of Cardiology, 49*(4), 403–414.

Goldich, G. (2006). Understanding the 12-lead ECG, Part I. *Nursing2006, 36*(11), 36–41.

Goldich, G. (2006). Understanding the 12-lead ECG, Part II. *Nursing2006, 36*(12), 36–41.

Hlatky, M.A., Boothroyd, D., Vittinghoff, E., et al. (2002). Lessons learned from the Womens Initiative Study. *Southern Medical Journal, 97,* 116–120.

King, J.E. (2004). Cardiac stress tests: Which one, why, and when? *Nursing2004, 34*(3), 28.

Kreiger, G. (2007). A basic guide to understanding plasma B-type naturiuretic peptide in the diagnosis of congestive heart failure. *Med/Surg Nursing,* 16(2), 75–78.

Luckowski, A. (2006). Marked for trouble (homocystine levels). *Nursing Made Incredibly Easy!, 5*(6), 64.

Mennick, F. (2004). Going up? Adolescents' blood pressure levels are rising along with their weight. *American Journal of Nursing, 104*(8), 22.

Moz, T. (2006). Solving the chest pain conundrum. *LPN2006,* 2(3), 39–43

Ozner, M.D. (2007). VAP Cholesterol Testing: Advanced technology uncovers hidden cardiovascular risks. *Life Extension, 13*(5), 67–71.

Pullen, R.L. (2006). The heart of the matter: Assessing hepatojugular reflux. *Nursing Made Incredibly Easy!, 5*(5), 17.

Rosenthal, K. (2004). The ins and outs of hemodynamic monitoring. *Nursing Made Incredibly Easy!, 2*(4), 6–9.

Rushing, J. (2004). Taking blood pressure accurately. *Nursing2004, 34*(11), 26.

Shichiri, M., Kishikawa, H., Ohkubo, Y. et al. (2001). Long-term results of the Kumamoto study on optimal diabetes control in Type 2 diabetic pattern. *Diabetes Care.* Retrived from http://journal.diabetes.org/diabetescare/FullText/Supplements/DiabestCare/Supplement 40

Stimke, C. (2006). Coronary artery calcium scoring. *American Journal of Nursing, 106*(6), 72AA–72GG.

Sunderlin, M.K. (2006). Keeping pace with cardiac devices. *RN, 69*(7), 40–43.

Turka, J. (2006). Deciphering diagnostics: Is this on the level? *Nursing Made Incredibly Easy!, 4*(4), 7–9.

Webb, M., Moody, L.E., & Mason, L.A. (2000). Dyspnea assessment and management in hospice patients with pulmonary disorders. *American Journal of Hospice and Palliative Medicine, 17*(4), 259–264.

Whittier, S. (2004). Cardiac assessment and disease management for home health nurses. *Geriatric Nursing, 2*(4), 248–249.

Woodruff, D.W. (2006). Just the facts: Statins and safety. *LPN2006, 2*(4), 11–12.

Zatsick, N.M. (2007). Fish oil: Getting to the heart of it. *Journal for Nurse Practitioners. 3*(2), 104–109.

Chapter 18

AACN News Eds. (2006). Deep vein thrombosis prevention. *AACN News, 23*(1), 4, 14.

Barja, J. (2005). Oral antiplatelet therapy in cerebrovascular disease, coronary artery disease, and peripheral arterial disease. *Journal of the American Medical Association, 293*(7), 793–795.

Bartley, M. (2006). Preventing venous embolism. *Nursing2006, 36*(1), 64cc1–64cc4.

Bauer, J. (2005). Clinical highlights: Few elderly patients have their BP under control. *RN, 68*(11), 24.

Beese-Bjurstrom, S. (2005). Hidden danger: Aortic aneurysms and dissections. *Nursing2004, 34*(2), 36–42

Calianno, C., & Holton, S.J. (2007). Fighting the triple threat of lower extremity ulcers. *Nursing2007, 37*(3), 57–63.

Chen, S. (2005). Treating HTN crisis: How long? how fast? *RN, 68*(6), 37–42.

Deedwania, P. (2005). Diabetes and hypertension: The deadly duet: Importance, therapeutic strategy, and selection of drug therapy. *Cardiology Clinics, 23*(2), 139–152.

Della Croce, H. (2007). Aortic dissection. *RN*, 70(3), 26–31.

Duggirala, M. (2005) Women with diabetes have poorer control of blood pressure than men. *Journal of Women's Health, 14*(5), 418–423

Federman, D. (2004). Peripheral arterial disease: A systematic disease extending beyond the affected extremity. *Geriatrics, 59*(4), 26, 29–30, 32.

Fletcher, L. (2006). Management of patients with intermittent claudication. *Nursing Standard, 20*(31), 59–66, 68.

Galvan, L. (2005). Wound and skin care: Assessing venous ulcers and venous insufficiency. *Nursing2005, 35*(11), 70.

Galvan, L. (2005). Wound and skin care: Using compression therapy for venous insufficiency. *Nursing2005, 35*(12), 24–25.

Gibbons, M. (2007). The bomb buried deep in the body: Many clinicians are unaware their patients are at risk for venous thromboembolism. *ADVANCE Newsmagazines for LPNs*. Retrieved from http://lpn.advanceweb.com/common/Edial/PrintFriendly.aspx?CC=92126

Gorski, L.A. (2007). A common and preventable condition: Venous thrombosis. *Home Healthcare Nurse*, 25(2), 94–100.

Gulczynski, B. (2007). Anticoagulation therapy. *ADVANCE for Nurses*, 4(11), 17–20.

Hall, G. (2006). Drug management of hypertension in primary care. *Primary Health Care, 16*(3), 27–31.

Hums, W. (2006). A comparative approach to deep vein thrombosis risk assessment. *Journal of Trauma Nursing, 13*(1), 28–30.

Irwin, G.H. (2007). How to protect a patient with aortic aneurysm. *Nursing2007, 37*(2), 36–42.

Johnson, S. (2006). Exercise and peripheral arterial disease. *Annals of Internal Medicine, 144*(9), 699–700.

Johnson, T.D. (2007). Pomegrante: Powerful protection for aging arteries—and much more. *Life Extension, 13*(5), 55-62.

Kelechi, T., & Edlund, B. (2007). Chronic venous insufficiency, *Advance Newmagazine for LPNs*. Retrieved from http://lpn.advanceweb.com/Edial/PrintFriendly.aspx?CC=84611

Klein, D. (2005). Thoracic aortic aneurysms. *Journal of Cardiovascular Nursing, 20*(4), 245–250.

Mayo Clinic Disease Overview. (2006). *Raynaud's disease.* Retrieved from www.mayoclinic.com/health/raynauds-disease/D500433

Mayo Clinic Health Letter. (2004). Peripheral artery disease: Are your legs at risk? *Mayo Clinic Health Letter, 22*(3), 1–3.

Mortality and Morbidity Weekly Report. (2006). Hypertension-related mortality among Hispanic subpopulations—United States 1995–2002. *MMWR 55*(7), 177–180.

National Heart, Lung, and Blood Institute Disease and Condition Index. (2006). *Deep vein thrombosis.* Retrieved from www.nhlb.nih.gov/health/dci/Disease/Dvt/DVT_All.html

Nursing2007 Eds. (2007). Fast facts about thiazides and thiazides-like diuretics. *Nursing2007*, 37(5), 56hn8.

Palmieri, R.L. (2006). Cerebral artery stenosis, *Nursing2006, 36*(6), 36-41.

Rankins, J. (2005) Dietary approaches to stop hypertension—intervention reduces blood pressure among hypertensive African American patients in a neighborhood health care center. *Journal of Nutrition Education and Behavior, 37*(5), 259–264.

Research Activities Eds. (2006). Management of chest pain in patients with hypertension differs in men, women, and ethnic groups. *Research Activities, Jan*(305), 5–6.

Research Activities Eds. (2005). Knowledge and beliefs about lifestyle changes may contribute to ethnic differences in blood pressure control. *Research Activities, Oct*(302), 8–9.

Research Activities Eds. (2005). Blacks and Latinos with hypertension have trouble adhering to recommended diets. *Research Activities, May*(297), 2–3.

Research Activities Eds. (2004). Greater severity of peripheral arterial disease among blacks may account for their higher rate of amputation. *Research Activities, May*(285), 13.

RN Eds. (2007). New type of BP treatment now available. *RN*, 70(4), 61.

Scheetz, L. (2006). Aortic dissection. *American Journal of Nursing, 106*(4), 55–59.

Sieggreen, M.Y. (2006). Getting a leg up on managing venous ulcers. *Nursing Made Incredibly Easy!*, 4(6), 52-60.

Smith, N. (2007). Peripheral artery disease interventions save lives and limbs. *NurseWeek, 20*(4), 12-13.

Spencer, A. (2005). Cardiovascular drug therapy in women. *Journal of Cardiovascular Nursing, 20*(5), 408–419.

Staffileno, B. (2005). Treating hypertension with cardioprotective therapies: The role of ACE inhibitors, ARBs, and β-blockers. *Journal of Cardiovascular Nursing, 20*(4), 354–364.

Summers, A. (2005). From white to blue to red: Raynaud's syndrome. *Emergency Nurse, 13*(7), 18–20

The Johns Hopkins Vasculitis Center. (2006). *Buerger's disease.* Retrieved from www.vasculitis_med.jhu.edu/typesofbuergers.html

Varga, J. (2004). Raynaud phenomenon, scleroderma, overlap syndromes, and other fibrosing syndromes. *Opinion in Rheumatology, 16*(6), 714–752.

Whitaker, C. (2004). Peripheral arterial disease in African Americans: Clinical characteristics, leg symptoms, and lower extremity functioning. *Journal of the American Geriatrics Society, 52*(6), 922–930.

Yang, J. (2005). Prevention and treatment of deep vein thrombosis and pulmonary embolism in critically ill patients. *Critical Care Nursing Quarterly, 28*(1), 72–79.

Zillich, A. (2006). ASHP therapeutic position statement on the treatment of hypertension. *American Journal of Health-System Pharmacy, 63*(11), 1074–1080.

Zolli, A. (2004). Foot ulceration due to arterial insufficiency: Role of cilostazol. *Journal of Wound Care, 13*(2), 45–47.

Chapter 19

Agency for Healthcare Research and Quality. (2006). *Program brief: Research on cardiovascular disease in women.* Retrieved from www.ahrq.gov/research/womheart.pdf

American Dietetic Association. (2006). *Disorders of lipid metabolism evidence-based nutrition practice guideline.* Retrieved from www.adaevidencelibrary.com/topic.cfm?

American Heart Association (2006a). *AHA/ACC guidelines for secondary prevention for patients with coronary and other atherosclerosis vascular disease: 2006.* Retrieved from http://circ.ahajournals.org/cgi/content/full/113/19/2363

American Heart Association. (2006b). *Intensive prevention key to fighting coronary heart disease.* Retrieved from http://americanheart.org/presenter.jhtml?identifier=3039477

Artinian, N. (2003). The psychosocial aspects of heart failure. *American Journal of Nursing, 103*(12), 32–42.

Ayers, D. (2005). Heart failure. *LPN2005, 1*(5), 24–28.

Barclay, L., & Lie, D. (2004). *ACCP revises guidelines for prevention of venous thromboembolism.* Retrieved from www.medscape.com/viewarticle/489427_print

Barsella, R.M. (2007). How to judge a failing heart. *NurseWeek,* 20(8), 8-9.

Breittenbach, J. (2007). Putting an end to perfusion confusion. *Nursing Made Incredibly Easy!,* 5(3), 50.

Brown, H. (2005). Cardiac tamponade. *Nursing2005, 35*(3), 88.

Bruce, J. (2005). Getting to the heart of cardiomyopathies. *Nursing2005, 35*(8), 44–47.

Della Rocca, J. (2007). Responding to fibrillation. *Nursing2007,* 37(4), 37–48.

Hays, D. (2005). Pacemaker malfunction. *Nursing2005, 35*(7), 88.

HeartCenterOnline. (2005). *Heart drug for US blacks can cut costs.* Retrieved from http://heart.healthcenteronline.com/newstories/newsprintfriendly.cfm?newsid=74104

HeartCenterOnline. (2006). *Type D personality boosts heart disease.* Retrieved from http://heart.healthcenteronline.com/newsstories/typedpersonaligyboostsheartdiseaserisk.cfm?general=NL_HEART

HeartCenterOnline. (2006). *Cocaine use linked to serious heart conditions.* Retrieved from http://heart.healthcenteronline.com/newsstories/cocaineuselinkedseriousheartconditioncfm?gener al=NL_HEART

HeartCenterOnline. (2006). *Diabetic heart disease: a major challenge.* Retrieved from http://heart.healthcenteronline.com/newsstories/diabeticheartdiseasemajorchallenge.cfm?general =NL_HEART

Heffelfinger, P.M. (2007). Cardiac resynchronization therapy. *Nursing2007,* 37(3), 53.

Heidenreich, P.A., McDonald, K.M., Hastie, T., et al. (1999). Meta-analysis of brials comparing beta-blockers, calcium antagonists, and nitrates for stable angina. *Journal of the American Medical Association, 281*(20), 1927–1936.

Holcomb, S. (2005). Recognizing and managing different types of carditis. *Travel Nursing2005, 1*(6), 6–11.

LPN2006 Eds. (2006). Keeping the pace with pacemakers. *LPN2006,* 2(1), 18–24.

Luckowski, A. (2007). Flat isn't where it's at (mystery rhythm). *Nursing Made Incredibly Easy!, 5*(3) 21–23.

MayoClinic.com. (2006). *Heart failure.* Retrieved from www.mayoclinic.com/health/heartfailure/DS00061/DSECTION=8

Medline Plus. (2006). *Medical encyclopedia: Cardiomyopathy.* Retrieved from www.nlm.nih.gov/medlineplus/encyclopedia/article/001105.htm

Miller, C. (2005). A heart failure case study in home health disease management. *Home Healthcare Nurse, 23*(9), 608–612.

Miller, J. (2007). Keeping your patient hemodynamically stable. *Nursing2007, 37*(5), 36–41.

Munson, B. (2005). About infective endocarditis. *Nursing2005, 35*(2), 71.

Neafsey, P. (2004). Of blood, bones, and broccoli: Warfarin–vitamin K interactions. *Home Healthcare Nurse, 22*(3), 178–182.

NHLBI. (2006). *Data fact sheet: Heart failure in the United States: A new epidemic.* Retrieved from http://library.advanced.org/27533/facts.html

Nursing Made Incredibly Easy! Eds. (2007). Cardioversion: Time to jump-start the heart. *5*(2), 26–27.

Quillen, T. (2005). About mitral valve prolapse. *Nursing2005, 35*(9), 71.

Sample, S. (2005). Left ventricular assist devices. *RN, 68*(11), 46–52.

Schrock, R., (2005). Keeping heart failure patients on the right path. *LPN2005, 1*(5), 18–24.

Sherrod, M. (2007) Heart disease: A woman's worst enemy. *American Nurse Today,* 2(2), 25–29

Taylor, A. (2005). Studying treatment of heart failure in blacks. *American Journal of Nursing, 105*(2), 20–21.

WebMD:Medical Tests. (2006). *Cardiac enzyme studies.* Retrieved from www.webmd.com/hw/heart_disease/hw224485.asp

Woodruff, D. W. (2005). Statins: They're safe, but… *Nursing Made Incredibly Easy!,* 3(4), 51–52.

Chapter 20

A-Z Health Guide from WebMD. (2005). *Medical tests cardiac enzyme studies.* Retrieved from www.webmd.com/hw/heart_disease/hw224485.asp

American Heart Association. (2002). *Aspirin in heart attack and stroke prevention.* Retrieved from www.americanheart.org/presenter.ajhtml?identifier=4456

American Heart Association. (2005). *Transmyocardial laser revascularization.* Retrieved from www.americanheart.org/presenter.ajhtml?identifier=4782

American Heart Association. (2006). *2006 Diet and lifestyle recommendations.* Retrieved from www.americanheart.org/presenter.ajhtml?identifier=851

Bates, E.R. (2001). Review: Aspirin reduces the incidence of coronary artery disease in patients at risk. *ACP Journal Club Nov-Dec 135*(3), 92.

Boden, W., O'Rourke, R., Teo, K., et al. (2007). Optimal medical therapy with or without PCI for stable coronary disease. *New England Journal of Medicine, 356*(15), 1503–1516.

Castle, N. (2006). Reperfusion therapy. *Emergency Nurse, 13*(9), 25–36.

Chapnick, M. (2005). Radiofrequency catheter ablation. *RN 2005, 68*(10), 40–44.

Columbia Hospital Department of Surgery. (2005). *Heart transplants.* Retrieved from www.Columbiasurgery.org/pat/hearttx/surgery.html

Eastwood, J., Doering, L.V. (2005). Gender differences in coronary artery disease. *Journal of Cardiovascular Nursing, 20*(5), 340–353.

Evangelista, L. (2005). Physical activity patterns in heart transplant women. *Journal of Cardiovascular Nursing, 20*(5), 334–339.

Heart Hospital Allegheny General Hospital. (2006). *Cardiomyoplasty.* Retrieved from www.wpahs.org/AGH/cardio/Services/Services_cardiomyo.html

HeartSite.Com. (2006). *Coronary stents.* Retrieved from www.heartsite.com/html/stent.html

Holcomb, S. (2004). Preventing CABG donor site infection. *Nursing2004, 34*(10), 68–69.

Hudson, K. (2006). Cardiac technology…the beat goes on. *Nursing Management, 37*(1), 50–52.

Katz, A. (2007). Sexuality and myocardial infarction: When it's safe to try again. *American Journal of Nursing, 107*(3), 49–52.

Lord, C. (2006). Preventing surgical site infections after coronary artery bypass graft. *Home Health Care Nurse, 24*(1), 28–37.

Lukkarinen, H. (2006). Treatment of coronary artery disease improves quality of life in long term. *Nursing Research, 55*(1), 26–33.

Metules, T. (2004). IABP therapy: Getting patients treatment fast. *RN, 66*(5), 56–62.

Moz, T. (2006). Solving the chest pain conundrum. *LPN2006,* 2(3), 38–43.

Moz, T. (2007). Cardiovascular disease: The heart of the matter. *LPN2007, 3*(2), 35–45.

Plomondon, M.E. (2003). Factors influencing risk-adjusted patient satisfaction after coronary artery bypass graft. *American Journal of Cardiology 92*(2), 206–208.

Plomondon, M.E., Casebeer, A.W., Schooley, L.M., et al. (2006). Exploring the volume-outcome relationship for off-pump coronary artery bypass graft procedures. *Annals of Thoracic Surgery 81,* 547–553.

Polick, T. (2007). Technology offers another chance: A cardiac assist device gives both patients and nurses opportunities to reach their potential. *2007 Spring Med/Surg Specialty Guide,* pp. 76–77.

Roman, L. & Metules, T. J. (2007). Door-to-balloon time: The race is on. *RN, 70*(2), 35–39.

Rosenfeld, A. (2005). Understanding treatment-seeking delay in women with acute myocardial infarction: Description of decision-making patterns. *Journal of Critical Care, 14*(4), 285–293.

Schultz, P. (2005). Gender differences in recovery after coronary artery bypass grafting. *Progress in Cardiovascular Nursing, 20*(2), 55–64.

Scordo, K. (2005). Noninvasive diagnosis of coronary artery disease in women. *Journal of Cardiovascular Nursing, 20*(6), 420–426.

Sehny, L. (2006). Off-pump coronary artery bypass graft: A case report. *AANA Journal, 74*(1), 39–44.

Stone, G. Moses, J. Ellis, S. et al. (2007) Safety and effectiveness of sirolimus and paclitaxel-eluting coronary stents. *New England Journal of Medicine, 356*(10), 998–1008.

Quigley, P. (2005). Valve jobs aren't just for '57 Chevys. *Nursing Made Incredibly Easy!, 3*(3), 20–23, 25–31, 33–37.

Young, L. (2004). Women and heart transplantation: An issue of gender equity? *Health Care for Women International, 25*(5), 436–453.

Chapter 21

Agency for Healthcare Research and Quality. (2001). *Treatment of Pulmonary Disease Following Cervical Spinal Cord Injury.* Number 27. Rockville, MD: U.S. Department of Heatlh and Human Services, Public Health Service.

Bodner, D.R. (2006). Evidence-based management of the neurogenic bladder: Clinical Practice Guideline. *Journal of Spinal Cord Medicine, 29*(5), 479.

Fischer, D. (2007). Is it upper or lower motor neuron disease? *Nursing Made Incredibly Easy!, 5*(2), 64.

Lower, J. (2007). Fearlessly facing neurologic evaluation. *LPN2007* 3(2), 11–15.

Mayo Clinic. (2005). *Mayo Clinic develops new coma measurement system.* Retrieved from www.mayoclinic.org/news2005-rst/3023.html

Meyers, S. (2007). Coma measurement system. *ADVANCE for Nurses 2007 Spring Med/Surg Specialy Guide.*

Miller, G. (2006). Risk of early onset of Parkinson's disease could be increased by pesticide exposure. Retrieved from *Medical News Today* at www.medicalnewstoday.com/printerfriendlynews.php?newsid=51960

Noah, P. (2004). Neurological assessment: A refresher. *RN,* TNT 18–23.

Nursing2005 Eds. (2005). New tool measures coma depth. *Nursing2005, 35*(12), 34–35.

Olsen, D.M., & Gambrell, M. (2005). Balancing sedation with bispectral index monitoring. *Nursing2005, 35*(5), 32cc1–32cc2.

Pullen, R.L. (2005a). Checking for oculocephalic reflex. *Nursing2005, 35*(5), 24.

Pullen, R.L. (2005b). Testing the corneal reflex. *Nursing2005, 35*(11), 68.

Royal-Evans, C. & Marcus, R. (2004). *A survey of the use of evidence-based practice in treatment of aphasia.* Presented at the Clinical Aphasiology Conference, Park City, UT, May 2004.

Spinal Cord Injury Association. (2006). *Autonomic dysreflexia.* Retrieved from www.spinalcord.org/html/factsheets/aut_dysreflexia.php

Suiter, D. M. (2007). Evidence-Based Practice for Dysphagia. Presented at MidSouth Conference on Communication Disorders, February 27, 2007.

Wijdicks, E.F., Bamlet, W.R., Maramattom, B.V., et al. (2005). Validation of a new coma scale: The FOUR scale. *Annals of Neurology, 58*(4), 585–593.

Chapter 22

Agency for Healthcare Research and Quality. (2007). *Acute management of autonomic dysreflexia: Individuals with spinal cord injury presenting to healthcare facilities.* Retrieved from www.guideline.gov/summary/summary.aspx?doc_id=2964&nbr=2190.

American Association of Neuroscience Nurses. (2007). *Guide to the Care of the Patient with Intracranial Pressure Monitoring.* Glenview, IL: American Association of Neuroscience Nurses.

Barker, E. (2005). SCI patients take a big step forward. *RN, 68*(7), 30–32.

Brain Injury Association of America. (2006). *Traumatic brain injury statistics.* Retrieved from www.biausa.org

Carpico, B. (2007). Suspected cervical spine injury. *Nursing2007, 37*(3), 88.

Castillo, D.A., Alvarez-Sabin, J., Secades, J.J., et al. (2002). *Oral citicoline in acute ischemic stroke: An individual patient data pooling analysis of clinical trials.* Retrieved from www.cdpcholine.com/ckpcholine-21.htm

Day, M.W. (2003). Epidural hematoma. *Nursing2003, 33*(8), 96.

Gibson, K.L. (2003). Caring for a patient who lives with a spinal cord injury. *Nursing2003, 33*(17), 36–41.

Hentschke, P. (2005). Autonomic dysreflexia crises. *ADVANCE for Nurses, 2*(21), 24–25.

Hilde, G., Hagen, K.B., Jamtvedt, G., et al. (2005). Advice to stay active as a single treatment for low-back pain and sciatica. Cochrane Back Group, *Cochrane Database System Review, 4,* CD001254.

Jones, T.S. (2005). A bolt out of the blue: Dealing with the aftermath of spinal cord injury. *Nursing Made Incredibly Easy!,* 3(6), 14–28.

Meaney, D.F. & Grady, M.S. (2005). Should corticosteroids be used to treat traumatic brain injury. *Nature Clinical Practice Neurology, 1*(10), 74–75.

National Center for Injury Prevention and Control. (2005). *Spinal cord injury (SCI: Fact Sheet.)* Retrieved from www.cdc.gov/ncipc/factsheets/scifacts.htm

National Institute of Health. (2006). *Spinal cord trauma.* Retrieved from www.nlm.nih.gov/medlineplus/print/ency/article 001066.htm

Perina, D. (2006). *Back pain, mechanical.* Retrieved from www.emedicine.com

Schollenberger, J., Rehwoldt, M., & Barnhill, B. (2006). Brain monitors. *RN, 69*(1), 44–49.

Spinal Cord Injury Association. (2006). *Autonomic dysreflexia.* Retrieved from www.spinalcord.org/htmll/factsheets/aut_dysreflexia.php

Vacca, V.M. (2006). Subdural hematoma. *Nursing2006, 36*(3), 88.

Vacca, V.M. (2007). Acute paraplegia. *Nursing2007, 37*(6), 64.

Vacca, V.M. (2007). Autonomic dysreflexia. *Nurisng2007, 37*(9), 72.

Wilensky, E.M., & Bloorm, S. (2005). Monitoring brain tissue oxygenation after severe brain injury. *Nursing2005, 35*(2), 32cc1–32cc4.

Yanagawa, T., Bunn, F., Roberts, I., et al. (2005). Nutritional support for head-injured patients. Cochrane Injuries Group. *Cochrane Database System Review, 4,* CD001530.

Zink, E.K., & McQuillan, K. (2005). Managing traumatic brain injury. *Nursing2005, 35*(9), 36–43.

Chapter 23

Adamow, S.M. (2005). Working miracles. *ADVANCE for Nurses,* 2(17), 15–17.

Adamow, S.M. Cowles, L., & Goulette, C. (Eds.). (2005). UCLA stroke study shows promise. *ADVANCE for Nurses,* 2(6), 7.

Agency for Healthcare Policy and Research. (1995). *Post-stroke rehabilitation: Assessment, referral, and patient management.* Rockville, MD: U.S. Department of Health and Human Services, Public Health Service.

Alexander, D.M. (2007). Facing the pain of trigeminal neuralgia. *Nursing2007, 37*(7), 18–19.

American Heart Association. (2005). *Going hot and cold can speed limb recovery in stroke survivors.* Retrieved from www.americanheart.org/presenter/jhtml?identifier=3035150

American Heart Association. (2006). *Stroke statistics.* Retrieved from www.americanheart.org/presenter.jhtml?identifier=4725

Baldwin, K.M. (2006). Stroke: It's a knock-out punch. *Nursing Made Incredibly Easy!, 4*(2), 10–25.

Barker, E. (2005). New hope for stroke patients. *RN, 68*(2), 39–43.

Barker, E. (2006). A new weapon to combat stroke. *RN, 69*(3), 26–29.

Bassett, J. (2007). A lifelong journey: Post-CVA patients who require rehab can find themselves on a continuous voyage of uncertainty. *Advance Newsmagazines for LPN*. Retrieved from http://lpn.advanceweb.com/common/editorial 3/9/07

Becker, K.J., & Trott, T.G. (2005). Approval of the MERCI clot retriever: A critical view. *Stroke, 36*, 400.

Bensing, K. (2006). Lifesaving technology: Patients diagnosed with AVMs benefit from surgical advances. *ADVANCE for Nurses, 3*(18), 23–24, 30.

Brain Tumor Society. (2006). *Brain tumor facts and statistics.* Retrieved from www.tbts.org/iemDetail.asp?categoryID=383itemID=16635

Cabaniss, R. (2005). Strokes related to drug use. *ADVANCE for Nurses, 2*(13), 17–20.

Castillo, D.A., Alvarez-Sabin, J., Secades, J.J., et al. (2002). *Oral citicoline in acute ischemic stroke: An individual patient data pooling analysis of clinical trials.* Retrieved from www.cdpcholine.com/ckpcholine-21.htm

Cohn, J.L., & Powers, J. (2005). Are you ready to manage patients with acute ischemic stroke? *LPN2005, 1*(4), 14–27.

Cowles, L. (2005). Brain attack. *ADVANCE for Nurses, 2*(7), 25–27.

Domrose, C. (2006). In search of seizures. *NurseWeek, 19*(5), 10–11.

Dunleavy, K. Finch, A., Overstreet, W., et al. (2005). Improving care for patients with subarachnoid hemorrhage. *Nursing2005, 35*(11), 26–27.

Emedicine.com. (2006). *Migraine headaches, vision effects.* Retrieved from www.emedicinehealth.com/fulltext/35023.htm

Fagley, M.U. (2007). Taking charge of seizure activity. *Nursing2007, 37*(9), 42–47.

Franges, E.Z. (2006). A sudden storm: Caring for seizure patients. *LPN2006, 2*(2), 28–36.

Gale, K. (2005). *Brain stimulation may aid stroke recovery.* Retrieved from news.yahoo.com/s/nm/20050524hl_nm/stimulation_stroke_dc&printer=1

Girard, P.S. (2007). Does syncope make you feel faint? *Nursing Made Incredibly Easy!, 5*(5), 64.

Grogan, P.M., & Gronseth, G.S. (2001). *Practice parameters: Steroids, acyclovir, and surgery for Bell's palsy (an evidence-based review).* Retrieved from www.neurology.org/cgi/content/abstract/56/7/830 4/17/07

Hacke, W., Donnan, G., Fieschi, C., et al.; ATLANTIS Trials Investigators; ECASS Trials Investigators; NINDS rt-PA Study Group Investigators. (2004). Association of outcome with early stroke treatment: Pooled analysis of ATLANTIS, ECASS, and NINDS rt-PA stroke trials. *Lancet, 363*, 768–774.

Hathaway, L.R. (2005). Stroke (brain attack). *Nursing2005, 35*(11), 49.

Haut, S. (2006). *Frontal lobe epilepsy.* Retrieved from www.emedicine.com/neuro/topic141.htm

Hayes, D.D. (2006). Viral meningitis in adults. *Nursing2006, 36*(2), 64.

Haymore, J. (2007). BIC for ICP. *ADVANCE for Nurses, 4*(9), 27–28.

Huff, J.S. (2005a). *Neoplasms, brain.* Retrieved from www.emedicine.com/emerg/topic334.htm

Huff, J.S. (2005b). *Trigeminal neuralgia.* Retrieved from www.emedicine.com/emerg/topic617.htm

Jia-Ching, C., & Liang, C.C. (2005). *Going hot and cold can speed limb recovery in stroke syndrome.* Retrieved from www.americanheart.org/presenter.jhtml?identifier=3035150

Lazoff, J. (2005). *Encephalitis.* Retrieved from www.emedicine.com/emerg/topic163.htm

Lites, D. (2006). *Supraorbital nerve stimulation.* Retrieved from www2.whdh.com/features/articles/healthcast/BOS2881

Louden, K. (2007). Primary headache primer. *NurseWeek, 20*(9), 8.

Maze, L.M. (2006). Under pressure: Caring for a patient with a brain bleed. *LPN2006, 2*(4), 36–41.

McCrory, D.C., Penzien, D.B., Hasselblad, V., et al. (2000). *Evidence report: Behavioral and physical treatments for tension-type and cervicogenic headache.* Duke University Evidence-based Practice Center. Retrieved from www.fcer.org/html/Research/DukeEvidenceReport.htm

Miller, J., & Elmore, S. (2005). Call a stroke code! *Nursing2005, 35*(3), 58–63.

Monnell, K. Zachariah, S.B., & Khoromi, S. (2005). *Bell palsy.* Retrieved from www.emedicine.com/neuro/topic413.htm

Nandalar, M. (2005). *Western equine encephalitis.* Retrieved from www.emedicine.com/med/topic3156.htm 4/17/07

NIH News Eds. (2007). *MRI more sensitive than CT in diagnosing most common form acute stroke, finds NIH study.* Retrieved from www.ninds.nih.gov/ 1/26/07

Nursing2006 Eds. (2006). Interleukin antagonist may help treat acute stroke. *Nursing2006, 36*(1), 26.

Nursing Made Incredibly Easy! Eds. (2005). Puzzled by "mini-strokes"? *Nursing Made Incredibly Easy!, 3*(5), 56–57.

Nursing Made Incredibly Easy! Eds. (2007). Don't let your head explode over increased ICP. *Nursing Made Incredibly Easy!, 5*(2), 21–25.

Peiffer, K.M.Z. (2007). Brain death and organ procurement. *American Journal of Nursing, 107*(3), 58–67.

Phillips, R.A. (2007). Treating carotid artery stenosis to prevent stroke. *Nursing Made Incredibly Easy!, 5*(1), 41–46.

Pope, W. (2002b). Cerebral vessel repair with coils & glue. *Nursing2002, 65*(7), 46–49.

Pullen, R.L. (2004). Assessing for signs of meningitis. *Nursing2004, 34*(5), 18.

Reddrop, C., Moldrich, R.X., Beart, P.M., et al. (2005). *Vampire bat salivary plasminogen activator (Desmoteplase) inhibits tissue-type plasminogen activator-induced potentiation of excitotoxic injury.* Retrieved from http://stroke.ahajournals.org/cgi/content/36/6/1241

Reed, N. (2007). Continuous electroencephalogram monitoring. *ADVANCE for Nurses, 4*(13), 27–28.

Rielo, D. (2006). *Vagus nerve stimulation.* Retrieved from www.emedicine.com/neuro/topic559.htm

Roach, A., & Roach, E. (2005). How to assess phenytoin levels. *Nursing2005, 35*(11), 18–19

Rush University. (2006). *Spinal cord stimulators tested as treatment for patients with migraine headaches.* Retrieved from www.emaxhealth.com/110/7599.html

Silberstein, S. D. (2000). *Evidence based guidelines for migraine headache.* Retrieved from www.neurology.org/cgi

Stringer, H. (2007). Cutting without a scalpel: Radiosurgery benefits patients with brain disorders. *NurseWeek, 20*(5), 8–9.

Towne, L.M. (2007) Relieving rebound headaches. *Nursing2007, 37*(6), 54.

UCLA Stroke Center. (2005). *Clinical trial: Field Administration of Stroke Therapy–Magnesium (FAST-MAG) Trial.* Retrieved from www.clinicaltrials.gov/ct/show/NCT00059332

Vacca, V.M. (2006). Acute ischemic stroke. *Nursing2006, 36*(9), 80.

Vacca, V.M. (2007). Status epilepticus. *Nursing2007, 37*(4), 80.

Vega, C. (2007). *Stimulant abuse may increase stroke among young adults. CME/CE presentation.* Retrieved from www.medscape.com/viewarticle/555229

Waknine, Y. (2005). FDA Approvals: Diastat AcuDial: Diazepam rectal gel delivery system for at-home seizure control. *Medscape Medical News*. Retrieved from www.medscape.com/viewarticle/514629

Wisniewski, A. (2007). Caring for the patient with hydrocephalus. *LPN2007, 3*(1), 41–45.

Wood, D.A. (2007). Seizures: Coming to a unit near you. *2007 Spring Med/Surg Specialty Guide* pp. 80–81.

Chapter 24

Agency for Healthcare Quality and Research. (2007). *Parkinson's disease.* Retrieved from www.ahrq.gov/clinic/tp/parktp.htm

Agency for Healthcare Quality and Research. (2007). Stimulation of the subthalamic nucleus of the brain improves quality of life for patients with advanced Parkinson's disease. *Agency for Healthcare Quality and Research Bulletin, 319*(3), 10–11.

Backer, J.H. (2006). The symptom experience of patients with Parkinson's disease. *Journal of Neuroscience Nursing, 38*(1), 51–57.

Blacker, J. (2005). *Parkinson disease.* Retrieved from www.emedicine.com/pmr/topic99.htm

Carroll, A., McDonnell, G., & Barnes, M. (2003). *A review of the management of Guillain-Barré syndrome in a regional neurological rehabilitation unit.* Retrieved from www.medscape.com/medline/abstract/14634364

Centers for Disease Control and Prevention. (2006). *Update: Guillain-Barré syndrome among recipients of Menactra meningococcal conjugate vaccine—United States, October 2005—February 2006.* Retrieved from www.cdc.gov/mmwr/preview/mmwrhtml/mm5513a2.htm?s_cid=mm5513a2_e

Dangond, F. (2005). *Multiple sclerosis.* Retrieved from www.emedicine.com/neuro/topic228.htm

Franges, E.Z. (2006). What you need to know about MS. *LPN2006, 2*(5), 24–33.

Gevitz, C. (2006). Managing postpolio syndrome pain. *Nursing2006, 36*(12), 17.

Healing with Nutrition Eds. (2006). *Parkinson's disease: Facts, disease prevention and treatment strategies.* Retrieved from www.healingwithnutrition.com/pdisease/parkinsons/parkinsons.html

Hughes, R.A.C., Wijdicks, E.F.M., Barohn, R., et al. (2007). *Practice parameter: Immunotherapy for Guillain-Barré syndrome.* Retrieved from www.neurology.org

Kaiser, L.R. (2006). *Thymectomy and myasthenia gravis.* Retrieved from www.medscape.com/viewarticle/524436

McCarron, K. (2006). The shakedown on Parkinson's disease. *Nursing Made Incredibly Easy!, 4*(6), 40–49.

Multiple Sclerosis Association of America. (2007). *Introduction: Multiple sclerosis.* Retrieved fromwww.msaa.com/publications/cooling/contnts.htm

National Institute of Neurological Diseases and Stroke. (2006). *How is ALS treated?* Retrieved from www.ninds.nih. gov/disorders/amyotrophiclateralsclerosis/detail_amyotrophiclaterals

National Institute of Neurological Diseases and Stroke. (2007). *NINCS deep brain stimulation for Parkinson's disease information page.* Retrieved from www.ninds.nih.gov/disorders/deep_brain_stimulation/deep_brain_stimulation.htm

National Institutes of Health. (2006). *Parkinson's disease research.* Retrieved from www.ninds.nih.gov/funding/research/parkinsonsweb/index.htm

New Scientist Eds. (2005). *Parkinson's drug prompts brain cell growth.* Retrieved from www.newscientist.com/article.ns?id=dn7619

Palmieri, R.L. (2005). Is it myasthenia gravis or Guillain-Barré syndrome? *Nursing2005, 35*(12), 32hn1–32hn4.

Palmieri, R.L. (2007). Unraveling the mystery of amyotrophic lateral sclerosis. *LPN2007, 3*(3), 28–34.

Reitbert, J.S. (2005). Multiple sclerosis and exercise. *Multiple Sclerosis Resource Center.* Retrieved from www.medscape.com/resources.ms

Thomure, A. (2006). Helping your patient manage Parkinson's disease. *Nursing2006, 36*(8), 20–21.

Wood, D.A. (2006). New Parkinson's guidelines emphasize quality of life. *NurseWeek, 19*(22), 21.

Chapter 25

Agency for Healthcare Quality and Research. (2005). *Screening for visual impairment.* Retrieved from www.ahrq.gov/clinic/2ndcps/visual.pdf

American Foundation for the Blind. (2005). *Blindness statistics.* Retrieved from www.afb.org/Section.asp?SectionID=15

Barclay, L., & Lie, D. (2006). *High dietary antioxidant intake may reduce risk for age-related macular degeneration.* Retrieved from www.medscape.com/viewarticle/520823

Boyd-Monk, H. (2005a). Bringing common eye emergencies into focus. *Nursing2005, 35*(12), 46–51.

Boyd-Monk, H. (2005b). The eyes have it: Understanding problems of the aging eye. *Nursing Made Incredibly Easy!, 3*(5), 34–45.

Boyd-Monk, H. (2006). Focus on the aging eye: Presbyopia and cataract. *LPN2006, 2*(6), 26–35.

Grant, P. (2005). *Sensorineural hearing loss.* Retrieved from www.medicineau.net.au/clinical/ent/SNHL.html 4-21-07

Gray, D.L., & Scott, P. (2005). Patient handout: Hearing aids. *ADVANCE for Nurses, 2*(16), 40.

LPN2006 Eds. (2006). Do you hear what I hear? Assessing your patient's hearing. *LPN2006, 2*(3), 6–10.

National Eye Institute. (2001). *Clinical advisory: Antioxidant vitamins and zinc reduce risk of vision loss from age-related macular degeneration.* Retrieved from www.nlm.nih.gov/databases/alerts/amd.html

National Institute on Deafness and Other Communication Disorders. (2005). *Statistics about hearing disorders, ear infections, and deafness.* Retrieved from www.nidcd.nih.gov/health/statistics/hearing.asp

National Institutes of Health. (2004). *U.S. Latinos have high rates of eye disease and visual impairment.* Retrieved from www.nih.gov.news/pr/aug2004/nei-09.htm 10-18-06

Pullen, R.L. (2006). Spin control: Caring for a patient with inner ear disease. *Nursing2006, 36*(5), 48–51.

Ross, M. (2005). *Rehabilitation engineering research center on hearing enhancement: Evidence-based audiology.* Retrieved from www.hearingresearch.org/Dr.Ross/Evidence-based_Audiology.htm. 4-21-07

Rushing, J. (2007). Administering eyedrops. *Nursing2007, 37*(5),18.

Spires, R.A. (2006). How you can help when older eyes fail. *RN, 69*(2), 38–43.

Wallhagen, M.I, Pettengill, E., & Whiteside, M. (2006). Sensory impairment in older adults: Part 1: Hearing loss. *American Journal of Nursing, 106*(10), 40–48.

Whiteside, M.M., Wallhagen, M.I., and Pettengill, E. (2006). Sensory impairment in older adults: Part 2: Vision loss. *American Journal of Nursing, 106*(11), 52–61.

Chapter 26

ADVANCE for Nurses Eds. (2004). Latinos and eye disease. *ADVANCE for Nurses, 1*(22), 38.

Agency for Healthcare Quality and Reseach. (2007). *Recommendation statement: Screening for glaucoma.* Retrieved from www.ahrq.gov/clinic/uspstf05/glaucoma/glaucrs.htm

Avery, R.L., Pieramici, D.J., Rabena, M.D., et al. (2007). Intravitreal bevacizumab (Avastin) for neovascular age-related macular degeneration. *Opthalmology, 113*(3), 363–372.

Bertsch, K., & Cristoph, S. B. (2006). Glaucoma: Living with a thief. *ADVANCE for Nurses, 3*(12), 15–17

Boyd-Monk, H. (2006). Focus on the aging eye: Presbyopia and cataract. *LPN2006, 2*(6), 27–35.

Boyd-Monk, H. (2007). Focus on the aging eye: Glaucoma degeneration. *LPN2007, 3*(1).47–53.

Chizek, M. (2007). The aging eye. *ADVANCE for Nurses, 4*(12), 21–23.

Claoue, C. (2004). Functional vision after cataract removal with multifocal and accommodating intraocular lens implantation: prospective comparative evaluation of Array multifocal and 1CU accommodating lenses. *Journal of Cataract Refraction Surgery, 30*(10), 2088–2091.

Covell, C.A., Graziano, J., Rich, D., et al. (2007). New outlook for age-related macular degeneration. *Nursing2007, 37*(3), 22–23.

Donaldson, J.D. (2004). *Middle ear, acute otitis media, medical treatment.* Retrieved from www.emedicine.com/ent/toppic212.htm

Duke Health. (2005). *Vestibular rehabilitation program.* Retrieved from http://dukehealth1.org/ptot/vestibular_rehab.asp

Eye Digest editor. (2006). *Lucentis (ranibizumab)—FDA approved drug for wet macular degeneration.* Retrieved from www.agingeye.net/mainnews/lucentis.php 4-22-07

Fleming, C., Whitlock, E.P., Beil, T., et al. (2005). *Screening for primary open-angle glaucoma in the primary care setting.* Retrieved from www. ahrq.gov/clinic/uspstf05/glaucoma/glaucup.htm

Glynn-Milley, C. (2005). Outlook positive for today's cataract patients. *NurseWeek, 18*(9), 17–19.
Halvorson, P. (2005). The silent thief. *RN, 68*(3), 41–45.
Haybach, P. J. (2004). The patient with Meniere's disease. *NurseWeek, 12*(12), 22–24.
Health Alliance. (2005). *Hearing loss—Incidence.* Retrieved from www.hearingalliance.com/incidence.htm
Larkin, G.L. (2005). *Retinal detachment.* Retrieved from www.medscape.com
Lorenzo, N. (2005). *Meniere's disease.* Retrieved from www.emedicine.com/emerg/topic308.htm
LPN2006 Eds. (2006). Understanding ocular drug delivery. *LPN2006,* 2(6), 12–14.
LPN2006 Eds. (2006). Do you hear what I hear? Assessing your patient's hearing. *LPN2006,* 2(3), 6–10.
Luggen, A.S. (2005). Gerontologic nurse practitioner care guidelines: Dry eyes. *Geriatric Nursing, 26*(5), 302–303.
Nursing2007 Eds. (2007). Focusing on eye emergencies. *Nursing2007, 37*(2), 46–47.
Porter, T.I. (2007). Eye shadow: Cataracts can make a patient's bright world go dark. *ADVANCE Newsmagazines for LPNs.* Retrieved from http://lpn.advanceweb.com/common/editorial/printFriendly.aspx?CC=83876
Rushing, J. (2007). Administering eyedrops. *Nursing2007, 37*(5), 18.
Whiteside, M.M., Wallhagen, M.I., & Pettengill, E. (2006). Sensory impairment in older adults: Part 2: Vision loss. *American Journal of Nursing, 106*(11), 52–61.

Chapter 27

Gendreau-Webb, R. (2007). Bone up on proton pump inhibitors and fracture risk. *Nursing2007, 37*(10), 60–61.
Kuszajewski, M.L. (2005). Prealbumin is best for nutritional monitoring. *Nursing2005, 35*(5), 70–71.
Lehrer, J.K. (Ed.). (2006). *Medical encyclopedia: Alcoholic liver disease.* Retrieved from www.nlm.nih.gov/medlineplus/print/ency/article/000281.htm.
Molle, E. (2005). Keep the upper GI tract from going downhill. *Nursing2005, 35*(10), 28–29.
National Digestive Diseases Information Clearinghouse. (2005). *Gallstones.* Retrieved from http://digestive.niddk.nih.gov/ddiseases/puts/gallstones
Nursing Made Incredibly Easy! Eds. (2007). Function junction: Testing your patient's liver function. *Nursing Made Incredibly Easy!, 5*(1), 17–18.
Pellegrino, A. (2006). Looking at liver cancer. *Nursing2006, 26*(10), 52–55.
Penharlow, C., & Spader, C. (2005). Liver function tests: Pieces of a complex diagnostic puzzle. *NurseWeek, 18*(3), 25–27.
Rushing, J. (2005). Assessing for ascites. *Nursing2005, 35*(2), 68.
Solan, M. (2006). Preventing disease by improving your oral health. *Life Extension, 12*(4), 71–75.
Walker, B.W. (2004). Assessing gastrointestinal infections. *Nursing2004, 34*(5), 48–52.

Chapter 28

American Cancer Society. (2006). *A new option for stomach cancer treatment.* Retrieved from www.cancer.org/docroot/NWS/content/NWS
Baker, B. (2006). Weight loss and diet plans. *American Journal of Nursing, 106*(6), 52–59.
Bowen, K. (2007). Bariatric surgery. *ADVANCE Newsmagazines for LPNs.* Retrieved from http://lpn.advanceweb.com/common/editorial/PrintFriendly.aspx?CC=85391
Chetney, R., & Waro, K. (2004). Swallowing disorders. *Home Healthcare Nurse, 22*(10), 703–710.
Daniels, J. (2006). Obesity: America's epidemic. *American Journal of Nursing, 106*(1), 40–50.
Fry, D.A. (2007). Exposing the source of peptic ulcer disease. *LPN2007, 3*(3), 6–7, 9–10.
Fujiwara, Y., Machida, A., Watanabe, Y., et. al. (2005). *Association between dinner-to-bed time and gastro-esophageal reflux disease.* Retrieved from www.medscape.com/viewarticle/518745
Gil-Montoya, J.A., Ferreiria de Mello, A.L., Cardenas, C.B., et al. (2006). Oral health protocol for the dependent institutionalized elderly. *Geriatric Nursing, 27,* 95–102.
Goldsmith, C. (2007). Periodontal disease is a systemwide risk. *NurseWeek, 20*(1), 14–16.
Holmes, S.L. (2006). Gastroesophageal reflux disease. *ADVANCE for Nurses,* 2(12), 33–35.
Hydock, C.M. (2005). A brief overview of bariatric surgical procedures currently being used to treat the obese patient. *Critical Care Quarterly, 28*(3), 217–226.
James, K.S., & Cook, L.M. (2006). Anorexia nervosa. *ADVANCE for Nurses,* 3(2), 16–19.
Keefe, S. (2006). Eating disorders in men. *ADVANCE for Nurses,* 3(13), 27–28.
Logsdon, B. (2006). Beyond dysphagia. *Advance Newsmagazines for LPNs.* Retrieved from http://lpn.advanceweb.com/common/editorial
Neafsey, P.J. (2004). Double trouble: Acetaminophen increases the risk of upper GI complications for people taking NSAIDs. *Home Healthcare Nurse, 22,* 641–642.
Nowlin, A. (2006). The dysphagia dilemma: How you can help. *RN, 69*(6), 45–48.
Overstreet, M. (2004). How does a PEG tube stay in? *Nursing2004, 34*(6), 21.
Patti, M., Tedesco, P., & Fisichella, P.M.A. (2005). *Gastroesophageal reflux disease.* Retrieved from www.emedicine.com/med/topic857.htm
Peters, V.L. (2006). Feeding patients with swallowing disorders. *LPN2006,* 2(2), 13–17.
Prateek, S. (2005). *Advances in GERD/liver disease.* Retrieved from www.medscape.com/viewprogram/2118_pnt
Qureshi, W.A., (2006). *Hiatal hernia.* Retrieved from www.emedicine.com/med/topic1012htm
Ramberan, H., & Petropoulos, P. (2005). *Ferri's Clinical Advisor: Instant Diagnosis and Treatment,* St. Louis: Elsevier Mosby.
Raythorn, N. (2004). Gastroesophageal reflux disease (GERD). *Nursing2004, 34*(7), 54–55.
Rodriguez, L.A.G., & Hernandez-Diaz, S. (2001). The risk of upper gastrointestinal complications associated with nonsteroidal anti-inflammatory drugs, glucocorticoids, acetaminophen, and combinations of these drugs. *Arthritis Research, 3,* 98–101.
Smith, B.L. (2005). Bariatric surgery: It's no easy fix. *RN, 68*(6), 58–63.
Smith, R., & Myers, S.A. (2005). 2 devices that unclog feeding tubes. *RN, 68*(1), 36–41.
Stoltey, J., Reeba, H., Ullah, N., et al. (2007). *Does Barrett's oesophagus develop over time in patients with chroic gastroesophageal reflux disease?* Retrieved from www.medscape.com/viewarticle/550714
Suiter, D.M. (2007). *Evidence-Based Practice for Dysphagia.* Presented at MidSouth Conference on Communicative Disorders. February 27, 2007.
Tabereaux, P.B. (2005). *Medical encyclopedia: Mouth sores.* Retrieved from www.nlm.nih.gov/medlineplus/ency/article/003059
Tozzo, M.A. (2007). Battling obesity: Small steps, big rewards. *Nursing2007, 37*(3), 68–69.
Tracey, D.L., & Patterson, G.E. (2006). Care of the gastrostomy tube in the home. *Home Healthcare Nurse, 24*(6), 381–387.
Walker, B.W. (2004). Assessing gastrointestinal infections. *Nursing2004, 34*(5), 48–52.
Woodruff, D.W. (2005). Slow the flow with proton pump inhibitors. *Nursing Made Incredibly Easy!,* 2(2), 50–52.
Woodruff, D.W. (2007). Safeguarding therapy with proton pump inhibitors. *Nursing2007, 37*(4), 64hn10–64hn12.
Yuan, Y., Padol, I.T., & Hunt, R.H. (2006). *Peptic ulcer disease today.* Retrieved from www.medscape.com/viewarticle/522900

RESOURCES

American Gastroenterological Association
www.gastro.org

Chapter 29

American Cancer Society (2007). *Colorectal cancer.* Retrieved from www.cancer.org/docroot/CRI/CRI_2_3xasp?dt=10 5/27/07

Amerine, E. (2006). Celiac disease goes against the grain. *Nursing2006, 36*(2), 46–48

Amerine, E. (2007). Preventing and managing acute diverticulitis. *Nursing2007*, 37(9), 56hn1–56hn2.

Boggs, W. (2005). High-fat dairy foods may reduce colorectal cancer risk. *American Journal of Clinical Nutrition, 82,* 894–900.

Clinical Nutrition Updates. (2006). *Probiotics and bowel inflammation.* Issue 247. Retrieved from www.arborcom.com

Della Rocca, J. (2007). Minimizing the perils of appendicitis. *Nursing2007, 37*(1), 64hn1–64hn2.

Figerote, R.J. (2005). *Colon cancer.* Retrieved from www.emedicine.com/fulltext/13703.htm

Freeman, L. C. (2007). Responding to small-bowel obstruction. *Nursing2007, 35*(5), 56hn1–56hn2.

Habel, M. (2006). Celiac disease demands a lifelong gluten-free diet. *NurseWeek, 19*(4), 15–16.

Hahn, J. (2007). The bottom line on hemorrhoids. *Nursing Made Incredibly Easy!*, 5(5), 13–17.

Harris, H. (2006). *C. difficile:* Attack of the killer diarrhea. *Nursing Made Incredibly Easy!*, *4*(3), 12–19.

Hill, R. (2007). Don't let constipation stop you up. *Nursing Made Incredibly Easy!*, 5(5), 40–43.

Kather, T.A. (2005). Colorectal cancer: Guidelines for prevention, screening and treatment. *ADVANCE for Nurses*, 2(5), 15–17.

Kent, V. (2007). Caring for a patient with a bowel obstruction. *LPN2007*, 3(5), 30–33.

King, J. F. (2007). Does my patient have ulcerative colitis or Crohn's disease? *Nursing2007, 37*(3), 30.

Lehrer, J. K., & Lichtenstein, G. R. (2005). *Irritable bowel syndrome.* Retrieved from www.emedicine.com/med/topic1190.htm

LPN2007 Eds. (2007). How to apply and change an ostomy pouch. *LPN2007, 3*(3), 20–22.

Louden, K. (2007). Don't ignore this gut feeling. *Spring Med/Surg Specialty Guide*, pp. 62–63.

Manning-Dimmitt, L.L., Dimmitt, S.G., & Wilson, G.R. (2005). Diagnosis of gastrointestinal bleeding in adults. *American Family Physician, 71,* 1339–1346.

Mayo Clinic. (2005). *Earlier screening for colorectal cancer recommended for African Americans.* Retrieved from www.mayoclinic.org/news2005-sct/2753.html

Mehta, M. (2003). Assessing the abdomen. *Nursing2003, 33*(5), 54–55.

Movius, M. (2006). What's causing that gut pain? *RN, 69*(7), 25–29.

Nursing2007 Eds. (2007). Managing inflammation. *Nursing2007, 37*(9), 56hn4–56hn6.

Nursing Made Incredibly Easy! Eds. (2005). There's trouble down below. *Nursing Made Incredibly Easy!*, *3*(1), 60–62.

Rowe, W.A. (2005). *Inflammatory bowel disease.* Retrieved from www.emedicine.com/med/topic 1169.htm 8/16/05

Thompson, J. (2000). A practical ostomy guide. *RN, 63*(11), 61–66.

Toth, P.E. (2006). Ostomy care and rehabilitation in colorectal cancer. *Seminars in Oncology Nursing, 22*(3), 174–177

Vega-Stromberg, T. (2005). Advances in colon cancer chemotherapy: Nursing implications. *Home Healthcare Nurse, 23*(3), 154–164.

RESOURCES

American Cancer Society
(800) 227-2345; www.cancer.org

Better Together Club
(800) 422-8811; www.convatec.com

Crohn's and Colitis Foundation of America
(800) 343-3637; www.ccfa.org

Hollister Incorporated
(800) 323-4060; www.hollister.com

United Ostomy Association
(800) 826-0826; www.uoa.org

Chapter 30

Aschenbrenner, D. S. (2006). Acetaminophen toxicity leading cause of liver failure. *American Journal of Nursing*, 106(6), 74–75.

Baltimore, J. J., & Deavidson, J. (2007). Caring for a patient with acute cholecystitis. *Nursing2007, 37*(3), 64hn1–64Hn4.

Buccolo, L.S. (2005). Viral hepatitis. *Clinics in Family Practice, 7*(1).

Burruss, N., & Holx, D. (2005). Understanding acute pancreatitis. *Nursing2005, 35*(3), 32hn1–32hn4.

Cancerbacup. (2005). *Primary liver cancer.* Retrieved from www.cancerbacup.org.uk/Cancertype/Liver/Primarylivercancer

Centers for Disease Control and Prevention. (2006*). National Center for Health Statistics: Chronic liver disease/cirrhosis.* Retrieved from www.cdc.gov/nchs/fastats/liverdis.htm

Despins, L. A., Kivlahan, C., & Cox, K. R. (2005). Acute pancreatitis: Diagnosis and treatment of a potentially fatal condition. *American Journal of Nursing, 105*(11), 54–57

Durston, S. (2004). The ABCs—and more of hepatitis. *Nursing Made Incredibly Easy!*, 2(4), 22–31.

Durston, S. (2005). Viral hepatitis. *Nursing2005, 35*(8), 26–41.

Holcomb, S.S. (2005). Gallstones. *Nursing2005, 35*(9), 45.

Holcomb, S.S. (2007). Stopping the destruction of acute pancreatitis. *Nursing2007, 37*(6), 43–47.

Johansson, M., Thune, A., Nelvin, L., et al. (2005). Randomized clinical trial of open versus laparoscopic cholecytectomy in the treatment of acute cholecystitis. *British Journal of Surgery*, 92(1):44–49.

Jones, S. (2003). When the liver fails: New help—and hope. *RN, 66*(11), 32–36.

Keeffe, E.B. (2006). *Treatment of chronic hepatitis B.* Highlights from the 41st Annual Meeting of the European Association for the Study of the Liver. Retrieved from www.medscape.com/viewarticle/533466

Krumberger, J.M. (2005). How to manage an acute upper GI bleed. *RN, 68*(3), 34–39.

McCarron, K. (2007). Jaundice: More than meets the eye. *Nursing Made Incredibly Easy!*, *5*(3), 25–27.

McMahon, B. J., Bruden, D. L., Petersen, K. M., et al. (2005). Antibody levels and protection after hepatitis B vaccination: results of a 15-year follow-up. *Annals of Internal Medicine, 142*(5), 333-341.

National Cancer Institute. (2005). *Milk thistle.* Retrieved from www.nci.nih.gov/cancertopics/pdq/cam/milkthistle/healthprofessional

National Digestive Diseases Information Clearinghouse. (2005). *Gallstones.* Retrieved from http://digestive.niddk.nih.gov/ddiseases/pubs/gallstones

Nursing2007 Eds. (2007). What are the options for managing ascites? *Nursing2007, 37*(3), 64hn6.

Nursing Made Incredibly Easy! Eds. (2005). A puzzling complication of liver disease. *Nursing Made Incredibly Easy!*, 3(3), 54–56.

Oettle, H., Post, S., Neuhaus, P. et al. (2007). Adjuvant chemotherapy with gemcitabine vs observation patients undergoing curative-intent resection of pancreatic cancer: A randomized controlled trial. *Journal of the American Medical Association, 297*(3), 267–277.

Pellegrino, A. (2006). Looking at liver cancer. *Nursing2006, 36*(10), 52.

Penharlow, C., & Spader, C. (2005). Liver function tests: Pieces of a complex diagnostic puzzle. *NurseWeek, 18*(3), 25–27.

Phillips, R. (2006). Acute pancreatitis: Inflammation gone wild. *Nursing Made Incredibly Easy!*, *64*(5), 18–28.

Polzien, G. (2007). Veterans' heathcare concerns: Hepatitis C. *Home Healthcare Nurse, 25*(5), 335–338.

Portal hypertension—new treatments. (2004). Retrieved from www.ccspublishing.om/journals51/portal_hypertension.htm

Riehl, M. (2007). Help your patient cope with pancreatic cancer. *Nursing2007, 37*(4), 54–57.

Rushing, J. (2005). Assessing for ascites. *Nursing2005, 35*(2), 68.

Rushing, J. (2006). Protect your patient during abdominal paracentesis. *Nursing2005, 35*(8), 14.

Sherker, A.H. (2005). *Hepatitis A, D, E, and G.* Retrieved from www.hepnet.com/uptate4.html

Stringer, H. (2007). Silent disease: GI nurses on the forefront of fighting hepatitis C. *NurseWeek, 20*(9), 24–25.

Whiteman, K., & McCormick, C. (2005). When your patient is in liver failure. *Nursing2005, 35*(4), 58–63.

RESOURCES

American Liver Foundation
www.liverfoundation.org

Centers for Disease Control and Prevention
Chronic Liver Diseases
www.cdc.gov/nchs/fastats/liverdis.htm

Hepatitis Central
http://hepatitis-central.com

National Center for Infectious Diseases
www.cdc.gov/ncidod/diseases/hepatitis/c

Chapter 31

Bennett, P.C. (2006). Foot care: Prevention of problems for optimal health. *Home Healthcare Nurse, 24*(5), 325–330.

Cancer Research UK. (2003). *HRT and breast cancer: Results of the million women study.* Retrieved from www.cancerresearchuk.org/news/presreleases/2003/august/39341

Domrose, C. (2006). No more waiting game: Joint replacements help boomers stay active. *NurseWeek, 19*(22), 8–9.

LPN2005 Eds. (2005). Maintaining mobility: Getting patients back on their feet. *LPN2005, 1*(4), 34–39.

Rooney, J. 2006). Oh, those aching joints! Helping patients manage arthritis. *LPN2006,* 27–34.

Sebba, A.I., Saag, K.G., Luckey, M.M., et al. (2006). Isteioirisus un 2005: A rheumatology perspective. *Journal of Rhematology.* Retrieved from www.medscape.com/viewprogram/5010

Veronesi, J.F. (2005). After the crash: Treating whiplash. *RN, 68*(9), 40–45.

Wagner, E. (2006). MSM improves pain, function in arthritis patients. *Life Extension, 12*(2), 14.

Chapter 32

American Association of Orthopedic Surgeons. (2000). *Smoking and musculoskeletal health.* Retrieved from http://orthoinfo.aaos.org/fact/thr_report.cfm?Thread_ID=240&topcategory=Wellness

Anderson, D.L. (2004). TNF inhibitors: A new age in rheumatoid arthritis treatment. *American Journal of Nursing, 104*(2), 60–67.

Bailey, M .M. (2005). Staying on your toes when managing pelvic fractures. *Nursing2005, 35*(10), 32cc1–32cc4.

Barclay, L., & Lie, D. (2006). *Acupuncture helps improve knee and hip osteoarthritis.* Retrieved from www.medscape.com/viewarticle/547162?src=mp

Bathon, J.M. (2005). Osteoarthritis treatments. *Johns Hopkins arthritis.* Retrieved from www.hopkins-arthritis.som.jhmi.edu/osteo/osteo_treat.html

Bennett, P. C. (2006). Foot care: Prevention of problems for optimal health. *Home Healthcare Nurse, 24*(5), 325–329.

Berman, B.M., Lao, L., Langenber, P., et al. (2004). Effectiveness of acupuncture as adjunctive therapy in osteoarthritis of the knee: A randomized, controlled trial. *Annals of Internal Medicine, 141*(12), 901–906.

Blakeley, J.A., & Ribeiro, V.E.S. (2004). Glucosamine & osteoarthritis. *American Journal of Nursing, 104*(2), 54–59.

Cooper, G., Lin, J., & Lane, J.M. (2005). *Nonoperative treatment of oseoporotic compression fractures.* Retrieved from www.emedicine.com/pmr/topic238.htm

D'Arcy, Y. (2005a). Following new guidelines to treat fibromyalgia pain. *Nursing2005, 35*(10), 17–18.

D'Arcy, Y. (2005b). Managing phantom limb pain. *Nursing2005, 35*(11), 17.

D'Arcy, Y. (2006a). Easing the pain after total joint replacement. *LPN2006, 2*(5), 7–8.

D'Arcy, Y. (2006b). Treating pain after a total knee replacement. *Nursing2006, 36*(5), 26–28.

D'Arcy, Y. (2006c). Treatment strategies for low back pain relief. *The Nurse Practioner: The American Journal of Primary Health Care, 31*(4), 16–25.

Durkin, S., & Durkin, M.E. (2007). Aging and sacropenia. *ADVANCE for Nurses, 4*(1), 29–30.

Family Doctor. (2005). *Cast care.* Retrieved from http://familydoctor.org/094.xml

Gaby, A.R. Borage seed oil effective against rheumatoid arthritis—Literature review and commentary. *Townsend Letter for Doctors and Patients.* Retrieved from www.findarticles.com/p/articles/mi_m0ISW/is_2002_May/ai_85131506

Gaines, J.M., Metter, E.J., & Talbot, L.A. (2004). The effect of neuromuscular electrical stimulation on arthritis knee pain in older adults with osteoarthritis of the knee. *Applied Nursing Research, 17*(3), 201–204.

Gore, T., & Lacey, S. (2005). Bone up on fat embolism. *Nursing2005, 35*(8), 32hn1–32hn4.

Gross, K. A. (2006). Solid advice on managing vertebral compression fractures. *Nursing2006, 36*(12), 64hn1–64hn4.

Habel, M. (2006a). Back in action with joint replacements, part 1.*NurseWeek, 19*(20), 15–16.

Habel, M. (2006b). Back in action with joint replacements, part 2. *NurseWeek, 19*(21), 21–22.

Habel, H. (2006c). Fibromyalgia—Looking good and feeling awful. *NurseWeek, 19*(12), 19–20.

Hobar, C. (2005). *Osteoporosis.* Retrieved from www.emedicine.com/med/topic1693.htm

Hohler, S.E. (2005). Looking into minimally invasive total hip arthroplasty. *Nursing2005, 35*(6), 54–57.

Holcomb, S.S. (2006). Osteoporosis. *Nursing2006, 36*(4), 48–49

Howell, B. (2007). Joint surgery: Paving the way to a smooth recovery. *RN, 70*(1), 32–37.

Jasniewski, J. (2006). Take steps to protect your patient from falls. *Nursing2006, 36*(4), 24–25.

Kent, V. P. (2006). Taking the puzzle out of carpal tunnel syndrome. *Nursing Made Incredibly Easy!, 4*(2), 4–5.

Kern, U., Alkemper, B., Kohl, M. (2006). Management of phantom pain with a textile, electromagnetically-acting stump liner: A randomized, double-blind, crossover study. *Journal of Pain Symptom Management, 32*(4), 352–360.

Landis, D.M. (2005). Fracture risk in postmenopausal women. *Nurse Practitioner, 30*(11), 48, 53–58.

Laskowski-Jones, L. (2006). First aid for amputations. *Nursing2006, 36*(4), 50–52.

LPN2005 Eds. (2005). Maintaining mobility: Getting patients back on their feet. *LPN2005, 1*(5), 15–16.

Munson, B. L. (2006). . . . About polymyalgia rheumatica. *Nursing2006, 36*(10), 28.

Nahhas, S. (2007). Back savers: A new lifting protocol reduces injuries to nurses. *ADVANCE for Nurses, 4*(12), 37.

Nursing Made Incredibly Easy! Eds. (2005). Strains and sprains explained. *Nursing Made Incredibly Easy!, 3*(6), 72/

Nursing Made Incredibly Easy! Eds. (2005). When the pressure's just too much. *Nursing Made Incredibly Easy!,*3(2), 53–54.

Nursing2006 Eds. (2006). Taking a closer look at costochondritis. *Nursing2006, 36*(11), 64cc1–64cc2.

Nursing2006 Eds. (2006). Traumatic amputation. *Nursing2006, 36*(10), 88.

Parson, K.S., Galinsky, T.L., & Waters, T. (2006). Preventing musculoskeletal disorders. *Home Healthcare Nurse, 24*(3), 158–164.

Polzien, G. (2006). Care after hip replacement. *Home Healthcare Nurse, 24*(7), 420–422.

Ricciuti, R. (2004). Cut gout out. *ADVANCE for Nurses Online.* Retrieved from http://nursing.advanceweb.com/common/editorial

Ruffolo, D. C. (2005). Life and limb: Understanding the challenges of crush injuries. *ADVANCE for Nurses, 2*(16), 25–27.

Schofied, C. (2004). What is osteonecrosis? *Nursing2004, 35*(1), 29.

Schultz, M., Hermandez, N., & Hernandez, J. (2004). Help patients cope with fibromyalgia. *RN, 67*(9), 46–50.

Sherman, K. J. (2005). Yoga more effective than exercise for low back pain. *Annals of Internal Medicine, 143*(12), 849–856.

Simon, A.M., & O'Connor, J.P. (2007). NSAIDs prevent proper fracture healing. *Journal of Bone and Joint Surgery, 89*, 500–511.

Smith, B.L. (2005). How to manage that pelvic fracture. *RN, 68*(8), 30–35.

Smith, H.R., & Smolen, J.S. (2006). *Rheumatoid arthritis.* Retrieved from www.emedicine.com/med/topic2024.htm

Spader, C. (2005). From sore to soothed: Managing bursitis. *NurseWeek, 18*(13), 16–17.

Wang, C.T., Lin, J., Chang, C.J., et. al. (2006). Therapeutic effects of hyaluronic acid on osteoarthritis of the knee. *Journal of Bone and Joint Surgery, 86* (5), 538–545.

Weil, A. (2003). Natural medicine for arthritis. *Prevention, 55*(4), 109–110.

Wilke, H.J., Mehnert, U., Claes, L.E., et al. (2006). *Spine, 31*(25), 2934–2941.

Zarowitz, B.J. (2007). Management of osteoporosis in older persons. *Geriatric Nursing, 27*(1), 26–27.

Chapter 33

Albo, M.E., Richter, H.E., Brubaker. L., et al.(2007). Burch colposuspension versus fascial sling to reduce urinary stress incontinence. *New England Journal of Medicine.* 356(21), 2143–2155.

Corbett, J.V. (2004). *Laboratory Tests and Diagnostic Procedures with Nursing Diagnosis* (6th ed.). Upper Saddle River, NJ: Prentice Hall.

Davis, K. (2004). Need urine from a catheter system? Forget the needle! *Nursing2004, 34*(12), 64.

Dougherty, M., Dwyer, J.W., Pendergast, J.F., et al. (2002). A randomized trial of behavioral management for continence with rural older women. *Research in Nursing and Health, 25*(1), 3–13.

Gray, M. (2005). Skin care of the incontinent patient. *Advances in Skin and Wound Care, 18*(3), 138–139.

Hoefler, P.A. (2004). *NCLEX-RN Exam Essentials Review* (11th ed.). Laurel, MD: Meds Publishing.

Lab Tests Online. (2006). *Cystatin C.* Retrieved from www.labtestsonline.org/understanding/analytes/cystatin_c/glance.html

MacDonald, C.D., & Butler, L. (2007). Silent no more: Elderly women's stories of living with urinary incontinence in long-term care. *Journal of Gerontological Nursing, 33*(1), 14–20.

Mason, D.J., Newman, D.K., Palmer, M.H. (2003). Bladder matters: Changing UI practice. *American Journal of Nursing, 103*(3), 129.

Mauk, K.L. (2005). Conservative therapy for urinary incontinence can help older adults. *Nursing2005, 35*(8), 20–21.

MedlinePlus. (2006). *Drugs and supplements.* Retrieved from www.nlm.nih.gov/medlineplus/druginfo/medmaster

Palmer, M. H. & Newman , D. K. (2007),. Urinary incontinence and estrogen. *American Journal of Nursing, 107*(3), 35–37.

Pomfret, I., & Holden, C. (2007). Implementing guidance on pelvic floor exercises. *Nursing Times, 103*(19), 40–41.

Pringle, J.K. (2005). Nine myths of incontinence in older adults. *American Journal of Nursing, 105*(6), 58–68.

Pullen, R.L. (2004). Inserting an indwelling urinary catheter in a male patient. *Nursing2004, 34*(7), 24.

Rushing, J. (2004). Inserting an indwelling urinary catheter in a female patient. *Nursing2004, 34*(8), 22.

Sampselle, C., Wyman, J.F., Thomas, K.K., et al. (2000). Continence for women: A test of AWHONN's evidence-based protocol in clinical practice. *Journal of Obstetric, Gynecologic, and Neonatal Nursing, 29*(1), 18–26.

Snyder, M., & Lindquist, R. (2006). *Complementary/Alternative Therapies in Nursing* (5th ed.). New York: Springer.

Toughill, E. (2005). Bladder matters: Indwelling urinary catheters. *American Journal of Nursing, 105*(5), 35–37.

Vasavada, S., & Rackley, R. (2006). How effective is pharmacology for overactive bladder? *Patient Care, 40*(1), 40–46.

Chapter 34

Borghi, L., Schianchi, T., Meschi, T., et al. (2002). Comparison of two diets for the prevention of recurrent stones in idiopathic hypercalciuria. *New England Journal of Medicine, 346*(2), 77–84.

Burrows-Hudson, S. (2005). Chronic kidney disease: An overview. *American Journal of Nursing, 105*(2), 40–50.

Campoy, S., & Elwell, R. (2005). Pharmacology & CKD. *American Journal of Nursing, 105*(9), 60–72.

Carson-Dewitt, R. (2006). *Other treatments for bladder cancer: Biologic therapy and photodynamic therapy.* Retrieved from www.swedish.org.

Castner, D., & Douglas, C. (2005). Onstage chronic kidney disease. *Nursing2005, 35*(12), 58–64.

Desai, A., & Hoenig, D. (2006). Improving the efficacy of ESWL. *Contemporary Urology*, April 2006, 16–25.

Emergency Nurses' Association. (2003). Newberry, L. (Ed.). *Sheehy's Emergency Nursing: Principles and Practice* (5th ed.). St. Louis: Mosby.

Fischbach, F., & Dunning, M.B. (2006). *Common Laboratory & Diagnostic Tests* (4th ed.). Philadelphia: Lippincott Williams & Wilkins.

Hayes, D.D. (2003). Performing peritoneal dialysis. *Nursing2003, 33*(3), 17.

Kear, T.M. (2006). Chronic kidney disease. *ADVANCE for Nurses, 4*(13), 19–22.

Kring, D. (2005). Get the lowdown on chronic kidney disease. *LPN, 1*(4), 28–34.

Kugler, C., Vlaminck, H., Haverich, A., et al. (2005). Nonadherence with diet and fluid restrictions among adults having hemodialysis. *Journal of Nursing Scholarship, 37*(1), 25–29.

LaCharity, L.A., Kumagai, C.K., & Bartz, B. (2006). *Prioritization, Delegation, & Assignment: Practice Exercises for Medical-Surgical Nursing.* St. Louis: Mosby.

Lameire, N. (2005). The pathophysiology of acute renal failure. *Critical Care Nursing Clinics of North America, 21*(2), 197–206.

Legg, V. (2005). Complications of chronic kidney disease. *American Journal of Nursing, 105*(6), 40–50.

Magee, C.C. (2006). Renal artery stenosis. *Medline Plus.* Retrieved from www.nlm.nih.gov/medlineplus/ency/article/001273.htm

Mahoney, C. (2007). Should patients eat during dialysis? *Nursing2007, 37*(10), 57–58.

Malecare (2006). *Men fighting cancer together. Cancer of the urinary bladder.* Retrieved from http://malecare.com/new_page_91.htm

Marguet, C.G., & Preminger, G.M. (2006). Renal stones. *Contemporary Urology,* March 2006, 34–39.

MayoClinic.com (2006). *Wilms' tumor.* Retrieved from www.mayoclinic.com/health/wilms-tumor/DS00436/DSECTION=9.

McCarley, P.B., & Salai, P.B. (2005). Cardiovascular disease in chronic kidney disease. *American Journal of Nursing, 105*(4), 40–53.

McDougall, G.J. (2005). The effect of acupressure with massage on fatigue and depression in patients with end-stage renal disease. *Geriatric Nursing, 26*(3), 164–165.

MedlinePlus. (2006). *Drugs and supplements.* Retrieved from www.nlm.nih.gov/medlineplus/druginfo/medmaster

Nursing2007 Eds. (2007). Fast facts about loop diuretics. *Nursing 2007, 37*(10), 56hn7–56hn8.

Pearce, J.M. (2007). Documenting peritoneal dialysis. *Nursing2007, 37*(10), 28.

Snyder, M., & Lindquist, R. (2006). *Complementary/Alternative Therapies in Nursing* (5th ed.). New York: Springer.

U.S. Food and Drug Administration.(2006). *FDA approves new treatment for gastrointestinal and kidney cancer.* Retrieved from www.fda.gov/bbs/topics/news/2006/NEW01302.html

Wilkinson, J.M. (2005). *Prentice Hall Nursing Diagnosis Handbook with NIC Interventions and NOC Outcomes* (8th ed.). Upper Saddle River, NJ: Prentice Hall.

Woods, A. (2005). Managing UTIs in older adults. *Nursing2005, 35*(3), 12.

Chapter 35

AGS Foundation for Health in Aging (2006). *Hormone disorders.* Retrieved from www.healthinaging.org/agingintheknow/chapters_print_ch_trial.asp?ch=48

Holcomb, S. S. (2007). A delicate balance: Keeping thyroid hormones in check. *LPN2007, 3*(2), 46–54.

Qatanani, M., Zhang, J., & Moore, D.D. (2005). Role of the constitutive androstane receptor in xenobiotic-induced thyroid hormone metabolism. *Endocrinology,* 146(3), 995–1002.

Samuels, M.H., Pillote, K., Asher, D. et al. (2003). Variable effects of nonsteroidal antiinflammatory agents on thyroid test results. *Journal of Clinical Endocrinology & Metabolism, 88*(12), 5710–5716.

Weinstock, R.S., & Zygmont, S.V. (2004). *Pancreatic islet function tests.* Retrieved from www.endotext.org/protocols/protocols5/protocols5.htm

Chapter 36

Agency for Healthcare Research and Quality (2005). *Women who smoke have nearly twice the risk of developing Graves' hyperthyroidism than nonsmokers.* Retrieved from www/ahrq.gov

Bass, A., Will, T., Todd, M., et al. (2007). The latest tools for patients with diabetes. *RN, 70*(6), 39–43.

Dulak, S.B. (2005). Thyroid storm: A medical emergency. *Travel Nursing Today,* April 2005. Retrieved from www.rnweb.com

Holcomb, S.S. (2005). Confronting Cushing's syndrome. *Nursing2005, 35*(9), 32hn1–32hn6.

Holcomb, S.S. (2005). Detecting thyroid disease. *Nursing2005, 35*(10-Supplement Travel Nursing2005), 4–8.

Kim, M.I., & Ladenson, P.W. (2004). *Hypothyroidism in the elderly.* Retrieved from www.endotext.org/aging/aging9/agingframe9.htm

Ratcliff, M. (2005). Treating thyroid cancer. *ADVANCE for Nurses, 22*(13), 21–22.

Chapter 37

Agins, A., & Agins, J. (2007). *Incretins, diabetes, and new drugs.* Retrieved from www.lexi.com/web/nursemailers.jsp?id=agins_oct06

American Diabetes Association (2005). Standards of medical care in diabetes. *Diabetes Care, 28,* S4–S36.

American Diabetes Association. (2006a). *Alcohol.* Retrieved from www.diabetes.org/type-1-diabetes/alcohol.jsp

American Diabetes Association. (2006b). *Complications of diabetes in the United States.* Retrieved from www.diabetes.org/diabetes-statistics/complications.jsp

American Diabetes Association. (2006c). *Kidney disease (nephropathy).* Retrieved from www.diabetes.org/type-1-diabetes/kidney-disease.jsp

American Diabetes Association. (2006d). *Make the link: diabetes, heart disease, and stroke.* Retrieved from www.diabetes.org/type-1-diabetes/well-being/heart-disease-and-stroke.jsp

American Diabetes Association and American Dietetic Association. (2003). *Exchange lists for meal planning.* Available for purchase at www.eatright.org/cps/rde/xchg/ada/hs.xsl/shop_378_ENU_HTML.htm.

Barclay, L. & Nghiem, H.T. (2006). *Metformin use increases vitamin B_{12} deficiency in patients with diabetes.* Retrieved from www.medscape.com/viewarticle/545792

Bass, A., Will, T., Todd, M., et al., (2007). The latest tools for patients with diabetes. *RN, 70*(6), 39–43.

Bonham, P.A. (2007). Healing the wounds: Assessing and managing diabetic neuropathy to avoid amputation. *ADVANCE for Nurses, 4*(4), 30–32.

Centers for Disease Control and Prevention. (2005). *National diabetes fact sheet, 2005.* Retrieved from http://ndep.nih.gov/diabetes/pubs/2005_National_Diabetes_Fact_Sheet.pdf

Cooperman, M. (2006). *Somogyi phenomenon.* Retrieved from www.emedicine.com/med/topic2098.htm

D'Arrigo, T. (2006). New products. *Diabetes Forecast: 2006 Resource Guide.* Retrieved from www.diabetes.org/uedocuments/rg06_newproducts.pdf

De la Cruz, G.J., Valente, S. & Brosnan, J. (2007). How to take care of your feet when you have diabetes. *Nursing2007, 37*(9), 14–15.

Diabetes Health (2007). *Your complete insulin reference guide.* Retrieved from www.DiabetesHealth.com

Diabetes Net. (2006). *Inhaled insulin.* Retrieved from www.diabetesnet.com/diabetes_treatments/insulin_inhaled.php

Eli Lilly and Company. (2005). *Glucagon for injection: Information for the physician.* Retrieved from http://pi.lilly.com/us/rglucagon-pi.pdf

Gates, B., Onufer, C., & Setter, S. (2007). Your complete type 2 medications reference guide. *Diabetes Health.* Retrieved from www.DiabetesHealth.com

Gattullo, B.A. (2007). Diabetic retinopathy. *Nursing2007, 37*(7), 51.

Hussar, D. (2007). Insulin glulisine and insulin detemir. *Nursing2007, 37*(2), 52.

Holmberg, M. (2006). An overview of insulin breakthroughs. *Pharmacy Times,* October 2006. Retrieved from www.pharmacytimes.com/Article.cfm?Menu=1+ID=3959

Institute for Safe Medication Practices (2006). *Pen injectors: Technology is not without impending risks.* Retrieved from www.ismp.org/Newsletters/acutecare/articles/20061130.asp

Krumholz, H.M. (2007). *Rosiglitazone associated with increased risk for MI.* Retrieved from www.medscape.com/viewarticle/558058

Lantus prescribing information. Retrieved from http://products.sanofi-aventis.us/lantus/lantus.html

Mayo Clinic Staff. (2005). *Islet cell transplantation: Emerging treatment for type 1 diabetes.* Retrieved from www.mayoclinic.com/health/islet-cell-transplant/DA00046

Medtronic Minimed. (2007). *Introducing the Guardian® Real-Time Continuous Glucose Monitoring System.* Retrieved from www.minimed.com/products/guardianrt/index.html

National Diabetes Information Clearinghouse. (2005). *National diabetes statistics.* Retrieved from http://diabetes.niddk.nih.gov/dm/pubs/statistics/index.htm#13

NDA-21-868. (2006). *Exubera US package insert.* Retrieved from www.pfizer.com/pfizer/download/uspi_exubera.pdf

Pavlovich-Danis, S. (2007). New horizons in diabetes treatment. *NurseWeek, 20*(12), 14–16.

Pavlovich-Danis, S. (2007). *Drug news: New combination pill for type 2 diabetes.* Retrieved from http://news.nurse.com/apps/pbcs.dll/article?AID=/20070707/CA09/70703002&SearchID=73287862412329

Ridge, R.A. (2007). Boosting insulin safety. *Nursing2007, 37*(2), 14–15.

Ryan, E.A., Paty, B.W., Senior, P.A., et al. (2005). Five-year follow-up after clinical islet transplantation. *Diabetes, 54*(7), 2060–2069.

Scemons, D. (2007). Are you up-to-date on diabetes medications? *Nursing2007, 37*(7), 45–49.

Seley, J.J., & Weinger, K. (2007). Executive summary: The state of the science on nursing best practices for diabetes self-management. *American Journal of Nursing, 107*(6), 73–78.

U.S. Department of Health and Human Services, Office of Public Affairs. (2000). *Rezulin to be withdrawn from the market.* Retrieved from www.fda.gov/bbs/topics/NEWS/NEW00721.html

U.S. Food and Drug Administration. (2006). *FDA approves first ever inhaled insulin combination product for treatment of diabetes.* January 27, 2006. Retrieved from www.fda.gov/bbs/topics/news/2006/NEW01304.html

U.S. Food and Drug Administration (2007). *Diabetes information: Insulin delivery devices.* Retrieved from www.fda.gov/diabetes/insulin.html

U.S. Food and Drug Administration (2007). *FDA News: FDA issues safety alert on Avandia.* Retrieved from www.fda.gov/bbs/topics/NEWS/2007/NEW01636.html

Vasudevan, A.R., Srinavasan, A.R., & Snow, K.J. (2006). *Hypoglycemia.* Retrieved from www.emedicine.com/MED/topic1123.htm

Walsh, J. (2006). *Insulin pumping: The latest advances.* PowerPoint presentation. Retrieved from www.diabetesnet.com/diabetes_technology/insulin-pumps-advanced.html

Zimkus, J., Cox, J.M., Tampellini, L., et al. (2007). Gestational diabetes: A danger to mother and baby. *LPN2007, 3*(3), 36–44.

Chapter 38

American College of Obstetricians and Gynecologists. (2005). Emergency contraception: ACOG Practice Bulletin: Clinical management guidelines for obstetrician-gynecologists, Number 69, December 2005. *Obstetrics and Gynecology, 106,* 1443–1451.

Anastasia, P. J. (2007). When the diagnosis is endometrial cancer. *NurseWeek,* 20(13)

Anderson, F.D, Gibbons, W., & Portman, D. (2006). Safety and efficacy of an extended regimen oral contraceptive utilizing continuous low-dose ethinyl estradiol. *Contraception, 73,* 229–234.

Baerwald, A.R., Olatunbosun, O.A., & Pierson, R.A. (2004). Ovarian follicular development is initiated during the hormone-free interval of oral contraceptive use. *Contraception, 70,* 371–377.

Bahamondes, L., Faundes, A., Sobreira-Lima, B., et al. (2005). TCu 380A IUD: A reversible permanent contraceptive method in women over 35 years of age. *Contraception, 72,* 337–341.

Berry, D.A., Cronin, K.A., Plevritis, S.K., et al. (2005). Effect of screening and adjustment therapy on mortality from breast cancer. *New England Journal of Medicine, 353,* 1784–1792.

Breslin, E.T., & Lucas, V.A. (2003). *Women's Health Nursing: Toward Evidence-Based Practice.* Philadelphia: Saunders.

Bucci, M.K., Bevan, A., & Roach, M. 3rd. (2005) Advances in radiation therapy: Conventional to 3D, to IMRT, to 4D, and beyond. *CA: A Cancer Journal for Clinicians, 55,* 117–134.

Carroll, C.M. (2006). Sorting out breast biopsy options. *Nursing2006, 36*(3), 70–71.

Carroll, D.G. (2006). Nonhormonal therapies for hot flashes in menopause. *American Family Physician, 73,* 457–468.

Cass, I., & Karlan, B. (2003). Neoplasms of the ovary & fallopian tube. In J. Scott, R. Gibbs, B., Karlan, & A. Haney (Eds.). *Danforth's Obstetrics and Gynecology* (9 ed., pp. 971–1006). Philadelphia: Lippincott, Williams & Wilkins.

Condon, M. (2004). *Women's Health: An Integrated Approach to Wellness & Illness.* Upper Saddle River, NJ: Prentice-Hall.

Cox, J.T. (2006). Cervical cancer guidelines: Making sense of the screening intervals. *Contemporary OB/GYN, 51*(4), 54–58.

Crossman, S. (2006). The challenge of pelvic inflammatory disease. *American Family Physician, 73,* 859–863.

Davis, A.R. (2006). Return to menses after continuous use of a low-dose oral contraceptive [Abstract]. *Obstetrics and Gynecology, 107*(35), 1–11.

Dell, D.D. (2005a). Battling breast cancer. *Nursing Made Incredibly Easy!, 3*(5), 4–20.

Dell, D.D. (2005b). Spread the word about breast cancer. *Nursing2005, 35*(10), 56–64.

Dershaw, D.D. (2005). Film or digital mammographic screening? *New England Journal of Medicine, 353,* 1846–1847.

Funk, S., Miller, M.M., Mishell, D.R. Jr., et al. (2005). Safety and efficacy of Implanon, a single-rod implantable contraceptive containing etonogestrel. *Contraception, 71,* 319–326.

Hacker, N.F., Moore, J.G., & Gambone, J.C. (Eds.). (2004). *Essentials of Obstetrics and Gynecology* (4 ed.). Philadelphia: Saunders.

Hiller, J.Y., Miller, M.J., & Stavas, J.M. (2005). Uterine artery embolization: A minimally invasive option to end fibroid symptoms. *ADVANCE for Nurse Practitioners, 13*(10), 20–25.

Horbach, N., Lee, T., Levy, B., et al. (2006). Laparoscopic supracervical hysterectomy. *Contemporary OB/GYN,* May 2006 Special Addendum, 1–11.

Hortobagyi, G.N. (2005). Trastuzumab in the treatment of breast cancer. *New England Journal of Medicine, 353,* 1734–1736.

Jenkins, T.R. (2004). Laparascopic supracervical hysterectomy. *American Journal of Obstetrics and Gynecology, 191,* 1875–1884.

Jick, S.S., Kaye, J.A., Russmann, S., et al. (2006). Risk of nonfatal venous thromboembolism in women using a contraceptive transdermal patch and oral contraceptives containing norgestimate and 35 microg of ethinyl estradiol. *Contraception, 73,* 223–228.

Kahn, J., & Hillard, P. (2006). What you can do to prevent cervical cancer and other HPV related diseases. *Contemporary Pediatrics, 23*(4), 55–74.

Katz, A. (2005). Do ask, do tell: Why do so many nurses avoid the topic of sexuality. *American Journal of Nursing, 105*(7), 66–68.

Katz, A. (2007). When sex hurts: Menopause-related dyspareunia. *American Journal of Nursing, 107*(7), 34–39.

Kaunitz, A.M. (2005). Beyond the pill: New data and options in hormonal and intrauterine contraception. *American Journal of Obstetrics and Gynecology, 192,* 998–1004.

Martin, V. (2006). Shining a light on ovarian cancer. *Nursing Made Incredibly Easy!, 4*(6), 28–37.

Master-Hunter, T., & Heiman, D.L. (2006). Amenorrhea: Evaluation and treatment. *American Family Physician, 73,* 1374.

Meyers, S. (2006). Contraceptive advancements provide more options, convenience. *NurseWeek, 19*(20), 19.

Miller, K.E. (2006). Diagnosis and treatment of *Chlamydia trachomatis* infection. *American Family Physician, 73,* 1411–1416.

Mischell, D.R. Jr. (2005). Rationale for decreasing the number of days of the hormone-free interval with use of low-dose oral contraceptive formulations. *Contraception, 71,* 304–305.

National Women's Health Resource Center. (2000). Genetic testing and women's health. *National Women's Health Report, 22*(6), 1–8.

Paik, S. (2006). Gene expression and benefit of chemotherapy in women with node-negative, estrogen receptor–positive breast cancer. *Journal of Clinical Oncology, 24,* 3726–3734.

Piccart-Gebhart, M.J., Procter, M., Leyland-Jones, B., et al. (2005). Trastuzumab after adjuvant chemotherapy in HER2-positive breast cancer. *New England Journal of Medicine, 353,* 1659–1672.

Schorge, J.O., & Rao, G.G. (2006). Chemoradiation: The new paradigm for invasive cervical cancer. *Contemporary OB/GYN, 51*(3), 48–50.

Schorn, M.N. (2006). How does oral emergency contraception work? *Nursing, 36*(2), 31

Spector, J.A., & Karp, N.S. (2005). A primer on breast reduction surgery. *Contemporary OB/GYN, 50*(11), 58–70.

Speroff, L. (2006). Using aromatase inhibitors to treat early breast cancer. *Contemporary OB/GYN, 51*(2), 60–66.

Stenchever, M.A. (2004). Physiology of micturition, diagnosis of voiding dysfunctions and incontinence, surgical and nonsurgical management. In Stenchever M.A., et al. (Eds.). *Comprehensive Gynecology* (5 ed.). St. Louis: Mosby.

Stewart, E.A., Rabinovici, J., Tempany, C.M., et al. (2006). Clinical outcomes of focused ultrasound surgery for the treatment of uterine fibroids. *Fertility and Sterility, 85,* 22–29.

Sutton, D. E. (2006). Uterine fibroid embolization. *ADVANCE for Nurses, 4*(11), 36.

Thiadens, S., & Anderson, L. (2006). On raising awareness of lymphedema. *NurseWeek, 19*(25), 31.

Tumolo, J. (2007). Kids, sex & the city. *ADVANCE for Nurses, 4*(3), 13, 24.

Vogel, V.G., Costantino, J.P., Wickerham, D.L., et al. (2002). The study of tamoxifen and raloxifene: Preliminary enrollment data from a randomized breast cancer risk reduction trial. *Clinical Breast Cancer, 3,* 153–159.

Williams, S. (2007). Herb helps relieve hot flashes: Cohosh is still a treatment option for menopausal symptoms. *NurseWeek, 20*(10), 39–40.

Yonkers, K.A., Brown, C., Pearlstein, T.B., et al. (2005). Efficacy of a new low-dose oral contraceptive with drospirenone in premenstrual dysphoric disorder. *Obstetrics and Gynecology, 106,* 492–501.

RESOURCES

Interactive website concerning contraception
www.ARHP.org/patienteducation/interactivetools/choosing/index.cfm?id=275

Planned Parenthood
www.plannedparenthood.org/birthcontrol-pregnancy/birthcontrol.htm

National Cancer networks
www.BreastCancer.org
www.ACCN.org

People Living With Cancer
www.PLWC.org

National Cancer Institute
www.cancer.gov

National Lymphedema network
www.lymphnet.org

Chapter 39

American Cancer Society. (2007) *Facts & Figures—2007*, Atlanta: Author.

Bent, S., Kane, C., Shinohara, K., et al. (2006). Saw palmetto for benign prostatic hyperplasia. *New England Journal of Medicine, 354*, 557–566.

Bhatnagar, V.,& Kaplan, R.M. (2005). Treatment options for prostate cancer: Evaluating the evidence. *American Family Physician, 71*, 1915–1934.

Burghart, G. (2006). The other ED. *ADVANCE for Nurses, 3*(11), 27–30.

Concato, J., Wells, C.K., Horwitz, R.I., et al. (2006) The effectiveness of screening for prostate cancer: A nested case-control survey. *Archives of Internal Medicine, 166*, 3.

Ficorelli, C.T. (2006). Facing up to prostate cancer. *Nursing2006, 36*(5), 66–68.

Gilchrist, K.L. (2005). Twin perils of prostate health. *Nursing Made Incredibly Easy!, 3*(6), 30–42.

Gray, M., & Sims, T. (2007). Prostate cancer: Prevention and management of localized disease. *The Nurse Practitioner: The American Journal of Primary Health Care, 31*(9), 14–29.

Katz, A. (2006). Erectile dysfunction and its discontents. *Amercian Journal of Nursing, 106*(12), 70–72.

Keefe, S. (2006). Andropause. *ADVANCE for Nurses, 3*(11), 29–30.

Margo, K., & Winn, R. (2006). Testosterone treatments: Why, when, and how? *American Family Physician, 73*, 1591–1603.

Micozzi, M.S. (2006). *Fundamentals of Complementary and Integrative Medicine* (3rd ed.). Philadelphia: Saunders.

Saigal, C.S., Wessells, H., Pace, J., et al. (2006). Predictors and prevalence of erectile dysfunction in a racially diverse population. *Archives of Internal Medicine, 166*, 207–212.

Thompson, I.M., Tangen, C.M., Goodman, P.J., et al. (2005). Erectile dysfunction and subsequent cardiovascular disease. *Journal of the American Medical Association, 294*, 2996–3002.

Wattendorf, D.J., & Muenke, M. (2005). Klinefelter syndrome. *American Family Physician, 72*, 2259–2262.

Weeks, B., & Ficorelli, C.T. (2006). Treating erectile dysfunction without first-line drugs. *Nursing2006, 36*(3), 26–27.

Chapter 40

Centers for Disease Control and Prevention. (2007). Update to CDC STD treatment guidelines. Sexually transmitted diseases treatment guidelines 2002. *MMWR: Morbidity and Mortality Weekly Report, 56*(4-13), 332–336. Retrieved from www.cdc.gov/std/treatment

Gardner, J. (2006). What you need to know about genital herpes. *Nursing2006, 36*(10), 26–27.

Mandell,G.L., Douglas, R.G., Bennett, J.E., et al. (2005). *Mandell, Douglas, and Bennett's Principles and Practice of Infectious Diseases* (6 ed.). Philadelphia: Elsevier Saunders.

Miller, K.E. (2006). Diagnosis and treatment of *Neisseria gonorrhoeae* infection. *American Family Physician, 73*, 1779–1784.

Morantz, C. (2006). Practice Guidelines: ACIP updates recommendations for prevention of hepatitis B virus transmission. *American Family Physician, 73*, 1839–1844.

Noonan, M. (2006). Is oral sex safe sex? No way! (2006). *ADVANCE for Nurses, 8*(8), 18.

NurseWeek Eds. (2007). New STD treatment guidelines. *NurseWeek, 20*(12), 21.

Raper, J.L. (2006). Anal pap screening in men with HIV. *ADVANCE for Nurse Practitioners, 14*(6), 30–35.

U.S. Department of Health and Human Services. (2000). *Healthy People 2010.* Washington, DC: Department of Health and Human Services.

Workowski, K., & Berman, S.M. (2006). Sexually transmitted diseases treatment guidelines, 2006. *MMWR: Recommended Reports, 55*(RR 11), 1–94. Retrieved from www.cdc.gov/STD/treatment/2006/rr5511.pdf

Chapter 41

Advances in Skin & Wound Care Eds. (2004). How aging affects wound healing. *Advances in Skin & Wound Care, 18*, 20–21.

Advances in Skin & Wound Care Eds. (2005). Identifying primary and secondary skin lesions. *Advances in Skin & Wound Care, 18*, 19.

American Cancer Society. (2006). *Skin cancer prevention: Be sun savvy.* Retrieved from www.cancer.org.docroot/PED/content/ped_7_1x_Protect_Your_Skin_From_UV.asp?sitearea=PED.

Anderson, J., Langemo, D., Hanson, D, et al. (2007). What you can learn from a comprehensive skin assessment. *Nursing2007, 37*(4), 65–66.

Ankrom, M.A., Bennett, R.G., Sprigle, S., et al. (2005). Pressure-related deep tissue injury under intact skin and the current pressure ulcer staging systems. *Advances in Skin & Wound Care, 18*, 35–41.

Ayello, E.A., & Lyder, D.H. (2007). Protecting patients from harm: Preventing pressure ulcers in hospital patients. *Nursing2007, 37*(10, 36–40.

Ayers, D.M.M. (2004). Melanoma. *Nursing2004, 34*(4), 52–53.

Baldwin, K.M. (2005). How to prevent and treat pressure ulcers. *LPN2005, 1*(2), 18–25.

Black, J. (2004). Preventing heel pressure ulcers. *Nursing2004, 34*(11), 17.

Braden, B.J., & Maklebust, J. (2005). Preventing pressure ulcers with the Braden scale. *American Journal of Nursing, 105*(6), 70–72.

Bresett, J. (2006). Would you suspect this skin-eating infection? *RN, 69*(3), 31–35.

Catania, K., Huang, C., James, P. & Ohr, M. (2007). PUPPI: The pressure ulcer prevention protocol interventions. *American Journal of Nursing, 107*(4), 44–52.

Chettle, C. C. (2006). Herpes—Common and sometimes dangerous. *NurseWeek, 19*(19),17–18.

Chicago Sun Times Eds. (2006). Aches & claims: Can you pop a pill for sun protection? [Edial]. *Chicago Sun Times*, June 4, 2006.

Courey, T.L. (2006). Addressing the physical and mental symptoms of shingles. *Journal for Nurse Practitioners, 2*(4), 229–235.

Fernandes, D. (2007). A closer look at sun protection: Sunscreens with high SPFs will not block out all UV light. *ADVANCE Newsmagazines for LPNs*. Retrieved from http:lpn.advanceweb.com/Common/Edial/PrintFriendly.aspx?CC=91389

Franck, P.A. (2004). Diagnosing ulcerative skin eruptions. *Advances in Skin & Wound Care, 17*, 260–262.

Giuliano, R., & Reintgen, D.S. (2004). Skin cancer. *ADVANCE for Nurses, 1*(1), 15–18.

Holcomb, S.S. (2006). Nonmelanoma skin cancer. *Nursing2006, 36*(6), 56–57.

Holcomb, S. S. (2007). Dodging the bullae: Stevens-Johnson syndrome: Lear now to turn the tables on this nasty rash. *Nursing2007, 37*(4), 64cc1–64cc3.

Lillis, K. (Ed.). (2006). Skin cancer: How to protect yourself. *ADVANCE for Nurses, 3*(11), 39.

Lorenz, J. M. (2007). Geriatric skin care. *ADVANCE for Nurses, 4*(11), 29–30.

Mascolo, L. (2006). Skin care team improves assessment and documentation. *Nursing2006,* 36(10), 66–67.

National Pressure Ulcer Advisory Panel. (2007). *Pressure ulcer stages revised by NPUAP.* Retrieved from www.npuap.org/pr2.htm

Nursing2006 Eds. (2006). Managing pruritus. *Nursing2006, 36*(7), 17.

Nursing Made Incredibly Easy!, Eds. (2007). Stop the fungus among us. *Nursing Made Incredibly Easy!, 5*(3), 9–10.

Ryan, J. M. (2006). Teamwork keeps the pressure off. *Home Healthcare Nurse, 24*(2), 97–101.

Sarvis, C. (2006). SJS and TEN leave their mark on the skin. *NurseWeek, 19*(25), 14–15.

Shields, J. (2007). Summer's Coming: Time to review skin cancer risk with patients. *NurseWeek, 20*(11), 12.

Stausberg, J., Kröger, K., Maier, I., et al. (2005). Pressure ulcers in secondary care: Incidence, prevalence, and relevance. *Advances in Skin & Wound Care, 18,* 140–145.

Zukowski, K., & Ratliff, C. (2007). Is it perineal dermatitis . . . or a pressure ulcer? *LPN2007, 3*(2), 19–21.

Chapter 42

ADVANCE for Nurses Ed. (2007). New T-shirt designed for wound & burn care. *ADVANCE for Nurses, 4*(13), 43.

Agency for Health Care Policy and Research. (1994). *Pressure ulcer treatment.* Rockville, MD: U.S. Department of Health and Human Services, Public Health Service.

American Cancer Society National Comprehensive Cancer Network. (2005). *Melanoma: Treatment guidelines for patients* (Part 2). Retrieved from www.medscape.com/viewarticle/507588

Ankrom, M.A., Bennett, R.G., Sprigle, S., et al. (2005). Pressure-related deep tissue injury under intact skin and the current pressure ulcer staging systems. *Advances in Wound & Skin Care, 18,* 35–42.

Baldwin, K.M.(2006). Damage control: Preventing and treatment pressure ulcers. *Nursing Made Incredibly Easy!, 4*(1), 13–26.

Bowles, D. (2005). Hope for the "heartbreak of psoriasis." *NurseWeek, 18*(13), 19–20.

Burn Survivor Resource Center. (2006). *Burn statistics.* Retrieved from www.burnsurvivor.com/burn_statistics.html

Chettle, C. C. (2006). Herpes—Common and sometimes dangerous. *NurseWeek, 19*(19), 17–18.

Combest, W. L. (2007). *Tea tree.* Retrieved from www.uspharmacist.com

D'Arcy, Y. (2006). Heading off the pain of postherpetic neuralgia. *Nursing2006, 36*(9), 25–26.

Easter, J.S. (2004). *Herpes zoster.* Retrieved from www.emedicine.com/derm/topic180.htm

Elston, D.M. (2005). *Lice.* Retrieved from www.emedicine.com/derm/topic229.htm

End of Life Palliative Education Resource Center. (2006). *Fast Fact and Concept #41: Pressure ulcer management: Debridement and dressings.* Retrieved from www.mywhatever.com/cifwriter/library/eperc/fastfact/ff41.html

Franck, P.A. (2004). Diagnosing ulcerative skin eruptions. *Advances in Skin & Wound Care, 17,* 260–263.

Guiliano, R., & Reintgen, D.S. (2004). Skin cancer: When prevention fails, treatment includes curettage and surgery. *ADVANCE for Nurses, 1*(1), 15–19.

Gupta, S., et al. (2004). Guidelines for managing pressure ulcers with negative pressure wound therapy. *Advances in Skin & Wound Care,* 17(Suppl 2), 1–16.

Heistein, J.B., & Ruberg, R.L. (2005). *Skin malignancies, melanoma.* Retrieved from www.emedicine.com/plastic/topic456.htm

Home Healthcare Nurse Eds. (2005). New best practice guidelines for managing pressure ulcers with negative pressure wound therapy published. *Home Healthcare Nurse, 23,* 469.

Kent, D.J. (2007). Getting misty over wound care. *Nursing2007,* 37(9), 36–37.

Laskowski-Jones, L. (2006). First aid for burns. *Nursing2006, 36*(1), 41–43.

Leatherman, M. (2005). What is causing a persistent skin boil? *Advances in Skin & Wound Care, 18,* 30–31.

Mayo Clinic. (2006). *Burns: First aid.* Retrieved from www.mayoclinic.com

National Guideline Clearing House. (2006). *Preventing pressure ulcers and skin tears.* Retrieved from www.guideline.gov/summary/summary.aspx?doc_id=3511

National Institute of Health. (2005). *Experimental shingles vaccine proves effective in nationwide study.* Retrieved from www.niaid.nih.gov/default.htm

National Institute of Health (2007). Tai Chi boosts immunity to shingles virus in older adults, NIH-sponsored study reports. *NIH News Press.* Retrieved from http://nccam.nih.gov

National Pressure Ulcer Advisory Panel. (2006a). *The facts about reverse staging in 2000. National Pressure Ulcer Advisory Panel.* Retrieved from http://222.npuap.org/positn5.html

National Pressure Ulcer Advisory Panel. (2006b). *PUSH tool 3.0.* Retrieved from http://222.npuap.org/positn5.html

Novatnack, E. (2007). Shingles: What you should know. *RN,* 79(6), 27–31.

Nowlin, A. (2006). The delicate business of burn care. *RN, 69*(1), 52–57.

Park, R. (2005). *Psoriasis.* Retrieved from www.emedicine.com/emerg/topic489.htm

Pavovich-Danis, S.J., & Etienne, M.O. (2005). Coping with the unwelcome surprise of shingles. *NurseWeek, 18*(7), 23–25.

Quillen, T.F. (2004). Easing the heartbreak of psoriasis. *Nursing2004, 34*(11), 18–19.

Santacroce, L., & Kennedy, A. (2005). *Epitheliomas, basal cell.* Retrieved from www.emedicine.com/med/topic722/htm

Santulli, E. R. (2007). For shingles. *ADVANCE for Nurses,* 4(11), 34.

Smith, M.C., Nederost, S., & Tackett, B. (2007). Facing up to withdrawal from topical steroids. *Nursing2007, 37*(9), 60–61.

Snow, M. (2007). The truth about scabies. *Nursing2007,* 37(2), 28, 30.

Supple, K.G. (2005). Burn injury care. *ADVANCE for Nurses,* 2(22), 17–21.

WoundHeal Eds. (2006). *Ulcer care.* Retrieved from www.woundheal.com/healing/clinical106.htm

Chapter 43

American Journal of Nursing Eds. (2005). On the road to disaster—and back. *American Journal of Nursing, 105*(11), 24–25.

American Red Cross (2005). *Blackouts.* Retrieved from www.redcross.org/services/diaster/0,1082,0_564_,00.html

American Red Cross (2006a). *Shelter-in-place in an emergency.* Retrieved from www.redcross.org/services/disaster/beprepared/shelterinplace.html

American Red Cross. (2006b). *Water treatment.* Retrieved from www.redcross.org/services/disaster/0,1082,0_563,00.html

Centers for Disease Control and Prevention. (2001). *How to handle anthrax and other biological agent threats.* Retrieved from www.cdc.gov/ncidod

Centers for Disease Control and Prevention. (2004). *Keep food and water safe after a natural disaster or power outage.* Retrieved from www.bt.cdc.gov/disasters/foodwater.asp

Centers for Disease Control and Prevention. (2006a). *Facts about ricin.* Retrieved from www.bt.cdc.gov/agent/ricin/facts.asp

Centers for Disease Control and Prevention. (2006b). *Viral hemorrhagic fevers.* Retrieved from www.cdc.gov/ncidod/dvrd/spb/mnpages/dispages/vhf.htm

Chaffee, M. (2006). Reality check: How prepared are we for disasters? *American Journal of Nursing, 106*(3), 13.

College of Nursing Art and Science, Hyogo. (2005). *Tips on nursing volunteer activities in the event of disaster (emergency and medium-term support for evacuees).* Retrieved from www.coe-cnas.jp/eng/group_network/nettowa-ku3hisaisya.asp

Couig, M.P., Martinelli, A., & Lavin, R.P. (2005). The National Response Plan: Health and Human Services takes the lead for emergency support function. *Disaster Management & Response, 3*(2), 34–40.

Employee Education System for the Office of Public Health and Environmental Hazards, Department of Veterans Affairs. (2003). *Pocket Guide for Responders to Ionizing Radiation Terrorism.* Bethesda, MD: Armed Forces Radiobiology Research Institute. Retrieved from www.afrri.usuhs.mil/www/outreach/pocketguide.htm

Fell-Carlson, D. (2003a). Terrorist danger: Nurses must be ready for radiological threat. *NurseWeek, 16*(2), 19–20.

Fell-Carlson, D. (2003b). Terrorist danger: The nurse's role in managing the radiological threat. *NurseWeek, 16*(3), 21–22.

Godyn, J.J., Reys, L., Siderits, R., et al. (2005). Cutaneous anthrax: Conservative or surgical treatment? *Advances in Skin & Wound Care, 18,* a46–a150.

Halpern, J.S., & Chaffee, M.W. (Eds.). (2005). Disaster management and response. *Nursing Clinics of North America, 40*(3).

Keefe, S. (2006). Responding to disaster. *ADVANCE for Nurses, 3*(1), 35–36.

National Oceanic and Atmospheric Administration. *Stay informed.* Retrieved from www.nhc/noaa.gov/HAV/english/disaster_prevention.shtml

Pattillo, M. (2005). Bioterrorism. *ADVANCE for Nurses, 2*(17), 19–23.

Persell, D.J., Arangie, P., Young, C., et al. (2002). Preparing for bioterrorism. *Nursing2002, 32*(2), 37–43.

Ross, K.L., & Bing, C.M. (2007). Emergency management: Expanding the disaster plan. *Home Healthcare Nurse, 25*(6), 370–377.

Sienkiewicz, J., Wilkinson, G., & Cubbage, B. (2007). Patient classification system for emergency events in home care. *Home Healthcare Nurse, 25*(6), 278–385.

Stopford, B.M. (2006). *Preparing for bioterrorism.* Retrieved from www.nursingconsult.com/das/news/body/2/cup/0/166321/1.html?pos=166321

Todd, R. (2006). Infection control and hurricane Katrina. *American Journal of Nursing, 106*(3), 29–31.

U.S. Department of Health and Human Services. (2002). *Disasters and emergencies.* Retrieved from www.hhs.gov/disasters/index.shtml

Waring, S.C., & Brown, B.J. (2005). The threat of communicable diseases following natural disasters: A public health response. *Disaster Management & Response, 3*(2), 41–47.

Wilshire, L., Hassmiller, S.B., & Wodicka, K.A. (2006). *Disaster preparedness and response for nurses (CE program).* American Red Cross and Sigma Theta Tau International. Retrieved from www.nursingsociety.org/education/case_studies/cases/SP0004.html

Chapter 44

Abella, B.S., Rhee, J.W., Huang, K.N., et al. (2005). Induced hypothermia is underused after resuscitation from cardiac arrest: A current practice survey. *Resuscitation, 64,* 181–186.

Beattie, S. (2006). In from the cold. *RN, 69*(11), 22–27.

Bridges, N., & Jarquin-Valdivia, A.A. (2005). Use of the Trendelenburg position as the resuscitation position: To T or not to T? *American Journal of Critical Care, 14,* 364–369.

Day, P. (2006). Hypothermia: A hazard for all seasons. *Nursing2006, 36*(12), 44–47.

Donnellan, M. (2007). Thwarting sepsis. *ADVANCE Newsmagazines for LPNs.* Retrieved from http://lpn.advanceweb.com/common/Edial/PrintFriendly.aspx?CC=88243

Dremsizov, T., Clermont, G., Kellum, J.A., et al. (2006). Severe sepsis in community-acquired pneumonia: When does it happen, and do systemic inflammatory response syndrome criteria help predict course? *Chest, 129,* 968.

Dreskin, A.C., & Palmer, G.W. (2005). *Anaphylaxis. WebMD.* Retrieved from www.emedicine.com/med/topic128.htm

Duhon, J., & Roman, L.M. (2006). When organs fail one by one. *RN, 69*(5), 44–49.

Fildes, J.J. (2005). *National Trauma Data Bank 2005.* Chicago: American College of Surgeons.

Hernandez, R.G., & Cohen, B.A. (2006). Insect bite-induced hypersensitivity and the SCRATCH principles: A new approach to papular urticaria. *Pediatrics, 118,* 380–382.

Holcomb, S.S. (2006). Black widow spider bite. *Nursing2006, 36*(5), 80.

Jacoby, S.F., Ackerson, T.H., & Richmond, T.S. (2006). Outcome from serious injury in older adults. *Journal of Nursing Scholarship, 38,* 133–141.

Jahan, A. (2006). Septic shock in the post operative patient: Three important management decisions. *Cleveland Clinic Journal of Medicine, 73*(Suppl 1), S67–S71.

Laskowski-Jones, L. (2006). Responding to trauma: Your priorities in the first hour. *Nursing2006, 36*(9), 52–58.

Louden, K. (2007). Nurses' detective work helps identify food poisoning. *NurseWeek, 20*(14), 8.

McArthur, B.J. (2006). Damage control surgery for the patient who has experienced multiple traumatic injuries. *AORN Journal, 84,* 991–992, 994, 996–1000.

Nunnelee, J. (2005). Summer injuries: Bites and stings. *RN, 68*(4), 56.

Ross, J.L. (2006). Near drowning. *RN, 68*(7), 36.

Sundeen, M. (2005). *Cell phones and highway safety: 2005 legislative update, National Conference of State Legislatures.* Retrieved from www.ncsl.org/programs/transportation/cellphoneupdate05.htm

Torpy, J.M., Lynm, C., & Glass, R.M. (2006). Automated external defibrillators. *Journal of the American Medical Association, 296,* 724.

Van den Berghe, G., Wilmer, A., Hermans, G., et al. (2006). Intensive insulin therapy in the medical ICU. *New England Journal of Medicine, 354,* 449–461.

Veronesi, J.F. (2004). Blunt chest injuries. *RN, 67*(3), 47.

Walsh, C.R. (2005). Multiple organ dysfunction syndrome after multiple trauma. *Orthopaedic Nursing, 24,* 324.

Wood, S., Lavieri, M.C., Durkin, T. (2007). What you need to know about sepsis. *Nursing2007, 37*(3), 46–50.

Woodruff, D.W. (2007). Saving lives with a rapid response team. *LPN2007, 3*(3), 23–27.

Chapter 45

Arnold, E. (2005). Sorting out the 3D's: Delirium, dementia, depression. *Holistic Nursing Practice, 19*(3), 99–105.

Blake, T. (2007). Tracking the ups and downs of antidepressants. *Nursing2007, 37*(4), 49–51.

Burgner, K. (2005). Musical intervention. *ADVANCE for Nurses, 3*(13), 15–17.

Chiocca, E.M. (2007). Suicidal ideation. *Nursing2007, 37*(5), 72.

Costell, S. (2003). Evidence-based treatment of mood disorders. *Nursing Clinics of North America, 38,* 21–33.

Crow, S. (2006). Suicide assessment in the ED. *ADVANCE for Nurses, 4*(4), 17–18.

Donoghue, K., Lomax, K. & Hall, J. (2007). Using group work to prevent relapse in bipolar disorder. *Nursing Times, 103*(19), 30–31.

Geffken, G.R., Storch, E.A., Gelfand, K.M., et al. (2004). Cognitive-behavioral therapy for obsessive-compulsive disorder. *Journal of Psychosocial Nursing, 42*(12), 44–51.

Haas, S.S. (2005). Adolescence and depresssion. *ADVANCE for Nurses, 3*(3), 33–34.

Harvard Medical School. (2007). Electroconvulsive therapy: with new methods and accumulated evidence, this treatment survives its critics. *Harvard Mental Health Letter, 23*(8), 1–4.

Howland, R.H. (2005a). Anticonvulsant drug therapies. *Journal of Psychosocial Nursing, 43*(6), 17–20.

Howland, R.H. (2005b). Therapeutic brain stimulation for mental disorders. *Journal of Psychosocial Nursing, 43*(2), 16–19.

James, K.S., & Cook, L.M. (2006). Anorexia nervosa. *ADVANCE for Nurses, 4*(2), 17–20.

Kneisl, C.R., Wilson, H.S., & Trigoboff, E. (2004). *Contemporary Psychiatric-Mental Health Nursing.* Upper Saddle River, NJ: Prentice Hall.

Murphy, K. (2005). Anxiety: When is it too much? *Nursing Made Incredibly Easy!, 3*(5), 22–31.

Murphy, K. (2007). A thin line: The lowdown on eating disorders. *LPN2007, 5,*10–23.

Parsons, C. (2005). Bipolar disorder. *ADVANCE for Nurses, 7*(2), 12.

Peden, A.R., Rayens, M.K., Hall, L.A., et al. (2005). Testing an intervention to reduce negative thinking, depressive symptoms and chronic stressors in low-income single mothers. *Journal of Nursing Scholarship, 37*(3), 268–274.

Psychiatric Nursing Made Incredibly Easy! (2004). Philadelphia: Lippincott.

Safety First. (2005). Patients at risk. *ADVANCE for Nurses, 3*(11), 43.

Wooten, J.M. (2006). Drug update. This drug fights depression within hours, not weeks. *RN, 69*(9), 69–70.

Zarate, C.A., Singh, J.B., Carlson, P.J., et al. (2006). A randomized trial of an *N*-methyl-d-aspartate antagonist in treatment-resistant major depression. *Archives of General Psychiatry, 63*(8), 856–864.

Chapter 46

Alcoholics Anonymous. (2005). *Twelve Steps.* New York: AA World Services.

American Cancer Society. (2006). *Questions about smoking, tobacco, and health.* Retrieved from www.cancer.org

Back, S.E. (2007). The role of nonpharmacologic therapy in alcohol dependence. *Medscape Psychiatry & Mental Health.* Retrieved from www.medscape.com/viewarticle/557742

Brown, J., & McColm, K. (2007). Raising nurses' awareness of alcohol use in older people. *Nursing Times, 103*(6), 30–31.

Bryan, R.H. (2007). Quitting the habit. *ADVANCE for Nurses, 8*(14), 11.

Buchanan, L.M., El-Banna, M., White, A., et al. (2005). An exploratory study of multicomponent treatment intervention for tobacco dependency. *Journal of Nursing Scholarship, 36*(4), 324–330.

Campral. (2006). *About Campral.* Retrieved from www.campral.com

Ellsworth, A.J., Witt, D.M., Dugdale, D.C., et al. (2004). *Mosby's Medical Drug Reference.* St. Louis: Mosby.

Ewing, J.A.(1984). Detecting alcoholism: The CAGE questionnaire. *JAMA, 252,* 1905–1907.

Foster, J., & Heather, N. (2005). Brief interventions for alcohol problems in hospital settings. *Nursing Times, 101*(26), 38–41.

Gendreau-Webb, R. (2004). Methadone overdose. *Nursing2004, 34*(11), 88.

Hughes, G., Moynes, P., & Jones, C. (2005). Engaging precontemplative dual diagnosis patients. *Nursing Times, 101*(20), 32–34.

Jennings-Ingle, S. (2007). Sobering up to alcohol withdrawal syndrome. *LPN2007, 3*(5), 40–48.

Lussier-Cushing, M., Repper-DelLisi, J., Mitchell, M.T., et al. (2007). Is your medical/surgical patient withdrawing from alcohol? *Nursing2007, 37*(10), 50–55.

Kneisl, C.R., Wilson, H.S., & Trigoboff, E. (2004). *Contemporary Psychiatric-Mental Health Nursing.* Upper Saddle River, NJ: Prentice Hall.

Letizia, M., & Reinholz, M. (2005). Identifying and managing acute alcohol withdrawal in the elderly. *Geriatric Nursing, 26,* 176–183.

Lussier-Cushing, M., Repper-DeLisi, J., Mitchell, M.T., et al. (2007). Is your medical-surgical patient withdrawing from alcohol? *Nursing2007, 37*(10), 50–55.

Nicotine replacement therapy. (2005). *Nursing Times, 101*(9), 32.

Patient Education Series. (2007). Smoking cessation. *Nursing2007, 37*(5), 57–58.

Shuttleworth, A. (2005). A key role in smoking cessation. *Nursing Times, 101*(30), 20–22.

Weiner, S.M. (2005). Perinatal substance abuse. *ADVANCE for Nurses, 3*(12), 19–21.

Wynd, C.A. (2005). Guided health imagery for smoking cessation and long-term abstinence. *Journal of Nursing Scholarship, 37*(3), 245–250.

Chapter 47

Abraham, I.L. (2006). Dementia and Alzheimer's disease: A practical orientation. *Nursing Clinics of North America, 41*(1), 119–127.

Aschenbrenner, D.S. (2005). Atypical antipsychotics: A warning. *American Journal of Nursing, 105*(8), 25.

Buettner, L.L, Lundegren, H., Lago, D., et al. (1996). Therapeutic recreation as an intervention for persons with dementia and agitation: An efficacy study. *American Journal of Alzheimer's Disease and Other Dementias, 11*(5), 4–12.

Bush, T. (2007). Use of cognitive assessment with Alzheimer's disease. *Nursing Times, 103*(2), 31–32.

Dubois, B., Feldman, H.H., Jacova, C., et al. (2007). Research criteria for the diagnosis of Alzheimer's disease revising the NINCDS-ADRDA criteria. *Lancet Neurology, 6*(8), 734–746.

Folstein, M.F., Folstein, S.E., & McHugh, P.R. (1975). A practical method of grading the cognitive state of patients for the clinician. *Journal of Psychiatric Research, 12*(3), 189–198.

Gray-Vickrey, P. (2005). What's behind acute delirium? *Nursing Made Incredibly Easy!, 3*(1), 20–28.

Hairon, N. (2007). The future of dementia care. *Nursing Times, 103*(10), 23–24.

Howland, R.H. (2005). Herbal therapies. *Journal of Psychosocial Nursing, 43*(4), 16–19.

Jeffery, S. (2007). Proposed new criteria for Alzheimer's diagnosis. *Medscape:Medical News.* Retrieved from www.medscape.com/viewarticle/559761

Kurlowicz, L.H. (2005). Depression in later life dispelling the myths. *Journal of Psychosocial Nursing, 43*(1), 16–19.

Milisen, K., Braes, T., Fick, D.M., et al. (2006). Cognitive assessment and differentiating the 3Ds (dementia, depression, delirium). *Nursing Clinics of North America, 41*(1), 1–22.

Oyama, K. (2005). When delirium takes hold. *RN, 68*(5), 52–56.

Patient Education Series. (2007). Alzheimer's disease. *Nursing2007, 37*(6), 50–51.

Patient Safety. (2007). Whither do they wander—and how can you intervene? *Nursing2007, 37*(4), 14–15.

Spires, R.A. (2006). Depression in the elderly. *RN, 69*(6), 38–42.

Stephan, S., & Phil, M. (2007). Successful seclusion and restraint reduction programs as quality indicators for psychiatric services. *Medscape:Medical News.* Retrieved from www.medscape.com/viewarticle /528949_1

Sundowner's Resource for Sundowner's Syndrome. *Treatment for sundowner's syndrome.* Retrieved from www.sundownerfacts.com/treatments.htm

Waknine, Y. (2007). FDA approvals: Exelon patch. *Medscape: Medical News.* Retrieved from www.medscape.com/viewarticle/559643

Williams, K., Kemper, S., & Hummert, M.L. (2005). Enhancing communication with older adults: Overcoming elderspeak. *Journal of Psychosocial Nursing, 43*(5), 12–16.

Wright, K.S. (2005). Mobility and safe handling of people with dementia. *Nursing Times, 101*(17), 38–40.

Chapter 48

FDA news. (2006). FDA approves Invega for long-term schizophrenia treatment. *Rx Trials Institute Drug Pipeline Alert,* 5(86) Retrieved from www. fdanews.com /newsletter / article?articleId =92633 &issueId=10097

Folstein, M.F., Folstein, S.E., & McHugh, P.R. (1975). A practical method of grading the cognitive state of patients for the clinician. *Journal of Psychiatric Research, 12*(3), 189–198.

Keltner, N.L. (2005). Genomic influences on schizophrenia-related neurotransmitter systems. *Journal of Nursing Scholarship, 37*(4), 322–328.

Lachman, V.D. (2006). Psychiatric advance directives. *ADVANCE for Nurses, 4*(3), 17–19.

Long, S.E. (2005). The validity of treating people with a personality disorder. *Nursing Times, 101*(15), 38–39.

Murphy, K. (2005). The separate reality of bipolar disorder and schizophrenia. *Nursing Made Incredibly Easy!, 3*(3), 6–18.

Psychiatric Nursing Made Incredibly Easy! (2004). Philadelphia: Lippincott.

Raynor, G., & Wilkins, T. (2005). Is personality disorder treatable? *Nursing Times, 101*(6), 20.

Ruiz, P. (2004). Addressing culture, race & ethnicity in psychiatric practice. *Psychiatric Annals, 34,* 527–532.

Savage, L. (2007). Prevention of schizophrenia relapse in secure settings. *Nursing Times, 103*(4), 30–31.

Stanton, K. (2007). Communicating with ED patients who have chronic mental illness. *American Journal of Nursing, 107*(2), 61–65.

Starr, D.L. (2004). Understanding those who self-mutilate. *Journal of Psychosocial Nursing, 42*(6), 33–40.

Strachan-Bennett, S. (2005). Managing violent patients. *Nursing Times, 101*(13), 19–20.

Townsend, M.C. (2006). *Psychiatric Mental Health Nursing: Concepts of Care in Evidenced-Based Practice.* (5 ed.). Philadelphia: F.A. Davis.

Ulrich, S.P., & Canale, S.W. (2005). *Nursing Care Planning Guides: For Adults in Acute, Extended and Home Care Settings.* Philadelphia: Elsevier Saunders.

Varcarolis, E.M. (2006). *Foundations of Psychiatric Mental Health Nursing: A Clinical Approach.* (5th ed.). Philadelphia: Saunders.

Ward, D. (2005). Improving physical health care in a mental health trust. *Nursing Times, 101*(7), 32–34.

Weiden, P.J., & Kane, J.M., (2006). Pharmacologic and psychosocial interventions in the treatment of schizophrenia. *Medscape Perspectives on the American Psychiatric Association 2006 Annual Meeting.* Retrieved from www.medscape.com/viewarticle /537387

Wilson, J.E.H., Hobbs, H., & Archie, S. (2005). The right stuff for early intervention in psychosis. *Journal of Psychosocial Nursing, 43*(6), 22–28.

Illustration Credits

Chapter 2

2–1, 2–2, 2–5 Courtesy Sheridan Memorial Hospital, Sheridan, WY. **2–3 A, B, 2–4, 2–5, A-B** from deWit, S.C. (2005). *Fundamental Concepts and Skills for Nursing* (2nd ed.). Philadelphia: Saunders.

Chapter 3

3–2 from Gould, B.E. (2002). *Pathophysiology for Health Professions* (2nd ed.). Philadelphia: Saunders. **3–3** from Jarvis, C. (2004). *Physical Examination and Health Assessment* (4th ed.). Philadelphia: Saunders. **3–5, 3–6** from Ignatavicius, D.D., & Workman, M.L. (2006). *Medical-Surgical Nursing: Critical Thinking for Collaborative Care* (5th ed.). Philadelphia: Saunders. **3–7, 3–8** from deWit, S.C. (2005). *Fundamental Concepts and Skills for Nursing* (2nd ed.). Philadelphia: Saunders. **3–9A** from Lewis, S.L., Heitkemper, M.M., Dirksen, S.R., et al. (2007). *Medical-Surgical Nursing: Assessment and Management of Clinical Problems* (7th ed.) St. Louis: Mosby. **3–9B** from Elkin, M.K., Perry, A.G., & Potter, A.G. (2004). *Nursing Interventions and Clinical Skills* (3rd ed.). St. Louis: Mosby.

Chapter 4

4–1, 4–5 courtesy Southwest Washington Medical Center, Vancouver, WA. **4–2** from Ignatavicius, D.D., & Workman, M.L. (2006). *Medical-Surgical Nursing: Critical Thinking for Collaborative Care* (5th ed.). Philadelphia: Saunders. **4–3** from deWit, S.C. (2005). *Fundamental Concepts and Skills for Nursing* (2nd ed.). Philadelphia: Saunders. **4–7** from Phipps, W.F., et al (2003). *Medical-Surgical Nursing: Health and Illness Perspective* (7th ed.). St. Louis: Mosby.

Chapter 5

5–1, 5–5 A-B, 5–6 from deWit, S.C. (2005). *Fundamental Concepts and Skills for Nursing* (2nd ed.). Philadelphia: Saunders. **5–2** from Black, J.M., & Hawks, J.H. (2005). *Medical-Surgical Nursing: Clinical Management for Positive Outcomes* (7th ed.). Philadelphia: Saunders.

Chapter 6

6–1 redrawn from Sattar, S.A., & Springthorpe, V.S. (2004) in Rutala, W.A. (Ed.). *Disinfection, Sterilization and Antisepsis.* Washington, DC: Association for Professionals in Infection Control and Epidemiology, Inc., (APIC). **6–2** from Applegate, E. (2006). *The Anatomy and Physiology Learning System* (3rd ed.) Philadelphia: Saunders. **6–3** from deWit, S.C. (2005). *Fundamental Concepts and Skills for Nursing* (2nd ed.). Philadelphia: Saunders.

Chapter 7

7–1 from deWit, S.C. (2005). *Fundamental Concepts and Skills for Nursing* (2nd ed.). Philadelphia: Saunders. **7–2, 7–6** from Lewis, S.L., Heitkemper, M.M., Dirksen, S.R., et al. (2007). *Medical-Surgical Nursing: Assessment and Management of Clinical Problems* (7th ed.) St. Louis: Mosby. **7–3** from Hockenberry, M.J., Wilson, D., & Winkelstein, M. (2005). *Wong's Essentials of Pediatric Nursing* (7th ed.). St. Louis: Mosby. **7–4** copyright © 2002, reprinted with permission from The Regents of the University of Michigan. **7–5** from Phipps, W.F., et al (2003). *Medical-Surgical Nursing: Health and Illness Perspective* (7th ed.). St. Louis: Mosby.

Chapter 8

8–1 copyright © The American Cancer Society, Inc., Atlanta, GA. **8–2** from Huether, S.E., & McCance, K.L. (2004). *Understanding Pathophysiology* (3rd ed.). St. Louis: Mosby. **8–3** from Phipps, W.F., et al (2003). *Medical-Surgical Nursing: Health and Illness Perspective* (7th ed.). St. Louis: Mosby. **8–4** courtesy the Cyberknife Center, Southwestern Washington Medical Center, Vancouver, WA.

Chapter 9

9–6 reprinted with permission, copyright © The Gerontological Society of America. **9–7** courtesy The Rehabilitation Institute at Santa Barbara, Santa Barbara, CA.

Chapter 10

10–3 from Huether, S.E., & McCance, K.L. (2004). *Understanding Pathophysiology* (3rd ed.). St. Louis: Mosby. **10–6** from Herlihy, B., & Maebius, N.K. (2003). *The Human Body in Health and Illness* (2nd ed.). Philadelphia: Saunders. **10–7** from Applegate, E. (2000). *The Anatomy and Physiology Learning System* (2nd ed.). Philadelphia: Saunders.

Chapter 11

11–1, 11–8 from Black, J.M., & Hawks, J.H. (2005). *Medical-Surgical Nursing: Clinical Management for Positive Outcomes* (7th ed.). Philadelphia: Saunders. **11–2, 11–4** from Gould, B.E. (2002). *Pathophysiology for Health Professions* (2nd ed.). Philadelphia: Saunders. **11–3** Herlihy, B., & Maebius, N.K. (2003). *The Human Body in Health and Illness* (2nd ed.). Philadelphia: Saunders. **11–5** from Ignatavicius, D.D., & Workman, M.L. (2006). *Medical-Surgical Nursing: Critical Thinking for Collaborative Care* (5th ed.). Philadelphia: Saunders. **11–6, 11–7** from Lewis, S.L., Heitkemper, M.M., Dirksen, S.R., et al. (2007). *Medical-Surgical Nursing: Assessment and Management of Clinical Problems* (7th ed.) St. Louis: Mosby.

Chapter 12

12–4 from Dorland (2003). *Dorland's Illustrated Medical Dictionary* (30th ed.). Philadelphia: Saunders. **12–12** from deWit, S.C. (2005). *Fundamental Concepts and Skills for Nursing* (2nd ed.). Philadelphia: Saunders.

Chapter 13

13–2, 13–8 from Lewis, S.L., Heitkemper, M.M., Dirksen, S.R., et al. (2007). *Medical-Surgical Nursing: Assessment and Management of Clinical Problems* (7th ed.) St. Louis: Mosby. **13–3, 13–4, 13–5, unnumbered 13–1, 13–2, 13–3, 13–4, 13–5** from deWit, S.C. (2005). *Fundamental Concepts and Skills for Nursing* (2nd ed.). Philadelphia: Saunders. **13–7** from Black, J.M., & Hawks, J.H. (2005). *Medical-Surgical Nursing: Clinical Management for Positive Outcomes* (7th ed.). Philadelphia: Saunders. **13–9** courtesy of Passey-Muir, Inc., Irvine, CA.

Chapter 14

14–6 from Harkreader, H., & Hogan, M.A. (2004). *Fundamentals of Nursing: Caring and Clinical Judgment* (2nd ed.). Philadelphia: Saunders. **14–7, 14–8** from deWit, S.C. (2005). *Fundamental Concepts and Skills for Nursing* (2nd ed.). Philadelphia: Saunders.

Chapter 15

15–1 from Thibodeau, G.A., & Patton, K.T. (2005). *The Human Body in Health and Disease* (4th ed.). St. Louis: Mosby. **15–2** from Applegate, E. (2006). *The Anatomy and Physiology Learning System* (3rd ed.) Philadelphia: Saunders.

Chapter 16

16–1 from Callen, W.B.S., et al (1993). *Color Atlas of Dermatology.* Philadelphia: Saunders. **16–4, 16–5, 16–6** from Lewis, S.L.,

Heitkemper, M.M., Dirksen, S.R., et al. (2007). *Medical-Surgical Nursing: Assessment and Management of Clinical Problems* (7th ed.) St. Louis: Mosby.

Chapter 17

17–1 from Ignatavicius, D.D., & Workman, M.L. (2006). *Medical-Surgical Nursing: Critical Thinking for Collaborative Care* (5th ed.). Philadelphia: Saunders. **17–6** from Huether, S.E., & McCance, K.L. (2004). *Understanding Pathophysiology* (3rd ed.). St. Louis: Mosby. **17–10** from Lewis, S.L., Heitkemper, M.M., Dirksen, S.R., et al. (2007). *Medical-Surgical Nursing: Assessment and Management of Clinical Problems* (7th ed.) St. Louis: Mosby. **17–12** from Jarvis, C. (2004). *Physical Examination and Health Assessment* (4th ed.). Philadelphia: Saunders.

Chapter 18

18–1, 18–3 from Mosby (2006). *Dictionary of Medicine, Nursing, and Health Professions* (7th ed.). St. Louis: Mosby. **18–2** courtesy Cameron Bangs, MD. **18–4** from Black, J.M., & Hawks, J.H. (2005). *Medical-Surgical Nursing: Clinical Management for Positive Outcomes* (7th ed.). Philadelphia: Saunders. **18–5** from Phipps, W.F., et al (2003). *Medical-Surgical Nursing: Health and Illness Perspective* (7th ed.). St. Louis: Mosby. **18–6, 18–10** from Kamal, A., & Brockelhurst, J.C. (1991). *Color Atlas of Geriatric Medicine* (2nd ed.). St. Louis: Mosby. **18–7** from Black, J.M., & Hawks, J.H. (2005). *Medical-Surgical Nursing: Clinical Management for Positive Outcomes* (7th ed.). Philadelphia: Saunders. **18–8** from Thibodeau, G.A., & Patton, K.T. (2005). *The Human Body in Health and Disease* (4th ed.). St. Louis: Mosby. **18–9** from Swartz, M. (2002). *Textbook of Physical Diagnosis: History and Examination* (4th ed.). Philadelphia: Saunders.

Chapter 19

19–1 from Bloom, A., Watkins, P.H., & Ireland, J. (1992). *Color Atlas of Diabetes* (2nd ed.). St. Louis: Mosby. **19–2** courtesy of Thoratec, Pleasanton, CA. **19–3** courtesy Datascope Corporation, Montvale, NJ. **19–4, 19–5, 19–6** from Aehlert, B. (2002). *EKGs Made Easy* (2nd ed.). St. Louis: Mosby. **19–7** from Lewis, S.L., Heitkemper, M.M., Dirksen, S.R., et al. (2007). *Medical-Surgical Nursing: Assessment and Management of Clinical Problems* (7th ed.) St. Louis: Mosby. **19–8** from Kumar, V., Abbas, A., & Fausto, N. (2005). *Robbins & Cotran's Pathologic Basis of Disease* (7th ed.). Philadelphia: Saunders. **19–9** from Gould, B.E. (2002). *Pathophysiology for Health Professions* (2nd ed.). Philadelphia: Saunders.

Chapter 20

20–2, 20–5 from Lewis, S.L., Heitkemper, M.M., Dirksen, S.R., et al. (2007). *Medical-Surgical Nursing: Assessment and Management of Clinical Problems* (7th ed.) St. Louis: Mosby. **20–3** from Chabner, D.A. (2001). *The Language of Medicine* (6th ed.). Philadelphia: Saunders. **20–7** courtesy of Medtronic, Inc., Minneapolis, MN. **20–8** from Ignatavicius, D.D., & Workman, M.L. (2006). *Medical-Surgical Nursing: Critical Thinking for Collaborative Care* (5th ed.). Philadelphia: Saunders.

Chapter 21

21–1 from Applegate, E. (2000). *The Anatomy and Physiology Learning System* (2nd ed.). Philadelphia: Saunders. **21–4** from Ignatavicius, D.D., & Workman, M.L. (2006). *Medical-Surgical Nursing: Critical Thinking for Collaborative Care* (5th ed.). Philadelphia: Saunders. **21–8** from deWit, S.C. (2005). *Fundamental Concepts and Skills for Nursing* (2nd ed.). Philadelphia: Saunders. **21–9** from Jarvis, C. (2004). *Physical Examination and Health Assessment* (4th ed.). Philadelphia: Saunders. **21–11** courtesy of Southwest Washington Medical Center, Vancouver, WA.

Chapter 22

22–2 from Black, J.M., & Hawks, J.H. (2005). *Medical-Surgical Nursing: Clinical Management for Positive Outcomes* (7th ed.). Philadelphia: Saunders. **22–3** from Bingham, B.J.B., Hawke, M., & Kwok, P. (1992). *Clinical Atlas of Otolaryngology.* St. Louis: Mosby. **22–5** from Chipps, E., Clanin, N., & Campbell, V. (1992). *Neurologic Disorders.* St. Louis: Mosby. **22–6, 22–7, 22–14** from Lewis, S.L., Heitkemper, M.M., Dirksen, S.R., et al. (2007). *Medical-Surgical Nursing: Assessment and Management of Clinical Problems* (7th ed.) St. Louis: Mosby. **22–8** from Thibodeau, G.A., & Patton, K.T. (2005). *The Human Body in Health and Disease* (4th ed.). St. Louis: Mosby. **22–9** from Ignatavicius, D.D., & Workman, M.L. (2006). *Medical-Surgical Nursing: Critical Thinking for Collaborative Care* (5th ed.). Philadelphia: Saunders. **22–10** courtesy Michael S. Clement, MD, Mesa, AZ. **22–11** courtesy of Acromed Corporation, Cleveland, OH. **22–12** courtesy of Kinetic Concepts, Inc., San Antonio, TX. **22–13** from deWit, S.C. (2005). *Fundamental Concepts and Skills for Nursing* (2nd ed.). Philadelphia: Saunders.

Chapter 23

23–3 from Cotran, R.S., Kumar, V., & Collins, T. (1999). *Robbins Pathologic Basis for Disease* (6th ed.). Philadelphia: Saunders. **23–5** from Black, J.M., & Hawks, J.H. (2005). *Medical-Surgical Nursing: Clinical Management for Positive Outcomes* (7th ed.). Philadelphia: Saunders.

Chapter 24

24–1, 24–4 from Lewis, S.L., Heitkemper, M.M., Dirksen, S.R., et al. (2007). *Medical-Surgical Nursing: Assessment and Management of Clinical Problems* (7th ed.) St. Louis: Mosby. **24–3** from Perkin, D.G. (2002). *Mosby's Color Atlas and Text of Neurology.* St. Louis: Mosby. **24–5** from Stevens, A., & Lowe, J. (2000). *Pathology: Illustrated Review in Color* (2nd ed.). London: Mosby. **24–6** courtesy of Heather Boyd-Monk and Wills Eye Hospital, Philadelphia. PA.

Chapter 25

25–3 from Swartz, M. (2002). *Textbook of Physical Diagnosis: History and Examination* (4th ed.). Philadelphia: Saunders. **25–4, 25–8** from Albert, D.M., & Jakobiec, F.A. (1994). *Principles and Practice of Ophthalmology,* vol. 3. Philadelphia: Saunders. **25–6, 25–11** from Ignatavicius, D.D., & Workman, M.L. (2006). *Medical-Surgical Nursing: Critical Thinking for Collaborative Care* (5th ed.). Philadelphia: Saunders. **25–10** from Jarvis, C. (2004). *Physical Examination and Health Assessment* (4th ed.). Philadelphia: Saunders. **25–13** from Black, J.M., & Hawks, J.H. (2005). *Medical-Surgical Nursing: Clinical Management for Positive Outcomes* (7th ed.). Philadelphia: Saunders.

Chapter 26

26–3, 26–5 courtesy of Ophthalmic Photography at the University of Michigan, W.K. Kellogg Eye Center, Ann Arbor, MI. **26–6** from Lehne, R.A. (2004). *Pharmacology for Nursing Care* (5th ed.). Philadelphia: Saunders. **26–7, 26–8** from Phipps, W.F., et al. (2003). *Medical-Surgical Nursing: Health and Illness Perspective* (7th ed.). St. Louis: Mosby. **26–10** courtesy of the Macula Foundation, Inc., New York.

Chapter 27

27–5 from deWit, S.C. (2005). *Fundamental Concepts and Skills for Nursing* (2nd ed.). Philadelphia: Saunders.

Chapter 28

28–6 from Lewis, S.L., Heitkemper, M.M., Dirksen, S.R., et al. (2007). *Medical-Surgical Nursing: Assessment and Management of Clinical Problems* (7th ed.) St. Louis: Mosby.

Chapter 29

29–1 from Swartz, M. (2002). *Textbook of Physical Diagnosis: History and Examination* (4th ed.). Philadelphia: Saunders. **29–7, 29–8, 29–9** from deWit, S.C. (2005). *Fundamental Concepts and Skills for Nursing* (2nd ed.). Philadelphia: Saunders.

Chapter 30

30–1 from Ignatavicius, D.D., & Workman, M.L. (2006). *Medical-Surgical Nursing: Critical Thinking for Collaborative Care* (5th ed.). Philadelphia: Saunders. **30–3** from Lewis, S.L., Heitkemper, M.M., Dirksen, S.R., et al. (2007). *Medical-Surgical Nursing: Assessment and Management of Clinical Problems* (7th ed.) St. Louis: Mosby.

Chapter 31

31–3 from Mourad, L.A. (1991). *Orthopedic Disorders*. St. Louis: Mosby. **31–6** courtesy of Hill-Rom Company, Batesville, IN.

Chapter 32

32–2, 32–6 from Black, J.M., & Hawks, J.H. (2005). *Medical-Surgical Nursing: Clinical Management for Positive Outcomes* (7th ed.). Philadelphia: Saunders. **32–8** from Ignatavicius, D.D., & Workman, M.L. (2006). *Medical-Surgical Nursing: Critical Thinking for Collaborative Care* (5th ed.). Philadelphia: Saunders. **32–9** courtesy of Otto Bock HealthCare, Minneapolis, MN.

Chapter 33

33–1, 33–3 from Ignatavicius, D.D., & Workman, M.L. (2006). *Medical-Surgical Nursing: Critical Thinking for Collaborative Care* (5th ed.). Philadelphia: Saunders. **33–2** from Lewis, S.L., Heitkemper, M.M., Dirksen, S.R., et al. (2007). *Medical-Surgical Nursing: Assessment and Management of Clinical Problems* (7th ed.) St. Louis: Mosby. **33–4** from Pagana, K.D., & Pagana, T.J. (2005). *Mosby's Diagnostic and Laboratory Test Reference* (7th ed.). St. Louis: Mosby.

Chapter 34

34–1, 34–3 from Lewis, S.L., Heitkemper, M.M., Dirksen, S.R., et al. (2007). *Medical-Surgical Nursing: Assessment and Management of Clinical Problems* (7th ed.) St. Louis: Mosby. **34–2, 34–5, 34–6** from Ignatavicius, D.D., & Workman, M.L. (2006). *Medical-Surgical Nursing: Critical Thinking for Collaborative Care* (5th ed.). Philadelphia: Saunders. **34–4, 34–7, 34–8** from Black, J.M., & Hawks, J.H. (2005). *Medical-Surgical Nursing: Clinical Management for Positive Outcomes* (7th ed.). Philadelphia: Saunders.

Chapter 35

35–4, 35–5, 35–6 from Applegate, E. (2000). *The Anatomy and Physiology Learning System* (2nd ed.). Philadelphia: Saunders. **35–7** from Lewis, S.L., Heitkemper, M.M., Dirksen, S.R., et al. (2007). *Medical-Surgical Nursing: Assessment and Management of Clinical Problems* (7th ed.) St. Louis: Mosby.

Chapter 36

36–1, 36–2, 36–3 from Ignatavicius, D.D., & Workman, M.L. (2006). *Medical-Surgical Nursing: Critical Thinking for Collaborative Care* (5th ed.). Philadelphia: Saunders. **36–4** from Lewis, S.L., Heitkemper, M.M., Dirksen, S.R., et al. (2007). *Medical-Surgical Nursing: Assessment and Management of Clinical Problems* (7th ed.) St. Louis: Mosby.

Chapter 37

37–1 from Ignatavicius, D.D., & Workman, M.L. (2006). *Medical-Surgical Nursing: Critical Thinking for Collaborative Care* (5th ed.). Philadelphia: Saunders. **37–3** courtesy of Medtronic MiniMed, Northridge, CA.

Chapter 38

38–2 modified from Leifer, G. (2007). *Introduction to Maternity and Pediatric Nursing* (5th ed.). Philadelphia: Saunders. **38–3** from McKinney, E.M., James, S., et al (2005). *Maternal-Child Nursing* (2nd ed.). Philadelphia: Saunders. **38–5, 38–6** from Lewis, S.L., Heitkemper, M.M., Dirksen, S.R., et al. (2007). *Medical-Surgical Nursing: Assessment and Management of Clinical Problems* (7th ed.) St. Louis: Mosby.

Chapter 39

39–1, 39–4, 39–5, 39–6 from Lewis, S.L., Heitkemper, M.M., Dirksen, S.R., et al. (2007). *Medical-Surgical Nursing: Assessment and Management of Clinical Problems* (7th ed.) St. Louis: Mosby. **39–2** courtesy of Coloplast Surgical Marketing, Minneapolis, MN. **39–7** from Black, J.M., & Hawks, J.H. (2005). *Medical-Surgical Nursing: Clinical Management for Positive Outcomes* (7th ed.). Philadelphia: Saunders.

Chapter 40

Unnumbered 40–1 and 40–4 from Morse, S., Moreland, A., & Holmes, K. (Eds.). (1996). *Atlas of Sexually Transmitted Diseases and AIDS*. London: Mosby-Wolfe. **Unnumbered 40–2** from Black, J.M., & Hawks, J.H. (2005). *Medical-Surgical Nursing: Clinical Management for Positive Outcomes* (7th ed.). Philadelphia: Saunders. **Unnumbered 40–3** reproduced with permission of GlaxoSmithKline, Research Triangle Park, NC. **Unnumbered 40–5** courtesy of U.S. Public Health Service, Washington, DC.

Chapter 41

41–1 from Lewis, S.L., Heitkemper, M.M., Dirksen, S.R., et al. (2007). *Medical-Surgical Nursing: Assessment and Management of Clinical Problems* (7th ed.). St. Louis: Mosby. **41–4** from Lookingbill, D.P., & Marks, J.G. (1993). *Principles of Dermatology* (2nd ed.). Philadelphia: Saunders. **41–5** copyright © 1998 Barbara Braden and Nancy Bergstrom. **41–6, 41–7, 41–8, 41–9** from Ignatavicius, D.D., & Workman, M.L. (2006). *Medical-Surgical Nursing: Critical Thinking for Collaborative Care* (5th ed.). Philadelphia: Saunders. **Unnumbered 41–1, A-F** from Thibodeau, G.A., & Patton, K.T.: *The Human Body in Health and Disease* (3rd ed.). St. Louis, 2002, Mosby

Chapter 42

42–1, 42–2, 42–6, 42–7, 42–8, 42–15 from Ignatavicius, D.D., & Workman, M.L. (2006). *Medical-Surgical Nursing: Critical Thinking for Collaborative Care* (5th ed.). Philadelphia: Saunders. **42–3** from Moschella, S.L., Hurley, H.J. (1992). *Dermatology* (3rd ed.). Philadelphia: Saunders. **42–9** Copyright © 1998 National Pressure Ulcer Advisory Panel. **42–11, 42–12, 42–13** from Black, J.M., & Hawks, J.H. (2005). *Medical-Surgical Nursing: Clinical Management for Positive Outcomes* (7th ed.). Philadelphia: Saunders. **42–14** from Lewis, S.L., Heitkemper, M.M., Dirksen, S.R., et al. (2007). *Medical-Surgical Nursing: Assessment and Management of Clinical Problems* (7th ed.). St. Louis: Mosby. **42–16** courtesy of Beiersdorf-Jobst, Inc., Charlotte, NC.

Chapter 43

43–1 courtesy of the American Red Cross, printed with permission. Copyright © The American Red Cross. **43–2** courtesy of Disaster Management Systems, Inc., Pomona, CA. **43–3** courtesy of Southwestern Medical Center, Vancouver, WA. **43–4, 43–5** courtesy of CDC, Public Images Library. CDC/Cheryl Tyron. **43–6** courtesy of AP/Wide World Photos.

Chapter 44

44–1, 44–4 from Elkin, M., Perry, A.M., & Potter, P.A. (2000). *Nursing Interventions and Clinical Skills* (2nd ed.). St. Louis: Mosby. **44–2, 44–6** from Black, J.M., & Hawks, J.H. (2005). *Medical-Surgical Nursing: Clinical Management for Positive Outcomes* (7th ed.). Philadelphia: Saunders.

Chapter 46

46–2 courtesy of Indiana Prevention Resource Center (IPRC) at Indiana University, Bloomington, IL.

Glossary

A

abduction Movement away from the midline of the body.

ablation The removal of a part, as by incision; eradication.

ablation therapy A treatment for hyperthyroidism using radioactive iodine (^{131}I).

abrasion A wound caused by rubbing or scraping the skin or mucous membrane.

absorption The passage of liquids or other substances through a body surface and into its tissues and fluids, as in absorption of the end products of digestion into the intestinal villi.

abuse Misuse; excessive or improper use.

acceptance Admission of reality, as in the reality of death; the final stage in the process of dealing with dying and death.

accommodation Adjustment, especially of the ocular lens for seeing objects at varying distances.

achlorhydria The absence of hydrochloric acid from maximally stimulated gastric secretions.

acid A substance that yields hydrogen ions in solution.

acid-base balance A normal condition in which the narrow range of normal pH and the normal ratio of carbonic acid to bicarbonate ions are maintained.

acidosis A condition in which the pH of body fluids is below normal range because of either a loss of base bicarbonate or an accumulation of acid.

acquired Occurring from factors outside the organism, as in response to the environment.

acquired immunity Immunity involving the functioning of the immune system acquired by natural infection or vaccination (active immunity) or transfer of antibody from an immune donor (passive immunity).

acquired immunodeficiency syndrome (AIDS) A group of symptoms believed to be caused by a virus (HIV) that infects and destroys T-lymphocytes.

acromegaly A chronic disease of adults caused by hypersecretion of the pituitary growth hormone and characterized by enlargement of many parts of the skeleton.

active immunity Immunity acquired by producing one's own antibody.

active transport Movement of substances from an area of lower concentration to an area of higher concentration.

acuity The degree of seriousness of illness or injury.

acupressure The application of digital pressure on a part of the body to relieve pain or produce anesthesia.

acupuncture A technique for treating certain painful conditions and for producing regional anesthesia by passing long, thin needles through the skin to specific points.

acute myocardial infarction Ischemic necrosis of an area of the heart muscle resulting from sudden occlusion of blood flow through one or more branches of the coronary arteries.

acute pain Sharp, severe pain.

addiction A psychological craving for alcohol or drugs with the presence of withdrawal symptoms if the substance cannot be obtained.

adduction Movement toward the midline of the body.

adenohypophysis The anterior lobe of the pituitary gland.

adhesion A fibrous band that binds together two parts that are normally separated; often occurs after surgery in the abdomen.

adjuvant That which assists, such as a drug added to a prescription that enhances the action of the principal ingredient.

adrenergic Having action that mimics that of the sympathetic nervous system.

adrenocortical Indicating the cortex of the adrenal gland.

adrenocorticotropic hormone (ACTH) A "tropic" hormone of the anterior pituitary gland. This hormone acts on the adrenal cortex.

adulthood A stage of life at which the individual has reached biologic maturity, usually at age 20.

advance directive A document prepared while an individual is alive and competent containing information for future health care.

adventitious Acquired; arising sporadically.

aerobe A microorganism that requires oxygen for survival.

aerobic Requiring oxygen to live.

aerosol A suspension of a drug or other substance that is dispensed in a cloud or mist.

affect The external expression; mood.

ageism Prejudice against aging and elderly people.

agent A party authorized to act on behalf of another.

agglutination One type of antigen-antibody reaction in which a solid antigen clumps together with a soluble antibody.

agnosia The loss of the power to recognize the significance of sensory stimuli.

agranulocytosis A condition of deficiency, or absolute lack, of granulocytic white blood cells.

airway The passage by which air enters and leaves the lungs; also, a device used to secure unobstructed respiration.

akathisia A condition of motor restlessness; a common extrapyramidal side effect of neuroleptic drugs.

albumin, serum A plasma protein formed principally in the liver and constituting about 60% of the protein concentration in the plasma.

aldosterone A mineralocorticoid steroid hormone produced by the adrenal cortex. Works in the renal tubules to retain sodium and conserve water by reabsorption; increases urinary potassium excretion.

From Chabner, D.E. (2004). *The Language of Medicine* (7th ed.). Philadelphia: Saunders.

Pronunciation Guide to Key Terms

The markings ¯ and ˘ above the vowels (a, e, i, o, and u) indicate the proper sounds of the vowels.

When ¯ is above a vowel its sound is long, that is, exactly like its name; for example:

ā as in āpe	ī as in īce	ū as in ūnit
ē as in ēven	ō as in ōpen	

The ˘ marking indicates a short vowel sound, as in the following examples:

ă as in ăpple	ĭ as in ĭnterest	ŭ as in ŭnder
ĕ as in ĕvery	ŏ as in pŏt	

alkalosis A condition in which the pH of body fluids is above normal because of either a loss of acid or an accumulation of base bicarbonate.
allergen(s) Any substance capable of triggering an exaggerated immune response.
allergy (allergies) An abnormal and individual hypersensitivity to a particular allergen; acquired by exposure to the allergen and manifested after reexposure.
alleviate To relieve; to make easier to bear.
alliance An agreement to cooperate made between a freestanding independent facility and a hospital.
allogeneic Having a different genetic constitution but belonging to the same species.
allograft Transplant tissue obtained from the same species.
alogia A psychiatric term meaning poverty of thoughts.
alopecia Baldness or loss of hair.
Alzheimer's disease (AD) The most common degenerative disease of the brain, with no known cause or cure. The disease causes loss of neurons in the frontal and temporal lobes and affects people over the age of 65, but can also strike younger people.
amenorrhea The absence of menstruation.
anabolic Constructive in nature; the opposite of catabolic.
anabolism The building up of the body substance; the constructive phase of metabolism.
anaerobe An organism that lives in an oxygen-free environment.
anaerobic Able to live in an oxygen-free environment.
analgesia The absence of normal sense of pain.
analgesic(s) A pain reliever.
anaphylaxis An unusual or exaggerated allergic reaction.
anasarca Generalized massive edema resulting from severe depletion of albumin.
anastomosis A communication between two tubular organs; also surgical, traumatic, or pathologic formation of a connection between two normally distinct structures.
androgen(s) Any steroid hormone that promotes male characteristics.
anemia(s) A condition in which there are too few functioning red blood cells to meet the oxygen needs of tissues.
anesthesia The loss of feeling or sensation.
aneurysm A sac formed by localized dilation of the wall of a blood vessel or the heart.
anger A feeling of hostility and bitterness against a situation or person; the second stage in acceptance of death.
angina pectoris Exertional chest pain caused by ischemia of the heart muscle and increased demand for oxygen.
angioedema A vascular reaction representing localized edema caused by dilation and characterized by development of giant wheals.
angiography X-ray studies of the arteries, veins, or lymph vessels of the body.
animate Alive.
anion A negatively charged atomic particle.
ankylosis Abnormal immobility and consolidation and obliteration of a joint.
anorexia A lack or loss of appetite for food.
anorexia nervosa An eating disorder in which there is an aberration of eating patterns, severe weight loss, and malnutrition.
anosmia The absence of the sense of smell; also called *anosphresia* and *olfactory anesthesia.*
anovulation Failure of the ovary to produce or release mature eggs.
antibiotic An agent that is capable of either killing or inhibiting the growth of microorganisms.
antibody (antibodies) An immunoglobulin molecule that is capable of adhering to and interacting only with the antigen that induced its synthesis.
anticoagulants Substances that suppress, delay, or nullify the coagulation of blood.
antidiuretic hormone A hormone that decreases the production of urine by increasing the reabsorption of water by the renal tubules. It is secreted by the hypothalamus and stored in the posterior lobe of the pituitary gland.
antidysrhythmic agents Substances that help return the heart rate and rhythm to more normal values and restore the origin of the heart's electrical activity to its natural pacemaker.
antiemetic An agent that prevents or relieves nausea and vomiting.
antifungal(s) An agent that is destructive to or inhibitive of the growth of fungi.
antigen(s) Any substance that can produce an antagonist.
antigen-antibody reaction An immune response that occurs when an antibody comes into contact with the specific antigen for which it was formed. In a transfusion reaction, the response is a clumping together, or agglutination, of the red blood cells carrying the antigens.
antihistamine An agent that counteracts the effects of histamine; used to relieve the symptoms of an allergic reaction.
antihypertensive A medication to prevent or control high blood pressure.
antimicrobial agent A substance capable of either killing or suppressing the multiplication and growth of microorganisms.
antineoplastic agent A substance that inhibits the maturation and proliferation of malignant cells.
antiseptic(s) Any substance that inhibits the growth of bacteria outside the body; in contrast, a germicide kills the bacteria outright.
antitoxin A specific kind of antibody produced in response to the presence of a toxin.
antitussive An agent that inhibits the cough reflex in the cough center in the brain.
antivenin A substance used to neutralize the venom of a poisonous animal.
anuria Diminished or absent production of urine by the kidney.
apathetic thyrotoxicosis Milder hyperthyroidism signs and symptoms seen in the elderly patient compared with symptoms seen in the typical adult patient.
aphakic eye An eye without a lens, as after a cataract extraction.
aphasia A defect in or loss of the power of expression by speech, writing, or signs or in the comprehension of spoken or written language.
aphonia The loss of the voice.
apical Pertaining to the apex of a structure; particularly the heart.
aplastic Having deficient or arrested development.
aplastic anemia Deficient red cell production due to a bone marrow disorder.
apnea Temporary cessation of breathing.
apraxia The loss or impairment of acquired motor skills.
arrhythmia (also dysrhythmia) Variation from the normal rhythm, especially of the heartbeat.
arteriosclerosis A group of diseases characterized by thickening and loss of elasticity of the arterial walls.
arthritis Inflammation of a joint.
arthrocentesis The surgical puncture of a joint cavity for aspiration of synovial fluid.
arthroplasty Surgery of a joint to increase mobility or decrease pain.
arthroscopy Endoscopic examination of the interior of a joint.

ascites The accumulation of edematous fluid within the peritoneal cavity.

asepsis, medical The destruction and containment of infectious agents after they leave the body of a patient with an infectious disease.

assessment, nursing Data-gathering activities for the purpose of collecting a complete, relevant database from which a nursing diagnosis can be made.

asterixis A motor disturbance marked by intermittent lapse of an assumed posture; a characteristic of hepatic coma. Also called "flapping tremor."

asthma A condition marked by recurrent attacks of paroxysmal dyspnea, with wheezing due to spasmodic contraction of the bronchi.

astigmatism An error of refraction in which light rays are not sharply focused on the retina because of abnormal curvature of the cornea or lens.

ataxia Uncoordinated motor movements.

atelectasis The collapsed or airless state of the lung.

atherosclerosis A disease process in which fibrinous plaques are laid down on the inner walls of the arteries, thus narrowing the lumens of the vessels and predisposing them to the development of intravascular clots.

atopy The tendency to develop allergies.

atrial fibrillation Rapid, irregular, and ineffective contractions of the atria.

atrial natriuretic peptide A hormone involved in the regulation of renal and cardiovascular homeostasis. It is produced in the atrium and helps to normalize blood pressure and volume.

atrophy Wasting, or a decrease in size, from lack of use.

atypical antipsychotics Newer medications used for treating schizophrenia with fewer side effects.

audiometry The measurement of sound perception.

audit An official examination of the record of all aspects of patient care.

aura A peculiar sensation preceding the appearance of more definite symptoms, especially a sensation, that occurs immediately before an epileptic seizure.

aural Pertaining to the ear.

auscultation Listening for sounds produced within the body, usually with a stethoscope.

autograft A graft transferred from one part of a patient's body to another.

autoimmune A defective cellular immune response in which antibodies are produced against normal parts of the person's body.

autoimmune disease A disease caused by the body's failure to recognize its own cells, thus rejecting them as it would a foreign substance.

autoinoculation Inoculation with microorganisms from one's own body.

autologous Indicating something that has its origin within an individual, as in transfusion with one's own blood.

automated external defibrillator (AED) A defibrillator found in many public places used to treat cardiac arrest.

automatisms Repetitive, automatic actions such as lip smacking.

autonomic dysreflexia Hyperreflexia, an uninhibited and exaggerated reflex response of the autonomic nervous system to some type of stimulation.

avolition A lack of motivation.

avulsion The tearing away of part or all of an organ or structure.

axon The projection, or process, of a neuron that transmits impulses away from the cell body.

azotemia Retention in the blood of urea, creatinine, and other nitrogenous protein metabolites that are normally eliminated in the urine.

B

Babinski's reflex A reflex action elicited by stimulating the sole of the foot and characterized by dorsiflexion of the great toe and flaring of the smaller toes. A positive Babinski reflex indicates an abnormality in the motor control pathways of the nervous system.

bacteria Microscopically small organisms belonging to the plant kingdom, some of which are capable of producing disease in humans.

bacterial vaginosis A bacterial disease of the vagina.

bactericidal Able to kill bacteria.

bacteriophage A virus that destroys bacteria by lysis. The virus is usually of a type specific for the particular kind of bacteria it attacks.

bacteriostatic Able to slow duplication of bacteria.

bargaining An attempt to make an arrangement whereby one gives something in order to gain something in return; the third stage in acceptance of death.

bariatrics The field of medicine that focuses on the treatment and control of obesity and diseases associated with obesity.

base A substance that combines with acids to form salts.

basement membrane The noncellular layer that secures the overlying epithelium to the underlying tissue.

behavior The manner in which one conducts oneself in response to social stimuli, an inner need, or a combination of the two.

belief A currently held idea or value derived from culture and experience.

benign Not very harmful; nonmalignant.

benign pituitary adenoma A benign tumor of the pituitary gland that secretes growth hormone (GH), leading to continued growth. It can also antagonize the effect of the hormone insulin, resulting in increased blood glucose.

bereaved Experiencing the reaction of grief and sadness on learning of the loss of a loved one.

biliary Pertaining to bile, the bile ducts, or the gallbladder.

biliary colic Acute pain resulting from obstruction of a bile duct, usually caused by cholelithiasis.

binder A broad bandage most commonly used as an encircling support of the abdomen or chest.

biofeedback A training program designed to develop one's ability to control the autonomic (involuntary) nervous system.

biologic dressing Materials obtained from a patient's intact skin, cadavers, or animals that is used to treat burn victims.

biologic response modifier (BRM) An agent that manipulates the immune system in hopes of controlling or curing a malignancy.

biomedicine Biologic medicine; focuses on the biologic aspects of medicine.

biopsy Removal of living cells for the purpose of examining them microscopically.

biosynthetic A biologic substance created by chemical processes. A term used for artificial skin that can be used as a temporary measure for grafting in burn victims.

bioterrorism An attack that involves the deliberate release of microorganisms or toxins derived from living organisms that cause disease or death to humans, animals, or plants on which we depend for food.

bipolar disorder A mood disorder in which manic and depressive episodes occur.

bisexual An individual who is sexually attracted to others of either sex.

bladder, cord A dysfunction of the urinary bladder caused by damage to the spinal cord.

bladder, neurogenic A dysfunction of the urinary bladder caused by a lesion of the central or peripheral nervous system and characterized by lack of awareness of the need to void.
blepharitis An infection of the glands and lash follicles along the margin of the eyelid.
blood gases, arterial (ABGs) The partial pressure exerted by oxygen and carbon dioxide in the arterial blood. ABGs reflect the ability of the lungs to exchange these gases, the effectiveness of the kidneys to retain and eliminate bicarbonate, and the efficiency of the heart as a pump.
B-lymphocyte A sensitized lymphocyte that is responsible for antibody formation and the development of humoral immunity.
borborygmi Gurgling, splashing sounds normally heard over the large intestine; rumbling in the bowels.
borderline personality disorder A mental disorder defined by the DSM-IV as "a pattern of instability in interpersonal relationships, self-image and affect, and marked impulsivity."
botulism Food poisoning caused by a neurotoxin produced by *Clostridium botulinum,* sometimes found in improperly canned or preserved foods.
bradycardia An abnormally slow heart rate, usually less than 60 beats per minute.
bradykinesia Slow movement; a symptom seen with Parkinson's disease.
bradypnea Abnormally slow breathing.
bronchiectasis Chronic dilation of the bronchi marked by fetid breath and paroxysmal coughing, with the expectoration of mucopurulent matter.
bronchodilator A drug that acts directly on the smooth muscles of the bronchi to relax them and relieve bronchospasm.
bronchogram A radiograph of the bronchial tree using a radiopaque substance that is introduced into the trachea.
bronchoscopy Insertion of an endoscope for diagnosis and treatment of disorders of the bronchi.
bruit An abnormal sound of venous or arterial origin heard on auscultation.
bulimia nervosa A mental disorder occurring predominantly in females characterized by episodes of binge eating that continue until terminated by abdominal pain, sleep, or self-induced vomiting.
bulla (bullae) A blister; a round, fluid-filled lesion of the skin, usually more than 5 mm in diameter.
burns, full-thickness Burns in which all of the epithelializing elements of the skin and those tissues lining the sweat glands, hair follicles, and sebaceous glands are destroyed.
burns, partial-thickness Burns in which the epithelializing elements remain intact.

C

cachexia A profound state of general ill health and malnutrition.
calculus (calculi) An abnormal concretion, usually of mineral salts, occurring mainly in hollow organs or their passages (e.g., renal calculus, or kidney stone).
callus A thickened area of the epidermis caused by pressure or friction.
caloric testing Testing to check the oculovestibular reflex. A patient's eye movements are observed while the external ear canal is irrigated with cold water. Absence of eye movement indicates a brainstem lesion.
candidiasis An infection with a fungus of the genus *Candida,* especially *C. albicans.* It is usually a superficial infection of the moist cutaneous areas of the body, although it becomes more severe in immunocompromised patients.
capitation A payment method wherein the health care provider is paid a monthly contracted rate for each member patient assigned regardless of the type or number of services provided.
capnography Measurement of inhaled and exhaled carbon dioxide as recorded on a capnogram.
caput medusa Dilated cutaneous veins around the umbilicus in patients suffering from cirrhosis of the liver.
carbuncles A collection of infected hair follicles. Most often occur on the back of the neck, the upper back, and the lateral thighs.
carcinogen Any substance or agent that produces or increases the risk of developing cancer in humans or lower animals.
carcinoma(s) A malignant growth made up of epithelial cells.
cardiac glycosides A group of compounds containing a carbohydrate molecule (e.g., digitalis) that affect the contractile force of the heart muscle.
cardiac tamponade Compression of the heart caused by collection of fluid in the pericardial sac.
cardiogenic shock A shock state caused by pump failure of the heart.
cardiomyopathy Disease of the myocardium, especially due to primary disease of the heart muscle.
cardiomyoplasty A procedure wherein the latissimus dorsi muscle is detached from its natural position, brought around to the front of the body and wrapped around the heart. A pacemaker, connected to the heart and back muscle, helps boost the heart's pumping action.
cardiopulmonary resuscitation The reestablishment of heart and lung action after they have suddenly stopped.
cardiotonic(s) An agent having the effect of strengthening contractions of the heart muscle.
cardioversion A mild electrical shock delivered to the heart at a specific time in the cardiac cycle to interrupt the abnormal rhythm and begin a new, normal rhythm of electrical impulse and contraction.
carpopedal spasm A spasm of the hand, thumbs, foot, or toes that accompanies tetany.
carriers People who harbor infectious organisms within their bodies without manifesting any outward symptoms of the infection.
catabolic Destructive in nature; the opposite of anabolic.
catabolism The phase of metabolism in which larger molecules are broken down and energy is released; the destructive phase of metabolism.
cataract(s) An opacity of the lens of the eye.
catecholamines One of a group of biogenic amines having a sympathomimetic action; examples are dopamine, norepinephrine, and epinephrine.
category-specific precautions A system of precautionary measures organized according to types of diseases (e.g., respiratory or enteric) and employed to prevent the spread of disease.
cations Positively charged atomic particles.
cauterize To burn with a cautery, or to apply one.
CD lymphocyte A type of lymphocyte that is the master regulator of the human immune system. It is the primary site of replication for HIV.
cell(s) The basic structural unit of living organisms.
cell-mediated immunity Immunity resulting from activation of sensitized lymphocytes.
cellulitis Inflammation of cellular or connective tissue.
central hearing loss Impaired perception of sound caused by pathology above the junction of the eighth cranial nerve and the brainstem (in the brain).

cerumen Earwax.
chalazion An infection of the meibomian gland of the eye; an internal stye.
chancre A primary syphilis skin lesion that begins as a papule and develops into a red, bloodless, painless ulcer with a scooped-out appearance.
chemonucleolysis Treatment of a herniated intervertebral disk by dissolution of a portion of the nucleus pulposus by injection of a chemolytic agent.
chemotherapy Use of chemicals, especially drugs, in the treatment of such diseases as cancer, infection, and some mental illnesses.
cholecystectomy The removal of the gallbladder.
cholecystitis An inflammation of the gallbladder.
choledocholithiasis The condition in which gallstones lodge in the common bile duct.
cholelithiasis The presence of stones within the gallbladder or biliary tract.
cholinergic An agent that produces the effect of acetylcholine.
chorea Involuntary muscle twitching.
chronic pain Pain of long duration showing little change or slowly progressive pain.
chronologic Occurring in a natural time sequence.
chyme The mixture of partly digested food and digestive secretions found in the stomach and small intestine during digestion of a meal.
cirrhosis A liver disease characterized by diffuse interlacing bands of fibrous tissue dividing the hepatic parenchyma into micronodular or macronodular areas.
cirrhosis of the liver A condition characterized by destruction of normal hepatic structures and their replacement with necrotic tissue and scarring.
claudication, intermittent A syndrome characterized by intensification of limb pain as exercise is increased; related to occlusion of arteries in the legs.
climacteric Endocrine, somatic, and psychic changes occurring at the end of the female reproductive period (menopause); also, normal diminution of testicular activity in the male.
clinical pathway A tool used to track patient progress along a set path in a managed care system.
clonic Alternating contraction and relaxation of muscles.
clonus Abnormal neuromuscular activity, characterized by rapidly alternating involuntary contraction and relaxation of skeletal muscle; occurs with epileptic seizure.
coarctation Narrowing (of the aorta).
code of ethics A set of rules governing one's conduct.
co-dependency A behavior pattern in which a family member or friend of a substance abuser attempts to control the behavior of the dependent person.
cognition The mental processes of perception, memory, judgment, and reasoning.
co-insurance Insurance in which both the insurer and the patient pay the medical bill.
coitus Sexual intercourse.
colectomy The removal of part of the colon.
colic A spasm causing pain; may be biliary, renal, intestinal, or uterine.
collaboration The act of working or cooperating with another.
collaborator One who works cooperatively with another.
collagen A fibrous protein found in skin, bone, cartilage, and ligaments.
colonization The process in which a group of organisms, especially bacteria, live together and multiply.
colostomy (colostomies) The surgical creation of an opening in the colon to allow fecal material to pass outside.
colporrhaphy The operation of suturing the vagina.
colposcopy The visual examination of the vagina and cervix with a specially designed endoscope that allows the detection of malignant growths in their early stages.
comedo (comedones) A plug of keratin and sebum in an enlarged pore; a blackhead.
communicable disease A disease that may be transmitted directly or indirectly from one individual to another.
complement system A complex series of enzymatic proteins that interact to combine with the antigen-antibody complex, producing lysis of intact antigen cells.
complement system of proteins A series of protective proteins that are activated in the inflammatory response.
complementary and alternative medicine (CAM) Types of treatments for medical disorders that do not rely on traditional medicine, but frequently are combined with traditional medical treatment for a disorder.
complete blood count (CBC) The number of each kind of cell in a sample of blood.
compliance An expression of the ability of lung tissue to distend when filled with air.
computed tomography (CT) scan A computer-aided technique in which small sections of tissue within an organ can be visualized by radiograph.
concept(s) An idea, thought, or notion derived from experiences and information acquired from one's external environment.
concussion A term used to describe a closed head injury in which the brain is compressed by a portion of the skull at the time of the blow and temporary ischemia of the brain tissue results.
conductive hearing loss Impaired perception of sound caused by a dysfunction of either the external or the middle ear.
confabulation A behavioral reaction to memory loss in which the patient fills in memory gaps with made-up facts and experiences.
confusion The state of not being aware of or oriented to time, place, or self.
congenital Present at birth.
congestive heart failure The exhaustion of the heart muscle and a resultant engorgement of the heart's chambers and the blood vessels. Eventually, sluggish blood flow leads to retention of fluid and edema in the lungs and elsewhere in the body.
conjugate Working in union; equally coupled.
conjunctivitis An inflammation of the membrane covering the eyeball and lining the eyelids.
consciousness Responsiveness of the mind to impressions made by the senses.
contactant A substance that produces an allergic or sensitivity response when in direct contact with the skin.
contamination The presence of a noxious agent, such as bacteria or radiation, in a place where it is not wanted.
contracture An adaptive shortening of skeletal muscle tissue that is not subjected to normal stretching and contraction.
contralateral On or affecting the opposite side of the body.
contusion A bruise; an injury of a part without a break in the skin.
conventional antipsychotics Neuroleptics used to treat the positive symptoms of schizophrenia. Cause serious and unpleasant side effects and are becoming less commonly prescribed.
convulsion A state of involuntary muscle contractions and relaxations.
copayment The amount a member of an HMO has to pay for each visit to the health care provider.
COPD Chronic obstructive pulmonary disease.

coronary artery bypass graft (CABG) Surgery in which a blood vessel is grafted onto the coronary artery to improve blood flow.
coronary insufficiency Decreased or insufficient blood flow in the coronary arteries.
coronary occlusion The closing off of a coronary artery and interruption of its blood flow.
cor pulmonale Heart disease characterized by hypertrophy of the right ventricle due to pulmonary hypertension.
corrosive Containing a destructive agent that produces disintegration or wearing away.
cost containment The need to hold costs to within fixed limits.
counterregulatory hormones Growth hormone, glucagons, and epinephrine that are released during the night that cause an increase in blood glucose. They act "counter" to insulin.
coup-contrecoup injury An injury that occurs when the head is moving rapidly and hits a stationary object. The contents within the cranium hit the inside of the skull (coup) and then bounce back and hit the opposite side, causing a second injury (contrecoup).
crackles An abnormal respiratory sound heard on auscultation during inspiration; can be a bubbling noise or a popping sound. Crackles do not clear with coughing.
creatinine A nonprotein substance that is formed in muscle in relatively small and constant amounts, passes into the bloodstream, and is eliminated by the kidneys. Urine creatinine levels are diminished when glomerular filtration is impaired.
Credé technique Exerting downward pressure with the open hand over the suprapubic area to facilitate emptying of the urinary bladder.
cremasteric reflex The retraction of the testicles when the inner thigh is stroked. This reflex is absent with testicular torsion.
crepitation A sound like that of hair rubbed between the fingers; occurs when bone fragments rub together.
cretinism A congenital condition due to lack of thyroid secretion, characterized by arrested physical and mental development, dystrophy of the bones and soft parts, and lowered basal metabolism.
criterion A standard for judging a condition or establishing a diagnosis.
critical thinking Purposeful, considered, organized cognitive processing used to examine a problem or situation or evaluate the thinking of others.
crust An outer layer of solid matter formed by dried exudate or secretion.
cryoprecipitate Any precipitate that forms as a result of cooling.
cryosurgery The destruction of tissue by application of extreme cold, as in removal of cataracts.
cryotherapy The therapeutic use of cold or freezing.
cryptorchidism (cryptorchism) The failure of one or both of the testes to descend into the scrotum during fetal life.
culdoscopy The direct inspection of the female viscera through an endoscope introduced into the pelvic cavity through the posterior vaginal fornix.
culture The propagation of microorganisms or living tissue cells in media conducive to their growth.
curettage Cleansing of a surface of an organ with a spoon-shaped instrument (curet).
cyanosis A bluish tinge to the skin caused by lack of oxygen and accumulation of carbon dioxide in the blood.
cystitis An inflammation of the urinary bladder.
cystocele A protrusion or herniation of the bladder through the wall of the vagina.
cystogram A radiograph of the urinary bladder using a contrast medium.
cystoscopy Endoscopic examination of the interior of the bladder.
cytokine A low-moleucular-weight protein secreted by various cell types and involved in cell-to-cell communication. It coordinates antibody and T-cell immune interactions and augments immune reactivity.
cytology The study of cells, their origin, structure, function, and pathology.
cytotoxic Destructive to cells.

D

dactylitis An inflammation of a finger or toe.
database A collection of facts and figures for analysis from which conclusions may be drawn.
data collection The systematic collection of physical and psychosocial data for a patient who is having a problem. Part of assessment within the nursing process.
dawn phenomenon A condition sometimes encountered in type 1 diabetes characterized by increased blood glucose in the morning caused by release of hormones during the night.
deaf Partially or completely lacking the sense of hearing.
death(s) The cessation of all physical and chemical processes that invariably occurs in all living organisms. *See also* Dying.
débride Peel away dead tissue.
débridement The removal of all foreign material and dead tissues from or adjacent to a traumatic or infected lesion until healthy tissue is exposed.
debriefing Questioning of personnel involved and obtaining knowledge about function and problems that occurred (during a disaster).
decerebrate posturing Extensor posturing; the arms are stiffly extended and held close to the body and the wrists are flexed outward. Indicates damage to the midbrain or brainstem.
decontamination The freeing of a person or an object of some contaminating substance such as radioactive material.
decorticate posturing Flexor posturing; extension of the legs and internal rotation and adduction of the arms with the elbows bent upward. Indicates damage to the cortex.
decubitus ulcer(s) A breakdown in the skin and underlying tissues caused by long-standing pressure, ischemia, and damage to the underlying tissue.
deductible The yearly amount an insured person must spend out-of-pocket before a health plan begins to pay its share.
defecate To evacuate the bowels; to have a bowel movement.
defibrillation Stopping fibrillation of the heart with electrical current.
dehiscence The separation of all layers of a surgical wound.
dehydration Excessive loss of water from tissues of the body.
delegate To authorize and send another as one's representative (to carry out a task).
delegation Allocation of patient care activities to team members.
delirium An altered state of consciousness that is usually acute and of short duration.
delusion A false, fixed belief that cannot be changed with rational explanation.
dementia A broad impairment of intellectual function that usually is progressive.
demyelination Destruction of the myelin sheath of nerve tissue.

demyelinization Demyelination.
dendrite Any of the thread-like extensions of the cytoplasm of a neuron.
denial A defense mechanism in which the existence of intolerable conditions is unconsciously rejected; the first stage in the acceptance of death.
denuded When the protective layer or covering is removed through surgery, trauma, or pathologic change.
deoxyribonucleic acid (DNA) The primary genetic material of all cellular organisms.
dependency The state of reliance on a substance; implies that there are physical and psychological symptoms of addiction. Term used to describe substance use disorder.
dependent (nursing action) Requiring an order from a health care provider.
dependent rubor The dusky-red color dangling feet soon take on after elevating the feet and legs above the heart for 1 to 2 minutes. This indicates arterial insufficiency.
depression A morbid sadness, dejection, or melancholy; a stage in the acceptance of death.
depression (of immune function) The decreased ability of the immune system to function normally.
dermabrasion Planing of the skin done by mechanical means to smooth the skin and remove scars.
dermatitis An inflammation of the skin.
dermatology The medical specialty concerned with diagnosing and treating skin disorders.
dermatome A nerve tract.
dermatophytosis Any superficial fungal infection caused by a dermatophyte and involving the stratum corneum of the skin, hair, and nails.
detoxification The process of ridding the body of a drug without causing harmful ill effects.
developmental task(s) A task that should be completed during a specific life period to ensure continuing psychosocial growth and maturity.
deviation Departure from normal.
diabetic neuropathy A disorder of the peripheral nerves that is associated with diabetes mellitus and is characterized by sexual impotence in the male, neurogenic bladder, and pain or loss of feeling in the lower extremities.
diabetogenic Causing diabetes.
diagnosis, nursing A concise statement of a patient's actual or potential health problems that nurses, by virtue of their education and experience, are able and licensed to treat.
diagnosis-related groups (DRGs) The classifications used to determine Medicare payments for patient care based on medical diagnoses.
dialysis The diffusion of solute molecules through a semipermeable membrane, the molecules passing from the more concentrated solution to the less concentrated one.
dialysis, peritoneal The use of the peritoneum as a dialyzing membrane to remove waste products that have accumulated in the body as a result of renal failure.
diaphoresis Excessive perspiration.
diastole The phase of the cardiac cycle in which the heart muscle relaxes between contractions; during this phase the two ventricles are dilated by blood flowing through them. Diastolic blood pressure is recorded as the bottom number in the pressure measurement.
diastolic blood pressure Arterial pressure during diastole.
diffusion The spontaneous mixing of the molecules or ions of two or more substances; the result of random thermal motion.
digital Pertaining to or resembling a finger or toe.
digitalization The initial administration of digitalis to build up a therapeutic blood level of the drug.
diplopia Double vision; seeing two images.
disability Difficulty in performing certain tasks because of impairment.
disaster A natural or man-made (bioterrorism or nuclear) event that overwhelms the community's existing emergency resources.
disease One possible outcome due to an infection.
disease-specific precautions A system of precautionary measures organized according to the specific infectious disease presented by the patient.
disinfectant(s) An agent that destroys infection-producing organisms.
dislocation Stretching or tearing of ligaments around a joint with complete displacement of a bone.
disseminated Widespread.
disseminated intravascular coagulation (DIC) A disorder characterized by reduction in the elements involved in blood coagulation due to their utilization in widespread blood clotting within the vessels; the activation of the clotting mechanism may arise from any of a number of disorders.
distal In a position farthest from the point of reference.
distraction Diversion of attention from present experience (i.e., pain).
diuresis The excretion of excess fluid in the urine.
diuretic(s) An agent that promotes secretion of urine.
diurnal Happening during daylight hours.
diverticulitis The inflammation of the diverticula.
diverticulosis The presence of diverticula, in the absence of diverticulitis.
diverticulum (diverticula) A small blind pouch resulting from a protrusion of the mucosa of a hollow organ through weakened areas in the organ's muscle wall.
documentation The recording of significant information on a patient's chart.
dowager's hump An abnormal backward curve of the cervical spine that is the result of osteoporosis and/or Cushing syndrome.
Down syndrome A congenital disorder characterized by physical malformations and some degree of mental retardation; also called *trisomy 21 syndrome* because there is a defect in chromosome 21.
DRGs *See* Diagnosis-related groups.
drusen Yellow exudates found beneath the retinal pigment epithelium, representing extracellular debris.
dual diagnosis The diagnosis of a patient with a substance abuse problem and a mental health disorder.
dumping syndrome A group of symptoms caused by too-rapid passage of food through the upper gastrointestinal tract.
dying A stage of life; a process that, from a medical point of view, begins when a person has a disease that is untreatable and inevitably ends in death; or the final stages of a fatal disease. *See also* Death(s).
dynamic Having vital force or inherent power.
dysarthria Slurring or indistinct speech articulation; difficulty speaking.
dyscrasia An imbalance of formed elements, as in blood dyscrasia.
dysfunctional uterine bleeding Uterine bleeding at times other than during normal menstruation.
dysmenorrhea Painful or difficult menstruation.
dyspareunia Difficult or painful coitus in women.
dyspepsia Impairment of the power or function of digestion; usually applied to epigastric discomfort following meals.
dysphagia Difficulty in swallowing.
dysphasia Difficulty speaking; usually caused by a brain lesion.
dyspnea Labored or difficult breathing.

dysrhythmia A variation from the normal rhythm, especially of the heartbeat.
dysthymia A disturbance in mood that may manifest in either depression or elation.
dystonic reactions Acute contractures of the tongue, face, neck, and back.
dysuria Painful urination.

E

eccentric Departing from conventional custom or practice; differing conspicuously in behavior, appearance, or opinions.
ecchymosis (ecchymoses) An irregularly shaped, blue-black skin discoloration caused by bleeding beneath the skin.
ECG (also EKG) *See* electrocardiogram.
ectopic Located away from normal position, as in ectopic pregnancy.
ectropion An outward turning of the eyelid.
edema An accumulation of fluid surrounding the cell.
edematous Pertaining to, or affected with, edema (abnormal fluid in the tissue).
EEG *See* Electroencephalogram.
effleurage A massage technique with long, light or firm strokes over the spine and back. May be circular strokes done with the fingertips.
effluent A discharge or outflow (i.e., the contents flowing out of an ileostomy or colostomy).
effusion An escape of fluid into a part or tissue, as an exudation or transudation.
ejaculation Ejection of the seminal fluid from the male urethra.
elastance The extent to which the lungs are able to return to their original position after being barely distended.
electrocardiogram The record produced by amplification of the electrical impulses normally generated by the heart.
electroconvulsive therapy (ECT) The oldest form of brain stimulation therapy, used for severe depression. Considered after several unsuccessful regimens of medication. Consists of electric shock to the brain via electrodes applied to the temples. This shock artificially induces a grand mal seizure lasting 30 to 90 seconds.
electroencephalogram A recording of changes in electric potentials in various areas of the brain.
electrolyte(s) A chemical substance that when dissolved in water dissociates into ions and thus is capable of conducting an electric current.
electromyography The recording and study of intrinsic electrical properties of skeletal muscle; useful in diagnosing neuromuscular disorders.
elimination Discharge from the body of indigestible materials and waste products of metabolism.
embolism A sudden obstruction of arterial blood flow by a blood clot or a mass that has been brought to the site in the bloodstream.
embolus A clot or plug of material (usually from a thrombus) carried by blood flow that lodges in a vessel and obstructs blood flow.
emesis Substance produced by vomiting.
empathy The ability to recognize and share the emotions and states of mind of another; understanding another's behavior.
emphysema A chronic pulmonary disease characterized by increase beyond normal in the size of air spaces distal to the terminal bronchiole with destructive changes in their walls.
empyema The presence of infected and purulent exudate within the pleural cavity.
enabling Doing something for a substance-dependent person that keeps the person from facing consequences. Term used with substance abuse.
encapsulated Surrounded by a fibrous capsule.
encephalopathy Any dysfunction of the brain.
endarterectomy The surgical removal of thickened atheromatous areas of the innermost layer of an artery.
endemic Present in a community at all times.
endocarditis An inflammation of the membrane lining the cavities of the heart and of the connective tissue bed on which it lies.
endocrine Secreting internally; refers to glandular function.
endogenous Coming from within.
endometriosis The presence of endometrial tissue in locations outside the uterus.
endorphin(s) Any of a group of opiate-like peptides naturally produced by the body.
endoscopy Examination with an endoscope that allows for direct visual inspection of the interior of hollow organs and body cavities.
endotoxin(s) A heat-stable toxin that is present in the intact bacterial cell wall, is pyrogenic, and is capable of increasing capillary permeability.
endotracheal intubation Airway management with a catheter or tube inserted through the mouth or nose into the trachea.
engraftment Successful establishment of the graft in bone marrow transplantation.
enteral feeding Feeding a patient by means of a tube passed into the stomach from the nasal passage.
enterocele A hernia containing intestines.
enterostomal Related to an abdominal stoma, or artificial opening of the intestine onto the surface of the body.
entropion Inversion of the eyelid margin.
enucleation Removal of an organ or other mass intact, as of the eyeball from the orbit.
environment All the physical and psychological factors that influence or affect the life or survival of a person.
enzyme Any protein that acts as a catalyst, increasing the rate at which chemical reaction occurs.
epidemic(s) A disease that simultaneously attacks many people in a geographic area, is widely diffused, and spreads rapidly.
epidermophytosis A fungal infection that most often affects the feet, especially between the toes; also called *athlete's foot* or *dermophytosis*.
epididymis A small oblong body resting on and beside the posterior surface of the testes that constitutes the first part of the excretory duct of each testis.
epidural Situated on or outside the dura mater.
epidural hematoma A hematoma caused by rapid leakage of blood from the middle meningeal artery, which quickly elevates intracranial pressure.
epigastric Pertaining to the region over the pit of the stomach.
epilepsy A group of neurologic disorders characterized by recurrent episodes of convulsive seizures, sensory disturbances, abnormal behaviors, loss of consciousness, or all of these.
epistaxis Nosebleed.
equilibrium Balance.
erection The state of swelling, hardness, and stiffness observed in the penis of the male and to a lesser extent in the clitoris of the female.
erythema Redness of the skin.
erythrasma A chronic bacterial infection of the major skinfolds, marked by red or brownish patches on the skin.

erythrocyte sedimentation rate The rate at which red blood cells settle out of unclotted blood in 1 hour.
erythropoiesis Formation of red blood cells, or erythrocytes.
eschar A castoff of dead tissue, as from a burn, corrosive application, or gangrene.
escharotomy Surgical incision of a constricting eschar in a burn victim, in order to permit the cut edges to separate and restore blood flow to unburned tissue.
esophageal varices Varicosities of branches of the azygous vein that connects with the portal vein in the lower esophagus; related to portal hypertension and cirrhosis of the liver.
estrogens The female sex hormones, including estradiol, estriol, and estrone.
etiology Study of the cause of disease; origin.
euthanasia An easy or painless death; active euthanasia, or mercy killing, is the deliberate ending of the life of a person who is incurably and terminally ill; passive euthanasia is the withholding of "heroic" measures and allowing the person to die.
euthymia A normal mood or feeling state.
evaluation, of outcome Appraisal of the patient's progress toward achievement of the goals and objectives stated in the nursing care plan.
evaluation, of process Appraisal of nursing activities and what has been done to assess, plan, and implement nursing care.
evaluation, of structure Appraisal of the physical facilities, equipment, staffing, and other characteristics of an agency that affect the quality of nursing care.
evisceration (1) extrusion of internal organs; (2) removal of the contents of the eyeball, leaving the sclera intact.
excess An amount beyond what is usual or necessary.
excoriation Any superficial loss of substance, such as that produced by scratching the skin.
excursion Range of movement (of the lungs).
exercises, isometric Active exercises performed against stable resistance, without change in the length of the muscle.
exfoliate To separate or peel off in scales, layers, or flakes.
exocrine Secreting externally via a duct.
exogenous Coming from outside.
exophthalmos Abnormal protrusion of the eyeball.
exotoxin A potent toxin formed and excreted by the bacterial cell.
Expanded Precautions Use of Standard Precaution techniques with additional protective actions specific to the organism and location involved.
expected outcomes Results expected to be achieved by the patient from health care provided and personal contributions.
expectorate To spit out saliva or cough up materials from the air passageways leading to the lungs.
extension A movement that brings a limb into or toward a straight position by increasing the angle between the bones forming a joint; opposite of flexion.
extracellular Outside of the cell.
extracellular fluids Body fluids outside the cell walls that constitute the environment of each cell.
extracorporeal Outside the body.
exudate Fluid that contains dead cells, serum, phagocytes, bacteria, or pus.

F

fecal impaction The accumulation of putty-like or hardened feces in the rectum or sigmoid colon.
feedback The process of providing a system with information about its output.
feedback, negative A corrective action in which a system is informed that its output is not satisfactory and a change is needed.
feedback, positive Information that tells a system its output is satisfactory.
fee-for-service Fee paid for services provided; a type of medical practice.
fetor hepaticus Foul-smelling breath associated with severe liver disease.
fibroid A thickened vascular mass in the uterus.
fibroma A fibrous, encapsulated connective tissue tumor.
fibrosis Fibrous tissue formation.
filtration Passage of a gas or liquid through a filter to separate out unwanted matter.
fistula(s) Any abnormal, tubelike passage within the body between two internal organs or leading from an internal organ to the body surface.
flaccid Limp, weak, or relaxed.
flatus Gas in the digestive tract.
flexion A movement that brings a limb into or toward a bent position by decreasing the angle between the bones forming a joint; opposite of extension.
flight of ideas Going from topic to topic in conversation with little or no connection.
flora Plant life, as distinguished from animal life.
fluid(s) The water and substances dissolved in it that form the internal environment.
fluid balance Equilibrium between the amount of fluid taken into the body and that lost through urine, feces, the lungs, skin, and possibly vomiting and fistulas.
fluid deficit(s) A fluid imbalance in which there is not enough fluid in one or more of the body's fluid compartments as a result of either inadequate intake or excessive loss.
fluid excess A fluid imbalance in which too much fluid accumulates in one or more of the body's fluid compartments as a result of either excessive intake or inadequate loss. *See also* Edema.
fluids, transcellular Body fluids that pass through cellular structures and eventually are eliminated from the body.
follicular pharyngitis An inflammation of the pharynx accompanied by purulent infection.
fracture(s) Interruption in the continuity of a bone.
friction rub A high-pitched, scratchy sound heard with the diaphragm of the stethoscope placed at the lower left sternal border of the chest; a symptom of pericarditis.
fructosamine assay A test that may be used to monitor control of glucose over a period of 2 to 3 weeks.
fulguration Destruction by electric cautery.
functional disorder A disorder that affects the function but not the structure of the body or body part.
fungus (fungi) A member of a group of organisms (mushrooms, yeasts, molds, etc.) that thrive in a warm, moist climate. Can cause infections that are difficult to eradicate because fungi tend to reproduce by means of spores that are resistant to ordinary disinfectants and antiseptics.
furuncles Inflammations of hair follicles. Also called *boils*.

G

galactosemia A genetic disorder in which there is a lack of the enzyme necessary for proper metabolism of galactose.
gangrene A necrosis, or death, of tissue, usually due to deficient or absent blood supply.
gastritis An inflammation of the mucous membrane lining the stomach.
gastrojejunostomy The surgical creation of an anastomosis between the stomach and jejunum.

gastroparesis Delayed gastric emptying.
gastrostomy The surgical creation of an opening into the stomach to administer food and liquids.
gate control theory The proposal that synapses in the dorsal horn of the spinal cord act as gates and that pain signals compete with signals of other kinds of stimuli for passage through the gate and transmission to the brain.
gene One of the self-reproducing biologic units of heredity that make up segments of the DNA molecule that controls cellular reproduction and function.
generalized anxiety disorder A persistent, unrealistic, or excessive worry about two or more life circumstances.
genital Pertaining to the genitals (reproductive organs).
geriatrics The medical treatment of diseases commonly associated with aging and elderly persons.
gerontology The study of the problems of aging in all its aspects.
gigantism Excessive size. Seen in children with excessive secretion of growth hormone.
gingivitis An inflammation of the gingivae.
glaucoma A group of diseases of the eye, characterized by increased intraocular pressure, that can produce blindness if not managed successfully.
global amnesia Irretrievable total loss of memory.
globulin(s) A general term for proteins; separated into five fractions by serum protein electrophoresis and classified in order of decreasing electrophoretic mobility. The fractions are $alpha_1$, $alpha_2$, $beta_1$, $beta_2$, and gamma globulins.
glucagon(s) A polypeptide hormone secreted by the alpha cells of the islets of Langerhans.
glucocorticoid Any hormone released from the adrenal cortex that increases glucogenesis and thus raises the level of liver glycogen and blood glucose.
glucogenesis The formation of glucose from glycogen.
glucose intolerance The inability to properly metabolize glucose.
glucose tolerance test A test to detect abnormal glucose metabolism; assists in diagnosis of diabetes mellitus.
glycemic Referring to the amount of glucose present in a substance.
glycosuria Glucose in the urine.
glycosylated hemoglobin (Hb A_{1c}) Hemoglobin with glucose attached to it; periodic measurements of hemoglobin A_{1c} can help determine a diabetic patient's average blood glucose level over a period of 3 to 4 months.
goal(s) A broad statement describing what is to be accomplished over a specified period.
goiter An enlargement of the thyroid gland.
gonads Gamete-producing glands; the ovaries and testicles.
goniometry The measurement of range of motion in a joint.
graft An implant or transplant of tissue or an organ.
gram negative Having the pink color of the counterstain used in Gram's method of staining microorganisms.
gram positive Retaining the violet color of the stain used in Gram's method of staining microorganisms.
granulocyte A leukocyte containing abundant granules in its cytoplasm; granulocytes include neutrophils, eosinophils, and basophils.
gynecomastia The development of abnormally large mammary glands in the male.

H

hallucination A sensory perception (touching, tasting, feeling, hearing, seeing) that occurs without external stimulation.
hand hygiene The primary intervention any health care provider can use to control the spread of infection; performed with soap and water, if the hands are visibly soiled, or an alcohol-based hand-sanitizing solution.
handicap A social disadvantage that exists because of a disability.
Haversian system A canal system that runs through the bones and contains the blood and lymph vessels.
health The ability to function well physically and mentally and to express the full range of one's potential.
health care–associated infection Formerly known as a *nosocomial* infection. Can occur when a patient is cared for in any kind of health care setting.
health maintenance organization (HMO) A type of group health care practice that provides basic and supplemental health maintenance and treatment services to enrollees who prepay a fixed periodic fee that is set without regard to the amount or kind of services received.
Healthy People 2010 A federal government mandate with goals for improving the health of the American people, with particular attention to minority groups' health.
hearing loss Impaired perception of sound.
heat exhaustion A disorder resulting from overexposure to heat or to the sun; also called *heat prostration.* It is caused by excessive perspiration and loss of body water and salt.
heatstroke A life-threatening condition resulting from prolonged exposure to environmental heat; also called *sunstroke.*
Helicobacter pylori A species of gram-negative, microaerophilic bacteria of the family Spirillaceae that causes gastritis and pyloric ulcers in humans.
helping relationship A relationship in which at least one of the parties intends to promote growth, development, maturity, improved functioning, and improved coping in the life of the other.
hemarthrosis A collection of blood in the joint space.
hematemesis Vomiting of blood.
hematocrit The volume percentage of red blood cells in whole blood.
hematoma(s) A localized collection of blood, usually clotted, that has leaked from adjacent blood vessels into an organ, space, or tissue.
hematuria Blood in the urine.
hemianopsia Blindness for half the field of vision in one or both eyes.
hemicolectomy Removal of part of the colon.
hemiparesis Weakness affecting only one side of the body.
hemiparesthesia Perverted sensation on one side of the body.
hemiplegia Paralysis of one half, or one side, of the body.
hemodialysis The removal of nitrogenous wastes from the blood by circulating arterial blood through a dialysate and returning it to the venous circulation.
hemodynamics The study of the movements of blood and the pressures being exerted in the blood vessels and the chambers of the heart.
hemoglobin The protein found in red blood cells that transports molecular oxygen in the blood; oxygenated hemoglobin (oxyhemoglobin) is bright red; unoxygenated hemoglobin is darker.
hemoglobinuria The presence of free hemoglobin in the urine.
hemolysis The rupture of red blood cells with release of hemoglobin into the plasma.
hemolytic Pertaining to the breakdown of red blood cells.
hemophilia An inherited disorder in which there is deficiency of one or more specific clotting factors in the blood.

hemoptysis Coughing and spitting of blood that can originate in the lungs, larynx, or trachea.
hemorrhoid A varicosity of a vein of the rectum. It may be internal (inside the sphincter muscles of the anus) or external (outside the sphincter muscles).
hemorrhoidectomy The removal of hemorrhoids.
hemothorax A collection of blood in the pleural cavity.
hepatic encephalopathy Degenerative changes in the brain associated with liver failure.
hepatitis An inflammation of the liver.
hernia The protrusion or projection of an organ or a part of an organ through the wall of the cavity that normally contains it.
hernioplasty The repair of a hernia.
herniorrhaphy The surgical repair of a hernia.
herpesvirus Any of a large group of DNA viruses found in many animal species. Type 1 herpes simplex virus (HSV) produces lesions that are primarily nongenital. Type 2 HSV lesions most often are genital.
heterosexual A person who is sexually attracted to a person of the opposite sex.
hiatal hernia Protrusion of a portion of the stomach through the opening in the diaphragm through which the esophagus passes.
hierarchy The arrangement of objects, elements, or values in a graduated series.
hirsutism The excessive growth of hair on the body.
HIV The causative agent for AIDS; *see* Human immunodeficiency virus.
HLA Human leukocyte antigen.
HMO *See* Health maintenance organization.
holism The belief that each person is a unified whole.
holistic health care Attention to the mental, social, spiritual, and physical aspects of health and illness.
Homans' sign Pain on passive dorsiflexion of the foot; a sign of thrombosis of deep calf veins.
homeopathy A practice based on the theory that substances that produce symptoms of a disease in healthy people in large doses will cure the same symptoms when administered in small amounts.
homeostasis A tendency of biologic systems to maintain stability in the internal environment while continually adjusting to changes necessary for survival.
homonymous hemianopia Blindness or defective vision in the right or left halves of the visual fields of both eyes.
homosexual A person who is sexually attracted to a person of the same sex.
homozygous Having inherited a genetic trait from both parents.
hordeolum An external stye.
hormone A chemical produced by the cells of the body and transported by the bloodstream to target cells and organs on which it has a regulatory effect.
hospice A program that provides a continuum of home and inpatient care for the terminally ill and their families.
host An organism in which another parasitic organism is nourished and harbored.
human immunodeficiency virus (HIV) A retrovirus that integrates itself into the genetic material of the cell it infects, changing the DNA of the host cell.
human needs Basic needs for survival and personal growth shared by all humans.
human needs theory The proposal that basic human needs act as stimuli to human behavior; Maslow postulated five levels of human needs: physiologic, safety and security, love and belonging, esteem, and self-actualization.
humoral Pertaining to body fluids or substances contained in them.
humoral immunity Antibody-mediated immunity, the result of B-cell action and the production of antibodies.
hydrocephalus Increased cerebrospinal fluid in the ventricles of the brain.
hydronephrosis Distention of the renal pelvis and calices with urine that cannot flow through obstructed ureters.
hydrostatic pressure The pressure or force due to the presence of a fluid.
hyperalimentation Total parenteral nutrition.
hypercalcemia An above-normal level of calcium in the blood (i.e., more than 5.5 mEq/L or 11 mg/dL).
hypercapnia A condition in which there is an abnormally high amount of carbon dioxide in the blood.
hyperchloremia An excess of chloride in the blood.
hyperesthesia Abnormal sensitivity to stimuli.
hyperglycemia An increase of blood sugar, as in diabetes.
hyperkalemia An excessive amount of potassium in the blood.
hyperlipidemia An excessive amount of lipids in the blood.
hypermagnesemia An abnormally large magnesium content in blood plasma.
hypernatremia An excess of sodium in the blood.
hyperopia A visual defect in which parallel light rays reaching the eye focus behind the retina; farsightedness.
hyperphosphatemia An excessive amount of phosphates in the blood.
hyperplasia An increase in the number of cells of an organ; extra cell growth.
hyperpyrexia An extremely elevated temperature.
hypersecretion Oversecretion.
hypersensitivity An exaggerated immune response to an agent perceived by the body to be foreign. *See also* Allergy (allergies).
hypersomnia Sleeping for long periods.
hypertension Persistently high blood pressure; in adults, a systolic pressure equal to or greater than 140 mm Hg and a diastolic pressure equal to or greater than 90 mm Hg.
hyperthermia Unusually high fever.
hypertonic Of greater concentration.
hypertonic solution A solution in which the osmotic pressure (concentration) is greater than that of body fluids.
hypertrophy An increase in size of a structure or organ.
hyperuricemia An excessive amount of uric acid in the urine.
hyperventilation An abnormal breathing pattern in which an above-normal amount of air is inhaled into the lungs.
hypervolemia An abnormal increase in the volume of circulating blood.
hypesthesia A dysesthesia consisting of abnormally decreased sensitivity, particularly to touch. Also called *hypoesthesia.*
hypnosis A subconscious condition, usually artificially induced, in which there is a response to suggestions and commands made by the hypnotist.
hypoalbuminemia A decreased level of albumin in the blood.
hypocalcemia A below-normal level of calcium in the blood (i.e., less than 4.5 mEq/L or 8.5 mg/dL).
hypocapnia A deficit of carbon dioxide in the blood resulting from hyperventilation.
hypochloremia An abnormally diminished level of chloride in the blood.
hypochromic Pertaining to a condition of the blood in which the red blood cells have a reduced hemoglobin content.
hypodermoclysis Injection of fluid into subcutaneous tissue via continuous infusion.
hypoesthesia *See* Hypesthesia.

hypogammaglobulinemia An immune deficiency characterized by abnormally low levels of generally all classes of serum gamma globulins with increased susceptibility to infectious diseases.
hypoglycemia A deficiency of sugar in the blood.
hypoglycemic agents Those agents that lower the blood glucose level (i.e., oral medications that are used to treat some forms of diabetes mellitus).
hypokalemia Extreme potassium depletion in the circulating blood.
hypomagnesemia An abnormally low magnesium content of the blood plasma.
hypomania Inflated or irritable mood for at least 4 days.
hyponatremia A decreased concentration of sodium in the blood.
hypophosphatemia An abnormally decreased amount of phosphates in the blood.
hypophysectomy Excision of the hypophysis cerebri.
hyposecretion Undersecretion.
hyposensitization A treatment used in managing hypersensitivity to a known allergen; the program involves regular injections of minute quantities of selected antigens over an extended period.
hypothalamus That portion of the diencephalon that lies beneath the thalamus at the base of the cerebrum; it activates, controls, and integrates many of the body's vital functions (e.g., regulation of metabolism, volume of body fluids, electrolyte content, and release of hormones).
hypothermia A serious loss of body heat caused by prolonged exposure to cold.
hypotonic Of less concentration.
hypotonic solution One in which the osmotic pressure (concentration) is less than that of body fluids.
hypotonic state Pertaining to abnormally decreased muscular tone or tension.
hypoventilation An abnormal breathing pattern in which insufficient amounts of air are inhaled into the lungs.
hypovolemia Diminished blood volume.
hypoxemia Insufficient oxygenation of the blood.
hypoxia Deficiency of oxygen.
hysterectomy Surgical removal of the uterus.

I

iatrogenic Caused by medical treatment or diagnostic procedure.
iatrogenic disorder An adverse condition induced by effects of treatment by a physician or surgeon.
icterus Bile pigmentation of the tissues, membranes, and secretions.
idiopathic Of unknown cause.
idiosyncrasy A special characteristic by which a person differs from others.
ileal conduit A surgically created passageway that uses a portion of the ileum to direct the flow of urine from the ureters to the outside of the body.
ileostomy (ileostomies) An artificial opening in the ileum, created surgically, to drain fecal material from the small intestine.
ileus Intestinal obstruction, especially failure of peristalsis.
illusion A misperception of an actual sensory perception; misinterpretation of reality.
imagery Imagination; the calling up of mental pictures or events.
immune deficiency A lack of immune bodies and resultant impairment of the immune response to foreign agents.
immunity Resistance to a specific disease.
immunity, active Immunity acquired by producing one's own antibody.
immunity, passive Immunity acquired from a source other than one's own body, such as by transfer of antibody or lymphocytes from an immune donor.
immunization The process of rendering an individual immune by passive immunity or of becoming immune by active immunity.
immunocompetence The capacity to develop an immune response after exposure to antigen.
immunoglobulin(s) A protein of animal origin with known antibody activity and a major component of humoral immunity. *See also* Antibody (antibodies).
immunoscintigraphy A radioactive scan of the immune structures.
immunosuppression The deliberate inhibition of antibody formation; used in transplantation to prevent rejection of the donor organ.
immunotherapy Development of passive immunity in a person by administration of preformed antibody; also, the administration of immunopotentiators and immunocompetent lymphoid tissue for cancer treatment.
impairment Dysfunction of a specific organ or body system.
impetigo An infection of the skin, usually by streptococci or staphylococci.
implementation A deliberate action performed to achieve a goal; carrying out of nursing interventions.
impotence Inability of the male to achieve or maintain an erection.
impulsive Acting in response to an impulse because the action brings emotional release or pleasure even though the action may be harmful to oneself or socially unacceptable.
inanimate Not alive; dull, lifeless.
incidence The rate at which certain events occur.
incontinence An alteration in the control of bowel or urinary elimination, or both.
incubation The interval between exposure to infection and the appearance of the first symptom.
induration An abnormally hard spot or place.
infarct A localized area of necrosis produced by ischemia caused by obstructed arterial supply or inadequate venous drainage.
infarction Occurrence of a localized area of dead tissue produced by inadequate blood flow.
infection The invasion and multiplication of pathogenic microorganisms in body tissue.
inference A deduction or conclusion.
infertility The condition of inability to produce offspring.
inflammation An immediate cellular response to any kind of injury to the cells and tissues.
ingestants Any substances taken orally, such as food or drink.
ingestion The taking of any substance, such as food, drugs, water, or chemicals, by mouth or through the digestive system.
inhalants Medication or compounds suitable for inhaling.
initial The beginning of a thing or process; the first.
injectables Fluids capable of being injected.
innate Belonging to the essential nature of something; existing in or belonging at birth.
innate immunity A person's natural (inborn) immunity to certain diseases.
inotropic Pertaining to the force or energy of muscular contractions, particularly of the heart.
insensible Unconscious; without feeling or consciousness.
inspection The process of visual examination.
insomnia A sleep disorder; an inability to sleep.
insufficiency The condition of being inadequate for a given purpose.

insulin A naturally occurring hormone secreted by the beta cells of the islets of Langerhans in the pancreas in response to increased levels of glucose in the blood.

insulin-dependent diabetes mellitus Type 1 diabetes; a form of the disease that requires replacement of endogenous insulin with regular injections of exogenous insulin.

intention tremor A tremor that occurs on attempt at voluntary movement.

interdisciplinary (collaborative) care plan A care plan composed through collaboration of all of the health care team members caring for a patient.

intermittent claudication Cramping pain in the muscles of the lower extremities brought on by exercise and relieved by rest. A common symptom of arterial insufficiency; pain usually occurs in the calves of the legs, but can also affect the muscles of the thighs and buttocks.

interstitial Placed or lying between.

interstitial fluids Body fluids that are located in the tissue spaces around the cells. *See also* Edema.

intervention Nursing activities performed by the nurse to meet the specified goals of a nursing care plan.

intracellular Within cells.

intracellular fluids Body fluids that are within cell walls.

intractable pain Hard-to-manage pain; pain not relieved by ordinary methods.

intraocular Within the eye.

intrathecal Injected into the subarachnoid space of the spinal cord via lumbar puncture.

intrathoracic Within the thoracic cavity.

intravascular fluids Body fluids within the blood vessels; they are composed of plasma and the substances it transports.

intravenous therapy The administration of fluids through a vein.

intussusception Telescoping of one part of the bowel into another.

ions Atoms or groups of atoms that have an electric charge through the gain or loss of an electron.

ipsilateral On or affecting the same side of the body.

iridectomy Excision of part of the iris.

ischemia A deficiency of blood supply to a part as a result of functional constriction of a blood vessel or of actual obstruction, as by a clot.

Islets of Langerhans Pancreatic cells. Beta cells, which secrete insulin, are found in these cells.

isolation technique Special precautionary procedures used to set apart a patient with a communicable disease; the purpose is to prevent the spread of infectious agents from the patient to others.

isometric Having equal dimensions; maintaining the same length.

isometric exercises Exercises that involve generating tension between two opposing sets of muscles.

isotonic Of equal solute concentration.

isotonic contraction A contraction that occurs when tension is developed in a muscle.

isotonic solution A solution in which the osmotic pressure is the same as that of intracellular fluid (e.g., normal saline [0.9% concentration]).

isotope One of a series of chemical elements that have nearly identical chemical properties but differ in their atomic weight and electric charge. Many isotopes are radioactive.

J

jaundice A yellowing of the skin and mucous membranes that reflects excessively high blood levels of bilirubin (bile pigment).

K

keloid Excessive, abnormal scar formation in the skin following trauma or surgical incision.

keratitis An inflammation of the cornea.

keratosis (keratoses) Any horny growth, such as a wart or callosity; usually either actinic keratosis or a seborrheic keratosis.

ketoacidosis The accumulation of ketone bodies in the blood because of incomplete metabolism of fats, resulting in metabolic acidosis.

ketonuria The presence of acetone bodies in the urine.

ketosis The accumulation in the body of the ketone bodies: acetone, beta-hydroxybutyric acid, and acetoacetic acid.

kinetic motion The motion of material bodies and the forces and energy associated with it.

Korsakoff syndrome Substance-induced persisting dementia.

Kupffer's cells Large, highly phagocytic cells in the liver; they form part of the reticuloendothelial system.

kyphosis An abnormally increased curvature of the thoracic spine, which gives a "hunchback" appearance.

L

labile Unsteady, not fixed; easily disarranged.

labyrinthitis An inflammation of the internal ear, including the vestibule, cochlea, and semicircular canal.

laparoscopy The examination of the peritoneal cavity with a fiberoptic instrument inserted through a small abdominal incision.

laryngectomy The partial or total removal of the larynx by surgical excision; the person who has had a laryngectomy is called a *laryngectomee.*

laryngitis An inflammation of the larynx.

laryngoscopy Direct or indirect visual examination of the larynx.

laser Stands for *l*ight *a*mplification by *s*timulated *e*mission of *r*adiation; converts light wavelengths into one small, intense unified beam of single-wavelength radiation; used for diagnosis and surgery.

latent Not obvious; hidden.

lesion A circumscribed area of pathologically altered tissue.

leukapheresis A process by which blood is withdrawn from a vein, white blood cells are removed, and the remaining blood is reinfused in the patient.

leukemia A malignant disease of the blood-forming organs, marked by abnormal proliferation and development of leukocytes and their precursors in the blood and bone marrow.

leukocyte A colorless blood cell whose chief function is to protect the body against pathogenic microorganisms.

leukocytosis An increase in the number of white blood cells, or leukocytes, in the blood.

leukopenia A reduction in the number of leukocytes in the blood to 5000 or less.

leukoplakia Patches of thickened, white tissue on mucous membrane; considered a precursor to cancer.

leukotrienes A class of biologically active compounds that occur naturally in leukocytes and produce allergic and inflammatory reactions similar to those of histamine.

level of consciousness (LOC) A standardized system to describe the state of consciousness (i.e., alert wakefulness, drowsiness, stupor, or coma).

Lhermitte sign An electric shock–like sensation felt along the spine when the neck is flexed.

libido The conscious or unconscious sexual drive.

lifestyle habits Entrenched practices related to work, recreation, diet, exercise, and other activities of daily living.

ligate To tie or bind.
lipodystrophy A disturbance of or defect in fat metabolism.
lipoma A fatty tumor.
lipoprotein Any of the macromolecular complexes that are transported in the blood.
lithiasis The formation of stones.
lithotripsy The crushing of a calculus in the kidney, bladder, urethra, or gallbladder.
loose associations Disordered thinking with little connection between thoughts.
lordosis An abnormal forward curvature of the spine.
lozenge(s) A medicated tablet or disk.
lucid Clear, especially applied to clarity of the mind.
lymphadenitis An inflammation of the lymph nodes.
lymphadenopathy A disease of the lymph nodes, often producing enlargement.
lymphangiography Radiography of lymphatic vessels after injection of a contrast medium.
lymphangitis An inflammation of the lymph vessels.
lymphatic system An accessory system by which fluids can flow from tissue spaces into the blood.
lymphedema The swelling of tissues drained by the lymphatic system.
lymph nodes Small bundles of lymphatic tissue containing lymphocytes, the functions of which are filtration and phagocytosis.
lymphocyte A mononuclear, nongranulous leukocyte that is chiefly a product of lymphoid tissue and is important in the development of immunity.
lymphocyte, sensitized A nongranular lymphocyte that has been processed either by the thymus (T lymphocyte) or an unknown processing area (B lymphocyte) and is responsible for either cellular or humoral immunity.
lymphocyte-transforming factor A protein mediator that causes transformation and clonal expansion of nonsensitized lymphocytes that produce a toxin destructive to antigen.
lymphoma Any neoplastic disorder of lymphoid tissue.
lyse To produce decomposition; to destroy.
lysis The gradual decline of a fever or disease; the opposite of crisis.

M

macrophage(s) A large, mononuclear phagocyte derived from monocytes; macrophages are components of the reticuloendothelial system.
macrophage-activating factor A mediator released by sensitized lymphocytes on contact with an antigen, the function of which is to induce in macrophages an increased content of lysosomal enzymes, more aggressive phagocytosis, and increased mitosis.
macrophage chemotaxis factor A protein mediator released by sensitized lymphocytes on contact with antigen, the function of which is to attract macrophages to the antigen site.
macule (macula) A discolored spot on the skin that is not raised above the surface.
major depressive disorder A mental disorder in which at least five symptoms characteristic of depression have been present for at least 2 weeks. Some of these symptoms include an overwhelming feeling of sadness, inability to feel pleasure or interest in daily activities, weight gain or loss not attributed to dieting, sleep disturbances, fatigue, difficulty concentrating, and suicidal thoughts.
malignancy *See* Carcinoma.
malignant Becoming progressively worse; resisting treatment and resulting in death; having the properties of anaplasia, invasiveness, and metastasis.
mammography The x-ray examination of the soft tissues of the breast.
mammoplasty Plastic surgery of the breast.
managed care Organization of health care delivery that coordinates care delivery by various health team members in a timely, cost-effective manner.
mania An elevation in mood characterized by feelings of elation, excitement, or extreme irritability.
mass casualties Casualties in such numbers that the normal health care system has difficulty providing adequate care.
mastication Chewing.
mean, mathematical An average (e.g., mean corpuscular hemoglobin concentration, which is the concentration of hemoglobin in the average erythrocyte).
measurable The ability to be expressed numerically, or to be described as to the extent or quantity (of a substance, energy, or time).
mediastinum The mass of tissues and organs separating the sternum in front and the vertebral column behind.
mediate To accomplish by indirect means; to act between two parties or sides.
Medicaid A federally funded state-operated program that provides medical assistance to eligible people with low incomes.
Medicare A federally funded national health insurance program in the United States for people over 65 years old.
meditation The act of contemplative thinking.
melanoma A malignant, darkly pigmented mole or tumor of the skin.
melena Black, tarry stools.
menarche The onset of menstruation.
Meniere's disease A group of symptoms produced by an increase in fluid in the labyrinthine spaces with swelling and congestion of the mucosa of the cochlea.
menopause The span of time during which the menstrual cycle wanes and gradually stops; *see* Climacteric.
menorrhagia Excessive menstruation.
menses The onset of the menstrual cycle.
menstruation The shedding of the uterine lining.
mentate To think.
MET Acronym for "metabolic equivalent of task," a measure of heat production by the body. This term is used with cardiac rehabilitation patients.
metabolic acidosis A condition in which the pH of body fluids is below 7.4 because of either an excessive production of carbonic acid through the oxidation of fats, or a loss of bicarbonate.
metabolic alkalosis A condition in which the pH of body fluids is above 7.4 because of either an excessive loss of acid, an above-normal intake or retention of base, or a low level of potassium in the blood.
metabolism The sum of the physical and chemical processes by which living tissue is formed and maintained and by which large molecules are disassembled to provide energy.
metastasis The movement of disease from one organ or body part to a distant location; for example, the migration of microorganisms and of malignant cells.
metrorrhagia Uterine bleeding occurring at irregular intervals and sometimes for prolonged periods.
microcytic Pertaining to a smaller-than-normal cell.
micron A unit of linear measure; equal to 0.001 mm.
micturition The voiding of urine.
milieu therapy Therapy in a structured environment of a hospital or group home setting to help patients participate as active members of the milieu community and practice social behaviors.

milliequivalent One-thousandth of a chemical equivalent, expressed as mEq; the concentration of electrolytes in a certain volume of solution is usually expressed as milliequivalents per liter (mEq/L).
mineralocorticoids A group of hormones elaborated by the adrenal cortex that have an effect on sodium, chloride, and potassium levels in extracellular fluid.
miotic A drug that constricts the pupil.
mitosis A type of cell division of somatic cells in which each daughter cell contains the same number of chromosomes as the parent cell. It is the process by which the body grows and by which somatic cells are replaced.
mittelschmerz A sharp pain in the right or left lower quadrant, sometimes felt at midcycle around the time of ovulation.
modulation The fourth of four phases associated with nociceptive pain wherein the brain sends signals back down the spinal cord by release of neurotransmitters.
monocytes Mononuclear phagocytic leukocytes.
monoparesis Weakness in one limb.
monoplegia Paralysis of one limb.
morphologic Related to the science of structures and forms without regard to function.
mucolytic Dissolving or destroying mucus.
mucorrhea The free discharge of mucus.
mucositis An inflammation of a mucous membrane.
multidrug-resistant organism (MDRO) A pathogen that has mutated due to inadequate dosages or delays in administration of antimicrobial medication and is now resistant to many medications.
multisystem organ dysfunction syndrome (MODS) A syndrome in which there is concurrent dysfunction of several organs.
muscle tone The readiness of a muscle to contract and relax normally.
mutation An unusual change in a gene occurring spontaneously or by induction. Mutation can occur in pathogenic organisms.
mycosis (mycoses) Any disease caused by a fungus.
mydriatic Dilating the pupil.
myocardial infarction (MI) Necrosis of the myocardium as a result of interruption of the blood supply to the area.
myocarditis An inflammation of the heart muscle.
myomectomy Surgical removal of a tumor from the uterine wall, accomplished by use of an endoscope.
myopia The error of refraction in which parallel light rays focus in front of the retina; nearsightedness.
myringotomy An incision into the eardrum.
myxedema A condition in the adult in which there are low thyroid levels.

N

nebulizer An atomizer; a device for delivering drugs or water to the respiratory tract by forcing air or oxygen through a solution.
necrosis The changes that occur as a result of death of cells; caused by enzymatic degradation.
necrotic Pertaining to death of a portion of tissue.
negative feedback In the endocrine system, if the hormonal need of a target tissue is being satisfied, production or secretion of the hormone will be inhibited.
negative symptoms One of the two divisions of signs and symptoms of schizophrenia; include apathy, social isolation, psychomotor retardation, and lack of motivation.
neologism(s) In psychiatry, a new word whose meaning may be known only to the person using it and may be related to his or her conflicts.
neoplasm A tumor; any new and abnormal growth.
nephron The structural and functional unit of the kidney, which consists of the renal corpuscle, the proximal convoluted tubule, limbs of the loop of Henle, the distal convoluted tubule, and the collecting tubule; thus each nephron is able to form urine independently.
nephrosclerosis Atherosclerotic disease of the small renal arteries related to hypertension and eventual destruction of renal cells.
nephrostomy Formation of an artificial fistula into the renal pelvis of the kidney.
nephrostomy tubes Tubes inserted to drain the renal pelvis.
networking Meeting people, exchanging phone numbers, expressing interest in other people and what they are doing, and establishing a business relationship that might be mutually beneficial.
neuroglycopenia A shortage of glucose in the brain.
neuron Any of the conducting cells of the nervous system; consists of a cell body containing the nucleus and cytoplasm and the axon and dendrites.
neuropathic pain Pain associated with a dysfunction of the nervous system; specifically, an abnormality in the processing of sensations.
neuropathy Any disease of the nerves.
neutropenia An abnormal decrease in the number of neutrophils in the blood.
neutrophilia An increase in the number of neutrophils in the blood.
neutrophils Granular leukocytes; also called *polymorphonuclear leukocytes.*
nociceptive pain Pain associated with pain stimuli from either somatic or visceral structures.
nocturia Excessive urination during the night.
nodules Small masses of tissue that can be detected by touch.
noncommunicable Cannot be carried from one person to another.
non–insulin-dependent diabetes mellitus Type 2 diabetes; a form of diabetes in which levels of endogenous insulin are adequate and control can be managed by diet and exercise and perhaps by an oral hypoglycemic agent.
nonjudgmental Avoiding judgment based on one's personal standards.
normal flora Flora most often found on or in body systems that have some form of contact with the outside environment. This flora prevents most harmful microorganisms from colonizing the body.
normo- A combining form indicating normal or usual.
North American Nursing Diagnosis Association International (NANDA-I) An organization that formulates and validates nursing diagnoses.
nosocomial Pertaining to or originating in a hospital.
nuchal rigidity Stiffness and pain in the neck from inflammation of the meninges.
nurse practice act A legal statute describing the parameters of nursing practice.
nursing The diagnosis and treatment of human responses to actual or potential health problems. *See also* Nursing process.
nursing care plans Written plans of care that serve to communicate to the nursing staff and others the specific nursing diagnoses and prescribed nursing orders for directing and evaluating the effectiveness of the care given.
nursing diagnosis A statement of a health problem or of a potential problem in the patient's health status that a nurse is licensed and competent to treat.
nursing interventions Acts by nurses that implement the nursing care plan.

nursing process A goal-directed series of activities whereby the practice of nursing accomplishes its goal of alleviating, minimizing, or preventing real or potential health problems.
nystagmus Involuntary, rapid rhythmic movement of the eyeball.

O

objective data Information obtained through the senses or measured by instruments.
objectives Well-defined steps toward the accomplishment of a goal; they should be realistic, be stated in measurable terms, and include the conditions under which they will be accomplished.
observation The act of watching carefully and attentively.
obsessive Having ideas, thoughts, or impulses that are persistent to an excessive degree.
obsessive-compulsive disorder A mental disorder characterized by recurrent or intrusive thoughts and rituals that can become overwhelming to the point of interfering with normal life.
obturator A device that is placed into a large-bore cannula during insertion to prevent potential blockage by tissues.
occult Obscure; concealed; hidden.
occult blood Hidden blood.
oculogyric crisis A side effect of antipyschotic medication characterized by uncontrolled rolling back of the eyes.
olfaction The act of smelling.
oligomenorrhea Decreased menstruation. Usually refers to menstrual periods that occur at an interval of 45 days or longer.
oliguria A diminished amount of urine formation.
oncogene A gene in a virus that has the ability to induce a cell to become malignant.
oncology The study of tumors.
onychomycosis A fungal infection of the fingernail or toenail.
oophoritis An inflammation of an ovary; ovaritis.
open access plan An insurance plan in which the patient can see any health care provider.
ophthalmologist A physician who specializes in treating eye disorders.
ophthalmoscope An instrument for examining the eye. The direct ophthalmoscope is used to inspect the back portion of the interior of the eyeball; the indirect ophthalmoscope permits stereoscopic inspection of the interior of the eye.
opportunistic infections (OIs) Infections that develop in an individual with a depressed immune system from organisms commonly found in the environment that are usually harmless.
opportunistic pathogen A fungus or bacterium, usually harmless, that causes infection in a person with a depressed immune system.
optic chiasm The part of the hypothalamus formed by the decussation, or crossing, of the fibers of the optic nerve from the medial half of each retina.
optician A specialist in the making of optical apparatus (e.g., eyeglasses).
optometrist A professional person trained to examine the eyes and prescribe eyeglasses to correct irregularities of vision.
orchiectomy The excision of one or both testes.
orchitis An inflammation of the testes.
orthopedic Referring to the correction of deformities of the musculoskeletal system.
orthopnea The ability to breathe easily only in the upright position.
orthopneic position Sitting up in bed with two or three pillows behind the back.
orthostatic hypotension A fall in blood pressure that occurs when standing up from a sitting or lying position or when standing in a fixed position; it is characterized by dizziness, syncope, and blurred vision.
oscilloscope An instrument that makes visible on a screen the nature of an electrical current.
osmolality The osmotic pressure of a solution, expressed in osmols or milliosmoles (mOsm) per kilogram of water.
osmosis The passage of solvent from a solution of lesser concentration to one of greater concentration through a selectively permeable membrane.
osmotic pressure Pressure that develops when two solutions of different concentrations are separated by a semipermeable membrane.
ossification Formation of or conversion into bone or a bony substance.
osteoporosis A porous condition of bone due to demineralization associated with aging.
otalgia Pain in the ear.
OTC Over the counter; available without a prescription.
otitis media An inflammation of the middle ear.
otorrhea An inflammation of the ear with purulent discharge.
otoscope An instrument for examining the ear canal and eardrum.
outcome The result of an action.
ovulation The periodic ripening and rupture of the mature graafian follicle and the discharge of the ovum from the cortex of the ovary.
oxidation The process by which a substance combines with oxygen.

P

pacemaker A mechanical device that provides electrical stimulation when an anatomic pacemaker fails; a cardiac pacemaker provides electrical stimulation when there is heart block.
pain A feeling of distress or suffering caused by stimulation of specialized nerve cells; considered to occur whenever a person says it is present.
pain threshold The point at which pain is perceived.
pain tolerance The length of time or intensity at which a person will endure pain before outwardly responding to it.
palliative Designed to relieve symptoms when a disease cannot be cured.
palliative care Comfort care.
palliative surgery Surgery performed to make a patient more comfortable.
palmar erythema A persistent redness of the palms, which may be seen in liver disease.
palpation A physical examination technique in which the texture, size, consistency, and location of body parts are felt with the hands.
palpitation A rapid, violent, or throbbing pulsation, as an abnormally rapid throbbing or fluttering of the heart.
pancreatitis An inflamed condition of the pancreas.
panhysterectomy The surgical removal of the entire uterus.
papule A small, round, solid, elevated lesion of the skin.
paracentesis The surgical puncture of a cavity to aspirate fluid.
paradoxical respirations Respirations in which, on inhalation, the traumatized portion of the chest wall moves inward rather than outward.
paralytic ileus The absence of peristalsis; paralysis of the intestines.
paranoia A mental disorder in which a person exhibits delusions of persecution or of grandeur or a combination of both.

paraplegia Paralysis of the lower extremities.
parathormone A hormone produced and secreted by the parathyroid gland.
parenteral Administered by a route other than the digestive tract.
paresthesia A feeling of tingling or numbness.
passive immunity Immunity acquired by transfer of antibody or lymphocytes from an immune donor.
patent Wide open.
pathogen A microorganism or substance capable of producing a disease.
pathologic Caused by a disease.
patient advocate A person who will advocate on the patient's behalf with the hospital, insurance company, or health care personnel.
PCA Patient-controlled analgesia.
pediculosis An infestation with lice.
pelvic inflammatory disease Any inflammation in the pelvis that occurs outside the uterus, uterine tubes, and ovaries.
peptic ulcer The loss of tissue lining the esophagus, stomach, or duodenum.
perception The recognition and interpretation of sensory stimuli that serve as a basis for comprehending, learning, and knowing or for motivating a particular action or reaction. Also, the third of four phases associated with nociceptive pain, during which impulses reach the brain and pain is recognized.
percussion The physical examination technique of tapping the body surface with the fingertips or fist to evaluate the size, borders, and consistency of some of the internal organs or to detect the presence of fluid in a body cavity.
percutaneous Through the skin.
perforation A hole or break in the retaining walls or membranes of an organ, as in perforated ulcer and perforated eardrum.
perfusion Supplying tissues and organs with nutrients and oxygen by blood flow through the arteries.
pericardial effusion A collection of serous or purulent exudate in the pericardial cavity.
pericardiocentesis The surgical puncture of the pericardial cavity for aspiration of fluid.
pericardiotomy The surgical incision of the pericardium.
pericarditis An inflammation of the sac that encloses the heart and the roots of the great vessels.
periodontal Located around a tooth.
perioperative Pertaining to the period extending from the time of hospitalization for surgery to the time of discharge.
periorbital Surrounding the socket of the eye.
periostomal Pertaining to the area around a stoma.
peripheral Pertaining to the area outside the central region or structure.
peristalsis Involuntary wavelike contraction of organs with both longitudinal and circular muscle fibers that passes along the organ and propels its contents, as in peristalsis of the digestive tract.
peritonitis An inflammation of the serous sac that lines the abdominal cavity and encloses the abdominal organs.
permeable Permitting passage of a substance.
personality disorder A mental disorder characterized by inflexible and maladaptive responses to life events, serious difficulty in personal and work relationships, a tendency to evoke interpersonal conflict, and a tendency to evoke a negative empathic response from others.
personal protective equipment (PPE) Equipment that forms some type of barrier to protect a person from exposure to blood-borne pathogens, body fluids, or other potentially infectious materials. Examples are gloves, covering gowns, and face masks.
pessary A hard rubber ring inserted in the vagina to help keep the abdominal organs in place.
petechiae Very small, nonraised, round, purplish spots, caused by intradermal or submucosal bleeding, that later turn blue or yellow.
pH The concentration of hydrogen (H) in a solution; the higher the concentration of hydrogen ions, the lower the pH of the solution.
phacoemulsification A technique of cataract extraction in which high-frequency vibrations are used to fragment the lens.
phagocytosis The engulfing of microorganisms and other foreign matter by phagocytes.
phantom pain A sensation of discomfort occurring where an extremity has been amputated.
pharyngitis An inflammation or infection of the pharynx that usually produces a sore throat.
phenylketonuria A genetic disorder in which there is a defect in the metabolism of phenylalanine resulting in the presence of this amino acid in the urine.
phlebitis An inflammation of a vein.
phlebotomy The surgical opening of a vein to draw blood, often done with a needle.
phobic disorder Excessive fear of a situation or object.
photocoagulation The alteration of proteins in tissue by the use of light energy in the form of ordinary light rays or a laser beam.
photodynamic therapy A type of chemotherapy in which the action of the drug is enhanced by exposure to light.
photophobia Difficulty tolerating light.
pilonidal Pertaining to, characterized by, or having a tuft of hairs.
pilonidal sinus A lesion located at the cleft of the buttocks in the sacrococcygeal region; also called *pilonidal cyst.*
placebo(s) A supposedly inactive substance or procedure that can have either positive or negative effects on the relief of symptoms and that is usually given under the guise of effective treatment or in clinical trials of new drugs.
planning A phase of the nursing process in which a plan is developed with the patient, family, or significant other to provide a blueprint for nursing intervention to achieve specified goals. *See also* Nursing care plans.
plaque A patch or flat area.
plasma The liquid portion of blood in which formed elements are suspended; it contains plasma proteins, inorganic salts, nutrients, gases, wastes from the cells, and various hormones and enzymes.
plasma cell A spherical or ellipsoidal cell involved in the synthesis, storage, and release of antibody.
plasmapheresis The separation of the cells and components of the blood.
platelets The smallest formed elements in the blood; important in coagulation and blood clotting.
plethora A general term denoting a red, florid complexion or an excess of blood.
pleurisy An inflammation of the pleura.
Pneumocystis jiroveci An opportunistic pathogen producing infection of the lung associated with acquired immunodeficiency syndrome (AIDS); formerly *Pneumocystis carinii.*
pneumonectomy The excision of lung tissue, especially of an entire lung.
pneumonia An inflammation of the lungs with consolidation.
pneumothorax The accumulation of air or gas in the pleural cavity, resulting in collapse of the lung on the affected side.

point-of-service (POS) option An option offered by some managed care plans in which a member pays an extra fee to see a desired physician outside of the care plan.
polyarteritis Multiple sites of inflammatory and destructive lesions in the arterial system.
polycystic ovarian syndrome An endocrine disturbance characterized by anovulation, amenorrhea, hirsutism, and infertility.
polycythemia An elevation in the total number of blood cells.
polydipsia Excessive thirst that results in drinking large quantities of water.
polymorphonuclear leukocytes The fully developed cells of the granulocyte series, especially neutrophils the nuclei of which contain three or more lobes.
polyphagia Increased hunger.
polyuria The production of an excessive amount of urine.
positive symptoms One of the two divisions of signs and symptoms seen with schizophrenia; includes hallucinations, delusions, and disordered thinking.
postictal state The condition of a person right after a seizure.
post-traumatic stress disorder A mental disorder characterized by recurrent symptoms of anxiety that some individuals may experience after encountering an extreme, life-threatening event. Nightmares or flashbacks may be part of the symptoms.
PPO *See* Preferred provider organization.
precancerous Term used to refer to a growth that is not yet, but probably will become, cancerous.
precipitate A deposit separated from a suspension or solution by precipitation; the reaction of a reagent that causes the deposit to fall to the bottom or float near the top.
preferred provider organization (PPO) An organization of physicians, hospitals, and pharmacists whose members discount their services to subscriber patients.
premenstrual syndrome A group of symptoms experienced by some women for several days before the onset of the menstrual period.
prepuce The foreskin or fold of skin over the glans penis in the male.
presbycusis Impairment of hearing in old age.
presbyopia Farsightedness that occurs normally with aging.
pressor A substance that causes a rise in blood pressure. Norepinephrine is an example of a "pressor" hormone. Norepinephrine maintains blood pressure.
pressure ulcer A sore caused by pressure from a splint or other appliance or from the body itself when it has remained immobile in bed for extended periods.
preventive Hindering the occurrence of something, especially disease.
priapism A prolonged penile erection resulting in a large, hard, and painful penis unrelated to sexual desire or activity.
primary union The joining of two edges of a wound that are close together, resulting in a thin scar after healing; also called *healing by first intention.*
priority Preference established on the basis of emergency or need.
priority setting Setting the sequence of actions according to importance or priority.
problem-oriented medical record (POMR) A system of documentation in which the information is arranged according to specific problems presented by the patient at the time of seeking health care. The four components are database, problem list, initial plan, and follow-up. *See also* Progress notes.
process A series of actions that move from one point to another on the way to completing a goal.
prodromal stage The early or very beginning stage of an illness.
prodrome An early sign of a developing condition or disease.
prognosis The predicted outcome of the course of a disease.
progress notes Entries in the medical record describing what has been done in the care of the patient and his or her response to the intervention.
prolapse The falling down or displacement of a part or all of an organ, as in prolapse of a stoma and prolapse of the uterus.
promoter(s) A type of epigenetic carcinogen that promotes neoplastic growth only after initiation by another substance; a cocarcinogen.
prophylactic Something done or used to prevent infection or disease.
prospective payment system A payment system for reimbursing hospitals for inpatient health care services in which a predetermined rate is set for treatment of specific illnesses.
prostaglandins A group of naturally occurring fatty acids that stimulate contraction of the uterine and other smooth-muscle tissue.
prostate-specific antigen (PSA) A protein produced by the prostate that is present in elevated levels in patients with cancer or other diseases of the prostate.
prosthesis An artificial substitute for a missing part, such as an eye, limb, or tooth, used for functional or cosmetic reasons, or both.
protease inhibitor A drug that works at the last stage of viral reproduction.
protective isolation Special precautionary procedures to minimize exposure to infectious agents in a patient who has an immune deficiency or who is otherwise susceptible to infection.
proteinuria An excess of serum proteins in the urine.
protocol The plan for a course of medical treatment.
Protozoa A phylum comprising the unicellular organisms; most are free-living, but some lead commensalistic, mutualistic, or parasitic existences.
provider Someone or an agency that provides health care services.
proximal Closest to a point of reference.
pruritus Itching.
pseudocyst An abnormal or dilated cavity resembling a true cyst but not lined with epithelium. Also called *adventitious cyst* or *false cyst.*
psychoactive substances Mind-altering agents capable of changing or altering a person's mood, behavior, cognition, arousal level, level of consciousness, and perceptions.
psychomotor retardation A slowing of speech, movement, and thought process often seen in the depressed patient.
psychotic features Hallucinations, delusions, and grossly disorganized behavior.
ptomaines Toxic substances produced by the action of putrefactive bacteria on proteins and amino acids.
ptosis The dropping of an organ below its usual position, for example, lowering of the eyelid so that it partially or completely covers the cornea.
pulmonary edema A diffuse accumulation of fluid in the tissues and air spaces of the lung.
pulmonary embolus A mass of clotted blood or other formed element in the lung.
pulse deficit The difference between the radial and apical pulse rates.

pulsus paradoxus A drop in systolic blood pressure of greater than 10 mm Hg on inspiration.
purpura Purplish areas caused by bleeding into the skin or mucous membranes.
purulence The condition of producing or discharging pus.
purulent Full of pus.
pus A liquid product of inflammation composed of albuminous substances, a thin fluid, and leukocytes; generally yellow.
pustule A small, round, pus-filled lesion of the skin.
pyelogram A radiograph of the kidney and ureters after injection of a contrast medium that may be administered intravenously (IV pyelogram) or by way of the ureters (retrograde pyelogram).
pyelonephritis An inflammation of the kidney and renal pelvis.
pyrogen Any agent that causes fever.
pyuria Pus in the urine.

Q

quadriplegia Paralysis of all four extremities.
quadriplegic A person with paralysis of all four limbs.

R

rad Radiation absorbed dose; the unit used for measuring doses of radiation.
radiation therapy The use of radiant energy from radioactive materials or high-voltage x-rays to treat disease.
radioimmunoassay A laboratory method for measuring minute quantities of specific antibodies or any antigen, such as a hormone or drug, against which antibodies have been produced.
radionuclide A radioactive substance given to the patient prior to radiography or scanning.
radiopaque Not penetrable by x-ray; appears white on radiograph.
rales Abnormal respiratory sounds heard on auscultation with a stethoscope indicating some pathologic condition.
range of motion The extent, measured in degrees of a circle, through which a joint can be extended and flexed.
rationalization A defense mechanism in which a patient finds logical reasons (justification) for his or her behavior while ignoring the real reasons.
realistic Attainable, based on the patient's condition and desire.
rectocele A protrusion of the rectum and posterior vaginal wall into the vagina.
recurrent Returning at intervals.
referred pain Pain felt in a part away from its point of origin.
reflex (reflexes) The sum of any particular autonomic (automatic) response mediated by the nervous system and not requiring conscious movement.
refraction The determination of refractive errors (inability to focus light rays on the retina) and their correction with eyeglasses.
regeneration The natural renewal of a structure.
regimen A prescribed scheme of diet, exercise, or activity to achieve certain ends.
rehabilitation The processes of treatment and education that help the disabled individual attain maximum function, a sense of well-being, and a personally satisfying level of independence.
remittent Having alternating periods of abating and returning, such as a fever that comes and goes.
replicate To duplicate, reproduce, or copy.
replication The process of duplicating or reproducing.
reservoir A passive host or carrier that harbors pathogenic organisms without harm to itself and is a source from which others can be infected.
residual urine Urine that remains in the bladder immediately after urination.
resorption Taking in or absorbing again.
respiration The taking in of oxygen, its utilization in the tissues, and the giving off of carbon dioxide.
respiratory acidosis A condition in which the pH of body fluids is below 7.4 because of failure of the lungs to remove sufficient amounts of carbon dioxide.
respiratory alkalosis A condition in which the pH of body fluids is above 7.4 because of excessive removal of carbon dioxide by the lungs, as in hyperventilation.
resuscitation Revival after apparent death.
reticuloendothelial system A network of cells and tissues found throughout the body, especially in the blood, connective tissue, spleen, liver, lungs, bone marrow, and lymph vessels; these cells play a role in blood cell formation and destruction and in inflammation and immunity.
retinopathy A pathologic condition of the retina associated with diabetes mellitus.
retrograde Moving backward; degenerating from a better to a worse state.
retrospective Dealing with the past.
retrospective payment system Medicare payment based on actual costs submitted to government. Used prior to 1983.
retrovirus A type of virus that contains RNA.
reverse transcriptase An enzyme that is present in retroviruses.
rhinitis An inflammation of the mucous membrane of the nose.
rhinoplasty A plastic surgical operation on the nose, either reconstructive, restorative, or cosmetic.
rhonchi Coarse rattling sounds in the bronchial tubes caused by a partial obstruction.
Rickettsia A genus of small, rod-shaped to round microorganisms found in tissue cells of lice, fleas, ticks, and mites and transmitted to humans by their bites.
rigor mortis The stiffness that occurs in dead bodies.
robotics The science of designing mechanical, computerized instruments for procedures.
Roux-en-Y Any Y-shaped anastomosis in which the small intestine is included.
rubor A dusky-red color seen in patients with arterial insufficiency.
rugae Ridges or folds on a mucous membrane.

S

safer sex Any sexual practice that is performed with the use of a barrier to prevent the exchange of body fluids.
salpingitis An inflammation of a uterine tube.
sarcoidosis A chronic, progressive, systemic granulomatous reticulosis of unknown etiology, involving almost any organ or tissue.
sarcoma A tumor, often highly malignant, composed of cells derived from connective tissue.
scabies An infestation with the mange mite.
scaling The shedding of small, thin, dry layers of skin.
scarring The replacement of damaged tissue with fibrous tissue.
schizophrenia A mental illness that causes unusual, bizarre behavior (hallucinations and delusions).
scleropathy The injection of a solution that causes the vessel to dry up and disintegrate.
scoliosis Lateral curvature of the spine.
scotoma An area of lost vision in the visual field.
sebaceous Containing or pertaining to sebum, an oily, fatty matter secreted by the sebaceous glands.

secondary union The healing of a wound in which the edges are far apart and cannot be brought together; the wound fills with granulation tissue and heals from the edges inward.
sedative(s) An agent that calms nervousness, irritability, and excitement.
seizure(s) An attack of uncontrollable muscular contractions; a convulsion.
self-care The process whereby one initiates and carries out certain health practices to maintain life, health, and personal well-being.
semen A thick, opalescent, viscid secretion discharged from the urethra of the male at the climax of sexual excitement (orgasm).
seminal Concerning the semen or seed.
senile lentigines Areas where melanocytes increase in production, producing brown age spots.
senile purpura Dark purplish red ecchymoses occurring on the forearms and backs of the hands in the elderly.
sensitivity reaction An exaggerated response to agents perceived by the body as foreign.
sensorineural hearing loss Impaired perception of sound caused by a dysfunction in the inner ear or the eighth cranial nerve.
sensory loss Impairment of acuity of sight, hearing, taste, touch, and smell.
sentinel infections Infections that may indicate an underlying immunosuppression.
sentinel node biopsy A biopsy of lymph nodes that receive drainage from the anatomic area of a breast cancer to determine spread of the disease.
sepsis Infection, contamination (refers to infection in the blood).
septicemia Invasion of the bloodstream by infective microorganisms.
sequela An abnormal condition that follows and is the result of a disease.
seroconversion The point at which antibodies to specific antigens are detectable in the blood.
seroma A collection of serum forming a tumor-like mass.
serosanguineous Containing both serum and blood.
serum (sera) The clear, liquid portion of blood that does not contain fibrinogen or blood cells. Immune serum is blood serum from the bodies of people or animals that have produced antibody; inoculation with such serum produces passive immunity.
serum sickness A hypersensitivity reaction to a foreign serum or other antigen.
sexually transmitted infection An infection that is transmitted by sexual intercourse.
shedding Losing or casting off by a natural process.
Sheehan syndrome A rare but serious postpartum complication that involves infarction of the pituitary gland secondary to postpartum hemorrhage.
shock Acute peripheral circulatory failure due to derangement of circulatory control or loss of circulating fluid.
shunting Physiologically bypassing, as when blood flows past the alveoli but the membrane is thickened and gases cannot cross into or out of the blood.
sickle cell disease All those genetic disorders in which sickle hemoglobin is found in the red cells.
slit lamp An instrument for examining the surface of the eye through a biomicroscopic lens.
smear A specimen for microscopic and cytologic study; the material is spread thinly and evenly across a slide with a swab or loop.
SOAP Acronym for *S*ubjective and *O*bjective data, *A*ssessment, and *P*lanning.
solute The substance that is dissolved in a solution.
Somogyi effect A rebound phenomenon due to overtreatment with insulin.
source-oriented record keeping A system of documentation in which information is arranged according to the person, department, or other source of information.
specific gravity The weight of a substance compared with the weight of an equal amount of another substance taken as a standard; for liquids, the standard usually is water (specific gravity of 1).
spermatozoa The mature male sex or germ cells formed within the seminiferous tubules of the testes.
spider angioma A form of telangiectasis with a central elevated red dot the size of a pinhead from which small blood vessels radiate; often occurs with liver disease.
spirochete Any organism that is a member of the order Spirochaetales.
spirometer An instrument for measuring air taken into and expelled from the lungs.
splenomegaly Enlargement of the spleen.
splitting A personality trait that involves initial idealization of a caregiver or friend, followed by a devaluing of that same person.
spores Reproductive cells, usually unicellular, produced by plants and some protozoa.
sprain The wrenching or twisting of a joint with partial or complete tearing of the ligaments.
sputum A substance expelled by coughing or clearing the throat.
Standard Precautions Precautions designed to prevent the transmission of microorganisms from one patient to another as well as to protect the health care worker from unnecessary exposure to infection.
stapedectomy The surgical removal of the stirrup of the middle ear and its replacement with a prosthetic device.
stasis Standing still; stagnation; usually refers to fluid.
status epilepticus A grave condition in which there is a rapid, unrelenting series of convulsive seizures without intervening periods of consciousness and with absence of respiration. Irreversible brain damage may occur if seizures are not controlled.
STD Sexually transmitted disease.
stem cells Generalized mother cells the descendants of which specialize, often in different functions; an example is an undifferentiated mesenchymal cell that is the progenitor of the blood and fixed-tissue cells of the bone marrow.
stenosis The narrowing or contraction of a passageway or opening.
stent A tubular device to give support to the interior of a vessel or tube, preventing its collapse.
stereotaxis A method of precisely locating areas in the brain.
stereotype(s) A simplification used to describe all members of a specific group without exception.
sterilization, microbe The process of rendering an article free of microorganisms and their pathogenic products.
Steri-Strips Small, reinforced, adhesive strips placed over a healing incision to hold it together after sutures are removed.
stoma(s) A mouth-like opening, especially one that is created surgically for the elimination of urine or fecal material.
stomatitis A generalized inflammation of the oral mucosa.
strabismus A deviation of the eye that cannot be controlled voluntarily.
strain The pulling or tearing of either muscle or tendon, or both.
stress incontinence The loss of urine during a sneeze of cough.

stridor A harsh, high-pitched respiratory sound such as the inspiratory sound often heard in acute laryngeal obstruction.

stromal cells Connective tissue cells of the supporting tissue or matrix of an organ.

stye An infected swelling near the margin of the eyelid.

subcutaneous Beneath or to be introduced beneath the skin.

subcutaneous emphysema Interstial emphysema characterized by the presence of air in the subcutaneous tissue, usually caused by intrathoracic injury.

subdural hematoma The accumulation of blood in the subdural space.

subjective data Data that the patient provides about a symptom that cannot be seen, felt, or heard by an examiner; pain is an example.

subluxation A partial or incomplete dislocation of a bone from its place in a joint.

substance use disorder A problem with alcoholism or drug abuse.

subsystem A system within a larger system.

"sucking" chest wound A wound in which the pleural cavity has been penetrated, allowing air and gas to enter the cavity and produce pneumothorax.

suicidal gestures Things done or said that indicate a patient is contemplating committing suicide.

sundowning The phenomenon of becoming confused and disoriented at night, although oriented during the day.

suppression Inhibition, such as interfering with immune response.

suprasystem A highly complex system.

susceptible Being predisposed or sensitive to the effects of an infectious disease, allergen, or other pathogenic agent; lacking immunity or resistance.

sympathectomy A surgical excision or interruption in some portion of the sympathetic nerve pathways.

syncope Fainting.

syndrome A combination of signs and symptoms associated with a pathologic process or disease.

synovial fluid The transparent viscid fluid found in joint cavities, bursae, and tendon sheaths.

synthesis The process or processes involved in the formation of a complex substance from simpler elements or compounds; opposite of decomposition.

synthesize To put together (data) into a logical whole.

system An organized whole composed of interacting parts.

systemic inflammatory response syndrome (SIRS) A condition in which the body's inflammatory response feedback mechanism fails, causing signs and symptoms (tachycardia, tachypnea, hypotension, oliguria, and fever) without a documented source of infection.

systole The phase of the cardiac cycle in which the ventricles contract and force blood into the aorta and pulmonary arteries; the systolic pressure is recorded as the top number in a blood pressure reading.

systolic blood pressure Arterial pressure during systole.

T

tachycardia An abnormally rapid heart rate, usually over 100 beats per minute.

tachypnea Abnormal rapidity of respiration.

tamponade The stoppage of blood flow to an organ or part of the body by pressure.

tardive dyskinesia A common extrapyramidal side effect seen with antipsychotics. Patients can exhibit lip-smacking, tongue protrusion, blinking, sucking, chewing, and lateral jaw movements.

target cells/tissues Cells and tissues that are affected by a specific hormone.

TENS *T*ranscutaneous *e*lectrical *n*erve *s*timulation.

tertiary Third in order or stage.

testis The male gonad. One of two reproductive glands located in the scrotum that produce the male reproductive cells and the male hormone, testosterone.

tetany The continuous tonic spasm of a muscle; associated with calcium deficit, vitamin D deficiency, and alkalosis.

tetraplegia Another term for quadraplegia (paralysis of all four extremities).

thalamus Either of two large structures composed of gray matter and situated at the base of the cerebrum that act as a relay station for impulses traveling from the spinal cord and brainstem to the cerebral cortex.

thanatologist One who studies death.

thanatology The medicolegal study of the dying process and death.

theory (theories) A belief, policy, or principle proposed or followed as the basis of action.

therapeutic Having medicinal or healing properties.

thermal Pertaining to heat.

thoracentesis The surgical puncture and drainage of the thoracic cavity.

thoracotomy The surgical incision of the wall of the chest.

thought disorder A mental disorder characterized by disorganized thought, behavior, and hallucinations. Mood and interpersonal relationships are altered.

thrombectomy The excision of a clot.

thrombocytopenia A decreased number of platelets.

thrombocytopenic purpura A bleeding disorder characterized by a marked decrease in the number of platelets, resulting in multiple bruises, petechiae, and hemorrhage into the tissues.

thrombolytic Dissolving or splitting up a thrombus.

thrombophlebitis An inflammation of a vein related to formation of a blood clot within the vessel.

thrombosis The formation, development, or presence of a blood clot within a blood vessel.

thrombus A blood clot that obstructs a blood vessel or a cavity of the heart.

thymus An endocrine gland that lies in the upper chest beneath the sternum and that, during fetal life, sensitizes certain stem cells that eventually become T lymphocytes.

thyrocalcitonin A hormone secreted by the thyroid gland.

thyroid crisis A sudden increase in the output of thyroxine and resultant extreme elevation of all body processes.

thyroid panel A group of tests performed to evaluate thyroid function.

thyroid storm *See* Thyroid crisis.

thyrotoxicosis A toxic condition due to hyperactivity of the thyroid gland.

thyroxine (T_4) A hormone secreted by the thyroid gland.

time-referenced Measured by an educated guess as to how long it will take to attain the outcome.

tinea Ringworm; a name applied to many different kinds of fungal infections of the skin. The specific type usually is designated by a modifying term (e.g., tinea capitis, or ringworm of the scalp).

tinea pedis A fungal infection of the foot; also called *athlete's foot.*

tinnitus A ringing, buzzing, or other continuous noise in the ear.

T lymphocytes Those white cells destined to provide cellular immunity that have passed through the thymus and migrated to the lymph nodes.

tolerance Increased resistance to a drug or substance that occurs when there is a need for increased amounts of substances to achieve the desired effect. Term used with substance use disorder.

tonic A state of rigid contraction of the muscles.
tonometer An instrument for measuring tension or pressure, especially intraocular pressure.
tophus (tophi) A deposit of sodium biurate in tissues near a joint, in the ear, or in bone, as occurs in gout.
topical Pertaining to the surface of a part of the body, as in topical medications applied to an area of the skin.
torsion The act of twisting or condition of being twisted.
total parenteral nutrition Intravenous feeding to provide all nutritional needs over time.
tourniquet A device for compressing an artery or vein; its use as an emergency measure to relieve hemorrhage is generally recommended only if the victim's life is threatened and other measures fail to stop massive blood loss.
toxin A poisonous substance.
tracheostomy A surgical incision into the trachea to insert a tube through which the patient can breathe.
traction The exertion of a pulling force, as that applied to a fractured bone or dislocated joint, to maintain proper positioning.
tranquilizers A group of agents that provide calm and relief from anxiety.
transcellular Between cells, but within an epithelial membrane.
transcellular fluid Secretions and excretions that move through cell membranes and eventually leave the body.
transduction The first of four phases associated with nociceptive pain. Tissue damage stimulates the nociceptors and initiates pain sensation.
transfer factor A factor occurring in sensitized lymphocytes that recruits additional lymphocytes and transfers to them the ability to confer cell-mediated immunity.
transformation A change to another form.
transfusion The administration of whole blood or blood components directly into the bloodstream.
transmission The second of four phases associated with nociceptive pain. Involves movement of sensation to the spinal cord.
triage The classification of casualties in an emergency room or location of a disaster by the gravity of the injury, urgency of treatment, and place for treatment.
triiodothyronine (T_3) A hormone secreted by the thyroid gland.
tuberculin test An evaluation of sensitivity to the tubercle bacillus; the most common method is intradermal injection of a purified protein derivative of tuberculin (the Mantoux test); a positive reaction indicates the need for further diagnostic procedures.
tuberculosis Any of the infectious diseases caused by species of *Mycobacterium* and characterized by the formation of tubercles and caseous necrosis in the tissues.
tumor marker A blood test to detect biochemical substances synthesized and released into the bloodstream by tumor cells; used mainly to confirm a diagnosis of cancer or response to cancer therapy.
tumor-node-metastasis (TNM) staging system A system for classifying cancers according to the extent to which the malignancy has spread.
turgor The normal tension of a cell; swelling, distention.
tympanoplasty An operative procedure on the eardrum or ossicles of the middle ear to restore or improve hearing in patients with a conductive hearing loss.

U

ultrasonography An imaging technique in which deep anatomic structures are recorded by depicting the echoes of ultrasonic waves that have been directed into the tissues; the echoes (reflections) returning from the structures are converted into electrical impulses that are displayed on a screen, thus presenting a "picture" of the tissues being examined.
unlicensed assistive personnel (UAP) Nursing assistants, technicians, unit secretaries, and aides who do not hold a professional license to perform some aspects of health care delivery and are hired to perform specific repetitive tasks.
urea nitrogen A major protein metabolite that is not recycled by the body but is excreted in the urine; blood urea nitrogen levels indicate the ability of the kidney to filtrate and excrete waste products.
uremia Retention in the blood of urea, creatinine, and other nitrogenous wastes normally eliminated in the urine; more correctly called *azotemia.*
ureterostomy (ureterostomies) Surgical creation of a stoma to divert urine to the outside.
urinalysis Analysis of a sample of urine, most often done to detect protein, glucose, acetone, blood, pus, and casts.
uroflowmetry Pressure flow studies of the bladder.
urticaria Hives.

V

vaccination The injection of a vaccine into the body to produce immunity to a specific disease.
vaccines Suspensions of attenuated or killed microorganisms administered by injection to provide active immunity to infectious disease.
vagotomy The interruption of impulses carried by the vagus nerve or nerves; may be done to reduce the production of gastric secretions and to inhibit gastric motility, as part of the treatment for peptic ulcer.
Valsalva maneuver An increase of thoracic pressure by forcible exhalation against the closed glottis, as in straining at stool.
value A personal belief about the worth of something that is cherished or held dear.
valvuloplasty A procedure in which a balloon catheter is threaded via the circulatory system through the heart and into the valve. The balloon is inflated to break open a stenosed valve.
varices Twisted and swollen veins.
varicose veins Enlarged and tortuous veins in which the distorted shape is the result of accumulations of pooled blood.
vascular dementia A broad term used to describe any type of dementia caused by vessel disease.
vascular disorders An abnormal functioning of blood vessels, either arterial or venous. Peripheral arterial disorders are most commonly caused by atherosclerosis. Peripheral venous problems are caused by defective valvular function.
vasectomy Excision of the vas (ductus) deferens, or a portion of it; bilateral vasectomy results in sterility.
vasoactive Tending to cause vasodilation or vasoconstriction.
vector(s) A carrier, usually one that transmits disease.
venereal Pertaining to or resulting from intercourse.
ventilation The movement of air from the external environment to the gas exchange units of the lung.
vertigo A sensation of movement of one's self or of one's surroundings.
vesicant Blistering; causing or forming blisters.
vesicle A small sac containing a serous liquid; a small blister.
vesicostomy The formation of an opening into the urinary bladder.
viable Capable of living.
virulence The degree of ability of an organism to cause disease.

viscera The internal organs contained within a cavity.
viscous Sticky, gummy, gelatinous; thicker than usual.
vitrectomy The removal of the contents of the vitreous chamber, and replacing them with a sterile physiologic saline solution.
volvulus A twisting of the bowel upon itself, causing obstruction.
vulvectomy The excision of the vulva.

W

wart An epidermal growth of viral origin.
Wernicke's encephalopathy Damage to brain cells caused by chronic alcohol abuse.
wheal A localized area of edema on the body surface.
wheeze A form of rhonchus characterized by a high-pitched or low-pitched musical quality caused by airflow through a narrowed airway.
withdrawal Symptoms that are the opposite of the symptoms caused by the ingestion of chemicals or drugs.
word salad A meaningless mixture of words and phrases characteristic of advanced schizophrenia.

X

xanthelasma A planar xanthoma involving the eyelid(s).
xanthoma A lipid deposit in the skin.
xenograft A surgical graft of tissue from an individual of one species to an individual of a different species.
xerostomia The lack of saliva; dry mouth.

Y

yeast A term for fungi that reproduce by budding.

Z

zygomatic Pertaining to the zygomatic bone.

Index

Page numbers followed by a *b* indicate boxes, *f*, figures; *t*, tables.

J

K

L

S

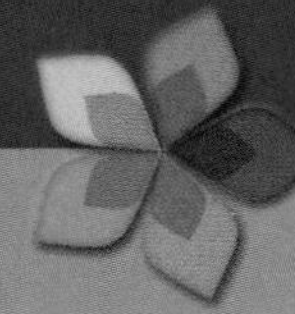

Answers to NCLEX-PN® Exam Style Review Questions

Chapter 1
1. **1**
2. **4**
3. **4**
4. **1**
5. **1**
6. **3**
7. **3**
8. **2**
9. **1, 2,** and **5**
10. **2, 3,** and **5**

Chapter 2
1. **2, 3, 4,** and **5**
2. **3**
3. **2**
4. **3**
5. **2**
6. **1, 2, 4,** and **5**
7. **4**
8. **1, 3, 4,** and **5**
9. **2**
10. **3**

Chapter 3
1. **2**
2. **2**
3. **1**
4. **2**
5. **1, 2,** and **5**
6. **1**
7. **3**
8. **1**
9. **1**
10. **2**

Chapter 4
1. **4**
2. **1** and **5**
3. **2**
4. **2**
5. **1**
6. **3**
7. **2**
8. **1**
9. **1** and **3**
10. **3**

Chapter 5
1. **4**
2. **3**
3. **2**
4. **2**
5. **3**
6. **2**
7. **1**
8. **2**
9. **1, 2,** and **3**
10. **2**

Chapter 6
1. **1**
2. **2**
3. **4**
4. **2, 3,** and **4**
5. **1**
6. **2**
7. **2**
8. **4**
9. **2**
10. **3**

Chapter 7
1. **1**
2. **1, 2, 3,** and **4**
3. **2**
4. **1**
5. **1**
6. **2**
7. **1, 3,** and **4**
8. **1**
9. **2**
10. **1**

Chapter 8
1. **3**
2. **1**
3. **4**
4. **2**
5. **1, 3,** and **4**
6. **3**
7. **3**
8. **1**
9. **1** and **5**
10. **3**

Chapter 9
1. **2**
2. **3**
3. **1, 3,** and **5**
4. **3**
5. **2**
6. **3**
7. **1**
8. **2, 3, 4,** and **5**
9. **1**
10. **1**

Chapter 10
1. **2**
2. **1**
3. **1**
4. **2**
5. **2**
6. **4**
7. **2**
8. **1**
9. **1**
10. **2**

Chapter 11
1. **1, 2,** and **4**
2. **2**
3. **4**
4. **3**
5. **1** and **3**
6. **2**
7. **1**
8. **2**
9. **2**
10. **1**

Chapter 12
1. **3**
2. Stridor
3. **2**
4. **2**
5. **1, 3,** and **5**
6. **3**
7. **2**
8. **2**
9. **2**
10. **3**

Chapter 13
1. **3**
2. **2**
3. **1** and **5**
4. **2**
5. Tracheostomy
6. **1, 3, 4,** and **5**
7. **2**
8. **2**
9. **2**
10. Epistaxis or nose bleed

Chapter 14
1. **4**
2. **2**
3. **2**
4. **1**
5. **2**
6. **1**
7. **3**
8. Directly observed therapy
9. **1, 3,** and **5**
10. **4**

Chapter 15
1. **3**
2. **1** and **2**
3. **2**
4. **1**
5. **1**
6. **4**
7. **3**
8. **1**
9. **2** and **4**
10. **1**

Chapter 16
1. **1**
2. **2**
3. **2**
4. Hand-foot syndrome
5. **3**
6. **4**
7. **3**
8. **2**
9. **1**
10. **3**

Chapter 17
1. **2, 4,** and **5**
2. **2**
3. Intermittent claudication
4. **1**
5. **2**
6. **1**
7. **3**
8. **2, 4,** and **5**
9. **3**
10. **1**

Chapter 18
1. **4**
2. **2**
3. **3**
4. **2**
5. **4**
6. **2**
7. **1**
8. **1**
9. **2**
10. **1, 3,** and **5**

Chapter 19
1. **1, 2,** and **4**
2. **3**
3. Cardioversion
4. **2**
5. **4**
6. **2**
7. **3**
8. **3**
9. **3**
10. **1**

Chapter 20
1. **1, 2,** and **4**
2. **2**
3. **3**
4. **1**
5. **1, 2, 4,** and **5**
6. **1**
7. **4**
8. **3**
9. **1, 2,** and **5**
10. **2**

Chapter 21
1. **2**
2. **3**
3. **2**
4. **1**
5. **3**
6. **2**
7. **3**
8. **1**
9. **2**
10. **2, 4,** and **5**

Chapter 22
1. **3**
2. **1, 3,** and **4**
3. **1**
4. **2**
5. **3**
6. Cushing's triad
7. **3**
8. **2, 3,** and **4**
9. **2**
10. **3**

Chapter 23
1. **2**
2. **3**
3. **1, 2, 3,** and **4**
4. **4**
5. Arterio-venous malformation
6. **1**
7. **2**
8. **4**
9. **3**
10. **3**

Chapter 24
1. **2**
2. **4**
3. **1**
4. **4**
5. **2**
6. **2**
7. **2**
8. **3**
9. **3**
10. **2, 3,** and **4**

Continued on next page

Chapter 25
1. Arcus senilis
2. **2**
3. **1, 3,** and **5**
4. **2**
5. **2**
6. **4**
7. **3**
8. **3**
9. **2**
10. **1, 4,** and **5**

Chapter 26
1. **2**
2. **2**
3. **1**
4. **2**
5. Glaucoma
6. **1, 2, 4,** and **5**
7. **1**
8. **2**
9. **2**
10. **1, 3,** and **4**

Chapter 27
1. Kupffer cells
2. **3**
3. **1, 2,** and **3**
4. **2**
5. **2**
6. **1, 2,** and **3**
7. **3**
8. **3**
9. **1**
10. **4**

Chapter 28
1. **2**
2. **1**
3. **2**
4. **1, 2, 3,** and **4**
5. Leukoplakia
6. **2**
7. **1**
8. **3**
9. **3**
10. **2** and **4**

Chapter 29
1. **2**
2. **2**
3. Intussusception
4. **1, 3,** and **5**
5. **2**
6. **1** and **3**
7. **4**
8. **3**
9. **3**
10. **2, 3,** and **4**

Chapter 30
1. **3**
2. Caput medusa
3. **1**
4. **2**
5. **2**
6. **3**
7. **2, 3,** and **4**
8. **3**
9. **2**
10. **2**

Chapter 31
1. **3**
2. Ankylosis
3. **2**
4. **2**
5. **2**
6. **2**
7. **3**
8. **2**
9. **3**
10. **2**

Chapter 32
1. **2**
2. **3**
3. **2**
4. **1**
5. **2**
6. **4**
7. **3**
8. **3**
9. **2**
10. **1** and **4**

Chapter 33
1. **3**
2. **4**
3. **1, 2,** and **5**
4. **2**
5. **3**
6. **2** and **3**
7. **4**
8. **2**
9. **1, 2,** and **5**
10. Creatinine

Chapter 34
1. Uremia
2. **1**
3. **1**
4. **2**
5. **3**
6. **2**
7. **3**
8. **1, 3, 4,** and **5**
9. **1, 3, 4,** and **5**
10. **4**

Chapter 35
1. **3**
2. **3**
3. **1, 2, 4,** and **5**
4. **1**
5. **2**
6. **2**
7. **1**
8. **2**
9. **2**
10. **2, 4,** and **5**

Chapter 36
1. **2**
2. **1**
3. **2**
4. **1** and **4**
5. **1, 3,** and **5**
6. **2**
7. **1**
8. **2**
9. **1, 2, 4,** and **5**
10. **2**

Chapter 37
1. **2**
2. **1**
3. **1, 2, 4,** and **5**
4. **3**
5. **3**
6. **4**
7. **3**
8. Dawn phenomenon
9. **2**
10. **4**

Chapter 38
1. **2**
2. **1, 3, 4,** and **5**
3. **2**
4. **3**
5. **1**
6. **1, 3,** and **4**
7. **2**
8. **2**
9. **2, 4,** and **5**
10. **1**

Chapter 39
1. **2**
2. **1, 2,** and **5**
3. **3**
4. **1**
5. **3**
6. **2**
7. **2**
8. Peyronie's disease
9. **2**
10. **2**

Chapter 40
1. **2**
2. **2, 3,** and **4**
3. **1**
4. **1, 2, 3,** and **4**
5. **2**
6. **2**
7. **2**
8. **1**
9. Ophthalmia neonatorum
10. **2**

Chapter 41
1. **2, 4,** and **5**
2. Senile lentigines
3. **2**
4. **1**
5. **2**
6. **4**
7. **1, 2, 3,** and **5**
8. **4**
9. **1** and **5**
10. **1, 2 , 3, 4,** and **5**

Chapter 42
1. **1**
2. **1, 2, 4,** and **5**
3. Acne rosacea
4. **1, 2, 3,** and **5**
5. **3**
6. **3**
7. **4**
8. **2**
9. **3, 4,** and **5**
10. **1, 2, 4,** and **5**

Chapter 43
1. Disaster
2. **1**
3. **4**
4. **2**
5. Bioterrorism
6. **3**
7. **3**
8. **2**
9. **1, 2, 3,** and **4**
10. **2**

Chapter 44
1. **2**
2. **3**
3. Ptomaine
4. **2**
5. **1, 2, 3,** and **5**
6. **2**
7. **2**
8. **4**
9. **2**
10. **3**

Chapter 45
1. **3**
2. **3**
3. **4**
4. **4**
5. **1**
6. **2**
7. **2**
8. **1, 2, 5, 7**
9. **1**
10. **4**

Chapter 46
1. **3**
2. **3**
3. **4**
4. **2**
5. **1**
6. **2**
7. **2**
8. **2**
9. **3**
10. **3**

Chapter 47
1. **1**
2. **3**
3. **3**
4. **3**
5. **2**
6. **1, 2, 6**
7. **4**
8. **2**
9. **3**
10. **1**

Chapter 48
1. **1**
2. **3**
3. **3**
4. **2**
5. **1**
6. **4**
7. **1, 3, 4,** and **5**
8. **2**
9. **3**
10. **3**